Recommended Dietary Allowances (RDA) and Adequate Intakes (A[illegible]

Age (yr)	Thiamin RDA (mg/day)	Riboflavin RDA (mg/day)	Niacin RDA (mg/day)[a]	Biotin AI (µg/day)	Pantothenic acid AI (mg/day)	Vitamin B_6 RDA (mg/day)	Folate RDA (µg/day)[b]	Vitamin B_{12} RDA (µg/day)	Choline AI (mg/day)	Vitamin C RDA (mg/day)	Vitamin A RDA (µg/day)[c] [illegible]	Vitamin D AI (µg/day)[d]	Vitamin E RDA (mg/day)[e] [illegible]	Vitamin K AI (µg/day)
Infants														
0–0.5	0.2	0.3	2	5	1.7	0.1	65	0.4	125	40	400	5	4	2.0
0.5–1	0.3	0.4	4	6	1.8	0.3	80	0.5	150	50	500	5	5	2.5
Children														
1–3	0.5	0.5	6	8	2	0.5	150	0.9	200	15	300	5	6	30
4–8	0.6	0.6	8	12	3	0.6	200	1.2	250	25	400	5	7	55
Males														
9–13	0.9	0.9	12	20	4	1.0	300	1.8	375	45	600	5	11	60
14–18	1.2	1.3	16	25	5	1.3	400	2.4	550	75	900	5	15	75
19–30	1.2	1.3	16	30	5	1.3	400	2.4	550	90	900	5	15	120
31–50	1.2	1.3	16	30	5	1.3	400	2.4	550	90	900	5	15	120
51–70	1.2	1.3	16	30	5	1.7	400	2.4	550	90	900	10	15	120
>70	1.2	1.3	16	30	5	1.7	400	2.4	550	90	900	15	15	120
Females														
9–13	0.9	0.9	12	20	4	1.0	300	1.8	375	45	600	5	11	60
14–18	1.0	1.0	14	25	5	1.2	400	2.4	400	65	700	5	15	75
19–30	1.1	1.1	14	30	5	1.3	400	2.4	425	75	700	5	15	90
31–50	1.1	1.1	14	30	5	1.3	400	2.4	425	75	700	5	15	90
51–70	1.1	1.1	14	30	5	1.5	400	2.4	425	75	700	10	15	90
>70	1.1	1.1	14	30	5	1.5	400	2.4	425	75	700	15	15	90
Pregnancy														
≤18	1.4	1.4	18	30	6	1.9	600	2.6	450	80	750	5	15	75
19–30	1.4	1.4	18	30	6	1.9	600	2.6	450	85	770	5	15	90
31–50	1.4	1.4	18	30	6	1.9	600	2.6	450	85	770	5	15	90
Lactation														
≤18	1.4	1.6	17	35	7	2.0	500	2.8	550	115	1200	5	19	75
19–30	1.4	1.6	17	35	7	2.0	500	2.8	550	120	1300	5	19	90
31–50	1.4	1.6	17	35	7	2.0	500	2.8	550	120	1300	5	19	90

NOTE: For all nutrients, values for infants are AI. The glossary on the inside back cover defines units of nutrient measure.

[a]Niacin recommendations are expressed as niacin equivalents (NE), except for recommendations for infants younger than 6 months, which are expressed as preformed niacin.

[b]Folate recommendations are expressed as dietary folate equivalents (DFE).

[c]Vitamin A recommendations are expressed as retinol activity equivalents (RAE).

[d]Vitamin D recommendations are expressed as cholecalciferol and assume an absence of adequate exposure to sunlight.

[e]Vitamin E recommendations are expressed as α-tocopherol.

Recommended Dietary Allowances (RDA) and Adequate Intakes (AI) for Minerals

Age (yr)	Sodium AI (mg/day)	Chloride AI (mg/day)	Potassium AI (mg/day)	Calcium AI (mg/day)	Phosphorus RDA (mg/day)	Magnesium RDA (mg/day)	Iron RDA (mg/day)	Zinc RDA (mg/day)	Iodine RDA (µg/day)	Selenium RDA (µg/day)	Copper RDA (µg/day)	Manganese AI (mg/day)	Fluoride AI (mg/day)	Chromium AI (µg/day)	Molybdenum RDA (µg/day)
Infants															
0–0.5	120	180	400	210	100	30	0.27	2	110	15	200	0.003	0.01	0.2	2
0.5–1	370	570	700	270	275	75	11	3	130	20	220	0.6	0.5	5.5	3
Children															
1–3	1000	1500	3000	500	460	80	7	3	90	20	340	1.2	0.7	11	17
4–8	1200	1900	3800	800	500	130	10	5	90	30	440	1.5	1.0	15	22
Males															
9–13	1500	2300	4500	1300	1250	240	8	8	120	40	700	1.9	2	25	34
14–18	1500	2300	4700	1300	1250	410	11	11	150	55	890	2.2	3	35	43
19–30	1500	2300	4700	1000	700	400	8	11	150	55	900	2.3	4	35	45
31–50	1500	2300	4700	1000	700	420	8	11	150	55	900	2.3	4	35	45
51–70	1300	2000	4700	1200	700	420	8	11	150	55	900	2.3	4	30	45
>70	1200	1800	4700	1200	700	420	8	11	150	55	900	2.3	4	30	45
Females															
9–13	1500	2300	4500	1300	1250	240	8	8	120	40	700	1.6	2	21	34
14–18	1500	2300	4700	1300	1250	360	15	9	150	55	890	1.6	3	24	43
19–30	1500	2300	4700	1000	700	310	18	8	150	55	900	1.8	3	25	45
31–50	1500	2300	4700	1000	700	320	18	8	150	55	900	1.8	3	25	45
51–70	1300	2000	4700	1200	700	320	8	8	150	55	900	1.8	3	20	45
>70	1200	1800	4700	1200	700	320	8	8	150	55	900	1.8	3	20	45
Pregnancy															
≤18	1500	2300	4700	1300	1250	400	27	12	220	60	1000	2.0	3	29	50
19–30	1500	2300	4700	1000	700	350	27	11	220	60	1000	2.0	3	30	50
31–50	1500	2300	4700	1000	700	360	27	11	220	60	1000	2.0	3	30	50
Lactation															
≤18	1500	2300	5100	1300	1250	360	10	14	290	70	1300	2.6	3	44	50
19–30	1500	2300	5100	1000	700	310	9	12	290	70	1300	2.6	3	45	50
31–50	1500	2300	5100	1000	700	320	9	12	290	70	1300	2.6	3	45	50

Tolerable Upper Intake Levels (UL) for Vitamins

Age (yr)	Niacin (mg/day)[a]	Vitamin B_6 (mg/day)	Folate (µg/day)[a]	Choline (mg/day)	Vitamin C (mg/day)	Vitamin A (µg/day)[b]	Vitamin D (µg/day)	Vitamin E (mg/day)[c]
Infants								
0–0.5	—	—	—	—	—	600	25	—
0.5–1	—	—	—	—	—	600	25	—
Children								
1–3	10	30	300	1000	400	600	50	200
4–8	15	40	400	1000	650	900	50	300
9–13	20	60	600	2000	1200	1700	50	600
Adolescents								
14–18	30	80	800	3000	1800	2800	50	800
Adults								
19–70	35	100	1000	3500	2000	3000	50	1000
>70	35	100	1000	3500	2000	3000	50	1000
Pregnancy								
≤18	30	80	800	3000	1800	2800	50	800
19–50	35	100	1000	3500	2000	3000	50	1000
Lactation								
≤18	30	80	800	3000	1800	2800	50	800
19–50	35	100	1000	3500	2000	3000	50	1000

[a]The UL for niacin and folate apply to synthetic forms obtained from supplements, fortified foods, or a combination of the two.

[b]The UL for vitamin A applies to the preformed vitamin only.

[c]The UL for vitamin E applies to any form of supplemental α-tocopherol, fortified foods, or a combination of the two.

Tolerable Upper Intake Levels (UL) for Minerals

Age (yr)	Sodium (mg/day)	Chloride (mg/day)	Calcium (mg/day)	Phosphorus (mg/day)	Magnesium (mg/day)[d]	Iron (mg/day)[b]	Zinc (mg/day)	Iodine (µg/day)	Selenium (µg/day)	Copper (µg/day)	Manganese (mg/day)	Fluoride (mg/day)	Molybdenum (µg/day)	Boron (mg/day)	Nickel (mg/day)	Vanadium (mg/day)
Infants																
0–0.5	—[e]	—[e]	—	—	—	40	4	—	45	—	—	0.7	—	—	—	—
0.5–1	—[e]	—[e]	—	—	—	40	5	—	60	—	—	0.9	—	—	—	—
Children																
1–3	1500	2300	2500	3000	65	40	7	200	90	1000	2	1.3	300	3	0.2	—
4–8	1900	2900	2500	3000	110	40	12	300	150	3000	3	2.2	600	6	0.3	—
9–13	2200	3400	2500	4000	350	40	23	600	280	5000	6	10	1100	11	0.6	—
Adolescents																
14–18	2300	3600	2500	4000	350	45	34	900	400	8000	9	10	1700	17	1.0	—
Adults																
19–70	2300	3600	2500	4000	350	45	40	1100	400	10,000	11	10	2000	20	1.0	1.8
>70	2300	3600	2500	3000	350	45	40	1100	400	10,000	11	10	2000	20	1.0	1.8
Pregnancy																
≤18	2300	3600	2500	3500	350	45	34	900	400	8000	9	10	1700	17	1.0	—
19–50	2300	3600	2500	3500	350	45	40	1100	400	10,000	11	10	2000	20	1.0	—
Lactation																
≤18	2300	3600	2500	4000	350	45	34	900	400	8000	9	10	1700	17	1.0	—
19–50	2300	3600	2500	4000	350	45	40	1100	400	10,000	11	10	2000	20	1.0	—

[d]The UL for magnesium applies to synthetic forms obtained from supplements or drugs only.

[e]Source of intake should be from human milk (or formula) and food only.

NOTE: An Upper Limit was not established for vitamins and minerals not listed and for those age groups listed with a dash (—) because of a lack of data, not because these nutrients are safe to consume at any level of intake. All nutrients can have adverse effects when intakes are excessive.

SOURCE: Adapted with permission from the *Dietary Reference Intakes* series, National Academy Press. Courtesy of the National Academy Press, Washington, D.C.

UNDERSTANDING NORMAL AND CLINICAL NUTRITION

SEVENTH EDITION

Sharon Rady Rolfes

Kathryn Pinna

Ellie Whitney

THOMSON

WADSWORTH

Australia • Brazil • Canada • Mexico • Singapore • Spain
United Kingdom • United States

THOMSON

WADSWORTH

Understanding Normal and Clinical Nutrition, **Seventh Edition**
Sharon Rady Rolfes, Kathryn Pinna, Ellie Whitney

Publisher: Peter Marshall
Development Editor: Elizabeth Howe
Assistant Editor: Elesha Feldman
Editorial Assistant: Lauren Vogelbaum
Technology Project Manager: Travis Metz
Marketing Manager: Jennifer Somerville
Marketing Assistant: Michele Colella
Marketing Communications Manager: Shemika Britt
Project Manager, Editorial Production: Sandra Craig
Creative Director: Rob Hugel
Art Director: Lee Friedman
Print Buyer: Barbara Britton
Permissions Editor: Stephanie Lee
Production Service: The Book Company
Text and Cover Designer: John Walker
Photo Researcher: Myrna Engler
Copy Editor: Patricia Lewis
Illustrator: Imagineering
Cover Image: © Brian Kuhlmann/Masterfile
Cover Printer: Phoenix Color Corp
Compositor: Parkwood Composition Service
Printer: Quebecor World/Dubuque

Printed in the United States of America
4 5 6 7 09 08 07

For more information about our products, contact us at:
Thomson Learning Academic Resource Center
1-800-423-0563

For permission to use material from this text or product, submit a request online at:
http://www.thomsonrights.com

Any additional questions about permissions can be submitted by e-mail to thomsonrights@thomson.com.

Library of Congress Control Number: 2005923766

Student Edition ISBN-13: 978-0-534-62208-4
ISBN-10: 0-534-62208-9

Thomson Higher Education
10 Davis Drive
Belmont, CA 94002–3098
USA

Asia (including India)
Thomson Learning
5 Shenton Way
#01-01 UIC Building
Singapore 068808

Australia/New Zealand
Thomson Learning Australia
102 Dodds Street
Southbank, Victoria 3006
Australia

Canada
Thomson Nelson
1120 Birchmount Road
Toronto, Ontario M1K 5G4
Canada

UK/Europe/Middle East/Africa
Thomson Learning
High Holborn House
50/51 Bedford Row
London WC1R 4LR
United Kingdom

Latin America
Thomson Learning
Seneca, 53
Colonia Polanco
11560 Mexico
D.F. Mexico

Spain (including Portugal)
Thomson Paraninfo
Calle Magallanes, 25
28015 Madrid, Spain

To my parents, Tom and Gladys Rady, whose love and guidance throughout the years enabled me to fulfill my dreams.

Sharon

To my mother and father, who inspired my love of books and learning from my earliest years.

Kathy

With gratitude to my co-author and friend, Sharon Rolfes, who for years has conscientiously and skillfully tended this book to make it as useful as possible both to recipients of diet therapy and to their caregivers.

Ellie

About the Authors

Sharon Rady Rolfes received her M.S. in nutrition and food science from the Florida State University. She is a founding member of Nutrition and Health Associates, an information resource center that maintains a research database on over 1000 nutrition-related topics. Her other publications include the college textbooks *Understanding Nutrition* and *Nutrition for Health and Health Care* and a multimedia CD-ROM called *Nutrition Interactive.* In addition to writing, she occasionally lectures at universities and at professional conferences and serves as a consultant for various educational projects. Her volunteer activities include coordinating meals for the hungry and homeless and serving as a partner in Stepping Toward Health, a community initiative that encourages individuals "to be more active and eat more nutritionally." She maintains her registration as a dietitian and membership in the American Dietetic Association.

Kathryn Pinna received her M.S. and Ph.D. in nutrition from the University of California at Berkeley. She has taught nutrition and food science courses in the San Francisco Bay Area for over 15 years, and currently teaches introductory nutrition classes at City College of San Francisco. She has also worked as an outpatient dietitian, Internet consultant, and freelance writer. She is a Registered Dietitian and member of the American Dietetic Association, American Society for Nutritional Sciences, and American Society for Clinical Nutrition.

Ellie Whitney grew up in New York City and received her B.A. and Ph.D. degrees in English and Biology at Radcliffe/Harvard University and Washington University, respectively. She has lived in Tallahassee since 1970, has taught at both the Florida State University and Florida A&M University, has written newspaper columns on environmental matters for the *Tallahassee Democrat,* and has authored almost a dozen college textbooks on nutrition, health, and related topics, some of which are in their seventh (or later) editions. In addition to teaching and writing, she has spent the past three-plus decades exploring outdoor Florida and studying its ecology. Her latest book is *Priceless Florida: The Natural Ecosystems* (Pineapple Press, 2004).

Brief Contents

Contents

BOXES

How to

Case Studies

Preface

Understanding Normal and Clinical Nutrition presents the core information of an introductory nutrition course for health care professionals. The early chapters focus on "normal" nutrition—the recommendations to maintain good health. The later chapters provide lessons in "clinical" nutrition—dietary strategies to manage various diseases.

This edition reflects the many advances in nutrition science and health care delivery that have developed since the last edition. Yet it maintains the same goals as earlier editions: to spark your enthusiasm for an understanding of nutrition so that your knowledge "will improve the quality of your life and the lives of those you serve as a health professional." As with previous editions, each chapter has been substantially revised and updated. New research topics, such as phytochemicals, ghrelin, and nutritional genomics, are introduced or more fully explored. Every chapter continues to include practical information and valuable resources to help readers apply nutrition knowledge and skills to their daily lives and the clinical setting.

The Chapters Chapter 1 first explores why we eat the foods we do and then continues with a brief overview of the nutrients, the science of nutrition, recommended nutrient intakes, assessment, and important relationships between diet and health. Chapter 2 describes the diet-planning principles and food guides used to create diets that support good health and includes instructions on how to read a food label, and thorough coverage of *Dietary Guidelines for Americans 2005*. In Chapter 3, readers follow the journey of digestion and absorption as the body transforms foods into nutrients. Chapters 4 through 6 describe carbohydrates, fats, and proteins—their chemistry, roles in the body, and places in the diet. Chapter 7 shows how the body derives energy from these three nutrients. Chapters 8 and 9 continue the story with a look at energy balance, the factors associated with overweight and underweight, and the benefits and dangers of weight loss and weight gain. Chapters 10 through 13 describe the vitamins, the minerals, and water—their roles in the body, deficiency and toxicity symptoms, and sources. Chapters 14 through 16 complete the "normal" chapters with a presentation of the special nutrient needs of people through the life cycle—pregnancy and lactation; infancy, childhood, and adolescence; and adulthood and the later years.

The remaining "clinical" chapters of the book focus on the nutrition care of individuals with health problems. Chapter 17 explains how illnesses and their treatments influence nutrient needs and describes the process of nutrition assessment. Chapter 18 discusses how nutrition care is implemented and introduces the different types of modified diets used in patient care. Chapter 19 explores the potential interactions between nutrients and medications and examines the benefits and risks associated with herbal remedies. Chapters 20 and 21 describe special ways of feeding people who cannot eat conventional foods. Chapter 22 describes the inflammatory process and explains how metabolic and respiratory stress influence nutrient needs. Chapters 23 through 29 explore the pathology, medical treatment, and nutrition care associated with specific diseases, including gastrointestinal disorders, liver disease, diabetes mellitus, cardiovascular diseases, renal disease, cancer, and HIV infection.

The Highlights Every chapter is followed by a highlight that provides readers with an in-depth look at a current, and often controversial, topic that relates to its companion chapter. New highlights in this edition feature a comparison of dietary guidelines from around the world, the benefits of (some) high-fat foods, the role of nutritional genomics in health care, the relationships between dental health and chronic illness, the development of anemia during illness, and the diagnosis and treatment of food allergies.

Special Features The art and layout in this edition have been redesigned to add visual appeal and enhance learning. In addition, special features help readers identify key concepts and apply nutrition knowledge. For example, a **definition** is provided whenever a new term is introduced. These definitions often include pronunciations and derivations to facilitate understanding. A glossary at the end of the book includes all defined terms.

definition (DEF-eh-NISH-en): the meaning of a word.
- **de** = from
- **finis** = boundary

Nutrition in Your Life

New to this edition are Nutrition in Your Life sections at the beginning and end of Chapters 1 through 16. The opening section introduces the essence of the chapter in a friendly and familiar scenario. The closing section revisits that message and prompts readers to consider whether their personal choices are meeting the dietary goals introduced in the chapter.

Nutrition in the Professional Setting

Similarly, Chapters 17 through 29 begin with Nutrition in the Professional Setting. These sections introduce the clinical chapters with real-life concerns often associated with diseases or their treatments.

NUTRITION ASSESSMENT CHECKLIST

Nutrition Assessment Checklist

The clinical chapters close with a Nutrition Assessment Checklist that helps readers evaluate how various disorders impair nutrition status. These sections highlight the medical, dietary, anthropometric, biochemical, and clinical findings most relevant to patients with specific diseases. Most of these chapters also include a section on Diet-Drug Interactions that describes the nutrition-related concerns associated with the medications commonly used to treat the disorders mentioned in the chapter.

IN SUMMARY Each major section within a chapter concludes with a summary paragraph that reviews the key concepts. Similarly, summary tables organize information in an easy-to-read format.

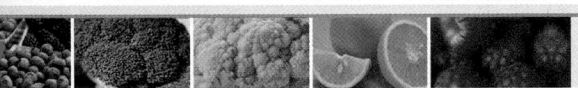

Also featured in this edition are the Healthy People 2010 nutrition-related priorities, which are presented whenever their subjects are discussed. Healthy People 2010 is a report developed by the U.S. Department of Health and Human Services that establishes national objectives in health promotion and disease prevention for the year 2010.

These nutrition-related priorities are presented throughout the text whenever their subjects are discussed.

HEALTHY PEOPLE 2010

HOW TO

Many of the chapters include "How to" sections that guide readers through problem-solving tasks. For example, the "How to" in Chapter 1 shows readers how to calculate energy intake from the grams of carbohydrate, fat, and protein in a food; another "How to" in Chapter 26 explains how to use the carbohydrate counting system in meal planning for people with diabetes.

NUTRITION CALCULATION

Several of the early chapters close with a "Nutrition Calculation" section. These sections often reinforce the "How to" lessons and provide practice in doing nutrition-related calculations. The problems enable readers to apply their skills to hypothetical situations and then check their answers (found at the end of the chapter). Readers who successfully master these exercises will be well prepared for "real-life" nutrition-related problems.

CASE STUDY

Similarly, the clinical chapters include case studies that present problems and pose questions that help readers apply chapter material to hypothetical situations. Readers who successfully master these exercises will be better prepared to face "real-life" challenges that arise in the clinical setting. Some clinical chapters also include a "Research Update" section, which briefly examines new discoveries or current controversies.

NUTRITION ON THE NET

Each chapter and many highlights also conclude with Nutrition on the Net—a list of websites for further study of topics covered in the accompanying text. These listings do not imply an endorsement of the organizations or their programs. We have tried to provide reputable sources, but cannot be responsible for the content of these sites. (Read Highlight 1 to learn how to find reliable information on the Internet.)

STUDY QUESTIONS

Each chapter ends with study questions in essay and multiple-choice format. Study questions offer readers the opportunity to review the major concepts presented in the chapters in preparation for exams. The page numbers after each essay question refer readers to discussions that answer the question; multiple-choice answers appear at the end of the chapter.

The Appendixes The appendixes are valuable references for a number of purposes. Appendix A summarizes background information on the hormonal and nervous systems, complementing Appendixes B and C on basic chemistry, the chemical structures of nutrients, and major metabolic pathways. Appendix D describes measures of protein quality. Appendix E provides detailed coverage on nutrition assessment, and Appendix F presents the estimated energy requirements for men and women at various levels of physical activity. Appendix G presents the 2003 U.S. Exchange System. Appendix H is a 2000-item food composition table compiled from the latest nutrient database. Appendix I presents recommendations from the World Health Organization (WHO) and information for Canadians—the Choice System and guidelines to healthy eating and physical activities. Appendix J provides examples of commercial enteral formulas commonly used in tube feedings or to supplement oral diets.

The Inside Covers The inside covers put commonly used information at your fingertips. The front covers (pp. A, B, and C) present the current nutrient recommendations; the inside back cover (p. Y on the left) features the Daily Values used on food labels and a glossary of nutrient measures; and the inside back cover (p. Z on the right) shows the suggested weight ranges for various heights. The pages just prior to the back cover (pp. W–X) assist readers with calculations and conversions.

Supplements A number of helpful teaching and learning resources are available. Students will find the online content to be a helpful review of chapter material, reiterating chapter objectives and key concepts. For instructors, the *Understanding Normal and Clinical Nutrition* Multimedia Manager makes it easy to assemble, edit, and present custom lectures—bringing together art, video clips and animations from this CD-ROM, the web, and your own material. JoinIn on TurningPoint provides book-specific instant response system content, which reinforces key concepts and tests students' comprehension with challenging questions. ExamView® Computerized Testing makes it possible to create custom tests and study guides (both print and online) in minutes. A printed test bank and instructor manual provides instructors with a complete and thorough test for each chapter of the text, and annotated lecture outlines, handouts, and helpful classroom activities.

Closing Comments We have tried to keep the number of references manageable. Many statements that have appeared in previous editions with references now appear without them, but every statement is backed by research, and the authors will supply references upon request. We have not provided a separate list of suggested readings, but have tried to include references that will provide readers with additional details or a good overview of the subject. Nutrition is a fascinating subject, and we hope our enthusiasm for it comes through on every page.

Sharon Rady Rolfes
Kathryn Pinna
Ellie Whitney
May 2005

Acknowledgments

To produce a book requires the coordinated effort of a team of people—and, no doubt, each team member has another team of support people as well. We salute, with a big round of applause, everyone who has worked so diligently to ensure the quality of this book.

We thank our partners and friends, Linda DeBruyne and Fran Webb, for their valuable consultations and contributions; working together over the past 20+ years has been a most wonderful experience. We especially appreciate Linda's research assistance on several chapters, and Margaret Hedley's attention to the Canadian information throughout the text and in Appendix I. A million thank-yous to Lynn Earnest for her careful attention to manuscript preparation and to Marni Jay Rolfes for her assistance in a multitude of other daily tasks. To Stephanie Lee and Kiely Sisk, a special thanks for their assistance in obtaining permissions. We also thank the many people who have prepared the ancillaries that accompany this text: Harry Sitren and Carrie Benton for writing and enhancing the Test Bank; Lori Turner, Mary Rhiner, Carrie Benton, and Margaret Hedley for preparing the Instructor's Manual; Thomas Castonguay, Steven Nizielski, and Richard Morel for developing the case studies and animations for the website; and Eugene Fenster and Connie Goff for gathering and creating slides for the Multimedia Manager. A big thank-you to Donna Kelley, Star MacKenzie Burruto, and the folks at FirstData Bank for compiling the food composition appendix, verifying the data in figures and tables, and developing the computerized diet analysis program that accompanies this book. Our special thanks to Peter Marshall for his continued support and insightful ideas; to Beth Howe for her brilliant suggestions for improvements and efficient coordination of reviews; to Sandra Craig for her guidance of this revision from conception to conclusion; to Dusty Friedman for her diligent attention to the innumerable details involved in production; to Jennifer Somerville and Shemika Britt for their enthusiastic efforts in marketing; to Travis Metz for his technology talents on our Website and CD products; to Elesha Feldman for her development and management of ancillaries; and to Lauren Vogelbaum for her willingness to fill in the gaps whenever the need arose. We also thank John Walker for the creative text design; Carolyn Deacy for styling the figures to add visual appeal and enhance learning; Lisa Sovran and the team of artists at Imagineering for creating accurate and attractive artwork to complement our writing; Myrna Engler for selecting photographs and coordinating photography sessions to deliver nutrition messages beautifully; Pat Lewis for sharing her grammar knowledge and copyediting over 2000 manuscript pages; Martha Ghent for proofreading close to 1000 final text pages; and Micki Taylor for composing a thorough and useful index. To the hundreds of others involved in production and sales, we tip our hats in appreciation.

We are especially grateful to our associates, friends, and families for their continued encouragement and support. We also thank our many reviewers for their comments and contributions.

Reviewers of *Understanding Normal and Clinical Nutrition*

Linda Armstrong
Normandale Community College

Natalie Caine-Bish
Kent State University

Nancy J. Cooley
University of Maine at Augusta

Elizabeth Coffman Butler
University of Central Arkansas

Cathy Cunningham
Tennessee Technological University

Mary L. Dundas
Idaho State University

Carol O. Eady
The University of Memphis

Jamie Erskine
University of Northern Colorado

Betty J. Forbes
West Virginia University

Mary Katheryn Gould
Marshall University

Pamela S. Hinton
University of Missouri-Columbia

Georgette Howell
SUNY Rockland Community College

Nancy H. Hunt
Lipscomb University

Clifford Lo, MD
Harvard University

Myrtle McCulloch
Georgetown University

Jaimette A. McCulley
Fontbonne University

Karen Meyers, MS
University of Central Oklahoma

Dawna Torres Mughal
Gannon University

Carmen L. Nochera
Grand Valley State University

Donna Jo Pruitt
Southwest Virginia Community College

Tonia Reinhard
Wayne State University

Karen K. Reilly
Daytona Beach Community College

Ruth A. Reilly
University of New Hampshire

Ruth Schneider
Idaho State University

Amy R. Shows
Lamar University

Debra Barone Sheats
College of St. Catherine, St. Paul, MN

Susan S. Swadener
California Polytechnic State University, San Luis Obispo

Glen P. Town
Westmont College

Barbara A. Troy
Marquette University

Katherine Vance
Idaho State University

Roxana Vlasceanu
Lorain County Community College

Threasia L. Witt
Alderson-Broaddus College

Patricia Zeabart
Ball State University

UNDERSTANDING NORMAL AND CLINICAL NUTRITION

Chapter 1

An Overview of Nutrition

Chapter Outline

Available Online

http://nutrition.wadsworth.com/uncn7

Nutrition Animation: *Consumer Concerns, Quackery and Sensationalism*

Student Practice Test

Glossary Terms

Nutrition on the Net

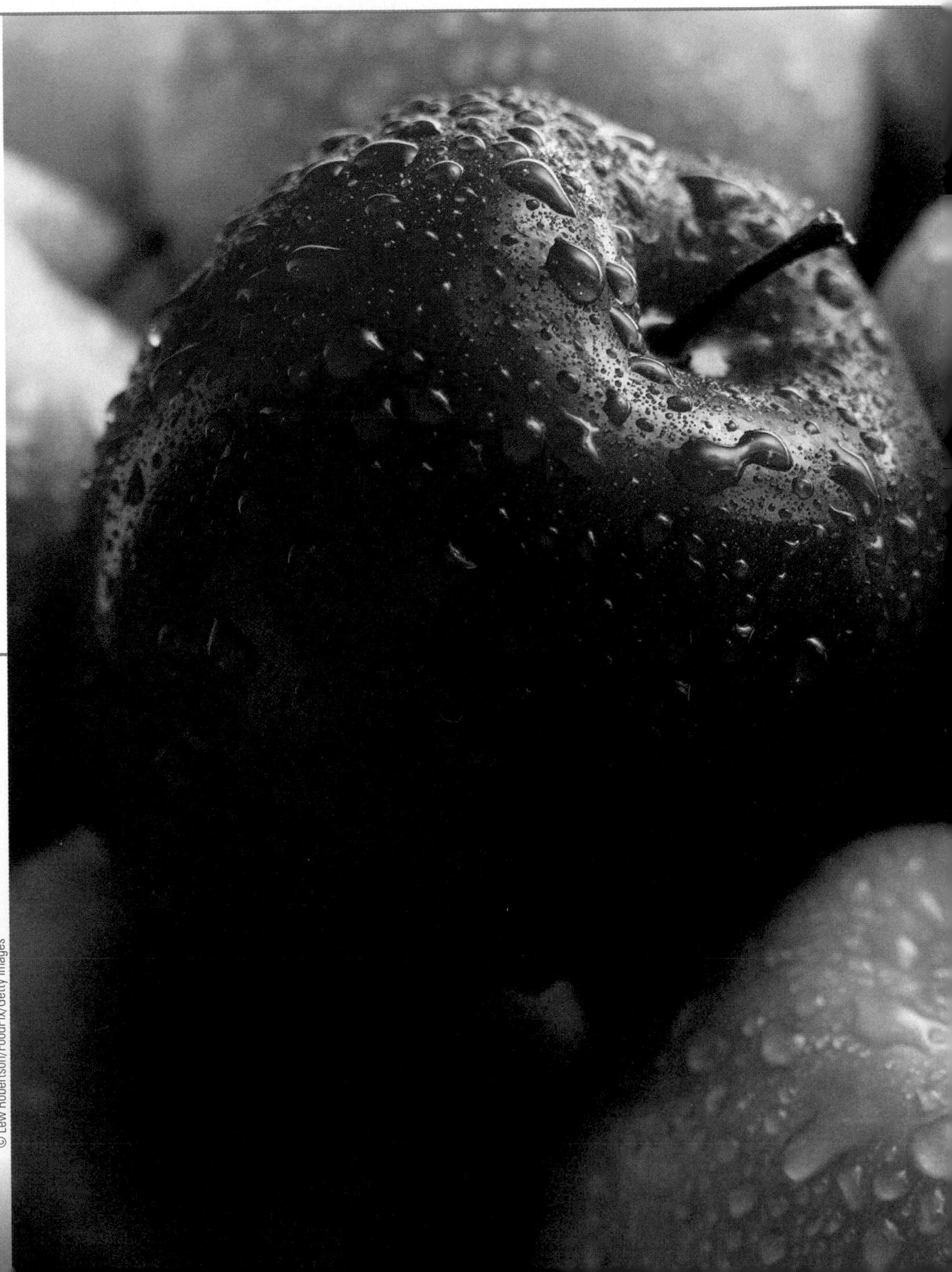

Nutrition in Your Life

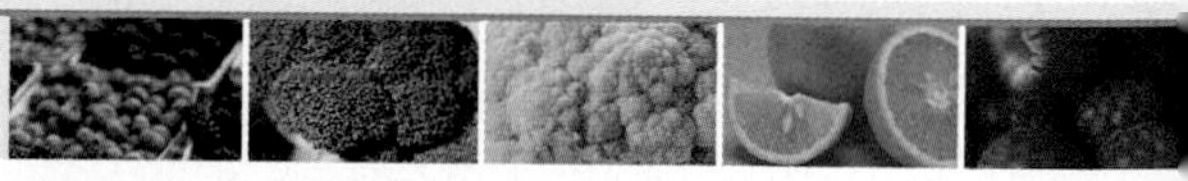

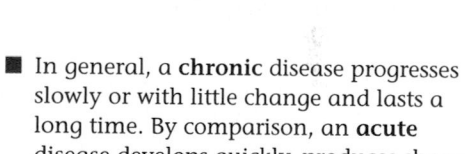

Believe it or not, you have probably eaten at least 20,000 meals in your life. Without any conscious effort on your part, your body uses the nutrients from those foods to make all its components, fuel all its activities, and defend itself against diseases. How successfully your body handles these tasks depends, in part, on your food choices. Nutritious food choices support healthy bodies.

Welcome to the world of **nutrition.** Nutrition has played a significant role in your life, even from before your birth, although you may not always have been aware of it. And it will continue to affect you in major ways, depending on the **foods** you select.

Every day, several times a day, you make food choices that influence your body's health for better or worse. Each day's choices may benefit or harm your health only a little, but when these choices are repeated over years and decades, the rewards or consequences become major. That being the case, close attention to good eating habits now can bring health benefits later. Conversely, carelessness about food choices from youth on can contribute to many chronic diseases■ prevalent in later life, including heart disease and cancer. Of course, some people will become ill or die young no matter what choices they make, and others will live long lives despite making poor choices. For the large majority, however, the food choices they make each and every day will benefit or impair their health in proportion to the wisdom of those choices.

Although most people realize that their food habits affect their health, they often choose foods for other reasons. After all, foods bring to the table a variety of pleasures, traditions, and associations as well as nourishment. The challenge, then, is to combine favorite foods and fun times with a nutritionally balanced **diet.**

■ In general, a **chronic** disease progresses slowly or with little change and lasts a long time. By comparison, an **acute** disease develops quickly, produces sharp symptoms, and runs a short course.
- **chronos** = time
- **acute** = sharp

nutrition: the science of foods and the nutrients and other substances they contain, and of their actions within the body (including ingestion, digestion, absorption, transport, metabolism, and excretion). A broader definition includes the social, economic, cultural, and psychological implications of food and eating.

foods: products derived from plants or animals that can be taken into the body to yield energy and nutrients for the maintenance of life and the growth and repair of tissues.

diet: the foods and beverages a person eats and drinks.

Food Choices

People decide what to eat, when to eat, and even whether to eat in highly personal ways, often based on behavioral or social motives rather than on awareness of nutrition's importance to health. Fortunately, many different food choices can be healthy ones, but nutrition awareness helps to make them so.

Personal Preference As you might expect, the number one reason people choose foods is taste—they like certain flavors. Two widely shared preferences are for the sweetness of sugar and the savoriness of salt. Liking high-fat foods appears to be another universally common preference. Other preferences might be for the hot peppers common in Mexican cooking or the curry spices of Indian cuisine. Some research suggests that genetics may influence people's food preferences.[1]

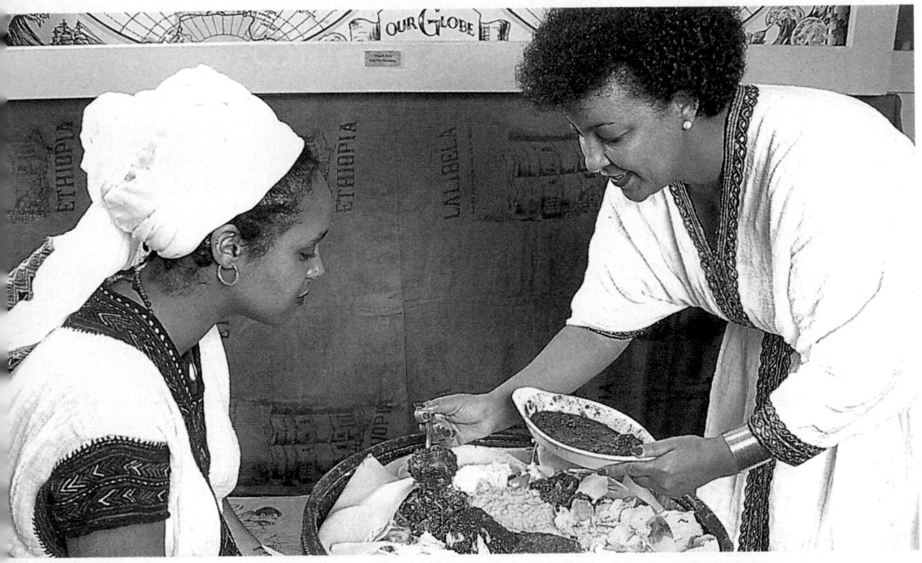
OUR GLOBE
ETHIOPIA
ETHIOPIA
LALIBELA
An enjoyable way to learn about other cultures is to taste their ethnic foods.

© Michael Newman/PhotoEdit

Habit People sometimes select foods out of habit. They eat cereal every morning, for example, simply because they have always eaten cereal for breakfast. Eating a familiar food and not having to make any decisions can be comforting.

Ethnic Heritage or Tradition Among the strongest influences on food choices are ethnic heritage and tradition. People eat the foods they grew up eating. Every country, and in fact every region of a country, has its own typical foods and ways of combining them into meals. The "American diet" includes many ethnic foods from various countries, all adding variety to the diet. This is most evident when eating out: 60 percent of U.S. restaurants (excluding fast-food places) have an ethnic emphasis, most commonly Chinese, Italian, or Mexican.

Social Interactions Most people enjoy companionship while eating. It's fun to join friends when they are ordering pizza or going out for ice cream. Meals are social events, and the sharing of food is part of hospitality. Social customs almost compel people to accept food or drink offered by a host or shared by a group.

Availability, Convenience, and Economy People eat foods that are accessible, quick and easy to prepare, and within their financial means. Consumers today value convenience highly and are willing to spend over half of their food budget on meals that require little, if any, further preparation.[2] They frequently eat out, bring home ready-to-eat meals, or have food delivered. Even when they venture into the kitchen, they want to prepare a meal in 15 to 20 minutes, using less than a half dozen ingredients—and those "ingredients" are often semiprepared foods, such as canned soups. Such emphasis on convenience limits food choices to the selections offered on menus and products designed for quick preparation. Whether decisions based on convenience meet a person's nutrition needs depends on the choices made. Eating a banana or a candy bar may be equally convenient, but the fruit offers more vitamins and minerals and less sugar and fat.

Positive and Negative Associations People tend to like foods with happy associations—such as hot dogs at ball games or cake and ice cream at birthday parties. By the same token, people can attach intense and unalterable dislikes to foods that they ate when they felt sick or that were forced on them when they weren't hungry. Parents may teach their children to like and dislike certain foods by using those foods as rewards or punishments.

Emotional Comfort Some people cannot eat when they are emotionally upset. Others may eat in response to a variety of emotional stimuli—for example, to relieve boredom or depression or to calm anxiety.[3] A depressed person may choose to eat chocolates rather than to call a friend. A person who has returned home from an exciting evening out may unwind with a late-night sandwich. These people may find emotional comfort, in part, because foods can influence the brain's chemistry and the mind's response. Carbohydrates and alcohol, for example, tend to calm, whereas proteins and caffeine are more likely to activate.[4] Eating in response to emotions can easily lead to overeating and obesity, but may be appropriate at times. For example, sharing food at times of bereavement serves both the giver's need to provide comfort and the receiver's need to be cared for and to interact with others, as well as to take nourishment.

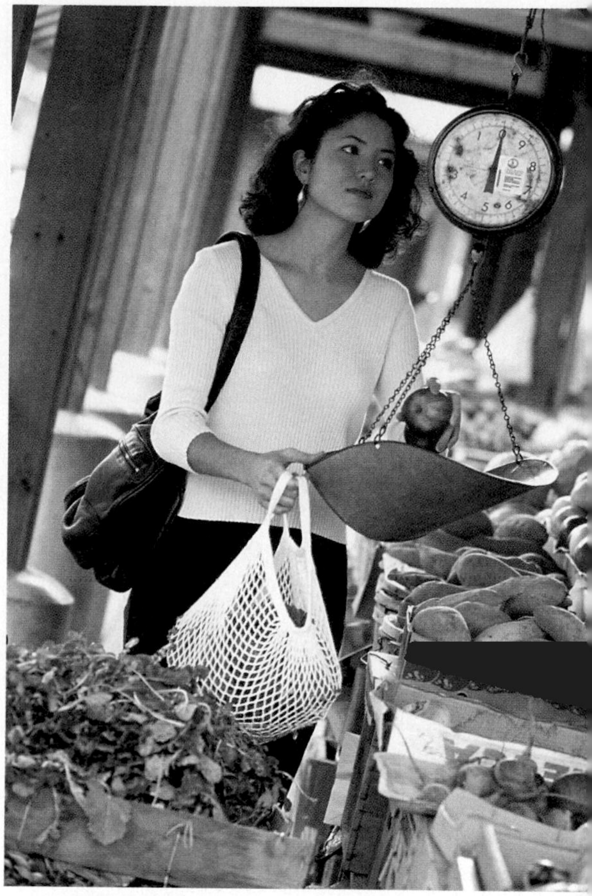

To enhance your health, keep nutrition in mind when selecting foods.

Values Food choices may reflect people's religious beliefs, political views, or environmental concerns. For example, many Christians forgo meat during Lent, the period prior to Easter, and Jewish law includes an extensive set of dietary rules that govern the use of foods derived from animals. Muslims fast between sunrise and sunset during Ramadan, the ninth month of the Islamic calendar. A concerned consumer may boycott fruit picked by migrant workers who have been exploited. People may buy vegetables from local farmers to save the fuel and environmental costs of foods shipped in from far away. They may also select foods packaged in containers that can be reused or recycled. Some consumers accept or reject foods that have been irradiated or genetically modified, depending on their approval of these processes.

Body Weight and Image Sometimes people select certain foods and supplements that they believe will improve their physical appearance and avoid those they believe might be detrimental. Such decisions can be beneficial when based on sound nutrition and fitness knowledge, but undermine good health when based on faddism or carried to extremes, as Highlight 9's discussion of eating disorders points out.

Nutrition and Health Benefits Finally, of course, many consumers make food choices that will benefit health. Food manufacturers and restaurant chefs have responded to scientific findings linking health with nutrition by offering an abundant selection of health-promoting foods and beverages. Foods that provide health benefits beyond their nutrient contributions are called **functional foods.** In some cases, functional foods are as natural and familiar as oatmeal or tomatoes. In other cases, the foods have been modified in a way that provides health benefits, perhaps by lowering the fat contents. In still other cases, manufacturers have fortified foods by adding nutrients or phytochemicals that provide health benefits (see Highlight 13). Examples of these functional foods include orange juice fortified with calcium to help build strong bones and margarine made with a plant sterol that lowers blood cholesterol.

Consumers welcome these new foods into their diets, provided that the foods are reasonably priced, clearly labeled, easy to find in the grocery store, and convenient to prepare. These foods must also taste good—as good as the traditional choices. Of course, a person need not eat any of these "special" foods to enjoy a healthy diet; many "regular" foods provide numerous health benefits as well. In fact, "regular" foods such as whole grains; vegetables and legumes; fruits; meats, fish, and poultry; and milk products are among the healthiest choices a person can make.

IN SUMMARY A person selects foods for a variety of reasons. Whatever those reasons may be, food choices influence health. Individual food selections neither make nor break a diet's healthfulness, but the balance of foods selected over time can make an important difference to health.[5] For this reason, people are wise to think "nutrition" when making their food choices.

functional foods: foods that provide health benefits beyond their nutrient contributions. Functional foods may include whole foods, fortified foods, and modified foods.

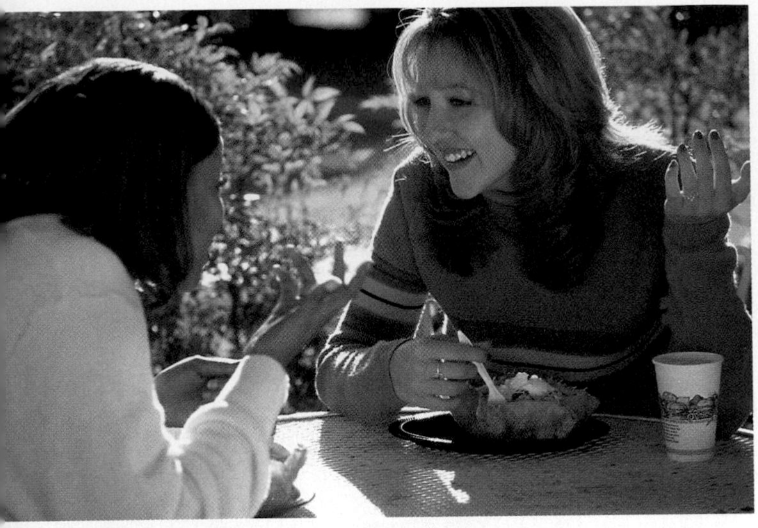

© SW Productions/Index Stock Imagery

Foods bring pleasure—and nutrients.

The Nutrients

Biologically speaking, people eat to receive nourishment. Do you ever think of yourself as a biological being made of carefully arranged atoms, molecules, cells, tissues, and organs? Are you aware of the activity going on within your body even as you sit still? The atoms, molecules, and cells of your body continually move and change, even though the structures of your tissues and organs and your external appearance remain relatively constant. Your skin, which has covered you since your birth, is replaced entirely by new cells every seven years. The fat beneath your skin is not the same fat that was there a year ago. Your oldest red blood cell is only 120 days old, and the entire lining of your digestive tract is renewed every 3 days. To maintain your "self," you must continually replenish, from foods, the **energy** and the **nutrients** you deplete in maintaining your body.

Nutrients in Foods and in the Body

Amazingly, the body can derive all the energy, structural materials, and regulating agents that it needs from the foods we eat. This section introduces the nutrients that foods deliver and shows how they participate in the dynamic processes that keep people alive and well.

■ As Chapter 5 explains, most lipids are fats.

Composition of Foods Chemical analysis of a food such as a tomato shows that it is composed primarily of water (95 percent). Most of the solid materials are carbohydrates, lipids,■ and proteins. If you could remove these materials, you would find a tiny residue of vitamins, minerals, and other compounds. Water, carbohydrates, lipids, proteins, vitamins, and some of the minerals found in foods are nutrients—substances the body uses for the growth, maintenance, and repair of its tissues.

This book focuses mostly on the nutrients, but foods contain other compounds as well—fibers, **phytochemicals**, pigments, additives, alcohols, and others. Some are beneficial, some are neutral, and a few are harmful. Later sections of the book touch on these **nonnutrients** and their significance.

Composition of the Body A complete chemical analysis of your body would show that it is made of materials similar to those found in foods (see Figure 1-1). A healthy 150-pound body contains about 90 pounds of water and about 20 to 45 pounds of fat. The remaining pounds are mostly protein, carbohydrate, and the major minerals of the bones. Vitamins, other minerals, and incidental extras constitute a fraction of a pound.

Chemical Composition of Nutrients The simplest of the nutrients are the minerals. Each mineral is a chemical element; its atoms are all alike. As a result, its identity never changes. Iron may change its form, for example, but it remains iron when a food is cooked, when a person eats the food, when iron becomes part of a red blood cell, when the cell is broken down, and when the iron is lost from the body by excretion. The next simplest nutrient is water, a compound made of two elements—hydrogen and oxygen. Minerals and water are **inorganic** nutrients—they contain no carbon.

The other four classes of nutrients (carbohydrates, lipids, proteins, and vitamins) are more complex. In addition to hydrogen and oxygen, they all contain carbon, an element found in all living things. They are therefore called **organic** compounds (meaning, literally, "alive"). Protein and some vitamins also contain nitrogen and may contain other elements as well (see Table 1-1).

energy: the capacity to do work. The energy in food is chemical energy. The body can convert this chemical energy to mechanical, electrical, or heat energy.

nutrients: chemical substances obtained from food and used in the body to provide energy, structural materials, and regulating agents to support growth, maintenance, and repair of the body's tissues. Nutrients may also reduce the risks of some diseases.

phytochemicals (FIE-toe-KEM-ih-cals): nonnutrient compounds found in plant-derived foods that have biological activity in the body.
- **phyto** = plant

nonnutrients: compounds in foods that do not fit within the six classes of nutrients.

inorganic: not containing carbon or pertaining to living things.
- **in** = not

organic: in chemistry, a substance or molecule containing carbon-carbon bonds or carbon-hydrogen bonds.* In agriculture, organic means growing crops and raising livestock according to U.S. Department of Agriculture (USDA) standards.

* This definition excludes coal, diamonds, and a few carbon-containing compounds that contain only a single carbon and no hydrogen, such as carbon dioxide (CO_2), calcium carbonate ($CaCO_3$), magnesium carbonate ($MgCO_3$), and sodium cyanide (NaCN).

FIGURE 1-1 Body Composition of Healthy-Weight Men and Women

The human body is made of compounds similar to those found in foods—mostly water (60 percent) and some fat (13 to 21 percent for young men, 23 to 31 percent for young women), with carbohydrate, protein, vitamins, minerals, and other minor constituents making up the remainder. (Chapter 8 describes the health hazards of too little or too much body fat.)

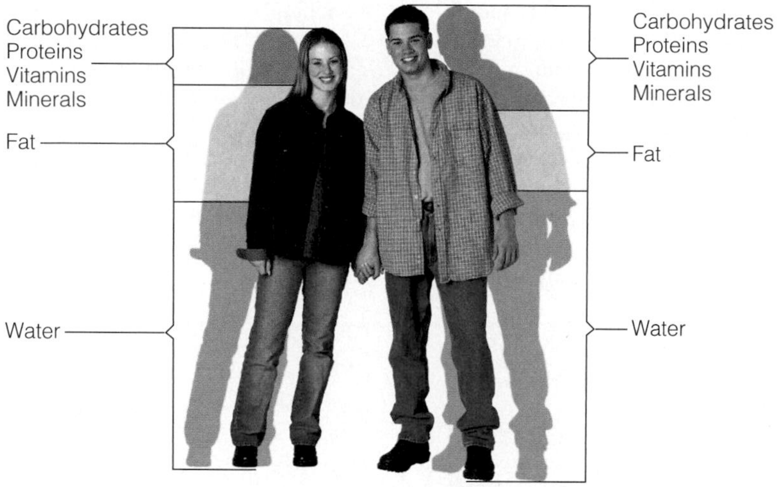
Carbohydrates
Proteins
Vitamins
Minerals
Fat
Water
Carbohydrates
Proteins
Vitamins
Minerals
Fat
Water

Essential Nutrients The body can make some nutrients, but it cannot make all of them, and it makes some in insufficient quantities to meet its needs. It must obtain these nutrients from foods. The nutrients that foods must supply are **essential nutrients.** When used to refer to nutrients, the word *essential* means more than just "necessary"; it means "needed from outside the body"—normally, from foods.

The Energy-Yielding Nutrients

In the body, three of the organic nutrients can be used to provide energy: carbohydrate, fat, and protein.■ In contrast to these **energy-yielding nutrients,** vitamins, minerals, and water do not yield energy in the human body.

■ Carbohydrate, fat, and protein are sometimes called **macronutrients** because they are required by the body in relatively large amounts (many grams daily). In contrast, vitamins and minerals are **micronutrients,** required in small amounts (milligrams or micrograms daily).

TABLE 1-1 Elements in the Six Classes of Nutrients

Notice that organic nutrients contain carbon.

	Carbon	Hydrogen	Oxygen	Nitrogen	Minerals
Inorganic nutrients					
Minerals					✓
Water		✓	✓		
Organic nutrients					
Carbohydrates	✓	✓	✓		
Lipids (fats)	✓	✓	✓		
Proteins[a]	✓	✓	✓	✓	
Vitamins[b]	✓	✓	✓		

[a]Some proteins also contain the mineral sulfur.
[b]Some vitamins contain nitrogen; some contain minerals.

essential nutrients: nutrients a person must obtain from food because the body cannot make them for itself in sufficient quantity to meet physiological needs; also called **indispensable nutrients.** About 40 nutrients are currently known to be essential for human beings.

energy-yielding nutrients: the nutrients that break down to yield energy the body can use:
- Carbohydrate.
- Fat.
- Protein.

HOW TO Think Metric

Like other scientists, nutrition scientists use metric units of measure. They measure food energy in kilocalories, people's height in centimeters, people's weight in kilograms, and the weights of foods and nutrients in grams, milligrams, or micrograms. For ease in using these measures, it helps to remember that the prefixes on the grams imply 1000. For example, a *kilo*gram is 1000 grams, a *milli*gram is 1/1000 of a gram, and a *micro*gram is 1/1000 of a milligram.

Most food labels and many recipe books provide "dual measures," listing both household measures, such as cups, quarts, and teaspoons, and metric measures, such as milliliters, liters, and grams. This practice gives people an opportunity to gradually learn to "think metric."

A person might begin to "think metric" by simply observing the measure—by noticing the amount of soda in a 2-liter bottle, for example. Through such experiences, a person can become familiar with a measure without having to do any conversions.

To facilitate communication, many members of the international scientific community have adopted a common system of measurement—the International System of Units (SI). In addition to using metric measures, the SI establishes common units of measurement. For example, the SI unit for measuring food energy is the joule (not the kcalorie). A joule is the amount of energy expended when 1 kilogram is moved 1 meter by a force of 1 newton. The joule is thus a measure of *work* energy, whereas the kcalorie is a measure of *heat* energy. While many scientists and journals report their findings in kilojoules (kJ), many others, particularly those in the United States, use kcalories. To convert energy measures from kcalories to kilojoules, multiply by 4.2. For example, a 50-kcalorie cookie provides 210 kilojoules:

$$50 \text{ kcal} \times 4.2 = 210 \text{ kJ}.$$

Exact conversion factors for these and other units of measure are in the Aids to Calculation section on the last two pages of the book.

Volume: Liters (L)

1L = 1000 milliliters (mL).
0.95 L = 1 quart.
1 mL = 0.03 fluid ounces.
240 mL = 1 cup.

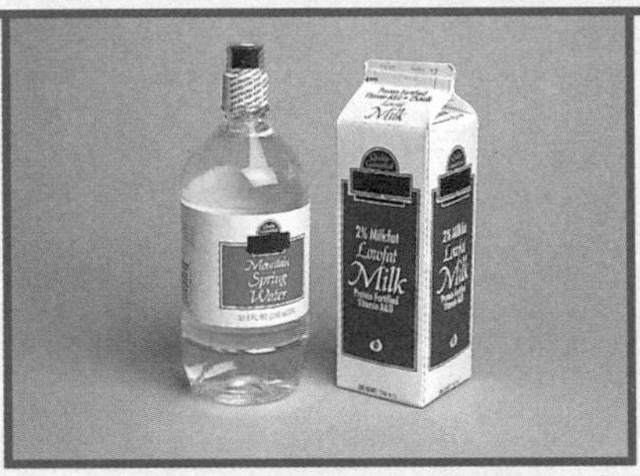

© Felicia Martinez/Photo Edit

A liter of liquid is approximately one U.S. quart. (Four liters are only about 5 percent more than a gallon.)

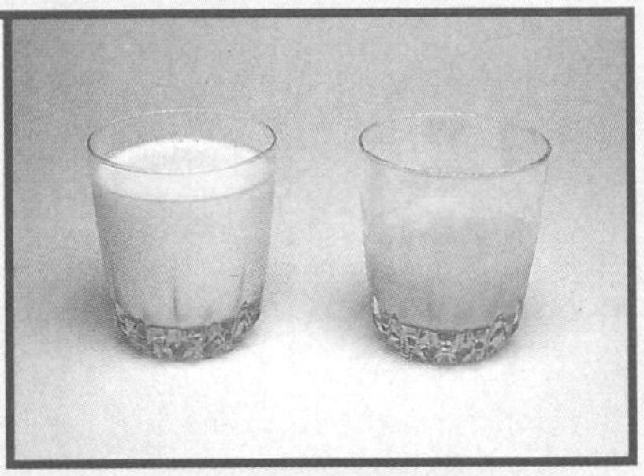

© PhotoEdit/Felicia Martinez

One cup is about 240 milliliters; a half-cup of liquid is about 120 milliliters.

Weight: Grams (g)

1 g = 1000 milligrams (mg).
1 g = 0.04 ounce (oz).
1 oz = 28.35 g or ≈ 30 g.
100 g ≈ 3½ oz.
1 kilogram (kg) = 1000 g.
1 kg = 2.2 pounds (lb).
454 g = 1 lb.

A kilogram is slightly more than 2 lb; conversely, a pound is about ½ kg.

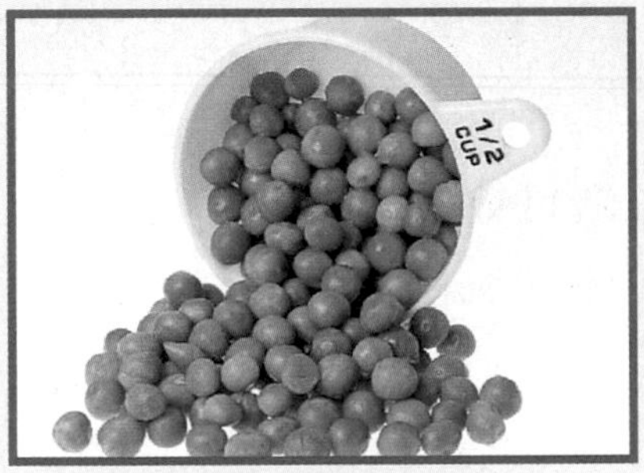
1/2
CUP

© Thomas Harm, Tom Peterson/Quest Photographic Inc.

A half-cup of vegetables weighs about 100 grams; one pea weighs about ½ gram.

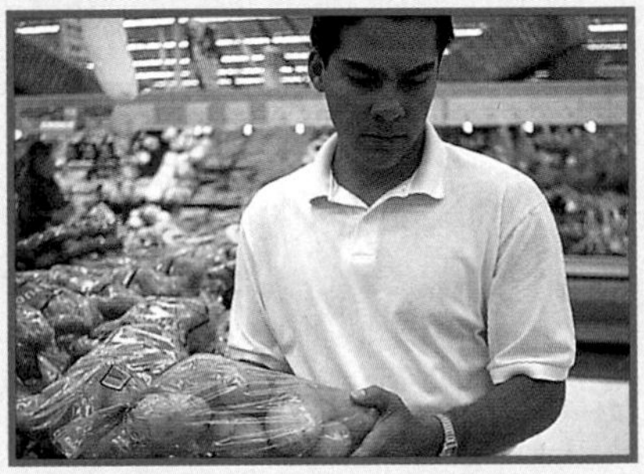

© Tony Freeman/Photo Edit

A 5-pound bag of potatoes weighs about 2 kilograms, and a 176-pound person weighs 80 kilograms.

calories: units by which energy is measured. Food energy is measured in **kilocalories** (1000 calories equal 1 kilocalorie), abbreviated **kcalories** or **kcal.** One kcalorie is the amount of heat necessary to raise the temperature of 1 kilogram (kg) of water 1°C. The scientific use of the term *kcalorie* is the same as the popular use of the term *calorie.*

Energy Measured in kCalories The energy released from carbohydrates, fats, and proteins can be measured in **calories**—tiny units of energy so small that a single apple provides tens of thousands of them. To ease calculations, energy is expressed in 1000-calorie metric units known as kilocalories (shortened to kcalories, but commonly called "calories"). When you read in popular books or magazines that an apple provides "100 calories," understand that it means 100 kcalories. This book uses the term *kcalorie* and its abbreviation *kcal* throughout, as do other scientific books and journals. The accompanying "How to" provides a few tips on how to "think metric."

Energy from Foods The amount of energy a food provides depends on how much carbohydrate, fat, and protein it contains. When completely broken down

HOW TO Calculate the Energy Available from Foods

To calculate the energy available from a food, multiply the number of grams of carbohydrate, protein, and fat by 4, 4, and 9, respectively. Then add the results together. For example, 1 slice of bread with 1 tablespoon of peanut butter on it contains 16 grams carbohydrate, 7 grams protein, and 9 grams fat:

$$16 \text{ g carbohydrate} \times 4 \text{ kcal/g} = 64 \text{ kcal.}$$
$$7 \text{ g protein} \times 4 \text{ kcal/g} = 28 \text{ kcal.}$$
$$9 \text{ g fat} \times 9 \text{ kcal/g} = 81 \text{ kcal.}$$
$$\text{Total} = 173 \text{ kcal.}$$

From this information, you can calculate the percentage of kcalories each of the energy nutrients contributes to the total. To determine the percentage of kcalories from fat, for example, divide the 81 fat kcalories by the total 173 kcalories:

$$81 \text{ fat kcal} \div 173 \text{ total kcal} = 0.468 \text{ (rounded to 0.47).}$$

Then multiply by 100 to get the percentage:

$$0.47 \times 100 = 47\%.$$

Dietary recommendations that urge people to limit fat intake to 20 to 35 percent of kcalories refer to the day's total energy intake, not to individual foods. Still, if the proportion of fat in each food choice throughout a day exceeds 35 percent of kcalories, then the day's total surely will, too. Knowing that this snack provides 47 percent of its kcalories from fat alerts a person to the need to make lower-fat selections at other times that day.

in the body, a gram of carbohydrate yields about 4 kcalories of energy; a gram of protein also yields 4 kcalories; and a gram of fat yields 9 kcalories (see Table 1-2). Fat, therefore, has a greater **energy density** than either carbohydrate or protein. Figure 1-2 (on p. 10) compares the energy density of two breakfast options, and later chapters describe how considering a food's energy density can help with weight management.■ The accompanying "How to" explains how to calculate the energy available from foods.

One other substance contributes energy: alcohol. Alcohol is not considered a nutrient because it interferes with the growth, maintenance, and repair of the body, but it does yield energy (7 kcalories per gram) when metabolized in the body. (Highlight 7 and later chapters present the potential harms and possible benefits of alcohol consumption.)

Most foods contain all three energy-yielding nutrients, as well as water, vitamins, minerals, and other substances. For example, meat contains water, fat, vitamins, and minerals as well as protein. Bread contains water, a trace of fat, a little protein, and some vitamins and minerals in addition to its carbohydrate. Only a few foods are exceptions to this rule, the common ones being sugar (pure carbohydrate) and oil (essentially pure fat).

Energy in the Body The body uses the energy-yielding nutrients to fuel all its activities. When the body uses carbohydrate, fat, or protein for energy, the bonds between the nutrient's atoms break. As the bonds break, they release energy.■ Some of this energy is released as heat, but some is used to send electrical impulses through the brain and nerves, to synthesize body compounds, and to move muscles. Thus the energy from food supports every activity from quiet thought to vigorous sports.

If the body does not use these nutrients to fuel its current activities, it rearranges them into storage compounds (such as body fat), to be used between meals and overnight when fresh energy supplies run low. If more energy is consumed than expended, the result is an increase in energy stores and weight gain. Similarly, if less energy is consumed than expended, the result is a decrease in energy stores and weight loss.

When consumed in excess of energy need, alcohol, too, can be converted to body fat and stored. When alcohol contributes a substantial portion of the energy in a person's diet, the harm it does far exceeds the problems of excess body fat. (Highlight 7 describes the effects of alcohol on health and nutrition.)

■ Foods with a high energy density help with weight gain, whereas those with a low energy density help with weight loss.

■ The processes by which nutrients are broken down to yield energy or used to make body structures are known as **metabolism** (defined and described further in Chapter 7).

TABLE 1-2 kCalorie Values of Energy Nutrients

Energy Nutrients	kCalories[a] (per gram)
Carbohydrate	4 kcal/g
Fat	9 kcal/g
Protein	4 kcal/g

NOTE: Alcohol contributes 7 kcalories per gram that can be used for energy, but it is not considered a nutrient because it interferes with the body's growth, maintenance, and repair.
[a] For those using kilojoules: 1 g carbohydrate = 17 kJ; 1 g protein = 17 kJ; 1 g fat = 37 kJ; and 1 g alcohol = 29 kJ.

energy density: a measure of the energy a food provides relative to the amount of food (kcalories per gram).

FIGURE 1-2 Energy Density of Two Breakfast Options Compared

Gram for gram, ounce for ounce, and bite for bite, foods with a high energy density deliver more kcalories than foods with a low energy density. Both of these breakfast options provide 500 kcalories, but the cereal with milk, fruit salad, scrambled egg, turkey sausage, and toast with jam offers three times as much food as the doughnuts (based on weight); it has a lower energy density than the doughnuts. Selecting a variety of foods also helps to ensure nutrient adequacy.

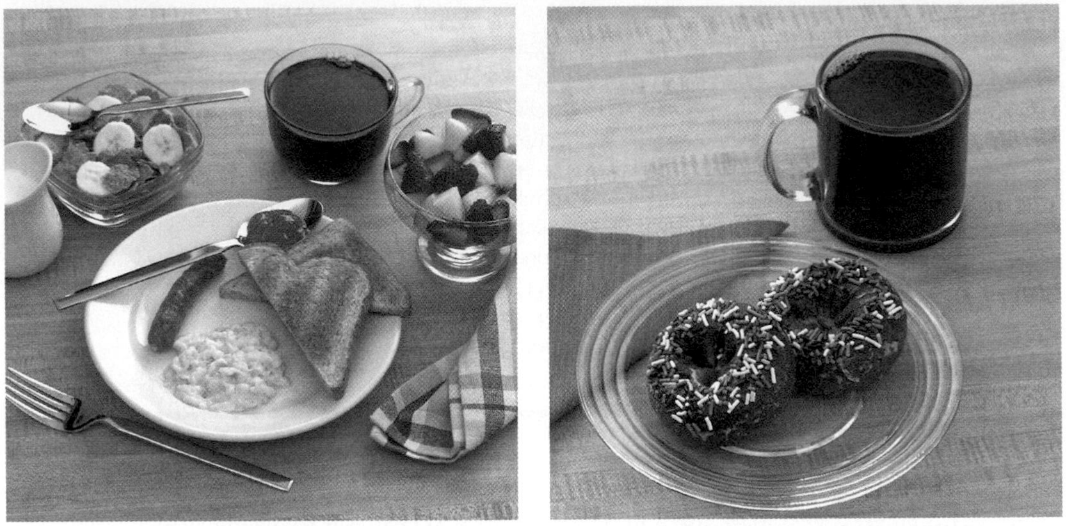

© Matthew Farruggio (both)

LOWER ENERGY DENSITY

This 450-gram breakfast delivers 500 kcalories, for an energy density of 1.1 (500 kcal ÷ 450 g = 1.1 kcal/g).

HIGHER ENERGY DENSITY

This 144-gram breakfast also delivers 500 kcalories, for an energy density of 3.5 (500 kcal ÷ 144 g = 3.5 kcal/g).

Other Roles of Energy-Yielding Nutrients In addition to providing energy, carbohydrates, fats, and proteins provide the raw materials for building the body's tissues and regulating its many activities. In fact, protein's role as a fuel source is relatively minor compared with both the other two nutrients and its other roles. Proteins are found in structures such as the muscles and skin and help to regulate activities such as digestion and energy metabolism.

The Vitamins

The **vitamins** are also organic, but they do not provide energy. Instead, they facilitate the release of energy from carbohydrate, fat, and protein and participate in numerous other activities throughout the body.

There are 13 different vitamins, each with its own special roles to play.* One vitamin enables the eyes to see in dim light, another helps protect the lungs from air pollution, and still another helps make the sex hormones—among other things. When you cut yourself, one vitamin helps stop the bleeding and another helps repair the skin. Vitamins busily help replace old red blood cells and the lining of the digestive tract. Almost every action in the body requires the assistance of vitamins.

Vitamins can function only if they are intact, but because they are complex organic molecules, they are vulnerable to destruction by heat, light, and chemical agents. This is why the body handles them carefully, and why nutrition-wise cooks do, too. The strategies of cooking vegetables at moderate temperatures, using small amounts of water, and for short times all help to preserve the vitamins.

vitamins: organic, essential nutrients required in small amounts by the body for health.

* The water-soluble vitamins are vitamin C and the eight B vitamins: thiamin, riboflavin, niacin, vitamins B_6 and B_{12}, folate, biotin, and pantothenic acid. The fat-soluble vitamins are vitamins A, D, E, and K. The water-soluble vitamins are the subject of Chapter 10 and the fat-soluble vitamins, of Chapter 11.

The Minerals

In the body, some **minerals** are put together in orderly arrays in such structures as bones and teeth. Minerals are also found in the fluids of the body and influence their properties. Whatever their roles, minerals do not yield energy.

Some 16 minerals are known to be essential in human nutrition.* Others are still being studied to determine whether they play significant roles in the human body. Still other minerals are *not* essential nutrients, but are important nevertheless because they are environmental contaminants that displace the nutrient minerals from their workplaces in the body, disrupting body functions. The problems caused by contaminant minerals are described in Chapter 13.

Because minerals are inorganic, they are indestructible and need not be handled with the special care that vitamins require. Minerals can, however, be bound by substances that interfere with the body's ability to absorb them. They can also be lost during food-refining processes or during cooking when they leach into water that is discarded.

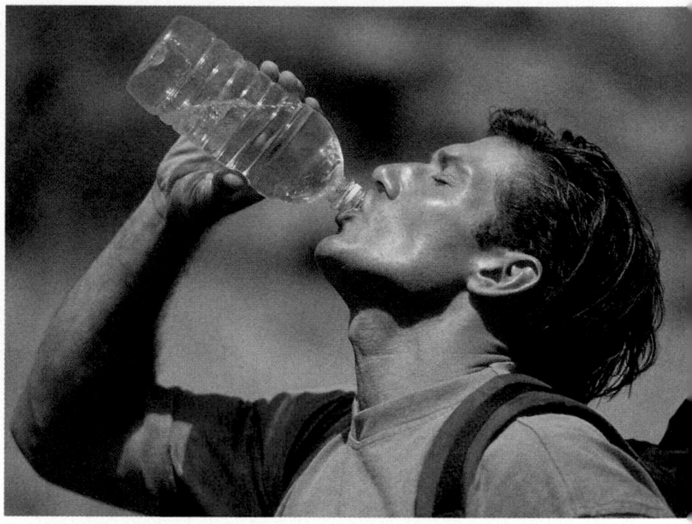

Water itself is an essential nutrient and naturally carries many minerals.

Water

Water, indispensable and abundant, provides the environment in which nearly all the body's activities are conducted. It participates in many metabolic reactions and supplies the medium for transporting vital materials to cells and waste products away from them. Water is discussed fully in Chapter 12, but it is mentioned in every chapter. If you watch for it, you cannot help but be impressed by water's participation in all life processes.

IN SUMMARY Foods provide nutrients—substances that support the growth, maintenance, and repair of the body's tissues. The six classes of nutrients include:

- Carbohydrates.
- Lipids (fats).
- Proteins.
- Vitamins.
- Minerals.
- Water.

Foods rich in the energy-yielding nutrients (carbohydrates, fats, and proteins) provide the major materials for building the body's tissues and yield energy for the body's use or storage. Energy is measured in kcalories. Vitamins, minerals, and water facilitate a variety of activities in the body. Without exaggeration, nutrients provide the physical and metabolic basis for nearly all that we are and all that we do.

The Science of Nutrition

The science of nutrition is the study of the nutrients and other substances in foods and the body's handling of them. Its foundation depends on several other sciences, including biology, biochemistry, and physiology. As sciences go, nutrition is a young one, but as you can see from the size of this book, much has happened in nutrition's short life. And it is currently entering a tremendous growth spurt as

minerals: inorganic elements. Some minerals are essential nutrients required in small amounts by the body for health.

* The major minerals are calcium, phosphorus, potassium, sodium, chloride, magnesium, and sulfur. The trace minerals are iron, iodine, zinc, chromium, selenium, fluoride, molybdenum, copper, and manganese. Chapters 12 and 13 are devoted to the major and trace minerals, respectively.

FIGURE 1-3 The Scientific Method

In conducting research, scientists follow the scientific method. Most often, research generates additional problems and questions. Thus the sequence begins anew, and research continues in a never-ending, somewhat cyclical way.

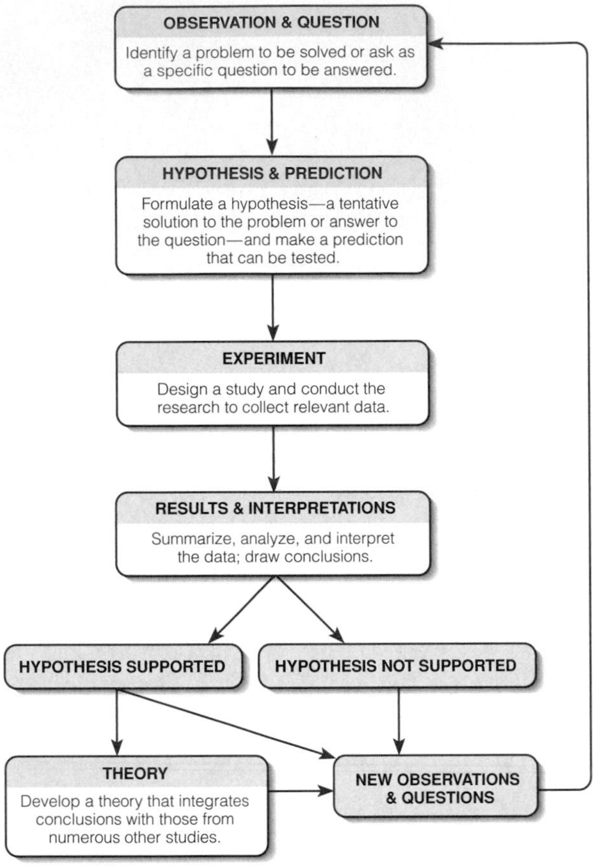
OBSERVATION & QUESTION
Identify a problem to be solved or ask as a specific question to be answered.
HYPOTHESIS & PREDICTION
Formulate a hypothesis—a tentative solution to the problem or answer to the question—and make a prediction that can be tested.
EXPERIMENT
Design a study and conduct the research to collect relevant data.
RESULTS & INTERPRETATIONS
Summarize, analyze, and interpret the data; draw conclusions.
HYPOTHESIS SUPPORTED
HYPOTHESIS NOT SUPPORTED
THEORY
Develop a theory that integrates conclusions with those from numerous other studies.
NEW OBSERVATIONS & QUESTIONS

scientists apply knowledge gained from sequencing the human **genome.** The integration of nutrition, genomics, and molecular biology has opened up a whole new world of study called **nutritional genomics**—the science of how nutrients affect the activities of genes and how genes affect the activities of nutrients.[6] Look for examples of these interactions and of how nutritional genomics is shaping the science of nutrition in later sections of the book.■ This section introduces the research methods scientists have used in uncovering the wonders of nutrition.

Nutrition Research

Researchers use the scientific method to guide their work (see Figure 1-3). As the figure shows, research always begins with a problem or a question. For example, "What foods or nutrients might protect against the common cold?" In search of an answer, scientists make an educated guess (hypothesis), such as "foods rich in vitamin C reduce the number of common colds." Then they systematically conduct research studies to collect data that will test the **hypothesis** (see the glossary on p. 14 for definitions of research terms). Some examples of various types of research designs are presented in Figure 1-4. Each type of study has strengths and weaknesses (see Table 1-3 on p. 14). Consequently, some provide stronger evidence than others. Findings must be analyzed and interpreted with an awareness of each study's limitations. Importantly, scientists must be cautious about drawing any conclusions until they have accumulated a body of evidence from multiple studies that have used various types of research designs. As evidence accumulates, scientists begin to develop a **theory** that integrates the various findings and explains the complex relationships. (See Highlight 1 for a discussion of how to evaluate research findings.)

In attempting to discover whether a nutrient relieves symptoms or cures a disease, researchers deliberately manipulate one variable (for example, the amount of vitamin C in the diet) and measure any observed changes (perhaps the number of colds). As much as possible, all other conditions are held constant. The following paragraphs illustrate how this is accomplished using research on vitamin C and the common cold as an example.

■ Highlight 18 features a complete discussion of nutritional genomics.

Controls In studies examining the effectiveness of vitamin C, researchers typically divide the **subjects** into two groups. One group (the **experimental group**) receives a vitamin C supplement, and the other (the **control group**) does not. Researchers observe both groups to determine whether the vitamin C group has fewer or shorter colds than the control group. A number of pitfalls are inherent in an experiment of this kind and must be avoided.

First, each person must have an equal chance of being assigned to either the experimental group or the control group. This is accomplished by **randomization;** that is, the members are chosen from the same population by flipping a coin or some other method involving chance.

Importantly, the two groups of people must be similar and must have the same track record with respect to colds to rule out the possibility that observed differences in the rate, severity, or duration of colds might have occurred anyway. If, for example, the control group would normally catch twice as many colds as the experimental group, then the findings prove nothing.

In experiments involving a nutrient, the diets of both groups must also be similar, especially with respect to the nutrient being studied. If those in the experimental group were receiving less vitamin C from their diet, then the effects of the supplement may not be apparent.

genome (GEE-nome): the full complement of genetic material (DNA) in the chromosomes of a cell. In human beings, the genome consists of 23 pairs of chromosomes. The study of genomes is **genomics.**

nutritional genomics: the science of how nutrients affect the activities of genes and how genes affect the activities of nutrients.

FIGURE 1-4 Examples of Research Designs

EPIDEMIOLOGICAL STUDIES

CROSS-SECTIONAL

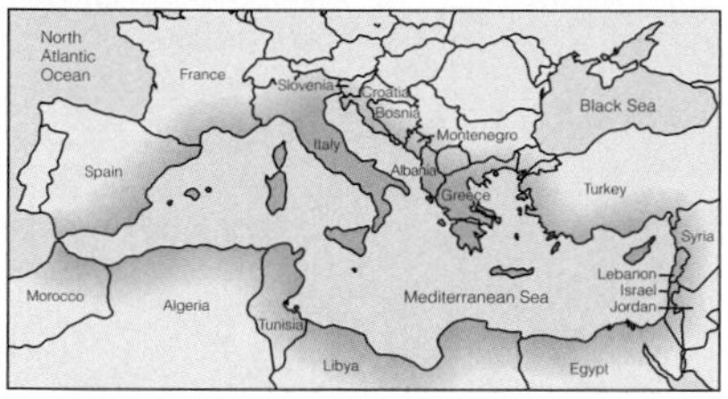
North Atlantic Ocean
France
Slovenia
Croatia
Bosnia
Montenegro
Black Sea
Spain
Italy
Albania
Greece
Turkey
Syria
Lebanon
Israel
Jordan
Morocco
Algeria
Tunisia
Mediterranean Sea
Libya
Egypt

Researchers observe how much and what kinds of foods a group of people eat and how healthy those people are. Their findings identify factors that might influence the incidence of a disease in various populations.

Example. The people of the Mediterranean region drink lots of wine, eat plenty of fat from olive oil, and have a lower incidence of heart disease than northern Europeans and North Americans.

CASE-CONTROL

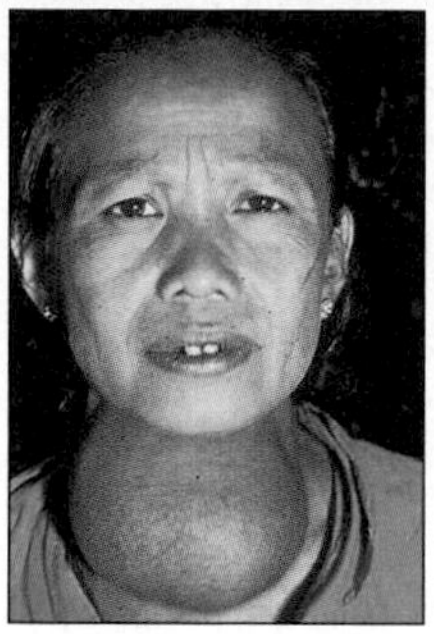

© L. V. Bergman and Associates Inc.

Researchers compare people who do and do not have a given condition such as a disease, closely matching them in age, gender, and other key variables so that differences in other factors will stand out. These differences may account for the condition in the group that has it.

Example. People with goiter lack iodine in their diets.

COHORT

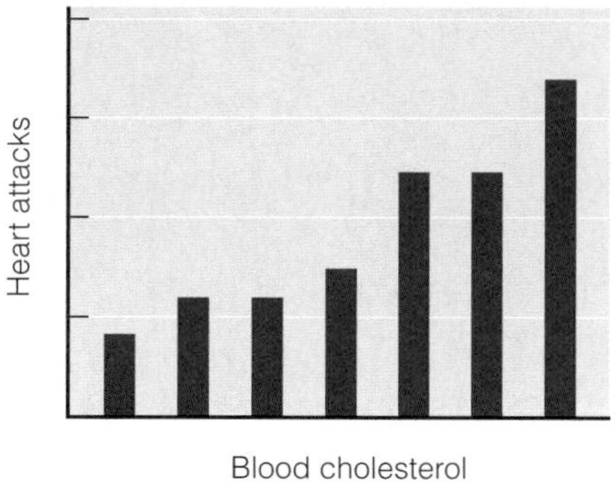
Heart attacks
Blood cholesterol

Researchers analyze data collected from a selected group of people (a cohort) at intervals over a certain period of time.

Example. Data collected periodically over the past several decades from over 5000 people randomly selected from the town of Framingham, Massachusetts, in 1948 have revealed that the risk of heart attack increases as blood cholesterol increases.

EXPERIMENTAL STUDIES

LABORATORY-BASED ANIMAL STUDIES

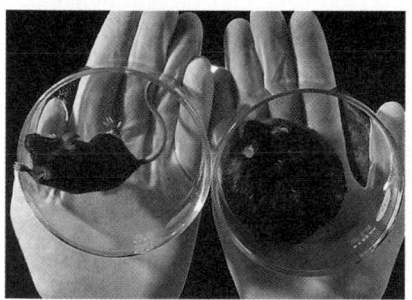

© R. Benali/Gamma

Researchers feed animals special diets that provide or omit specific nutrients and then observe any changes in health. Such studies test possible disease causes and treatments in a laboratory where all conditions can be controlled.

Example. Mice fed a high-fat diet eat less food than mice given a lower-fat diet, so they receive the same number of kcalories—but the mice eating the fat-rich diet become severely obese.

LABORATORY-BASED IN VITRO STUDIES

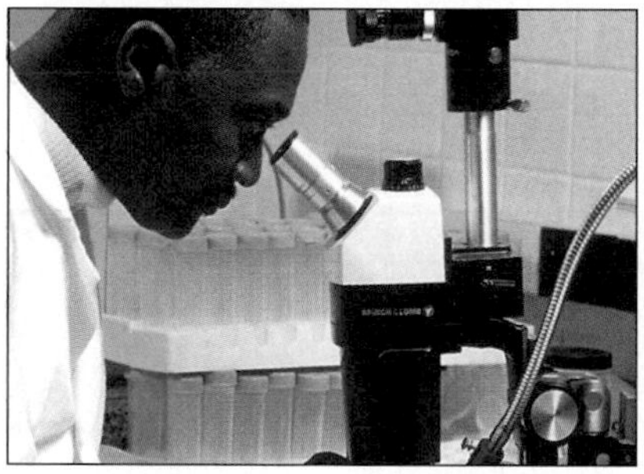

USDA Agricultural Research Service

Researchers examine the effects of a specific variable on a tissue, cell, or molecule isolated from a living organism.

Example. Laboratory studies find that fish oils inhibit the growth and activity of the bacteria implicated in ulcer formation.

HUMAN INTERVENTION (OR CLINICAL) TRIALS

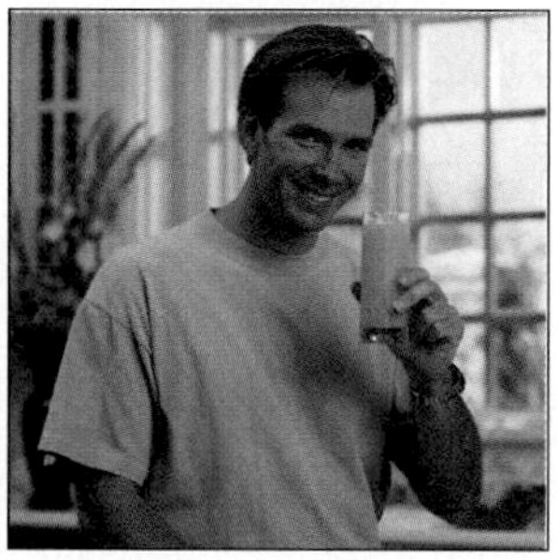

© 2001 Photo Disc Inc.

Researchers ask people to adopt a new behavior (for example, eat a citrus fruit, take a vitamin C supplement, or exercise daily). These trials help determine the effectiveness of such interventions on the development or prevention of disease.

Example. Heart disease risk factors improve when men receive fresh-squeezed orange juice daily for two months compared with those on a diet low in vitamin C—even when both groups follow a diet high in saturated fat.

Sample Size To ensure that chance variation between the two groups does not influence the results, the groups must be large. If one member of a group of five people catches a bad cold by chance, he will pull the whole group's average toward bad colds; but if one member of a group of 500 catches a bad cold, she will not unduly affect the group average. Statistical methods are used to determine whether differences between groups of various sizes support a hypothesis.

TABLE 1-3 Strengths and Weaknesses of Research Designs

Type of Research	Strengths	Weaknesses
Epidemiological studies determine the incidence and distribution of diseases in a population. Epidemiological studies include cross-sectional, case-control, and cohort (see Figure 1-4).	• Can narrow down the list of possible causes • Can raise questions to pursue through other types of studies	• Cannot control variables that may influence the development or the prevention of a disease • Cannot prove cause and effect
Laboratory-based studies explore the effects of a specific variable on a tissue, cell, or molecule. Laboratory-based studies are often conducted in test tubes (in vitro) or on animals.	• Can control conditions • Can determine effects of a variable	• Cannot apply results from test tubes or animals to human beings
Human intervention or **clinical trials** involve human beings who follow a specified regimen.	• Can control conditions (for the most part) • Can apply findings to some groups of human beings	• Cannot generalize findings to all human beings • Cannot use certain treatments for clinical or ethical reasons

Placebos If people take vitamin C for colds and *believe* it will cure them, their chances of recovery may improve. Taking anything believed to be beneficial may hasten recovery. This phenomenon, the result of expectations, is known as the **placebo effect.** In experiments designed to determine vitamin C's effect on colds, this mind-body effect must be rigorously controlled. Severity of symptoms is often a subjective measure, and people who believe they are receiving treatment may report less severe symptoms.

GLOSSARY OF RESEARCH TERMS

blind experiment: an experiment in which the subjects do not know whether they are members of the experimental group or the control group.

control group: a group of individuals similar in all possible respects to the experimental group except for the treatment. Ideally, the control group receives a placebo while the experimental group receives a real treatment.

correlation (CORE-ee-LAY-shun): the simultaneous increase, decrease, or change in two variables. If A increases as B increases, or if A decreases as B decreases, the correlation is **positive.** (This does not mean that A causes B or vice versa.) If A increases as B decreases, or if A decreases as B increases, the correlation is **negative.** (This does not mean that A prevents B or vice versa.) Some third factor may account for both A and B.

double-blind experiment: an experiment in which neither the subjects nor the researchers know which subjects are members of the experimental group and which are serving as control subjects, until after the experiment is over.

experimental group: a group of individuals similar in all possible respects to the control group except for the treatment. The experimental group receives the real treatment.

hypothesis (hi-POTH-eh-sis): an unproven statement that tentatively explains the relationships between two or more variables.

peer review: a process in which a panel of scientists rigorously evaluates a research study to assure that the scientific method was followed.

placebo (pla-SEE-bo): an inert, harmless medication given to provide comfort and hope; a sham treatment used in controlled research studies.

placebo effect: the result of expectations in the effectiveness of a medicine, even medicine without pharmaceutical effects.

randomization (RAN-dom-ih-ZAY-shun): a process of choosing the members of the experimental and control groups without bias.

replication (REP-lee-KAY-shun): repeating an experiment and getting the same results. The skeptical scientist, on hearing of a new, exciting finding, will ask, "Has it been replicated yet?" If it hasn't, the scientist will withhold judgment regarding the finding's validity.

subjects: the people or animals participating in a research project.

theory: a tentative explanation that integrates many and diverse findings to further the understanding of a defined topic.

validity (va-LID-ih-tee): having the quality of being founded on fact or evidence.

variables: factors that change. A variable may depend on another variable (for example, a child's height depends on his age), or it may be independent (for example, a child's height does not depend on the color of her eyes). Sometimes both variables correlate with a third variable (a child's height and eye color both depend on genetics).

One way experimenters control for the placebo effect is to give pills to all participants; those in the experimental group receive pills containing vitamin C, and those in the control group receive a **placebo,** pills of similar appearance and taste containing an inactive ingredient. This way, the expectations of both groups will be equivalent. It is not necessary to convince all subjects that they are receiving vitamin C, but the extent of belief or unbelief must be the same in both groups. A study conducted under these conditions is called a **blind experiment**—that is, the subjects do not know (are blind to) whether they are members of the experimental group (receiving treatment) or the control group (receiving the placebo).

Double Blind When both the subjects and the researchers do not know which subjects are in which group, the study is called a **double-blind experiment.** Being fallible human beings and having an emotional and sometimes financial investment in a successful outcome, researchers might record and interpret results with a bias in the expected direction. To prevent such bias, the pills are coded by a third party, who does not reveal to the experimenters which subjects were in which group until all results have been recorded.

Correlations and Causes Researchers often examine the relationships between two or more **variables**—for example, daily vitamin C intake and the number of colds or the duration and severity of cold symptoms. Importantly, researchers must be able to observe, measure, or verify the variables selected. Findings sometimes suggest no **correlation** between the two variables (regardless of the amount of vitamin C consumed, the number of colds remains the same). Other times, studies find either a **positive correlation** (the more vitamin C, the more colds) or a **negative correlation** (the more vitamin C, the fewer colds). Correlational evidence proves only that two variables are associated, not that one is the cause of the other. People often jump to conclusions when they learn of correlations, but the conclusions are often wrong. To prove that A causes B, scientists have to find evidence of the *mechanism*—that is, to catch A in the act of causing B, so to speak. Furthermore, other scientists must confirm or disprove the findings through **replication** before the results are accepted into the body of nutrition knowledge. Before the findings are published, they are subjected to **peer review**—a process whereby a panel of scientists critically evaluates the study to confirm that it followed standard scientific methods.

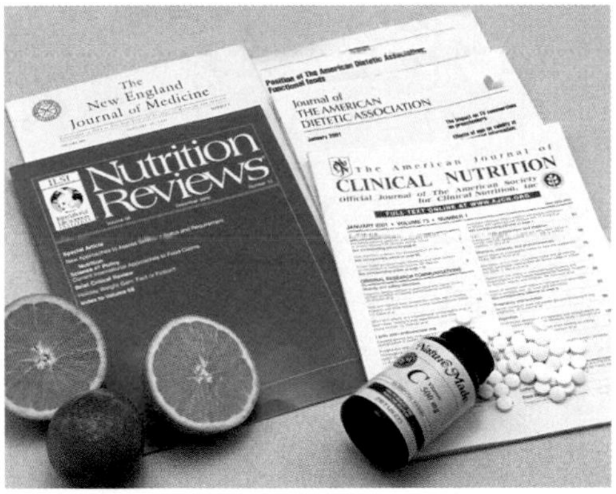
The New England Journal of Medicine
Nutrition Reviews
Journal of THE AMERICAN DIETETIC ASSOCIATION
The American Journal of CLINICAL NUTRITION

© Craig M. Moore

Knowledge about the nutrients and their effects on health comes from scientific study.

Research versus Rumors

In discussing these subtleties of experimental design, our intent is to show you what a far cry scientific **validity** is from the experience of your neighbor Sarah (sample size, one; no control group), who says she takes vitamin C when she feels a cold coming on and "it works every time."■ She knows what she is taking, she believes in its effectiveness, and she tends not to notice when it doesn't work. Before concluding that an experiment has shown that a nutrient cures a disease or alleviates a symptom, ask these questions:

- Who participated in the study, and how were participants selected?
- Were the control group and the experimental group similar?
- Was the sample size large enough to rule out chance variation?
- Was a placebo effectively administered (blind)?
- Was the experiment double blind?
- Were the variables selected appropriately and measured accurately?
- Do the data support the conclusions?

These characteristics of well-designed research have enabled scientists to study the actions of nutrients in the body. Such research has laid the foundation for quantifying how much of each nutrient the body needs.

■ A personal account of an experience or event is an **anecdote** and is not accepted as reliable scientific information.
- **anekdotos** = unpublished

IN SUMMARY Scientists learn about nutrition by conducting experiments that follow the protocol of scientific research. Researchers take care to establish similar control and experimental groups, large sample sizes, placebos, and blind treatments. Their findings must be reviewed and replicated by other scientists before being accepted as valid.

Dietary Reference Intakes

Nutrition experts have produced a set of standards that define the amounts of energy, nutrients, other dietary components, and physical activity that best support health. These recommendations are called **Dietary Reference Intakes (DRI)** and reflect the collaborative efforts of researchers in both the United States and Canada.*[7] The inside front covers provide a handy reference for DRI values.

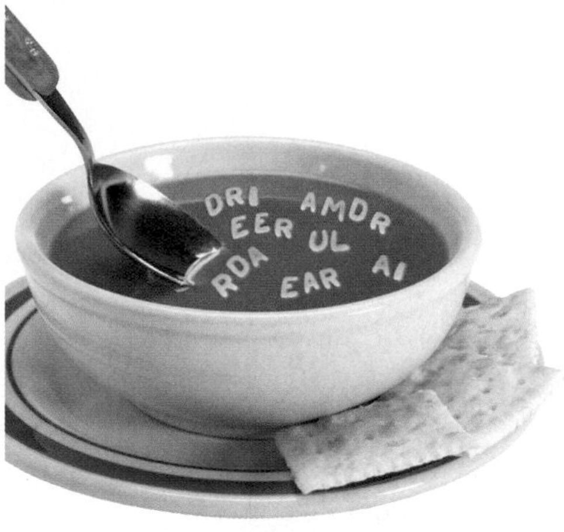
DRI
AMDR
EER
UL
RDA
EAR
AI

Don't let the DRI's "alphabet soup" of nutrient intake standards confuse you. Their names make sense when you learn their purposes.

Establishing Nutrient Recommendations

The DRI Committee consists of highly qualified scientists who base their estimates of nutrient needs on careful examination and interpretation of scientific evidence. These recommendations apply to healthy people and may not be appropriate for people with diseases that increase or decrease nutrient needs. The next several paragraphs discuss specific aspects of how the committee goes about establishing the values that make up the DRI:

- Estimated Average Requirements (EAR).
- Recommended Dietary Allowances (RDA).
- Adequate Intakes (AI).
- Tolerable Upper Intake Levels (UL).

Estimated Average Requirements (EAR) The committee reviews hundreds of research studies to determine the **requirement** for a nutrient—how much is needed in the diet. The committee selects a different criterion for each nutrient based on its roles both in performing activities in the body and in reducing disease risks.■ From this information, the committee determines an **Estimated Average Requirement (EAR)** for the nutrient—the average amount that appears sufficient to maintain a specific body function in half of the population.

■ Research in nutritional genomics is expected to identify specific nutrient-gene interactions that will help estimate nutrient requirements more precisely.

An examination of all the available data reveals that each person's body is unique and has its own set of requirements. Men differ from women, and needs change as a person grows from infancy through old age. For this reason, the committee clusters its recommendations for people into groups by age and gender. Even so, the exact requirements of people the same age and gender are likely to be different. For example, person A might need 40 units of the nutrient each day; person B might need 35; person C, 57. A look at enough individuals might reveal that their requirements fall into a symmetrical distribution, with most near the midpoint (shown in Figure 1-5 as 45 units) and only a few at the extremes.

Recommended Dietary Allowances (RDA) Then the committee must decide what intake to recommend for everybody—the **Recommended Dietary Allowance (RDA)**. Assuming the distribution shown in Figure 1-5, the Estimated Average Requirement (shown in the figure as 45 units) for each nutrient is probably closest to everyone's need. But if people consumed exactly the average requirement of a given nutrient each day, half of the population would develop deficiencies of that nutrient; in Figure 1-5, person C would be among them. Recommendations should be set high enough above the Estimated Average Requirement to meet the needs of most healthy people.

Dietary Reference Intakes (DRI): a set of nutrient intake values for healthy people in the United States and Canada. These values are used for planning and assessing diets and include:
- Estimated Average Requirements (EAR).
- Recommended Dietary Allowances (RDA).
- Adequate Intakes (AI).
- Tolerable Upper Intake Levels (UL).

requirement: the lowest continuing intake of a nutrient that will maintain a specified criterion of adequacy.

Estimated Average Requirement (EAR): the average daily amount of a nutrient that will maintain a specific biochemical or physiological function in half the healthy people of a given age and gender group.

Recommended Dietary Allowance (RDA): the average daily amount of a nutrient considered adequate to meet the known nutrient needs of practically all healthy people; a goal for dietary intake by individuals.

* The DRI reports are produced by the Food and Nutrition Board, Institute of Medicine of the National Academies, with active involvement of scientists from Canada.

FIGURE 1-5 Estimated Average Requirements and Recommended Dietary Allowances Compared

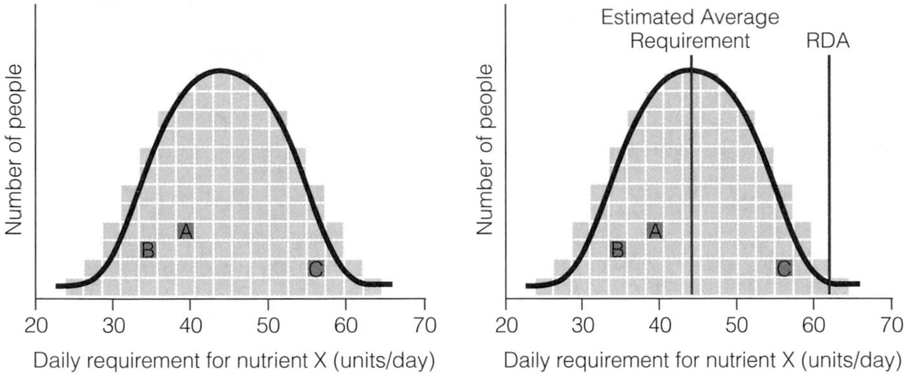
Number of people
A
B
C
20 30 40 50 60 70
Daily requirement for nutrient X (units/day)
Estimated Average Requirement
RDA
Number of people
A
B
C
20 30 40 50 60 70
Daily requirement for nutrient X (units/day)

Each square represents a person. Some people require only a small amount of the nutrient, and some require a lot, but most fall somewhere near the middle. The text discusses three of these people: A, B, and C.

The RDA for a nutrient is set well above the Estimated Average Requirement. It covers about 98% of the population.

Small amounts above the daily requirement do no harm, whereas amounts below the requirement lead to health problems. When people's nutrient intakes are consistently **deficient** (less than the requirement), their nutrient stores decline, and over time this decline leads to poor health and deficiency symptoms. Therefore, to ensure that the nutrient RDA meet the needs of as many people as possible, the RDA are set near the top end of the range of the population's estimated requirements.

In this example, a reasonable RDA might be 63 units a day (see Figure 1-5). Such a point can be calculated mathematically so that it covers about 98 percent of a population. Almost everybody—including person C whose needs were higher than the average—would be covered if they met this dietary goal. Relatively few people's requirements would exceed this recommendation, and even then, they wouldn't exceed by much.

Adequate Intakes (AI) For some nutrients, there is insufficient scientific evidence to determine an Estimated Average Requirement (which is needed to set an RDA). In these cases, the committee establishes an **Adequate Intake (AI)** instead of an RDA. An AI reflects the average amount of a nutrient that a group of healthy people consumes. Like the RDA, the AI may be used as nutrient goals for individuals.

Although both the RDA and the AI serve as nutrient intake goals for individuals, their differences are noteworthy. An RDA for a given nutrient is based on enough scientific evidence to expect that the needs of almost all healthy people will be met. An AI, on the other hand, must rely more heavily on scientific judgments because sufficient evidence is lacking. The percentage of people covered by an AI is unknown; an AI is expected to exceed average requirements, but it may cover more or fewer people than an RDA would (if an RDA could be determined). For these reasons, AI values are more tentative than RDA. The table on the inside front cover identifies which nutrients have an RDA and which have an AI. Later chapters present the RDA and AI values for the vitamins and minerals.

Tolerable Upper Intake Levels (UL) As mentioned earlier, the recommended intakes for nutrients are generous, and although they do not necessarily cover every individual for every nutrient, they probably should not be exceeded by much. People's tolerances for high doses of nutrients vary, and somewhere above

deficient: the amount of a nutrient below which almost all healthy people can be expected, over time, to experience deficiency symptoms.

Adequate Intake (AI): the average daily amount of a nutrient that appears sufficient to maintain a specified criterion; a value used as a guide for nutrient intake when an RDA cannot be determined.

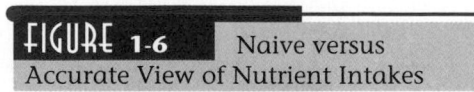

FIGURE 1-6 Naive versus Accurate View of Nutrient Intakes

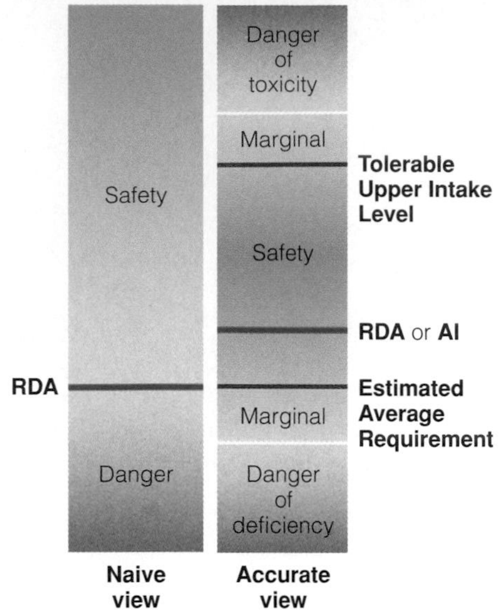
Safety
Danger
RDA
Danger of toxicity
Marginal
Tolerable Upper Intake Level
Safety
RDA or AI
Estimated Average Requirement
Marginal
Danger of deficiency
Naive view
Accurate view

The RDA or AI for a given nutrient represents a point that lies within a range of appropriate and reasonable intakes between toxicity and deficiency. Both of these recommendations are high enough to provide reserves in times of short-term dietary inadequacies, but not so high as to approach toxicity. Nutrient intakes above or below this range may be equally harmful.

■ Reference adults:
- Men: 19–30 yr, 5 ft 10 in, 154 lb.
- Women: 19–30 yr, 5 ft 4 in, 126 lb.

Tolerable Upper Intake Level (UL): the maximum daily amount of a nutrient that appears safe for most healthy people and beyond which there is an increased risk of adverse health effects.

Estimated Energy Requirement (EER): the average dietary energy intake that maintains energy balance and good health in a person of a given age, gender, weight, height, and level of physical activity.

Acceptable Macronutrient Distribution Ranges (AMDR): ranges of intakes for the energy nutrients that provide adequate energy and nutrients and reduce the risk of chronic diseases.

the recommended intake is a **Tolerable Upper Intake Level (UL)** beyond which a nutrient is likely to become toxic. It is naive—and inaccurate—to think of recommendations as minimum amounts. A more accurate view is to see a person's nutrient needs as falling within a range, with marginal and danger zones both below and above it (see Figure 1-6).

Upper levels are particularly useful in guarding against the overconsumption of nutrients, which may occur when people use large-dose supplements and fortified foods regularly. Later chapters discuss the dangers associated with excessively high intakes of vitamins and minerals, and the inside front cover presents a table that includes the upper-level values for selected nutrients.

Establishing Energy Recommendations

In contrast to the RDA and AI values for nutrients, the recommendation for energy is not generous. Energy's recommendation—called the **Estimated Energy Requirement (EER)**—is similar to the Estimated Average Requirement in that it is set at the *average* of the population's estimated requirements (see Figure 1-7).

Estimated Energy Requirement (EER) The Estimated Energy Requirement represents the average dietary energy intake (kcalories per day) that will maintain energy balance in a healthy person of a given age, gender, weight, height, and physical activity level.■ Balance is key to the energy recommendation. Enough energy is needed to sustain a healthy and active life, but too much energy can lead to weight gain and obesity. Because any amount in excess of needs results in weight gain, there is no upper level for energy.

Acceptable Macronutrient Distribution Ranges (AMDR) People don't eat energy directly; they derive energy from foods containing carbohydrate, fat, and protein. Each of these three energy-yielding nutrients contributes to the total energy intake, and those contributions vary in relation to each other. The DRI committee has determined that the composition of a diet that provides adequate energy and nutrients and reduces the risk of chronic diseases is:

- 45 to 65 percent from carbohydrate.
- 20 to 35 percent from fat.
- 10 to 35 percent from protein.

These values are known as **Acceptable Macronutrient Distribution Ranges (AMDR).**

FIGURE 1-7 Recommended Intakes of Nutrients and Energy Compared

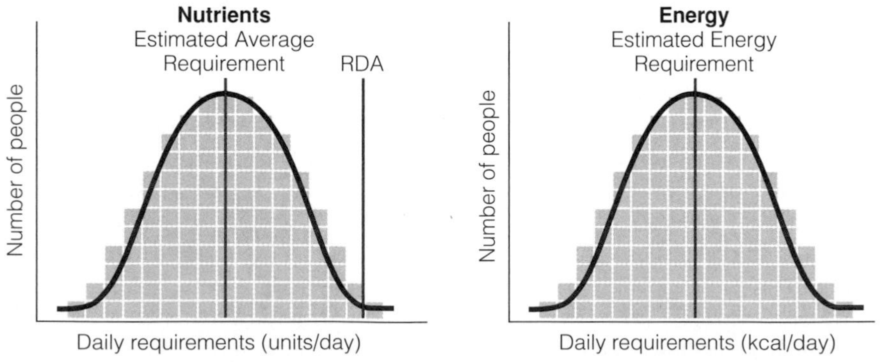
Nutrients
Estimated Average Requirement
RDA
Number of people
Daily requirements (units/day)
Energy
Estimated Energy Requirement
Number of people
Daily requirements (kcal/day)

The nutrient intake recommendations are set high enough to cover nearly everyone's requirements (the boxes represent people).

The recommended intake for energy is set at the average that will maintain energy balance in a healthy person of desirable body weight.

Using Nutrient Recommendations

Although the intent of nutrient recommendations may seem simple enough, they are the subject of much misunderstanding and controversy. Perhaps the following facts will help put them in perspective. First, estimates of adequate energy and nutrient intakes apply to *healthy* people. They need to be adjusted for malnourished people or those with medical problems who may require supplemented or restricted intakes.

Second, these *recommendations* are not minimum requirements, nor are they necessarily optimal intakes for all individuals. Recommendations can only target "most" of the people and cannot account for individual variations in nutrient needs—yet. Given the recent explosion of knowledge about genetics, the day may be fast approaching when nutrition scientists will be able to determine an individual's optimal nutrient needs.[8] Until then, registered dietitians■ and other qualified health professionals can help determine whether recommendations should be adjusted to meet individual needs.

■ A **registered dietitian** is a college-educated food and nutrition specialist who is qualified to evaluate people's nutritional health and needs. See Highlight 1 for more on what constitutes a nutrition expert.

Third, most nutrient goals are intended to be met through diets composed of a variety of *foods* whenever possible. Because foods contain mixtures of nutrients and nonnutrients, they deliver more than just those nutrients covered by the recommendations. Excess intakes of vitamins and minerals are unlikely when their sources are foods rather than supplements.

Fourth, recommendations apply to *average* daily intakes. Meeting recommendations for every nutrient every day is difficult and unnecessary. The length of time over which a person's intake can deviate from the average without risk of deficiency or overdose varies for each nutrient, depending on the body's use and storage of the nutrient. For most nutrients (such as thiamin and vitamin C), deprivation would lead to rapid development of deficiency symptoms (within days or weeks); for others (such as vitamin A and vitamin B_{12}), deficiencies would develop more slowly (over months or years).

Fifth, each of the DRI categories serves a unique purpose. For example, the Estimated Average Requirements are most appropriately used to develop and evaluate nutrition programs for *groups* such as schoolchildren or military personnel. The RDA (or AI if an RDA is not available) can be used to set goals for *individuals*. Tolerable Upper Intake Levels help to keep nutrient intakes below the amounts that increase the risk of toxicity. With these understandings, professionals can use the DRI for a variety of purposes.

Comparing Nutrient Recommendations

At least 40 different nations and international organizations have published nutrient standards similar to those used in the United States and Canada. Slight differences may be apparent, reflecting differences both in the interpretation of the data from which the standards were derived and in the food habits and physical activities of the populations they serve.

Many countries use the recommendations developed by two international groups: FAO (Food and Agriculture Organization) and WHO (World Health Organization).■ The FAO/WHO recommendations are considered sufficient to maintain health in nearly all healthy people worldwide.

■ Nutrient recommendations from FAO/WHO are provided in Appendix I.

IN SUMMARY The Dietary Reference Intakes (DRI) are a set of nutrient intake values that can be used to plan and evaluate diets for healthy people. The Estimated Average Requirement defines the amount of a nutrient that supports a specific function in the body for half of the population. The Recommended Dietary Allowance (RDA) is based on the Estimated Average Requirement and establishes a goal for dietary intake that will meet the needs of almost all healthy people. An Adequate Intake (AI) serves a similar purpose when an RDA cannot be determined. The Estimated Energy Requirement defines the average amount of energy intake needed to maintain energy balance, and the Acceptable Macronutrient Distribution Ranges define the proportions contributed by carbohydrate, fat, and protein to a healthy diet. The Tolerable Upper Intake Level establishes the highest amount that appears safe for regular consumption.

Nutrition Assessment

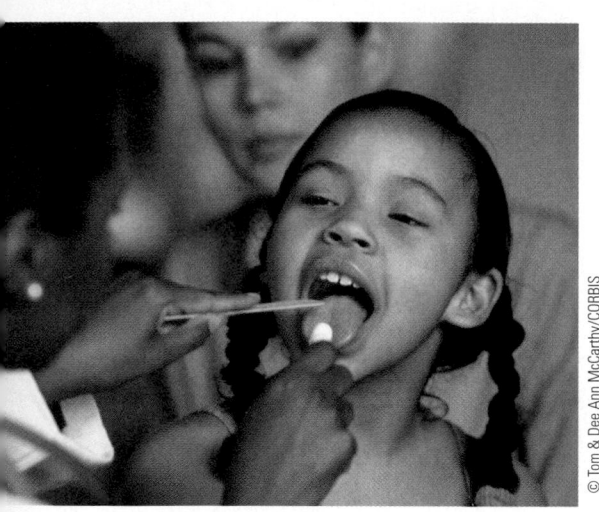

© Tom & Dee Ann McCarthy/CORBIS

A peek inside the mouth provides clues to a person's nutrition status—an inflamed tongue indicating a B vitamin deficiency or mottled teeth revealing fluoride toxicity, for example.

What happens when a person doesn't get enough or gets too much of a nutrient or energy? If the deficiency or excess is significant over time, the person exhibits signs of **malnutrition.** With a deficiency of energy, the person may display the symptoms of **undernutrition** by becoming extremely thin, losing muscle tissue, and becoming prone to infection and disease. With a deficiency of a nutrient, the person may experience skin rashes, depression, hair loss, bleeding gums, muscle spasms, night blindness, or other symptoms. With an excess of energy, the person may become obese and vulnerable to diseases associated with **overnutrition** such as heart disease and diabetes. With a sudden nutrient overdose, the person may experience hot flashes, yellowing skin, a rapid heart rate, low blood pressure, or other symptoms. Similarly, regular intakes in excess of needs may also have adverse effects.

Malnutrition symptoms are easy to miss. They resemble the symptoms of other diseases: diarrhea, skin rashes, pain, and the like. But a person who has learned how to use assessment techniques to detect malnutrition can tell when these conditions are caused by poor nutrition and can take steps to correct it. This discussion presents the basics of nutrition assessment; many more details are offered in later chapters and in Appendix E.

Nutrition Assessment of Individuals

To prepare a **nutrition assessment,** a registered dietitian or other trained health care professional uses:

- Historical information.
- Anthropometric data.
- Physical examinations.
- Laboratory tests.

Each of these methods involves collecting data in various ways and interpreting each finding in relation to the others to create a total picture.

Historical Information One step in evaluating nutrition status is to obtain information about a person's history with respect to health status, socioeconomic status, drug use, and diet. The health history reflects a person's medical record and may reveal a disease that interferes with the person's ability to eat or the body's use of nutrients. The person's family history of major diseases is also noteworthy, especially for conditions such as heart disease that have a genetic tendency to run in families. Economic circumstances may show a financial inability to buy foods or inadequate kitchen facilities in which to prepare them. Social factors such as marital status, ethnic background, and educational level also influence food choices and nutrition status. A drug history may highlight possible diet-medication interactions that lead to nutrient deficiencies (as described in Chapter 19). A diet history can indicate whether the diet may be under- or oversupplying nutrients or energy.

malnutrition: any condition caused by excess or deficient food energy or nutrient intake or by an imbalance of nutrients.
- **mal** = bad

undernutrition: deficient energy or nutrients.

overnutrition: excess energy or nutrients.

nutrition assessment: a comprehensive analysis of a person's nutrition status that uses health, socioeconomic, drug, and diet histories; anthropometric measurements; physical examinations; and laboratory tests.

To take a diet history, the assessor collects data about the foods a person eats. The data may be collected by recording the foods the person has eaten over a period of 24 hours, three days, or a week or more or by asking what foods the person typically eats and how much of each. The days in the record have to be fairly typical of the person's diet, and portion sizes must be recorded accurately. To determine the amounts of nutrients consumed, the assessor usually enters the foods and their portion sizes into a computer using a diet analysis program. This step can also be done manually by looking up each food in a table of food composition such as Appendix H in this book. Then the assessor compares the calculated nutrient intakes with the DRI to determine the probability of adequacy (see Figure 1-8).[9] Alternatively, the diet history might be compared against standards such as the USDA Food Guide or the 2005 *Dietary Guidelines* (described in Chapter 2).

An estimate of energy and nutrient intakes from a diet history, combined with other sources of information, can help confirm or rule out the *possibility* of suspected nutrition problems. A sufficient intake of a nutrient does not guarantee adequacy, and an insufficient intake does not always indicate a deficiency, but such findings warn of possible problems.

FIGURE 1-8 Using the DRI to Assess the Dietary Intake of a Healthy Individual

If a person's usual intake falls above the RDA, the intake is probably adequate because the RDA covers the needs of almost all people. A usual intake that falls between the RDA and the Estimated Average Requirement is more difficult to assess; the intake may be adequate, but the chances are greater or equal that it is inadequate. If the usual intake falls below the Estimated Average Requirement, it is probably inadequate.

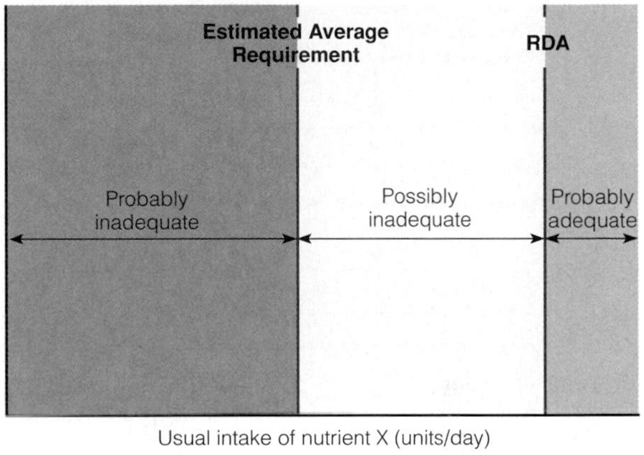
Estimated Average Requirement
RDA
Probably inadequate
Possibly inadequate
Probably adequate
Usual intake of nutrient X (units/day)

Anthropometric Data A second technique that may help to reveal nutrition problems is the taking of **anthropometric** measures such as height and weight. The assessor compares measurements taken on an individual with standards specific for gender and age or with previous measures on the same individual. (Chapter 8 presents information on body weight and its standards.)

Measurements taken periodically and compared with previous measurements reveal patterns and indicate trends in a person's overall nutrition status, but they provide little information about specific nutrients. Instead, measurements out of line with expectations may reveal such problems as growth failure in children, wasting or swelling of body tissues in adults, and obesity—conditions that may reflect energy or nutrient deficiencies or excesses.

Physical Examinations A third nutrition assessment technique is a physical examination that looks for clues to poor nutrition status. Every part of the body that can be inspected can offer such clues: the hair, eyes, skin, posture, tongue, fingernails, and others. The examination requires skill, for many physical signs can reflect more than one nutrient deficiency or toxicity or even nonnutrition conditions. Like the other assessment techniques, a physical examination does not by itself point to firm conclusions. Instead, it reveals possible nutrient imbalances for other assessment techniques to confirm, or it confirms data collected from other assessment measures.

Laboratory Tests A fourth way to detect a developing deficiency, imbalance, or toxicity is to take samples of blood or urine, analyze them in the laboratory, and compare the results with normal values for a similar population.■ A goal of nutrition assessment is to uncover early signs of malnutrition before symptoms appear, and laboratory tests are most useful for this purpose. In addition, they can confirm suspicions raised by other assessment methods.

■ Assessment may one day depend on measures of how a nutrient influences genetic activity within the cells, instead of quantities in the blood or other tissues.

Iron, for Example The mineral iron can be used to illustrate the stages in the development of a nutrient deficiency and the assessment techniques useful in detecting them. The **overt,** or outward, signs of an iron deficiency appear at the end of a long sequence of events. Figure 1-9 describes what happens in the body as a nutrient deficiency progresses and shows which assessment methods can reveal those changes.

anthropometric (AN-throw-poe-MET-rick): relating to measurement of the physical characteristics of the body, such as height and weight.
- **anthropos** = human
- **metric** = measuring

overt (oh-VERT): out in the open and easy to observe.
- **ouvrir** = to open

FIGURE 1-9 Stages in the Development of a Nutrient Deficiency

Internal changes precede outward signs of deficiencies. As a corollary, signs of sickness need not appear before a person takes corrective measures. Tests can either reveal the presence of problems in the early stages or confirm that nutrient stores are adequate.

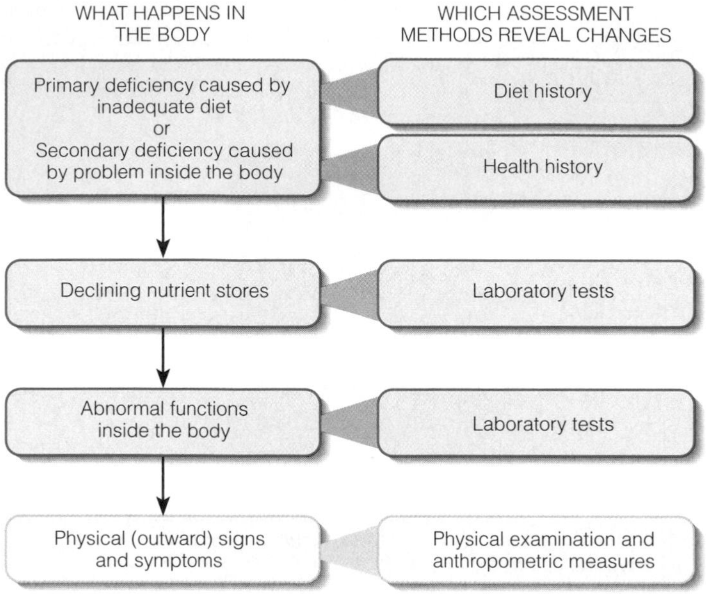
WHAT HAPPENS IN THE BODY
WHICH ASSESSMENT METHODS REVEAL CHANGES
Primary deficiency caused by inadequate diet or Secondary deficiency caused by problem inside the body
Diet history
Health history
Declining nutrient stores
Laboratory tests
Abnormal functions inside the body
Laboratory tests
Physical (outward) signs and symptoms
Physical examination and anthropometric measures

First, the body has too little iron—either because iron is lacking in the person's diet (a **primary deficiency**) or because the person's body doesn't absorb enough, excretes too much, or uses iron inefficiently (a **secondary deficiency**). A diet history provides clues to primary deficiencies; a health history provides clues to secondary deficiencies.

Then the body begins to use up its stores of iron. At this stage, the deficiency might be described as **subclinical.** It exists as a **covert** condition and might be detected by laboratory tests, but outward signs have not yet appeared.

Finally, iron stores are exhausted. Now, the body cannot make enough iron-containing red blood cells to replace those that are aging and dying. The iron in red blood cells normally carries oxygen to all the body's tissues. When iron is lacking, fewer red blood cells are made, the new ones are pale and small, and every part of the body feels the effects of an oxygen shortage. Now the overt symptoms of deficiency appear—weakness, fatigue, pallor, and headaches, reflecting the iron-deficient state of the blood. Physical examination would reveal these symptoms.

HEALTHY PEOPLE 2010

Increase the proportion of primary health care providers who provide nutrition assessment when appropriate and formulate a diet plan for those who need intervention.

■ Healthy People 2010 is described on p. 23.

Nutrition Assessment of Populations

To assess a population's nutrition status, researchers conduct surveys using techniques similar to those used on individuals. The data collected are then used by various agencies for numerous purposes, including the development of national health goals.

National Nutrition Surveys The National Nutrition Monitoring program coordinates the many nutrition-related activities of various federal agencies. One of its most recent projects is the integration of two major national surveys to provide comprehensive data efficiently.[10] One portion of the survey collects data on the kinds and amounts of foods people eat.* Then researchers calculate the energy and nutrients in the foods and compare the amounts consumed with a standard. The other portion examines the people themselves, using anthropometric measurements, physical examinations, and laboratory tests.†[11] The data provide valuable information on several nutrition-related conditions, such as growth retardation, heart disease, and nutrient deficiencies. National nutrition surveys often oversample high-risk groups (low-income families, pregnant women, adolescents, the elderly, African Americans, and Mexican Americans) in order to glean an accurate estimate of their health and nutrition status.

The resulting wealth of information from the national nutrition surveys is used for a variety of purposes. For example, Congress uses this information to establish

primary deficiency: a nutrient deficiency caused by inadequate dietary intake of a nutrient.

secondary deficiency: a nutrient deficiency caused by something other than an inadequate intake such as a disease condition or drug interaction that reduces absorption, accelerates use, hastens excretion, or destroys the nutrient.

subclinical deficiency: a deficiency in the early stages, before the outward signs have appeared.

covert (KOH-vert): hidden, as if under covers.
- **couvrir** = to cover

* This portion of the survey was formerly called the Continuing Survey of Food Intakes by Individuals (CSFII), popularly known as *What We Eat in America*.

† This portion of the survey is known as the National Health and Nutrition Examination Survey (NHANES).

public policy on nutrition education, food assistance programs, and the regulation of the food supply. Scientists use the information to establish research priorities. The food industry uses these data to guide decisions in public relations and product development.[12] The Dietary Reference Intakes and other major reports that examine the relationships between diet and health depend on information collected from these nutrition surveys. These data also provide the basis for developing and monitoring national health goals.

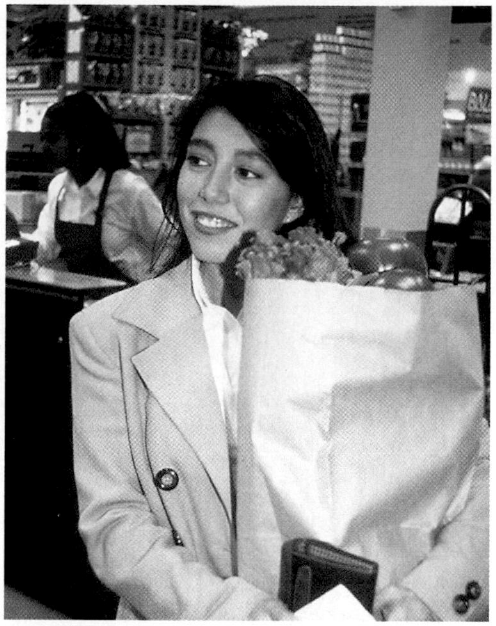

© Burke-Triolo Productions/FoodPix/Getty Images

Surveys provide valuable information about the kinds of foods people are eating.

National Health Goals **Healthy People,** a program that identifies the nation's health priorities and guides policies that promote health and prevent disease, was initiated over 20 years ago. At the start of each decade, the program sets goals for improving the nation's health during the following ten years. The goals of Healthy People 2010 focus on "improving the quality of life and eliminating disparity in health among racial and ethnic groups."[13] Nutrition is one of many focus areas, each with numerous objectives. Table 1-4 lists the nutrition objectives for 2010. These and other nutrition-related objectives appear throughout the text where their subjects are discussed.

At the close of the twentieth century, the nation's progress toward meeting its Healthy People 2000 goals was mixed.[14] For almost 60 percent of the objectives, the population either met the target or was moving in the right direction. Successes included reductions in the incidence of food- and water-borne infections, oral and breast cancer, and infant mortality, for example. On the downside, the population was moving in the opposite direction of several key objectives, most notably for reducing overweight and increasing physical activity.

TABLE 1-4 Healthy People 2010 Nutrition and Overweight Objectives

HEALTHY PEOPLE 2010

- Increase the proportion of adults who are at a *healthy weight.*
- Reduce the proportion of adults who are *obese.*
- Reduce the proportion of children and adolescents who are *overweight* or *obese.*
- Reduce *growth retardation* among low-income children under age 5 years.
- Increase the proportion of persons aged 2 years and older who consume at least two daily servings of *fruit.*
- Increase the proportion of persons aged 2 years and older who consume at least three daily servings of *vegetables,* with at least one-third being dark green or orange vegetables.
- Increase the proportion of persons aged 2 years and older who consume at least six daily servings of *grain products,* with at least three being whole grains.
- Increase the proportion of persons aged 2 years and older who consume less than 10 percent of kcalories from *saturated fat.*
- Increase the proportion of persons aged 2 years and older who consume no more than 30 percent of kcalories from *total fat.*
- Increase the proportion of persons aged 2 years and older who consume 2400 mg or less of *sodium.*
- Increase the proportion of persons aged 2 years and older who meet dietary recommendations for *calcium.*
- Reduce *iron deficiency* among young children, females of childbearing age, and pregnant females.
- Reduce *anemia* among low-income pregnant females in their third trimester.
- Increase the proportion of children and adolescents aged 6 to 19 years whose intake of *meals and snacks at school* contributes to good overall dietary quality.
- Increase the proportion of schools that teach all essential *nutrition education* topics in one course.
- Increase the proportion of worksites that offer *nutrition or weight management classes or counseling.*
- Increase the proportion of primary care providers who provide nutrition *assessment* when appropriate and who formulate a diet plan for those who need *intervention.*
- Increase the proportion of physician office visits made by patients with a diagnosis of cardiovascular disease, diabetes, or hyperlipidemia that include *counseling or education related to diet and nutrition.*
- Increase *food security* among U.S. households and in so doing reduce hunger.

NOTE: "Nutrition and Overweight" is one of 28 focus areas, each with numerous objectives. Several of the other focus areas have nutrition-related objectives, and these are presented in later chapters.

SOURCE: Healthy People 2010, **www.healthypeople.gov**

Healthy People: a national public health initiative under the jurisdiction of the U.S. Department of Health and Human Services (DHHS) that identifies the most significant preventable threats to health and focuses efforts toward eliminating them.

IN SUMMARY People become malnourished when they get too little or too much energy or nutrients. Deficiencies, excesses, and imbalances of nutrients lead to malnutrition diseases. To detect malnutrition in individuals, health care professionals use four nutrition assessment methods. Reviewing dietary data and health information may suggest a nutrition problem in its earliest stages. Laboratory tests may detect it before it becomes overt, whereas anthropometrics and physical examinations pick up on the problem only after it is causing symptoms. Similar assessment methods are used in national surveys to measure people's food consumption and to evaluate the nutrition status of populations.

Diet and Health

Diet has always played a vital role in supporting health.■ Early nutrition research focused on identifying the nutrients in foods that would prevent such common diseases as rickets and scurvy, the vitamin D– and vitamin C–deficiency diseases. With this knowledge, developed countries have been successful in protecting against nutrient deficiency diseases. World hunger and nutrient deficiency diseases still pose a major health threat in developing countries, but not because of a lack of nutrition knowledge. More recently, nutrition research has focused on **chronic diseases** associated with energy and nutrient excesses. Once thought to be "rich countries' problems," chronic diseases have become epidemic in developing countries as well—contributing to three out of five deaths worldwide.[15]

■ Nutritional genomics will provide a better understanding of the relationships among genes, foods, and health.

Chronic Diseases

Table 1-5 lists the ten leading causes of death in the United States. These "causes" are stated as if a single condition such as heart disease caused death, but most chronic diseases arise from multiple factors over many years. A person who died of heart disease may have been overweight, had high blood pressure, been a cigarette smoker, and spent years eating a diet high in saturated fat and getting too little exercise.

Of course, not all people who die of heart disease fit this description, nor do all people with these characteristics die of heart disease. People who are overweight might die from the complications of diabetes instead, or those who smoke might die of cancer. They might even die from something totally unrelated to any of these factors, such as an automobile accident. Still, statistical studies have shown that certain conditions and behaviors are linked to certain diseases.

TABLE 1-5 Leading Causes of Death in the United States

	Percentage of Total Deaths
1. Heart disease	28.9
2. Cancers	22.9
3. Strokes	6.8
4. Chronic lung diseases	5.1
5. Accidents	4.0
6. Diabetes mellitus	2.9
7. Pneumonia and influenza	2.6
8. Alzheimer's disease	2.2
9. Kidney diseases	1.6
10. Blood infections	1.3

NOTE: The diseases highlighted in green have relationships with diet; yellow indicates a relationship with alcohol.

Risk Factors for Chronic Diseases

Factors that increase or reduce the *risk* of developing chronic diseases are identified by analyzing statistical data. A strong association between a **risk factor** and a disease means that when the factor is present, the *likelihood* of developing the disease increases. It does not mean that all people with the risk factor will develop the disease. Similarly, a lack of risk factors does not guarantee freedom from a given disease. On the average, though, the more risk factors in a person's life, the greater that person's chances of developing the disease. Conversely, the fewer risk factors in a person's life, the better the chances for good health.

Risk Factors Persist Risk factors tend to persist over time. Without intervention, a young adult with high blood pressure will most likely continue to have

chronic diseases: diseases characterized by a slow progression and long duration. Examples include heart disease, cancer, and diabetes.

risk factor: a condition or behavior associated with an elevated frequency of a disease but not proved to be causal. Leading risk factors for chronic diseases include obesity, cigarette smoking, high blood pressure, high blood cholesterol, physical inactivity, and a diet high in saturated fats and low in vegetables, fruits, and whole grains.

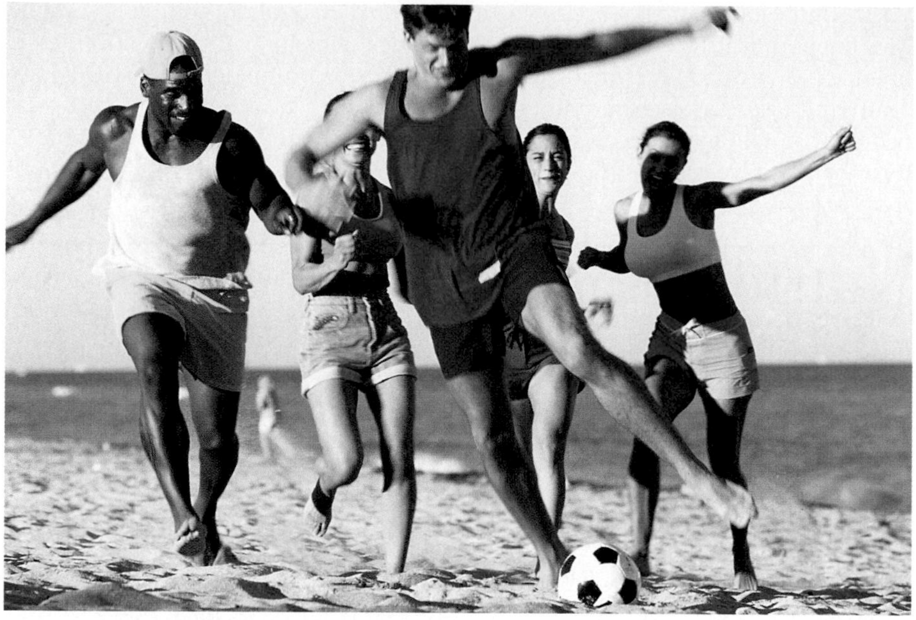

© Ray Morsch/CORBIS

Physical activity can be both fun and beneficial.

TABLE 1-6 Factors Contributing to Deaths in the United States

Factors	Percentage of Deaths
Tobacco	20
Poor diet/inactivity	14
Alcohol	6
Microbial agents	4
Pollutants/toxins	3
Firearms	2
Sexual behavior	1
Motor vehicles	1
Illicit drugs	1

SOURCE: Centers for Disease Control, **www.cdc.gov**.

high blood pressure as an older adult, for example. Thus, to minimize the damage, early intervention is most effective.

Risk Factors Cluster Risk factors also tend to cluster. For example, a person who is obese may be physically inactive, have high blood pressure, and have high blood cholesterol—all risk factors associated with heart disease. Intervention that focuses on one risk factor often benefits the others as well. For example, physical activity can help reduce weight. Then both physical activity and weight loss will help to lower blood pressure and blood cholesterol.

Risk Factors in Perspective The most prominent factor contributing to death in the United States is tobacco use,■ followed by diet and activity patterns, and alcohol use (see Table 1-6). Risk factors such as smoking, poor dietary habits, physical inactivity, and alcohol consumption are personal behaviors that can be changed. Decisions to not smoke, to eat a well-balanced diet, to engage in regular physical activity, and to drink alcohol in moderation (if at all) improve the likelihood that a person will enjoy good health. Other risk factors, such as genetics,■ gender, and age, also play important roles in the development of chronic diseases, but they cannot be changed. Health recommendations acknowledge the influence of such factors on the development of disease, but must focus on those that are changeable. For the two out of three Americans who do not smoke or drink alcohol excessively, the one choice that can influence long-term health prospects more than any other is diet.[16]

■ Cigarette smoking is responsible for almost one of every five deaths each year.

■ Highlight 18 considers how findings from the Human Genome Project will influence health care.

IN SUMMARY Within the range set by genetics, a person's choice of diet influences long-term health. Diet has no influence on some diseases, but is linked closely to others. Personal life choices, such as engaging in physical activity and using tobacco or alcohol, also affect health for the better or worse.

Increase the proportion of persons appropriately counseled about health behaviors.

HEALTHY PEOPLE 2010

The next several chapters will provide many more details about nutrients and how they support health. Whenever appropriate, the discussion will show how diet influences each of today's major diseases. Dietary recommendations will appear again and again, as each nutrient's relationships with health are explored. Most people who follow the recommendations will benefit and can enjoy good health into their later years.

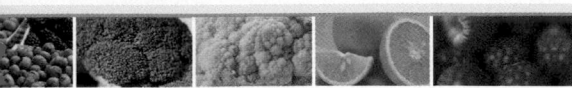

Nutrition in Your Life

Your food choices play a key role in keeping you healthy and reducing your risk of chronic diseases.

- **What factors most influence your food choices? How often do you think of health and nutrition when choosing foods?**
- **Do you or members of your family have any of the chronic disease risk factors and conditions (listed on p. 24 in the definition)? If so, which ones?**
- **What lifestyle changes could you make to improve your chances of enjoying good health?**

NUTRITION ON THE NET

Access these websites for further study of topics covered in this chapter.

- Find updates and quick links to these and other nutrition-related sites at our website: **www.wadsworth.com/nutrition**
- Search for "nutrition" at the U.S. Government health and nutrition information sites: **www.healthfinder.gov** or **www.nutrition.gov**
- Learn more about basic science research from the National Science Foundation and Research!America: **www.nsf.gov** and **researchamerica.org**
- Review the Dietary Reference Intakes: **www.nap.edu**
- Review nutrition recommendations from the Food and Agriculture Organization and the World Health Organization: **www.fao.org** and **www.who.org**
- View Healthy People 2010: **www.healthypeople.gov**
- Visit the Food and Nutrition section of the Healthy Living area in Health Canada: **www.hc-sc.gc.ca**
- Learn about the national nutrition survey: **www.cdc.gov/nchs/nhanes.htm**
- Get information from the Food Surveys Research Group: **www.barc.usda.gov/bhnrc/foodsurvey**
- Visit the food and nutrition center of the Mayo Clinic: **www.mayohealth.org**
- Find reviews of, and links to, nutrition and health websites by Tufts University Nutrition Navigator: **navigator.tufts.edu**

NUTRITION CALCULATIONS

Several chapters end with problems to give you practice in doing simple nutrition-related calculations. Although the situations are hypothetical, the numbers are real, and calculating the answers (check them on p. 29) provides a valuable nutrition lesson. Once you have mastered these examples, you will be prepared to examine your own food choices. Be sure to show your calculations for each problem.

1. Calculate the energy provided by a food's energy-nutrient contents. A cup of fried rice contains 5 grams protein, 30 grams carbohydrate, and 11 grams fat.
   a. How many kcalories does the rice provide from these energy nutrients?
      ________ = ___ kcal protein.
      ________ = ___ kcal carbohydrate.
      ________ = ___ kcal fat.
      Total = ___ kcal.
   b. What percentage of the energy in the fried rice comes from each of the energy-yielding nutrients?
      ________ = ___ % kcal from protein.
      ________ = ___ % kcal from carbohydrate.
      ________ = ___ % kcal from fat.
      Total = ___ %
      Note: The total should add up to 100%; 99% or 101% due to rounding is also acceptable.
   c. Calculate how many of the 146 kcalories provided by a 12-ounce can of beer come from alcohol, if the beer contains 1 gram protein and 13 grams carbohydrate. (Note: The remaining kcalories derive from alcohol.)
      1 g protein = ___ kcal protein.
      13 g carbohydrate = ___ kcal carbohydrate.
      = ___ kcal alcohol.
      How many grams of alcohol does this represent? ___ g alcohol.
2. Even a little nutrition knowledge can help you identify some bogus claims. Consider an advertisement for a new "super supplement" that claims the product provides 15 grams protein and 10 kcalories per dose. Is this possible? ___ Why or why not? ________ = ___ kcal.

STUDY QUESTIONS

These questions will help you review this chapter. You will find the answers in the discussions on the pages provided.

1. Give several reasons (and examples) why people make the food choices that they do. (pp. 4–5)
2. What is a nutrient? Name the six classes of nutrients found in foods. What is an essential nutrient? (pp. 6–7)
3. Which nutrients are inorganic, and which are organic? Discuss the significance of that distinction. (pp. 6, 10–11)
4. Which nutrients yield energy, and how much energy do they yield per gram? How is energy measured? (pp. 7–9)
5. Describe how alcohol resembles nutrients. Why is alcohol not considered a nutrient? (p. 9)
6. What is the science of nutrition? Describe the types of research studies and methods used in acquiring nutrition information. (pp. 11–15)
7. Explain how variables might be correlational but not causal. (p. 15)
8. What are the DRI? Who develops the DRI? To whom do they apply? How are they used? In your description, identify the categories of DRI and indicate how they are related. (pp. 16–19)
9. What judgment factors are involved in setting the energy and nutrient recommendations? (pp. 17–18)
10. What happens when people get either too little or too much energy or nutrients? Define malnutrition, undernutrition, and overnutrition. Describe the four methods used to detect energy and nutrient deficiencies and excesses. (pp. 20–21)
11. What methods are used in nutrition surveys? What kinds of information can these surveys provide? (pp. 22–23)
12. Describe risk factors and their relationships to disease. (pp. 24–25)

These multiple choice questions will help you prepare for an exam. Answers can be found on p. 29.

1. When people eat the foods typical of their families or geographic region, their choices are influenced by:
   a. habit.
   b. nutrition.
   c. personal preference.
   d. ethnic heritage or tradition.
2. Both the human body and many foods are composed mostly of:
   a. fat.
   b. water.
   c. minerals.
   d. proteins.

3. The inorganic nutrients are:
   a. proteins and fats.
   b. vitamins and minerals.
   c. minerals and water.
   d. vitamins and proteins.
4. The energy-yielding nutrients are:
   a. fats, minerals, and water.
   b. minerals, proteins, and vitamins.
   c. carbohydrates, fats, and vitamins.
   d. carbohydrates, fats, and proteins.
5. Studies of populations that reveal correlations between dietary habits and disease incidence are:
   a. clinical trials.
   b. laboratory studies.
   c. case-control studies.
   d. epidemiological studies.
6. An experiment in which neither the researchers nor the subjects know who is receiving the treatment is known as:
   a. double blind.
   b. double control.
   c. blind variable.
   d. placebo control.
7. An RDA represents the:
   a. highest amount of a nutrient that appears safe for most healthy people.
   b. lowest amount of a nutrient that will maintain a specified criterion of adequacy.
   c. average amount of a nutrient considered adequate to meet the known nutrient needs of practically all healthy people.
   d. average amount of a nutrient that will maintain a specific biochemical or physiological function in half the people.
8. Historical information, physical examinations, laboratory tests, and anthropometric measures are:
   a. techniques used in diet planning.
   b. steps used in the scientific method.
   c. approaches used in disease prevention.
   d. methods used in a nutrition assessment.
9. A deficiency caused by an inadequate dietary intake is a(n):
   a. overt deficiency.
   b. covert deficiency.
   c. primary deficiency.
   d. secondary deficiency.
10. Behaviors such as smoking, dietary habits, physical activity, and alcohol consumption that influence the development of disease are known as:
    a. risk factors.
    b. chronic causes.
    c. preventive agents.
    d. disease descriptors.

REFERENCES

1. L. L. Birch, Development of food preferences, *Annual Review of Nutrition* 19 (1999): 41–62; M. B. M. van den Bree, L. J. Eaves, and J. T. Dwyer, Genetic and environmental influences on eating patterns of twins aged ≥ 50 y, *American Journal of Clinical Nutrition* 70 (1999): 456–465.
2. J. E. Tillotson, Our ready-prepared, ready-to-eat nation, *Nutrition Today* 37 (2002): 36–38; F. Katz, "How nutritious?" meets "How convenient?" *Food Technology* 53 (1999): 44–50.
3. L. Canetti, E. Bachar, and E. M. Berry, Food and emotion, *Behavioural Processes* 60 (2002): 157–164.
4. J. D. Fernstrom, Diet, neurochemicals, and mental energy, *Nutrition Reviews* 59 (2001): S22–S24.
5. Position of the American Dietetic Association: Total diet approach to communicating food and nutrition information, *Journal of the American Dietetic Association* 102 (2002): 100–108.
6. D. Shattuck, Nutritional genomics, *Journal of the American Dietetic Association* 103 (2003): 16, 18; P. Trayhurn, Nutritional genomics—"Nutrigenom-ics," *British Journal of Nutrition* 89 (2003): 1–2; F. P. Guengerich, Functional genomics and proteomics applied to the study of nutritional metabolism, *Nutrition Reviews* 59 (2001): 259–263.
7. Committee on Dietary Reference Intakes, *Dietary Reference Intakes for Energy, Carbohydrate, Fiber, Fat, Fatty Acids, Cholesterol, Protein, and Amino Acids* (Washington, D.C.: National Academies Press, 2002); Committee on Dietary Reference Intakes, *Dietary Reference Intakes for Vitamin A, Vitamin K, Arsenic, Boron, Chromium, Copper, Iodine, Iron, Manganese, Molybdenum, Nickel, Silicon, Vanadium, and Zinc* (Washington, D.C.: National Academy Press, 2001); Committee on Dietary Reference Intakes, *Dietary Reference Intakes for Vitamin C, Vitamin E, Selenium, and Carotenoids* (Washington, D.C.: National Academy Press, 2000); Committee on Dietary Reference Intakes, *Dietary Reference Intakes for Thiamin, Riboflavin, Niacin, Vitamin B_6, Folate, Vitamin B_{12}, Pantothenic Acid, Biotin, and Choline* (Washington, D.C.: National Academy Press, 1998); Committee on Dietary Reference Intakes, *Dietary Reference Intakes for Calcium, Phosphorus, Magnesium, Vitamin D, and Fluoride* (Washington, D.C.: National Academy Press, 1997).
8. C. D. Berndanier, Nutrient-gene interactions, *Nutrition Today* 35 (2000): 8–17.
9. S. P. Murphy, S. I. Barr, and M. I. Poos, Using the new Dietary Reference Intakes to assess diets: A map to the maze, *Nutrition Reviews* 60 (2002): 267–275.
10. J. Dwyer and coauthors, Integration of the Continuing Survey of Food Intakes by Individuals and the National Health and Nutrition Examination Survey, *Journal of the American Dietetic Association* 101 (2001): 1142–1143.
11. S. S. Smith, NCHS launches latest National Health and Nutrition Examination Survey, *Public Health Reports* 114 (1999): 190–192.
12. S. J. Crockett and coauthors, Nutrition monitoring application in the food industry, *Nutrition Today* 37 (2002): 130–135.
13. U.S. Department of Health and Human Services, *Healthy People 2010: Understanding and Improving Health,* January 2000.
14. D. S. Satcher, Healthy People at 2000, *Public Health Reports* 114 (1999): 563–564.
15. Joint WHO/FAO expert report on diet, nutrition and the prevention of chronic disease, available at **www.who.int/hpr/nutrition/expertconsultationge.htm**.
16. *The Surgeon General's Report on Nutrition and Health: Summary and Recommendations,* DHHS (PHS) publication no. 88-50211 (Washington, D.C.: Government Printing Office, 1988).

ANSWERS

Nutrition Calculations

1. a. 5 g protein × 4 kcal/g = 20 kcal protein.
30 g carbohydrate × 4 kcal/g = 120 kcal carbohydrate.
11 g fat × 9 kcal/g = 99 kcal fat.
Total = 239 kcal.

b. 20 kcal ÷ 239 kcal × 100 = 8.4% kcal from protein.
120 kcal ÷ 239 kcal × 100 = 50.2% kcal from carbohydrate.
99 kcal ÷ 239 kcal × 100 = 41.4% kcal from fat.
Total = 100%.

c. 1 g protein = 4 kcal protein.
13 g carbohydrate = 52 kcal carbohydrate.
146 total kcal − 56 kcal (protein + carbohydrate) = 90 kcal alcohol.
90 kcal alcohol ÷ 7 g/kcal = 12.9 g alcohol.

2. No. 15 g protein × 4 kcal/g = 60 kcal.

Study Questions (multiple choice)

1. d 2. b 3. c 4. d 5. d 6. a 7. c 8. d
9. c 10. a

HIGHLIGHT

Nutrition Information and Misinformation—On the Net and in the News

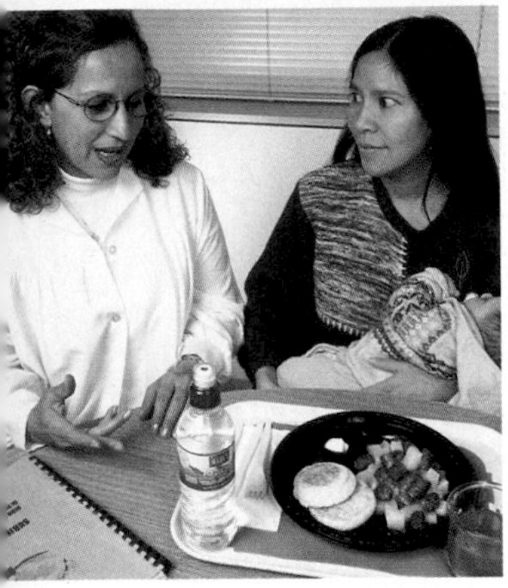
© USDA, Agricultural Research Service

People learn about nutrition daily as they watch television, read newspapers, turn the pages of magazines, talk with friends, and search the Internet. They want to know how best to take care of themselves. In some cases, they are seeking miracles: tricks to help them lose weight, foods to forestall aging, and supplements to build muscles. People's heightened interest in nutrition and health translates into billions of dollars spent on services and products sold by both legitimate and fraudulent businesses. Although consumers who obtain legitimate products can improve their health, those enticed by **fraud** may lose their health, their savings, or both.[1] Ironically, nutrition **quackery** prevents people from attaining the health they seek by giving them false hope and delaying the implementation of effective strategies (boldface terms are defined in the glossary on p. 31). Furthermore, the conflicting information that results from a mixture of science and quackery confuses consumers.

Science and quackery may be easy to tell apart at the extremes, but much nutrition information lies between the extremes. How can people distinguish valid nutrition information from misinformation? One excellent approach is to notice *who* is purveying the information. The "who" behind the information is not always evident, though, especially in the world of electronic media. Consumers need to keep in mind that *people* develop CD-ROMs and create websites on the Internet, just as people write books and report the news.

This highlight begins by examining the unique potential and problems of relying on the Internet and the media for nutrition information. It continues with a discussion of how to identify reliable nutrition information that applies to all resources, including the Internet and the news.

Nutrition on the Net

Got a question? The **Internet** has an answer. The Internet offers endless opportunities to obtain high-quality information, but it also delivers an abundance of incomplete, misleading, or inaccurate information. Simply put: anyone can publish anything.

For experienced users who know which sources are reliable, results are just a mouse click away; not only is access easy, but the information is often more current than that obtainable from other sources. For others, though, answers lie tangled in a web of information overload and questionable reliability.

With hundreds of millions of **websites** on the **World Wide Web,** searching for nutrition information can be an overwhelming experience—much like walking into an enormous bookstore with millions of books, magazines, newspapers, and videos. And like a bookstore, the Internet offers no guarantees of the accuracy of the information found there—and much of it is pure fiction.

When using the Internet, keep in mind that the quality of health-related information available covers a broad range.[2] Just because you find it on the Net doesn't make it true. Websites must be evaluated for their accuracy, just like every other source. The accompanying "How to" provides tips for determining whether a website is reliable.

> HEALTHY PEOPLE 2010
>
> Increase the proportion of health-related World Wide Web sites that disclose information that can be used to assess the quality of the site.

To help users find reliable nutrition information on the Internet, Tufts University maintains an online rating and review guide called the Nutrition Navigator (**navigator.tufts.edu**). The ratings reflect the opinions of a panel of nutrition experts who have scored selected websites on the basis of their accuracy, depth, and ease of use. In addition to a rating, the Nutrition Navigator provides a review of the website's content and links to recommended sites. The Nutrition Navigator is an excellent site from which to launch your ventures into nutrition **cyberspace.** Similarly, the Health on the Net Foundation (**www.hon.ch**) provides guidance in finding useful and reliable health information online.[3]

Nutrition in the News

Consumers get most of their nutrition information from television news and magazine reports, which have heightened awareness of how diet influences the development of diseases.

Consumers benefit from news coverage of nutrition when they learn to make lifestyle changes that will improve their health. Sometimes, however, magazine articles or television programs reporting on nutrition trends mislead consumers and create confusion. The high-protein diet craze, for example, was featured numerous times in national news magazines and on all major networks. No doubt, it was a hot topic and people wanted to know all about it (see Highlight 8 for coverage of the high-protein weight-loss diets). Unfortunately, many of these reports told a lopsided story based on a few testimonials. They did not present the results of research studies or a balance of expert opinions. Telling the whole story might not have been as entertaining, but it would have been more informative.

Tight deadlines and limited understanding sometimes make it difficult to provide a thorough report. Hungry for the latest news, the media often report scientific findings prematurely—without benefit of careful interpretation, replication, and peer review.[4] Usually, the reports present findings from a single, recently released study, making the news current and controversial.[5] Consequently, the public receives diet and health news

HOW TO Determine Whether a Website Is Reliable

To determine whether a website offers reliable nutrition information, ask the following questions:

- **Who?** Who is responsible for the site? Is it staffed by qualified professionals? Look for the authors' names and credentials. Have experts reviewed the content for accuracy?
- **When?** When was the site last updated? Because nutrition is an ever-changing science, sites need to be dated and updated frequently.
- **Where?** Where is the information coming from? The three letters following the dot in a Web address identify the site's affiliation. Addresses ending in "gov" (government), "edu" (educational institute), and "org" (organization) generally provide reliable information; "com" (commercial) sites represent businesses and, depending on their qualifications and integrity, may or may not offer dependable information.
- **Why?** Why is the site giving you this information? Is the site providing a public service or selling a product? Many commercial sites provide accurate information, but some do not. When money is the prime motivation, be aware that the information may be biased.

If you are satisfied with the answers to all of the above questions, then ask this final question:

- **What?** What is the message, and is it in line with other reliable sources? Information that contradicts common knowledge should be questioned. Many reliable sites provide links to other sites to facilitate your quest for knowledge, but this provision alone does not guarantee a reputable intention. Be aware that any site can link to any other site without permission.

GLOSSARY

accredited: approved; in the case of medical centers or universities, certified by an agency recognized by the U.S. Department of Education.

American Dietetic Association (ADA): the professional organization of dietitians in the United States. The Canadian equivalent is Dietitians of Canada, which operates similarly.

correspondence schools: schools that offer courses and degrees by mail. Some correspondence schools are accredited; others are not.

cyberspace: a term coined by William Gibson referring to the nonphysical place where all Internet activity occurs.

dietetic technician: a person who has completed a minimum of an associate's degree from an accredited university or college and an approved dietetic technician program that includes a supervised practice experience. See also *dietetic technician, registered (DTR).*

dietetic technician, registered (DTR): a dietetic technician who has passed a national examination and maintains registration through continuing professional education.

dietitian: a person trained in nutrition, food science, and diet planning. See also *registered dietitian.*

DTR: see *dietetic technician, registered.*

fraud or **quackery:** the promotion, for financial gain, of devices, treatments, services, plans, or products (including diets and supplements) that alter or claim to alter a human condition without proof of safety or effectiveness. (The word *quackery* comes from the term *quacksalver,* meaning a person who quacks loudly about a miracle product—a lotion or a salve.)

Internet (the Net): a worldwide network of millions of computers linked together to share information.

license to practice: permission under state or federal law, granted on meeting specified criteria, to use a certain title (such as dietitian) and offer certain services. **Licensed dietitians** may use the initials **LD** after their names.

misinformation: false or misleading information.

nutritionist: a person who specializes in the study of nutrition. Note that this definition does not specify qualifications and may apply not only to registered dietitians but also to self-described experts whose training is questionable. Most states have licensing laws that define the scope of practice for those calling themselves nutritionists.

public health dietitians: dietitians who specialize in providing nutrition services through organized community efforts.

RD: see *registered dietitian.*

registered dietitian (RD): a person who has completed a minimum of a bachelor's degree from an accredited university or college, has completed approved course work and a supervised practice program, has passed a national examination, and maintains registration through continuing professional education.

registration: listing; with respect to health professionals, listing with a professional organization that requires specific course work, experience, and passing of an examination.

websites: Internet resources composed of text and graphic files, each with a unique URL (Uniform Resource Locator) that names the site (for example, www.usda.gov).

World Wide Web (the Web, commonly abbreviated **www**): a graphical subset of the Internet.

quickly, but not always in perspective. Pressure to write catchy headlines and sensational stories twists inconclusive findings into "meaningful discoveries."

As a result, "surprising new findings" seem to contradict one another, and consumers feel frustrated and betrayed. Occasionally, the reports are downright erroneous, but sometimes the apparent contradictions are simply the normal result of science at work. A single study contributes to the big picture, but when viewed alone, the image is distorted. To be meaningful, its conclusions must be presented cautiously within the context of other research findings.

People who do not understand how science operates may become distrustful as they try to learn nutrition from current news reports: "How am I supposed to know what to eat when the scientists themselves don't know?" General background knowledge about the science of nutrition is the best foundation a person can have for judging the validity of new nutrition information. (Congratulations on your decision to take this course.)

Identifying Nutrition Experts

Regardless of whether the medium is electronic, print, or video, consumers need to ask whether the person behind the information is qualified to speak on nutrition. If the creator of a website on the Internet recommends eating three pineapples a day to lose weight, a trainer at the gym praises a high-protein diet, or a health-store clerk suggests an herbal supplement, should you believe these people? Can you distinguish between accurate news reports and sensational programs on television? Have you noticed that many televised nutrition messages are presented by celebrities, fitness experts, psychologists, food editors, and chefs—that is, almost anyone except a **dietitian**? When you are confused or need sound dietary advice, whom should you ask?

Physicians and Other Health Care Professionals

Many people turn to physicians or other health care professionals for dietary advice, expecting them to know all about health-related matters. But are they the best sources of accurate and current information on nutrition? Only about one-fourth of all medical schools in the United States require students to take even one nutrition course; less than half provide an elective nutrition course.[6] Students attending these classes receive an average of 20 hours of nutrition instruction—an amount they themselves consider inadequate. By comparison, most students reading this text are taking a nutrition class that provides an average of 45 hours of instruction.

The **American Dietetic Association (ADA)** asserts that standardized nutrition education should be included in the curricula for all health care professionals: physicians, nurses, physician's assistants, dental hygienists, physical and occupational therapists, social workers, and all others who provide services directly to clients.[7] When these professionals understand the relevance of nutrition in the treatment and prevention of disease and have command of reliable nutrition information, then all the people they serve will also be better informed.[8]

Most health care professionals appreciate the connections between health and nutrition. Those who have specialized in clinical nutrition are especially well qualified to speak on the subject. Few, however, have the time or experience to develop diet plans and provide detailed diet instructions for clients. Often they wisely refer clients to a qualified nutrition expert—a **registered dietitian (RD)**.

HEALTHY PEOPLE 2010

Increase the proportion of physician office visits that provide or order nutrition counseling and educational services.

Registered Dietitians (RD)

A registered dietitian (RD) has the educational background necessary to deliver reliable nutrition advice and care. To become an RD, a person must earn an undergraduate degree requiring some 60 or so semester hours in nutrition, food science, and other related subjects; complete a year's clinical internship or the equivalent; pass a national examination administered by the ADA; and maintain up-to-date knowledge and **registration** by participating in required continuing education activities such as attending seminars, taking courses, or writing professional papers.

Some states allow anyone to use the title dietitian or **nutritionist**, but others allow only RDs or people with certain graduate degrees to call themselves dietitians. Many states provide a further guarantee: a certification or **license to practice.** By requiring dietitians to be licensed, states identify people who have met minimal standards of education and experience.

Dietitians perform a multitude of duties in many settings in most communities. They work in the food industry, pharmaceutical companies, home health agencies, long-term care institutions, private practice, public health departments, research centers, education settings, fitness centers, and hospitals. Depending on their work settings, dietitians can assume a number of different job responsibilities and positions. In hospitals, administrative dietitians manage the foodservice system; clinical dietitians provide client care (see Table H1-1); and nutrition support team dietitians coordinate nutrition care with other health care professionals. In the food industry, dietitians conduct research, develop products, and market services.

Public health dietitians who work in government-funded agencies play a key role in delivering nutrition services to people in the community.[9] Among their many roles, public health dietitians help plan, coordinate, and evaluate food assistance programs; act as consultants to other agencies; manage finances; and much more.

TABLE H1-1 Responsibilities of a Clinical Dietitian

- Assesses clients' nutrition status.
- Determines clients' nutrient requirements.
- Monitors clients' nutrient intakes.
- Develops, implements, and evaluates clients' nutrition care plans.
- Counsels clients to cope with unique diet plans.
- Teaches clients and their families about nutrition needs and diet plans.
- Provides training for other dietitians, nurses, interns, and dietetics students.
- Serves as liaison between clients and the foodservice department.
- Communicates with physicians, nurses, pharmacists, and other health care professionals about clients' progress, needs, and treatments.
- Participates in professional activities to enhance knowledge and skill.

Other Dietary Employees

In some facilities, a **dietetic technician** assists registered dietitians in both administrative and clinical responsibilities. A dietetic technician has been educated and trained to work under the guidance of a registered dietitian; upon passing a national examination, the person's title changes to **dietetic technician, registered (DTR)**.

In addition to the dietetic technician, dietary employees may include clerks, aides, cooks, porters, and other assistants. These dietary employees do not have extensive formal training in nutrition, and their ability to provide accurate information may be limited.

Identifying Fake Credentials

In contrast to registered dietitians, thousands of people possess fake nutrition degrees and claim to be nutrition consultants or doctors of "nutrimedicine." These and other such titles may sound meaningful, but most of these people lack the established credentials and training of an ADA-sanctioned dietitian. If you look closely, you can see signs of their fake expertise.

Consider educational background, for example. The minimal standards of education for a dietitian specify a bachelor of science (BS) degree in food science and human nutrition or related fields from an **accredited** college or university. Such a degree generally requires four to five years of study. In contrast, a fake nutrition expert may display a degree from a six-month correspondence course. Such a degree simply falls short. In some cases, businesses posing as legitimate **correspondence schools** offer even less—they sell certificates to anyone who pays the fees. To obtain these "degrees," a candidate need not attend any classes, read any books, or pass any examinations.

To guard educational quality, an accrediting agency recognized by the U.S. Department of Education (DOE) certifies that certain schools meet criteria established to ensure that an institution provides complete and accurate schooling. Unfortunately, fake nutrition degrees are available from schools "accredited" by more than 30 phony accrediting agencies.

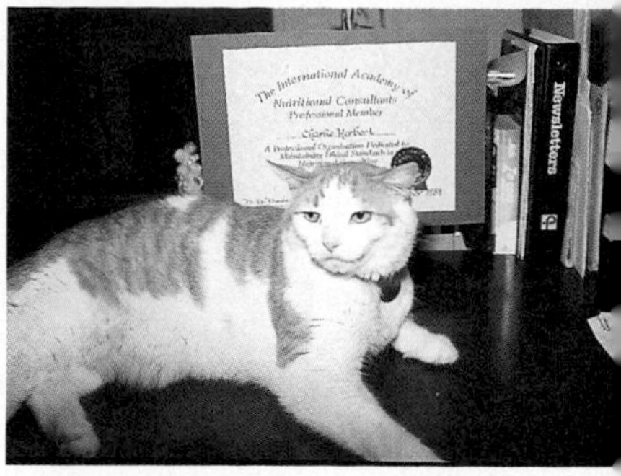

© Marilyn Herbert/Photography

Charlie displays his professional credentials.

To dramatize the ease with which anyone can obtain a fake nutrition degree, one writer enrolled in a correspondence course for a fee of $82. She made every attempt to fail, intentionally answering all examination questions incorrectly. Even so, she received a "nutritionist" certificate at the end of the course. The "school" explained that it was sure she must have just misread the test.

In a similar stunt, Ms. Sassafras Herbert was named a "professional member" of a professional association. For her efforts, Sassafras has received a wallet card and is listed in a *Who's Who* publication that is distributed at health fairs and trade shows nationwide. Sassafras is a poodle; her master, Victor Herbert, MD, paid $50 to prove that she could be awarded these honors merely by sending in her name. Mr. Charlie Herbert, who is also a professional member of such an organization, is a cat. Admittedly, these examples are dated, but acquiring false credentials is still easy—perhaps even more so, thanks to the Internet.

By knowing what qualifies someone to speak on nutrition, consumers can determine whether that person's advice might be harmful or helpful. Don't be afraid to ask for credentials. Does the personal trainer at the gym have a degree in nutrition from an accredited university? Is the creator of a nutrition website an RD or otherwise qualified to write on nutrition? Have you seen the health-store clerk's license to practice as a dietitian? If not, seek a better-qualified source for your nutrition information. After all, your health depends on it.

Identifying Valid Information

Where do nutrition experts get their information? As Chapter 1 explained, nutrition knowledge derives from scientific research.

Researchers conduct experiments and then record and analyze their results, exercising caution in their interpretation of the findings. For example, in an epidemiological study, scientists may use a specific segment of the population—say, men 18 to 30 years old. When the scientists draw conclusions, they are careful not to generalize the findings to all people. Similarly, scientists performing research studies using animals are cautious in applying their findings to human beings. Conclusions from any one research study are always tentative and take into account findings from studies conducted by other scientists as well. As evidence accumulates, scientists gain confidence about making recommendations that affect people's health and lives. Still, their statements are worded cautiously, as in "A diet high in fruits and vegetables *may* protect against *some* cancers."

Quite often, as they approach an answer to one research question, scientists raise several more questions, so future research projects are never lacking. Further scientific investigation then seeks to answer questions such as "What substance or substances within fruits and vegetables provide protection?" If those substances turn out to be the vitamins found so abundantly in fresh produce, then, "How much is needed to offer protection?" "How do these vitamins protect against cancer?" "Is it their action as antioxidant nutrients?" "If not, might it be another action or even another substance that accounts for the protection fruits and vegetables provide against cancer?" (Highlight 11 explores the answers to these questions and reviews recent research on antioxidant nutrients and disease.)

The findings from a research study are submitted to a board of reviewers composed of other scientists who rigorously evaluate the study to assure that the scientific method was followed—a process known as peer review. The reviewers critique the study's hypothesis, methodology, statistical significance, and conclusions (Table H1-2 describes the parts of a research article). If the reviewers consider the conclusions to be well supported by the evidence, they endorse the work for publication in a scientific journal where others can read it. This raises an important point regarding information found on the Internet: much gets published without the rigorous scrutiny of peer review. Consequently, readers must assume greater responsibility for examining the data and conclusions presented—often without the benefit of journal citations. Until you feel confident in critically evaluating nutrition information, you would be wise to restrict your research to one of the many online peer-reviewed journals (see the accompanying "How to" for selected website addresses).

Regardless of whether an article is presented on the Internet, on television, or in print, readers must evaluate the study and assess the findings in light of knowledge gleaned from other studies. Figure H1-1 provides examples of reliable nutrition information.

Even when a new finding is published or released to the media, it is still only preliminary and not very meaningful by itself. Other scientists will need to confirm or disprove the findings through replication. To be accepted into the body of nutrition knowledge, a finding must stand up to rigorous, repeated testing in experiments performed by several different researchers. What we "know" in nutrition results from years of replicating study findings. Communicating the latest finding in its proper context without distorting or oversimplifying the message is a challenge for scientists and journalists alike.

With each report from scientists, the field of nutrition changes a little—each finding contributes another piece to the whole body of knowledge. People who know how science works understand that single findings, like single frames in a movie, are just small parts of a larger story. Over years, the pic-

HOW TO Find Credible Sources of Nutrition Information

Government agencies, volunteer associations, consumer groups, and professional organizations provide consumers with reliable health and nutrition information. Credible sources of nutrition information include:

- Nutrition and food science departments at a university or community college.
- Local agencies such as the health department or County Cooperative Extension Service.
- Government health agencies such as:
  - Department of Agriculture (USDA) — **www.usda.gov**
  - Department of Health and Human Services (DHHS) — **www.os.dhhs.gov**
  - Food and Drug Administration (FDA) — **www.fda.gov**
  - Health Canada — **www.hc-sc.gc.ca/nutrition**
- Volunteer health agencies such as:
  - American Cancer Society — **www.cancer.org**
  - American Diabetes Association — **www.diabetes.org**
  - American Heart Association — **www.americanheart.org**
- Reputable consumer groups such as:
  - American Council on Science and Health — **www.acsh.org**
  - Federal Citizen Information Center — **www.pueblo.gsa.gov**
  - International Food Information Council — **ific.org**
- Professional health organizations such as:
  - American Dietetic Assocation — **www.eatright.org**
  - American Medical Association — **www.ama-assn.org**
  - Dietitians of Canada — **www.dietitians.ca**
- Journals such as:
  - *American Journal of Clinical Nutrition* — **www.faseb.org/ajcn**
  - *New England Journal of Medicine* — **www.nejm.org**
  - *Nutrition Reviews* — **www.ilsi.org/publications**

TABLE H1-2 Parts of a Research Article

- *Abstract.* The abstract provides a brief overview of the article.
- *Introduction.* The introduction clearly states the purpose of the current study by proposing a hypothesis.
- *Review of literature.* A comprehensive review of the literature reveals all that science has uncovered on the subject to date.
- *Methodology.* The methodology section defines key terms and describes the instruments and procedures used in conducting the study.
- *Results.* The results report the findings and may include tables and figures that summarize the information.
- *Conclusions.* The conclusions drawn are those supported by the data and reflect the original purpose as stated in the introduction. Usually, they answer a few questions and raise several more.
- *References.* The references reflect the investigator's knowledge of the subject and should include an extensive list of relevant studies (including key studies several years old as well as current ones).

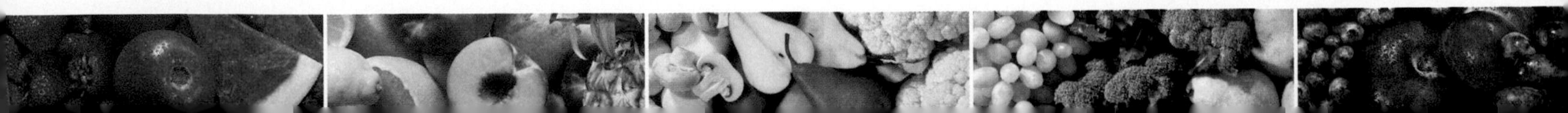

FIGURE H1-1 Sources of Reliable Nutrition Information

REVIEWS

Articles that examine all the major work on a subject are published in review journals like *Nutrition Reviews*. These articles provide references to all of the original work reviewed.

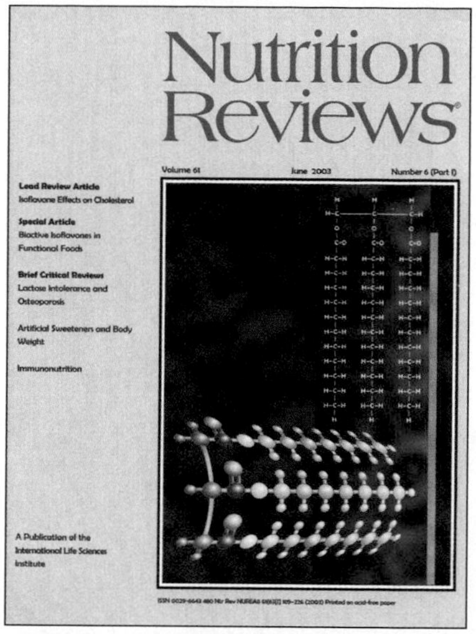
Nutrition Reviews
Volume 61
June 2003
Number 6 (Part I)
Lead Review Article
Isoflavone Effects on Cholesterol
Special Article
Bioactive Isoflavones in Functional Foods
Brief Critical Reviews
Lactose Intolerance and Osteoporosis
Artificial Sweeteners and Body Weight
Immunonutrition
A Publication of the International Life Sciences Institute

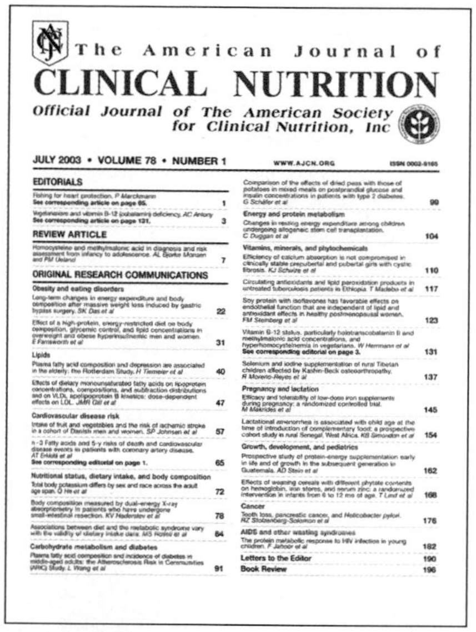
The American Journal of
CLINICAL NUTRITION
Official Journal of The American Society for Clinical Nutrition, Inc
JULY 2003 • VOLUME 78 • NUMBER 1
EDITORIALS
REVIEW ARTICLE
ORIGINAL RESEARCH COMMUNICATIONS

JOURNALS

Articles that present all the details of the methods, results, and conclusions of a particular study are published in journals like the *American Journal of Clinical Nutrition.*

INDEXES

Indexes provide a listing of research articles on a given subject. Several online indexes are available, but one of the best for nutrition research is PubMed, a service of the National Library of Medicine. For free access, visit www.pubmed.gov

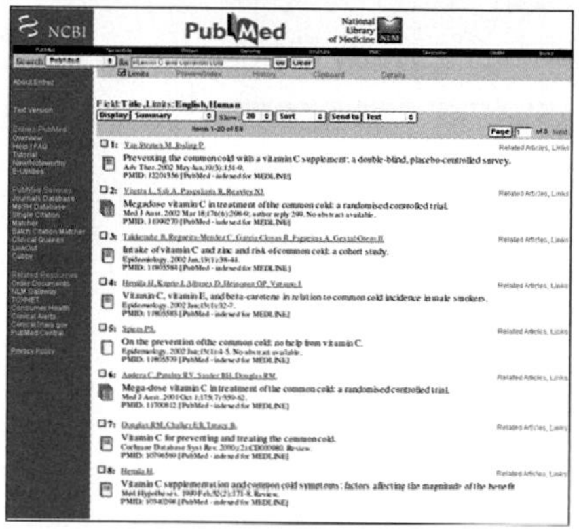
NCBI
PubMed
National Library of Medicine

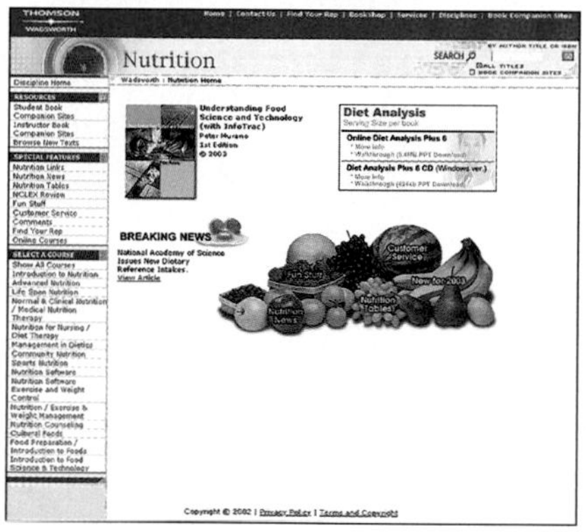
Nutrition
Diet Analysis
BREAKING NEWS

WEBSITES

Websites on the Internet developed by credible sources, such as those listed on p. 34, can provide valuable nutrition information and direct users to other resources. A quick link to many of these nutrition resources is available when you visit www.wadsworth.com/nutrition

ture of what is "true" in nutrition gradually changes, and modifications in recommendations then follow. Highlight 5 provides an example in presenting a detailed look at how dietary fat recommendations have evolved over the past several decades as researchers have uncovered the relationships between the various kinds of fat and their roles in supporting or harming health.

Because science is a step-by-step, information-gathering and testing process, old research still has value. A hypothesis first advanced in 1960 that stands up to decades of validation has real strength. When it comes to scientific information, "new" does not necessarily mean "improved." In fact, any science report based on all new references is suspect, for truly strong research is based on a body of work conducted over many years. This is why, even in books published just this year, you will see references to old reports. Some studies have become classics: they were exciting when they first appeared, and they have stood up to the test of time.

Identifying Misinformation

Did you receive the e-mail warning about Costa Rican bananas causing the disease "necrotizing fasciitis"? If so, you've been scammed by Internet misinformation. Nutrition is a hot topic, and scattered among the valid research findings are thousands of misleading and unfounded claims. How can a person identify nutrition **misinformation** and quackery—on the Net and in the news? Once upon a time, quacks rode into town in wooden wagons hawking snake oil for 50 cents a bottle to "cure what ails you," but those days are gone. Today's purveyors approach consumers in less obvious ways. They deliver their messages via the Internet, on glossy pages of magazines, in televised infomercials, and at social gatherings. The claims may look slick and sound logical, but they lack the research support found in nutrition science. Figure H1-2 presents red flags that alert consumers to nutrition misinformation.[10]

FIGURE H1-2 Red Flags of Nutrition Quackery

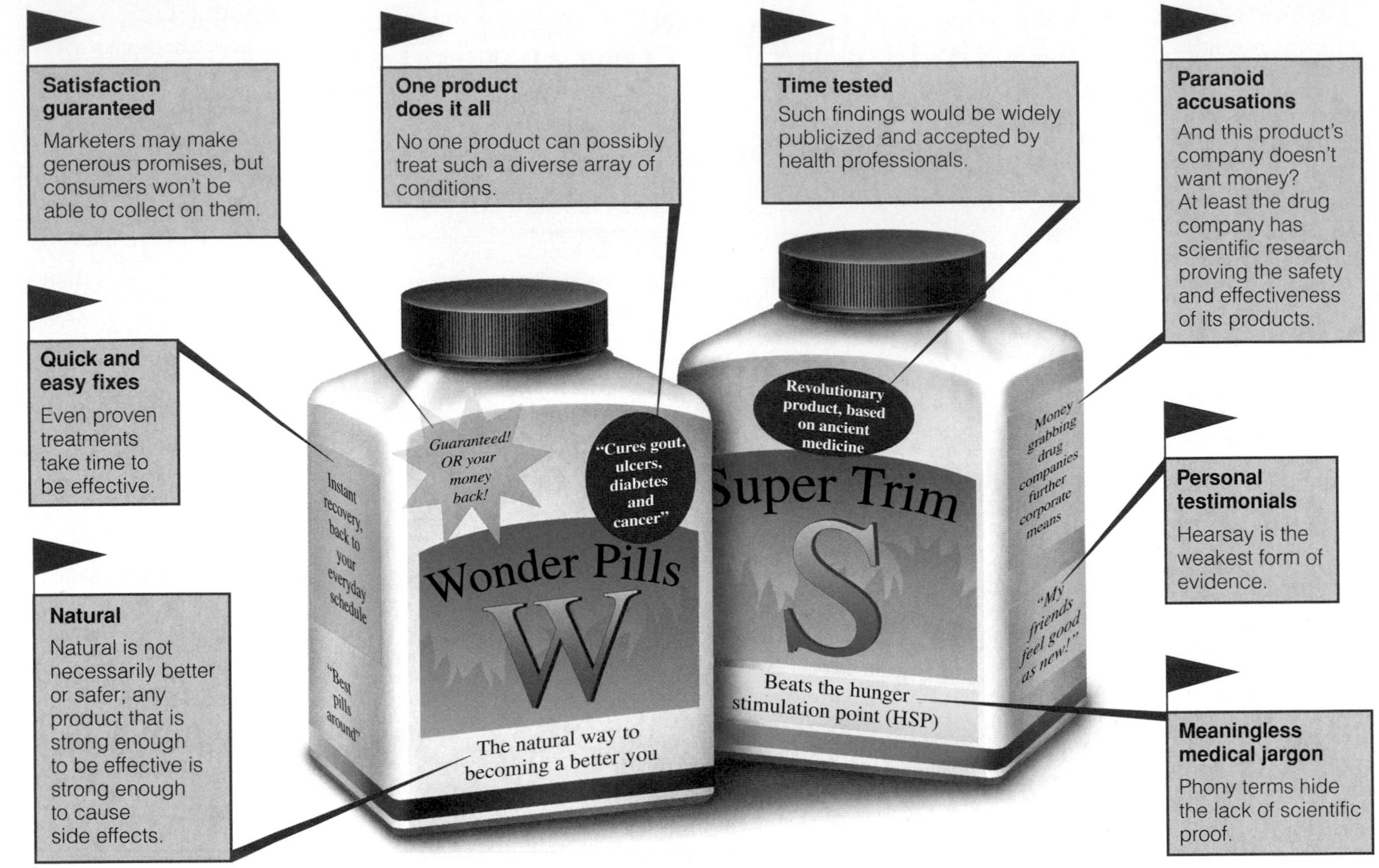
Satisfaction guaranteed
Marketers may make generous promises, but consumers won't be able to collect on them.
One product does it all
No one product can possibly treat such a diverse array of conditions.
Time tested
Such findings would be widely publicized and accepted by health professionals.
Paranoid accusations
And this product's company doesn't want money? At least the drug company has scientific research proving the safety and effectiveness of its products.
Quick and easy fixes
Even proven treatments take time to be effective.
Natural
Natural is not necessarily better or safer; any product that is strong enough to be effective is strong enough to cause side effects.
Personal testimonials
Hearsay is the weakest form of evidence.
Meaningless medical jargon
Phony terms hide the lack of scientific proof.
Guaranteed! OR your money back!
"Cures gout, ulcers, diabetes and cancer"
Instant recovery, back to your everyday schedule
"Best pills around"
Wonder Pills
W
The natural way to becoming a better you
Revolutionary product, based on ancient medicine
Super Trim
S
Money grabbing drug companies further corporate means
"My friends feel good as new!"
Beats the hunger stimulation point (HSP)

Sales of unproven and dangerous products have always been a concern, but the Internet now provides merchants with an easy and inexpensive way to reach millions of customers around the world. Because of the difficulty in regulating the Internet, fraudulent and illegal sales of medical products have hit a bonanza. As is the case with the air, no one owns the Internet, and similarly, no one has control over the pollution. Countries have different laws regarding sales of drugs, dietary supplements, and other health products, but applying these laws to the Internet marketplace is almost impossible. Even if illegal activities could be defined and identified, finding the person responsible for a particular website is not always possible. Websites can open and close in a blink of a cursor. Now, more than ever, consumers must heed the caution "Buyer beware."

In summary, when you hear nutrition news, consider its source. Ask yourself these two questions: Is the person purveying the information qualified to speak on nutrition? Is the information based on valid scientific research? If not, find a better source, for your health is your most precious asset.

NUTRITION ON THE NET

Access these websites for further study of topics covered in this highlight.

- Find updates and quick links to these and other nutrition-related sites at our website: **www.wadsworth.com/nutrition**
- Visit the National Council Against Health Fraud: **www.ncahf.org**
- Check the ratings and reviews of websites by Tufts University Nutrition Navigator: **navigator.tufts.edu**

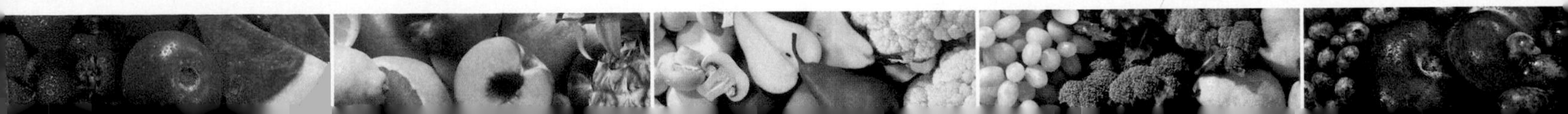

- Find a registered dietitian in your area from the American Dietetic Association: **www.eatright.org**
- Find a nutrition professional in Canada from the Dietitians of Canada: **www.dietitians.ca**
- Find out whether a correspondence school is accredited from the Distance Education and Training Council's Accrediting Commission: **www.detc.org**
- Find out whether a school is properly accredited for a dietetics degree from the American Dietetic Association: **www.eatright.org/cade**
- Obtain a listing of accredited institutions, professionally accredited programs, and candidates for accreditation from the American Council on Education: **www.acenet.edu**
- Learn more about quackery from Stephen Barrett's Quackwatch: **www.quackwatch.com**
- Search "quackery" at the U.S. Government health information site: **www.healthfinder.gov**
- Check out health-related hoaxes and rumors: **www.cdc.gov/hoax_rumors.htm** and **www.urbanlegends.com/ulz**
- Find reliable research articles: **www.pubmed.gov**

REFERENCES

1. Position of the American Dietetic Association: Food and nutrition misinformation, *Journal of the American Dietetic Association* 102 (2002): 260–266.
2. G. Eysenbach and coauthors, Empirical studies assessing the quality of health information for consumers on the World Wide Web: A systematic review, *Journal of the American Medical Association* 287 (2002): 2691–2700.
3. S. M. Dorman, Health on the Net Foundation: Advocating for quality health information, *Journal of School Health* 72 (2002): 86.
4. L. M. Schwartz, S. Woloshin, and L. Baczek, Media coverage of scientific meetings: Too much, too soon? *Journal of the American Medical Association* 287 (2002): 2859–2863.
5. N. S. Wellman and coauthors, Do we facilitate the scientific process and the development of dietary guidance when findings from single studies are publicized? An American Society for Nutritional Sciences Controversy Session Report, *American Journal of Clinical Nutrition* 70 (1999): 802–805.
6. J. A. Schulman, Nutrition education in medical schools: Trends and implications for health educators, *Med Ed Online,* **www.med-ed-Online.org/ f0000015.htm** (accessed October 24, 2000).
7. Position of the American Dietetic Association: Nutrition education for health care professionals, *Journal of the American Dietetic Association* 98 (1998): 343–346.
8. Intersociety Professional Nutrition Education Consortium, Bringing nutrition specialists into the mainstream: Rationale for the Intersociety Professional Nutrition Education Consortium, *American Journal of Clinical Nutrition* 68 (1998): 894–898.
9. D. B. Johnson and coauthors, Public health nutrition practice in the United States, *Journal of the American Dietetic Association* 101 (2001): 529–534.
10. Adapted from P. Kurtzweil, How to spot health fraud, *FDA Consumer,* November/-December 1999, pp. 22–26.

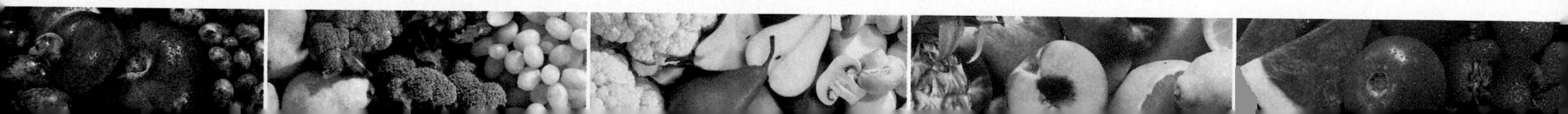

Chapter 2

Planning a Healthy Diet

Chapter Outline

Principles and Guidelines: *Diet-Planning Principles • Dietary Guidelines for Americans*

Diet-Planning Guides: *USDA Food Guide • Exchange Lists • Putting the Plan into Action • From Guidelines to Groceries*

Food Labels: *The Ingredient List • Serving Sizes • Nutrition Facts • The Daily Values • Nutrient Claims • Health Claims • Structure-Function Claims • Consumer Education*

Highlight: *A World Tour of Pyramids, Pagodas, and Plates*

Available Online

http://nutrition.wadsworth.com/uncn7

Nutrition Animation: *Diet Planning Using the Healthy Eating Index*

Student Practice Test

Glossary Terms

Nutrition on the Net

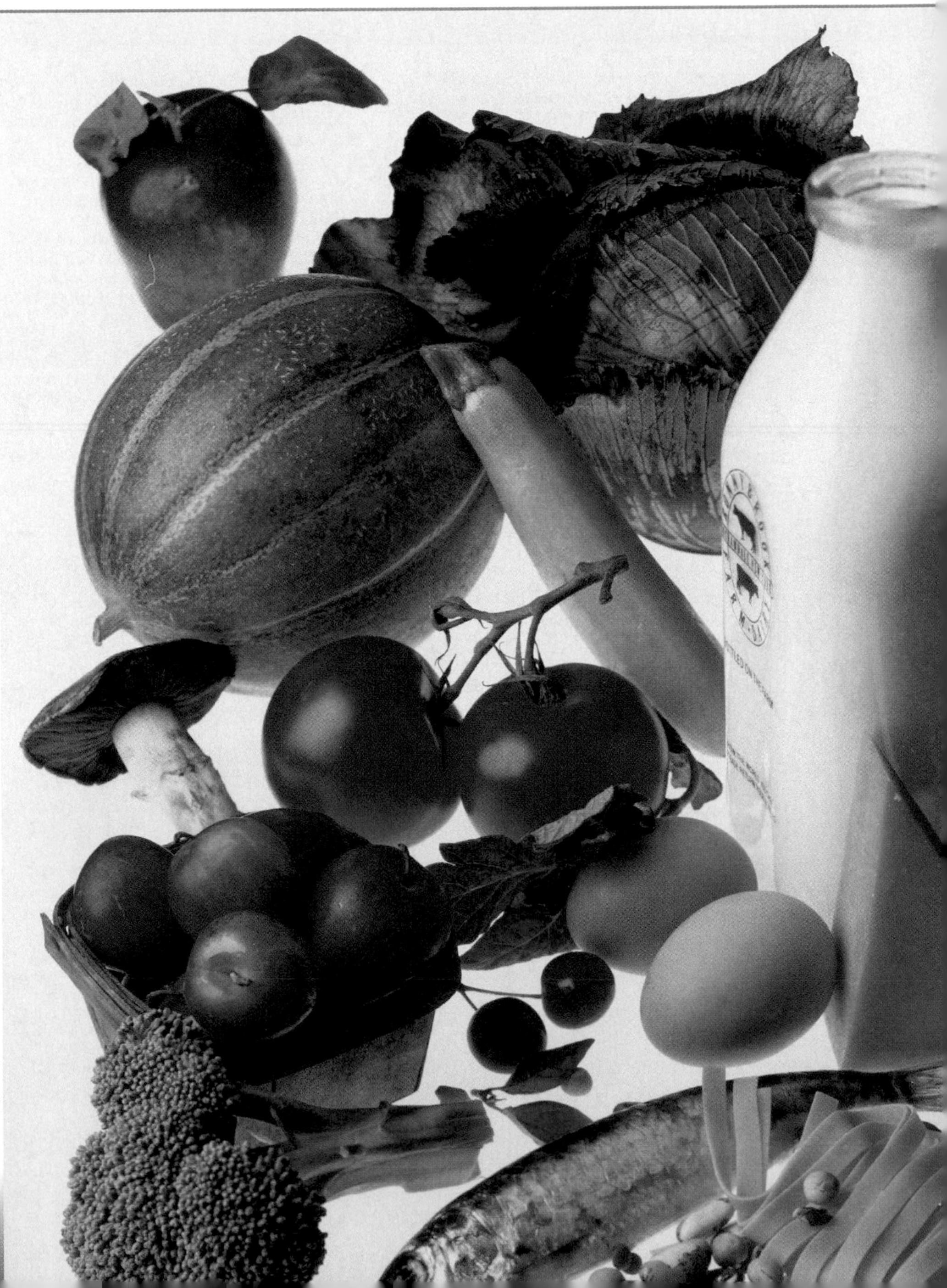

Nutrition in Your Life

You make food choices—deciding what to eat and how much to eat—more than 1000 times every year. We eat so frequently that it's easy for us to choose a meal without giving its nutrient contributions or health consequences any thought. Even when we want to make healthy choices, we may not know which foods to select or what quantity to consume. Given a few tools and tips, you can learn to plan a healthy diet.

Chapter 1 explained that the body's many activities are supported by the nutrients delivered by the foods people eat. Food choices made over years influence the body's health, and consistently poor choices increase the risks of developing chronic diseases. This chapter shows how a person can select from the tens of thousands of foods available to create a diet that supports health. Fortunately, most foods provide several nutrients, so one trick for wise diet planning is to select a combination of foods that deliver a full array of nutrients. This chapter begins by introducing the diet-planning principles and dietary guidelines that assist people in selecting foods that will deliver nutrients without excess energy.

Principles and Guidelines

How well you nourish yourself does not depend on the selection of any one food. Instead it depends on the selection of many different foods at numerous meals over days, months, and years. Diet-planning principles and dietary guidelines are key concepts to keep in mind whenever you are selecting foods—whether shopping at the grocery store, choosing from a restaurant menu, or preparing a home-cooked meal.

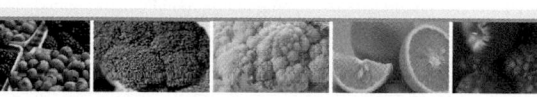

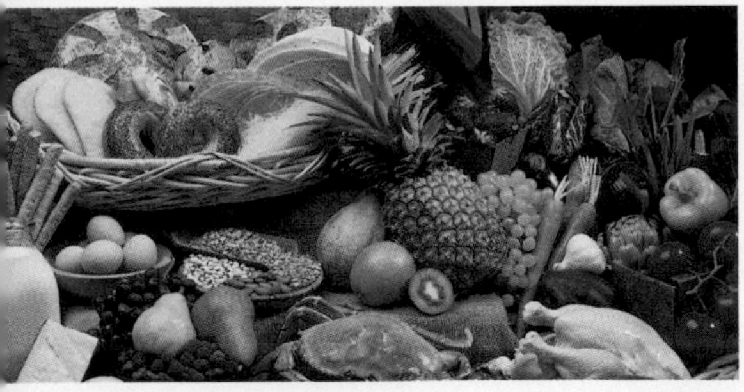
© Polara Studios Inc.

To ensure an adequate and balanced diet, eat a variety of foods daily, choosing different foods from each group.

■ Diet-planning principles:
- **A**dequacy.
- **B**alance.
- k**C**alorie (energy) control.
- Nutrient **D**ensity.
- **M**oderation.
- **V**ariety.

■ Balance in the diet helps to ensure adequacy.

■ Nutrient density promotes adequacy and kcalorie control.

adequacy (dietary): providing all the essential nutrients, fiber, and energy in amounts sufficient to maintain health.

balance (dietary): providing foods in proportion to each other and in proportion to the body's needs.

kcalorie (energy) control: management of food energy intake.

nutrient density: a measure of the nutrients a food provides relative to the energy it provides. The more nutrients and the fewer kcalories, the higher the nutrient density.

empty-kcalorie foods: a popular term used to denote foods that contribute energy but lack protein, vitamins, and minerals.

Diet-Planning Principles

Diet planners have developed several ways to select foods. Whatever plan or combination of plans they use, though, they keep in mind the six basic diet-planning principles■ listed in the margin.

Adequacy **Adequacy** means that the diet provides sufficient energy and enough of all the nutrients to meet the needs of healthy people. Take the essential nutrient iron, for example. Each day the body loses some iron, so people have to replace it by eating foods that contain iron. A person whose diet fails to provide enough iron-rich foods may develop the symptoms of iron-deficiency anemia: the person may feel weak, tired, and listless; have frequent headaches; and find that even the smallest amount of muscular work brings disabling fatigue. To prevent these deficiency symptoms, a person must include foods that supply adequate iron. The same is true for all the other essential nutrients introduced in Chapter 1.

Balance The art of balancing the diet involves consuming enough—but not too much—of each type of food. The essential minerals calcium and iron, taken together, illustrate the importance of dietary **balance.** Meats, fish, and poultry are rich in iron but poor in calcium. Conversely, milk and milk products are rich in calcium but poor in iron. Use some meat or meat alternates for iron; use some milk and milk products for calcium; and save some space for other foods, too, since a diet consisting of milk and meat alone would not be adequate.■ For the other nutrients, people need whole grains, vegetables, and fruits.

kCalorie (Energy) Control Designing an adequate diet without overeating requires careful planning. Once again, balance plays a key role. The amount of energy coming into the body from foods should balance with the amount of energy being used by the body to sustain its metabolic and physical activities. Upsetting this balance leads to gains or losses in body weight. The discussion of weight control in Chapter 9 examines this issue in more detail, but the key to **kcalorie control** is to select foods of high **nutrient density.**

Nutrient Density To eat well without overeating, select foods that deliver the most nutrients for the least food energy. Consider foods containing calcium, for example. You can get about 300 milligrams of calcium from either 1½ ounces of cheddar cheese or 1 cup of fat-free milk, but the cheese delivers about twice as much food energy (kcalories) as the milk. The fat-free milk, then, is twice as calcium dense as the cheddar cheese; it offers the same amount of calcium for half the kcalories. Both foods are excellent choices for adequacy's sake alone, but to achieve adequacy while controlling kcalories,■ the fat-free milk is the better choice. (Alternatively, a person could select a low-fat cheddar cheese.) The many bar graphs that appear in Chapters 10 through 13 highlight the most nutrient-dense choices, and the accompanying "How to" describes how to compare foods based on nutrient density.

Just like a person who has to pay for rent, food, clothes, and tuition on a tight budget, a person whose energy allowance is limited has to obtain iron, calcium, and all the other essential nutrients on a tight energy budget. To succeed, the person has to get many nutrients for each kcalorie "dollar." In the cola and grapes example in the margin on p. 41, both provide about the same number of kcalories, but the grapes deliver many more nutrients. A person who makes nutrient-dense choices such as fruit over cola can meet daily nutrient needs on a lower energy budget. Such choices support good health.

Foods that are notably low in nutrient density—such as potato chips, candies, and colas—are sometimes called **empty-kcalorie foods.** The kcalories these foods provide are "empty" in that they deliver only energy (from sugar, fat, or both) with little, or no, protein, vitamins, or minerals.

Moderation Foods rich in fat and sugar provide enjoyment and energy but relatively few nutrients. In addition, they promote weight gain when eaten in excess.

HOW TO Compare Foods Based on Nutrient Density

One way to evaluate foods is simply to notice their nutrient contribution *per serving:* 1 cup of milk provides about 300 milligrams of calcium, and ½ cup of fresh, cooked turnip greens provides about 100 milligrams. Thus a serving of milk offers three times as much calcium as a serving of turnip greens. To get 300 milligrams of calcium, a person could choose either 1 cup of milk or 1½ cups of turnip greens.

Another valuable way to evaluate foods is to consider their nutrient density—their nutrient contribution *per kcalorie.* Fat-free milk delivers about 85 kcalories with its 300 milligrams of calcium. To calculate the nutrient density, divide milligrams by kcalories:

$$\frac{300 \text{ mg calcium}}{85 \text{ kcal}} = 3.5 \text{ mg per kcal.}$$

Do the same for the fresh turnip greens, which provide 15 kcalories with the 100 milligrams of calcium:

$$\frac{100 \text{ mg calcium}}{15 \text{ kcal}} = 6.7 \text{ mg per kcal.}$$

The more milligrams per kcalorie, the greater the nutrient density. Turnip greens are more calcium dense than milk. They provide more calcium *per kcalorie* than milk, but milk offers more calcium *per serving.* Both approaches offer valuable information, especially when combined with a realistic appraisal. What matters most is which are you more likely to consume—1½ cups of turnip greens or 1 cup of milk? You can get 300 milligrams of calcium from either, but the greens will save you about 40 kcalories (the savings would be even greater if you usually use whole milk).

Keep in mind, too, that calcium is only one of the many nutrients that foods provide. Similar calculations for protein, for example, would show that fat-free milk provides more protein both *per kcalorie* and *per serving* than turnip greens—that is, milk is more protein dense. Combining variety with nutrient density helps to ensure the adequacy of all nutrients.

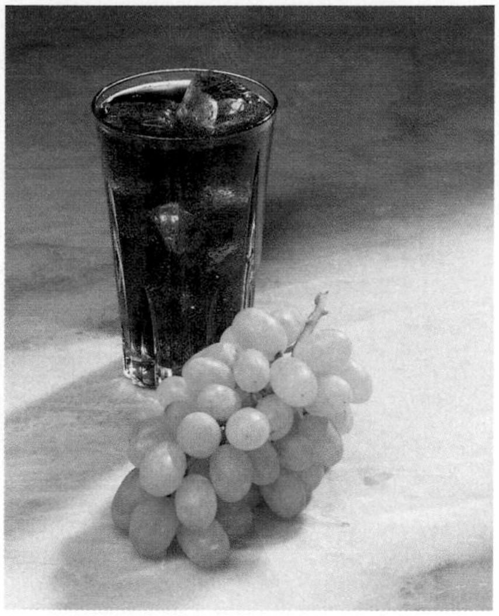

© Polara Studios Inc.

This cola and bunch of grapes illustrate nutrient density. Each provides about 150 kcalories, but the grapes offer a trace of protein, some vitamins, minerals, phytochemicals, and fiber along with the energy; the cola beverage offers only "empty" kcalories from sugar without any other nutrients. Grapes, or any fruit for that matter, are more nutrient dense than cola beverages.

A person practicing **moderation**■ would eat such foods only on occasion and would regularly select foods low in fat and sugar, a practice that automatically improves nutrient density. Returning to the example of cheddar cheese and fat-free milk, the fat-free milk not only offers the same amount of calcium for less energy, but it contains far less fat than the cheese.

■ Moderation contributes to adequacy, balance, and kcalorie control.

Variety A diet may have all of the virtues just described and still lack **variety,** if a person eats the same foods day after day. People should select foods from each of the food groups daily and vary their choices within each food group from day to day for several reasons. First, different foods within the same group contain different arrays of nutrients. Among the fruits, for example, strawberries are especially rich in vitamin C while apricots are rich in vitamin A. Second, no food is guaranteed entirely free of substances that, in excess, could be harmful. The strawberries might contain trace amounts of one contaminant, the apricots another. By alternating fruit choices, a person will ingest very little of either contaminant. Third, as the adage goes, variety is the spice of life. Even if a person eats beans frequently, the person can enjoy pinto beans in Mexican burritos today, garbanzo beans in Greek salad tomorrow, and baked beans with barbecued chicken on the weekend. Eating nutritious meals need never be boring.

Dietary Guidelines for Americans

What should a person eat to stay healthy? The *Dietary Guidelines for Americans 2005* provide the answer based on a "preponderance of scientific evidence for promoting health and reducing risk of chronic diseases through diet and physical activity."[1] Table 2-1 presents the nine *Guideline* topics with their key recommendations. The first three topics focus on choosing nutrient-dense foods within energy needs, maintaining a healthy body weight, and engaging in regular physical activity. The fourth

moderation (dietary): providing enough but not too much of a substance.

variety (dietary): eating a wide selection of foods within and among the major food groups.

TABLE 2-1 Key Recommendations of the *Dietary Guidelines for Americans 2005*

Adequate Nutrients within Energy Needs

- Consume a variety of nutrient-dense foods and beverages within and among the basic food groups; limit intakes of saturated and *trans* fats, cholesterol, added sugars, salt, and alcohol.
- Meet recommended intakes within energy needs by adopting a balanced eating pattern, such as the USDA Food Guide (see pp. 44–45).

Weight Management

- To maintain body weight in a healthy range, balance kcalories from foods and beverages with kcalories expended (see Chapters 8 and 9).
- To prevent gradual weight gain over time, make small decreases in food and beverage kcalories and increase physical activity.

Physical Activity

- Engage in regular physical activity and reduce sedentary activities to promote health, psychological well-being, and a healthy body weight.
- Achieve physical fitness by including cardiovascular conditioning, stretching exercises for flexibility, and resistance exercises or calisthenics for muscle strength and endurance.

Food Groups to Encourage

- Consume a sufficient amount of fruits, vegetables, milk and milk products, and whole grains while staying within energy needs.
- Select a variety of fruits and vegetables each day, including selections from all five vegetable subgroups (dark green, orange, legumes, starchy vegetables, and other vegetables) several times a week. Make at least half of the grain selections whole grains. Select fat-free or low-fat milk products.

Fats

- Consume less than 10 percent of kcalories from saturated fats and less than 300 milligrams of cholesterol per day, and keep *trans* fats consumption as low as possible (see Chapter 5).
- Keep total fat intake between 20 and 35 percent of kcalories; choose from mostly polyunsaturated and monounsaturated fat sources such as fish, nuts, and vegetable oils.
- Select and prepare foods that are lean, low fat, or fat-free and low in saturated and/or *trans* fats.

Carbohydrates

- Choose fiber-rich fruits, vegetables, and whole grains often.
- Choose and prepare foods and beverages with little added sugars (see Chapter 4).
- Reduce the incidence of dental caries by practicing good oral hygiene and consuming sugar- and starch-containing foods and beverages less frequently.

Sodium and Potassium

- Choose and prepare foods with little salt (less than 2300 milligrams sodium or approximately 1 teaspoon salt). At the same time, consume potassium-rich foods, such as fruits and vegetables (see Chapter 12).

Alcoholic Beverages

- Those who choose to drink alcoholic beverages should do so sensibly and in moderation (up to one drink per day for women and up to two drinks per day for men).
- Some individuals should not consume alcoholic beverages (see Highlight 7).

Food Safety

- To avoid microbial foodborne illness, keep foods safe: clean hands, food contact surfaces, and fruits and vegetables; separate raw, cooked, and ready-to-eat foods; cook foods to a safe internal temperature; chill perishable food promptly; and defrost food properly.
- Avoid unpasteurized milk and products made from it; raw or undercooked eggs, meat, poultry, fish, and shellfish; unpasteurized juices; raw sprouts.

NOTE: These guidelines are intended for adults and healthy children ages 2 and older.
SOURCE: The *Dietary Guidelines for Americans 2005*, available at **www.healthierus.gov/dietaryguidelines**.

topic, "Food Groups to Encourage," focuses on the selection of a variety of fruits and vegetables, whole grains, and milk. The next four topics advise people to choose sensibly in their use of fats, carbohydrates, salt, and alcoholic beverages for those who partake. Finally, consumers are reminded to keep food safe. Together, the *Dietary Guidelines* point the way toward better health. Table 2-2 presents *Canada's Guidelines for Healthy Eating,* and Highlight 2 examines dietary guidelines from several countries around the world, as well as those from the United States and Canada.

IN SUMMARY A well-planned diet delivers adequate nutrients, a balanced array of nutrients, and an appropriate amount of energy. It is based on nutrient-dense foods, moderate in substances that can be detrimental to health, and varied in its selections. The 2005 *Dietary Guidelines* apply these principles, offering practical advice on how to eat for good health.

TABLE 2-2 *Canada's Guidelines for Healthy Eating*

- Enjoy a variety of foods.
- Emphasize cereals, breads, other grain products, vegetables, and fruits.
- Choose lower-fat dairy products, leaner meats, and foods prepared with little or no fat.
- Achieve and maintain a healthy body weight by enjoying regular physical activity and healthy eating.
- Limit salt, alcohol, and caffeine.

SOURCE: These guidelines derive from *Action Towards Healthy Eating—Canada's Guidelines for Healthy Eating and Recommended Strategies for Implementation.*

Diet-Planning Guides

To plan a diet that achieves all of the dietary ideals just outlined, a person needs tools as well as knowledge. Among the most widely used tools for diet planning are **food group plans** that build a diet from clusters of foods that are similar in nutrient content. Thus each group represents a set of nutrients that differs somewhat from the nutrients supplied by the other groups. Selecting foods from each of the groups eases the task of creating an adequate and balanced diet.

USDA Food Guide

The 2005 *Dietary Guidelines* encourage consumers to adopt a balanced eating plan, such as the USDA's Food Guide (see Figure 2-1 on pp. 44–45).■ The USDA Food Guide assigns foods to five major food groups■ and recommends daily amounts of foods from each group to meet nutrient needs. In addition to presenting the food groups, the figure lists the most notable nutrients of each group, the serving sizes, and the foods within each group sorted by nutrient density. Chapter 15 provides a food guide for young children, and Appendix I presents Canada's food group plan, the *Food Guide to Healthy Eating.*

■ The DASH Eating Plan, another dietary pattern that exemplifies the 2005 *Dietary Guidelines,* is presented in Chapter 27.

■ Five food groups:
- Fruits.
- Vegetables.
- Grains.
- Meat and legumes.
- Milk.

Recommended Amounts All food groups offer valuable nutrients, and people should make selections from each group daily. Table 2-3 (on p. 46 top) specifies the amounts of foods from each group needed daily to create a healthful diet for several energy (kcalorie) levels.■ Estimated daily kcalorie needs for sedentary and active men and women are shown in Table 2-4 (on p. 46 bottom). A sedentary young woman needing 2000 kcalories a day for example, would select 2 cups of fruit; 2½ cups of vegetables (dispersed among the vegetable subgroups); 6 ounces of grain foods (with at least half coming from whole grains); 5½ ounces of meat, poultry, or fish, or the equivalent of **legumes,** eggs, seeds, or nuts; and 3 cups of milk or yogurt, or the equivalent of cheese or fortified soy products. Additionally, a small amount of unsaturated oil, such as vegetable oil, or the oils of nuts, olives, or fatty fish, is required to supply needed nutrients.

■ Chapter 8 explains how to determine energy needs. For an approximation, turn to the DRI Estimated Energy Requirement on the inside front cover.

All vegetables provide an array of vitamins, fiber, and the mineral potassium, but some vegetables are especially good sources of certain nutrients and beneficial phytochemicals.■ For this reason, the USDA Food Guide sorts the vegetable group into five subgroups. The dark green vegetables deliver the B vitamin folate; the orange vegetables provide abundant vitamin A; legumes supply iron and protein; the starchy vegetables contribute abundant carbohydrate energy; and the other vegetables fill in the gaps and add more of these same nutrients.

■ Reminder: *Phytochemicals* are the nonnutrient compounds found in plant-derived foods that have biological activity in the body.

In a 2000-kcalorie diet, then, the recommended 2½ cups of daily vegetables should be varied among the subgroups over a week's time, as shown in Table 2-5 (p. 47). In

food group plans: diet-planning tools that sort foods into groups based on nutrient content and specify the amounts of foods that people should eat from each group.

legumes (lay-GYOOMS, LEG-yooms): plants of the bean and pea family, with seeds that are rich in protein compared with other plant-derived foods.

FIGURE 2-1 USDA Food Guide, 2005

Key:
- ● Foods generally high in nutrient density (choose most often)
- △ Foods lower in nutrient density (limit selections)

GRAINS

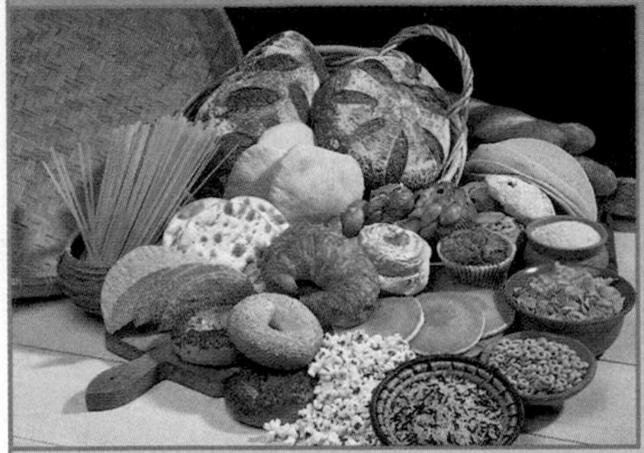

© Polara Studios, Inc.

Make at least half of the grain selections whole grains.

These foods contribute folate, niacin, riboflavin, thiamin, iron, magnesium, selenium, and fiber.

1 oz grains is equivalent to 1 slice bread; ½ c cooked rice, pasta, or cereal; 1 oz dry pasta or rice; 1 c ready-to-eat cereal; 3 c popped popcorn.

- ● Whole grains (barley, brown rice, bulgur, millet, oats, rye, wheat) and whole-grain, low-fat breads, cereals, crackers, and pastas; popcorn.
- ● Enriched bagels, breads, cereals, pastas (couscous, macaroni, spaghetti), pretzels, rice, rolls, tortillas.
- △ Biscuits, cakes, cookies, cornbread, crackers, croissants, doughnuts, french toast, fried rice, granola, muffins, pancakes, pastries, pies, presweetened cereals, taco shells, waffles.

VEGETABLES

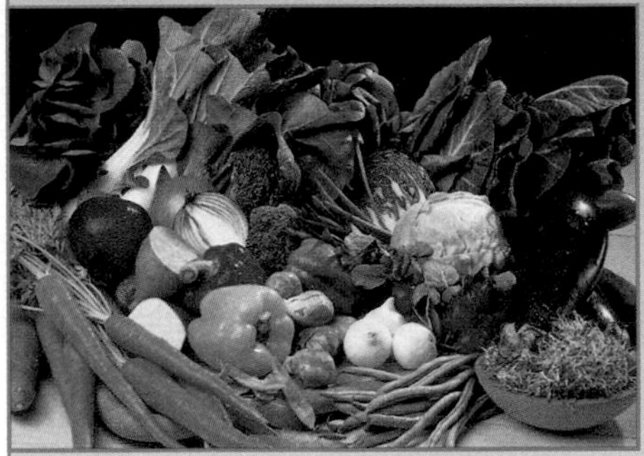

© Polara Studios, Inc.

Choose a variety of vegetables from all five subgroups several times a week.

These foods contribute folate, vitamin A, vitamin C, vitamin E, magnesium, potassium, and fiber.

½ c vegetables is equivalent to ½ c cut-up raw or cooked vegetables; ½ c cooked legumes; ½ c vegetable juice; 1 c raw, leafy greens.

- ● Dark green vegetables: Broccoli and leafy greens such as arugula, beet greens, bok choy, collard greens, kale, mustard greens, romaine lettuce, spinach, and turnip greens.
- ● Orange and deep yellow vegetables: Carrots, carrot juice, pumpkin, sweet potatoes, and winter squash (acorn, butternut).
- ● Legumes: Black beans, black-eyed peas, garbanzo beans (chickpeas), kidney beans, lentils, navy beans, pinto beans, soybeans and soy products such as tofu, and split peas.
- ● Starchy vegetables: Cassava, corn, green peas, hominy, lima beans, and potatoes.
- ● Other vegetables: Artichokes, asparagus, bamboo shoots, bean sprouts, beets, brussels sprouts, cabbages, cactus, cauliflower, celery, cucumbers, eggplant, green beans, iceberg lettuce, mushrooms, okra, onions, peppers, seaweed, snow peas, tomatoes, vegetable juices, zucchini.
- △ Baked beans, candied sweet potatoes, coleslaw, french fries, potato salad, refried beans, scalloped potatoes, tempura vegetables.

FRUITS

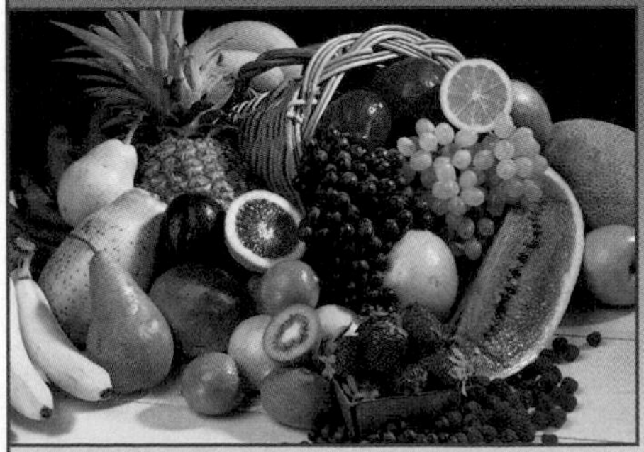

© Polara Studios, Inc.

Consume a variety of fruits and no more than one-third of the recommended intake as fruit juice.

These foods contribute folate, vitamin A, vitamin C, potassium, and fiber.

½ c fruit is equivalent to ½ c fresh, frozen, or canned fruit; 1 small fruit; ¼ c dried fruit; ½ c fruit juice.

- ● Apples, apricots, avocados, bananas, blueberries, cantaloupe, cherries, grapefruit, grapes, guava, kiwi, mango, oranges, papaya, peaches, pears, pineapples, plums, raspberries, strawberries, watermelon; dried fruit; unsweetened juices.
- △ Canned or frozen fruit in syrup; juices, punches, ades, and fruit drinks with added sugars; fried plantains.

FIGURE 2-1 USDA Food Guide, 2005—continued

MILK, YOGURT, AND CHEESE

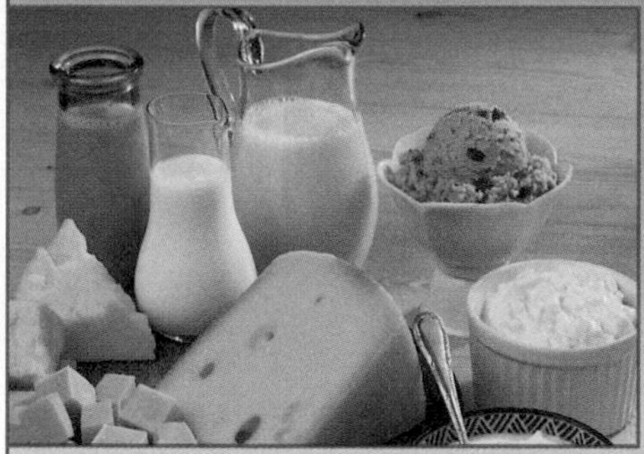

© Polara Studios, Inc.

Make fat-free or low-fat choices. Choose lactose-free products or other calcium-rich foods if you don't consume milk.

These foods contribute protein, riboflavin, vitamin B_{12}, calcium, magnesium, potassium, and, when fortified, vitamin A and vitamin D.

1 c milk is equivalent to 1 c fat-free milk or yogurt; 1½ oz fat-free natural cheese; 2 oz fat-free processed cheese.

- ● Fat-free milk and fat-free milk products such as buttermilk, cheeses, cottage cheese, yogurt; fat-free fortified soy milk.
- ▲ 1% low-fat milk, 2% reduced-fat milk, and whole milk; low-fat, reduced-fat, and whole-milk products such as cheeses, cottage cheese, and yogurt; milk products with added sugars such as chocolate milk, custard, ice cream, ice milk, milk shakes, pudding, sherbet; fortified soy milk.

MEAT, POULTRY, FISH, LEGUMES, EGGS, AND NUTS

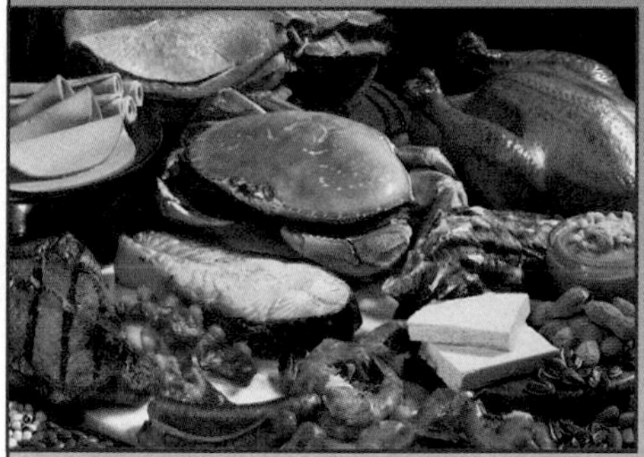

© Polara Studios, Inc.

Make lean or low-fat choices. Prepare them with little, or no, added fat.

Meat, poultry, fish, and eggs contribute protein, niacin, thiamin, vitamin B_6, vitamin B_{12}, iron, magnesium, potassium, and zinc; legumes and nuts are notable for their protein, folate, thiamin, vitamin E, iron, magnesium, potassium, zinc, and fiber.

1 oz meat is equivalent to 1 oz cooked lean meat, poultry, or fish; 1 egg; ¼ c cooked legumes or tofu; 1 tbs peanut butter; ½ oz nuts or seeds.

- ● Poultry (no skin), fish, shellfish, legumes, eggs, lean meat (fat-trimmed beef, game, ham, lamb, pork); low-fat tofu, tempeh, peanut butter, nuts or seeds.
- ▲ Bacon; baked beans; fried meat, fish, poultry, eggs, or tofu; refried beans; ground beef; hot dogs; luncheon meats; marbled steaks; poultry with skin; sausages; spare ribs.

OILS

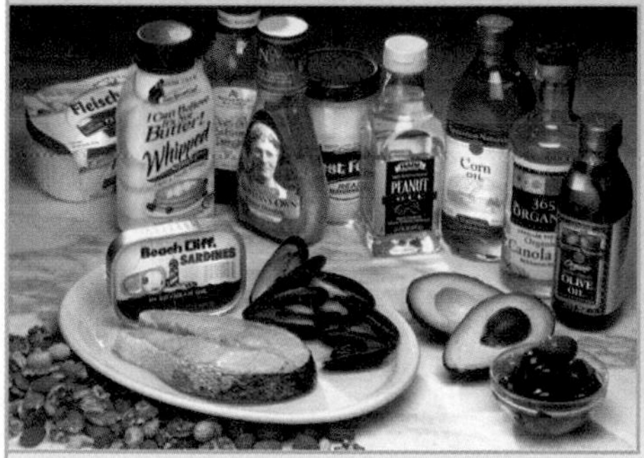

Matthew Farruggio

Select the recommended amounts of oils from among these sources.

These foods contribute vitamin E and essential fatty acids (see Chapter 5), along with abundant calories.

1 tsp oil is equivalent to 1 tbs low-fat mayonnaise; 2 tbs light salad dressing; 1 tsp vegetable oil; 1 tsp soft margarine.

- ● Liquid vegetable oils such as canola, corn, flaxseed, nut, olive, peanut, safflower, sesame, soybean, and sunflower oils; mayonnaise, oil-based salad dressing, soft *trans*-free margarine.
- ● Unsaturated oils that occur naturally in foods such as avocados, fatty fish, nuts, olives, and shellfish.

SOLID FATS AND ADDED SUGARS

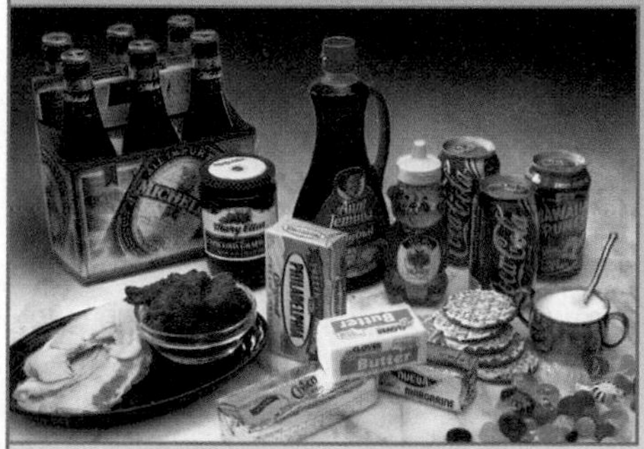

Matthew Farruggio

Limit intakes of food and beverages with solid fats and added sugars.

Solid fats deliver saturated fat and *trans* fat, and intake should be kept low. Solid fats and added sugars contribute abundant calories but few nutrients, and intakes should not exceed the discretionary calorie allowance—calories to meet energy needs after all nutrient needs have been met with nutrient-dense foods. Alcohol also contributes abundant calories but few nutrients, and its calories are counted among discretionary calories. See Table 2-3 for some discretionary calorie allowances; Table I-1 of Appendix I includes others.

- ▲ Solid fats that occur in foods naturally such as milk fat and meat fat (see ▲ in previous lists).
- ▲ Solid fats that are often added to foods such as butter, cream cheese, hard margarine, lard, sour cream, and shortening.
- ▲ Added sugars such as brown sugar, candy, honey, jelly, molasses, soft drinks, sugar, and syrup.
- ▲ Alcoholic beverages include beer, wine, and liquor.

TABLE 2-3 Recommended Daily Amounts from Each Food Group

	1600 kcal	1800 kcal	2000 kcal	2200 kcal	2400 kcal	2600 kcal	2800 kcal	3000 kcal
Fruits	1½ c	1½ c	2 c	2 c	2 c	2 c	2½ c	2½ c
Vegetables	2 c	2½ c	2½ c	3 c	3 c	3½ c	3½ c	4 c
Grains	5 oz	6 oz	6 oz	7 oz	8 oz	9 oz	10 oz	10 oz
Meat and legumes	5 oz	5 oz	5½ oz	6 oz	6½ oz	6½ oz	7 oz	7 oz
Milk	3 c	3 c	3 c	3 c	3 c	3 c	3 c	3 c
Oils	5 tsp	5 tsp	6 tsp	6 tsp	7 tsp	8 tsp	8 tsp	10 tsp
Discretionary kcalorie allowance	132 kcal	195 kcal	267 kcal	290 kcal	362 kcal	410 kcal	426 kcal	512 kcal

other words, consuming 2½ cups of potatoes or even spinach every day for seven days does *not* meet the recommended vegetable intakes. Potatoes and spinach make excellent choices when consumed in balance with other vegetables from other subgroups. Intakes of vegetables are appropriately averaged over a week's time—it is not necessary to include every subgroup every day.

HEALTHY PEOPLE 2010

Increase the proportion of persons aged 2 years and older who consume at least two daily servings of fruit; at least three daily servings of vegetables, with at least one-third being dark green or orange vegetables; and at least six daily servings of grain products, with at least three being whole grains.

Notable Nutrients As Figure 2-1 notes, each food group contributes key nutrients. This feature provides flexibility in diet planning: a person can select any food from a food group and receive similar nutrients. For example, a person can choose milk, cheese, or yogurt and receive the same key nutrients. Importantly, foods provide not only the nutrients for which each group is noted, but small amounts of other nutrients and phytochemicals as well.

The USDA Food Guide encourages greater consumption from certain food groups to provide the nutrients most often lacking■ in the diets of Americans. In general, most people need to eat:

- *More* dark green vegetables, orange vegetables, legumes, fruits, whole grains, and low-fat milk and milk products.
- *Less* refined grains, total fats (especially saturated fat, *trans* fat, and cholesterol), added sugars, and total kcalories.

■ The USDA nutrients of concern are fiber, vitamin A, vitamin C, vitamin E, and the minerals calcium, magnesium, and potassium.

Nutrient Density The USDA Food Guide provides a foundation for a healthy diet by emphasizing nutrient-dense options within each food group. By consistently selecting nutrient-dense foods, a person can both obtain all the nutrients needed and keep kcalories under control. In contrast, eating foods that are low in nutrient density makes it difficult to get enough nutrients without exceeding energy needs and gaining weight. For this reason, consumers should select low-fat foods from each group and foods without added fats or sugars—for example, fat-free milk instead of whole milk, baked chicken without the skin instead of hot dogs, green beans instead of french fries, orange juice instead of fruit punch, and whole-wheat bread instead of biscuits. Notice that Figure 2-1 provides a key indicating which foods *within each group* are high or low in nutrient density. Oil is a notable exception: even though oil is pure fat and therefore rich in kcalories, a small amount of oil from sources such as nuts, fish, or vegetable oils is necessary every day to provide nutrients lacking from other foods. Consequently these high-fat foods are listed among the nutrient-dense foods (see Highlight 5 to learn why).

Discretionary kCalorie Allowance At each kcalorie level, people who consistently choose nutrient-dense foods may be able to meet their nutrient needs with-

TABLE 2-4 Estimated Daily kCalorie Needs for Adults

	Sedentary[a]	Active[b]
Women		
19–30 yr	2000	2400
31–50 yr	1800	2200
51+ yr	1600	2100
Men		
19–30 yr	2400	3000
31–50 yr	2200	2900
51+ yr	2000	2600

[a] Sedentary describes a lifestyle that includes only the activities typical of day-to-day life.
[b] Active describes a lifestyle that includes physical activity equivalent to walking more than 3 miles per day at a rate of 3 to 4 miles per hour, in addition to the activities typical of day-to-day life. kCalorie values for active people reflect the midpoint of the range appropriate for age and gender, but within each group, older adults may need fewer kcalories and younger adults may need more.
NOTE: In addition to gender, age, and activity level, energy needs vary with height and weight (see Chapter 8 and Appendix F).

TABLE 2-5 Recommended Weekly Amounts from the Vegetable Subgroups

Table 2-3 specifies the recommended amounts of total vegetables per *day*. This table shows those amounts dispersed among five vegetable subgroups per *week*.

Vegetable Subgroups	1600 kcal	1800 kcal	2000 kcal	2200 kcal	2400 kcal	2600 kcal	2800 kcal	3000 kcal
Dark green	2 c	3 c	3 c	3 c	3 c	3 c	3 c	3 c
Orange and deep yellow	1½ c	2 c	2 c	2 c	2 c	2½ c	2½ c	2½ c
Legumes	2½ c	3 c	3 c	3 c	3 c	3½ c	3½ c	3½ c
Starchy	2½ c	3 c	3 c	6 c	6 c	7 c	7 c	9 c
Other	5½ c	6½ c	6½ c	7 c	7 c	8½ c	8½ c	10 c

out consuming their full allotment of kcalories. This difference between the kcalories needed to supply nutrients and those needed for energy—known as the **discretionary kcalorie allowance**—is illustrated in Figure 2-2.

Table 2-3 (on p. 46 top) includes the discretionary kcalorie allowance for several kcalorie levels. A person with discretionary kcalories available might choose to:

- Eat additional nutrient-dense foods, such as an extra serving of skinless chicken or a second ear of corn.
- Select a few foods with fats or added sugars, such as reduced-fat milk or sweetened cereal.
- Add a little fat or sugar to foods, such as butter or jelly on toast.
- Consume some alcohol. (Highlight 7 explains why this may not be a good choice for some individuals.)

Alternatively, a person wanting to lose weight might choose to:

- *Not* use the kcalories available from the discretionary kcalorie allowance.

Added fats and sugars are always counted as discretionary kcalories. The kcalories from the fat in higher-fat milks and meats are also counted among discretionary kcalories. It helps to think of fat-free milk as "milk" and whole milk or reduced-fat milk as "milk with added fat." Similarly, "meats" should be the leanest; other cuts are "meats with added fat." Puddings and other desserts made from whole milk provide discretionary kcalories from both the sugar added to sweeten them and the naturally occurring fat in the whole milk they contain. Even fruits, vegetables, and grains can carry discretionary kcalories into the diet in the form of peaches canned in syrup, scalloped potatoes, or high-fat crackers.

Discretionary kcalories must be counted separately from the kcalories of the nutrient-dense foods of which they may be a part. A fried chicken leg, for example, provides discretionary kcalories from two sources: the naturally occurring fat of the chicken skin and the added fat absorbed during frying. The kcalories of the skinless chicken underneath are not discretionary kcalories—they are necessary to provide the nutrients of chicken.

Serving Equivalents Recommended amounts for fruits, vegetables, and milk are given in cups and those for grains and meats, in ounces. Figure 2-1 provides equivalent measures among the foods in each group specifying, for example, that 1 ounce of grains is equivalent to 1 slice of bread or ½ cup of cooked rice.

A person using the USDA Food Guide can become more familiar with measured portions by determining the answers to questions such as these:■ What portion of a cup is a small handful of raisins? Is a "helping" of mashed potatoes more or less than a half-cup? How many ounces of cereal do you typically pour into the bowl? How many ounces is the steak at your favorite restaurant? How many cups of milk does your glass hold? Figure 2-1 (on pp. 44–45) includes the serving sizes and equivalent amounts for foods within each group.

FIGURE 2-2 Discretionary kCalorie Allowance for a 2000-kCalorie Diet Plan

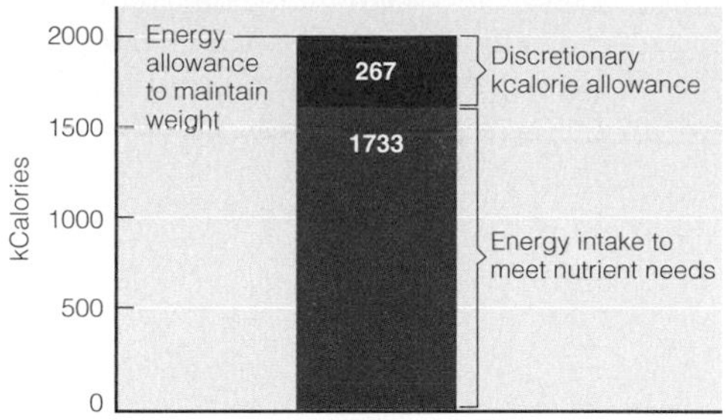
2000
1500
1000
500
0
kCalories
Energy allowance to maintain weight
267
1733
Discretionary kcalorie allowance
Energy intake to meet nutrient needs

■ For quick and easy estimates, visualize each portion as being about the size of a common object:
- 1 c fruit or vegetables = a baseball.
- ¼ c dried fruit = a golf ball.
- 3 oz meat = a deck of cards.
- 2 tbs peanut butter = a marshmallow.
- 1½ oz cheese = 6 stacked dice.
- ½ c ice cream = a racquetball.
- 4 small cookies = 4 poker chips.

discretionary kcalorie allowance: the kcalories remaining in a person's energy allowance after consuming enough nutrient-dense foods to meet all nutrient needs for a day.

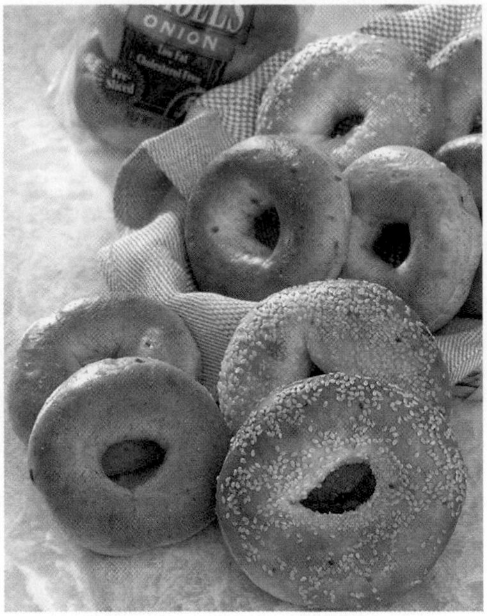
ONION

© Matthew Farruggio

Most bagels today weigh in at 4 ounces or more—meaning that a person eating one of these large bagels for breakfast is actually getting four or more grain servings, not one.

Mixtures of Foods Some foods—such as casseroles, soups, and sandwiches—fall into two or more food groups. With a little practice, users can begin to divide these foods into food groups. From the USDA Food Guide point of view, a taco represents four different food groups: the taco shell from the grains group; the onions, lettuce, and tomatoes from the "other vegetables" group; the ground beef from the meat group; and the cheese from the milk group.

Vegetarian Food Guide Vegetarian diets rely mainly on plant foods: grains, vegetables, legumes, fruits, seeds, and nuts. Some vegetarian diets include eggs, milk products, or both. People who do not eat meats or milk products can still use the USDA Food Guide to create an adequate diet.[2] The food groups are similar, and the amounts of foods remain the same. Vegetarians select *meat alternates* from the meat group—foods such as legumes, seeds, nuts, tofu, and, for those who eat them, eggs. Legumes and at least one cup of dark green leafy vegetables help to supply the iron that meats usually provide. Vegetarians who do not drink cow's milk can use soy "milk"—a product made from soybeans that provides similar nutrients if it has been fortified with calcium, vitamin D, and vitamin B_{12}. Highlight 6 presents a Food Guide for Vegetarians, defines vegetarian terms, and provides more information on vegetarian diet planning.

Ethnic Food Choices People can use the USDA Food Guide and still enjoy a diverse array of culinary styles by sorting ethnic foods into their appropriate food groups. For example, a person eating Mexican foods would find tortillas in the grains group, jicama in the vegetable group, and guava in the fruit group. Table 2-6 features ethnic food choices, and Highlight 2 presents food guides from selected countries.

MyPyramid—Steps to a Healthier You The USDA created an educational tool called MyPyramid to illustrate the concepts presented in the *Dietary Guidelines* and USDA Food Guide. Figure 2-3 presents a graphic image of MyPyramid, which was de-

TABLE 2-6 Ethnic Food Choices

	Grains	Vegetables	Fruits	Meats and Alternates	Milk
Asian 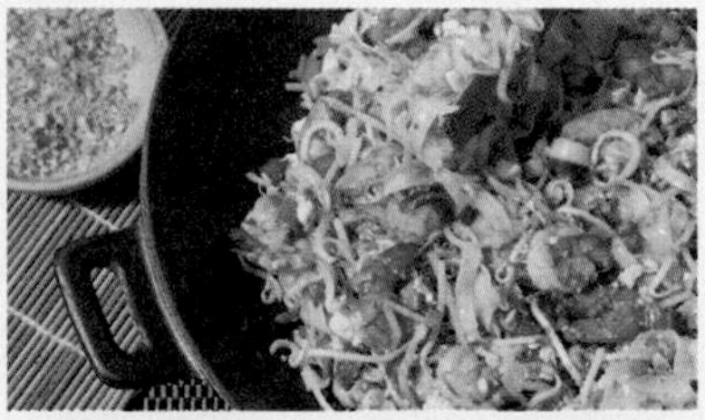 © Becky Luigart-Stayner/Corbis	Rice, noodles, millet	Amaranth, baby corn, bamboo shoots, chayote, bok choy, mung bean sprouts, sugar peas, straw mushrooms, water chestnuts, kelp	Carambola, guava, kumquat, lychee, persimmon, melons, mandarin orange	Soybeans, squid, tofu, duck eggs, pork, poultry, fish and other seafood, peanuts, cashews	Soy milk
Mediterranean 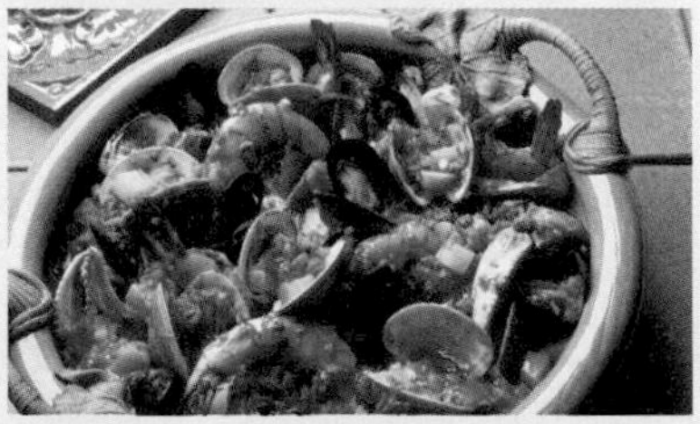 © PhotoDisc Inc.	Pita pocket bread, pastas, rice, couscous, polenta, bulgur, focaccia, Italian bread	Eggplant, tomatoes, peppers, cucumbers, grape leaves	Olives, grapes, figs	Fish and other seafood, gyros, lamb, chicken, beef, pork, sausage, lentils, fava beans	Ricotta, provolone, parmesan, feta, mozzarella, and goat cheeses; yogurt
Mexican 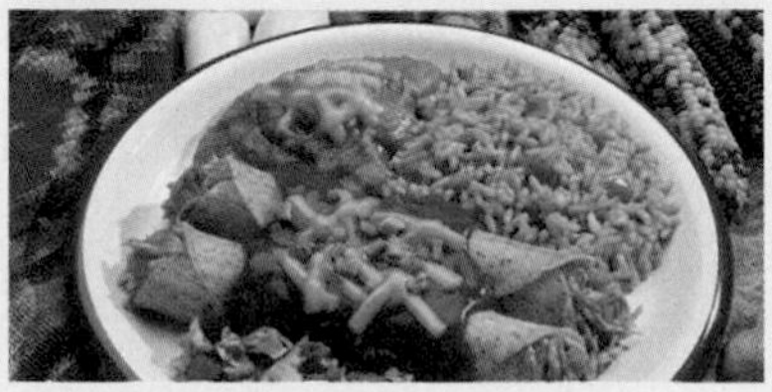 © PhotoDisc Inc.	Tortillas (corn or flour), taco shells, rice	Chayote, corn, jicama, tomato salsa, cactus, cassava, tomatoes, yams, chilies	Guava, mango, papaya, avocado, plantain, bananas, oranges	Refried beans, fish, chicken, chorizo, beef, eggs	Cheese, custard

FIGURE 2-3 MyPyramid

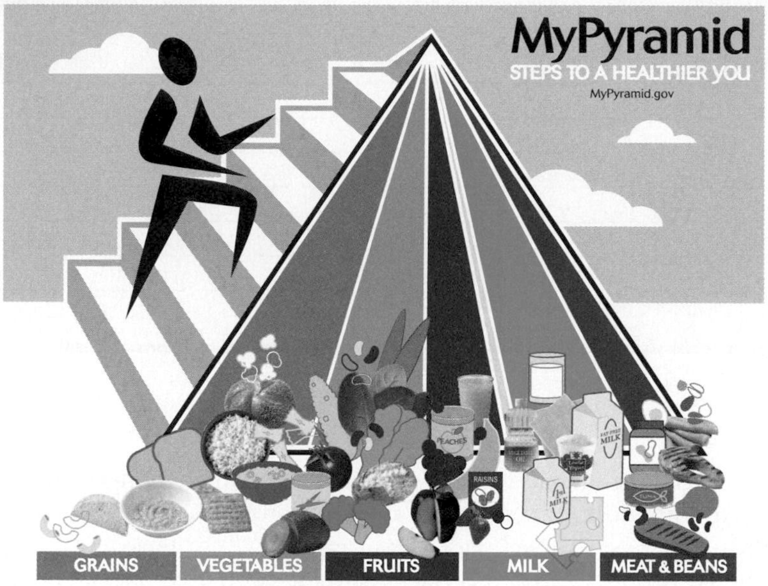
MyPyramid
STEPS TO A HEALTHIER YOU
MyPyramid.gov
GRAINS
VEGETABLES
FRUITS
MILK
MEAT & BEANS

FIGURE 2-4 Healthy Eating Index Components

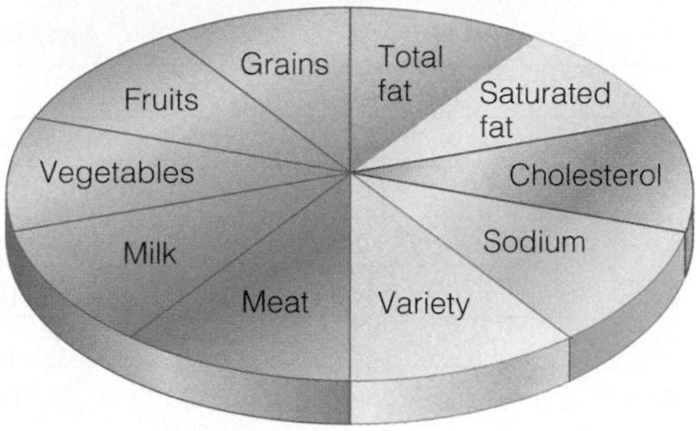
Grains
Total fat
Fruits
Saturated fat
Vegetables
Cholesterol
Milk
Sodium
Meat
Variety

signed to encourage consumers to make healthy food and physical activity choices every day. A person climbing steps reminds consumers to be physically active each day. The multiple colors of the pyramid illustrate variety, with each color representing one of the five food groups, plus one for oils. The different widths of the colors suggest the proportion each food group contributes to a healthy diet. The wideness of orange, green, red, and blue emphasizes the dietary guideline to encourage foods from the grain, vegetable, fruit, and milk groups, respectively. The colors also gradually narrow from the bottom to the top, suggesting moderation. The wide bottom indicates that nutrient-dense foods should be selected often and the narrow top implies that those with solid fats and added sugars should be limited.

An abundance of material supporting MyPyramid is available to consumers who want to find the kinds and amounts of foods to eat each day (**MyPyramid.gov**). In addition to creating a personal plan, consumers can find tips to help them improve their diet and lifestyle by taking small steps each day.

Healthy Eating Index How can a person know whether his or her diet is doing its share to support good health? To measure how well a diet meets the recommendations of the *Dietary Guidelines* and the USDA Food Guide, the USDA developed the **Healthy Eating Index.** Meeting the recommendations of the *Dietary Guidelines* for total fat, saturated fat, cholesterol, sodium, and variety can each provide up to 10 points as can sufficient selections from each of the five food groups of the USDA Food Guide—for a possible total of 100 points. Figure 2-4 shows how these dietary components contribute to the overall score.

Exchange Lists

Food group plans are particularly well suited to help a person achieve dietary adequacy, balance, and variety. **Exchange lists** provide additional help in achieving kcalorie control and moderation. Originally developed for people with diabetes, exchange systems have proved useful for general diet planning as well.

Unlike the USDA Food Guide, which sorts foods primarily by their vitamin and mineral contents, the exchange system sorts foods according to their energy-nutrient contents. Consequently, foods do not always appear on the exchange list where you might first expect to find them. For example, cheeses are grouped with meats because, like meats, cheeses contribute energy from protein and fat but

Healthy Eating Index: a measure developed by the USDA for assessing how well a diet conforms to the recommendations of the USDA Food Guide and the *Dietary Guidelines for Americans.*

exchange lists: diet-planning tools that organize foods by their proportions of carbohydrate, fat, and protein. Foods on any single list can be used interchangeably.

TABLE 2-7 Diet Planning Using the USDA Food Guide

This diet plan is one of many possibilities. It follows the amounts of foods suggested for a 2000-kcalorie diet as shown in Table 2-3 on p. 46 (with an extra ½ cup of vegetables).

Food Group	Amounts	Breakfast	Lunch	Snack	Dinner	Snack
Fruits	2 c	½ c		½ c	1 c	
Vegetables	2½ c		1 c		2 c	
Grains	6 oz	1 oz	2 oz	½ oz	2 oz	½ oz
Meat and legumes	5½ oz		2 oz		3½ oz	
Milk	3 c	1 c		1 c		1 c
Oils	5½ tsp		1½ tsp		4 tsp	
Discretionary kcalorie allowance	267 kcal					

provide negligible carbohydrate. (In the food group plan presented earlier, cheeses are classed with milk because they are milk products with similar calcium contents.)

For similar reasons, starchy vegetables such as corn, green peas, and potatoes are listed with grains on the starch list in the exchange system, rather than with the vegetables. Likewise, olives are not classed as a "fruit" as a botanist would claim; they are classified as a "fat" because their fat content makes them more similar to butter than to berries. Bacon and nuts are also on the fat list to remind users of their high fat content. These groupings highlight the characteristics of foods that are significant to energy intake. To learn more about this useful diet-planning tool, study Appendix G, which gives complete details of the major exchange system used in the United States, and Appendix I, which provides details of the choice system used in Canada.

Putting the Plan into Action

Table 2-7 shows how to use the USDA Food Guide to plan a diet. The USDA Food Guide ensures that a certain amount is chosen from each of the five food groups (see the second column of the table). The next step in diet planning is to assign the food groups to meals (and snacks), as in the remaining columns of Table 2-7.

Next, a person could begin to fill in the plan with real foods to create a menu. For example, the breakfast calls for 1 ounce grain, ½ cup fruit, and 1 cup milk. A person might select a bowl of cereal with banana slices and milk:

1 cup cereal = 1 ounce grain.
1 small banana = ½ cup fruit.
1 cup fat-free milk = 1 cup milk.

Or ½ bagel and a bowl of cantaloupe pieces topped with yogurt:

½ small bagel = 1 ounce grain.
½ cup melon pieces = ½ cup fruit.
1 cup fat-free plain yogurt = 1 cup milk.

Then the person could move on to complete the menus for lunch, dinner, and snacks. The final plan might look like the one in Figure 2-5. With the addition of a small amount of oils, this sample diet plan provides about 1850 kcalories and adequate amounts of the essential nutrients.

As you can see, we all make countless food-related decisions daily—whether we have a plan or not. Following a plan, like the USDA Food Guide, that incorporates health recommendations and diet-planning principles helps a person to make wise decisions.

FIGURE 2-5 A Sample Diet Plan and Menu

This sample menu provides about 1850 kcalories and meets dietary recommendations to provide 45 to 65 percent of its kcalories from carbohydrate, 20 to 35 percent from fat, and 10 to 35 percent from protein. Some discretionary kcalories were spent on the fat in the low-fat cheese and in the sugar added to the graham crackers; about 150 discretionary kcalories remain available in this 2000-kcalorie diet plan.

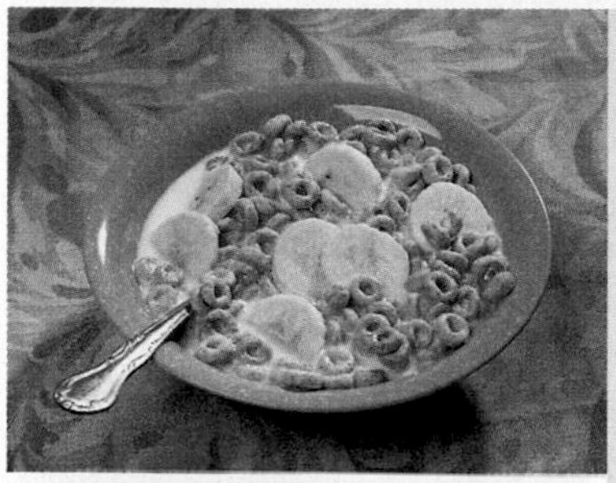
© Polara Studios, Inc.

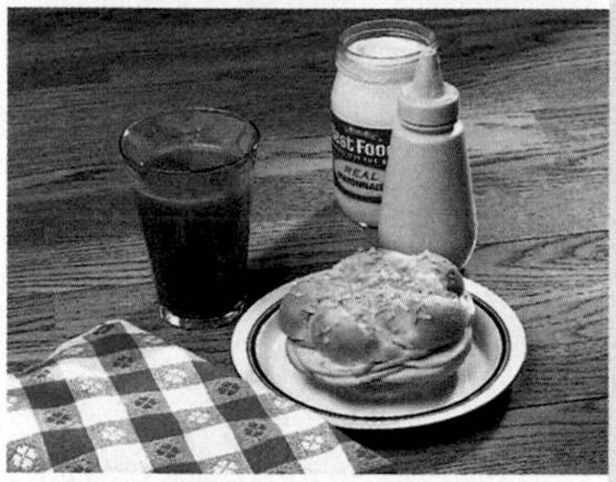
© Polara Studios, Inc.

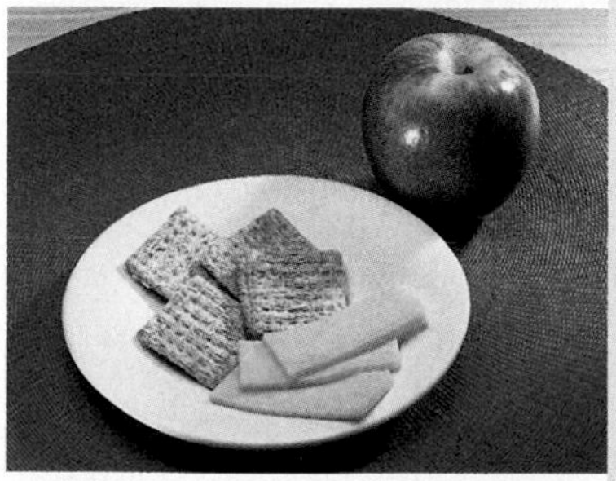
© Quest

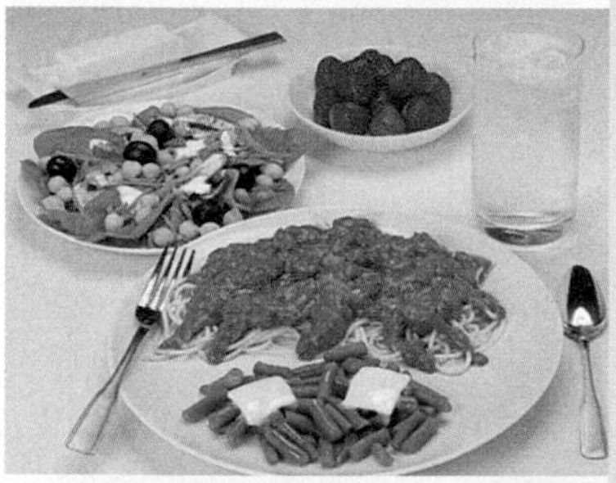
© Quest

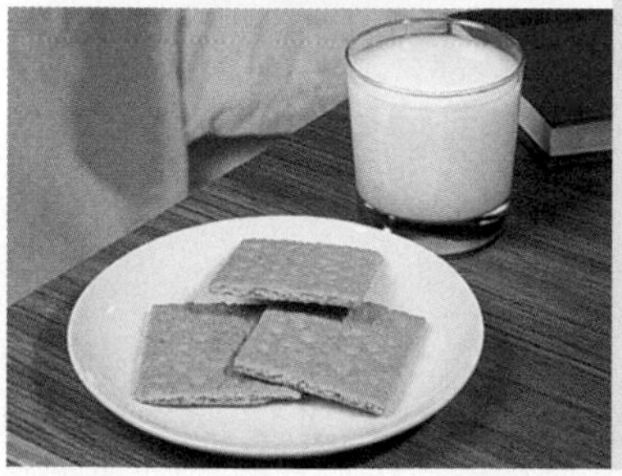
© Polara Studios, Inc.

Amounts	SAMPLE MENU	Energy (kcal)
	Breakfast	
1 oz whole grains	1 c whole-grain cereal	108
1 c milk	1 c fat-free milk	83
1/2 c fruit	1 medium banana (sliced)	105
	Lunch	
2 oz whole grains, 2 oz meats	1 turkey sandwich on roll	272
1 1/2 tsp oils	1 1/2 tbs low-fat mayonnaise	75
1 c vegetables	1 c vegetable juice	53
	Snack	
1/2 oz whole grains	4 whole-wheat, reduced-fat crackers	86
1 c milk	1 1/2 oz low-fat cheddar cheese	74
1/2 c fruit	1 medium apple	72
	Dinner	
1/2 c vegetables	1 c raw spinach leaves	8
1/4 c vegetables	1/4 c shredded carrots	11
1 oz meats	1/4 c garbanzo beans	71
2 tsp oils	2 tbs oil-based salad dressing and olives	81
3/4 c vegetables, 2 1/2 oz meats, 2 oz enriched grains	Spaghetti with meat sauce	425
1/2 c vegetables	1/2 c green beans	22
2 tsp oils	2 tsp soft margarine	67
1 c fruit	1 c strawberries	49
	Snack	
1/2 oz whole grains	3 graham crackers	90
1 c milk	1 c fat-free milk	83

From Guidelines to Groceries

Dietary recommendations emphasize nutrient-rich foods such as whole grains, fruits, vegetables, lean meats, fish, poultry, and low-fat milk products. You can design such a diet for yourself, but how do you begin? Start with the foods you enjoy eating. Then try to make improvements, little by little. When shopping, think of the food groups, and choose nutrient-dense foods within each group.

Be aware that many of the 50,000 food options available today are **processed foods** that have lost valuable nutrients and gained sugar, fat, and salt as they were transformed from farm-fresh foods to those found in the bags, boxes, and cans that line grocery-store shelves. Their value in the diet depends on the starting food and the type of processing. Sometimes these foods have been **fortified** to improve their nutrient contents.

Grains When shopping for grain products, you will find them described as *refined, enriched,* or *whole grain.* These terms refer to the milling process and the making of grain products, and they have different nutrition implications (see Figure 2-6). **Refined** foods may have lost many nutrients during processing; **enriched** products may have had some nutrients added back; and **whole-grain** products may be rich in fiber and all the nutrients found in the original grain. As such, whole-grain products support good health and should account for at least half of the grains daily.

When it became a common practice to refine the wheat flour used for bread by milling it and removing the bran and the germ, consumers suffered a tragic loss of many nutrients.[3] As a consequence, in the early 1940s Congress passed legislation

processed foods: foods that have been treated to change their physical, chemical, microbiological, or sensory properties.

fortified: the addition to a food of nutrients that were either not originally present or present in insignificant amounts. Fortification can be used to correct or prevent a widespread nutrient deficiency or to balance the total nutrient profile of a food.

refined: the process by which the coarse parts of a food are removed. When wheat is refined into flour, the bran, germ, and husk are removed, leaving only the endosperm.

enriched: the addition to a food of nutrients that were lost during processing so that the food will meet a specified standard.

whole grain: a grain milled in its entirety (all but the husk), not refined.

FIGURE 2-6 A Wheat Plant

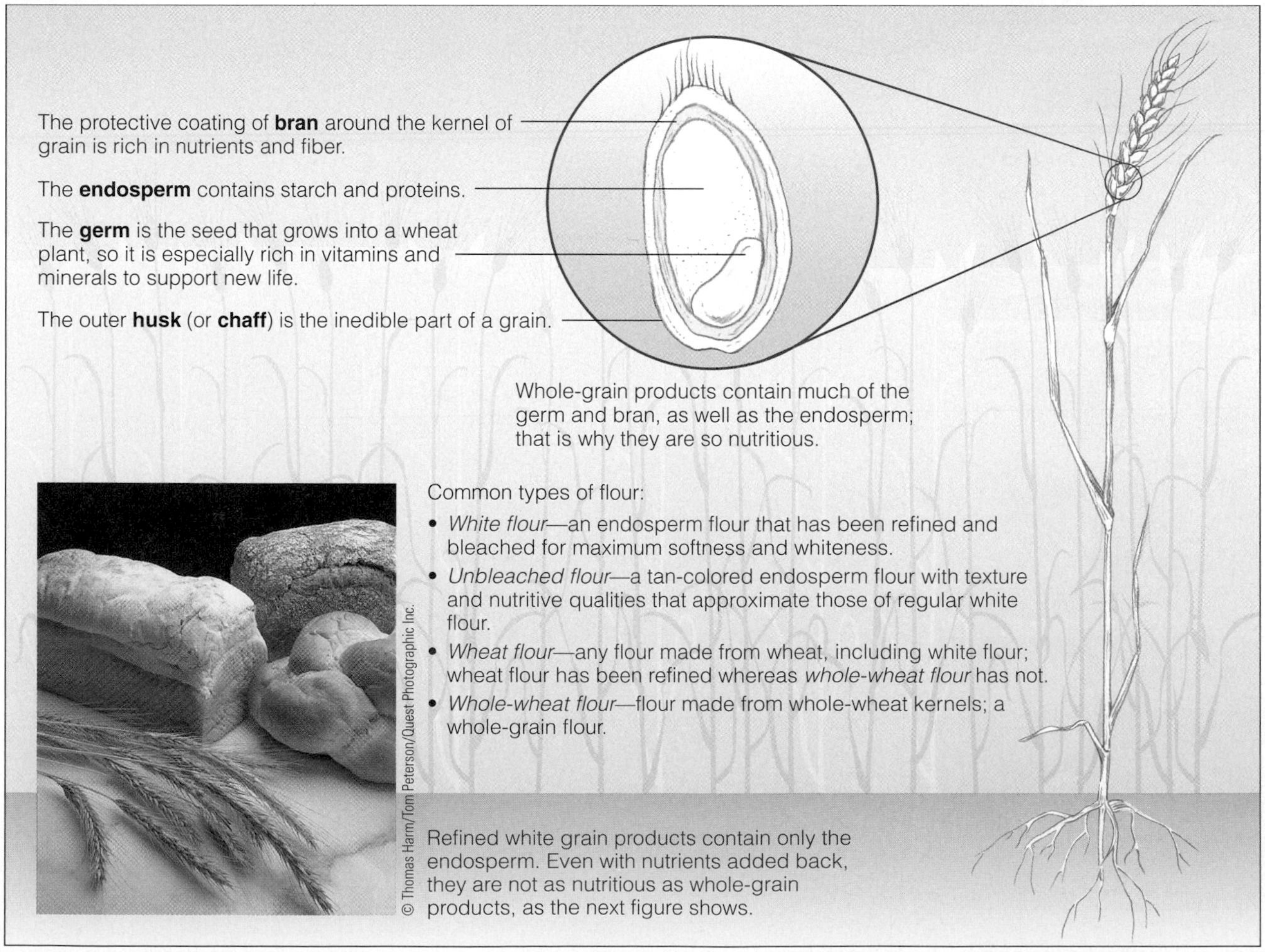
The protective coating of **bran** around the kernel of grain is rich in nutrients and fiber.
The **endosperm** contains starch and proteins.
The **germ** is the seed that grows into a wheat plant, so it is especially rich in vitamins and minerals to support new life.
The outer **husk** (or **chaff**) is the inedible part of a grain.
Whole-grain products contain much of the germ and bran, as well as the endosperm; that is why they are so nutritious.
Common types of flour:
• *White flour*—an endosperm flour that has been refined and bleached for maximum softness and whiteness.
• *Unbleached flour*—a tan-colored endosperm flour with texture and nutritive qualities that approximate those of regular white flour.
• *Wheat flour*—any flour made from wheat, including white flour; wheat flour has been refined whereas *whole-wheat flour* has not.
• *Whole-wheat flour*—flour made from whole-wheat kernels; a whole-grain flour.
Refined white grain products contain only the endosperm. Even with nutrients added back, they are not as nutritious as whole-grain products, as the next figure shows.
© Thomas Harm/Tom Peterson/Quest Photographic Inc.

requiring that all grain products that cross state lines be enriched with iron, thiamin, riboflavin, and niacin. In 1996, this legislation was amended to include folate, a vitamin considered essential in the prevention of some birth defects. Most grain products that have been refined, such as rice, wheat pastas like macaroni and spaghetti, and cereals (both cooked and ready-to-eat types), have subsequently been enriched,■ and their labels say so.

Enrichment doesn't make a slice of bread rich in these added nutrients, but people who eat several slices a day obtain significantly more of these nutrients than they would from unenriched white bread. To a great extent, the enrichment of white flour helps to prevent deficiencies of these nutrients, but it fails to compensate for losses of many other nutrients and fiber. As Figure 2-7 shows, whole-grain items still outshine the enriched ones. Only *whole-grain* flour contains all of the nutritive portions of the grain. Whole-grain products, such as brown rice or oatmeal, not only provide more nutrients and fiber, but often do not contain the added salt and sugar of flavored, processed rice or sweetened cereals.

Speaking of cereals, ready-to-eat breakfast cereals are the most highly fortified foods on the market. Like an enriched food, a *fortified* food has had nutrients added during processing, but in a fortified food, the added nutrients may not have been present in the original product. (The terms *fortified* and *enriched* may be used interchangeably.)[4] Some breakfast cereals made from refined flour and fortified with high doses of vitamins and minerals are actually more like supplements disguised as cereals than they are like whole grains. They may be nutritious—with respect to the nutrients added—but they still may fail to convey the full spectrum of nutrients that a whole-grain food or a mixture of such foods might provide. Still, fortified foods help people meet their vitamin and mineral needs.[5]

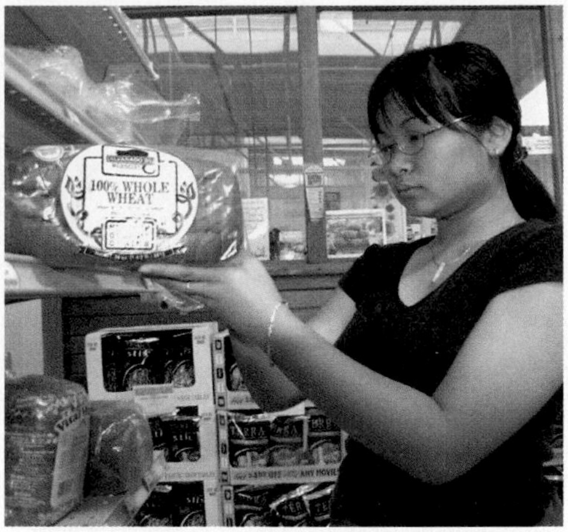
100% WHOLE WHEAT

© Geri Engberg Photography

When shopping for bread, look for the descriptive words *whole grain* or *whole wheat* and check the fiber contents on the Nutrition Facts panel of the label—the more fiber, the more likely the bread is a whole-grain product.

■ Grain enrichment nutrients:
- Iron.
- Thiamin.
- Riboflavin.
- Niacin.
- Folate.

FIGURE 2-7 Nutrients in Bread

Whole-grain bread is more nutritious than other breads, even enriched bread. For iron, thiamin, riboflavin, niacin, and folate, enriched bread provides about the same quantities as whole-grain bread and significantly more than unenriched bread. For fiber and the other nutrients (both those shown here and those not shown), enriched bread provides less than whole-grain bread.

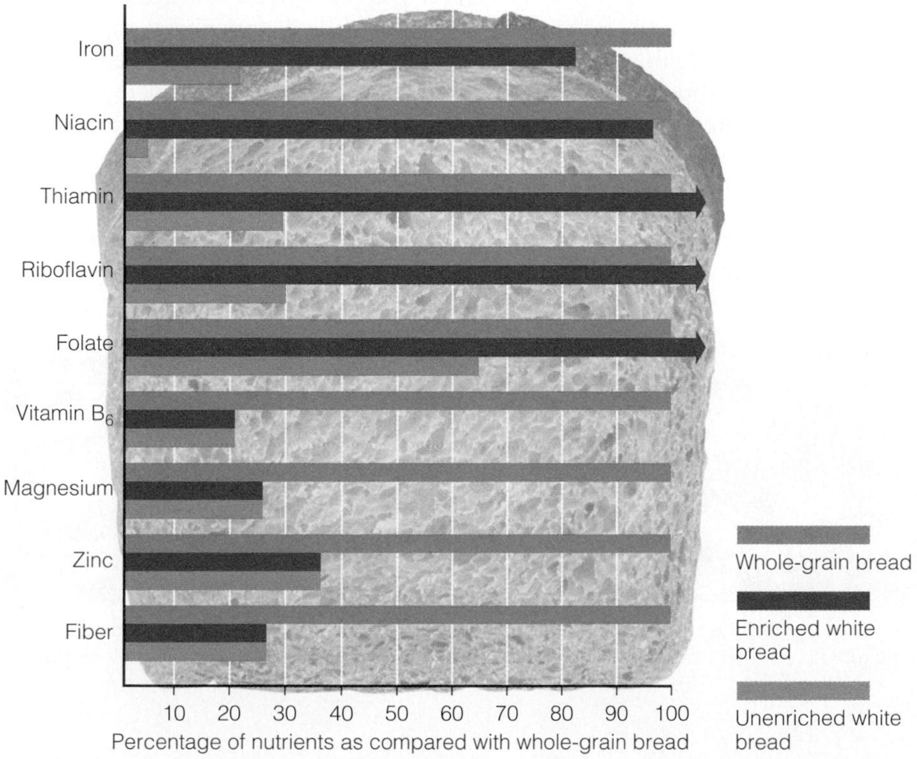
Iron
Niacin
Thiamin
Riboflavin
Folate
Vitamin B_6
Magnesium
Zinc
Fiber
10 20 30 40 50 60 70 80 90 100
Percentage of nutrients as compared with whole-grain bread
Whole-grain bread
Enriched white bread
Unenriched white bread

FIGURE 2-8 Eat 5 to 9 a Day for Better Health

The "5 to 9 a Day" campaign (**www.5aday.gov**) encourages consumers to eat a variety of fruits and vegetables by selecting a serving or two from each of five colors.

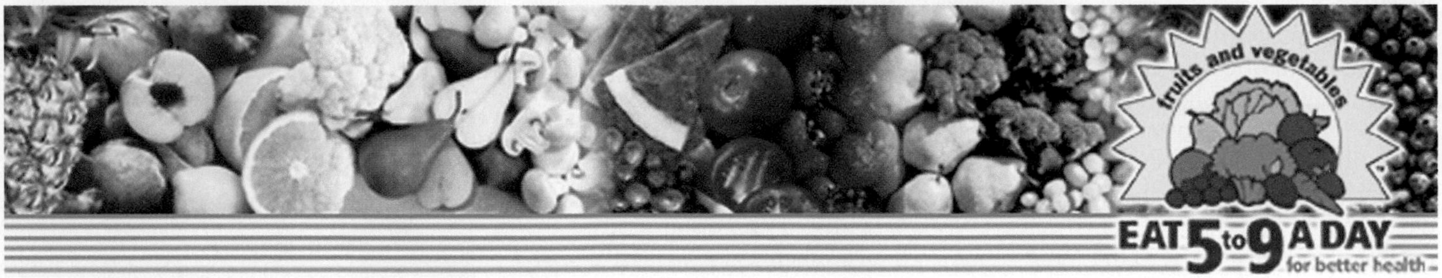
fruits and vegetables
EAT 5 to 9 A DAY
for better health

Vegetables Posters in the produce section of grocery stores encourage consumers to "eat 5 a day." Such efforts are part of a national educational campaign to increase fruit and vegetable consumption to 5 to 9 servings every day (see Figure 2-8). To help consumers remember to eat a variety of fruits and vegetables, the campaign provides practical tips, such as selecting from each of five colors.

Choose fresh vegetables often, especially dark green leafy and yellow-orange vegetables like spinach, broccoli, and sweet potatoes. Cooked or raw, vegetables are good sources of vitamins, minerals, and fiber. Frozen and canned vegetables without added salt are acceptable alternatives to fresh. To control fat, energy, and sodium intakes, limit butter and salt on vegetables.

■ Legumes include a variety of beans and peas:
- Black beans.
- Black-eyed peas.
- Garbanzo beans.
- Great northern beans.
- Kidney beans.
- Lentils.
- Navy beans.
- Peanuts.
- Pinto beans.
- Soybeans.
- Split peas.

Legumes Choose often from the variety of legumes available.■ They are an economical, low-fat, nutrient- and fiber-rich food choice.

Fruit Choose fresh fruits often, especially citrus fruits and yellow-orange fruits like cantaloupes and peaches. Frozen, dried, and canned fruits without added sugar are acceptable alternatives to fresh. Fruits supply valuable vitamins, minerals, fibers, and phytochemicals. They add flavors, colors, and textures to meals, and their natural sweetness makes them enjoyable as snacks or desserts.

Fruit juices are healthy beverages, but contain little dietary fiber compared with whole fruits. Whole fruits satisfy the appetite better than juices, thereby helping people to limit food energy intakes. For people who need extra food energy, though, juices are a good choice. Be aware that sweetened fruit "drinks" or "ades" contain mostly water, sugar, and a little juice for flavor. Some may have been fortified with vitamin C, but lack any other significant nutritional value.

Meat, Fish, and Poultry Meat, fish, and poultry provide essential minerals, such as iron and zinc, and abundant B vitamins as well as protein. To buy and

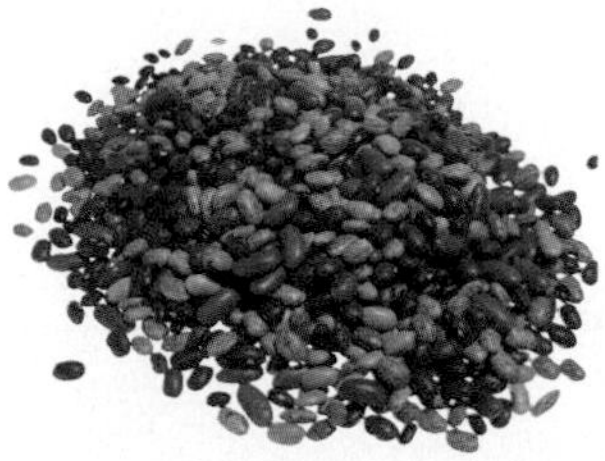

Combining legumes with foods from other food groups creates delicious meals.

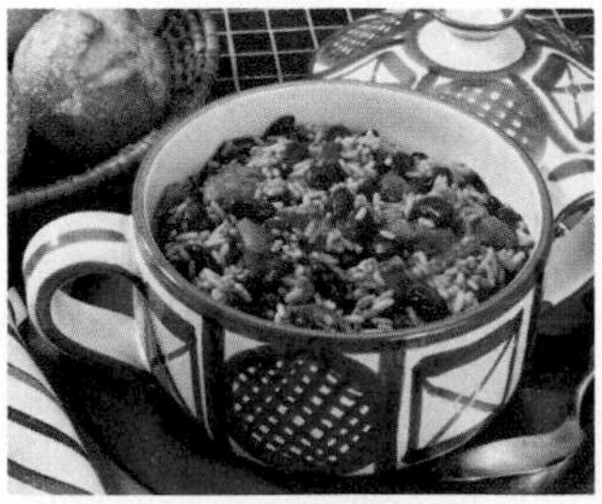

© 1998 Photo Disc Inc.

Add rice to red beans for a hearty meal.

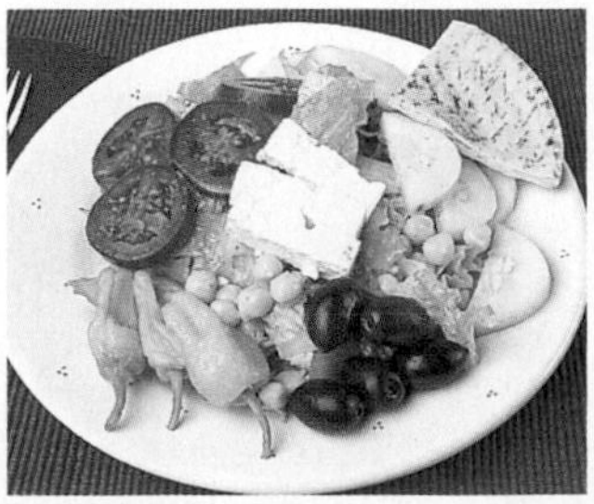

© 1998 Photo Disc Inc.

Enjoy a Greek salad topped with garbanzo beans for a little ethnic diversity.

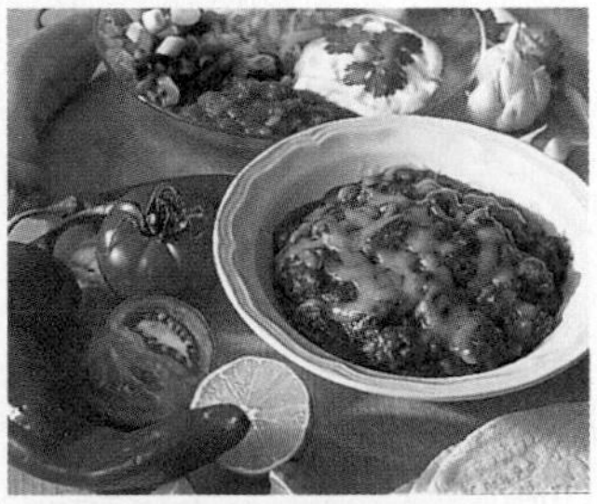

© Felicia Martinez/PhotoEdit

A bit of meat and lots of spices turn kidney beans into chili con carne.

© Michael Newman/PhotoEdit

prepare these foods without excess energy, fat, and sodium takes a little knowledge and planning. When shopping in the meat department, choose fish, poultry, and lean cuts of beef and pork named "round" or "loin" (as in top round or pork tenderloin). As a guide, "prime" and "choice" cuts generally have more fat than "select" cuts. Restaurants usually serve prime cuts. Ground beef, even "lean" ground beef, derives most of its food energy from fat. Have the butcher trim and grind a lean round steak instead. Alternatively, **textured vegetable protein** can be used instead of ground beef in a casserole, spaghetti sauce, or chili, saving fat kcalories.

Weigh meat after it is cooked and the bones and fat are removed. In general, 4 ounces of raw meat is equal to about 3 ounces of cooked meat. Some examples of 3-ounce portions of meat include 1 medium pork chop, ½ chicken breast, or 1 steak or hamburger about the size of a deck of cards. To keep fat intake moderate, bake, roast, broil, grill, or braise meats (but do not fry them in fat); remove the skin from poultry after cooking; trim visible fat before cooking; and drain fat after cooking. Chapter 5 offers many additional strategies for moderating fat intake.

Milk Shoppers will find a variety of fortified foods in the dairy case. Examples are milk, to which vitamins A and D have been added, and soy milk,■ to which calcium, vitamin D, and vitamin B_{12} have been added. In addition, shoppers may find **imitation foods** (such as cheese products), **food substitutes** (such as egg substitutes), and functional foods■ (such as margarine with plant sterols added). As food technology advances, many such foods offer alternatives to traditional choices that may help people who want to reduce their fat and cholesterol intakes. Chapter 5 gives other examples.

When shopping, choose fat-free■ or low-fat milk, yogurt, and cheeses. Such selections help consumers obtain adequate nutrients within energy needs. Milk products are important sources of calcium, but can provide too much sodium and fat if not selected with care.

■ Be aware that not all soy milks have been fortified. Read labels carefully.

■ Reminder: *Functional foods* contain physiologically active compounds that provide health benefits beyond basic nutrition.

■
- **Fat-free** milk may also be called **nonfat, skim, zero-fat,** or **no-fat.**
- **Low-fat** milk refers to 1% milk.
- **Reduced-fat** milk refers to 2% milk; it may also be called **less-fat.**

IN SUMMARY Food group plans select from different families of similar foods to provide adequacy, balance, and variety in the diet. They make it easier to plan a diet that includes abundant grains, vegetables, legumes, and fruits and moderate amounts of meats and milk products. In making any food choice, remember to view the food in the context of your total diet. It is the combination of many different foods that provides the abundance of nutrients so essential to a healthy diet.

Food Labels

Many consumers read food labels to help them select foods with less saturated fat, *trans* fat, cholesterol, and sodium and more vitamins, minerals, and dietary fiber. Food labels appear on virtually all processed foods, and posters or brochures provide similar nutrition information for fresh meats, fruits, and vegetables (see Figure 2-9). A few foods need not carry nutrition labels: those contributing few nutrients, such as plain coffee, tea, and spices; those produced by small businesses; and those prepared and sold in the same establishment. Producers of some of these items, however, voluntarily use labels. Even markets selling nonpackaged items voluntarily present nutrient information, either in brochures or on signs posted at the point of purchase. Restaurants need not supply complete nutrition information for menu items unless claims such as "low fat" or "heart healthy" have been made. When ordering such items, keep in mind that restaurants tend to serve extra-large portions—two to three times standard serving sizes. A "low-fat" ice cream, for example, may have only 3 grams of fat per ½ cup, but you may be served 2 cups for a total of 12 grams of fat and all their accompanying kcalories.

textured vegetable protein: processed soybean protein used in vegetarian products such as soy burgers.

imitation foods: foods that substitute for and resemble another food, but are nutritionally inferior to it with respect to vitamin, mineral, or protein content. If the substitute is not inferior to the food it resembles and if its name provides an accurate description of the product, it need not be labeled "imitation."

food substitutes: foods that are designed to replace other foods.

FIGURE 2-9 Example of a Food Label

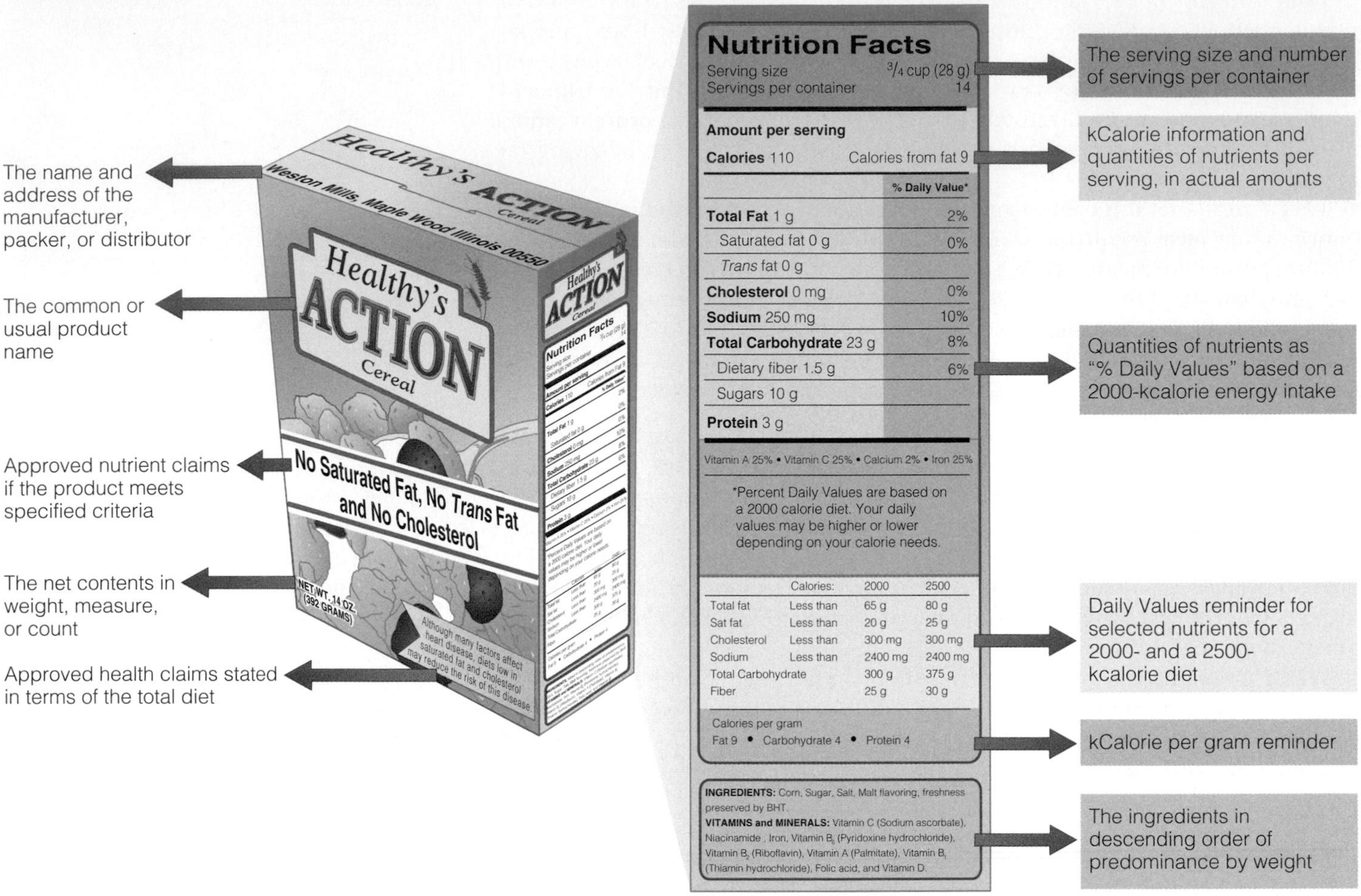
The name and address of the manufacturer, packer, or distributor
The common or usual product name
Approved nutrient claims if the product meets specified criteria
The net contents in weight, measure, or count
Approved health claims stated in terms of the total diet
Healthy's ACTION Cereal
Weston Mills, Maple Wood Illinois 00550
No Saturated Fat, No Trans Fat and No Cholesterol
NET WT. 14 OZ. (392 GRAMS)
Although many factors affect heart disease, diets low in saturated fat and cholesterol may reduce the risk of this disease.
Nutrition Facts
Serving size 3/4 cup (28 g)
Servings per container 14
Amount per serving
Calories 110 Calories from fat 9
% Daily Value*
Total Fat 1 g 2%
Saturated fat 0 g 0%
Trans fat 0 g
Cholesterol 0 mg 0%
Sodium 250 mg 10%
Total Carbohydrate 23 g 8%
Dietary fiber 1.5 g 6%
Sugars 10 g
Protein 3 g
Vitamin A 25% • Vitamin C 25% • Calcium 2% • Iron 25%
*Percent Daily Values are based on a 2000 calorie diet. Your daily values may be higher or lower depending on your calorie needs.
Calories: 2000 2500
Total fat Less than 65 g 80 g
Sat fat Less than 20 g 25 g
Cholesterol Less than 300 mg 300 mg
Sodium Less than 2400 mg 2400 mg
Total Carbohydrate 300 g 375 g
Fiber 25 g 30 g
Calories per gram
Fat 9 • Carbohydrate 4 • Protein 4
INGREDIENTS: Corn, Sugar, Salt, Malt flavoring, freshness preserved by BHT.
VITAMINS and MINERALS: Vitamin C (Sodium ascorbate), Niacinamide, Iron, Vitamin B6 (Pyridoxine hydrochloride), Vitamin B2 (Riboflavin), Vitamin A (Palmitate), Vitamin B1 (Thiamin hydrochloride), Folic acid, and Vitamin D.
The serving size and number of servings per container
kCalorie information and quantities of nutrients per serving, in actual amounts
Quantities of nutrients as "% Daily Values" based on a 2000-kcalorie energy intake
Daily Values reminder for selected nutrients for a 2000- and a 2500-kcalorie diet
kCalorie per gram reminder
The ingredients in descending order of predominance by weight

The Ingredient List

All packaged foods must list all ingredients on the label in descending order of predominance by weight. Knowing that the first ingredient predominates by weight, consumers can glean much information. Compare these products, for example:

- A beverage powder that contains "sugar, citric acid, natural flavors . . ." versus a juice that contains "water, tomato concentrate, concentrated juices of carrots, celery. . . ."
- A cereal that contains "puffed milled corn, sugar, corn syrup, molasses, salt . . ." versus one that contains "100 percent rolled oats."
- A canned fruit that contains "sugar, apples, water" versus one that contains simply "apples, water."

In each comparison, consumers can tell that the second product is the more nutrient dense.

Serving Sizes

Because labels present nutrient information per serving, they must identify the size of a serving. The Food and Drug Administration (FDA) has established specific serving sizes for various foods and requires that all labels for a given product use the same serving size. For example, the serving size for all ice creams is ½ cup and for all beverages, 8 fluid ounces. This facilitates comparison shopping. Consumers can see at a glance which brand has more or fewer kcalories or grams of fat, for example. Standard serving sizes are expressed in both common household measures, such as cups, and metric measures, such as milliliters, to accommodate users of both types of measures (see Table 2-8).

When examining the nutrition facts on a food label, consumers need to consider how the serving size compares with the actual quantity eaten. If it is not the same, they will need to adjust the quantities accordingly. For example, if the serving size is four cookies and you only eat two, then you need to cut the nutrient and kcalorie values in half; similarly, if you eat eight cookies, then you need to double the values. Notice, too, that small bags or individually wrapped items, such as chips or candy bars, may contain more than a single serving. The number of servings per container is listed just below the serving size.

Be aware that serving sizes on food labels are not always the same as those of the USDA Food Guide.[6] For example, a serving of rice on a food label is 1 cup, whereas in the USDA Food Guide it is ½ cup. Unfortunately, this discrepancy, coupled with each person's own perception (oftentimes misperception) of standard serving sizes, sometimes creates confusion for consumers trying to follow recommendations.

TABLE 2-8 Household and Metric Measures

- 1 teaspoon (tsp) = 5 milliliters (mL)
- 1 tablespoon (tbs) = 15 mL
- 1 cup (c) = 240 mL
- 1 fluid ounce (fl oz) = 30 mL
- 1 ounce (oz) = 28 grams (g)

NOTE: The Aids to Calculation section at the back of the book provides additional weights and measures.

Nutrition Facts

In addition to the serving size and the servings per container, the FDA requires that the "Nutrition Facts" panel on a label present nutrient information in two ways—in quantities (such as grams) and as percentages of standards called the **Daily Values.** The Nutrition Facts panel must provide the nutrient amount, percent Daily Value, or both for the following:

- Total food energy (kcalories).
- Food energy from fat (kcalories).
- Total fat (grams and percent Daily Value).
- Saturated fat (grams and percent Daily Value).
- *Trans* fat (grams).*
- Cholesterol (milligrams and percent Daily Value).
- Sodium (milligrams and percent Daily Value).
- Total carbohydrate, including starch, sugar, and fiber (grams and percent Daily Value).
- Dietary fiber (grams and percent Daily Value).
- Sugars (grams), including both those naturally present in and those added to the food.
- Protein (grams).

The labels must also present nutrient content information as a percentage of the Daily Values for the following vitamins and minerals:

- Vitamin A.
- Vitamin C.
- Iron.
- Calcium.

The FDA developed the Daily Values for use on food labels because comparing nutrient amounts against a standard helps make them meaningful to consumers. A person might wonder, for example, whether 1 milligram of iron or calcium is a little or a lot. Well, as Table 2-9 shows, the Daily Value for iron is 18 milligrams, so 1 milligram of iron is enough to take notice of: it is over 5 percent. But the Daily

* *Trans* fats are required on food labels by January 1, 2006.

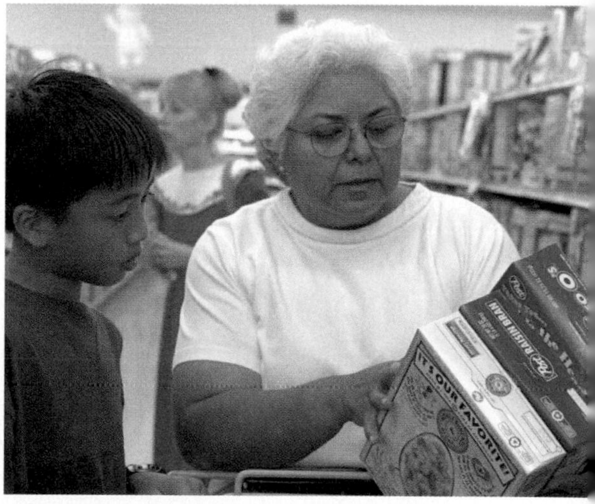

© Bob Daemmrich Photography

Consumers read food labels to learn about the nutrient contents of a food or to compare similar foods.

Daily Values (DV): reference values developed by the FDA specifically for use on food labels.

TABLE 2-9 Daily Values for Food Labels

Food labels must present the "% Daily Value" for these nutrients.

Food Component	Daily Value	Calculation Factors
Fat	65 g	30% of kcalories
Saturated fat	20 g	10% of kcalories
Cholesterol	300 mg	—
Carbohydrate (total)	300 g	60% of kcalories
Fiber	25 g	11.5 g per 1000 kcalories
Protein	50 g	10% of kcalories
Sodium	2400 mg	—
Potassium	3500 mg	—
Vitamin C	60 mg	—
Vitamin A	1500 μg	—
Calcium	1000 mg	—
Iron	18 mg	—

NOTE: Daily Values were established for adults and children over 4 years old. The values for energy-yielding nutrients are based on 2000 kcalories a day. For fiber, the Daily Value was rounded up from 23.

■ % Daily Values:
≥20% = high or excellent source.
10–19% = good source.

nutrient claims: statements that characterize the quantity of a nutrient in a food.

Value for calcium on food labels is 1000 milligrams, so 1 milligram of calcium is essentially nothing.

The Daily Values

The Daily Values reflect dietary recommendations for nutrients and dietary components that have important relationships with health. The "% Daily Value" column on a label provides a ballpark estimate of how individual foods contribute to the total diet. It compares key nutrients in a serving of food with the daily goals of a person consuming 2000 kcalories. A 2000-kcalorie diet is considered about right for sedentary younger women, active older women, and sedentary older men. Young children and sedentary women may need fewer kcalories. Most labels list, at the bottom, Daily Values for both a 2000-kcalorie and a 2500-kcalorie diet, but the "% Daily Value" column on all labels applies only to a 2000-kcalorie diet. A 2500-kcalorie diet is considered about right for many men, teenage boys, and active younger women. People who are exceptionally active may have still higher energy needs. Labels may also provide a reminder of the kcalories in a gram of carbohydrate, fat, and protein below the Daily Value information (review Figure 2-9).

A person who consumes 2000 kcalories a day can simply add up all the "% Daily Values" for a particular nutrient to see if the day's diet fits with recommendations. People who require more or less than 2000 kcalories daily must do some calculations to see how foods compare with their personal nutrition goals. They can use the calculation column in Table 2-9 or the suggestions presented in the accompanying "How to" feature.

Daily Values help consumers see easily whether a food contributes "a little" or "a lot" of a nutrient.■ For example, the "% Daily Value" column on a label of macaroni and cheese may say 20 percent for fat. This tells the consumer that each serving of this food contains about 20 percent of the day's allotted 65 grams of fat. A person consuming 2000 kcalories a day could simply keep track of the percentages of Daily Values from foods eaten in a day and try not to exceed 100 percent. Be aware that for some nutrients (such as fat and sodium) you will want to select foods with a low "% Daily Value" and for others (such as calcium and fiber) you will want a high "% Daily Value." To determine whether a particular food is a wise choice, a consumer needs to consider its place in the diet among all the other foods eaten during the day.

Daily Values also make it easy to compare foods. For example, a consumer might discover that frozen macaroni and cheese has a Daily Value for fat of 20 percent, whereas macaroni and cheese prepared from a boxed mix has a Daily Value of 15 percent. By comparing labels, consumers who are concerned about their fat intakes will be able to make informed decisions.

Nutrient Claims

Have you noticed phrases such as "good source of fiber" on a box of cereal or "rich in calcium" on a package of cheese? These and other **nutrient claims** may be used on labels as long as they meet FDA definitions, which include the conditions under which each term can be used (see the glossary on p. 60 for these definitions). For example, in addition to having less than 2 milligrams of cholesterol, a "cholesterol-free" product may not contain more than 2 grams of saturated fat and *trans* fat combined per serving.

Some descriptions *imply* that a food contains, or does not contain, a nutrient. Implied claims are prohibited unless they meet specified criteria. For example, a claim that a product "contains no oil" *implies* that the food contains no fat. If the product is truly fat-free, then it may make the no-oil claim, but if it contains another source of fat, such as butter, it may not.

HOW TO Calculate Personal Daily Values

The Daily Values on food labels are designed for a 2000-kcalorie intake, but you can calculate a personal set of Daily Values based on your energy allowance. Consider a person with a 1500-kcalorie intake, for example. To calculate a daily goal for fat, multiply energy intake by 30 percent:

$$1500 \text{ kcal} \times 0.30 \text{ kcal from fat} = 450 \text{ kcal from fat.}$$

The "kcalories from fat" are listed on food labels, so a person could then add all the "kcalories from fat" values for a day, using 450 as an upper limit. A person who preferred to count grams of fat could divide this 450 kcalories from fat by 9 kcalories per gram to determine the goal in grams:

$$450 \text{ kcal from fat} \div 9 \text{ kcal/g} = 50 \text{ g fat.}$$

Alternatively, a person could calculate that 1500 kcalories is 75 percent of the 2000-kcalorie intake used for Daily Values:

$$1500 \text{ kcal} \div 2000 \text{ kcal} = 0.75.$$
$$0.75 \times 100 = 75\%.$$

Then, instead of trying to achieve 100 percent of the Daily Value, a person consuming 1500 kcalories would aim for 75 percent. Similarly, a person consuming 2800 kcalories would aim for 140 percent:

$$2800 \text{ kcal} \div 2000 \text{ kcal} = 1.40 \text{ or } 140\%.$$

Table 2-9 includes a calculation column that can help you estimate your personal daily value for several nutrients.

Health Claims

Until recently, the FDA held manufacturers to the highest standards of scientific evidence before approving **health claims** on food labels. Consumers reading "Diets low in sodium may reduce the risk of high blood pressure," for example, knew that the FDA had examined enough scientific evidence to establish a clear link between diet and health. Such reliable health claims make up the FDA's "A" list (see Table 2-10).

These reliable health claims still appear on some food labels, but finding them may be difficult now that the FDA has created three additional categories of claims based on scientific evidence that is less conclusive (see Table 2-11 on p. 60). These categories were added after a court ruled that "holding only the highest scientific standard for claims interferes with commercial free speech."[7] Food manufacturers had argued that they should be allowed to inform consumers about possible benefits based on less than clear and convincing evidence. The FDA states that the new rules will enable consumers to receive more information about nutrients and foods that show preliminary promise in preventing disease. Consumer groups argue that such information is confusing. Even with required disclaimers for health claims graded "B," "C," or "D," distinguishing "A" claims from others is difficult, as the next section shows. (Health claims on supplement labels are presented in Highlight 10.)

TABLE 2-10 Food Label Health Claims—The "A" List

- Calcium and reduced risk of osteoporosis
- Sodium and reduced risk of hypertension
- Dietary saturated fat and cholesterol and reduced risk of coronary heart disease
- Dietary fat and reduced risk of cancer
- Fiber-containing grain products, fruits, and vegetables and reduced risk of cancer
- Fruits, vegetables, and grain products that contain fiber, particularly soluble fiber, and reduced risk of coronary heart disease
- Fruits and vegetables and reduced risk of cancer
- Folate and reduced risk of neural tube defects
- Sugar alcohols and reduced risk of tooth decay
- Soluble fiber from whole oats and from psyllium seed husk and reduced risk of heart disease
- Soy protein and reduced risk of heart disease
- Whole grains and reduced risk of heart disease and certain cancers
- Plant sterol and plant stanol esters and heart disease
- Potassium and reduced risk of hypertension and stroke

Structure-Function Claims

Unlike health claims, which require food manufacturers to collect scientific evidence and petition the FDA, **structure-function claims** can be made without any FDA approval. Products can claim to "slow aging," "improve memory," and "build strong bones" without any proof. The only criterion for a structure-function claim is that it must not mention a disease or symptom. Unfortunately, structure-function claims can be deceptively similar to health claims. Consider these statements:

- "May reduce the risk of heart disease."
- "Promotes a healthy heart."

Most consumers would argue that these two claims say the same thing. In fact, the first is a health claim that requires FDA approval and the second is an unproven,

health claims: statements that characterize the relationship between a nutrient or other substance in a food and a disease or health-related condition.

structure-function claims: statements that characterize the relationship between a nutrient or other substance in a food and its role in the body.

TABLE 2-11 The FDA's Health Claims Report Card

Grade	Level of Confidence in Health Claim	Required Label Disclaimers
A	High: Significant scientific agreement	These health claims do not require disclaimers; see Table 2-10 for examples.
B	Moderate: Evidence is supportive, but not conclusive	"[Health claim.] Although there is scientific evidence supporting this claim, the evidence is not conclusive."
C	Low: Evidence is limited and not conclusive	"Some scientific evidence suggests [health claim]. However, FDA has determined that this evidence is limited and not conclusive."
D	Very low: Little scientific evidence supporting this claim	"Very limited and preliminary scientific research suggests [health claim]. FDA concludes that there is little scientific evidence supporting this claim."

GLOSSARY OF TERMS ON FOOD LABELS

GENERAL TERMS

free: "nutritionally trivial" and unlikely to have a physiological consequence; synonyms include "without," "no," and "zero." A food that does not contain a nutrient naturally may make such a claim, but only as it applies to all similar foods (for example, "applesauce, a fat-free food").

good source of: the product provides between 10 and 19% of the Daily Value for a given nutrient per serving.

healthy: a food that is low in fat, saturated fat, cholesterol, and sodium and that contains at least 10% of the Daily Values for vitamin A, vitamin C, iron, calcium, protein, or fiber.

high: 20% or more of the Daily Value for a given nutrient per serving; synonyms include "rich in" or "excellent source."

less: at least 25% less of a given nutrient or kcalories than the comparison food (see individual nutrients); synonyms include "fewer" and "reduced."

light or **lite:** any use of the term other than as defined must specify what it is referring to (for example, "light in color" or "light in texture").

low: an amount that would allow frequent consumption of a food without exceeding the Daily Value for the nutrient. A food that is naturally low in a nutrient may make such a claim, but only as it applies to all similar foods (for example, "fresh cauliflower, a low-sodium food"); synonyms include "little," "few," and "low source of."

more: at least 10% more of the Daily Value for a given nutrient than the comparison food; synonyms include "added" and "extra."

organic: on food labels, that at least 95% of the product's ingredients have been grown and processsed according to USDA regulations defining the use of fertilizers, herbicides, insecticides, fungicides, preservatives, and other chemical ingredients.

ENERGY

kcalorie-free: fewer than 5 kcal per serving.

light: one-third fewer kcalories than the comparison food.

low kcalorie: 40 kcal or less per serving.

reduced kcalorie: at least 25% fewer kcalories per serving than the comparison food.

FAT AND CHOLESTEROL[a]

percent fat-free: may be used only if the product meets the definition of *low fat* or *fat-free* and must reflect the amount of fat in 100 g (for example, a food that contains 2.5 g of fat per 50 g can claim to be "95 percent fat free").

fat-free: less than 0.5 g of fat per serving (and no added fat or oil); synonyms include "zero-fat," "no-fat," and "nonfat."

low fat: 3 g or less fat per serving.

less fat: 25% or less fat than the comparison food.

saturated fat-free: less than 0.5 g of saturated fat and 0.5 g of *trans* fat per serving.

low saturated fat: 1 g or less saturated fat and less than 0.5 g of *trans* fat per serving.

less saturated fat: 25% or less saturated fat and *trans* fat combined than the comparison food.

***trans* fat-free:** less than 0.5 g of *trans* fat and less than 0.5 g of saturated fat per serving.

cholesterol-free: less than 2 mg cholesterol per serving and 2 g or less saturated fat and *trans* fat combined per serving.

low cholesterol: 20 mg or less cholesterol per serving and 2 g or less saturated fat and *trans* fat combined per serving.

less cholesterol: 25% or less cholesterol than the comparison food (reflecting a reduction of at least 20 mg per serving), and 2 g or less saturated fat and *trans* fat combined per serving.

extra lean: less than 5 g of fat, 2 g of saturated fat and *trans* fat combined, and 95 mg of cholesterol per serving and per 100 g of meat, poultry, and seafood.

lean: less than 10 g of fat, 4.5 g of saturated fat and *trans* fat combined, and 95 mg of cholesterol per serving and per 100 g of meat, poultry, and seafood.

light: 50% or less of the fat than in the comparison food (for example, 50% less fat than our regular cookies).

CARBOHYDRATES: FIBER AND SUGAR

high fiber: 5 g or more fiber per serving. A high-fiber claim made on a food that contains more than 3 g fat per serving and per 100 g of food must also declare total fat.

sugar-free: less than 0.5 g of sugar per serving.

SODIUM

sodium-free and **salt-free:** less than 5 mg of sodium per serving.

low sodium: 140 mg or less per serving.

light: a low-kcalorie, low-fat food with a 50% reduction in sodium.

light in sodium: no more than 50% of the sodium of the comparison food.

very low sodium: 35 mg or less per serving.

[a]Foods containing more than 13 grams total fat per serving or per 50 grams of food must indicate those contents immediately after a cholesterol claim. As you can see, all cholesterol claims are prohibited when the food contains more than 2 grams saturated fat and *trans* fat combined per serving.

but legal, structure-function claim. Table 2-12 lists examples of structure-function claims.

Consumer Education

Labels are valuable only if people know how to use them, so the FDA has designed several programs to educate consumers. Consumers who understand how to read labels will be best able to apply the information to achieve and maintain healthful dietary practices.

Table 2-13 (on p. 62) shows how the messages from the 2005 *Dietary Guidelines,* the USDA Food Guide, and food labels coordinate with each other. To help consumers understand and coordinate these messages, an alliance of health organizations, the food industry, and government agencies has developed an educational program called "It's All About You." The program is designed to deliver simple messages that will motivate consumers to think positively about making reasonable changes in their eating and physical activity habits.

IN SUMMARY Food labels provide consumers with information they need to select foods that will help them meet their nutrition and health goals. Given labels with relevant information presented in a standardized, easy-to-read format, consumers are well prepared to plan and create healthful diets.

TABLE 2-12 Examples of Structure-Function Claims

- Builds strong bones
- Defends your health
- Promotes relaxation
- Slows aging
- Improves memory
- Guards against colds
- Boosts the immune system
- Lifts your spirits
- Supports heart health

NOTE: Structure-function claims cannot make statements about diseases. See Table 2-10 on p. 59 for examples of health claims.

TABLE 2-13 From Guidelines to Groceries

Dietary Guidelines	USDA Food Guide	Food Labels
Adequate nutrients within energy needs	Select the recommended amounts from each food group at the energy level appropriate for your energy needs.	Look for foods that describe their vitamin, mineral, or fiber contents as a *good source* or *high.*
Weight management	Select nutrient-dense foods and beverages within and among the food groups. Limit high-fat foods and foods and beverages with added fats and sugars. Use appropriate portion sizes.	Look for foods that describe their kcalorie contents as *free, low, reduced, light,* or *less.*
Physical activity		
Food groups to encourage	Select a variety of fruits each day. Include vegetables from all five subgroups (dark green, orange, legumes, starchy vegetables, and other vegetables) several times a week. Make at least half of the grain selections whole grains. Select fat-free or low-fat milk products.	Look for foods that describe their fiber contents as *good source* or *high.* Look for foods that provide at least 10% of the Daily Value for fiber, vitamin A, vitamin C, iron, and calcium from a variety of sources.
Fats	Choose foods within each group that are lean, low fat, or fat-free. Choose foods within each group that have little added fat.	Look for foods that describe their fat, saturated fat, *trans* fat, and cholesterol contents as *free, less, low, light, reduced, lean,* or *extra lean.* Look for foods that provide no more than 5% of the Daily Value for fat, saturated fat, and cholesterol.
Carbohydrates	Choose fiber-rich fruits, vegetables, and whole grains often. Choose foods and beverages within each group that have little added sugars.	Look for foods that describe their sugar contents as *free* or *reduced.* A food may be high in sugar if its ingredients list begins with or contains several of the following: *sugar, sucrose, fructose, maltose, lactose, honey, syrup, corn syrup, high-fructose corn syrup, molasses, evaporated cane juice,* or *fruit juice concentrate.*
Sodium and potassium	Choose foods within each group that are low in salt or sodium. Choose potassium-rich foods such as fruits and vegetables.	Look for foods that describe their salt and sodium contents as *free, low,* or *reduced.* Look for foods that provide no more than 5% of the Daily Value for sodium. Look for foods that provide at least 10% of the Daily Value for potassium.
Alcoholic beverages	Use sensibly and in moderation (no more than one drink a day for women and two drinks a day for men).	*Light* beverages contain fewer kcalories and less alcohol than regular versions.
Food safety		Follow the *safe handling instructions* on packages of meat and other safety instructions, such as *keep refrigerated,* on packages of perishable foods.

Nutrition in Your Life

The secret to making healthy food choices is learning to incorporate the 2005 *Dietary Guidelines* and the USDA Food Guide into your decisions.

- Do you eat the amounts recommended for your energy needs from each of the five food groups daily?
- Do you try to vary your choices within each food group from day to day? If not, why not?
- What dietary changes could you make to improve your chances of enjoying good health?

NUTRITION ON THE NET

Access these websites for further study of topics covered in this chapter.

- Find updates and quick links to these and other nutrition-related sites at our website: **www.wadsworth.com/nutrition**
- Search for "diet" and "food labels" at the U.S. Government health information site: **www.healthfinder.gov**
- Learn more about the *Dietary Guidelines for Americans:* **www.healthierus.gov/dietaryguidelines**
- Find Canadian information on nutrition guidelines and food labels at: **www.hc-sc.gc.ca**
- Visit the USDA Food Guide section (including its ethnic/cultural versions) of the U.S. Department of Agriculture: **www.nal.usda.gov/fnic**
- Learn more about the USDA Food Guide and MyPyramid: **mypyramid.gov**
- Visit the Traditional Diet Pyramids for various ethnic groups at Oldways Preservation and Exchange Trust: **www.oldwayspt.org**
- Search for "exchange lists" at the American Diabetes Association: **www.diabetes.org**
- Learn more about food labeling from the Food and Drug Administration: **www.cfsan.fda.gov**
- Search for "food labels" at the International Food Information Council: **www.ific.org**
- Assess your diet at the CNPP Interactive Healthy Eating Index: **www.usda.gov/cnpp**
- Get healthy eating tips from the "5 a day" programs: **www.5aday.gov** or **www.5aday.org**

NUTRITION CALCULATIONS

These problems will give you practice in doing simple nutrition-related calculations. Although the situations are hypothetical, the numbers are real, and calculating the answers (check them on p. 65) provides a valuable nutrition lesson. Be sure to show your calculations for each problem.

1. *Read a food label.* Look at the cereal label in Figure 2-9 and answer the following questions:
    a. What is the size of a serving of cereal?
    b. How many kcalories are in a serving?
    c. How much fat is in a serving?
    d. How many kcalories does this represent?
    e. What percentage of the kcalories in this product comes from fat?
    f. What does this tell you?
    g. What is the % Daily Value for fat?
    h. What does this tell you?
    i. Does this cereal meet the criteria for a low-fat product (refer to the glossary on p. 60)?
    j. How much fiber is in a serving?
    k. Read the Daily Value chart on the lower section of the label. What is the Daily Value for fiber?
    l. What percentage of the Daily Value for fiber does a serving of the cereal contribute? Show the calculation the label-makers used to come up with the % Daily Value for fiber.
    m. What is the predominant ingredient in the cereal?
    n. Have any nutrients been added to this cereal (is it fortified)?

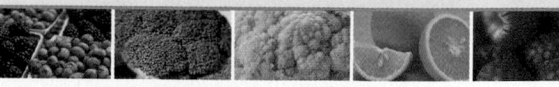

2. *Calculate a personal Daily Value.* The Daily Values on food labels are for people with a 2000-kcalorie intake.
   a. Suppose a person has a 1600-kcalorie energy allowance. Use the calculation factors listed in Table 2-8 to calculate a set of personal "Daily Values" based on 1600 kcalories. Show your calculations.
   b. Revise the % Daily Value chart of the cereal label in Figure 2-9 based on your "Daily Values" for a 1600-kcalorie diet.

STUDY QUESTIONS

These questions will help you review this chapter. You will find the answers in the discussions on the pages provided.

1. Name the diet-planning principles and briefly describe how each principle helps in diet planning. (pp. 39–41)
2. What recommendations appear in the *Dietary Guidelines for Americans*? (pp. 41–43)
3. Name the five food groups in the USDA Food Guide and identify several foods typical of each group. Explain how such plans group foods and what diet-planning principles the plans best accommodate. How are food group plans used, and what are some of their strengths and weaknesses? (pp. 43–49)
4. Review the *Dietary Guidelines*. What types of grocery selections would you make to achieve those recommendations? (pp. 42, 52–55)
5. What information can you expect to find on a food label? How can this information help you choose between two similar products? (pp. 55–58)
6. What are the Daily Values? How can they help you meet health recommendations? (p. 57–58)
7. Describe the differences between nutrient claims, health claims, and structure-function claims. (pp. 58–59, 61)

These multiple choice questions will help you prepare for an exam. Answers can be found on p. 65.

1. The diet-planning principle that provides all the essential nutrients in sufficient amounts to support health is:
   a. balance.
   b. variety.
   c. adequacy.
   d. moderation.
2. A person who chooses a chicken leg that provides 0.5 milligram of iron and 95 kcalories instead of two tablespoons of peanut butter that also provide 0.5 milligram of iron but 188 kcalories is using the principle of nutrient:
   a. control.
   b. density.
   c. adequacy.
   d. moderation.
3. Which of the following is consistent with the *Dietary Guidelines for Americans*?
   a. Choose a diet restricted in fat and cholesterol.
   b. Balance the food you eat with physical activity.
   c. Choose a diet with plenty of milk products and meats.
   d. Eat an abundance of foods to ensure nutrient adequacy.
4. According to the USDA Food Guide, added fats and sugars are counted as:
   a. meats and grains.
   b. nutrient-dense foods.
   c. discretionary kcalories.
   d. oils and carbohydrates.
5. Foods within a given food group of the USDA Food Guide are similar in their contents of:
   a. energy.
   b. proteins and fibers.
   c. vitamins and minerals.
   d. carbohydrates and fats.
6. In the exchange system, each portion of food on any given list provides about the same amount of:
   a. energy.
   b. satiety.
   c. vitamins.
   d. minerals.
7. Enriched grain products are fortified with:
   a. fiber, folate, iron, niacin, and zinc.
   b. thiamin, iron, calcium, zinc, and sodium.
   c. iron, thiamin, riboflavin, niacin, and folate.
   d. folate, magnesium, vitamin B_6, zinc, and fiber.
8. Food labels list ingredients in:
   a. alphabetical order.
   b. ascending order of predominance by weight.
   c. descending order of predominance by weight.
   d. manufacturer's order of preference.
9. "Milk builds strong bones" is an example of a:
   a. health claim.
   b. nutrition fact.
   c. nutrient content claim.
   d. structure-function claim.
10. Daily Values on food labels are based on a:
    a. 1500-kcalorie diet.
    b. 2000-kcalorie diet.
    c. 2500-kcalorie diet.
    d. 3000-kcalorie diet.

REFERENCES

1. U.S. Department of Agriculture and U.S. Department of Health and Human Services, *Dietary Guidelines for Americans* (Washington, D.C.: 2005).
2. Position of the American Dietetic Association and Dietitians of Canada: Vegetarian diets, *Journal of the American Dietetic Association* 103 (2003): 748–765.
3. J. R. Backstrand, The history and future of food fortification in the United States: A public health perspective, *Nutrition Reviews* 60 (2002): 15–26; Y. K. Park and coauthors, History of cereal-grain product fortification in the United States, *Nutrition Today* 36 (2001): 124–137.
4. As cited in 21 Code of Federal Regulations—Food and Drugs, Section 104.20, 45 *Federal Register* 6323, January 25, 1980, as amended in 58 *Federal Register* 2228, January 6, 1993.
5. Position of the American Dietetic Association: Food fortification and dietary supplements, *Journal of the American Dietetic Association* 101 (2001): 115–125.
6. D. Herring and coauthors, Serving sizes in the Food Guide Pyramid and on the nutrition facts label: What's different and why? *Family Economics and Nutrition Review* 14 (2002): 71–73; M. B. Hogbin and M. A. Hess, Public confusion over food portions and servings, *Journal of the American Dietetic Association* 99 (1999): 1209–1211.
7. N. Hellmich, FDA to allow qualified health claims on foods, *USA Today,* 11 July 2003, available at **www.USATODAY.com**.

ANSWERS

Nutrition Calculations

1. a. ¾ cup (28 g).
   b. 110 kcalories.
   c. 1 g fat.
   d. 9 kcalories.
   e. 9 kcal ÷ 110 kcal = 0.08.
      0.08 × 100 = 8%.
   f. This cereal derives 8 percent of its kcalories from fat.
   g. 2%.
   h. A serving of this cereal provides 2 percent of the 65 grams of fat recommended for a 2000-kcalorie diet.
   i. Yes.
   j. 1.5 g fiber.
   k. 25 g.
   l. 1.5 g ÷ 25 g = 0.06.
      0.06 × 100 = 6%.
   m. Corn.
   n. Yes.

2. a. Daily Values for 1600-kcalorie diet:

Fat: 1600 kcal × 0.30 = 480 kcal from fat.
   480 kcal ÷ 9 kcal/g = 53 g fat.

Saturated fat: 1600 kcal × 0.10 = 160 kcal from saturated fat.
   160 kcal ÷ 9 kcal/g = 18 g saturated fat.

Cholesterol: 300 mg.

Carbohydrate: 1600 kcal × 0.60 = 960 kcal from carbohydrate.
   960 kcal ÷ 4 kcal/g = 240 g carbohydrate.

Fiber: 1600 kcal ÷ 1000 kcal = 1.6.
   1.6 × 11.5 g = 18.4 g fiber.

Protein: 1600 kcal × 0.10 = 160 kcal from protein.
   160 kcal ÷ 4 kcal/g = 40 g protein.

Sodium: 2400 mg.

Potassium: 3500 mg.

b.

Total fat	2%	(1 g ÷ 53 g)
Saturated fat	0%	(0 g ÷ 18 g)
Cholesterol	0%	(no calculation needed)
Sodium	10%	(no calculation needed)
Total carbohydrate	10%	(23 g ÷ 240 g)
Dietary fiber	8%	(1.5 g ÷ 18.4 g)

Study Questions (multiple choice)

1. c 2. b 3. b 4. c 5. c 6. a 7. c 8. c
9. d 10. b

HIGHLIGHT

A World Tour of Pyramids, Pagodas, and Plates

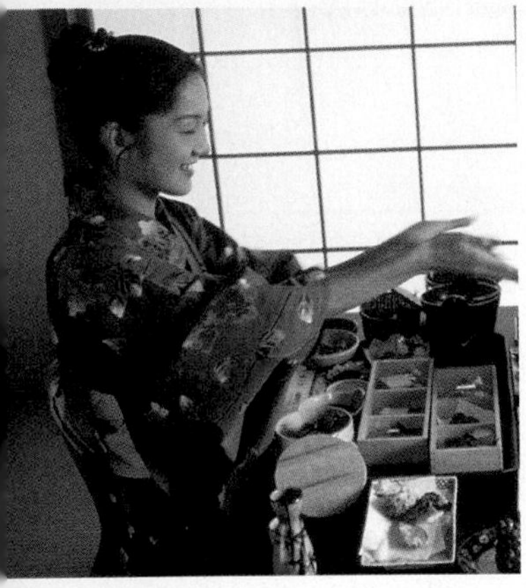

© Michael S. Yamashita/CORBIS

In China, a family's meal may include horse meat or fried scorpion; in Great Britain, people traditionally drink a pot of tea and eat a scone between lunch and dinner; and in India, those with a reverence for life called *ahimsa* espouse a vegetarian diet.[1] The food supplies, eating habits, and cultural beliefs of people living in diverse regions of the world are different, but their needs are similar in fundamental ways. People from every corner of the world need foods—whether cheeseburgers or grasshoppers—to provide the nutrients necessary to maintain life and defend against disease.

How should a person select foods to maintain good health? In the United States, the *Dietary Guidelines for Americans 2005* offer direction. Other countries provide similar guidelines, and it can be enlightening to see how U.S. guidelines compare with those from other countries. A tour of dietary guidelines from around the world finds they are similar in many ways and different in a few. This highlight elaborates on the *Dietary Guidelines for Americans 2005* that were introduced in Chapter 2 and compares them with guidelines from around the world.

Dietary Guidelines

Governments develop dietary guidelines based on the nutrition problems, food supplies, eating habits, and cultural beliefs of their populations. These guidelines offer practical suggestions for making food choices that will support good health and reduce the risk of chronic diseases. They also provide the basis for many policy and education decisions. Although each set of guidelines reflects the people and foodways of a specific country, guidelines from around the world exhibit more similarities than differences.

Adequate Nutrients within Energy Needs

Each food provides a unique assortment of nutrients. To get all the nutrients in the right amounts without exceeding energy needs, a person needs to eat a variety of nutrient-dense foods in appropriate quantities. The *Dietary Guidelines for Americans 2005* depend on the USDA Food Guide to direct daily food choices. Not all nations use the USDA Food Guide, of course, but most consistently feature "variety" in their message, quite often as the premier guideline. To achieve variety, guidelines in Japan, for example, recommend "incorporating new and different dishes."

Figure H2-1 (on pp. 68–69) features shapes of various food guide plans from selected nations.[2] Most food guide plans classify foods into the following groups: grains, vegetables, fruits, meats, and milk products, with a few minor variations. For example, Canada, China, and Portugal cluster fruits and vegetables into one group; Mexico and the Philippines group milk products with meats.

Potatoes and legumes appear in all food guides, but their locations vary. In the United States, potatoes are grouped with vegetables, but in Great Britain, Mexico, and Korea, potatoes are listed with the grains. Sweden separates potatoes and other tubers into their own group, featuring them as a "base food," providing a "foundation for a nutritious and inexpensive diet." As for legumes, the United States includes them in both the meat and the vegetable groups; Sweden, Germany, and Australia put them in the vegetable group; and China places them in the milk group.

Most food guide plans describe the recommended number of servings and serving sizes for each food group. Some, such as Mexico, do not quantify recommendations, but instead offer general guidelines—"muchas verduras y frutas" (many vegetables and fruits) and "pocos alimentos de origen animal" (little food of animal origin). In all cases, the guidelines emphasize abundant grains, vegetables, and fruits and moderate meats and milks.

Weight Management

Healthy body weight plays a key role in reducing the risk of chronic diseases. To that end, the *Dietary Guidelines for Americans 2005* encourage people to maintain body weight in a healthy range by balancing kcalories from foods and beverages with kcalories expended. Canada, Germany, Australia, and dozens of other developed countries also advise consumers to "watch your weight and stay active."

A notable difference is apparent in developing countries, such as Indonesia, where undernutrition threatens health as much or more than overnutrition does. The focus there is on consuming "foods to provide sufficient energy."

Physical Activity

Physical activity not only helps with weight management and disease prevention, but it also improves cardiovascular fitness, strengthens bones and muscles, controls blood pressure, and promotes psychological well-being. Furthermore, a person who is physically active can afford to eat more, which makes it easier to get the nutrients the body needs to stay fit. The *Dietary Guidelines for Americans 2005* recommend participating in at least 30 minutes of moderately intense physical activity on most days. This amount of activity offers some health benefits, but it is not enough to maintain a healthy body weight. To prevent weight gain and to accrue additional health benefits, most adults need to engage in 60 minutes of moderate- to vigorous-intensity activity on most days. To sustain weight loss may require even more—at least 60 to 90 minutes of moderate-intensity physical activity daily. (Chapter 8 includes a table showing energy expenditures for a variety of activities.)

Many of the guidelines from around the world that encourage a healthy body weight mention balancing physical activity with food intake. For example, Japan's guideline says to "balance the kcalories you eat with physical activity."

Food Groups to Encourage

The USDA Food Guide encourages greater consumption of fruits, vegetables, milk and milk products, and whole grains to provide the nutrients most often missing from the diets of Americans. These food groups help to supply the diet with fiber, vitamin A, vitamin C, vitamin E, calcium, magnesium, and potassium.

As Chapter 2 mentioned, the campaign to "eat 5 to 9 a day" reflects the recommendation to select a variety of fruits and vegetables each day. Not only do fruits and vegetables supply vitamins and minerals in abundance, but their phytochemicals and fibers help to maintain good health and protect against diseases such as heart disease and cancer. Because different fruits and vegetables deliver different nutrients, it is especially important to select a variety and to include dark green vegetables, orange vegetables, legumes, starchy vegetables, other vegetables, citrus fruits, melons, and berries weekly. Several nations have a guideline that encourages consumers to "eat plenty of fruits and vegetables." Many have adopted a "5 a day" recommendation.

Another food group the USDA Food Guide encourages is milk and milk products. Consumers are advised to select 3 cups of fat-free or low-fat milk or the equivalent in milk products daily. Food guides in Canada and Australia suggest similar amounts, whereas countries such as China, Korea, and Germany advise the equivalent of 1 cup or less.

The USDA Food Guide also encourages consumers to make at least half of their grain selections whole grains such as whole wheat, brown rice, and oats. Canada, Australia, Germany, and Great Britain also mention the need to "eat plenty of foods rich in starch and fiber," such as bread and cereals. Guidelines from Greece suggest that people "prefer whole grain breads and pastas." Other countries, such as Indonesia, recommend that consumers "obtain about half of total energy from complex carbohydrate–rich foods."

Fats

Some fat in the diet is essential to good health, but certain kinds of fat, most notably saturated and *trans* fats, can be detrimental to heart health as Highlight 5 explains. For this reason, the *Dietary Guidelines for Americans 2005* encourage people to limit saturated fat intake to less than 10 percent of total kcalories, *trans* fat to as low as possible, cholesterol intake to less than 300 milligrams a day, and total fat intake to between 20 and 35 percent of total kcalories.

Most countries make some statement about not eating "too many foods that contain a lot of fat," but the recommended limitations vary. Canada, for example, agrees with the United States. Korea suggests "keeping fat intake at 20 percent of energy intake," and the Netherlands allows "up to 35 percent." Interestingly, both Korea and the Netherlands have lower rates of heart disease than the United States and Canada.[3] Germany does not mention "percent kcalories from fat," but instead restricts dietary fat to 70 to 90 grams per day, which is equivalent to 30 to 40 percent of a 2000-kcalorie diet. The German fat message adds a preference for fats of plant origin and cautions that meat, sausages, and eggs should be eaten in moderation. China—a country with a relatively low rate of heart disease—also advises consumers to "eat more vegetable oils than animal fat."

Carbohydrates

Foods and beverages containing sugar promote tooth decay. In addition, they frequently deliver many kcalories with few, if any, nutrients. For these reasons, the *Dietary Guidelines for Americans 2005* encourage people to choose and prepare foods and beverages with little added sugars. (Chapter 4 presents additional dietary strategies to limit tooth decay, and Highlight 23 describes the relationships between dental problems and chronic illnesses.)

Many nations take a similar approach, saying "don't have sugary foods and drinks too often" or "eat only a moderate amount of sugars and foods containing added sugars." Greek guidelines do not address sugar directly, but urge consumers to "prefer fruits and nuts as snacks, instead of sweets or candy bars" and to "prefer water over soft drinks"—suggestions that reflect traditional Greek foodways. Other nations, including Canada, Korea, China, the Philippines, and Japan, do not mention sugars in their dietary guidelines.

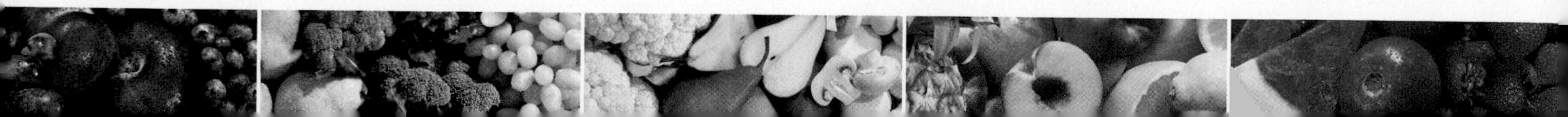

FIGURE H2-1 A Comparison of Food Guide Designs from Selected Nations

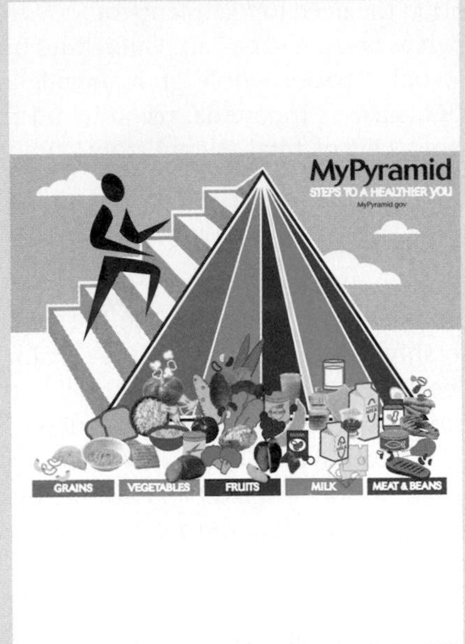
MyPyramid
STEPS TO A HEALTHIER YOU
GRAINS
VEGETABLES
FRUITS
MILK
MEAT & BEANS

The United States uses a pyramid to convey the messages of proportionality, variety, moderation, and activity. (Interestingly, Thailand inverts the pyramid to convey the same message of proportionality, putting the largest amounts at the top and the smaller amounts at the bottom.)

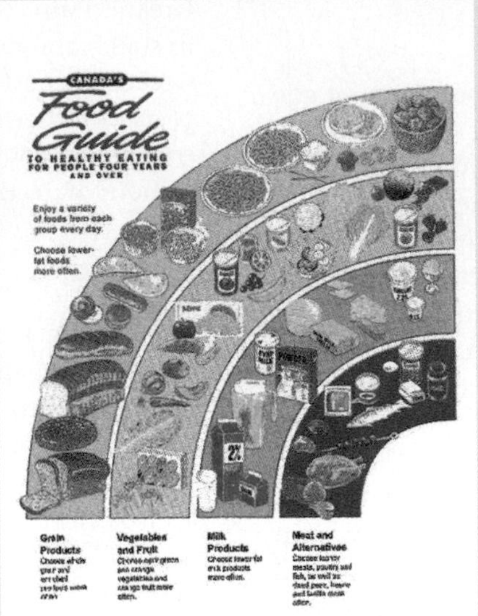
CANADA'S
Food Guide
TO HEALTHY EATING FOR PEOPLE FOUR YEARS AND OVER
Grain Products
Vegetables and Fruit
Milk Products
Meat and Alternatives

Canada

Canada's unique rainbow design also illustrates proportionality.

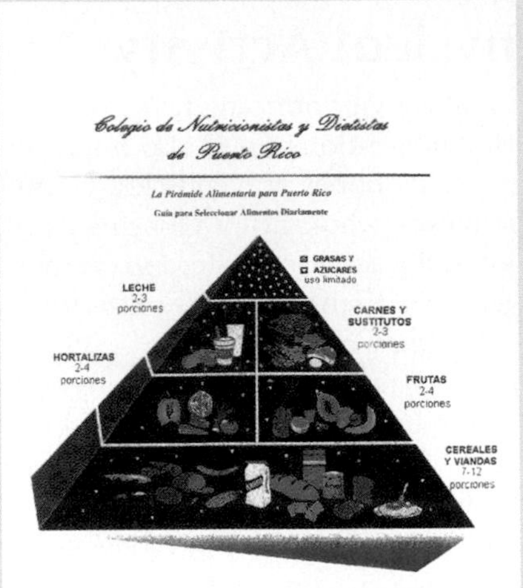
Colegio de Nutricionistas y Dietistas de Puerto Rico
LECHE
2-3
porciones
CARNES Y SUSTITUTOS
2-3
porciones
HORTALIZAS
2-4
porciones
FRUTAS
2-4
porciones
CEREALES Y VIANDAS
7-12
porciones

Puerto Rico

Puerto Rico (and the Philippines) adopted the pyramid design and then made modifications. Notably, Puerto Rico adds a blue shadow to illustrate water, and the Philippines combines the milk and meat groups into one group of animal foods.

SOURCE: *Journal of the American Dietetic Association.* April 2002, pp. 484–485.

Sodium and Potassium

Because of the link between salt intake and high blood pressure, the *Dietary Guidelines for Americans 2005* suggest that consumers choose and prepare foods with little salt. "A little salt" means less than 2300 milligrams of sodium or about one teaspoon of salt (6 grams). Because potassium intake helps to prevent high blood pressure, consumers are also encouraged to eat potassium-rich foods such as fruits and vegetables.

Japan is one of the few countries to specify a quantity, and its upper limit on salt is almost twice that of the U.S. guideline—10 grams a day. Most nations address salt intake without specifying quantities. Canada states that "the sodium content of the diet should be reduced"; Australia advises that you "choose low salt foods and use salt sparingly"; and Great Britain suggests that you "minimize salt use." Indonesia and Germany—two countries whose iodine status is less than sufficient—do not limit salt intake, but instead remind consumers to use iodized salt.[4]

Alcoholic Beverages

Because alcohol consumed in excess is detrimental to health in many ways, the *Dietary Guidelines for Americans 2005* advise adults who drink alcoholic beverages to do so sensibly and in moderation. *Moderation* is defined as one drink a day for women and two a day for men—and the size of "a drink" is specified (see Highlight 7).

Most countries agree: "if you drink alcohol, limit your intake." Canada's limit on alcohol is "no more than 5 percent of energy intake as alcohol, or two drinks daily, whichever is less." Greece cautions those who drink alcohol to do so only occasionally and in small quantities—specified as 25 milliliters of pure alcohol (equivalent to a little less than one ounce of pure alcohol, or about two drinks). Great Britain is less specific and simply suggests that "if you drink, keep within sensible limits." Some countries, such as Indonesia, restrict consumption altogether, advising consumers to "avoid drinking alcoholic beverages." In Hungary, "alcohol is forbidden for children and

FIGURE H2-1 A Comparison of Food Guide Designs from Selected Nations—continued

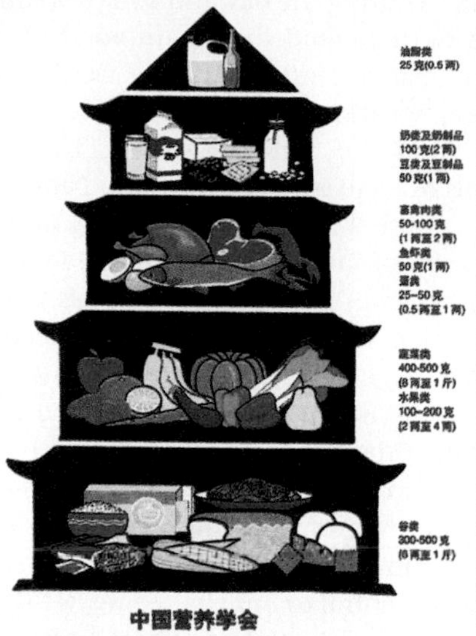
中国营养学会

China

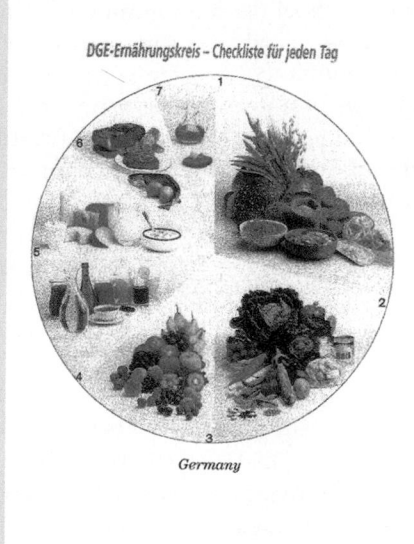

In China (and Korea), a pagoda is used to depict the food guide.

DGE-Ernährungskreis - Checkliste für jeden Tag
1
2
3
4
5
6
7

Germany

In Germany (and most other European countries, as well as Australia), the food guide is illustrated with a circle.

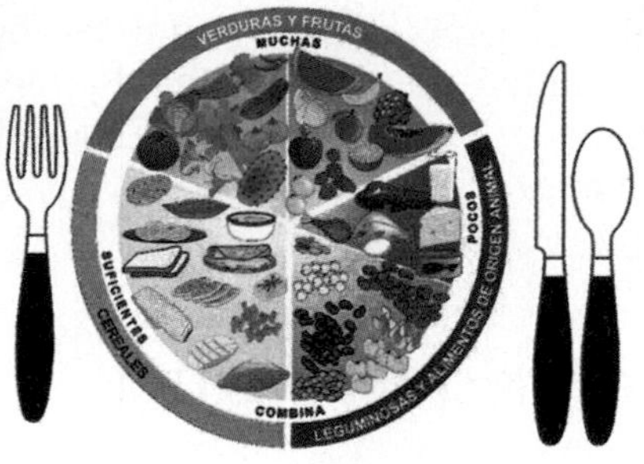
VERDURAS Y FRUTAS
MUCHAS
POCOS
SUFICIENTES
CEREALES
COMBINA
LEGUMINOSAS Y ALIMENTOS DE ORIGEN ANIMAL

Mexico

In Mexico (and Great Britain), a circular food guide is transformed into a sectioned plate of foods.

SOURCE: *Journal of the American Dietetic Association.* April 2002, pp. 484–485.

pregnant women." The Netherlands simply acknowledges "that current alcohol consumption is far too high in many cases."

Keep Foods Safe to Eat

Maintaining a healthy weight, exercising daily, and selecting a variety of grains, legumes, fruits, and vegetables protect a person's health over a lifetime. Foods can also affect immediate health. Foods that are tainted with harmful bacteria, viruses, parasites, or chemical contaminants can make people sick with flu-like symptoms of nausea and diarrhea—or worse. Keeping foods safe requires washing hands and food preparation surfaces often; separating raw, cooked, and prepared foods while shopping, cooking, and storing; cooking foods to the appropriate temperature; and refrigerating perishable foods promptly.

The developing countries of Southeast Asia have among the highest prevalence and risks of foodborne illnesses in the world.[5] Many of these countries include a guideline advising their people to "eat clean and safe food." The message in Indonesia and Thailand is to "consume food which is prepared hygienically." The Philippine guideline goes on to explain that eating clean and safe food "will prevent foodborne diseases."

Additional Comments

As you can see, dietary guidelines from around the world look a little different on the surface, but on close examination their messages agree with each other. They all support good health.

Guidelines from other countries sometimes address issues that are not covered in the *Dietary Guidelines for Americans 2005*. For example, Indonesia encourages its people to "eat breakfast." Several countries specify guidelines for iron and calcium. Most of these make general statements, such as "consume iron rich foods." Some countries offer suggestions for specific groups of people, most commonly, pregnant or breastfeeding women. In Indonesia, mothers are advised to "breast feed your baby exclusively for four months," and in Australia, guidelines "encourage and support breastfeeding."

Water and fluid intakes are addressed in several sets of dietary guidelines. People of Indonesia are advised to "drink adequate quantities of fluids that are free from contaminants," and those in Greece are told to drink about 1.5 liters of water daily. Canada's comment on water addresses its fluoride content, rather than intake. In addition, Canada advises consumers to limit caffeine to no more than the equivalent of four cups of regular coffee a day.

Eating Pleasure

The *Dietary Guidelines for Americans 2005* do not specifically acknowledge that "eating is one of life's greatest pleasures," but the guidelines of many nations do. Clearly, eating provides more than just food to the body. Foods bring pleasure through their flavors and promote social interactions, ethnic traditions, and family time together. Great Britain's first guideline says simply, "enjoy your food." The Netherlands also presents a simple message: "food + joy = health." French guidelines also emphasize enjoyment and suggest that you eat "three good meals a day." Greek guidelines advocate that you "eat slowly, preferably at regular times during the day and in a pleasant environment." Similarly, German guidelines want you to "make sure your dishes are prepared gently and taste well" and to "take your time and enjoy eating." Japan's guidelines capture the spirit of enjoying food and family together: "Have delicious and healthy meals that are good for your mind and body. Enjoy communication at the table with your family and participate in the preparation of meals." Vietnam's guideline delivers a similar message—serve "healthy family meals that are delicious, wholesome, economical, and served with affection."

We agree. Eating should be a pleasure. In this fast-paced world of drive-through restaurants and packaged meals, we sometimes forget to take time to enjoy foods. Eating has become another time-consuming task in our busy days—one that is undertaken with little thought of how the foods eaten will nourish the body or how the time spent will nourish the mind. Because eating is so central to our well-being, we should pay attention and do it well. Take time to select fresh foods. Prepare them creatively. Give thanks for the bounty. Share meals with others. Savor the flavors. Enjoy conversations. Experience the pleasure of nourishing yourself well.

NUTRITION ON THE NET

Access these websites for further study of topics covered in this highlight.

- Find updates and quick links to these and other nutrition-related sites at our website: **www.wadsworth.com/nutrition**
- Link to dietary guidelines from around the world from the USDA: **www.nal.usda.gov/fnic/dga**

REFERENCES

1. P. G. Kittler and K. P. Sucher, *Cultural Foods* (Belmont, Calif.: Wadsworth/Thomson Learning, 2002).
2. J. Painter, J. Rah, and Y. Lee, Comparison of international food guide pictorial representations, *Journal of the American Dietetic Association* 102 (2002): 483–489.
3. World Health Organization, **www.who.int/whosis**, visited June 2003.
4. International Council for the Control of Iodine Deficiency Disorder, **www.people.virginia.edu/~jtd/iccidd/mi/regions/americas_map.htm**, visited June 2003.
5. M. D. Miliotis and J. W. Bier, *International Handbook of Foodborne Pathogens* (New York: Marcel Dekker, 2003).

Chapter 3

Digestion, Absorption, and Transport

Chapter Outline

Digestion: *Anatomy of the Digestive Tract • The Muscular Action of Digestion • The Secretions of Digestion • The Final Stage*

Absorption: *Anatomy of the Absorptive System • A Closer Look at the Intestinal Cells*

The Circulatory Systems: *The Vascular System • The Lymphatic System*

Regulation of Digestion and Absorption: *Gastrointestinal Hormones and Nerve Pathways • The System at Its Best*

Highlight: *Common Digestive Problems*

Available Online

http://nutrition.wadsworth.com/uncn7

Nutrition Animation: *Digestion and Absorption*

Student Practice Test

Glossary Terms

Nutrition on the Net

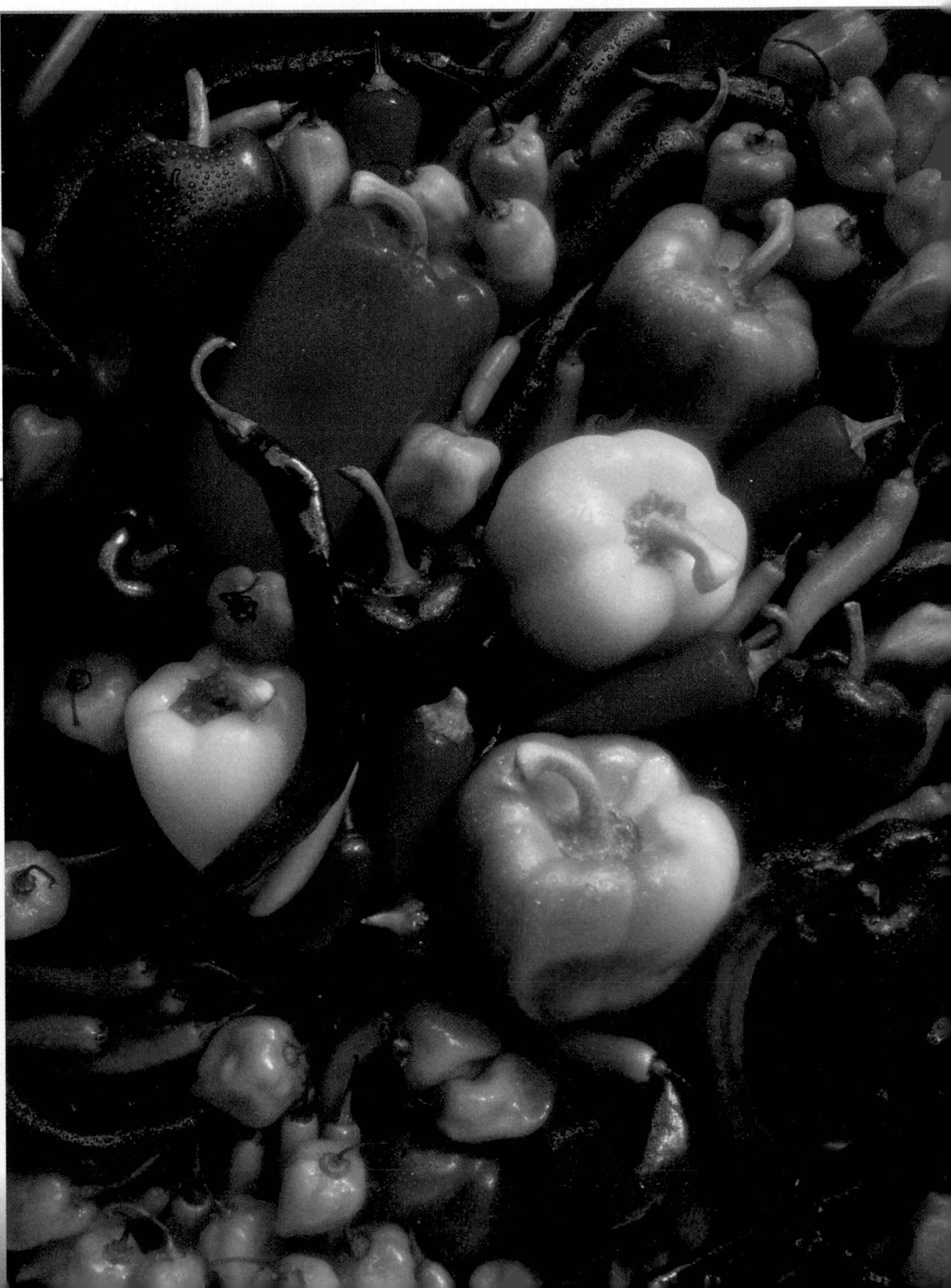

Nutrition in Your Life

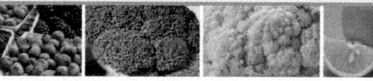

Have you ever wondered what happens to the food you eat after you swallow it? Or how your body extracts nutrients from food? Have you ever marveled at how it all just seems to happen? Follow foods as they travel through the digestive system. Learn how a healthy digestive system transforms whatever food you give it—whether sirloin steak and potatoes or tofu and brussels sprouts—into the nutrients that will nourish the cells of your body.

This chapter takes you on the journey that transforms the foods you eat into the nutrients featured in the later chapters. Then it follows the nutrients as they travel through the intestinal cells and into the body to do their work. This introduction presents a general overview of the processes common to all nutrients; later chapters discuss the specifics of digesting and absorbing individual nutrients.

Digestion

Digestion is the body's ingenious way of breaking down foods into nutrients in preparation for **absorption.** In the process, it overcomes many obstacles for you without any conscious effort on your part. Consider these obstacles:

1. Human beings breathe, eat, and drink through their mouths. Air taken in through the mouth must go to the lungs; food and liquid must go to the stomach. The throat must be arranged so that swallowing and breathing don't interfere with each other.
2. Below the lungs lies the diaphragm, a dome of muscle that separates the upper half of the major body cavity from the lower half. Food must pass through this wall to reach the stomach.
3. The materials within the tract should be kept moving forward, slowly but steadily, at a pace that permits all reactions to reach completion.

digestion: the process by which food is broken down into absorbable units.
- **digestion** = take apart

absorption: the uptake of nutrients by the cells of the small intestine for transport into either the blood or the lymph.
- **absorb** = suck in

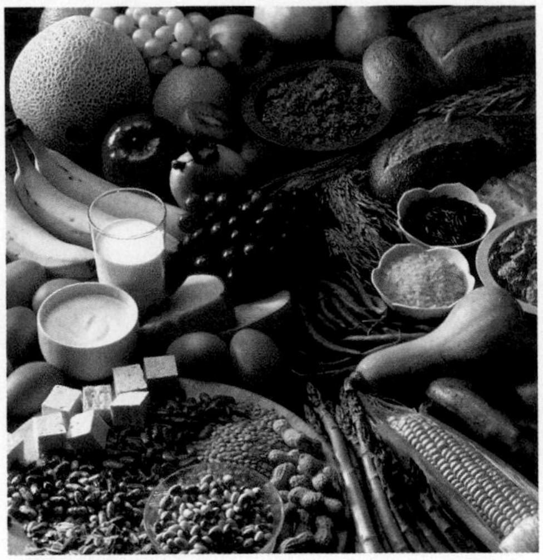
© Joe Pellegrini/FoodPix/Getty Images

The process of digestion transforms all kinds of *foods* into *nutrients.*

4. To move through the system, food must be lubricated with fluids. Too much would form a liquid that would flow too rapidly; too little would form a paste too dry and compact to move at all. The amount of fluids must be regulated to keep the intestinal contents at the right consistency to move smoothly along.
5. When the digestive enzymes are breaking food down, they need it in finely divided form, suspended in enough liquid so that every particle is accessible. Once digestion is complete and the needed nutrients have been absorbed out of the tract into the body, the system must excrete the residue that remains, but excreting all the water along with the solid residue would be both wasteful and messy. Some water should be withdrawn, leaving a paste just solid enough to be smooth and easy to pass.
6. The enzymes of the digestive tract are designed to digest carbohydrate, fat, and protein. The walls of the tract, composed of living cells, are also made of carbohydrate, fat, and protein. These cells need protection against the action of the powerful digestive juices that they secrete.
7. Once waste matter has reached the end of the tract, it must be excreted, but it would be inconvenient and embarrassing if this function occurred continuously. Provision must be made for periodic, voluntary evacuation.

The following sections show how the body elegantly and efficiently handles these obstacles.

Anatomy of the Digestive Tract

The **gastrointestinal (GI) tract** is a flexible muscular tube from the mouth, through the esophagus, stomach, small intestine, large intestine, and rectum to the anus. Figure 3-1 traces the path followed by food from one end to the other. In a sense, the human body surrounds the GI tract. The inner space within the GI tract, called the **lumen,** is continuous from one end to the other (GI anatomy terms appear in boldface type and are defined in the glossary below). Only when a nutrient or other substance penetrates the GI tract's wall does it enter the body proper; many materials pass through the GI tract without being digested or absorbed.

gastrointestinal (GI) tract: the digestive tract. The principal organs are the stomach and intestines.
- **gastro** = stomach
- **intestinalis** = intestine

GLOSSARY OF GI ANATOMY TERMS

These terms are listed in order from start to end of the digestive tract.

mouth: the oral cavity containing the tongue and teeth.

pharynx (FAIR-inks): the passageway leading from the nose and mouth to the larynx and esophagus, respectively.

epiglottis (epp-ee-GLOTT-iss): cartilage in the throat that guards the entrance to the trachea and prevents fluid or food from entering it when a person swallows.
- **epi** = upon (over)
- **glottis** = back of tongue

esophagus (ee-SOFF-ah-gus): the food pipe; the conduit from the mouth to the stomach.

sphincter (SFINK-ter): a circular muscle surrounding, and able to close, a body opening. Sphincters are found at specific points along the GI tract and regulate the flow of food particles.
- **sphincter** = band (binder)

esophageal (ee-SOF-ah-GEE-al) **sphincter:** a sphincter muscle at the upper or lower end of the esophagus. The *lower esophageal sphincter* is also called the *cardiac sphincter.*

stomach: a muscular, elastic, saclike portion of the digestive tract that grinds and churns swallowed food, mixing it with acid and enzymes to form chyme.

pyloric (pie-LORE-ic) **sphincter:** the circular muscle that separates the stomach from the small intestine and regulates the flow of partially digested food into the small intestine; also called *pylorus* or *pyloric valve.*
- **pylorus** = gatekeeper

gallbladder: the organ that stores and concentrates bile. When it receives the signal that fat is present in the duodenum, the gallbladder contracts and squirts bile through the bile duct into the duodenum.

pancreas: a gland that secretes digestive enzymes and juices into the duodenum.

small intestine: a 10-foot length of small-diameter intestine that is the major site of digestion of food and absorption of nutrients. Its segments are the duodenum, jejunum, and ileum.

lumen (LOO-men): the space within a vessel, such as the intestine.

duodenum (doo-oh-DEEN-um, doo-ODD-num): the top portion of the small intestine (about "12 fingers' breadth" long in ancient terminology).
- **duodecim** = twelve

jejunum (je-JOON-um): the first two-fifths of the small intestine beyond the duodenum.

ileum (ILL-ee-um): the last segment of the small intestine.

ileocecal (ill-ee-oh-SEEK-ul) **valve:** the sphincter separating the small and large intestines.

large intestine or **colon** (COAL-un): the lower portion of intestine that completes the digestive process. Its segments are the ascending colon, the transverse colon, the descending colon, and the sigmoid colon.
- **sigmoid** = shaped like the letter S (sigma in Greek)

appendix: a narrow blind sac extending from the beginning of the colon that stores lymph cells.

rectum: the muscular terminal part of the intestine, extending from the sigmoid colon to the anus.

anus (AY-nus): the terminal outlet of the GI tract.

FIGURE 3-1 The Gastrointestinal Tract

INGESTION ↓

Mouth
Chews and mixes food with saliva.

Pharynx
Directs food from mouth to esophagus.

Salivary glands
Secrete saliva (contains starch-digesting enzymes).

Epiglottis
Protects airway during swallowing.

Trachea
Allows air to pass to and from lungs.

Esophagus
Passes food from the mouth to the stomach.

Esophageal sphincters
Allow passage from mouth to esophagus and from esophagus to stomach. Prevent backflow from stomach to esophagus and from esophagus to mouth.

Stomach
Adds acid, enzymes, and fluid. Churns, mixes, and grinds food to a liquid mass.

Pyloric sphincter
Allows passage from stomach to small intestine. Prevents backflow from small intestine.

Liver
Manufactures bile salts, detergent-like substances, to help digest fats.

Gallbladder
Stores bile until needed.

Bile duct
Conducts bile from the gallbladder to the small intestine.

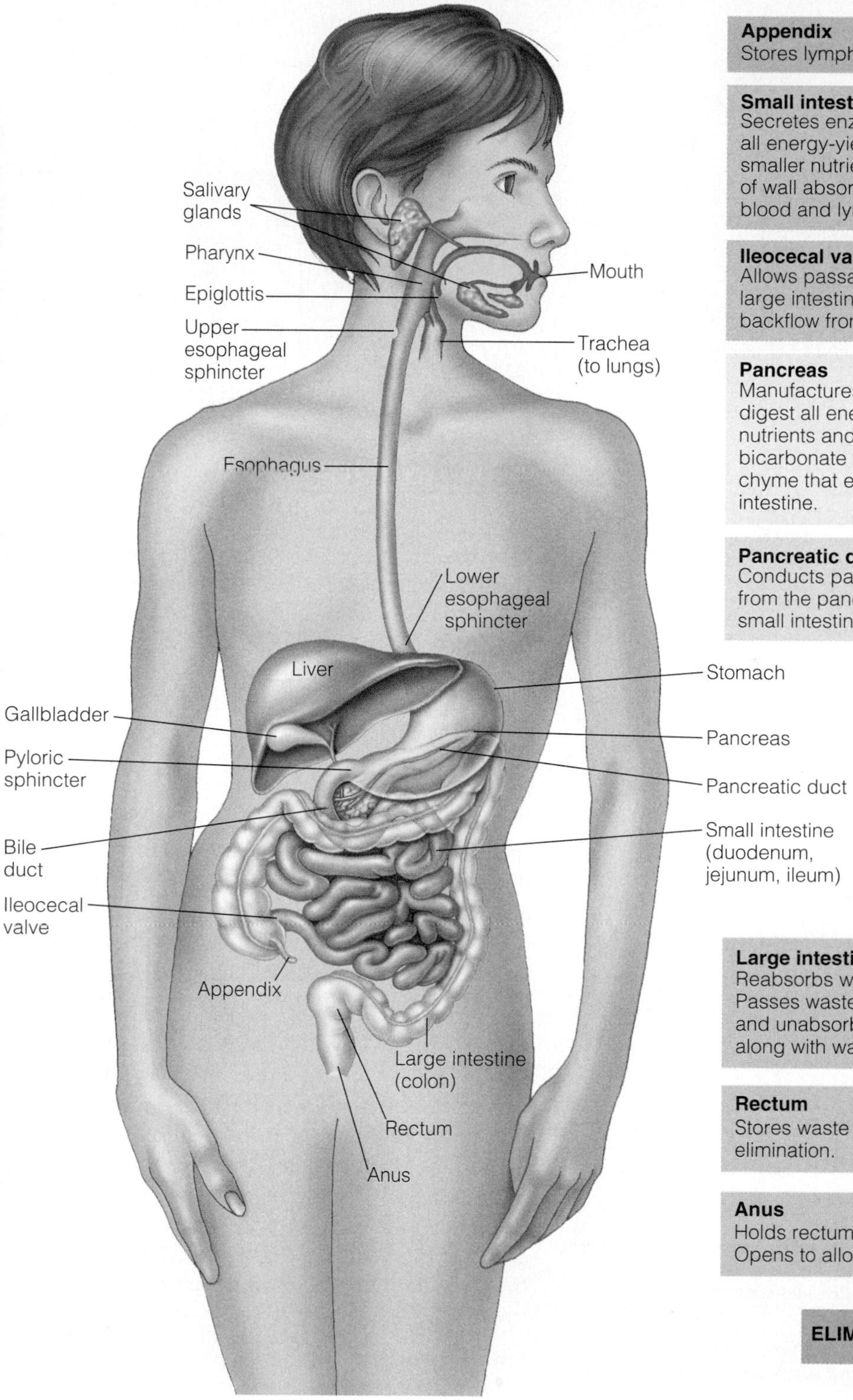

Salivary glands
Pharynx
Epiglottis
Upper esophageal sphincter
Mouth
Trachea (to lungs)
Esophagus
Lower esophageal sphincter
Liver
Gallbladder
Pyloric sphincter
Bile duct
Ileocecal valve
Appendix
Stomach
Pancreas
Pancreatic duct
Small intestine (duodenum, jejunum, ileum)
Large intestine (colon)
Rectum
Anus

Appendix
Stores lymph cells.

Small intestine
Secretes enzymes that digest all energy-yielding nutrients to smaller nutrient particles. Cells of wall absorb nutrients into blood and lymph.

Ileocecal valve (sphincter)
Allows passage from small to large intestine. Prevents backflow from large intestine.

Pancreas
Manufactures enzymes to digest all energy-yielding nutrients and releases bicarbonate to neutralize acid chyme that enters the small intestine.

Pancreatic duct
Conducts pancreatic juice from the pancreas to the small intestine.

Large intestine (colon)
Reabsorbs water and minerals. Passes waste (fiber, bacteria, and unabsorbed nutrients) along with water to the rectum.

Rectum
Stores waste prior to elimination.

Anus
Holds rectum closed. Opens to allow elimination.

ELIMINATION ↓

FIGURE 3-2 The Teeth

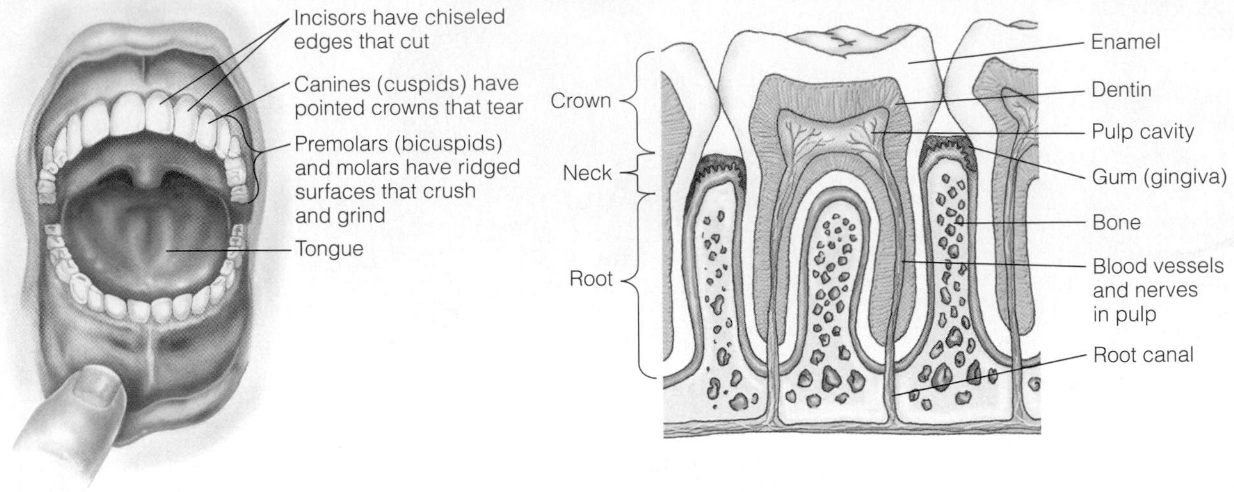
Incisors have chiseled edges that cut
Canines (cuspids) have pointed crowns that tear
Premolars (bicuspids) and molars have ridged surfaces that crush and grind
Tongue
Crown
Neck
Root
Enamel
Dentin
Pulp cavity
Gum (gingiva)
Bone
Blood vessels and nerves in pulp
Root canal

■ The process of chewing is called **mastication** (mass-tih-KAY-shun).

Mouth The process of digestion begins in the **mouth.** As you chew,■ your teeth crush large pieces of food into smaller ones (see Figure 3-2), and fluids blend with these pieces to ease swallowing. Fluids also help dissolve the food so that you can taste it; only particles in solution can react with taste buds. When stimulated, the taste buds detect one, or a combination, of the four basic taste sensations: sweet, sour, bitter, and salty. Some scientists also include the flavor associated with monosodium glutamate, sometimes called *savory* or its Asian name *umami* (ooh-MOM-ee). In addition to these chemical triggers, aroma, texture, and temperature also affect a food's flavor. In fact, the sense of smell is thousands of times more sensitive than the sense of taste.

The tongue allows you not only to taste food, but also to move food around the mouth, facilitating chewing and swallowing. When you swallow a mouthful of food, it passes through the **pharynx,** a short tube that is shared by both the **digestive system** and the respiration system. To bypass the entrance to your lungs, the **epiglottis** closes off your air passages so that you don't choke when you swallow, thus resolving obstacle 1. (Choking is discussed on pp. 94–95.) After a mouthful of food has been swallowed, it is called a **bolus.**

Esophagus to the Stomach The **esophagus** has a **sphincter** muscle at each end. During a swallow, the upper **esophageal sphincter** opens. The bolus then slides down the esophagus, which passes through a hole in the diaphragm (obstacle 2) to the **stomach.** The lower esophageal sphincter at the entrance to the stomach closes behind the bolus so that it proceeds forward and doesn't slip back into the esophagus (obstacle 3). The stomach retains the bolus for a while in its upper portion. Little by little, the stomach transfers the food to its lower portion, adds juices to it, and grinds it to a semiliquid mass called **chyme.** Then, bit by bit, the stomach releases the chyme through the **pyloric sphincter,** which opens into the **small intestine** and then closes behind the chyme.

Small Intestine At the top of the small intestine, the chyme bypasses the opening from the common bile duct, which is dripping fluids (obstacle 4) into the small intestine from two organs outside the GI tract—the **gallbladder** and the **pancreas.** The chyme travels on down the small intestine through its three segments—the **duodenum,** the **jejunum,** and the **ileum**—almost 10 feet of tubing coiled within the abdomen.*

digestive system: all the organs and glands associated with the ingestion and digestion of food.

bolus (BOH-lus): a portion; with respect to food, the amount swallowed at one time.
- **bolos** = lump

chyme (KIME): the semiliquid mass of partly digested food expelled by the stomach into the duodenum.
- **chymos** = juice

*The small intestine is almost two and a half times shorter in living adults than it is at death, when muscles are relaxed and elongated.

Large Intestine (Colon) Having traveled the length of the small intestine, what remains of the chyme arrives at another sphincter (obstacle 3 again): the **ileocecal valve,** at the beginning of the **large intestine (colon)** in the lower right-hand side of the abdomen. As the chyme enters the colon, it passes another opening. Had it slipped into this opening, it would have ended up in the **appendix,** a blind sac about the size of your little finger. The chyme bypasses this opening, however, and travels along the large intestine up the right-hand side of the abdomen, across the front to the left-hand side, down to the lower left-hand side, and finally below the other folds of the intestines to the back side of the body, above the **rectum.**

During the chyme's passage to the rectum, the colon withdraws water from it, leaving semisolid waste (obstacle 5). The strong muscles of the rectum and anal canal hold back this waste until it is time to defecate. Then the rectal muscles relax (obstacle 7), and the two sphincters of the **anus** open to allow passage of the waste.

The Muscular Action of Digestion

The first step in the reduction of food to a liquid takes place in the mouth, where chewing, the addition of saliva, and the action of the tongue reduce the food to a coarse mash. Then you swallow, and thereafter, you are generally unaware of all the activity that follows. As is the case with so much else that happens in the body, the muscles of the digestive tract meet internal needs without your having to exert any conscious effort. They keep things moving■ at just the right pace, slow enough to get the job done and fast enough to make progress.

■ The ability of the GI tract muscles to move is called their **motility** (moh-TIL-ah-tee).

Peristalsis The entire GI tract is ringed with circular muscles that can squeeze it tightly. Surrounding these rings of muscle are longitudinal muscles. When the rings tighten and the long muscles relax, the tube is constricted. When the rings relax and the long muscles tighten, the tube bulges. This action—called **peristalsis**—occurs continuously and pushes the intestinal contents along (obstacle 3 again). (If you have ever watched a lump of food pass along the body of a snake, you have a good picture of how these muscles work.)

The waves of contraction ripple along the GI tract at varying rates and intensities depending on the part of the GI tract and on whether food is present. For example, waves occur three times per minute in the stomach, but speed up to ten times per minute when chyme reaches the small intestine. When you have just eaten a meal, the waves are slow and continuous; when the GI tract is empty, the intestine is quiet except for periodic bursts of powerful rhythmic waves. Peristalsis, along with the sphincter muscles that surround the digestive tract at key places, keeps things moving along.

FIGURE 3-3 Stomach Muscles

The stomach has three layers of muscles.

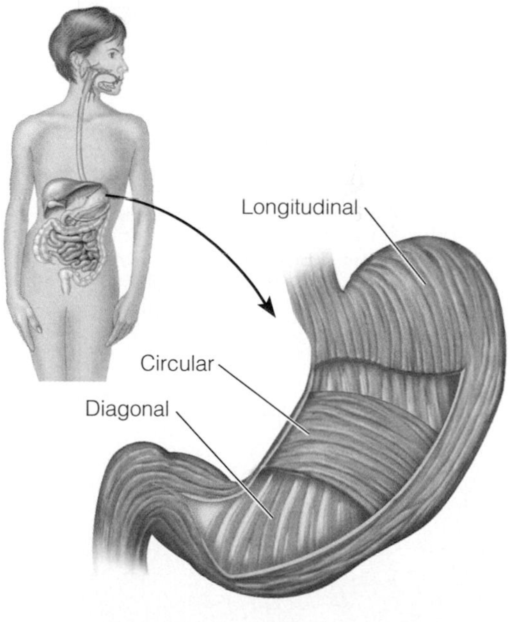
Longitudinal
Circular
Diagonal

Stomach Action The stomach has the thickest walls and strongest muscles of all the GI tract organs. In addition to the circular and longitudinal muscles, it has a third layer of diagonal muscles that also alternately contract and relax (see Figure 3-3). These three sets of muscles work to force the chyme downward, but the pyloric sphincter usually remains tightly closed, preventing the chyme from passing into the duodenum of the small intestine. As a result, the chyme is churned and forced down, hits the pyloric sphincter, and remains in the stomach. Meanwhile, the stomach wall releases gastric juices. When the chyme is completely liquefied, the pyloric sphincter opens briefly, about three times a minute, to allow small portions of chyme through. At this point, the chyme no longer resembles food in the least.

Segmentation The circular muscles of the intestines rhythmically contract and squeeze their contents. These contractions, called **segmentation,** mix the chyme and promote close contact with the digestive juices and the absorbing cells of the intestinal walls before letting the contents move slowly along. Figure 3-4 illustrates peristalsis and segmentation.

peristalsis (per-ih-STALL-sis): wavelike muscular contractions of the GI tract that push its contents along.
- **peri** = around
- **stellein** = wrap

segmentation (SEG-men-TAY-shun): a periodic squeezing or partitioning of the intestine at intervals along its length by its circular muscles.

FIGURE 3-4 Peristalsis & Segmentation

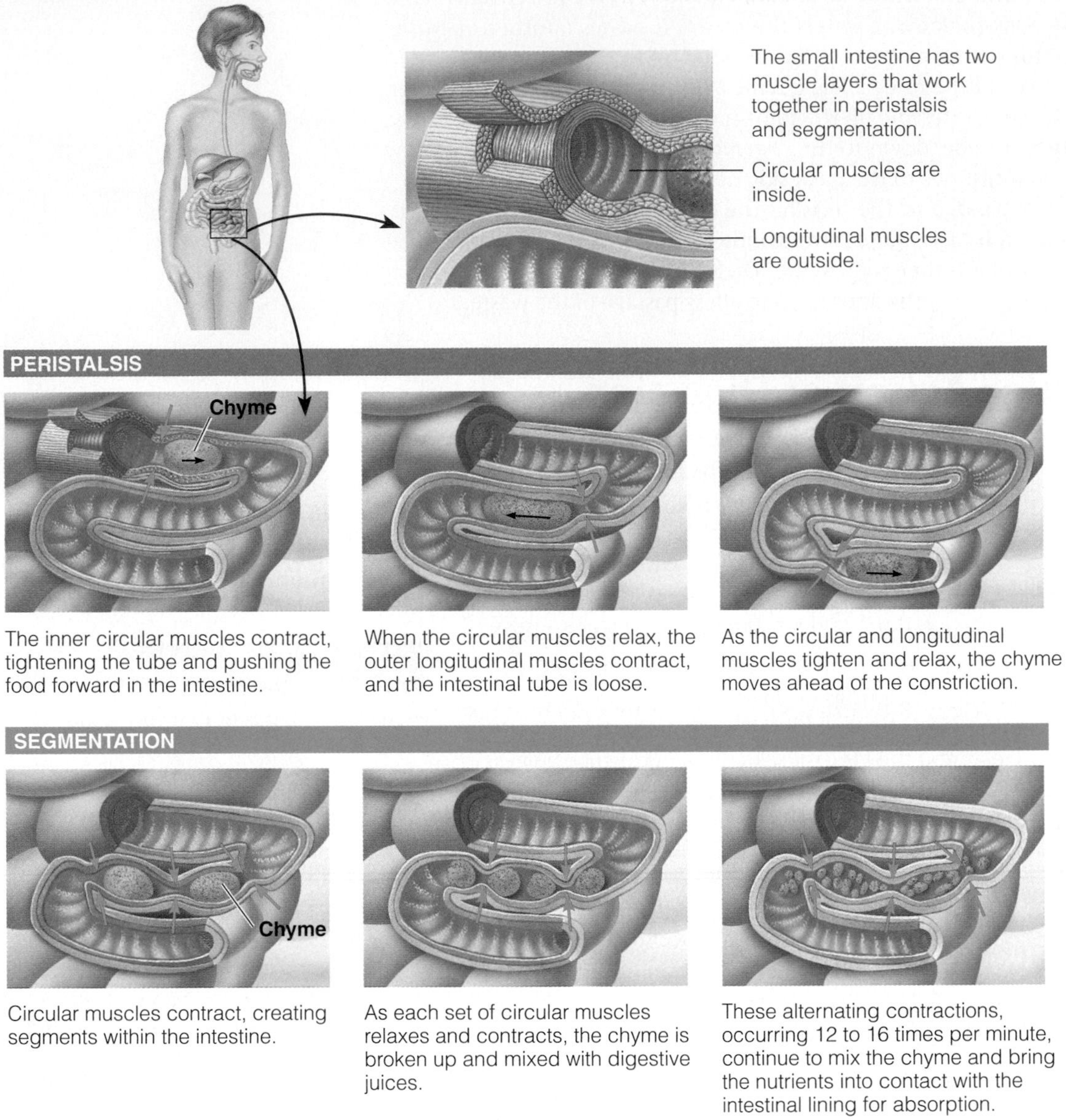
The small intestine has two muscle layers that work together in peristalsis and segmentation.
Circular muscles are inside.
Longitudinal muscles are outside.
PERISTALSIS
Chyme
The inner circular muscles contract, tightening the tube and pushing the food forward in the intestine.
When the circular muscles relax, the outer longitudinal muscles contract, and the intestinal tube is loose.
As the circular and longitudinal muscles tighten and relax, the chyme moves ahead of the constriction.
SEGMENTATION
Chyme
Circular muscles contract, creating segments within the intestine.
As each set of circular muscles relaxes and contracts, the chyme is broken up and mixed with digestive juices.
These alternating contractions, occurring 12 to 16 times per minute, continue to mix the chyme and bring the nutrients into contact with the intestinal lining for absorption.

Sphincter Contractions Sphincter muscles periodically open and close, allowing the contents of the GI tract to move along at a controlled pace (obstacle 3 again). At the top of the esophagus, the upper esophageal sphincter opens in response to swallowing. At the bottom of the esophagus, the lower esophageal sphincter (sometimes called the cardiac sphincter because of its proximity to the heart) prevents **reflux** of the stomach contents. At the bottom of the stomach, the pyloric sphincter, which stays closed most of the time, holds the chyme in the stomach long enough for it to be thoroughly mixed with gastric juice and liquefied. The pyloric sphincter also prevents the intestinal contents from backing up into the stomach. At the end of the small intestine, the ileocecal valve performs a similar function, emptying the contents of the small intestine into the large intestine. Finally, the tightness of the rectal muscle is a kind of safety device; together with the two sphincters of the anus, it prevents elimination until you choose to perform

reflux: a backward flow.
- **re** = back
- **flux** = flow

FIGURE 3-5 An Example of a Sphincter Muscle

When the circular muscles of a sphincter contract, the passage closes; when they relax, the passage opens.

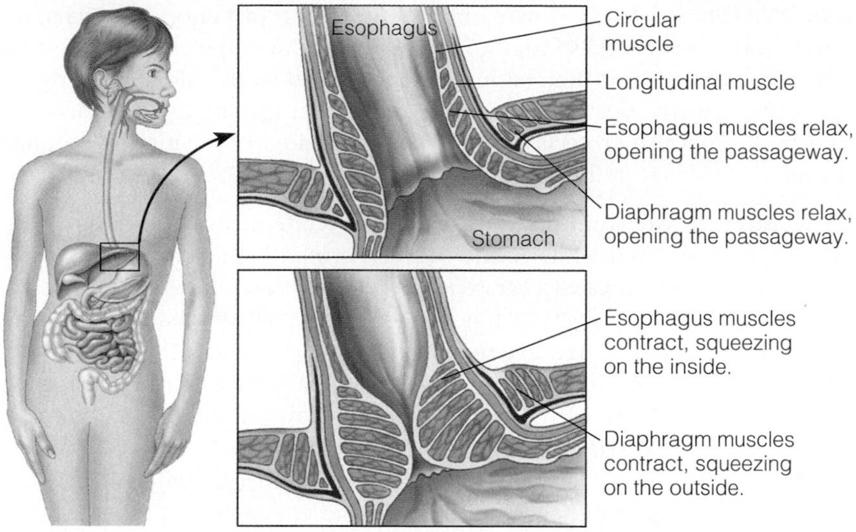
Esophagus
Circular muscle
Longitudinal muscle
Esophagus muscles relax, opening the passageway.
Diaphragm muscles relax, opening the passageway.
Stomach
Esophagus muscles contract, squeezing on the inside.
Diaphragm muscles contract, squeezing on the outside.

it voluntarily (obstacle 7). Figure 3-5 illustrates how sphincter muscles contract and relax to close and open passageways.

The Secretions of Digestion

To break down food into small nutrients that the body can absorb, five different organs produce secretions: the salivary glands, the stomach, the pancreas, the liver (via the gallbladder), and the small intestine. These secretions enter the GI tract at various points along the way, bringing an abundance of water (obstacle 3 again) and a variety of enzymes.

Enzymes■ are formally introduced in Chapter 6, but for now a simple definition will suffice. An enzyme is a protein that facilitates a chemical reaction—making a molecule, breaking a molecule, changing the arrangement of a molecule, or exchanging parts of molecules. As a **catalyst,** the enzyme itself remains unchanged. The enzymes involved in digestion facilitate a chemical reaction known as **hydrolysis**—the addition of water *(hydro)* to break *(lysis)* a molecule into smaller pieces. The glossary below identifies some of the common **digestive enzymes** and related terms; later chapters introduce specific enzymes. When learning about enzymes, it

■ All enzymes and some hormones are proteins, but enzymes are not hormones. Enzymes facilitate the making and breaking of bonds in chemical reactions; hormones act as chemical messengers, sometimes regulating enzyme action.

catalyst (CAT-uh-list): a compound that facilitates chemical reactions without itself being changed in the process.

GLOSSARY OF DIGESTIVE ENZYMES

digestive enzymes: proteins found in digestive juices that act on food substances, causing them to break down into simpler compounds.

-ase (ACE): a word ending denoting an enzyme. The word beginning often identifies the compounds the enzyme works on. Examples include:
- **carbohydrase** (KAR-boe-HIGH-drase), an enzyme that hydrolyzes carbohydrates.
- **lipase** (LYE-pase), an enzyme that hydrolyzes lipids (fats).
- **protease** (PRO-tee-ase), an enzyme that hydrolyzes proteins.

hydrolysis (high-DROL-ih-sis): a chemical reaction in which a major reactant is split into two products, with the addition of a hydrogen atom (H) to one and a hydroxyl group (OH) to the other (from water, H_2O). (The noun is **hydrolysis;** the verb is **hydrolyze.**)
- **hydro** = water
- **lysis** = breaking

FIGURE 3-6 The Salivary Glands

The salivary glands secrete saliva into the mouth and begin the digestive process. Given the short time food is in the mouth, salivary enzymes contribute little to digestion.

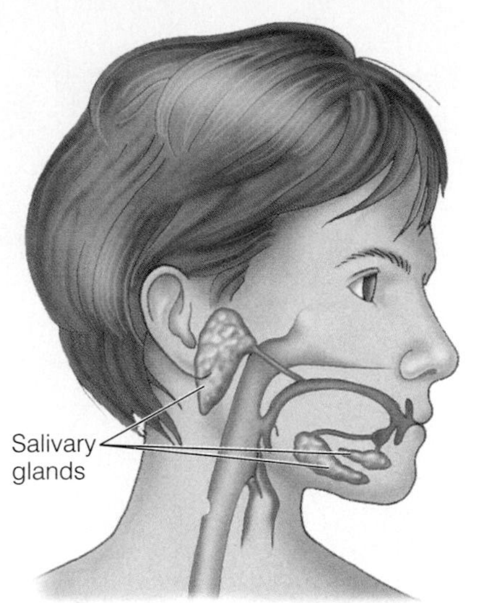
Salivary
glands

helps to know that the word ending *-ase* denotes an enzyme. Enzymes are often identified by the organ they come from and the compounds they work on; *gastric lipase,* for example, is a stomach enzyme that acts on lipids, whereas *pancreatic lipase* comes from the pancreas (and also works on lipids).

Saliva The **salivary glands,** shown in Figure 3-6, squirt just enough **saliva** to moisten each mouthful of food so that it can pass easily down the esophagus (obstacle 4). (Digestive glands and their secretions are defined in the glossary below.) The saliva contains water, salts, mucus, and enzymes that initiate the digestion of carbohydrates. Saliva also protects the teeth and the linings of the mouth, esophagus, and stomach from attack by substances that might harm them.

Gastric Juice In the stomach, **gastric glands** secrete **gastric juice,** a mixture of water, enzymes, and **hydrochloric acid** that acts primarily in protein digestion. The acid is so strong that it causes the sensation of heartburn if it happens to reflux into the esophagus. Highlight 3, following this chapter, discusses heartburn, ulcers, and other common digestive problems.■

The strong acidity of the stomach prevents bacterial growth and kills most bacteria that enter the body with food. It would destroy the cells of the stomach as well, but for their natural defenses. To protect themselves from gastric juice, the cells of the stomach wall secrete **mucus,** a thick, slippery, white substance that coats the cells, protecting them from the acid and enzymes that might otherwise harm them (obstacle 6).

Figure 3-7 shows how the strength of acids is measured—in **pH** units. Note that the acidity of gastric juice registers below "2" on the pH scale—stronger than vinegar. The stomach enzymes work most efficiently in the stomach's strong acid, but the salivary enzymes, which are swallowed with food, do not work in acid this strong. Consequently, the salivary digestion of carbohydrate gradually ceases as the stomach acid penetrates each newly swallowed bolus of food. In fact, salivary enzymes become just other proteins to be digested.

■ Chapters 23 and 24 describe medical conditions that impair GI functions and dietary approaches that ease symptoms and prevent malnutrition.

pH: the unit of measure expressing a substance's acidity or alkalinity (Chapter 12 provides a more detailed definition).

Pancreatic Juice and Intestinal Enzymes By the time food leaves the stomach, digestion of all three energy nutrients (carbohydrates, fats, and proteins) has begun, and the action gains momentum in the small intestine. There the pancreas contributes digestive juices by way of ducts leading into the duodenum. The **pancreatic juice** contains enzymes that act on all three energy nutrients, and the cells of the intestinal wall also possess digestive enzymes on their surfaces.

GLOSSARY OF DIGESTIVE GLANDS AND THEIR SECRETIONS

These terms are listed in order from start to end of the digestive tract.

gland: a cell or group of cells that secretes materials for special uses in the body. Glands may be **exocrine** (EKS-oh-crin) **glands,** secreting their materials "out" (into the digestive tract or onto the surface of the skin), or **endocrine** (EN-doe-crin) **glands,** secreting their materials "in" (into the blood).
- **exo** = outside
- **endo** = inside
- **krine** = to separate

salivary glands: exocrine glands that secrete saliva into the mouth.

saliva: the secretion of the salivary glands. Its principal enzyme begins carbohydrate digestion.

gastric glands: exocrine glands in the stomach wall that secrete gastric juice into the stomach.
- **gastro** = stomach

gastric juice: the digestive secretion of the gastric glands of the stomach.

hydrochloric acid: an acid composed of hydrogen and chloride atoms (HCl). The gastric glands normally produce this acid.

mucus (MYOO-kus): a slippery substance secreted by cells of the GI lining (and other body linings) that protects the cells from exposure to digestive juices (and other destructive agents). The lining of the GI tract with its coat of mucus is a **mucous membrane.** (The noun is **mucus;** the adjective is **mucous.**)

liver: the organ that manufactures bile. (The liver's many other functions are described in Chapter 7.)

bile: an emulsifier that prepares fats and oils for digestion; an exocrine secretion made by the liver, stored in the gallbladder, and released into the small intestine when needed.

emulsifier (ee-MUL-sih-fire): a substance with both water-soluble and fat-soluble portions that promotes the mixing of oils and fats in a watery solution.

pancreatic (pank-ree-AT-ic) **juice:** the exocrine secretion of the pancreas, containing enzymes for the digestion of carbohydrate, fat, and protein as well as bicarbonate, a neutralizing agent. The juice flows from the pancreas into the small intestine through the pancreatic duct. (The pancreas also has an endocrine function, the secretion of insulin and other hormones.)

bicarbonate: an alkaline secretion of the pancreas, part of the pancreatic juice. (Bicarbonate also occurs widely in all cell fluids.)

In addition to enzymes, the pancreatic juice contains sodium **bicarbonate,** which is basic or alkaline—the opposite of the stomach's acid (review Figure 3-7). The pancreatic juice thus neutralizes the acid chyme arriving in the small intestine from the stomach. From this point on, the chyme remains at a neutral or slightly alkaline pH. The enzymes of both the intestine and the pancreas work best in this environment.

Bile **Bile** also flows into the duodenum. The **liver** continuously produces bile, which is then concentrated and stored in the gallbladder. The gallbladder squirts the bile into the duodenum when fat arrives there. Bile is not an enzyme, but an **emulsifier** that brings fats into suspension in water so that enzymes can break them down into their component parts. Thanks to all these secretions, the three energy-yielding nutrients are digested in the small intestine (the summary on p. 82 provides a table of digestive secretions and their actions).

Protective Factors Both the small and the large intestine, being neutral in pH, permit the growth of bacteria (known as the intestinal flora). In fact, a healthy intestinal tract supports a thriving bacterial population that normally does the body no harm and may actually do some good. Bacteria in the GI tract produce several vitamins,■ including a significant amount of vitamin K, although the amount is insufficient to meet the body's total need for that vitamin.

Provided that the normal intestinal flora are thriving, infectious bacteria have a hard time getting established and launching an attack on the system. Diet is one of several factors that influence the bacterial population and its environment. For example, GI bacteria digest some dietary fibers and produce short fragments of fat that the cells of the colon use for energy.* In addition to diet, secretions from the GI tract—saliva, mucus, gastric acid, and digestive enzymes—not only help with digestion, but also defend against foreign invaders. The GI tract also maintains several different kinds of defending cells that confer specific immunity against intestinal diseases such as inflammatory bowel disease.

FIGURE 3-7 The pH Scale

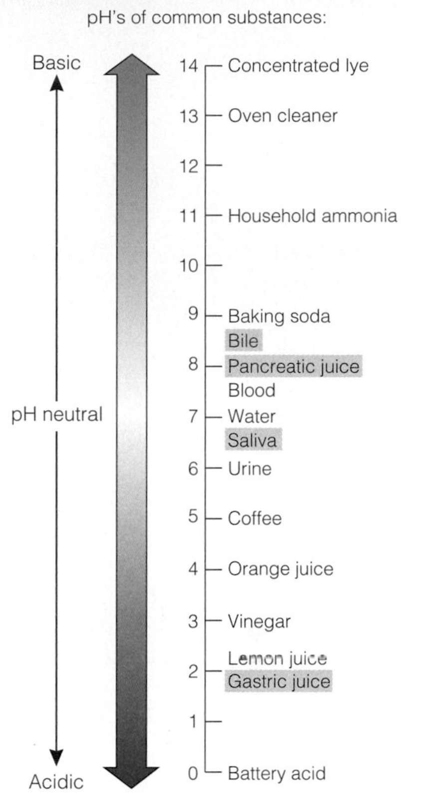
pH's of common substances:
Basic
pH neutral
Acidic
14 Concentrated lye
13 Oven cleaner
12
11 Household ammonia
10
9 Baking soda
Bile
8 Pancreatic juice
Blood
7 Water
Saliva
6 Urine
5 Coffee
4 Orange juice
3 Vinegar
Lemon juice
2 Gastric juice
1
0 Battery acid

A substance's acidity or alkalinity is measured in pH units. The pH is the negative logarithm of the hydrogen ion concentration. Each increment presents a tenfold increase in concentration of hydrogen particles. For example, a pH of 2 is 1000 times stronger than a pH of 5.

■ Vitamins produced by bacteria include:
- Biotin.
- Folate.
- Vitamin B_6.
- Vitamin B_{12}.
- Vitamin K.

The Final Stage

At this point, the three energy-yielding nutrients—carbohydrate, fat, and protein—have been disassembled and are ready to be absorbed. Most of the other nutrients—vitamins, minerals, and water—need no such disassembly; some vitamins and minerals are altered slightly during digestion, but most are absorbed as they are. Undigested residues, such as some fibers, are not absorbed, but continue through the digestive tract, providing a semisolid mass that helps exercise the muscles and keep them strong enough to perform peristalsis efficiently. Fiber also retains water, accounting for the pasty consistency of **stools,** and carries some bile acids, some minerals, and some additives and contaminants with it out of the body.

By the time the contents of the GI tract reach the end of the small intestine, little remains but water, a few dissolved salts and body secretions, and undigested materials such as fiber. These enter the large intestine (colon).

In the colon, intestinal bacteria ferment some fibers, producing water, gas, and small fragments of fat that provide energy for the cells of the colon. The colon itself retrieves all materials that the body can recycle—water and dissolved salts (see Figure 3-8). The waste that is finally excreted has little or nothing of value left in it. The body has extracted all that it can use from the food. Figure 3-9 summarizes digestion by following a sandwich through the GI tract and into the body.

stools: waste matter discharged from the colon; also called **feces** (FEE-seez).

*These small fragments of fat are short-chain fatty acids, described in Chapter 5.

FIGURE 3-8 The Colon

The colon begins with the ascending colon rising upward toward the liver. It becomes the transverse colon as it turns and crosses the body toward the spleen. The descending colon turns downward and becomes the sigmoid colon, which extends to the rectum. Along the way, the colon mixes the intestinal contents, absorbs water and salts, and forms stools.

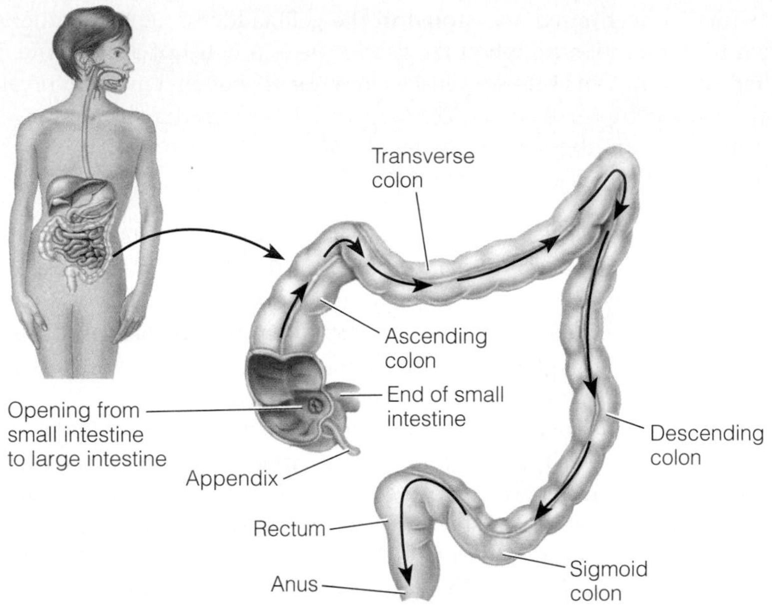
Transverse colon
Ascending colon
End of small intestine
Opening from small intestine to large intestine
Appendix
Descending colon
Rectum
Anus
Sigmoid colon

Available Online

http://nutrition.wadsworth.com/uncn7
Follow the movement of a bolus of food as it moves through the GI tract. Along the way the functions of the primary organs involved in digestion are illustrated.

IN SUMMARY As Figure 3-1 shows, food enters the mouth and travels down the esophagus and through the upper and lower esophageal sphincters to the stomach, then through the pyloric sphincter to the small intestine, on through the ileocecal valve to the large intestine, past the appendix to the rectum, ending at the anus. The wavelike contractions of peristalsis and the periodic squeezing of segmentation keep things moving at a reasonable pace. Along the way, secretions from the salivary glands, stomach, pancreas, liver (via the gallbladder), and small intestine deliver fluids and digestive enzymes.

Summary of Digestive Secretions and Their Actions

Organ or Gland	Target Organ	Secretion	Action
Salivary glands	Mouth	Saliva	Fluid eases swallowing; salivary enzyme breaks down **carbohydrate.**
Gastric glands	Stomach	Gastric juice	Fluid mixes with bolus; hydrochloric acid uncoils **proteins;** enzymes break down proteins; mucus protects stomach cells.
Pancreas	Small intestine	Pancreatic juice	Bicarbonate neutralizes acidic gastric juices; pancreatic enzymes break down **carbohydrates, fats,** and **proteins.**
Liver	Gallbladder	Bile	Bile stored until needed.
Gallbladder	Small intestine	Bile	Bile emulsifies **fat** so enzymes can attack.
Intestinal glands	Small intestine	Intestinal juice	Intestinal enzymes break down **carbohydrate, fat,** and **protein** fragments; mucus protects the intestinal wall.

FIGURE 3-9 The Digestive Fate of a Sandwich

To review the digestive processes, follow a peanut butter and banana sandwich on whole-wheat, seasame seed bread through the GI tract.

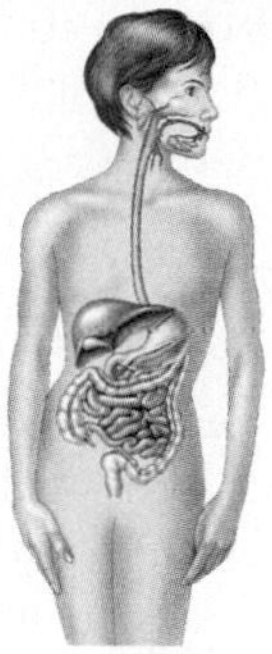

MOUTH: CHEWING AND SWALLOWING, WITH LITTLE DIGESTION

Carbohydrate digestion begins as the salivary enzyme starts to break down the starch from bread and peanut butter.
Fiber covering on the sesame seeds is crushed by the teeth, which exposes the nutrients inside the seeds to the upcoming digestive enzymes.

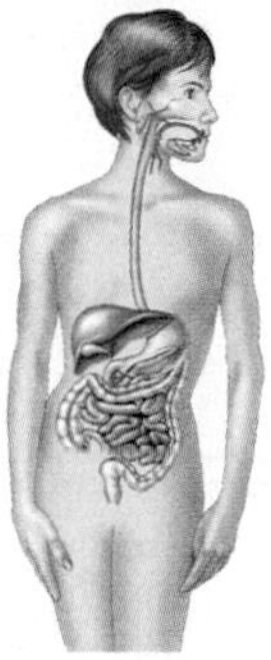

STOMACH: COLLECTING AND CHURNING, WITH SOME DIGESTION

Carbohydrate digestion continues until the mashed sandwich has been mixed with the gastric juices; the stomach acid of the gastric juices inactivates the salivary enzyme, and carbohydrate digestion ceases.
Proteins from the bread, seeds, and peanut butter begin to uncoil when they mix with the gastric acid, making them available to the gastric protease enzymes that begin to digest proteins.
Fat from the peanut butter forms a separate layer on top of the watery mixture.

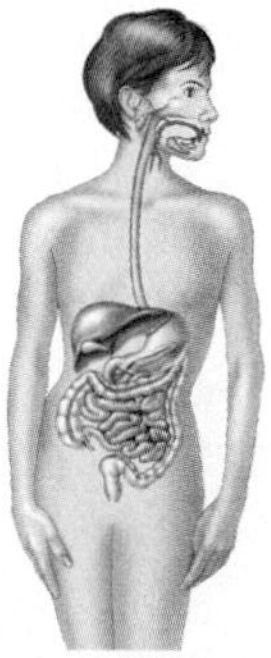

SMALL INTESTINE: DIGESTING AND ABSORBING

Sugars from the banana require so little digestion that they begin to traverse the intestinal cells immediately on contact.
Starch digestion picks up when the pancreas sends pancreatic enzymes to the small intestine via the pancreatic duct. Enzymes on the surfaces of the small intestinal cells complete the process of breaking down starch into small fragments that can be absorbed through the intestinal cell walls and into the portal vein.
Fat from the peanut butter and seeds is emulsified with the watery digestive fluids by bile. Now the pancreatic and intestinal lipases can begin to break down the fat to smaller fragments that can be absorbed through the cells of the small intestinal wall and into the lymph.
Protein digestion depends on the pancreatic and intestinal proteases. Small fragments of protein are liberated and absorbed through the cells of the small intestinal wall and into the portal vein.
Vitamins and minerals are absorbed.

Note: Sugars and starches are members of the carbohydrate family.

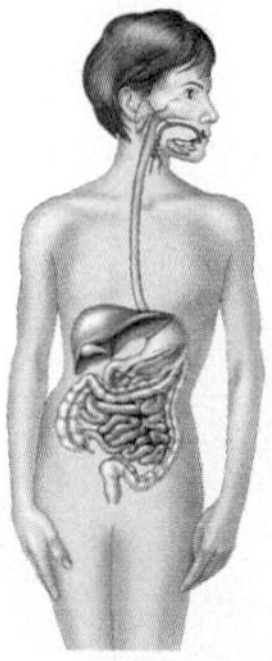

LARGE INTESTINE: REABSORBING AND ELIMINATING

Fluids and some minerals are absorbed.
Some fibers from the seeds, whole-wheat bread, peanut butter, and banana are partly digested by the bacteria living there, and some of these products are absorbed.
Most fibers pass through the large intestine and are excreted as feces; some fat, cholesterol, and minerals bind to fiber and are also excreted.

Absorption

Within three or four hours after you have eaten a dinner of beans and rice (or spinach lasagna, or steak and potatoes) with vegetable, salad, beverage, and dessert, your body must find a way to absorb the molecules derived from carbohydrate, protein, and fat digestion—and the vitamin and mineral molecules as well. Most absorption takes place in the small intestine, one of the most elegantly designed organ systems in the

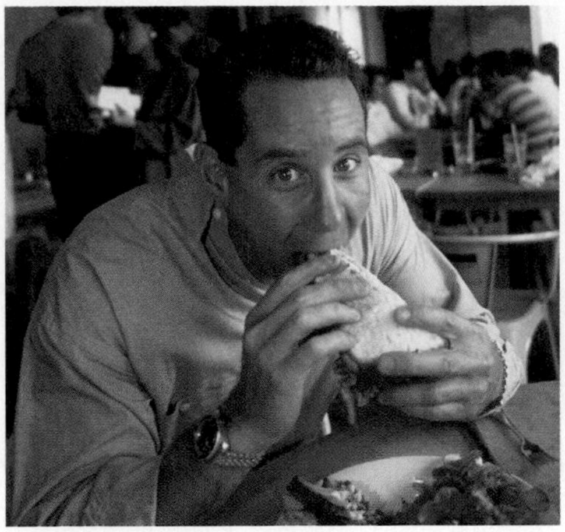

Food must be digested and absorbed before the body can use it.

body. Within its 10-foot length, which provides a surface area equivalent to a tennis court, the small intestine engulfs and absorbs the nutrient molecules. To remove the molecules rapidly and provide room for more to be absorbed, a rush of circulating blood continuously washes the underside of this surface, carrying the absorbed nutrients away to the liver and other parts of the body. Figure 3-10 describes how nutrients are absorbed by simple diffusion, facilitated diffusion, or active transport. Later chapters provide details on specific nutrients. Before following nutrients through the body, we must look more closely at the anatomy of the absorptive system.

Anatomy of the Absorptive System

The inner surface of the small intestine looks smooth and slippery, but viewed through a microscope, it turns out to be wrinkled into hundreds of folds. Each fold in turn is contoured into thousands of fingerlike projections, as numerous as the hairs on velvet fabric. These small intestinal projections are the **villi.** A single villus, magnified still more, turns out to be composed of hundreds of cells, each covered with its own microscopic hairs, the **microvilli** (see Figure 3-11). In the crevices between the villi lie the **crypts**—tubular glands that secrete the intestinal juices into the small intestine. Near by **goblet cells** secrete mucus.

The villi are in constant motion. Each villus is lined by a thin sheet of muscle, so it can wave, squirm, and wriggle like the tentacles of a sea anemone. Any nutrient molecule small enough to be absorbed is trapped among the microvilli that coat the cells and then drawn into the cells. Some partially digested nutrients are caught in the microvilli, digested further by enzymes there, and then absorbed into the cells.

villi (VILL-ee, VILL-eye): fingerlike projections from the folds of the small intestine; singular **villus.**

microvilli (MY-cro-VILL-ee, MY-cro-VILL-eye): tiny, hairlike projections on each cell of every villus that can trap nutrient particles and transport them into the cells; singular **microvillus.**

crypts (KRIPTS): tubular glands that lie between the intestinal villi and secrete intestinal juices into the small intestine.

goblet cells: cells of the GI tract (and lungs) that secrete mucus.

A Closer Look at the Intestinal Cells

The cells of the villi are among the most amazing in the body, for they recognize and select the nutrients the body needs and regulate their absorption. As already described, each cell of a villus is coated with thousands of microvilli, which project from the cell's membrane (review Figure 3-11). In these microvilli and in the membrane lie hundreds of different kinds of enzymes and "pumps," which recognize

FIGURE 3-10 Absorption of Nutrients

Absorption of nutrients into intestinal cells typically occurs by simple diffusion, facilitated diffusion, or active transport.

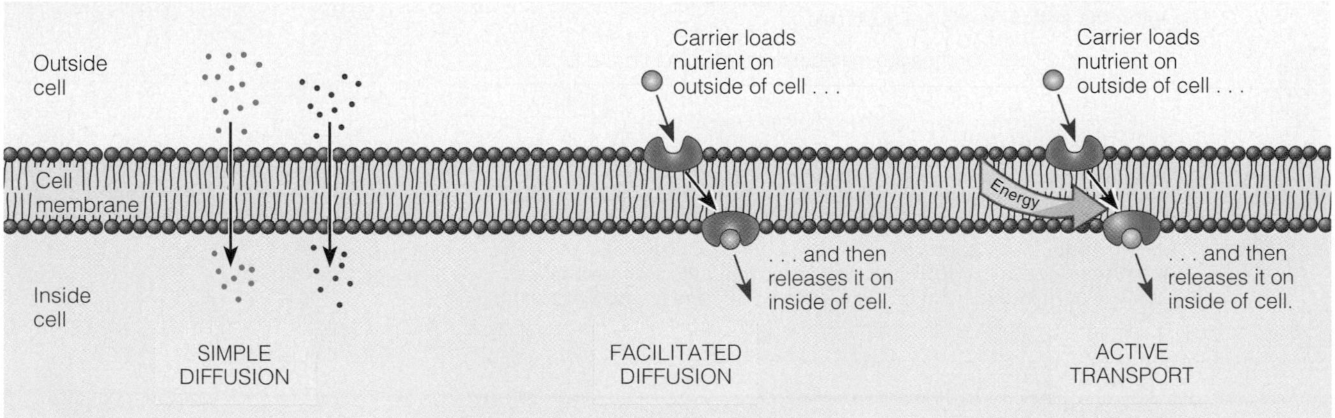
Outside cell
Cell membrane
Inside cell
SIMPLE DIFFUSION
Carrier loads nutrient on outside of cell . . .
. . . and then releases it on inside of cell.
FACILITATED DIFFUSION
Carrier loads nutrient on outside of cell . . .
Energy
. . . and then releases it on inside of cell.
ACTIVE TRANSPORT

Some nutrients (such as water and small lipids) are absorbed by simple diffusion. They cross into intestinal cells freely.

Some nutrients (such as the water-soluble vitamins) are absorbed by facilitated diffusion. They need a specific carrier to transport them from one side of the cell membrane to the other. (Alternatively, facilitated diffusion may occur when the carrier changes the cell membrane in such a way that the nutrients can pass through.)

Some nutrients (such as glucose and amino acids) must be absorbed actively. These nutrients move against a concentration gradient, which requires energy.

FIGURE 3-11 The Small Intestinal Villi

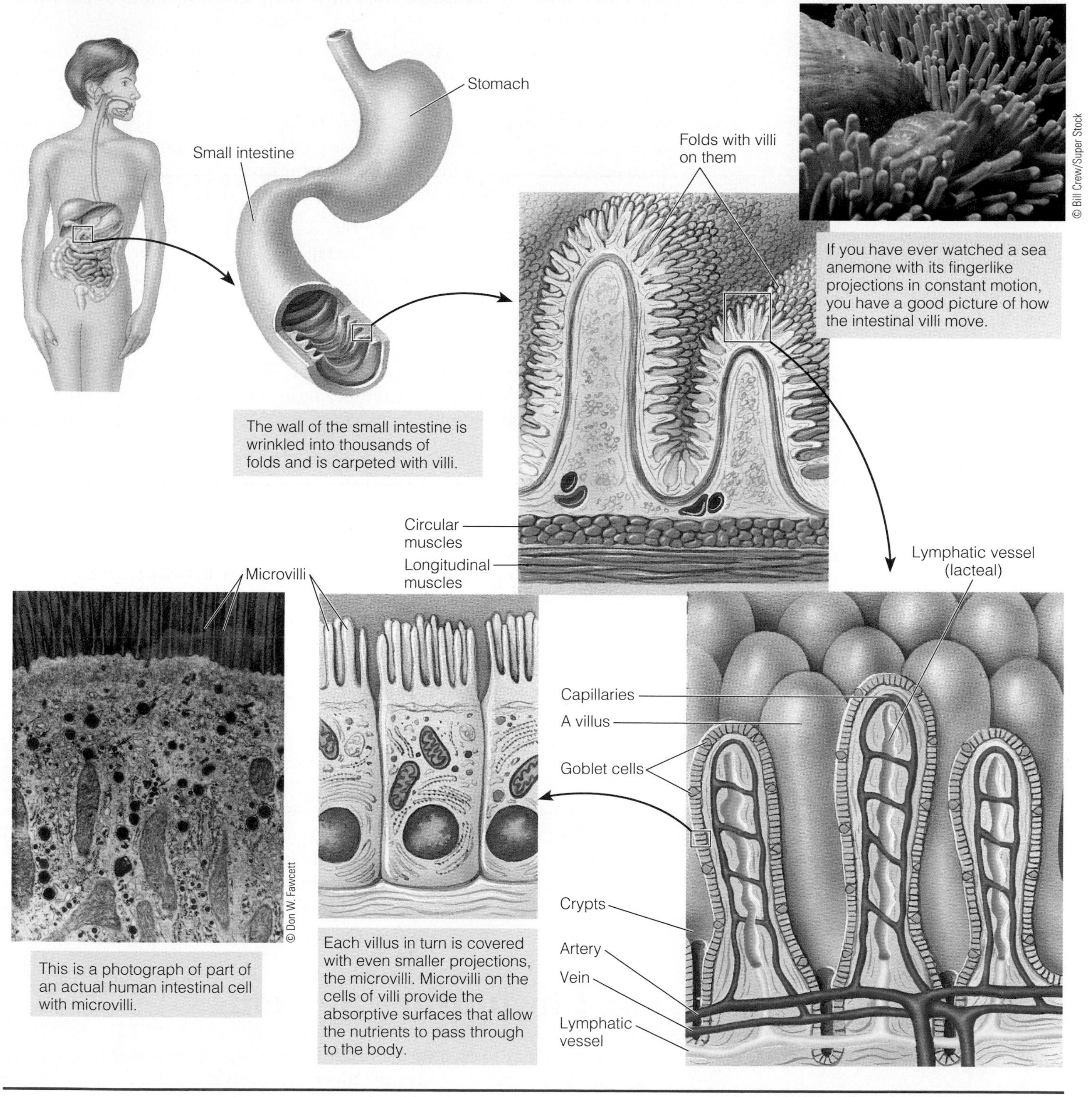
Stomach
Small intestine
Folds with villi on them
© Bill Crew/Super Stock
If you have ever watched a sea anemone with its fingerlike projections in constant motion, you have a good picture of how the intestinal villi move.
The wall of the small intestine is wrinkled into thousands of folds and is carpeted with villi.
Circular muscles
Longitudinal muscles
Lymphatic vessel (lacteal)
Microvilli
Microvilli
Capillaries
A villus
Goblet cells
Crypts
Artery
Vein
Lymphatic vessel
© Don W. Fawcett
This is a photograph of part of an actual human intestinal cell with microvilli.
Each villus in turn is covered with even smaller projections, the microvilli. Microvilli on the cells of villi provide the absorptive surfaces that allow the nutrients to pass through to the body.

and act on different nutrients. Descriptions of specific enzymes and "pumps" for each nutrient are presented in the following chapters where appropriate, but the point here is that the cells are equipped to handle all kinds and combinations of foods and nutrients.

Specialization in the GI Tract A further refinement of the system is that the cells of successive portions of the intestinal tract are specialized to absorb different nutrients. The nutrients that are ready for absorption early are absorbed near the top of the tract; those that take longer to be digested are absorbed farther down. Registered dietitians and medical professionals who treat digestive disorders learn the specialized absorptive functions of different parts of the GI tract so that if one part becomes dysfunctional, the diet can be adjusted accordingly.

The Myth of "Food Combining" The idea that people should not eat certain food combinations (for example, fruit and meat) at the same meal, because the digestive system cannot handle more than one task at a time, is a myth. The art of "food combining" (which actually emphasizes "food separating") is based on this idea, and it represents faulty logic and a gross underestimation of the body's capabilities. In fact, the contrary is often true; foods eaten together can enhance each other's use by the body. For example, vitamin C in a pineapple or other citrus fruit can enhance the absorption of iron from a meal of chicken and rice or other iron-containing foods. Many other instances of mutually beneficial interactions are presented in later chapters.

Preparing Nutrients for Transport When a nutrient molecule has crossed the cell of a villus, it enters either the bloodstream or the lymphatic system. Both transport systems supply vessels to each villus, as shown in Figure 3-11. The water-soluble nutrients and the smaller products of fat digestion are released directly into the bloodstream and guided directly to the liver where their fate and destination will be determined. The larger fats and the fat-soluble vitamins are insoluble in water, however, and blood is mostly water. The intestinal cells assemble many of the products of fat digestion into larger molecules. These larger molecules cluster together with special proteins, forming chylomicrons.■ These chylomicrons cannot pass into the capillaries and are released into the lymphatic system instead; the chylomicrons move through the lymph and later enter the bloodstream at a point near the heart, thus bypassing the liver at first. Details follow.

■ Chylomicrons (kye-lo-MY-cronz) are described in Chapter 5.

IN SUMMARY The many folds and villi of the small intestine dramatically increase its surface area, facilitating nutrient absorption. Nutrients pass through the cells of the villi and enter either the blood (if they are water soluble or small fat fragments) or the lymph (if they are fat soluble).

The Circulatory Systems

Once a nutrient has entered the bloodstream, it may be transported to any of the cells in the body, from the tips of the toes to the roots of the hair. The circulatory systems deliver nutrients wherever they are needed.

The Vascular System

The vascular, or blood circulatory, system is a closed system of vessels through which blood flows continuously, with the heart serving as the pump (see Figure 3-12). As the blood circulates through this system, it picks up and delivers materials as needed.

FIGURE 3-12 The Vascular System

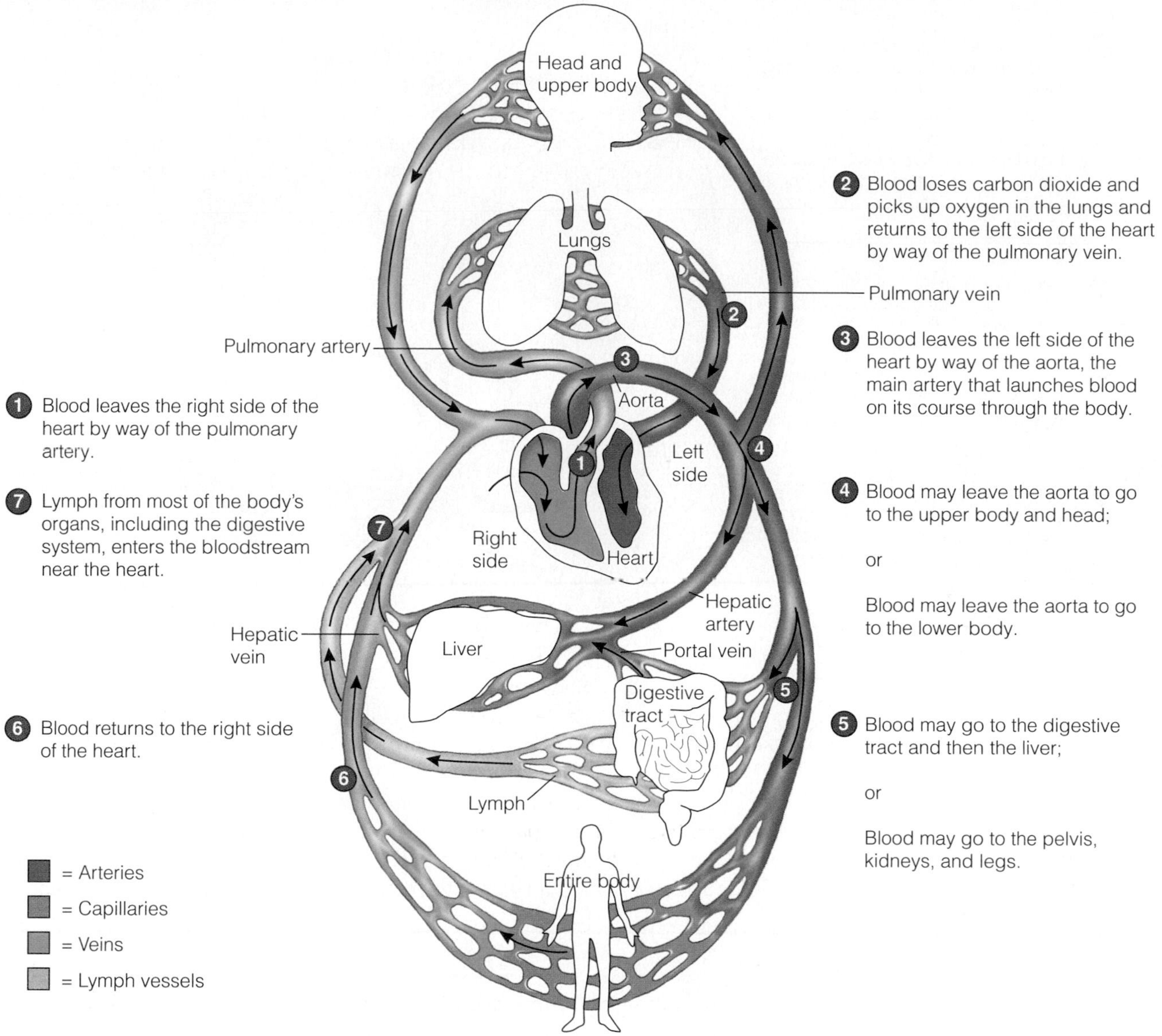
Head and upper body
Lungs
Pulmonary artery
Pulmonary vein
Aorta
Left side
Right side
Heart
Hepatic artery
Hepatic vein
Liver
Portal vein
Digestive tract
Lymph
Entire body
2 Blood loses carbon dioxide and picks up oxygen in the lungs and returns to the left side of the heart by way of the pulmonary vein.
3 Blood leaves the left side of the heart by way of the aorta, the main artery that launches blood on its course through the body.
1 Blood leaves the right side of the heart by way of the pulmonary artery.
7 Lymph from most of the body's organs, including the digestive system, enters the bloodstream near the heart.
4 Blood may leave the aorta to go to the upper body and head;
or
Blood may leave the aorta to go to the lower body.
6 Blood returns to the right side of the heart.
5 Blood may go to the digestive tract and then the liver;
or
Blood may go to the pelvis, kidneys, and legs.
= Arteries
= Capillaries
= Veins
= Lymph vessels

All the body tissues derive oxygen and nutrients from the blood and deposit carbon dioxide and other wastes into it. The lungs exchange carbon dioxide (which leaves the blood to be exhaled) and oxygen (which enters the blood to be delivered to all cells). The digestive system supplies the nutrients to be picked up. In the kidneys, wastes other than carbon dioxide are filtered out of the blood to be excreted in the urine.

Blood leaving the right side of the heart circulates through the lungs and then back to the left side of the heart. The left side of the heart then pumps the blood out through **arteries** to all systems of the body. The blood circulates in the **capillaries,** where it exchanges material with the cells, and then collects into **veins,** which return it again to the right side of the heart. In short, blood travels this simple route:

- Heart to arteries to capillaries to veins to heart.

arteries: vessels that carry blood from the heart to the tissues.

capillaries (CAP-ill-aries): small vessels that branch from an artery. Capillaries connect arteries to veins. Exchange of oxygen, nutrients, and waste materials takes place across capillary walls.

veins (VANES): vessels that carry blood to the heart.

FIGURE 3-13 The Liver

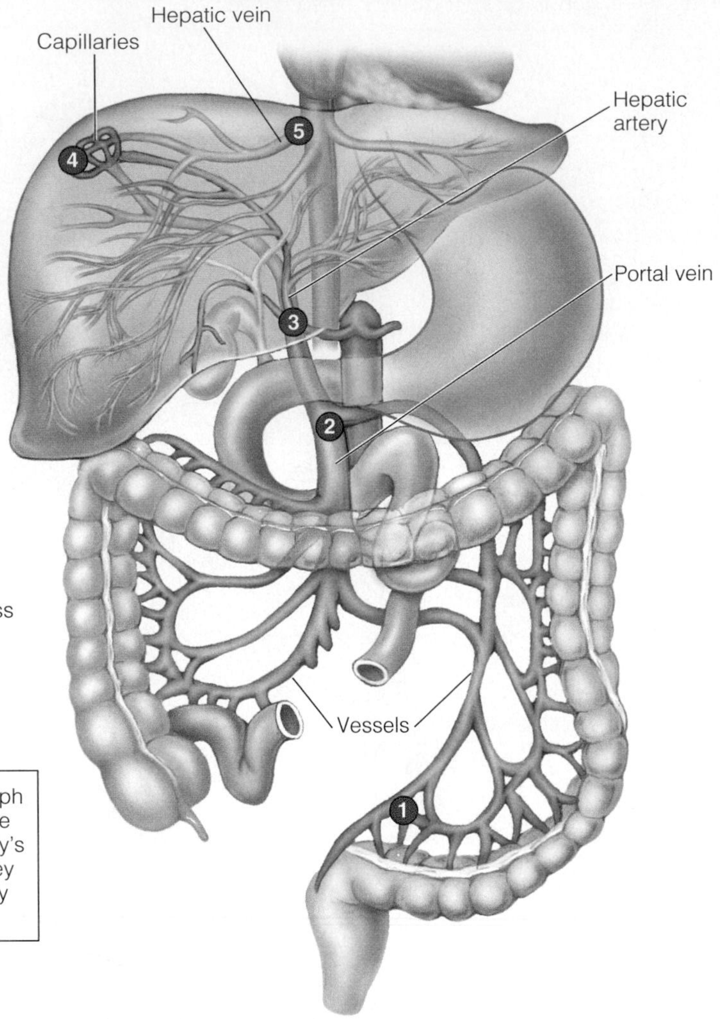
Hepatic vein
Capillaries
Hepatic artery
Portal vein
Vessels
1
2
3
4
5

1. Vessels gather up nutrients and reabsorbed water and salts from all over the digestive tract.

Not shown here:
Parallel to these vessels (veins) are other vessels (arteries) that carry oxygen-rich blood from the heart to the intestines.

2. The vessels merge into the portal vein, which conducts all absorbed materials to the liver.

3. The hepatic artery brings a supply of freshly oxygenated blood (not loaded with nutrients) from the lungs to supply oxygen to the liver's own cells.

4. Capillaries branch all over the liver, making nutrients and oxygen available to all its cells and giving the cells access to blood from the digestive system.

5. The hepatic vein gathers up blood in the liver and returns it to the heart.

In contrast, nutrients absorbed into lymph do not go to the liver first. They go to the heart, which pumps them to all the body's cells. The cells remove the nutrients they need, and the liver then has to deal only with the remnants.

The routing of the blood past the digestive system has a special feature. The blood is carried to the digestive system (as to all organs) by way of an artery, which (as in all organs) branches into capillaries to reach every cell. Blood leaving the digestive system, however, goes by way of a vein. The **portal vein** directs blood not back to the heart, but to another organ—the liver. This vein *again* branches into *capillaries* so that every cell of the liver has access to the blood. Blood leaving the liver then *again* collects into a vein, called the **hepatic vein,** which returns blood to the heart.

The route is:

- Heart to arteries to capillaries (in intestines) to vein to capillaries (in liver) to vein to heart.

Figure 3-13 shows the liver's key position in nutrient transport. An anatomist studying this system knows there must be a reason for this special arrangement. The liver's placement ensures that it will be first to receive the materials absorbed from the GI tract. In fact, the liver has many jobs to do in preparing the absorbed nutrients for use by the body. It is the body's major metabolic organ.

You might guess that, in addition, the liver serves as a gatekeeper to defend against substances that might harm the heart or brain. This is why, when people ingest poisons that succeed in passing the first barrier (the intestinal cells), the liver quite often suffers the damage—from viruses such as hepatitis, from drugs

portal vein: the vein that collects blood from the GI tract and conducts it to capillaries in the liver.
- **portal** = gateway

hepatic vein: the vein that collects blood from the liver capillaries and returns it to the heart.
- **hepatic** = liver

such as barbiturates or alcohol, from toxins such as pesticide residues, and from contaminants such as mercury. Perhaps, in fact, you have been undervaluing your liver, not knowing what heroic tasks it quietly performs for you.

The Lymphatic System

The **lymphatic system** provides a one-way route for fluid from the tissue spaces to enter the blood. Unlike the vascular system, the lymphatic system has no pump; instead, **lymph** circulates between the cells of the body and collects into tiny vessels. The fluid moves from one portion of the body to another as muscles contract and create pressure here and there. Ultimately, much of the lymph collects in a large duct behind the heart. This duct terminates in a vein that moves the lymph toward the heart.■ Thus materials from the GI tract that enter lymphatic vessels■ (large fats and fat-soluble vitamins) ultimately enter the bloodstream, circulating through arteries, capillaries, and veins like the other nutrients, with a notable exception—they bypass the liver at first.

Once inside the vascular system, the nutrients can travel freely to any destination and can be taken into cells and used as needed. What becomes of them is described in later chapters.

■ The duct that conveys lymph toward the heart is the **thoracic** (thor-ASS-ic) **duct.** The **subclavian** (sub-KLAY-vee-an) **vein** connects this duct with the right upper chamber of the heart, providing a passageway by which lymph can be returned to the vascular system.

■ The lymphatic vessels of the intestine that take up nutrients and pass them to the lymph circulation are called **lacteals** (LACK-tee-als).

IN SUMMARY Nutrients leaving the digestive system via the blood are routed directly to the liver before being transported to the body's cells. Those leaving via the lymphatic system eventually enter the vascular system, but bypass the liver at first.

Regulation of Digestion and Absorption

There is nothing random about digestion and absorption; they are coordinated in every detail. The ability of the digestive tract to handle its ever-changing contents routinely illustrates an important physiological principle that governs the way all living things function—the principle of **homeostasis.** Simply stated, conditions have to stay about the same for an organism to survive; if they deviate too far from the norm, the organism must "do something" to bring them back to normal. The body's regulation of digestion is one example of homeostatic regulation. The body also regulates its temperature, its blood pressure, and all other aspects of its blood chemistry in similar ways.

The following paragraphs describe the regulation of digestion and absorption in healthy adults, but many factors■ can influence normal GI function. For example, peristalsis and sphincter action are poorly coordinated in newborns, so infants tend to "spit up" during the first several months of life. Older adults often experience constipation, in part because the intestinal wall loses strength and elasticity with age, which slows GI motility. Diseases can also interfere with digestion and absorption and often lead to malnutrition. Lack of nourishment, in general, and lack of certain dietary constituents such as fiber, in particular, alter the structure and function of GI cells. Quite simply, GI tract health depends on adequate nutrition.

■ Factors influencing GI function:
- Physical immaturity.
- Aging.
- Illness.
- Nutrition.

lymphatic (lim-FAT-ic) **system:** a loosely organized system of vessels and ducts that convey fluids toward the heart. The GI part of the lymphatic system carries the products of fat digestion into the bloodstream.

lymph (LIMF): a clear yellowish fluid that is almost identical to blood except that it contains no red blood cells or platelets. Lymph from the GI tract transports fat and fat-soluble vitamins to the bloodstream via lymphatic vessels.

homeostasis (HOME-ee-oh-STAY-sis): the maintenance of constant internal conditions (such as blood chemistry, temperature, and blood pressure) by the body's control systems. A homeostatic system is constantly reacting to external forces so as to maintain limits set by the body's needs.
- **homeo** = the same
- **stasis** = staying

Gastrointestinal Hormones and Nerve Pathways

Two intricate and sensitive systems coordinate all the digestive and absorptive processes: the hormonal (or endocrine) system and the nervous system. Even before the first bite of food is taken, the mere thought, sight, or smell of food can trigger a response from these systems. Then, as food travels through the GI tract, it either stimulates or inhibits digestive secretions by way of messages that are carried from one section of the GI tract to another by both **hormones** and nerve pathways. (Appendix A presents a brief summary of the body's hormonal system and nervous system.)

Notice that the kinds of regulation that will be described are all examples of *feedback* mechanisms. A certain condition demands a response. The response changes that condition, and the change then cuts off the response. Thus the system is self-corrective. Examples follow:

- *The stomach normally maintains a pH between 1.5 and 1.7. How does it stay that way?* Food entering the stomach stimulates cells in the stomach wall to release the hormone **gastrin.** Gastrin, in turn, stimulates the stomach glands to secrete the components of hydrochloric acid. When pH 1.5 is reached, the acid itself turns off the gastrin-producing cells. They stop releasing gastrin, and the glands stop producing hydrochloric acid. Thus the system adjusts itself.

  Nerve receptors in the stomach wall also respond to the presence of food and stimulate both the gastric glands to secrete juices and the muscles to contract. As the stomach empties, the receptors are no longer stimulated, the flow of juices slows, and the stomach quiets down.
- *The pyloric sphincter opens to let out a little chyme, then closes again. How does it know when to open and close?* When the pyloric sphincter relaxes, acidic chyme slips through. The cells of the pyloric muscle on the intestinal side sense the acid, causing the pyloric sphincter to close tightly. Only after the chyme has been neutralized by pancreatic bicarbonate and the juices surrounding the pyloric sphincter have become alkaline can the muscle relax again. This process ensures that the chyme will be released slowly enough to be neutralized as it flows through the small intestine. This is important because the small intestine has less of a mucous coating than the stomach does and so is not as well protected from acid.
- *As the chyme enters the intestine, the pancreas adds bicarbonate to it so that the intestinal contents always remain at a slightly alkaline pH. How does the pancreas know how much to add?* The presence of chyme stimulates the cells of the duodenum wall to release the hormone **secretin** into the blood. When secretin reaches the pancreas, it stimulates the pancreas to release its bicarbonate-rich juices. Thus, whenever the duodenum signals that acidic chyme is present, the pancreas responds by sending bicarbonate to neutralize it. When the need has been met, the cells of the duodenal wall are no longer stimulated to release secretin, the hormone no longer flows through the blood, the pancreas no longer receives the message, and it stops sending pancreatic juice. Nerves also regulate pancreatic secretions.
- *Pancreatic secretions contain a mixture of enzymes to digest carbohydrate, fat, and protein. How does the pancreas know how much of each type of enzyme to provide?* This is one of the most interesting questions physiologists have asked. Clearly, the pancreas does know what its owner has been eating, and it secretes enzyme mixtures tailored to handle the food mixtures that have been arriving lately (over the last several days). Enzyme activity changes proportionately in response to the amounts of carbohydrate, fat, and protein in the diet. If a person has been eating mostly carbohydrates, the pancreas makes and secretes mostly carbohydrases; if the person's diet has been high in fat, the pancreas produces more lipases; and so forth. Presumably, hormones from the GI tract, secreted in response to meals, keep the pancreas informed as to its digestive tasks. The day or two lag between the time a person's diet changes dramatically and the time digestion of the new diet becomes efficient explains why dietary changes can "upset digestion" and should be made gradually.
- *Why don't the digestive enzymes damage the pancreas?* The pancreas protects itself from harm by producing an inactive form of the enzymes.■ Then it releases these proteins into the small intestine where they are activated to

■ The inactive precursor of an enzyme is called a **proenzyme** or **zymogen** (ZYE-mo-jen).
- **pro** = before
- **zym** = concerning enzymes
- **gen** = to produce

hormones: chemical messengers. Hormones are secreted by a variety of glands in response to altered conditions in the body. Each hormone travels to one or more specific target tissues or organs, where it elicits a specific response to maintain homeostasis. In general, any gastrointestinal hormone may be called an **enterogastrone** (EN-ter-oh-GAS-trone), but the term refers specifically to any hormone that slows motility and inhibits gastric secretions.

gastrin: a hormone secreted by cells in the stomach wall. Target organ: the glands of the stomach. Response: secretion of gastric acid.

secretin (see-CREET-in): a hormone produced by cells in the duodenum wall. Target organ: the pancreas. Response: secretion of bicarbonate-rich pancreatic juice.

become enzymes. In pancreatitis, the digestive enzymes somehow become active within the pancreas itself, causing inflammation and damaging the delicate pancreatic tissues.

- *When fat is present in the intestine, the gallbladder contracts to squirt bile into the intestine to emulsify the fat. How does the gallbladder get the message that fat is present?* Fat in the intestine stimulates cells of the intestinal wall to release the hormone **cholecystokinin (CCK).** This hormone, traveling by way of the blood to the gallbladder, stimulates it to contract, releasing bile into the small intestine. Once the fat in the intestine is emulsified and enzymes have begun to work on it, the fat no longer provokes release of the hormone, and the message to contract is canceled. (By the way, fat emulsification can continue even after a diseased gallbladder has been surgically removed because the liver can deliver bile directly to the small intestine.)
- *Fat takes longer to digest than carbohydrate does. When fat is present, intestinal motility slows to allow time for its digestion. How does the intestine know when to slow down?* Cholecystokinin and **gastric-inhibitory peptide** slow GI tract motility. By slowing the digestive process, fat helps to maintain a pace that will allow all reactions to reach completion. Gastric-inhibitory peptide also inhibits gastric acid secretion. Hormonal and nervous mechanisms like these account for much of the body's ability to adapt to changing conditions.

Once a person has started to learn the answers to questions like these, it may be hard to stop. Some people devote their whole lives to the study of physiology. For now, however, these few examples will be enough to illustrate how all the processes throughout the digestive system are precisely and automatically regulated without any conscious effort.

IN SUMMARY Digestion and absorption depend on the coordinated efforts of the hormonal system and the nervous system. Together, they regulate the processes of transforming foods into nutrients.

The System at Its Best

This chapter has described the anatomy of the digestive tract on several levels: the sequence of digestive organs, the cells and structures of the villi, and the selective machinery of the cell membranes. The intricate architecture of the digestive system makes it sensitive and responsive to conditions in its environment. Knowing the optimal conditions will help you to promote the best functioning of the system.

One indispensable condition is good health of the digestive tract itself. This health is affected by such lifestyle factors as sleep, physical activity, and state of mind. Adequate sleep allows for repair and maintenance of tissue and removal of wastes that might impair efficient functioning. Activity promotes healthy muscle tone. Mental state influences the activity of regulatory nerves and hormones; for healthy digestion, you should be relaxed and tranquil at mealtimes.

Another factor is the kind of meals you eat. Among the characteristics of meals that promote optimal absorption of nutrients are those mentioned in Chapter 2: balance, moderation, variety, and adequacy. Balance and moderation require having neither too much nor too little of anything. For example, too much fat can be harmful, but some fat is beneficial in slowing down intestinal motility and providing time for absorption of some of the nutrients that are slow to be absorbed.

Variety is important for many reasons, but one is that some food constituents interfere with nutrient absorption. For example, some compounds common in high-fiber foods such as whole-grain cereals, certain leafy green vegetables, and legumes bind with minerals. To some extent, then, the minerals in those foods may become unavailable for absorption. These high-fiber foods are still valuable, but need to be balanced with a variety of other foods that can provide the minerals.

cholecystokinin (coal-ee-sis-toe-KINE-in), or **CCK:** a hormone produced by cells of the intestinal wall. Target organ: the gallbladder. Response: release of bile and slowing of GI motility.

gastric-inhibitory peptide: a hormone produced by the intestine. Target organ: the stomach. Response: slowing of the secretion of gastric juices and of GI motility.

As for adequacy—in a sense, this entire book is about dietary adequacy. But here, at the end of this chapter, is a good place to underline the interdependence of the nutrients. It could almost be said that every nutrient depends on every other. All the nutrients work together, and all are present in the cells of a healthy digestive tract. To maintain health and promote the functions of the GI tract, you should make balance, moderation, variety, and adequacy features of every day's menus.

Nutrition in Your Life

A healthy digestive system can adjust to almost any diet and can handle any combination of foods with ease.

- **Do you usually enjoy meals without overeating to the point of discomfort?**
- **Do you experience GI distress regularly?**
- **What changes can you make in your eating habits to promote GI health?**

NUTRITION ON THE NET

Access these websites for further study of topics covered in this chapter.

- Find updates and quick links to these and other nutrition-related sites at our website: **www.wadsworth.com/nutrition**
- Visit the Center for Digestive Health and Nutrition: **www.gihealth.com**
- Visit the Digest This! section of the American College of Gastroenterology: **www.acg.gi.org**

STUDY QUESTIONS

These questions will help you review this chapter. You will find the answers in the discussions on the pages provided.

1. Describe the obstacles associated with digesting food and the solutions offered by the human body. (pp. 73–80)
2. Describe the path food follows as it travels through the digestive system. Summarize the muscular actions that take place along the way. (pp. 74–79)
3. Name five organs that secrete digestive juices. How do the juices and enzymes facilitate digestion? (pp. 79–81)
4. Describe the problems associated with absorbing nutrients and the solutions offered by the small intestine. (pp. 83–86)
5. How is blood routed through the digestive system? Which nutrients enter the bloodstream directly? Which are first absorbed into the lymph? (pp. 86–89)
6. Describe how the body coordinates and regulates the processes of digestion and absorption. (pp. 89–91)
7. How does the composition of the diet influence the functioning of the GI tract? (pp. 90–91)
8. What steps can you take to help your GI tract function at its best? (pp. 91–92)

These multiple choice questions will help you prepare for an exam. Answers can be found on p. 93.

1. The semiliquid, partially digested food that travels through the intestinal tract is called:
   a. bile.
   b. lymph.
   c. chyme.
   d. secretin.
2. The muscular contractions that move food through the GI tract are called:
   a. hydrolysis.
   b. sphincters.
   c. peristalsis.
   d. bowel movements.

3. The main function of bile is to:
   a. emulsify fats.
   b. catalyze hydrolysis.
   c. slow protein digestion.
   d. neutralize stomach acidity.
4. The pancreas neutralizes stomach acid in the small intestine by secreting:
   a. bile.
   b. mucus.
   c. enzymes.
   d. bicarbonate.
5. Which nutrient passes through the GI tract mostly undigested and unabsorbed?
   a. fat
   b. fiber
   c. protein
   d. carbohydrate
6. Absorption occurs primarily in the:
   a. mouth.
   b. stomach.
   c. small intestine.
   d. large intestine.
7. All blood leaving the GI tract travels first to the:
   a. heart.
   b. liver.
   c. kidneys.
   d. pancreas.
8. Which nutrients leave the GI tract by way of the lymphatic system?
   a. water and minerals
   b. proteins and minerals
   c. all vitamins and minerals
   d. fats and fat-soluble vitamins
9. Digestion and absorption are coordinated by the:
   a. pancreas and kidneys.
   b. liver and gallbladder.
   c. hormonal system and the nervous system.
   d. vascular system and the lymphatic system.
10. Gastrin, secretin, and cholecystokinin are examples of:
   a. crypts.
   b. enzymes.
   c. hormones.
   d. goblet cells.

ANSWERS

Study Questions (multiple choice)

1. c   2. c   3. a   4. d   5. b   6. c   7. b   8. d
9. c   10. c

HIGHLIGHT

Common Digestive Problems

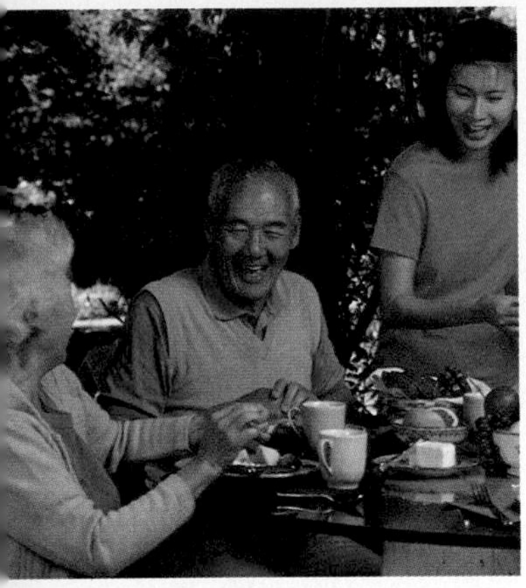

The facts of anatomy and physiology presented in Chapter 3 permit easy understanding of some common problems that occasionally arise in the digestive tract. Food may slip into the air passages instead of the esophagus, causing choking. Bowel movements may be loose and watery, as in diarrhea, or painful and hard, as in constipation. Some people complain about belching, while others are bothered by intestinal gas. Sometimes people develop medical problems such as an ulcer. This highlight describes some of the symptoms of these common digestive problems and suggests strategies for preventing them (the glossary on p. 96 defines the relevant terms).

Choking

A person chokes when a piece of food slips into the **trachea** and becomes lodged so securely that it cuts off breathing (see Figure H3-1). Without oxygen, the person may suffer brain damage or die. For this reason, it is imperative that everyone learn to recognize the international signal for choking (shown in Figure H3-2) and act promptly.

The choking scenario might read like this. A person is dining in a restaurant with friends. A chunk of food, usually meat, becomes lodged in his trachea so firmly that he cannot make a sound. No sound can be made because the **larynx** is in the trachea and makes sounds only when air is pushed across it. Often he chooses to suffer alone rather than "make a scene in public." If he tries to communicate distress to his friends, he must depend on pantomime. The friends are bewildered by his antics and become terribly worried when he "faints" after a few minutes without air. They call for an ambulance, but by the time it arrives, he is dead from suffocation.

To help a person who is choking, first ask this critical question: "Can you make any sound at all?" If so, relax. You have time to decide what you can do to help. Whatever you do, don't hit him on the back—the particle may become lodged more firmly in his air passage. If the person cannot make a sound, shout for help and perform the **Heimlich maneuver** (described in Figure H3-2). You would do well to take a life-saving course and practice these techniques, for you will have no time for hesitation once you are called on to perform this death-defying act.

Almost any food can cause choking, although some are cited more often than others: chunks of meat, hot dogs, nuts, whole grapes, raw carrots, marshmallows, hard or sticky candies, gum, popcorn, and peanut butter. These foods are particularly difficult for young children to safely chew and swallow. In 2000, more than 17,500 children (under 15 years old) in the United States choked; most of them choked on food, and 160 of them choked to death.[1] Always remain alert to the dangers of choking whenever young children are eating. To prevent choking, cut food into small pieces, chew thoroughly

FIGURE H3-1 Normal Swallowing and Choking

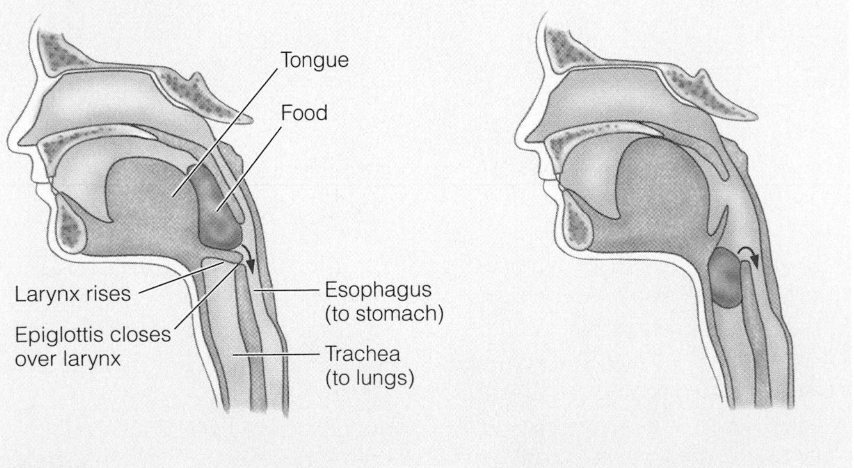
Tongue
Food
Larynx rises
Epiglottis closes over larynx
Esophagus (to stomach)
Trachea (to lungs)

Swallowing. The epiglottis closes over the larynx, blocking entrance to the lungs via the trachea. The red arrow shows that food is heading down the esophagus normally.

Choking. A choking person cannot speak or gasp because food lodged in the trachea blocks the passage of air. The red arrow points to where the food should have gone to prevent choking.

FIGURE H3-2 First Aid for Choking

The strategy most likely to succeed is abdominal thrusts, sometimes called the Heimlich maneuver. Only if all else fails, open the mouth by grasping both the tongue and lower jaw and lifting. Then, and only if you can see the object, use your finger to sweep it out and begin rescue breathing.

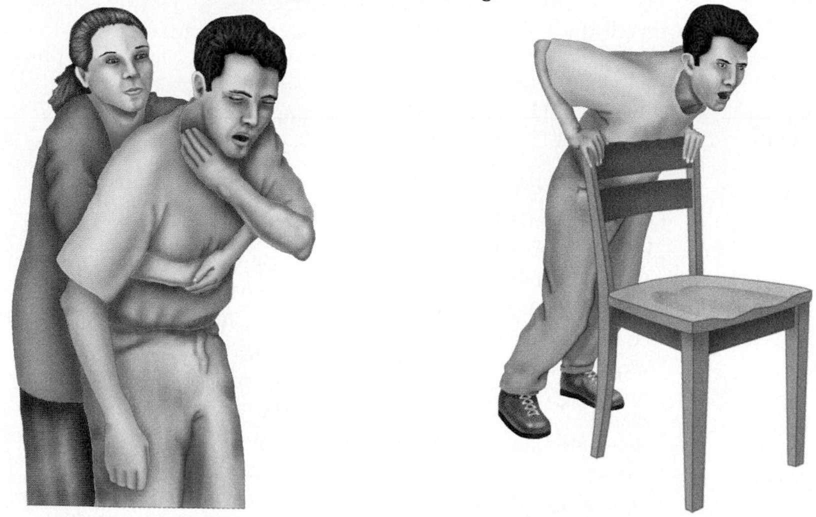

This universal signal for choking alerts others to the need for assistance. Stand behind the person, and wrap your arms around him. Place the thumb side of one fist snugly against his body, slightly above the navel and below the rib cage. Grasp your fist with your other hand and give him a sudden strong hug inward and upward. Repeat thrusts as necessary.

To self-administer first aid, place the thumb side of one fist slightly above the navel and below the rib cage, grasp the fist with your other hand, and then press inward and upward with a quick motion. If this is unsuccessful, quickly press your upper abdomen over any firm surface such as the back of a chair, a countertop, or a railing.

before swallowing, don't talk or laugh with food in your mouth, and don't eat when breathing hard.

Vomiting

Another common digestive mishap is **vomiting.** Vomiting can be a symptom of many different diseases or may arise in situations that upset the body's equilibrium, such as air or sea travel. For whatever reason, the waves of peristalsis reverse direction, and the contents of the stomach are propelled up through the esophagus to the mouth and expelled.

If vomiting continues long enough or is severe enough, the reverse peristalsis will extend beyond the stomach and carry the contents of the duodenum, with its green bile, into the stomach and then up the esophagus. Although certainly unpleasant and wearying for the nauseated person, vomiting such as this is no cause for alarm. Vomiting is one of the body's adaptive mechanisms to rid itself of something irritating. The best advice is to rest and drink small amounts of liquids as tolerated until the nausea subsides.

A physician's care may be needed, however, when large quantities of fluid are lost from the GI tract, causing dehydration. With massive fluid loss from the GI tract, all of the body's other fluids redistribute themselves so that, eventually, fluid is taken from every cell of the body. Leaving the cells with the fluid are salts that are absolutely essential to the life of the cells, and they must be replaced, which is difficult while the vomiting continues. Intravenous feedings of saline and glucose are frequently necessary while the physician is diagnosing the cause of the vomiting and instituting corrective therapy.

In an infant, vomiting is likely to become serious early in its course, and a physician should be contacted soon after onset. Infants have more fluid between their body cells than adults do, so more fluid can move readily into the digestive tract and be lost from the body. Consequently, the body water of infants becomes depleted and their body salt balance upset faster than in adults.

Self-induced vomiting, such as occurs in bulimia nervosa, also has serious consequences. In addition to fluid and salt imbalances, repeated vomiting can cause irritation and infection of the pharynx, esophagus, and salivary glands; erosion of the teeth and gums; and dental caries. The esophagus may rupture or tear, as may the stomach. Sometimes the eyes become red from pressure during vomiting. Bulimic behavior reflects underlying psychological problems that require intervention. (Bulimia nervosa is discussed fully in Highlight 9.)

Projectile vomiting is also serious. The contents of the stomach are expelled with such force that they leave the mouth in a wide arc like a bullet leaving a gun. This type of vomiting requires immediate medical attention.

Diarrhea

Diarrhea is characterized by frequent, loose, watery stools. Such stools indicate that the intestinal contents have moved too quickly through the intestines for fluid absorption to take place, or that water has been drawn from the cells lining the intestinal tract and added to the food residue. Like vomiting, diarrhea can lead to considerable fluid and salt losses, but the composition of the fluids is different. Stomach fluids lost in vomiting are highly acidic, whereas intestinal fluids lost in diarrhea are nearly neutral. When fluid losses require medical attention, correct replacement is crucial.

Diarrhea is a symptom of a variety of medical conditions and treatments. It may occur abruptly in a healthy person as a result

GLOSSARY

acid controllers: medications used to prevent or relieve indigestion by suppressing production of acid in the stomach; also called **H2 blockers.** Common brands include Pepcid AC, Tagamet HB, Zantac 75, and Axid AR.

antacids: medications used to relieve indigestion by neutralizing acid in the stomach. Common brands include Alka-Seltzer, Maalox, Rolaids, and Tums.

belching: the expulsion of gas from the stomach through the mouth.

colitis (ko-LYE-tis): inflammation of the colon.

colonic irrigation: the popular, but potentially harmful practice of "washing" the large intestine with a powerful enema machine.

constipation: the condition of having infrequent or difficult bowel movements.

defecate (DEF-uh-cate): to move the bowels and eliminate waste.
- **defaecare** = to remove dregs

diarrhea: the frequent passage of watery bowel movements.

diverticula (dye-ver-TIC-you-la): sacs or pouches that develop in the weakened areas of the intestinal wall (like bulges in an inner tube where the tire wall is weak).
- **divertir** = to turn aside

diverticulitis (DYE-ver-tic-you-LYE-tis): infected or inflamed diverticula.
- **itis** = infection or inflammation

diverticulosis (DYE-ver-tic-you-LOH-sis): the condition of having diverticula. About one in every six people in Western countries develops diverticulosis in middle or later life.
- **osis** = condition

enemas: solutions inserted into the rectum and colon to stimulate a bowel movement and empty the lower large intestine.

gastroesophageal reflux: the backflow of stomach acid into the esophagus, causing damage to the cells of the esophagus and the sensation of heartburn. **Gastroesophageal reflux disease (GERD)** is characterized by symptoms of reflux occurring two or more times a week.

heartburn: a burning sensation in the chest area caused by backflow of stomach acid into the esophagus.

Heimlich (HIME-lick) **maneuver (abdominal thrust maneuver):** a technique for dislodging an object from the trachea of a choking person (see Figure H3-2); named for the physician who developed it.

hemorrhoids (HEM-oh-royds): painful swelling of the veins surrounding the rectum.

hiccups (HICK-ups): repeated cough-like sounds and jerks that are produced when an involuntary spasm of the diaphragm muscle sucks air down the windpipe; also spelled *hiccoughs.*

indigestion: incomplete or uncomfortable digestion, usually accompanied by pain, nausea, vomiting, heartburn, intestinal gas, or belching.
- **in** = not

irritable bowel syndrome: an intestinal disorder of unknown cause. Symptoms include abdominal discomfort and cramping, diarrhea, constipation, or alternating diarrhea and constipation.

larynx: the voice box (see Figure H3-1).

laxatives: substances that loosen the bowels and thereby prevent or treat constipation.

mineral oil: a purified liquid derived from petroleum and used to treat constipation.

peptic ulcer: a lesion in the mucous membrane of either the stomach (a gastric ulcer) or the duodenum (a duodenal ulcer).
- **peptic** = concerning digestion

trachea (TRAKE-ee-uh): the windpipe; the passageway from the mouth and nose to the lungs.

ulcer: a lesion of the skin or mucous membranes characterized by inflammation and damaged tissues. See also *peptic ulcer.*

vomiting: expulsion of the contents of the stomach up through the esophagus to the mouth.

of infections (such as food poisoning) or as a side effect of medications. When used in large quantities, food ingredients such as the sugar alternative sorbitol and the fat alternative olestra may also cause diarrhea in some people. If a food is responsible, then that food must be omitted from the diet, at least temporarily. If medication is responsible, a different medicine, when possible, or a different form (injectable versus oral, for example) may alleviate the problem.

Diarrhea may also occur as a result of disorders of the GI tract, such as irritable bowel syndrome or colitis. **Irritable bowel syndrome** is one of the most common GI disorders and is characterized by a disturbance in the motility of the GI tract.[2] Dietary treatment hinges on identifying and avoiding individual foods that cause intolerance. For most people, a low-fat diet provided in small meals, with a gradual increase in fiber, is helpful. People with **colitis,** an inflammation of the large intestine, may also suffer from severe diarrhea. They often benefit from complete bowel rest and medication. If treatment fails, surgery to remove the colon and rectum may be necessary.

As you can see, treatment for diarrhea depends on its cause and its severity. Mild diarrhea may remit without treatment; simply rest and drink extra liquids to replace fluid losses. If diarrhea persists, though, especially in an infant, young child, or elderly person, call a physician. Severe diarrhea can be life-threatening when it leads to dehydration and electrolyte imbalances. (Chapter 12 provides more information on dehydration and its therapy.)

Constipation

Like diarrhea, **constipation** describes a symptom, not a disease. Each person's GI tract has its own cycle of waste elimination, which depends on its owner's health, the type of food eaten, when it was eaten, and when the person takes time to **defecate.** What's normal for some people may not be normal for others. Some people have bowel movements three times a day; others may have them three times a week. Only when people pass stools that are difficult or painful to expel or when they experience a reduced frequency of bowel movements from their typical pattern are they constipated. Abdominal discomfort, headaches, backaches, and the passing of gas sometimes accompany constipation.

Often a person's lifestyle may cause constipation. Being too busy to respond to the defecation signal is a common complaint. If a person receives the signal to defecate and ignores it, the signal may not return for several hours. In the meantime, water continues to be withdrawn from the fecal matter, so when the person does defecate, the bowel movement is dry and hard. In such a case, a person's daily regimen may need to be revised to allow time to have a bowel movement when the body sends its signal. One possibility is to go to bed earlier in order to rise earlier, allowing ample time for a leisurely breakfast and a movement.

Another cause of constipation is lack of physical activity. Physical activity improves muscle tone, not just of the outer body, but also of the digestive tract. As little as 30 minutes of physical activity a day can help prevent or alleviate constipation.

Although constipation usually reflects lifestyle habits, in some cases it may be a side effect of medication or may reflect a medical problem such as tumors that are obstructing the passage of waste. If discomfort is associated with passing fecal matter, seek medical advice to rule out disease. Once this has been done, dietary or other measures for correction can be considered.

One dietary measure that may be appropriate is to increase dietary fiber. Fibers found in cereal products help to prevent constipation by increasing fecal mass. In the GI tract, fiber attracts water, creating soft, bulky stools that stimulate bowel contractions to push the contents along. These contractions strengthen the intestinal muscles. The improved muscle tone, together with the water content of the stools, eases elimination, reducing the pressure in the rectal veins and helping to prevent **hemorrhoids.** Chapter 4 provides more information on fiber's role in maintaining a healthy colon and reducing the risks of colon cancer and diverticulosis. **Diverticulosis** is a condition in which the intestinal walls develop bulges in weakened areas, most commonly in the colon (see Figure H3-3). These bulging pockets, known as **diverticula,** can worsen constipation, entrap feces, and become painfully infected and inflamed **(diverticulitis).** Treatment may require hospitalization, antibiotics, or surgery.

Drinking plenty of water in conjunction with eating high-fiber foods also helps with constipation. The increased bulk physically stimulates the upper GI tract, promoting peristalsis throughout.

Eating prunes—or "dried plums" as some have renamed them—can also be helpful. Prunes are high in fiber and also contain a laxative substance.* If a morning defecation is desired, a person can drink prune juice at bedtime; if the evening is preferred, the person can drink prune juice with breakfast.

Honey can also have a laxative effect due to its incomplete absorption. Although this characteristic may cause problems for people with irritable bowel syndrome, eating honey may be an easy and effective treatment for those who are constipated. Honey should never be fed to infants, however, because of the risk of botulism (as explained in Chapter 15).

FIGURE H3-3 Diverticula in the Colon

Diverticula may develop anywhere along the GI tract, but are most common in the colon.

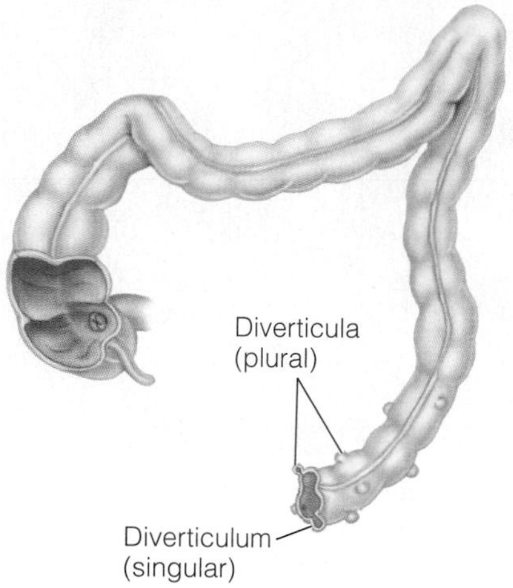
Diverticula
(plural)
Diverticulum
(singular)

Adding fat to the diet can relieve some constipation by stimulating the hormone cholecystokinin, which summons bile into the duodenum. Bile's high salt content draws water from the intestinal wall, which stimulates peristalsis and softens the fecal matter.

These suggested changes in lifestyle or diet should correct chronic constipation without the use of **laxatives, enemas,** or **mineral oil,** although television commercials often try to persuade people otherwise. One of the fallacies often perpetrated by advertisements is that one person's successful use of a product is a good recommendation for others to use that product.

As a matter of fact, diet changes that relieve constipation for one person may increase the constipation of another. For instance, increasing fiber intake stimulates peristalsis and helps the person with a sluggish colon. Some people, though, have a spastic type of constipation, in which peristalsis promotes strong contractions that close off a segment of the colon and prevent passage; for these people, increasing fiber intake would be exactly the wrong thing to do.

A person who seems to need products such as laxatives should seek a physician's advice. Opinions from friends or alternative medicine practitioners may cause more harm than good. One potentially harmful but currently popular practice that is being promoted by some alternative medicine practitioners is **colonic irrigation**—the internal washing of the large intestine with a powerful enema machine. Such an extreme cleansing is not only unnecessary, but can be hazardous, causing illness and death from equipment contamination, electrolyte depletion,

*This substance is dihydroxyphenyl isatin.

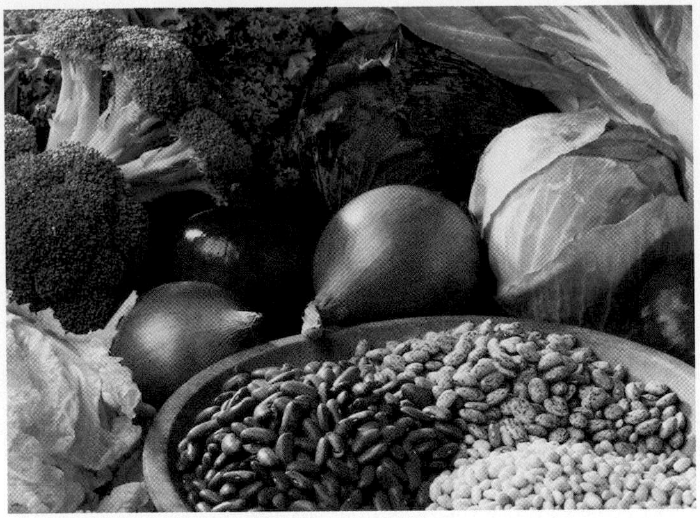
© Polara Studios Inc.

Beans, broccoli, cabbage, and onions produce gas in many people. People troubled by gas need to determine which foods bother them and then eat those foods in moderation.

and intestinal perforation. Less extreme practices can cause problems, too. Frequent use of laxatives and enemas can lead to dependency; upset the body's fluid, salt, and mineral balances; and, in the case of mineral oil, interfere with the absorption of fat-soluble vitamins. (Mineral oil dissolves the vitamins, but is not itself absorbed; instead, it leaves the body, carrying the vitamins with it.)

Belching and Gas

Many people complain of problems that they attribute to excessive gas. For some, **belching** is the complaint. Others blame intestinal gas for abdominal discomforts and embarrassment. Most people believe that the problems occur after they eat certain foods. This may be the case with intestinal gas, but belching results from swallowing air. The best advice for belching seems to be to eat slowly, chew thoroughly, and relax while eating.

Everyone swallows a little bit of air with each mouthful of food, but people who eat too fast may swallow too much air and then have to belch. Ill-fitting dentures, carbonated beverages, and chewing gum can also contribute to the swallowing of air with resultant belching. Occasionally, belching can be a sign of a more serious disorder, such as gallbladder disease or a peptic ulcer.

People who eat or drink too fast may also trigger **hiccups,** the repeated spasms that produce a cough-like sound and jerky movement. Normally, hiccups soon subside and are of no medical significance, but they can be bothersome. The most effective cure is to hold the breath for as long as possible, which helps to relieve the spasms of the diaphragm.

While expelling gas can be a humiliating experience, it is quite normal. (People experiencing painful bloating from malabsorption diseases, however, require medical treatment.) Healthy people expel several hundred milliliters of gas several times a day. Almost all (99 percent) of the gases expelled—nitrogen, oxygen, hydrogen, methane, and carbon dioxide—are odorless. The remaining "volatile" gases are the infamous ones.

Foods that produce gas usually must be determined individually. The most common offenders are foods rich in the carbohydrates—sugars, starches, and fibers. When partially digested carbohydrates reach the large intestine, bacteria digest them, giving off gas as a by-product. People can test foods suspected of forming gas by omitting them individually for a trial period and seeing if there is any improvement.

Heartburn and "Acid Indigestion"

Almost everyone has experienced **heartburn** at one time or another, usually soon after eating a meal. Medically known as **gastroesophageal reflux,** heartburn is the painful sensation a person feels behind the breastbone when the lower esophageal sphincter allows the stomach contents to reflux into the esophagus (see Figure H3-4). This may happen if a person eats or drinks too much (or both). Tight clothing and even changes of position (lying down, bending over) can cause it, too, as can some medications and smoking. A defect of the sphincter muscle itself is a possible, but less common cause.

If the heartburn is not caused by an anatomical defect, treatment is fairly simple. To avoid such misery in the future, the person needs to learn to eat less at a sitting, chew food more thoroughly, and eat it more slowly. Additional strategies are presented in Table H3-1 at the end of this highlight.

As far as "acid indigestion" is concerned, recall from Chapter 3 that the strong acidity of the stomach is a desirable condition—television commercials for **antacids** and **acid controllers** notwithstanding. People who overeat or eat too quickly are likely to suffer from **indigestion.** The muscular reaction of the stomach to unchewed lumps or to being overfilled may be so violent that it causes regurgitation (reverse peristalsis). When this happens, overeaters may taste the stomach acid and feel pain. Responding to advertisements, they may reach for antacids or acid controllers. Both of these drugs were originally designed to treat GI illnesses such as ulcers. As is true of most over-the-counter medicines, antacids and acid controllers should be used only infrequently for occasional heartburn; they may mask or cause problems if used regularly, as the next section explains. Instead of self-

FIGURE H3-4 Gastroesophageal Reflux

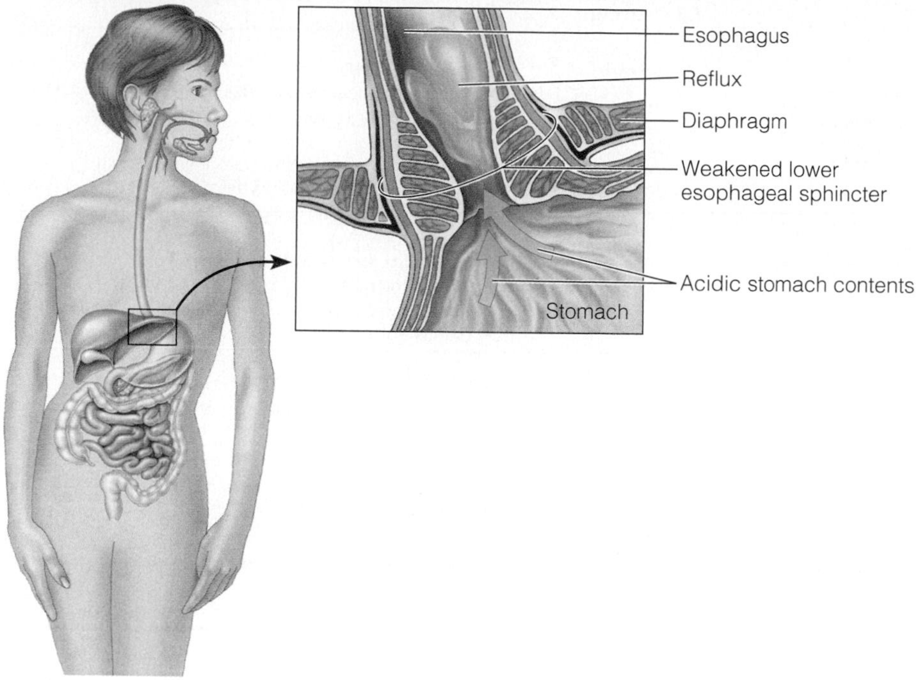
Esophagus
Reflux
Diaphragm
Weakened lower esophageal sphincter
Acidic stomach contents
Stomach

medicating, people who suffer from frequent and regular bouts of heartburn and indigestion need to see a physician, who can prescribe specific medication to control gastroesophageal reflux. Without treatment, the repeated splashes of acid can severely damage the cells of the esophagus, creating a condition known as Barrett's esophagus.[3] At that stage, the risk of cancer in the throat or esophagus increases dramatically. To repeat, if symptoms persist, see a doctor—don't self-medicate.

Ulcers

Ulcers of the stomach (gastric ulcers) or the duodenum of the small intestine (duodenal ulcers) are another common digestive problem. (The term **peptic ulcer** includes both types.) An **ulcer** is an erosion of the top layer of cells from an area, such as the wall of the stomach or duodenum. This erosion leaves the underlying layers of cells unprotected and exposed to gastric juices. The erosion may proceed until the gastric juices reach the capillaries that feed the area, leading to bleeding, and reach the nerves, causing pain. If GI bleeding is excessive, iron deficiency may develop. If the erosion penetrates all the way through the GI lining, a life-threatening infection can develop.

Many people naively believe that an ulcer is caused by stress or spicy foods, but this is not the case. The stomach lining in a healthy person is well protected by its mucous coat. What, then, causes ulcers to form?

Three major causes of ulcers have been identified: bacterial infection with *Helicobacter pylori* (commonly abbreviated *H. pylori*); the use of certain anti-inflammatory drugs such as aspirin, ibuprofen, and naproxen; and disorders that cause excessive gastric acid secretion. Most commonly, ulcers develop in response to *H. pylori* infection.[4] The cause of the ulcer dictates the type of medication used in treatment. For example, people with ulcers caused by infection receive antibiotics, whereas those with ulcers caused by medicines discontinue their use. In addition, all treatment plans aim to relieve pain, heal the ulcer, and prevent recurrence.

Diet therapy once played a major role in ulcer treatment, but it no longer does. Current practice is simply to treat for infection, eliminate any food that routinely causes indigestion or pain, and avoid coffee and caffeine- and alcohol-containing beverages. Both regular and decaffeinated coffee stimulate acid secretion and so aggravate *existing* ulcers.

Ulcers and their treatments highlight the importance of not self-medicating when symptoms persist. People with *H. pylori* infection often take over-the-counter acid controllers to relieve the pain of their ulcers when they need physician-prescribed antibiotics instead. Suppressing gastric acidity not only fails to heal the ulcer, but actually worsens inflammation during an *H. pylori* infection. Furthermore, *H. pylori* infection has been linked with stomach cancer as well, making prompt diagnosis and appropriate treatment essential.[5]

Table H3-1 (on p. 100) summarizes strategies to prevent or alleviate common GI problems. Many of these problems reflect hurried lifestyles. For this reason, many of their remedies require that people slow down and take the time to eat leisurely; chew food thoroughly to prevent choking, heartburn, and acid indigestion; rest until vomiting and diarrhea subside; and heed the urge to defecate. In addition, learn how to handle life's day-to-day problems and challenges without overreacting and becoming upset; learn how to relax, to get enough sleep, and to enjoy life. Remember, "what's eating you" may cause more GI distress than what you eat.

TABLE H3-1 Strategies to Prevent or Alleviate Common GI Problems

GI Problem	Strategies
Choking	• Take small bites of food. • Chew thoroughly before swallowing. • Don't talk or laugh with food in your mouth. • Don't eat when breathing hard.
Diarrhea	• Rest. • Drink fluids to replace losses. • Call for medical help if diarrhea persists.
Constipation	• Eat a high-fiber diet. • Drink plenty of fluids. • Exercise regularly. • Respond promptly to the urge to defecate.
Belching	• Eat slowly. • Chew thoroughly. • Relax while eating.
Intestinal gas	• Eat bothersome foods in moderation.
Heartburn	• Eat small meals. • Drink liquids between meals. • Sit up while eating; elevate your head when lying down. • Wait 1 hour after eating before lying down. • Wait 2 hours after eating before exercising. • Refrain from wearing tight-fitting clothing. • Avoid foods, beverages, and medications that aggravate your heartburn. • Refrain from smoking cigarettes or using tobacco products. • Lose weight if overweight.
Ulcer	• Take medicine as prescribed by your physician. • Avoid coffee and caffeine- and alcohol-containing beverages. • Avoid foods that aggravate your ulcer. • Minimize aspirin, ibuprofen, and naproxen use. • Refrain from smoking cigarettes.

NUTRITION ON THE NET

Access these websites for further study of topics covered in this highlight.

- Find updates and quick links to these and other nutrition-related sites at our website: **www.wadsworth.com/nutrition**
- Search for "choking," "vomiting," "diarrhea," "constipation," "heartburn," "indigestion," and "ulcers" at the U.S. Government health information site: **www.healthfinder.gov**
- Visit the Center for Digestive Health and Nutrition: **www.gihealth.com**
- Visit the Digestive Diseases section of the National Institute of Diabetes, Digestive, and Kidney Diseases: **www.niddk.nih.gov/health/health.htm**
- Visit the Digest This! section of the American College of Gastroenterology: **www.acg.gi.org**
- Learn more about *H. pylori* from the Helicobacter Foundation: **www.helico.com**

REFERENCES

1. K. Gotsch, J. L. Annest, and P. Holmgreen, Nonfatal choking-related episodes among children—United States, 2001, *Morbidity and Mortality Weekly Report* 51 (2002): 945–948.
2. B. J. Horwitz and R. S. Fisher, The irritable bowel syndrome, *New England Journal of Medicine* 344 (2001): 1846–1850.
3. N. Shaheen and D. F. Ransohoff, Gastroesophageal reflux, Barrett's esophagus, and esophageal cancer: Scientific review, *Journal of the American Medical Association* 287 (2002): 1972–1981.
4. S. Suerbaum and P. Michetti, *Helicobacter pylori* infection, *New England Journal of Medicine* 347 (2002): 1175–1186.
5. N. Uemura and coauthors, *Helicobacter pylori* infection and the developoment of gastric cancer, *New England Journal of Medicine* 345 (2001): 784–789.

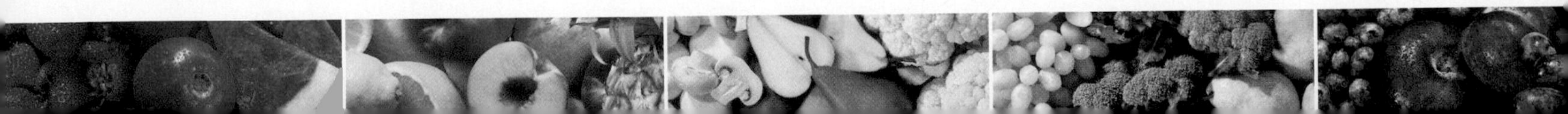

Chapter 4

The Carbohydrates: Sugars, Starches, and Fibers

Chapter Outline

Available Online

http://nutrition.wadsworth.com/uncn7

Nutrition Animation: *Carbohydrate Digestion*

Student Practice Test

Glossary Terms

Nutrition on the Net

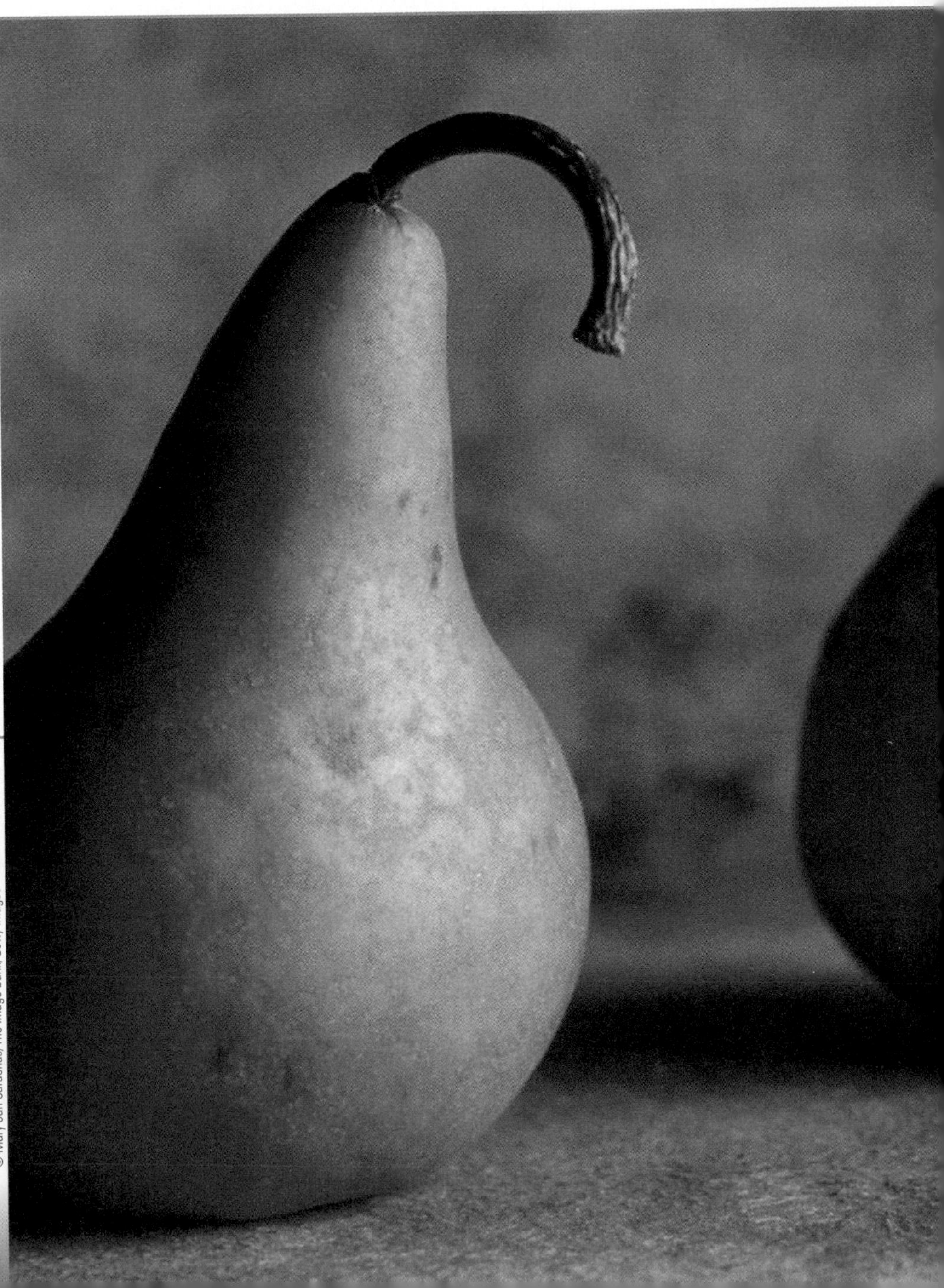

Nutrition in Your Life

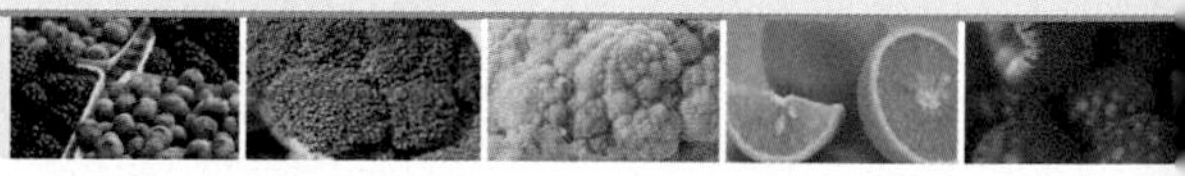

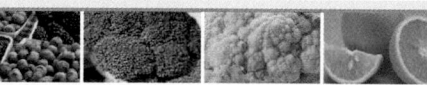

Whether you are cramming for an exam or daydreaming about your next vacation, your brain needs carbohydrate to power its activities. Your muscles need carbohydrate to fuel their work, too, whether you are racing up the stairs to class or moving on the dance floor to your favorite music. Where can you get carbohydrate? And are some foods healthier choices than others? As you will learn from this chapter, whole grains, vegetables, legumes, and fruits naturally deliver ample carbohydrate and fiber with valuable vitamins and minerals and little or no fat. Milk products typically lack fiber, but they also provide carbohydrate along with an assortment of vitamins and minerals.

A student, quietly studying a textbook, is seldom aware that within his brain cells, billions of glucose molecules are splitting to provide the energy that permits him to learn. Yet glucose provides nearly all of the energy the human brain uses daily. Similarly, a marathon runner, bursting across the finish line in an explosion of sweat and triumph, seldom gives thanks to the glycogen fuel her muscles have devoured to help her finish the race. Yet, together, glucose and its storage form glycogen provide about half of all the energy muscles and other body tissues use. The other half of the body's energy comes mostly from fat.

People don't eat glucose and glycogen directly; they eat foods rich in **carbohydrates.** Then their bodies convert the carbohydrates mostly into glucose for immediate energy and into glycogen for reserve energy. All plant foods—whole grains, vegetables, legumes, and fruits—provide ample carbohydrate. Milk also contains carbohydrates.

carbohydrates: compounds composed of carbon, oxygen, and hydrogen arranged as monosaccharides or multiples of monosaccharides. Most, but not all, carbohydrates have a ratio of one carbon molecule to one water molecule: $(CH_2O)_n$.
- **carbo** = carbon (C)
- **hydrate** = with water (H_2O)

Many people mistakenly think of carbohydrates as "fattening" and avoid them when trying to lose weight. Such a strategy may be helpful if the carbohydrates are the simple sugars of candy bars and cookies, but counterproductive if the carbohydrates are the complex carbohydrates of whole grains, vegetables, and legumes. As the next section explains, not all carbohydrates are created equal.

The Chemist's View of Carbohydrates

The dietary carbohydrate family includes the **simple carbohydrates** (the sugars) and the **complex carbohydrates** (the starches and fibers). The simple carbohydrates are those that chemists describe as:

- Monosaccharides—single sugars.
- Disaccharides—sugars composed of pairs of monosaccharides.

The complex carbohydrates are:

- Polysaccharides—large molecules composed of chains of monosaccharides.

To understand the structure of carbohydrates, look at the units of which they are made. The monosaccharides most important in nutrition are the 6-carbon hexoses.■ Each contains 6 carbon atoms, 12 hydrogens, and 6 oxygens (written in shorthand as $C_6H_{12}O_6$).

■ Most of the monosaccharides important in nutrition are **hexoses,** simple sugars with six atoms of carbon and the formula $C_6H_{12}O_6$.
- **hex** = six

Each atom can form a certain number of chemical bonds with other atoms:

- Carbon atoms can form four bonds.
- Nitrogen atoms, three.
- Oxygen atoms, two.
- Hydrogen atoms, only one.

Chemists represent the bonds as lines between the chemical symbols (such as C, N, O, and H) that stand for the atoms (see Figure 4-1).

Atoms form molecules in ways that satisfy the bonding requirements of each atom. Figure 4-1 includes the structure of ethyl alcohol, the active ingredient of alcoholic beverages, as an example. The two carbons each have four bonds represented by lines; the oxygen has two; and each hydrogen has one bond connecting it to other atoms. Chemical structures obey these bonding rules because the laws of nature demand it.

FIGURE 4-1 Atoms and Their Bonds

The four main types of atoms found in nutrients are hydrogen (H), oxygen (O), nitrogen (N), and carbon (C).

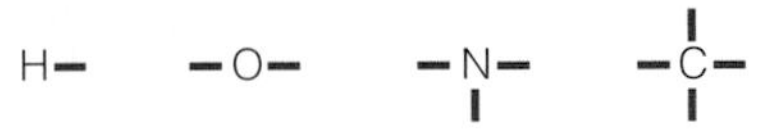
H
O
N
C

1 2 3 4

Each atom has a characteristic number of bonds it can form with other atoms.

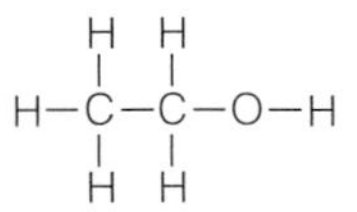
H H
H C C O H
H H

Notice that in this simple molecule of ethyl alcohol, each H has one bond, O has two, and each C has four.

IN SUMMARY The carbohydrates are made of carbon (C), oxygen (O), and hydrogen (H). Each of these atoms can form a specified number of chemical bonds: carbon forms four, oxygen forms two, and hydrogen forms one.

simple carbohydrates (sugars): monosaccharides and disaccharides.

complex carbohydrates (starches and fibers): polysaccharides composed of straight or branched chains of monosaccharides.

The Simple Carbohydrates

The following list of the simple carbohydrates most important in nutrition symbolizes them as hexagons and pentagons of different colors.* Three are monosaccharides:

- Glucose.
- Fructose.
- Galactose.

*Fructose is shown as a pentagon, but like the other monosaccharides, it has six carbons (as you will see in Figure 4-4).

Three are disaccharides:

- Maltose (glucose + glucose). 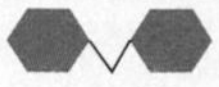
- Sucrose (glucose + fructose). 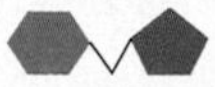
- Lactose (glucose + galactose). 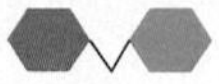

Monosaccharides

The three **monosaccharides** important in nutrition all have the same numbers and kinds of atoms, but in different arrangements. These chemical differences account for the differing sweetness of the monosaccharides. A pinch of purified glucose on the tongue gives only a mild sweet flavor, and galactose hardly tastes sweet at all, but fructose is as intensely sweet as honey and, in fact, is the sugar primarily responsible for honey's sweetness.

Glucose Chemically, **glucose** is a larger and more complicated molecule than the ethyl alcohol shown in Figure 4-1, but it obeys the same rules of chemistry: each carbon atom has four bonds; each oxygen, two bonds; and each hydrogen, one bond. Figure 4-2 illustrates the chemical structure of a glucose molecule.

The diagram of a glucose molecule shows all the relationships between the atoms and proves simple on examination, but chemists have adopted even simpler ways to depict chemical structures. Figure 4-3 shows how the chemical structure of glucose can be simplified by combining or omitting several symbols and still convey the same information.

Commonly known as blood sugar, glucose serves as an essential energy source for all the body's activities. Its significance to nutrition is tremendous. Later sections will explain that glucose is one of the two sugars in every disaccharide and the unit from which the polysaccharides are made almost exclusively. One of these polysaccharides, starch, is the chief food source of energy for the world's people; another, glycogen, is an important storage form of energy in the body. Glucose reappears frequently throughout this chapter and all those that follow.

Fructose **Fructose** is the sweetest of the sugars. Curiously, fructose has exactly the same chemical *formula* as glucose—$C_6H_{12}O_6$—but its *structure* differs (see Figure 4-4). The arrangement of the atoms in fructose stimulates the taste buds on the tongue to produce the sweet sensation. Fructose occurs naturally in fruits and honey; other sources include products such as soft drinks, ready-to-cereals, and desserts that have been sweetened with high-fructose corn syrup (defined on p. 120).

Galactose The monosaccharide **galactose** rarely occurs naturally as a single sugar. Galactose has the same numbers and kinds of atoms as glucose and fructose in yet another arrangement. Figure 4-5 shows galactose beside a molecule of glucose for comparison.

FIGURE 4-2 Chemical Structure of Glucose

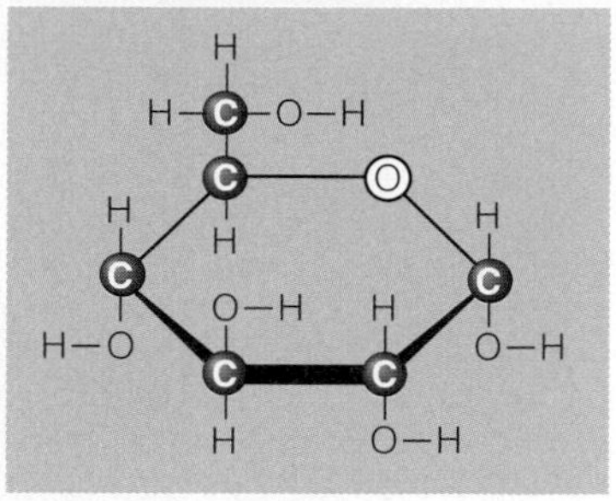
H
H—C—O—H
C
O
H
H
C
H
O—H
H
C
H—O
O—H
C
C
H
O—H

On paper, the structure of glucose has to be drawn flat, but in nature the five carbons and oxygen are roughly in a plane. The atoms attached to the ring carbons extend above and below the plane.

monosaccharides (mon-oh-SACK-uh-rides): carbohydrates of the general formula $C_nH_{2n}O_n$ that consist of a single ring. See Appendix C for the chemical structures of the monosaccharides.
- **mono** = one
- **saccharide** = sugar

glucose (GLOO-kose): a monosaccharide; sometimes known as blood sugar or **dextrose.**
- **ose** = carbohydrate
-  = glucose

fructose (FRUK-tose or FROOK-tose): a monosaccharide. Sometimes known as fruit sugar or **levulose,** fructose is found abundantly in fruits, honey, and saps.
- **fruct** = fruit
- 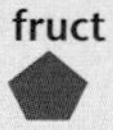 = fructose

galactose (ga-LAK-tose): a monosaccharide; part of the disaccharide lactose.
-  = galactose

FIGURE 4-3 Simplified Diagrams of Glucose

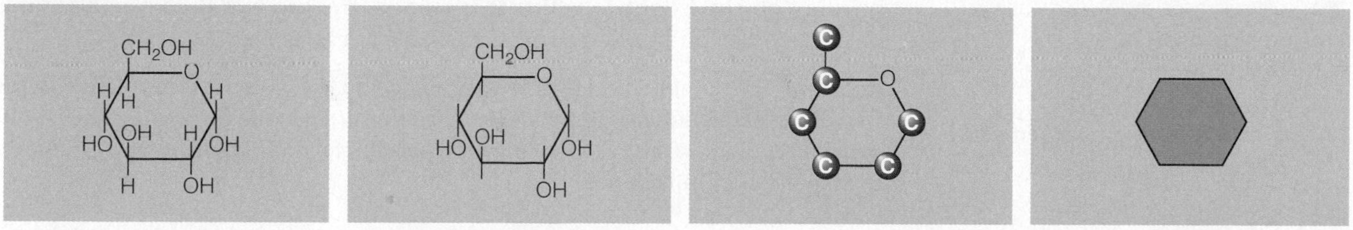
CH₂OH
O
H
H
H
HO
OH
H
OH
H
OH
CH₂OH
O
HO
OH
OH
OH
C
C
O
C
C
C
C

The lines representing some of the bonds and the carbons at the corners are not shown.

Now the single hydrogens are not shown, but lines still extend upward or downward from the ring to show where they belong.

Another way to look at glucose is to notice that its six carbon atoms are all connected.

In this and other illustrations throughout this book, glucose is represented as a blue hexagon.

FIGURE 4-4 Two Monosaccharides: Glucose and Fructose

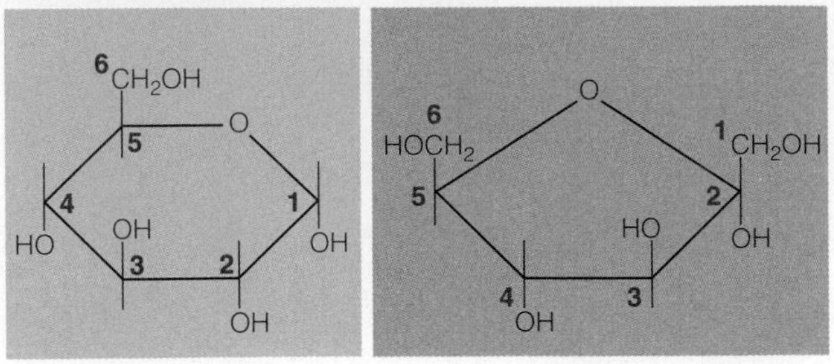
6CH2OH
O
5
4
1
HO
OH
OH
3
2
OH
O
6
HOCH2
1CH2OH
5
2
HO
OH
4
3
OH

Glucose Fructose

Can you see the similarities? If you learned the rules in Figure 4-3, you will be able to "see" 6 carbons (numbered), 12 hydrogens (those shown plus one at the end of each single line), and 6 oxygens in both these compounds.

FIGURE 4-5 Two Monosaccharides: Glucose and Galactose

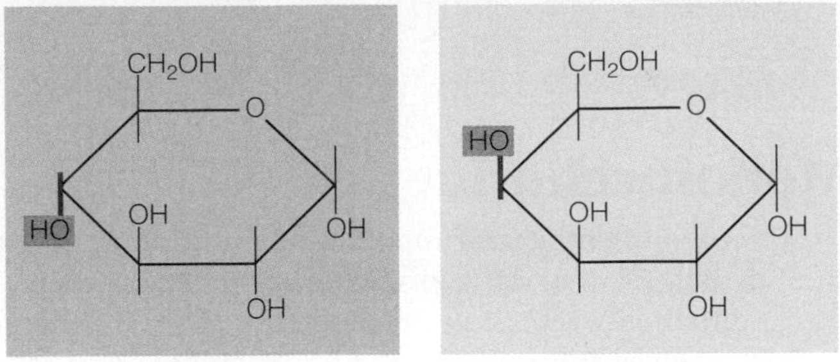
CH2OH
O
HO
OH
OH
OH
CH2OH
O
HO
OH
OH
OH

Glucose Galactose

Notice the similarities and the difference (highlighted in red).

Disaccharides

The **disaccharides** are pairs of the three monosaccharides just described. Glucose occurs in all three; the second member of the pair is either fructose, galactose, or another glucose. These carbohydrates—and all the other energy nutrients—are put together and taken apart by similar chemical reactions: condensation and hydrolysis.

Condensation To make a disaccharide, a chemical reaction known as **condensation** links two monosaccharides together (see Figure 4-6). A hydroxyl (OH) group from one monosaccharide and a hydrogen atom (H) from the other combine to create a molecule of water (H_2O). The two originally separate monosaccharides link together with a single oxygen (O).

Hydrolysis To break a disaccharide in two, a chemical reaction known as hydrolysis■ occurs (see Figure 4-7). A molecule of water splits to provide the H and OH needed to complete the resulting monosaccharides. Hydrolysis reactions commonly occur during digestion.

■ Reminder: A *hydrolysis* reaction splits a molecule into two, with H added to one and OH to the other (from water); Chapter 3 explained that hydrolysis reactions break down molecules during digestion.

Maltose The disaccharide **maltose** consists of two glucose units. Maltose is produced whenever starch breaks down—as happens in plants when seeds germinate and in human beings during carbohydrate digestion. It also occurs during the fermentation process that yields alcohol. Maltose is only a minor constituent of a few foods, most notably barley.

Sucrose Fructose and glucose together form **sucrose.** Because the fructose is in a position accessible to the taste receptors, sucrose tastes sweet, accounting for some of the natural sweetness of fruits, vegetables, and grains. To make table sugar, sucrose is refined from the juices of sugarcane and sugar beets, then granulated. Depending on the extent to which it is refined, the product becomes the familiar brown, white, and powdered sugars available at grocery stores.

Lactose The combination of galactose and glucose makes the disaccharide **lactose,** the principal carbohydrate of milk. Known as milk sugar, lactose contributes about 5 percent of milk's weight. Depending on the milk's fat content, lactose contributes 30 to 50 percent of milk's energy.

disaccharides (dye-SACK-uh-rides): pairs of monosaccharides linked together. See Appendix C for the chemical structures of the disaccharides.
- **di** = two

condensation: a chemical reaction in which two reactants combine to yield a larger product.

maltose (MAWL-tose): a disaccharide composed of two glucose units; sometimes known as malt sugar.
- 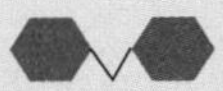 = maltose

sucrose (SUE-krose): a disaccharide composed of glucose and fructose; commonly known as table sugar, beet sugar, or cane sugar. Sucrose also occurs in many fruits and some vegetables and grains.
- sucro = sugar
- 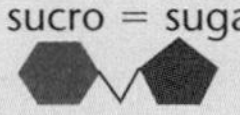 = sucrose

lactose (LAK-tose): a disaccharide composed of glucose and galactose; commonly known as milk sugar.
- **lact** = milk
- 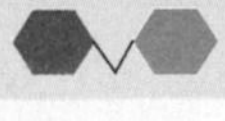 = lactose

IN SUMMARY Six simple carbohydrates, or sugars, are important in nutrition. The three monosaccharides (glucose, fructose, and galactose) all have the same chemical formula ($C_6H_{12}O_6$), but their structures differ. The three disaccharides (maltose, sucrose, and lactose) are pairs of monosaccharides, each

FIGURE 4-6 Condensation of Two Monosaccharides to Form a Disaccharide

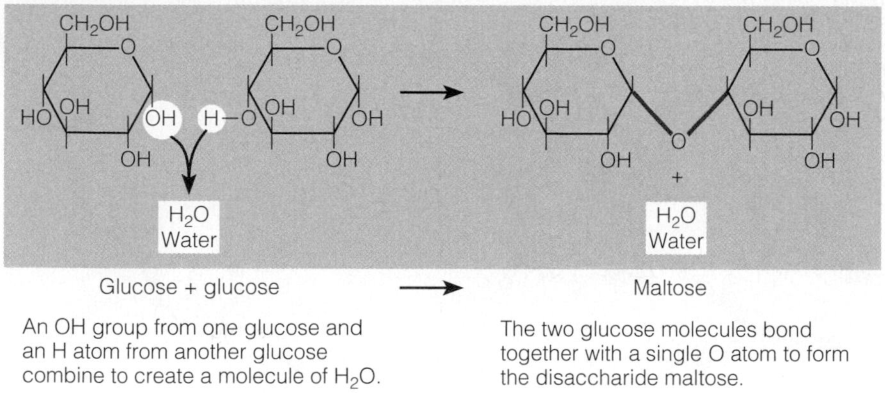
CH2OH
O
HO
OH
OH
OH
H—O
OH
OH
H2O
Water
+
Glucose + glucose
Maltose
An OH group from one glucose and an H atom from another glucose combine to create a molecule of H2O.
The two glucose molecules bond together with a single O atom to form the disaccharide maltose.

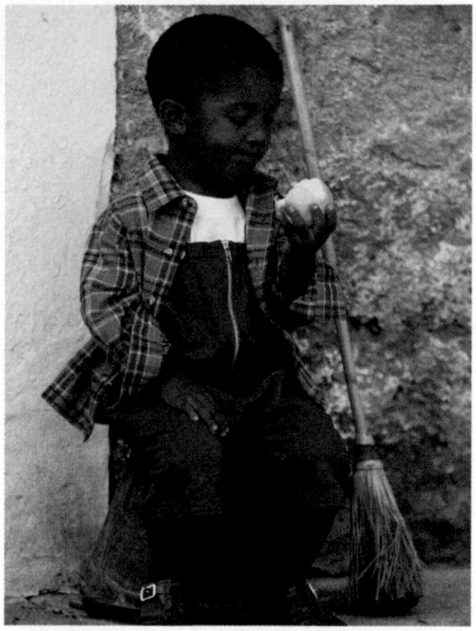

© Wartenberg/Picture Press/Corbis

Fruits package their simple sugars with fibers, vitamins, and minerals, making them a sweet and healthy snack.

containing a glucose paired with one of the three monosaccharides. The sugars derive primarily from plants, except for lactose and its component galactose, which come from milk and milk products. Two monosaccharides can be linked together by a condensation reaction to form a disaccharide and water. A disaccharide, in turn, can be broken into its two monosaccharides by a hydrolysis reaction using water.

The Complex Carbohydrates

The simple carbohydrates are the sugars just mentioned—the monosaccharides glucose, fructose, and galactose and the disaccharides maltose, sucrose, and lactose. In contrast, the complex carbohydrates contain many glucose units and, in some cases, a few other monosaccharides strung together as **polysaccharides.** Three types of polysaccharides are important in nutrition: glycogen, starches, and fibers.

Glycogen is a storage form of energy in the animal body; starches play that role in plants; and fibers provide structure in stems, trunks, roots, leaves, and skins of plants. Both glycogen and starch are built of glucose units; fibers are composed of a variety of monosaccharides and other carbohydrate derivatives.

FIGURE 4-7 Hydrolysis of a Disaccharide

Hydrolysis occurs during digestion.

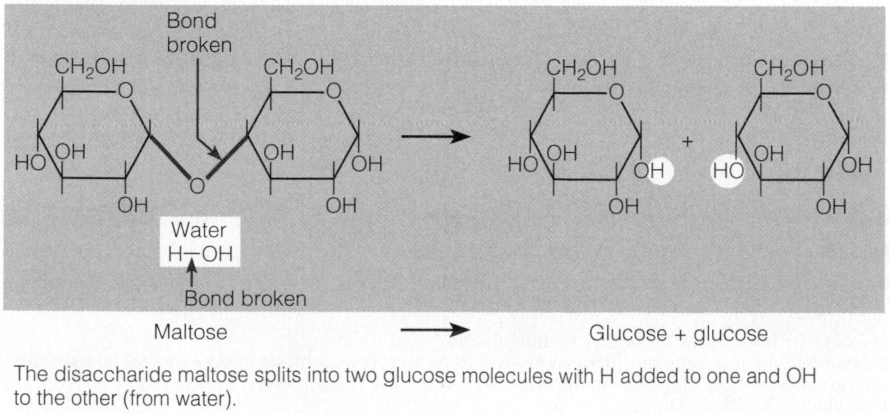
Bond broken
CH2OH
O
HO
OH
Water
H—OH
Bond broken
+
Maltose
Glucose + glucose
The disaccharide maltose splits into two glucose molecules with H added to one and OH to the other (from water).

polysaccharides: compounds composed of many monosaccharides linked together. An intermediate string of three to ten monosaccharides is an **oligosaccharide.**

- **poly** = many
- **oligo** = few

FIGURE 4-8 Glycogen and Starch Molecules Compared (Small Segments)

Notice the more highly branched the structure, the greater the number of ends from which glucose can be released. (These units would have to be magnified millions of times to appear at the size shown in this figure. For details of the chemical structures, see Appendix C.)

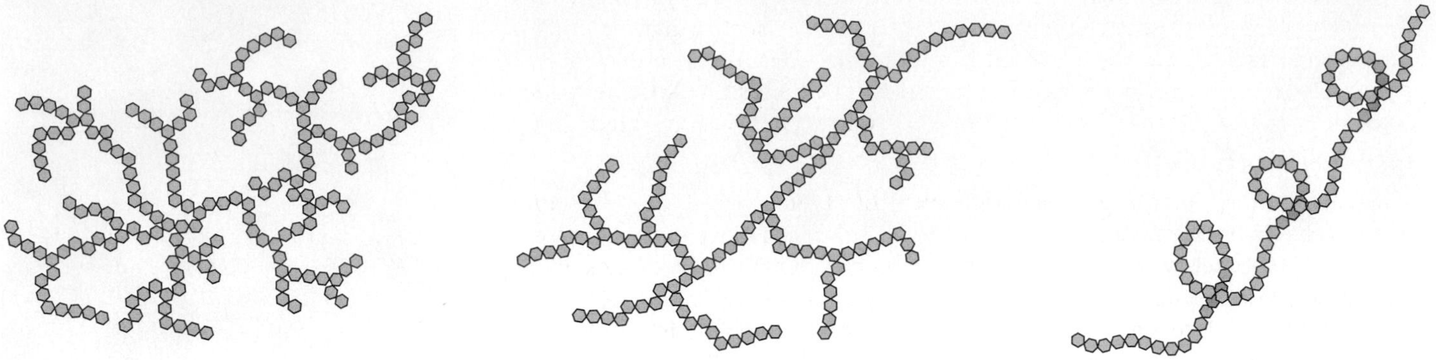

Glycogen

A glycogen molecule contains hundreds of glucose units in long, highly branched chains.

Starch (amylopectin) Starch (amylose)

A starch molecule contains hundreds of glucose molecules in either occasionally branched chains (amylopectin) or unbranched chains (amylose).

Glycogen

Glycogen is found to only a limited extent in meats and not at all in plants.* For this reason, glycogen is not a significant food source of carbohydrate, but it does perform an important role in the body. The human body stores much of its glucose as glycogen—many glucose molecules linked together in highly branched chains (see the left side of Figure 4-8). This arrangement permits rapid hydrolysis. When the hormonal message "Release energy" arrives at the storage sites in a liver or muscle cell, enzymes respond by attacking all the many branches of each glycogen simultaneously, making a surge of glucose available.†

Starches

Just as the human body stores glucose as glycogen, plant cells store glucose as **starches**—long, branched or unbranched chains of hundreds or thousands of glucose molecules linked together (see the middle and right side of Figure 4-8). These giant starch molecules are packed side by side in grains such as wheat or rice, in root crops and tubers such as yams and potatoes, and in legumes such as peas and beans. When you eat the plant, your body hydrolyzes the starch to glucose and uses the glucose for its own energy purposes.

All starchy foods come from plants. Grains are the richest food source of starch, providing much of the food energy for people all over the world—rice in Asia; wheat in Canada, the United States, and Europe; corn in much of Central and South America; and millet, rye, barley, and oats elsewhere. Legumes and tubers are also important sources of starch.

Fibers

Fibers are the structural parts of plants and thus are found in all plant-derived foods—vegetables, fruits, grains, and legumes. Most fibers are polysaccharides. As mentioned earlier, starches are also polysacharides, but fibers differ from starches

*Glycogen in animal muscles rapidly hydrolyzes after slaughter.

†Normally, only liver cells can produce glucose from glycogen to be sent *directly* to the blood; muscle cells can also produce glucose from glycogen, but must use it themselves. Muscle cells can restore the blood glucose level *indirectly*, however, as Chapter 7 explains.

glycogen (GLY-co-gen): an animal polysaccharide composed of glucose; manufactured and stored in the liver and muscles as a storage form of glucose. Glycogen is not a significant food source of carbohydrate and is not counted as one of the complex carbohydrates in foods.
- **glyco** = glucose
- **gen** = gives rise to

starches: plant polysaccharides composed of glucose.

fibers: in plant foods, the *nonstarch polysaccharides* that are not digested by human digestive enzymes, although some are digested by GI tract bacteria. Fibers include cellulose, hemicelluloses, pectins, gums, and mucilages and the nonpolysaccharides lignins, cutins, and tannins.

in that the bonds between their monosaccharides cannot be broken down by digestive enzymes in the body. Consequently, fibers contribute no monosaccharides, and therefore little or no energy, to the body.

For these reasons, fibers are often described as *nonstarch polysaccharides*. The nonstarch polysaccharide fibers include cellulose, hemicelluloses, pectins, gums, and mucilages. Fibers also include some *nonpolysaccharides* such as lignins, cutins, and tannins. Each of the fibers has a different structure. Most contain monosaccharides, but differ in the types they contain and in the bonds that link the monosaccharides to each other. These differences produce diverse health effects as explained later.

Cellulose Cellulose is the primary constituent of plant cell walls and therefore occurs naturally in all vegetables, fruits, and legumes. Cellulose can also be extracted from wood pulp or cotton and added to foods as an anticaking, thickening, and texturizing agent during processing.

Like starch, cellulose is composed of glucose molecules connected in long chains. Unlike starch, however, the chains do not branch, and the bonds linking the glucose molecules together cannot be broken by human enzymes (see Figure 4-9).

Hemicelluloses The hemicelluloses are the main constituent of cereal fibers. They are composed of various monosaccharide backbones with branching side chains of monosaccharides.*

Pectins All pectins consist of a backbone of one type of monosaccharide; some are unbranched, whereas others have side chains of various monosaccharides.† Commonly found in vegetables and fruits (especially citrus fruits and apples), pectins may be isolated and used by the food industry to thicken jelly, keep salad dressings from separating, and otherwise control texture and consistency. Pectins can perform these functions because they readily form gels in water.

Gums and Mucilages When cut, a plant secretes gums from the site of the injury. Like the other fibers, gums are composed of various monosaccharides and their derivatives. Gums such as *guar gum* and *gum arabic* are used as additives by the food industry to thicken processed foods. Mucilages are similar to gums in structure; they include *psyllium* and *carrageenan,* which are added to foods as stabilizers.

Lignin This *nonpolysaccharide* fiber has a three-dimensional structure that gives it strength.‡ Because of its toughness, few of the foods that people eat contain much lignin. It occurs in the woody parts of vegetables such as carrots and the small seeds of fruits such as strawberries.

Resistant Starches A few starches are classified as fibers. Known as **resistant starches,** these starches escape digestion and absorption in the small intestine. Starch may resist digestion for several reasons, including the individual's efficiency in digesting starches and the food's physical properties. Resistant starch is common in whole legumes, raw potatoes, and unripe bananas.

Fiber Characteristics The previous paragraphs described fibers according to their chemistry, but their physical characteristics may better explain their actions in the body. Fibers do not sort neatly into groups, but a few generalizations can be made. Some fibers dissolve in water **(soluble fibers),** form gels **(viscous),** and are easily digested by bacteria in the colon **(fermentable).** Commonly found in legumes and fruits, these fibers are most often associated with protecting against heart disease and diabetes by lowering blood cholesterol and glucose levels, respectively.[1]

*In hemicelluloses, the most common backbone monosaccharides are xylose, mannose, and galactose; the common side chains are arabinose, glucuronic acid, and galactose (see Appendix C for structures).
†In pectins, the backbone is usually made of galacturonic acid units.
‡Lignins are polymers of several dozen molecules of phenol (an alcohol), with strong internal bonds that make them impervious to digestive enzymes.

FIGURE 4-9 Starch and Cellulose Molecules Compared (Small Segments)

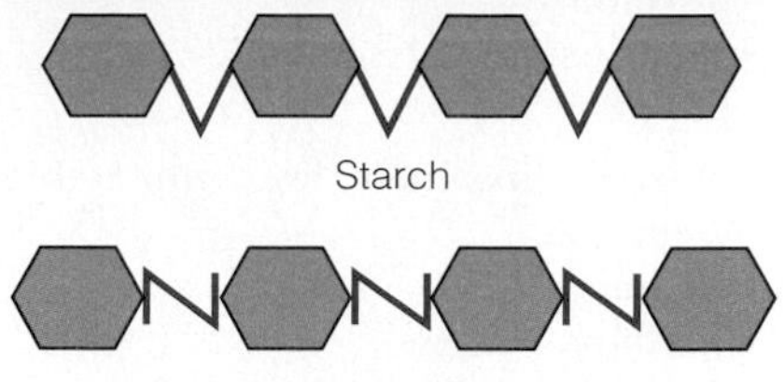
Starch
Cellulose

The bonds that link the glucose molecules together in cellulose are different from the bonds in starch (and glycogen). Human enzymes cannot digest cellulose. See Appendix C for chemical structures and descriptions of linkages.

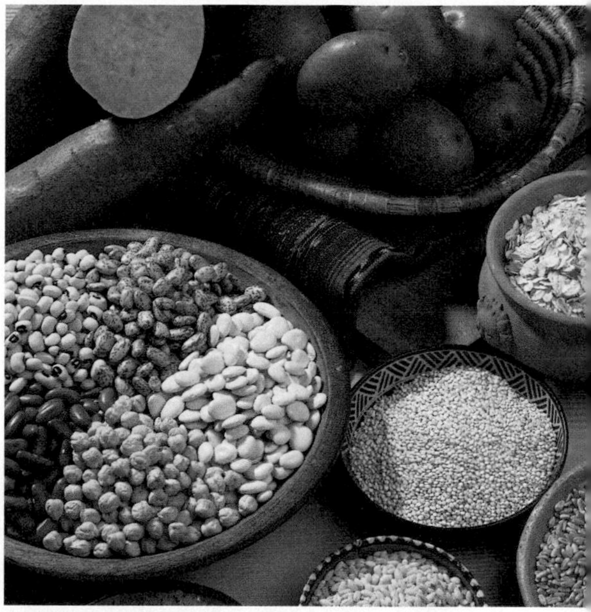

© Polara Studios Inc.

Major sources of starch include grains, (such as rice, wheat, millet, rye, barley, and oats), legumes (such as kidney beans, black-eyed peas, pinto beans, navy beans, and garbanzo beans), tubers (such as potatoes), and root crops (such as yams and cassava).

resistant starches: starches that escape digestion and absorption in the small intestine of healthy people.

soluble fibers: indigestible food components that dissolve in water to form a gel. An example is pectin from fruit, which is used to thicken jellies.

viscous: a gel-like consistency.

fermentable: the extent to which bacteria in the GI tract can break down fibers to fragments that the body can use.*

*Dietary fibers are fermented by bacteria in the colon to short-chain fatty acids, which are absorbed and metabolized by cells in the GI tract and liver (Chapter 5 describes fatty acids).

Other fibers do not dissolve in water **(insoluble fibers),** do not form gels (nonviscous), and are less readily fermented. Found mostly in grains and vegetables, these fibers promote bowel movements and alleviate constipation. These generalizations between viscous■ and nonviscous■ fibers are useful, but exceptions occur. For example, insoluble rice bran also lowers blood cholesterol, and the soluble fiber of the psyllium plant effectively promotes bowel movements.

- Viscous (soluble, more fermentable):
  - Gums and mucilages.
  - Pectins.
  - Psyllium.
  - Some hemicelluloses.

- Nonviscous (insoluble, less fermentable):
  - Cellulose.
  - Lignins.
  - Psyllium.
  - Resistant starch.
  - Many hemicelluloses.

Recently, the committee on Dietary Reference Intakes (DRI) proposed terms that distinguish fibers not by their chemical or physical properties, but by their source. Fibers that occur naturally in intact plants are called *dietary fibers,* whereas fibers that have been extracted from plants or manufactured and have beneficial health effects are called *functional fibers. Total fiber* refers to the sum of dietary fibers and functional fibers. These definitions■ were created to accommodate the labeling of products that may contain new fiber sources that prove to have beneficial effects.

- *Dietary fibers* occur naturally in intact plants. *Functional fibers* have been extracted from plants or manufactured and have beneficial effects in human beings. *Total fiber* is the sum of dietary fibers and functional fibers.

A compound not classed as a fiber but often found with it in foods is **phytic acid.** Because of this close association, researchers have been unable to determine whether it is the fiber, the phytic acid, or both, that binds with minerals, preventing their absorption. This binding presents a risk of mineral deficiencies, but the risk is minimal when fiber intake is reasonable and mineral intake adequate. The nutrition consequences of such mineral losses are described further in Chapters 12 and 13.

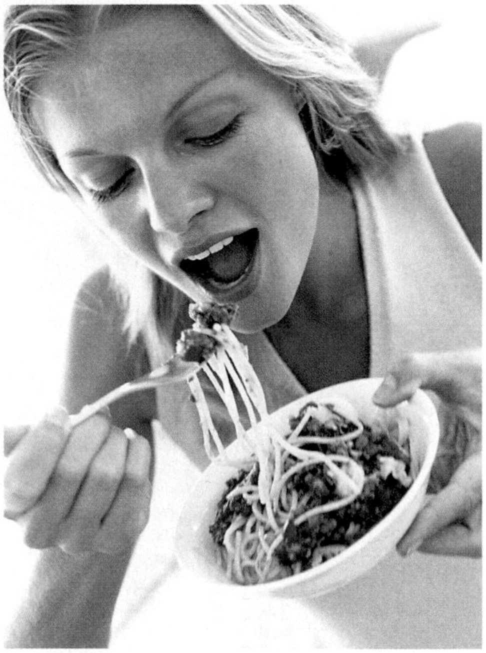

© Banana Stock/SuperStock

When a person eats carbohydrate-rich foods, the body receives a valuable commodity—glucose.

IN SUMMARY The complex carbohydrates are the polysaccharides (chains of monosaccharides): glycogen, starches, and fibers. Both glycogen and starch are storage forms of glucose—glycogen in the body, and starch in plants—and both yield energy for human use. The fibers also contain glucose (and other monosaccharides), but their bonds cannot be broken by human digestive enzymes, so they yield little, if any, energy. The accompanying table summarizes the carbohydrate family of compounds.

The Carbohydrate Family

Simple Carbohydrates (sugars)	Complex Carbohydrates
• Monosaccharides	• Polysaccharides
Glucose	Glycogen[a]
Fructose	Starches
Galactose	Fibers
• Disaccharides	
Maltose	
Sucrose	
Lactose	

[a]Glycogen is a complex carbohydrate (a polysaccharide), but not a *dietary* source of carbohydrate.

insoluble fibers: indigestible food components that do not dissolve in water. Examples include the tough, fibrous structures found in the strings of celery and the skins of corn kernels.

phytic (FYE-tick) **acid:** a nonnutrient component of plant seeds; also called **phytate** (FYE-tate). Phytic acid occurs in the husks of grains, legumes, and seeds and is capable of binding minerals such as zinc, iron, calcium, magnesium, and copper in insoluble complexes in the intestine, which the body excretes unused.

Digestion and Absorption of Carbohydrates

The ultimate goal of digestion and absorption of sugars and starches is to dismantle them into small molecules—chiefly glucose—that the body can absorb and use. The large starch molecules require extensive breakdown; the disaccharides need only be broken once and the monosaccharides not at all. The initial splitting begins in the mouth; the final splitting and absorption occur in the small intestine; and conversion to a common energy currency (glucose) takes place in the liver. The details follow.

Carbohydrate Digestion

Figure 4-10 (on p. 112) traces the digestion of carbohydrates through the GI tract. When a person eats foods containing starch, enzymes hydrolyze the long chains to shorter chains,■ the short chains to disaccharides, and, finally, the disaccharides to monosaccharides. This process begins in the mouth.

■ The short chains of glucose units that result from the breakdown of starch are known as **dextrins.** The word sometimes appears on food labels because dextrins can be used as thickening agents in foods.

In the Mouth In the mouth, thoroughly chewing high-fiber foods slows eating and stimulates the flow of saliva. The salivary enzyme **amylase** starts to work, hydrolyzing starch to shorter polysaccharides and to maltose. In fact, you can taste the change if you hold a piece of starchy food like a cracker in your mouth for a few minutes without swallowing it—the cracker begins tasting sweeter as the enzyme acts on it. Because food is in the mouth for only a short time, very little carbohydrate digestion takes place there. That digestive activity temporarily ceases is of no consequence, however; it picks up again further down the tract.

In the Stomach The swallowed bolus■ mixes with the stomach's acid and protein-digesting enzymes, which inactivate salivary amylase. Thus the role of salivary amylase in starch digestion is relatively minor. To a small extent, the stomach's acid continues breaking down starch, but its juices contain no enzymes to digest carbohydrate. Fibers linger in the stomach and delay gastric emptying, thereby providing a feeling of fullness and **satiety.**

■ Reminder: A *bolus* is a portion of food swallowed at one time.

In the Small Intestine The small intestine performs most of the work of carbohydrate digestion. A major carbohydrate-digesting enzyme, pancreatic amylase, enters the intestine via the pancreatic duct and continues breaking down the polysaccharides to shorter glucose chains and disaccharides. The final step takes place on the outer membranes of the intestinal cells. There specific enzymes■ dismantle specific disaccharides:

- **Maltase** breaks maltose into two glucose molecules.
- **Sucrase** breaks sucrose into one glucose and one fructose molecule.
- **Lactase** breaks lactose into one glucose and one galactose molecule.

■ Reminder: In general, the word ending *–ase* identifies an enzyme, and the word beginning identifies the molecule that the enzyme works on.

At this point, all polysaccharides and disaccharides have been broken down to monosaccharides—mostly glucose molecules, with some fructose and galactose molecules as well.

In the Large Intestine Within one to four hours after a meal, all the sugars and most of the starches have been digested.■ Only the fibers remain in the digestive tract. Fibers in the large intestine attract water, which softens the stools for passage without straining. Also, bacteria in the GI tract ferment some fibers. This process generates water, gas, and short-chain fatty acids (described in Chapter 5).* The colon uses these small fat molecules for energy. Metabolism of short-chain fatty acids also occurs in the cells of the liver. Fibers, therefore, can contribute some energy (1.5 to 2.5 kcalories per gram), depending on the extent to which they are broken down by bacteria and the fatty acids are absorbed.

■ Starches and sugars are called **available carbohydrates** because human digestive enzymes break them down for the body's use. In contrast, fibers are called **unavailable carbohydrates** because human digestive enzymes cannot break their bonds.

Carbohydrate Absorption

Glucose is unique in that it can be absorbed to some extent through the lining of the mouth, but for the most part, nutrient absorption takes place in the small intestine. Glucose and galactose traverse the cells lining the small intestine by active transport; fructose is absorbed by facilitated diffusion, which slows its entry and produces a smaller rise in blood glucose. Likewise, unbranched chains of starch are digested slowly and produce a smaller rise in blood glucose than branched chains, which have many more places for enzymes to attack and release glucose rapidly.

amylase (AM-ih-lace): an enzyme that hydrolyzes amylose (a form of starch). Amylase is a *carbohydrase,* an enzyme that breaks down carbohydrates.

satiety (sah-TIE-eh-tee): the feeling of fullness and satisfaction that food brings (Chapter 8 provides a more detailed description).
- **sate** = to fill

maltase: an enzyme that hydrolyzes maltose.

sucrase: an enzyme that hydrolyzes sucrose.

lactase: an enzyme that hydrolyzes lactose.

*The short-chain fatty acids produced by GI bacteria are primarily acetic acid, propionic acid, and butyric acid.

FIGURE 4-10 Carbohydrate Digestion in the GI Tract

STARCH

Mouth and salivary glands
The salivary glands secrete saliva into the mouth to moisten the food. The salivary enzyme amylase begins digestion:

Starch $\xrightarrow{\text{amylase}}$ small polysaccharides, maltose

Stomach
Stomach acid inactivates salivary enzymes, halting starch digestion.

Small intestine and pancreas
The pancreas produces an amylase that is released through the pancreatic duct into the small intestine:

Starch $\xrightarrow{\text{Pancreatic amylase}}$ Small polysaccharides, maltose

Then disaccharidase enzymes on the surface of the small intestinal cells hydrolyze the disaccharides into monosaccharides:

Maltose $\xrightarrow{\text{maltase}}$ glucose + glucose

Sucrose $\xrightarrow{\text{sucrase}}$ fructose + glucose

Lactose $\xrightarrow{\text{lactase}}$ galactose + glucose

Intestinal cells absorb these monosaccharides.

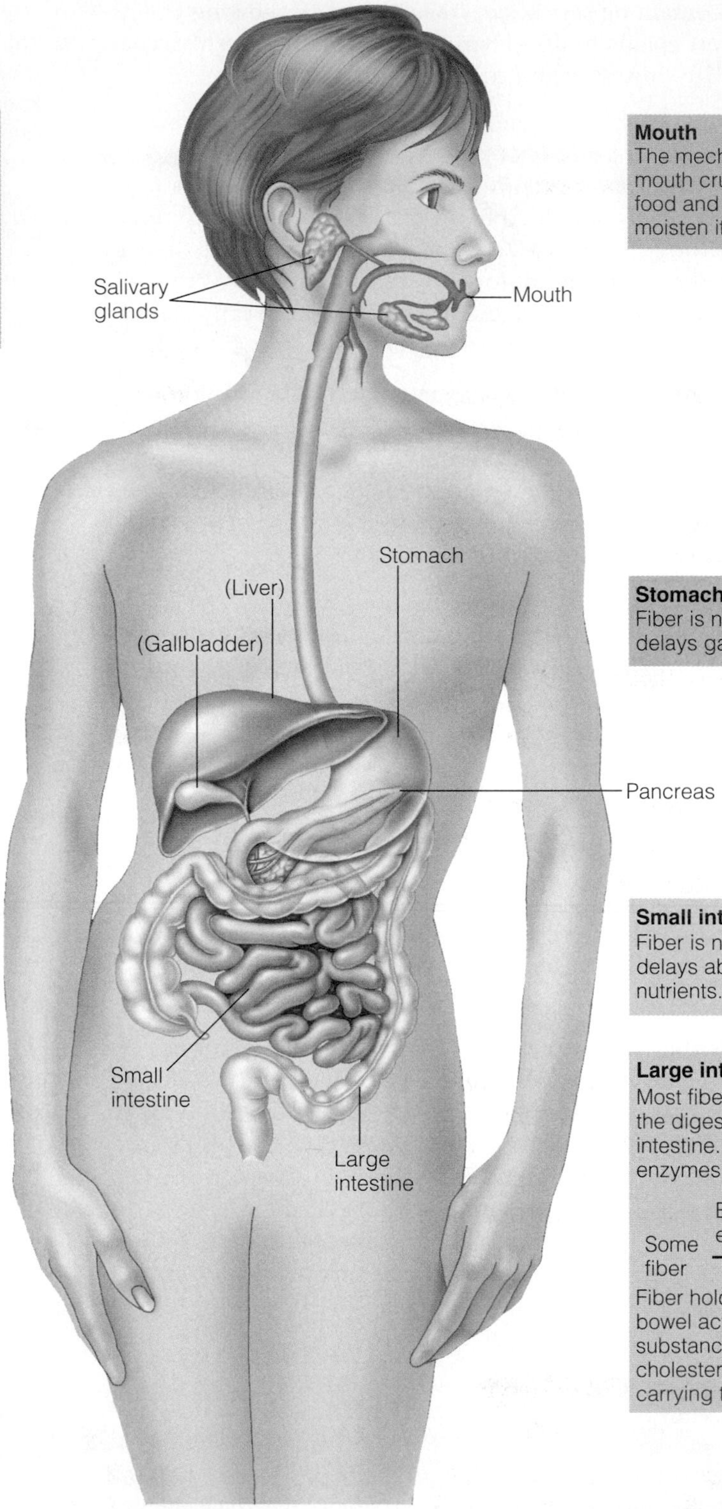
Salivary glands
Mouth
Stomach
(Liver)
(Gallbladder)
Pancreas
Small intestine
Large intestine

FIBER

Mouth
The mechanical action of the mouth crushes and tears fiber in food and mixes it with saliva to moisten it for swallowing.

Stomach
Fiber is not digested, and it delays gastric emptying.

Small intestine
Fiber is not digested, and it delays absorption of other nutrients.

Large intestine
Most fiber passes intact through the digestive tract to the large intestine. Here, bacterial enzymes digest fiber:

Some fiber $\xrightarrow{\text{Bacterial enzymes}}$ Fatty acids, gas

Fiber holds water; regulates bowel activity; and binds substances such as bile, cholesterol, and some minerals, carrying them out of the body.

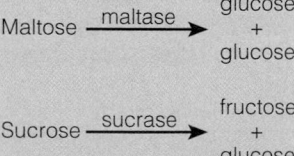

Available Online

http://nutrition.wadsworth.com/uncn7
Follow the digestion of starch as it begins in the mouth, and is completed in the small intestine with the release of glucose.

FIGURE 4-11 Absorption of Monosaccharides

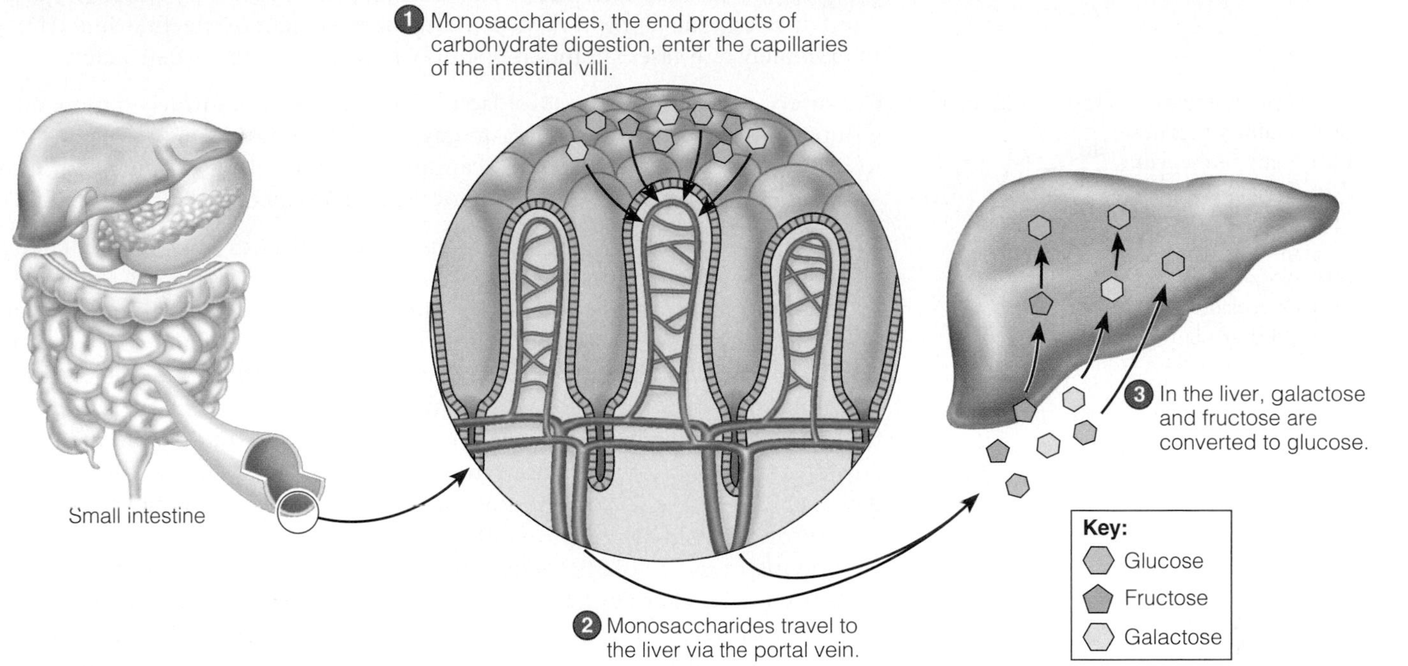
1 Monosaccharides, the end products of carbohydrate digestion, enter the capillaries of the intestinal villi.
Small intestine
2 Monosaccharides travel to the liver via the portal vein.
3 In the liver, galactose and fructose are converted to glucose.
Key:
Glucose
Fructose
Galactose

As the blood from the intestines circulates through the liver, cells there take up fructose and galactose and convert them to other compounds, most often to glucose, as shown in Figure 4-11. Thus all disaccharides provide at least one glucose molecule directly, and they can provide another one indirectly—through the conversion of fructose and galactose to glucose.

IN SUMMARY In the digestion and absorption of carbohydrates, the body breaks down starches into disaccharides and disaccharides into monosaccharides; it then converts monosaccharides mostly to glucose to provide energy for the cells' work. The fibers help to regulate the passage of food through the GI system and slow the absorption of glucose, but contribute little, if any, energy.

Lactose Intolerance

Normally, the intestinal cells produce enough of the enzyme lactase to ensure that the disaccharide lactose found in milk is both digested and absorbed efficiently. Lactase activity is highest immediately after birth, as befits an infant whose first and only food for a while will be breast milk or infant formula. In the great majority of the world's populations, lactase activity declines dramatically during childhood and adolescence to about 5 to 10 percent of the activity at birth. Only a relatively small percentage (about 30 percent) of the people in the world retain enough lactase to digest and absorb lactose efficiently throughout adult life.

Symptoms When more lactose is consumed than the available lactase can handle, lactose molecules remain in the intestine undigested, attracting water and causing bloating, abdominal discomfort, and diarrhea—the symptoms of **lactose intolerance.** The undigested lactose becomes food for intestinal bacteria, which multiply and produce irritating acid and gas, further contributing to the discomfort and diarrhea.

lactose intolerance: a condition that results from inability to digest the milk sugar lactose; characterized by bloating, gas, abdominal discomfort, and diarrhea. Lactose intolerance differs from milk allergy, which is caused by an immune reaction to the protein in milk.

Causes As mentioned, lactase activity commonly declines with age. **Lactase deficiency** may also develop when the intestinal villi are damaged by disease, certain medicines, prolonged diarrhea, or malnutrition; this can lead to temporary or permanent lactose malabsorption, depending on the extent of the intestinal damage. In extremely rare cases, an infant is simply born with a lactase deficiency.

Prevalence The prevalence■ of lactose intolerance varies widely among ethnic groups, indicating that the trait is genetically determined. The prevalence of lactose intolerance is lowest among Scandinavians and other northern Europeans and highest among native North Americans and Southeast Asians.

■ Estimated prevalence of lactose intolerance:
- >80% Southeast Asians.
- 80% Native Americans.
- 75% African Americans.
- 70% Mediterranean peoples.
- 60% Inuits.
- 50% Hispanics.
- 20% Caucasians.
- <10% Northern Europeans.

Dietary Changes Managing lactose intolerance requires some dietary changes, although total elimination of milk products usually is not necessary. Excluding all milk products from the diet can lead to nutrient deficiencies, for these foods are a major source of several nutrients, notably the mineral calcium, the B vitamin riboflavin, and vitamin D. Fortunately, many people with lactose intolerance can consume foods containing up to 6 grams of lactose (½ cup milk) without symptoms. The most successful strategies are to increase intake of milk products gradually, take them with other foods in meals, and spread their intake throughout the day. A change in the GI bacteria, not the reappearance of the missing enzyme, accounts for the ability to adapt to milk products.

In many cases, lactose-intolerant people can tolerate fermented milk products such as yogurt and **acidophilus milk.**[2] The bacteria in these products digest lactose for their own use, thus reducing the lactose content. Even when the lactose content is equivalent to milk's, yogurt produces fewer symptoms. Hard cheeses and cottage cheese are often well tolerated because most of the lactose is removed with the whey during manufacturing. Lactose continues to diminish as the cheese ages.

Many lactose-intolerant people use commercially prepared milk products that have been treated with an enzyme that breaks down the lactose. Alternatively, they take enzyme tablets with meals or add enzyme drops to their milk. The enzyme hydrolyzes much of the lactose in milk to glucose and galactose, which lactose-intolerant people can absorb without ill effects.

Because people's tolerance to lactose varies widely, lactose-restricted diets must be highly individualized. A completely lactose-free diet can be difficult because lactose appears not only in milk and milk products but also as an ingredient in many nondairy foods■ such as breads, cereals, breakfast drinks, salad dressings, and cake mixes. People on strict lactose-free diets need to read labels and avoid foods that include milk, milk solids, whey (milk liquid), and casein (milk protein, which may contain traces of lactose). They also need to check all medications with the pharmacist because 20 percent of prescription drugs and 5 percent of over-the-counter drugs contain lactose as a filler.

■ Lactose in selected foods:

Whole-wheat bread, 1 slice	0.5 g
Dinner roll, 1	0.5 g
Cheese, 1 oz	
Cheddar or American	0.5 g
Parmesan or cream	0.8 g
Doughnut (cake type), 1	1.2 g
Chocolate candy, 1 oz	2.3 g
Sherbet, 1 c	4.0 g
Cottage cheese (low-fat), 1 c	7.5 g
Ice cream, 1 c	9.0 g
Milk, 1 c	12.0 g
Yogurt (low-fat), 1 c	15.0 g

Note: Yogurt is often enriched with nonfat milk solids, which increase its lactose content to a level higher than milk's.

People who consume few or no milk products must take care to meet riboflavin, vitamin D, and calcium needs. Later chapters on the vitamins and minerals offer help with finding good nonmilk sources of these nutrients.

IN SUMMARY Lactose intolerance is a common condition that occurs when there is insufficient lactase to digest the disaccharide lactose found in milk and milk products. Symptoms include GI distress. Because treatment requires limiting milk intake, other sources of riboflavin, vitamin D, and calcium must be included in the diet.

lactase deficiency: a lack of the enzyme required to digest the disaccharide lactose into its component monosaccharides (glucose and galactose).

acidophilus (ASS-ih-DOF-ih-lus) **milk:** a cultured milk created by adding *Lactobacillus acidophilus,* a bacterium that breaks down lactose to glucose and galactose, producing a sweet, lactose-free product.

Glucose in the Body

The primary role of the available carbohydrates in human nutrition is to supply the body's cells with glucose to deliver the indispensable commodity, energy. Starch contributes most to the body's glucose supply, but as explained earlier, any of the monosaccharides can also provide glucose.

Scientists have long known that providing energy is glucose's primary role in the body, but only recently uncovered additional roles glucose and other sugars perform in the body.[3]■ Sugar molecules dangle from many of the body's protein and fat molecules, with dramatic consequences. Sugars attached to a protein change the protein's shape and function; when they bind to lipids in a cell's membranes, sugars alter the way cells recognize each other.■ Cancer cells coated with sugar molecules, for example, are able to sneak by the cells of the immune system. Armed with this knowledge, scientists are now trying to use sugar molecules to create an anticancer vaccine. Further advances in knowledge are sure to reveal numerous ways these simple, yet remarkable, sugar molecules influence the health of the body.

■ The study of sugars is known as *glycobiology.*

■ These combination molecules are known as *glycoproteins* and *glycolipids,* respectively.

A Preview of Carbohydrate Metabolism

Glucose plays the central role in carbohydrate metabolism. This brief discussion provides just enough information about carbohydrate metabolism to illustrate that the body needs and uses glucose as a chief energy nutrient. Chapter 7 provides a full description of energy metabolism, and Chapter 10 shows how the B vitamins participate.

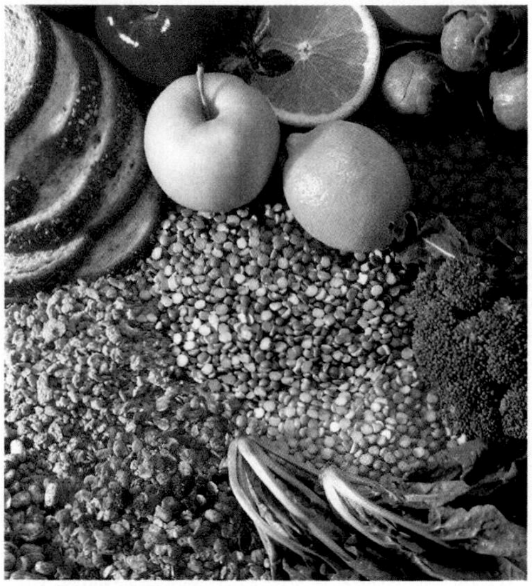

© Brian Leatart/FoodPix/Getty Images

The carbohydrates of grains, vegetables, fruits, and legumes supply most of the energy in a healthful diet.

Storing Glucose as Glycogen The liver stores about one-third of the body's total glycogen and releases glucose into the bloodstream as needed. After a meal, blood glucose rises, and liver cells link the excess glucose molecules by condensation reactions into long, branching chains of glycogen. When blood glucose falls, the liver cells dismantle the glycogen by hydrolysis reactions into single molecules of glucose and release them into the bloodstream. Thus glucose becomes available to supply energy to the brain and other tissues regardless of whether the person has eaten recently. Muscle cells can also store glucose as glycogen (the other two-thirds), but they hoard most of their supply, using it just for themselves during exercise.

Glycogen holds water and therefore is rather bulky. The body can store only enough glycogen to provide energy for relatively short periods of time—less than a day during rest and a few hours at most during exercise. For its long-term energy reserves, for use over days or weeks of food deprivation, the body uses its abundant, water-free fuel, fat, as Chapter 5 describes.

Using Glucose for Energy Glucose fuels the work of most of the body's cells. Inside a cell, enzymes break glucose in half. These halves can be put back together to make glucose, or they can be further broken down into smaller fragments (never again to be reassembled to form glucose). The small fragments can yield energy when broken down completely to carbon dioxide and water.

As mentioned, the liver's glycogen stores last only for hours, not for days. To keep providing glucose to meet the body's energy needs, a person has to eat dietary carbohydrate frequently. Yet people who do not always attend faithfully to their bodies' carbohydrate needs still survive. How do they manage without glucose from dietary carbohydrate? Do they simply draw energy from the other two energy-yielding nutrients, fat and protein? They do draw energy, but not simply.

Making Glucose from Protein Glucose is the preferred energy source for brain cells, other nerve cells, and developing red blood cells. Body protein can be converted to glucose to some extent, but protein has jobs of its own that no other nutrient can do. Body fat cannot be converted to glucose to any significant extent. Thus, when a person does not replenish depleted glycogen stores by eating carbohydrate, body proteins are dismantled to make glucose to fuel these special cells.

The conversion of protein to glucose is called **gluconeogenesis**—literally, the making of new glucose. Only adequate dietary carbohydrate can prevent this use of protein for energy, and this role of carbohydrate is known as its **protein-sparing action.**

gluconeogenesis (gloo-co-nee-oh-GEN-ih-sis): the making of glucose from a noncarbohydrate source (described in more detail in Chapter 7).
- **gluco** = glucose
- **neo** = new
- **genesis** = making

protein-sparing action: the action of carbohydrate (and fat) in providing energy that allows protein to be used for other purposes.

Making Ketone Bodies from Fat Fragments An inadequate supply of carbohydrate can shift the body's energy metabolism in a precarious direction. With less carbohydrate providing glucose to meet the brain's energy needs, fat takes an alternative metabolic pathway; instead of entering the main energy pathway, fat fragments combine with each other, forming **ketone bodies.** Ketone bodies provide an alternate fuel source during starvation, but when their production exceeds their use, they accumulate in the blood, causing **ketosis,** a condition that disturbs the body's normal **acid-base balance,** as Chapter 7 describes. (Highlight 8 explores ketosis and the health consequences of low-carbohydrate diets further.)

To spare body protein and prevent ketosis, the body needs at least 50 to 100 grams of carbohydrate a day. Dietary recommendations urge people to select abundantly from carbohydrate-rich foods to provide for considerably more.

Using Glucose to Make Fat After meeting its energy needs and filling its glycogen stores to capacity, the body must find a way to store any extra glucose. The liver breaks it into smaller molecules and puts them together into the more permanent energy-storage compound—fat. Then the fat travels to the fatty tissues of the body for storage. Unlike the liver cells, which can store only enough glycogen to meet less than a day's worth of energy needs, fat cells can store unlimited quantities of fat.

Even though excess carbohydrate can be converted to fat and stored, this is a relatively minor pathway under normal conditions. Storing carbohydrate as body fat is energetically expensive; the body uses more energy to convert dietary carbohydrate to body fat than it does to convert dietary fat to body fat.

The Constancy of Blood Glucose

Every body cell depends on glucose for its fuel to some extent, and the cells of the brain and the rest of the nervous system depend almost exclusively on glucose for their energy. The activities of these cells never cease, and they do not have the ability to store glucose. Day and night they continually draw on the supply of glucose in the fluid surrounding them. To maintain the supply, a steady stream of blood moves past these cells bringing more glucose from either the intestines (food) or the liver (via glycogen breakdown or glucose synthesis).

Maintaining Glucose Homeostasis To function optimally, the body must maintain blood glucose within limits that permit the cells to nourish themselves. If blood glucose falls below normal,■ the person may become dizzy and weak; if it rises above normal, the person may become fatigued. Left untreated, fluctuations to the extremes—either high or low—can be fatal.

The Regulating Hormones Blood glucose homeostasis■ is regulated primarily by two hormones: insulin, which moves glucose from the blood into the cells, and glucagon, which brings glucose out of storage when necessary. Figure 4-12 depicts these hormonal regulators at work.

After a meal, as blood glucose rises, special cells of the pancreas respond by secreting **insulin** into the blood.* In general, the amount of insulin secreted corresponds with the rise in glucose. As the circulating insulin contacts the receptors on the body's other cells, the receptors respond by ushering glucose from the blood into the cells. Most of the cells take only the glucose they can use for energy right away, but the liver and muscle cells can assemble the small glucose units into long, branching chains of glycogen for storage. The liver cells can also convert glucose to fat for export to other cells. Thus elevated blood glucose returns to normal as excess glucose is stored as glycogen (which can be converted back to glucose) and fat (which cannot be).

When blood glucose falls (as occurs between meals), other special cells of the pancreas respond by secreting **glucagon** into the blood.† Glucagon raises blood glucose by signaling the liver to dismantle its glycogen stores and release glucose into the blood for use by all the other body cells.

■ Normal blood glucose (fasting): 70 to 110 mg/dL.

■ Reminder: *Homeostasis* is the maintenance of constant internal conditions by the body's control systems.

ketone (KEE-tone) **bodies:** the product of the incomplete breakdown of fat when glucose is not available in the cells.

ketosis (kee-TOE-sis): an undesirably high concentration of ketone bodies in the blood and urine.

acid-base balance: the equilibrium in the body between acid and base concentrations (see Chapter 12).

insulin (IN-suh-lin): a hormone secreted by special cells in the pancreas in response to (among other things) increased blood glucose concentration. The primary role of insulin is to control the transport of glucose from the bloodstream into the muscle and fat cells.

glucagon (GLOO-ka-gon): a hormone that is secreted by special cells in the pancreas in response to low blood glucose concentration and elicits release of glucose from liver glycogen stores.

*The *beta* (BAY-tuh) *cells,* one of several types of cells in the pancreas, secrete insulin in response to elevated blood glucose concentration.

†The *alpha cells* of the pancreas secrete glucagon in response to low blood glucose.

FIGURE 4-12 Maintaining Blood Glucose Homeostasis

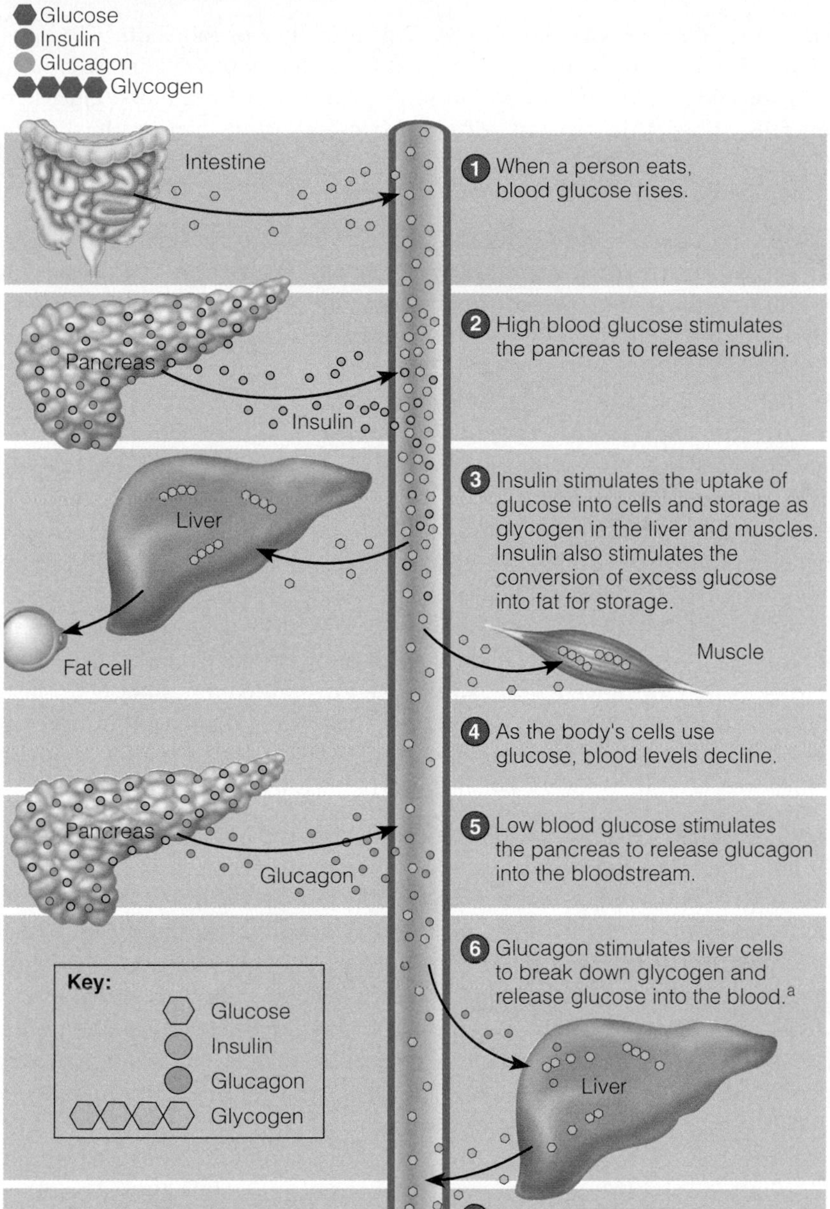

Glucose
Insulin
Glucagon
Glycogen
Intestine
1 When a person eats, blood glucose rises.
Pancreas
Insulin
2 High blood glucose stimulates the pancreas to release insulin.
Liver
3 Insulin stimulates the uptake of glucose into cells and storage as glycogen in the liver and muscles. Insulin also stimulates the conversion of excess glucose into fat for storage.
Fat cell
Muscle
4 As the body's cells use glucose, blood levels decline.
Pancreas
Glucagon
5 Low blood glucose stimulates the pancreas to release glucagon into the bloodstream.
6 Glucagon stimulates liver cells to break down glycogen and release glucose into the blood.a
Key:
Glucose
Insulin
Glucagon
Glycogen
Liver
7 Blood glucose begins to rise.

[a]The stress hormone epinephrine and other hormones also bring glucose out of storage.

Another hormone that calls glucose from the liver cells is the "fight-or-flight" hormone, **epinephrine.** When a person experiences stress, epinephrine acts quickly, ensuring that all the body cells have energy fuel in emergencies. Among its many roles in the body, epinephrine works to release glucose from liver glycogen to the blood.

Balancing within the Normal Range The maintenance of normal blood glucose ordinarily depends on two processes. When blood glucose falls below normal, food can replenish it, or in the absence of food, glucagon can signal the liver to break down glycogen stores. When blood glucose rises above normal, insulin can signal the cells to take in glucose for energy. Eating balanced meals at regular intervals helps the body maintain a happy medium between the extremes. Balanced

epinephrine (EP-ih-NEFF-rin): a hormone of the adrenal gland that modulates the stress response; formerly called **adrenaline.**

meals that provide abundant complex carbohydrates, including fibers, and a little fat help to slow down the digestion and absorption of carbohydrate so that glucose enters the blood gradually, providing a steady, ongoing supply.

Falling outside the Normal Range This influence of foods on blood glucose has given rise to the oversimplification that foods *govern* blood glucose concentrations. Foods do not; the body does. In some people, however, blood glucose regulation fails. When this happens, either of two conditions can result: diabetes or hypoglycemia. People with these conditions often plan their diets to help maintain their blood glucose within a normal range.

Diabetes In **diabetes,** blood glucose surges after a meal and remains above normal levels■ because insulin is either inadequate or ineffective. Thus *blood* glucose is central to diabetes, but *dietary* carbohydrates do not cause diabetes.

■ Blood glucose (fasting):
- Prediabetes: 110 to 125 mg/dL.
- Diabetes: ≥126 mg/dL.

There are two main types of diabetes. In **type 1 diabetes,** the less common type, the pancreas fails to make insulin; the exact cause is unclear. Some research suggests that in genetically susceptible people, certain viruses activate the immune system to attack and destroy cells in the pancreas as if they were foreign cells. In **type 2 diabetes,** the more common type of diabetes, the cells fail to respond to insulin;■ this condition tends to occur as a consequence of obesity. As the incidence of obesity in the United States has risen in recent decades, the incidence of diabetes has followed. This trend is most notable among children and adolescents, as obesity among the nation's youth reaches epidemic proportions. Because obesity can precipitate type 2 diabetes, the best preventive measure is to maintain a healthy body weight. Concentrated sweets are not strictly excluded from the diabetic diet as they once were, but can be eaten in limited amounts with meals as part of a healthy diet. Chapter 14 describes the type of diabetes that develops in some women during pregnancy (gestational diabetes), and Chapter 26 gives full coverage to type 1 and type 2 diabetes and their associated problems.

■ The condition of having blood glucose levels higher than normal, but below the diagnosis of diabetes is sometimes called **prediabetes.**

Hypoglycemia In healthy people, blood glucose rises after eating and then gradually falls back into the normal range. The transition occurs without notice. In people with **hypoglycemia,** however, blood glucose drops dramatically, producing symptoms that mimic an anxiety attack: weakness, rapid heartbeat, sweating, anxiety, hunger, and trembling. Most commonly, hypoglycemia occurs as a consequence of poorly managed diabetes. Too much insulin, strenuous physical activity, inadequate food intake, or illness can cause blood glucose levels to plummet.

Hypoglycemia in healthy people is rare. Most people who experience hypoglycemia need only adjust their diets by replacing refined carbohydrates with fiber-rich carbohydrates and ensuring an adequate protein intake.[4] In addition, smaller meals eaten more frequently may help. Hypoglycemia caused by certain medications, pancreatic tumors, overuse of insulin, alcohol abuse, or other illnesses requires medical intervention.

The Glycemic Response The **glycemic response** refers to how quickly glucose is absorbed after a person eats, how high blood glucose rises, and how quickly it returns to normal. Slow absorption, a modest rise in blood glucose, and a smooth return to normal are desirable (a low glycemic response); fast absorption, a surge in blood glucose, and an overreaction that plunges glucose below normal are less desirable (a high glycemic response). Different foods have different effects on blood glucose.

The rate of glucose absorption is particularly important to people with diabetes, who may benefit from limiting foods that produce too great a rise, or too sudden a fall, in blood glucose. To aid their choices, such people may be able to use the **glycemic index,** a method of classifying foods according to their potential to raise blood glucose. Figure 4-13 ranks selected foods by their glycemic index.[5] Some studies have shown that selecting foods with a low glycemic index is a practical way to improve glucose control.[6]

Lowering the glycemic index of the *diet* may improve lipid metabolism and prevent heart disease as well.[7] It may also help with weight management.[8] Fibers and

diabetes (DYE-ah-BEE-teez): a disorder of carbohydrate metabolism resulting from inadequate or ineffective insulin.

type 1 diabetes: the less common type of diabetes in which the person produces no insulin at all; formerly known as **insulin-dependent diabetes mellitus (IDDM)** or **juvenile-onset diabetes** (because it frequently develops in childhood), although some cases arise in adulthood.

type 2 diabetes: the more common type of diabetes in which the fat cells resist insulin; formerly called **noninsulin-dependent diabetes mellitus (NIDDM)** or **adult-onset diabetes.** Type 2 usually progresses more slowly than type 1.

hypoglycemia (HIGH-po-gligh-SEE-me-ah): an abnormally low blood glucose concentration.

glycemic (gligh-SEEM-ic) **response:** the extent to which a food raises the blood glucose concentration and elicits an insulin response.

glycemic index: a method of classifying foods according to their potential for raising blood glucose.

other slowly digested carbohydrates prolong the presence of foods in the digestive tract, thus providing greater satiety and diminishing the insulin response, which can help with weight control.[9] In contrast, the rapid absorption of glucose from a high-glycemic diet seems to increase the risk of heart disease and promote overeating in some overweight people.[10]

Despite these possible benefits, the usefulness of the glycemic index is surrounded by controversy as researchers debate whether selecting foods based on the glycemic index is practical or offers any real health benefits.[11] Those opposing the use of the glycemic index argue that it is not well enough supported by scientific research.[12] Relatively few foods have had their glycemic index determined, and when the glycemic index has been established, it is based on an average of multiple tests that often result in wide variations. Values vary because of differences in the physical and chemical characteristics of foods, testing methods of laboratories, and digestive processes of individuals.

Furthermore, the practical utility of the glycemic index is limited because this information is nether provided on food labels nor intuitively apparent. Indeed, a food's glycemic index is not always what one might expect. Ice cream, for example, is a high-sugar food, but it produces less of a response than baked potatoes, a high-starch food, most likely because the fat in the ice cream slows GI motility and thus the rate of glucose absorption. Mashed potatoes produce more of a response than honey, probably because the honey's fructose content has little effect on blood glucose. Perhaps most relevant to real life, a food's glycemic effect differs depending on how it is prepared and whether it is eaten alone or with other foods. Most people eat a variety of foods, cooked and raw, that provide different amounts of carbohydrate, fat, and protein—all of which influence the glycemic index of a meal.

Paying attention to the glycemic index may not be necessary because current guidelines already suggest many low glycemic index choices: whole grains, legumes, vegetables, fruits, and milk products.[13] In addition, eating frequent, small meals spreads glucose absorption across the day and thus offers similar metabolic advantages to eating foods with a low glycemic response. People wanting to follow a low-glycemic diet should be careful not to adopt a low-carbohydrate diet.[14] The problems associated with a low-carbohydrate diet are addressed in Highlight 8.

FIGURE 4-13 Glycemic Index of Selected Foods

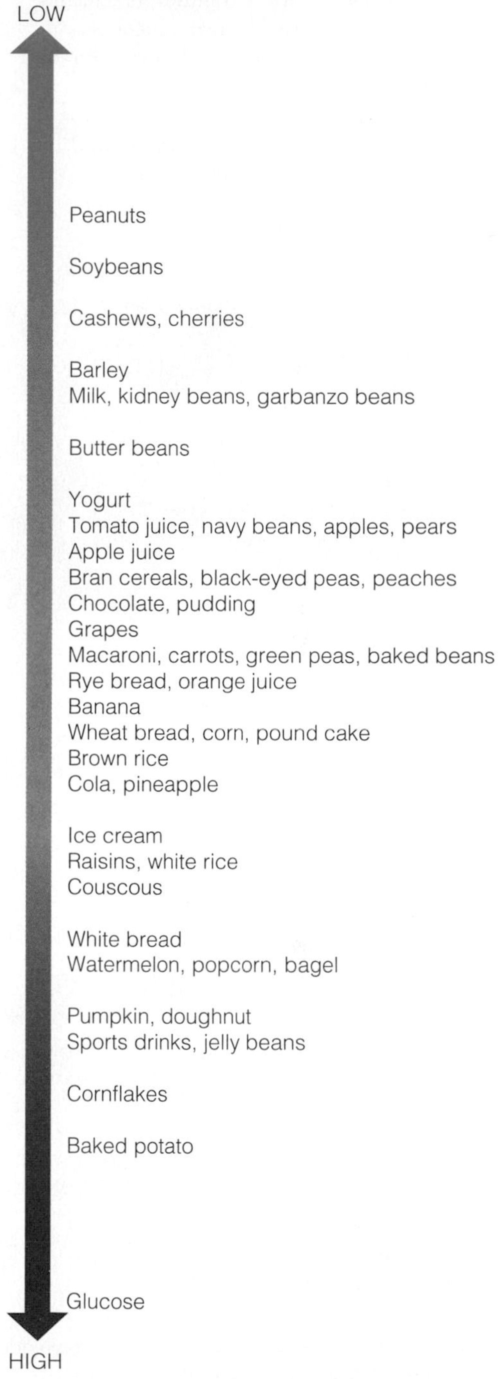
LOW
Peanuts
Soybeans
Cashews, cherries
Barley
Milk, kidney beans, garbanzo beans
Butter beans
Yogurt
Tomato juice, navy beans, apples, pears
Apple juice
Bran cereals, black-eyed peas, peaches
Chocolate, pudding
Grapes
Macaroni, carrots, green peas, baked beans
Rye bread, orange juice
Banana
Wheat bread, corn, pound cake
Brown rice
Cola, pineapple
Ice cream
Raisins, white rice
Couscous
White bread
Watermelon, popcorn, bagel
Pumpkin, doughnut
Sports drinks, jelly beans
Cornflakes
Baked potato
Glucose
HIGH

IN SUMMARY Dietary carbohydrates provide glucose that can be used by the cells for energy, stored by the liver and muscles as glycogen, or converted into fat if intakes exceed needs. All of the body's cells depend on glucose; those of the central nervous system are especially dependent on it. Without glucose, the body is forced to break down its protein tissues to make glucose and to alter energy metabolism to make ketone bodies from fats. Blood glucose regulation depends primarily on two pancreatic hormones: insulin to remove glucose from the blood into the cells when levels are high and glucagon to free glucose from glycogen stores and release it into the blood when levels are low. The glycemic index measures how blood glucose responds to foods.

Health Effects and Recommended Intakes of Sugars

Ever since people first discovered honey and dates, they have enjoyed the sweetness of sugars. In the United States, the natural sugars of milk, fruits, vegetables, and grains account for about half of the sugar intake; the other half consists of sugars that have been refined and added to foods for a variety of purposes (see p. 120 margin).■ The use of sweeteners in food manufacturing has risen steadily over the past several decades. These **added sugars** assume various names on food labels: sucrose, invert sugar, corn sugar, corn syrups and solids, high-fructose corn syrup, and honey. A food

added sugars: sugars and syrups used as an ingredient in the processing and preparation of foods such as breads, cakes, beverages, jellies, and ice cream as well as sugars eaten separately or added to foods at the table.

- As an additive, sugar:
  - Enhances flavor.
  - Supplies texture and color to baked goods.
  - Provides fuel for fermentation, causing bread to rise or producing alcohol.
  - Acts as a bulking agent in ice cream and baked goods.
  - Acts as a preservative in jams.
  - Balances the acidity of tomato- and vinegar-based products.

is likely to be high in added sugars if its ingredient list starts with any of the sugars named in the accompanying glossary or if it includes several of them.

Health Effects of Sugars

In moderate amounts, sugars add pleasure to meals without harming health. In excess, however, they can be detrimental in two ways. One, sugars can contribute to nutrient deficiencies by supplying energy (kcalories) without providing nutrients. Two, sugars contribute to tooth decay.

Nutrient Deficiencies Empty-kcalorie foods that contain lots of added sugar such as cakes, candies, and sodas deliver glucose and energy with few, if any, other nutrients. By comparison, foods such as whole grains, vegetables, legumes, and fruits that contain some natural sugars and lots of starches and fibers deliver protein, vitamins, and minerals along with their glucose and energy.

A person spending 200 kcalories of a day's energy allowance on a 16-ounce soda gets little of value for those kcaloric "dollars." In contrast, a person using 200 kcalories on three slices of whole-wheat bread gets 9 grams of protein, 6 grams of fiber, plus several of the B vitamins with those kcalories. For the person who wants something sweet, perhaps a reasonable compromise would be to have two slices of bread with a teaspoon of jam on each. The amount of sugar a person can afford to eat depends on how many kcalories are available beyond those needed to deliver indispensable vitamins and minerals.

With careful food selections, a person can obtain all the needed nutrients within an allowance of about 1500 kcalories. Some people have more generous energy allowances with which to "purchase" nutrients. For example, an active teenage boy may need as many as 4000 kcalories a day. If he eats mostly nutritious foods, then the "empty kcalories" of cola beverages may be an acceptable addition to his diet. In contrast, an inactive older woman who is limited to fewer than 1500 kcalories a day can afford only the most nutrient-dense foods.

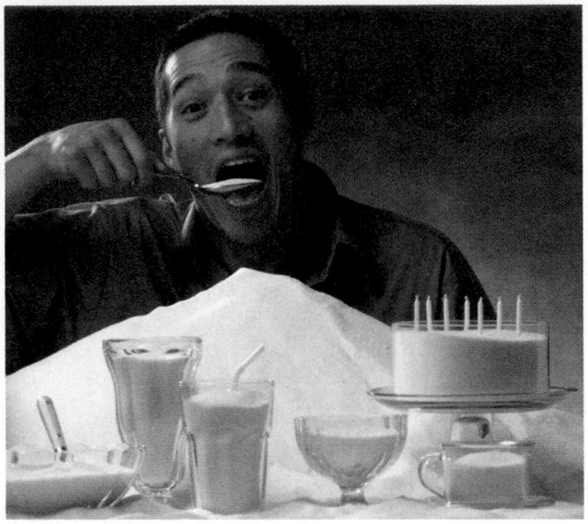

Over half of the added sugars in our diet come from soft drinks and table sugar, but baked goods, fruit drinks, ice cream, candy, and breakfast cereals also make substantial contributions.

GLOSSARY OF ADDED SUGARS

brown sugar: refined white sugar crystals to which manufacturers have added molasses syrup with natural flavor and color; 91 to 96% pure sucrose.

confectioners' sugar: finely powdered sucrose, 99.9% pure.

corn sweeteners: corn syrup and sugars derived from corn.

corn syrup: a syrup made from cornstarch that has been treated with acid, high temperatures, and enzymes that produce glucose, maltose, and dextrins. See also *high-fructose corn syrup (HFCS).*

dextrose: an older name for glucose.

granulated sugar: crystalline sucrose; 99.9% pure.

high-fructose corn syrup (HFCS): a syrup made from cornstarch that has been treated with an enzyme that converts some of the glucose to the sweeter fructose; made especially for use in processed foods and beverages, where it is the predominant sweetener. With a chemical structure similar to sucrose, HFCS has a fructose content of 42, 55, or 90%, with glucose making up the remainder.

honey: sugar (mostly sucrose) formed from nectar gathered by bees. An enzyme splits the sucrose into glucose and fructose. Composition and flavor vary, but honey always contains a mixture of sucrose, fructose, and glucose.

invert sugar: a mixture of glucose and fructose formed by the hydrolysis of sucrose in a chemical process; sold only in liquid form and sweeter than sucrose. Invert sugar is used as a food additive to help preserve freshness and prevent shrinkage.

levulose: an older name for fructose.

maple sugar: a sugar (mostly sucrose) purified from the concentrated sap of the sugar maple tree.

molasses: the thick brown syrup produced during sugar refining. Molasses retains residual sugar and other by-products and a few minerals; blackstrap molasses contains significant amounts of calcium and iron—the iron comes from the *machinery* used to process the sugar.

raw sugar: the first crop of crystals harvested during sugar processing. Raw sugar cannot be sold in the United States because it contains too much filth (dirt, insect fragments, and the like). Sugar sold as "raw sugar" domestically has actually gone through over half of the refining steps.

turbinado (ter-bih-NOD-oh) **sugar:** sugar produced using the same refining process as white sugar, but without the bleaching and anti-caking treatment. Traces of molasses give turbinado its sandy color.

white sugar: pure sucrose or "table sugar," produced by dissolving, concentrating, and recrystallizing raw sugar.

TABLE 4-1 Sample Nutrients in Sugar and Other Foods

The indicated portion of any of these foods provides approximately 100 kcalories. Notice that for a similar number of kcalories and grams of carbohydrate, milk, legumes, fruits, grains, and vegetables offer more of the other nutrients than do the sugars.

	Size of 100 kcal Portion	Carbohydrate (g)	Protein (g)	Calcium (mg)	Iron (mg)	Vitamin A (µg)	Vitamin C (mg)
Foods							
Milk, 1% low-fat	1 c	12	8	300	0.1	144	2
Kidney beans	½ c	20	7	30	1.6	0	2
Apricots	6	24	2	30	1.1	554	22
Bread, whole wheat	1½ slices	20	4	30	1.9	0	0
Broccoli, cooked	2 c	20	12	188	2.2	696	148
Sugars							
Sugar, white	2 tbs	24	0	trace	trace	0	0
Molasses, blackstrap	2½ tbs	28	0	343	12.6	0	0.1
Cola beverage	1 c	26	0	6	trace	0	0
Honey	1½ tbs	26	trace	2	0.2	0	trace

Some people believe that because honey is a natural food, it is nutritious—or, at least, more nutritious than sugar.* A look at their chemical structures reveals the truth. Honey, like table sugar, contains glucose and fructose. The primary difference is that in table sugar the two monosaccharides are bonded together as a disaccharide, whereas in honey some of them are free. Whether a person eats monosaccharides individually, as in honey, or linked together, as in table sugar, they end up the same way in the body: as glucose and fructose.

Honey does contain a few vitamins and minerals, but not many, as Table 4-1 shows. Honey is denser than crystalline sugar, too, so it provides more energy per spoonful.

This is not to say that all sugar sources are alike, for some are more nutritious than others. Consider a fruit, say, an orange. The fruit may give you the same amounts of fructose and glucose and the same number of kcalories as a dose of sugar or honey, but the packaging is more valuable nutritionally. The fruit's sugars arrive in the body diluted in a large volume of water, packaged in fiber, and mixed with valuable minerals, vitamins, and phytochemicals.

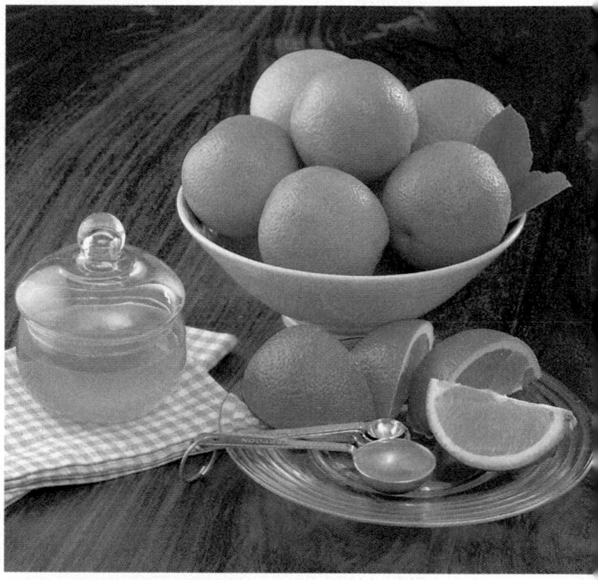

Matthew Farruggio

You receive about the same amount and kinds of sugars from an orange as from a tablespoon of honey, but the packaging makes a big nutrition difference.

As these comparisons illustrate, the significant difference between sugar sources is not between "natural" honey and "purified" sugar but between concentrated sweets and the dilute, naturally occurring sugars that sweeten foods. You can suspect an exaggerated nutrition claim when someone asserts that one product is more nutritious than another because it contains honey.

Sugar can contribute to nutrient deficiencies only by displacing nutrients. For nutrition's sake, the appropriate attitude to take is not that sugar is "bad" and must be avoided, but that nutritious foods must come first. If the nutritious foods end up crowding sugar out of the diet, that is fine—but not the other way around. As always, the goals to seek are balance, variety, and moderation.

Dental Caries Both sugars and starches begin breaking down to sugars in the mouth and so can contribute to tooth decay.■ Bacteria in the mouth ferment the sugars and in the process produce an acid that dissolves tooth enamel (see Figure 4-14). People can eat sugar without this happening, though, for much depends on how long foods stay in the mouth. Sticky foods stay on the teeth longer and keep yielding acid longer than foods that are readily cleared from the mouth. For that reason, sugar in a juice consumed quickly, for example, is less likely to cause **dental caries** than sugar in a pastry. By the same token, the sugar in sticky foods such as dried fruits is more detrimental than its quantity alone would suggest.

■ Highlight 23 presents the relationships between dental health and chronic illness.

dental caries: decay of teeth.
- **caries** = rottenness

*Honey should never be fed to infants because of the risk of botulism. Chapter 15 provides more details.

FIGURE 4-14 Dental Caries

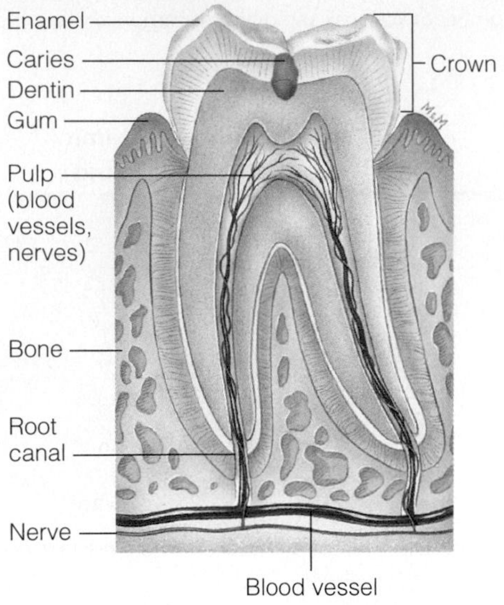
Enamel
Caries
Dentin
Gum
Pulp (blood vessels, nerves)
Bone
Root canal
Nerve
Crown
Blood vessel

Dental caries begins when acid dissolves the enamel that covers the tooth. If not repaired, the decay may penetrate the dentin and spread into the pulp of the tooth, causing inflammation and an abscess.

■ To prevent dental caries:
- Limit between-meal snacks containing sugars and starches.
- Brush and floss teeth regularly.
- If brushing and flossing are not possible, at least rinse with water.

■ 2005 *Dietary Guidelines:*
- Reduce the incidence of dental caries by practicing good oral hygiene and consuming sugar- and starch-containing foods and beverages less frequently.

dental plaque: a gummy mass of bacteria that grows on teeth and can lead to dental caries and gum disease.

serotonin (SER-oh-tone-in): a neurotransmitter important in sleep regulation, appetite control, and sensory perception among other roles.

Another concern is how often people eat sugar. Bacteria produce acid for 20 to 30 minutes after each exposure. If a person eats three pieces of candy at one time, the teeth will be exposed to approximately 30 minutes of acid destruction. But, if the person eats three pieces at half-hour intervals, the time of exposure increases to 90 minutes. Likewise, slowly sipping a sugary soft drink may be more harmful than drinking quickly and clearing the mouth of sugar. Nonsugary foods can help remove sugar from tooth surfaces; hence, it is better to eat sugar with meals than between meals. Foods such as milk and cheese may be particularly helpful in minimizing the effects of the acids and in restoring the lost enamel.[15]

The development of caries depends on several factors: the bacteria that reside in **dental plaque,** the saliva that cleanses the mouth, the minerals that form the teeth, and the foods that remain after swallowing. For most people, good oral hygiene will prevent■ dental caries. In fact, regular brushing (twice a day, with a fluoride toothpaste) and flossing may be more effective in preventing dental caries than restricting sugary foods.[16]■

Accusations against Sugars

Sugars have been blamed for a variety of other health problems.[17] The following paragraphs evaluate some of these accusations.

Accusation: Sugar Causes Obesity Foods high in added sugars deliver a lot of energy (kcalories). When they are high in fat too, both total energy and fat intakes increase. Exceeding energy needs contributes to weight gain, but sugar is not the sole cause of obesity—and obesity can occur without a high-sugar diet. The notion that eating sweet foods stimulates appetite and promotes overeating has not been supported by research.

Limiting selections of foods and beverages high in added sugars can be an effective weight-loss strategy, however, especially for people whose excess kcalories derive primarily from added sugars. Replacing a can of cola with a glass of water every day, for example, can help a person lose a pound (or at least not gain a pound) in a month. That may not sound like much, but it adds up to over 10 pounds a year, for very little effort.

Accusation: Sugar Causes Heart Disease A diet high in added sugars can alter blood lipids to favor heart disease.[18] (Lipids include fats and cholesterol, as Chapter 5 explains.) This effect is most dramatic in people who respond to sucrose with abnormally high insulin secretions, which promote the making of excess fat.[19] For most people, though, moderate sugar intakes do *not* elevate blood lipids.[20] To keep these findings in perspective, consider that heart disease correlates most closely with factors that have nothing to do with nutrition, such as smoking and genetics. Among dietary risk factors, several—such as saturated fats, *trans* fats, and obesity—have much stronger associations with heart disease than do sugar intakes.

Accusation: Sugar Causes Misbehavior in Children and Criminal Behavior in Adults Sugar has been blamed for the misbehaviors of hyperactive children, delinquent adolescents, and lawbreaking adults. Such speculations have been based on personal stories and have not been confirmed by scientific research. No scientific evidence supports a relationship between sugar and hyperactivity or other misbehaviors. Chapter 15 provides accurate information on diet and children's behavior.

Accusation: Sugar Causes Cravings and Addictions Foods in general, and carbohydrates and sugars more specifically, are not addictive in the biological ways that drugs are. Yet some people describe themselves as having "carbohydrate cravings" or being "sugar addicts." One frequently noted theory is that people seek carbohydrates as a way to increase their levels of the brain neurotransmitter

serotonin, which elevates mood. Interestingly, when those with self-described carbohydrate cravings indulge, they tend to eat more of everything, but the percentage of energy from carbohydrates remains unchanged.[21] Alcohol also raises serotonin levels, and alcohol-dependent people who crave carbohydrates seem to handle sobriety better when given a high-carbohydrate diet.[22]

One reasonable explanation for the carbohydrate cravings that some people experience involves the self-imposed labeling of a food as both "good" and "bad"—that is, one that is desirable but should be eaten with restraint.[23] Chocolate is a familiar example. Restricting intake heightens the desire further (a "craving"). Then "addiction" is used to explain why resisting the food is so difficult and, sometimes, even impossible. But the "addiction" is not pharmacological; a capsule of the psychoactive substances commonly found in chocolate, for example, does not satisfy the craving.

Recommended Intakes of Sugars

Because added sugars deliver kcalories but few or no nutrients, the 2005 *Dietary Guidelines*■ urge consumers to "choose and prepare foods and beverages with little added sugars." The USDA Food Guide counts these sugar kcalories (and those from solid fats and alcohol) as discretionary kcalories. Most people can afford only a little added sugar.■ Estimates indicate that, on average, each person in the United States consumes about 105 pounds of added sugar per year, or about 30 teaspoons of added sugar a day, an amount that exceeds these guidelines.[24]

Estimating the *added* sugars in a diet is not always easy for consumers. Food labels list the total grams of sugar a food provides, but this total reflects both added sugars and those occurring naturally in foods. To help estimate sugar and energy intakes accurately, the list in the margin■ shows the amounts of concentrated sweets that are equivalent to 1 teaspoon of white sugar. These sugars all provide about 5 grams of carbohydrate and about 20 kcalories per teaspoon. Some are lower (16 kcalories for table sugar), while others are higher (22 kcalories for honey), but a 20-kcalorie average is an acceptable approximation. For a person who uses catsup liberally, it may help to remember that 1 tablespoon of catsup supplies about 1 teaspoon of sugar.

The DRI committee did not set an upper limit for sugar, but as mentioned, excessive intakes can interfere with sound nutrition and dental health. Few people can eat lots of sugary treats and still meet all of their nutrient needs without exceeding their kcalorie allowance. Specifically, the DRI suggests that added sugars should account for no more than 25 percent of the day's total energy intake.[25] When added sugars occupy this much of a diet, intakes from the five food groups fall below recommendations.[26] For a person consuming 2000 kcalories a day, 25 percent represents 500 kcalories (that is, 125 grams or 31 teaspoons) from concentrated sugars—and that's a lot of sugar.■ Perhaps an athlete in training whose energy needs are high can afford the added sugars from sports drinks without compromising nutrient intake, but most people would do better limiting their use of added sugars. The World Health Organization (WHO) and the Food and Agriculture Organization (FAO) suggest restricting consumption of added sugars to less than 10 percent of total energy.

■ 2005 *Dietary Guidelines:*
- Choose and prepare foods and beverages with little added sugars.

■ USDA Food Guide amounts of added sugars that can be included as discretionary kcalories when food choices are nutrient-dense and fat ≤30% total kcalories:
- 3 tsp for a 1600 kcal diet.
- 5 tsp for a 1800 kcal diet.
- 8 tsp for a 2000 kcal diet.
- 9 tsp for a 2200 kcal diet.
- 12 tsp for a 2400 kcal diet.

■ 1 tsp white sugar =
- 1 tsp brown sugar.
- 1 tsp candy.
- 1 tsp corn sweetener or corn syrup.
- 1 tsp honey.
- 1 tsp jam or jelly.
- 1 tsp maple sugar or maple syrup.
- 1 tsp molasses.
- 1½ oz carbonated soda.
- 1 tbs catsup.

■ For perspective, each of these concentrated sugars provides about 500 kcal:
- 40 oz cola.
- ½ c honey.
- 125 jelly beans.
- 23 marshmallows.
- 30 tsp sugar.

How many kcalories from sugar does your favorite beverage or snack provide?

IN SUMMARY Sugars pose no major health threat except for an increased risk of dental caries. Excessive intakes may displace needed nutrients and fiber and may contribute to obesity when energy intake exceeds needs. A person deciding to limit daily sugar intake should recognize that not all sugars need to be restricted, just concentrated sweets, which are relatively empty of other nutrients and high in kcalories. Sugars that occur naturally in fruits, vegetables, and milk are acceptable.

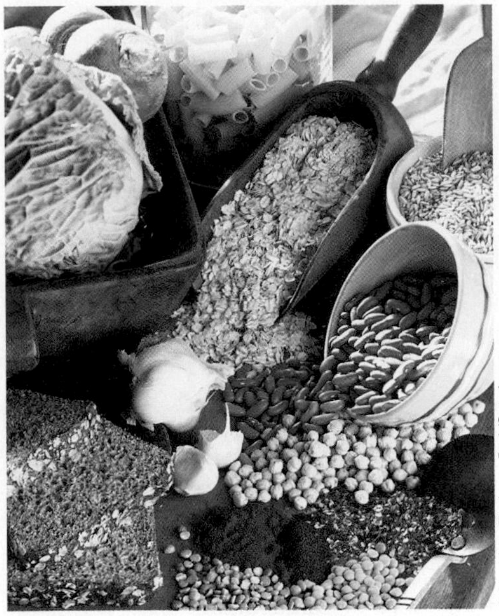
© Rita Maas/The Image Bank/Getty Images

Foods rich in starch and fiber offer many health benefits.

Health Effects and Recommended Intakes of Starch and Fibers

Carbohydrates and fats are the two major sources of energy in the diet. When one is high, the other is usually low—and vice versa. A diet that provides abundant carbohydrate (45 to 65 percent of energy intake) and some fat (20 to 35 percent of energy intake) within a reasonable energy allowance best supports good health. To increase carbohydrate, focus on whole grains, vegetables, legumes, and fruits—foods noted for their starch, fibers, and naturally occurring sugars.

Health Effects of Starch and Fibers

In addition to starch, fibers, and natural sugars, whole grains, vegetables, legumes, and fruits supply valuable vitamins and minerals and little or no fat. The following paragraphs describe some of the health benefits of diets that include a variety of these foods daily.

Heart Disease High-carbohydrate diets, especially those rich in whole grains, may protect against heart disease and stroke, although sorting out the exact reasons why can be difficult.[27] Such diets are low in animal fat and cholesterol and high in fibers, vegetable proteins, and phytochemicals—all factors associated with a lower risk of heart disease. (The role of animal fat and cholesterol in heart disease is discussed in Chapter 5. The role of vegetable proteins in heart disease is presented in Chapter 6. The benefits of phytochemicals in disease prevention are featured in Highlight 13.)

Foods rich in viscous fibers (such as oat bran, barley, and legumes) lower blood cholesterol■ by binding with bile acids and thereby increasing their excretion.[28] Consequently, the liver must use its cholesterol to make new bile acids. In addition, the bacterial by-products of fiber fermentation in the colon also inhibit cholesterol synthesis in the liver.[29] The net result is lower blood cholesterol.[30]

■ Consuming 5 to 10 g of viscous fiber daily reduces blood cholesterol by 3 to 5%. For perspective, ½ c dry oat bran provides 8 g of fiber, and 1 c cooked barley or ½ c cooked legumes provides about 6 g of fiber.

Several researchers have speculated that fiber may also exert its effect by displacing fats in the diet. While this is certainly helpful, even when dietary fat is low, high intakes of fibers exert a separate and significant cholesterol-lowering effect. In other words, a high-fiber diet helps to prevent heart disease independent of fat intake.

Diabetes High-fiber foods play a key role in reducing the risk of type 2 diabetes.[31] When viscous fibers trap nutrients and delay their transit through the GI tract, glucose absorption is slowed, and this helps to prevent the glucose surge and rebound that seem to be associated with diabetes onset.

GI Health Dietary fibers enhance the health of the large intestine. The healthier the intestinal walls, the better they can block absorption of unwanted constituents. Fibers such as cellulose (as in cereal brans, fruits, and vegetables) increase stool weight, easing passage, and reduce transit time. In this way, the fibers help to alleviate or prevent constipation.

Taken with ample fluids, fibers help to prevent several GI disorders. Large, soft stools ease elimination for the rectal muscles and reduce the pressure in the lower bowel, making it less likely that rectal veins will swell (hemorrhoids). Fiber prevents compaction of the intestinal contents, which could obstruct the appendix and permit bacteria to invade and infect it (appendicitis). In addition, fiber stimulates the GI tract muscles so that they retain their strength and resist bulging out into pouches known as diverticula (illustrated in Figure H3-3 on p. 97).[32]

Cancer Many, but not all, research studies suggest that increasing dietary fiber protects against colon cancer.[33] When the largest study of diet and cancer to date examined the diets of over a half million people in ten countries for four and a half years, the researchers found an inverse association between dietary fiber and colon cancer.[34] People who ate the most dietary fiber (35 grams per day) reduced their risk of colon cancer by 40 percent compared with those who ate the least fiber (15 grams per day). Importantly, the study focused on dietary fiber, not fiber supplements or additives, which lack valuable nutrients and phytochemicals that also help protect against cancer.

Fibers help prevent colon cancer by diluting, binding, and rapidly removing potentially cancer-causing agents from the colon. In addition, some fibers stimulate bacterial fermentation of resistant starch and fiber in the colon, a process that produces short-chain fatty acids that lower the pH.[35] These small fat molecules and the lower pH inhibit cancer growth in the colon.[36]

Discrepancies in research findings may reflect the delay between eating low-fiber diets and developing colon cancer decades later or the differences in effectiveness between various types and sources of fiber. Despite the inconclusive evidence, health care professionals continue to recommend a high-fiber diet that includes at least five servings of vegetables and fruits and generous portions of whole grains and legumes.[37]

Weight Management Foods rich in complex carbohydrates tend to be low in fat and added sugars and can therefore promote weight loss by delivering less energy■ per bite. In addition, as fibers absorb water from the digestive juices, they swell, creating feelings of fullness and delaying hunger.[38]

■ Reminder:
- Carbohydrate: 4 kcal/g.
- Fat: 9 kcal/g.

Many weight-loss products on the market today contain bulk-inducing fibers such as methylcellulose, but buying pure fiber compounds like this is neither necessary nor advisable. To use fiber in a weight-loss plan, select fresh fruits, vegetables, legumes, and whole-grain foods. High-fiber foods not only add bulk to the diet, but are economical and nutritious.

Most experts agree that the health benefits attributed to fiber may come from other constituents of fiber-containing foods, and not from fiber alone.[39] For this reason, consumers should select whole grains, legumes, fruits, and vegetables instead of fiber supplements. Table 4-2 summarizes fibers and their health benefits.

Harmful Effects of Excessive Fiber Intake Despite fiber's benefits to health, a diet high in fiber also has a few drawbacks. A person who has a small capacity and eats mostly high-fiber foods may not be able to take in enough food to meet

TABLE 4-2 Fibers: Their Characteristics, Food Sources, and Health Effects in the Body

Fiber Characteristics	Major Food Sources	Actions in the Body	Health Benefits
Viscous, soluble, more fermentable • Gums and mucilages • Pectins • Psyllium[a] • Some hemicelluloses	Whole-grain products (barley, oats, oat bran, rye), fruits (apples, citrus), legumes, seeds and husks, vegetables; also extracted and used as food additives.	• Lower blood cholesterol by binding bile. • Slow glucose absorption. • Slow transit of food through upper GI tract. • Hold moisture in stools, softening them. • Yield small fat molecules after fermentation that the colon can use for energy.	• Lower risk of heart disease. • Lower risk of diabetes.
Nonviscous, insoluble, less fermentable • Cellulose • Lignins • Psyllium[a] • Resistant starch • Many hemicelluloses	Brown rice, fruits, legumes, seeds, vegetables (cabbage, carrots, brussels sprouts), wheat bran, whole grains; also extracted and used as food additives.	• Increase fecal weight and speed fecal passage through colon. • Provide bulk and feelings of fullness.	• Alleviate constipation. • Lower risks of diverticulosis, hemorrhoids, and appendicitis. • May help with weight management.

[a]Psyllium, a fiber laxative and cereal additive, has both soluble and insoluble properties.

energy or nutrient needs. The malnourished, the elderly, and young children adhering to all-plant (vegan) diets are especially vulnerable to this problem.

Launching suddenly into a high-fiber diet can cause temporary bouts of abdominal discomfort, gas, and diarrhea and, more seriously, can obstruct the GI tract. To prevent such complications, a person adopting a high-fiber diet is advised to:

- Increase fiber intake gradually over several weeks to give the GI tract time to adapt.
- Drink lots of liquids to soften the fiber as it moves through the GI tract.
- Select fiber-rich foods from a variety of sources—fruits, vegetables, legumes, and whole-grain breads and cereals.

Some fibers can limit the absorption of nutrients by speeding the transit of foods through the GI tract and by binding to minerals. When mineral intake is adequate, however, a reasonable intake of high-fiber foods does not seem to compromise mineral balance.

Clearly, fiber is like all the nutrients in that "more" is "better" only up to a point. Again, the key words are balance, moderation, and variety.

IN SUMMARY An adequate intake of fiber:
- Fosters weight management.
- Lowers blood cholesterol.
- May help prevent colon cancer.
- Helps prevent and control diabetes.
- Helps prevent and alleviate hemorrhoids.
- Helps prevent appendicitis.
- Helps prevent diverticulosis.

An excessive intake of fiber:
- Displaces energy- and nutrient-dense foods.
- Causes intestinal discomfort and distention.
- May interfere with mineral absorption.

Recommended Intakes of Starch and Fibers

Dietary recommendations suggest that carbohydrates provide about half (45 to 65 percent) of the energy requirement. A person consuming 2000 kcalories a day should therefore have 900 to 1300 kcalories of carbohydrate, or about 225 to 325 grams.■ This amount is more than adequate to meet the RDA■ for carbohydrate, which is set at 130 grams per day, based on the average minimum amount of glucose used by the brain.[40]

When it established the Daily Values that appear on food labels, the Food and Drug Administration (FDA) used a 60 percent of kcalories guideline in setting the Daily Value■ for carbohydrate at 300 grams per day. For most people, this means increasing total carbohydrate intake. To this end, the *Dietary Guidelines*■ encourage people to choose a variety of whole grains, vegetables, fruits, and legumes daily.

■ • 45% of 2000 kcal:

$$\frac{45}{100} = \frac{x}{2000\text{ kcal.}}$$

$$100x = 90{,}000\text{ kcal.}$$

$$x = 900\text{ kcal.}$$

$$900\text{ kcal} \div 4\text{ kcal/g} = 225\text{ g.}$$

• 65% of 2000 kcal:

$$\frac{65}{100} = \frac{x}{2000\text{ kcal.}}$$

$$100x = 130{,}000\text{ kcal.}$$

$$x = 1300\text{ kcal.}$$

$$1300\text{ kcal} \div 4\text{ kcal/g} = 325\text{ g.}$$

■ RDA for carbohydrate:
- 130 g/day.
- 45 to 65% of energy intake.

■ Daily Values:
- 300 g carbohydrate (based on 60% of 2000 kcal diet).

■ 2005 *Dietary Guidelines:*
- Choose fiber-rich fruits, vegetables, and whole grains often.

■ To increase your fiber intake:
- Eat whole-grain cereals that contain ≥5 g fiber per serving for breakfast.
- Eat raw vegetables.
- Eat fruits (such as pears) and vegetables (such as potatoes) with their skins.
- Add legumes to soups, salads, and casseroles.
- Eat fresh and dried fruit for snacks.

HEALTHY PEOPLE 2010

Increase the proportion of people who meet the *Dietary Guidlines* daily goal of at least six servings of grain products and at least five servings of vegetables and fruits.

Recommendations for fiber■ suggest the same foods just mentioned: whole grains, vegetables, fruits, and legumes, which also provide minerals and vitamins. The FDA set the Daily Value■ for fiber at 25 grams for a 2000-kcalorie diet, rounded

■ Daily Values:
- 25 g fiber/2000 kcal (based on 11.5 g/1000 kcal).

TABLE 4-3 Fiber in Selected Foods

Grains

Whole-grain products provide about 1 to 2 grams (or more) of fiber per serving:

- 1 slice whole-wheat, pumpernickel, rye bread.
- 1 oz ready-to-eat cereal (100% bran cereals contain 10 grams or more).
- ½ c cooked barley, bulgur, grits, oatmeal.

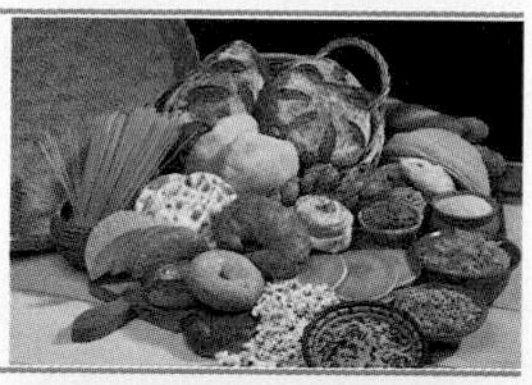

© Polara Studios, Inc.

Vegetables

Most vegetables contain about 2 to 3 grams of fiber per serving:

- 1 c raw bean sprouts.
- ½ c cooked broccoli, brussels sprouts, cabbage, carrots, cauliflower, collards, corn, eggplant, green beans, green peas, kale, mushrooms, okra, parsnips, potatoes, pumpkin, spinach, sweet potatoes, swiss chard, winter squash.
- ½ c chopped raw carrots, peppers.

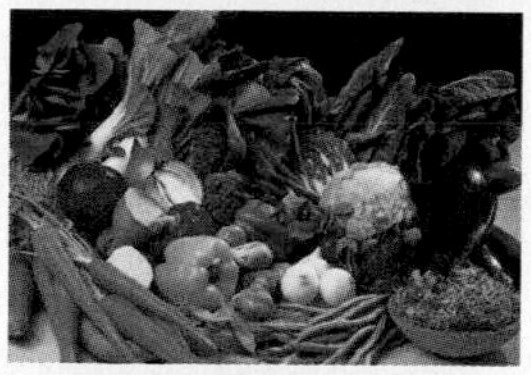

© Polara Studios, Inc.

Fruits

Fresh, frozen, and dried fruits have about 2 grams of fiber per serving:

- 1 medium apple, banana, kiwi, nectarine, orange, pear.
- ½ c applesauce, blackberries, blueberries, raspberries, strawberries.
- Fruit juices contain very little fiber.

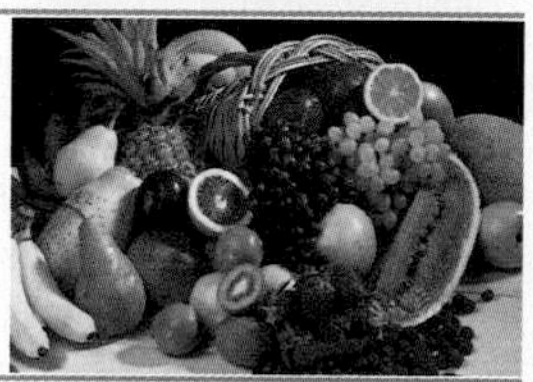

© Polara Studios, Inc.

Legumes

Many legumes provide about 6 to 8 grams of fiber per serving:

- ½ c cooked baked beans, black beans, black-eyed peas, kidney beans, navy beans, pinto beans.

Some legumes provide about 5 grams of fiber per serving:

- ½ c cooked garbanzo beans, great northern beans, lentils, lima beans, split peas.

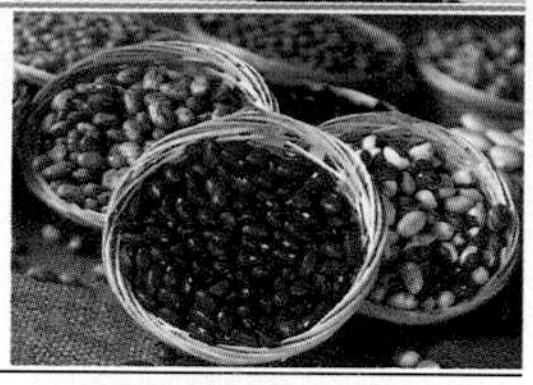

© Photo Disc Blue/Getty Images

NOTE: Appendix H provides fiber grams for over 2000 foods.

up from 11.5 grams per 1000-kcalorie intake. The DRI recommendation■ is slightly higher, at 14 grams per 1000-kcalorie intake. Similarly, the American Dietetic Association suggests 20 to 35 grams of dietary fiber daily, which is about two times higher than the average intake in the United States.[41] An effective way to add fiber while lowering fat is to substitute plant sources of proteins (legumes) for animal sources (meats). Table 4-3 presents a list of fiber sources.

■ Fiber AI:
- 14 g/1000 kcal/day.
- Men:
  19–50 yr: 38 g/day.
  51+ yr: 30 g/day.
- Women:
  19–50 yr: 25 g/day.
  51+ yr: 21 g/day.

Reminder: An *AI (Adequate Intake)* is used as a guide for nutrient intake when an RDA cannot be established (see Chapter 1).

As mentioned earlier, too much fiber is no better than too little. The World Health Organization recommends an upper limit of 40 grams of dietary fiber a day.

From Guidelines to Groceries

A diet following the USDA Food Guide, which includes several servings of fruits, vegetables, and grains daily, can easily supply the recommended amount of carbohydrates and fiber. In selecting high-fiber foods, keep in mind the principle of variety. The fibers in oats lower cholesterol, whereas those in bran help promote GI tract health. (Review Table 4-2 to see the diverse health effects of various fibers.)

Grains A serving of most foods in the grain group provides about 15 grams of carbohydrate, mostly as starch. Be aware that some foods in this group, especially snack crackers and baked goods such as biscuits, croissants, and muffins, contain added sugars, added fat, or both. When selecting from the grain group, be sure to include at least half as whole-grain products (see Figure 4-15). The "3 are Key" message may help consumers to remember to choose a whole-grain cereal for breakfast, a whole-grain bread for lunch, and a whole-grain pasta or rice for dinner.[42]

FIGURE 4-15 Bread Labels Compared

Food labels provide the quantities of total carbohydrate, dietary fiber, and sugars. Total carbohydrate and dietary fiber are also stated as "% Daily Values." A close look at these two labels reveals that bread made from whole wheat flour provides almost three times as much fiber as the one made mostly from refined wheat flour. When the words whole wheat or whole grain appear on the label, the bread inside contains all of the nutrients that bread can provide.

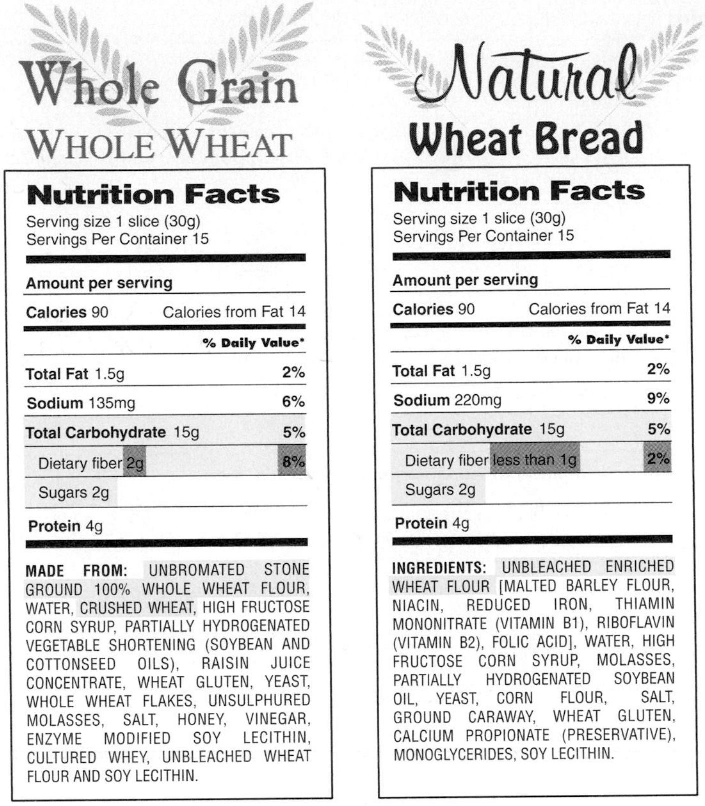
Whole Grain
WHOLE WHEAT
Nutrition Facts
Serving size 1 slice (30g)
Servings Per Container 15
Amount per serving
Calories 90 Calories from Fat 14
% Daily Value*
Total Fat 1.5g 2%
Sodium 135mg 6%
Total Carbohydrate 15g 5%
Dietary fiber 2g 8%
Sugars 2g
Protein 4g
MADE FROM: UNBROMATED STONE GROUND 100% WHOLE WHEAT FLOUR, WATER, CRUSHED WHEAT, HIGH FRUCTOSE CORN SYRUP, PARTIALLY HYDROGENATED VEGETABLE SHORTENING (SOYBEAN AND COTTONSEED OILS), RAISIN JUICE CONCENTRATE, WHEAT GLUTEN, YEAST, WHOLE WHEAT FLAKES, UNSULPHURED MOLASSES, SALT, HONEY, VINEGAR, ENZYME MODIFIED SOY LECITHIN, CULTURED WHEY, UNBLEACHED WHEAT FLOUR AND SOY LECITHIN.
Natural
Wheat Bread
Nutrition Facts
Serving size 1 slice (30g)
Servings Per Container 15
Amount per serving
Calories 90 Calories from Fat 14
% Daily Value*
Total Fat 1.5g 2%
Sodium 220mg 9%
Total Carbohydrate 15g 5%
Dietary fiber less than 1g 2%
Sugars 2g
Protein 4g
INGREDIENTS: UNBLEACHED ENRICHED WHEAT FLOUR [MALTED BARLEY FLOUR, NIACIN, REDUCED IRON, THIAMIN MONONITRATE (VITAMIN B1), RIBOFLAVIN (VITAMIN B2), FOLIC ACID], WATER, HIGH FRUCTOSE CORN SYRUP, MOLASSES, PARTIALLY HYDROGENATED SOYBEAN OIL, YEAST, CORN FLOUR, SALT, GROUND CARAWAY, WHEAT GLUTEN, CALCIUM PROPIONATE (PRESERVATIVE), MONOGLYCERIDES, SOY LECITHIN.

Vegetables The amount of carbohydrate a serving of vegetables provides depends primarily on its starch content. Starchy vegetables—a half-cup of cooked corn, peas, plantain, potatoes, or sweet potatoes—provide about 15 grams of carbohydrate per serving. A serving of most other *nonstarchy* vegetables—such as a half-cup of carrots, broccoli, tomatoes, or squash or a cup of salad greens—provides about 5 grams.

Fruits A typical fruit serving—a small banana, apple, or orange, or a half-cup of most canned or fresh fruit—contains an average of about 15 grams of carbohydrate, mostly as sugars, including the fruit sugar fructose. Fruits vary greatly in their water and fiber contents and, therefore, in their sugar concentrations.

Milks and Milk Products A serving (a cup) of milk or yogurt provides about 12 grams of carbohydrate. Cottage cheese provides about 6 grams of carbohydrate per cup, but most other cheeses contain little, if any, carbohydrate.

Meats and Meat Alternates With two exceptions, foods in the meats and meat alternates group deliver almost no carbohydrate to the diet. The exceptions are nuts, which provide a little starch and fiber along with their abundant fat, and legumes, which provide an abundance of both starch and fiber. Just a half-cup serving of legumes provides about 20 grams of carbohydrate, a third from fiber.

Read Food Labels Food labels list the amount, in grams, of *total* carbohydrate—including starch, fibers, and sugars—per serving (review Figure 4-15). Fiber grams are also listed separately, as are the grams of sugars. (With this information, you can calculate starch grams■ by subtracting the grams of fibers and sugars from the total carbohydrate.) Sugars reflect both added sugars and those that occur naturally in foods. Total carbohydrate and dietary fiber are also expressed as "% Daily Values" for a person consuming 2000 kcalories; there is no Daily Value for sugars.

■ To calculate starch grams using the first label in Figure 4-15: 15 g total − 4 g (dietary fiber + sugars) = 11 g starch.

IN SUMMARY Clearly, a diet rich in complex carbohydrates—starches and fibers—supports efforts to control body weight and prevent heart disease, cancer, diabetes, and GI disorders. For these reasons, recommendations urge people to eat plenty of whole grains, vegetables, legumes, and fruits—enough to provide 45 to 65 percent of the daily energy intake from carbohydrate.

In today's world, there is one other reason why plant foods rich in complex carbohydrates and natural sugars are a better choice than animal foods or foods high in concentrated sweets. In general, less energy and resources are required to grow and process plant foods than to produce sugar or foods derived from animals.

Nutrition in Your Life

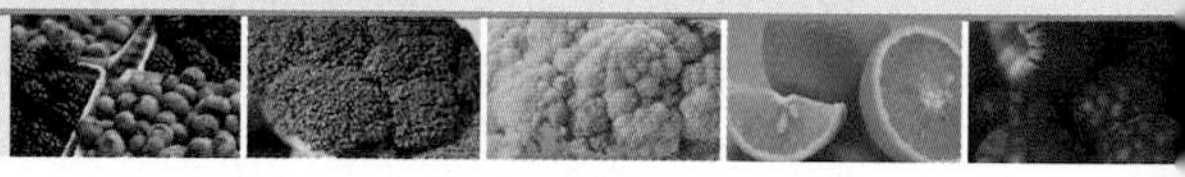

Foods that derive from plants—whole grains, vegetables, legumes, and fruits—naturally provide ample carbohydrates and fiber with little or no fat. Refined foods often contain added sugars and fat.

- **Do you eat the equivalent of at least 5 ounces of grain products daily, making sure to include at least half as whole-grain foods?**
- **Do you eat the equivalent of at least 1½ cups of fruits and 2 cups of vegetables daily, making sure to include a variety of dark green and orange vegetables as well as legumes?**
- **Do you choose and prepare foods and beverages with little added sugars?**

NUTRITION ON THE NET

Access these websites for further study of topics covered in this chapter.

- Find updates and quick links to these and other nutrition-related sites at our website: **www.wadsworth.com/nutrition**
- Search for "lactose intolerance" at the U.S. Government health information site: **www.healthfinder.gov**
- Search for "sugars" and "fiber" at the International Food Information Council site: **www.ific.org**
- Learn more about dental caries from the American Dental Association and the National Institute of Dental and Craniofacial Research: **www.ada.org** and **www.nidcr.nih.gov**
- Learn more about diabetes from the American Diabetes Association, the Canadian Diabetes Association, and the National Institute of Diabetes and Digestive and Kidney Diseases: **www.diabetes.org**, **www.diabetes.ca**, and **www.niddk.nih.gov**

NUTRITION CALCULATIONS

These problems will give you practice in doing simple nutrition-related calculations. Although the situations are hypothetical, the numbers are real, and calculating the answers (check them on p. 132) provides a valuable lesson. Be sure to show your calculations for each problem.

Health recommendations suggest that 45 to 65 percent of the daily energy intake come from carbohydrates. Stating recommendations in terms of percentage of energy intake is meaningful only if energy intake is known. The following exercises illustrate this concept.

1. Calculate the carbohydrate intake (in grams) for a student who has a high carbohydrate intake (70 percent of energy intake) and a moderate energy intake (2000 kcalories a day).
   How does this carbohydrate intake compare to the Daily Value of 300 grams? To the 45 to 65 percent recommendation?
2. Now consider a professor who eats half as much carbohydrate as the student (in grams) and has the same energy intake. What percentage does carbohydrate contribute to the daily intake?
   How does carbohydrate intake compare to the Daily Value of 300 grams? To the 45 to 65 percent recommendation?
3. Now consider an athlete who eats twice as much carbohydrate (in grams) as the student and has a much higher energy intake (6000 kcalories a day). What percentage does carbohydrate contribute to this person's daily intake?
   How does carbohydrate intake compare to the Daily Value of 300 grams? To the 45 to 65 percent recommendation?
4. One more example. In an attempt to lose weight, a person adopts a diet that provides 150 grams of carbohydrate per day and limits energy intake to 1000 kcalories. What percentage does carbohydrate contribute to this person's daily intake?
   How does this carbohydrate intake compare to the Daily Value of 300 grams? To the 45 to 65 percent recommendation?

These exercises should convince you of the importance of examining actual intake as well the percentage of energy intake.

STUDY QUESTIONS

These questions will help you review this chapter. You will find the answers in the discussions on the pages provided.

1. Which carbohydrates are described as simple, and which are complex? (p. 104)
2. Describe the structure of a monosaccharide and name the three monosaccharides important in nutrition. Name the three disaccharides commonly found in foods and their component monosaccharides. In what foods are these sugars found? (pp. 105–106)
3. What happens in a condensation reaction? In a hydrolysis reaction? (pp. 106–107)
4. Describe the structure of polysaccharides and name the ones important in nutrition. How are starch and glycogen similar, and how do they differ? How do the fibers differ from the other polysaccharides? (pp. 107–110)
5. Describe carbohydrate digestion and absorption. What role does fiber play in the process? (pp. 110–113)
6. What are the possible fates of glucose in the body? What is the protein-sparing action of carbohydrate? (pp. 114–115)
7. How does the body maintain its blood glucose concentration? What happens when the blood glucose concentration rises too high or falls too low? (pp. 116–118)
8. What are the health effects of sugars? What are the dietary recommendations regarding concentrated sugar intakes? (pp. 120–122)
9. What are the health effects of starches and fibers? What are the dietary recommendations regarding these complex carbohydrates? (pp. 124–127)
10. What foods provide starches and fibers? (pp. 127–128)

These multiple choice questions will help you prepare for an exam. Answers can be found on p. 132.

1. Carbohydrates are found in virtually all foods except:
   a. milks.
   b. meats.
   c. breads.
   d. fruits.
2. Disaccharides include:
   a. starch, glycogen, and fiber.
   b. amylose, pectin, and dextrose.
   c. sucrose, maltose, and lactose.
   d. glucose, galactose, and fructose.
3. The making of a disaccharide from two monosaccharides is an example of:
   a. digestion.
   b. hydrolysis.
   c. condensation.
   d. gluconeogenesis.
4. The storage form of glucose in the body is:
   a. insulin.
   b. maltose.
   c. glucagon.
   d. glycogen.

5. The significant difference between starch and cellulose is that:
   a. starch is a polysaccharide, but cellulose is not.
   b. animals can store glucose as starch, but not as cellulose.
   c. hormones can make glucose from cellulose, but not from starch.
   d. digestive enzymes can break the bonds in starch, but not in cellulose.
6. The ultimate goal of carbohydrate digestion and absorption is to yield:
   a. fibers.
   b. glucose.
   c. enzymes.
   d. amylase.
7. The enzyme that breaks a disaccharide into glucose and galactose is:
   a. amylase.
   b. maltase.
   c. sucrase.
   d. lactase.
8. With insufficient glucose in metabolism, fat fragments combine to form:
   a. dextrins.
   b. mucilages.
   c. phytic acids.
   d. ketone bodies.
9. What does the pancreas secrete when blood glucose rises? When blood glucose falls?
   a. insulin; glucagon
   b. glucagon; insulin
   c. insulin; glycogen
   d. glycogen; epinephrine
10. What percentage of the daily energy intake should come from carbohydrates?
    a. 15 to 20
    b. 25 to 30
    c. 45 to 50
    d. 45 to 65

REFERENCES

1. B. M. Davy and C. L. Melby, The effect of fiber-rich carbohydrates on features of Syndrome X, *Journal of the American Dietetic Association* 103 (2003): 86–96.
2. S. W. Rizkalla and coauthors, Chronic consumption of fresh but not heated yogurt improves breath-hydrogen status and short-chain fatty acid profiles: A controlled study in healthy men with or without lactose maldigestion, *American Journal of Clinical Nutrition* 72 (2000): 1474–1479.
3. T. Maeder, Sweet medicines, *Scientific American* 287 (2002): 40–47; J. Travis, The true sweet science—Researchers develop a taster for the study of sugars, *Science News* 161 (2002): 232–233; multiple articles in Carbohydrates and glycobiology—Searching for medicine's sweet spot, *Science* 291 (2001): 2338–2378.
4. G. Pourmotabbed and A. E. Kitabchi, Hypoglycemia, *Obstetrics and Gynecology Clinics of North America* 28 (2001): 383–400.
5. K. Foster-Powell, S. H. A. Holt, and J. C. Brand-Miller, International table of glycemic index and glycemic load values: 2002, *American Journal of Clinical Nutrition* 76 (2002): 5–56.
6. A. E. Buyken and coauthors, Glycemic index in the diet of European outpatients with type 1 diabetes: Relations to glycated hemoglobin and serum lipids, *American Journal of Clinical Nutrition* 73 (2001): 574–581.
7. T. M. S. Wolever, Carbohydrate and the regulation of blood glucose and metabolism, *Nutrition Reviews* 61 (2003): S40–S48; D. J. A. Jenkins and coauthors, Glycemic index: Overview of implications in health and disease, *American Journal of Clinical Nutrition* 76 (2002): 266S–273S; S. Liu and coauthors, Dietary glycemic load assessed by food-frequency questionnaire in relation to plasma high-density lipoprotein cholesterol and fasting plasma triacylglycerols in postmenopausal women, *American Journal of Clinical Nutrition* 73 (2001): 560–566; S. Liu and coauthors, A prospective study of dietary glycemic load, carbohydrate intake, and risk of coronary heart disease in US women, *American Journal of Clinical Nutrition* 71 (2000): 1455–1461; K. L. Morris and M. B. Zemel, Glycemic index, cardiovascular disease, and obesity, *Nutrition Reviews* 57 (1999): 273–276.
8. L. E. Spieth and coauthors, A low-glycemic index diet in the treatment of pediatric obesity, *Archives of Pediatrics and Adolescent Medicine* 154 (2000): 947–951.
9. S. B. Roberts, Glycemic index and satiety, *Nutrition in Clinical Care* 6 (2003): 20–26; D. S. Ludwig and coauthors, Dietary fiber, weight gain, and cardiovascular disease risk factors in young adults, *Journal of the American Medical Association* 282 (1999): 1539–1546.
10. S. Liu and coauthors, Relation between a diet with a high glycemic load and plasma concentrations of high-sensitivity C-reactive protein in middle-aged women, *American Journal of Clinical Nutrition* 75 (2002): 492–498; D. S. Ludwig and coauthors, High glycemic index foods, overeating, and obesity, *Pediatrics* 103 (1999): e26 (**www.pediatrics.org**).
11. D. S. Ludwig, The glycemic index—Physiological mechanisms relating to obesity, diabetes, and cardiovascular disease, *Journal of the American Medical Association* 287 (2002): 2414–2423.
12. F. X. Pi-Sunyer, Glycemic index and disease, *American Journal of Clinical Nutrition* 76 (2002): 290S–298S.
13. C. Beebe, Diets with a low glycemic index: Not ready for practice yet! *Nutrition Today* 34 (1999): 82–86.
14. E. Saltzman, The low glycemic index diet: Not yet ready for prime time, *Nutrition Reviews* 57 (1999): 297.
15. S. Kashket and D. P. DePaola, Cheese consumption and the development and progression of dental caries, *Nutrition Reviews* 60 (2002): 97–103; Department of Health and Human Services, *Oral Health in America: A Report of the Surgeon General* (Rockville, Md.: National Institutes of Health, 2000), pp. 250–251.
16. S. Gibson and S. Williams, Dental caries in pre-school children: Associations with social class, toothbrushing habit and consumption of sugars and sugar-containing foods. Further analysis of data from the National Diet and Nutrition Survey of children aged 1.5–4.5 years, *Caries Research* 33 (1999): 101–113.
17. J. M. Jones and K. Elam, Sugars and health: Is there an issue? *Journal of the American Dietetic Association* 103 (2003): 1058–1060.
18. B. V. Howard and J. Wylie-Rosett, AHA Scientific Statement: Sugar and cardiovascular disease, *Circulation* 106 (2002): 523.
19. J. M. Schwarz and coauthors, Hepatic de novo lipogenesis in normoinsulinemic and hyperinsulinemic subjects consuming high-fat, low-carbohydrate and low-fat, high-carbohydrate isoenergetic diets, *American Journal of Clinical Nutrition* 77 (2003): 43–50.
20. E. J. Parks and M. K. Hellerstein, Carbohydrate-induced hypertriacylglycerolemia: Historical perspective and review of biological mechanisms, *American Journal of Clinical Nutrition* 71 (2000): 412–433.
21. S. Yanovski, Sugar and fat: Cravings and aversions, *Journal of Nutrition* 133 (2003): 835S–837S.
22. M. Moorhouse and coauthors, Carbohydrate craving by alcohol-dependent men during sobriety: Relationship to nutrition and serotonergic function, *Alcoholism, Clinical and Experimental Research* 24 (2000): 635–643.
23. P. J. Rogers and H. J. Smit, Food craving and food "addiction": A critical review of the evidence from a biopsychosocial perspective, *Pharmacology, Biochemistry, and Behavior* 66 (2000): 3–14.

24. Economic Research Service, Farm Service Agency, and Foreign Agricultural Service, USDA, 2001.
25. Committee on Dietary Reference Intakes, *Dietary Reference Intakes for Energy, Carbohydrate, Fiber, Fat, Fatty Acids, Cholesterol, Protein, and Amino Acids* (Washington, D.C.: National Academies Press, 2002).
26. S. A. Bowman, Diets of individuals based on energy intakes from added sugars, *Family Economics and Nutrition Review* 12 (1999): 31–38.
27. F. B. Hu and W. C. Willett, Optimal diets for prevention of coronary heart disease, *Journal of the American Medical Association* 288 (2002): 2569–2578; N. M. McKeown and coauthors, Whole-grain intake is favorably associated with metabolic risk factors for type 2 diabetes and cardiovascular disease in the Framingham Offspring Study, *American Journal of Clinical Nutrition* 76 (2002): 390–398; S. Liu and coauthors, Whole-grain consumption and risk of coronary heart disease: Results from the Nurses' Health Study, *American Journal of Clinical Nutrition* 70 (1999): 412–419; A. Wolk and coauthors, Long-term intake of dietary fiber and decreased risk of coronary heart disease among women, *Journal of the American Medical Association* 281 (1999): 1998–2004; J. L. Slavin and coauthors, Plausible mechanisms for the protectiveness of whole grains, *American Journal of Clinical Nutrition* 70 (1999): 459S–463S.
28. L. Van Horn and N. Ernst, A summary of the science supporting the new National Cholesterol Education program dietary recommendations: What dietitians should know, *Journal of the American Dietetic Association* 101 (2001): 1148–1154; L. Brown and coauthors, Cholesterol-lowering effects of dietary fiber: A meta-analysis, *American Journal of Clinical Nutrition* 69 (1999): 30–42.
29. M. L. Fernandez, Soluble fiber and nondigestible carbohydrate effects on plasma lipids and cardiovascular risk, *Current Opinion in Lipidology* 12 (2001): 35–40; Brown and coauthors, 1999.
30. B. M. Davy and coauthors, High-fiber oat cereal compared with wheat cereal consumption favorably alters LDL-cholesterol subclass and particle numbers in middle-aged and older men, *American Journal of Clinical Nutrition* 76 (2002): 351–358; D. J. A. Jenkins and coauthors, Soluble fiber intake at a dose approved by the US Food and Drug Administration for a claim of health benefits: Serum lipid risk factors for cardiovascular disease assessed in a randomized controlled crossover trial, *American Journal of Clinical Nutrition* 75 (2002): 834–839; J. W. Anderson and coauthors, Cholesterol-lowering effects of psyllium intake adjunctive to diet therapy in men and women with hypercholesterolemia: A meta-analysis of 8 controlled trials, *American Journal of Clinical Nutrition* 71 (2000): 472–479; Brown and coauthors, 1999.
31. T. T. Fung and coauthors, Whole-grain intake and the risk of type 2 diabetes: A prospective study in men, *American Journal of Clinical Nutrition* 76 (2002): 535–540.
32. W. Aldoori and M. Ryan-Harshman, Preventing diverticular disease: Review of recent evidence on high-fibre diets, *Canadian Family Physician* 48 (2002): 1632–1637.
33. A. Schatzkin and coauthors, Lack of effect of a low-fat, high-fiber diet on the recurrence of colorectal adenomas, *New England Journal of Medicine* 342 (2000): 1149–1155; D. S. Alberts and coauthors, Lack of effect of a high-fiber cereal supplement on the recurrence of colorectal adenomas, *New England Journal of Medicine* 342 (2000): 1156–1162; F. Macrae, Wheat bran fiber and development of adenomatous polyps: Evidence from randomized, controlled clinical trials, *American Journal of Medicine* 106 (1999): 38S–42S; D. Kritchevsky, Protective role of wheat bran fiber: Preclinical data, *American Journal of Medicine* 106 (1999): 28S–31S; C. S. Fuchs and coauthors, Dietary fiber and risk of colorectal cancer and adenoma in women, *New England Journal of Medicine* 340 (1999): 169–176.
34. S. A. Bingham and coauthors, Dietary fibre in food and protection against colorectal cancer in the European Prospective Investigation into Cancer and Nutrition (EPIC): An observational study, *Lancet* 361 (2003): 1496–1501.
35. J. L. Slavin, Mechanisms for the impact of whole grain foods on cancer risk, *Journal of the American College of Nutrition* 19 (2000): 300S–307S.
36. N. J. Emenaker and coauthors, Short-chain fatty acids inhibit invasive human colon cancer by modulating uPA, TIMP-1, TIMP-2, Mutant p53, Bcl-2, Bax, p21, and PCNA protein expression in an in vitro cell culture model, *Journal of Nutrition* 131 (2001): 3041S–3046S.
37. American Gastroenterological Association medical position statement: Impact of dietary fiber on colon cancer occurrence, *Gastroenterology* 118 (2000): 1233–1234.
38. N. C. Howarth, E. Saltzman, and S. B. Roberts, Dietary fiber and weight regulation, *Nutrition Reviews* 59 (2001): 129–139; A. Sparti and coauthors, Effect of diets high or low in unavailable and slowly digestible carbohydrates on the pattern of 24-h substrate oxidation and feelings of hunger in humans, *American Journal of Clinical Nutrition* 72 (2000): 1461–1468.
39. Committee on Dietary Reference Intakes, 2002, p. 7-4.
40. Committee on Dietary Reference Intakes, 2002.
41. Position of the American Dietetic Association: Health implications of dietary fiber, *Journal of the American Dietetic Association* 102 (2002): 993–999.
42. J. L. Slavin and coauthors, The role of whole grains in disease prevention, *Journal of the American Dietetic Association* 101 (2001): 780–785.

ANSWERS

Nutrition Calculations

1. 0.7×2000 total kcal/day = 1400 kcal from carbohydrate/day.
   1400 kcal from carbohydrate ÷ 4 kcal/g = 350 g carbohydrate.

This carbohydrate intake is higher than the Daily Value and higher than the 45 to 65 percent recommendation.

2. 350 g carbohydrate ÷ 2 = 175 g carbohydrate/day.
   175 g carbohydrate × 4 kcal/g = 700 kcal from carbohydrate.
   700 kcal from carbohydrate ÷ 2000 total kcal/day = 0.35.
   0.35×100 = 35% kcal from carbohydrate.

This carbohydrate intake is lower than the Daily Value and lower than the 45 to 65 percent recommendation.

3. 350 g carbohydrate × 2 = 700 g carbohydrate/day.
   700 g carbohydrate × 4 kcal/g = 2800 kcal from carbohydrate.
   2800 kcal from carbohydrate ÷ 6000 total kcal/day = 0.466 (rounded to 0.47)
   0.47×100 = 47% kcal from carbohydrate.

This carbohydrate intake is higher than the Daily Value and meets the 45 to 65 percent recommendation.

4. 150 g carbohydrate × 4 kcal/g = 600 kcal from carbohydrate.
   600 kcal from carbohydrate ÷ 1000 total kcal/day = 0.60.
   0.60×100 = 60% kcal from carbohydrate.

This carbohydrate intake is lower than the Daily Value and meets the 45 to 65 percent recommendation.

Study Questions (multiple choice)

1. b 2. c 3. c 4. d 5. d
6. b 7. d 8. d 9. a 10. d

HIGHLIGHT

Alternatives to Sugar

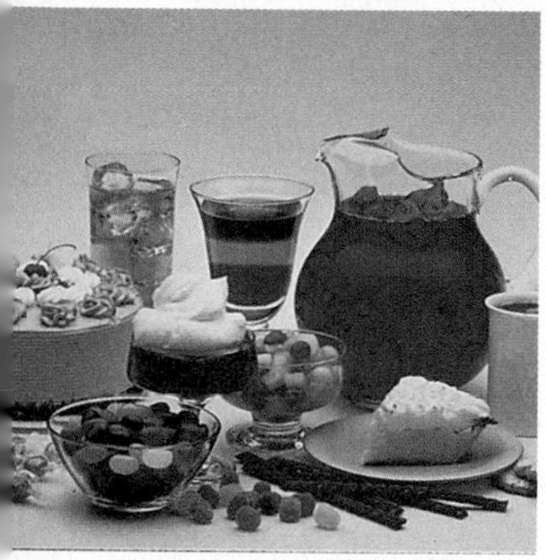

Funnette Division, Hoechst Celanese Corp.

Almost everyone finds sweet tastes pleasing—after all, a preference for sweets is inborn. To a child's taste, the sweeter the food, the better. In adults, the preference for sweets is somewhat diminished, but most still enjoy an occasional sweet food or beverage. Facing the health concerns of overweight and obesity, many consumers turn to alternative sweeteners to help them control kcalories and limit their use of sugar. In doing so, they encounter two sets of alternative sweeteners. One set, the **artificial sweeteners**, provide virtually no energy and are sometimes referred to as nonnutritive sweeteners. The other set, the **sugar replacers,** yield energy and are sometimes referred to as **nutritive sweeteners.**

Artificial Sweeteners

Artificial sweeteners permit people to keep their sugar and energy intakes down, yet still enjoy the delicious sweet tastes of their favorite foods and beverages. The Food and Drug Administration (FDA) has approved the use of several artificial sweeteners—saccharin, aspartame, acesulfame potassium (acesulfame-K), sucralose, and neotame. Two others have petitioned the FDA and are awaiting approval—alitame and cyclamate. Table H4-1 and the glossary below provide general details about each of these sweeteners.

Saccharin, acesulfame-K, and sucralose are not metabolized in the body; in contrast, the body digests aspartame as a protein. In fact, aspartame is *technically* classified as a nutritive sweetener because it yields energy (4 kcalories per gram, as does protein). But because so little is used, its energy contribution is negligible.

Some consumers have challenged the safety of using artificial sweeteners. Considering that all substances are toxic at

GLOSSARY

Acceptable Daily Intake (ADI): the estimated amount of a sweetener that individuals can safely consume each day over the course of a lifetime without adverse effect.

acesulfame (AY-sul-fame) **potassium:** an artificial sweetener composed of an organic salt that has been approved for use in both the United States and Canada; also known as **acesulfame-K** because K is the chemical symbol for potassium.

alitame (AL-ih-tame): an artificial sweetener composed of two amino acids (alanine and aspartic acid); FDA approval pending.

artificial sweeteners: sugar substitutes that provide negligible, if any, energy; sometimes called **nonnutritive sweeteners.**

aspartame (ah-SPAR-tame or ASS-par-tame): an artificial sweetener composed of two amino acids (phenylalanine and aspartic acid); approved for use in both the United States and Canada.

cyclamate (SIGH-kla-mate): an artificial sweetener that is being considered for approval in the United States and is available in Canada as a tabletop sweetener, but not as an additive.

neotame (NEE-oh-tame): an artificial sweetener composed of two amino acids (phenylalanine and aspartic acid); approved for use in the United States.

nutritive sweeteners: sweeteners that yield energy, including both sugars and sugar replacers.

saccharin (SAK-ah-ren): an artificial sweetener that has been approved for use in the United States. In Canada, approval for use in foods and beverages is pending; currently available only in pharmacies and only as a tabletop sweetener, not as an additive.

stevia (STEE-vee-ah): a South American shrub whose leaves are used as a sweetener; sold in the United States as a dietary supplement that provides sweetness without kcalories.

sucralose (SUE-kra-lose): an artificial sweetener approved for use in the United States and Canada.

sugar replacers: sugarlike compounds that can be derived from fruits or commercially produced from dextrose; also called **sugar alcohols** or **polyols.** Sugar alcohols are absorbed more slowly than other sugars and metabolized differently in the human body; they are not readily utilized by ordinary mouth bacteria. Examples are **maltitol, mannitol, sorbitol, xylitol, isomalt,** and **lactitol.**

tagatose (TAG-ah-tose): a monosaccharide structurally similar to fructose that is incompletely absorbed and thus provides only 1.5 kcalories per gram; approved for use as a "generally recognized as safe" ingredient.

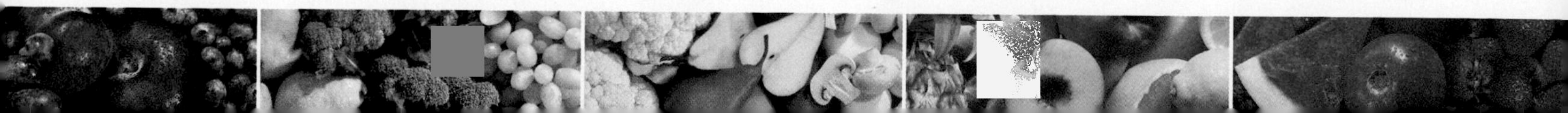

TABLE H4-1 Sweeteners

Sweeteners	Relative Sweetness[a]	Energy (kcal/g)	Acceptable Daily Intake	Average Amount to Replace 1 tsp Sugar	Approved Uses
Approved Sweeteners					
Saccharin	450	0	5 mg/kg body weight	12 mg	Tabletop sweeteners, wide range of foods, beverages, cosmetics, and pharmaceutical products
Aspartame	200	4[b]	50 mg/kg body weight[c] Warning to people with PKU: Contains phenylalanine	18 mg	General purpose sweetener in all foods and beverages
Acesulfame-K	200	0	15 mg/kg body weight[d]	25 mg	Tabletop sweeteners, puddings, gelatins, chewing gum, candies, baked goods, desserts, alcoholic beverages
Sucralose	600	0	5 mg/kg body weight	6 mg	Carbonated beverages, dairy products, baked goods, coffee and tea, fruit spreads, syrups, tabletop sweeteners, chewing gum, frozen desserts, salad dressing
Neotame	8000	0	18 mg/day	0.5µg	Baked goods, nonalcoholic beverages, chewing gum, candies, frostings, frozen desserts, gelatins, puddings, jams and jellies, syrups
Tagatose	0.8	1.5	7.5 g/day	1 tsp	Baked goods, beverages, cereals, chewing gum, confections, dairy products, dietary supplements, health bars, tabletop sweetener
Sweeteners with Approval Pending					**Proposed Uses**
Alitame	2000	4[e]	—		Beverages, baked goods, tabletop sweeteners, frozen desserts
Cyclamate	30	0	—		Tabletop sweeteners, baked goods

[a] Relative sweetness is determined by comparing the approximate sweetness of a sugar substitute with the sweetness of pure sucrose, which has been defined as 1.0. Chemical structure, temperature, acidity, and other flavors of the foods in which the substance occurs all influence relative sweetness.

[b] Aspartame provides 4 kcalories per gram, as does protein, but because so little is used, its energy contribution is negligible. In powdered form it is sometimes mixed with lactose, however, so a 1-gram packet may provide 4 kcalories.

[c] Recommendations from the World Health Organization and in Europe and Canada limit aspartame intake to 40 milligrams per kilogram of body weight.

[d] Recommendations from the World Health Organization limit acesulfame-K intake to 9 milligrams per kilogram of body weight.

[e] Alitame provides 4 kcalories per gram, as does protein, but because so little is used, its energy contribution is negligible.

some dose, it is little surprise that large doses of artificial sweeteners (or their components or metabolic by-products) have toxic effects. The question to ask is whether their ingestion is safe for human beings in quantities people normally use (and potentially abuse). The answer is yes, except in the special case described later for aspartame.

Saccharin

Saccharin, used for over 100 years in the United States, is currently used by some 50 million people—primarily in soft drinks, secondarily as a tabletop sweetener. Saccharin is rapidly excreted in the urine and does not accumulate in the body.

Questions about saccharin's safety surfaced in 1977, when experiments suggested that large doses of saccharin (equivalent to hundreds of cans of diet soda daily for a lifetime) increased the risk of bladder cancer in rats. The FDA proposed banning saccharin as a result. Public outcry in favor of saccharin was so loud, however, that Congress imposed a moratorium on the ban—a moratorium that was repeatedly extended until 1991, when the FDA withdrew its proposal to ban saccharin. Products containing saccharin were required to carry a warning label: "Use of this product may be hazardous to your health. This product contains saccharin, which has been determined to cause cancer in laboratory animals."

Does saccharin cause cancer? The largest population study to date, involving 9000 men and women, showed that overall saccharin use did not increase the risk of cancer. Among certain small groups of the population, however, such as those who both smoked heavily and used saccharin, the risk of bladder cancer was slightly greater. Other studies involving more than 5000 people with bladder cancer showed no association between bladder cancer and saccharin use.[1] In 2000, saccharin was removed from the list of suspected cancer-causing substances. Warning labels are no longer required.

Common sense dictates that consuming large amounts of any substance is probably not wise, but at current, moderate intake levels, saccharin appears to be safe for most people. It has been approved for use in more than 100 countries.

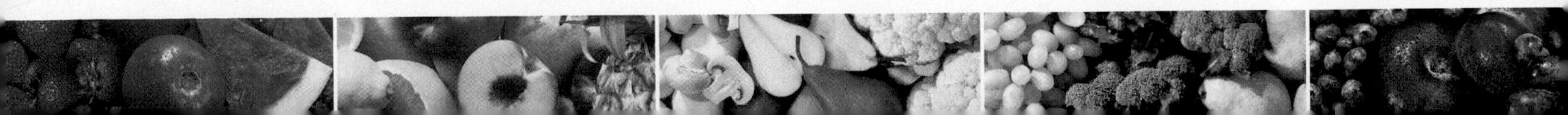

FIGURE H4-1 Structure of Aspartame

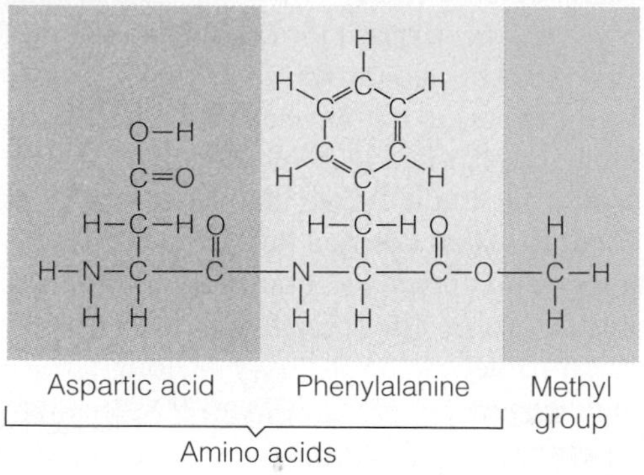
Aspartic acid
Phenylalanine
Methyl group
Amino acids

FIGURE H4-2 Metabolism of Aspartame

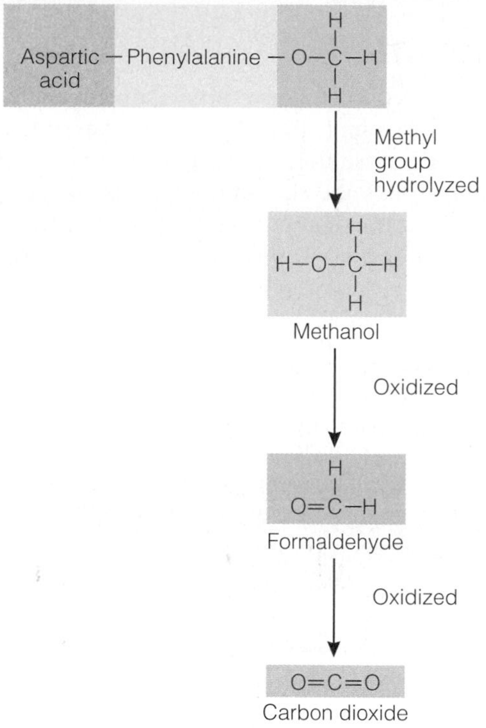
Aspartic acid
Phenylalanine
Methyl group hydrolyzed
Methanol
Oxidized
Formaldehyde
Oxidized
Carbon dioxide

Aspartame

Aspartame is one of the most studied of all food additives; extensive animal and human studies document its safety. Long-term consumption of aspartame is not associated with any adverse health effects.

The nutrients in aspartame may present a problem for certain people, however, and for this reason, aspartame carries a warning on its label. Aspartame is a simple chemical compound made of components common to a many foods: two amino acids (phenylalanine and aspartic acid) and a methyl group (CH_3). Figure H4-1 shows its chemical structure. The flavors of the components give no clue to the combined effect; one of them tastes bitter, and the other is tasteless, but the combination creates a product that is 200 times sweeter than sucrose.

In the digestive tract, enzymes split aspartame into its three component parts. The body absorbs the two amino acids and uses them just as if they had come from food protein, which is made entirely of amino acids including these two.

Because this sweetener contributes phenylalanine, products containing aspartame must bear a warning label for people with the inherited disease phenylketonuria (PKU). People with PKU are unable to dispose of any excess phenylalanine. The accumulation of phenylalanine and its by-products is toxic to the developing nervous system, causing irreversible brain damage. For this reason, all newborns in the United States are screened for PKU. The treatment for PKU is a special diet that must strike a balance, providing enough phenylalanine to support normal growth and health but not enough to cause harm. The question is, does aspartame raise blood phenylalanine high enough to be toxic to people with PKU? Apparently not. The little extra phenylalanine from aspartame poses only a small risk, even in heavy users.

Still, there is a compelling reason why children with PKU need to get all their phenylalanine from foods, and not from an artificial sweetener. The PKU diet excludes such protein- and nutrient-rich foods as milk, meat, fish, poultry, cheese, eggs, nuts, legumes, and many bread products. Only with difficulty can these children obtain the many essential nutrients—such as calcium, iron, and the B vitamins—found along with phenylalanine in these foods. To suggest that children with PKU squander any of their limited phenylalanine allowance on the purified phenylalanine of aspartame, which contributes none of the associated vitamins or minerals essential for good health and normal growth, would open the way for poor nutrition.

Setting aside the special case of PKU, is there any reason to be concerned about the products aspartame yields in the body? During metabolism, the methyl group momentarily becomes methyl alcohol (methanol)—a potentially toxic compound (see Figure H4-2). This breakdown also occurs when aspartame-sweetened beverages are stored at warm temperatures over time. The amount of methanol produced may be safe to consume, but a person may not want to, considering that the beverage has lost its sweetness. In the body, enzymes convert methanol to formaldehyde, another toxic compound. Finally, formaldehyde is broken down to carbon dioxide. Before aspartame could be approved, the quantities of these products generated during metabolism had to be determined; they were found to fall below the threshold at which they would cause harm. In fact, ounce for ounce, tomato juice yields six times as much methanol as a diet soda.

In conclusion, except for people with PKU, aspartame is safe. Some individuals may exhibit vague, but not dangerous, symptoms due to unusual sensitivity to aspartame, but it is generally safe. Like saccharin, aspartame has been approved for use in more than 100 countries.

Acesulfame-K

The FDA approved **acesulfame potassium (acesulfame-K)** in 1988 after reviewing more than 90 safety studies conducted over 15 years. Some consumer groups believe that acesulfame-K causes tumors in rats and should not have been approved. The FDA counters that the tumors were not caused by the sweetener, but were typical of those commonly found in rat studies. Acesulfame-K has been approved for use in more than 60 countries.

Sucralose

Sucralose received FDA approval in 1998 after a review of over 110 safety studies conducted on both animals and human beings. Sucralose is unique among the artificial sweeteners in that it is made from sugar that has had three of its hydroxyl (OH) groups replaced by chlorine atoms. The result is an exceptionally stable molecule that is 600 times sweeter than sugar. Because the body does not recognize sucralose as a carbohydrate, it passes through the GI tract undigested and unabsorbed.

Neotame

Neotame is the most recent artificial sweetener to hit the markets. The FDA approved neotame in 2002 after reviewing more than 110 safety studies conducted on both animals and human beings. Neotame is so intensely sweet—about 8000 times sweeter than sugar—that very little is needed.

Like aspartame, neotame also contains the amino acids phenylalanine and aspartic acid and a methyl group. Unlike aspartame, however, neotame has an additional side group attached. This simple difference makes all the difference to people with PKU because it blocks the digestive enzymes that normally separate phenylalanine and aspartic acid. Consequently, the amino acids are not absorbed and neotame need not carry a warning for people with PKU.

Tagatose

The FDA recently granted the fructose relative **tagatose** the status of generally recognized as safe, making it available as a low-kcalorie sweetener for a variety of foods and beverages. This monosaccharide is naturally found in only a few foods, but it can be derived from lactose. Unlike fructose or lactose, however, 80 percent of tagatose remains unabsorbed until it reaches the large intestine. There, bacteria ferment tagatose, releasing gases and short chain fatty acids that are absorbed. As a result, tagatose provides only 1.5 kcalories per gram. At high doses, tagatose causes flatulence, rumbling, and loose stools; otherwise, no adverse side effects have been noted. Unlike other sugars, tagatose does not promote dental caries and may carry a dental caries health claim.

Alitame and Cyclamate

FDA approval for **alitame** and **cyclamate** is still pending. To date, no safety issues have been raised for alitame, and it has been approved for use in other countries. In contrast, cyclamate has been battling safety issues for 50 years. Approved by the FDA in 1949, cyclamate was banned in 1969 principally on the basis of one study indicating that it caused bladder cancer in rats.

The National Research Council has reviewed dozens of studies on cyclamate and concluded that neither cyclamate nor its metabolites cause cancer. The council did, however, recommend further research to determine if heavy or long-term use poses risks. Although cyclamate does not *initiate* cancer, it may *promote* cancer development once it is started. The FDA currently has no policy on substances that enhance the cancer-causing activities of other substances, but it is unlikely to approve cyclamate soon, if at all. Agencies in more than 50 other countries, including Canada, have approved cyclamate.

Stevia—An Herbal Alternative

The FDA has backed its approval or denial of artificial sweeteners with decades of extensive research. Such research is lacking for the herb **stevia**, a shrub whose leaves have long been used by the people of South America to sweeten their beverages. In the United States, stevia is sold in health-food stores as a dietary supplement. The FDA has reviewed the limited research on the use of stevia as an alternative to artificial sweeteners and found concerns regarding its effect on reproduction, cancer development, and energy metabolism. Used sparingly, stevia may do little harm, but the FDA could not approve its extensive and widespread use in the U.S. market. Canada, the European Union, and the United Nations have reached similar conclusions. That stevia can be sold as a dietary supplement, but not used as a food additive in the United States, highlights key differences in FDA regulations. Food additives must prove their safety and effectiveness before receiving FDA approval, whereas dietary supplements are not required to submit to any testing or receive any approval. (See Highlight 10 and Chapter 19 for information on dietary supplements.)

Acceptable Daily Intake

The amount of artificial sweetener considered safe for daily use is called the **Acceptable Daily Intake (ADI).** The ADI represents the level of consumption that, if maintained every day throughout a person's life, would still be considered safe by a wide margin.

For example, the ADI for aspartame is 50 milligrams per kilogram of body weight. That is, the FDA approved aspartame based on the assumption that no one would consume more than 50 milligrams per kilogram of body weight in a day. This maximum daily intake is indeed a lot: for a 150-pound adult, it adds up to 97 packets of Equal or 20 cans of soft drinks sweetened only with aspartame. The company that produces aspartame estimates that if all the sugar and saccharin in the U.S. diet were replaced with

TABLE H4-2 Average Aspartame Contents of Selected Foods

Food	Aspartame (mg)
12 oz diet soft drink	170
8 oz powdered drink	100
8 oz sugar-free fruit yogurt	124
4 oz gelatin dessert	80
1 packet sweetener	35

aspartame, 1 percent of the population would be consuming the FDA maximum. Most people who use aspartame consume less than 5 milligrams per kilogram of body weight per day. But a young child who drinks four glasses of aspartame-sweetened beverages on a hot day and has five servings of other products with aspartame that day (such as pudding, chewing gum, cereal, gelatin, and frozen desserts) takes in the FDA maximum level. Although this presents no proven hazard, it seems wise to offer children other foods so as not to exceed the limit. Table H4-2 lists the average amounts of aspartame in some common foods.

For persons choosing to use artificial sweeteners, the American Dietetic Association wisely advises that they be used in moderation and only as part of a well-balanced nutritious diet.[2] The dietary principles of both moderation and variety help to reduce the possible risks associated with any food.

Artificial Sweeteners and Weight Control

The rate of obesity in the United States has been rising for decades. Foods and beverages sweetened with artificial sweeteners were among the first products developed to help people control their weight. Ironically, a few studies have reported that intense sweeteners, such as aspartame, may stimulate appetite, which could lead to weight gain.[3] Contradicting these reports, most studies find no change in feelings of hunger and no change in food intakes or body weight.[4] Adding to the confusion, some studies report lower energy intakes and greater weight losses when people eat or drink artificially sweetened products.[5]

When studying the effects of artificial sweeteners on food intake and body weight, researchers ask different questions and take different approaches. It matters, for example, whether the people used in a study are of a healthy weight and whether they are following a weight-loss diet. Motivations for using sweeteners differ, too, and this influences a person's actions. For example, one person might drink an artificially sweetened beverage now so as to be able to eat a high-kcalorie food later. This person's energy intake might stay the same or increase. Another person trying to control food energy intake might drink an artificially sweetened beverage now and then choose a low-kcalorie food later. This plan would help reduce the person's energy intake.

TABLE H4-3 Sugar Replacers

Sugar Alcohols	Relative Sweetness[a]	Energy (kcal/g)	Approved Uses
Isomalt	0.5	2.0	Candies, chewing gum, ice cream, jams and jellies, frostings, beverages, baked goods
Lactitol	0.4	2.0	Candies, chewing gum, frozen dairy desserts, jams and jellies, frostings, baked goods
Maltitol	0.9	2.1	Particularly good for candy coating
Mannitol	0.7	1.6	Bulking agent, chewing gum
Sorbitol	0.5	2.6	Special dietary foods, candies, gums
Xylitol	1.0	2.4	Chewing gum, candies, pharmaceutical and oral health products

[a] Relative sweetness is determined by comparing the approximate sweetness of a sugar replacer with the sweetness of pure sucrose, which has been defined as 1.0. Chemical structure, temperature, acidity, and other flavors of the foods in which the substance occurs all influence relative sweetness.

In designing experiments on artificial sweeteners, researchers have to distinguish between the effects of sweetness and the effects of a particular substance. If a person is hungry shortly after eating an artificially sweetened snack, is that because the sweet taste (of all sweeteners, including sugars) stimulates appetite? Or is it because the artificial sweetener itself stimulates appetite? Research must also distinguish between the effects of food energy and the effects of the substance. If a person is hungry shortly after eating an artificially sweetened snack, is that because less food energy was available to satisfy hunger? Or is it because the artificial sweetener itself triggers hunger? Furthermore, if appetite is stimulated and a person feels hungry, does that actually lead to increased food intake?

Whether a person compensates for the energy reduction of artificial sweeteners either partially or fully depends on several factors. Using artificial sweeteners will not automatically lower energy intake; to control energy intake successfully, a person needs to make informed diet and activity decisions throughout the day (as Chapter 9 explains).

Sugar Replacers

Some "sugar-free" or reduced-kcalorie products contain sugar replacers.* The term *sugar replacers* describes the sugar alcohols—familiar examples include mannitol, sorbitol, xylitol,

*To minimize confusion, the American Diebetes Association prefers the term *sugar replacers* instead of "sugar alcohols" (which connotes alcohol), "bulk sweeteners" (which connotes fiber), or "sugar substitutes" (which connotes aspartame and saccharin).

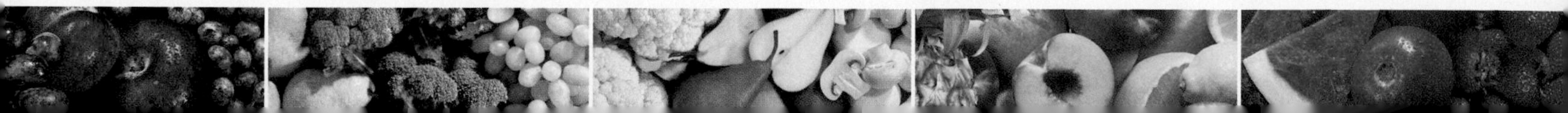

FIGURE H4-3 Sugar Alternatives on Food Labels

FOR STRONG HEALTHY TEETH
Trident
FOR KIDS
SUGARLESS GUM
Recaldent
MILK DERIVED
Berry Bubble Gum
LONG LASTING FLAVOR!
Wrigley's
Extra
Does not promote tooth decay
Trident
GOOD FOR YOUR TEETH
VAL-U-PAK
18 STICKS
Spearmint

© Craig Moore

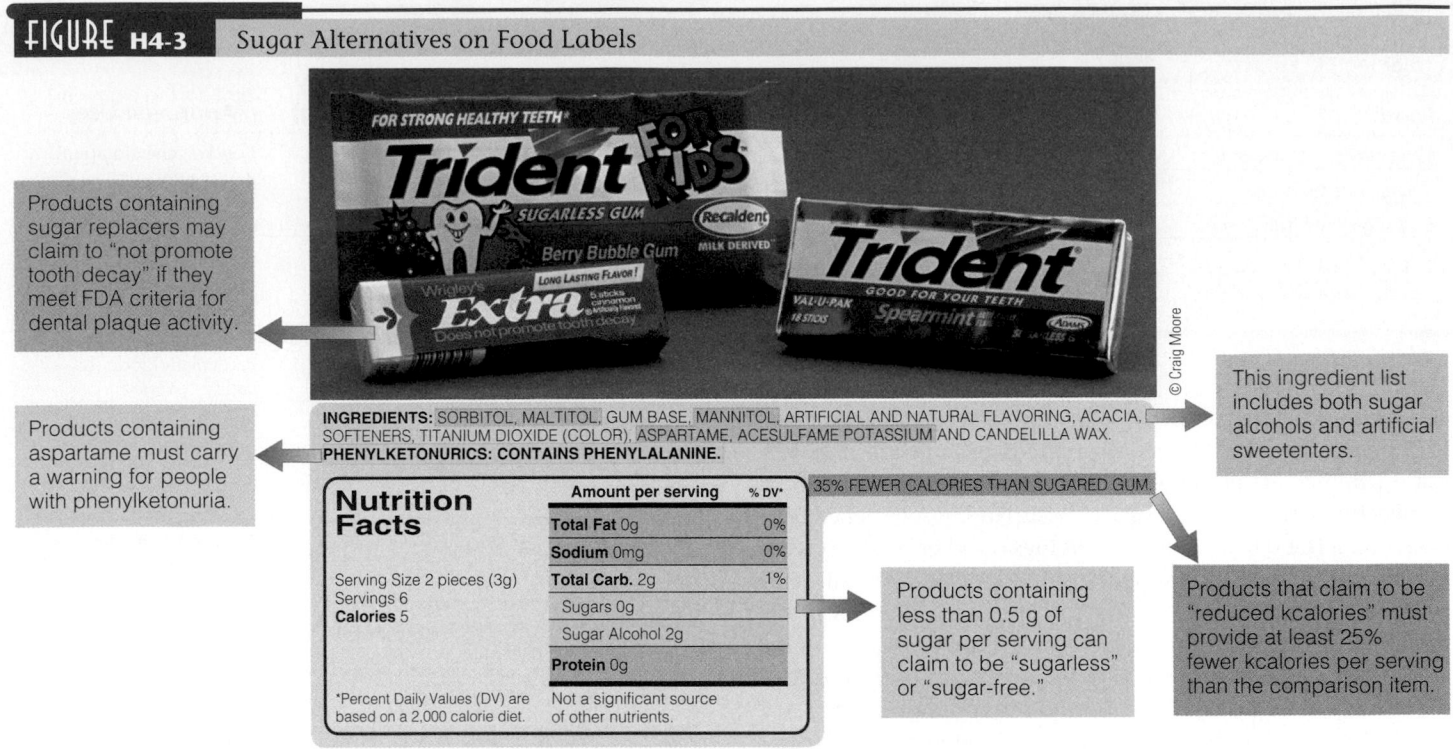

Products containing sugar replacers may claim to "not promote tooth decay" if they meet FDA criteria for dental plaque activity.

INGREDIENTS: SORBITOL, MALTITOL, GUM BASE, MANNITOL, ARTIFICIAL AND NATURAL FLAVORING, ACACIA, SOFTENERS, TITANIUM DIOXIDE (COLOR), ASPARTAME, ACESULFAME POTASSIUM AND CANDELILLA WAX.
PHENYLKETONURICS: CONTAINS PHENYLALANINE.

This ingredient list includes both sugar alcohols and artificial sweeteners.

Products containing aspartame must carry a warning for people with phenylketonuria.

35% FEWER CALORIES THAN SUGARED GUM.

Nutrition Facts

Serving Size 2 pieces (3g)
Servings 6
Calories 5

Amount per serving	**% DV***
Total Fat 0g	0%
Sodium 0mg	0%
Total Carb. 2g	1%
Sugars 0g	
Sugar Alcohol 2g	
Protein 0g	

*Percent Daily Values (DV) are based on a 2,000 calorie diet.

Not a significant source of other nutrients.

Products containing less than 0.5 g of sugar per serving can claim to be "sugarless" or "sugar-free."

Products that claim to be "reduced kcalories" must provide at least 25% fewer kcalories per serving than the comparison item.

maltitol, isomalt, and lactitol—that provide bulk and sweetness in cookies, hard candies, sugarless gums, jams, and jellies. These products claim to be "sugar-free" on their labels, but in this case, "sugar-free" does not mean free of kcalories. Sugar replacers do provide kcalories, but fewer than their carbohydrate cousins, the sugars. Table H4-3 includes their energy values, but a simple estimate can help consumers: divide grams by 2.[6] Sugar alcohols occur naturally in fruits and vegetables; they are also used by manufacturers as a low-energy bulk ingredient in many products.

Sugar alcohols evoke a low glycemic response. The body absorbs sugar alcohols slowly; consequently, they are slower to enter the bloodstream than other sugars. Side effects such as gas, abdominal discomfort, and diarrhea, however, make them less attractive than the artificial sweeteners. For this reason, regulations require food labels to state that "Excess consumption may have a laxative effect" if reasonable consumption of that food could result in the daily ingestion of 50 grams of a sugar alcohol.

The real benefit of using sugar replacers is that they do not contribute to dental caries. Bacteria in the mouth cannot metabolize sugar alcohols as rapidly as sugar. They are therefore valuable in chewing gums, breath mints, and other products that people keep in their mouths for a while. Figure H4-3 presents labeling information for products using alternatives to sugar.

The sugar replacers, like the artificial sweeteners, can occupy a place in the diet, and provided they are used in moderation, they will do no harm. In fact, they can help, both by providing an alternative to sugar for people with diabetes and by inhibiting caries-causing bacteria. People may find it appropriate to use all three sweeteners at times: artificial sweeteners, sugar replacers, and sugar itself.

NUTRITION ON THE NET

Access these websites for further study of topics covered in this highlight.

- Find updates and quick links to these and other nutrition-related sites at our website: **www.wadsworth.com/nutrition**
- Search for "artificial sweeteners" at the U.S. Government health information site: **www.healthfinder.gov**
- Search for "sweeteners" at the International Food Information Council site: **www.ific.org**

REFERENCES

1. Position of the American Dietetic Association: Use of nutritive and nonnutritive sweeteners, *Journal of the American Dietetic Association* 98 (1998): 580–587.
2. Position of the American Dietetic Association, 1998.
3. J. E. Blundell and P. J. Rogers, Sweet carbohydrate substitutes (intense sweeteners) and the control of appetite: Scientific issues, in *Appetites and Body Weight Regulation: Sugar, Fat, and Macronutrient Substitutes,* ed. J. D. Fernstrom and G. D. Miller (Boca Raton, Fla,: CRC Press, 1994), pp. 113–124.
4. S. J. Gatenby and coauthors, Extended use of foods modified in fat and sugar content: Nutrition implications in a free-living female population, *American Journal of Clinical Nutrition* 65 (1997): 1867–1873; A. Drewnowski, Intense sweeteners and the control of appetite, *Nutrition Reviews* 53 (1995): 1–7.
5. A. Raben and coauthors, Sucrose compared with artificial sweeteners: Different effects on ad libitum food intake and body weight after 10 wk of supplementation in overweight subjects, *American Journal of Clinical Nutrition* 76 (2002): 721–729; G. L. Blackburn and coauthors, The effect of aspartame as part of a multidisciplinary weight-control program on short- and long-term control of body weight, *American Journal of Clinical Nutrition* 65 (1997): 409–418.
6. K. McNutt, What clients need to know about sugar replacers, *Journal of the American Dietetic Association* 100 (2000): 466–469.

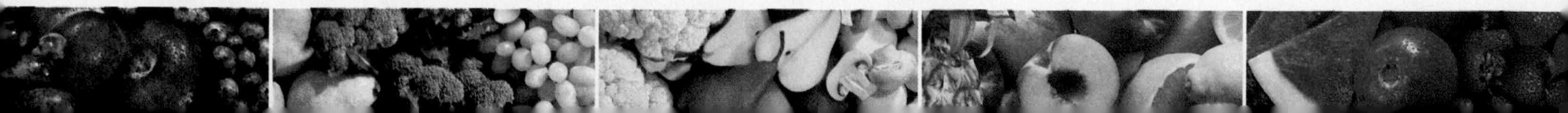

Chapter 5

The Lipids: Triglycerides, Phospholipids, and Sterols

Chapter Outline

Available Online

http://nutrition.wadsworth.com/uncn7

Nutrition Animation: *Lipids in the Body*

Student Practice Test

Glossary Terms

Nutrition on the Net

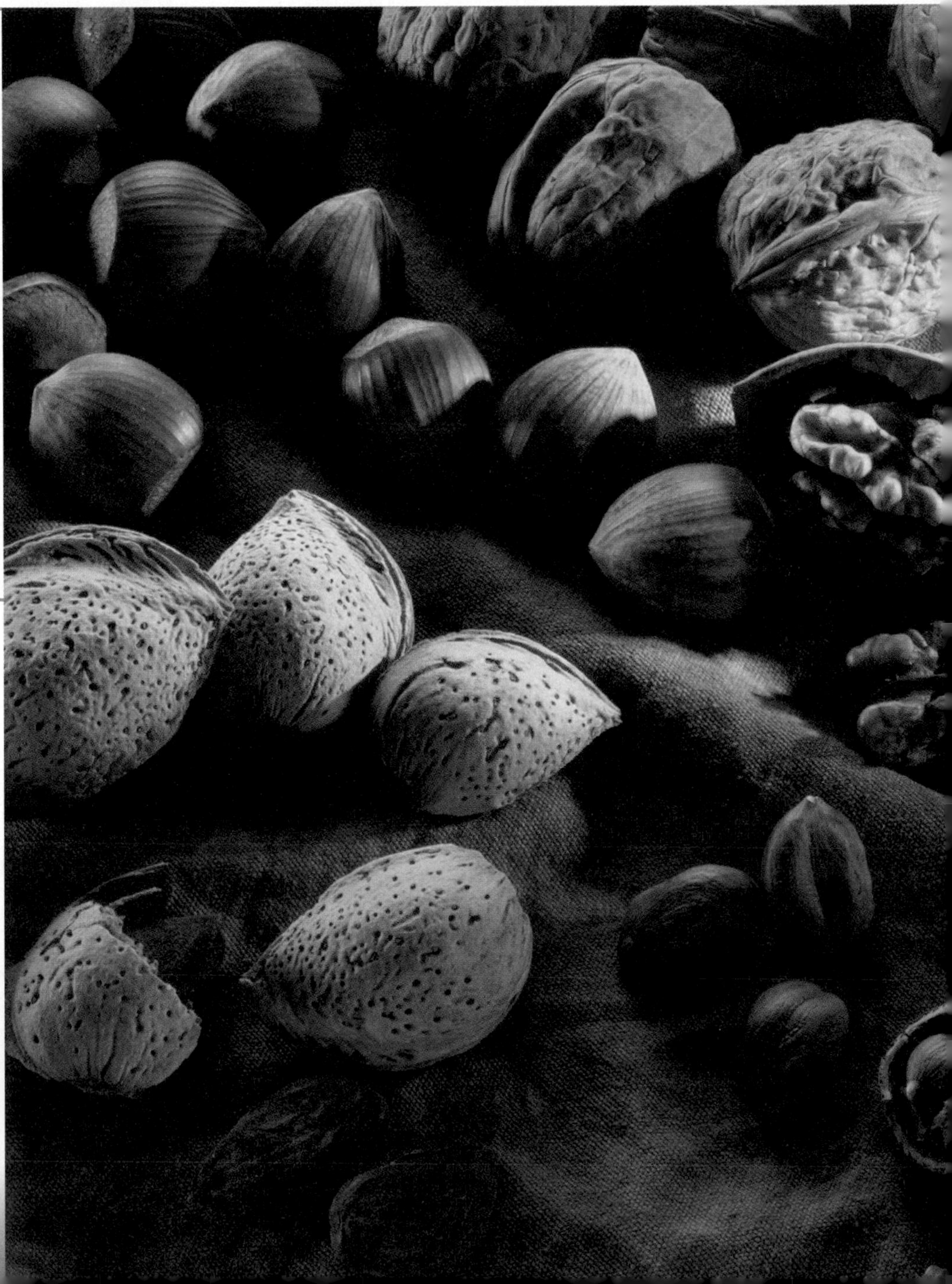

© Luc Hautecoeur/Stone/Getty Images

Nutrition in Your Life

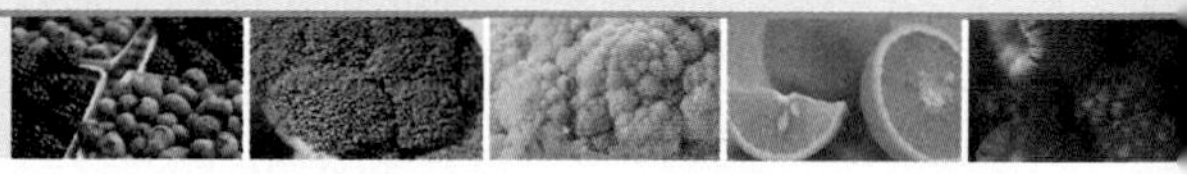

Most likely, you know what you don't like about body fat, but do you appreciate how it insulates you against the cold or powers your hike around a lake? And what about food fat? You're right to thank fat for providing the delicious flavors and aromas of buttered popcorn and fried chicken—and to curse it for contributing to the weight gain and heart disease so common today. The challenge is to strike a healthy balance of enjoying some fat, but not too much. Learning which kinds of fats are most harmful will also serve you well.

Most people are surprised to learn that fat has some virtues. Only when people consume either too much or too little fat, or too much of some kinds of fat, does ill health follow. It is true, though, that in our society of abundance, people are likely to encounter too much fat.

Fat refers to the class of nutrients known as **lipids**. The lipid family includes triglycerides (**fats** and **oils**), phospholipids, and sterols. The triglycerides■ predominate, both in foods and in the body.

■ Of the lipids in foods, 95% are fats and oils (triglycerides); of the lipids stored in the body, 99% are triglycerides.

The Chemist's View of Fatty Acids and Triglycerides

Like carbohydrates, fatty acids and triglycerides are composed of carbon (C), hydrogen (H), and oxygen (O). These lipids have many more carbons and hydrogens in proportion to their oxygens, however, and so can supply more energy per gram (Chapter 7 provides details).

The many names and relationships in the lipid family can seem overwhelming—like meeting a friend's extended family for the first time. To ease the introductions,

lipids: a family of compounds that includes triglycerides, phospholipids, and sterols. Lipids are characterized by their insolubility in water. (Lipids also include the fat-soluble vitamins, described in Chapter 11.)

fats: lipids that are solid at room temperature (70°F or 25°C).

oils: lipids that are liquid at room temperature (70°F or 25°C).

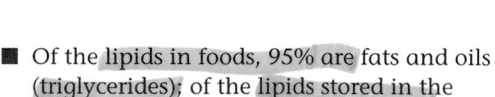

this chapter first presents each of the lipids from a chemist's point of view using both words and diagrams. Then the chapter follows the lipids through digestion and absorption and into the body to examine their roles in health and disease. For people who think more easily in words than in chemical symbols, this *preview* of the upcoming chemistry may be helpful:

1. Every triglyceride contains one molecule of glycerol and three fatty acids (basically, chains of carbon atoms).
2. Fatty acids may be 4 to 24 (even numbers of) carbons long, the 18-carbon ones being the most common in foods and especially noteworthy in nutrition.
3. Fatty acids may be saturated or unsaturated. Unsaturated fatty acids may have one or more points of unsaturation (that is, they may be monounsaturated or polyunsaturated).
4. Of special importance in nutrition are the polyunsaturated fatty acids whose *first* point of unsaturation is next to the third carbon (known as omega-3 fatty acids) or next to the sixth carbon (omega-6).
5. The 18-carbon fatty acids that fit this description are linolenic acid (omega-3) and linoleic acid (omega-6). Each is the primary member of a family of longer-chain fatty acids that help to regulate blood pressure, blood clotting, and other body functions important to health.

The paragraphs, definitions, and diagrams that follow present this information again in much more detail.

Fatty Acids

A **fatty acid** is an organic acid—a chain of carbon atoms with hydrogens attached—that has an acid group (COOH) at one end and a methyl group (CH_3) at the other end. The organic acid shown in Figure 5-1 is acetic acid, the compound that gives vinegar its sour taste. Acetic acid is the shortest such acid, with a "chain" only two carbon atoms long.

FIGURE 5-1 Acetic Acid

Acetic acid is a two-carbon organic acid.

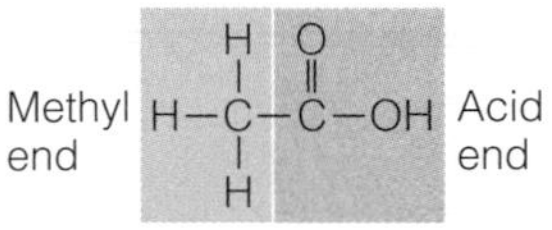
Methyl end
Acid end

The Length of the Carbon Chain Most naturally occurring fatty acids contain even numbers of carbons in their chains—up to 24 carbons in length. This discussion begins with the 18-carbon fatty acids, which are abundant in our food supply. Stearic acid is the simplest of the 18-carbon fatty acids; the bonds between its carbons are all alike:

Stearic acid, an 18-carbon saturated fatty acid.

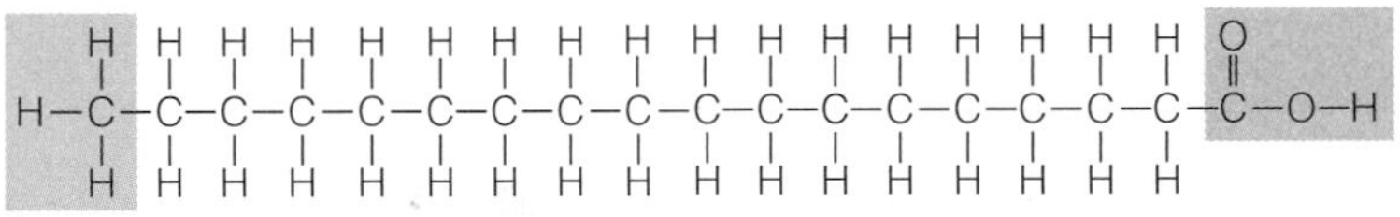

As you can see, stearic acid is 18 carbons long, and each atom meets the rules of chemical bonding described in Figure 4-1 on p. 104. The following structure also depicts stearic acid, but in a simpler way, with each "corner" on the zigzag line representing a carbon atom with two attached hydrogens:

Stearic acid (simplified structure).

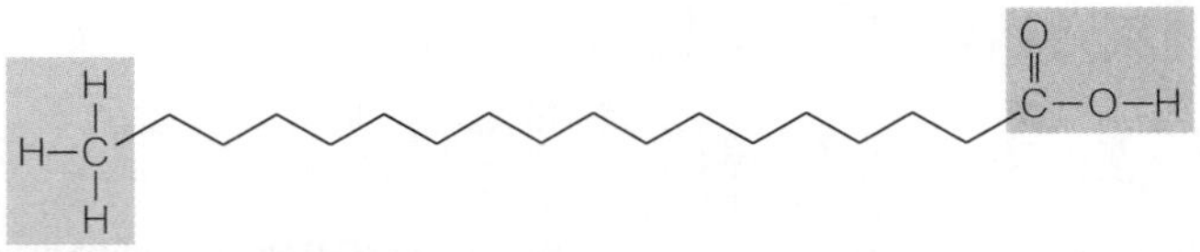

As mentioned, the carbon chains of fatty acids vary in length. The long-chain (12 to 24 carbons) fatty acids of meats, fish, and vegetable oils are most common in the diet. Smaller amounts of medium-chain (6 to 10 carbons) and short-chain (fewer than 6 carbons) fatty acids also occur, primarily in dairy products. (Tables C-1 and C-2 in Appendix C provide the names, chain lengths, and sources of fatty acids commonly found in foods.)

fatty acid: an organic compound composed of a carbon chain with hydrogens attached and an acid group (COOH) at one end and a methyl group (CH_3) at the other end.

GLOSSARY OF SATURATION TERMS

These terms are listed in order from the most saturated to the most unsaturated.

saturated fatty acid: a fatty acid carrying the maximum possible number of hydrogen atoms—for example, stearic acid. A **saturated fat** is composed of triglycerides in which most of the fatty acids are saturated.

point of unsaturation: the double bond of a fatty acid, where hydrogen atoms can easily be added to the structure.

unsaturated fatty acid: a fatty acid that lacks hydrogen atoms and has at least one double bond between carbons (includes monounsaturated and polyunsaturated fatty acids). An **unsaturated fat** is composed of triglycerides in which most of the fatty acids are unsaturated.

monounsaturated fatty acid: a fatty acid that lacks two hydrogen atoms and has one double bond between carbons—for example, oleic acid. A **monounsaturated fat** is composed of triglycerides in which most of the fatty acids are monounsaturated.

- **mono** = one

polyunsaturated fatty acid (PUFA): a fatty acid that lacks four or more hydrogen atoms and has two or more double bonds between carbons—for example, linoleic acid (two double bonds) and linolenic acid (three double bonds). A **polyunsaturated fat** is composed of triglycerides in which most of the fatty acids are polyunsaturated.

- **poly** = many

The Degree of Unsaturation Stearic acid is a **saturated fatty acid**, (terms that describe the saturation of fatty acids are defined in the glossary above). A saturated fatty acid is fully loaded with hydrogen atoms and contains only single bonds between its carbon atoms. If two hydrogens were missing from the middle of the carbon chain, the remaining structure might be:

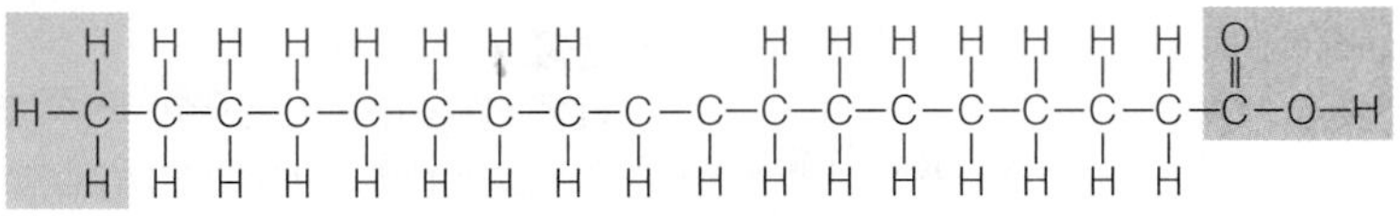

An impossible chemical structure.

Such a compound cannot exist, however, because two of the carbons have only three bonds each, and nature requires that every carbon have four bonds. The two carbons therefore form a double bond:

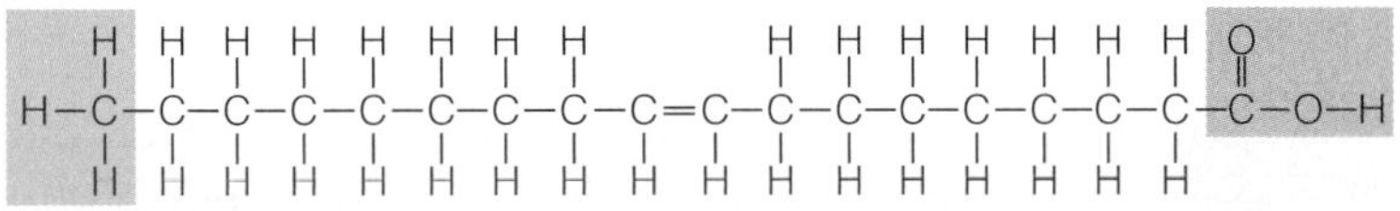

Oleic acid, an 18-carbon monounsaturated fatty acid.

The same structure drawn more simply looks like this:*

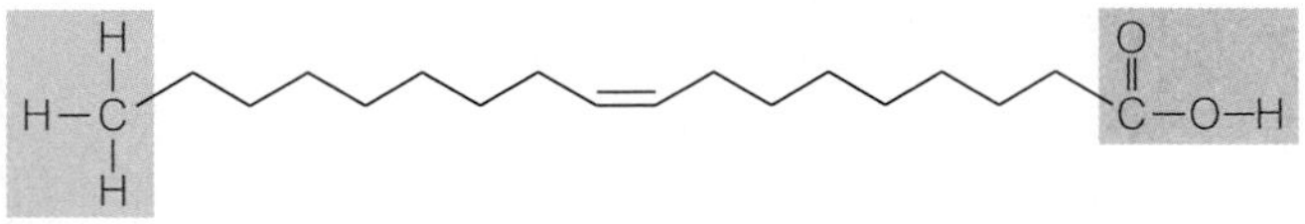

Oleic acid (simplified structure).

The double bond is a **point of unsaturation.** Hence, a fatty acid like this—with two hydrogens missing and a double bond—is an ***un*saturated fatty acid.** This one is the 18-carbon ***mono*unsaturated fatty acid** oleic acid, which is abundant in olive oil and canola oil.

A ***poly*unsaturated fatty acid** has two or more carbon-to-carbon double bonds. **Linoleic acid**, the 18-carbon fatty acid common in vegetable oils, lacks four hydrogens and has two double bonds:

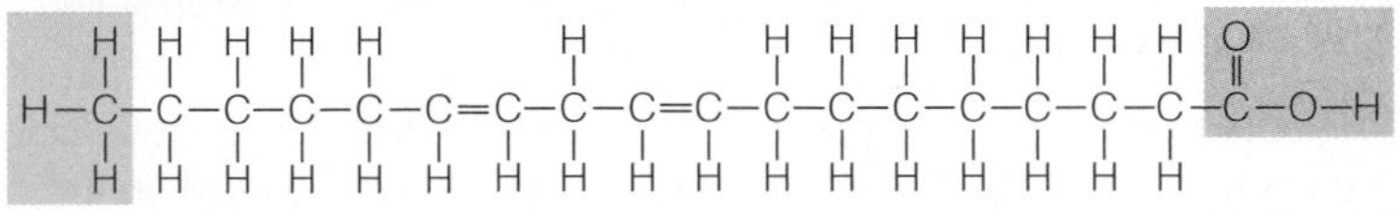

Linoleic acid, an 18-carbon polyunsaturated fatty acid.

*Remember that each "corner" on the zigzag line represents a carbon atom with two attached hydrogens. In addition, although drawn straight here, the actual shape kinks at the double bonds (as shown in the left side of Figure 5-8).

linoleic (lin-oh-LAY-ick) **acid:** an essential fatty acid with 18 carbons and two double bonds.

TABLE 5-1 18-Carbon Fatty Acids

Name	Number of Carbon Atoms	Number of Double Bonds	Saturation	Common Food Sources
Stearic acid	18	0	Saturated	Most animal fats
Oleic acid	18	1	Monounsaturated	Olive, canola oils
Linoleic acid	18	2	Polyunsaturated	Sunflower, safflower, corn, and soybean oils
Linolenic acid	18	3	Polyunsaturated	Soybean and canola oils, flaxseed, walnuts

Drawn more simply, linoleic acid looks like this (though the actual shape would kink at the double bonds):

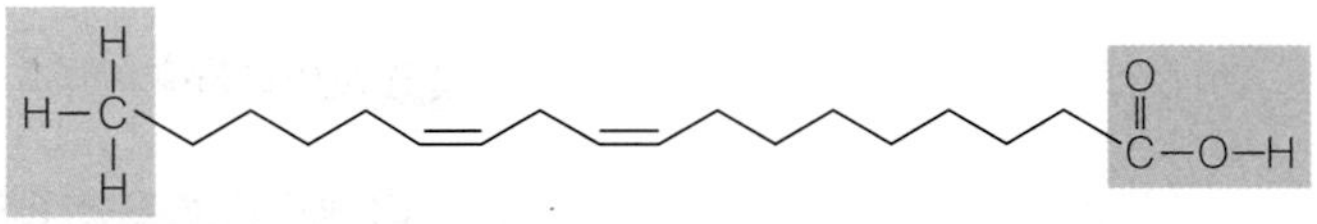

Linoleic acid (simplified structure).

A fourth 18-carbon fatty acid is **linolenic acid**, which has three double bonds. Table 5-1 presents the 18-carbon fatty acids.■

■ Chemists use a shorthand notation to describe fatty acids. The first number indicates the number of carbon atoms; the second, the number of double bonds. For example, the notation for stearic acid is 18:0.

The Location of Double Bonds Fatty acids differ not only in the length of their chains and their degree of saturation, but also in the locations of their double bonds (see Figure 5-2). Chemists identify polyunsaturated fatty acids by the position of the double bond nearest the methyl (CH_3) end of the carbon chain, which is described by an **omega** number. A polyunsaturated fatty acid with its first double bond three carbons away from the methyl end is an **omega-3 fatty acid**. Similarly, an **omega-6 fatty acid** is a polyunsaturated fatty acid with its first double bond six carbons away

FIGURE 5-2 Omega-3 and Omega-6 Fatty Acids Compared

Linolenic acid, an omega-3 fatty acid

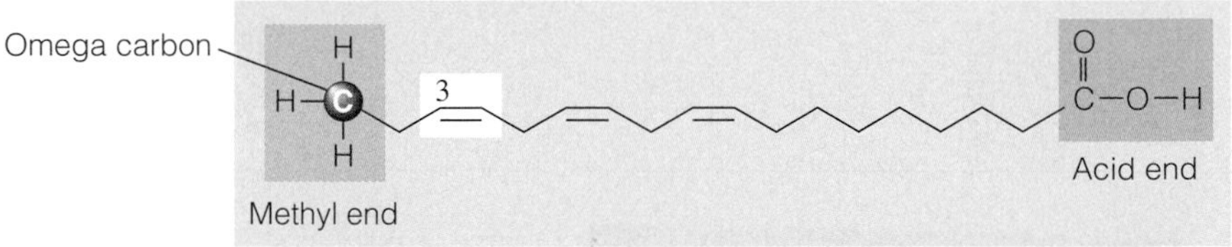
Omega carbon
3
Methyl end
Acid end

Linoleic acid, an omega-6 fatty acid

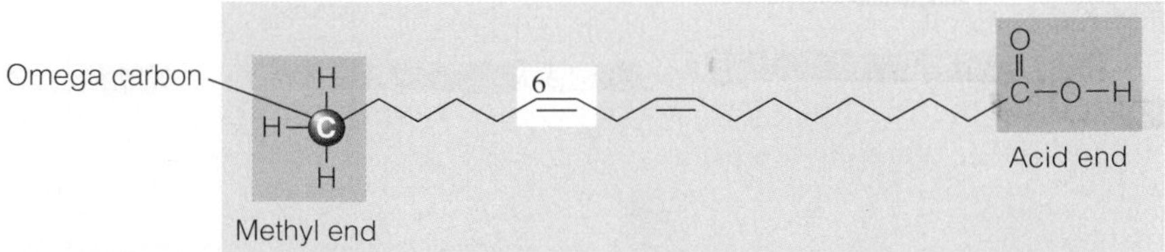
Omega carbon
6
Methyl end
Acid end

The omega number indicates the position of the first double bond in a fatty acid, counting from the methyl (CH_3) end. Thus an omega-3 fatty acid's first double bond occurs three carbons from the methyl end, and an omega-6 fatty acid's first double bond occurs six carbons from the methyl end. The members of an omega family may have different lengths and different numbers of double bonds, but the first double bond occurs at the same point in all of them. These structures are drawn linearly here to ease counting carbons and locating double bonds, but their shapes actually bend at the double bonds, as shown in Figure 5-8.

linolenic (lin-oh-LEN-ick) **acid:** an essential fatty acid with 18 carbons and three double bonds.

omega: the last letter of the Greek alphabet (ω), used by chemists to refer to the position of the first double bond from the methyl end of a fatty acid.

omega-3 fatty acid: a polyunsaturated fatty acid in which the first double bond is three carbons away from the methyl (CH_3) end of the carbon chain.

omega-6 fatty acid: a polyunsaturated fatty acid in which the first double bond is six carbons from the methyl (CH_3) end of the carbon chain.

from the methyl end. Figure 5-2 compares two 18-carbon fatty acids—linolenic acid (an omega-3 fatty acid) and linoleic acid (an omega-6 fatty acid).

Triglycerides

Few fatty acids occur free in foods or in the body. Most often, they are incorporated into **triglycerides**—lipids composed of three fatty acids attached to a **glycerol**. (Figure 5-3 presents a glycerol molecule.) To make a triglyceride, a series of condensation reactions combine a hydrogen atom (H) from the glycerol and a hydroxyl (OH) group from a fatty acid, forming a molecule of water (H_2O) and leaving a bond between the other two molecules (see Figure 5-4). Most triglycerides contain a mixture of more than one type of fatty acid (see Figure 5-5 on p. 146).

FIGURE 5-3 Glycerol

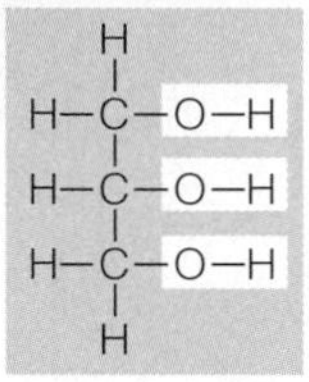

When glycerol is free, an OH group is attached to each carbon. When glycerol is part of a triglyceride, each carbon is attached to a fatty acid by a carbon-oxygen bond.

Degree of Unsaturation Revisited

The chemistry of a fatty acid—whether it is short or long, saturated or unsaturated, with its first double bond here or there—influences the characteristics of foods and the health of the body. A later section of this chapter explains how these features affect health; this section describes how the degree of unsaturation influences the fats and oils in foods.

Firmness The degree of unsaturation influences the firmness of fats at room temperature. Generally speaking, the polyunsaturated vegetable oils are liquid at room temperature, and the more saturated animal fats are solid. Not all vegetable oils are polyunsaturated, however. Cocoa butter, palm oil, palm kernel oil, and coconut oil■ are saturated even though they are of vegetable origin; they are firmer than most vegetable oils because of their saturation, but softer than most animal fats because of their short carbon chains (8 to 14 carbons long). Generally, the shorter the carbon chain, the softer the fat is at room temperature. Fatty acid compositions of selected fats and oils are shown in Figure 5-6 (on p. 146), and Appendix H provides the fat and fatty acid contents of many other foods.

Stability Saturation also influences stability. All fats can become rancid when exposed to oxygen. Polyunsaturated fats spoil most readily because their double bonds are unstable; monounsaturated fats are slightly less susceptible. Saturated

■ The food industry often refers to these saturated vegetable oils as the "tropical oils."

triglycerides (try-GLISS-er-rides): the chief form of fat in the diet and the major storage form of fat in the body; composed of a molecule of glycerol with three fatty acids attached; also called **triacylglycerols** (try-ay-seel-GLISS-er-ols).*
- **tri** = three
- **glyceride** = of glycerol
- **acyl** = a carbon chain

*Research scientists commonly use the term *triacylglycerols;* this book continues to use the more familiar term *triglycerides,* as do many other health and nutrition books and journals.

glycerol (GLISS-er-ol): an alcohol composed of a three-carbon chain, which can serve as the backbone for a triglyceride.
- **ol** = alcohol

FIGURE 5-4 Condensation of Glycerol and Fatty Acids to Form a Triglyceride

To make a triglyceride, three fatty acids attach to glycerol in condensation reactions:

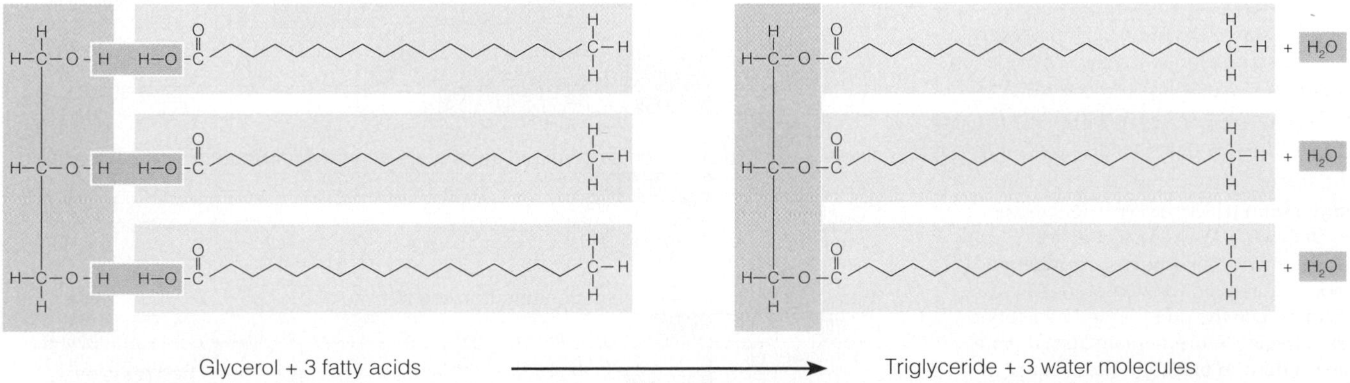
Glycerol + 3 fatty acids
Triglyceride + 3 water molecules

An H atom from glycerol and an OH group from a fatty acid combine to create water, leaving the O on the glycerol and the C at the acid end of each fatty acid to form a bond.

Three fatty acids attached to a glycerol form a triglyceride and yield water. In this example, all three fatty acids are stearic acid, but most often triglycerides contain mixtures of fatty acids (as shown in Figure 5-5).

FIGURE 5-5 A Mixed Triglyceride

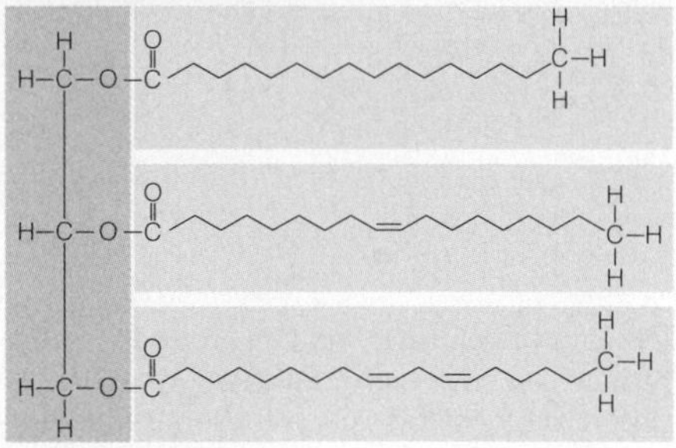

This mixed triglyceride includes a saturated fatty acid, a monounsaturated fatty acid, and a polyunsaturated fatty acid.

fats are most resistant to **oxidation** and thus least likely to become rancid. The oxidation of fats produces a variety of compounds that smell and taste rancid; other types of spoilage can occur due to microbial growth.

Manufacturers can protect fat-containing products against rancidity in three ways—none of them perfect. First, products may be sealed air-tight in nonmetallic containers, protected from light, and refrigerated—an expensive and inconvenient storage system. Second, manufacturers may add **antioxidants** to compete for the oxygen and thus protect the oil (examples are the additives BHA and BHT and vitamin E). Third, manufacturers may saturate some or all of the points of unsaturation by adding hydrogen molecules—a process known as hydrogenation.

Hydrogenation **Hydrogenation** offers two advantages. First, it protects against oxidation (thereby prolonging shelf life) by making polyunsaturated fats more saturated (see Figure 5-7). Second, it alters the texture of foods by making liquid vegetable oils more solid (as in margarine and shortening). Hydrogenated fats make margarine spreadable, pie crusts flaky, and puddings creamy.

***Trans*-Fatty Acids** Figure 5-7 illustrates the total hydrogenation of a polyunsaturated fatty acid to a saturated fatty acid, which rarely occurs during food processing. Most often, a fat is partially hydrogenated, and some of the double bonds that remain after processing change from *cis* to *trans*. In nature, most double bonds are *cis*—meaning that the hydrogens next to the double bonds are on the same side of the carbon chain. Only a few fatty acids (notably those found in milk and meat products) are ***trans*-fatty acids**—meaning that the hydrogens next to the double bonds are on opposite sides of the carbon chain (see Figure 5-8). These arrangements result in different configurations for the fatty acids, and this difference affects function: in the body, *trans*-fatty acids behave more like saturated fats than like unsaturated fats. The relationship between *trans*-fatty acids and heart disease has been the subject of much recent research, as a later section describes.

FIGURE 5-6 Comparison of Dietary Fats

Most fats are a mixture of saturated, monounsaturated, and polyunsaturated fatty acids.

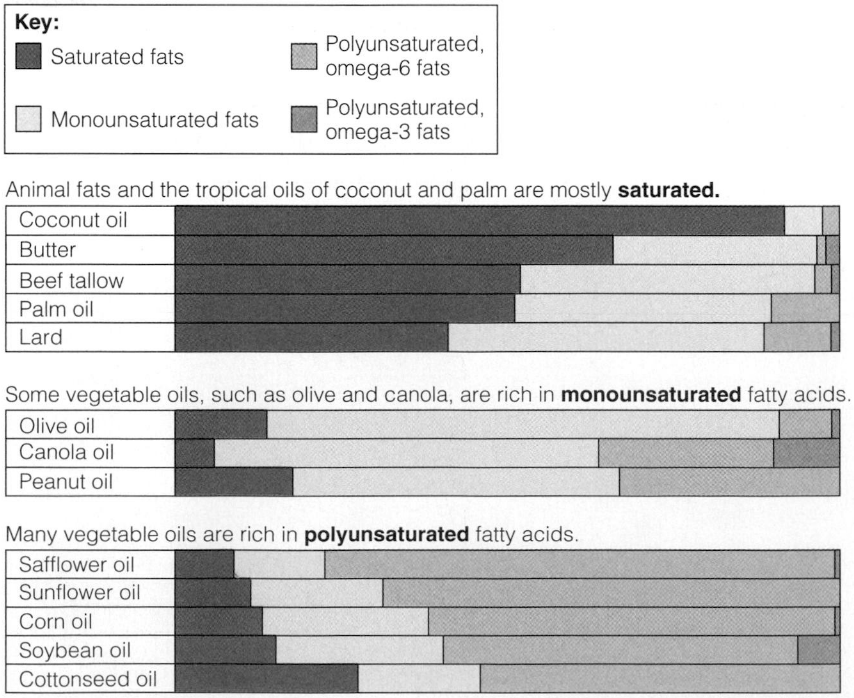
Key:
Saturated fats
Polyunsaturated, omega-6 fats
Monounsaturated fats
Polyunsaturated, omega-3 fats
Animal fats and the tropical oils of coconut and palm are mostly **saturated.**
Coconut oil
Butter
Beef tallow
Palm oil
Lard
Some vegetable oils, such as olive and canola, are rich in **monounsaturated** fatty acids.
Olive oil
Canola oil
Peanut oil
Many vegetable oils are rich in **polyunsaturated** fatty acids.
Safflower oil
Sunflower oil
Corn oil
Soybean oil
Cottonseed oil

oxidation (OKS-ee-day-shun): the process of a substance combining with oxygen; oxidation reactions involve the loss of electrons.

antioxidants: compounds that protect others from oxidation by being oxidized themselves.

hydrogenation (HIGH-dro-gen-AY-shun or high-DROJ-eh-NAY-shun): a chemical process by which hydrogens are added to monounsaturated or polyunsaturated fatty acids to reduce the number of double bonds, making the fats more saturated (solid) and more resistant to oxidation (protecting against rancidity). Hydrogenation produces *trans*-fatty acids.

***trans*-fatty acids:** fatty acids with hydrogens on opposite sides of the double bond.

FIGURE 5-7 Hydrogenation

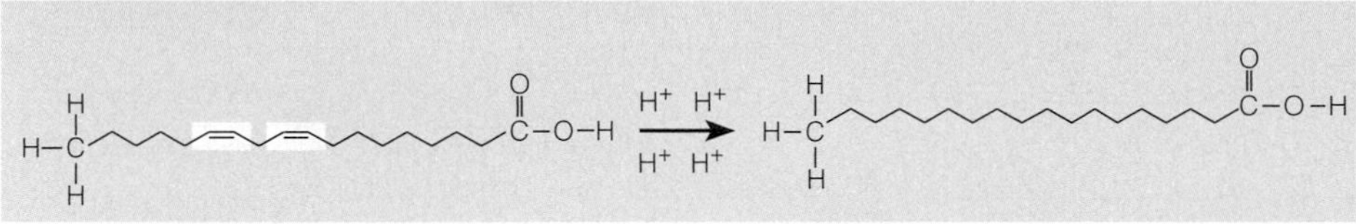

Polyunsaturated fatty acid — Hydrogenated (saturated) fatty acid

Double bonds carry a slightly negative charge and readily accept positively charged hydrogen atoms, creating a saturated fatty acid. Most often, fat is partially hydrogenated, creating a *trans*-fatty acid (shown in Figure 5-8).

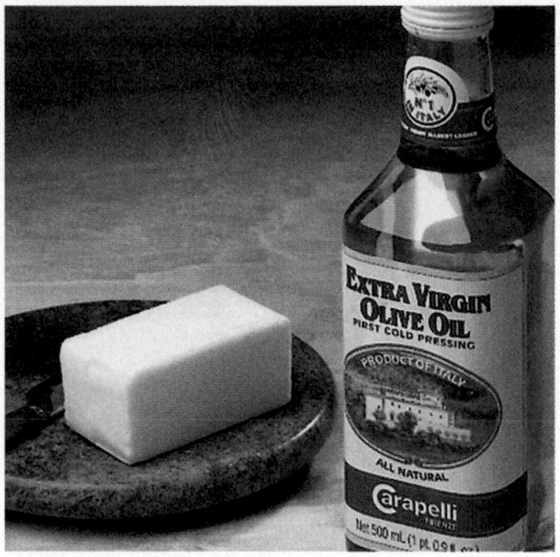

Extra Virgin Olive Oil
First Cold Pressing
All Natural
Carapelli

© Polara Studios Inc.

At room temperature, saturated fats (such as those found in butter and other animal fats) are solid, whereas unsaturated fats (such as those found in oil) are usually liquid.

IN SUMMARY The predominant lipids both in foods and in the body are triglycerides: glycerol backbones with three fatty acids attached. Fatty acids vary in the length of their carbon chains, their degrees of unsaturation, and the location of their double bond(s). Those that are fully loaded with hydrogens are saturated; those that are missing hydrogens and therefore have double bonds are unsaturated (monounsaturated or polyunsaturated). The vast majority of triglycerides contain more than one type of fatty acid. Fatty acid saturation affects fats' physical characteristics and storage properties. Hydrogenation, which makes polyunsaturated fats more saturated, gives rise to *trans*-fatty acids, altered fatty acids that may have health effects similar to those of saturated fatty acids.

The Chemist's View of Phospholipids and Sterols

The preceding pages have been devoted to one of the three classes of lipids, the triglycerides, and their component parts, the fatty acids. The other two classes of lipids, the phospholipids and sterols, make up only 5 percent of the lipids in the diet.

FIGURE 5-8 *Cis*- and *Trans*-Fatty Acids Compared

This example shows the *cis* configuration for an 18-carbon monounsaturated fatty acid (oleic acid) and its corresponding *trans* configuration (elaidic acid).

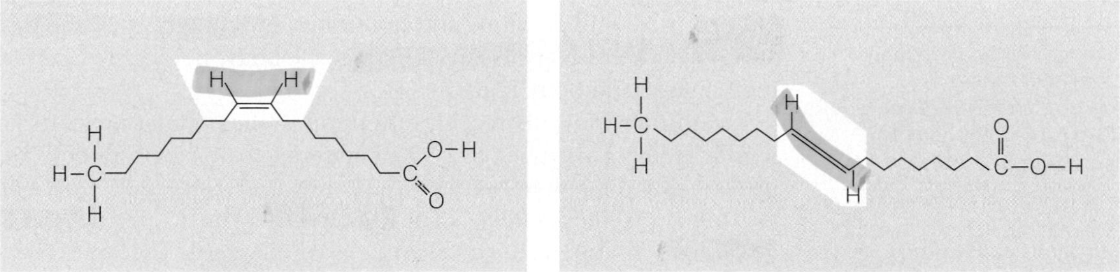

cis-fatty acid

A *cis*-fatty acid has its hydrogens on the same side of the double bond; *cis* molecules fold back into a U-like formation. Most naturally occuring unsaturated fatty acids in foods are *cis*.

trans-fatty acid

A *trans*-fatty acid has its hydrogens on the opposite sides of the double bond; *trans* molecules are more linear. The *trans* form typically occurs in partially hydrogenated foods when hydrogen atoms shift around some double bonds and change the configuration from *cis* to *trans*.

FIGURE 5-9 Lecithin

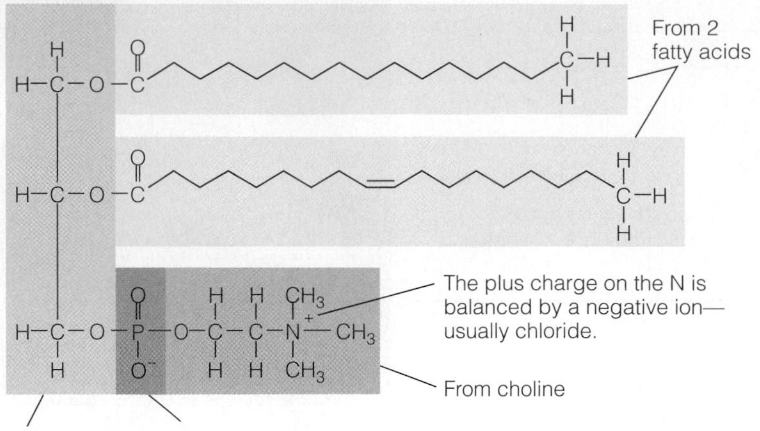
From 2 fatty acids
The plus charge on the N is balanced by a negative ion—usually chloride.
From choline
From glycerol
From phosphate

Lecithin is one of the phospholipids. Other phospholipids have different fatty acids at the upper two positions and different groups attached to phosphate. Notice that a molecule of lecithin is similar to a triglyceride but contains only two fatty acids. The third position is occupied by a phosphate group and a molecule of choline.

FIGURE 5-10 Phospholipids of a Cell Membrane

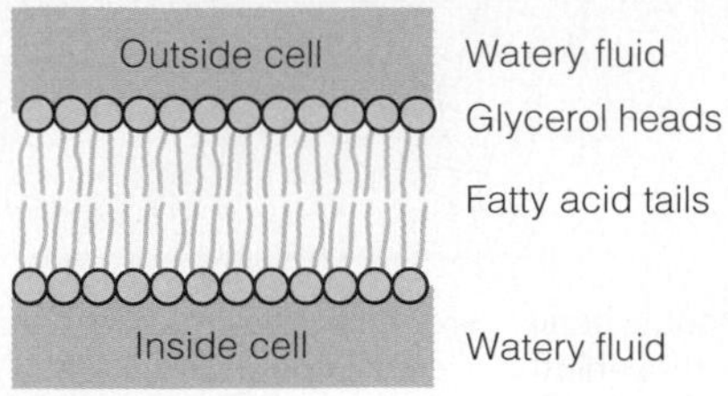
Outside cell
Inside cell
Watery fluid
Glycerol heads
Fatty acid tails
Watery fluid

A cell membrane is made of phospholipids assembled into an orderly formation called a bilayer. The fatty acid "tails" orient themselves away from the watery fluid inside and outside of the cell. The glycerol and phosphate "heads" are attracted to the watery fluid.

Phospholipids

The best-known **phospholipid** is **lecithin.** A diagram of a lecithin molecule is shown in Figure 5-9. Notice that lecithin has a backbone of glycerol with two of its three attachment sites occupied by fatty acids like those in triglycerides. The third site is occupied by a phosphate group and a molecule of **choline.** The fatty acids make phospholipids soluble in fat; the phosphate group allows them to dissolve in water. Such versatility enables the food industry to use phospholipids as emulsifiers■ to mix fats with water in such products as mayonnaise and candy bars.

■ Reminder: *Emulsifiers* are substances with both water-soluble and fat-soluble portions that promote the mixing of oils and fats in watery solutions.

Phospholipids in Foods In addition to the phospholipids used by the food industry as emulsifiers, phospholipids are also found naturally in foods. The richest food sources of lecithin are eggs, liver, soybeans, wheat germ, and peanuts.

Roles of Phospholipids The lecithins and other phospholipids are important constituents of cell membranes (see Figure 5-10). Because phospholipids are soluble in both water and fat, they can help lipids move back and forth across the cell membranes into the watery fluids on both sides. Thus they enable fat-soluble substances, including vitamins and hormones, to pass easily in and out of cells. The phospholipids also act as emulsifiers in the body, helping to keep fats suspended in the blood and body fluids.

Lecithin periodically receives attention in the popular press. Its fans claim that it is a major constituent of cell membranes (true), that all cells depend on the integrity of their membranes (true), and that consumers must therefore take lecithin supplements (false). The liver makes from scratch all the lecithin a person needs. As for lecithin taken as a supplement, the digestive enzyme lecithinase■ in the intestine hydrolyzes most of it before it passes into the body, so little lecithin reaches the tissues intact. In other words, the lecithins are *not essential nutrients;* they are just another lipid. Like other lipids, they contribute 9 kcalories per gram to the body's energy economy—an unexpected "bonus" many people taking lecithin supplements fail to realize. Furthermore, large doses of lecithin may cause GI distress, sweating, and loss of appetite. Perhaps these symp-

■ Reminder: The word ending *-ase* denotes an enzyme. Hence, lecithinase is an enzyme that works on lecithin.

phospholipid (FOS-foe-LIP-id): a compound similar to a triglyceride but having a phosphate group (a phosphorus-containing salt) and choline (or another nitrogen-containing compound) in place of one of the fatty acids.

lecithin (LESS-uh-thin): one of the phospholipids. Both nature and the food industry use lecithin as an emulsifier to combine water-soluble and fat-soluble ingredients that do not ordinarily mix, such as water and oil.

choline (KOH-leen): a nitrogen-containing compound found in foods as part of lecithin and other phospholipids.

toms are beneficial because they may warn people to stop self-dosing with lecithin.

IN SUMMARY Phospholipids, including lecithin, have a unique chemical structure that allows them to be soluble in both water and fat. In the body, phospholipids are part of cell membranes; the food industry uses phospholipids as emulsifiers to mix fats with water.

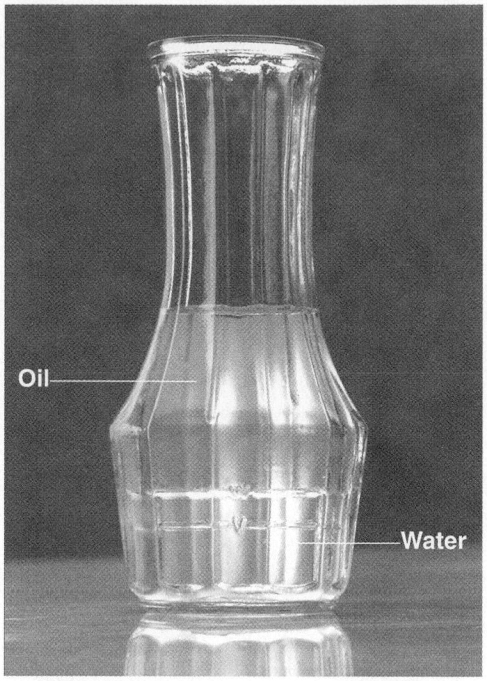
Oil
Water

Matthew Farruggio

Without help from emulsifiers, fats and water don't mix.

Sterols

In addition to triglycerides and phospholipids, the lipids include the **sterols,** compounds with a multiple-ring structure.[*] The most famous sterol is **cholesterol;** Figure 5-11 (on p. 150) shows its chemical structure.

Sterols in Foods Foods derived from both plants and animals contain sterols, but only those from animals contain cholesterol: meats, eggs, fish, poultry, and dairy products. Some people, confused about the distinction between dietary and blood cholesterol, have asked which foods contain the "good" cholesterol. "Good" cholesterol is not a type of cholesterol found in foods, but refers to the way the body transports cholesterol in the blood, as explained later (p. 154).

Roles of Sterols Many vitally important body compounds are sterols. Among them are bile acids, the sex hormones (such as testosterone), the adrenal hormones (such as cortisol), and vitamin D, as well as cholesterol itself. Cholesterol in the body can serve as the starting material for the synthesis of these compounds or as a structural component of cell membranes; more than 90 percent of all the body's cholesterol resides in the cells. Despite popular impressions to the contrary, cholesterol is not a villain lurking in some evil foods—it is a compound the body makes and uses.■ Right now, as you read, your liver is manufacturing cholesterol from fragments of carbohydrate, protein, and fat. In fact, the liver makes about 800 to 1500 milligrams of cholesterol per day,■ thus contributing much more to the body's total than does the diet.

Cholesterol's harmful effects in the body occur when it forms deposits in the artery walls. These deposits lead to **atherosclerosis,** a disease that causes heart attacks and strokes (Chapter 27 provides many more details).

■ The chemical structure is the same, but cholesterol that is made in the body is called **endogenous** (en-DOGDE-eh-nus), whereas cholesterol from outside the body (from foods) is called **exogenous** (eks-ODGE-eh-nus).
- **endo** = within
- **gen** = arising
- **exo** = outside (the body)

■ For perspective, the Daily Value for cholesterol is 300 mg/day.

IN SUMMARY Sterols have a multiple-ring structure that differs from the structure of other lipids. In the body, sterols include cholesterol, bile, vitamin D, and some hormones. Only animal-derived foods contain cholesterol. To summarize, the members of the lipid family include:

- **Triglycerides** (fats and oils), which are made of:
  - Glycerol (1 per triglyceride) and
  - Fatty acids (3 per triglyceride). Depending on the number of double bonds, fatty acids may be:
    - *Saturated* (no double bonds).
    - *Monounsaturated* (one double bond).
    - *Polyunsaturated* (more than one double bond). Depending on the location of the double bonds, polyunsaturated fatty acids may be:
      - *Omega-3* (first double bond 3 carbons away from methyl end).
      - *Omega-6* (first double bond 6 carbons away from methyl end).
- **Phospholipids** (such as lecithin).
- **Sterols** (such as cholesterol).

sterols (STARE-ols or STEER-ols): compounds containing a four-carbon ring structure with any of a variety of side chains attached.

cholesterol (koh-LESS-ter-ol): one of the sterols containing a four-carbon ring structure with a carbon side chain.

atherosclerosis (ath-er-oh-scler-OH-sis): a type of artery disease characterized by accumulations of cholesterol-containing material on the inner walls of the arteries (see Chapter 27).
- **athero** = porridge or soft
- **scleros** = hard
- **osis** = condition

[*]The four-ring core structure identifies a steroid; sterols are alcohol derivatives with a steroid ring structure.

FIGURE 5-11 Cholesterol

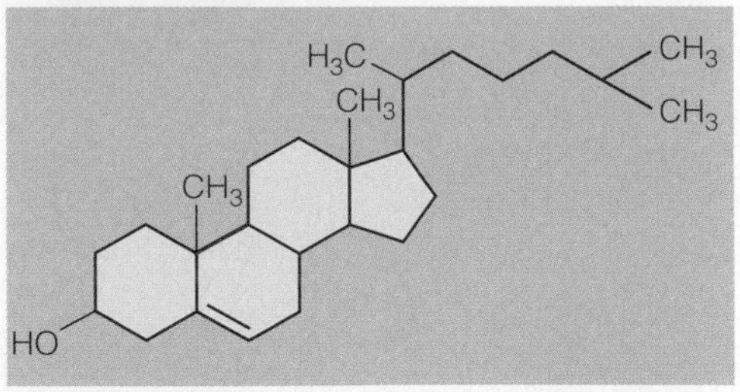
H3C
CH3
CH3
CH3
CH3
HO

Cholesterol

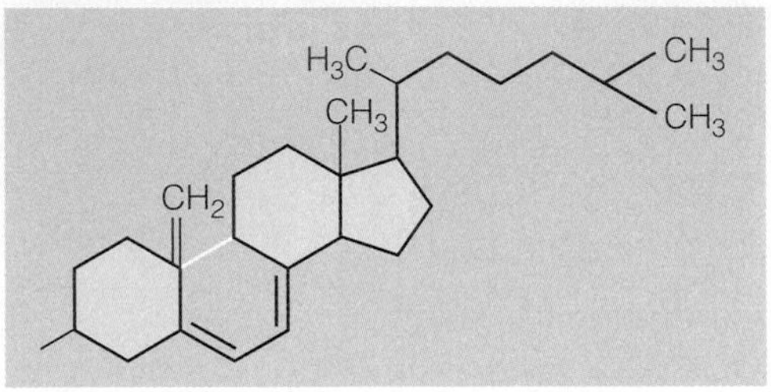
H3C
CH3
CH3
CH3
CH2

Vitamin D_3

The fat-soluble vitamin D is synthesized from cholesterol; notice the many similarities. The only difference is that cholesterol has a closed ring (highlighted in color), whereas vitamin D's is open, accounting for its vitamin activity. Notice, too, how different cholesterol is from the triglycerides and phospholipids.

Digestion, Absorption, and Transport of Lipids

Each day, the GI tract receives, on average, 50 to 100 grams of triglycerides, 4 to 8 grams of phospholipids, and 200 to 350 milligrams of cholesterol. The body faces a challenge in digesting and absorbing these lipids: getting at them. Fats are **hydrophobic**—that is, they tend to separate from the watery fluids of the GI tract—whereas the enzymes for digesting fats are **hydrophilic.** The challenge is keeping the fats mixed in the watery fluids of the GI tract.

Lipid Digestion

The goal of fat digestion is to dismantle triglycerides into small molecules that the body can absorb and use—namely, **monoglycerides,** fatty acids, and glycerol. Figure 5-12 traces the digestion of triglycerides through the GI tract, and the following paragraphs provide the details.

In the Mouth Fat digestion starts off slowly in the mouth, with some hard fats beginning to melt when they reach body temperature. A salivary gland at the base of the tongue releases an enzyme (lingual lipase)■ that plays a minor role in fat digestion in adults and an active role in infants. In infants, this enzyme efficiently digests the short- and medium-chain fatty acids found in milk.

In the Stomach In a quiet stomach, fat would float as a layer above the other components of swallowed food. But the strong muscle contractions of the stomach propel the stomach contents toward the pyloric sphincter. Some chyme passes through the pyloric sphincter periodically, but the remaining partially digested food is propelled back into the body of the stomach. This churning grinds the solid pieces to finer particles, mixes the chyme, and disperses the fat into smaller droplets. These actions help to expose the fat for attack by the gastric lipase enzyme—an enzyme that performs best in the acidic environment of the stomach.[1] Still, little fat digestion takes place in the stomach; most of the action occurs in the small intestine.

In the Small Intestine Fat in the small intestine triggers the release of the hormone cholecystokinin (CCK), which signals the gallbladder to release its stores of bile. (Remember that the liver makes bile, and the gallbladder stores it until it is needed.) Among bile's many ingredients■ are bile acids, which are made in the liver from cholesterol and have a similar structure. In addition, they often pair up with an amino acid (a building block of protein). The amino acid end is attracted to water, and the sterol end is attracted to fat (see Figure 5-13 on p. 152). This structure improves bile's ability to act as an emulsifier, drawing fat molecules into the surrounding watery fluids. There the fats are fully digested as they encounter lipase enzymes from the pancreas and small intestine. The process of emulsification is diagrammed in Figure 5-14 (on p. 152).

Most of the hydrolysis of triglycerides occurs in the small intestine. The major fat-digesting enzymes are pancreatic lipases; some intestinal lipases are also active. These enzymes remove one, then the other, of each triglyceride's outer fatty acids, leaving a monoglyceride. Occasionally, enzymes remove all three fatty acids, leaving a free molecule of glycerol. Hydrolysis of a triglyceride is shown in Figure 5-15 (on p. 153).

Phospholipids are digested similarly—that is, their fatty acids are removed by hydrolysis. The two fatty acids and the remaining phospholipid fragment are then absorbed. Most sterols can be absorbed as is; if any fatty acids are attached, they are first hydrolyzed off.

Bile's Routes After bile has entered the small intestine and emulsified fat, it has two possible destinations, illustrated in Figure 5-16 (on p. 153). Most of the bile is reabsorbed from the intestine and recycled. The other possibility is that some of the bile can be trapped by fibers in the large intestine and carried out of the body

■ Reminder: An enzyme that hydrolyzes lipids is called a *lipase; lingual* refers to the tongue.

■ In addition to bile acids and bile salts, bile contains cholesterol, phospholipids (especially lecithin), antibodies, water, electrolytes, and bilirubin and biliverdin (pigments resulting from the breakdown of heme).

hydrophobic (high-dro-FOE-bick): a term referring to water-fearing, or non-water-soluble, substances; also known as **lipophilic** (fat loving).
- **hydro** = water
- **phobia** = fear
- **lipo** = lipid
- **phile** = love

hydrophilic (high-dro-FIL-ick): a term referring to water-loving, or water-soluble, substances.

monoglycerides: molecules of glycerol with one fatty acid attached. A molecule of glycerol with two fatty acids attached is a **diglyceride.**
- **mono** = one
- **di** = two

FIGURE 5-12 Fat Digestion in the GI Tract

FAT

Mouth and salivary glands
Some hard fats begin to melt as they reach body temperature. Sublingual salivary gland in the base of the tongue secretes lingual lipase.

Stomach
The acid-stable lingual lipase initiates lipid digestion by hydrolyzing one bond of triglycerides to produce diglycerides and fatty acids. The degree of hydrolysis by lingual lipase is slight for most fats but may be appreciable for milk fats. The stomach's churning action mixes fat with water and acid. A gastric lipase accesses and hydrolyzes (only a very small amount of) fat.

Small intestine
Bile flows in from the gallbladder (via the common bile duct):

Fat —(bile)→ emulsified fat

Pancreatic lipase flows in from the pancreas (via the pancreatic duct):

Emulsified fat (triglycerides) —(Pancreatic (and intestinal) lipase)→ monoglycerides, glycerol, fatty acids (absorbed)

Large intestine
Some fat and cholesterol trapped in fiber, exit in feces.

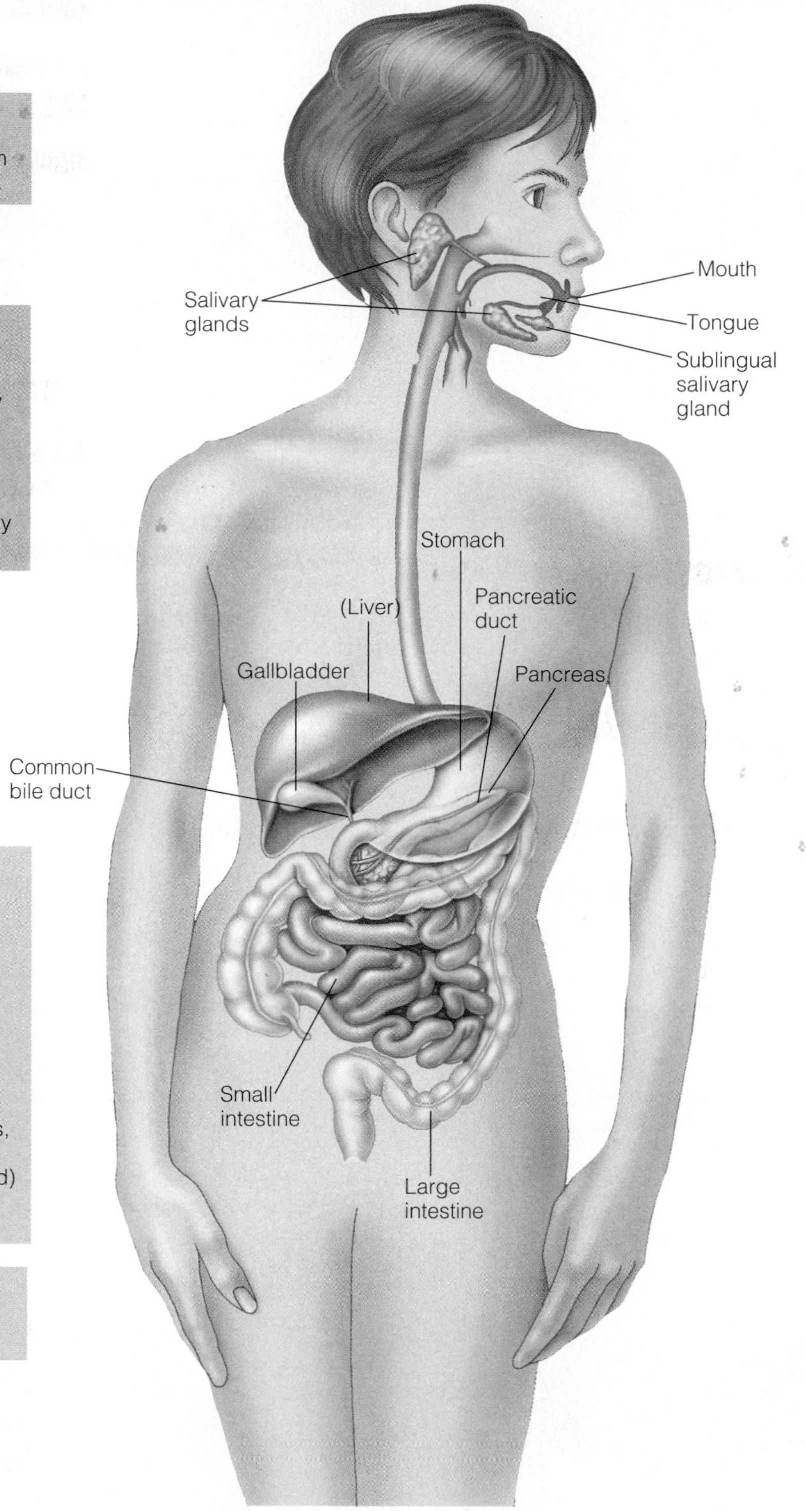
Salivary glands
Mouth
Tongue
Sublingual salivary gland
Stomach
(Liver)
Pancreatic duct
Gallbladder
Pancreas
Common bile duct
Small intestine
Large intestine

with the feces. Because cholesterol is needed to make bile, the excretion of bile effectively reduces blood cholesterol. As Chapter 4 explains, the fibers most effective at lowering blood cholesterol this way are the pectins and gums commonly found in fruits, oats, and legumes.[2]

FIGURE 5-13 A Bile Acid

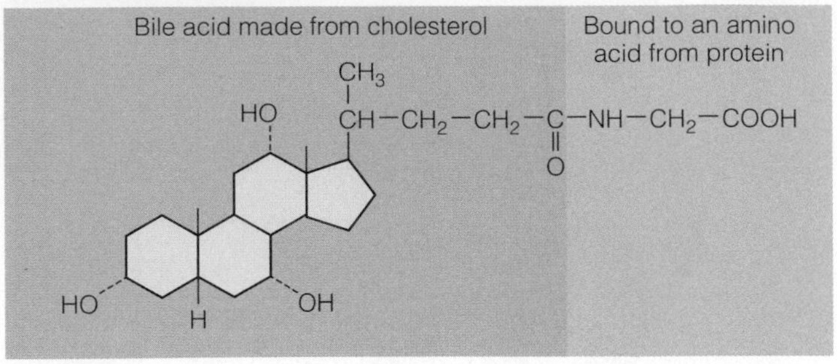
Bile acid made from cholesterol
Bound to an amino acid from protein
CH3
HO
CH—CH2—CH2—C—NH—CH2—COOH
O
HO
H
OH

This is one of several bile acids the liver makes from cholesterol. It is then bound to an amino acid to improve its ability to form micelles, spherical complexes of emulsified fat. Most bile acids occur as bile salts, usually in association with sodium, but sometimes with potassium or calcium.

Lipid Absorption

Figure 5-17 (on p. 154) illustrates the absorption of lipids. Small molecules of digested triglycerides (glycerol and short- and medium-chain fatty acids) can diffuse easily into the intestinal cells; they are absorbed directly into the bloodstream. Larger molecules (the monoglycerides and long-chain fatty acids) merge into spherical complexes, known as **micelles.** Micelles are emulsified fat droplets formed by molecules of bile surrounding monoglycerides and fatty acids. This configuration permits solubility in the watery digestive fluids and transportation to the intestinal cells. Upon arrival, the lipid contents of the micelles diffuse into the intestinal cells. Once inside, the monoglycerides and long-chain fatty acids are reassembled into new triglycerides.

Within the intestinal cells, the newly made triglycerides and other lipids (cholesterol and phospholipids) are packed with protein into transport vehicles known as **chylomicrons.** The intestinal cells then release the chylomicrons into the lymphatic system. The chylomicrons glide through the lymph until they reach a point of entry into the bloodstream at the thoracic duct near the heart. (Recall from Chapter 3 that nutrients from the GI tract that enter the lymph system bypass the liver at first.) The blood carries these lipids to the rest of the body for immediate use or storage. A look at these lipids in the body reveals the kinds of fat the diet has been delivering.[3] The fat stores and muscle cells of people who eat a diet rich in unsaturated fats, for example, contain more unsaturated fats than those of people who select a diet high in saturated fats.

micelles (MY-cells): tiny spherical complexes of emulsified fat that arise during digestion; most contain bile salts and the products of lipid digestion, including fatty acids, monoglycerides, and cholesterol.

chylomicrons (kye-lo-MY-cronz): the class of lipoproteins that transport lipids from the intestinal cells to the rest of the body.

lipoproteins (LIP-oh-PRO-teenz): clusters of lipids associated with proteins that serve as transport vehicles for lipids in the lymph and blood.

VLDL (very-low-density lipoprotein): the type of lipoprotein made primarily by liver cells to transport lipids to various tissues in the body; composed primarily of triglycerides.

IN SUMMARY The body makes special arrangements to digest and absorb lipids. It provides the emulsifier bile to make them accessible to the fat-digesting lipases that dismantle triglycerides, mostly to monoglycerides and fatty acids, for absorption by the intestinal cells. The intestinal cells assemble freshly absorbed lipids into chylomicrons, lipid packages with protein escorts, for transport so that cells all over the body may select needed lipids from them.

FIGURE 5-14 Emulsification of Fat by Bile

Like bile, detergents are emulsifiers and work the same way, which is why they are effective in removing grease spots from clothes. Molecule by molecule, the grease is dissolved out of the spot and suspended in the water, where it can be rinsed away.

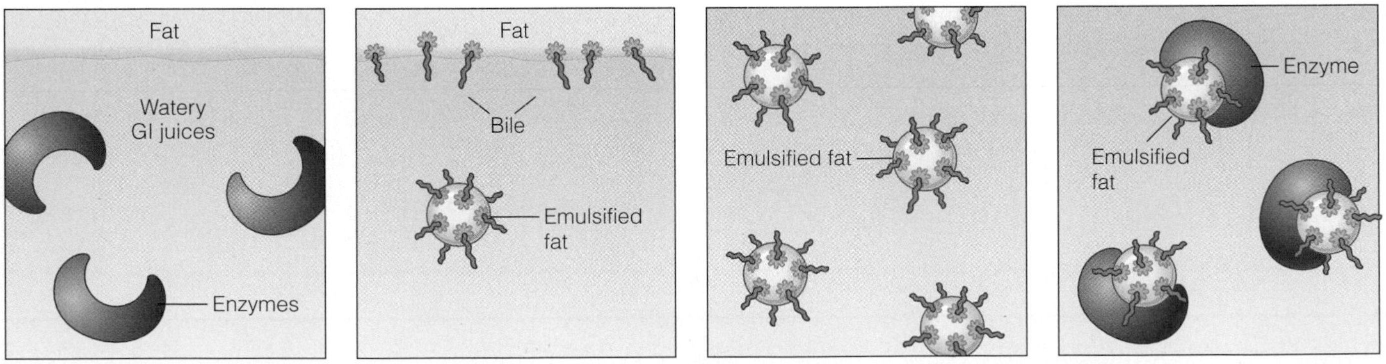
Fat
Watery GI juices
Enzymes
Fat
Bile
Emulsified fat
Emulsified fat
Enzyme
Emulsified fat

In the stomach, the fat and watery GI juices tend to separate. The enzymes in the GI juices can't get at the fat.

When fat enters the small intestine, the gallbladder secretes bile. Bile has an affinity for both fat and water, so it can bring the fat into the water.

Bile's emulsifying action converts large fat globules into small droplets that repel each other.

After emulsification, more fat is exposed to the enzymes, making fat digestion more efficient.

FIGURE 5-15 Digestion (Hydrolysis) of a Triglyceride

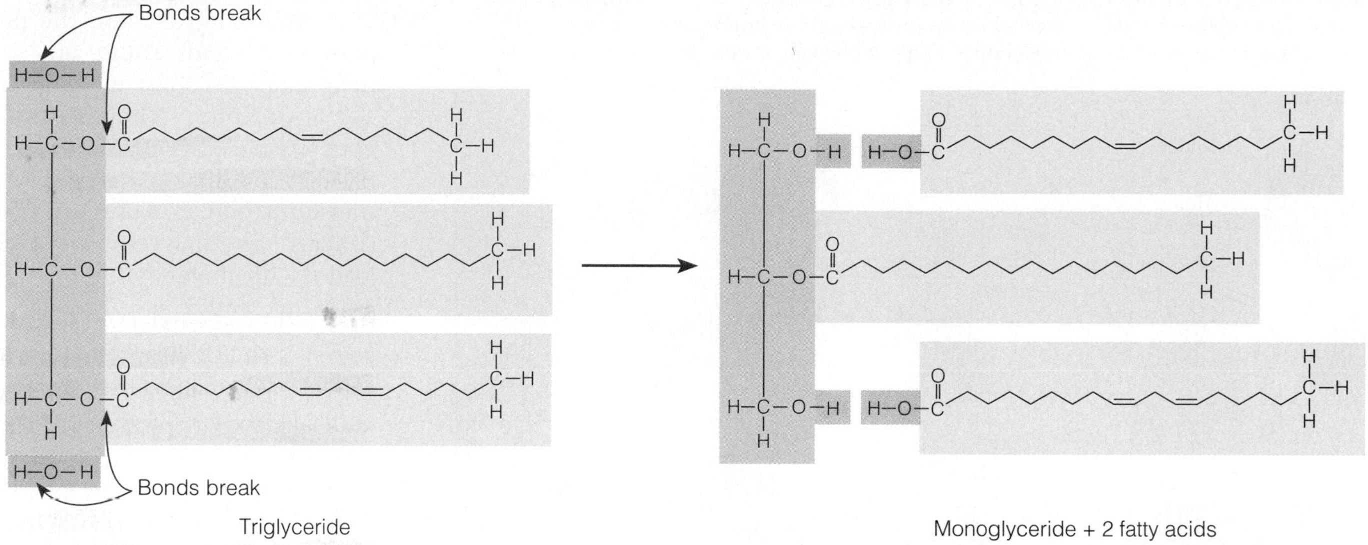
Bonds break
Bonds break
Triglyceride
Monoglyceride + 2 fatty acids

The triglyceride and two molecules of water are split. The H and OH from water complete the structures of two fatty acids and leave a monoglyceride.

These products may pass into the intestinal cells, but sometimes the monoglyceride is split with another molecule of water to give a third fatty acid and glycerol. Fatty acids, monoglycerides, and glycerol are absorbed into intestinal cells.

Lipid Transport

The chylomicrons are only one of several clusters of lipids and proteins that are used as transport vehicles for fats. As a group, these vehicles are known as **lipoproteins**, and they solve the body's problem of transporting fatty materials through the watery bloodstream. The body makes four main types of lipoproteins, distinguished by their size and density.* Each type contains different kinds and amounts of lipids and proteins.■ Figure 5-18 on p. 155 shows the relative compositions and sizes of the lipoproteins.

Chylomicrons The chylomicrons are the largest and least dense of the lipoproteins. They transport *diet*-derived lipids (mostly triglycerides) from the intestine (via the lymph system) to the rest of the body. Cells all over the body remove triglycerides from the chylomicrons as they pass by, so the chylomicrons get smaller and smaller. Within 14 hours after absorption, most of the triglycerides have been depleted, and only a few remnants of protein, cholesterol, and phospholipid remain. Special protein receptors on the membranes of the liver cells recognize and remove these chylomicron remnants from the blood. After collecting the remnants, the liver cells first dismantle them and then either use or recycle the pieces.

VLDL (Very-Low-Density Lipoproteins) Meanwhile, in the liver, the most active site of lipid synthesis, the cells are synthesizing other lipids. The liver cells use fatty acids arriving in the blood to make cholesterol, other fatty acids, and other compounds. At the same time, the liver cells may be making lipids from carbohydrates, proteins, or alcohol. Ultimately, the lipids made in the liver and those collected from chylomicron remnants are packaged with proteins as **VLDL (very-low-density lipoproteins)**■ and shipped to other parts of the body.

*Chemists can identify the various lipoproteins by their density by layering a blood sample below a thick fluid in a test tube and spinning the tube in a centrifuge. The most buoyant particles (highest in lipids) rise to the top and have the lowest density; the densest particles (highest in proteins) remain at the bottom and have the highest density. Others distribute themselves in between.

■ The more lipids, the lower the density; the more proteins, the higher the density.

■ Chylomicrons and VLDL transport triglycerides.

FIGURE 5-16 Enterohepatic Circulation

Most of the bile released into the small intestine is reabsorbed and sent back to the liver to be reused. This cycle is called the **enterohepatic circulation** of bile. Some bile is excreted.

- **enteron** = intestine
- **hepat** = liver

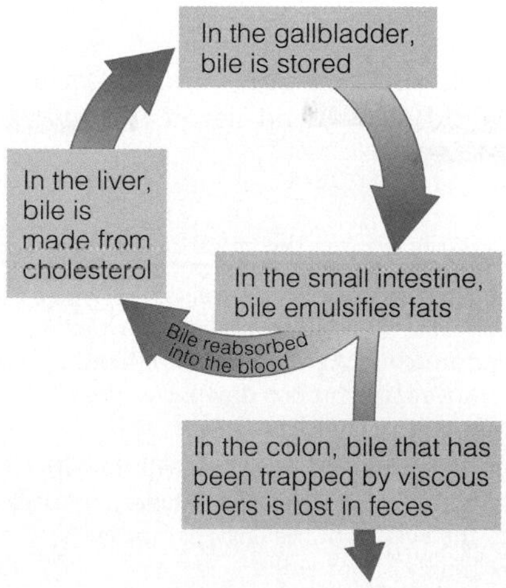
In the gallbladder, bile is stored
In the liver, bile is made from cholesterol
In the small intestine, bile emulsifies fats
Bile reabsorbed into the blood
In the colon, bile that has been trapped by viscous fibers is lost in feces

FIGURE 5-17 Absorption of Fat

The end products of fat digestion are mostly monoglycerides, some fatty acids, and very little glycerol. Their absorption differs depending on their size. (In reality, molecules of fatty acid are too small to see without a powerful microscope, while villi are visible to the naked eye.)

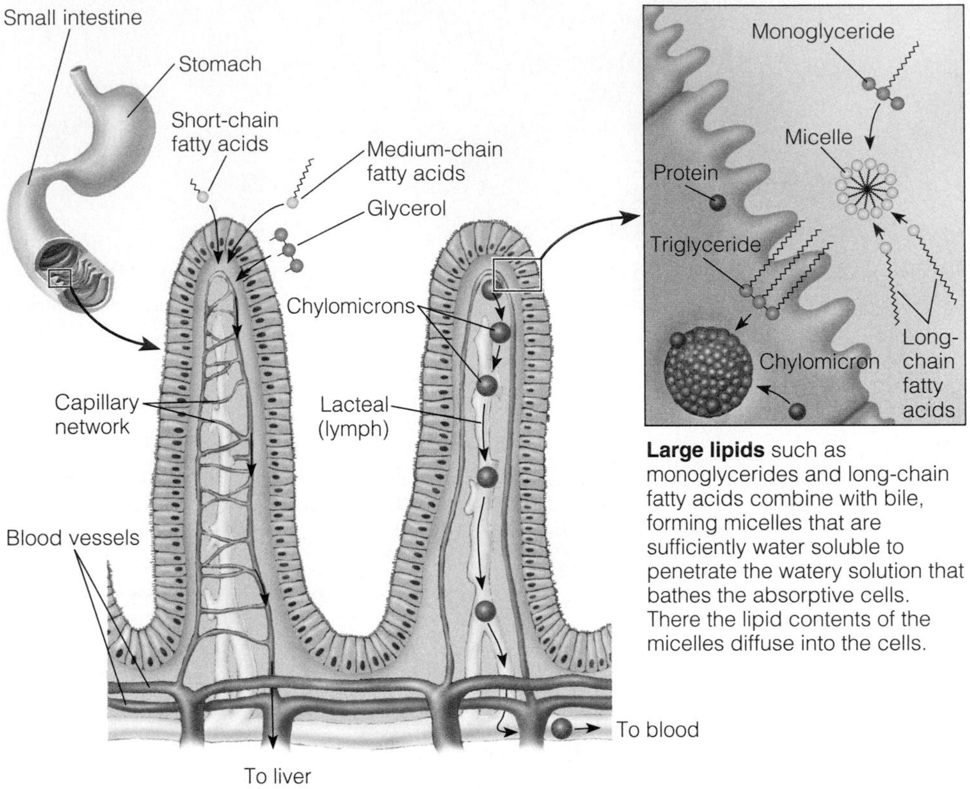

Small intestine
Stomach
Short-chain fatty acids
Medium-chain fatty acids
Glycerol
Chylomicrons
Capillary network
Lacteal (lymph)
Blood vessels
To liver
To blood
Monoglyceride
Micelle
Protein
Triglyceride
Chylomicron
Long-chain fatty acids

Large lipids such as monoglycerides and long-chain fatty acids combine with bile, forming micelles that are sufficiently water soluble to penetrate the watery solution that bathes the absorptive cells. There the lipid contents of the micelles diffuse into the cells.

Glycerol and small lipids such as short- and medium-chain fatty acids can move directly into the bloodstream.

As the VLDL travel through the body, cells remove triglycerides, causing the VLDL to shrink. As a VLDL loses triglycerides, the proportion of lipids shifts, and the lipoprotein becomes more dense. The remaining cholesterol-rich lipoprotein eventually becomes an **LDL (low-density lipoprotein).*** This transformation explains why LDL contain few triglycerides but are loaded with cholesterol.

LDL (Low-Density Lipoproteins) The LDL circulate throughout the body, making their contents available to the cells of all tissues—muscles, including the heart muscle; fat stores; the mammary glands; and others. The cells take triglycerides, cholesterol, and phospholipids to build new membranes, make hormones or other compounds, or store for later use. Special LDL receptors on the liver cells play a crucial role in the control of blood cholesterol concentrations by removing LDL from circulation.

HDL (High-Density Lipoproteins) Fat cells may release glycerol, fatty acids, cholesterol, and phospholipids to the blood. The liver makes **HDL (high-density lipoprotein)** to carry cholesterol■ from the cells back to the liver for recycling or disposal.

■ LDL and HDL transport cholesterol.

■ The transport of cholesterol from the tissues to the liver is sometimes called the *scavenger pathway.*

■ To help you remember, think of elevated HDL as Healthy and elevated LDL as Less healthy.

LDL (low-density lipoprotein): the type of lipoprotein derived from very-low-density lipoproteins (VLDL) as VLDL triglycerides are removed and broken down; composed primarily of cholesterol.

HDL (high-density lipoprotein): the type of lipoprotein that transports cholesterol back to the liver from the cells; composed primarily of protein.

Health Implications The distinction between LDL and HDL has implications for the health of the heart and blood vessels. The blood cholesterol linked to heart disease is LDL cholesterol. HDL also carry cholesterol, but elevated HDL represent cholesterol returning■ from the rest of the body to the liver for breakdown and excretion.[4] High LDL cholesterol is associated with a high risk of heart attack, whereas high HDL cholesterol seems to have a protective effect. This is why some people refer to LDL as "bad," and HDL as "good," cholesterol.■ Keep in mind that the cholesterol itself is the same, and that the differences between LDL and HDL reflect the *proportions* and *types* of lipids and proteins within them—not the type of cholesterol. The margin on p. 155■ lists factors that influence LDL and HDL, and Chapter 27 provides many more details.

Not too surprisingly, numerous genes influence how the body handles the uptake, synthesis, transport, and degradation of the lipoproteins.[5] Much research is currently focusing on how nutrient-gene interactions may direct the progression of heart disease.

*Before becoming LDL, the VLDL are first transformed into intermediate-density lipoproteins (IDL), sometimes called VLDL remnants. Some IDL may be picked up by the liver and rapidly broken down; those IDL that remain in circulation continue to deliver triglycerides to the cells and eventually become LDL. Researchers debate whether IDL are simply transitional particles or a separate class of lipoproteins; normally, IDL do not accumulate in the blood. Measures of blood lipids include IDL and LDL.

FIGURE 5-18 Size and Compositions of the Lipoproteins

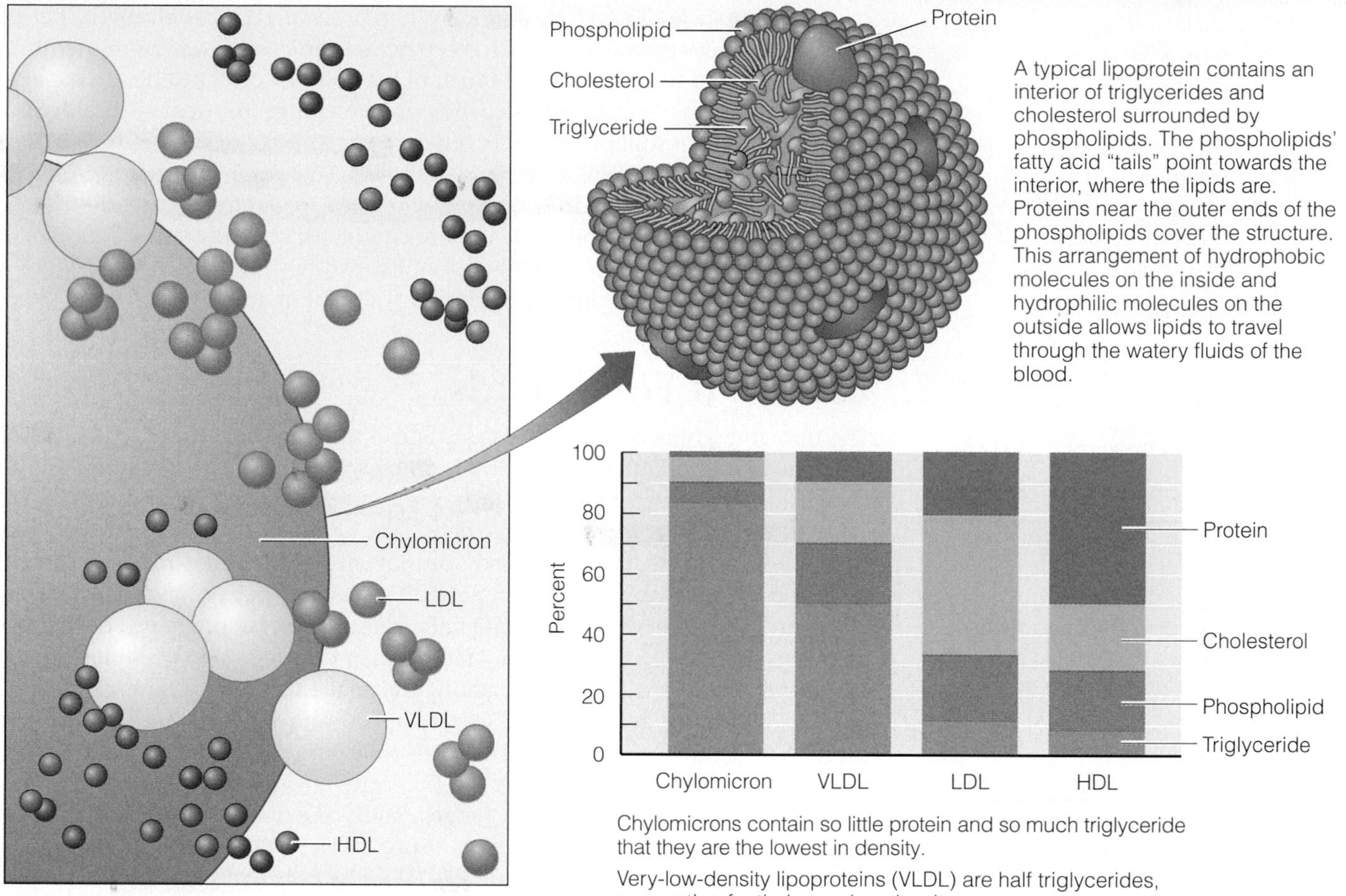

Chylomicron
LDL
VLDL
HDL
Phospholipid
Protein
Cholesterol
Triglyceride
A typical lipoprotein contains an interior of triglycerides and cholesterol surrounded by phospholipids. The phospholipids' fatty acid "tails" point towards the interior, where the lipids are. Proteins near the outer ends of the phospholipids cover the structure. This arrangement of hydrophobic molecules on the inside and hydrophilic molecules on the outside allows lipids to travel through the watery fluids of the blood.
100
80
60
40
20
0
Percent
Protein
Cholesterol
Phospholipid
Triglyceride
Chylomicron
VLDL
LDL
HDL

This solar system of lipoproteins shows their relative sizes. Notice how large the fat-filled chylomicron is compared with the others and how the others get progressively smaller as their proportion of fat declines and protein increases.

Chylomicrons contain so little protein and so much triglyceride that they are the lowest in density.

Very-low-density lipoproteins (VLDL) are half triglycerides, accounting for their very low density.

Low-density lipoproteins (LDL) are half cholesterol, accounting for their implication in heart disease.

High-density lipoproteins (HDL) are half protein, accounting for their high density.

Available Online

http://nutrition.wadsworth.com/uncn7
View the various types of lipoproteins as they leave their tissue of origin, and follow their metabolism as they deliver their cargo of lipids to specific destinations throughout the body.

IN SUMMARY The liver packages lipids with proteins into lipoproteins for transport around the body. All four types of lipoproteins carry all classes of lipids (triglycerides, phospholipids, and cholesterol), but the chylomicrons are the largest and the highest in triglycerides; VLDL are smaller and are about half triglycerides; LDL are smaller still and are high in cholesterol; and HDL are the smallest and are rich in protein.

■ Factors that lower LDL or raise HDL:
- Weight control.
- Monounsaturated or polyunsaturated, instead of saturated, fat in the diet.
- Soluble, viscous fibers (see Chapter 4).
- Phytochemicals (see Highlight 13).
- *Moderate* alcohol consumption.
- Physical activity.

Lipids in the Body

The blood carries lipids to various sites around the body. Once they arrive at their destinations, the lipids can get to work providing energy, insulating against temperature extremes, protecting against shock, and maintaining cell membranes. This section provides an overview first of the roles of triglycerides and fatty acids and then of the metabolic pathways they can follow within the body's cells.

FIGURE 5-19 The Pathway from One Omega-6 Fatty Acid to Another

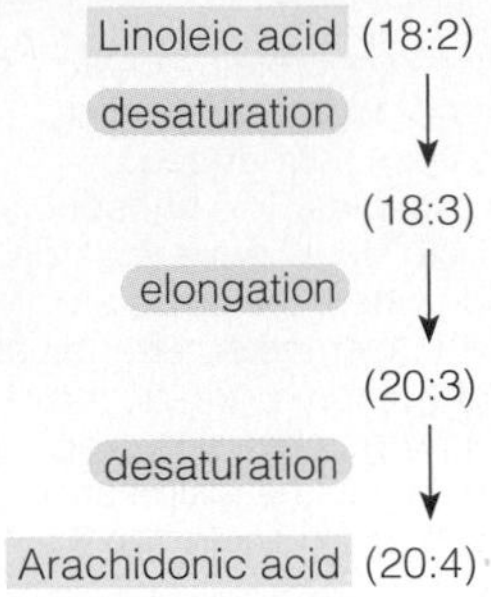
Linoleic acid (18:2)
desaturation
(18:3)
elongation
(20:3)
desaturation
Arachidonic acid (20:4)

Note: The first number indicates the number of carbons and the second, the number of double bonds. Similar reactions occur when the body makes EPA and DHA from linolenic acid.

■ A nonessential nutrient (such as arachidonic acid) that must be supplied by the diet in special circumstances (as in a linoleic acid deficiency) is considered *conditionally* essential.

essential fatty acids: fatty acids needed by the body, but not made by it in amounts sufficient to meet physiological needs.

arachidonic (a-RACK-ih-DON-ic) **acid:** an omega-6 polyunsaturated fatty acid with 20 carbons and four double bonds; present in small amounts in meat and other animal products and synthesized in the body from linoleic acid.

EPA, or **eicosapentaenoic** (EYE-cossa-PENTA-ee-NO-ick) **acid:** an omega-3 polyunsaturated fatty acid with 20 carbons and five double bonds; present in fish and synthesized in limited amounts in the body from linolenic acid.

DHA, or **docosahexaenoic** (DOE-cossa-HEXA-ee-NO-ick) **acid:** an omega-3 polyunsaturated fatty acid with 22 carbons and six double bonds; present in fish and synthesized in limited amounts in the body from linolenic acid.

eicosanoids (eye-COSS-uh-noyds): derivatives of 20-carbon fatty acids; biologically active compounds that help to regulate blood pressure, blood clotting, and other body functions. They include *prostaglandins* (PROS-tah-GLAND-ins), *thromboxanes* (throm-BOX-ains), and *leukotrienes* (LOO-ko-TRY-eens).

Roles of Triglycerides

First and foremost, the triglycerides—either from food or from the body's fat stores—provide the body with energy. When a person dances all night, her dinner's triglycerides provide the fuel to keep her moving; when a person loses his appetite, his stored triglycerides fuel much of his body's work until he can eat again.

Efficient energy metabolism depends on the energy nutrients—carbohydrate, fat, and protein—supporting each other. Glucose fragments combine with fat fragments during energy metabolism, and fat and carbohydrate help spare protein, providing energy so that protein can be used for other important tasks.

Fat also insulates the body. Fat is a poor conductor of heat, so the layer of fat beneath the skin helps keep the body warm. Fat pads also serve as natural shock absorbers, providing a cushion for the bones and vital organs.

Essential Fatty Acids

The human body needs fatty acids, and it can make all but two of them—linoleic acid (the 18-carbon omega-6 fatty acid) and linolenic acid (the 18-carbon omega-3 fatty acid). These two fatty acids must be supplied by the diet and are therefore called **essential fatty acids.** A simple definition of an essential nutrient has already been given: a nutrient that the body cannot make, or cannot make in sufficient quantities to meet its physiological needs. The cells do not possess the enzymes to make any of the omega-6 or omega-3 fatty acids from scratch; nor can they convert an omega-6 fatty acid to an omega-3 fatty acid or vice versa. They *can* start with the 18-carbon member of an omega family and make the longer fatty acids of that family by forming double bonds (desaturation) and lengthening the chain two carbons at a time (elongation), as shown in Figure 5-19. This is a slow process because the two families compete for the same enzymes. Too much of one can create a deficiency of the other's longer family members, which is critical only when the diet fails to deliver adequate supplies. Therefore, the most effective way to maintain body supplies of all the omega-6 and omega-3 fatty acids is to obtain them directly from foods—most notably, from vegetable oils, seeds, nuts, fish, and other marine foods.

Linoleic Acid and the Omega-6 Family Linoleic acid is the primary member of the omega-6 family. Given linoleic acid, the body can make other members of the omega-6 family—such as the 20-carbon polyunsaturated fatty acid, **arachidonic acid.** Should a linoleic acid deficiency develop, arachidonic acid, and all other fatty acids that derive from linoleic acid, would also become essential and have to be obtained from the diet.■ Normally, vegetable oils and meats supply enough omega-6 fatty acids to meet the body's needs.

Linolenic Acid and the Omega-3 Family Linolenic acid is the primary member of the omega-3 family.* Like linoleic acid, this 18-carbon fatty acid cannot be made in the body and must be supplied by foods. Given dietary linolenic acid, the body can make small amounts of the 20- and 22-carbon members of the omega-3 series, **EPA (eicosapentaenoic acid)** and **DHA (docosahexaenoic acid).** These omega-3 fatty acids are essential for normal growth and development, especially in the eyes and brain.[6] They may also play an important role in the prevention and treatment of heart disease.

Eicosanoids The body uses arachidonic acid and EPA to make substances known as **eicosanoids.** Eicosanoids are a diverse group of compounds that are sometimes described as "hormonelike," but they differ from hormones in important ways. For one, hormones are secreted in one location and travel to affect cells all over the

*This omega-3 linolenic acid is known as alpha-linolenic acid and is the fatty acid referred to in this chapter. Another fatty acid, also with 18 carbons and three double bonds, belongs to the omega-6 family and is known as gamma-linolenic acid.

body, whereas eicosanoids appear to affect only the cells in which they are made or nearby cells in the same localized environment. For another, hormones elicit the same response from all their target cells, whereas eicosanoids often have different effects on different cells.

The actions of various eicosanoids sometimes oppose each other. One causes muscles to relax and blood vessels to dilate, while another causes muscles to contract and blood vessels to constrict, for example. Certain eicosanoids participate in the immune response to injury and infection, producing fever, inflammation, and pain.[7] One of the ways aspirin works to relieve these symptoms is by slowing the synthesis of these eicosanoids.

Eicosanoids that derive from EPA differ slightly from those that derive from arachidonic acid, with those from EPA providing greater health benefits. The EPA eicosanoids help lower blood pressure, prevent blood clot formation, protect against irregular heartbeats, and reduce inflammation. Because the omega-6 and omega-3 fatty acids compete for the same enzymes to make arachidonic acid and EPA and to make the eicosanoids, the body needs these long-chain polyunsaturated fatty acids from the diet to make eicosanoids in sufficient quantities.

Fatty Acid Deficiencies Most diets in the United States and Canada meet the essential fatty acid requirement adequately. Historically, deficiencies have developed only in infants and young children fed fat-free milk and low-fat diets or in hospital clients mistakenly fed formulas that provided no polyunsaturated fatty acids for long periods of time. Classic deficiency symptoms include growth retardation, reproductive failure, skin lesions, kidney and liver disorders, and subtle neurological and visual problems.

Interestingly, a deficiency of omega-3 fatty acids (EPA and DHA) may be associated with depression.[8] Some neurochemical pathways in the brain become more active and others become less active.[9] It is unclear, however, which comes first—whether inadequate intake alters brain activity or depression alters fatty acid metabolism. To find the answers, researchers must untangle a multitude of confounding factors.

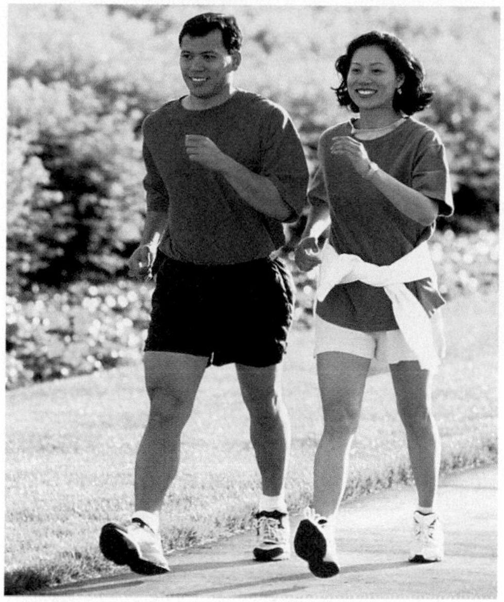

© Jim Cummins/Taxi/Getty Images

Double thanks: The body's fat stores provide energy for a walk, and the heel's fat pads cushion against the hard pavement.

IN SUMMARY In the body, triglycerides:

- Provide an energy reserve when stored in the body's fat tissue.
- Insulate against temperature extremes.
- Protect against shock.
- Help the body use carbohydrate and protein efficiently.

Linoleic acid (18 carbons, omega-6) and linolenic acid (18 carbons, omega-3) are essential nutrients. They serve as structural parts of cell membranes and as precursors to the longer fatty acids that can make eicosanoids—powerful compounds that participate in blood pressure regulation, blood clot formation, and the immune response to injury and infection, among other functions. Because essential fatty acids are common in the diet and stored in the body, deficiencies are unlikely.

FIGURE 5-20 An Adipose Cell

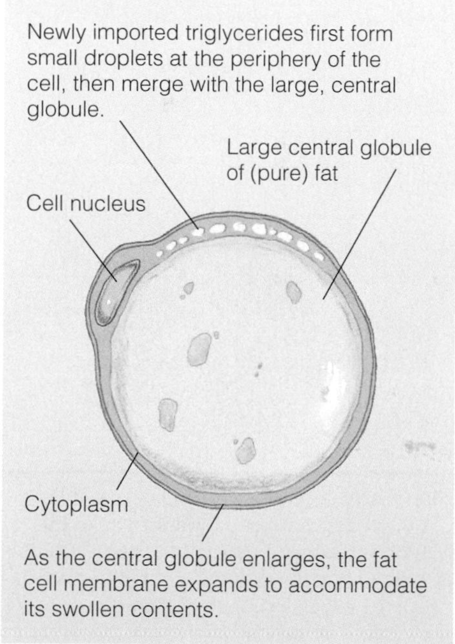
Newly imported triglycerides first form small droplets at the periphery of the cell, then merge with the large, central globule.
Large central globule of (pure) fat
Cell nucleus
Cytoplasm
As the central globule enlarges, the fat cell membrane expands to accommodate its swollen contents.

A Preview of Lipid Metabolism

The blood delivers triglycerides to the cells for their use. This is a preview of how the cells store and release energy from fat; Chapter 7 provides details.

Storing Fat as Fat The triglycerides, familiar as the fat in foods and as body fat, serve the body primarily as a source of fuel. Fat provides more than twice the energy of carbohydrate and protein,■ making it an extremely efficient storage form of energy. Unlike the liver's glycogen stores, the body's fat stores have virtually unlimited capacity, thanks to the special cells of the **adipose tissue**. Unlike most body cells, which can store only limited amounts of fat, the fat cells of the adipose tissue readily take up and store fat. An adipose cell is depicted in Figure 5-20.

■ 1 g fat = 9 kcal.

adipose (ADD-ih-poce) **tissue:** the body's fat tissue; consists of masses of triglyceride-storing cells.

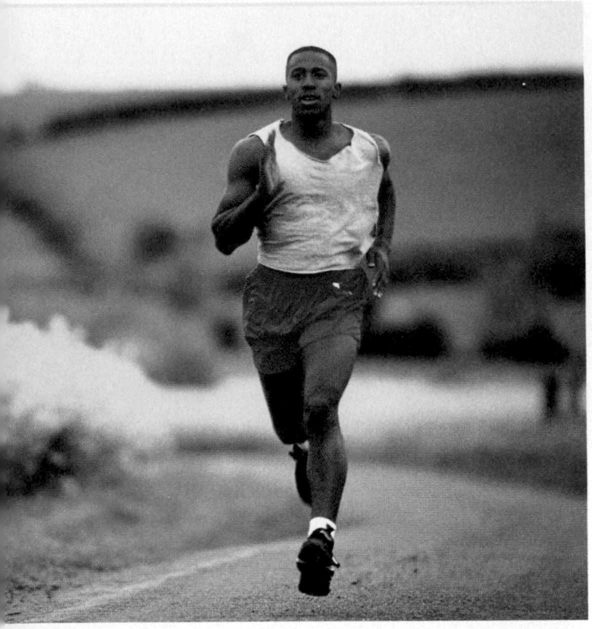

© Bob Thomas/Stone/Getty Images

Fat supplies most of the energy during a long-distance run.

■ Reminder: Gram for gram, fat provides more than twice as much energy as carbohydrate or protein.

■ 1 lb body fat = 3500 kcal.

To convert food fats to body fat, the body simply absorbs the parts and puts them (and others) together again in storage. It requires very little energy to do this. An enzyme—**lipoprotein lipase (LPL)**—hydrolyzes triglycerides from lipoproteins, producing glycerol, fatty acids and monoglycerides that enter the adipose cells. Inside the cells, other enzymes reassemble the pieces into triglycerides again for storage. Earlier, Figure 5-4 (on p. 145) showed how the body can make a triglyceride from glycerol and fatty acids. Triglycerides fill the adipose cells, storing a lot of energy in a relatively small space.■ Adipose cells store fat after meals when a heavy traffic of chylomicrons and VLDL loaded with triglycerides passes by; they release it later whenever the blood needs replenishing.

Using Fat for Energy Fat supplies 60 percent of the body's ongoing energy needs during rest. During prolonged light to moderately intense exercise or extended periods of food deprivation, fat stores may make a slightly greater contribution to energy needs.

When cells demand energy, an enzyme **(hormone-sensitive lipase)** inside the adipose cells responds by dismantling stored triglycerides and releasing the glycerol and fatty acids directly into the blood. Energy-hungry cells anywhere in the body can then capture these compounds and take them through a series of chemical reactions to yield energy, carbon dioxide, and water.

A person who fasts (drinking only water) will rapidly metabolize body fat. A pound of body fat provides 3500 kcalories,■ so you might think a fasting person who expends 2000 kcalories a day could lose more than half a pound of body fat each day.* Actually, the person has to obtain some energy from lean tissue because the brain, nerves, and red blood cells need glucose. Also, the complete breakdown of fat requires carbohydrate or protein. Even on a total fast, a person cannot lose more than half a pound of pure fat per day. Still, in conditions of enforced starvation—say, during a siege or a famine—a fatter person can survive longer than a thinner person thanks to this energy reserve.

Although fat provides energy during a fast, it can provide very little glucose to give energy to the brain and nerves. Only the small glycerol molecule can be converted to glucose; fatty acids cannot be. (Figure 7-12 on p. 226 illustrates how only 3 of the 50 or so carbon atoms in a molecule of fat can yield glucose.) After prolonged glucose deprivation, brain and nerve cells develop the ability to derive about two-thirds of their minimum energy needs from the ketone bodies that the body makes from fat fragments. Ketone bodies cannot sustain life by themselves, however. As Chapter 7 explains, fasting for too long will cause death, even if the person still has ample body fat.

IN SUMMARY The body can easily store unlimited amounts of fat if given excesses, and this body fat is used for energy when needed. The liver can also convert excess carbohydrate and protein into fat. Fat breakdown requires simultaneous carbohydrate breakdown for maximum efficiency; without carbohydrate, fats break down to ketone bodies.

lipoprotein lipase (LPL): an enzyme that hydrolyzes triglycerides passing by in the bloodstream and directs their parts into the cells, where they can be metabolized for energy or reassembled for storage.

hormone-sensitive lipase: an enzyme inside adipose cells that responds to the body's need for fuel by hydrolyzing triglycerides so that their parts (glycerol and fatty acids) escape into the general circulation and thus become available to other cells for fuel. The signals to which this enzyme responds include epinephrine and glucagon, which oppose insulin (see Chapter 4).

Health Effects and Recommended Intakes of Lipids

Of all the nutrients, fat is most often linked with heart disease, some types of cancer, and obesity. Fortunately, the same recommendation can help with all of these health problems: choose a diet that is low in saturated fats, *trans* fats, and cholesterol and moderate in total fat.

*The reader who knows that 1 pound = 454 grams and that 1 gram of fat = 9 kcalories may wonder why a pound of body fat does not equal 4086 (9 × 454) kcalories. The reason is that body fat contains some cell water and other minerals; it is not quite pure fat.

Health Effects of Lipids

Hearing a physician say, "Your blood lipid profile looks fine," is reassuring. The **blood lipid profile**■ reveals the concentrations of various lipids in the blood, notably triglycerides and cholesterol, and their lipoprotein carriers (VLDL, LDL, and HDL). This information alerts people to their disease risks and their need to change eating habits.

Heart Disease Most people realize that elevated blood cholesterol is a major risk factor for **cardiovascular disease.** Cholesterol accumulates in the arteries, restricting blood flow and raising blood pressure. The consequences are deadly; in fact, heart disease is the nation's number one killer of adults. Blood cholesterol is often used to predict the likelihood of a person's suffering a heart attack or stroke; the higher the cholesterol, the earlier and more likely the tragedy. Efforts to prevent heart disease focus on lowering blood cholesterol.[10]

Commercials advertise products that are low in cholesterol, and magazine articles tell readers how to cut the cholesterol in their favorite recipes. What most people don't realize, though, is that *food* cholesterol does not raise *blood* cholesterol as dramatically as *saturated fat* does.

Risks from Saturated Fats Recall that LDL cholesterol raises the risk of heart disease. Most often implicated in raising LDL cholesterol are the saturated fats. In general, the more saturated fat in the diet, the more LDL cholesterol in the body. Not all saturated fats have the same cholesterol-raising effect, however. Most notable among the saturated fatty acids that raise blood cholesterol are lauric, myristic, and palmitic acids (12, 14, and 16 carbons, respectively). In contrast, stearic acid (18 carbons) does not seem to raise blood cholesterol, but making such distinctions may be impractical in diet planning because these saturated fatty acids typically appear together in the same foods.[11]

Fats from animal sources are the main sources of saturated fats■ in most people's diets (see Figure 5-21). Some vegetable fats (coconut and palm) and hydrogenated fats provide smaller amounts of saturated fats. Selecting poultry or fish and fat-free milk products helps to lower saturated fat intake and heart disease risk.[12] Using nonhydrogenated margarine and unsaturated cooking oil is another simple change that can dramatically lower saturated fat intake.

Risks from *Trans* Fats Research also suggests an association between dietary *trans*-fatty acids and heart disease.[13] In the body, *trans*-fatty acids alter blood cholesterol the same way some saturated fats do: they raise LDL cholesterol.[14] Limiting the intake of *trans*-fatty acids can improve blood cholesterol. *Trans*-fatty acids make up approximately 7 percent of the fat intake (or 2 percent of the energy intake) in the U.S. diet.[15]■

Reports on *trans*-fatty acids have raised consumer doubts about whether margarine is, after all, a better choice than butter for heart health. The American Heart Association has stated that because butter is rich in both saturated fat and cholesterol while margarine is made from vegetable fat with no dietary cholesterol, margarine is still preferable to butter. Be aware that soft margarines (liquid or tub) ■ are less hydrogenated and relatively lower in *trans*-fatty acids; consequently, they do not raise blood cholesterol as the saturated fats of butter or the *trans* fats of hard (stick) margarines do.[16] Some manufacturers are now offering nonhydrogenated margarines that are "*trans* fat free." The last section of this chapter describes how to read food labels and compares butter and margarines; whichever you decide to use, remember to use them sparingly.

Risks from Cholesterol Dietary cholesterol has also been implicated in raising blood cholesterol and increasing the risk of heart disease, although its effect is not as strong as that of saturated fat or *trans* fat. Still, health experts advise limiting cholesterol intake.

Recall that cholesterol is found only in foods derived from animals. Consequently, eating less fat from meats, eggs, and milk products helps lower dietary

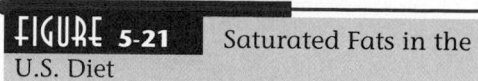

FIGURE 5-21 Saturated Fats in the U.S. Diet

Fruits, grains, and vegetables are insignificant sources, unless saturated fats are intentionally added to them during preparation.

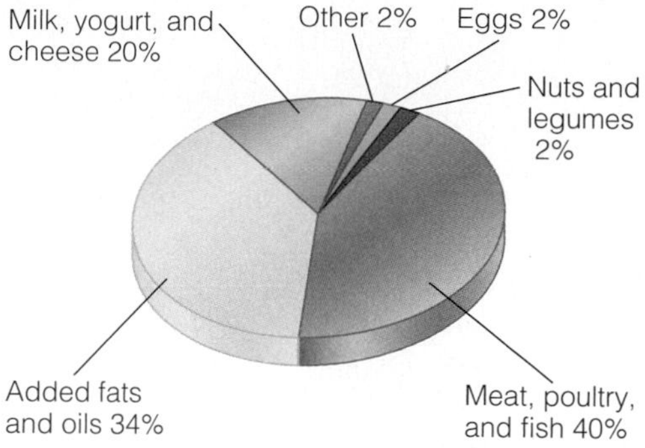
Milk, yogurt, and cheese 20%
Other 2%
Eggs 2%
Nuts and legumes 2%
Added fats and oils 34%
Meat, poultry, and fish 40%

■ Desirable blood lipid profile:
- Total cholesterol: <200 mg/dL.
- LDL cholesterol: <100 mg/dL.
- HDL cholesterol: ≥60 mg/dL.
- Triglycerides: <150 mg/dL.

■ Major sources of saturated fats:
- Whole milk, cream, butter, cheese.
- Fatty cuts of beef and pork.
- Coconut, palm, and palm kernel oils (and products containing them such as candies, pastries, pies, doughnuts, and cookies).

■ Major sources of *trans* fats:
- Deep-fried foods (vegetable shortening).
- Cakes, cookies, doughnuts, pastry, crackers.
- Snack chips.
- Margarine.
- Imitation cheese.
- Meat and dairy products.

■ When selecting margarine, look for:
- Soft (liquid or tub) instead of hard (stick).
- ≤2 g saturated fat.
- Liquid vegetable oil (not hydrogenated or partially hydrogenated) as first ingredient.
- "*Trans* fat free."

blood lipid profile: results of blood tests that reveal a person's total cholesterol, triglycerides, and various lipoproteins.

cardiovascular disease (CVD): a general term for all diseases of the heart and blood vessels. Atherosclerosis is the main cause of CVD. When arteries that carry blood to the heart muscle become blocked, the heart suffers damage known as **coronary heart disease (CHD).**
- **cardio** = heart
- **vascular** = blood vessels

■ Major sources of cholesterol:
- Eggs.
- Milk products.
- Meat, poultry, shellfish.

cholesterol intake■ (as well as total and saturated fat intakes). Figure 5-22 shows the cholesterol contents of selected foods. Many more foods, with their cholesterol contents, appear in Appendix H. For most people trying to lower blood cholesterol, however, limiting saturated fat is more effective than limiting cholesterol intake.

An egg contains just over 200 milligrams of cholesterol, all of it in the yolk. A person on a strict low-cholesterol diet must curtail the use of egg yolks, but for people with a healthy lipid profile, eating up to one egg a day is not detrimental.[17] Eggs are a valuable part of the diet because they are inexpensive, useful in cooking, and a source of high-quality protein and other nutrients.[18] Food manufacturers have produced several fat-free, no-cholesterol egg substitutes. Alternatively, a person could use the whites of a fresh egg.

■ Sources of monounsaturated fats:
- Olive oil, canola oil, peanut oil.
- Avocados.

■ Sources of polyunsaturated fats:
- Vegetable oils (safflower, sesame, soy, corn, sunflower).
- Nuts and seeds.

Benefits from Monounsaturated Fats and Polyunsaturated Fats Replacing both saturated and *trans* fats with monounsaturated■ and polyunsaturated■ fats may be the most effective dietary strategy in preventing heart disease.[19] The lower rates of heart disease among people in the Mediterranean region of the world are often attributed to their liberal use of olive oil, a rich source of monounsaturated fatty acids.[20] Olive oil also delivers valuable phytochemicals that help to protect against heart disease.[21] Replacing saturated fats with the polyunsaturated fatty acids of other vegetable oils also lowers blood cholesterol. Highlight 5 examines various types of fats and their roles in supporting or harming heart health.

■ Major sources of omega-3 fats:
- Vegetable oils (canola, soybean, flaxseed).
- Walnuts, flaxseeds.
- Fatty fish (mackerel, salmon, sardines).

Benefits from Omega-3 Fats Research on the different types of fats has spotlighted the beneficial effects of the omega-3■ polyunsaturated fatty acids in reducing the risks of heart disease.[22] Regular consumption of omega-3 fatty acids helps to prevent blood clots, protect against irregular heartbeats, and lower blood pressure, espeically in people with hypertension or atherosclerosis.[23]

Fatty fish are among the best sources of omega-3 fatty acids, and Highlight 5 features their role in supporting heart health. Chapter 27 presents more details on the roles of omega-3 fatty acids in heart disease and discusses the adverse consequences of mercury, an environmental contaminant common in some fish that may diminish the health benefits of omega-3 fatty acids.[24]

FIGURE 5-22 Cholesterol in Selected Foods

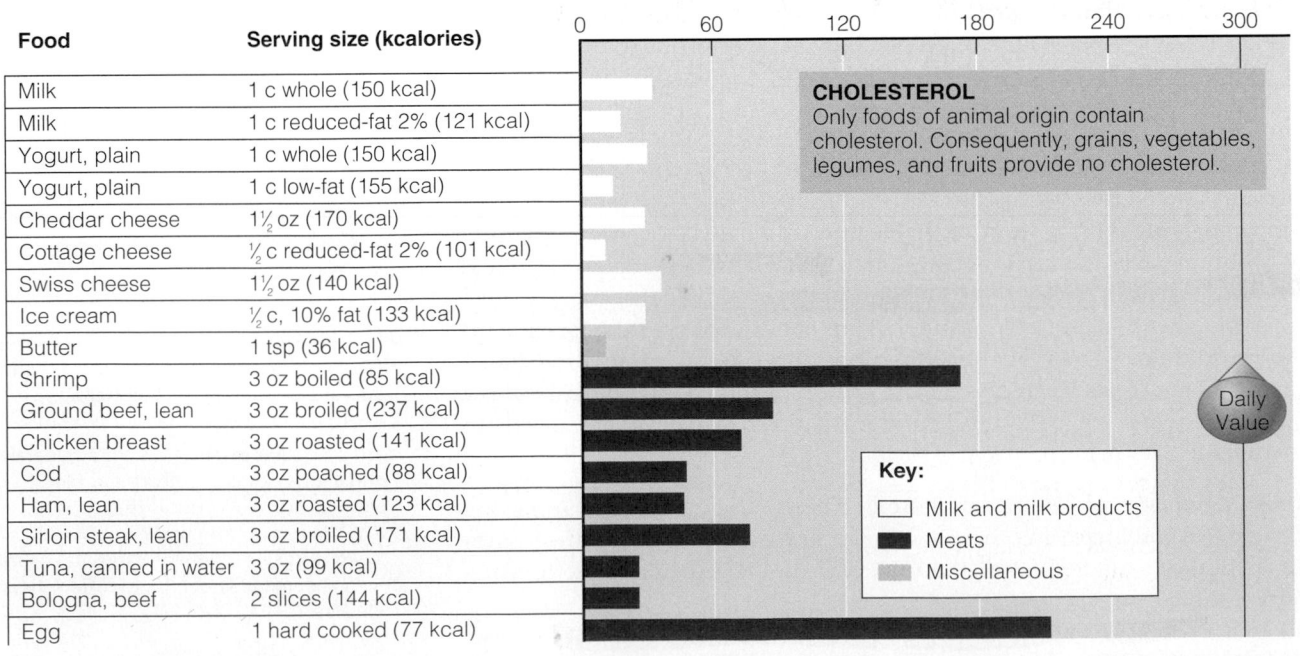

Food	Serving size (kcalories)
Milk	1 c whole (150 kcal)
Milk	1 c reduced-fat 2% (121 kcal)
Yogurt, plain	1 c whole (150 kcal)
Yogurt, plain	1 c low-fat (155 kcal)
Cheddar cheese	1½ oz (170 kcal)
Cottage cheese	½ c reduced-fat 2% (101 kcal)
Swiss cheese	1½ oz (140 kcal)
Ice cream	½ c, 10% fat (133 kcal)
Butter	1 tsp (36 kcal)
Shrimp	3 oz boiled (85 kcal)
Ground beef, lean	3 oz broiled (237 kcal)
Chicken breast	3 oz roasted (141 kcal)
Cod	3 oz poached (88 kcal)
Ham, lean	3 oz roasted (123 kcal)
Sirloin steak, lean	3 oz broiled (171 kcal)
Tuna, canned in water	3 oz (99 kcal)
Bologna, beef	2 slices (144 kcal)
Egg	1 hard cooked (77 kcal)

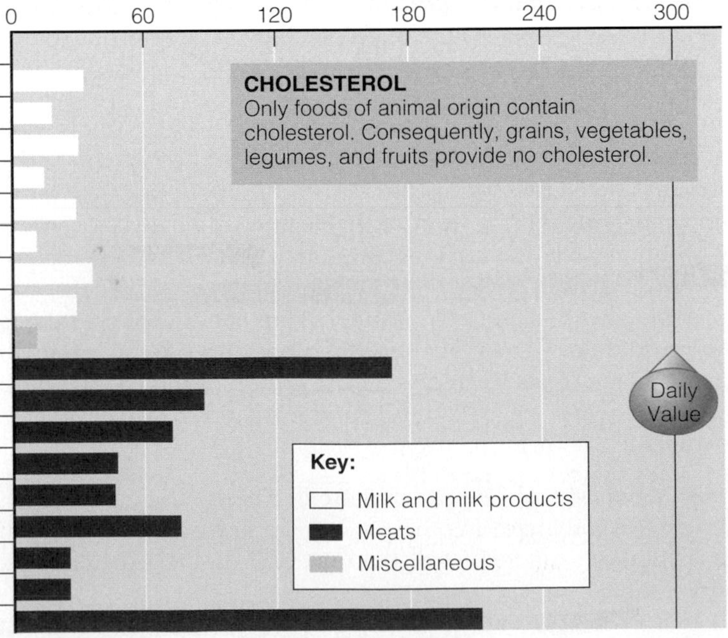

0
60
120
180
240
300
CHOLESTEROL
Only foods of animal origin contain cholesterol. Consequently, grains, vegetables, legumes, and fruits provide no cholesterol.
Daily Value
Key:
Milk and milk products
Meats
Miscellaneous

TABLE 5-2 Sources of Omega Fatty Acids

Omega-6	
Linoleic acid	Vegetable oils (corn, sunflower, safflower, soybean, cottonseed), poultry fat, nuts, seeds
Arachidonic acid	Meats, poultry, eggs (or can be made from linoleic acid)
Omega-3	
Linolenic acid	Oils (flaxseed, canola, walnut, wheat germ, soybean) Nuts and seeds (butternuts, flaxseeds, walnuts, soybean kernels) Vegetables (soybeans)
EPA and DHA	Human milk Pacific oysters and fish[a] (mackerel, salmon, bluefish, mullet, sablefish, menhaden, anchovy, herring, lake trout, sardines, tuna) (or can be made from linolenic acid)

[a]All fish contain some EPA and DHA; the amounts vary among species and within a species depending on such factors as diet, season, and environment. The fish listed here except tuna provide at least 1 gram of omega-3 fatty acids in 100 grams of fish (3.5 ounces). Tuna provides fewer omega-3 fatty acids, but because it is commonly consumed, its contribution can be significant.

Balance Omega-6 and Omega-3 Intakes Table 5-2 provides sources of omega-6 and omega-3 fatty acids. To obtain the right balance between omega-6 and omega-3 fatty acids, most people need to eat more fish and less meat. The American Heart Association recommends two 3-ounce servings of fish a week, with an emphasis on fatty fish (salmon, herring, and mackerel, for example).[25] Eating fish instead of meat supports heart health, especially when combined with physical activity. Even one fish meal a month may be enough to make a difference.[26] When preparing fish, grill, bake, or broil, but do not fry. Fried fish from fast-food restaurants and frozen fried fish products are often low in omega-3 fatty acids and high in *trans*- and saturated fatty acids. Fish provides many minerals (except iron) and vitamins and is leaner than most other animal-protein sources. When used in a weight-loss program, eating fish improves blood lipids even more effectively than either measure alone.[27]

In addition to fish, other functional foods■ are being developed to help consumers improve their omega-3 fatty acid intake. For example, hens fed flaxseed produce eggs rich in omega-3 fatty acids. Including even one enriched egg in the diet daily can significantly increase a person's intake of omega-3 fatty acids. Another option may be to select wild game or pasture-fed cattle, which provide more omega-3 fatty acids and less saturated fat than grain-fed cattle.[28]

■ Reminder: *Functional foods* contain physiologically active compounds that provide health benefits beyond basic nutrition (see Highlight 13 for a full discussion).

For most people, fish oil should come from fish, and omega-3 fatty acids should come from foods, not from supplements.[29] Routine supplementation is not recommended for a number of reasons.* Perhaps most importantly, high intakes of omega-3 polyunsaturated fatty acids may increase bleeding time, interfere with wound healing, raise LDL cholesterol, and suppress immune function.[30] Fish oil supplements are made from fish skins and livers, which may contain environmental contaminants. Some fish oils also naturally contain large amounts of the two most potentially toxic vitamins, A and D. Lastly, supplements are expensive; money is better spent on foods that can provide a full array of nutrients. People with heart disease, however, may benefit from doses greater than can be achieved through diet alone; they should consult a physician about including supplements as part of their treatment plan.[31]

Cancer The evidence for links between dietary fats and cancer■ is less convincing than for heart disease, but it does suggest a possible association between fat and some types of cancers.[32] Dietary fat seems not to *initiate* cancer development but to *promote* cancer once it has arisen.

■ Other risk factors for cancer include smoking, alcohol, and environmental contaminants. Chapter 29 provides many more details about these risk factors and the development of cancer.

*In Canada, fish oil supplements require a physician's prescription.

The relationship between dietary fat and the risk of cancer differs for various types of cancers. In the case of breast cancer, evidence has been weak and inconclusive.[33] Some studies indicate little or no association between dietary fat and breast cancer; others find that total *energy* intake and obesity are better predictors than percentage of kcalories from fat.[34] In the case of prostate cancer, there appears to be a harmful association with fat, although a specific type of fat has not yet been implicated.[35]

The relationship between dietary fat and the risk of cancer differs for various types of fats as well. The association between cancer and fat appears to be due primarily to saturated fats or dietary fat from meats (which is mostly saturated). Fat from milk or fish has not been implicated in cancer risk. In fact, eating fish rich in omega-3 fatty acids seems to protect against some cancers.[36] Thus health advice to reduce cancer risks parallels that given to reduce heart disease risks: reduce saturated fats and increase omega-3 fatty acids.

■ Reminder: Fat is a more concentrated energy source than the other energy nutrients: 1 g carbohydrate or protein = 4 kcal, but 1 g fat = 9 kcal.

Obesity Fat contributes more than twice as many kcalories■ per gram as either carbohydrate or protein. Consequently, people who eat high-fat diets regularly may exceed their energy needs and gain weight, especially if they are inactive.[37] Because fat boosts energy intake, cutting fat can be an effective strategy in cutting kcalories. In some cases, though, choosing a fat-free food offers no kcalorie savings. Fat-free frozen desserts, for example, often have so much sugar added that the kcalorie count can be as high as in the regular-fat product. In that case, cutting fat and adding carbohydrate offers no kcalorie savings or weight-loss advantage. In fact, it may even raise energy intake and exacerbate weight problems. Later chapters revisit the role of dietary fat in the development of obesity.

IN SUMMARY High blood LDL cholesterol poses a risk of heart disease, and high intakes of saturated and *trans* fats, specifically, contribute most to high LDL. Cholesterol in foods presents less of a risk. Omega-3 fatty acids appear to be protective.

Recommended Intakes of Fat

■ DRI and 2005 *Dietary Guidelines* for total fat:
- 20 to 35% of energy intake (from mostly polyunsaturated and monounsaturated fat sources such as fish, nuts, and vegetable oils).

■ Linoleic acid AI:
- 5 to 10% of energy intake.

Men:
- 19–50 yr: 17 g/day.
- 51+ yr: 14 g/day.

Women:
- 19–50 yr: 12 g/day.
- 51+ yr: 11 g/day.

■ Linolenic acid AI:
- 0.6 to 1.2% energy intake.

Men: 1.6 g/day.
Women: 1.1 g/day.

■ Daily Values:
- 65 g fat (based on 30% of 2000 kcal diet).
- 20 g saturated fat (based on 10% of 2000 kcal diet).
- 300 mg cholesterol.

Some fat in the diet is essential for good health, but too much fat, especially saturated fat, increases the risks for chronic diseases. Defining the exact amount of fat, saturated fat, or cholesterol that benefits health or begins to harm health, however, is not possible; for this reason, no RDA or upper limit has been set. Instead, the DRI and 2005 *Dietary Guidelines* suggest a diet that is low in saturated fat, *trans* fat, and cholesterol and provides 20 to 35 percent of the daily energy intake from fat.■ The top end of this range is slightly higher than previous recommendations. This revision recognizes that diets with up to 35 percent of kcalories from fat can be compatible with good health if energy intake is reasonable and saturated fat intake is low. When total fat exceeds 35 percent, saturated fat increases to unhealthy levels.[38] For a 2000-kcalorie diet, 20 to 35 percent represents 400 to 700 kcalories from fat (roughly 45 to 75 grams). Part of this fat allowance should provide for the essential fatty acids—linoleic acid and linolenic acid. Recommendations suggest that linoleic acid■ provide 5 to 10 percent of the daily energy intake and linolenic acid,■ 0.6 to 1.2 percent.[39]

To help consumers meet the dietary fat goals, the Food and Drug Administration (FDA) established Daily Values■ on food labels using 30 percent of energy intake as the guideline for fat and 10 percent for saturated fat; the Daily Value for cholesterol is 300 milligrams regardless of energy intake. There is no Daily Value for *trans* fat, but consumers should try to keep intakes within the 10 percent allotted for saturated fat. According to surveys, adults in the United States receive about 35 percent of their total energy from fat, with saturated fat contributing about 12 percent of the total; cholesterol intakes in the United States average 250 milligrams a day for women and 350 for men.[40]

Increase the proportion of people who consume less than 10 percent of kcalories from saturated fat and no more than 30 percent of kcalories from total fat.

HEALTHY PEOPLE 2010

The fats of fish, nuts, and vegetable oils are not counted as discretionary kcalories because they provide valuable omega-3 fatty acids, essential fatty acids, and vitamin E.* In contrast, solid fats■ deliver an abundance of saturated fatty acids; the USDA Food Guide counts them as discretionary kcalories. Discretionary kcalories may be used to add fats in cooking or at the table, or to select higher fat items from the food groups.■

Although it is very difficult to do, some people actually manage to eat too little fat—to their detriment. Among them are people with eating disorders, described in Highlight 9, and athletes. Athletes following a diet too low in fat (15 percent of total kcalories) fall short on energy, vitamins, minerals, and essential fatty acids as well as on performance.[41] Trained athletes have greater endurance on a high-fat diet (42 to 55 percent) than on a low-fat diet (10 to 15 percent)—even when energy intake is the same.[42] As mentioned earlier, most adults should consume at least 20 percent of their energy intake from fat, but athletes need at least 30 percent.[43] As a practical guideline, it is wise to include the equivalent of at least a teaspoon of fat in every meal—a little peanut butter on toast or mayonnaise on tuna, for example. Dietary recommendations that limit fat were developed for healthy people over age two; Chapter 15 discusses the fat needs of infants and young children.

As the photos in Figure 5-23 (p. 164) show, fat accounts for a lot of the energy in foods, and removing the fat from foods cuts energy and saturated fat intakes dramatically. To reduce dietary fat, eliminate fat as a seasoning and in cooking; remove the fat from high-fat foods; replace high-fat foods with low-fat alternatives; and emphasize grains, fruits, and vegetables. The remainder of the chapter identifies sources of fat in the diet, food group by food group.

■ Solid fats include meat and poultry fats (as in poultry skin, luncheon meats, sausage); milk fat (as in whole milk, cheese, butter); shortenings (as in fried foods and baked goods); and hard margarines.

■ USDA Food Guide amounts of fats that can be included as discretionary kcalories when most food choices are nutrient-dense and fat ≤30% total kcalories:
- 11 g for 1600 kcal diet.
- 15 g for 1800 kcal diet.
- 18 g for 2000 kcal diet.
- 19 g for 2200 kcal diet.
- 22 g for 2400 kcal diet.

For perspective, 1 tsp oil = 5 g fat and provides about 45 kcal.

From Guidelines to Groceries

Fats accompany protein in foods derived from animals,■ such as meat, fish, poultry, and eggs, and carbohydrate in foods derived from plants, such as avocados and coconuts. Fats carry with them the four fat-soluble vitamins—A, D, E, and K—together with many of the compounds that give foods their flavor, texture, and palatability. Fat is responsible for the delicious aromas associated with sizzling bacon and hamburgers on the grill, onions being sautéed, or vegetables in a stir-fry. Of course, these wonderful characteristics lure people into eating too much from time to time. With careful selections, a diet following the USDA Food Guide can both support good health and meet fat recommendations (see the "How to" feature on p. 165).

Meats and Meat Alternates Many meats and meat alternates■ contain fat, saturated fat, and cholesterol, but also provide high-quality protein and valuable vitamins and minerals. They can be included in a healthy diet if a person makes lean choices and prepares them using the suggestions outlined in the box on p. 165. Another strategy to lower blood cholesterol is to prepare meals using soy protein instead of animal protein.[44]

Milks and Milk Products Like meats, milks and milk products■ should also be selected with an awareness of their fat, saturated fat, and cholesterol contents. Fat-free and low-fat milk products provide as much or more protein, calcium, and other nutrients as their whole-milk versions—but with little or no saturated fat. Preliminary research suggests that selecting fermented milk products, such as yogurt, may also help to lower blood cholesterol.[45] These foods increase the population and

■ 2005 *Dietary Guidelines:*
- When selecting and preparing meat, poultry, and milk or milk products, make choices that are lean, low fat, or fat-free.

■ Very lean options:
- Chicken (white meat, no skin); cod, flounder, trout; tuna (canned in water); legumes.

Lean options:
- Beef or pork "round" or "loin" cuts; chicken (dark meat, no skin); herring or salmon; tuna (canned in oil).

Medium-fat options:
- Ground beef; eggs, tofu.

High-fat options:
- Sausage, bacon; luncheon meats; hot dogs; peanut butter, nuts.

■ Fat-free and low-fat options:
- Fat-free or 1% milk or yogurt (plain); fat-free and low-fat cheeses.

Reduced-fat options:
- 2% milk, low-fat yogurt (plain).

High-fat options:
- Whole milk, regular cheeses.

*A new diglyceride-rich oil, brand name Enova, is similar in kcalories and nutrients to soybean oil, but makes health and weight-loss claims that remain to be proven.

FIGURE 5-23 Cutting Fat Cuts kCalories—and Saturated Fat

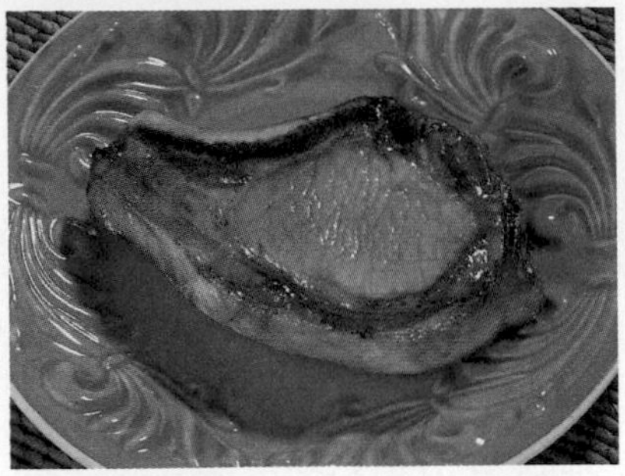

Pork chop with fat (340 kcal, 19 g fat, 7 g saturated fat).

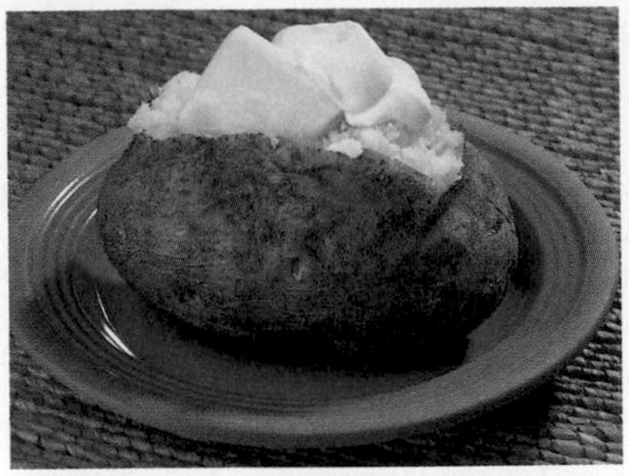

Potato with 1 tbs butter and 1 tbs sour cream (350 kcal, 14 g fat, 10 g saturated fat).

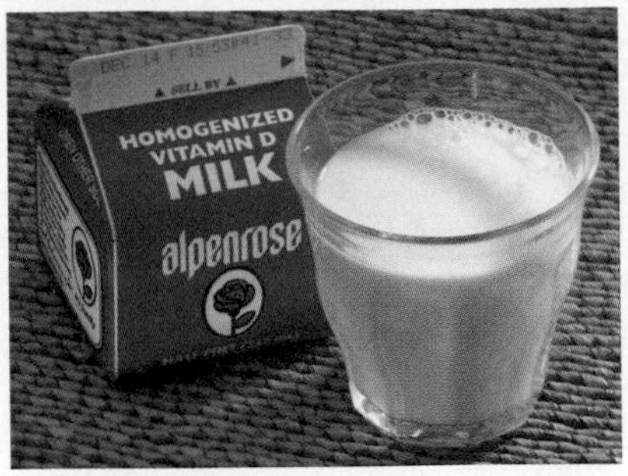
HOMOGENIZED VITAMIN D
MILK
alpenrose

Whole milk, 1 c (150 kcal, 8 g fat, 5 g saturated fat).

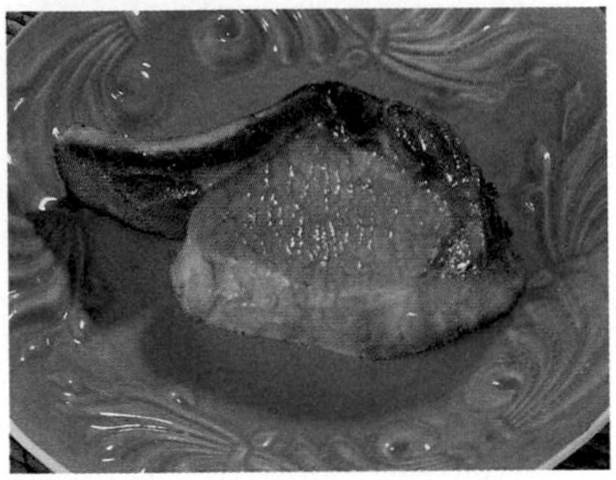

Pork chop with fat trimmed off (230 kcal, 9 g fat, 3 g saturated fat).

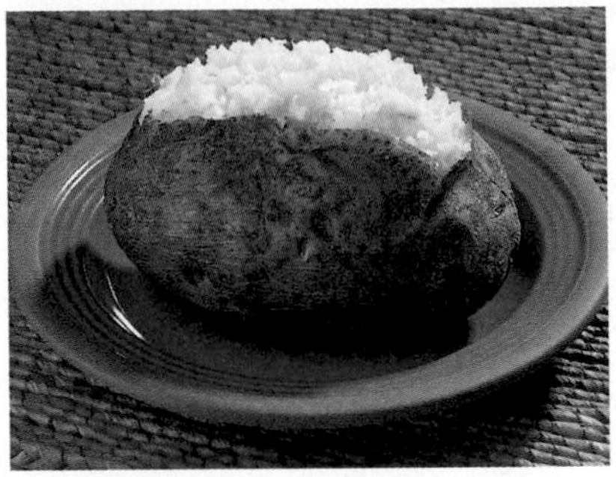

Plain potato (200 kcal, <1 g fat, 0 g saturated fat).

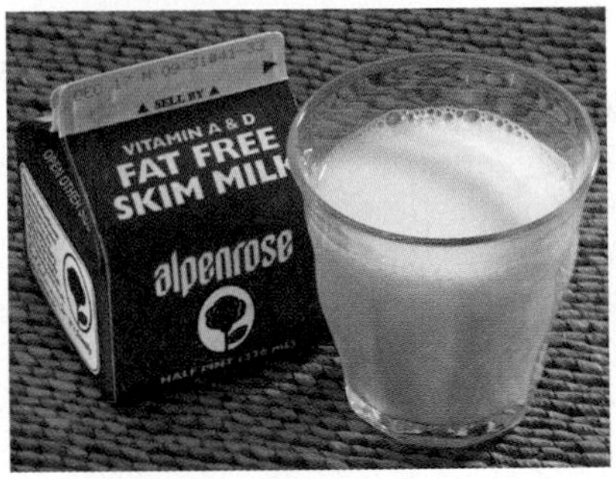
VITAMIN A & D
FAT FREE
SKIM MILK
alpenrose

Fat-free milk, 1 c (90 kcal, <1 g fat, <1 g saturated fat).

activity of bacteria in the colon that ferment fibers. As Chapter 4 explained, this action lowers blood cholesterol by excreting bile and producing short-chain fatty acids that inhibit cholesterol synthesis in the liver.[46]

Vegetables, Fruits, and Grains Choosing vegetables, fruits, whole grains, and legumes also helps lower the saturated fat, cholesterol, and total fat content of the diet. Most vegetables and fruits naturally contain little or no fat; avocados and olives are exceptions, but most of their fat is unsaturated, which is not harmful to heart health. Most grains contain only trace amounts of fat. Some grain *products* such as fried taco shells, croissants, and biscuits are high in saturated fat, though, so consumers need to read food labels. Similarly, many people add butter, margarine, or cheese sauce to grains and vegetables, which raises their saturated and *trans* fat contents. Because fruits are often eaten without added fat, a diet that includes several servings of fruit daily can help a person meet the dietary recommendations for fat.

A diet rich in vegetables, fruits, whole grains, and legumes offers abundant vitamin C, folate, vitamin A, vitamin E, and dietary fiber—all important in supporting health. Consequently, such a diet protects against disease by both reducing saturated fat, cholesterol, and total fat and by increasing nutrients. It also provides valuable phytochemicals that help defend against heart disease.

Invisible Fat *Visible* fat, such as butter and the fat trimmed from meat, is easy to see. *Invisible* fat is less apparent and can be present in foods in surprising amounts.[47] Invisible fat "marbles" a steak or is hidden in foods like cheese. Any *fried* food contains abundant fat: potato chips, french fries, fried wontons, and fried fish. Many *baked* goods, too, are high in fat: pie crusts, pastries, crackers, biscuits, cornbread, doughnuts, sweet rolls, cookies, and cakes. Most chocolate bars deliver more kcalories from fat than from sugar. Even cream-of-mushroom soup prepared with water derives 66 percent of its energy from fat. Keep invisible fats in mind when making food selections.

HOW TO Make Heart-Healthy Choices—by Food Group

Grains

- Select breads, cereals, and crackers that are low in saturated and *trans* fat (for example, bagels instead of croissants).
- Prepare pasta with a tomato sauce instead of a cheese or cream sauce.

Vegetables and Fruits

- Enjoy the natural flavor of steamed vegetables for dinner and fruits for dessert.
- Eat at least two vegetables (in addition to a salad) with dinner.
- Snack on raw vegetables or fruits instead of high-fat items like potato chips.
- Buy frozen vegetables without sauce.

Milk and Milk Products

- Switch from whole milk to reduced-fat, from reduced-fat to low-fat, and from low-fat to fat-free (nonfat).
- Use fat-free and low-fat cheeses (such as part-skim ricotta and low-fat mozzarella) instead of regular cheeses.
- Use fat-free or low-fat yogurt or sour cream instead of regular sour cream.
- Use evaporated fat-free milk instead of cream.
- Enjoy fat-free frozen yogurt, sherbet, or ice milk instead of ice cream.

Meats and Legumes

- Fat adds up quickly, even with lean meat; limit intake to about 6 ounces (cooked weight) daily.
- Eat at least two servings of fish per week (particularly fish such as mackerel, lake trout, herring, sardines, and salmon).
- Choose fish, poultry, or lean cuts of pork or beef; look for unmarbled cuts named *round* or *loin* (eye of round, top round, bottom round, round tip, tenderloin, sirloin, center loin, and top loin).
- Choose processed meats such as lunch meats and hot dogs that are low in saturated fat and cholesterol.
- Trim the fat from pork and beef; remove the skin from poultry.
- Grill, roast, broil, bake, stir-fry, stew, or braise meats; don't fry. When possible, place food on a rack so that fat can drain.
- Use lean ground turkey or lean ground beef in recipes; brown ground meats without added fat, then drain off fat.
- Select tuna, sardines, and other canned meats packed in water; rinse oil-packed items with hot water to remove much of the fat.
- Fill kabob skewers with lots of vegetables and slivers of meat; create main dishes and casseroles by combining a little meat, fish, or poultry with a lot of pasta, rice, or vegetables.
- Use legumes often.
- Eat a meatless meal or two daily.
- Use egg substitutes in recipes instead of whole eggs or use two egg whites in place of each whole egg.

Fats and Oils

- Use butter or margarine sparingly; select soft margarines instead of hard margarines.
- Limit use of lard and meat fat.
- Limit use of products made with coconut oil, palm kernel oil, and palm oil (read labels on bakery goods, processed foods, popcorn oils, and nondairy creamers).
- Reduce use of hydrogenated shortenings and margarines and products that contain them (read labels on crackers, cookies, and other commercially prepared baked goods).

Miscellaneous

- Use a nonstick pan or coat the pan lightly with vegetable oil.
- Refrigerate soups and stews; when the fat solidifies, remove it.
- Use wine; lemon, orange, or tomato juice; herbs; spices; fruits; or broth instead of butter or margarine when cooking.
- Stir-fry in a small amount of oil; add moisture and flavor with broth, tomato juice, or wine.
- Use variety to enhance enjoyment of the meal: vary colors, textures, and temperatures—hot cooked versus cool raw foods—and use garnishes to complement food.

SOURCE: Adapted from Third Report of the National Cholesterol Education Program (NCEP) Expert Panel on Detection, Evaluation, and Treatment of High Blood Cholesterol in Adults (Adult Treatment Panel III), NIH publication no. 02-5215 (Bethesda, Md.: National Heart, Lung, and Blood Institute, 2002), pp. V-25–V-27.

Choose Wisely Consumers can find an abundant array of foods that are low in saturated fat, *trans* fat,■ cholesterol, and total fat. In many cases, they are familiar foods prepared with less fat. For example, fat can be removed by skimming milk or trimming meats. Manufacturers can dilute fat by adding water or whipping in air. They use fat-free milk in creamy desserts and lean meats in frozen entrées. Sometimes they simply prepare the products differently. For example, fat-free potato chips may be baked instead of fried. Beyond lowering the fat content, manufacturers have developed margarines fortified with phytochemicals that lower blood cholesterol.*[48] (Highlight 13 explores these and other functional foods designed to support health.) Such choices make heart-healthy eating easy.

■ 2005 *Dietary Guidelines*:
- Limit intakes of fats and oils high in saturated and/or *trans*-fatty acids, and choose products low in such fats and oils.

Fat Replacers Some foods are made with **fat replacers**—ingredients derived from carbohydrate, protein, or fat that replace some or all of the fat in foods. The body may digest and absorb some of these substances, so they may contribute some energy, although significantly less than fat's 9 kcalories per gram.

Some foods are made with **artificial fats**—fat replacers that offer the sensory and cooking qualities of fats, but none of the kcalories. A familiar example of an artificial fat that has been approved for use in snack foods such as potato chips, crackers,

fat replacers: ingredients that replace some or all of the functions of fat and may or may not provide energy.

artificial fats: zero-energy fat replacers that are chemically synthesized to mimic the sensory and cooking qualities of naturally occurring fats, but are totally or partially resistant to digestion.

*Margarines that lower blood cholesterol contain plant sterols and are marketed under the brand names Benecol and Take Control.

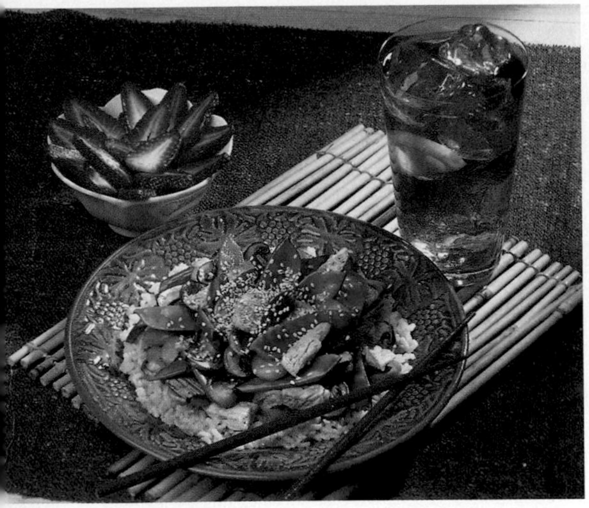

Well-balanced, healthy meals provide some fat with an emphasis on monounsaturated and polyunsaturated fats.

and tortilla chips is **olestra.** Olestra's chemical structure is similar to that of a regular fat (a triglyceride) but with important differences. A triglyceride is composed of a glycerol molecule with three fatty acids attached, whereas olestra is made of a sucrose molecule with six to eight fatty acids attached. Enzymes in the digestive tract cannot break the bonds of olestra, so unlike sucrose or fatty acids, olestra passes through the system unabsorbed.

The FDA's evaluation of olestra's safety addressed two questions. First, is olestra toxic? Research on both animals and human beings supports the safety of olestra as a partial replacement for dietary fats and oils, with no reports of cancer or birth defects. Second, does olestra affect either nutrient absorption or the health of the digestive tract? When olestra passes through the digestive tract unabsorbed, it binds with some of the fat-soluble vitamins A, D, E, and K and carries them out of the body, robbing the person of these valuable nutrients. To compensate for these losses, the FDA requires the manufacturer to fortify olestra with vitamins A, D, E, and K. Saturating olestra with these vitamins does not make the product a good source of vitamins, but it does block olestra's ability to bind with the vitamins from other foods. An asterisk in the ingredients list informs consumers that these added vitamins are "dietarily insignificant."

Some consumers of olestra experience digestive distress: cramps, gas, bloating, and diarrhea. The FDA initially required a label warning stating that "olestra may cause abdominal cramping and loose stools" and that it "inhibits the absorption of some vitamins and other nutrients," but recently concluded that such a statement is no longer warranted.

Consumers need to keep in mind that low-fat and fat-free foods still deliver kcalories. Decades ago, consumers hailed the arrival of artificial sweeteners as a weight-loss wonder, but in reality, kcalories saved by using artificial sweeteners were readily replaced by kcalories from other foods. Alternatives to fat can help to lower energy intake and support weight loss only when they actually *replace* fat and energy in the diet.

Read Food Labels Labels list total fat, saturated fat, and cholesterol contents of foods in addition to fat kcalories per serving (see Figure 5-24). Because each package provides information for a single serving and serving sizes are standardized, consumers can easily compare similar products. By 2006 labels will provide content information on *trans*-fatty acids as well.[49] In the meantime, keep in mind that a food that lists partially hydrogenated oils among its first three ingredients usually contains substantial amounts of *trans*-fatty acids, as well as some saturated fat. Figure 5-24 includes tips on finding the *trans* fats on food labels.

Total fat, saturated fat, and cholesterol are also expressed as "% Daily Values" for a person consuming 2000 kcalories. People who are consuming more or less than 2000 kcalories daily can calculate their personal Daily Value for fat as described in the "How to" on p. 168 (top). *Trans* fats do not have a Daily Value.

Be aware that the "% Daily Value" for fat is not the same as "% kcalories from fat." This important distinction is explained in the "How to" feature on p. 168 (bottom). Because recommendations apply to average daily intakes and not to individual food items, food labels do not provide "% kcalories from fat." Still, you can get an idea of whether a particular food is high or low in fat.

IN SUMMARY In foods, triglycerides:

- Deliver fat-soluble vitamins, energy, and essential fatty acids.
- Contribute to the sensory appeal of foods and stimulate appetite.

While some fat in the diet is necessary, health authorities recommend a diet moderate in total fat and low in saturated fat, *trans* fat, and cholesterol. They also recommend replacing saturated fats with monounsaturated and polyunsaturated fats, particularly omega-3 fatty acids from foods such as fish, not from supplements. Many selection and preparation strategies can help bring these goals within reach, and food labels help to identify foods consistent with these guidelines.

olestra: a synthetic fat made from sucrose and fatty acids that provides 0 kcalories per gram; also known as **sucrose polyester.**

FIGURE 5-24 Butter and Margarine Labels Compared

Food labels list the kcalories from fat and the quantities and Daily Values for fat, saturated fat, and cholesterol. Information on polyunsaturated and monounsaturated fats is optional, but if it is provided, you can add the three types of fat together and subtract from the total to calculate *trans* fat. In this example, stick margarine has 3 g *trans* fat, tub margarine has 1 g *trans* fat, and liquid margarine has 0.5 g *trans* fat. Products that contain 0.5 g or less of *trans* fat and 0.5 g or less of saturated fat may claim "no *trans* fat." Similarly, products that contain 2 mg or less of cholesterol and 2 g or less of saturated fat may claim to be "cholesterol-free."

If the list of ingredients includes hydrogenated oils, you know the food contains *trans* fat. Chapter 2 explained that foods list their ingredients in descending order of predominance by weight. As you can see from this example, the closer "partially hydrogenated oils" is to the beginning of the ingredients list, the more *trans* fats the product contains.

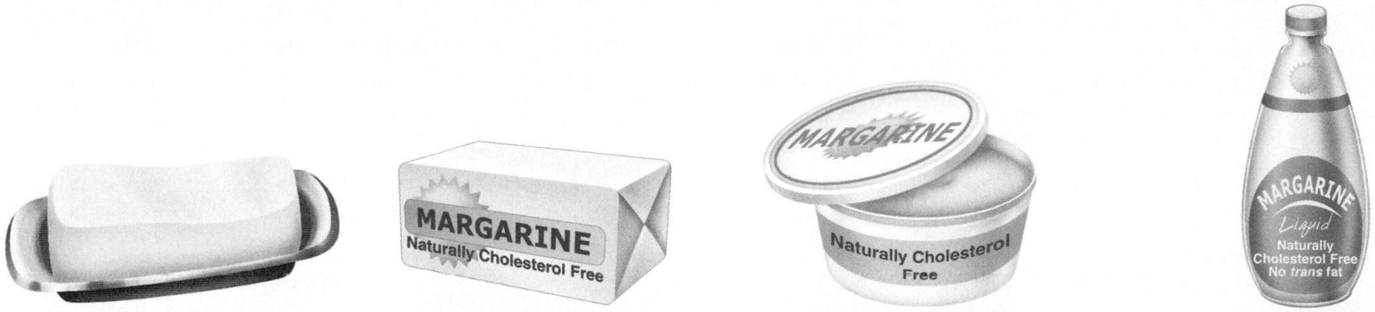

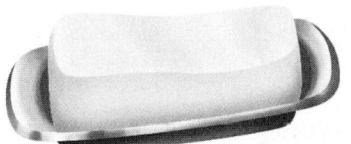

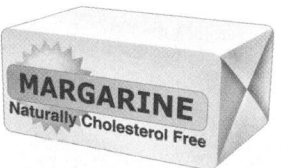

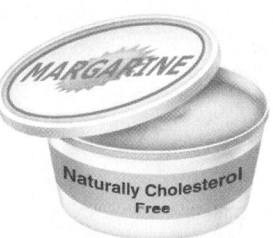
MARGARINE
Naturally Cholesterol Free
MARGARINE
Naturally Cholesterol Free
MARGARINE
Liquid
Naturally Cholesterol Free
No trans fat

Butter

Nutrition Facts
Serving size 1 Tbsp (14g)
Servings Per Container 32

Amount per serving	
Calories 100 Calories from Fat 100	
	%Daily Value*
Total Fat 11g	17%
Saturated Fat 7g	36%
Cholesterol 30mg	10%
Sodium 90mg	4%
Total Carbohydrate 0g	0%
Protein 0g	
Vitamin A 8%	
Not a significant source of dietary fiber, sugars, vitamin C, calcium, and iron.	
*Percent Daily Values are based on a 2,000 calorie diet.	

INGREDIENTS: Cream, salt.

Margarine (stick)

Nutrition Facts
Serving size 1 Tbsp (14g)
Servings Per Container 32

Amount per serving	
Calories 90	Calories from Fat 90
	%Daily Value*
Total Fat 10g	15%
Saturated Fat 2g	10%
Polyunsaturated Fat 2g	
Monounsaturated Fat 3g	
Cholesterol 0mg	0%
Sodium 95mg	4%
Total Carbohydrate 0g	0%
Protein 0g	
Vitamin A 10%	
Not a significant source of dietary fiber, sugars, vitamin C, calcium, and iron.	
*Percent Daily Values are based on a 2,000 calorie diet.	

INGREDIENTS: Vegetable oil blend (partially hydrogenated and liquid soybean oils), water, sweet cream buttermilk, salt, vegetable mono- and diglycerides, soy lecithin, citric acid, artificial flavor, vitamin A, colored with beta carotene.

Margarine (tub)

Nutrition Facts
Serving size 1 Tbsp (14g)
Servings Per Container 32

Amount per serving	
Calories 90	Calories from Fat 90
	%Daily Value*
Total Fat 10g	15%
Saturated Fat 2g	10%
Polyunsaturated Fat 4.5g	
Monounsaturated Fat 2.5g	
Cholesterol 0mg	0%
Sodium 95mg	4%
Total Carbohydrate 0g	0%
Protein 0g	
Vitamin A 10%	
Not a significant source of dietary fiber, sugars, vitamin C, calcium, and iron.	
*Percent Daily Values are based on a 2,000 calorie diet.	

INGREDIENTS: Water, liquid soybean oil, partially hydrogenated soybean oil, sweet cream, buttermilk, gelatin, salt, vegetable mono- and diglycerides, soy lecithin, lactic acid, artificial flavor, vitamin A, colored with beta carotene.

Margarine (liquid)

Nutrition Facts
Serving size 1 Tbsp (14g)
Servings Per Container 32

Amount per serving	
Calories 60	Calories from Fat 60
	%Daily Value*
Total Fat 7g	10%
Saturated Fat 1g	6%
Polyunsaturated Fat 4g	
Monounsaturated Fat 1.5g	
Cholesterol 0mg	0%
Sodium 85mg	3%
Total Carbohydrate 0g	0%
Protein 0g	
Vitamin A 10%	
Not a significant source of dietary fiber, sugars, vitamin C, calcium, and iron.	
*Percent Daily Values are based on a 2,000 calorie diet.	

INGREDIENTS: Liquid soybean oil, water, sweet cream buttermilk, salt, partially hydrogenated cottonseed oil, vegetable mono- and diglycerides, soy lecithin, citric acid, artificial flavor, vitamin A, colored with beta carotene.

If people were to make only one change in their diets, they would be wise to limit their intakes of saturated fat. Sometimes these choices can be difficult, though, because fats make foods taste delicious. To maintain good health, must a person give up all high-fat foods forever—never again to eat marbled steak, hollandaise sauce, or gooey chocolate cake? Not at all. These foods bring pleasure to a meal and can be enjoyed as part of a healthy diet when eaten in small quantities on occasion, but it is true that they are not everyday foods. The key word for fat is not deprivation, but moderation: Appreciate the energy and enjoyment that fat provides, but take care not to exceed your needs.

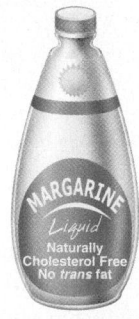

HOW TO Calculate a Personal Daily Value for Fat

The % Daily Value for fat on food labels is based on 65 grams. To know how your intake compares with this recommendation, you can either count grams until you reach 65, or add the "% Daily Values" until you reach 100 percent—if your energy intake is 2000 kcalories a day. If your energy intake is more or less, you have a couple of options.

You can calculate your personal daily fat allowance in grams. Suppose your energy intake is 1800 kcalories per day and your goal is 30 percent kcalories from fat. Multiply your total energy intake by 30 percent, then divide by 9:

$$1800 \text{ total kcal} \times 0.30 \text{ from fat} = 540 \text{ fat kcal.}$$
$$540 \text{ fat kcal} \div 9 \text{ kcal/g} = 60 \text{ g fat.}$$

Another way to calculate your personal fat allowance is to cross out the last digit of your energy intake and divide by 3. For example, 1800 kcalories becomes 180; then you divide by 3:

$$180 \div 3 = 60 \text{ g fat/day.}$$

(In familiar measures, 60 grams of fat is about the same as ⅔ stick of butter or ¼ cup of oil.)

The accompanying table shows the numbers of grams of fat allowed per day for various energy intakes. With one of these numbers in mind, you can quickly evaluate the number of fat grams in foods you are considering eating.

Energy (kcal/day)	20% kCalories from Fat	35% kCalories from Fat	Fat (g/day)
1200	240	420	27–47
1400	280	490	31–54
1600	320	560	36–62
1800	360	630	40–70
2000	400	700	44–78
2200	440	770	49–86
2400	480	840	53–93
2600	520	910	58–101
2800	560	980	62–109
3000	600	1050	67–117

HOW TO Understand "% Daily Value" and "% kCalories from Fat"

The "% Daily Value" that is used on food labels to describe the amount of fat in a food is not the same as the "% kcalories from fat" that is used in dietary recommendations to describe the amount of fat in the diet. They may appear similar, but their difference is worth understanding. Consider, for example, a piece of lemon meringue pie that provides 140 kcalories and 12 grams of fat. Because the Daily Value for fat is 65 grams for a 2000-kcalorie intake, 12 grams represent about 18 percent:

$$12 \text{ g} \div 65 \text{ g} = 0.18.$$
$$0.18 \times 100 = 18\%.$$

The pie's "% Daily Value" is 18 percent, or almost one-fifth, of the day's fat allowance.

Uninformed consumers may mistakenly believe that this food meets recommendations to limit fat to "20 to 35 percent kcalories,"but it doesn't—for two reasons. First, the pie's 12 grams of fat contribute 108 of the 140 kcalories, for a total of 77 percent kcalories from fat:

$$12 \text{ g fat} \times 9 \text{ kcal/g} = 108 \text{ kcal.}$$
$$108 \text{ kcal} \div 140 \text{ kcal} = 77\%.$$

Second, the "percent kcalories from fat" guideline applies to a day's total intake, not to an individual food. Of course, if every selection throughout the day exceeds 35 percent kcalories from fat, you can be certain that the day's total intake will, too.

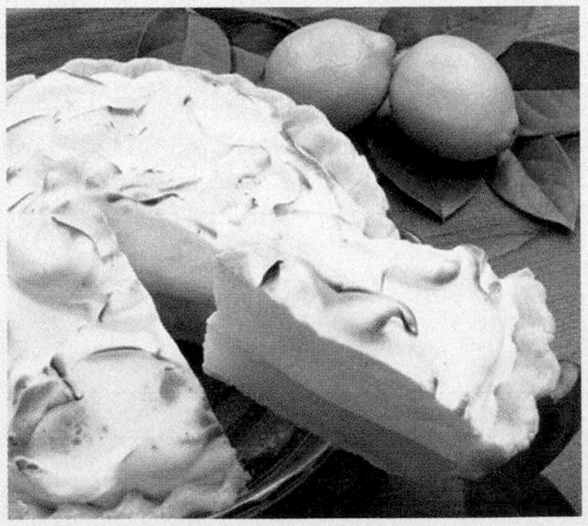

Whether a person's energy and fat allowance can afford a piece of lemon meringue pie depends on the other food and activity choices made that day.

Nutrition in Your Life

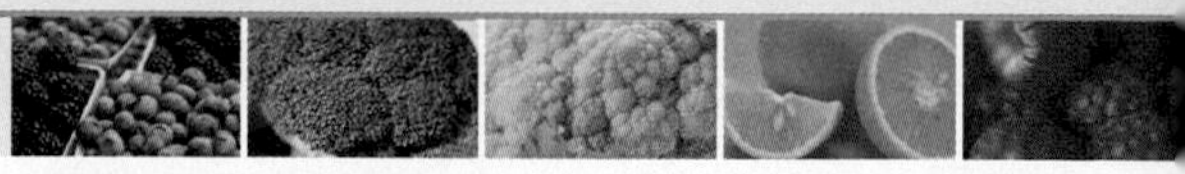

To maintain good health, eat enough, but not too much, fat and select the right kinds.

- **Do you use polyunsaturated and monounsaturated vegetable oils instead of animal fats, hard margarine, and partially hydrogenated shortenings?**
- **Do you choose fat-free or low-fat milk products and lean meats, fish, and poultry?**
- **Do you eat fish at least twice a week? If not, does your diet include other sources of omega-3 fatty acids?**

NUTRITION ON THE NET

Access these websites for further study of topics covered in this chapter.

- Find updates and quick links to these and other nutrition-related sites at our website: **www.wadsworth.com/nutrition**
- Search for "cholesterol" and "dietary fat" at the U.S. Government health information site: **www.healthfinder.gov**
- Review the American Dietetic Association's *ABC's of Fats, Oils, and Cholesterol:* **www.eatright.org/nfs2.html**
- Search for "fat" at the International Food Information Council site: **www.ific.org**
- Find dietary strategies to prevent heart disease at the American Heart Association: **www.americanheart.org**

NUTRITION CALCULATIONS

These problems will give you practice in doing simple nutrition-related calculations (see p. 172 for answers). Show your calculations for each problem.

1. Be aware of the fats in milks. Following are four categories of milk.

	Wt (g)	Fat (g)	Prot (g)	Carb (g)
Milk A (1 c)	244	8	8	12
Milk B (1 c)	244	5	8	12
Milk C (1 c)	244	3	8	12
Milk D (1 c)	244	0	8	12

   a. Based on *weight,* what percentage of each milk is fat (round off to a whole number)?

   b. How much energy from fat will a person receive from drinking 1 cup of each milk?

   c. How much total energy will the person receive from 1 cup of each milk?

   d. What percentage of the energy in each milk comes from fat?

   e. In the grocery store, how is each milk labeled?

2. Judge foods' fat contents by their labels.

   a. A food label says that one serving of the food contains 6.5 grams fat. What would the % Daily Value for fat be? What does the Daily Value you just calculated mean?

   b. How many kcalories from fat does a serving contain? (Round off to the nearest whole number.)

   c. If a *serving* of the food contains 200 kcalories, what percentage of the energy is from fat?

This example should show you how easy it is to evaluate foods' fat contents by reading labels and to see the difference between the % Daily Value and the percentage of kcalories from fat.

3. Now consider a piece of carrot cake. Remember that the Daily Value suggests 65 grams of fat as acceptable within a 2000-kcalorie diet. A serving of carrot cake provides 30 grams of fat. What percentage of the Daily Value is that? What does this mean?

STUDY QUESTIONS

These questions will help you review this chapter. You will find the answers in the discussions on the pages provided.

1. Name three classes of lipids found in the body and in foods. What are some of their functions in the body? What features do fats bring to foods? (pp. 141, 155–157)
2. What features distinguish fatty acids from each other? (pp. 142–145)
3. What does the term *omega* mean with respect to fatty acids? Describe the roles of the omega fatty acids in disease prevention. (pp. 144,160–161)
4. What are the differences between saturated, unsaturated, monounsaturated, and polyunsaturated fatty acids? Describe the structure of a triglyceride. (pp. 142–145)
5. What does hydrogenation do to fats? What are *trans*-fatty acids, and how do they influence heart disease? (pp. 146, 159)
6. How do phospholipids differ from triglycerides in structure? How does cholesterol differ? How do these differences in structure affect function? (pp. 148–149)
7. What roles do phospholipids perform in the body? What roles does cholesterol play in the body? (pp. 148–149)
8. Trace the steps in fat digestion, absorption, and transport. Describe the routes cholesterol takes in the body. (pp. 150–153)
9. What do lipoproteins do? What are the differences among the chylomicrons, VLDL, LDL, and HDL? (pp. 153–154)
10. Which of the fatty acids are essential? Name their chief dietary sources. (pp. 156–157)
11. How does excessive fat intake influence health? What factors influence LDL, HDL, and total blood cholesterol? (pp. 159–162)
12. What are the dietary recommendations regarding fat and cholesterol intake? List ways to reduce intake. (pp. 162–166)
13. What is the Daily Value for fat (for a 2000-kcalorie diet)? What does this number represent? (pp. 162, 168)

These multiple choice questions will help you prepare for an exam. Answers can be found on p. 172.

1. Saturated fatty acids:
   a. are always 18 carbons long.
   b. have at least one double bond.
   c. are fully loaded with hydrogens.
   d. are always liquid at room temperature.
2. A triglyceride consists of:
   a. three glycerols attached to a lipid.
   b. three fatty acids attached to a glucose.
   c. three fatty acids attached to a glycerol.
   d. three phospholipids attached to a cholesterol.
3. The difference between *cis*- and *trans*-fatty acids is:
   a. the number of double bonds.
   b. the length of their carbon chains.
   c. the location of the first double bond.
   d. the configuration around the double bond.
4. Which of the following is *not* true? Lecithin is:
   a. an emulsifier.
   b. a phospholipid.
   c. an essential nutrient.
   d. a constituent of cell membranes.
5. Chylomicrons are produced in the:
   a. liver.
   b. pancreas.
   c. gallbladder.
   d. small intestine.
6. Transport vehicles for lipids are called:
   a. micelles.
   b. lipoproteins.
   c. blood vessels.
   d. monoglycerides.
7. The lipoprotein most associated with a high risk of heart disease is:
   a. CHD.
   b. HDL.
   c. LDL.
   d. LPL.
8. Which of the following is not true? Fats:
   a. contain glucose.
   b. provide energy.
   c. protect against organ shock.
   d. carry vitamins A, D, E, and K.
9. The essential fatty acids include:
   a. stearic acid and oleic acid.
   b. oleic acid and linoleic acid.
   c. palmitic acid and linolenic acid.
   d. linoleic acid and linolenic acid.
10. A person consuming 2200 kcalories a day who wants to meet health recommendations should limit daily fat intake to:
    a. 20 to 35 grams.
    b. 50 to 85 grams.
    c. 75 to 100 grams.
    d. 90 to 130 grams.

REFERENCES

1. C. T. Phan and P. Tso, Intestinal lipid absorption and transport, *Frontiers in Bioscience* 6 (2001): 299–319.
2. L. Brown and coauthors, Cholesterol-lowering effects of dietary fiber: A meta-analysis, *American Journal of Clinical Nutrition* 69 (1999): 30–42.
3. A. Andersson and coauthors, Fatty acid composition of skeletal muscle reflects dietary fat composition in humans, *American Journal of Clinical Nutrition* 76 (2002): 1222–1229; A. Baylin and coauthors, Adipose tissue biomarkers of fatty acid intake, *American Journal of Clinical Nutrition* 76 (2002): 750–757.
4. C. Bruce, R. A. Chouinard, Jr., and A. R. Tall, Plasma lipid transfer proteins, high-density lipoproteins, and reverse cholesterol transport, *Annual Review of Nutrition* 18 (1998): 297–330.
5. C. D. Berdanier, *Advanced Nutrition: Macronutrients* (Boca Raton, Fla.: CRC Press, 2000), pp. 273–280.
6. R. Uauy and P. Mena, Lipids and neurodevelopment, *Nutrition Reviews* 59 (2001): S34–S48.
7. D. Hwang, Fatty acids and immune responses—A new perspective in searching for clues to mechanism, *Annual Review of Nutrition* 20 (2000): 431–456; O. Morteau, Prostaglandins and inflammation: The cyclooxygenase controversy, *Archivum Immunologiae et Therapiae Experimentalis* 48 (2000): 473–480.
8. J. R. Hibbeln, Seafood consumption, the DHA content of mothers' milk and prevalence rates of postpartum depression: A cross-national, ecological analysis, *Journal of Affective Disorders* 69 (2002): 15–29; K. A. Bruinsma and D. L. Taren, Dieting, essential fatty acid intake, and depression, *Nutrition Reviews* 58 (2000): 98–108; A. L. Stoll and coauthors, Omega 3 fatty acids in bipolar disorder: A preliminary double-blind placebo-controlled trial, *Archives of General Psychiatry* 56 (1999): 407–412.
9. L. Zimmer and coauthors, The dopamine mesocorticolimbic pathway is affected by deficiency in n-3 polyunsaturated fatty acids, *American Journal of Clinical Nutrition* 75 (2002): 662–667.
10. J. Stamler and coauthors, Relationship of baseline serum cholesterol levels in 3 large cohorts of younger men to long-term coronary, cardiovascular, and all-cause mortality and to longevity, *Journal of the American Medical Association* 284 (2000): 311–318; D. Steinberg and A. M. Gotto, Preventing coronary artery disease by lowering cholesterol levels, *Journal of the American Medical Association* 282 (1999): 2043–2050.
11. F. D. Kelly and coauthors, A stearic acid–rich diet improves thrombogenic and atherogenic risk factor profiles in healthy males, *European Journal of Clinical Nutrition* 55 (2001): 88–96; F. B. Hu and coauthors, Dietary saturated fats and their food sources in relation to the risk of coronary heart disease in women, *American Journal of Clinical Nutrition* 70 (1999): 1001–1008; W. E. Connor, Harbingers of coronary heart disease: Dietary saturated fatty acids and cholesterol—Is chocolate benign because of its stearic acid content? *American Journal of Clinical Nutrition* 70 (1999): 951–952.
12. Hu and coauthors, 1999.
13. J. I. Pederson and coauthors, Adipose tissue fatty acids and risk of myocardial infarction, *European Journal of Clinical Nutrition* 54 (2000): 618–625.
14. M. B. Katan, *Trans* fatty acids and plasma lipoproteins, *Nutrition Reviews* 58 (2000): 188–191.
15. D. B. Allison and coauthors, Estimated intakes of *trans* fatty and other fatty acids in the US population, *Journal of the American Dietetic Association* 99 (1999): 166–174.
16. M. A. Denke, B. Adams-Huet, and A. T. Nguyen, Individual cholesterol variation in response to a margarine- or butter-based diet: A study in families, *Journal of the American Medical Association* 284 (2000): 2740–2747; A. H. Lichtenstein and coauthors, Effects of different forms of dietary hydrogenated fats on serum lipoprotein cholesterol levels, *New England Journal of Medicine* 340 (1999): 1933–1940.
17. W. D. Song and J. M. Kerver, Nutritional contribution of eggs to American diets, *Journal of the American College of Nutrition* 19 (2000): 556S–562S; S. B. Kritchevsky and D. Kritchevsky, Egg consumption and coronary heart disease: An epidemiologic review, *Journal of the American College of Nutrition* 19 (2000): 549S–555S; F. B. Hu and coauthors, A prospective study of egg consumption and risk of cardiovascular disease in men and women, *Journal of the American Medical Association* 281 (1999): 1387–1394.
18. Song and Kerver, 2000.
19. Lichtenstein and coauthors, 1999.
20. C. Thomsen and coauthors, Differential effects of saturated and monounsaturated fatty acids on postprandial lipemia and incretin responses in healthy subjects, *American Journal of Clinical Nutrition* 69 (1999): 1135–1143.
21. A. H. Stark and Z. Madar, Olive oil as a functional food: Epidemiology and nutritional approaches, *Nutrition Reviews* 60 (2002): 170–176.
22. F. B. Hu and coauthors, Fish and omega-3 fatty acid intake and risk of coronary heart disease in women, *Journal of the American Medical Association* 287 (2002): 1815–1821; C. M. Albert and coauthors, Blood levels of long-chain n-3 fatty acids and the risk of sudden death, *New England Journal of Medicine* 346 (2002): 1113–1118; C. von Schacky, n-3 Fatty acids and the prevention of coronary atherosclerosis, *American Journal of Clinical Nutrition* 71 (2000): 224S–227S.
23. P. J. H. Jones and V. W. Y. Lau, Effect of n-3 polyunsaturated fatty acids on risk reduction of sudden death, *Nutrition Reviews* 60 (2002): 407–413; P. J. Nestel, Fish oil and cardiovascular disease: Lipids and arterial function, *American Journal of Clinical Nutrition* 71 (2000): 228S–231S.
24. E. Guallar and coauthors, Mercury, fish oils, and the risk of myocardial infarction, *New England Journal of Medicine* 347 (2002): 1747–1754.
25. AHA Dietary Guidelines, published online on October 5, 2000, **http://circ.ahajournals.org/cgi/content/full/4304635102**.
26. K. He and coauthors, Fish consumption and risk of stroke in men, *Journal of the American Medical Association* 288 (2002): 3130–3136.
27. T. A. Mori and coauthors, Dietary fish as a major component of a weight-loss diet: Effect on serum lipids, glucose, and insulin metabolism in overweight hypertensive subjects, *American Journal of Clinical Nutrition* 70 (1999): 817–825.
28. L. Cordain and coauthors, Fatty acid analysis of wild ruminant tissues: Evolutionary implications for reducing diet-related chronic disease, *European Journal of Clinical Nutrition* 56 (2002): 181–191.
29. T. A. Mori and L. J. Beilin, Long-chain omega 3 fatty acids, blood lipids and cardiovascular risk reduction, *Current Opinion in Lipidology* 12 (2001): 11–17.
30. S. Bechoua and coauthors, Influence of very low dietary intake of marine oil on some functional aspects of immune cells in healthy elderly people, *British Journal of Nutrition* 89 (2003): 523–532; F. Thies and coauthors, Dietary supplementation with eicosapentaenoic acid, but not with other long-chain n-3 or n-6 polyunsaturated fatty acids, decreases natural killer cell activity in healthy subjects aged >55 y, *American Journal of Clinical Nutrition* 73 (2001): 539–548; V. M. Montori and coauthors, Fish oil supplementation in type 2 diabetes: A quantitative systematic review, *Diabetes Care* 23 (2000): 1407–1415.
31. P. M. Kris-Etherton and coauthors, AHA Scientific Statement: Fish consumption, fish oil, omega-3 fatty acids, and cardiovascular disease, *Circulation* 106 (2002): 2747–2757.
32. P. L. Zock, Dietary fats and cancer, *Current Opinion in Lipidology* 12 (2001): 5–10.
33. M. M. Lee and S. S. Lin, Dietary fat and breast cancer, *Annual Review of Nutrition* 20 (2000): 221–248; E. B. Feldman, Breast cancer risk and intake of fat, *Nutrition Reviews* 57 (1999): 353–356.
34. M. D. Holmes and coauthors, Association of dietary intake of fat and fatty acids with risk of breast cancer, *Journal of the American Medical Association* 281 (1999): 914–920.
35. A. R. Kristal and coauthors, Associations of energy, fat, calcium, and vitamin D with prostate cancer risk, *Cancer Epidemiology, Biomarkers and Prevention* 11 (2002): 719–725; L. N. Kolonel, A. M. Nomura, and R. V. Cooney, Dietary fat and prostate cancer: Current status, *Journal of the National Cancer Institute* 91 (1999): 414–428; J. A. Thomas, Diet, micronutrients, and the prostate gland, *Nutrition Reviews* 57 (1999): 95–103.
36. R. F. Gimble and coauthors, The ability of fish oil to suppress tumor necrosis factor α production by peripheral blood mononuclear cells in healthy men is associated with polymorphisms in genes that influence tumor necrosis factor α production, *American Journal of Clinical Nutrition* 76 (2002): 454–459; L. Guangming and coauthors, Omega 3 but not omega 6 fatty acids inhibit AP-1 activity and cell transformation in JB6 cells, *Proceedings of the National Academy of Sciences* 98 (2001): 7510–7515; P. Terry and coauthors, Fatty fish consumption and risk of prostate cancer, *Lancet* 357 (2001): 1764–1766; E. D. Collett and coauthors, n-6 and n-3 polyunsaturated fatty acids differentially modulate oncogenic Ras activation in colonocytes, *American Journal of Physiology: Cell Physiology* 280 (2001): C1066–C1075; E. Fernandez and coauthors, Fish consumption and cancer risk, *American Journal of Clinical Nutrition* 70 (1999): 85–90.
37. Committee on Dietary Reference Intakes, *Dietary Reference Intakes for Energy, Carbohydrate, Fiber, Fat, Fatty Acids, Cholesterol, Protein, and Amino Acids* (Washington, D.C.: National Academies Press, 2002).
38. Committee on Dietary Reference Intakes, 2002.
39. Committee on Dietary Reference Intakes, 2002.
40. N. D. Ernst and coauthors, Consistency between US dietary fat intake and serum

total cholesterol concentrations: The National Health and Nutrition Examination Surveys, *American Journal of Clinical Nutrition* 66 (1997): 965S–972S; National Center for Health Statistics, www.cdc.gov/nchs, site visited on November 6, 2000.
41. P. J. Horvath and coauthors, The effects of varying dietary fat on performance and metabolism in trained male and female runners, *Journal of the American College of Nutrition* 19 (2000): 52–60; P. J. Horvath and coauthors, The effects of varying dietary fat on the nutrient intake in trained male and female runners, *Journal of the American College of Nutrition* 19 (2000): 42–51.
42. D. R. Pendergast, J. J. Leddy, and J. T. Venkatraman, A perspective on fat intake in athletes, *Journal of the American College of Nutrition* 19 (2000): 345–350.
43. Committee on Dietary Reference Intakes, 2002; Pendergast, 2000.
44. S. Tonstad, K. Smerud, and L. Høie, A comparison of the effects of 2 doses of soy protein or casein on serum lipids, serum lipoproteins, and plasma total homocysteine in hyper-cholesterolemic subjects, *American Journal of Clinical Nutrition* 76 (2002): 78–84; S. R. Teixeira and coauthors, Effects of feeding 4 levels of soy protein for 3 and 6 wk on blood lipids and apolipoproteins in moderately hypercholesterolemic men, *American Journal of Clinical Nutrition* 71 (2000): 1077–1084.
45. M. Pfeuffer and J. Schrezenmeir, Bioactive substances in milk with properties decreasing risk of cardiovascular diseases, *British Journal of Nutrition* 84 (2000): S155–S159.
46. B. M. Davy and coauthors, High-fiber oat cereal compared with wheat cereal consumption favorably alters LDL-cholesterol subclass and particle numbers in middle-aged and older men, *American Journal of Clinical Nutrition* 76 (2002): 351–358; D. J. A. Jenkins and coauthors, Soluble fiber intake at a dose approved by the US Food and Drug Administration for a claim of health benefits: Serum lipid risk factors for cardiovascular disease assessed in a randomized controlled crossover trial, *American Journal of Clinical Nutrition* 75 (2002): 834–839; L. Van Horn and N. Ernst, A summary of the science supporting the new National Cholesterol Education program dietary recommendations: What dietitians should know, *Journal of the American Dietetic Association* 101 (2001): 1148–1154; M. L. Fernandez, Soluble fiber and nondigestible carbohydrate effects on plasma lipids and cardiovascular risk, *Current Opinion in Lipidology* 12 (2001): 35–40; J. W. Anderson and coauthors, Cholesterol-lowering effects of psyllium intake adjunctive to diet therapy in men and women with hypercholesterolemia: A meta-analysis of 8 controlled trials, *American Journal of Clinical Nutrition* 71 (2000): 472–479; M. P. St. Onge, E. R. Farnworth, and P. J. H. Jones, Consumption of fermented and nonfermented dairy products: Effects on cholesterol concentrations and metabolism, *American Journal of Clinical Nutrition* 71 (2000): 674–681; Brown and coauthors, 1999.
47. B. M. Popkin and coauthors, Where's the fat? Trends in U.S. diets 1965–1996, *Preventive Medicine* 32 (2001): 245–254.
48. P. J. H. Jones and coauthors, Cholesterol-lowering efficacy of a sitostanol-containing phytosterol mixture with a prudent diet in hyperlipidemic men, *American Journal of Clinical Nutrition* 69 (1999): 1144–1150; M. A. Hallikainen and M. I. J. Uusitupa, Effects of 2 low-fat stanol ester-containing margarines on serum cholesterol concentrations as part of a low-fat diet in hypercholesterolemic subjects, *American Journal of Clinical Nutrition* 69 (1999): 403–410.
49. J. G. Dausch, Trans-fatty acids: A regulatory update, *Journal of the American Dietetic Association* 102 (2002): 18.

ANSWERS

Nutrition Calculations

1. a. Milk A: 8 g fat ÷ 244 g total = 0.03; 0.03 × 100 = 3%.
   Milk B: 5 g fat ÷ 244 g total = 0.02; 0.02 × 100 = 2%.
   Milk C: 3 g fat ÷ 244 g total = 0.01; 0.01 × 100 = 1%.
   Milk D: 0 g fat ÷ 244 g total = 0.00; 0.00 × 100 = 0%.
   b. Milk A: 8 g fat × 9 kcal/g = 72 kcal from fat.
   Milk B: 5 g fat × 9 kcal/g = 45 kcal from fat.
   Milk C: 3 g fat × 9 kcal/g = 27 kcal from fat.
   Milk D: 0 g fat × 9 kcal/g = 0 kcal from fat.
   c. Milk A: (8 g fat × 9 kcal/g) + (8 g prot × 4 kcal/g) + (12 g carb × 4 kcal/g) = 152 kcal.
   Milk B: (5 g fat × 9 kcal/g) + (8 g prot × 4 kcal/g) + (12 g carb × 4 kcal/g) = 125 kcal.
   Milk C: (3 g fat × 9 kcal/g) + (8 g prot × 4 kcal/g) + (12 g carb × 4 kcal/g) = 107 kcal.
   Milk D: (0 g fat × 9 kcal/g) + (8 g prot × 4 kcal/g) + (12 g carb × 4 kcal/g) = 80 kcal.
   d. Milk A: 72 kcal from fat ÷ 152 total kcal = 0.47; 0.47 × 100 = 47%.
   Milk B: 45 kcal from fat ÷ 125 total kcal = 0.36; 0.36 × 100 = 36%.
   Milk C: 27 kcal from fat ÷ 107 total kcal = 0.25; 0.25 × 100 = 25%.
   Milk D: 0 kcal from fat ÷ 80 total kcal = 0.00; 0.00 × 100 = 0%.
   e. Milk A: whole.
   Milk B: reduced-fat, 2%, or less-fat.
   Milk C: low-fat or 1%.
   Milk D: fat-free, nonfat, skim, zero-fat, or no-fat.
2. a. 6.5 g ÷ 65 g = 0.1; 0.1 × 100 = 10%. A Daily Value of 10% means that one serving of this food contributes about 1⁄10 of the day's fat allotment.
   b. 6.5 g × 9 kcal/g = 58.5, rounded to 59 kcal from fat.
   c. (59 kcal from fat ÷ 200 kcal) × 100 = 30% kcalories from fat.
3. (30 g fat ÷ 65 g fat) × 100 = 46% of the Daily Value for fat; this means that almost half of the day's fat allotment would be used in this one dessert.

Study Questions (multiple choice)

1. c 2. c 3. d 4. c 5. d 6. b 7. c 8. a 9. d 10. b

HIGHLIGHT

High-Fat Foods—Friend or Foe?

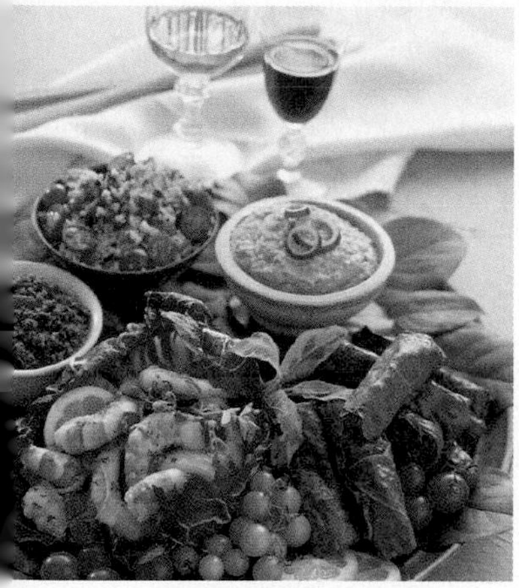

© Philip Salavery/FoodPix/Getty Images

Eat less fat. Eat more fatty fish. Give up butter. Use margarine. Give up margarine. Use olive oil. Steer clear of saturated. Seek out omega-3. Stay away from *trans*. Stick with mono- and polyunsaturated. Keep fat intake moderate. Today's fat messages seem to be forever multiplying and changing. No wonder people feel confused about dietary fat. The confusion stems in part from the complexities of fat and in part from the nature of recommendations. As Chapter 5 explained, "dietary fat" refers to several kinds of fats, some fats support health whereas others damage it, and foods typically provide a mixture of fats in varying proportions. It has taken researchers decades to sort through the relationships between the various kinds of fat and their roles in supporting or harming health. Translating these research findings into dietary recommendations is a challenging process. Too little information can mislead consumers, but too much detail can overwhelm them. As research findings accumulate, recommendations slowly evolve and become more refined. That's where we are with fat recommendations today—refining them from the general to the specific. Though they may seem to be "forever multiplying and changing," in fact, they are becoming more meaningful.

This highlight begins with a look at these changing guidelines. It continues by identifying which foods provide which fats and presenting the Mediterranean diet, an example of a food plan that embraces the heart-healthy fats. It closes with strategies to help consumers choose the right amounts of the right kinds of fats for a healthy diet.

Changing Guidelines for Fat Intake

Dietary recommendations for fat have changed in recent years, shifting the emphasis from lowering total fat, in general, to limiting saturated and *trans* fat, specifically. For decades, health experts advised limiting intakes of total fat to 30 percent or less of energy intake. They recognized that saturated fats and *trans* fats were the ones that raise blood cholesterol, but reasoned that by limiting total fat intake, saturated and *trans* fat intake would decline as well. People were simply advised to cut back on all fat so that they would cut back on saturated and *trans* fat. Such advice may have oversimplified the message and unnecessarily restricted total fat.

Low-fat diets have a place in treatment plans for people with elevated blood lipids or heart disease, but researchers question the wisdom of such diets for healthy people as a means of controlling weight and preventing diseases.[1] Several problems accompany low-fat diets. For one, many people find low-fat diets difficult to maintain over time.[2] For another, low-fat diets are not necessarily low-kcalorie diets; if energy intake exceeds energy needs, weight gain follows, and obesity brings a host of health problems, including heart disease. For still another, diets extremely low in fat may exclude fatty fish, nuts, seeds, and vegetable oils—all valuable sources of many essential fatty acids, phytochemicals, vitamins, and minerals. Importantly, the fats from these sources protect against heart disease, as later sections of this highlight explain.

Today, health experts have revised dietary recommendations to acknowledge that not all fats have damaging health consequences. In fact, higher intakes of some kinds of fats (for example, the omega-3 fatty acids) support good health. Instead of urging people to cut back on all fats, current recommendations suggest carefully replacing the "bad" saturated fats with the "good" unsaturated fats and enjoying them in moderation.[3] The goal is to create a diet moderate in kcalories that provides enough of the fats that support good health, but not too much of those that harm health. (Turn to pp. 159–160 for a review of the health consequences of each type of fat.)

With these findings and goals in mind, the DRI committee recently established a healthy range of 20 to 35 percent of energy intake from fat. This range appears to be compatible with low rates of heart disease, diabetes, obesity, and cancer.[4] Heart-healthy recommendations suggest that within this range, consumers should try to minimize their intakes of saturated fat, *trans* fat, and cholesterol and use monounsaturated and polyunsaturated fats instead.[5]

Asking consumers to limit their total fat intake was less than perfect advice, but it was straightforward—find the fat and cut back. Asking consumers to keep their intakes of saturated fats, *trans* fats, and cholesterol low and to use monounsaturated and polyunsaturated fats instead may be more on target with heart health, but it also makes diet planning more complicated. To make appropriate selections, consumers must first learn which foods contain which fats.

High-Fat Foods and Heart Health

Avocados, bacon, walnuts, potato chips, and mackerel are all high-fat foods, yet some of these foods have detrimental effects on heart health when consumed in excess, while others seem neutral or even beneficial. This section presents some of the accumulating evidence that helped to distinguish which high-fat foods belong in a healthy diet and which ones need to be kept to a minimum. As you will see, a little more fat in the diet may be compatible with heart health, but only if the great majority of it is the unsaturated kind.

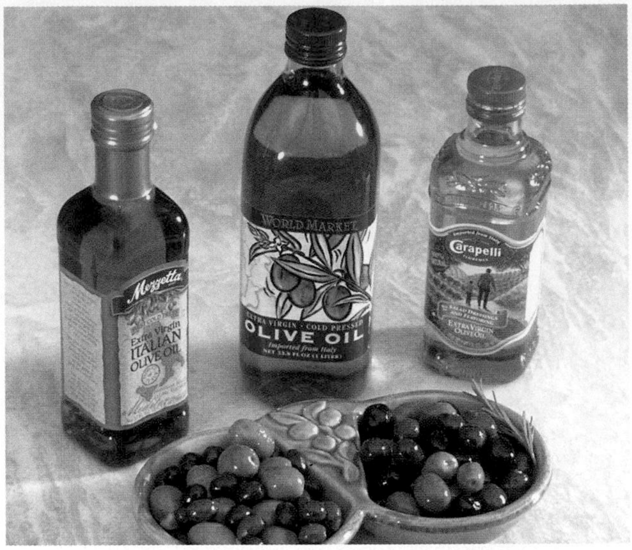
WORLD MARKET
OLIVE OIL
Carapelli
Matthew Farruggio

Olives and their oil may benefit heart health.

Cook with Olive Oil

As it turns out, the traditional diets of Greece and other countries in the Mediterranean region offer an excellent example of eating patterns that use "good" fats liberally. Often, these diets are rich in olives and their oil. A classic study of the world's people, the Seven Countries Study, found that death rates from heart disease were strongly associated with diets high in saturated fats, but only weakly linked with total fat.[6] In fact, the two countries with the highest fat intakes, Finland and the Greek island of Crete, had the highest (Finland) and lowest (Crete) rates of heart disease deaths. In both countries, the people consumed 40 percent or more of their kcalories from fat. Clearly, a high-fat diet was not the primary problem, so researchers refocused their attention on the type of fat. They began to notice the benefits of olive oil.

A diet that uses olive oil instead of other cooking fats, especially butter, stick margarine, and meat fats, may offer numerous health benefits.[7] Olive oil helps to protect against heart disease by:

- Lowering total and LDL cholesterol and not lowering HDL cholesterol or raising triglycerides.[8]
- Lowering LDL cholesterol susceptibility to oxidation.[9]
- Lowering blood-clotting factors.[10]
- Providing phytochemicals that act as antioxidants (see Highlight 11).[11]
- Lowering blood pressure.[12]

When compared with other fats, olive oil seems to be a wise choice, but controlled clinical trials are too scarce to support population-wide recommendations to switch to a high-fat diet rich in olive oil.[13] Importantly, olive oil is not a magic potion; drizzling it on foods does not make them healthier. Like other fats, olive oil delivers 9 kcalories per gram, which can contribute to weight gain in people who fail to balance their energy intake with their energy output. Its role in a healthy diet is to *replace* the saturated fats. Other vegetable oils, such as canola or safflower oil, in their liquid unhydrogenated states, are also generally low in saturated fats and high in unsaturated fats. For this reason, heart-healthy diets use these unsaturated vegetable oils as substitutes for the more saturated fats of butter, hydrogenated stick margarine, lard, or shortening. (Remember that the tropical oils—coconut, palm, and palm kernel—are too saturated to be included with the heart-healthy vegetable oils.)

Nibble on Nuts

Tree nuts and peanuts are traditionally excluded from low-fat diets, and for good reasons. Nuts provide up to 80 percent of their kcalories from fat, and a quarter cup (about an ounce) of mixed nuts provides over 200 kcalories. In a recent review of the literature, however, researchers found that people who ate a one-ounce serving of nuts on five or more days a week had a reduced risk of heart disease compared with people consuming no nuts.[14] A smaller positive association was noted for any amount greater than one serving of nuts a week. The nuts were those commonly eaten in the United States: almonds, Brazil nuts, cashews, hazelnuts, macadamia nuts, pecans, pistachios, walnuts, and even peanuts. On average, these nuts contain mostly monounsaturated fat (59 percent), some polyunsaturated fat (27 percent), and little saturated fat (14 percent).[15]

Research has shown a benefit from walnuts and almonds in particular. In study after study, walnuts, when substituted for other fats in the diet, produce favorable effects on blood lipids—even in people with elevated total and LDL cholesterol.[16] Results are similar for almonds. In one study, researchers gave men and women one of three kinds of snacks, all of equal kcalories: whole-wheat muffins, almonds (about 2½ ounces), or half muffins and half almonds.[17] At the end of a month, people receiving the full almond snack had the greatest drop in blood LDL cholesterol; those eating the half almond snack had a lesser, but still significant drop in blood lipids; and those eating the muffin-only snack had no change.

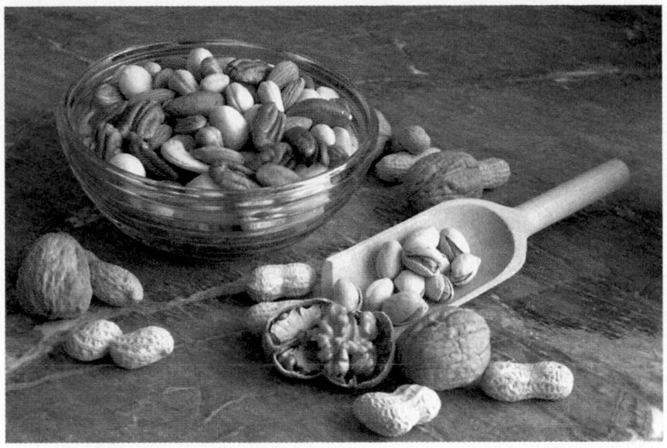
Matthew Farruggio

For heart health, snack on nuts instead of potato chips.

Studies on peanuts, macadamia nuts, pecans, and pistachios follow suit, indicating that including nuts may be a wise strategy against heart disease. Nuts may protect against heart disease because they provide:

- Monounsaturated and polyunsaturated fats in abundance, but few saturated fats.
- Fiber, vegetable protein, and other valuable nutrients, including the antioxidant vitamin E (see Highlight 11).
- Phytochemicals that act as antioxidants (see Highlight 13).

Before advising consumers to include nuts in their diets, a caution is in order. As mentioned, most of the energy nuts provide comes from fats. Consequently, they deliver many kcalories per bite. In studies examining the effects of nuts on heart disease, researchers carefully adjust diets to make room for the nuts without increasing the total kcalories—that is, they use nuts *instead of, not in addition to,* other foods (such as meats, potato chips, oils, margarine, and butter). Consumers who do not make similar replacements could end up gaining weight if they simply add nuts on top of their regular diets. Weight gain, in turn, elevates blood lipids and raises the risks of heart disease.

Feast on Fish

Research into the health benefits of the long-chain omega-3 polyunsaturated fatty acids began with a simple observation: The native peoples of Alaska, northern Canada, and Greenland, who eat a diet rich in omega-3 fatty acids, notably EPA and DHA, have a remarkably low rate of heart disease even though their diets are relatively high in fat.[18] These omega-3 fatty acids help to protect against heart disease by:[19]

- Reducing blood triglycerides.
- Preventing blood clots.
- Protecting against irregular heartbeats.
- Lowering blood pressure.
- Defending against inflammation.
- Serving as precursors to eicosanoids.

For people with hypertension or atherosclerosis, these actions can be life saving. (Chapter 27 presents more details on the action of omega-3 fatty acids in preventing heart disease.)

Research studies have provided strong evidence that increasing omega-3 fatty acids in the diet supports heart health and lowers the rate of deaths from heart disease.[20] For this reason, the American Heart Association recommends including fish in a heart-healthy diet. People who eat some fish each week can lower their risks of heart attack and stroke.[21] Table 5-2 on p. 161 lists fish that provide at least 1 gram of omega-3 fatty acids per serving.

Fish is the best source of EPA and DHA in the diet, but it is also a major source of mercury, an environmental contaminant. Most fish contain at least trace amounts of mercury, but tilefish, swordfish, king mackerel, marlin, and shark have especially high levels. For this reason, the FDA advises pregnant and lactating women, women of childbearing age who may become pregnant, and young children to avoid:

- Tilefish, swordfish, king mackeral, marlin, and shark.

And to limit average weekly consumption of:

- Ocean, coastal, and other commercial fish to 12 ounces (cooked or canned) *or* freshwater fish caught by family and friends to 6 ounces (cooked).

Others may want to adopt this advice as well. In addition to the direct toxic effects of mercury, some (but not all) research suggests that mercury may diminish the health benefits of omega-3 fatty acids.[22] Such findings serve as a reminder that our health depends on the health of our planet. The protective effect of fish in the diet is available, provided that the fish and their surrounding waters are not heavily contaminated. (As Chapter 27 explains, the environmental contaminant mercury, which is common in some fish, may diminish the health benefits of omega-3 fatty acids.)

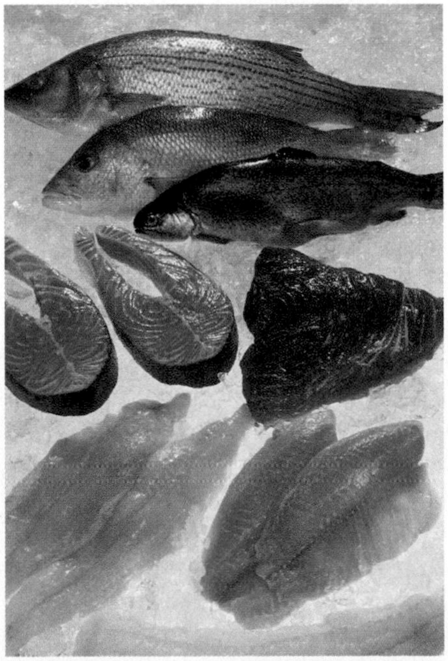
© www.comstock.com

Fish is a good source of the omega-3 fatty acids.

In an effort to limit exposure to pollutants, some consumers choose farm-raised fish. Compared with fish caught in the wild, farm-raised fish do tend to be lower in mercury, but they are also lower in

FIGURE H5-1 Potential Relationships among Dietary Saturated Fatty Acids, LDL Cholesterol, and Heart Disease Risk

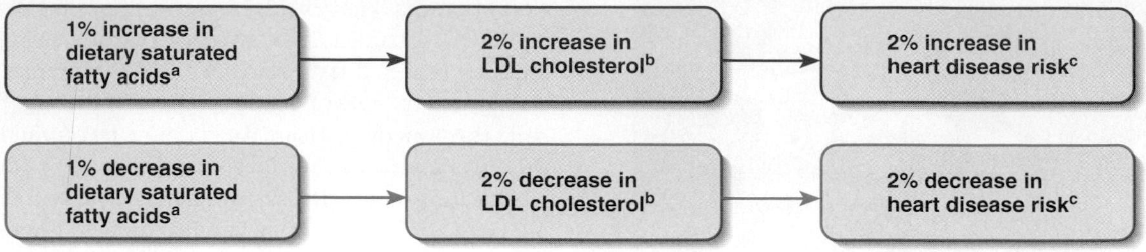
1% increase in dietary saturated fatty acids[a]
2% increase in LDL cholesterol[b]
2% increase in heart disease risk[c]
1% decrease in dietary saturated fatty acids[a]
2% decrease in LDL cholesterol[b]
2% decrease in heart disease risk[c]

[a]Percentage of change in total dietary energy from saturated fatty acids.
[b]Percentage of change in blood LDL cholesterol.
[c]Percentage of change in an individual's risk of heart disease; the percentage of change in risk may increase when blood lipid changes are sustained over time.

SOURCE: Third Report of the National Cholesterol Education Program (NCEP) Expert Panel on Detection, Evaluation, and Treatment of High Blood Cholesterol in Adults (Adult Treatment Panel III), NIH publication no. 02-5215 (Bethesda, Md.: National Heart, Lung, and Blood Institute, 2002), p. V-8 and II-4.

omega-3 fatty acids. When selecting fish, keep the diet strategies of variety and moderation in mind. Varying choices and eating moderate amounts helps to limit the intake of contaminants such as mercury.

High-Fat Foods and Heart Disease

The number one dietary determinant of LDL cholesterol is saturated fat. Figure H5-1 shows that each 1 percent increase in energy from saturated fatty acids in the diet may produce a 2 percent jump in heart disease risk by elevating blood LDL cholesterol. Conversely, reducing saturated fat intake by 1 percent can be expected to produce a 2 percent drop in heart disease risk by the same mechanism. Even a 2 percent drop in LDL represents a significant improvement for the health of the heart.[23] Like saturated fats, *trans* fats also raise heart disease risk by elevating LDL cholesterol. A heart-healthy diet limits foods rich in these two types of fat.

Limit Fatty Meats, Whole-Milk Products, and Tropical Oils

The major sources of saturated fats in the U.S. diet are fatty meats, whole-milk products, tropical oils, and products made from any of these foods. To limit saturated fat intake, consumers must choose carefully among these high-fat foods. Over a third of the fat in most meats is saturated. Similarly, over half of the fat is saturated in whole milk and other high-fat dairy products, such as cheese, butter, cream, half-and-half, cream cheese, sour cream, and ice cream. The tropical oils of palm, palm kernel, and coconut are rarely used by consumers in the kitchen, but are used heavily by food manufacturers and so are commonly found in many commercially prepared foods.

When choosing meats, milk products, and commercially prepared foods, look for those lowest in saturated fat. Labels provide a useful guide for comparing products in this regard, and Appendix H lists the saturated fat in several thousand foods.

Even with careful selections, a nutritionally adequate diet will provide some saturated fat. Zero saturated fat is not possible even when experts design menus with the mission to keep saturated fat as low as possible.[24] Because most saturated fats come from animal foods, vegetarian diets can, and usually do, deliver fewer saturated fats than mixed diets.

Limit Hydrogenated Foods

Chapter 5 explained that solid shortening and margarine are made from vegetable oil that has been hardened through hydrogenation. This process both saturates some of the unsaturated fatty acids and introduces *trans*-fatty acids. Many convenience foods contain *trans* fats, including:

- Fried foods such as french fries, chicken, and other commercially fried foods.
- Commercial baked goods such as cookies, doughnuts, pastries, breads, and crackers.
- Snack foods such as chips.
- Imitation cheeses.

To keep *trans* fat intake low, use these foods sparingly as an occasional taste treat. Chapter 5 describes current labeling regulations for *trans* fats and provides tips for reading food labels.

Table H5-1 summarizes which foods provide which fats. Substituting unsaturated fats for saturated fats at each meal and snack can help protect against heart disease. Table H5-2 provides several examples and shows how such substitutions can lower saturated fat and raise unsaturated fat—even when total fat and kcalories remain unchanged.

TABLE H5-1 Major Sources of Various Fatty Acids

Healthful Fatty Acids

Monounsaturated	Omega-6 Polyunsaturated	Omega-3 Polyunsaturated
Avocado	Margarine (nonyhydrogenated)	Fatty fish (herring, mackerel, salmon, tuna)
Oils (canola, olive, peanut, sesame)	Oils (corn, cottonseed, safflower, soybean)	Flaxseed
Nuts (almonds, cashews, filberts, hazelnuts, macadamia nuts, peanuts, pecans, pistachios)	Nuts (walnuts)	Nuts
Olives	Mayonnaise	
Peanut butter	Salad dressing	
Seeds (sesame)	Seeds (pumpkin, sunflower)	

Harmful Fatty Acids

Saturated	*Trans*
Bacon	Fried foods (hydrogenated shortening)
Butter	Margarine (hydrogenated or partially hydrogenated)
Chocolate	Nondairy creamers
Coconut	Many fast foods
Cream cheese	Shortening
Cream, half-and-half	Commercial baked goods (including doughnuts, cakes, cookies)
Lard	Many snack foods (including microwave popcorn, chips, crackers)
Meat	
Milk and milk products (whole)	
Oils (coconut, palm, palm kernel)	
Shortening	
Sour cream	

NOTE: Keep in mind that foods contain a mixture of fatty acids.

TABLE H5-2 Replacing Saturated Fat with Unsaturated Fat

Examples of ways to replace saturated fats with unsaturated fats include sautéing foods in olive oil instead of butter, garnishing salads with sunflower seeds instead of bacon, snacking on mixed nuts instead of potato chips, using avocado instead of cheese on a sandwich, and eating salmon instead of steak. Portion sizes have been adjusted so that each of these foods provides approximately 100 kcalories. Notice that for a similar number of kcalories and grams of fat, the first choices offer less saturated fat and more unsaturated fat.

	Total Fat (g)	Saturated Fat (g)	Unsaturated Fat (g)
Olive oil vs. butter	11 vs. 11	2 vs. 7	9 vs. 4
Sunflower seeds vs. bacon	8 vs. 9	1 vs. 3	7 vs. 6
Mixed nuts vs. potato chips	9 vs. 7	1 vs. 2	8 vs. 5
Avocado vs. cheese	10 vs. 8	2 vs. 4	8 vs. 4
Salmon vs. steak	4 vs. 5	1 vs. 2	3 vs. 3
Totals	**42 vs. 40**	**7 vs. 18**	**35 vs. 22**

NOTE: Portion sizes that provide approximately 100 kcalories: 1 tbs olive oil, 1 tbs butter, 2 tbs dry roasted sunflower seeds, 2 slices cooked bacon, 2 tbs dry roasted mixed nuts, 10 potato chips, 6 slices avocado, 1 slice cheddar cheese, 2 oz salmon, and 1½ oz steak.

The Mediterranean Diet

The links between good health and traditional Mediterranean diets of the mid-1900s and health were introduced earlier with regard to olive oil.[25] For people who eat these diets, the incidence of heart disease, some cancers, and other chronic diseases is low, and life expectancy is high.[26]

Although each of the many countries that border the Mediterranean Sea has its own culture, traditions, and dietary habits, their similarities are much greater than the use of olive oil alone. In fact, according to a recent study, no one factor alone can be credited with reducing disease risks—the association holds true only when the overall diet pattern is present.[27] Apparently, each of the foods contributes small benefits that harmonize to produce either a substantial cumulative or a synergistic effect.

The Mediterranean people focus their diets on crusty breads, whole grains, potatoes, and pastas; a variety of vegetables (including wild greens) and legumes; feta and mozzarella cheeses and yogurt; nuts; and fruits (especially grapes and figs). They eat some fish, other seafood, poultry, a few eggs, and little meat.

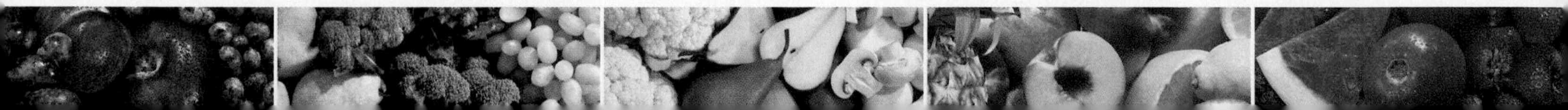

Along with olives and olive oil, their principal sources of fat are nuts and fish; they rarely use butter or encounter hydrogenated fats. Consequently, traditional Mediterranean diets are:

- Low in saturated fat.
- Very low in *trans* fat.
- Rich in unsaturated fat.
- Rich in complex carbohydrate and fiber.
- Rich in nutrients and phytochemicals that support good health.

People following the traditional Mediterranean diet can receive as much as 40 percent of a day's kcalories from fat, but their limited consumption of dairy products and meats provides less than 10 percent from saturated fats. In addition, because the animals graze, the meat, dairy products, and eggs are richer in omega-3 fatty acids than those from animals fed grain. Other foods typical of the Mediterranean, such as wild plants and snails, provide omega-3 fatty acids as well. All in all, the traditional Mediterranean diet has gained a reputation for its health benefits as well as its delicious flavors, but beware of the typical Mediterranean-style cuisine available in U.S. restaurants. It has been adjusted to popular tastes, meaning that it is often much higher in saturated fats and meats, and much lower in the potentially beneficial constituents, than the traditional fare.

Conclusion

Are some fats "good" and others "bad" from the body's point of view? The saturated and *trans* fats indeed seem mostly bad for the health of the heart. Aside from providing energy, which unsaturated fats can do equally well, saturated and *trans* fats bring no indispensable benefits to the body. Furthermore, no harm can come from consuming diets low in them. Still, foods rich in these fats are often delicious, giving them a special place in the diet.

In contrast, the unsaturated fats are mostly good for the health of the heart when consumed in moderation. To date, their one proven fault seems to be that they, like all fats, provide abundant energy to the body and so may promote obesity if they drive kcalorie intakes higher than energy needs.[28] Obesity, in turn, often begets many body ills, as Chapter 8 makes clear.

When judging foods by their fatty acids, keep in mind that the fat in foods is a mixture of "good" and "bad," providing both saturated and unsaturated fatty acids. Even predominantly monounsaturated olive oil delivers some saturated fat. Consequently, even when a person chooses foods with mostly unsaturated fats, saturated fat can still add up if total fat is high. For this reason, fat must be kept below 35 percent of total kcalories if the diet is to be moderate in saturated fat. Even experts run into difficulty when attempting to create nutritious diets from a variety of foods that are low in saturated fats when kcalories from fat exceed 35 percent of the total.[29]

Does this mean that you must forever go without favorite cheeses, ice cream cones, or a grilled steak? The famous French chef Julia Child makes this point about moderation:

> An imaginary shelf labeled INDULGENCES is a good idea. It contains the best butter, jumbo-size eggs, heavy cream, marbled steaks, sausages and pâtés, hollandaise and butter sauces, French butter-cream fillings, gooey chocolate cakes, and all those lovely items that demand disciplined rationing. Thus, with these items high up and almost out of reach, we are ever conscious that they are not everyday foods. They are for special occasions, and when that occasion comes we can enjoy every mouthful.
>
> —Julia Child, *The Way to Cook,* 1989.

Additionally, food manufacturers may come to the assistance of consumers wishing to avoid the health threats from saturated and *trans* fats. A margarine maker has announced that it will no longer offer products containing *trans* fats; a major snack manufacturer will soon reduce the saturated and *trans* fats in some of its products and offer snack foods in single-serving packages. Other companies are likely to follow if consumers respond favorably.

Another idea is to adopt some of the Mediterranean eating habits and simply enjoy a high-fat diet. Including vegetables, fruits, and legumes as part of a balanced daily diet is a good idea, as is *replacing* saturated fats such as butter, shortening, and meat fat with unsaturated fats like olive oil and the oils from nuts and fish. These foods provide vitamins, minerals, and phytochemicals—all valuable in protecting the body's health. The authors of this book would not stop there, however. They would urge you to reduce fats from convenience foods and fast foods; choose small portions of meats, fish, and poultry; and include fresh foods from all the groups each day. Take care to select portion sizes that will best meet your energy needs. Also, exercise daily.

REFERENCES

1. F. B. Hu, J. E. Manson, and W. C. Willett, Types of dietary fat and risk of coronary heart disease: A critical review, *Journal of the American College of Nutrition* 20 (2001): 5–19.
2. M. de Lorgeril and coauthors, Mediterranean diet, traditional risk factors, and the rate of cardiovascular complications after myocardial infarction: Final report of the Lyon Diet Heart Study, *Circulation* 99 (1999): 779–785.
3. Third Report of the National Cholesterol Education Program (NCEP) Expert Panel on Detection, Evaluation, and Treatment of High Blood Cholesterol in Adults (Adult Treatment Panel III), NIH publication no.

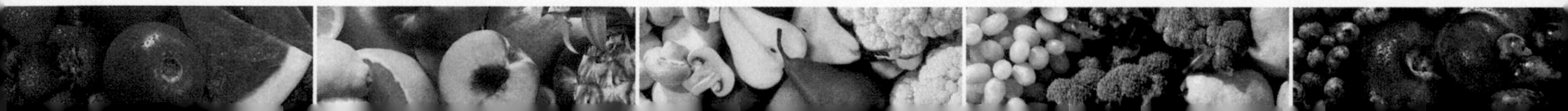

02-5215 (Bethesda, Md.: National Heart, Lung, and Blood Institute, 2002); Committee on Dietary Reference Intakes, *Dietary Reference Intakes for Energy, Carbohydrate, Fiber, Fat, Fatty Acids, Cholesterol, Protein, and Amino Acids* (Washington, D.C.: National Academies Press, 2002).

4. Committee on Dietary Reference Intakes, 2002, p. 11–3.
5. Third Report of the National Cholesterol Education Program (NCEP) Expert Panel on Detection, Evaluation, and Treatment of High Blood Cholesterol in Adults (Adult Treatment Panel III), 2002.
6. A. Keys, *Seven Countries: A Multivariate Analysis of Death and Coronary Heart Disease* (Cambridge, Mass.: Harvard University Press, 1980).
7. A. H. Stark and Z. Madar, Olive oil as a functional food: Epidemiology and nutritional approaches, *Nutrition Reviews* 60 (2002): 170–176.
8. P. M. Kris-Etherton and coauthors, High-monounsaturated fatty acid diets lower both plasma cholesterol and triacyglycerol concentrations, *American Journal of Clinical Nutrition* 70 (1999): 1009–1015.
9. R. L. Hargrove and coauthors, Low fat and high monounsaturated fat diets decrease human low density lipoprotein oxidative susceptibility in vitro, *Journal of Nutrition* 131 (2001): 1758–1763.
10. C. M. Williams, Beneficial nutritional properties of olive oil: Implications for postprandial lipoproteins and factor VII, *Nutrition, Metabolism, and Cardiovascular Diseases* 11 (2001): 51–56; J. P. De La Cruz and coauthors, Antithrombotic potential of olive oil administration in rabbits with elevated cholesterol, *Thrombosis Research* 100 (2000): 305–315; L. F. Larsen, J. Jespersen, and P. Marckmann, Are olive oil diets antithrombotic? Diets enriched with olive, rapeseed, or sunflower oil affect postprandial factor VII differently, *American Journal of Clinical Nutrition* 70 (1999): 976–982.
11. F. Visiol and C. Galli, Biological properties of olive oil phytochemicals, *Critical Reviews in Food Science and Nutrition* 42 (2002): 209–221; M. N. Vissers and coauthors, Olive oil phenols are absorbed in humans, *Journal of Nutrition* 132 (2002): 409–417; M. Fito and coauthors, Protective effect of olive oil and its phenolic compounds against low density lipoprotein oxidation, *Lipids* 35 (2000): 633–638; R. W. Owen and coauthors, The antioxidant/anticancer potential of phenolic compounds isolated from olive oil, *European Journal of Cancer* 36 (2000): 1235–1247.
12. L. A. Ferrara and coauthors, Olive oil and reduced need for antihypertensive medications, *Archives of Internal Medicine* 160 (2000): 837–842.
13. L. Van Horn and N. Ernst, A summary of the science supporting the new National Cholesterol Education program dietary recommendations: What dietitians should know, *Journal of the American Dietetic Association* 101 (2001): 1148–1154.
14. P. M. Kris-Etherton and coauthors, The effects of nuts on coronary heart disease risk, *Nutrition Reviews* 59 (2001): 103–111.
15. F. B. Hu and M. J. Stampfer, Nut consumption and risk of coronary heart disease: A review of epidemiologic evidence, *Current Atherosclerosis Reports* 1 (1999): 204–209.
16. E. B. Feldman, The scientific evidence for a beneficial health relationship between walnuts and coronary heart disease, *Journal of Nutrition* 132 (2002): 1062S–1101S; D. Zambón and coauthors, Substituting walnuts for monounsaturated fat improves the serum lipid profile of hypercholesterolemic men and women: A randomized crossover trial, *Annals of Internal Medicine* 132 (2000): 538–546.
17. D. J. Jenkins and coauthors, Dose response of almonds on coronary heart disease risk factors: Blood lipids, oxidized low-density lipoproteins, lipoprotein (a), homocysteine, and pulmonary nitric oxide: A randomized, controlled, crossover trial, *Circulation* 106 (2002): 1327–1332.
18. E. Dewailly and coauthors, Cardiovascular disease risk factors and n-3 fatty acid status in the adult population of James Bay Cree, *American Journal of Clinical Nutrition* 76 (2002): 85–92; E. Dewailly and coauthors, n-3 fatty acids and cardiovascular disease risk factors among the Inuit of Nunavik, *American Journal of Clinical Nutrition* 74 (2001): 464–473.
19. P. J. H. Jones and V. W. Y. Lau, Effect of n-3 polyunsaturated fatty acids on risk reduction of sudden death, *Nutrition Reviews* 60 (2002): 407–413; W. E. Connor, Importance of n-3 fatty acids in health and disease, *American Journal of Clinical Nutrition* 71 (2000): 171S–175S; P. J. Nestel, Fish oil and cardiovascular disease: Lipids and arterial function, *American Journal of Clinical Nutrition* 71 (2000): 228S–231S; C. von Schacky, n-3 fatty acids and the prevention of coronary atherosclerosis, *American Journal of Clinical Nutrition* 71 (2000): 224S–227S.
20. F. B. Hu and coauthors, Fish and omega-3 fatty acid intake and risk of coronary heart disease in women, *Journal of the American Medical Association* 287 (2002): 1815–1821; C. M. Albert and coauthors, Blood levels of long-chain n-3 fatty acids and the risk of sudden death, *New England Journal of Medicine* 346 (2002): 1113–1118; von Schacky, 2000.
21. H. Iso and coauthors, Intake of fish and omega-3 acids and risk of stroke in women, *Journal of the American Medical Association* 285 (2001): 304–312.
22. E. Guallar and coauthors, Mercury, fish oils, and the risk of myocardial infarction, *New England Journal of Medicine* 347 (2002): 1747–1754; K. Yoshizawa and coauthors, Mercury and the risk of coronary heart disease in man, *New England Journal of Medicine* 347 (2002): 1755–1760.
23. Third Report of the National Cholesterol Education Program (NCEP) Expert Panel on Detection, Evaluation, and Treatment of High Blood Cholesterol in Adults (Adult Treatment Panel III), 2002, p.V-8.
24. Committee on Dietary Reference Intakes, 2002, pp. 11–46 and G-1.
25. A. P. Simopoulos, The Mediterranean diets: What is so special about the diet of Greece? The scientific evidence, *Journal of Nutrition* 131 (2001): 3065S–3073S.
26. A. Trichopoulou and coauthors, Cancer and Mediterranean dietary traditions, *Cancer Epidemiology, Biomarkers and Prevention* 9 (2000): 869–873; C. Lasheras, S. Fernandez, and A. M. Patterson, Mediterranean diet and age with respect to overall survival in institutionalized, nonsmoking elderly people, *American Journal of Clinical Nutrition* 71 (2000): 987–992; A. Trichopoulou and E. Vasilopoulou, Mediterranean diet and longevity, *British Journal of Nutrition* 84 (2000): 205–209.
27. A. Trichopoulou and coauthors, Adherence to a Mediterranean diet and survival in a Greek population, *New England Journal of Medicine* 348 (2003): 2599–2608.
28. Committee on Dietary Reference Intakes, 2002, pp. 11–19.
29. Committee on Dietary Reference Intakes, 2002, pp. 11–22.

Chapter 6

Protein: Amino Acids

Chapter Outline

Available Online

http://nutrition.wadsworth.com/uncn7

Nutrition Animation: *Protein Digestion*

Student Practice Test

Glossary Terms

Nutrition on the Net

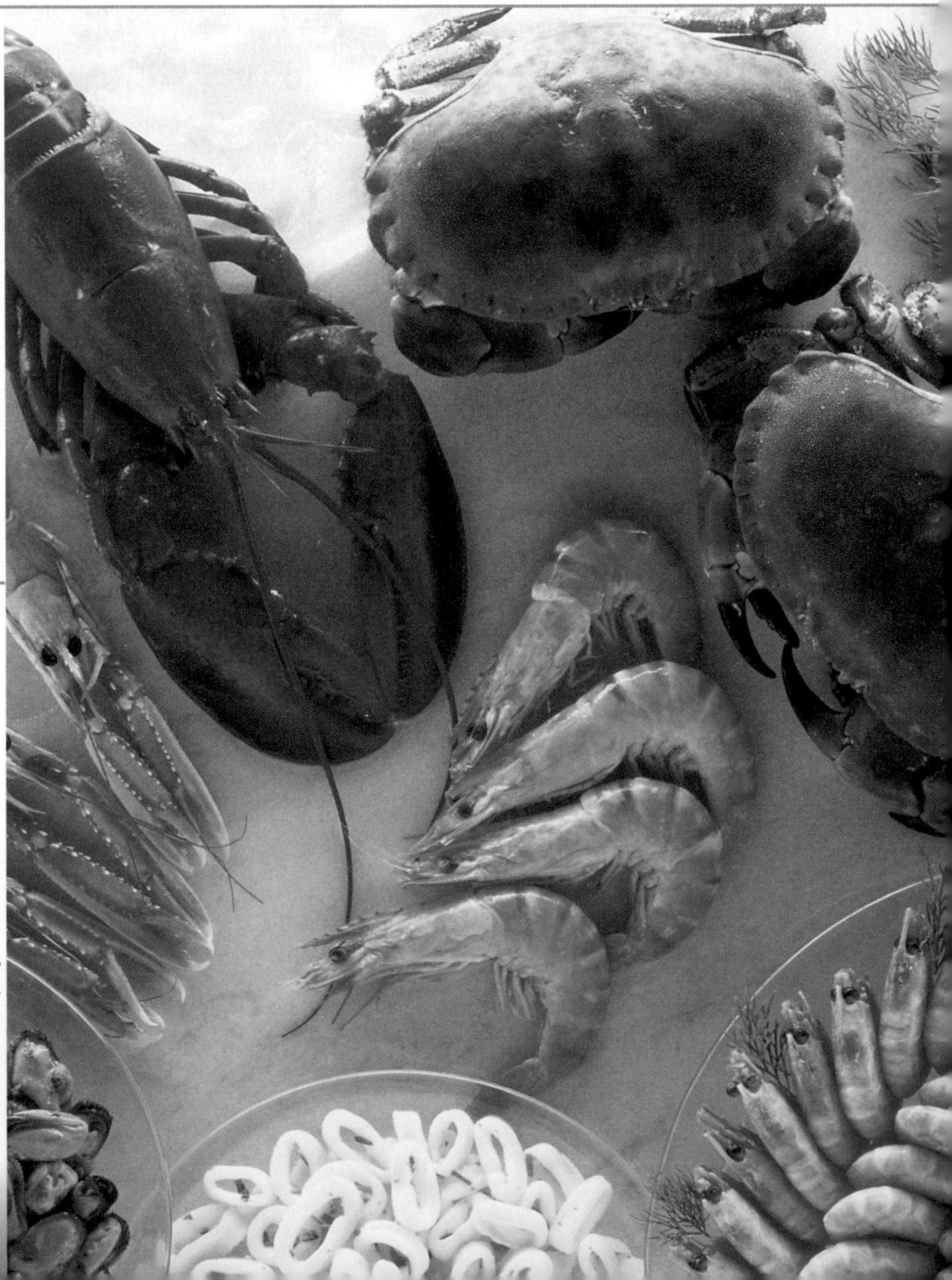

© James Jackson/Stone/Getty Images

Nutrition in Your Life

Their versatility in the body is impressive. They help your muscles to contract, your blood to clot, and your eyes to see. They keep you alive and well by facilitating chemical reactions and defending against infections. Without them, your bones, skin, and hair would have no structure. No wonder they were named *proteins,* meaning "of prime importance." Does that mean proteins deserve top billing in your diet as well? Are the best sources of protein beef, beans, or broccoli? Learn which foods will supply you with enough, but not too much, high-quality protein.

People commonly associate protein with strength and meat with protein. Consequently, they eat steak to build their muscles, but their thinking is only partly correct. Protein is a vital structural and working substance in all cells, not just muscle cells. Meat is a good source of protein, but so are milk, eggs, legumes, and many grains and vegetables. People who overvalue protein may overemphasize meat in their diets, sometimes at the expense of other, equally important nutrients and foods. Protein is important, but it is only one of the nutrients needed to maintain the body's health.

The Chemist's View of Proteins

Chemically, **proteins** contain the same atoms as carbohydrates and lipids—carbon (C), hydrogen (H), and oxygen (O)—but proteins also contain nitrogen (N) atoms. These nitrogen atoms give the name *amino* (nitrogen containing) to the amino acids—the links in the chains of proteins.

proteins: compounds composed of carbon, hydrogen, oxygen, and nitrogen atoms, arranged into amino acids linked in a chain. Some amino acids also contain sulfur atoms.

FIGURE 6-1 Amino Acid Structure

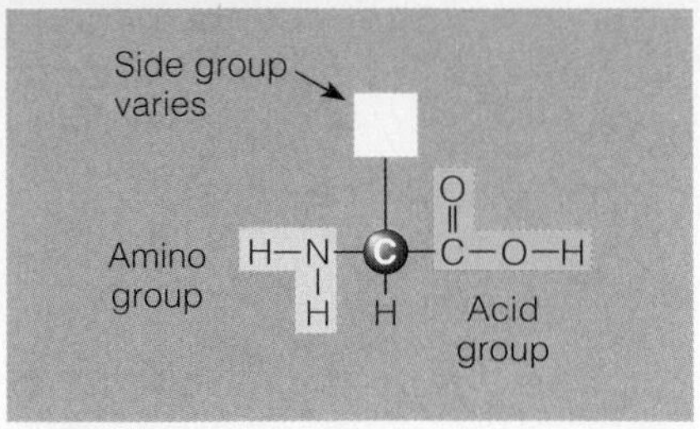
Side group varies
Amino group
H—N—C—C—O—H
O
H H
Acid group

All amino acids have a carbon (known as the alpha-carbon), with an amino group (NH_2), an acid group (COOH), a hydrogen (H), and a side group attached. The side group is a unique chemical structure that differentiates one amino acid from another.

■ Reminder:
- H forms 1 bond.
- O forms 2 bonds.
- N forms 3 bonds.
- C forms 4 bonds.

■ Some researchers refer to essential amino acids as **indispensable** and to nonessential amino acids as **dispensable.**

amino (a-MEEN-oh) **acids:** building blocks of proteins. Each contains an amino group, an acid group, a hydrogen atom, and a distinctive side group, all attached to a central carbon atom.
- **amino** = containing nitrogen

nonessential amino acids: amino acids that the body can synthesize (see Table 6-1).

essential amino acids: amino acids that the body cannot synthesize in amounts sufficient to meet physiological needs (see Table 6-1).

Amino Acids

All **amino acids** have the same basic structure—a central carbon (C) atom with a hydrogen (H), an amino group (NH_2), and an acid group (COOH) attached to it. Carbon atoms need to form four bonds,■ though, so a fourth attachment is necessary. It is this fourth site that distinguishes each amino acid from the others. Attached to the carbon atom at the fourth bond is a distinct atom, or group of atoms, known as the *side group* or *side chain* (see Figure 6-1).

Unique Side Groups The side groups on amino acids vary from one amino acid to the next, making proteins more complex than either carbohydrates or lipids. A polysaccharide (starch, for example) may be several thousand units long, but every unit is a glucose molecule just like all the others. A protein, on the other hand, is made up of about 20 different amino acids, each with a different side group. Table 6-1 lists the amino acids most common in proteins.*

The simplest amino acid, glycine, has a hydrogen atom as its side group. A slightly more complex amino acid, alanine, has an extra carbon with three hydrogen atoms. Other amino acids have more complex side groups (see Figure 6-2 for examples). Thus, although all amino acids share a common structure, they differ in size, shape, electrical charge, and other characteristics because of differences in these side groups.

Nonessential Amino Acids More than half of the amino acids are **nonessential,** meaning that the body can synthesize them for itself. Proteins in foods usually deliver these amino acids, but it is not essential that they do so. The body can make any nonessential amino acid, given nitrogen to form the amino group and fragments from carbohydrate or fat to form the rest of the structure.

Essential Amino Acids There are nine amino acids that the human body either cannot make at all or cannot make in sufficient quantity to meet its needs. These nine amino acids must be supplied by the diet; they are **essential.**■ The first column in Table 6-1 presents the essential amino acids.

Conditionally Essential Amino Acids Sometimes a nonessential amino acid becomes essential under special circumstances. For example, the body normally

* Besides the 20 common amino acids, which can all be components of proteins, others do not occur in proteins, but can be found individually (for example, taurine and ornithine). Some amino acids occur in related forms (for example, proline can acquire an OH group to become hydroxyproline).

TABLE 6-1 Amino Acids

Proteins are made up of about 20 common amino acids. The first column lists the essential amino acids for human beings (those the body cannot make—that must be provided in the diet). The second column lists the nonessential amino acids. In special cases, some nonessential amino acids may become conditionally essential (see the text). In a newborn, for example, only five amino acids are truly nonessential; the other nonessential amino acids are conditionally essential until the metabolic pathways are developed enough to make those amino acids in adequate amounts.

Essential Amino Acids		Nonessential Amino Acids	
Histidine	(HISS-tuh-deen)	Alanine	(AL-ah-neen)
Isoleucine	(eye-so-LOO-seen)	Arginine	(ARJ-ih-neen)
Leucine	(LOO-seen)	Asparagine	(ah-SPAR-ah-geen)
Lysine	(LYE-seen)	Aspartic acid	(ah-SPAR-tic acid)
Methionine	(meh-THIGH-oh-neen)	Cysteine	(SIS-teh-een)
Phenylalanine	(fen-il-AL-ah-neen)	Glutamic acid	(GLU-tam-ic acid)
Threonine	(THREE-oh-neen)	Glutamine	(GLU-tah-meen)
Tryptophan	(TRIP-toe-fan,	Glycine	(GLY-seen)
	TRIP-toe-fane)	Proline	(PRO-leen)
Valine	(VAY-leen)	Serine	(SEER-een)
		Tyrosine	(TIE-roe-seen)

FIGURE 6-2 Examples of Amino Acids

Note that all amino acids have a common chemical structure but that each has a different side group. Appendix C presents the chemical structures of the 20 amino acids most common in proteins.

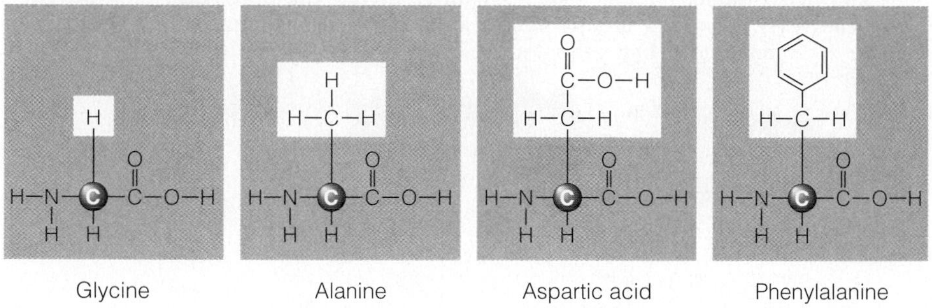
Glycine
Alanine
Aspartic acid
Phenylalanine

uses the essential amino acid phenylalanine to make tyrosine (a nonessential amino acid). But if the diet fails to supply enough phenylalanine, or if the body cannot make the conversion for some reason (as happens in the inherited disease phenylketonuria), then tyrosine becomes **conditionally essential.**

Proteins

Cells link amino acids end-to-end in a variety of sequences to form thousands of different proteins. A **peptide bond** unites each amino acid to the next.

Amino Acid Chains Condensation reactions connect amino acids, just as they combine monosaccharides to form disaccharides, and fatty acids with glycerol to form triglycerides. Two amino acids bonded together form a **dipeptide** (see Figure 6-3). By another such reaction, a third amino acid can be added to the chain to form a **tripeptide.** As additional amino acids join the chain, a **polypeptide** is formed. Most proteins are a few dozen to several hundred amino acids long. Figure 6-4 (on p. 184) provides an example—insulin.

Amino Acid Sequences If a person could walk along a carbohydrate molecule like starch, the first stepping stone would be a glucose. The next stepping stone would also be a glucose, and it would be followed by a glucose, and yet another glucose. But if a person were to walk along a polypeptide chain, each stepping stone would be one of 20 different amino acids. The first stepping stone might be the amino acid methionine. The second might be an alanine. The third might be a glycine, and the fourth a tryptophan, and so on. Walking along another

FIGURE 6-3 Condensation of Two Amino Acids to Form a Dipeptide

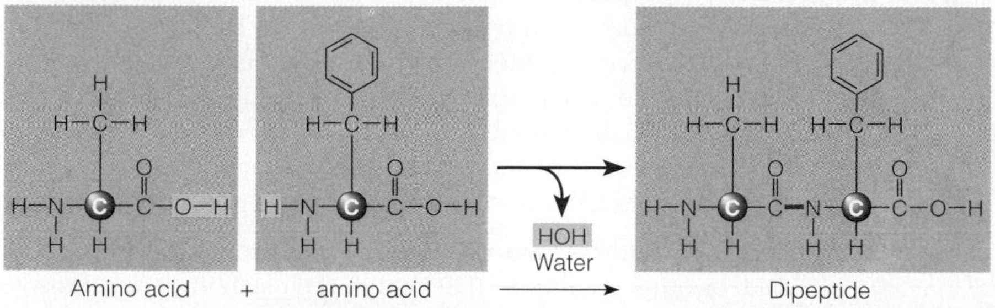
HOH
Water
Amino acid + amino acid
Dipeptide

An OH group from the acid end of one amino acid and an H atom from the amino group of another join to form a molecule of water.

A peptide bond (highlighted in red) forms between the two amino acids, creating a dipeptide.

conditionally essential amino acid: an amino acid that is normally nonessential, but must be supplied by the diet in special circumstances when the need for it exceeds the body's ability to produce it.

peptide bond: a bond that connects the acid end of one amino acid with the amino end of another, forming a link in a protein chain.

dipeptide (dye-PEP-tide): two amino acids bonded together.
- **di** = two
- **peptide** = amino acid

tripeptide: three amino acids bonded together.
- **tri** = three

polypeptide: many (ten or more) amino acids bonded together.
- **poly** = many

FIGURE 6-4 Amino Acid Sequence of Human Insulin

Human insulin is a relatively small protein that consists of 51 amino acids in two short polypeptide chains. (For amino acid abbreviations, see Appendix C.) Two bridges link the two chains. A third bridge spans a section within the short chain.

Known as disulfide bridges, these links always involve the amino acid cysteine (Cys), whose side group contains sulfur (S). Cysteines connect to each other when bonds form between these side groups.

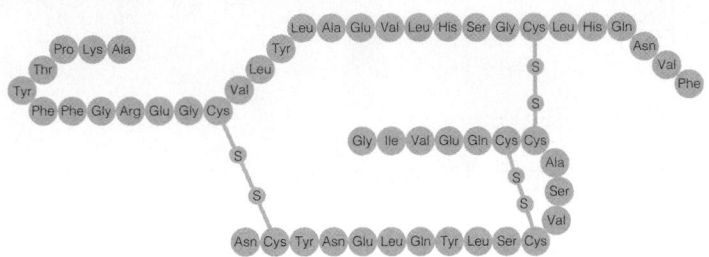
Pro Lys Ala
Thr
Tyr
Phe Phe Gly Arg Glu Gly Cys
Val
Leu
Tyr
Leu Ala Glu Val Leu His Ser Gly Cys Leu His Gln
Asn
Val
Phe
S
S
Gly Ile Val Glu Gln Cys Cys
Ala
Ser
Val
S
S
S
S
Asn Cys Tyr Asn Glu Leu Gln Tyr Leu Ser Cys

polypeptide path, a person might step on a phenylalanine, then a valine, and a glutamine. In other words, amino acid sequences within proteins vary.

The amino acids can act somewhat like the letters in an alphabet. If you had only the letter G, all you could write would be a string of Gs: G–G–G–G–G–G–G. But with 20 different letters available, you could create poems, songs, or novels. Similarly, the 20 amino acids can be linked together in a variety of sequences—even more than are possible for letters in a word or words in a sentence. Thus the variety of possible sequences for polypeptide chains is tremendous.

hemoglobin (HE-moh-GLOW-bin): the globular protein of the red blood cells that carries oxygen from the lungs to the cells throughout the body.
- **hemo** = blood
- **globin** = globular protein

denaturation (dee-NAY-chur-AY-shun): the change in a protein's shape and consequent loss of its function brought about by heat, agitation, acid, base, alcohol, heavy metals, or other agents.

Protein Shapes Polypeptide chains twist into a variety of complex, tangled shapes, depending on their amino acid sequences. The unique side group of each amino acid gives it characteristics that attract it to, or repel it from, the surrounding fluids and other amino acids. Some amino acid side groups carry electrical charges that are attracted to water molecules (they are hydrophilic). Other side groups are neutral and are repelled by water (they are hydrophobic). As amino acids are strung together to make a polypeptide, the chain folds so that its charged hydrophilic side groups are on the outer surface near water; the neutral hydrophobic groups tuck themselves inside, away from water. The intricate, coiled shape the polypeptide finally assumes gives it maximum stability.

FIGURE 6-5 The Structure of Hemoglobin

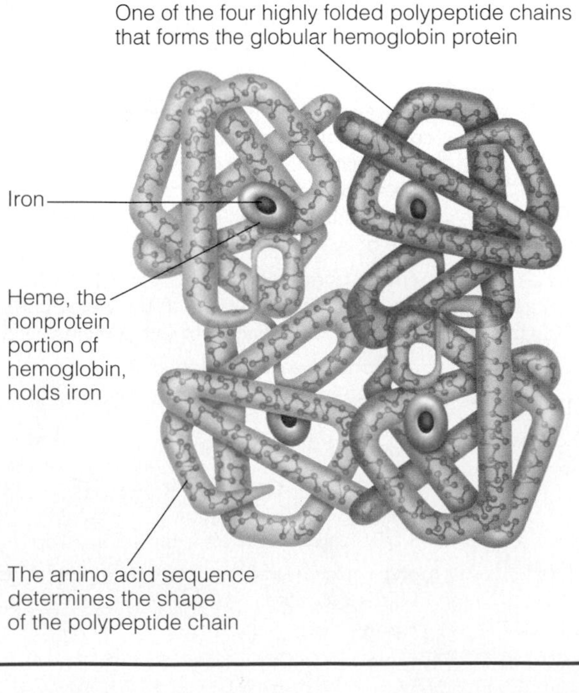
One of the four highly folded polypeptide chains that forms the globular hemoglobin protein
Iron
Heme, the nonprotein portion of hemoglobin, holds iron
The amino acid sequence determines the shape of the polypeptide chain

Protein Functions The extraordinary and unique shapes of proteins enable them to perform their various tasks in the body. Some form hollow balls that can carry and store materials within them, and some, such as those of tendons, are more than ten times as long as they are wide, forming strong, rodlike structures. Some polypeptides are functioning proteins as they are; others need to associate with other polypeptides to form larger working complexes. Some proteins require minerals to activate them. One molecule of **hemoglobin**—the large, globular protein molecule that, by the billions, packs the red blood cells and carries oxygen—is made of four associated polypeptide chains, each holding the mineral iron (see Figure 6-5).

Protein Denaturation When proteins are subjected to heat, acid, or other conditions that disturb their stability, they undergo **denaturation**—that is, they uncoil and lose their shapes and, consequently, their ability to function. Past a certain point, denaturation is irreversible. Familiar examples of denaturation include the hardening of an egg when it is cooked, the curdling of milk when acid is added, and the stiffening of egg whites when they are whipped.

IN SUMMARY Chemically speaking, proteins are more complex than carbohydrates or lipids, being made of some 20 different amino acids, 9 of which the body cannot make (they are essential). Each amino acid contains an amino group, an acid group, a hydrogen atom, and a distinctive side group. Cells link amino acids together in a series of condensation reactions to create proteins. The distinctive sequence of amino acids in each protein determines its unique shape and function.

Digestion and Absorption of Protein

Proteins in foods do not become body proteins directly. Instead, they supply the amino acids from which the body makes its own proteins. When a person eats foods containing protein, enzymes break the long polypeptide strands into shorter strands, the short strands into tripeptides and dipeptides, and, finally, the tripeptides and dipeptides into amino acids.

Protein Digestion

Figure 6-6 (on p. 186) illustrates the digestion of protein through the GI tract. Proteins are crushed and moistened in the mouth, but the real action begins in the stomach.

In the Stomach The major event in the stomach is the partial breakdown (hydrolysis) of proteins. Hydrochloric acid uncoils (denatures) each protein's tangled strands so that digestive enzymes can attack the peptide bonds. The hydrochloric acid also converts the inactive form■ of the enzyme pepsinogen to its active form, **pepsin.** Pepsin cleaves proteins—large polypeptides—into smaller polypeptides and some amino acids.

■ The inactive form of an enzyme is called a **proenzyme** or a **zymogen** (ZYE-moh-jen).

In the Small Intestine When polypeptides enter the small intestine, several pancreatic and intestinal **proteases** hydrolyze them further into short peptide chains,■ tripeptides, dipeptides, and amino acids. Then **peptidase** enzymes on the membrane surfaces of the intestinal cells split most of the dipeptides and tripeptides into single amino acids. Only a few peptides escape digestion and enter the blood intact. Figure 6-6 includes names of the digestive enzymes for protein and describes their actions.

■ A string of four to nine amino acids is an **oligopeptide** (OL-ee-go-PEP-tide).
- **oligo** = few

Protein Absorption

A number of specific carriers transport amino acids (and some dipeptides and tripeptides) into the intestinal cells. Once inside the intestinal cells, amino acids may be used for energy or to synthesize needed compounds. Those not used by the intestinal cells are transported across the cell membrane into the surrounding fluid where they enter the capillaries on their way to the liver.

Some nutrition faddists fail to realize that most proteins are broken down to amino acids before absorption. They urge consumers to "Eat enzyme A. It will help you digest your food." Or "Don't eat food B. It contains enzyme C, which will digest cells in your body." In reality, though, enzymes in foods are digested, just as all proteins are. Even the digestive enzymes—which function optimally at their specific pH—are denatured and digested when the pH of their environment changes. (For example, the enzyme pepsin, which works best in the low pH of the stomach becomes inactive and is digested when it enters the higher pH of the small intestine.)

Another misconception is that eating predigested proteins (amino acid supplements) saves the body from having to digest proteins and keeps the digestive system

pepsin: a gastric enzyme that hydrolyzes protein. Pepsin is secreted in an inactive form, **pepsinogen,** which is activated by hydrochloric acid in the stomach.

proteases (PRO-tee-aces): enzymes that hydrolyze protein.

peptidase: a digestive enzyme that hydrolyzes peptide bonds. *Tripeptidases* cleave tripeptides; *dipeptidases* cleave dipeptides. *Endopeptidases* cleave peptide bonds within the chain to create smaller fragments, whereas *exopeptidases* cleave bonds at the ends to release free amino acids.
- **tri** = three
- **di** = two
- **endo** = within
- **exo** = outside

FIGURE 6-6 Protein Digestion in the GI Tract

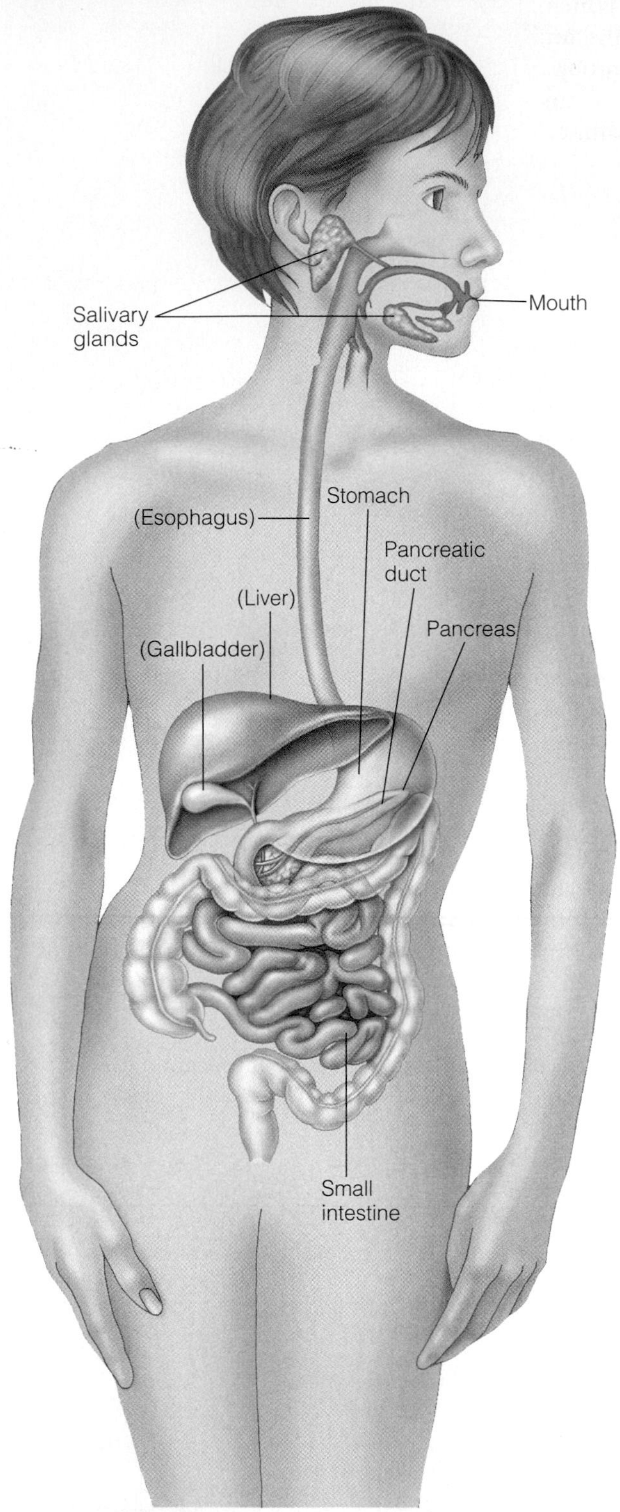
Salivary glands
Mouth
(Esophagus)
Stomach
Pancreatic duct
(Liver)
Pancreas
(Gallbladder)
Small intestine

PROTEIN

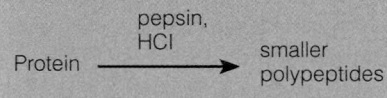

Mouth and salivary glands

Chewing and crushing moisten protein-rich foods and mix them with saliva to be swallowed.

Stomach

Hydrochloric acid (HCl) uncoils protein strands and activates stomach enzymes:

Protein —(pepsin, HCl)→ smaller polypeptides

In the Stomach:

Hydrochloric acid (HCl)
- Denatures protein structure.
- Activates pepsinogen to pepsin.

Pepsin
- Cleaves proteins to smaller polypeptides and some free amino acids.
- Inhibits pepsinogen synthesis.

Small intestine and pancreas

Pancreatic and small intestinal enzymes split polypeptides further:

Polypeptides —(pancreatic and intestinal proteases)→ tripeptides, dipeptides, amino acids

Then enzymes on the surface of the small intestinal cells hydrolyze these peptides and the cells absorb them:

Peptides —(intestinal tripeptidases and dipeptidases)→ amino acids (absorbed)

In the Small Intestine:

Enteropeptidase[a]
- Converts pancreatic trypsinogen to trypsin.

Trypsin
- Inhibits trypsinogen synthesis.
- Cleaves peptide bonds next to the amino acids lysine and arginine.
- Converts pancreatic procarboxypeptidases to carboxypeptidases.
- Converts pancreatic chymotrypsinogen to chymotrypsin.

Chymotrypsin
- Cleaves peptide bonds next to the amino acids phenylalanine, tyrosine, tryptophan, methionine, asparagine, and histidine.

Carboxypeptidases
- Cleave amino acids from the acid (carboxyl) ends of polypeptides.

Elastase and collagenase
- Cleave polypeptides into smaller polypeptides and tripeptides.

Intestinal tripeptidases
- Cleave tripeptides to dipeptides and amino acids.

Intestinal dipeptidases
- Cleave dipeptides to amino acids.

Intestinal aminopeptidases
- Cleave amino acids from the amino ends of small polypeptides (oligopeptides).

[a]Enteropeptidase was formerly known as *enterokinase*.

Available Online **http://nutrition.wadsworth.com/uncn7**
View the digestion of proteins in the stomach and small intestine as they are denatured and their peptide bonds are subsequently hydrolyzed.

from "overworking." Such a belief grossly underestimates the body's abilities. As a matter of fact, the digestive system handles whole proteins *better* than predigested ones because it dismantles and absorbs the amino acids at rates that are optimal for the body's use. (The last section of this chapter discusses amino acid supplements further.)

IN SUMMARY Digestion is facilitated mostly by the stomach's acid and enzymes, which first denature dietary proteins, then cleave them into smaller polypeptides and some amino acids. Pancreatic and intestinal enzymes split these polypeptides further, to oligo-, tri-, and dipeptides, and then split most of these to single amino acids. Then carriers in the membranes of intestinal cells transport the amino acids into the cells, where they are released into the bloodstream.

Proteins in the Body

The human body contains an estimated 10,000 to 50,000 different kinds of proteins. Of these, about 1000 have been studied,■ although with the recent surge in knowledge gained from sequencing the human genome,■ this number is sure to grow rapidly. Only about 10 are described in this chapter—but these should be enough to illustrate the versatility, uniqueness, and importance of proteins. As you will see, each protein has a specific function and that function is determined during protein synthesis.

■ The study of the body's proteins is called **proteomics.**

■ Reminder: The human genome is the full set of chromosomes, including all of the genes and associated DNA.

Protein Synthesis

Each human being is unique because of minute differences in the body's proteins. These differences are determined by the amino acid sequences of proteins, which, in turn, are determined by genes. The following paragraphs describe in words the ways cells synthesize proteins; Figure 6-7 (on p. 188) provides a pictorial description.

The instructions for making every protein in a person's body are transmitted by way of the genetic information received at conception. This body of knowledge, which is filed in the DNA (deoxyribonucleic acid) within the nucleus of every cell, never leaves the nucleus.

Delivering the Instructions To inform a cell of the sequence of amino acids for a needed protein, a stretch of DNA serves as a template for making a strand of RNA (ribonucleic acid) that carries a code. Known as messenger RNA, this molecule escapes through the nuclear membrane. Messenger RNA seeks out and attaches itself to one of the ribosomes (a protein-making machine, which is itself composed of RNA and protein). Thus situated, messenger RNA presents its list, specifying the sequence in which the amino acids are to line up to make a strand of protein.

Lining Up the Amino Acids Other forms of RNA, called transfer RNA, collect amino acids from the cell fluid and bring them to the messenger. Each of the 20 amino acids has a specific transfer RNA. Thousands of transfer RNA, each carrying its amino acid, cluster around the ribosomes, awaiting their turn to unload. When the messenger's list calls for a specific amino acid, the transfer RNA carrying that amino acid moves into position. Then the next loaded transfer RNA moves into place and then the next and the next. In this way, the amino acids line up in the sequence that is called for, and enzymes bind them together. Finally, the completed protein strand is released, the messenger is degraded, and the transfer RNA are freed to return for other loads of amino acids.

■ Anemia is not a disease, but a symptom of various diseases. In the case of sickle-cell anemia, a defect in the hemoglobin molecule changes the shape of the red blood cells. Later chapters describe how vitamin and mineral deficiencies affect the size and color of the red blood cells. In all cases, the abnormal blood cells are unable to meet the body's oxygen demands.

Sequencing Errors The sequence of amino acids in each protein determines its shape, which supports a specific function. If a genetic error alters the amino acid sequence of a protein, or if a mistake is made in copying the sequence, an altered protein will result, sometimes with dramatic consequences. The protein hemoglobin offers one example of such a genetic variation. In a person with **sickle-cell anemia,**■ two of hemoglobin's four polypeptide chains (described earlier on p. 184) have the normal sequence of amino acids, but the other two chains do not—they have the amino acid valine in a position that is normally occupied by glutamic acid (see

sickle-cell anemia: a hereditary form of anemia characterized by abnormal sickle- or crescent-shaped red blood cells. Sickled cells interfere with oxygen transport and blood flow. Symptoms are precipitated by dehydration and insufficient oxygen (as may occur at high altitudes) and include hemolytic anemia (red blood cells burst), fever, and severe pain in the joints and abdomen.

FIGURE 6-7 Protein Synthesis

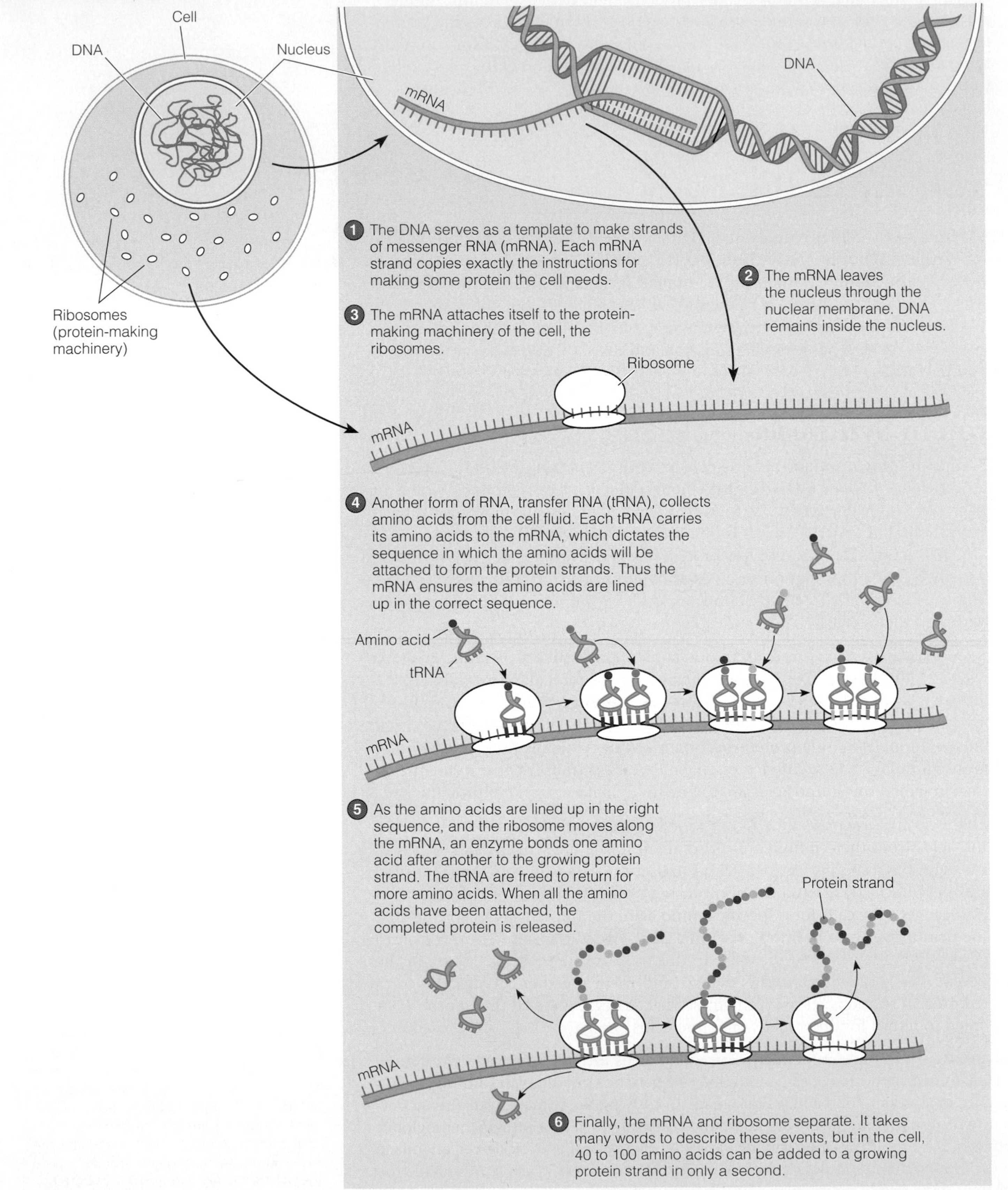
Cell
DNA
Nucleus
Ribosomes (protein-making machinery)
mRNA
DNA
1 The DNA serves as a template to make strands of messenger RNA (mRNA). Each mRNA strand copies exactly the instructions for making some protein the cell needs.
2 The mRNA leaves the nucleus through the nuclear membrane. DNA remains inside the nucleus.
3 The mRNA attaches itself to the protein-making machinery of the cell, the ribosomes.
Ribosome
mRNA
4 Another form of RNA, transfer RNA (tRNA), collects amino acids from the cell fluid. Each tRNA carries its amino acids to the mRNA, which dictates the sequence in which the amino acids will be attached to form the protein strands. Thus the mRNA ensures the amino acids are lined up in the correct sequence.
Amino acid
tRNA
mRNA
5 As the amino acids are lined up in the right sequence, and the ribosome moves along the mRNA, an enzyme bonds one amino acid after another to the growing protein strand. The tRNA are freed to return for more amino acids. When all the amino acids have been attached, the completed protein is released.
Protein strand
mRNA
6 Finally, the mRNA and ribosome separate. It takes many words to describe these events, but in the cell, 40 to 100 amino acids can be added to a growing protein strand in only a second.

Figure 6-8). This single alteration in the amino acid sequence changes the character and shape of hemoglobin so much that it loses its ability to carry oxygen effectively. The red blood cells filled with this abnormal hemoglobin stiffen into elongated sickle, or crescent, shapes instead of maintaining their normal pliable disc shape—hence the name, sickle-cell anemia. Sickle-cell anemia raises energy needs, causes many medical problems, and can be fatal.[1] Caring for children with sickle-cell anemia includes diligent attention to their water needs; dehydration can trigger a crisis.

Nutrients and Gene Expression When a cell makes a protein as described earlier, scientists say that the gene for that protein has been "expressed." Cells can regulate gene expression to make the type of protein, in the amounts and at the rate, they need. Nearly all of the body's cells possess the genes for making all human proteins, but each type of cell makes only the proteins it needs. For example, cells of the pancreas express the gene for insulin; in other cells, that gene is idle. Similarly, the cells of the pancreas do not make the protein hemoglobin, which is needed only by the red blood cells.

Recent research has unveiled some of the fascinating ways nutrients regulate gene expression and protein synthesis.■ These discoveries have begun to explain some of the relationships among nutrients, genes, and disease development. The benefits of polyunsaturated fatty acids in defending against heart disease, for example, are partially explained by their role in influencing gene expression for lipid enzymes. Later chapters provide additional examples of how nutrients influence gene expression.

FIGURE 6-8 Sickle Cells Compared with Normal Red Blood Cells

Normally, red blood cells are disc-shaped; in the inherited disorder sickle-cell anemia, red blood cells are sickle- or crescent-shaped. This alteration in shape occurs because valine replaces glutamic acid in the amino acid sequence of two of hemoglobin's polypeptide chains. As a result of this one alteration, the hemoglobin has a diminished capacity to carry oxygen.

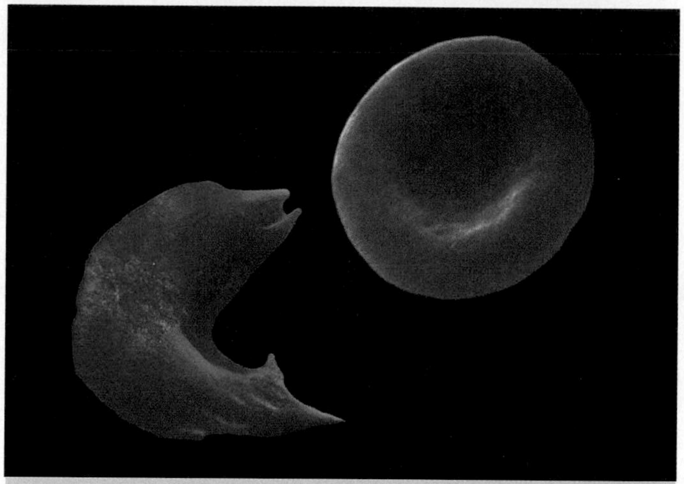
Sickle-shaped blood cells
Normal red blood cells

Amino acid sequence of normal hemoglobin:
Val–His–Leu–Thr–Pro–Glu–Glu

Amino acid sequence of sickle-cell hemoglobin:
Val–His–Leu–Thr–Pro–Val–Glu

IN SUMMARY Cells synthesize proteins according to the genetic information provided by the DNA in the nucleus of each cell. This information dictates the order in which amino acids must be linked together to form a given protein. Sequencing errors occasionally occur, sometimes with significant consequences.

■ Nutrients can play key roles in activating or silencing genes. Switching genes on and off, without changing the genetic sequence itself, is known as **epigenetics.**
- **epi** = among

Roles of Proteins

Whenever the body is growing, repairing, or replacing tissue, proteins are involved. Sometimes their role is to facilitate or to regulate; other times it is to become part of a structure. Versatility is a key feature of proteins.

As Building Materials for Growth and Maintenance From the moment of conception, proteins form the building blocks of muscles, blood, and skin—in fact, of most body structures. For example, to build a bone or a tooth, cells first lay down a **matrix** of the protein **collagen** and then fill it with crystals of calcium, phosphorus, magnesium, fluoride, and other minerals.

Collagen also provides the material of ligaments and tendons and the strengthening glue between the cells of the artery walls that enables the arteries to withstand the pressure of the blood surging through them with each heartbeat. Also made of collagen are scars that knit the separated parts of torn tissues together.

Proteins are also needed for replacement. The life span of a skin cell is only about 30 days. As old skin cells are shed, new cells made largely of protein grow from underneath to compensate. Cells in the deeper skin layers synthesize new proteins to go into hair and fingernails. Muscle cells make new proteins to grow larger and stronger in response to exercise. Cells of the GI tract are replaced every

matrix (MAY-tricks): the basic substance that gives form to a developing structure; in the body, the formative cells from which teeth and bones grow.

collagen (KOL-ah-jen): the protein from which connective tissues such as scars, tendons, ligaments, and the foundations of bones and teeth are made.

FIGURE 6-9 Enzyme Action

Each enzyme facilitates a specific chemical reaction. In this diagram, an enzyme enables two compounds to make a more complex structure, but the enzyme itself remains unchanged.

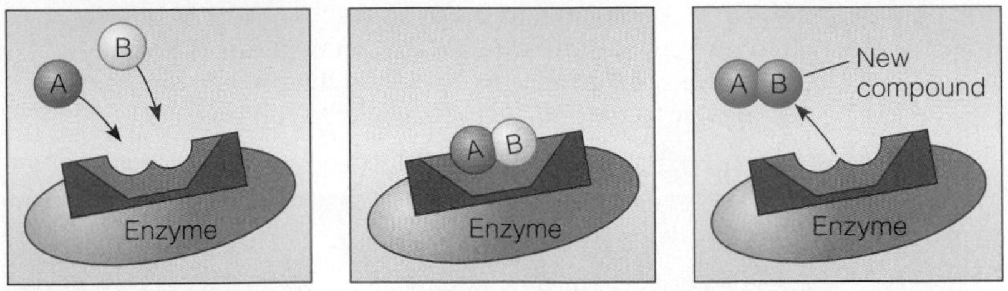
A
B
Enzyme
A B
Enzyme
A B
New compound
Enzyme

The separate compounds, A and B, are attracted to the enzyme's active site, making a reaction likely.

The enzyme forms a complex with A and B.

The enzyme is unchanged, but A and B have formed a new compound, AB.

three days. Both inside and outside, then, the body continuously deposits protein into new cells that replace those that have been lost.

As Enzymes Some proteins act as **enzymes.** Digestive enzymes have appeared in every chapter since Chapter 3, but digestion is only one of the many processes enzymes facilitate. Enzymes not only break down substances, they also build substances (such as bone)■ and transform one substance into another (amino acids into glucose, for example). Figure 6-9 diagrams a synthesis reaction.

■ Breaking down reactions are **catabolic,** whereas building up reactions are **anabolic** (Chapter 7 provides more details).

An analogy may help to clarify the role of enzymes. Enzymes are comparable to the clergy and judges who make and dissolve marriages. When a minister marries two people, they become a couple, with a new bond between them. They are joined together—but the minister remains unchanged. The minister represents enzymes that synthesize large compounds from smaller ones. One minister can perform thousands of marriage ceremonies, just as one enzyme can perform billions of synthetic reactions.

Similarly, a judge who lets married couples separate may decree many divorces before retiring or dying. The judge represents enzymes that hydrolyze larger compounds to smaller ones; for example, the digestive enzymes. The point is that, like the minister and the judge, enzymes themselves are not altered by the reactions they facilitate. They are catalysts, permitting reactions to occur more quickly and efficiently than if substances depended on chance encounters alone.

As Hormones Cells can switch their protein machinery on or off in response to the body's needs. Often hormones do the switching, with marvelous precision. The body's many hormones are messenger molecules, and *some* hormones are proteins. Various endocrine glands in the body release hormones in response to changes that challenge the body. The blood carries the hormones from these glands to their target tissues, where they elicit the appropriate responses to restore normal conditions.

The hormone insulin provides a familiar example. When blood glucose rises, the pancreas releases its insulin. Insulin stimulates the transport proteins of the muscles and adipose tissue to pump glucose into the cells faster than it can leak out. (After acting on the message, the cells destroy the insulin.) Then, as blood glucose falls, the pancreas slows its release of insulin. Many other proteins act as hormones, regulating a variety of actions in the body (see Table 6-2 for examples).

TABLE 6-2 Examples of Hormones and Their Actions

Hormones	Actions
Growth hormone	Promotes growth.
Insulin and glucagon	Regulate blood glucose (see Chapter 4).
Thyroxin	Regulates the body's metabolic rate (see Chapter 8).
Calcitonin and parathormone	Regulate blood calcium (see Chapter 12).
Antidiuretic hormone	Regulates fluid and electrolyte balance (see Chapter 12).

NOTE: *Hormones* are chemical messengers that are secreted by endocrine glands in response to altered conditions in the body. Each travels to one or more specific target tissues or organs, where it elicits a specific response. For descriptions of many hormones important in nutrition, see Appendix A.

As Regulators of Fluid Balance Proteins help to maintain the body's **fluid balance.** Figure 12-1 in Chapter 12 illustrates a cell and its associated fluids. As the figure explains, the body's fluids are contained inside the cells (intracellular) or outside the cells (extracellular). Extracellular fluids, in turn, can be found either in the spaces between the cells (interstitial) or within the blood vessels (intravascular). The fluid within the intravascular spaces is called plasma (essentially blood without its red blood cells). Fluids can flow freely between these compartments, but being large, proteins cannot. Proteins are trapped primarily within the cells and to a lesser extent in the plasma. Wherever proteins are, they attract water.

The exchange of materials between the blood and the cells takes place across the capillary walls, which allow the passage of fluids and a variety of materials—but usually not plasma proteins. Still some plasma proteins leak out of the capillaries into the interstitial fluid between the cells. These proteins cannot be reabsorbed back into the plasma; they normally reenter circulation via the lymph system. If plasma proteins enter the interstitial spaces faster than they can be cleared, fluid accumulates (because proteins attract water) and causes swelling. Swelling due to an excess of interstitial fluid is known as **edema.** The protein-related causes of edema include:

- Excessive protein losses caused by kidney disease or large wounds (such as extensive burns).

enzymes: proteins that facilitate chemical reactions without being changed in the process; protein catalysts.

fluid balance: maintenance of the proper types and amounts of fluid in each compartment of the body fluids (see also Chapter 12).

edema (eh-DEEM-uh): the swelling of body tissue caused by excessive amounts of fluid in the interstitial spaces; seen in protein deficiency (among other conditions).

- Inadequate protein synthesis caused by liver disease.
- Inadequate dietary intake of protein.

Whatever the cause of edema, the result is the same: a diminished capacity to deliver nutrients and oxygen to the cells and to remove wastes from them. As a consequence, cells fail to function adequately.

As Acid-Base Regulators Proteins also help to maintain the balance between **acids** and **bases** within the body fluids. Normal body processes continually produce acids and bases, which the blood carries to the kidneys and lungs for excretion. The challenge is to do this without upsetting the blood's acid-base balance.

In an acid solution, hydrogen ions abound; the more hydrogen ions, the more concentrated the acid. Proteins, which have negative charges on their surfaces, attract hydrogen ions, which have positive charges. By accepting and releasing hydrogen ions,■ proteins maintain the acid-base balance of the blood and body fluids.

■ Compounds that help keep a solution's acidity or alkalinity constant are called **buffers.**

The blood's acid-base balance is tightly controlled. The extremes of **acidosis** and **alkalosis** lead to coma and death, largely because they denature working proteins. Disturbing a protein's shape renders it useless. To give just one example, denatured hemoglobin loses its capacity to carry oxygen.

As Transporters Some proteins move about in the body fluids, carrying nutrients and other molecules. The protein hemoglobin carries oxygen from the lungs to the cells. The lipoproteins transport lipids around the body. Special transport proteins carry vitamins and minerals.

The transport of the mineral iron provides an especially good illustration of these proteins' specificity and precision. When iron enters an intestinal cell after a meal has been digested and absorbed, it is captured by a protein. Before leaving the intestinal cell, iron is attached to another protein that carries it though the bloodstream to the cells. Once iron enters a cell, it is attached to a storage protein that will hold the iron until it is needed. When it is needed, iron is incorporated into proteins in the red blood cells and muscles that assist in oxygen transport and use. (Chapter 13 provides more details on how these protein carriers transport and store iron.)

Some transport proteins reside in cell membranes and act as "pumps," picking up compounds on one side of the membrane and releasing them on the other as needed. Each transport protein is specific for a certain compound or group of related compounds. Figure 6-10 illustrates how a membrane-bound transport protein

acids: compounds that release hydrogen ions in a solution.

bases: compounds that accept hydrogen ions in a solution.

acidosis (assi-DOE-sis): above-normal acidity in the blood and body fluids.

alkalosis (alka-LOE-sis): above-normal alkalinity (base) in the blood and body fluids.

FIGURE 6-10 An Example of Protein Transport

This transport protein resides within a cell membrane and acts as a two-door passageway. Molecules enter on one side of the membrane and exit on the other, but the protein doesn't leave the membrane. This example shows how the transport protein moves sodium and potassium in opposite directions across the membrane to maintain a high concentration of potassium and a low concentration of sodium within the cell. This active transport system requires energy.

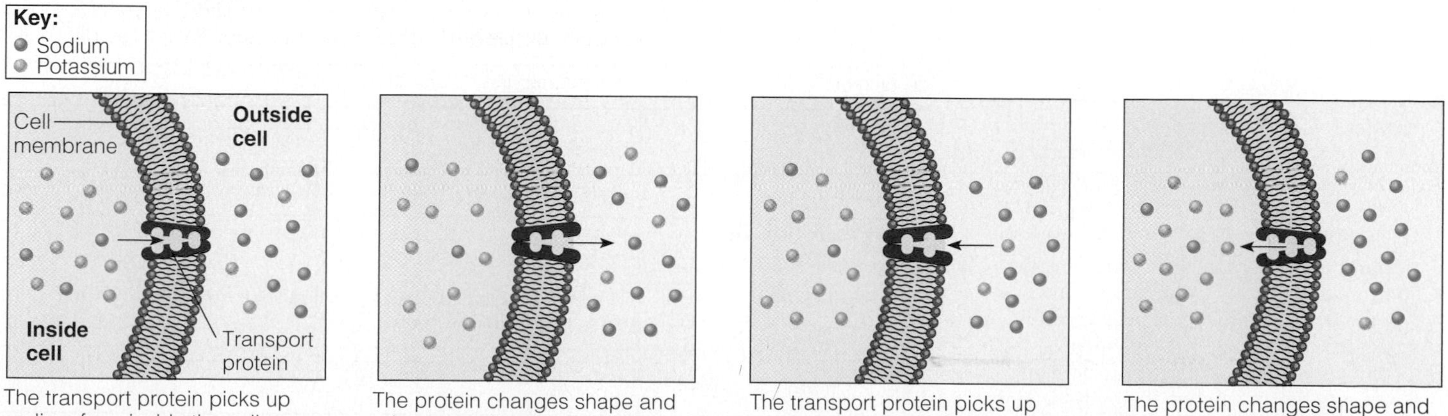
Key:
Sodium
Potassium
Cell membrane
Outside cell
Inside cell
Transport protein

The transport protein picks up sodium from inside the cell. The protein changes shape and releases sodium outside the cell. The transport protein picks up potassium from outside the cell. The protein changes shape and releases potassium inside the cell.

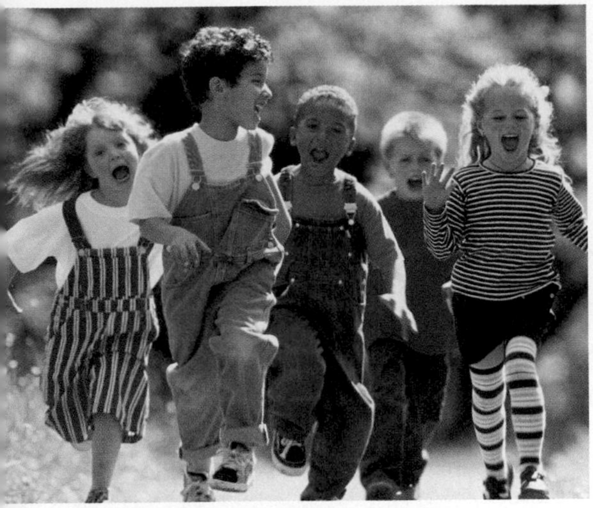

Growing children end each day with more bone, blood, muscle, and skin cells than they had at the beginning of the day.

helps to maintain the sodium and potassium concentrations in the fluids inside and outside cells. The balance of these two minerals is critical to nerve transmissions and muscle contractions; imbalances can cause irregular heartbeats, muscular weakness, kidney failure, and even death.

As Antibodies Proteins also defend the body against disease. A virus—whether it is one that causes flu, smallpox, measles, or the common cold—enters the cells and multiplies there. One virus may produce 100 replicas of itself within an hour or so. Each replica can then burst out and invade 100 different cells, soon yielding 10,000 virus particles, which invade 10,000 cells. Left free to do their worst, they will soon overwhelm the body with disease.

Fortunately, when the body detects these invading **antigens,** it manufactures **antibodies,** giant protein molecules designed specifically to combat them. The antibodies work so swiftly and efficiently that in a normal, healthy individual, most diseases never have a chance to get started. Without sufficient protein, though, the body cannot maintain its army of antibodies to resist infectious diseases.

Each antibody is designed to destroy just one antigen. Once the body has manufactured antibodies against a particular antigen (such as the measles virus), it remembers how to make them. Consequently, the next time the body encounters that same antigen, it will produce antibodies even more quickly. In other words, the body develops a molecular memory, known as **immunity.** (Chapter 15 and Highlight 24 describe food allergies—the immune system's response to food antigens.)

As a Source of Energy and Glucose Even though proteins are needed to do the work that only they can perform, they will be sacrificed to provide energy■ and glucose■ if need be. Without energy, cells die; without glucose, the brain and nervous system falter. Chapter 7 provides many more details on energy metabolism.

- ■ Reminder: Protein provides 4 kcal/g. Return to p. 9 for a refresher on how to calculate the protein kcalories from foods.
- ■ Reminder: The making of glucose from noncarbohydrate sources such as amino acids is *gluconeogenesis.*

Other Roles As mentioned earlier, proteins form integral parts of most body structures such as skin, muscles, and bones. They also participate in some of the body's most amazing activities such as blood clotting and vision. When a tissue is injured, a rapid chain of events leads to the production of fibrin, a stringy, insoluble mass of protein fibers that forms a clot from liquid blood. Later, more slowly, the protein collagen forms a scar to replace the clot and permanently heal the wound. The light-sensitive pigments in the cells of the retina are molecules of the protein opsin. Opsin responds to light by changing its shape, thus initiating the nerve impulses that convey the sense of sight to the brain.

IN SUMMARY The protein functions discussed here are summarized in the table below. They are only a few of the many roles proteins play, but they convey some sense of the immense variety of proteins and their importance in the body.

Growth and maintenance	Proteins form integral parts of most body structures such as skin, tendons, membranes, muscles, organs, and bones. As such, they support the growth and repair of body tissues.
Enzymes	Proteins facilitate chemical reactions.
Hormones	Proteins regulate body processes. (Some, but not all, hormones are proteins.)
Fluid balance	Proteins help to maintain the volume and composition of body fluids.
Acid-base balance	Proteins help maintain the acid-base balance of body fluids by acting as buffers.
Transportation	Proteins transport substances, such as lipids, vitamins, minerals, and oxygen, around the body.
Antibodies	Proteins inactivate foreign invaders, thus protecting the body against diseases.
Energy	Proteins provide some fuel for the body's energy needs.

antigens: substances that elicit the formation of antibodies or an inflammation reaction from the immune system. A bacterium, a virus, a toxin, and a protein in food that causes allergy are all examples of antigens.

antibodies: large proteins produced by the immune system in response to the invasion of the body by foreign molecules (usually proteins called antigens). Antibodies combine with and inactivate the foreign invaders, thus protecting the body.

immunity: the body's ability to defend itself against diseases; see Highlight 17.

A Preview of Protein Metabolism

This section previews protein metabolism; Chapter 7 provides a full description. Cells have several metabolic options, depending on their protein and energy needs.

Protein Turnover and the Amino Acid Pool Within each cell, proteins are continually being made and broken down, a process known as **protein turnover.** When proteins break down, they free amino acids to join the general circulation.■ These amino acids mix with amino acids from dietary protein to form an **"amino acid pool"** within the cells and circulating blood. The rate of protein degradation and the amount of protein intake may vary, but the pattern of amino acids within the pool remains fairly constant. Regardless of their source, any of these amino acids can be used to make body proteins or other nitrogen-containing compounds, or they can be stripped of their nitrogen and used for energy (either immediately or stored as fat for later use).

■ Amino acids (or proteins) that derive from within the body are **endogenous** (en-DODGE-eh-nus). In contrast, those that derive from foods are **exogenous** (eks-ODGE-eh-nus).
- **endo** = within
- **gen** = arising
- **exo** = outside (the body)

Nitrogen Balance Protein turnover and **nitrogen balance** go hand in hand. In healthy adults, protein synthesis balances with degradation, and protein intake from food balances with nitrogen excretion in the urine, feces, and sweat. When nitrogen intake equals nitrogen output, the person is in nitrogen equilibrium,■ or zero nitrogen balance. Researchers use nitrogen balance studies to estimate protein requirements.[2]

■ Nitrogen equilibrium (zero nitrogen balance): N in = N out.

If the body synthesizes more than it degrades and adds protein, nitrogen status becomes positive.■ Nitrogen status is positive in growing infants and children, pregnant women, and people recovering from protein deficiency or illness; their nitrogen intake exceeds their nitrogen output. They are retaining protein in new tissues as they add blood, bone, skin, and muscle cells to their bodies.

■ Positive nitrogen: N in > N out.

If the body degrades more than it synthesizes and loses protein, nitrogen status becomes negative.■ Nitrogen status is negative in people who are starving or suffering other severe stresses such as burns, injuries, infections, and fever; their nitrogen output exceeds their nitrogen intake. During these times, the body loses nitrogen as it breaks down muscle and other body proteins for energy.

■ Negative nitrogen: N in < N out.

Using Amino Acids to Make Proteins or Nonessential Amino Acids As mentioned, cells can assemble amino acids into the proteins they need to do their work. If a particular nonessential amino acid is not readily available, cells can make it from another amino acid. If an essential amino acid is missing, the body may break down some of its own proteins to obtain it.

Using Amino Acids to Make Other Compounds Cells can also use amino acids to make other compounds. For example, the amino acid tyrosine is used to make the **neurotransmitters** norepinephrine and epinephrine, which relay nervous system messages throughout the body. Tyrosine can also be made into the pigment melanin, which is responsible for brown hair, eye, and skin color, or into the hormone thyroxin, which helps to regulate the metabolic rate. For another example, the amino acid tryptophan serves as a precursor for the vitamin niacin and for serotonin, a neurotransmitter important in sleep regulation, appetite control, and sensory perception.[3]

Using Amino Acids for Energy and Glucose As mentioned earlier, when glucose or fatty acids are limited, cells are forced to use amino acids for energy and glucose. The body does not make a specialized storage form of protein as it does for carbohydrate and fat. Glucose is stored as glycogen in the liver and fat as triglycerides in adipose tissue, but protein in the body is available only as the working and structural components of the tissues. When the need arises, the body dismantles its tissue proteins and uses them for energy. Thus, over time, energy deprivation (starvation) always causes wasting of lean body tissue as well as fat loss. An adequate supply of carbohydrates and fats spares amino acids from being used for energy and allows them to perform their unique roles.

protein turnover: the degradation and synthesis of protein.

amino acid pool: the supply of amino acids derived from either food proteins or body proteins that collect in the cells and circulating blood and stand ready to be incorporated in proteins and other compounds or used for energy.

nitrogen balance: the amount of nitrogen consumed (N in) as compared with the amount of nitrogen excreted (N out) in a given period of time.*

neurotransmitters: chemicals that are released at the end of a nerve cell when a nerve impulse arrives there. They diffuse across the gap to the next cell and alter the membrane of that second cell to either inhibit or excite it.

* The genetic materials DNA and RNA contain nitrogen, but the quantity is insignificant compared with the amount in protein. The average amino acid weighs about 6.25 times as much as the nitrogen it contains, so scientists can estimate the amount of protein in a sample of food, body tissue, or other material by multiplying the weight of the nitrogen in it by 6.25.

Deaminating Amino Acids When amino acids are broken down (as occurs when they are used for energy), they are first deaminated—stripped of their nitrogen-containing amino groups. **Deamination** produces ammonia, which the cells release into the bloodstream. The liver picks up the ammonia, converts it into urea (a less toxic compound), and returns the urea to the blood. (Urea metabolism is described in Chapter 7.) The kidneys filter urea out of the blood; thus the amino nitrogen ends up in the urine. The remaining carbon fragments of the deaminated amino acids may enter a number of metabolic pathways—for example, they may be used for energy or for the production of glucose, ketones, cholesterol, or fat.*

Using Amino Acids to Make Fat Amino acids may be used to make fat when energy and protein intakes exceed needs and carbohydrate intake is adequate. The amino acids are deaminated, the nitrogen is excreted, and the remaining carbon fragments are converted to fat and stored for later use. In this way, protein-rich foods can contribute to weight gain.

IN SUMMARY Proteins are constantly being synthesized and broken down as needed. The body's assimilation of amino acids into proteins and its release of amino acids via protein degradation and excretion can be tracked by measuring nitrogen balance, which should be positive during growth and steady in adulthood. An energy deficit or an inadequate protein intake may force the body to use amino acids as fuel, creating a negative nitrogen balance. Protein eaten in excess of need is degraded and stored as body fat.

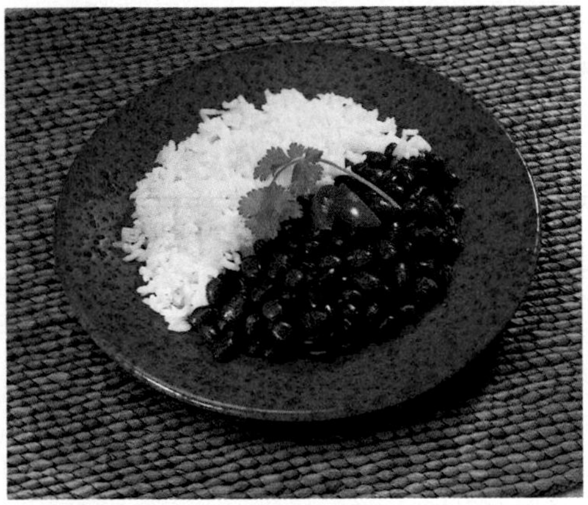
© Polara Studios Inc.

Black beans and rice, a favorite Hispanic combination, together provide a balanced array of amino acids.

Protein in Foods

In the United States and Canada, where nutritious foods are abundant, most people eat protein in such large quantities that they receive all the amino acids they need. In countries where food is scarce and the people eat only marginal amounts of protein-rich foods, however, the *quality* of the protein becomes crucial.

Protein Quality

The protein quality of the diet determines, in large part, how well children grow and how well adults maintain their health. Put simply, **high-quality proteins** provide enough of all the essential amino acids needed to support the body's work, and low-quality proteins don't. Two factors influence protein quality—the protein's digestibility and its amino acid composition.

Digestibility As explained earlier, proteins must be digested before they can provide amino acids. **Protein digestibility** depends on such factors as the protein's source and the other foods eaten with it. The digestibility of most animal proteins is high (90 to 99 percent); plant proteins are less digestible (70 to 90 percent for most, but over 90 percent for soy and legumes).

Amino Acid Composition To make proteins, a cell must have all the needed amino acids available simultaneously. The liver can produce any nonessential amino acid that may be in short supply so that the cells can continue linking amino acids into protein strands. If an essential amino acid is missing, though, a cell must dismantle its own proteins to obtain it. Therefore, to prevent protein breakdown, dietary protein must supply at least the nine essential amino acids

*Chemists sometimes classify amino acids according to the destinations of their carbon fragments after deamination. If the fragment leads to the production of glucose, the amino acid is called "glucogenic"; if it leads to the formation of ketone bodies, fats, and sterols, the amino acid is called "ketogenic." There is no sharp distinction between glucogenic and ketogenic amino acids, however. A few are both; most are considered glucogenic; only one (leucine) is clearly ketogenic.

deamination (dee-AM-eh-NAY-shun): removal of the amino (NH_2) group from a compound such as an amino acid.

high-quality proteins: dietary proteins containing all the essential amino acids in relatively the same amounts that human beings require. They may also contain nonessential amino acids.

protein digestibility: a measure of the amount of amino acids absorbed from a given protein intake.

plus enough nitrogen-containing amino groups and energy for the synthesis of the others. If the diet supplies too little of any essential amino acid, protein synthesis will be limited. The body makes whole proteins only; if one amino acid is missing, the others cannot form a "partial" protein. An essential amino acid supplied in less than the amount needed to support protein synthesis is called a **limiting amino acid.**

Reference Protein The quality of food proteins is determined based on how they compare with the essential amino acid requirements of preschool-age children. Such a standard is called a **reference protein.**■ The rationale behind using the requirements of this age group is that if a protein will effectively support a young child's growth and development, then it will meet or exceed the requirements of older children and adults.

High-Quality Proteins As mentioned earlier, a high-quality protein contains all the essential amino acids in relatively the same amounts as human beings require; it may or may not contain all the nonessential amino acids. Proteins that are low in an essential amino acid cannot, by themselves, support protein synthesis. Generally, foods derived from animals (meat, fish, poultry, cheese, eggs, yogurt, and milk) provide high-quality proteins, although gelatin is an exception (it lacks tryptophan and cannot support growth and health as a diet's sole protein). Proteins from plants (vegetables, nuts, seeds, grains, and legumes) have more diverse amino acid patterns and tend to be limiting in one or more essential amino acids. Some plant proteins (for example, corn protein) are notoriously low quality. A few others (for example, soy protein) are high quality.

Complementary Proteins In general, plant proteins are of lower quality than animal proteins, and plants also offer less protein (per weight or measure of food). For this reason, many vegetarians improve the quality of proteins in their diets by combining plant-protein foods that have different but complementary amino acid patterns. This strategy yields **complementary proteins** that together contain all the essential amino acids in quantities sufficient to support health. The protein quality of the combination is greater than for either food alone (see Figure 6-11).

Many people have long believed that combining plant proteins at every meal is critical to protein nutrition. For most healthy vegetarians, though, it is not necessary to balance amino acids at each meal when protein intake is varied and energy intake is sufficient.[4] Vegetarians can receive all the amino acids they need over the course of a day, if they eat a variety of grains, legumes, seeds, nuts, and vegetables. Protein deficiency will develop, however, when fruits and certain vegetables make up the core of the diet, severely limiting both the *quantity* and *quality* of protein. Highlight 6 shows how to plan a nutritious vegetarian diet.

A Measure of Protein Quality—PDCAAS Researchers have developed several methods for evaluating the quality of food proteins and identifying high-quality proteins. The following paragraph briefly describes the measure used by the Committee on Dietary Reference Intakes to evaluate protein quality. Appendix D provides details on other measures.

The **protein digestibility–corrected amino acid score,** or **PDCAAS,** compares the amino acid composition of a protein with human amino acid requirements and corrects for digestibility. First the protein's amino acid composition is determined, and then it is compared against the amino acid requirements of preschool-age children. This comparison reveals the most limiting amino acid—the one that falls shortest compared with the reference. If a food protein's limiting amino acid is 70 percent of the amount found in the reference protein, it receives a score of 70. The amino acid score is multiplied by the food's protein digestibility percentage to determine the PDCAAS. The box on the next page provides an example of how to calculate the PDCAAS, and Table 6-3 lists the PDCAAS values of selected foods.

■ In the past, egg protein was commonly used as the reference protein. Table D-1 in Appendix D presents the amino acid profile of egg. As the reference protein, egg was assigned the value of 100; Table D-2 includes scores of other food proteins for comparison.

FIGURE 6-11 Complementary Proteins

In general, legumes provide plenty of isoleucine (Ile) and lysine (Lys), but fall short in methionine (Met) and tryptophan (Trp). Grains have the opposite strengths and weaknesses, making them a perfect match for legumes.

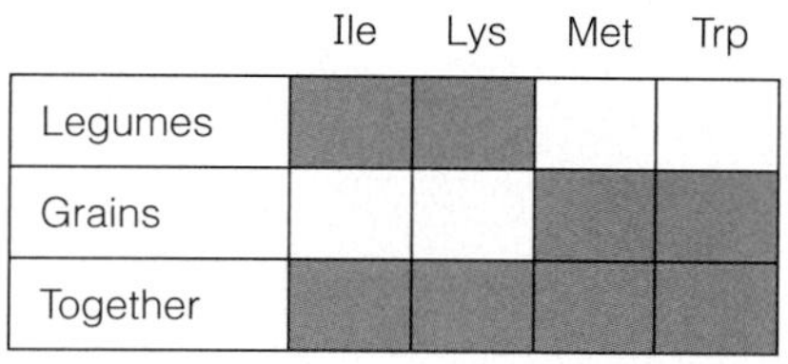

	Ile	Lys	Met	Trp
Legumes	■	■		
Grains			■	■
Together	■	■	■	■

limiting amino acid: the essential amino acid found in the shortest supply relative to the amounts needed for protein synthesis in the body. Four amino acids are most likely to be limiting:
- Lysine.
- Methionine.
- Threonine.
- Tryptophan.

reference protein: a standard against which to measure the quality of other proteins.

complementary proteins: two or more dietary proteins whose amino acid assortments complement each other in such a way that the essential amino acids missing from one are supplied by the other.

protein digestibility–corrected amino acid score (PDCAAS): a measure of protein quality assessed by comparing the amino acid score of a food protein with the amino acid requirements of preschool-age children and then correcting for the true digestibility of the protein.

TABLE 6-3 PDCAAS Values of Selected Foods

Casein (milk protein)	1.00
Egg white	1.00
Soybean (isolate)	.99
Beef	.92
Pea flour	.69
Kidney beans (canned)	.68
Chickpeas (canned)	.66
Pinto beans (canned)	.66
Rolled oats	.57
Lentils (canned)	.52
Peanut meal	.52
Whole wheat	.40

NOTE: 1.0 is the maximum PDCAAS a food protein can receive.

HOW TO Measure Protein Quality Using PDCAAS

To calculate the PDCAAS (protein digestibility–corrected amino acid score), researchers first determine the amino acid profile of the test protein (in this example, pinto beans). The second column of the table below presents the essential amino acid profile for pinto beans. The third column presents the amino acid reference pattern.

To determine how well the food protein meets human needs, researchers calculate the ratio by dividing the second column by the third column (for example, $30 \div 18 = 1.67$). The amino acid with the lowest ratio is the most limiting amino acid—in this case, methionine. Its ratio is the amino acid score for the protein—in this case, 0.84.

The amino acid score alone, however, does not account for digestibility. Protein digestibility, as determined by rat studies, yields a value of 79 percent for pinto beans. Together, the amino acid score and the digestibility value determine the PDCAAS:

$$\text{PDCAAS} = \text{protein digestibility} \times \text{amino acid score.}$$
$$\text{PDCAAS for pinto beans} = 0.79 \times 0.84 = 0.66.$$

Thus the PDCAAS for pinto beans is 0.66. Table 6-3 lists the PDCAAS values of selected foods.

The PDCAAS is used to determine the % Daily Value on food labels. To calculate the % Daily Value for protein for canned pinto beans, multiply the number of grams of protein in a standard serving (in the case of pinto beans, 7 grams per ½ cup) by the PDCAAS:

$$7\text{ g} \times 0.66 = 4.62.$$

This value is then divided by the recommended standard for protein (for children over age four and adults, 50 grams):

$$4.62 \div 50 = 0.09 \text{ (or 9\%)}.$$

The food label for this can of pinto beans would declare that one serving provides 7 grams protein, and if the label included a % Daily Value for protein (which is optional), the value would be 9 percent.

Essential Amino Acids	Amino Acid Profile of Pinto Beans (mg/g protein)	Amino Acid Reference Pattern (mg/g protein)	Amino Acid Score
Histidine	30.0	18	1.67
Isoleucine	42.5	25	1.70
Leucine	80.4	55	1.46
Lysine	69.0	51	1.35
Methionine (+ cystine)	21.1	25	0.84
Phenylalanine (+ tyrosine)	90.5	47	1.93
Threonine	43.7	27	1.62
Tryptophan	8.8	7	1.26
Valine	50.1	32	1.57

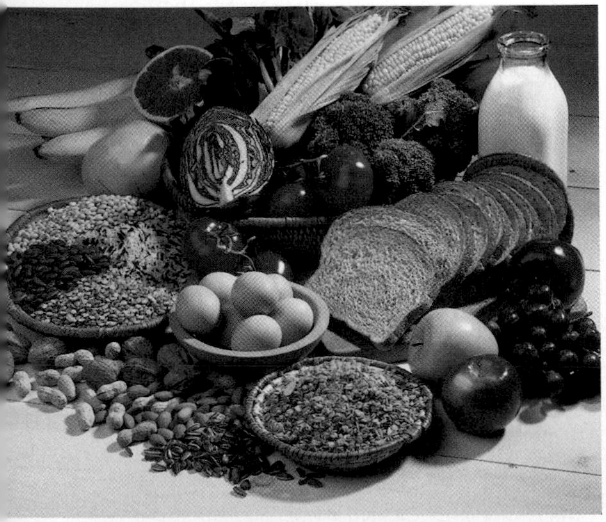

Vegetarians obtain their protein from whole grains, legumes, nuts, vegetables, and, in some cases, eggs and milk products.

IN SUMMARY A diet inadequate in any of the essential amino acids limits protein synthesis. The best guarantee of amino acid adequacy is to eat foods containing high-quality proteins or mixtures of foods containing incomplete but complementary proteins so that each can supply the amino acids missing in the other. Vegetarians can meet their protein needs by eating a variety of whole grains, legumes, seeds, nuts, and vegetables.

Protein Regulations for Food Labels

All food labels must state the *quantity* of protein in grams. The "% Daily Value"■ for protein is not mandatory on all labels, but is required whenever a food makes a protein claim or is intended for consumption by children under four years old.* Whenever the Daily Value percentage is declared, researchers must determine the *quality* of the protein by using the PDCAAS method. Thus, when a % Daily Value is stated for protein, it reflects both quantity and quality.

■ Daily Values:
- 50 g protein (based on 10% of 2000 kcal diet).

IN SUMMARY The quality of protein is measured by its amino acid content, its digestibility, and its ability to support growth. Such measures are of great importance in dealing with malnutrition worldwide, but in the United States and Canada, where protein deficiency is not common, protein quality scores of individual foods deserve little emphasis.

Health Effects and Recommended Intakes of Protein

As you know by now, protein is indispensable to life. It should come as no surprise that protein deficiency can have devastating effects on people's health. But, like the other nutrients, protein in excess can also be harmful. This section examines the health effects and recommended intakes of protein.

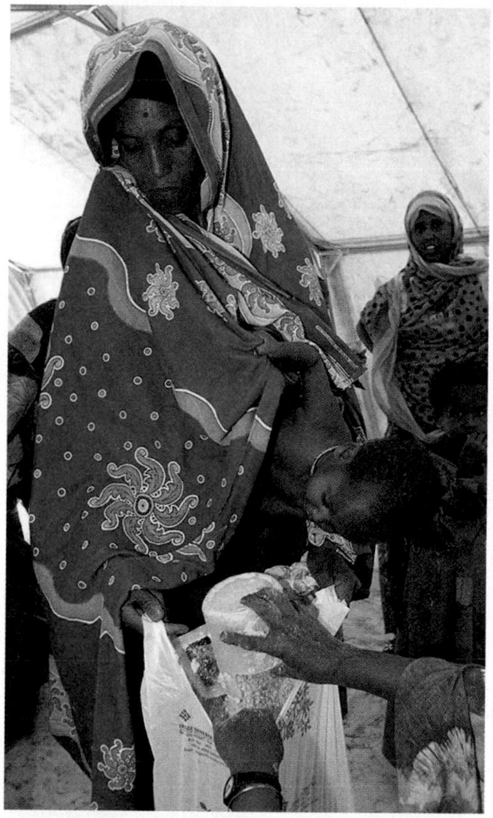

AP/Wide World Photos

Donated food saves some people from starvation, but it is usually insufficient to meet nutrient needs or even to provide a full belly for every person who is hungry.

Protein-Energy Malnutrition

When people are deprived of protein, energy, or both, the result is **protein-energy malnutrition (PEM).** Although PEM touches many adult lives, it most often strikes early in childhood. It is one of the most prevalent and devastating forms of malnutrition in the world, afflicting over 500 million children. Most of the 33,000 children who die each day are malnourished.

Inadequate food intake leads to poor growth in children and to weight loss and wasting in adults. Children who are thin for their height may be suffering from **acute PEM** (recent severe food deprivation), whereas children who are short for their age have experienced **chronic PEM** (long-term food deprivation). Poor growth due to PEM is easy to overlook because a small child may look quite normal, but it is the most common sign of malnutrition.

PEM is most prevalent in Africa, Central America, South America, the Middle East, and East and Southeast Asia. In the United States, homeless people and those living in substandard housing in inner cities and rural areas have been diagnosed with PEM. In addition to those living in poverty, elderly people who live alone and adults who are addicted to drugs and alcohol are frequently victims of PEM. PEM develops in young children when parents mistakenly provide "health-food beverages"■ that lack adequate energy or protein instead of milk, most commonly because of nutritional ignorance, perceived milk intolerance, or food faddism.[5] Adult PEM is also seen in people hospitalized with infections such as AIDS or tuberculosis; these infections deplete body proteins, demand extra energy, induce nutrient losses, and alter metabolic pathways. Furthermore, poor nutrient intake during hospitalization worsens malnutrition and impairs recovery, whereas nutrition intervention often improves the body's response to other treatments and the chances of survival.[6] PEM is also common in those suffering from the eating disorder anorexia nervosa

■ Rice drinks are often sold as milk alternatives, but fail to provide adequate protein, vitamins, and minerals.

protein-energy malnutrition (PEM), also called **protein-kcalorie malnutrition (PCM)**: a deficiency of protein, energy, or both, including kwashiorkor, marasmus, and instances in which they overlap (see p. 198).

acute PEM: protein-energy malnutrition caused by recent severe food restriction; characterized in children by thinness for height (wasting).

chronic PEM: protein-energy malnutrition caused by long-term food deprivation; characterized in children by short height for age (stunting).

*For labeling purposes, the Daily Values for protein are as follows: for infants, 14 grams; for children under age four, 16 grams; for older children and adults, 50 grams; for pregnant women, 60 grams; and for lactating women, 65 grams.

TABLE 6-4 Features of Marasmus and Kwashiorkor in Children

Separating PEM into two classifications oversimplifies the condition, but at the extremes, marasmus and kwashiorkor exhibit marked differences. Marasmus-kwashiorkor mix presents symptoms common to both marasmus and kwashiorkor. In all cases, children are likely to develop diarrhea, infections, and multiple nutrient deficiencies.

Marasmus	Kwashiorkor
Infancy (less than 2 yr)	Older infants and young children (1 to 3 yr)
Severe deprivation, or impaired absorption, of protein, energy, vitamins, and minerals	Inadequate protein intake or, more commonly, infections
Develops slowly; chronic PEM	Rapid onset; acute PEM
Severe weight loss	Some weight loss
Severe muscle wasting, with no body fat	Some muscle wasting, with retention of some body fat
Growth: <60% weight-for-age	Growth: 60 to 80% weight-for-age
No detectable edema	Edema
No fatty liver	Enlarged fatty liver
Anxiety, apathy	Apathy, misery, irritability, sadness
Good appetite possible	Loss of appetite
Hair is sparse, thin, and dry; easily pulled out	Hair is dry and brittle; easily pulled out; changes color; becomes straight
Skin is dry, thin, and easily wrinkles	Skin develops lesions

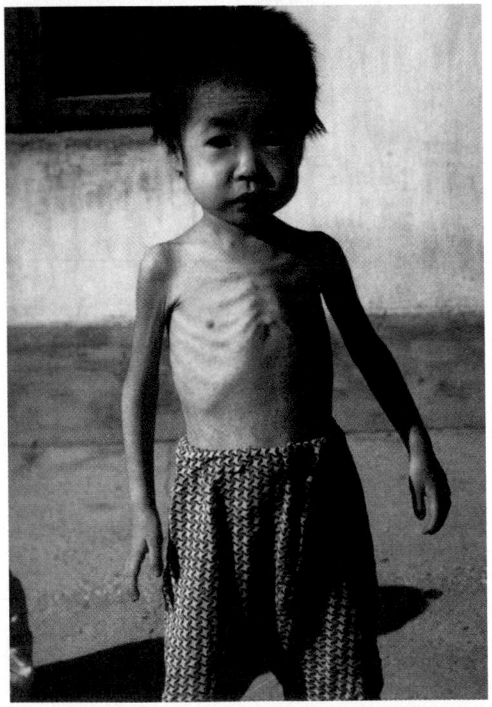
AP/Wide World Photos

The extreme loss of muscle and fat characteristic of marasmus is apparent in this child's "matchstick" arms.

(discussed in Highlight 9). Prevention emphasizes frequent, nutrient-dense, energy-dense meals and, equally important, resolution of the underlying causes of PEM—poverty, infections, and illness.

Classifying PEM PEM occurs in two forms: marasmus and kwashiorkor, which differ in their clinical features (see Table 6-4). The following paragraphs present three clinical syndromes—marasmus, kwashiorkor, and the combination of the two.

Marasmus Appropriately named from the Greek word meaning "dying away," **marasmus** reflects a severe deprivation of food over a long time (chronic PEM). Put simply, the person is starving and suffering from an inadequate energy *and* protein intake (and inadequate essential fatty acids, vitamins, and minerals as well). Marasmus occurs most commonly in children from 6 to 18 months of age in all the overpopulated urban slums of the world. Children in impoverished nations simply do not have enough to eat and subsist on diluted cereal drinks that supply scant energy and protein of low quality; such food can barely sustain life, much less support growth. Consequently, marasmic children look like little old people—just skin and bones.

Without adequate nutrition, muscles, including the heart, waste and weaken.[7] Because the brain normally grows to almost its full adult size within the first two years of life, marasmus impairs brain development and learning ability. Reduced synthesis of key hormones slows metabolism and lowers body temperature. There is little or no fat under the skin to insulate against cold. Hospital workers find that children with marasmus need to be clothed, covered, and kept warm. Because these children often suffer delays in their mental and behavioral development, they also need loving care, a stimulating environment, and parental attention.

The starving child faces this threat to life by engaging in as little activity as possible—not even crying for food. The body musters all its forces to meet the crisis, so it cuts down on any expenditure of protein not needed for the functioning of the heart, lungs, and brain. Growth ceases; the child is no larger at age four than at age two. Enzymes are in short supply and the GI tract lining deteriorates. Consequently, the child can't digest and absorb what little food is eaten.

Kwashiorkor **Kwashiorkor** typically reflects a sudden and recent deprivation of food (acute PEM). Kwashiorkor was originally a Ghanaian word meaning "the illness that develops in the first child when the second child is born." When a

marasmus (ma-RAZ-mus): a form of PEM that results from a severe deprivation, or impaired absorption, of energy, protein, vitamins, and minerals.

kwashiorkor (kwash-ee-OR-core, kwash-ee-or-CORE): a form of PEM that results either from inadequate protein intake or, more commonly, from infections.

mother who has been nursing her first child bears a second child, she weans the first child and puts the second one on the breast. The first child, suddenly switched from nutrient-dense, protein-rich breast milk to a starchy, protein-poor cereal, soon begins to sicken and die. Kwashiorkor typically sets in between 18 months and two years.

Kwashiorkor usually develops rapidly as a result of protein deficiency or, more commonly, is precipitated by an illness such as measles or other infection. Other factors may also contribute to the symptoms that accompany kwashiorkor.

The loss of weight and body fat is usually not as severe in kwashiorkor as in marasmus, but there may be some muscle wasting. Proteins and hormones that previously maintained fluid balance diminish, and fluid leaks into the interstitial spaces. The child's limbs and face become swollen with edema, a distinguishing feature of kwashiorkor. The lack of the protein carriers that transport fat out of the liver causes the belly to bulge with a fatty liver. The fatty liver lacks enzymes to clear metabolic toxins from the body, so their harmful effects are prolonged. Inflammation in response to these toxins and to infections further contributes to the edema that accompanies kwashiorkor. Without sufficient tyrosine to make melanin, the child's hair loses its color; inadequate protein synthesis leaves the skin patchy and scaly, often with sores that fail to heal. The lack of proteins to carry or store iron leaves iron free. Unbound iron is common in children with kwashiorkor and may contribute to their illnesses and deaths by promoting bacterial growth and free-radical damage. (Free-radical damage is discussed fully in Highlight 11.)

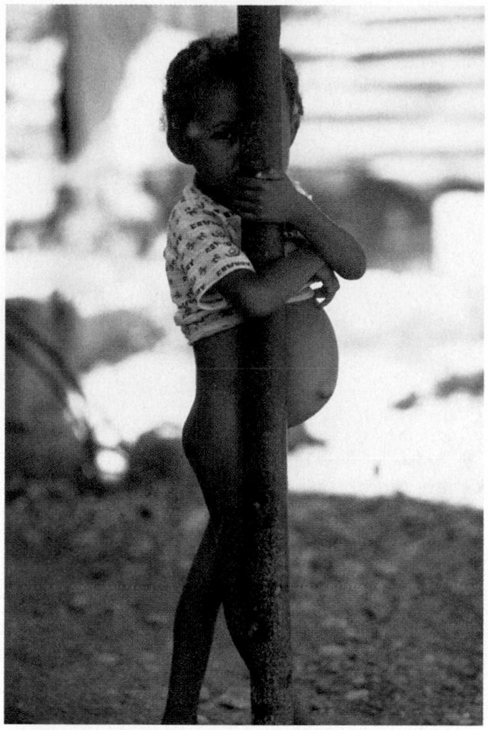

© Paul A. Souders/Corbis

The edema and enlarged liver characteristic of kwashiorkor are apparent in this child's swollen belly. Malnourished children commonly have an enlarged abdomen from parasites as well.

Marasmus-Kwashiorkor Mix The combination of marasmus and kwashiorkor is characterized by the edema of kwashiorkor with the wasting of marasmus. Most often, the child is suffering the effects of both malnutrition and infections. Some researchers believe that kwashiorkor and marasmus are two stages of the same disease. They point out that kwashiorkor and marasmus often exist side by side in the same community where children consume the same diet. They note that a child who has marasmus can later develop kwashiorkor. Some research indicates that marasmus represents the body's adaptation to starvation and that kwashiorkor develops when adaptation fails.

Infections In PEM, antibodies to fight off invading bacteria are degraded to provide amino acids for other uses, leaving the malnourished child vulnerable to infections. Blood proteins, including hemoglobin, are no longer synthesized, so the child becomes anemic and weak. **Dysentery,** an infection of the digestive tract, causes diarrhea, further depleting the body of nutrients. In the marasmic child, once infection sets in, kwashiorkor often follows and the immune response weakens further.[8]

The combination of infections, fever, fluid imbalances, and anemia often leads to heart failure and occasionally sudden death. Infections combined with malnutrition are responsible for two-thirds of the deaths of young children in developing countries. Measles, which might make a healthy child sick for a week or two, kills a child with PEM within two or three days.

Rehabilitation If caught in time, the life of a starving child may be saved with nutrition intervention. Diarrhea will have incurred dramatic fluid and mineral losses that will require careful correction to help raise the blood pressure and strengthen the heartbeat. After the first 24 to 48 hours, protein and food energy may be given in *small* quantities, with intakes *gradually* increased as tolerated. Severely malnourished people, especially those with edema, recover better with an initial diet that is relatively low in protein (10 percent kcalories from protein).[9]

Experts assure us that we possess the knowledge, technology, and resources to end hunger. Programs that tailor interventions to the local people and involve them in the process of identifying problems and devising solutions have the most success.[10] To win the war on hunger, those who have the food, technology, and resources must make fighting hunger a priority (see Highlight 16 for more on hunger).

dysentery (DISS-en-terry): an infection of the digestive tract that causes diarrhea.

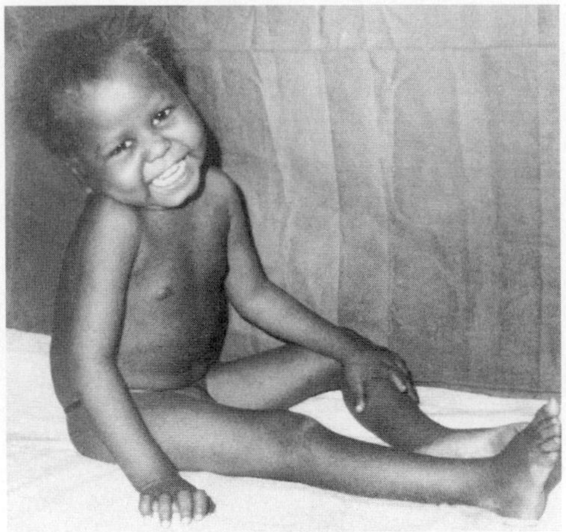

Given appropriate nutrition care, this child has successfully recovered from kwashiorkor.

Health Effects of Protein

While many of the world's people struggle to obtain enough food energy and protein, in developed countries both are so abundant that problems of excess are seen. Overconsumption of protein offers no benefits and may pose health risks. High-protein diets have been implicated in several chronic diseases, including heart disease, cancer, osteoporosis, obesity, and kidney stones, but evidence is insufficient to establish an upper limit.[11]

Researchers attempting to clarify the relationships between excess protein and chronic diseases face several obstacles. Population studies have difficulty determining whether diseases correlate with animal proteins or with their accompanying saturated fats, for example. Studies that rely on data from vegetarians must sort out the many lifestyle factors, other than a "no-meat diet," that might explain relationships between protein and health.

Heart Disease As Chapter 5 mentioned, foods rich in animal protein tend to be rich in saturated fats. Consequently, it is not surprising to find a correlation between animal-protein intake and heart disease, although no independent effect has been demonstrated. On the other hand, substituting soy protein for animal protein lowers blood cholesterol, especially in those with high blood cholesterol.[12]

Research suggests that elevated levels of the amino acid homocysteine may be an independent risk factor for heart disease.[13] Researchers do not yet fully understand the many factors that can raise homocysteine in the blood or whether elevated levels are a cause or an effect of heart disease.[14] Until they can determine the exact role homocysteine plays in heart disease, they are following several leads in pursuit of the answers.[15] Coffee's role in heart disease has been controversial, but research suggests it is among the most influential factors in raising homocysteine, which may explain some of the adverse health effects of heavy consumption.[16] Elevated homocysteine levels are among the many adverse health consequences of smoking cigarettes and drinking alcohol as well.[17] Homocysteine is also elevated with suboptimal intakes of B vitamins and can usually be lowered with supplements of vitamin B_{12}, vitamin B_6, and folate.[18] Such research suggests that a high intake of these vitamins may reduce the risk of heart disease.[19]

In contrast to homocysteine, the amino acid arginine may be a protective factor for heart disease, slowing the progression of atherosclerosis. The exact amount of arginine needed to defend against heart disease has not yet been determined, but it appears to be much greater than a healthy diet or a reasonable quantity of supplements alone can provide. If research confirms the benefits of arginine, look for manufacturers to begin producing functional foods enriched with this amino acid. In the meantime, it would be unwise for consumers to use supplements of arginine, or any other amino acid for that matter (as p. 203 explains).

Cancer As in heart disease, the effects of protein and fats on cancers cannot be easily separated. Population studies suggest a correlation between high intakes of animal proteins and some types of cancer (notably, cancer of the colon, breast, kidneys, pancreas, and prostate).

Adult Bone Loss (Osteoporosis) Chapter 12 presents calcium metabolism, and Highlight 12 elaborates on the main factors that influence osteoporosis. This section briefly describes the relationships between protein intake and bone loss. When protein intake is high, calcium excretion rises. Whether excess protein depletes the bones of their chief mineral may depend upon the ratio of calcium intake to protein intake. After all, bones need both protein and calcium. An ideal ratio has not been determined, but a young woman whose intake meets recommendations for both nutrients has a calcium-to-protein ratio of more than 20 to 1 (milligrams to grams), which probably provides adequate protection for the bones. For most women in the United States, however, average calcium intakes are lower and protein intakes are higher, yielding a 9-to-1 ratio, which may produce calcium losses significant enough to compromise bone health. In other words, the problem may reflect too little calcium, not too much protein. In establishing recommendations, the DRI Committee considered protein's effect on calcium metabolism and bone health, but did not find sufficient evidence to warrant an adjustment for calcium or an upper limit for protein.[20]

Inadequate intakes of protein may also compromise bone health. Osteoporosis is particularly common in elderly women and in adolescents with anorexia nervosa—groups who typically receive less protein than they need. For these people, increasing protein intake may be just what they need to protect their bones.[21]

Weight Control Protein-rich foods are often fat-rich foods that contribute to weight gain with its accompanying health risks. As Highlight 8 explains, weight-loss gimmicks that encourage a high-protein diet may be effective, but only because they are low-kcalorie diets. Diets that provide adequate protein, moderate fat, and sufficient energy from carbohydrates can better support weight loss and good health. Including protein at each meal may help with weight loss by providing satiety; selecting too many protein-rich foods, such as meat and milk, may crowd out fruits, vegetables, and grains, making the diet inadequate in other nutrients.

Kidney Disease Excretion of the end products of protein metabolism depends, in part, on an adequate fluid intake and healthy kidneys. A high protein intake increases the work of the kidneys, but does not appear to cause kidney disease. Restricting dietary protein, however, may help to slow the progression of kidney disease and limit the formation of kidney stones in people who have these conditions.

IN SUMMARY Protein deficiencies arise from both energy-poor and protein-poor diets and lead to the devastating diseases of marasmus and kwashiorkor. Together, these diseases are known as PEM (protein-energy malnutrition), a major form of malnutrition causing death in children worldwide. Excesses of protein offer no advantage; in fact, overconsumption of protein-rich foods may incur health problems as well.

Recommended Intakes of Protein

As mentioned earlier, the body continuously breaks down and loses some protein and cannot store amino acids. To replace protein, the body needs dietary protein for two reasons: first, food protein is the only source of the *essential* amino acids; and second, it is the only practical source of *nitrogen* with which to build the nonessential amino acids and other nitrogen-containing compounds the body needs.

Given recommendations that people's fat intakes should contribute 20 to 35 percent of total food energy, and carbohydrate, 45 to 65 percent, that leaves 10 to 35 percent for protein. In a 2000-kcalorie diet, that represents 200 to 700 kcalories from protein, or 50 to 175 grams. Average intakes in the United States and Canada fall within this range.

Protein RDA The protein RDA■ for adults is 0.8 gram per kilogram of healthy body weight per day. For infants and children, the RDA is slightly higher. The table on the inside front cover lists the RDA for males and females at various ages in two ways—grams per day based on reference body weights and grams per kilogram per day.

The RDA generously covers the needs for replacing worn-out tissue, so it increases for larger people; it also covers the needs for building new tissue during growth, so it increases for infants, children, and pregnant women. The protein RDA is the same for athletes as for others, although some fitness authorities recommend a slightly higher intake.[22] The accompanying "How to" shows how to calculate your RDA for protein.

■ RDA for protein:
- 0.8 g/kg/day.
- 10 to 35% of energy intake.

HOW TO Calculate Recommended Protein Intakes

To figure your protein RDA:
- Look up the healthy weight for a person of your height (inside back cover). If your present weight falls within that range, use it for the following calculations. If your present weight falls outside the range, use the midpoint of the healthy weight range as your reference weight.
- Convert pounds to kilograms, if necessary (pounds divided by 2.2 equals kilograms).
- Multiply kilograms by 0.8 to get your RDA in grams per day. (Older teens 14 to 18 years old, multiply by 0.85.) Example:

Weight = 150 lb.

150 lb ÷ 2.2 lb/kg = 68 kg (rounded off).

68 kg × 0.8 g/kg= 54 g protein (rounded off).

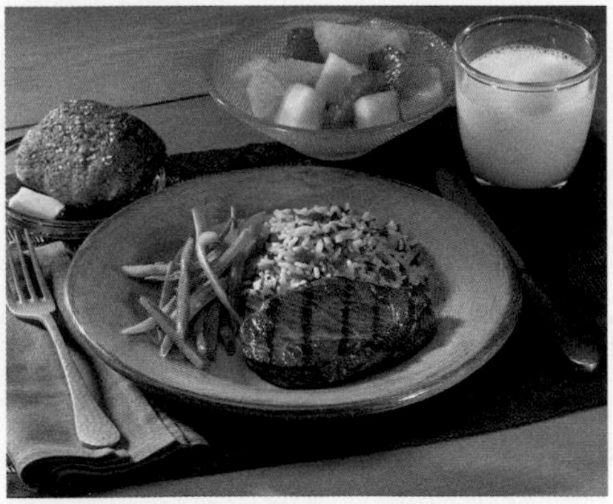
© Polara Studios, Inc.

This 5-ounce steak provides almost all of the meat recommended for a day's intake in a 2000-kcalorie diet.

In setting the RDA, the committee assumes that people are healthy and do not have unusual metabolic needs for protein; that the protein eaten will be of mixed quality (from both high- and low-quality sources); and that the body will use the protein efficiently. In addition, the committee assumes that the protein is consumed along with sufficient carbohydrate and fat to provide adequate energy and that other nutrients in the diet are adequate.

Adequate Energy Note the qualification "adequate energy" in the preceding statement, and consider what happens if energy intake falls short of needs. An intake of 50 grams of protein provides 200 kcalories, which represents 10 percent of the total energy from protein, if the person receives 2000 kcalories a day. But if the person cuts energy intake drastically—to, say, 800 kcalories a day—then an intake of 200 kcalories from protein is suddenly 25 percent of the total; yet it's still the same amount of protein (number of grams). The protein intake is reasonable, but the energy intake is not; the low energy intake will force the body to use the protein to meet energy needs rather than to replace lost body protein. Similarly, if the person's energy intake is high—say, 4000 kcalories—the 50-gram protein intake will represent only 5 percent of the total; yet it *still* is a reasonable protein intake. Again, the energy intake is unreasonable for most people, but in this case, it will permit the protein to be used to meet the body's needs.

Be careful when judging protein (or carbohydrate or fat) intake as a percentage of energy. Always ascertain the number of grams as well, and compare it with the RDA or another standard stated in grams. A recommendation stated as a percentage of energy intake is useful only if the energy intake is within reason.

Protein in Abundance Most people in the United States and Canada receive much more protein than they need. Even athletes in training typically don't need to increase their protein intakes because the additional foods they eat to meet their high energy needs deliver protein as well. That protein intake is high is not surprising considering the abundance of food eaten and the central role meats hold in the North American diet. A single ounce of meat (or ½ cup legumes) delivers about 7 grams of protein, so 8 ounces of meat alone supplies more than the RDA for an average-sized person. Besides meat, well-fed people eat many other nutritious foods, many of which also provide protein. A cup of milk provides 8 grams of protein. Grains and vegetables provide small amounts of protein, but they can add up to significant quantities; fruits and fats provide no protein.

To illustrate how easy it is to overconsume protein, consider the amounts recommended by the USDA Food Guide for a 2000-kcalorie diet. Six ounces of grains provide about 18 grams of protein; 2½ cups of vegetables deliver about 10 grams; 3 cups of milk offer 24 grams; and 5½ ounces of meat supply 38 grams. This totals 90 grams of protein—higher than recommendations for most people and yet still lower than the average intake of people in the United States.

Most people in the United States and Canada get more protein than they need. If they have an adequate *food* intake, they have a more-than-adequate protein intake. The key diet-planning principle to emphasize for protein is moderation. Even though most people receive plenty of protein, some feel compelled to take supplements as well, as the next section describes.

IN SUMMARY Optimally, the diet will be adequate in energy from carbohydrate and fat and will deliver 0.8 gram of protein per kilogram of healthy body weight each day. U.S. and Canadian diets are typically more than adequate in this respect.

Protein and Amino Acid Supplements

Websites, health-food stores, and popular magazine articles advertise a wide variety of protein supplements, and people take these supplements for many different reasons, all of them unfounded. Athletes take protein supplements to build muscle. Dieters take them to spare their bodies' protein while losing weight. Women take them to strengthen their fingernails. People take individual amino acids, too—to cure herpes, to make themselves sleep better, to lose weight, and to relieve pain and depression.* Like many other magic solutions to health problems, protein and amino acid■ supplements don't work these miracles. Furthermore, they may be harmful.[23]

Muscle work builds muscle; protein supplements do not, and athletes do not need them. Instead, athletes need a well-balanced diet that provides sufficient dietary protein and adequate food energy. Food energy spares body protein; carbohydrate and fat serve this purpose equally well. Fingernails are not affected by protein supplements, provided the diet is adequate. Furthermore, protein supplements are expensive, less completely digested than protein-rich foods, and, when used as replacements for such foods, often downright dangerous.

Single amino acids do not occur naturally in foods and offer no benefit to the body; in fact, they may be harmful. The body was not designed to handle the high concentrations and unusual combinations of amino acids found in supplements. An excess of one amino acid can create such a demand for a carrier that it limits the absorption of another amino acid, presenting the possibility of a deficiency. Those amino acids winning the competition enter in excess, creating the possibility of a toxicity. Toxicity of single amino acids in animal studies raises concerns about their use in human beings. Anyone considering taking amino acid supplements should check with a registered dietitian or physician first.

In two cases, recommendations for single amino acid supplements have led to widespread public use—lysine to prevent or relieve the infections that cause herpes cold sores on the mouth or genital organs, and tryptophan to relieve pain, depression, and insomnia. In both cases, enthusiastic popular reports preceded careful scientific experiments and health recommendations. A review of the research indicates that lysine may suppress herpes infections in some individuals and appears safe (up to 3 grams per day) when taken in divided doses with meals.[24]

Tryptophan is also effective with respect to pain and sleep, but its use for these purposes is still experimental. More than 1500 people who elected to take tryptophan supplements developed a rare blood disorder known as eosinophilia-myalgia syndrome (EMS). EMS is characterized by severe muscle and joint pain, extremely high fever, and, in over three dozen cases, death. Treatment for EMS usually involves physical therapy and low doses of corticosteroids to relieve symptoms temporarily. The Food and Drug Administration determined that contaminants caused the disease and issued a recall of all products containing manufactured tryptophan.

■ Use of amino acids as dietary supplements is *inappropriate,* especially for:
- All women of childbearing age.
- Pregnant or lactating women.
- Infants, children, and adolescents.
- Elderly people.
- People with inborn errors of metabolism that affect their bodies' handling of amino acids.
- Smokers.
- People on low-protein diets.
- People with chronic or acute mental or physical illnesses who take amino acids without medical supervision.

IN SUMMARY Normal, healthy people never need protein or amino acid supplements. It is safest to obtain lysine, tryptophan, and all other amino acids from protein-rich foods, eaten with abundant carbohydrate and some fat to facilitate their use in the body. With all that we know about science, it is hard to improve on nature.

*Canada only allows single amino acid supplements to be sold as drugs or used as food additives.

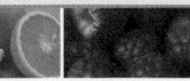

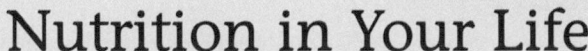

Nutrition in Your Life

Foods that derive from animals—meats, fish, poultry, eggs, and milk products—provide plenty of protein, but are often accompanied by fat. Those that derive from plants—whole grains, vegetables, and legumes—may provide less protein, but also less fat.

- **Calculate your daily protein needs. Do you receive enough, but not too much, protein daily?**
- **What are your dietary sources of proteins? Do you use mostly plant-based or animal-based protein foods in your diet?**
- **Do you take protein or amino acid supplements?**

NUTRITION ON THE NET

Access these websites for further study of topics covered in this chapter.

- Find updates and quick links to these and other nutrition-related sites at our website: **www.wadsworth.com/nutrition**
- Learn more about sickle-cell anemia from the National Heart, Lung, and Blood Institute or the Sickle Cell Disease Association of America: **www.nhlbi.nih.gov** or **www.sicklecelldisease.org**
- Learn more about protein-energy malnutrition and world hunger from the World Health Organization Nutrition Programme: **www.who.int/nut**
- Highlight 16 offers many more websites on malnutrition and world hunger.

NUTRITION CALCULATIONS

These problems will give you practice in doing simple nutrition-related calculations using hypothetical situations (see p. 207 for answers). Once you have mastered these examples, you will be prepared to examine your own protein needs. Be sure to show your calculations for each problem.

1. Compute recommended protein intakes for people of different sizes. Refer to the "How to" on p. 201 and compute the protein recommendation for the following people. The intake for a woman who weighs 144 pounds is computed for you as an example.

$$144 \text{ lb} \div 2.2 \text{ lb/kg} = 65 \text{ kg}.$$

$$0.8 \text{ g/kg} \times 65 \text{ kg} = 52 \text{ g protein per day}.$$

   a. A woman who weighs 116 pounds.
   b. A man (18 years) who weighs 180 pounds.

2. The chapter warns that recommendations based on percentage of energy intake are not always appropriate. Consider a woman 26 years old who weighs 165 pounds. Her diet provides 1500 kcalories/day with 50 grams carbohydrate and 100 grams fat.
   a. What is this woman's protein intake? Show your calculations.
   b. Is her protein intake appropriate? Justify your answer.
   c. Are her carbohydrate and fat intakes appropriate? Justify your answer.

This exercise should help you develop a perspective on protein recommendations.

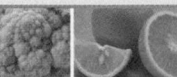

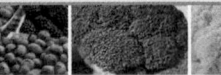

STUDY QUESTIONS

These questions will help you review the chapter. You will find the answers in the discussions on the pages provided.

1. How does the chemical structure of proteins differ from the structures of carbohydrates and fats? (pp. 181–182)
2. Describe the structure of amino acids, and explain how their sequence in proteins affects the proteins' shapes. What are essential amino acids? (pp. 182–184)
3. Describe protein digestion and absorption. (pp. 185–186)
4. Describe protein synthesis. (pp. 187–189)
5. Describe some of the roles proteins play in the human body. (pp. 189–192)
6. What are enzymes? What roles do they play in chemical reactions? Describe the differences between enzymes and hormones. (p. 190)
7. How does the body use amino acids? What is deamination? Define nitrogen balance. What conditions are associated with zero, positive, and negative balance? (pp. 193–194)
8. What factors affect the quality of dietary protein? What is a high-quality protein? (pp. 194–195)
9. How can vegetarians meet their protein needs without eating meat? (p. 195)
10. What are the health consequences of ingesting inadequate protein and energy? Describe marasmus and kwashiorkor. How can the two conditions be distinguished, and in what ways do they overlap? (pp. 197–199)
11. How might protein excess, or the type of protein eaten, influence health? (pp. 200–201)
12. What factors are considered in establishing recommended protein intakes? (pp. 201–202)
13. What are the benefits and risks of taking protein and amino acid supplements? (p. 203)

These multiple choice questions will help you prepare for an exam. Answers can be found on p. 207.

1. Which part of its chemical structure differentiates one amino acid from another?
   a. its side group
   b. its acid group
   c. its amino group
   d. its double bonds
2. Isoleucine, leucine, and lysine are:
   a. proteases.
   b. polypeptides.
   c. essential amino acids.
   d. complementary proteins.
3. In the stomach, hydrochloric acid:
   a. denatures proteins and activates pepsin.
   b. hydrolyzes proteins and denatures pepsin.
   c. emulsifies proteins and releases peptidase.
   d. condenses proteins and facilitates digestion.
4. Proteins that facilitate chemical reactions are:
   a. buffers.
   b. enzymes.
   c. hormones.
   d. antigens.
5. If an essential amino acid that is needed to make a protein is unavailable, the cells must:
   a. deaminate another amino acid.
   b. substitute a similar amino acid.
   c. break down proteins to obtain it.
   d. synthesize the amino acid from glucose and nitrogen.
6. Protein turnover describes the amount of protein:
   a. found in foods and the body.
   b. absorbed from the diet.
   c. synthesized and degraded.
   d. used to make glucose.
7. The PDCAAS is used to:
   a. determine protein quality.
   b. assess protein-energy malnutrition.
   c. estimate the weight of nitrogen in a food.
   d. calculate the percentage kcalories from protein.
8. Marasmus develops from:
   a. too much fat clogging the liver.
   b. megadoses of amino acid supplements.
   c. inadequate protein and energy intake.
   d. excessive fluid intake causing edema.
9. The protein RDA for a healthy adult who weighs 180 pounds is:
   a. 50 milligrams/day.
   b. 65 grams/day.
   c. 180 grams/day.
   d. 2000 milligrams/day.
10. Which of these foods has the least protein per ½ cup?
   a. rice
   b. broccoli
   c. pinto beans
   d. orange juice

REFERENCES

1. M. S. Buchowski and coauthors, Equation to estimate resting energy expenditure in adolescents with sickle cell anemia, *American Journal of Clinical Nutrition* 76 (2002): 1335–1344; Committee on Genetics, Health supervision for children with sickle cell disease, *Pediatrics* 109 (2002): 526–535; S. T. Miller and coauthors, Prediction of adverse outcomes in children with sickle cell disease, *New England Journal of Medicine* 342 (2000): 83–89.
2. W. M. Rand, P. L. Pellett, and V. R. Young, Meta-analysis of nitrogen balance studies for estimating protein requirements in healthy adults, *American Journal of Clinical Nutrition* 77 (2003): 109–127.
3. J. Hernández-Rodriguez and G. Manjarrez-Guitiérrez, Macronutrients and neurotransmitter formation during brain development, *Nutrition Reviews* 59 (2001): S49–S59.
4. Position of the American Dietetic Association: Vegetarian diets, *Journal of the American Dietetic Association* 97 (1997): 1317–1321.
5. T. Liu and coauthors, Kwashiorkor in the United States: Fad diets, perceived and true milk allergy, and nutritional ignorance, *Archives of Dermatology* 137 (2001): 630–636; G. Massa, Protein malnutrition due to replacement of milk by rice drink, *European Journal of Pediatrics* 160 (2001): 382–384; N. F. Carvalho and coauthors, Severe nutritional deficiencies in toddlers resulting from health food milk alternatives, *Pediatrics* 107 (2001): e46.
6. G. Akner and T. Cederholm, Treatment of protein-energy malnutrition in chronic nonmalignant disorders, *American Journal of Clinical Nutrition* 74 (2001): 6–24; D. H. Sullivan, S. Sun, and R. C. Walls, Protein-energy undernutrition among elderly hospitalized patients: A prospective study, *Journal of the American Medical Association* 281 (1999): 2013–2019.
7. L. Combaret, D. Taillandier, and D. Attaix, Nutritional and hormonal control of protein breakdown, *American Journal of Kidney Diseases* 37 (2001): S108–S111.
8. M. Reid and coauthors, The acute-phase protein response to infection in edematous and nonedematous protein-energy malnutrition, *American Journal of Clinical Nutrition* 76 (2002): 1409–1415.
9. V. Scherbaum and P. Furst, New concepts on nutritional management of severe malnutrition: The role of protein, *Current Opinion in Clinical Nutrition and Metabolic Care* 3 (2000): 31–38.
10. B. A. Underwood and S. Smitasiri, Micronutrient malnutrition: Policies and programs for control and their implications, *Annual Review of Nutrition* 19 (1999): 303–324; C. G. Victora and coauthors, Potential interventions for the prevention of childhood pneumonia in developing countries: Improving nutrition, *American Journal of Clinical Nutrition* 70 (1999): 309–320.
11. Committee on Dietary Reference Intakes, *Dietary Reference Intakes for Energy, Carbohydrate, Fiber, Fat, Fatty Acids, Cholesterol, Protein, and Amino Acids* (Washington, D.C.: National Academies Press, 2002), p. 10–77.
12. S. Tonstad, K. Smerud, and L. Høie, A comparison of the effects of 2 doses of soy protein or casein on serum lipids, serum lipoproteins, and plasma total homocysteine in hypercholesterolemic subjects, *American Journal of Clinical Nutrition* 76 (2002): 78–84; S. R. Teixeira and coauthors, Effects of feeding 4 levels of soy protein for 3 and 6 wk on blood lipids and apolipoproteins in moderately hypercholesterolemic men, *American Journal of Clinical Nutrition* 71 (2000): 1077–1084.
13. D. S. Wald, M. Law, and J. K. Morris, Homocysteine and cardiovascular disease: Evidence on causality from a meta-analysis, *British Medical Journal* 325 (2002): 1202–1217; The Homocysteine Studies Collaboration, Homocysteine and risk of ischemic heart disease and stroke, *Journal of the American Medical Association* 288 (2002): 2015–2022; P. M. Ridker, Homocysteine and risk of cardiovascular disease among postmenopausal women, *Journal of the American Medical Association* 281 (1999): 1817–1821.
14. L. Brattström and D. E. L. Wilcken, Homocysteine and cardiovascular disease: Cause or effect? *American Journal of Clinical Nutrition* 72 (2000): 315–323; R. Meleady and I. Graham, Plasma homocysteine as a cardiovascular risk factor: Causal, consequential, or of no consequence? *Nutrition Reviews* 57 (1999): 299–305.
15. J. Selhub, Homocysteine metabolism, *Annual Review of Nutrition* 19 (1999): 217–246.
16. P. Verhoef and coauthors, Contribution of caffeine to the homocysteine-raising effect of coffee: A randomized controlled trial in humans, *American Journal of Clinical Nutrition* 76 (2002): 1244–1248; M. J. Grubben and coauthors, Unfiltered coffee increases plasma homocysteine concentrations in healthy volunteers: A randomized trial, *American Journal of Clinical Nutrition* 71 (2000): 480–484.
17. L. I. Mennen and coauthors, Homocysteine, cardiovascular disease risk factors, and habitual diet in the French Supplementation and Antioxidant Vitamins and Minerals Study, *American Journal of Clinical Nutrition* 76 (2002): 1279–1289; A. DeBree and coauthors, Lifestyle factors and plasma homocysteine concentrations in a general population sample, *American Journal of Epidemiology* 153 (2001): 150–154.
18. G. Schnyder and coauthors, Decreased rate of coronary restenosis after lowering of plasma homocysteine levels, *New England Journal of Medicine* 345 (2001): 1539–1600; P. F. Jacques and coauthors, The effect of folic acid fortification on plasma folate and total homocysteine concentrations, *New England Journal of Medicine* 340 (1999): 1449–1454; A. Chait and coauthors, Increased dietary micronutrients decrease serum homocysteine concentrations in patients at high risk of cardiovascular disease, *American Journal of Clinical Nutrition* 70 (1999): 881–887; I. A. Brouwer and coauthors, Low-dose folic acid supplementation decreases plasma homocysteine concentrations: A randomized trial, *American Journal of Clinical Nutrition* 69 (1999): 99–104.
19. G. Schnyder and coauthors, Effect of homocysteine-lowering therapy with folic acid, vitamin B_{12}, and vitamin B_6 on clinical outcome after percutaneous coronary intervention—The Swiss Heart Study: A randomized controlled trial, *Journal of the American Medical Association* 288 (2002): 973–979; B. J. Venn and coauthors, Dietary counseling to increase natural folate intake: A randomized, placebo-controlled trial in free-living subjects to assess effects on serum folate and plasma total homocysteine, *American Journal of Clinical Nutrition* 76 (2002): 758–765; E. B. Rimm and coauthors, Folate and vitamin B_6 from diet and supplements in relation to risk of coronary heart disease among women, *Journal of the American Medical Association* 279 (1998): 359–364.
20. Committee on Dietary Reference Intakes, 2002, pp. 11-50–11-51; Committee on Dietary Reference Intakes, *Dietary Reference Intakes for Calcium, Phosphorus, Magnesium, Vitamin D, and Fluoride* (Washington, D.C.: National Academy Press, 1997), pp. 75–76.
21. J. Bell and S. J. Whiting, Elderly women need dietary protein to maintain bone mass, *Nutrition Reviews* 60 (2002): 337–341; M. T. Munoz and J. Argente, Anorexia nervosa in female adolescents: Endocrine and bone mineral density disturbances, *European Journal of Endocrinology* 147 (2002): 275–286.
22. Position of the American Dietetic Association, Dietitians of Canada, and the American College of Sports Nutrition, Nutrition and athletic performance, *Journal of the American Dietetic Association* 100 (2000): 1543–1556.
23. P. J. Garlick, Assessment of the safety of glutamine and other amino acids, *Journal of Nutrition* 131 (2001): 2556S–2561S.
24. N. W. Flodin, The metabolic roles, pharmacology, and toxicology of lysine, *Journal of the American College of Nutrition* 16 (1997): 7–21.

ANSWERS

Nutrition Calculations

1. a. 116 lb ÷ 2.2 lb/kg = 53 kg.
   0.8 g/kg × 53 kg = 42 g protein per day.
   b. 180 lb ÷ 2.2 lb/kg = 82 kg.
   He is 18 years old, so use 0.85 g/kg. 0.85 g/kg × 82 kg = 70 g protein per day.

2. a. 50 g carbohydrate × 4 kcal/g = 200 kcal from carbohydrate.
   100 g fat × 9 kcal/g = 900 kcal from fat.
   1500 kcal − (200 + 900 kcal) = 400 kcal from protein.
   400 kcal ÷ 4 kcal/g = 100 g protein.
   b. Using the RDA guideline of 0.8 g/kg, an appropriate protein intake for this woman would be 60 g protein/day (165 lb ÷ 2.2 lb/kg = 75 kg; 0.8 g/kg × 75 = 60 g/day). Her intake is higher than her RDA. Using the guideline that protein should contribute 10 to 35% of energy intake, her intake of 100 g protein on a 1500 kcal diet falls within the suggested range (400 kcal protein ÷ 1500 total kcal = 27%).
   c. Using the guideline that carbohydrate should contribute 45 to 65% and fat should contribute 20 to 35% of energy intake, her intake of 50 g carbohydrate is low (200 kcal carbohydrate ÷ 1500 total kcal = 13%), and her intake of 100 g fat is high (900 kcal fat ÷ 1500 total kcal = 60%).

Study Questions (multiple choice)

1. a 2. c 3. a 4. b 5. c 6. c 7. a
8. c 9. b 10. d

HIGHLIGHT

Vegetarian Diets

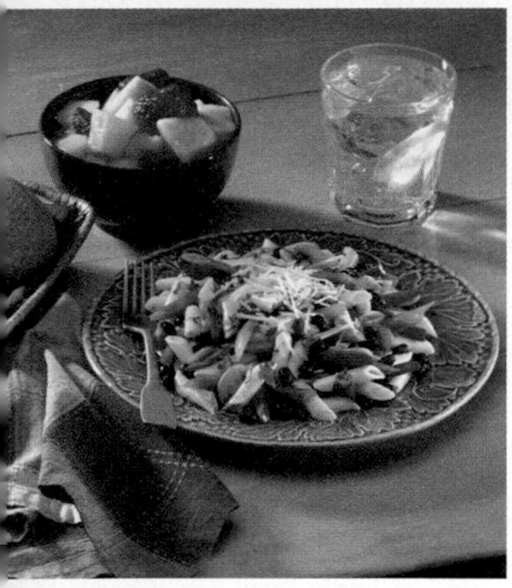

© Polara Studios, Inc.

The waiter presents this evening's specials: a fresh spinach salad topped with mandarin oranges, raisins, and sunflower seeds, served with a bowl of pasta smothered in a mushroom and tomato sauce and topped with grated parmesan cheese. Then this one: a salad made of chopped parsley, scallions, celery, and tomatoes mixed with bulgur wheat and dressed with olive oil and lemon juice, served with a spinach and feta cheese pie. Do these meals sound good to you? Or is something missing . . . a pork chop or ribeye, perhaps?

Would vegetarian fare be acceptable to you some of the time? Most of the time? Ever? Perhaps it is helpful to recognize that dietary choices fall along a continuum—from one end, where people eat no meat or foods of animal origin, to the other end, where they eat generous quantities daily. Meat's place in the diet has been the subject of much research and controversy, as this highlight will reveal. One of the missions of this highlight, in fact, is to identify the *range* of meat intakes most compatible with health.

People who choose to exclude meat and other animal-derived foods from their diets today do so for many of the same reasons the Greek philosopher Pythagoras cited in the sixth century B.C.: physical health, ecological responsibility, and philosophical concerns. They might also cite world hunger issues, economic reasons, ethical concerns, or religious beliefs as motivating factors. Whatever their reasons—and even if they don't have a particular reason—people who exclude meat will be better prepared to plan well-balanced meals if they understand the nutrition and health implications of vegetarian diets.

Vegetarians generally are categorized, not by their motivations, but by the foods they choose to exclude (see the glossary below). Some exclude red meat only; some also exclude chicken or fish; others also exclude eggs; and still others exclude milk and milk products as well. In fact, finding agreement on the definition of the term *vegetarian* is a challenge.[1]

As you will see, though, the foods a person *excludes* are not nearly as important as the foods a person *includes* in the diet. Vegetarian diets that include a variety of whole grains, vegetables, legumes, seeds, nuts, and fruits offer abundant complex carbohydrates and fibers, an assortment of vitamins and minerals, and little fat—characteristics that reflect current dietary recommendations aimed at promoting health and reducing obesity. This highlight examines the health benefits and potential problems of vegetarian diets and shows how to plan a well-balanced vegetarian diet.

Health Benefits of Vegetarian Diets

Research on the health impacts of vegetarianism would be relatively easy if vegetarians differed from other people only in not eating meat. Many vegetarians, however, have adopted lifestyles

GLOSSARY

lactovegetarians: people who include milk and milk products, but exclude meat, poultry, fish, seafood, and eggs from their diets.
- **lacto** = milk

lacto-ovo-vegetarians: people who include milk, milk products, and eggs, but exclude meat, poultry, fish, and seafood from their diets.
- **ovo** = egg

macrobiotic diets: extremely restrictive diets limited to a few grains and vegetables; based on metaphysical beliefs and not on nutrition.

meat replacements: products formulated to look and taste like meat, fish, or poultry; usually made of textured vegetable protein.

omnivores: people who have no formal restriction on the eating of any foods.
- **omni** = all
- **vores** = to eat

tempeh (TEM-pay): a fermented soybean food, rich in protein and fiber.

textured vegetable protein: processed soybean protein used in vegetarian products such as soy burgers; see also *meat replacements.*

tofu (TOE-foo): a curd made from soybeans, rich in protein and often fortified with calcium; used in many Asian and vegetarian dishes in place of meat.

vegans (VEE-guns, VAY-guns, or VEJ-ans): people who exclude all animal-derived foods (including meat, poultry, fish, eggs, and dairy products) from their diets; also called **pure vegetarians, strict vegetarians,** or **total vegetarians.**

vegetarians: a general term used to describe people who exclude meat, poultry, fish, or other animal-derived foods from their diets.

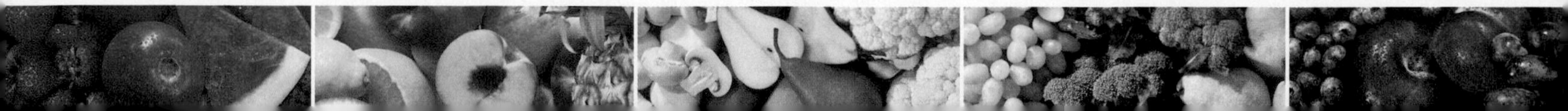

that differ from others: they typically maintain a healthy weight, use no tobacco or illicit drugs, use little (if any) alcohol, and are physically active. Researchers must account for these lifestyle differences before they can determine which aspects of health correlate just with diet. Even then, *correlations* merely reveal what health factors *go with* the vegetarian diet, not what health effects may be *caused by* the diet. Without more evidence, conclusions remain tentative. Still, with all these qualifications, research findings suggest that well-planned vegetarian diets offer sound nutrition and health benefits to adults.[2]

In general, vegetarians maintain a healthier body weight than nonvegetarians.[3] Studies report higher weights among people eating a mixed diet compared with vegetarians and that body weight increases as frequency of meat consumption increases.[4] Vegetarians' lower body weights correlate with their high intakes of fiber and low intakes of fat. Since obesity impairs health in a number of ways, this gives vegetarians a health advantage.

Vegetarians tend to have lower blood pressure and lower rates of hypertension than nonvegetarians. Appropriate body weight helps to maintain a healthy blood pressure, as does a diet low in total fat and saturated fat and high in fiber, fruits, and vegetables. Lifestyle factors also seem to influence blood pressure: smoking and alcohol intake raise blood pressure, and physical activity lowers it.

The incidence of heart disease and related deaths is much lower for vegetarians than for meat eaters. The dietary factor most directly related to heart disease is saturated animal fat, and in general, vegetarian diets are lower in total fat, saturated fat, and cholesterol than typical meat-based diets. The fats common in plant-based diets—the monounsaturated fats of olives, seeds, and nuts and the polyunsaturated fats of vegetable oils—are associated with a decreased risk of heart disease.[5] Furthermore, vegetarian diets are generally higher in dietary fiber, another factor that helps control blood lipids and protect against heart disease.

Many vegetarians include soy products such as **tofu** in their diets, and these foods offer additional benefits. Even when their intakes of energy, protein, carbohydrate, total fat, saturated fat, unsaturated fat, alcohol, and fiber are the same, people eating meals based on tofu have lower blood cholesterol and triglyceride levels than those eating meat.[6] Soy products, such as tofu, contain phytochemicals that may be responsible for their ability to lower blood cholesterol (as Highlight 13 explains in greater detail).[7]

Vegetarians have a significantly lower rate of cancer than the general population. Their low cancer rates may be due to their high intakes of fruits and vegetables.

Some scientific findings indicate that vegetarian diets are associated not only with lower cancer mortality in general, but with lower incidence of cancer at specific sites as well, most notably, colon cancer. People with colon cancer seem to eat more meat, more saturated fat, and fewer vegetables than others without cancer. High-protein, high-fat, low-fiber diets create an environment in the colon that promotes the development of cancer in some people. A high-meat diet has been associated with stomach cancer as well.[8]

Vegetarian Diet Planning

The vegetarian has the same meal-planning task as any other person—using a variety of foods that will deliver all the needed nutrients within an energy allowance that maintains a healthy body weight (as discussed in Chapter 2). An added challenge is to do so with fewer options.

Vegetarians who include milk products and eggs can meet recommendations for most nutrients about as easily as nonvegetarians. Such diets provide enough energy, protein, and other nutrients to support the health of adults and the growth of children and adolescents.

Vegetarians are often advised to follow the USDA Food Guide presented in Chapter 2 with a few modifications. Those who include milk products and eggs can follow the regular plan, using legumes, nuts, and seeds and products made from them, such as peanut butter, **tempeh,** and tofu, in place of meat. Those who do not use milk can use soy milk and tofu fortified with calcium, vitamin D, and vitamin B_{12}. Dark green vegetables and legumes help meet iron and zinc needs.

Several food guides have been developed specifically for vegetarian diets.[9] They all address the particular nutrition concerns of vegetarians, but differ slightly. Figure H6-1 presents one version. The vegetable and fruit groups have subgroups that emphasize particularly good sources of calcium and iron, respectively. Green leafy vegetables are featured in the vegetable group because they provide almost five times as much calcium per serving as other vegetables. Similarly, dried fruits receive special notice in the fruit group because they deliver six times as much iron as other fruits. A separate group for nuts and seeds provides additional sources of protein, iron, zinc, and essential fatty acids. A group for oils at the tip encourages the use of vegetable oils rich in unsaturated fats and omega-3 fatty acids. The meat and legumes group has been revised and renamed "beans and protein foods," and soy milks are found in the dairy group. To ensure adequate intakes of vitamin B_{12}, vitamin D, and calcium, vegetarians need to select fortified foods or use supplements daily. This design is flexible enough that a variety of people can use it: people who have adopted various vegetarian diets, those who want to make the transition to a vegetarian diet, and those who simply want to include more plant-based meals in their diets. This vegetarian food guide also includes other lifestyle factors that contribute to good health: physical activity and water intake.

Most vegetarians easily obtain large quantities of the nutrients that are abundant in plant foods: thiamin, folate, and vitamins B_6, C, A, and E. Vegetarian food guides help to ensure adequate intakes of the main nutrients vegetarian diets might otherwise lack: iron, zinc, calcium, vitamin B_{12}, and vitamin D.

FIGURE H6-1 Vegetarian Food Pyramid

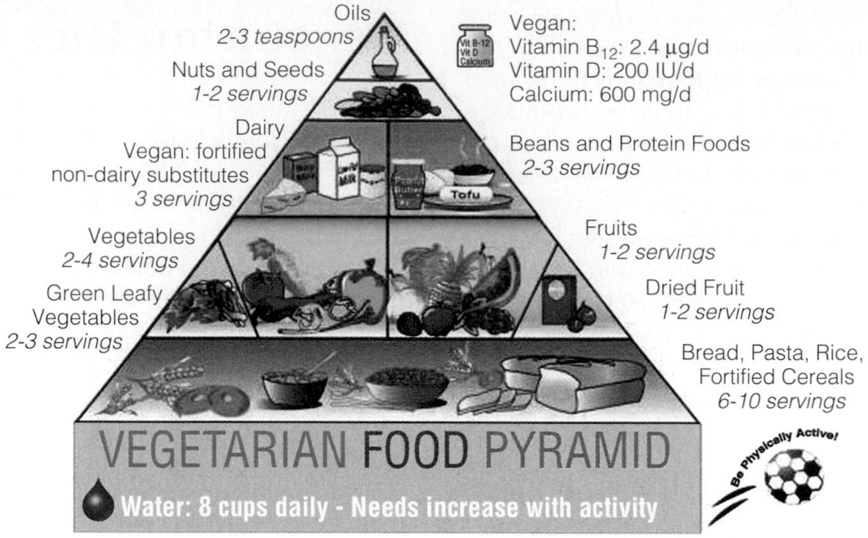
Oils
2-3 teaspoons
Nuts and Seeds
1-2 servings
Dairy
Vegan: fortified
non-dairy substitutes
3 servings
Vegetables
2-4 servings
Green Leafy
Vegetables
2-3 servings
Vegan:
Vitamin B12: 2.4 µg/d
Vitamin D: 200 IU/d
Calcium: 600 mg/d
Beans and Protein Foods
2-3 servings
Tofu
Fruits
1-2 servings
Dried Fruit
1-2 servings
Bread, Pasta, Rice,
Fortified Cereals
6-10 servings
VEGETARIAN FOOD PYRAMID
Water: 8 cups daily - Needs increase with activity
Be Physically Active!

SOURCE: C. A. Venti and C. S. Johnston, Modifiied food guide pyramid for lactovegetarians and vegans *Journal of Nutrition* 132 (2002): 1050–1054.

Protein

The protein RDA for vegetarians is the same as for others, although some have suggested that it should be higher because of the lower digestibility of plant proteins.[11] **Lacto-ovo-vegetarians** who use animal-derived foods such as milk and eggs receive high-quality proteins and are likely to meet their protein needs. Even those who adopt only plant-based diets are likely to meet protein needs provided that energy intakes are adequate and the protein sources varied.[12] The proteins of whole grains, legumes, seeds, nuts, and vegetables can provide adequate amounts of all the amino acids. An advantage of many vegetarian protein foods is that they are generally lower in saturated fat than meats and are often higher in fiber and richer in some vitamins and minerals.

To ease meal preparation, vegetarians sometimes use **meat replacements** made of **textured vegetable protein** (soy protein). These foods are formulated to look and taste like meat, fish, or poultry. Many of these products are fortified to provide the known nutrient contents of animal-protein foods, but sometimes they fall short. A wise vegetarian learns to use a variety of whole, unrefined foods often and commercially prepared foods less frequently. Vegetarians may also use soybeans in the form of tofu to bolster protein intake.

Vitamins and Minerals

Getting enough iron can be a problem even for meat eaters, and those who eat no meat must pay special attention to their iron intake. The iron in plant foods such as legumes, dark green leafy vegetables, iron-fortified cereals, and whole-grain breads and cereals is poorly absorbed.[13] Because the bioavailability of iron from a vegetarian diet is low, the iron RDA for vegetarians is higher than for others (see Chapter 13 for more details).

Fortunately, the body seems to adapt to a vegetarian diet by absorbing iron more efficiently.[14] Furthermore, iron absorption is enhanced by vitamin C, and vegetarians typically eat many vitamin C–rich fruits and vegetables. Consequently, vegetarians suffer no more iron deficiency than other people do.[15]

Zinc is similar to iron in that meat is its richest food source and zinc from plant sources is not well absorbed.[16] In addition, soy, which is commonly used as a meat alternate in vegetarian meals, interferes with zinc absorption. Nevertheless, most vegetarian adults are not zinc deficient. Perhaps the best advice to vegetarians regarding zinc is to eat a variety of nutrient-dense foods; include whole grains, nuts, and legumes such as black-eyed peas, pinto beans, and kidney beans; and maintain an adequate energy intake. For those who include seafood in their diets, oysters, crabmeat, and shrimp are rich in zinc.

The calcium intakes of **lactovegetarians** are similar to those of the general population, but people who use no milk products risk deficiency. Careful planners select calcium-rich foods, such as calcium-fortified juices, soy milk, and breakfast cereals, in ample quantities regularly. This is especially important for children and adolescents. Soy formulas for infants are fortified with calcium and can be used in cooking, even for adults. Other good calcium sources include figs, some legumes, some green vegetables such as broccoli and turnip greens, some nuts such as almonds, certain seeds such as sesame seeds, and calcium-set tofu.* The choices should be

*Calcium salts are often added during processing to coagulate the tofu.

varied because calcium absorption from some plant foods may be limited (as Chapter 12 explains).

The requirement for vitamin B_{12} is small, but this vitamin is found only in animal-derived foods. Fermented soy products such as tempeh may contain some vitamin B_{12} from the bacteria that did the fermenting, but unfortunately, much of the vitamin B_{12} found in these products may be an inactive form. Seaweeds such as nori and chlorella supply some vitamin B_{12}, but not much, and excessive intakes of these foods can lead to iodine toxicity. To defend against vitamin B_{12} deficiency, **vegans** must rely on vitamin B_{12}–fortified sources (such as soy milk or breakfast cereals) or supplements. Without vitamin B_{12}, the nerves suffer damage, leading to such health consequences as loss of vision.[17]

People who do not use vitamin D–fortified foods and do not receive enough exposure to sunlight to synthesize adequate vitamin D may need supplements to defend against bone loss.[18] This is particularly important for infants, children, and older adults. In northern climates during winter months, young children on vegan diets can readily develop rickets, the vitamin D–deficiency disease.

Omega-3 Fatty Acids

Vegetarian diets typically provide enough omega-6 fatty acids, but lack omega-3 fatty acids. This imbalance slows production of EPA and DHA in the body, and without fish, eggs, or sea vegetables in the diet, intake of EPA and DHA falls short as well. To compensate for this inadequacy, vegetarians need to include good sources of linolenic acid, such as flaxseed, walnuts, soybeans, and their oils, in their diets daily.

Vegetarian Diets through the Life Span

Vegetarians who plan their diets carefully easily obtain all the nutrients they need to support good health. Achieving adequate energy and nutrient intakes may be difficult, however, for the vegan who excludes all animal products, and particularly for growing children and pregnant and lactating women. Foods of plant origin generally offer much less energy per bite than foods of animal origin. While a diet that delivers a lot of food with relatively little energy may be advantageous for overweight adults wanting to lose weight, it can be detrimental during stages of the life span involving growth. Diet planning during pregnancy, lactation, infancy, childhood, and adolescence must provide for the increases in energy and nutrients needed during those times—when the consequences of poor nutrition can be great.

Pregnancy and Lactation

In general, a vegetarian diet favors a healthy pregnancy and successful lactation if it provides adequate energy; includes milk and milk products; and contains a wide variety of legumes, cereals, fruits, and vegetables.[19] Many vegetarian women are well nourished, with nutrient intakes from diet alone exceeding the RDA for all vitamins and minerals except iron, which is low for most women. In contrast, vegan women who restrict themselves to an exclusively plant-based diet generally have low food energy intakes and are thin; for pregnant women, this can be a problem. Women with low prepregnancy weights and small weight gains during pregnancy jeopardize a healthy pregnancy.

Vegan diets, which exclude all foods of animal origin, may require supplementation with vitamin B_{12}, calcium, and vitamin D, or the addition of foods fortified with these nutrients. Infants of vegan parents may suffer spinal cord damage and develop severe psychomotor retardation due to a lack of vitamin B_{12} in the mother's diet during pregnancy. Breastfed infants of vegan mothers have been reported to develop vitamin B_{12} deficiency and severe movement disorders. Giving the infants vitamin B_{12} supplements corrects the blood and neurological symptoms of deficiency, as well as the structural abnormalities, but cognitive and language development delays may persist. A vegan mother needs a regular source of vitamin B_{12}–fortified foods or a supplement that provides 2.6 micrograms daily.

A pregnant woman who cannot meet her calcium needs through diet alone may need 600 milligrams of supplemental calcium daily, taken with meals. Pregnant women who do not receive sufficient dietary vitamin D or enough exposure to sunlight may need a supplement that provides 10 micrograms daily.

Infancy

The newborn infant is a lactovegetarian. As long as the infant has access to sunlight as a source of vitamin D and to sufficient quantities of either infant formulas or breast milk from a mother who eats an adequate diet, the infant will thrive during the early months. "Health-food beverages," such as rice milk, are inappropriate choices because they lack the protein, vitamins, and minerals infants and toddlers need; in fact, their use can lead to severe nutritional deficiencies.[20]

Infants beyond about four months of age present a greater challenge in terms of meeting nutrient needs by way of vegetarian and, especially, vegan diets. Continued breastfeeding or formula feeding is recommended, but supplementary feedings are necessary to ensure adequate energy and iron intakes. Infants and young children in vegetarian families should be given iron-fortified infant cereals well into the second year of life. Mashed or pureed legumes, tofu, and cooked eggs can be added to their diets in place of meat.

The risks of poor nutrition status in infants increase with weaning and reliance on table foods. Infants who receive a

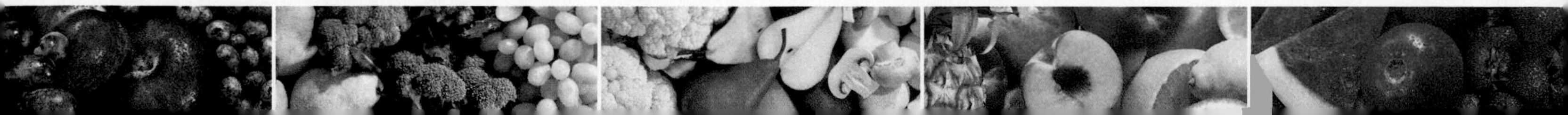

well-balanced vegetarian diet that includes milk products and a variety of other foods can easily meet their nutritional requirements for growth. This is not always true for vegan infants. Restrictive vegan diets pose a threat to infants' health. Parents or caregivers who choose to feed their infants vegan diets should consult with their pediatrician and a registered dietitian to ensure a nutritionally adequate diet that will support growth.[21]

The growth of vegan infants slows significantly around the time of transition from breast milk to solid foods. Protein-energy malnutrition and deficiencies of vitamin D, vitamin B_{12}, iron, and calcium have been reported in infants fed vegan diets. Vegan diets that are high in fiber, other complex carbohydrates, and water fill an infant's stomach before meeting energy needs. This problem can be partially alleviated by providing more energy-dense foods: nut butters, legumes, dried fruit spreads, and mashed avocado. Using soy formulas (or milk) fortified with calcium, vitamin B_{12}, and vitamin D and including vitamin C–containing foods at meals to enhance iron absorption will help prevent other nutrient deficiencies in vegan diets.

Childhood and Adolescence

Well-planned vegetarian diets, especially those that include eggs, milk, and milk products, can easily provide adequate nutrient intakes for growing children. The growth of vegetarian children is similar to that of their peers.[22]

Vegan diets, on the other hand, can fail to provide sufficient energy to support the growth of a child within a quantity of food small enough for the child to eat. A child's small stomach can hold only so much food, and a vegan child may feel full before eating enough to meet nutrient and energy needs. A vegan child's diet should emphasize cereals, legumes, and nuts to meet protein and energy needs in a small volume. Meat, which contains abundant protein, iron, and food energy in less bulk, supports the growth of children more efficiently. Compared with meat-eating children, vegan children tend to be shorter in height and lighter in weight; their low energy intakes can impair growth.

When vegan children get their protein only from plant foods, they may need protein intakes higher than the RDA for normal growth and health. The standard protein recommendations may be inadequate to support the growth of vegan children, but specific recommendations have not been established.

Other nutritional concerns for vegans include vitamin B_{12}, calcium, and vitamin D. Children who were raised on vegan diets and then switched to more liberal diets have difficulty achieving an adequate vitamin B_{12} status even with a moderate consumption of animal products.[23] Adolescents following a vegan diet low in calcium and vitamin D have a reduced bone density, which may have implications for bone health later in life. Numerous fortified animal-free foods are now available to help meet the nutrient needs of growing children on a vegan diet.[24]

For many adolescents, vegetarian diets offer the advantages of more fruits and vegetables and fewer sweets, fast foods, and salty snacks. As a result, these teens meet many of the Healthy People 2010 objectives and enjoy good growth and health.[25] Some teens, however, use vegetarian diets as a camouflage for eating disorders.[26] By hiding behind a vegetarian diet, these teens can greatly limit their food choices while distracting their parents from an eating disorder that threatens growth and health (see Highlight 9 for more details).

Healthy Food Choices

In general, adults who eat vegetarian diets have lowered their risks of mortality and several chronic diseases, including obesity, high blood pressure, heart disease, and cancer.[26] But there is nothing mysterious or magical about the vegetarian diet; vegetarianism is not a religion like Buddhism or Hinduism, but merely an eating plan that selects plant foods to deliver needed nutrients. The quality of the diet depends not on whether it includes meat, but on whether the other food choices are nutritionally sound. A diet that includes ample fruits, vegetables, whole grains, legumes, nuts, and seeds is higher in fiber, antioxidant vitamins, and phytochemicals, and lower in saturated fats than meat-based diets. Variety is key to nutritional adequacy in a vegetarian diet. Restrictive plans, such as **macrobiotic diets,** that limit selections to a few grains and vegetables cannot possibly deliver a full array of nutrients.

Having learned some of the relationships between diet and health, many people may discover that their strategies for planning meals need to change. In the past, they decided what cut of beef, ham, pork, lamb, poultry, or fish to prepare and then filled in the menu with an accompanying "starch" (potato, rice, or noodles), salad or other vegetable, and bread. Now they fill their dinner plates with legumes, whole grains, vegetables, and fruits. Then they may add small quantities of milk products, eggs, lean meat, fish, or poultry. They have decreased their use of animal products and increased their consumption of plant foods without any intention of "becoming a vegetarian." Such a plan offers many of the same health advantages of a vegetarian diet if it limits meat intake to the recommended 5 to 7 ounces daily and includes lean cuts, as well as abundant whole grains, fruits, and vegetables.

For the most part, it seems that nonmeat and low-meat diets can both support good health. Conversely, both plant-based and meat-based diets can be detrimental to health when overloaded with fat. Vegetarians who dine on cheddar cheese, butter sauces, sour cream, and deep-fried vegetables invite the same health hazards as **omnivores** who overeat high-fat meats. And both diets, if not properly balanced, can lack nutrients. Poorly planned vegetarian diets typically lack iron, zinc, calcium, vitamin B_{12}, and vitamin D; without planning, the meat eater's diet may lack vitamin A, vitamin C, folate, and fiber, among others. Quite simply, the negative health aspects of any diet, including vegetarian diets, reflect poor diet planning. Careful attention to energy intake and specific problem nutrients can ensure adequacy.

Keep in mind, too, that diet is only one factor influencing health. Whatever a diet consists of, its context is also important: no smoking, alcohol consumption in moderation (if at all), regular physical activity, adequate rest, and medical attention when needed all contribute to a healthy life. Establishing these healthy habits early in life seems to be the most important step one can take to reduce the risks of later diseases (as Highlight 15 explains).

NUTRITION ON THE NET

Access these websites for further study of topics covered in this highlight.

- Find updates and quick links to these and other nutrition-related sites at our website: **www.wadsworth.com/nutrition**
- Search for "vegetarian" at the Food and Drug Administration's site: **www.fda.gov**
- Visit the Vegetarian Resource Group: **www.vrg.org**
- Review another vegetarian diet pyramid developed by Oldways Preservation & Exchange Trust: **www.oldwayspt.org**

REFERENCES

1. S. I. Barr and G. E. Chapman, Perceptions and practices of self-defined current vegetarian, former vegetarian, and nonvegetarian women, *Journal of the American Dietetic Association* 102 (2002): 354–360; R. Weinsier, Use of the term vegetarian, *American Journal of Clinical Nutrition* 71 (2000): 1211–1212; P. K. Johnston and J. Sabate, Reply to R. Weinsier, *American Journal of Clinical Nutrition* 71 (2000): 1212–1213.
2. Position of the American Dietetic Association and Dietitians of Canada: Vegetarian diets, *Journal of the American Dietetic Association* 103 (2003): 748–765; T. J. Key, G. K. Davey, and P. N. Appleby, Health benefits of a vegetarian diet, *The Proceedings of the Nutrition Society* 58 (1999): 271–273; T. J. Key and coauthors, Mortality in vegetarians and nonvegetarians: Detailed findings from a collaborative analysis of 5 prospective studies, *American Journal of Clinical Nutrition* 70 (1999): 516S–524S.
3. Key, Davey, and Appleby, 1999.
4. G. E. Fraser, Associations between diet and cancer, ischemic heart disease, and all-cause mortality in non-Hispanic white California Seventh-day Adventists, *American Journal of Clinical Nutrition* 70 (1999): 532S–538S; P. N. Appleby and coauthors, The Oxford vegetarian study: An overview, *American Journal of Clinical Nutrition* 70 (1999): 525S–531S.
5. Third Report of the National Cholesterol Education Program (NCEP) Expert Panel on Detection, Evaluation, and Treatment of High Blood Cholesterol in Adults (Adult Treatment Panel III), NIH publication no. 02-5215 (Bethesda, Md.: National Heart, Lung, and Blood Institute, 2002); A. M. Coulston, The role of dietary fats in plant-based diets, *American Journal of Clinical Nutrition* 70 (1999): 512S–515S.
6. E. L. Ashton, F. S. Dalais, and M. J. Ball, Effect of meat replacement by tofu on CHD risk factors including copper induced LDL oxidation, *Journal of the American College of Nutrition* 19 (2000): 761–767.
7. C. D. Gardner and coauthors, The effect of soy protein with or without isoflavones relative to milk protein on plasma lipids in hypercholesterolemic postmenopausal women, *American Journal of Clinical Nutrition* 73 (2001): 667–668.
8. H. Chen and coauthors. Dietary patterns and adenocarcinoma of the esophagus and distal stomach, *American Journal of Clinical Nutrition* 75 (2002): 137–144.
9. M. Virginia, V. Melina, and A. R. Mangels, A new food guide for North American vegetarians, *Journal of the American Dietetic Association* 103 (2003): 771–775; C. A. Venti and C. S. Johnston, Modified food guide pyramid for lactovegetarians and vegans, *Journal of Nutrition* 132 (2002): 1050–1054; E. H. Haddad, J. Sabaté, and C. G. Whitten, Vegetarian food guide pyramid: A conceptual framework, *American Journal of Clinical Nutrition* 70 (1999): 615S–619S.
10. Venti and Johnston, 2002.
11. Venti and Johnston, 2002; V. Messina and A. R. Mangels, Considerations in planning vegan diets: Children, *Journal of the American Dietetic Association* 101 (2001): 661–669.
12. Position of the American Dietetic Association and Dietitians of Canada, 2003.
13. J. R. Hunt, Moving toward a plant-based diet: Are iron and zinc at risk? *Nutrition Reviews* 60 (2002): 127–134.
14. J. R. Hunt and Z. K. Roughead, Nonheme-iron absorption, fecal ferritin excretion, and blood indexes of iron status in women consuming controlled lactoovovegetarian diets for 8 wk, *American Journal of Clinical Nutrition* 69 (1999): 944–952.
15. C. L. Larsson and G. K. Johansson, Dietary intake and nutritional status of young vegans and omnivores in Sweden, *American Journal of Clinical Nutrition* 76 (2002): 100–106; M. J. Ball and M. A. Bartlett, Dietary intake and iron status of Australian vegetarian women, *American Journal of Clinical Nutrition* 70 (1999): 353–358.
16. Hunt, 2002.
17. D. Milea, N. Cassoux, and P. LeHoang, Blindness in a strict vegan, *New England Journal of Medicine* 342 (2000): 897–898.
18. T. A. Outila and coauthors, Dietary intake of vitamin D in premenopausal, healthy vegans was insufficient to maintain concentrations of serum 25-hydroxyvitamin D and intact parathyroid hormone within normal ranges during the winter in Finland, *Journal of the American Dietetic Association* 100 (2000): 434–441.
19. Position of the American Dietetic Association and Dietitians of Canada, 2003.
20. T. Liu and coauthors, Kwashiorkor in the United States: Fad diets, perceived and true milk allergy, and nutritional ignorance, *Archives of Dermatology* 137 (2001): 630–636; G. Massa, Protein malnutrition due to replacement of milk by rice drink, *European Journal of Pediatrics* 160 (2001): 382–384; N. F. Carvalho and coauthors, Severe nutritional deficiencies in toddlers resulting from health food milk alternatives, *Pediatrics* 107 (2001): e46.
21. A. R. Mangels and V. Messina, Considerations in planning vegan diets: Infants, *Journal of the American Dietetic Association* 101 (2001): 670–677.
22. M. Hebbelinck, P. Clarys, and A. DeMalsche, Growth, development, and physical fitness of Flemish vegetarian children, adolescents, young adults, *American Journal of Clinical Nutrition* 70 (1999): 579S–585S.
23. M. van Dusseldorp and coauthors, Risk of persistent cobalamin deficiency in adolescents fed a macrobiotic diet in early life, *American Journal of Clinical Nutrition* 69 (1999): 664–671.
24. Messina and Mangels, 2001.
25. C. L. Perry and coauthors, Adolescent vegetarians: How well do their dietary patterns meet the Healthy People 2010 objectives? *Archives of Pediatrics and Adolescent Medicine* 156 (2002): 431–437.
26. Y. Martins, P. Pliner, and R. O'Connor, Restrained eating among vegetarians: Does a vegetarian eating style mask concerns about weight? *Appetite* 32 (1999): 145–154.
27. Fraser, 1999.

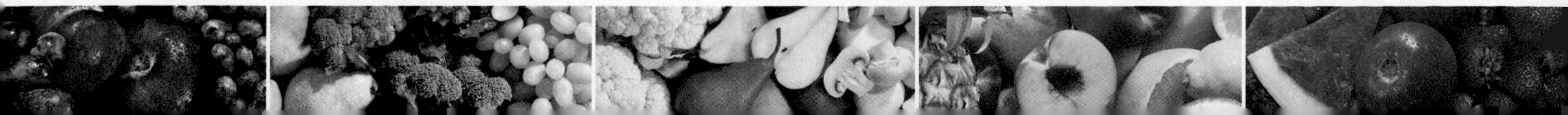

Chapter 7

Metabolism: Transformations and Interactions

Chapter Outline

Available Online

http://nutrition.wadsworth.com/uncn7

Nutrition Animations:

1. *Metabolism: Glucose to Pyruvate/Lactate and on to Acetyl CoA*
2. *Metabolism: Fatty Acids to Acetyl CoA*
3. *Metabolism: The TCA Cycle*
4. *Metabolism: The Electron Transport Chain and ATP Synthesis*

Student Practice Test

Glossary Terms

Nutrition on the Net

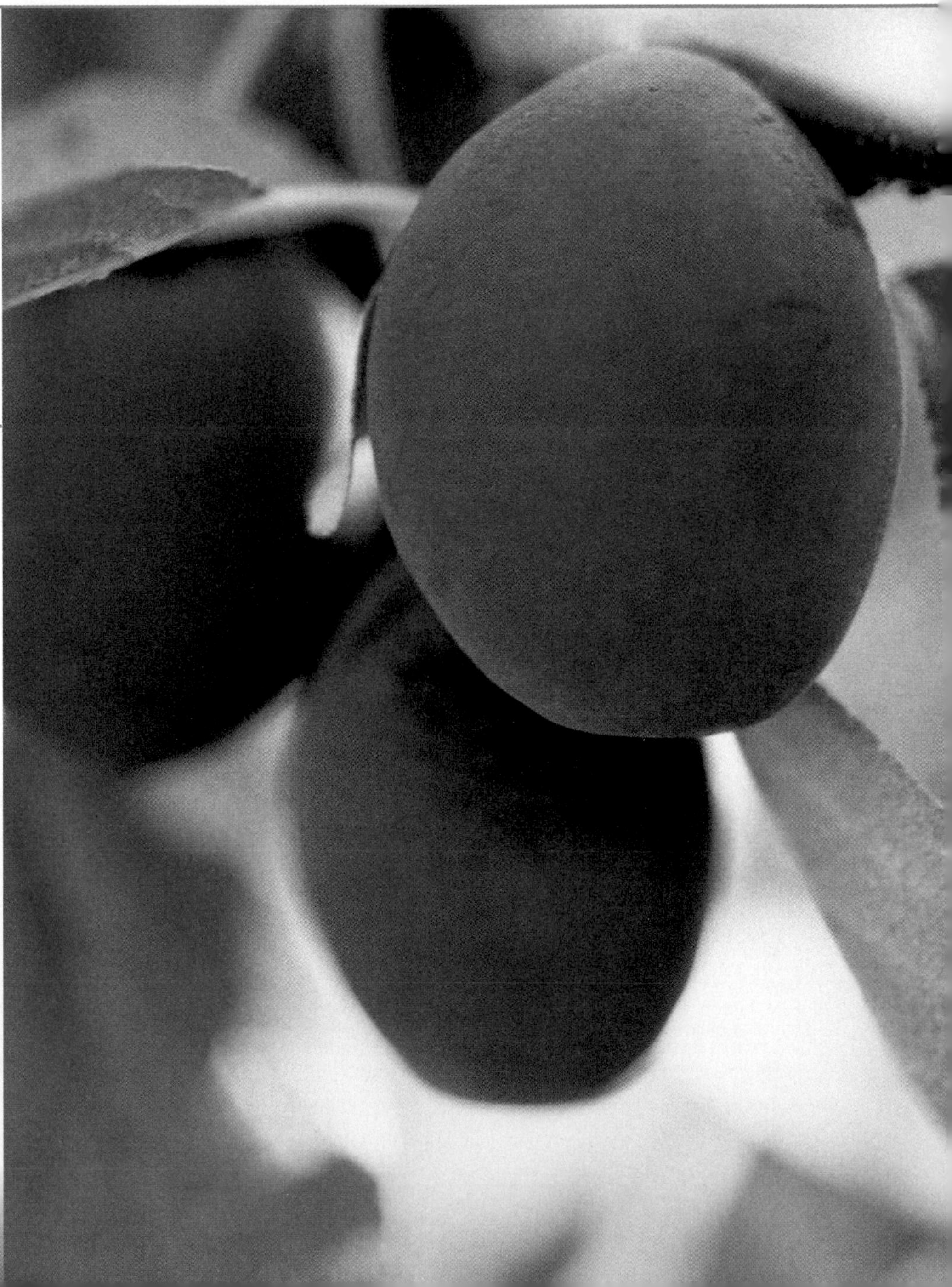

Nutrition in Your Life

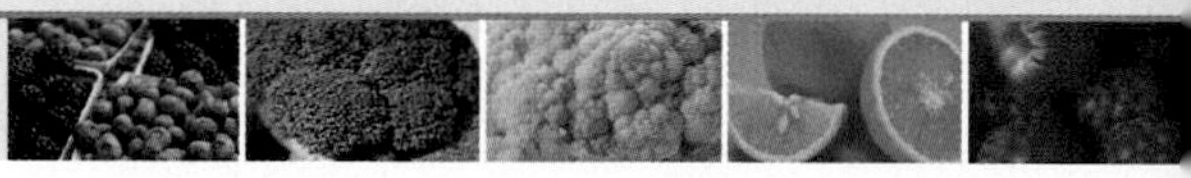

You eat breakfast and hustle off to class. After lunch, you study for tomorrow's exam. Dinner is followed by an evening of dancing. Do you ever think about how the food you eat powers the activities of your life? What happens when you don't eat—or when you eat too much? Learn how the cells of your body transform carbohydrates, fats, and proteins into energy—and what happens when you give your cells too much or too little of any of these nutrients. Discover the metabolic pathways that lead to body fat and those that support physical activity. It's really quite fascinating.

Energy enables people to breathe, ride bicycles, compose music, and do everything else they do. All the energy that sustains human life initially comes from the sun. During **photosynthesis,** plants make simple sugars from carbon dioxide and capture the sun's light energy in the chemical bonds of those sugars. Then human beings eat either the plants or animals that have eaten the plants. These foods provide energy, but how does the body obtain that energy from foods? This chapter presents the nutrients that provide the body with **fuel** and follows them through a series of reactions that release energy from their chemical bonds. As the bonds break, they release energy in a controlled version of the process by which wood burns in a fire. Both wood and food have the potential to provide energy. When wood burns in the presence of oxygen, it generates heat and light (energy), steam (water), and some carbon dioxide and ash (waste). Similarly, during the body's **metabolism,** energy, water, and carbon dioxide are released.

By studying metabolism, you will understand how the body uses foods to meet its needs and why some foods meet those needs better than others. Readers who are interested in weight control will discover which foods contribute most to body fat and which to select when trying to gain or lose weight safely. Physically active readers

photosynthesis: the process by which green plants use the sun's energy to make carbohydrates from carbon dioxide and water.
- **photo** = light
- **synthesis** = put together (making)

fuel: compounds that cells can use for energy. The major fuels include glucose, fatty acids, and amino acids; other fuels include ketone bodies, lactic acid, glycerol, and alcohol.

metabolism: the sum total of all the chemical reactions that go on in living cells. Energy metabolism includes all the reactions by which the body obtains and spends the energy from food.
- **metaballein** = change

will discover which foods best support endurance activities and which to select when trying to build lean body mass.

Chemical Reactions in the Body

Earlier chapters introduced some of the body's chemical reactions: the making and breaking of the bonds in carbohydrates, lipids, and proteins. Metabolism is the sum of these and all the other chemical reactions that go on in living cells; *energy metabolism* includes all the ways the body obtains and uses energy from food.

Chapters 4, 5, and 6 laid the groundwork for the study of metabolism; a brief review may be helpful. During digestion, the body breaks down the three energy-yielding nutrients—carbohydrates, lipids, and proteins—into four basic units that can be absorbed into the blood:

- From carbohydrates—glucose (and other monosaccharides).
- From fats (triglycerides)—glycerol and fatty acids.
- From proteins—amino acids.

The body uses carbohydrates and fats for most of its energy needs; amino acids are used primarily as building blocks for proteins, but they also enter energy pathways, contributing about 10 to 15 percent of the day's energy use.

Look for these four basic units to appear again and again in the metabolic reactions described in this chapter. Alcohol also enters many of the metabolic pathways; Highlight 7 focuses on how alcohol disrupts metabolism and how the body handles it.

Building Reactions—Anabolism Earlier chapters described how condensation reactions combine the basic units of energy-yielding nutrients to build body compounds. Glucose molecules may be joined together to make glycogen chains. Glycerol and fatty acids may be assembled into triglycerides. Amino acids may be linked together to make proteins. Each of these reactions starts with small, simple compounds and uses them as building blocks to form larger, more complex structures. Such reactions involve doing work and so require energy. The building up of body compounds is known as **anabolism;** this book represents anabolic reactions, wherever possible, with "up" arrows in chemical diagrams (such as those shown in Figure 7-1).

Breakdown Reactions—Catabolism The breaking down of body compounds is known as **catabolism;** catabolic reactions release energy and are represented, wherever possible, by "down" arrows in chemical diagrams (as in Figure 7-1). Earlier chapters described how hydrolysis reactions break down glycogen to glucose, triglycerides to fatty acids and glycerol, and proteins to amino acids. When the body needs energy, it breaks down any or all of these four basic units into even smaller units, as described later.

The Transfer of Energy in Reactions As Chapter 1 explained, *energy* is the capacity to do work. The concept of energy can be difficult to grasp because although every aspect of our lives depends on energy, it cannot be seen or touched and it manifests in various forms, including heat, mechanical, electrical, and chemical energy. In the body, heat energy maintains a constant body temperature, and electrical energy sends nerve impulses, for example. Energy is stored in foods and in the body as chemical energy.

Some of the energy released during the breakdown of glucose, glycerol, fatty acids, and amino acids from foods is captured by "high-energy storage compounds" in the body. One such compound is **ATP (adenosine triphosphate).** ATP, as its name indicates, contains three phosphate groups (see Figure 7-2).■ The bonds connecting the phosphate groups are often described as "high-energy" bonds, referring to the bonds'

■ ATP = A-P~P~P.
(Each ~ denotes a "high-energy" bond.)

anabolism (an-ABB-o-lism): reactions in which small molecules are put together to build larger ones. Anabolic reactions require energy.
- **ana** = up

catabolism (ca-TAB-o-lism): reactions in which large molecules are broken down to smaller ones. Catabolic reactions release energy.
- **kata** = down

ATP or **adenosine** (ah-DEN-oh-seen) **triphosphate** (try-FOS-fate): a common high-energy compound composed of a purine (adenine), a sugar (ribose), and three phosphate groups.

FIGURE 7-1 Anabolic and Catabolic Reactions Compared

NOTE: You need not memorize a color code to understand the figures in this chapter, but you may find it helpful to know that blue is used for carbohydrates, yellow for fats, and red for proteins.

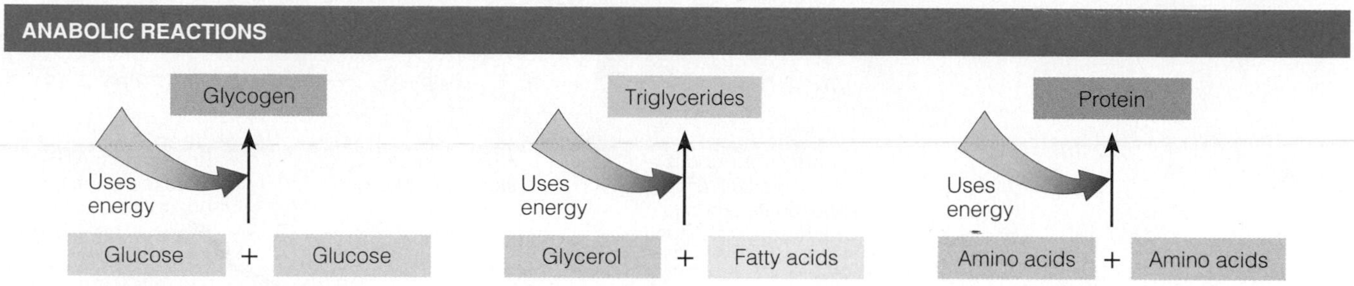
ANABOLIC REACTIONS
Glycogen
Uses energy
Glucose
+
Glucose
Triglycerides
Uses energy
Glycerol
+
Fatty acids
Protein
Uses energy
Amino acids
+
Amino acids

Anabolic reactions include the making of glycogen, triglycerides, and protein; these reactions require differing amounts of energy.

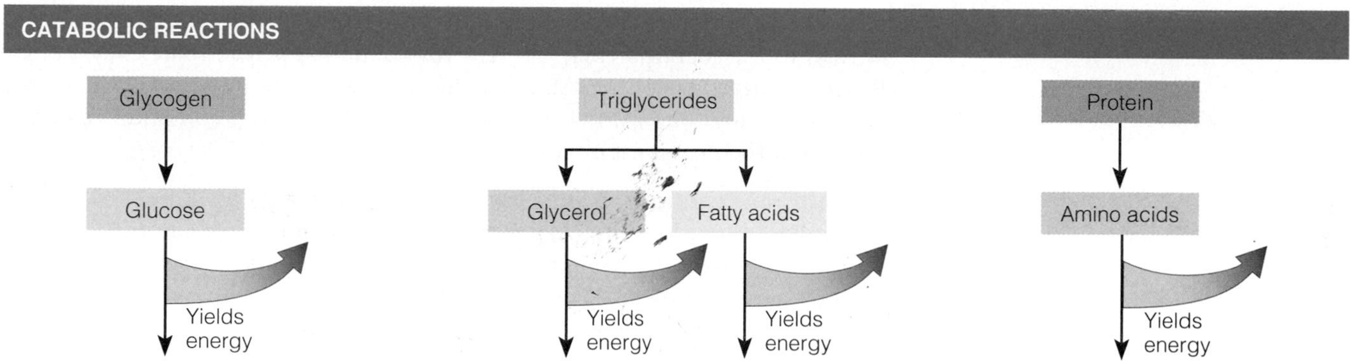
CATABOLIC REACTIONS
Glycogen
Glucose
Yields energy
Triglycerides
Glycerol
Fatty acids
Yields energy
Yields energy
Protein
Amino acids
Yields energy

Catabolic reactions include the breakdown of glycogen, triglycerides, and protein; the further catabolism of glucose, glycerol, fatty acids, and amino acids releases differing amounts of energy. Much of the energy released is captured in the bonds of adenosine triphosphate (ATP), introduced on p. 216.

readiness to release their energy. The negative charges on the phosphate groups make ATP vulnerable to hydrolysis. Whenever cells do any work that requires energy, hydrolysis reactions readily break these high-energy bonds of ATP, splitting off one or two phosphate groups and releasing their energy. Quite often, the hydrolysis of ATP occurs simultaneously with reactions that will use that energy—a metabolic duet known as **coupled reactions.**

Figure 7-3 illustrates how the body captures and releases energy in the bonds of ATP. In essence, the body uses ATP to transfer the energy released during catabolic

FIGURE 7-2 ATP (Adenosine Triphosphate)

ATP is one of the body's quick-energy molecules. Notice that the bonds connecting the three phosphate groups have been drawn as wavy lines, indicating a high-energy bond. When these bonds are broken, energy is released.

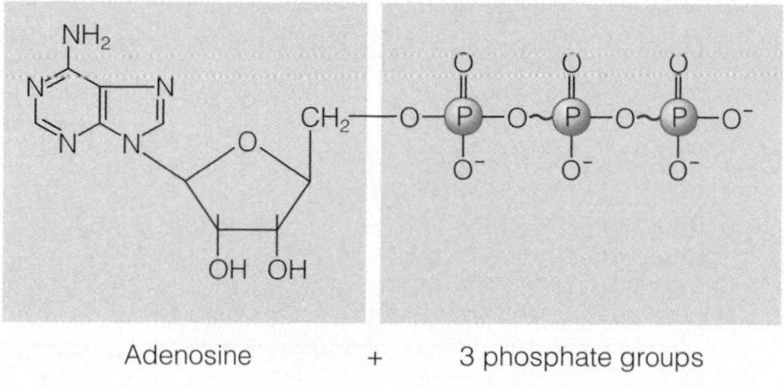
Adenosine
+
3 phosphate groups

coupled reactions: pairs of chemical reactions in which some of the energy released from the breakdown of one compound is used to create a bond in the formation of another compound.

FIGURE 7-3 Transfer of Energy by ATP

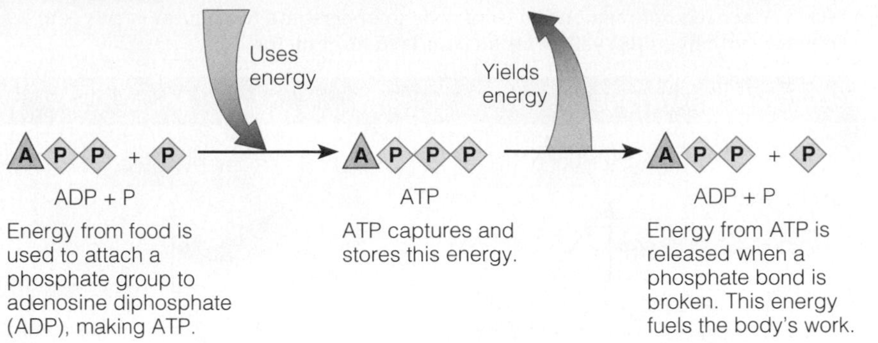
Uses energy
Yields energy
ADP + P
Energy from food is used to attach a phosphate group to adenosine diphosphate (ADP), making ATP.
ATP
ATP captures and stores this energy.
ADP + P
Energy from ATP is released when a phosphate bond is broken. This energy fuels the body's work.

reactions to power its anabolic reactions. The body converts the chemical energy of food to the chemical energy of ATP with about 40 percent efficiency, radiating the rest as heat.[1] Energy is lost as heat again when the body uses the chemical energy of ATP to do its work—moving muscles, synthesizing compounds, or transporting nutrients, for example.

The Site of Reactions—Cells Metabolic work is going on all the time within all the body's trillions of cells. (Appendix A presents a brief summary of the structure and function of the cell.) Figure 7-4 depicts a typical cell and shows where the major reactions of energy metabolism take place. The type and extent of metabolic activity

FIGURE 7-4 A Typical Cell (Simplified Diagram)

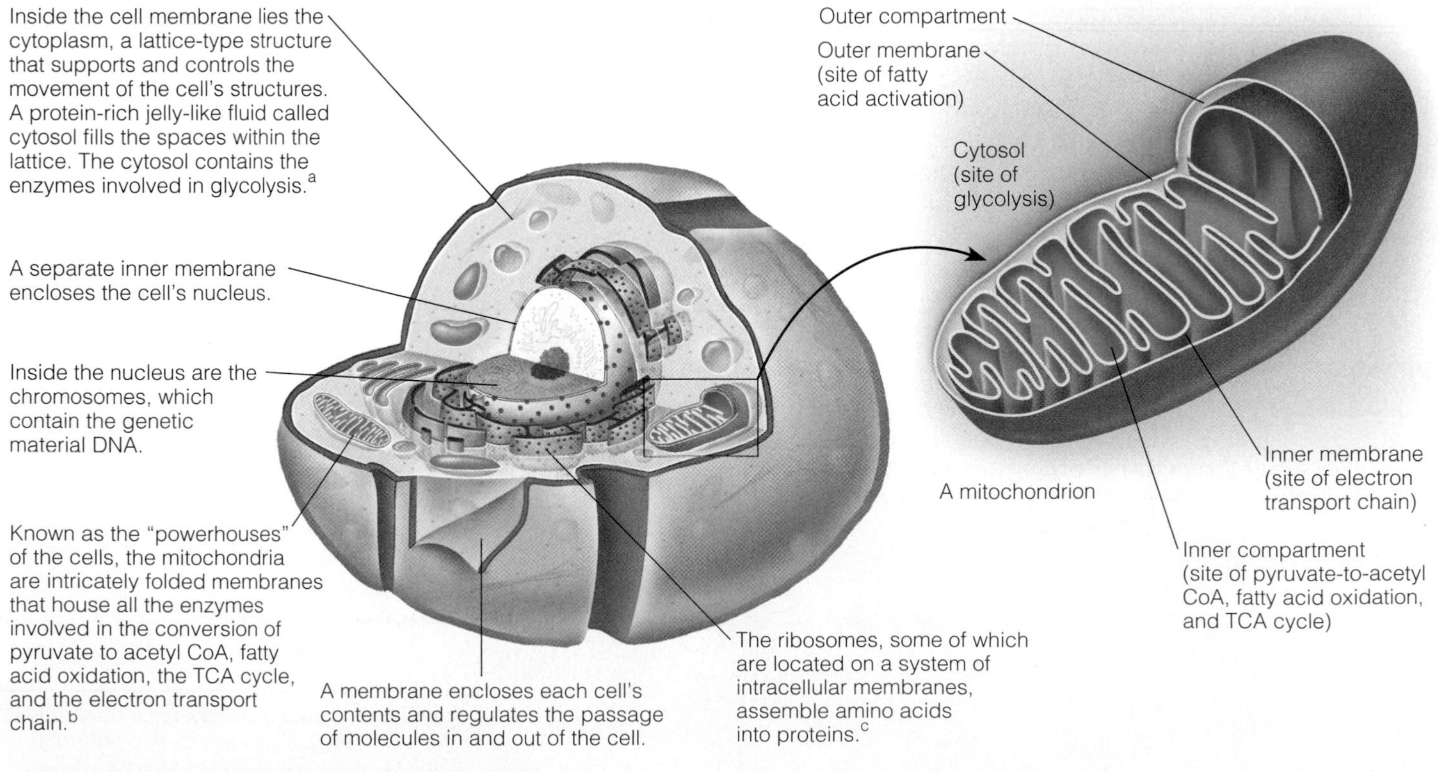
Inside the cell membrane lies the cytoplasm, a lattice-type structure that supports and controls the movement of the cell's structures. A protein-rich jelly-like fluid called cytosol fills the spaces within the lattice. The cytosol contains the enzymes involved in glycolysis.[a]
A separate inner membrane encloses the cell's nucleus.
Inside the nucleus are the chromosomes, which contain the genetic material DNA.
Known as the "powerhouses" of the cells, the mitochondria are intricately folded membranes that house all the enzymes involved in the conversion of pyruvate to acetyl CoA, fatty acid oxidation, the TCA cycle, and the electron transport chain.[b]
A membrane encloses each cell's contents and regulates the passage of molecules in and out of the cell.
The ribosomes, some of which are located on a system of intracellular membranes, assemble amino acids into proteins.[c]
Outer compartment
Outer membrane (site of fatty acid activation)
Cytosol (site of glycolysis)
A mitochondrion
Inner membrane (site of electron transport chain)
Inner compartment (site of pyruvate-to-acetyl CoA, fatty acid oxidation, and TCA cycle)

[a]Glycolysis is described on p. 221.
[b]The conversion of pyruvate to acetyl CoA, fatty acid oxidation, the TCA cycle, and the electron transport chain are described on pp. 223, 224–225, 229, 230–231.
[c]Figure 6-7 on p. 188 describes protein synthesis.

TABLE 7-1 Metabolic Work of the Liver

The liver is the most active processing center in the body. When nutrients enter the body, the liver receives them first; then it metabolizes, packages, stores, or ships them out for use by other organs. When alcohol, drugs, or poisons enter the body, they are also sent directly to the liver; here they are detoxified and their by-products shipped out for excretion. An enthusiastic anatomy and physiology professor once remarked that given the many vital activities of the liver, we should express our feelings for others by saying, "I love you with all my liver," instead of with all my heart. Granted, this declaration lacks romance, but it makes a valid point. Here are just some of the many jobs performed by the liver.

Carbohydrates:

- Converts fructose and galactose to glucose.
- Makes and stores glycogen.
- Breaks down glycogen and releases glucose.
- Breaks down glucose for energy when needed.
- Makes glucose from some amino acids and glycerol when needed.
- Converts excess glucose to fatty acids.

Lipids:

- Builds and breaks down triglycerides, phospholipids, and cholesterol as needed.
- Breaks down fatty acids for energy when needed.
- Packages extra lipids in lipoproteins for transport to other body organs.
- Manufactures bile to send to the gallbladder for use in fat digestion.
- Makes ketone bodies when necessary.

Proteins:

- Manufactures nonessential amino acids that are in short supply.
- Removes from circulation amino acids that are present in excess of need and deaminates them or converts them to other amino acids.
- Removes ammonia from the blood and converts it to urea to be sent to the kidneys for excretion.
- Makes other nitrogen-containing compounds the body needs (such as bases used in DNA and RNA).
- Makes plasma proteins such as clotting factors.

Other:

- Detoxifies alcohol, other drugs, and poisons; prepares waste products for excretion.
- Helps dismantle old red blood cells and captures the iron for recycling.
- Stores most vitamins and many minerals.

To renew your appreciation for this remarkable organ, you might want to review Figure 3-13 on p. 88.

vary depending on the type of cell, but of all the body's cells, the liver cells are the most versatile and metabolically active. Table 7-1 offers insights into the liver's work.

The Helpers in Reactions—Enzymes and Coenzymes Metabolic reactions almost always require enzymes■ to facilitate their action. In many cases, the enzymes need assistants to help them. Enzyme helpers are called **coenzymes.**■

Coenzymes are complex organic molecules that associate closely with most enzymes, but are not proteins themselves. The relationships between various coenzymes and their respective enzymes may differ in detail, but one thing is true of all: without its coenzyme, an enzyme cannot function. Some of the B vitamins serve as coenzymes that participate in the energy metabolism of glucose, glycerol, fatty acids, and amino acids (Chapter 10 provides more details).

■ Reminder: *Enzymes* are protein catalysts—proteins that facilitate chemical reactions without being changed in the process.

■ The general term for substances that facilitate enzyme action is **cofactors;** they include both organic coenzymes such as vitamins and inorganic substances such as minerals.

IN SUMMARY During digestion the energy-yielding nutrients—carbohydrates, lipids, and proteins—are broken down to glucose (and other monosaccharides), glycerol, fatty acids, and amino acids. Aided by enzymes and coenzymes, the cells use these products of digestion to build more complex compounds (anabolism) or break them down further to release energy (catabolism). The energy released during catabolism may be captured by high-energy compounds such as ATP.

coenzymes: complex organic molecules that work with enzymes to facilitate the enzymes' activity. Many coenzymes have B vitamins as part of their structures (Figure 10-1 in Chapter 10 illustrates coenzyme action).
• **co** = with

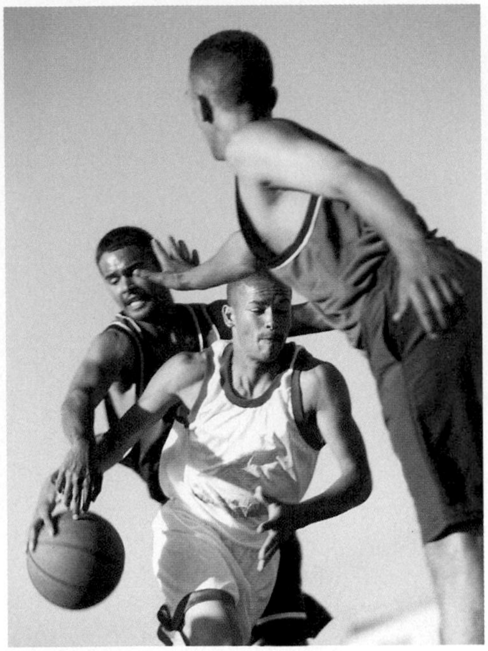

All the energy used to keep the heart beating, the brain thinking, and the legs running comes from the carbohydrates, fats, and proteins in foods.

Breaking Down Nutrients for Energy

Glucose, glycerol, fatty acids, and amino acids are the basic units derived from food, but a molecule of each of these compounds is made of still smaller units, the atoms—carbons, nitrogens, oxygens, and hydrogens. During catabolism, the body separates these atoms from one another. To follow this action, recall how many carbons are in the "backbones" of these compounds:

- Glucose has 6 carbons:

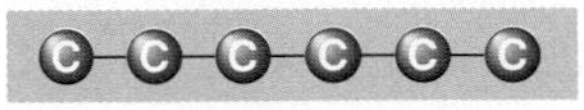

- Glycerol has 3 carbons:

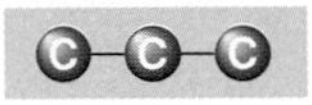

- A fatty acid usually has an even number of carbons, commonly 16 or 18 carbons:*

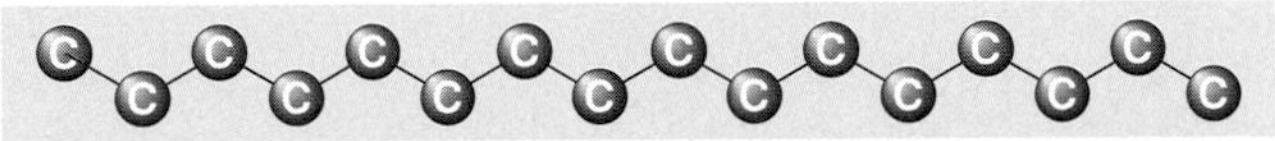

- An amino acid has 2, 3, or more carbons with a nitrogen attached:†

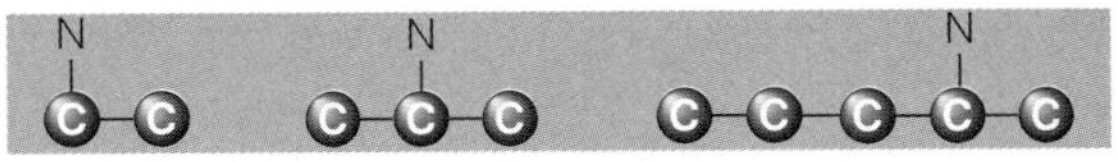

Full chemical structures and reactions appear both in the earlier chapters and in Appendix C; this chapter diagrams the reactions using just the compounds' carbon and nitrogen backbones.

As you will see, each of the compounds—glucose, glycerol, fatty acids, and amino acids—starts down a different path. Along the way, two new names appear—**pyruvate** (a 3-carbon structure) and **acetyl CoA** (a 2-carbon structure with a coenzyme, **CoA,** attached)—and the rest of the story falls into place around them.§ Two major points to notice in the following discussion:

- Pyruvate can be used to make glucose.
- Acetyl CoA cannot be used to make glucose.

Eventually, all of the energy-yielding nutrients can enter the common pathways of the **TCA cycle** and the **electron transport chain.** (Similarly, people from three different locations can all enter an interstate highway and travel to the same destination.) The TCA cycle and electron transport chain have central roles in energy metabolism and receive full attention later in the chapter, but first the text describes how each of the energy-yielding nutrients is broken down to acetyl CoA and other compounds in preparation for their entrance into these final energy pathways.

Glucose

What happens to glucose, glycerol, fatty acids, and amino acids during energy metabolism can best be understood by starting with glucose. This discussion features glucose because of its central role in carbohydrate metabolism and because liver cells convert the other monosaccharides (fructose and galactose) to compounds that enter the same energy pathways.

pyruvate (PIE-roo-vate): a 3-carbon compound that plays a key role in energy metabolism.

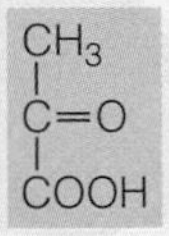
CH3
C=O
COOH

acetyl CoA (ASS-eh-teel, or ah-SEET-il, coh-AY): a 2-carbon compound (**acetate,** or **acetic acid,** shown in Figure 5-1 on p. 142) to which a molecule of CoA is attached.

CoA (coh-AY): coenzyme A; the coenzyme derived from the B vitamin pantothenic acid and central to energy metabolism.

TCA cycle or **tricarboxylic** (try-car-box-ILL-ick) **acid cycle:** a series of metabolic reactions that break down molecules of acetyl CoA to carbon dioxide and hydrogen atoms; also called the **Kreb's cycle** after the biochemist who elucidated its reactions.

electron transport chain: the final pathway in energy metabolism that transports electrons from hydrogen to oxygen and captures the energy released in the bonds of ATP.

*The figures in this chapter show 16- or 18-carbon fatty acids. Fatty acids may have 4 to 20 or more carbons, with chain lengths of 16 and 18 carbons most prevalent.

†The figures in this chapter usually show amino acids as compounds of 2, 3, or 5 carbons arranged in a straight line, but in reality amino acids may contain other numbers of carbons and assume other structural shapes (see Appendix C).

§The term *pyruvate* means a salt of *pyruvic acid.* (Throughout this book, the ending *-ate* is used interchangeably with *-ic acid;* for our purposes they mean the same thing.)

FIGURE 7-5 Glycolysis: Glucose-to-Pyruvate

A little ATP is used to start the splitting of the 6-carbon compound glucose into two interchangeable 3-carbon compounds. These compounds are converted to pyruvate in a series of reactions.

Any of the monosaccharides can enter the glycolysis pathway at various points.

A little ATP is produced, and coenzymes carry the hydrogens and their electrons to the electron transport chain.

Glycolysis of one molecule of glucose produces two molecules of pyruvate.

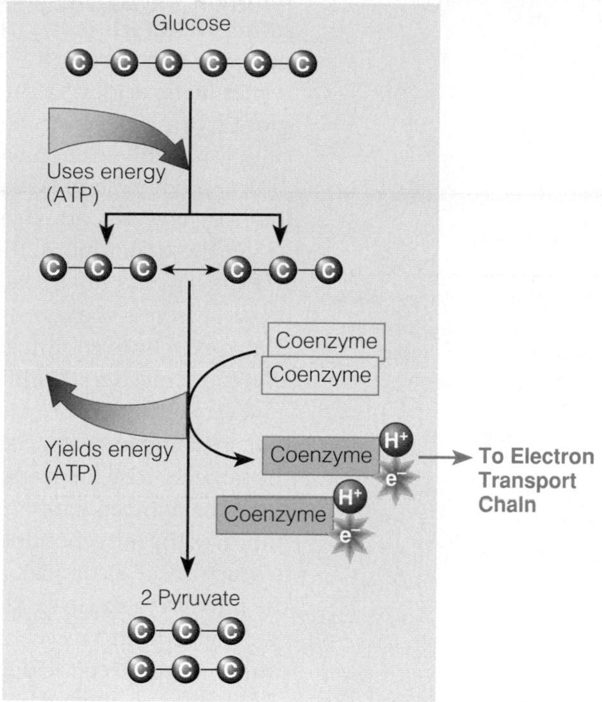
Glucose
Uses energy (ATP)
Coenzyme
Coenzyme
Yields energy (ATP)
Coenzyme
Coenzyme
H+
e−
To Electron Transport Chain
2 Pyruvate

NOTE: These arrows point down indicating the breakdown of glucose to pyruvate during energy metabolism. Alternatively, the arrows could point up indicating the making of glucose from pyruvate, but that is not the focus of this discussion.

Available Online

Watch an animated explanation of the first pathway glucose takes on its way to yield energy.

Glucose-to-Pyruvate The first pathway glucose takes on its way to yield energy is called **glycolysis** (glucose splitting).[*] Figure 7-5 shows a simplified drawing of glycolysis. (This pathway actually involves several steps and several enzymes, which are shown in Appendix C.) In glycolysis, the 6-carbon glucose is split in half, forming two 3-carbon compounds. These 3-carbon compounds continue along the pathway until they are converted to pyruvate. Thus the net yield of one glucose molecule is two pyruvate molecules. The net yield of energy at this point is small; to start glycolysis, the cell uses a little energy and then produces only a little more than it had to invest initially.[†] In addition, as glucose breaks down to pyruvate, hydrogen atoms with their electrons are released and carried to the electron transport chain by coenzymes made from the B vitamin niacin. A later section of the chapter explains how oxygen accepts the electrons and combines with the hydrogens to form water and how the process captures energy in the bonds of ATP.

This discussion focuses primarily on the breakdown of glucose for energy, but if needed, cells in the liver (and to some extent, the kidneys) can make glucose again from pyruvate in a process similar to the reversal of glycolysis. Making glucose requires energy, however, and a few different enzymes. Still, glucose can be made from pyruvate, so the arrows between glucose and pyruvate could point up as well as down.■

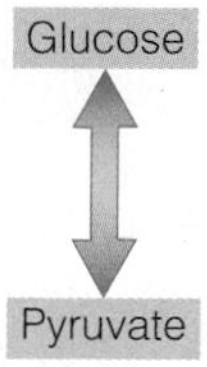
Glucose
Pyruvate

■ Glucose may go "down" to make pyruvate, or pyruvate may go "up" to make glucose, depending on the cell's needs.

Pyruvate's Options Pyruvate may enter either an anaerobic or an aerobic energy pathway. When the body needs energy quickly—as occurs when you run a quarter mile as fast as you can—pyruvate is converted to lactic acid in an **anaerobic** pathway. When energy expenditure proceeds at a slower pace—as occurs when you ride a bike for an hour—pyruvate breaks down to acetyl CoA in an **aerobic** pathway. The following paragraphs explain these pathways.

glycolysis (gligh-COLL-ih-sis): the metabolic breakdown of glucose to pyruvate. Glycolysis does not require oxygen (anaerobic).
- **glyco** = glucose
- **lysis** = breakdown

anaerobic (AN-air-ROE-bic): not requiring oxygen.
- **an** = not

aerobic (air-ROE-bic): requiring oxygen.

[*] Glycolysis takes place in the cytosol of the cell (see Figure 7-4).
[†] The cell uses 2 ATP to begin the breakdown of glucose to pyruvate, but then gains 4 ATP for a net gain of 2 ATP.

Pyruvate-to-Lactic Acid As mentioned earlier, coenzymes carry the hydrogens from glucose breakdown to the electron transport chain. If the electron transport chain is unable to accept these hydrogens, as may occur when cells lack sufficient **mitochondria** (review Figure 7-4) or in the absence of sufficient oxygen, pyruvate can accept the hydrogens. By accepting the hydrogens, pyruvate becomes **lactic acid,** and the coenzymes are freed to return to glycolysis to pick up more hydrogens. In this way, glucose can continue providing energy anaerobically for a while (see the left side of Figure 7-6).

The production of lactic acid occurs to a limited extent even at rest. During high-intensity exercise, however, the concentration of lactic acid increases dramatically. Under these conditions, the muscles rely heavily on anaerobic glycolysis to produce ATP quickly. The rapid rate of glycolysis produces abundant pyruvate and releases hydrogen-carrying coenzymes more rapidly than the mitochondria can handle them. To enable exercise to continue at this intensity, pyruvate is converted to lactic acid, which allows glycolysis to continue (as mentioned earlier). The accumulation of lactic acid (and the subsequent drop in pH) in the muscles produces the burning pain and fatigue that are commonly associated with intense exercise. In contrast, a person performing the same exercise following endurance training experiences less discomfort in part because the number of mitochondria in the muscle cells have increased. This adaptation improves the mitochondria's ability to keep pace with the rapid rate of glycolysis, and less lactic acid accumulates. One possible fate of lactic acid is to be transported from the muscles to the liver. There the liver can convert the lactic acid produced in muscles to glucose in a recycling process called the **Cori cycle** (see Figure 7-6). (Muscle cells cannot recycle lactic acid to glucose because they lack a necessary enzyme.)

Whenever carbohydrates, fats, or proteins are broken down to provide energy, oxygen is always ultimately involved in the process. The role of oxygen in metabolism is worth noticing, for it helps our understanding of physiology and metabolic reactions. The breakdown of glucose-to-pyruvate-to-lactic acid proceeds without oxygen (it is anaerobic). This anaerobic pathway yields energy quickly, but it cannot be sustained

mitochondria (my-toh-KON-dree-uh): the cellular organelles responsible for producing ATP aerobically; made of membranes (lipid and protein) with enzymes mounted on them.

- **mitos** = thread (referring to their slender shape)
- **chondros** = cartilage (referring to their external appearance)

lactic acid: a 3-carbon compound produced from pyruvate during anaerobic metabolism.

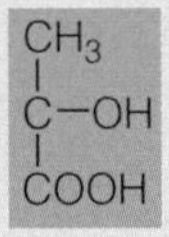

CH_3
C—OH
COOH

Cori cycle: the path from muscle lactic acid (which travels to the liver) to glucose (which can travel back to the muscle); named after the scientist who elucidated this pathway.

FIGURE 7-6 Pyruvate-to-Lactic Acid (Anaerobic)

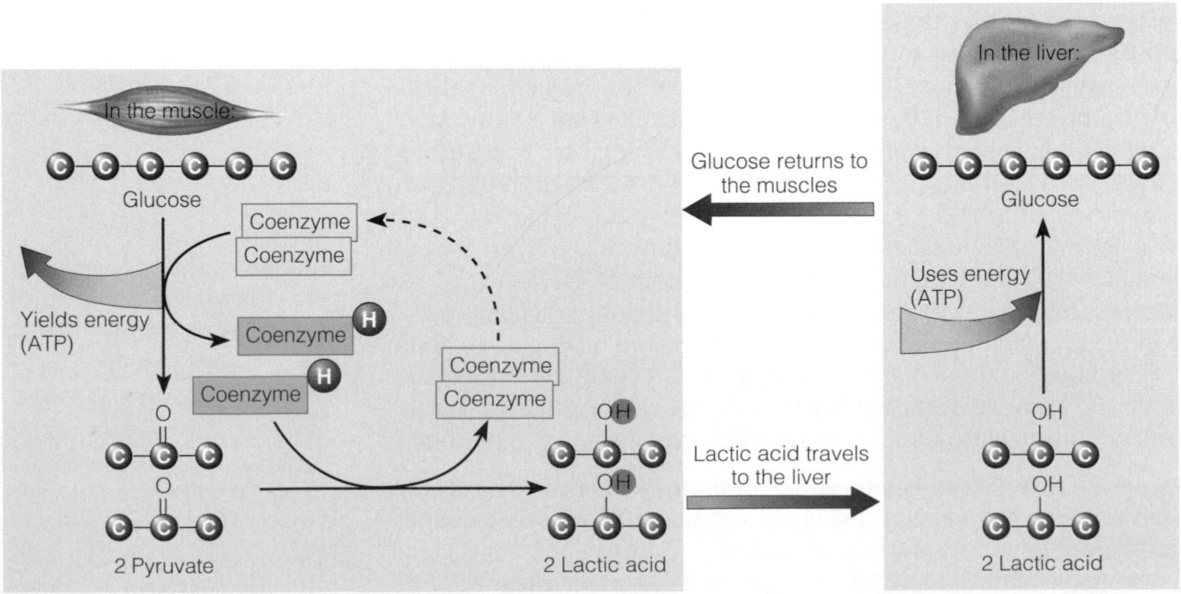

In the muscle:
Glucose
Coenzyme
Coenzyme
Yields energy (ATP)
Coenzyme H
Coenzyme H
Coenzyme
Coenzyme
2 Pyruvate
2 Lactic acid
Glucose returns to the muscles
Lactic acid travels to the liver
In the liver:
Glucose
Uses energy (ATP)
OH
OH
2 Lactic acid

Working muscles break down most of their glucose molecules anaerobically to pyruvate. If the cells lack sufficient mitochondria or in the absence of sufficient oxygen, pyruvate can accept the hydrogens from glucose breakdown and become lactic acid. This conversion frees the coenzymes so that glycolysis can continue.

Liver enzymes can convert lactic acid to glucose, but this reaction requires energy. The recycling of glucose from lactic acid is known as the Cori cycle.

for long—a couple of minutes at most. Conversely, the aerobic pathways produce energy more slowly, but because they can be sustained for a long time, their total energy yield is greater.

Pyruvate-to-Acetyl CoA If the cell needs energy and oxygen is available, pyruvate molecules enter the mitochondria of the cell where they will be converted to acetyl CoA. A carbon group (COOH) from the 3-carbon pyruvate is removed to produce a 2-carbon compound that bonds with a molecule of CoA, becoming acetyl CoA. The carbon group from pyruvate becomes carbon dioxide, which is released into the blood, circulated to the lungs, and breathed out. Figure 7-7 diagrams the pyruvate-to-acetyl CoA reaction.

The step from pyruvate to acetyl CoA is metabolically irreversible: a cell cannot retrieve the shed carbons from carbon dioxide to remake pyruvate and then glucose. It is a one-way step and is therefore shown with only a "down" arrow in Figure 7-8.

Acetyl CoA's Options Acetyl CoA has two main options—it may be used to synthesize fats or to generate ATP. When ATP is abundant, acetyl CoA makes fat, the most efficient way to store energy for later use when energy may be needed. Thus any molecule that can make acetyl CoA—including glucose, glycerol, fatty acids, and amino acids—can make fat. In reviewing Figure 7-8, notice that acetyl CoA can be used as a building block for fatty acids, but it cannot be used to make glucose or amino acids.

When ATP is low and the cell needs energy, acetyl CoA may proceed through the TCA cycle, releasing hydrogens with their electrons to the electron transport chain. The story of acetyl CoA continues on p. 229 after a discussion of how fat and protein arrive at the same crossroads. For now, know that when acetyl CoA from the breakdown of glucose enters the aerobic pathways of the TCA cycle and electron transport chain, much more ATP is produced than during glycolysis. The role of glycolysis is to provide energy for short bursts of activity and to prepare glucose for later energy pathways.

FIGURE 7-7 Pyruvate-to-Acetyl CoA (Aerobic)

Each pyruvate loses a carbon as carbon dioxide and picks up a molecule of CoA, becoming acetyl CoA. The arrow goes only one way (down), because the step is not reversible. Result from 1 glucose: 2 carbon dioxide and 2 acetyl CoA.

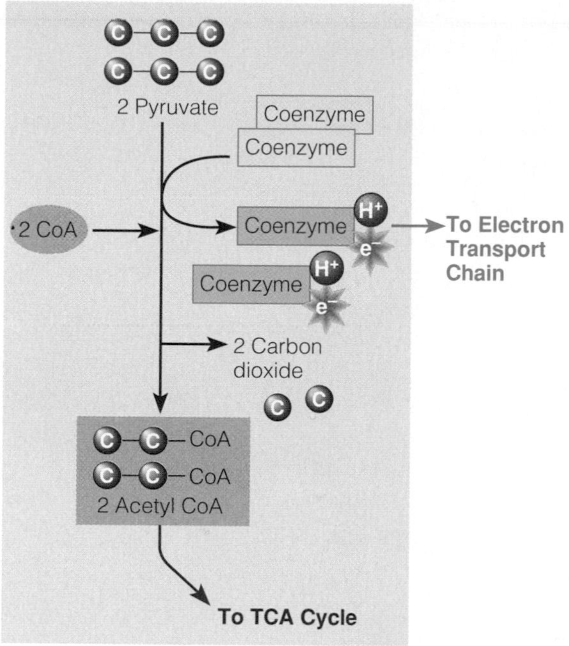

C C C
C C C
2 Pyruvate
Coenzyme
Coenzyme
2 CoA
Coenzyme
H+
e-
To Electron Transport Chain
Coenzyme
H+
e-
2 Carbon dioxide
C C
C C CoA
C C CoA
2 Acetyl CoA
To TCA Cycle

IN SUMMARY The breakdown of glucose to energy begins with glycolysis, a pathway that produces pyruvate. Keep in mind that glucose can be synthesized only from pyruvate or compounds earlier in the pathway. Pyruvate may be converted to lactic acid anaerobically or to acetyl CoA aerobically. Once the commitment to acetyl CoA is made, glucose is not retrievable; acetyl CoA cannot go back to glucose. Figure 7-9 summarizes the breakdown of glucose.

FIGURE 7-8 The Paths of Pyruvate and Acetyl CoA

Pyruvate may follow several reversible paths, but the path from pyruvate to acetyl CoA is irreversible.

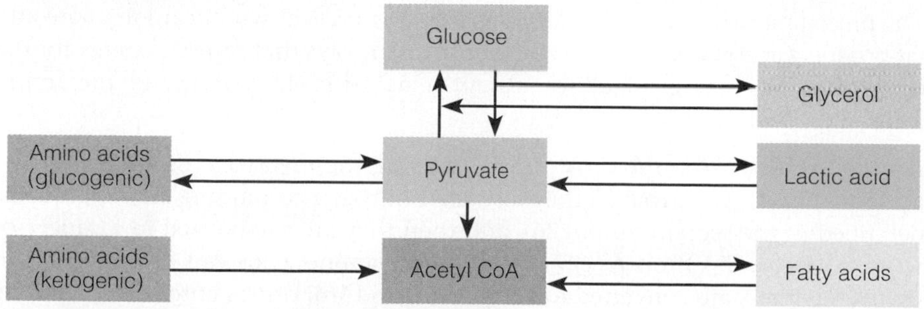

Glucose
Glycerol
Amino acids (glucogenic)
Pyruvate
Lactic acid
Amino acids (ketogenic)
Acetyl CoA
Fatty acids

NOTE: Amino acids that can be used to make glucose are called *glucogenic;* amino acids that are converted to acetyl CoA are called *ketogenic.*

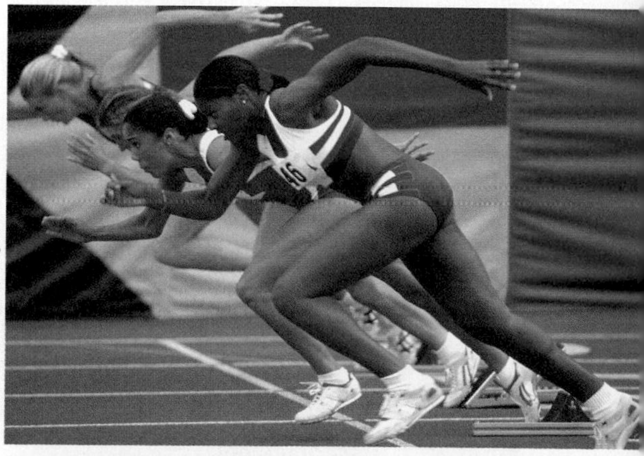

© Jim Cummins/Taxi/Getty Images

The anaerobic breakdown of glucose-to-pyruvate-to-lactic acid is the major source of energy for short, intense exercise.

FIGURE 7-9 Glucose Enters the Energy Pathway

This figure combines Figure 7-5 and Figure 7-7 to show the breakdown of glucose-to-pyruvate-to-acetyl CoA. Details of the TCA cycle and the electron transport chain are given later and in Appendix C.

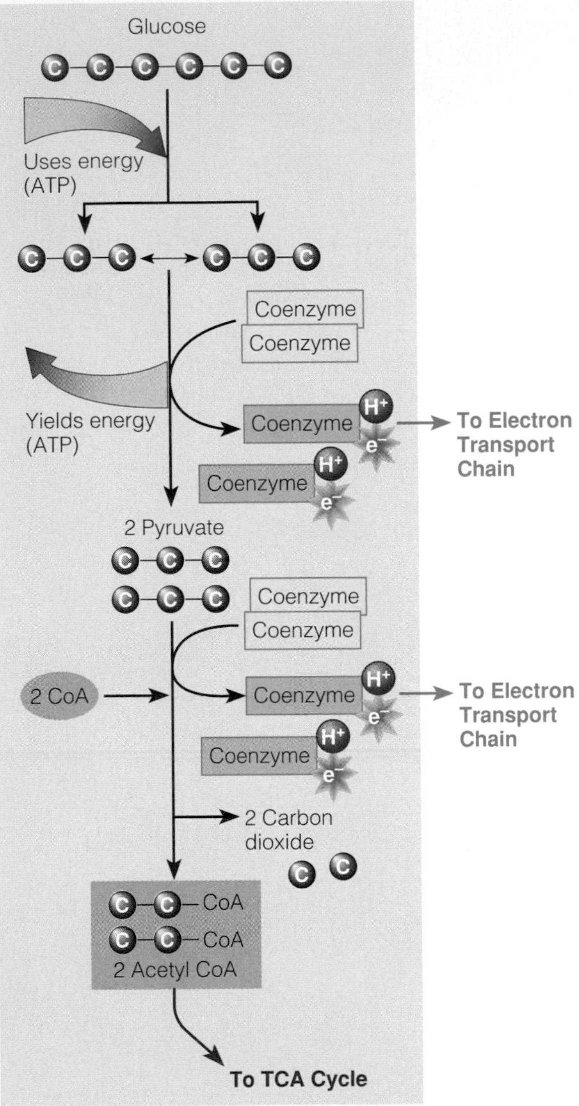
Glucose
C C C C C C
Uses energy (ATP)
C C C
C C C
Coenzyme
Coenzyme
Yields energy (ATP)
Coenzyme
H+
e−
To Electron Transport Chain
Coenzyme
H+
e−
2 Pyruvate
C C C
C C C
Coenzyme
Coenzyme
2 CoA
Coenzyme
H+
e−
To Electron Transport Chain
Coenzyme
H+
e−
2 Carbon dioxide
C C
C C CoA
C C CoA
2 Acetyl CoA
To TCA Cycle

- Note: The *oxidation* of energy nutrients refers to the metabolic reactions that lead to the release of energy.

- Reminder: The making of glucose from noncarbohydrate sources is called *gluconeogenesis*. The glycerol portion of a triglyceride and most amino acids can be used to make glucose (review Figure 7-8). The liver is the major site of gluconeogenesis, but the kidneys become increasingly involved under certain circumstances, such as starvation.

fatty acid oxidation: the metabolic breakdown of fatty acids to acetyl CoA; also called **beta oxidation.**

Glycerol and Fatty Acids

Once glucose breakdown is understood, fat and protein breakdown are easily learned, for all three eventually enter the same metabolic pathways. Recall that triglycerides can break down to glycerol and fatty acids.

Glycerol-to-Pyruvate Glycerol (a 3-carbon compound like pyruvate, but with a different arrangement of H and OH on the C) is easily converted to another 3-carbon compound. This compound may go either "up" the pathway to form glucose or "down" to form pyruvate and then acetyl CoA (review Figure 7-8 on p. 223).

Fatty Acids-to-Acetyl CoA Fatty acids are taken apart 2 carbons at a time in a series of reactions known as **fatty acid oxidation.***■ Figure 7-10 illustrates fatty acid oxidation and shows that in the process, each 2-carbon fragment splits off and combines with a molecule of CoA to make acetyl CoA. As each 2-carbon fragment breaks off from a fatty acid during oxidation, hydrogens and their electrons are released and carried to the electron transport chain by coenzymes made from the B vitamins riboflavin and niacin. Figure 7-11 (on p. 226) summarizes the breakdown of fats.

Fatty Acids Cannot Be Used to Synthesize Glucose When carbohydrate is unavailable, the liver cells can make glucose from pyruvate and other 3-carbon compounds, such as glycerol,■ but they cannot make glucose from the 2-carbon fragments of fatty acids. In chemical diagrams, the arrow between pyruvate and acetyl CoA always points only one way—down—and fatty acid fragments enter the metabolic path below this arrow (review Figure 7-8). Thus fatty acids cannot be used to make glucose.

The significance of this is that red blood cells and the brain and nervous system depend primarily on glucose as fuel. Remember that almost all dietary fats are triglycerides and that triglycerides contain only one small molecule of glycerol with three fatty acids. The glycerol can yield glucose, but that represents only 3 of the 50 or so carbon atoms in a triglyceride—about 5 percent of its weight (see Figure 7-12 on p. 226). The other 95 percent cannot be converted to glucose.

IN SUMMARY The body can convert the small glycerol portion of a triglyceride to either pyruvate (and then glucose) or acetyl CoA. The fatty acids of a triglyceride, on the other hand, cannot make glucose, but they can provide abundant acetyl CoA. Acetyl CoA from either source may then enter the TCA cycle to release energy or combine with other molecules of acetyl CoA to make body fat.

Amino Acids

The preceding two sections have shown how the breakdown of carbohydrate and fat produces acetyl CoA, which can enter the pathways that provide energy for the body's use. One energy-yielding nutrient remains: protein or, rather, the amino acids of protein.

Amino Acids-to-Acetyl CoA Before entering the metabolic pathways, amino acids are deaminated (that is, they lose their nitrogen-containing amino group as described in the section on p. 226), and then they are catabolized in a variety of ways. As Figure 7-13 (on p. 227) shows, some amino acids can be converted to pyruvate; others are converted to acetyl CoA; and still others enter the TCA cycle directly as compounds other than acetyl CoA.

*Oxidation of fatty acids occurs in the mitochondria of the cells (see Figure 7-4).

FIGURE 7-10 Fatty Acid to Acetyl CoA

Fatty acids are taken apart to 2-carbon fragments that combine with CoA to make acetyl CoA.

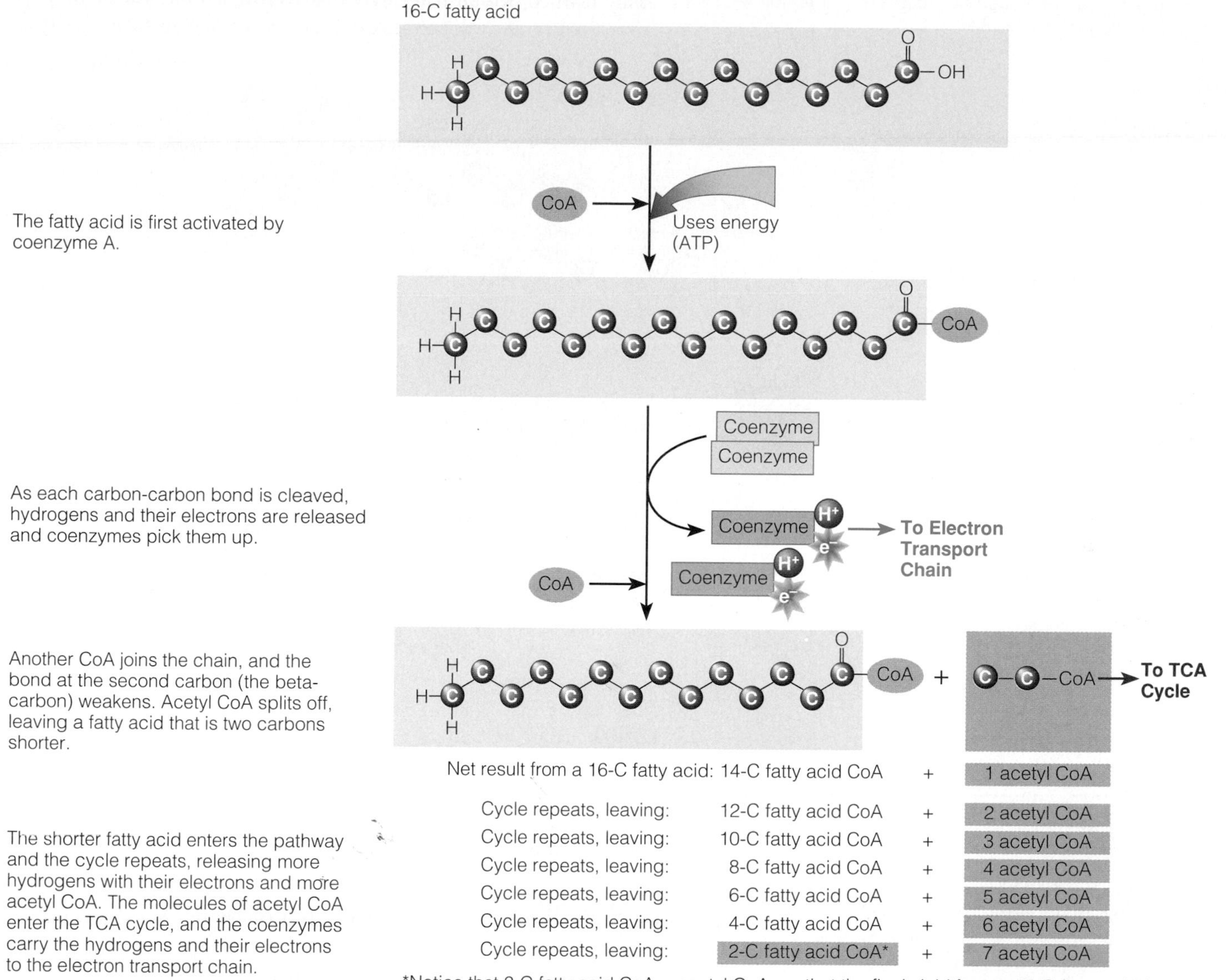
16-C fatty acid
OH
CoA
Uses energy (ATP)
The fatty acid is first activated by coenzyme A.
CoA
Coenzyme
Coenzyme
Coenzyme
Coenzyme
H+
e-
To Electron Transport Chain
As each carbon-carbon bond is cleaved, hydrogens and their electrons are released and coenzymes pick them up.
CoA
Another CoA joins the chain, and the bond at the second carbon (the beta-carbon) weakens. Acetyl CoA splits off, leaving a fatty acid that is two carbons shorter.
CoA +
C–C–CoA
To TCA Cycle
Net result from a 16-C fatty acid: 14-C fatty acid CoA + 1 acetyl CoA
Cycle repeats, leaving: 12-C fatty acid CoA + 2 acetyl CoA
Cycle repeats, leaving: 10-C fatty acid CoA + 3 acetyl CoA
Cycle repeats, leaving: 8-C fatty acid CoA + 4 acetyl CoA
Cycle repeats, leaving: 6-C fatty acid CoA + 5 acetyl CoA
Cycle repeats, leaving: 4-C fatty acid CoA + 6 acetyl CoA
Cycle repeats, leaving: 2-C fatty acid CoA* + 7 acetyl CoA
The shorter fatty acid enters the pathway and the cycle repeats, releasing more hydrogens with their electrons and more acetyl CoA. The molecules of acetyl CoA enter the TCA cycle, and the coenzymes carry the hydrogens and their electrons to the electron transport chain.

*Notice that 2-C fatty acid CoA = acetyl CoA, so that the final yield from a 16-C fatty acid is 8 acetyl CoA.

Available Online

Watch as fatty acids are taken apart two carbons at a time in a series of aerobic reactions known as fatty acid oxidation.

Amino Acids-to-Glucose As you might expect, amino acids that are used to make pyruvate can provide glucose, whereas those used to make acetyl CoA can provide additional energy or make body fat but cannot make glucose.■ Amino acids entering the TCA cycle directly can continue in the cycle and generate energy; alternatively, they can generate glucose.[2] Thus protein, unlike fat, is a fairly good source of glucose when carbohydrate is not available.

■ Amino acids that can make glucose via either pyruvate or TCA cycle intermediates are *glucogenic;* amino acids that are degraded to acetyl CoA are *ketogenic.*

A key to understanding these metabolic pathways is learning which fuels can be converted to glucose and which cannot. The parts of protein and fat that can be converted to pyruvate *can* provide glucose for the body, whereas the parts that are converted to acetyl CoA *cannot* provide glucose, but can readily provide fat. The body must have glucose to fuel the activities of the central nervous system and red blood cells. Without glucose from food, the body will devour its own lean (protein-containing) tissue to provide the amino acids to make glucose. Therefore, to keep this from happening, the body needs foods that can provide glucose—primarily carbohydrate. Giving the body only fat, which delivers mostly acetyl CoA, puts it in the position of having to break down protein tissue to make glucose. Giving the

FIGURE 7-11 Fats Enter the Energy Pathway

Glycerol enters the glycolysis pathway about midway between glucose and pyruvate and can be converted to either; fatty acids are broken down into 2-carbon fragments that combine with CoA to form acetyl CoA (shown in Figure 7-10). Net from a 16-carbon fatty acid: 8 acetyl CoA molecules.

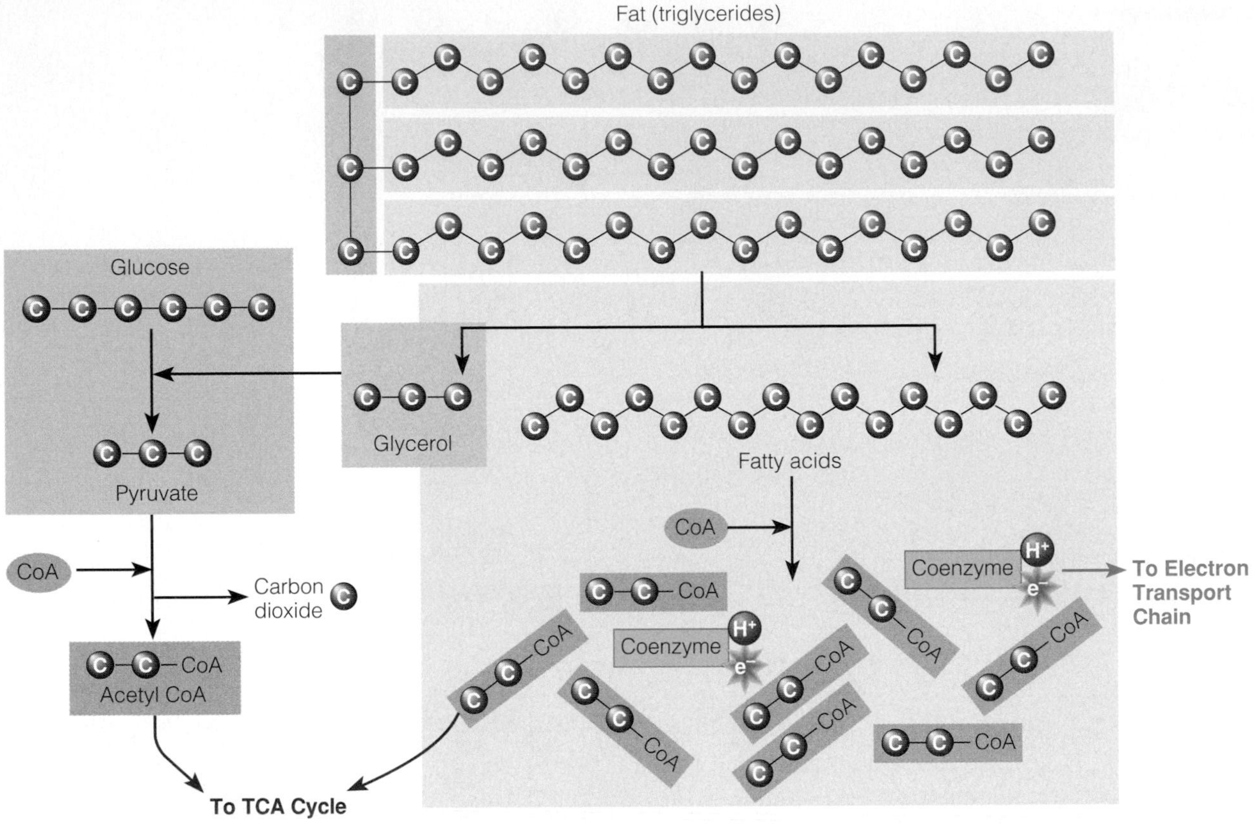

Fat (triglycerides)
Glucose
Pyruvate
Glycerol
Fatty acids
CoA
Carbon dioxide
Acetyl CoA
Coenzyme
To Electron Transport Chain
To TCA Cycle

■ A healthy diet provides:
- 45–65% kcalories from carbohydrate.
- 10–35% kcalories from protein.
- 20–35% kcalories from fat.

body only protein puts it in the position of having to convert protein to glucose. Clearly, the best diet■ supplies ample carbohydrate, adequate protein, and some fat.

Deamination When amino acids are metabolized for energy or used to make fat, they must be deaminated first. Two products result from deamination. One is the carbon structure without its amino group—often a **keto acid** (see Figure 7-14). The other

FIGURE 7-12 The Carbons of a Typical Triglyceride

A typical triglyceride contains only one small molecule of glycerol (3 C), but has three fatty acids (each commonly 16 C or 18 C, or about 48 C to 54 C in total). Only the glycerol portion of a triglyceride can yield glucose

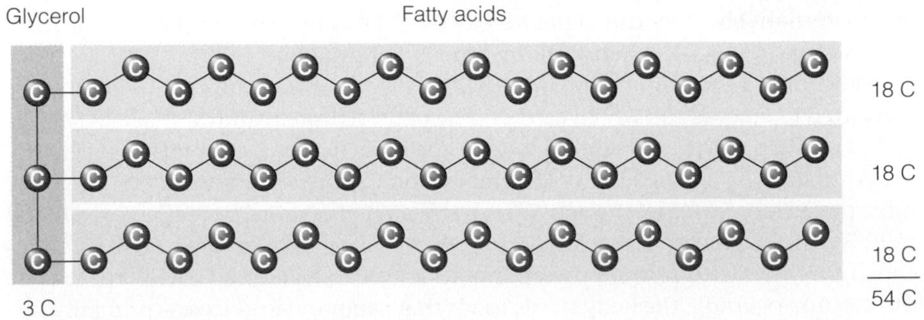

Glycerol
Fatty acids
18 C
18 C
18 C
3 C
54 C

keto (KEY-toe) **acid:** an organic acid that contains a carbonyl group (C=O).

FIGURE 7-13 Amino Acids Enter the Energy Pathway

NOTE: The arrows from pyruvate and the TCA cycle to amino acids are possible only for *nonessential* amino acids; remember, the body cannot make essential amino acids.

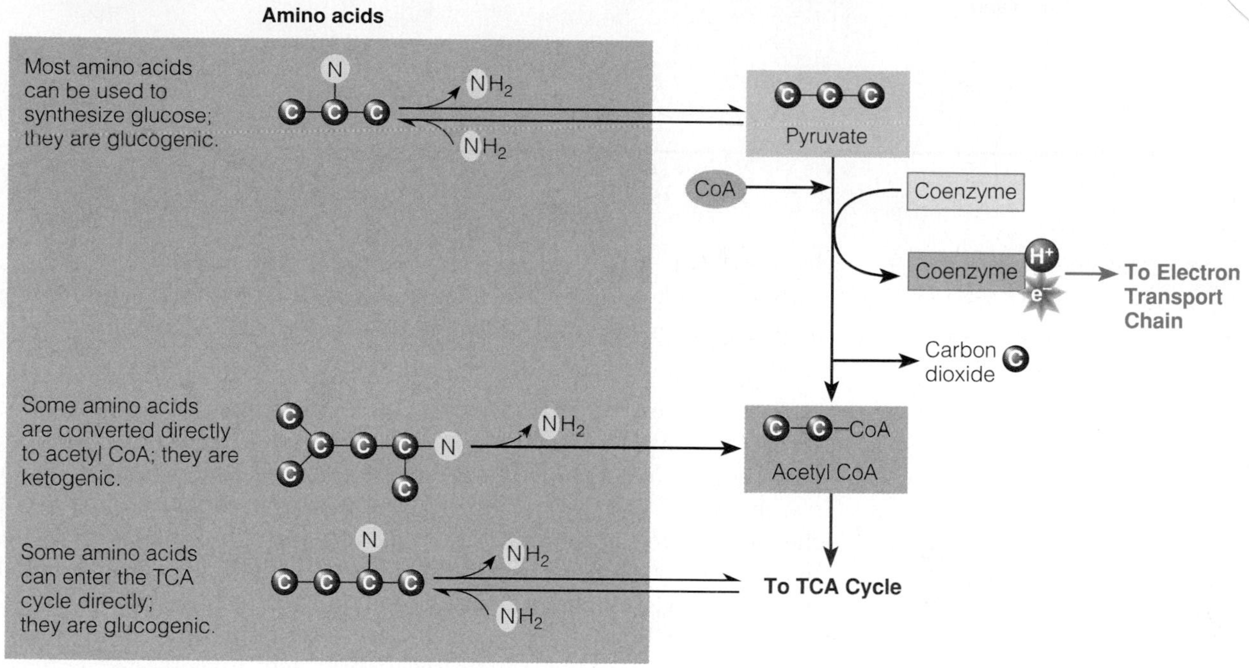

Amino acids
Most amino acids can be used to synthesize glucose; they are glucogenic.
N
C C C
NH2
NH2
C C C
Pyruvate
CoA
Coenzyme
Coenzyme
H+
e-
To Electron Transport Chain
Carbon dioxide
C
Some amino acids are converted directly to acetyl CoA; they are ketogenic.
C C C C N
NH2
C C —CoA
Acetyl CoA
Some amino acids can enter the TCA cycle directly; they are glucogenic.
N
C C C C
NH2
NH2
To TCA Cycle

product is **ammonia** (NH_3), a toxic compound chemically identical to the strong-smelling ammonia in bottled cleaning solutions. Ammonia is a base, and if the body produces larger quantities than it can handle, the blood's critical acid-base balance becomes upset.

Transamination As the discussion of protein in Chapter 6 pointed out, only some amino acids are essential; others can be made in the body, given a source of nitrogen. By transferring an amino group from one amino acid to its corresponding keto acid, cells can make a new amino acid and a new keto acid, as shown in Figure 7-15 (on p. 228). Through many such **transamination** reactions, involving many different keto acids, the liver cells can synthesize the nonessential amino acids.

Ammonia-to-Urea in the Liver The liver continuously produces small amounts of ammonia in deamination reactions. Some of this ammonia provides the nitrogen needed for the synthesis of nonessential amino acids (review

FIGURE 7-14 Deamination and Synthesis of a Nonessential Amino Acid

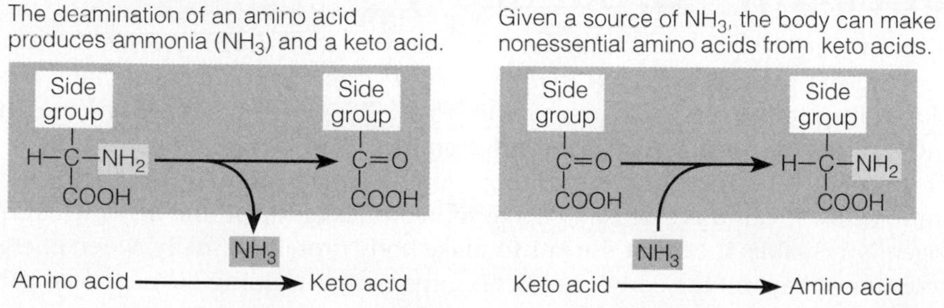

The deamination of an amino acid produces ammonia (NH3) and a keto acid.
Side group
H—C—NH2
COOH
Side group
C=O
COOH
NH3
Amino acid
Keto acid
Given a source of NH3, the body can make nonessential amino acids from keto acids.
Side group
C=O
COOH
Side group
H—C—NH2
COOH
NH3
Keto acid
Amino acid

ammonia: a compound with the chemical formula NH_3; produced during the deamination of amino acids.

transamination (TRANS-am-ih-NAY-shun): the transfer of an amino group from one amino acid to a keto acid, producing a new nonessential amino acid and a new keto acid.

FIGURE 7-15 Transamination and Synthesis of a Nonessential Amino Acid

The body can transfer amino groups (NH_2) from an amino acid to a keto acid, forming a new *nonessential* amino acid and a new keto acid.

Transamination reactions require the vitamin B_6 coenzyme.

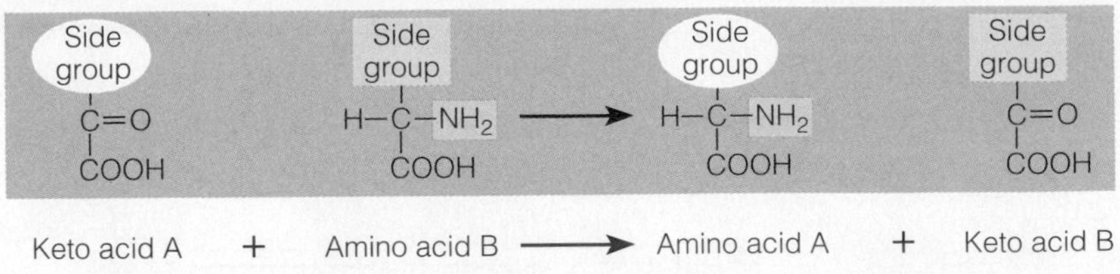
Side group
C=O
COOH
Side group
H—C—NH2
COOH
Side group
H—C—NH2
COOH
Side group
C=O
COOH
Keto acid A
+
Amino acid B
Amino acid A
+
Keto acid B

FIGURE 7-16 Urea Synthesis

When amino nitrogen is stripped from amino acids, ammonia is produced. The liver detoxifies ammonia before releasing it into the bloodstream by combining it with another waste product, carbon dioxide, to produce urea. See Appendix C for details.

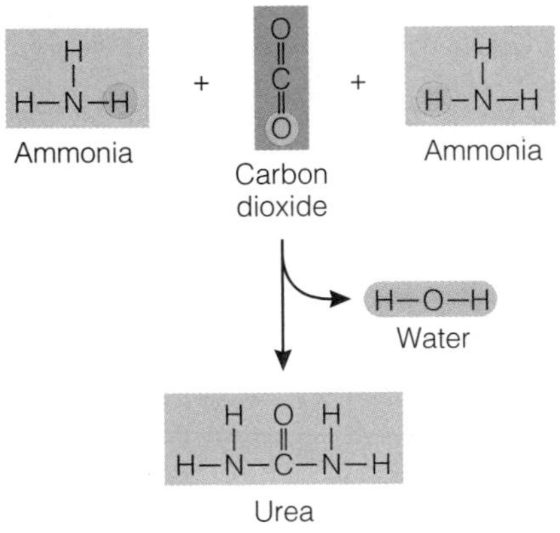
Ammonia
Carbon dioxide
Ammonia
H—O—H
Water
Urea

Figure 7-14). The liver quickly combines any remaining ammonia with carbon dioxide to make **urea**, a much less toxic compound. Figure 7-16 provides a greatly oversimplified diagram of urea synthesis; details are shown in Appendix C.

Urea Excretion via the Kidneys Liver cells release urea into the blood, where it circulates until it passes through the kidneys (see Figure 7-17). The kidneys then remove urea from the blood for excretion in the urine. Normally, the liver efficiently captures all the ammonia, makes urea from it, and releases the urea into the blood; then the kidneys clear all the urea from the blood. This division of labor allows easy diagnosis of diseases of both organs. In liver disease, blood ammonia will be high; in kidney disease, blood urea will be high.

Urea is the body's principal vehicle for excreting unused nitrogen, and the amount of urea produced increases with protein intake. To keep urea in solution, the body needs water. For this reason, a person who regularly consumes a high-protein diet (say, 100 grams a day or more) must drink plenty of water to dilute and excrete urea from the body. Without extra water, a person on a high-protein diet risks dehydration because the body uses its water to rid itself of urea. This explains some of the water loss that accompanies high-protein diets. Such losses may make high-protein diets *appear* to be effective, but water loss, of course, is of no value to the person who wants to lose body fat (as Highlight 8 explains).

IN SUMMARY The body can use some amino acids to produce glucose, while others can be used either to generate energy or to make fat. Before an amino acid enters one of these metabolic pathways, its nitrogen-containing amino group must be removed through deamination. Some of the nitrogen may be used to make nonessential amino acids and other nitrogen-containing compounds; the rest is cleared from the body via urea synthesis in the liver and excretion in the kidneys.

Breaking Down Nutrients for Energy—In Summary

To review the ways the body can use the energy-yielding nutrients, see the summary table at the top of p. 229. To obtain energy, the body uses glucose and fatty acids as its primary fuels, and amino acids to a lesser extent. To make glucose, the body can use all carbohydrates and most amino acids, but it can convert only 5 percent of fat (the glycerol portion) to glucose. To make proteins, the body needs amino acids. It can use glucose to make some nonessential amino acids when nitrogen is available; it cannot use fats to make body proteins. Finally, when energy is consumed beyond the body's needs, all three energy-yielding nutrients can contribute to fat storage.

urea (you-REE-uh): the principal nitrogen-excretion product of protein metabolism. Two ammonia fragments are combined with carbon dioxide to form urea.

IN SUMMARY

Nutrient	Yields Energy?	Yields Glucose?	Yields Amino Acids and Body Proteins?	Yields Fat Stores?[a]
Carbohydrates (glucose)	Yes	Yes	Yes—when nitrogen is available, can yield *nonessential* amino acids	Yes
Lipids (fatty acids)	Yes	No	No	Yes
Lipids (glycerol)	Yes	Yes—when carbohydrate is unavailable	Yes—when nitrogen is available, can yield *nonessential* amino acids	Yes
Proteins (amino acids)	Yes	Yes—when carbohydrate is unavailable	Yes	Yes

[a]When energy intake exceeds needs, any of the energy-yielding nutrients can contribute to body fat stores.

FIGURE 7-17 Urea Excretion

The liver and kidneys both play a role in disposing of excess nitrogen. Can you see why the person with liver disease has high blood ammonia, while the person with kidney disease has high blood urea? (Figure 12-2 provides details of how the kidneys work.)

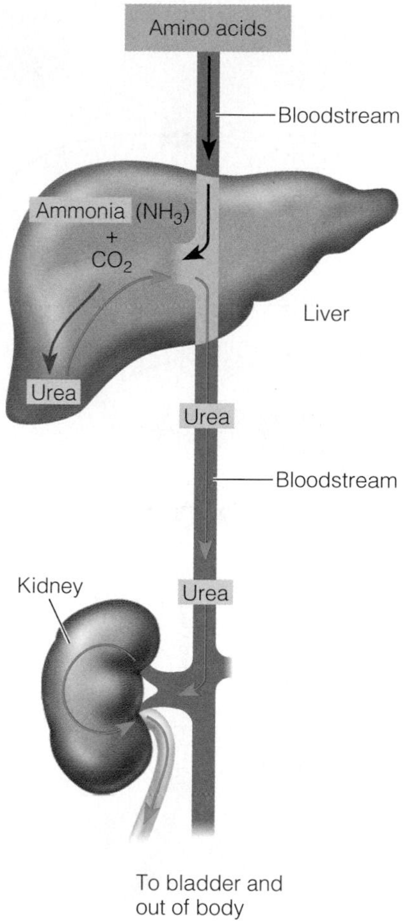
Amino acids
Bloodstream
Ammonia (NH_3)
+
CO_2
Liver
Urea
Urea
Bloodstream
Kidney
Urea
To bladder and out of body

The Final Steps of Catabolism

Thus far the discussion has followed each of the energy-yielding nutrients down three different pathways. All lead to the point where acetyl CoA enters the TCA cycle. The TCA cycle reactions take place in the inner compartment of the mitochondria (see Figure 7-4 on p. 218). The significance of this location will become evident as details unfold.

The TCA Cycle Acetyl CoA enters the TCA cycle, a busy metabolic traffic center. The TCA cycle is called a cycle, but that doesn't mean it regenerates acetyl CoA. Acetyl CoA goes one way only—down to two carbon dioxide molecules and a coenzyme (CoA). The TCA cycle is a circular path, though, in the sense that a 4-carbon compound known as **oxaloacetate** is needed in the first step and synthesized in the last step.

Oxaloacetate's role in replenishing the TCA cycle is critical. When oxaloacetate is insufficient, the TCA cycle slows down, and the cells face an energy crisis. Oxaloacetate is made primarily from pyruvate, although it can be made from certain amino acids. Importantly, oxaloacetate cannot be made from fat. That oxaloacetate must be available for acetyl CoA to enter the TCA cycle underscores the importance of carbohydrates in the diet. A diet that provides ample carbohydrate ensures an adequate supply of oxaloacetate (because glucose produces pyruvate during glycolysis). (Highlight 8 presents more information on the consequences of low-carbohydrate diets.)

As Figure 7-18 shows, oxaloacetate is the first 4-carbon compound to enter the TCA cycle. Oxaloacetate picks up acetyl CoA (a 2-carbon compound), drops off one carbon (as carbon dioxide), then another carbon (as carbon dioxide), and returns to pick up another acetyl CoA. As for the acetyl CoA, its carbons go only one way—to carbon dioxide (see Appendix C for additional details).*

As acetyl CoA molecules break down to carbon dioxide, hydrogen atoms with their electrons are removed from the compounds in the cycle. Each turn of the TCA cycle loses a total of eight electrons. Coenzymes made from the B vitamins niacin and riboflavin receive the hydrogens and their electrons from the TCA cycle

oxaloacetate (OKS-ah-low-AS-eh-tate): a carbohydrate intermediate of the TCA cycle.

*Actually, the carbons that enter the cycle in acetyl CoA may not be the exact ones that are given off as carbon dioxide. In one of the steps of the cycle, a 6-carbon compound of the cycle becomes symmetrical, both ends being identical. Thereafter it loses carbons to carbon dioxide at one end or the other. Thus only half of the carbons from acetyl CoA are given off as carbon dioxide in any one turn of the cycle; the other half become part of the compound that returns to pick up another acetyl CoA. It is true to say, though, that for each acetyl CoA that enters the TCA cycle, 2 carbons are given off as carbon dioxide. It is also true that with each turn of the cycle the energy equivalent of one acetyl CoA is released.

FIGURE 7-18 The TCA Cycle

Oxaloacetate, a compound made primarily from pyruvate, starts the TCA cycle. (Knowing that glucose produces pyruvate during glycolysis and that oxaloacetate must be available to start the TCA cycle, you can understand why the complete oxidation of fat requires carbohydrate.) The 4-carbon oxaloacetate joins with the 2-carbon acetyl CoA. The new 6-carbon compound releases carbons as carbon dioxide, becoming a 5- and then a 4-carbon compound. Each reaction changes the structure slightly until finally the original 4-carbon oxaloacetate forms again and picks up another acetyl CoA—from the breakdown of glucose, glycerol, fatty acids, and amino acids—and starts the cycle over again. The breakdown of acetyl CoA releases hydrogens with their electrons, which are carried by coenzymes made from the B vitamins niacin and riboflavin to the electron transport chain. (For more details, see Appendix C.)

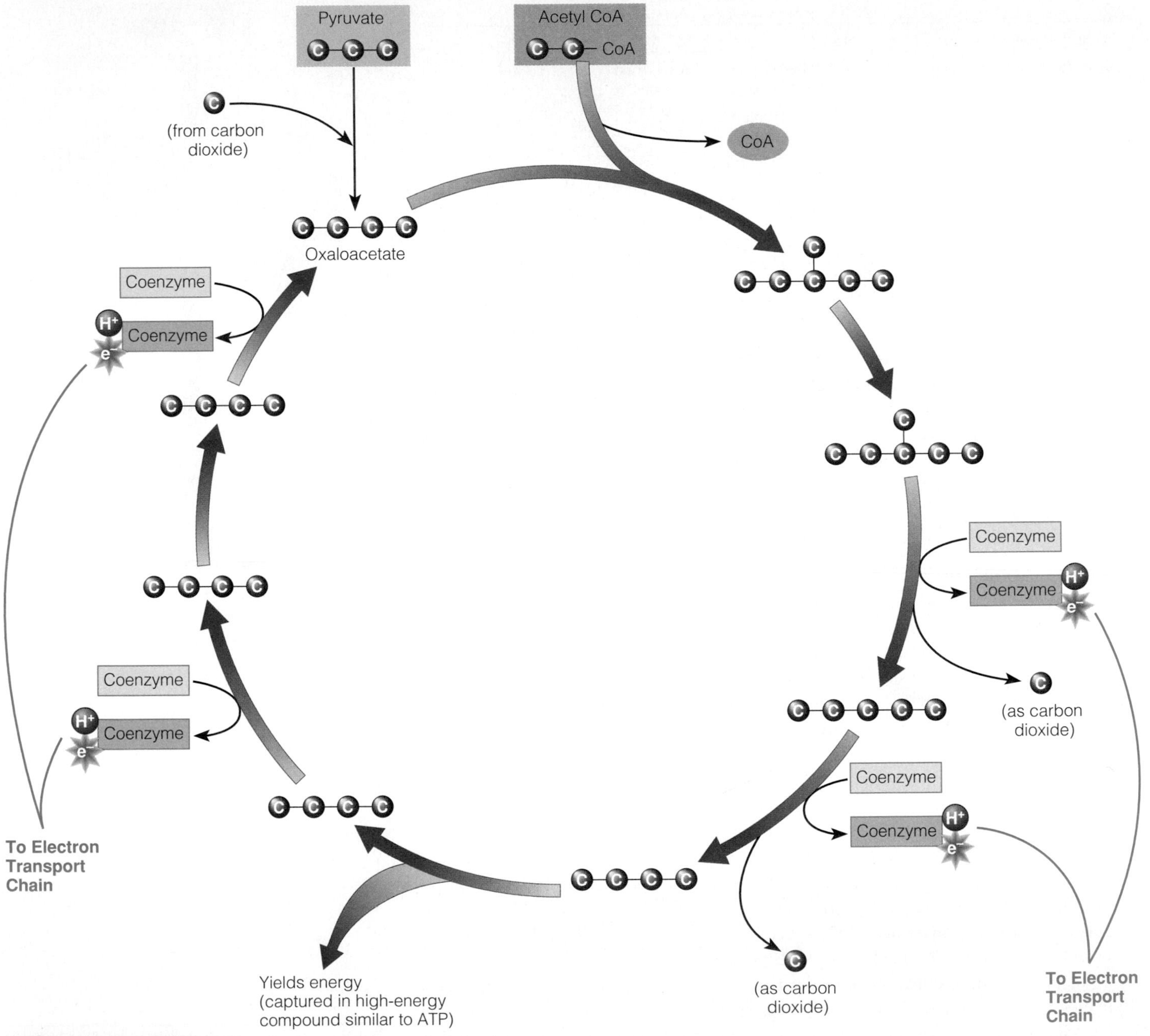
Pyruvate
C C C
Acetyl CoA
C C CoA
C
(from carbon dioxide)
CoA
C C C C
Oxaloacetate
Coenzyme
H+
e−
Coenzyme
(as carbon dioxide)
Coenzyme
Coenzyme
To Electron Transport Chain
Yields energy (captured in high-energy compound similar to ATP)
(as carbon dioxide)
To Electron Transport Chain

Available Online

Watch as a series of metabolic reactions break down molecules of acetyl CoA to carbon dioxide and hydrogen atoms.

and transfer them to the electron transport chain—much like a taxi cab that picks up passengers in one location and drops them off in another.

The Electron Transport Chain In the final pathway, the electron transport chain, energy is captured in the high-energy bonds of ATP. The electron transport chain consists of a series of proteins that serve as electron "carriers." These carriers are mounted in sequence on the inner membrane of the mitochondria (review Figure 7-4 on p. 218). As the coenzymes deliver their electrons from the TCA cycle, glycolysis, and fatty acid oxidation to the electron transport chain, each carrier receives the electrons and then passes them on to the next carrier. These electron carriers continue passing the electrons down until they reach oxygen at the end of the chain. Oxygen (O) accepts the electrons and combines with hydrogen atoms (H) to form water (H_2O).■ That oxygen must be available for energy metabolism explains why it is essential to life.

■ The results of the electron transport chain:
- O_2 consumed.
- H_2O and CO_2 produced.
- Energy captured in ATP.

As electrons are passed from carrier to carrier, enough energy is released to pump hydrogen ions across the membrane to the outer compartment of the mitochondria. The rush of hydrogen ions back into the inner compartment powers the synthesis of ATP. In this way, energy is captured in the bonds of ATP. The ATP leaves the mitochondria and enters the cytoplasm, where it can be used for energy. Figure 7-19 provides a simple diagram of the electron transport chain; see Appendix C for details.

The kCalories-per-Gram Secret Revealed Of the three energy-yielding nutrients, fat provides the most energy per gram.■ The reason may be apparent from Figure 7-20, which compares a fatty acid with a glucose molecule. Notice that nearly all the bonds in a the fatty acid are between carbons and hydrogens. Oxygen can be added to all of them (forming carbon dioxide with the carbons, and water with the hydrogens). As this happens, hydrogens are released to coenzymes heading for the electron transport chain. In glucose, on the other hand, an oxygen is already bonded to each carbon; thus there is less potential for oxidation, and fewer hydrogens released when the remaining bonds are broken.

■ Fat = 9 kcal/g.
Carbohydrate = 4 kcal/g.
Protein = 4 kcal/g.

Available Online

Watch an animated explanation of the electron transport chain, the final pathway in energy metabolism where electrons from hydrogen are passed to oxygen and the energy released is trapped in the bonds of ATP.

FIGURE 7-19 Electron Transport Chain and ATP Synthesis

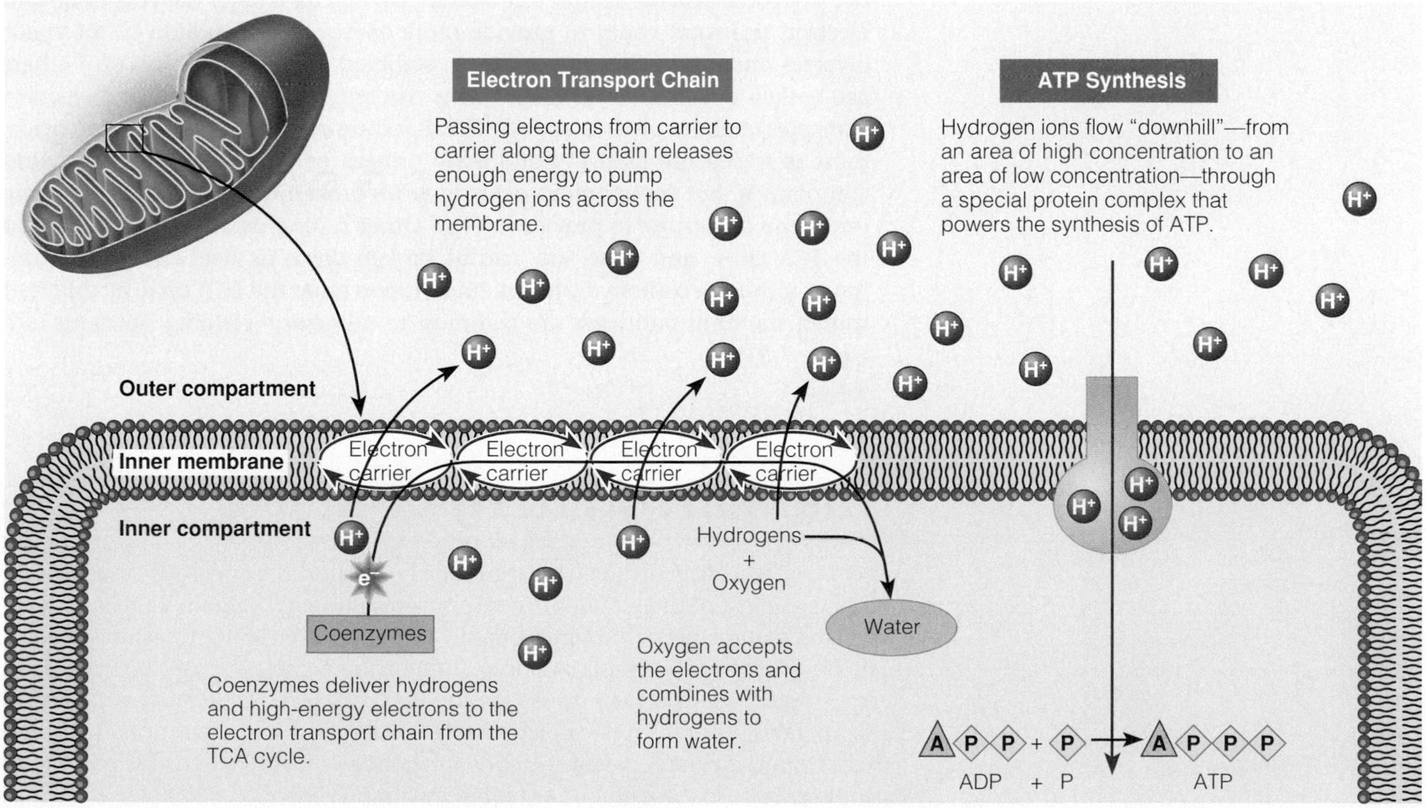
Electron Transport Chain
Passing electrons from carrier to carrier along the chain releases enough energy to pump hydrogen ions across the membrane.
ATP Synthesis
Hydrogen ions flow "downhill"—from an area of high concentration to an area of low concentration—through a special protein complex that powers the synthesis of ATP.
Outer compartment
Inner membrane
Inner compartment
Electron carrier
Electron carrier
Electron carrier
Electron carrier
H+
e−
Coenzymes
Hydrogens + Oxygen
Water
Coenzymes deliver hydrogens and high-energy electrons to the electron transport chain from the TCA cycle.
Oxygen accepts the electrons and combines with hydrogens to form water.
A P P + P → A P P P
ADP + P
ATP

FIGURE 7-20 Chemical Structures of a Fatty Acid and Glucose Compared

To ease comparison, the structure shown here for glucose is not the ring structure shown in Chapter 4, but an alternative way of drawing its chemical structure.

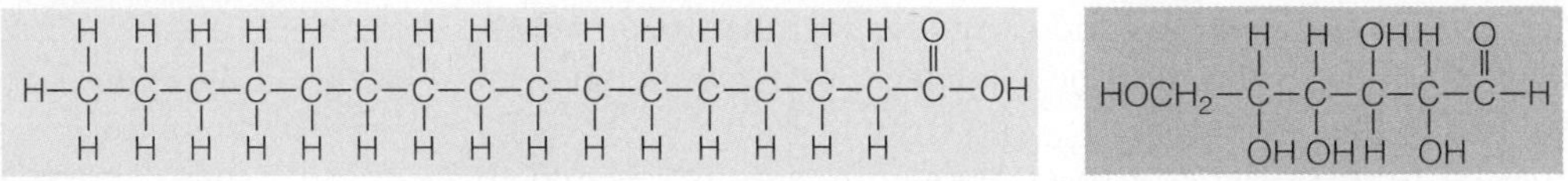
Fatty acid
Glucose

Because fat contains many carbon-hydrogen bonds that can be readily oxidized, it sends numerous coenzymes with their hydrogens and electrons to the electron transport chain where that energy can be captured in the bonds of ATP. This explains why fat yields more kcalories per gram than carbohydrate or protein. (Remember that each ATP holds energy and that kcalories measure energy; thus the more ATP generated, the more kcalories have been collected.) For example, one glucose molecule will yield 36 to 38 ATP when completely oxidized. In comparison, one 16-carbon fatty acid molecule will yield 129 ATP when completely oxidized. Fat is a more efficient fuel source. Gram for gram, fat can provide much more energy than either of the other two energy-yielding nutrients, making it the body's preferred form of energy storage. (Similarly, you might prefer to fill your car with a fuel that provides 130 miles per gallon versus one that provides 35 miles per gallon.)

IN SUMMARY After a balanced meal, the body handles the nutrients as follows. The digestion of carbohydrate yields glucose (and other monosaccharides); some is stored as glycogen, and some is broken down to pyruvate and acetyl CoA to provide energy. The acetyl CoA can then enter the TCA cycle and electron transport chain to provide more energy. The digestion of fat yields glycerol and fatty acids; some are reassembled and stored as fat, and others are broken down to acetyl CoA, which can enter the TCA cycle and electron transport chain to provide energy. The digestion of protein yields amino acids, most of which are used to build body protein or other nitrogen-containing compounds, but some amino acids may be broken down through the same pathways as glucose to provide energy. Other amino acids enter directly into the TCA cycle, and these, too, can be broken down to yield energy. In summary, although carbohydrate, fat, and protein enter the TCA cycle by different routes, the final pathways are common to all energy-yielding nutrients (see Figure 7-21).

The Body's Energy Budget

Every day, a healthy diet delivers thousands of kcalories from foods, and the active body uses most of them to do its work. As a result, body weight changes little, if at all. This remarkable achievement could be called the economy of maintenance. The body's energy budget is balanced. Some people, however, eat too much or exercise too little and get fat; others eat too little or exercise too much and get thin. The metabolic details have already been described; the next sections will review them from the perspective of the body fat gained or lost. The possible reasons why people gain or lose weight are explored in Chapter 8.

FIGURE 7-21 The Central Pathways of Energy Metabolism

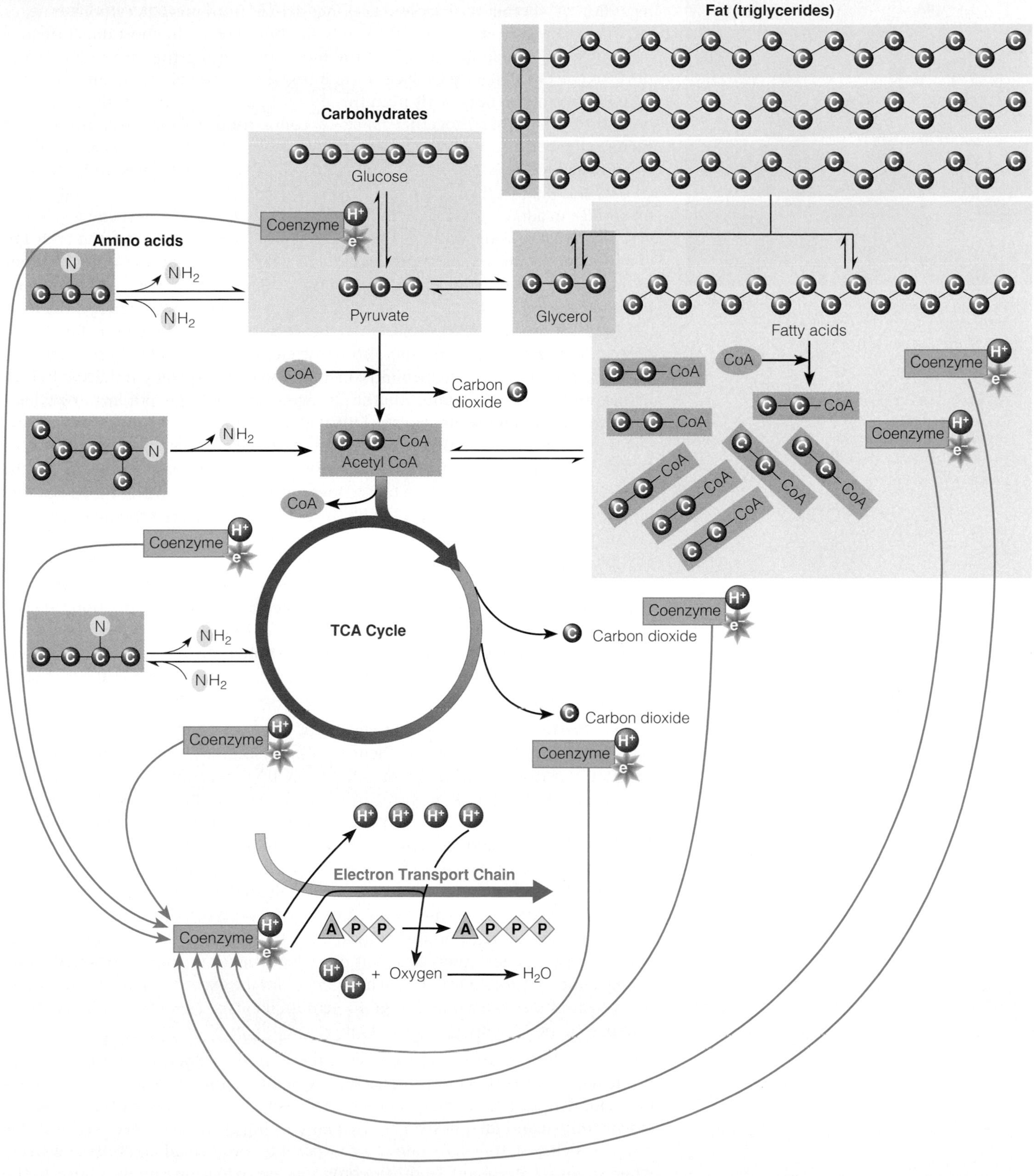

Fat (triglycerides)
Carbohydrates
Glucose
Coenzyme
Amino acids
NH_2
NH_2
Pyruvate
Glycerol
Fatty acids
CoA
Carbon dioxide
CoA
Acetyl CoA
CoA
Coenzyme
TCA Cycle
Carbon dioxide
Carbon dioxide
Coenzyme
Electron Transport Chain
+ Oxygen
H_2O

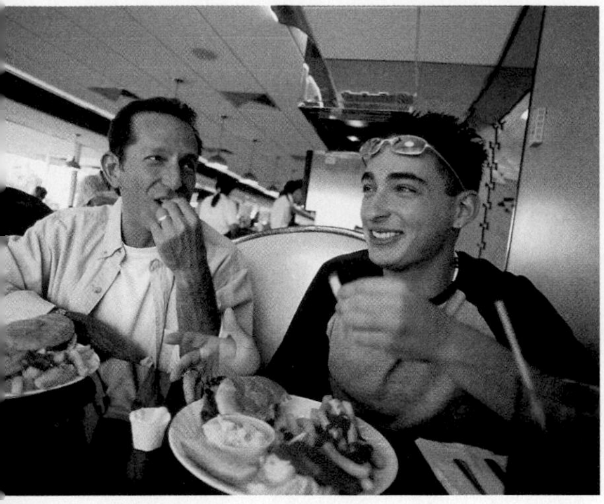

People can enjoy bountiful meals such as this without storing body fat, provided that they spend as much energy as they take in.

The Economics of Feasting

When a person eats too much, metabolism favors fat formation. Fat cells enlarge regardless of whether the excess in kcalories derives from protein, carbohydrate, or fat. The pathway from dietary fat to body fat, however, is the most direct (requiring only a few metabolic steps) and the most efficient (costing only a few kcalories). To convert a dietary triglyceride to a triglyceride in adipose tissue, the body removes two of the fatty acids from the glycerol backbone, absorbs the parts, and puts them (and others) together again. By comparison, to convert a molecule of sucrose, the body has to split glucose from fructose, absorb them, dismantle them to pyruvate and acetyl CoA, assemble many acetyl CoA molecules into fatty acid chains, and finally attach fatty acids to a glycerol backbone to make a triglyceride for storage in adipose tissue. Quite simply, the body uses much less energy to convert dietary fat to body fat than it does to convert dietary carbohydrate to body fat. On average, storing excess energy from dietary fat in body fat uses only 5 percent of the ingested energy intake, but storing excess energy from dietary carbohydrate in body fat requires an expenditure of 25 percent of the ingested energy intake.

The pathways from excess protein and excess carbohydrate to body fat are not only indirect and inefficient, but also less preferred (having other priorities). Before entering fat storage, protein must first tend to its many roles in the body's lean tissues, and carbohydrate must fill the glycogen stores. Simply put, making fat is a low priority for these two nutrients. Still, if eaten in abundance, any of the energy-yielding nutrients can make fat.

This chapter has described each of the energy-yielding nutrients individually, but cells use a mixture of these fuels. How much of which nutrient is in the fuel mix depends, in part, on its availability from the diet. Dietary protein and dietary carbohydrate influence the mixture of fuel used during energy metabolism. Usually, protein's contribution to the fuel mix is relatively minor and fairly constant, but protein oxidation does increase when protein is eaten in excess. Similarly, carbohydrate eaten in excess significantly enhances carbohydrate oxidation. In contrast, fat oxidation does *not* respond to dietary fat intake, especially when dietary changes occur abruptly. The more protein or carbohydrate in the fuel mix, the less fat contributes to the fuel mix. Instead of being oxidized, fat accumulates in storage. Details follow.

Excess Protein Recall from Chapter 6 that the body cannot store excess amino acids as such; it has to convert them to other compounds. Contrary to popular opinion, a person cannot grow muscle simply by overeating protein. Lean tissue such as muscle develops in response to a stimulus such as hormones or physical activity. When a person overeats protein, the body uses the surplus first by replacing normal daily losses and then by increasing protein oxidation. The body achieves protein balance this way, but any increase in protein oxidation displaces fat in the fuel mix. Any additional protein is then deaminated and the remaining carbons used to make fatty acids. Thus a person can grow fat by eating too much protein.

People who eat huge portions of meat and other protein-rich foods may wonder why they have weight problems. Not only does the fat in those foods lead to fat storage, but the protein can, too, when energy intake exceeds energy needs. Many fad weight-loss diets encourage high protein intakes based on the false assumption that protein builds only muscle, not fat (see Highlight 8 for more details).

Excess Carbohydrate Compared with protein, the proportion of carbohydrate in the fuel mix changes more dramatically when a person overeats. The body handles abundant carbohydrate by first storing it as glycogen, but glycogen storage areas are limited and fill quickly. Because maintaining glucose balance is critical, the body uses glucose frugally when the diet provides only small amounts and freely when stores are abundant. In other words, glucose oxidation rapidly adjusts to the dietary intake of carbohydrate.

Excess glucose can be converted to fat directly, but this is a minor pathway.[3] As mentioned earlier, converting glucose to fat is energetically expensive and does not occur until after glycogen stores have been filled. Even then, only a little, if any, new fat is made from carbohydrate.[4]

Nevertheless, excess dietary carbohydrate can lead to weight gain when extra carbohydrate displaces fat in the fuel mix. When this occurs, carbohydrate spares both dietary fat and body fat from oxidation—an effect that may be more pronounced in overweight people than in lean people.[5] The net result: excess carbohydrate contributes to obesity or at least to the maintenance of an overweight body.

Excess Fat Unlike excess protein and carbohydrate, which both enhance their own oxidation, eating too much fat does not promote fat oxidation. Instead, excess dietary fat moves efficiently into the body's fat stores; almost all of the excess is stored.

IN SUMMARY If energy intake exceeds the body's energy needs, the result will be weight gain—regardless of whether the excess intake is from protein, carbohydrate, or fat. The difference is that the body is much more efficient at storing energy when the excess derives from dietary fat.

The Transition from Feasting to Fasting

Figure 7-22 shows the metabolic pathways operating in the body as it shifts from feasting (part A) to fasting (parts B and C). After a meal, glucose, glycerol, and fatty acids from foods are used as needed and then stored. Later, as the body shifts from

FIGURE 7-22 Feasting and Fasting

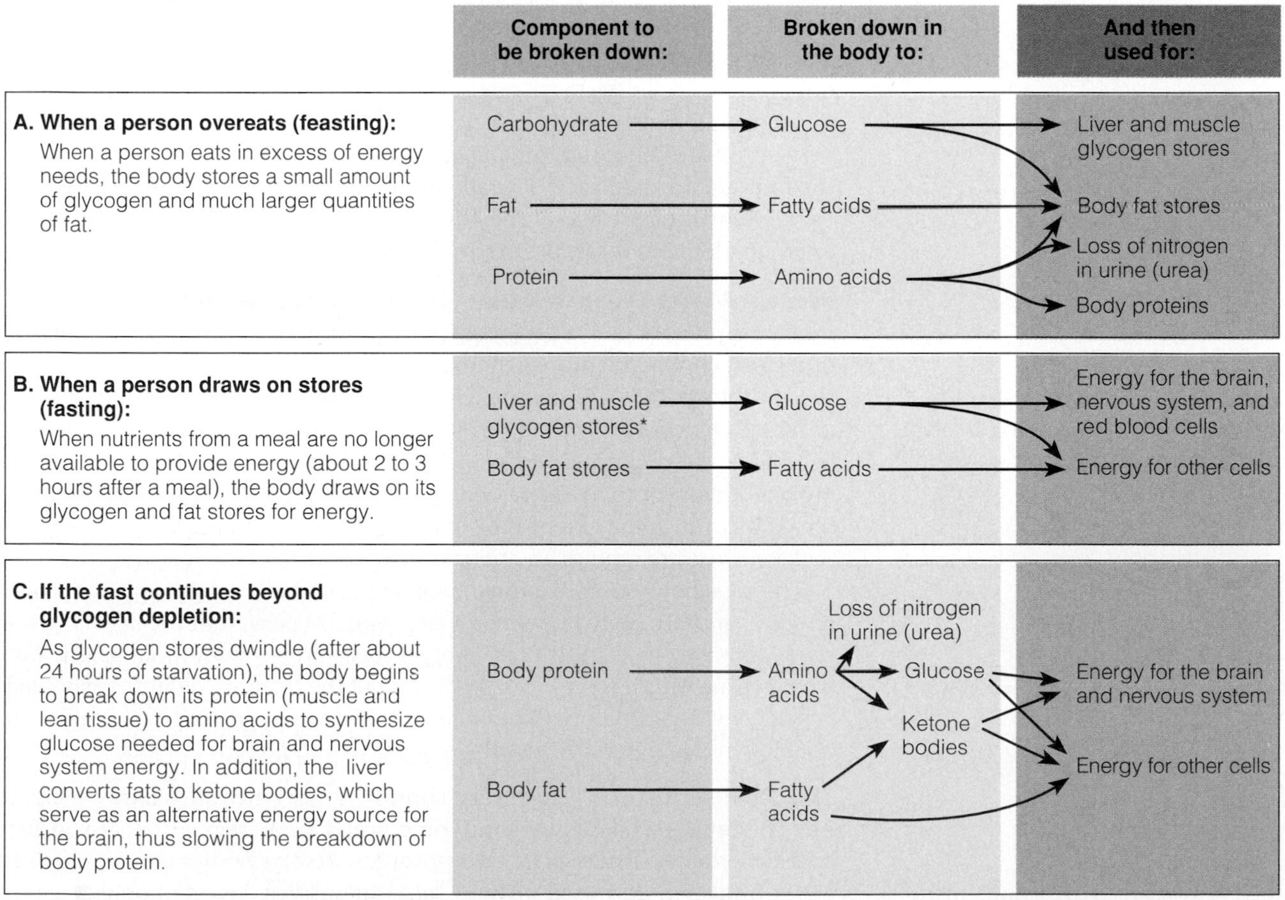
Component to be broken down:
Broken down in the body to:
And then used for:
A. When a person overeats (feasting):
When a person eats in excess of energy needs, the body stores a small amount of glycogen and much larger quantities of fat.
Carbohydrate
Glucose
Liver and muscle glycogen stores
Fat
Fatty acids
Body fat stores
Protein
Amino acids
Loss of nitrogen in urine (urea)
Body proteins
B. When a person draws on stores (fasting):
When nutrients from a meal are no longer available to provide energy (about 2 to 3 hours after a meal), the body draws on its glycogen and fat stores for energy.
Liver and muscle glycogen stores*
Glucose
Energy for the brain, nervous system, and red blood cells
Body fat stores
Fatty acids
Energy for other cells
C. If the fast continues beyond glycogen depletion:
As glycogen stores dwindle (after about 24 hours of starvation), the body begins to break down its protein (muscle and lean tissue) to amino acids to synthesize glucose needed for brain and nervous system energy. In addition, the liver converts fats to ketone bodies, which serve as an alternative energy source for the brain, thus slowing the breakdown of body protein.
Loss of nitrogen in urine (urea)
Body protein
Amino acids
Glucose
Energy for the brain and nervous system
Ketone bodies
Energy for other cells
Body fat
Fatty acids

*The muscles' stored glycogen provides glucose only for the muscle in which the glycogen is stored.

a fed state to a fasting one, it begins drawing on these stores. Glycogen and fat are released from storage to provide more glucose, glycerol, and fatty acids for energy.

Energy is needed all the time. Even when a person is asleep and totally relaxed, the cells of many organs are hard at work. In fact, this work—the cells' work that maintains all life processes■ without any conscious effort—represents about two-thirds to three-fourths of the total energy a person spends in a day. The small remainder is the work that a person's muscles perform voluntarily during waking hours.

■ The cells' work that maintains all life processes refers to the body's *basal metabolism,* which is described in Chapter 8.

The body's top priority is to meet the cells' needs for energy, and it normally does this by periodic refueling—that is, by eating several times a day. When food is not available, the body turns to its own tissues for other fuel sources. If people choose not to eat, we say they are fasting; if they have no choice, we say they are starving. The body makes no such distinction. In either case, the body is forced to switch to a wasting metabolism, drawing on its reserves of carbohydrate and fat and, within a day or so, on its vital protein tissues as well.

The Economics of Fasting

During fasting, carbohydrate, fat, and protein are all eventually used for energy—fuel must be delivered to every cell. As the fast begins, glucose from the liver's stored glycogen and fatty acids from the adipose tissue's stored fat are both flowing into cells, then breaking down to yield acetyl CoA, and delivering energy to power the cells' work. Several hours later, however, most of the glucose is used up—liver glycogen is exhausted and blood glucose begins to fall. Low blood glucose serves as a signal that promotes further fat breakdown and release of amino acids from muscles.

Glucose Needed for the Brain At this point, most of the cells are depending on fatty acids to continue providing their fuel. But red blood cells and the cells of the nervous system need glucose. Glucose is their major energy fuel, and even when other energy fuels are available, glucose must be present to permit the energy-metabolizing machinery of the nervous system to work. Normally, the brain and nerve cells—which weigh only about three pounds—consume about two-thirds of the total *glucose* used each day (about 400 to 600 kcalories' worth). About one-fifth to one-fourth of the *energy* the adult body uses when it is at rest is spent by the brain; in children, it can be up to one-half.

Protein Meets Glucose Needs The red blood cells' and brain's special requirements for glucose pose a problem for the fasting body. The body can use its stores of fat, which may be quite generous, to furnish most of its cells with energy, but the red blood cells are completely dependent on glucose,■ and the brain and nerves prefer energy in the form of glucose. Amino acids that yield pyruvate can be used to make glucose; and to obtain the amino acids, body proteins must be broken down. For this reason, body protein tissues such as muscle and liver always break down to some extent during fasting. The amino acids that can't be used to make glucose are used as an energy source for other body cells.

■ Red blood cells contain no mitochondria. Review Figure 7-4 to fully appreciate why red blood cells must depend on glucose for energy.

The breakdown of body protein is an expensive way to obtain glucose. In the first few days of a fast, body protein provides about 90 percent of the needed glucose; glycerol, about 10 percent. If body protein losses were to continue at this rate, death would ensue within three weeks, regardless of the quantity of fat a person had stored. Fortunately, fat breakdown also increases with fasting—in fact, fat breakdown almost doubles, providing energy for other body cells and glycerol for glucose production.

The Shift to Ketosis As the fast continues, the body finds a way to use its fat to fuel the brain. It adapts by combining acetyl CoA fragments derived from fatty acids to produce an alternate energy source, ketone bodies (see Figure 7-23). Normally produced and used only in small quantities, ketone bodies■ can provide fuel for some brain cells. Ketone body production rises until, after about ten days of fasting, it is meeting much of the nervous system's energy needs. Still, many ar-

■ Reminder: *Ketone bodies* are compounds produced during the incomplete breakdown of fat when glucose is not available.

FIGURE 7-23 Ketone Body Formation

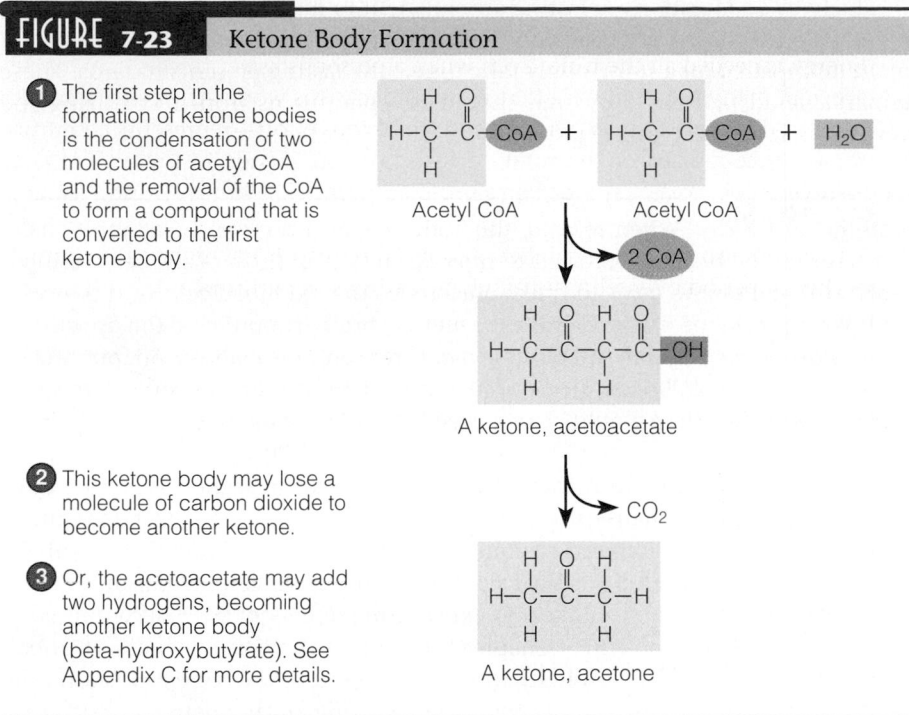

1. The first step in the formation of ketone bodies is the condensation of two molecules of acetyl CoA and the removal of the CoA to form a compound that is converted to the first ketone body.
2. This ketone body may lose a molecule of carbon dioxide to become another ketone.
3. Or, the acetoacetate may add two hydrogens, becoming another ketone body (beta-hydroxybutyrate). See Appendix C for more details.

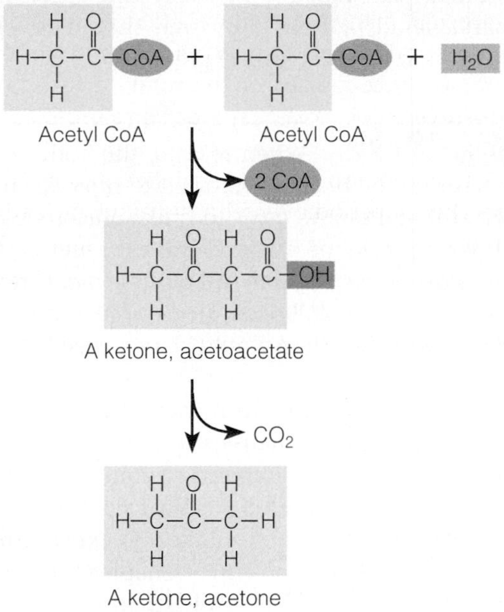
Acetyl CoA
Acetyl CoA
H_2O
2 CoA
A ketone, acetoacetate
CO_2
A ketone, acetone

eas of the brain rely exclusively on glucose, and to produce it, the body continues to sacrifice protein—albeit at a slower rate than in the early days of fasting.

When ketone bodies contain an acid group (COOH), they are called keto acids. Small amounts of keto acids are a normal part of the blood chemistry, but when their concentration rises, the pH of the blood drops. This is ketosis, a sign that the body's chemistry is going awry. Elevated blood ketones (ketonemia) are excreted in the urine (ketonuria). A fruity odor on the breath (known as acetone breath) develops, reflecting the presence of the ketone acetone.

Suppression of Appetite Ketosis also induces a loss of appetite. As starvation continues, this loss of appetite becomes an advantage to a person without access to food, because the search for food would be a waste of energy. When the person finds food and eats again, the body shifts out of ketosis, the hunger center gets the message that food is again available, and the appetite returns. Highlight 8 includes a discussion of the risks of ketosis-producing diets in its review of popular weight-loss diets.

Slowing of Metabolism In an effort to conserve body tissues for as long as possible, the hormones of fasting slow metabolism. As the body shifts to the use of ketone bodies, it simultaneously reduces its energy output and conserves both its fat and its lean tissue. Still the lean (protein-containing) organ tissues shrink in mass and perform less metabolic work, reducing energy expenditures. As the muscles waste, they can do less work and so demand less energy, reducing expenditures further. Because of the slowed metabolism, the loss of fat falls to a bare minimum—less, in fact, than the fat that would be lost on a low-kcalorie diet. Thus, although *weight* loss during fasting may be quite dramatic, *fat* loss may be less than when at least some food is eaten.

Symptoms of Starvation The adaptations just described—slowing of energy output and reduction in fat loss—occur in the starving child, the hungry homeless adult, the fasting religious person, the adolescent with anorexia nervosa, and the malnourished hospital patient. Such adaptations help to prolong their lives and explain the physical symptoms of energy deprivation: wasting, slowed metabolism, lowered body temperature, and reduced resistance to disease.

The body's adaptations to fasting are sufficient to maintain life for a long time. Mental alertness need not be diminished, and even some physical energy may remain unimpaired for a surprisingly long time. Still, fasting presents hazards. These remarkable adaptations, however, should not prevent us from recognizing the very real hazards that fasting presents.

IN SUMMARY When fasting, the body makes a number of adaptations: increasing the breakdown of fat to provide energy for most of the cells, using glycerol and amino acids to make glucose for the red blood cells and central nervous system, producing ketones to fuel the brain, suppressing the appetite, and slowing metabolism. All of these measures conserve energy and minimize losses. In fact, metabolism slows to such an extent that the loss of fat eventually slows to less than would be achieved with a low-kcalorie diet.

This chapter has probed the intricate details of metabolism at the level of the cells, exploring the transformations of nutrients to energy and to storage compounds. Several chapters and highlights to come build on this information. The highlight that follows this chapter shows how alcohol disrupts normal metabolism. Chapter 8 describes how a person's intake and expenditure of energy are reflected in body weight and body composition. Chapter 9 examines the consequences of unbalanced energy budgets—overweight and underweight. And Chapter 10 shows the vital roles the B vitamins play as coenzymes assisting all the metabolic pathways described here.

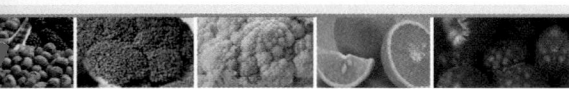

Nutrition in Your Life

All day, every day, your cells dismantle carbohydrates, fats, and proteins, with the help of vitamins, minerals, and water, releasing energy to meet your body's immediate needs or storing it as fat for later use.

- **What types of foods best support aerobic and anaerobic activities?**
- **Do you eat more protein, carbohydrate, or fat than your body needs?**
- **Do you follow a low-carbohydrate diet that forces your body into ketosis?**

STUDY QUESTIONS

These questions will help you review the chapter. You will find the answers in the discussions on the pages provided.

1. Define metabolism, anabolism, and catabolism; give an example of each. (pp. 215–216)
2. Name one of the body's high-energy molecules, and describe how it is used. (pp. 216–218)
3. What are coenzymes, and what service do they provide in metabolism? (p. 219)
4. Name the four basic units, derived from foods, that are used by the body in metabolic transformations. How many carbons are in the "backbones" of each? (p. 220)
5. Define aerobic and anaerobic metabolism. How does insufficient oxygen influence metabolism? (pp. 221–223)
6. How does the body dispose of excess nitrogen? (pp. 227–229)
7. Summarize the main steps in the metabolism of glucose, glycerol, fatty acids, and amino acids. (pp. 228–229)
8. Describe how a surplus of the three energy nutrients contributes to body fat stores. (pp. 234–235)

9. What adaptations does the body make during a fast? What are ketone bodies? Define ketosis. (pp. 236–237)
10. Distinguish between a loss of *fat* and a loss of *weight,* and describe how each might happen. (pp. 237–238)

These multiple choice questions will help you prepare for an exam. Answers can be found below.

1. Hydrolysis is an example of a(n):
   a. coupled reaction.
   b. anabolic reaction.
   c. catabolic reaction.
   d. synthesis reaction.
2. During metabolism, released energy is captured and transferred by:
   a. enzymes.
   b. pyruvate.
   c. acetyl CoA.
   d. adenosine triphosphate.
3. Glycolysis:
   a. requires oxygen.
   b. generates abundant energy.
   c. converts glucose to pyruvate.
   d. produces ammonia as a by-product.
4. The pathway from pyruvate to acetyl CoA:
   a. produces lactic acid.
   b. is known as gluconeogenesis.
   c. is metabolically irreversible.
   d. requires more energy than it produces.
5. For complete oxidation, acetyl CoA enters:
   a. glycolysis.
   b. the TCA cycle.
   c. the Cori cycle.
   d. the electron transport chain.
6. Deamination of an amino acid produces:
   a. vitamin B_6 and energy.
   b. pyruvate and acetyl CoA.
   c. ammonia and a keto acid.
   d. carbon dioxide and water.
7. Before entering the TCA cycle, each of the energy-yielding nutrients is broken down to:
   a. ammonia.
   b. pyruvate.
   c. electrons.
   d. acetyl CoA.
8. The body stores energy for future use in:
   a. proteins.
   b. acetyl CoA.
   c. triglycerides.
   d. ketone bodies.
9. During a fast, when glycogen stores have been depleted, the body begins to synthesize glucose from:
   a. acetyl CoA.
   b. amino acids.
   c. fatty acids.
   d. ketone bodies.
10. During a fast, the body produces ketone bodies by:
   a. hydrolyzing glycogen.
   b. condensing acetyl CoA.
   c. transaminating keto acids.
   d. converting ammonia to urea.

REFERENCES

1. J. H. Wilmore and D. L. Costill, Physical energy: Fuel metabolism, *Nutrition Reviews* 59 (2001): S13–S16; A. D. Kriketos, J. C. Peters, and J. O. Hill, Cellular and whole-animal energetics, in *Biochemical and Physiological Aspects of Human Nutrition,* ed. M. H. Stipanuk (Philadelphia: W. B. Saunders, 2000), pp. 411–424.
2. J. L. Groff and S. S. Gropper, *Advanced Nutrition and Human Metabolism* (Belmont, Calif.: Wadsworth/Thomson Learning, 2000), p. 188.
3. M. K. Hellerstein, De novo lipogenesis in humans: Metabolic and regulatory aspects, *European Journal of Clinical Nutrition* 53 (1999): S53–S65.
4. R. M. Devitt and coauthors, De novo lipogenesis during controlled overfeeding with sucrose or glucose in lean and obese women, *American Journal of Clinical Nutrition* 74 (2001): 707–708.
5. I. Marques-Lopes and coauthors, Postprandial de novo lipogenesis and metabolic changes induced by a high-carbohydrate, low-fat meal in lean and overweight men, *American Journal of Clinical Nutrition* 73 (2001): 253–261.

ANSWERS

Study Questions (multiple choice)

1. c 2. d 3. c 4. c 5. b 6. c 7. d 8. c 9. b 10. b

HIGHLIGHT

Alcohol and Nutrition

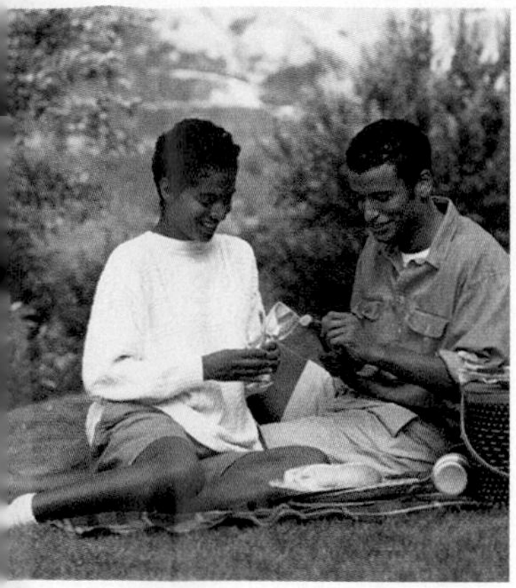

With the understanding of metabolism gained from Chapter 7, you are in a position to understand how the body handles alcohol, how alcohol interferes with metabolism, and how alcohol impairs health and nutrition. The potential health benefits of drinking alcohol in *moderation* are presented in Chapter 27.

FIGURE H7-1 Two Alcohols: Glycerol and Ethanol

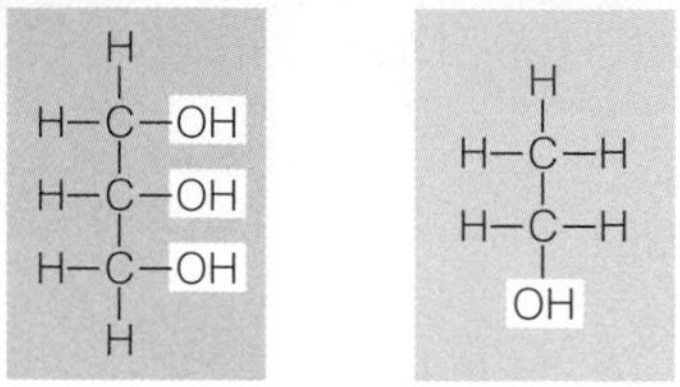
H
H—C—OH
H—C—OH
H—C—OH
H
H
H—C—H
H—C—H
OH

Glycerol is the alcohol used to make triglycerides.

Ethanol is the alcohol in beer, wine, and distilled liquor.

Alcohol in Beverages

To the chemist, **alcohol** refers to a class of organic compounds containing hydroxyl (OH) groups (the accompanying glossary defines alcohol and related terms). The glycerol to which fatty acids are attached in triglycerides is an example of an alcohol to a chemist. To most people, though, *alcohol* refers to the intoxicating ingredient in **beer, wine,** and **distilled liquor (hard liquor).** The chemist's name for this particular alcohol is *ethyl alcohol,* or **ethanol.** Glycerol has 3 carbons with 3 hydroxyl groups attached; ethanol has only 2 carbons and 1 hydroxyl group (see Figure H7-1). The remainder of this highlight talks about the particular alcohol, ethanol, but refers to it simply as *alcohol.*

Alcohols affect living things profoundly, partly because they act as lipid solvents. Their ability to dissolve lipids out of cell membranes allows alcohols to penetrate rapidly into cells, destroying cell structures and thereby killing the cells. For this reason, most alcohols are toxic in relatively small amounts; by the same token, because they kill microbial cells, they are useful as disinfectants.

Ethanol is less toxic than the other alcohols. Sufficiently diluted and taken in small enough doses, its action in the brain produces an effect that people seek—not with zero risk, but with a low enough risk (if the doses are low enough) to be tolerable. Used in this way, alcohol is a **drug**—that is, a substance that modifies body functions. Like all drugs, alcohol both offers benefits and poses hazards. The 2005 *Dietary Guidelines* advise "those who choose to drink alcoholic beverages to do so sensibly and in moderation."

The term **moderation** is important in describing alcohol use. How many drinks constitute moderate use, and how much is "a drink"? First, a **drink** is any alcoholic beverage that delivers ½ ounce of *pure ethanol:*

- 5 ounces of wine.
- 10 ounces of wine cooler.
- 12 ounces of beer.
- 1½ ounces of distilled liquor (80 proof whiskey, scotch, rum, or vodka).

Beer, wine, and liquor deliver different amounts of alcohol. The amount of alcohol in distilled liquor is stated as **proof:** 100 proof liquor is 50 percent alcohol, 80 proof is 40 percent alcohol, and so forth. Wine and beer have less alcohol than distilled liquor, although some fortified wines and beers have more alcohol than the regular varieties (see photo caption on p. 241).

Second, because people have different tolerances for alcohol, it is impossible to name an exact daily amount of alcohol that is appropriate for everyone. Authorities have attempted to identify amounts that are acceptable for most healthy people. An accepted definition of moderation is not more than two drinks a day for the average-sized man and not more than one drink a day for the average-sized woman. (Pregnant women are advised to ab-

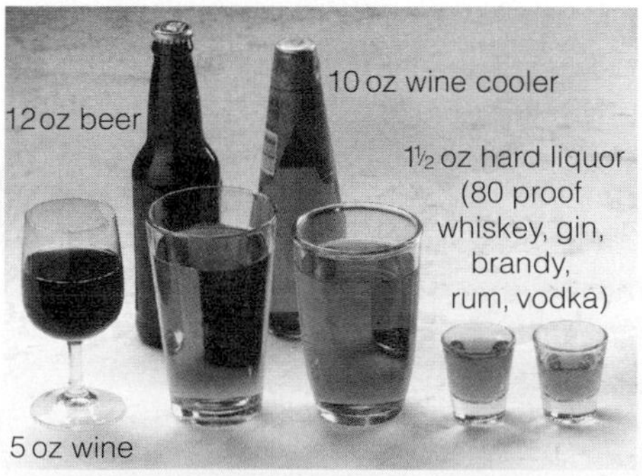
12oz beer
10 oz wine cooler
1½ oz hard liquor (80 proof whiskey, gin, brandy, rum, vodka)
5 oz wine

Each of these servings equals one drink.

GLOSSARY

acetaldehyde (ass-et-AL-duh-hide): an intermediate in alcohol metabolism.

alcohol: a class of organic compounds containing hydroxyl (OH) groups.

alcohol abuse: a pattern of drinking that includes failure to fulfill work, school, or home responsibilities; drinking in situations that are physically dangerous (as in driving while intoxicated); recurring alcohol-related legal problems (as in aggravated assault charges); or continued drinking despite ongoing social problems that are caused by or worsened by alcohol.

alcohol dehydrogenase (dee-high-DROJ-eh-nayz): an enzyme active in the stomach and the liver that converts ethanol to acetaldehyde.

alcoholism: a pattern of drinking that includes a strong craving for alcohol, a loss of control and an inability to stop drinking once begun, withdrawal symptoms (nausea, sweating, shakiness, and anxiety) after heavy drinking, and the need for increasing amounts of alcohol in order to feel "high."

antidiuretic hormone (ADH): a hormone produced by the pituitary gland in response to dehydration (or a high sodium concentration in the blood). It stimulates the kidneys to reabsorb more water and therefore to excrete less. This ADH should not be confused with the enzyme alcohol dehydrogenase, which is also sometimes abbreviated ADH.

beer: an alcoholic beverage brewed by fermenting malt and hops.

cirrhosis (seer-OH-sis): advanced liver disease in which liver cells turn orange, die, and harden, permanently losing their function; often associated with alcoholism.
- **cirrhos** = an orange

distilled liquor or **hard liquor:** an alcoholic beverage made by fermenting and distilling grains; sometimes called *distilled spirits.*

drink: a dose of any alcoholic beverage that delivers ½ oz of pure ethanol:
- 5 oz of wine.
- 10 oz of wine cooler.
- 12 oz of beer.
- 1½ oz of hard liquor (80 proof whiskey, scotch, rum, or vodka).

drug: a substance that can modify one or more of the body's functions.

ethanol: a particular type of alcohol found in beer, wine, and distilled liquor; also called *ethyl alcohol* (see Figure H7-1). Ethanol is the most widely used—and abused—drug in our society. It is also the only legal, nonprescription drug that produces euphoria.

fatty liver: an early stage of liver deterioration seen in several diseases, including kwashiorkor and alcoholic liver disease. Fatty liver is characterized by an accumulation of fat in the liver cells.

fibrosis (fye-BROH-sis): an intermediate stage of liver deterioration seen in several diseases, including viral hepatitis and alcoholic liver disease. In fibrosis, the liver cells lose their function and assume the characteristics of connective tissue cells (fibers).

MEOS or **microsomal** (my-krow-SO-mal) **ethanol-oxidizing system:** a system of enzymes in the liver that oxidize not only alcohol, but also several classes of drugs.

moderation: in relation to alcohol consumption, not more than two drinks a day for the average-sized man and not more than one drink a day for the average-sized woman.

NAD (nicotinamide adenine dinucleotide): the main coenzyme form of the vitamin niacin. Its reduced form is NADH.

narcotic (nar-KOT-ic): a drug that dulls the senses, induces sleep, and becomes addictive with prolonged use.

proof: a way of stating the percentage of alcohol in distilled liquor. Liquor that is 100 proof is 50% alcohol; 90 proof is 45%, and so forth.

Wernicke-Korsakoff (VER-nee-key KORE-sah-kof) **syndrome:** a neurological disorder typically associated with chronic alcoholism and caused by a deficiency of the B vitamin thiamin; also called *alcohol-related dementia.*

wine: an alcoholic beverage made by fermenting grape juice.

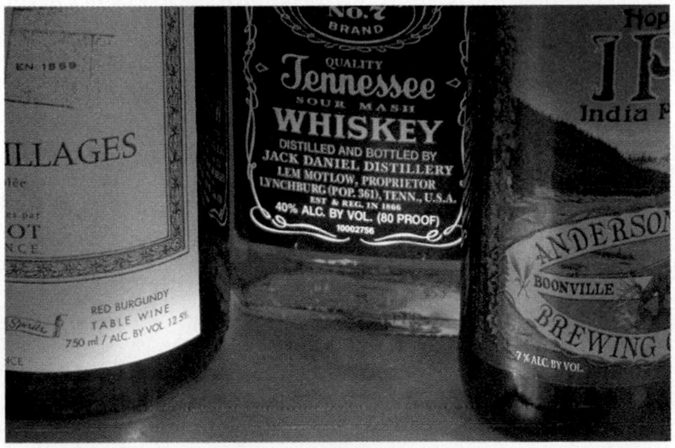
BRAND
QUALITY
Tennessee
SOUR MASH
WHISKEY
DISTILLED AND BOTTLED BY
JACK DANIEL DISTILLERY
LEM MOTLOW, PROPRIETOR
LYNCHBURG (POP. 361), TENN., U.S.A.
40% ALC. BY VOL. (80 PROOF)
ILLAGES
RED BURGUNDY
TABLE WINE
India
ANDERSON
BOONVILLE
BREWING

Matthew Farruggio

Wines contain 7 to 24 percent alcohol by volume; those containing 14 percent or more must state their alcohol content on the label, whereas those with less than 14 percent may simply state "table wine" or "light wine." Beers typically contain less than 5 percent alcohol by volume and malt liquors, 5 to 8 percent; regulations vary, with some states requiring beer labels to show the alcohol content and others prohibiting such statements.

stain from alcohol, as Highlight 14 explains.) Notice that this advice is stated as a maximum, not as an average; seven drinks one night a week would not be considered moderate, even though one a day would be. Doubtless some people could consume slightly more; others could not handle nearly so much without risk. The amount a person can drink safely is highly individual, depending on genetics, health, gender, body composition, age, and family history.

Reduce average annual alcohol consumption. HEALTHY PEOPLE 2010

Alcohol in the Body

From the moment an alcoholic beverage enters the body, alcohol is treated as if it has special privileges. Unlike foods, which require time for digestion, alcohol needs no digestion and is quickly absorbed. About 20 percent is absorbed directly across the walls of an empty stomach and can reach the brain within a minute. Consequently, a person can immediately feel euphoric when drinking, especially on an empty stomach.

When the stomach is full of food, alcohol has less chance of touching the walls and diffusing through, so its influence on the brain is slightly delayed. This information leads to a practical tip: eat snacks when drinking alcoholic beverages. Carbohydrate snacks slow alcohol absorption and high-fat snacks slow peristalsis, keeping the alcohol in the stomach longer. Salty snacks make a person thirsty; to quench thirst, drink water instead of more alcohol.

The stomach begins to break down alcohol with its **alcohol dehydrogenase** enzyme. This action can reduce the amount of alcohol entering the blood by about 20 percent. Women produce less of this stomach enzyme than men; consequently, more alcohol reaches the intestine for absorption into the bloodstream. As a result, women absorb about one-third more alcohol than men of the same size who drink the same amount of alcohol. Consequently, they are more likely to become more intoxicated on less alcohol than men. These differences between men and women help explain why women have a lower alcohol tolerance and a lower recommendation for moderate intake.

In the small intestine, alcohol is rapidly absorbed. From this point on, alcohol receives priority treatment: it gets absorbed and metabolized before most nutrients. Alcohol's priority status helps to ensure a speedy disposal and reflects two facts: alcohol cannot be stored in the body, and it is potentially toxic.

Alcohol Arrives in the Liver

The capillaries of the digestive tract merge into veins that carry the alcohol-laden blood to the liver. These veins branch and rebranch into capillaries that touch every liver cell. Liver cells are the only other cells in the body that can make enough of the alcohol dehydrogenase enzyme to oxidize alcohol at an appreciable rate. The routing of blood through the liver cells gives them the chance to dispose of some alcohol before it moves on.

Alcohol affects every organ of the body, but the most dramatic evidence of its disruptive behavior appears in the liver. If liver cells could talk, they would describe alcohol as demanding, egocentric, and disruptive of the liver's efficient way of running its business. For example, liver cells normally prefer fatty acids as their fuel, and they like to package excess fatty acids into triglycerides and ship them out to other tissues. When alcohol is present, however, the liver cells are forced to metabolize alcohol and let the fatty acids accumulate, sometimes in huge stockpiles. Alcohol metabolism can also permanently change liver cell structure, impairing the liver's ability to metabolize fats. This explains why heavy drinkers develop fatty livers.

The liver can process about ½ ounce *ethanol* per hour (the amount in a typical drink), depending on the person's body size, previous drinking experience, food intake, and general health. This maximum rate of alcohol breakdown is set by the amount of alcohol dehydrogenase available. If more alcohol arrives at the liver than the enzymes can handle, the extra alcohol travels to all parts of the body, circulating again and again until liver enzymes are finally available to process it. Another practical tip derives from this information: drink slowly enough to allow the liver to keep up—no more than one drink per hour.

The amount of alcohol dehydrogenase enzyme present in the liver varies with individuals, depending on the genes they have inherited and on how recently they have eaten. Fasting for as little as a day forces the body to degrade its proteins, including the alcohol-processing enzymes, and this can slow the rate of alcohol metabolism by half. Drinking after not eating all day thus causes the drinker to feel the effects more promptly for two reasons: rapid absorption and slowed breakdown. By maintaining higher blood alcohol concentrations for longer times, alcohol can anesthetize the brain more completely (as described later in this highlight).

The alcohol dehydrogenase enzyme breaks down alcohol by removing hydrogens in two steps. (Figure H7-2 provides a simplified diagram of alcohol metabolism; Appendix C provides the chemical details.) In the first step, alcohol dehydrogenase oxidizes alcohol to **acetaldehyde.** High concentrations of acetaldehyde in the brain and other tissues are responsible for many of the damaging effects of **alcohol abuse.**

In the second step, a related enzyme, acetaldehyde dehydrogenase, converts acetaldehyde to acetate, which is then converted to acetyl CoA—the "crossroads" compound introduced in Chapter 7 that can enter the TCA cycle to generate energy. These

FIGURE H7-2 Alcohol Metabolism

The conversion of alcohol to acetyl CoA requires the B vitamin niacin in its role as the coenzyme NAD. When the enzymes oxidize alcohol, they remove H atoms and attach them to NAD. Thus NAD is used up, and NADH accumulates. (Note: More accurately, NAD+ is converted to NADH + H+.)

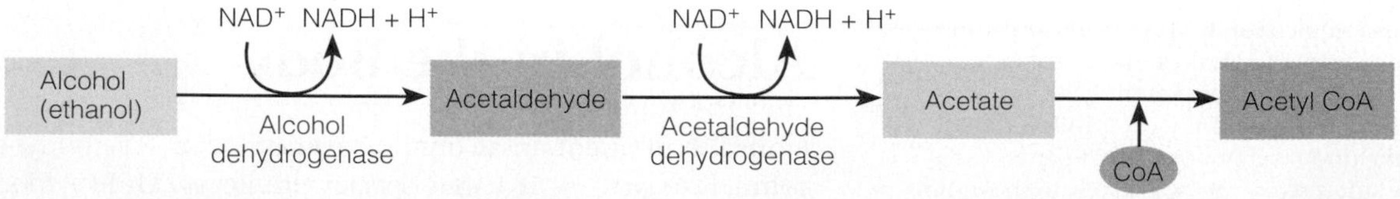
NAD+ NADH + H+
Alcohol (ethanol)
Alcohol dehydrogenase
Acetaldehyde
NAD+ NADH + H+
Acetaldehyde dehydrogenase
Acetate
CoA
Acetyl CoA

FIGURE H7-3 Alternate Route for Acetyl CoA: To Fat

Acetyl CoA molecules are blocked from getting into the TCA cycle by the high level of NADH. Instead of being used for energy, the acetyl CoA molecules become building blocks for fatty acids.

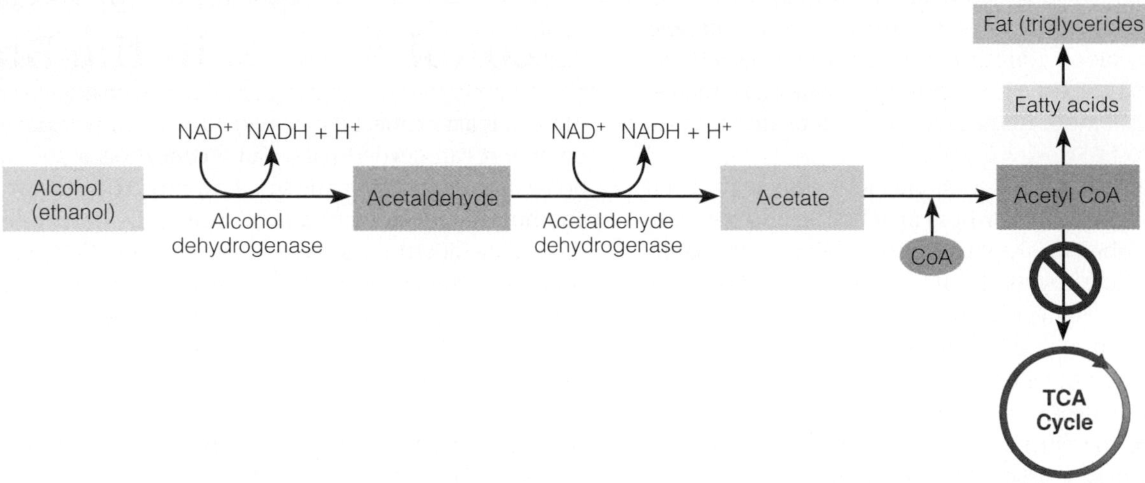

Fat (triglycerides)
Fatty acids
NAD^+ $NADH + H^+$
NAD^+ $NADH + H^+$
Alcohol (ethanol)
Alcohol dehydrogenase
Acetaldehyde
Acetaldehyde dehydrogenase
Acetate
CoA
Acetyl CoA
TCA Cycle

reactions produce hydrogen ions (H^+). The B vitamin niacin, in its role as the coenzyme **NAD** (nicotinamide adenine dinucleotide), helpfully picks up these hydrogen ions (becoming NADH). Thus, whenever the body breaks down alcohol, NAD diminishes and NADH accumulates. (Chapter 10 presents information on NAD and the other coenzyme roles of the B vitamins.)

Alcohol Disrupts the Liver

During alcohol metabolism, the multitude of other metabolic processes for which NAD is required, including glycolysis, the TCA cycle, and the electron transport chain, falter. Its presence is sorely missed in these energy pathways because it is the chief carrier of the hydrogens that travel with their electrons along the electron transport chain. Without adequate NAD, these energy pathways cannot function. Traffic either backs up, or an alternate route is taken. Such changes in the normal flow of energy pathways have striking physical consequences.

For one, the accumulation of hydrogen ions during alcohol metabolism shifts the body's acid-base balance toward acid. For another, the accumulation of NADH slows the TCA cycle, so pyruvate and acetyl CoA build up. Excess acetyl CoA then takes the route to fatty acid synthesis (as Figure H7-3 illustrates), and fat clogs the liver.

As you might expect, a liver overburdened with fat cannot function properly. Liver cells become less efficient at performing a number of tasks. Much of this inefficiency impairs a person's nutritional health in ways that cannot be corrected by diet alone. For example, the liver has difficulty activating vitamin D, as well as producing and releasing bile. To overcome such problems, a person needs to stop drinking alcohol.

The synthesis of fatty acids accelerates with exposure to alcohol. Fat accumulation can be seen in the liver after a single night of heavy drinking. **Fatty liver,** the first stage of liver deterioration seen in heavy drinkers, interferes with the distribution of nutrients and oxygen to the liver cells. Fatty liver is reversible with abstinence from alcohol. If fatty liver lasts long enough, however, the liver cells will die and form fibrous scar tissue. This second stage of liver deterioration is called **fibrosis.** Some liver cells can regenerate with good nutrition and abstinence from alcohol, but in the most advanced stage, **cirrhosis,** damage is the least reversible.

The fatty liver has difficulty generating glucose from protein. The lack of glucose together with the overabundance of acetyl CoA sets the stage for ketosis. The body uses the acetyl CoA to make ketone bodies; their acidity pushes the acid-base balance further toward acid and suppresses nervous system activity.

Excess NADH also promotes the making of lactic acid from pyruvate. The conversion of pyruvate to lactic acid uses the hydrogens from NADH and restores some NAD, but a lactic acid buildup has serious consequences of its own—it adds still further to the body's acid burden and interferes with the excretion of another acid, uric acid, causing inflammation of the joints.

Alcohol alters both amino acid and protein metabolism. Synthesis of proteins important in the immune system slows down, weakening the body's defenses against infection. Protein deficiency can develop, both from a diminished synthesis of protein and from a poor diet. Normally, the cells would at least use the amino acids from the protein foods a person eats, but the drinker's liver deaminates the amino acids and uses the carbon fragments primarily to make fat or ketones. Eating well does not protect the drinker from protein depletion; a person has to stop drinking alcohol.

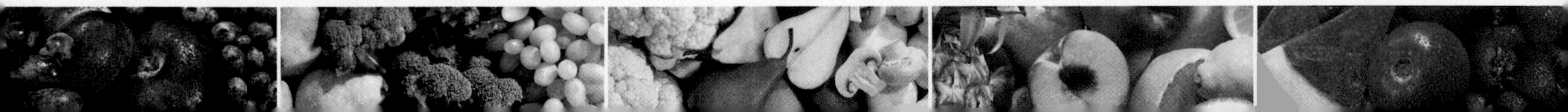

The liver's priority treatment of alcohol affects its handling of drugs as well as nutrients. In addition to the dehydrogenase enzyme already described, the liver possesses an enzyme system that metabolizes *both* alcohol and several other types of drugs. Called the **MEOS (microsomal ethanol-oxidizing system),** this system handles about one-fifth of the total alcohol a person consumes. At high blood concentrations or with repeated exposures, alcohol stimulates the synthesis of enzymes in the MEOS. The result is a more efficient metabolism of alcohol and tolerance to its effects.

As a person's blood alcohol rises, alcohol competes with—and wins out over—other drugs whose metabolism also relies on the MEOS. If a person drinks and uses another drug at the same time, the MEOS will dispose of the alcohol first and metabolize the drug more slowly. While the drug waits to be handled later, the dose may build up so that its effects are greatly amplified—sometimes to the point of being fatal.

In contrast, once a heavy drinker stops drinking and alcohol is no longer competing with other drugs, the enhanced MEOS metabolizes drugs much faster than before. As a result, determining the correct dosages of medications can be challenging.

This discussion has emphasized the major way that the blood is cleared of alcohol—metabolism by the liver—but there is another way. About 10 percent of the alcohol leaves the body through the breath and in the urine. This is the basis for the breath and urine tests for drunkenness. The amounts of alcohol in the breath and in the urine are in proportion to the amount still in the bloodstream and brain. In nearly all states, legal drunkenness is set at 0.10 percent or less, reflecting the relationship between alcohol use and traffic and other accidents.

Alcohol Arrives in the Brain

Alcohol is a **narcotic.** People used it for centuries as an anesthetic because it can deaden pain. But alcohol was a poor anesthetic because one could never be sure how much a person would need and how much would be a fatal dose. Consequently, new, more predictable anesthetics have replaced alcohol. Nonetheless, alcohol continues to be used today as a kind of social anesthetic to help people relax or to relieve anxiety. People think that alcohol is a stimulant because it seems to relieve inhibitions. Actually, though, it accomplishes this by sedating *inhibitory* nerves, which are more numerous than excitatory nerves. Ultimately, alcohol acts as a depressant and affects all the nerve cells. Figure H7-4 describes alcohol's effects on the brain.

It is lucky that the brain centers respond to a rising blood alcohol concentration in the order described in Figure H7-4 because a person usually passes out before managing to drink a lethal dose. It is possible, though, to drink so fast that the effects of alcohol continue to accelerate after the person has passed out. Occasionally, a person dies from drinking enough to stop the heart before passing out. Table H7-1 shows the

FIGURE H7-4 Alcohol's Effects on the Brain

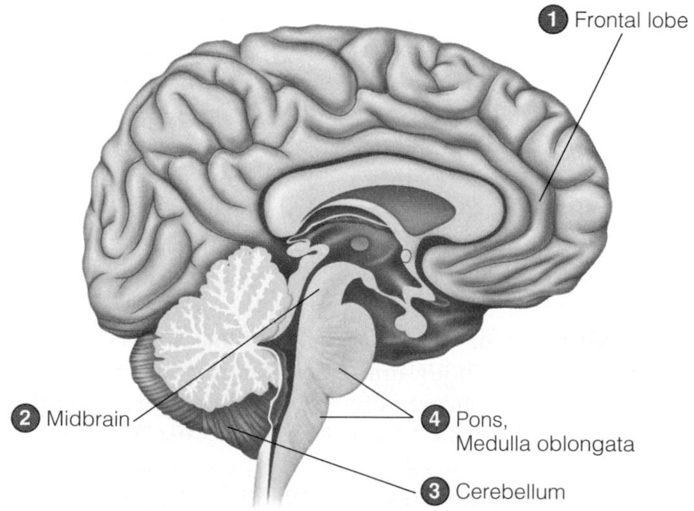

1 Frontal lobe
2 Midbrain
4 Pons, Medulla oblongata
3 Cerebellum

1. Judgment and reasoning centers are most sensitive to alcohol. When alcohol flows to the brain, it first sedates the frontal lobe, the center of all conscious activity. As the alcohol molecules diffuse into the cells of these lobes, they interfere with reasoning and judgment.

2. Speech and vision centers in the midbrain are affected next. If the drinker drinks faster than the rate at which the liver can oxidize the alcohol, blood alcohol concentrations rise: the speech and vision centers of the brain become sedated.

3. Voluntary muscular control is then affected. At still higher concentrations, the cells in the cerebellum responsible for coordination of voluntary muscles are affected, including those used in speech, eye-hand coordination, and limb movements. At this point people under the influence stagger or weave when they try to walk, or they may slur their speech.

4. Respiration and heart action are the last to be affected. Finally, the conscious brain is completely subdued, and the person passes out. Now the person can drink no more; this is fortunate because higher doses would anesthetize the deepest brain centers that control breathing and heartbeat, causing death.

TABLE H7-1 Alcohol Doses and Blood Levels

Number of Drinks[a]	Percentage of Blood Alcohol by Body Weight				
	100 lb	120 lb	150 lb	180 lb	200 lb
2	0.08	0.06	0.05	0.04	0.04
4	0.15	0.13	0.10	0.08	0.08
6	0.23	0.19	0.15	0.13	0.11
8	0.30	0.25	0.20	0.17	0.15
12	0.45	0.36	0.30	0.25	0.23
14	0.52	0.42	0.35	0.34	0.27

NOTE: In some states driving under the influence is proved when an adult's blood contains 0.08 percent alcohol, and in others, 0.10. Many states have adopted a "zero-tolerance" policy for drivers under age 21, using 0.02 percent as the limit.

[a]Taken within an hour or so; each drink equivalent to ½ ounce pure ethanol.

TABLE H7-2 Alcohol Blood Levels and Brain Responses

Blood Alcohol Concentration	Effect on Brain
0.05	Impaired judgment, relaxed inhibitions, altered mood, increased heart rate
0.10	Impaired coordination, delayed reaction time, exaggerated emotions, impaired peripheral vision, impaired ability to operate a vehicle
0.15	Slurred speech, blurred vision, staggered walk, seriously impaired coordination and judgment
0.20	Double vision, inability to walk
0.30	Uninhibited behavior, stupor, confusion, inability to comprehend
0.40 to 0.60	Unconsciousness, shock, coma, death (cardiac or respiratory failure)

NOTE: Blood alcohol concentration depends on a number of factors, including alcohol in the beverage, the rate of consumption, the person's gender, and body weight. For example, a 100-pound female can become legally drunk (0.10 concentration) by drinking three beers in an hour, whereas a 220-pound male consuming that amount at the same rate would have a 0.05 blood alcohol concentration.

blood alcohol levels that correspond to progressively greater intoxication, and Table H7-2 shows the brain responses that occur at these blood levels.

Like liver cells, brain cells die with excessive exposure to alcohol. Liver cells may be replaced, but not all brain cells can regenerate. Thus some heavy drinkers suffer permanent brain damage. Whether alcohol impairs cognition in moderate drinkers is unclear.[1]

People who drink alcoholic beverages may notice that they urinate more, but they may be unaware of the vicious cycle that results. Alcohol depresses production of **antidiuretic hormone (ADH),** a hormone produced by the pituitary gland that retains water. Loss of body water leads to thirst, and thirst leads to more drinking. Water will relieve dehydration, but the thirsty drinker may drink alcohol instead, which only worsens the problem. Such information provides another practical tip: drink water when thirsty and before each alcoholic drink. Drink an extra glass or two before going to bed. This strategy will help lessen the effects of a hangover.

Water loss is accompanied by the loss of important minerals. As Chapters 12 and 13 will explain, these minerals are vital to the body's fluid balance and to many chemical reactions in the cells, including muscle action. Detoxification treatment includes restoration of mineral balance as quickly as possible.

Alcohol and Malnutrition

For many moderate drinkers, alcohol does not suppress food intake and may actually stimulate appetite.[2] Moderate drinkers usually consume alcohol as *added* energy—on top of their normal food intake. In addition, alcohol in moderate doses is efficiently metabolized. Consequently, alcohol can contribute to body fat and weight gain.[3] Metabolically, alcohol is almost as efficient as fat in promoting obesity; each ounce of alcohol represents about a half-ounce of fat. Alcohol's contribution to body fat is most evident in the central obesity that commonly accompanies alcohol consumption, popularly—and appropriately—known as the "beer belly." Alcohol in heavy doses, though, is not efficiently metabolized, generating more heat than fat. Heavy drinkers usually consume alcohol as *substituted* energy—instead of their normal food intake. They tend to eat poorly and suffer malnutrition.

Alcohol is rich in energy (7 kcalories per gram), but as with pure sugar or fat, the kcalories are empty of nutrients. The more alcohol people drink, the less likely that they will eat enough food to obtain adequate nutrients. The more kcalories spent on alcohol, the fewer kcalories available to spend on nutritious foods. Table H7-3 shows the kcalorie amounts of typical alcoholic beverages.

Chronic alcohol abuse not only displaces nutrients from the diet, but also interferes with the body's metabolism of nutrients.[4] Most dramatic is alcohol's effect on the B vitamin folate. The liver loses its ability to retain folate, and the kidneys increase their excretion of it. Alcohol abuse creates a folate deficiency that devastates digestive system function. The intestine normally releases and retrieves folate continuously, but it becomes damaged by folate deficiency and alcohol toxicity, so it fails to retrieve its own folate and misses any that may trickle in from food as well. Alcohol also interferes with the action of folate in converting homocysteine to methionine. The result is an excess of homocysteine, which has been linked to heart disease, and an inadequate supply of methionine, which slows the production of new cells, especially the rapidly dividing cells of the intestine and the blood. The combination of poor folate status and alcohol consumption has also been implicated in promoting colorectal cancer.

The inadequate food intake and impaired nutrient absorption that accompany chronic alcohol abuse frequently lead to

TABLE H7-3 kCalories in Alcoholic Beverages and Mixers

Beverage	Amount (oz)	Energy (kcal)
Beer		
Regular	12	150
Light	12	78–131
Nonalcoholic	12	32–82
Distilled liquor (gin, rum, vodka, whiskey)		
80 proof	1½	100
86 proof	1½	105
90 proof	1½	110
Liqueurs		
Coffee liqueur, 53 proof	1½	175
Coffee and cream liqueur, 34 proof	1½	155
Crème de menthe, 72 proof	1½	185
Mixers		
Club soda	12	0
Cola	12	150
Cranberry juice cocktail	8	145
Diet drinks	12	2
Ginger ale or tonic	12	125
Grapefruit juice	8	95
Orange juice	8	110
Tomato or vegetable juice	8	45
Wine		
Dessert	3½	110–135
Nonalcoholic	8	14
Red or rosé	3½	75
White	3½	70
Wine cooler	12	170

a deficiency of another B vitamin—thiamin. In fact, the cluster of thiamin-deficiency symptoms commonly seen in chronic **alcoholism** has its own name—the **Wernicke-Korsakoff syndrome.** This syndrome is characterized by paralysis of the eye muscles, poor muscle coordination, impaired memory, and damaged nerves; it and other alcohol-related memory problems may respond to thiamin supplements.[5]

Acetaldehyde, an intermediate in alcohol metabolism (review Figure H7-2 on p. 242), interferes with nutrient use, too. For example, acetaldehyde dislodges vitamin B_6 from its protective binding protein so that it is destroyed, causing a vitamin B_6 deficiency and, thereby, lowered production of red blood cells.

Malnutrition occurs not only because of lack of intake and altered metabolism, but because of direct toxic effects as well. Alcohol causes stomach cells to oversecrete both gastric acid and histamine, an immune system agent that produces inflammation. Beer in particular stimulates gastric acid secretion, irritating the linings of the stomach and esophagus and making them vulnerable to ulcer formation.

Overall, nutrient deficiencies are virtually inevitable in alcohol abuse, not only because alcohol displaces food but also because alcohol directly interferes with the body's use of nutrients, making them ineffective even if they are present. Intestinal cells fail to absorb B vitamins, notably, thiamin, folate, and vitamin B_{12}. Liver cells lose efficiency in activating vitamin D. Cells in the retina of the eye, which normally process the alcohol form of vitamin A (retinol) to its aldehyde form needed in vision (retinal), find themselves processing ethanol to acetaldehyde instead. Likewise, the liver cannot convert the aldehyde form of vitamin A to its acid form (retinoic acid), which is needed to support the growth of its (and all) cells.[6]

Regardless of dietary intake, excessive drinking over a lifetime creates deficits of all the nutrients mentioned in this discussion and more. No diet can compensate for the damage caused by heavy alcohol consumption.

Alcohol's Short-Term Effects

The effects of abusing alcohol may be apparent immediately, or they may not become evident for years to come. Among the immediate consequences, all of the following involve alcohol use:[7]

- One-quarter of all emergency-room admissions.
- One-third of all suicides.
- One-half of all homicides.
- One-half of all domestic violence incidents.
- One-half of all traffic fatalities.
- One-half of all fire victim fatalities.

These statistics are sobering. The consequences of heavy drinking touch all elements of society—men and women, black and white, young and old, rich and poor. One group particularly hard hit by heavy drinking is college students—not because they are prone to alcoholism, but because they are living in an environment and during a developmental stage of life in which heavy drinking is considered acceptable.[8]

Heavy or binge drinking (defined as at least four drinks in a row for women and five drinks in a row for men) is widespread on college campuses and poses serious health and social consequences to drinkers and nondrinkers alike.[*9] In fact, binge drinking can kill: the respiratory center of the brain becomes anesthetized, and breathing stops. Acute alcohol intoxication can cause coronary artery spasms, leading to heart attacks.

Binge drinking is especially common among college students who live in a fraternity or sorority house, attend parties frequently, engage in other risky behaviors, and have a history of binge drinking in high school.[10] Compared with nondrinkers or moderate drinkers, people who frequently binge drink (at least three times within two weeks) are more likely to

HEALTHY PEOPLE 2010 Reduce the proportion of persons engaging in binge drinking of alcoholic beverages.

*This definition of binge drinking, without specification of time elapsed, is consistent with standard practice in alcohol research.

TABLE H7-4 Signs of Alcoholism

- Tolerance—the person needs higher and higher intakes of alcohol to achieve intoxication.
- Withdrawal—the person who stops drinking experiences anxiety, agitation, increased blood pressure, or seizures, or seeks alcohol to relieve these symptoms.
- Impaired control—the person intends to have 1 or 2 drinks, but has 9 or 10 instead, or the person tries to control or quit drinking, but fails.
- Disinterest—the person neglects important social, family, job, or school activities because of drinking.
- Time—the person spends a great deal of time obtaining and drinking alcohol or recovering from excessive drinking.
- Impaired ability—the person's intoxication or withdrawal symptoms interfere with work, school, or home.
- Problems—the person continues drinking despite physical hazards or medical, legal, psychological, family, employment, or school problems.

The presence of three or more of these conditions is required to make a diagnosis.

SOURCE: Adapted with permission from *Diagnostic and Statistical Manual of Mental Disorders,* 4th ed. Text Revision (Washington, D.C.: American Psychiatric Association, 2000).

engage in unprotected sex, have multiple sex partners, damage property, and assault others.[11] On average, *every day* alcohol is involved in the:[12]

- Death of 4 college students.
- Sexual assault of 192 college students.
- Injury of 1370 college students.
- Assault of 1644 college students.

Binge drinkers skew the statistics on college students' alcohol use. The median number of drinks consumed by college students is 1.5 per week, but for binge drinkers, it is 14.5. Nationally, only 20 percent of all students are frequent binge drinkers; yet they account for two-thirds of all the alcohol students report consuming and most of the alcohol-related problems.[13]

Binge drinking is not limited to college campuses, of course, but that environment seems most accepting of such behavior despite its problems. Social acceptance may make it difficult for binge drinkers to recognize themselves as problem drinkers. For this reason, interventions must focus both on educating individuals and on changing the campus social environment.[14] The damage alcohol causes only becomes worse if the pattern is not broken. Alcohol abuse sets in much more quickly in young people than in adults. Those who start drinking at an early age more often suffer from alcoholism than people who start later on. Table H7-4 lists the key signs of alcoholism.

Alcohol's Long-Term Effects

The most devastating long-term effect of alcohol is the damage done to a child whose mother abused alcohol during pregnancy. The effects of alcohol on the unborn, and the message that pregnant women should not drink alcohol, are presented in Highlight 14.

For nonpregnant adults, a drink or two sets in motion many destructive processes in the body, but the next day's abstinence reverses them. As long as the doses are moderate, the time between them is ample, and nutrition is adequate, recovery is probably complete.

If the doses of alcohol are heavy and the time between them short, complete recovery cannot take place. Repeated onslaughts of alcohol gradually take a toll on all parts of the body (see Table H7-5). Compared with nondrinkers and moderate drinkers, heavy drinkers—especially those under age 35—have significantly greater risks of dying from all causes.[15]

Personal Strategies

One obvious option available to people attending social gatherings is to enjoy the conversation, eat the food, and drink nonalcoholic beverages. Several nonalcoholic beverages are available that mimic the look and taste of their alcoholic counterparts. For those who enjoy champagne or beer, sparkling ciders and beers without alcohol are available. Instead of drinking a cocktail, a person can sip tomato juice with a slice of lime and a stalk of celery or just a plain cola beverage. Any of these drinks can ease conversation.

The person who chooses to drink alcohol should sip each drink slowly with food. The alcohol should arrive at the liver cells slowly enough that the enzymes can handle the load. It is best to space drinks, too, allowing about an hour or so to metabolize each drink.

If you want to help sober up a friend who has had too much to drink, don't bother walking arm in arm around the block. Walking muscles have to work harder, but muscle cells can't metabolize alcohol; only liver cells can. Remember that each person has a limited amount of the alcohol dehydrogenase enzyme that clears the blood at a steady rate. Time alone will do the job.

Nor will it help to give your friend a cup of coffee. Caffeine is a stimulant, but it won't speed up alcohol metabolism. The police say ruefully, "If you give a drunk a cup of coffee, you'll just have a wide-awake drunk on your hands." Table H7-6 presents other alcohol myths.

TABLE H7-5 Health Effects of Heavy Alcohol Consumption

Health Problem	Effects of Alcohol
Arthritis	Increases the risk of inflamed joints.
Cancer	Increases the risk of cancer of the liver, pancreas, rectum, and breast; increases the risk of cancer of the mouth, pharynx, larynx, and esophagus, where alcohol interacts synergistically with tobacco.
Fetal alcohol syndrome	Causes physical and behavioral abnormalities in the fetus (see Highlight 14).
Heart disease	In heavy drinkers, raises blood pressure, blood lipids, and the risk of stroke and heart disease; when compared with those who abstain, heart disease risk is generally lower in light-to-moderate drinkers (see Chapter 27).
Hyperglycemia	Raises blood glucose.
Hypoglycemia	Lowers blood glucose, especially in people with diabetes.
Infertility	Increases the risks of menstrual disorders and spontaneous abortions (in women); suppresses luteinizing hormone (in women) and testosterone (in men).
Kidney disease	Enlarges the kidneys, alters hormone functions, and increases the risk of kidney failure.
Liver disease	Causes fatty liver, alcoholic hepatitis, and cirrhosis.
Malnutrition	Increases the risk of protein-energy malnutrition; low intakes of protein, calcium, iron, vitamin A, vitamin C, thiamin, vitamin B_6, and riboflavin; and impaired absorption of calcium, phosphorus, vitamin D, and zinc.
Nervous disorders	Causes neuropathy and dementia; impairs balance and memory.
Obesity	Increases energy intake, but is not a primary cause of obesity.
Psychological disturbances	Causes depression, anxiety, and insomnia.

NOTE: This list is by no means all-inclusive. Alcohol has direct toxic effects on all body systems.

TABLE H7-6 Myths and Truths concerning Alcohol

Myth:	Hard liquors such as rum, vodka, and tequila are more harmful than wine and beer.
Truth:	The damage caused by alcohol depends largely on the amount consumed. Compared with hard liquor, beer and wine have relatively low percentages of alcohol, but they are often consumed in larger quantities.
Myth:	Consuming alcohol with raw seafood diminishes the likelihood of getting hepatitis.
Truth:	People have eaten contaminated oysters while drinking alcoholic beverages and not gotten as sick as those who were not drinking. But do not be misled: hepatitis is too serious an illness for anyone to depend on alcohol for protection.
Myth:	Alcohol stimulates the appetite.
Truth:	For some people, alcohol may stimulate appetite, but it seems to have the opposite effect in heavy drinkers. Heavy drinkers tend to eat poorly and suffer malnutrition.
Myth:	Drinking alcohol is healthy.
Truth:	Moderate alcohol consumption is associated with a lower risk for heart disease (see Chapter 27 for more details). Higher intakes, however, raise the risks for high blood pressure, stroke, heart disease, some cancers, accidents, violence, suicide, birth defects, and deaths in general. Furthermore, excessive alcohol consumption damages the liver, pancreas, brain, and heart. No authority recommends that nondrinkers begin drinking alcoholic beverages to obtain health benefits.
Myth:	Wine increases the body's absorption of minerals.
Truth:	Wine may increase the body's absorption of potassium, calcium, phosphorus, magnesium, and zinc, but the alcohol in wine also promotes the body's excretion of these minerals, so no benefit is gained.
Myth:	Alcohol is legal and, therefore, not a drug.
Truth:	Alcohol is legal for adults 21 years old and older, but it is also a drug—a substance that alters one or more of the body's functions.
Myth:	A shot of alcohol warms you up.
Truth:	Alcohol diverts blood flow to the skin making you feel warmer, but it actually cools the body.
Myth:	Wine and beer are mild; they do not lead to alcoholism.
Truth:	Alcoholism is not related to the kind of beverage, but rather to the quantity and frequency of consumption.
Myth:	Mixing different types of drinks gives you a hangover.
Truth:	Too much alcohol in any form produces a hangover.
Myth:	Alcohol is a stimulant.
Truth:	People think alcohol is a stimulant because it seems to relieve inhibitions, but it does so by depressing the activity of the brain. Alcohol is medically defined as a depressant drug.
Myth:	Beer is a great source of carbohydrate, vitamins, minerals, and fluids.
Truth:	Beer does provide some carbohydrate, but most of its kcalories come from alcohol. The few vitamins and minerals in beer cannot compete with rich food sources. And the diuretic effect of alcohol causes the body to lose more fluid in urine than is provided by the beer.

People who have passed out from drinking need 24 hours to sober up completely. Let them sleep, but watch over them. Encourage them to lie on their sides, instead of their backs. That way, if they vomit, they won't choke.

Don't drive too soon after drinking. The lack of glucose for the brain's function and the length of time needed to clear the blood of alcohol make alcohol's adverse effects linger long after its blood concentration has fallen. Driving coordination is still impaired the morning *after* a night of drinking, even if the drinking was moderate. Responsible aircraft pilots know that they must allow 24 hours for their bodies to clear alcohol completely, and they refuse to fly any sooner. The Federal Aviation Administration and major airlines enforce this rule.

Reduce deaths and injuries caused by alcohol- and drug-related motor vehicle crashes. HEALTHY PEOPLE 2010

Look again at the drawing of the brain in Figure H7-4 and note that when someone drinks, judgment fails first. Judgment might tell a person to limit alcohol consumption to two drinks at a party, but if the first drink takes judgment away, many more drinks may follow. The failure to stop drinking as planned, on repeated occasions, is a danger sign warning that the person should not drink at all. The accompanying Nutrition on the Net provides websites for organizations that offer information about alcohol and alcohol abuse.

Ethanol interferes with a multitude of chemical and hormonal reactions in the body—many more than have been enumerated here. With heavy alcohol consumption, the potential for harm is great. The best way to escape the harmful effects of alcohol is, of course, to refuse alcohol altogether. If you do drink alcoholic beverages, do so with care, and in moderation.

NUTRITION ON THE NET

Access these websites for further study of topics covered in this highlight.

- Find updates and quick links to these and other nutrition-related sites at our website: **www.wadsworth.com/nutrition**
- Search for "alcohol" at the U.S. Government health site: **www.healthfinder.gov**
- Gather information on alcohol and drug abuse from the National Clearinghouse for Alcohol and Drug Information (NCADI): **www.health.org**
- Learn more about alcoholism and drug dependence from the National Council on Alcoholism and Drug Dependence (NCADD): **www.ncadd.org**
- Find help for a family alcohol problem from Alateen and Al-Anon Family support groups: **www.al-anon.alateen.org**
- Find help for an alcohol or drug problem from Alcoholics Anonymous (AA) or Narcotics Anonymous: **www.aa.org** or **www.wsoinc.com**
- Search for "party" to find tips for hosting a safe party from Mothers Against Drunk Driving (MADD): **www.madd.org**

REFERENCES

1. D. Krahn and coauthors, Alcohol use and cognition at mid-life: The importance of adjusting for baseline cognitive ability and educational attainment, *Alcoholism: Clinical and Experimental Research* 27 (2003): 1162–1166.
2. M. S. Westerterp-Plantenga and C. R. Verwegen, The appetizing effect of an aperitif in overweight and normal-weight humans, *American Journal of Clinical Nutrition* 69 (1999): 205–212.
3. S. G. Wannamethee and A. G. Shaper, Alcohol, body weight, and weight gain in middle-aged men, *American Journal of Clinical Nutrition* 77 (2003): 1312–1317.
4. C. S. Lieber, Alcohol: Its metabolism and interaction with nutrients, *Annual Review of Nutrition* 20 (2000): 395–430.
5. M. L. Ambrose, S. C. Bowden, and G. Whelan, Thiamin treatment and working memory function of alcohol-dependent people: Preliminary findings, *Alcoholism: Clinical and Experimental Research* 25 (2001): 112–116.
6. X.-D. Wang, Chronic alcohol intake interferes with retinoid metabolism and signaling, *Nutrition Reviews* 57 (1999): 51–59.
7. Position paper on drug policy: Physician Leadership on National Drug Policy (PLNDP), Brown University Center for Alcohol and Addiction Studies, 2000.
8. A. M. Brower, Are college students alcoholics? *Journal of American College Health* 50 (2002): 253–255.
9. H. Wechsler and coauthors, Trends in college binge drinking during a period of increased prevention efforts—Findings from Harvard School of Public Health College Alcohol Study Surveys: 1993–2001, *Journal of American College Health* 50 (2002): 203–217.
10. P. W. Meilman, J. S. Leichliter, and C. A. Presley, Greeks and athletes: Who drinks more? *Journal of American College Health* 47 (1999): 187–190; B. E. Borsari and K. B. Carey, Understanding fraternity drinking: Five recurring themes in the literature, 1980–1998, *Journal of American College Health* 48 (1999): 30–37.
11. Wechsler and coauthors, 2002.
12. R. W. Hingson and coauthors, Magnitude of alcohol-related mortality and morbidity among U.S. college students ages 18–24, *Journal of Studies on Alcohol* 63 (2002): 136–144; National Institute of Alcohol Abuse and Alcoholism, *A Call to Action: Changing the Culture of Drinking at U.S. Colleges, 2002,* available from **www.collegedrinkingprevention.gov**.
13. H. Wechsler and coauthors, College alcohol use: A full or empty glass? *Journal of American College Health* 47 (1999): 247–252.
14. A. Ziemelis, R. B. Bucknam, and A. M. Elfessi, Prevention efforts underlying decreases in binge drinking at institutions of higher learning, *Journal of American College Health* 50 (2002): 238–252.
15. I. R. White, D. R. Altmann, and K. Nanchahal, Alcohol consumption and mortality: Modeling risks for men and women at different ages, *British Medical Journal* 325 (2002): 191–197.

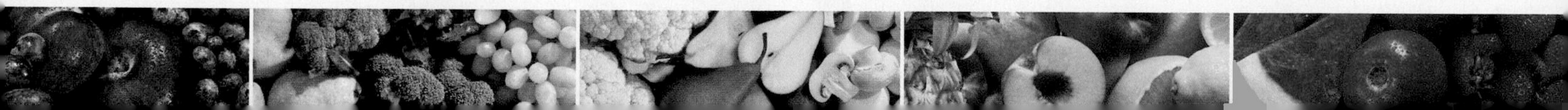

Chapter 8

Energy Balance and Body Composition

Chapter Outline

Available Online

http://nutrition.wadsworth.com/uncn7

Nutrition Animation: *Energy Balance and Body Composition*

Student Practice Test

Glossary Terms

Nutrition on the Net

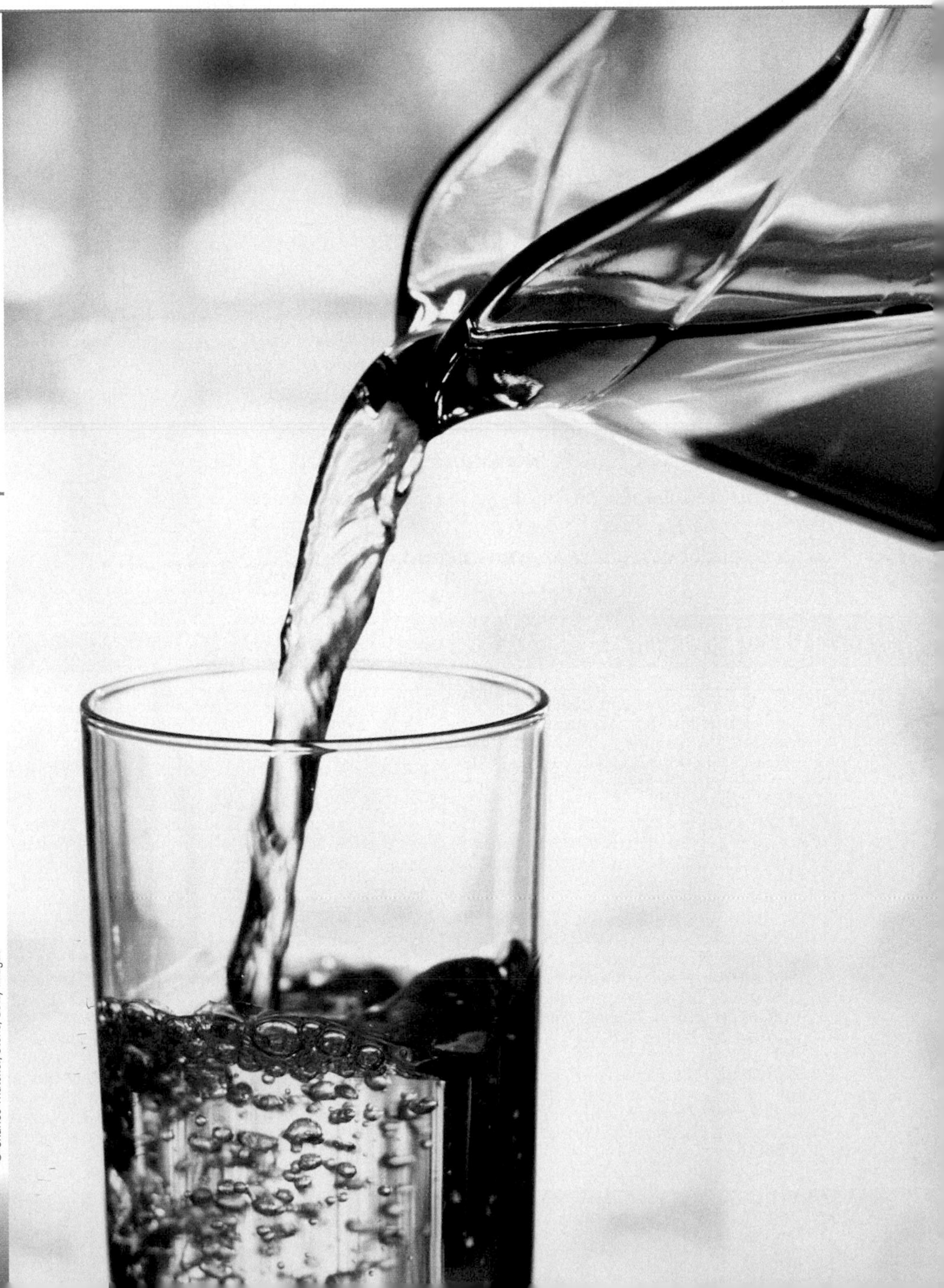

© Charles Thatcher/Stone/Getty Images

Nutrition in Your Life

It's a simple mathematical equation: energy in + energy out = energy balance. The reality, of course, is much more complex. One day you may devour a dozen doughnuts at midnight and sleep through your morning workout—tipping the scales toward weight gain. Another day you may snack on veggies and train for this weekend's 10K race—shifting the balance toward weight loss. Your body weight—especially as it relates to your body fat—and your level of fitness have consequences for your health. So, how are you doing? Are you ready to see how your "energy in" and "energy out" balance and whether your body weight and fat measures are consistent with good health?

The body's remarkable machinery can cope with many extremes of diet. As Chapter 7 explained, both excess carbohydrate (glucose) and excess protein (amino acids) can contribute to body fat. To some extent, amino acids can be used to make glucose. To a very limited extent, even fat (the glycerol portion) can be used to make glucose. But a grossly unbalanced diet imposes hardships on the body. If energy intake is too low or if too little carbohydrate or protein is supplied, the body must degrade its own lean tissue to meet its glucose and protein needs. If energy intake is too high, the body stores fat.

Both excessive and deficient body fat result from unbalanced energy budgets. The simple picture is as follows. People who have consumed more food energy than they have spent bank the surplus as body fat. To reduce body fat, they need to expend more energy than they take in from food. In contrast, people who have consumed too little food energy to support their bodies' activities have relied on their bodies' fat stores and possibly some of their lean tissues as well. To gain

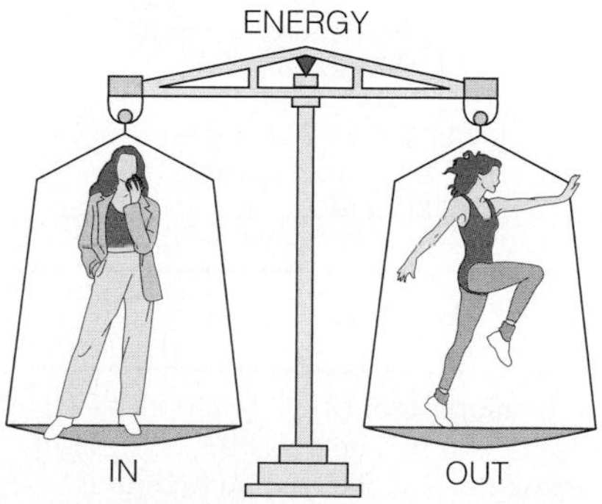
ENERGY
IN
OUT
When energy in balances with energy out, a person's body weight is stable.

weight, these people need to take in more food energy than they expend. As you will see, though, the details of the body's weight regulation are quite complex. This chapter describes energy balance and body composition and examines the health problems associated with having too much or too little body fat; the next chapter presents strategies toward resolving these problems.

Energy Balance

People expend energy continuously and eat periodically to refuel. Ideally, their energy intakes cover their energy expenditures without too much excess. Excess energy is stored as fat, and stored fat is used for energy between meals. The amount of body fat a person deposits in, or withdraws from, "storage" on any given day depends on the energy balance for that day—the amount consumed (energy in) versus the amount expended (energy out). When a person is maintaining weight, energy in equals energy out. When the balance shifts, weight changes. For each 3500 kcalories■ eaten in excess, a pound of body fat is stored; similarly, a pound of fat is lost for each 3500 kcalories expended beyond those consumed. The fat stores of even a healthy-weight adult represent an ample reserve of energy—50,000 to 200,000 kcalories.

■ 1 lb body fat = 3500 kcal.
Body fat, or adipose tissue, is composed of a mixture of mostly fat, some protein, and water. A pound of body fat (454 g) is approximately 87% fat, or (454 × 0.87) 395 g, and 395 g × 9 kcal/g = 3555 kcal.

Quick changes in body weight are not simple changes in fat stores. Weight gained or lost rapidly includes some fat, large amounts of fluid, and some lean tissues such as muscles and bone minerals. (Because water constitutes about 60 percent of an adult's body weight, retention or loss of water influences body weight significantly.) Even over the long term, the composition of weight gained or lost is normally about 75 percent fat and 25 percent lean. During starvation, losses of fat and lean are about equal. (Recall from Chapter 7 that without adequate carbohydrate, protein-rich lean tissues break down to provide glucose.) Invariably, though, *fat* gains and losses are gradual. The next two sections examine the two sides of the energy-balance equation: energy in and energy out.

FIGURE 8-1 Bomb Calorimeter

When food is burned, the chemical bonds between the carbons and hydrogens are broken, and energy is released in the form of heat. The amount of heat generated provides a direct measure of the amount of energy stored in the food's chemical bonds.

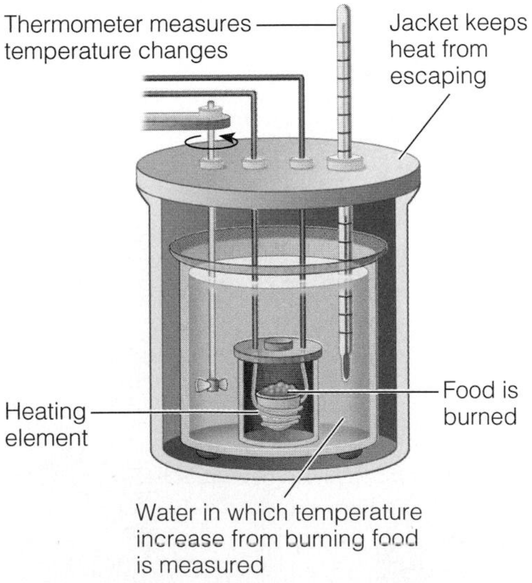
Thermometer measures temperature changes
Jacket keeps heat from escaping
Heating element
Food is burned
Water in which temperature increase from burning food is measured

IN SUMMARY When the energy consumed equals the energy expended, a person is in energy balance and body weight is stable. If more energy is taken in than is expended, a person gains weight. If more energy is spent than is taken in, a person loses weight.

Energy In: The kCalories Foods Provide

Foods and beverages provide the "energy in" part of the energy-balance equation. How much energy a person receives depends on the composition of the foods and beverages and on the amount the person eats and drinks.

Food Composition

To find out how many kcalories a food provides, a scientist can burn the food in a **bomb calorimeter** (see Figure 8-1). When the food burns, the chemical bonds between the carbon and hydrogen atoms break, releasing energy in the form of heat. The amount of heat given off provides a *direct* measure of the food's energy value (remember that kcalories are units of heat energy). In addition to releasing heat, these reactions generate carbon dioxide and water—just as the body's cells do when they metabolize the energy-yielding nutrients. When the food burns and

bomb calorimeter (KAL-oh-RIM-eh-ter): an instrument that measures the heat energy released when foods are burned, thus providing an estimate of the potential energy of the foods.
- **calor** = heat
- **metron** = measure

the chemical bonds break, the carbons (C) and hydrogens (H) combine with oxygen (O) to form carbon dioxide (CO_2) and water (H_2O). The amount of oxygen consumed gives an *indirect* measure■ of the amount of energy released.

A bomb calorimeter measures the available energy in foods, but overstates the amount of energy that the human body■ derives from foods. The body is less efficient than a calorimeter and cannot metabolize all of a food's energy-yielding nutrients all the way to carbon dioxide and water. Researchers can correct for this discrepancy mathematically to create useful tables of the energy values of foods (such as Appendix H). These values provide reasonable estimates, but do not reflect the *precise* amount of energy a person will derive from the foods consumed.

The energy values of foods can also be computed from the amounts of carbohydrate, fat, and protein (and alcohol, if present) in the foods.* For example, a food■ containing 12 grams of carbohydrate, 5 grams of fat, and 8 grams of protein would provide 48 carbohydrate kcalories, 45 fat kcalories, and 32 protein kcalories, for a total of 125 kcalories. (To review how to calculate the energy available from foods, turn to p. 9.)

■ Food energy values can be determined by:
- **Direct calorimetry**, which measures the amount of heat released.
- **Indirect calorimetry**, which measures the amount of oxygen consumed.

■ The number of kcalories that the body derives from a food, as contrasted with the number of kcalories determined by calorimetry, is the **physiological fuel value.**

■ Reminder:
- 1 g carbohydrate = 4 kcal.
- 1 g fat = 9 kcal.
- 1 g protein = 4 kcal.
- 1 g alcohol = 7 kcal.

As Chapter 1 mentioned, many scientists measure food energy in kilojoules instead. Conversion factors for these and other measures are in the Aids to Calculation section on the last two pages of the book.

Food Intake

To achieve energy balance, the body must meet its needs without taking in too much or too little energy. Somehow the body decides how much and how often to eat—when to start eating and when to stop. As you will see, many signals initiate or delay eating.

Hunger People eat for a variety of reasons, most obviously (although not necessarily most commonly) because they are hungry. Most people recognize **hunger** as an irritating feeling that prompts thoughts of food and motivates them to start eating. In the body, hunger is the physiological response to a need for food triggered by chemical messengers originating and acting in the brain, primarily in the **hypothalamus.**[1] Hunger can be influenced by the presence or absence of nutrients in the bloodstream, the size and composition of the preceding meal, customary eating patterns, climate (heat reduces food intake; cold increases it), exercise, hormones, and physical and mental illnesses.

The stomach is ideally designed to handle periodic batches of food, and people typically eat meals at roughly four-hour intervals. Four hours after a meal, most, if not all, of the food has left the stomach. Most people do not feel like eating again until the stomach is either empty or almost so. Even then, a person may not feel hungry for quite a while.

Appetite Hunger is only one of the signals determining whether a person will eat. **Appetite** also initiates eating. A person may experience appetite without hunger, for example, when presented with a hot piece of apple pie after having eaten a large dinner. The sight and smell of the pie, not hunger, trigger appetite. In contrast, a person may feel hungry but have no appetite for food when faced with unfamiliar foods, a stressful situation, or illness; in such circumstances, eating becomes a chore.

Satiation During the course of a meal, as food enters the GI tract and hunger diminishes, **satiation** develops. Receptors in the stomach stretch, and the person begins to feel full. The response: satiation occurs and the person stops eating.

Satiety After a meal, the feeling of **satiety** continues to suppress hunger and allows a person to not eat again for a while. Whereas *satiation* tells us to "stop eating," *satiety* reminds us to "not start eating again." Figure 8-2 summarizes the relationships among hunger, satiation, and satiety. Of course, people can override these signals, especially when presented with stressful situations or favorite foods.

hunger: the painful sensation caused by a lack of food that initiates food-seeking behavior.

hypothalamus (high-po-THAL-ah-mus): a brain center that controls activities such as maintenance of water balance, regulation of body temperature, and control of appetite.

appetite: the integrated response to the sight, smell, thought, or taste of food that initiates or delays eating.

satiation (say-she-AY-shun): the feeling of satisfaction and fullness that occurs during a meal and halts eating. Satiation determines how much food is consumed during a meal.

satiety (sah-TIE-eh-tee): the feeling of satisfaction that occurs after a meal and inhibits eating until the next meal. Satiety determines how much time passes between meals.

*Some of the food energy values in the table of food composition in Appendix H were derived by bomb calorimetry, and many were calculated from their energy-yielding nutrient contents.

FIGURE 8-2 Hunger, Satiation, and Satiety

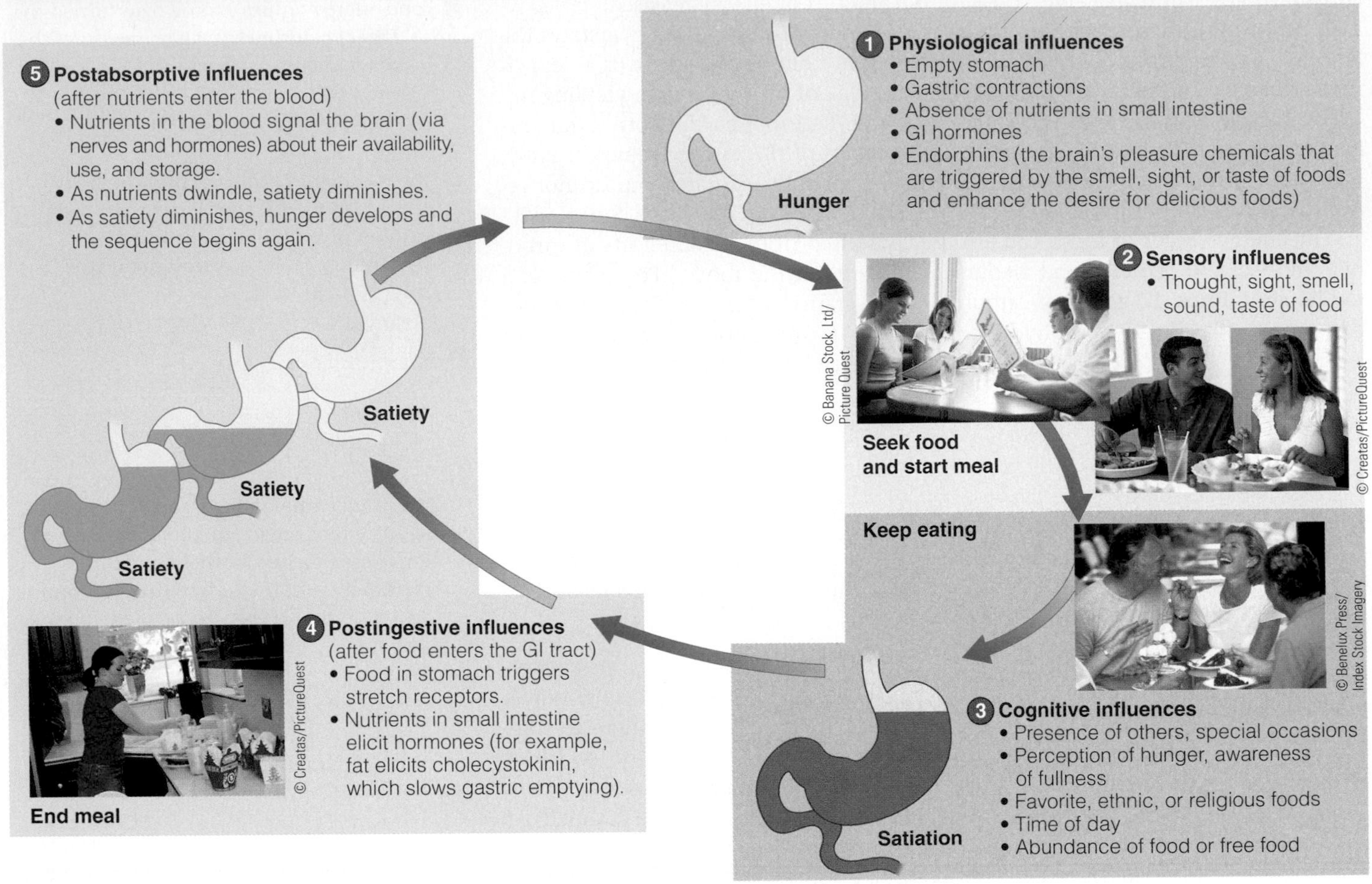

1 Physiological influences
• Empty stomach
• Gastric contractions
• Absence of nutrients in small intestine
• GI hormones
• Endorphins (the brain's pleasure chemicals that are triggered by the smell, sight, or taste of foods and enhance the desire for delicious foods)
Hunger
2 Sensory influences
• Thought, sight, smell, sound, taste of food
Seek food and start meal
© Banana Stock, Ltd/ Picture Quest
© Creatas/PictureQuest
Keep eating
© Benelux Press/ Index Stock Imagery
3 Cognitive influences
• Presence of others, special occasions
• Perception of hunger, awareness of fullness
• Favorite, ethnic, or religious foods
• Time of day
• Abundance of food or free food
Satiation
4 Postingestive influences
(after food enters the GI tract)
• Food in stomach triggers stretch receptors.
• Nutrients in small intestine elicit hormones (for example, fat elicits cholecystokinin, which slows gastric emptying).
© Creatas/PictureQuest
End meal
5 Postabsorptive influences
(after nutrients enter the blood)
• Nutrients in the blood signal the brain (via nerves and hormones) about their availability, use, and storage.
• As nutrients dwindle, satiety diminishes.
• As satiety diminishes, hunger develops and the sequence begins again.
Satiety
Satiety
Satiety

■ Eating in response to arousal is called **stress eating.**

■ Cognitive influences include perceptions, memories, intellect, and social interactions.

satiating: having the power to suppress hunger and inhibit eating.

Overriding Hunger and Satiety Not surprisingly, eating can be triggered by signals other than hunger, even when the body does not need food. Some people experience food cravings when they are bored or anxious. In fact, they may eat in response to any kind of stress,■ negative or positive. ("What do I do when I'm grieving? Eat. What do I do when I'm celebrating? Eat!") Some people respond to external cues such as the time of day ("It's time to eat") or the availability, sight, and taste of food ("I'd love a piece of chocolate even though I'm stuffed"). Being presented with large portion sizes, favorite foods, or an abundance or variety of foods also stimulates eating and increases energy intake.[2] These cognitive influences■ can easily lead to weight gain.

Eating can also be suppressed by signals other than satiety, even when a person is hungry. People with the eating disorder anorexia nervosa, for example, use tremendous discipline to ignore the pangs of hunger. Some people simply cannot eat during times of stress, negative or positive. ("I'm too sad to eat. I'm too excited to eat!") Why some people overeat in response to stress and others cannot eat at all remains a bit of a mystery. Factors that appear to be involved include how the person perceives the stress and whether usual eating behaviors are restrained. (Highlight 9 features anorexia nervosa and other eating disorders.)

Sustaining Satiation and Satiety The extent to which foods produce satiation and sustain satiety depends in part on the nutrient composition of a meal.[3] Of the three energy-yielding nutrients, protein is the most **satiating.** Foods rich in complex carbohydrates and fibers also effectively provide satiation by filling the stomach and delaying the absorption of nutrients. In contrast, fat has a weak effect on satiation; consequently, eating high-fat foods may lead to passive overconsumption. High-fat foods are flavorful, which stimulates the appetite and entices people to eat more. High-fat foods are also energy dense; consequently, they deliver more kcalories per bite. (Chapter 1 introduced the concept of energy density, and Chapter 9 describes how considering a food's energy density can help with weight management.) Although fat provides little satiation during a meal, it produces strong satiety signals once it enters the intestine. Fat in the intestine triggers the release of cholecystokinin—a hormone that signals satiety and inhibits food intake.[4]

Eating high-fat foods while trying to limit energy intake requires small portion sizes, which can leave a person feeling unsatisfied. By comparison, simple, whole foods such as potatoes, apples, oranges, whole-grain pastas, fish, and steak are highly satiating—and they provide a rich array of nutrients. Instead of feeling deprived eating small portions of high-fat foods, a person can feel satisfied eating large portions of high-protein and high-fiber foods. Portion size correlates directly with a food's satiety.[5] Figure 8-3 illustrates how fat influences portion size.

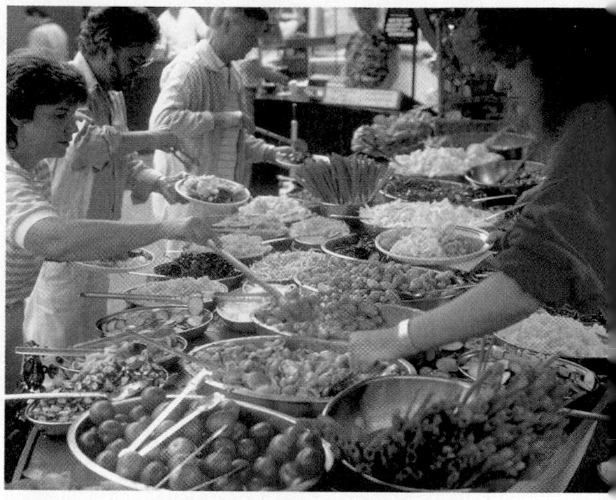

© Owen Franken/CORBIS

Regardless of hunger, people typically overeat when offered the abundance and variety of an "all you can eat" buffet.

Message Central—The Hypothalamus As you can see, eating is a complex behavior controlled by a variety of psychological, social, metabolic, and physiological factors. The hypothalamus appears to be the control center, integrating messages about energy intake, expenditure, and storage from other parts of the brain and from the mouth, GI tract, and liver. Some of these messages influence satiation, controlling the size of a meal; others influence satiety, determining the frequency of meals.

Dozens of chemicals in the brain participate in appetite control and energy balance.[6] By understanding the action of these brain chemicals, researchers may one day be able to control appetite. The greatest challenge now is in sorting out the many actions of these brain chemicals. For example, one of these chemicals, **neuropeptide Y,** causes carbohydrate cravings, initiates eating, decreases energy expenditure, and increases fat storage—all factors favoring a positive energy balance and weight gain.

neuropeptide Y: a chemical produced in the brain that stimulates appetite, diminishes energy expenditure, and increases fat storage.

FIGURE 8-3 How Fat Influences Portion Sizes

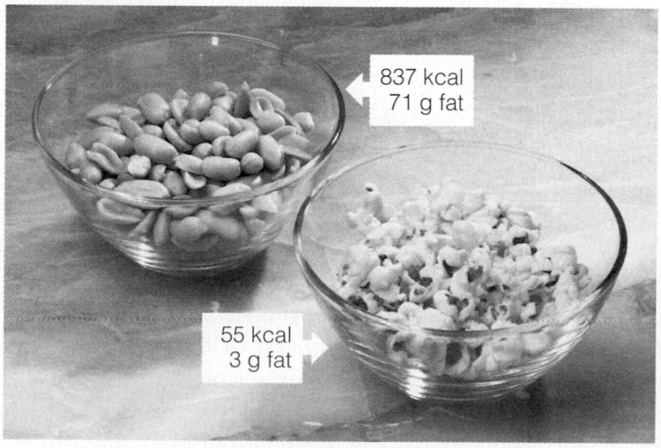
837 kcal
71 g fat
55 kcal
3 g fat

For the same size portion, peanuts deliver more than 15 times the kcalories and 20 times the fat of popcorn.

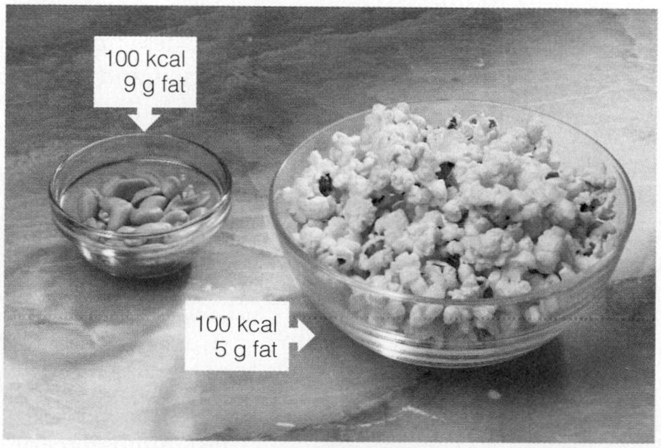
100 kcal
9 g fat
100 kcal
5 g fat

© Polarra Studios Inc. (both)

For the same number of kcalories, a person can have a few high-fat peanuts or almost 2 cups of high-fiber popcorn. (This comparison used oil-based popcorn; using air-popped popcorn would double the amount of popcorn in this example.)

IN SUMMARY A mixture of signals governs a person's eating behaviors. Hunger and appetite initiate eating, whereas satiation and satiety stop and delay eating. Each responds to messages from the nervous and hormonal systems. Superimposed on these are complex factors involving emotions, habits, and other aspects of human behavior.

Energy Out: The kCalories the Body Expends

Chapter 7 explained that heat is released whenever the body breaks down carbohydrate, fat, or protein for energy and again when that energy is used to do work. The work itself, as it is done, generates heat as well. The body's generation of heat is known as **thermogenesis,** and it can be measured to determine the amount of energy expended.■ The total energy a body expends reflects three main categories of thermogenesis:

- Energy expended for basal metabolism.
- Energy expended for physical activity.
- Energy expended for food consumption.

A fourth category is sometimes involved:

- Energy expended for adaptation.

■ Energy expenditure, like food energy, can be determined by:
- **Direct calorimetry**, which measures the amount of heat released.
- **Indirect calorimetry**, which measures the amount of oxygen consumed and carbon dioxide expelled.

FIGURE 8-4 Components of Energy Expenditure

The amount of energy spent in a day differs for each individual, but in general, basal metabolism is the largest component of energy expenditure (60 to 65 percent), and the thermic effect of food is the smallest (only 10 percent). The amount spent in voluntary physical activities has the greatest variability, depending on a person's activity patterns. For a sedentary person, physical activities may account for less than half as much energy as basal metabolism, whereas an extremely active person may expend as much on activity as for basal metabolism.

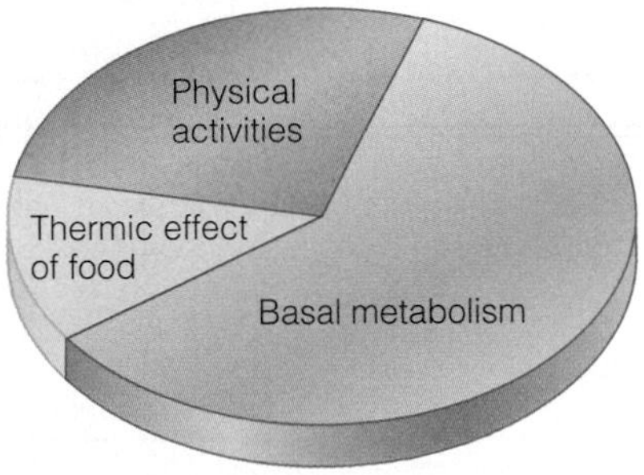
Physical activities
Thermic effect of food
Basal metabolism

Components of Energy Expenditure

People expend energy when they are physically active, of course, but they also expend energy when they are resting quietly. In fact, quiet metabolic activities account for the lion's share of most people's energy expenditures, as Figure 8-4 shows.

Basal Metabolism About two-thirds of the energy the average person expends in a day supports the body's **basal metabolism.** Metabolic activities maintain the body temperature, keep the lungs inhaling and exhaling air, the bone marrow making new red blood cells, the heart beating 100,000 times a day, and the kidneys filtering wastes—in short, they support all the basic processes of life.

The **basal metabolic rate (BMR)** is the rate at which the body expends energy for these maintenance activities.■ The rate may vary dramatically from person to person and may vary for the same individual with a change in circumstance or physical condition. The rate is slowest when a person is sleeping undisturbed, but it is usually measured in a room with a comfortable temperature when the person is awake, but lying still, after a restful sleep and an overnight (12- to 14-hour) fast. A similar measure of energy output—called the **resting metabolic rate (RMR)**—is slightly higher than the BMR because its criteria for recent food intake and physical activity are not as strict.

In general, the more a person weighs, the more *total* energy is expended on basal metabolism, but the amount of energy *per pound* of body weight may be lower. For example, an adult's BMR might be 1500 kcalories per day and an infant's only 500, but compared to body weight, the infant's BMR is more than twice as fast. Similarly, a normal-weight adult may have a metabolic rate one and a half times that of an obese adult when compared to body weight because lean tissue is metabolically more active than body fat.

Table 8-1 summarizes the factors that raise and lower the BMR. For the most part, the BMR is highest in people who are growing (children and pregnant women) and in those with considerable **lean body mass** (physically fit people and

■ Quick and easy estimates for basal energy needs:
- Men: Slightly >1 kcal/min (1.1 to 1.3 kcal/min) or 24 kcal/kg/day.
- Women: Slightly <1 kcal/min (0.8 to 1.0 kcal/min) or 23 kcal/kg/day.

For perspective, a burning candle or a 75-watt light bulb releases about 1 kcal/min.

thermogenesis: the generation of heat; used in physiology and nutrition studies as an index of how much energy the body is expending.

basal metabolism: the energy needed to maintain life when a body is at complete digestive, physical, and emotional rest.

males). One way to increase the BMR then is to participate in endurance and strength-training activities regularly to maximize lean body mass.[7] The BMR is also high in people with fever or under stress and in people with highly active thyroid glands. The BMR slows down with a loss of lean body mass and during fasting and malnutrition.

Physical Activity The second component of a person's energy output is physical activity: voluntary movement of the skeletal muscles and support systems. Physical activity is the most variable—and the most changeable—component of energy expenditure. Consequently, its influence on both weight gain and weight loss can be significant.

During physical activity, the muscles need extra energy to move, and the heart and lungs need extra energy to deliver nutrients and oxygen and dispose of wastes. The amount of energy needed for any activity, whether playing tennis or studying for an exam, depends on three factors: muscle mass, body weight, and activity. The larger the muscle mass required and the heavier the weight of the body part being moved, the more energy is spent. Table 8-2 (on p. 258) gives average energy expenditures for people of different body weights engaged in various activities and shows that a heavy person usually uses more energy per minute to perform a task than a light person does. The activity's duration, frequency, and intensity also influence energy expenditure: the longer, the more frequent, and the more intense the activity, the more kcalories spent.

Thermic Effect of Food When a person eats, the GI tract muscles speed up their rhythmic contractions, the cells that manufacture and secrete digestive juices begin their tasks, and some nutrients are absorbed by active transport. This acceleration

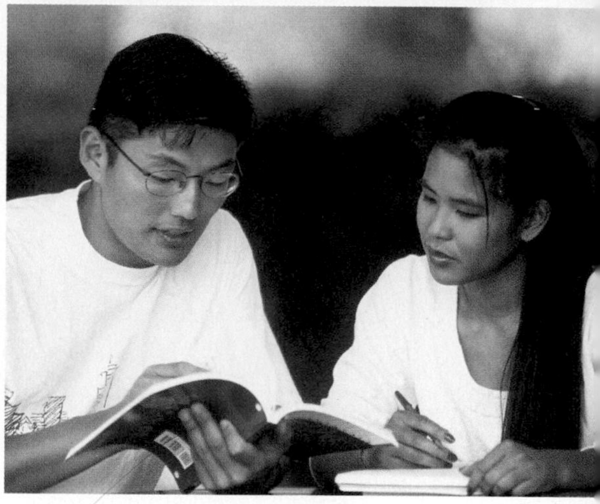

© Bob Torrez/Stone/Getty Images

It feels like work and it may make you tired, but studying requires only a kcalorie or two per minute.

Available Online

Examine the effect of too much or too little energy on body composition.

TABLE 8-1 Factors That Affect the BMR

Factor	Effect on BMR
Age	Lean body mass diminishes with age, slowing the BMR.[a]
Height	In tall, thin people, the BMR is higher.[b]
Growth	In children and pregnant women, the BMR is higher.
Body composition (gender)	The more lean tissue, the higher the BMR (which is why males usually have a higher BMR than females). The more fat tissue, the lower the BMR.
Fever	Fever raises the BMR.[c]
Stresses	Stresses (including many diseases and certain drugs) raise the BMR.
Environmental temperature	Both heat and cold raise the BMR.
Fasting/starvation	Fasting/starvation lowers the BMR.[d]
Malnutrition	Malnutrition lowers the BMR.
Hormones (gender)	The thyroid hormone thyroxin, for example, can speed up or slow down the BMR.[e] Premenstrual hormones slightly raise the BMR.
Smoking	Nicotine increases energy expenditure.
Caffeine	Caffeine increases energy expenditure.
Sleep	BMR is lowest when sleeping.

[a] The BMR begins to decrease in early adulthood (after growth and development cease) at a rate of about 2 percent/decade. A reduction in voluntary activity as well brings the total decline in energy expenditure to 5 percent/decade.
[b] If two people weigh the same, the taller, thinner person will have the faster metabolic rate, reflecting the greater skin surface, through which heat is lost by radiation, in proportion to the body's volume (see the margin drawing on p. 259).
[c] Fever raises the BMR by 7 percent for each degree Fahrenheit.
[d] Prolonged starvation reduces the total amount of metabolically active lean tissue in the body, although the decline occurs sooner and to a greater extent than body losses alone can explain. More likely, the neural and hormonal changes that accompany fasting are responsible for changes in the BMR.
[e] The thyroid gland releases hormones that travel to the cells and influence cellular metabolism. Thyroid hormone activity can speed up or slow down the rate of metabolism by as much as 50 percent.

basal metabolic rate (BMR): the rate of energy use for metabolism under specified conditions: after a 12-hour fast and restful sleep, without any physical activity or emotional excitement, and in a comfortable setting. It is usually expressed as kcalories per kilogram body weight per hour.

resting metabolic rate (RMR): similar to the BMR, a measure of the energy use of a person at rest in a comfortable setting, but with less stringent criteria for recent food intake and physical activity. Consequently, the RMR is slightly higher than the BMR.

lean body mass: the weight of the body minus the fat content.

TABLE 8-2 Energy Spent on Various Activities

The values listed in this table reflect both the energy spent in physical activity *and* the amount used for BMR.

Activity	kCal/lb/min[a]	kCalories per Minute at Different Body Weights				
		110 lb	125 lb	150 lb	175 lb	200 lb
Aerobic dance (vigorous)	.062	6.8	7.8	9.3	10.9	12.4
Basketball (vigorous, full court)	.097	10.7	12.1	14.6	17.0	19.4
Bicycling						
13 mph	.045	5.0	5.6	6.8	7.9	9.0
15 mph	.049	5.4	6.1	7.4	8.6	9.8
17 mph	.057	6.3	7.1	8.6	10.0	11.4
19 mph	.076	8.4	9.5	11.4	13.3	15.2
21 mph	.090	9.9	11.3	13.5	15.8	18.0
23 mph	.109	12.0	13.6	16.4	19.0	21.8
25 mph	.139	15.3	17.4	20.9	24.3	27.8
Canoeing, flat water, moderate pace	.045	5.0	5.6	6.8	7.9	9.0
Cross-country skiing						
8 mph	.104	11.4	13.0	15.6	18.2	20.8
Golf (carrying clubs)	.045	5.0	5.6	6.8	7.9	9.0
Handball	.078	8.6	9.8	11.7	13.7	15.6
Horseback riding (trot)	.052	5.7	6.5	7.8	9.1	10.4
Rowing (vigorous)	.097	10.7	12.1	14.6	17.0	19.4
Running						
5 mph	.061	6.7	7.6	9.2	10.7	12.2
6 mph	.074	8.1	9.2	11.1	13.0	14.8
7.5 mph	.094	10.3	11.8	14.1	16.4	18.8
9 mph	.103	11.3	12.9	15.5	18.0	20.6
10 mph	.114	12.5	14.3	17.1	20.0	22.9
11 mph	.131	14.4	16.4	19.7	22.9	26.2
Soccer (vigorous)	.097	10.7	12.1	14.6	17.0	19.4
Studying	.011	1.2	1.4	1.7	1.9	2.2
Swimming						
20 yd/min	.032	3.5	4.0	4.8	5.6	6.4
45 yd/min	.058	6.4	7.3	8.7	10.2	11.6
50 yd/min	.070	7.7	8.8	10.5	12.3	14.0
Table tennis (skilled)	.045	5.0	5.6	6.8	7.9	9.0
Tennis (beginner)	.032	3.5	4.0	4.8	5.6	6.4
Walking (brisk pace)						
3.5 mph	.035	3.9	4.4	5.2	6.1	7.0
4.5 mph	.048	5.3	6.0	7.2	8.4	9.6
Weight lifting						
light-to-moderate effort	.024	2.6	3.0	3.6	4.2	4.8
vigorous effort	.048	5.2	6.0	7.2	8.4	9.6
Wheelchair basketball	.084	9.2	10.5	12.6	14.7	16.8
Wheeling self in wheelchair	.030	3.3	3.8	4.5	5.3	6.0

[a]To calculate kcalories spent per minute of activity for your own body weight, multiply kcal/lb/min by your exact weight and then multiply that number by the number of minutes spent in the activity. For example, if you weigh 142 pounds, and you want to know how many kcalories you spent doing 30 minutes of vigorous aerobic dance: $0.062 \times 142 = 8.8$ kcalories per minute; 8.8×30 (minutes) $= 264$ total kcalories spent.

SOURCE: Reprinted with permission of Ross Laboratories.

of activity requires energy and produces heat; it is known as the **thermic effect of food (TEF).**

The thermic effect of food is proportional to the food energy taken in and is usually estimated at 10 percent of energy intake. Thus a person who ingests 2000 kcalories probably expends about 200 kcalories on the thermic effect of food. The proportions vary for different foods, however, and are also influenced by factors such as meal size and frequency. In general, the thermic effect of food is greater for high-protein foods than for high-fat foods■ and for a meal eaten all at once rather than spread out over a couple of hours. Some research suggests that the thermic effect of food is reduced in obese people and may contribute to their efficient storage of fat.[8] For most purposes, however, the thermic effect of food can be ignored when estimating energy expenditure because its contribution to total energy output is smaller than the probable errors involved in estimating overall energy intake and output.

Adaptive Thermogenesis Some additional energy is spent when a person must adapt to dramatically changed circumstances **(adaptive thermogenesis).** When the body has to adapt to physical conditioning, extreme cold, overfeeding, starvation, trauma, or other types of stress, it has extra work to do, building the tissues and producing the enzymes and hormones necessary to cope with the demand. In some circumstances, this energy makes a considerable difference in the total energy spent. Because this component of energy expenditure is so variable and specific to individuals, it is not included when calculating energy requirements.

Estimating Energy Requirements

In estimating energy requirements, the DRI Committee developed equations that consider how the following factors influence energy expenditure:■

- *Gender.* In general, women have a lower BMR than men, in large part because men typically have more lean body mass. In addition, menstrual hormones influence the BMR in women, raising it just prior to menstruation. Two sets of energy equations—one for men and one for women—were developed to accommodate the influence of gender on energy expenditure.
- *Growth.* The BMR is high in people who are growing. For this reason, pregnant women and children have their own sets of energy equations.
- *Age.* The BMR declines during adulthood as lean body mass diminishes.[9] This change in body composition occurs, in part, because some hormones that influence metabolism become more, or less, active with age. Physical activities tend to decline as well, bringing the average reduction in energy expenditure to about 5 percent per decade. The decline in the BMR that occurs when a person becomes less active reflects the loss of lean body mass and may be prevented with ongoing physical activity. Because age influences energy expenditure, it is also factored into the energy equations.
- *Physical activity.* Using individual values for various physical activities (as in Table 8-2) is time-consuming and impractical for estimating the energy needs of a population. Instead, various activities are clustered according to the typical intensity of a day's efforts. Energy equations include a physical activity factor for various levels of intensity for each gender.
- *Body composition and body size.* The BMR is high in people who are tall and so have a large surface area.■ Similarly, the more a person weighs, the more energy is expended on basal metabolism. For these reasons, the energy equations include a factor for both height and weight.

As just explained, energy needs vary between individuals depending on such factors as gender, growth, age, physical activity, and body composition. Even when two people are similarly matched, however, their energy needs will still differ because of genetic differences. Perhaps one day genetic research will reveal how to estimate

■ Thermic effect of foods:
- Carbohydrate: 5–10%.
- Fat: 0–5%.
- Protein: 20–30%.
- Alcohol: 20%.

The percentages are calculated by dividing the energy expended during digestion and absorption (above basal) by the energy content of the food.

■ Note that Table 8-1 (p. 257) listed these factors among those that influence BMR and consequently energy expenditure.

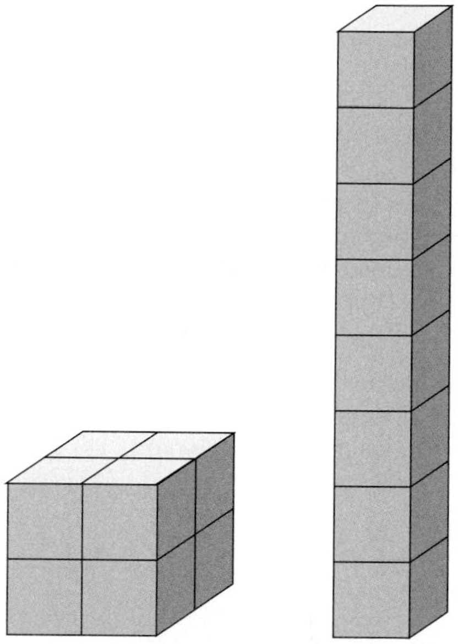

■ Each of these structures is made of 8 blocks. They weigh the same, but they are arranged differently. The short, wide structure has 24 sides and the tall, thin one has 34. Because the tall, thin structure has a greater surface area, it will lose more heat (expend more energy) than the short, wide one. Similarly, two people of different heights might weigh the same, but the taller, thin one will have a higher BMR (expending more energy) because of the greater skin surface.

thermic effect of food (TEF): an estimation of the energy required to process food (digest, absorb, transport, metabolize, and store ingested nutrients); also called the **specific dynamic effect (SDE)** of food or the **specific dynamic activity (SDA)** of food. The sum of the TEF and any increase in the metabolic rate due to overeating is known as **diet-induced thermogenesis (DIT).**

adaptive thermogenesis: adjustments in energy expenditure related to changes in environment such as extreme cold and to physiological events such as overfeeding, trauma, and changes in hormone status.

HOW TO Estimate Energy Requirements

To determine your estimated energy requirements (EER), use the appropriate equation, inserting your age in years, weight (wt) in kilograms, height (ht) in meters, and physical activity (PA) factor from the accompanying table. (To convert pounds to kilograms, divide by 2.2; to convert inches to meters, divide by 39.37.)

- For men 19 years and older:
  EER = 662 − 9.53 × age + PA × [(15.91 × wt) + (539.6 × ht)].
- For women 19 years and older:
  EER = 354 − 6.91 × age + PA × [(9.36 × wt) + (726 × ht)].

For example, consider an active 30-year-old male who is 5 feet 11 inches tall and weighs 178 pounds. First, he converts his weight from pounds to kilograms and his height from inches to meters, if necessary:

178 lb ÷ 2.2 = 80.9 kg.
71 in ÷ 39.37 = 1.8 m.

Next, he considers his level of daily physical activity and selects the appropriate PA factor from the accompanying table (in this example, 1.25 for an active male). Then, he inserts his age, PA factor, weight, and height into the appropriate equation:

EER = 662 − 9.53 × 30 + 1.25 × [(15.91 × 80.9) + (539.6 × 1.8)].

(A reminder: do calculations within the parentheses first, and multiplication before addition and subtraction.) He calculates:

EER = 662 − 9.53 × 30 + 1.25 × (1287 + 971).
EER = 662 − 9.53 × 30 + 1.25 × 2258.
EER = 662 − 286 + 2823.
EER = 3199.

The estimated energy requirement for an active 30-year-old male who is 5 feet 11 inches tall and weighs 178 pounds is about 3200 kcalories/day. His actual requirement probably falls within a range■ of 200 kcalories above and below this estimate.

Physical Activity (PA) Factors for EER Equations

	Men	Women	Physical Activity
Sedentary	1.0	1.0	Only those physical activities required for normal independent living
			For an average-weight person, activities equivalent to walking at a pace of 2–4 mph for the following distances:
Low active	1.11	1.12	1.5 to 3.0 miles/day
Active	1.25	1.27	3 to 10 miles/day
Very active	1.48	1.45	10 or more miles/day

■ For *most* people, the actual energy requirement falls within these ranges:
- For men, EER ± 200 kcal.
- For women, EER ± 160 kcal.

For *almost all* people, the actual energy requirement falls within these ranges:
- For men, EER ± 400 kcal.
- For women, EER ± 320 kcal.

requirements for each individual. For now, the accompanying "How to" provides instructions on calculating your estimated energy requirements using the DRI equations and physical activity factors.■

■ Appendix F presents tables that provide a shortcut to estimating total energy expenditure and instructions to help you determine the appropriate physical activity factor to use in the equation.

IN SUMMARY A person in energy balance takes in energy from food and expends most of it on basal metabolic activities, some of it on physical activities, and a little on the thermic effect of food. Because energy requirements vary from person to person, such factors as gender, age, weight, and height as well as the intensity and duration of physical activity must be considered when estimating energy requirements.

Body Weight, Body Composition, and Health

A person 5 feet 10 inches tall who weighs 150 pounds may carry only about 30 of those pounds as fat. The rest is mostly water and lean tissues—muscles, organs such as the heart and liver, and the bones of the skeleton. Direct measures of

Available Online

http://nutrition.wadsworth.com/uncn7
Examine the effect of too much or too little energy on body composition.

body composition are impossible in living human beings; instead, researchers assess body composition indirectly based on the following assumption:

Body weight = fat + lean tissue (including water).

Weight gains and losses tell us nothing about how the body's composition may have changed, yet weight is the measure most people use to judge their "fatness." For many people, overweight means overfat, but this is not always the case. Athletes with dense bones and well-developed muscles may be overweight by some standards, but have little body fat. Conversely, inactive people may seem to have acceptable weights, when, in fact, they may have too much body fat.

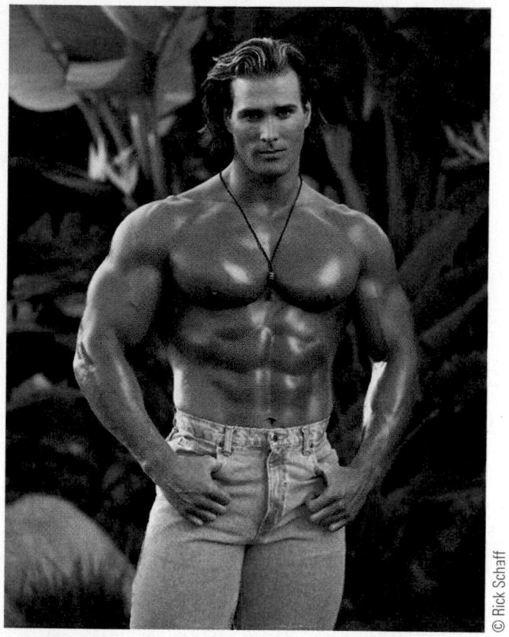
© Rick Schaff
At 6 feet 3 inches tall and 245 pounds, Mike O'Hearn would be considered over*weight* by most standards. Yet he is clearly not over*fat*.

Defining Healthy Body Weight

How much should a person weigh? How can a person know if her weight is appropriate for her height? How can a person know if his weight is jeopardizing his health? Such questions seem so simple, yet the answers can be complex—and quite different depending on whom you ask.

The Criterion of Fashion In asking what is ideal, people often mistakenly turn to fashion for the answer. No doubt our society sets unrealistic ideals for body weight, especially for women. Miss America, our nation's icon of beauty, has never been overweight, and she has grown progressively thinner over the years (see Figure 8-5).[10] Magazines, movies, and television all convey the message that to be thin is to be beautiful and happy. As a result, the media have a great influence on the weight concerns and dieting patterns of people of all ages, but most tragically on young, impressionable children and adolescents.[11] Even five-year-olds are concerned about their body weight.[12] One-half of preteen girls and one-third of preteen boys are dissatisfied with their body weight and shape.[13]

Importantly, perceived body image has little to do with actual body weight or size. People of all shapes, sizes, and ages—including extremely thin fashion models with anorexia nervosa and fitness instructors with ideal body composition—have learned to be unhappy with their "overweight" bodies. Such dissatisfaction can lead to damaging behaviors, such as starvation diets, diet pill abuse, and health care avoidance.[14] The first step toward making healthy changes may be self-acceptance.

body composition: the proportions of muscle, bone, fat, and other tissue that make up a person's total body weight.

FIGURE 8-5 The Declining Weight of Miss America

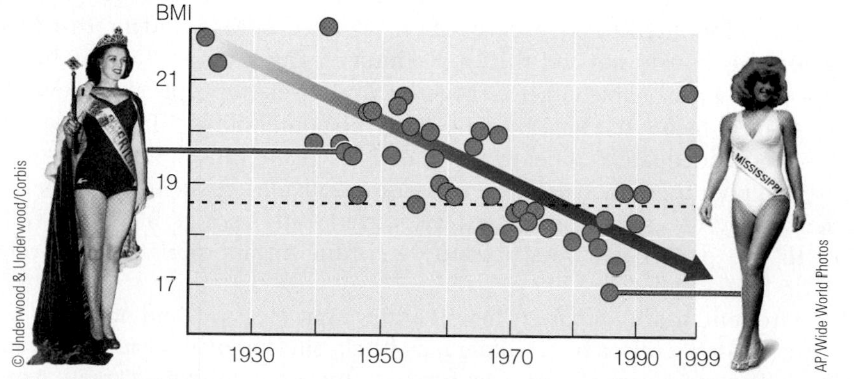
BMI
21
19
17
1930
1950
1970
1990
1999
MISSISSIPPI
© Underwood & Underwood/Corbis
AP/Wide World Photos
Miss America 1944
Miss America 1986

As explained on p. 262, the body mass index (BMI) describes relative weight for height. Over the years, the BMI of Miss America has declined steadily. Since the mid-1960s, most have fallen below 18.5, the cutoff point indicating underweight with its associated health problems.

SOURCE: S. Rubenstein and B. Caballero, Is Miss America an undernourished role model? *Journal of the American Medical Association* 283 (2000): 1569. Used with permission.

TABLE 8-3 Tips for Accepting a Healthy Body Weight

- Value yourself and others for human attributes other than body weight. Realize that prejudging people by weight is as harmful as prejudging them by race, religion, or gender.
- Use positive, nonjudgmental descriptions of your body.
- Accept positive comments from others.
- Focus on your whole self including your intelligence, social grace, and professional and scholastic achievements.
- Accept that no magic diet exists.
- Stop dieting to lose weight. Adopt a lifestyle of healthy eating and physical activity permanently.
- Follow the USDA Food Guide. Never restrict food intake below the minimum levels that meet nutrient needs.
- Become physically active, not because it will help you get thin but because it will make you feel good and enhance your health.
- Seek support from loved ones. Tell them of your plan for a healthy life in the body you have been given.
- Seek professional counseling, *not* from a weight-loss counselor, but from someone who can help you make gains in self-esteem without weight as a factor.
- Join with others to fight weight discrimination and fashion stereotypes. (Search your local paper, or see p. 304 for names of support groups.)

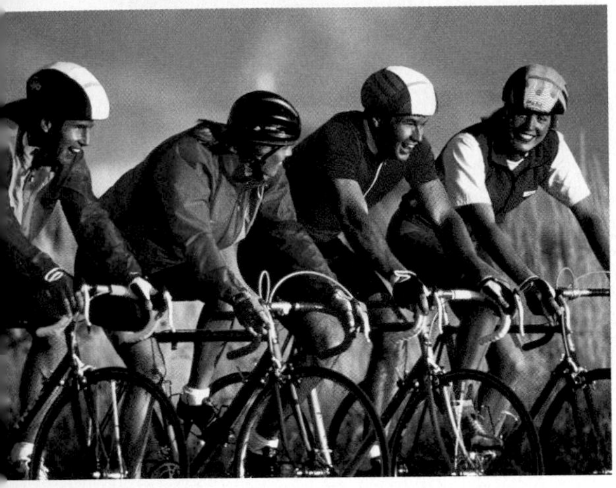

A healthy body contains enough lean tissue to support health and the right amount of fat to meet body needs.

Keep in mind that fashion is fickle; body shapes that our society values change with time. Furthermore, body shapes that our society values differ from those of other societies. The standards defining "ideal" are subjective and frequently have little in common with health. Table 8-3 offers some tips for adopting health as an ideal, rather than society's misconceived image of beauty.

The Criterion of Health Even if our society were to accept fat as beautiful, obesity would still be a major risk factor for several life-threatening diseases. For this reason, the most important criterion for determining how much a person should weigh and how much body fat a person needs is not appearance but good health and longevity. Ideally, a person has enough fat to meet basic needs but not so much as to incur health risks. This range of healthy body weights has been identified using a common measure of weight and height—the body mass index.[15]

Body Mass Index The **body mass index (BMI)** describes relative weight for height:■

$$\text{BMI} = \frac{\text{weight (kg)}}{\text{height (m)}^2} \quad \text{or} \quad \frac{\text{weight (lb)} \times 703.}{\text{height (in)}^2}$$

■ To convert pounds to kilograms:
lb ÷ 2.2 lb/kg = kg.
To convert inches to meters:
in ÷ 39.37 in/m = m.

Weight classifications based on BMI are presented in Figure 8-6. Notice that healthy weight falls between a BMI of 18.5 and 24.9, with **underweight** below 18.5, **overweight** above 25, and obese above 30. Well over half of adults in the United States have a BMI greater than 25, as Figure 8-7 shows.[16]

A BMI of 25 for adults represents a healthy target either for overweight people to achieve or for others to not exceed. Obesity-related diseases and increased mortality become evident beyond this upper limit.[17] The lower end of the healthy range may be a reasonable target for severely underweight people to achieve. BMI values slightly below the healthy range may be compatible with good health if food intake is adequate, but below a BMI of 17, signs of illness, reduced work capacity, and poor reproductive function become apparent.[18] The inside back cover pre-sents weights and visual images associated with various BMI values. The "How to" on p. 264 describes how to determine an appropriate body weight based on BMI.

Keep in mind that BMI reflects height and weight measures and not body composition. Consequently, a bodybuilder may be classified as over*weight* by BMI standards and not be over*fat*. At the peak of his bodybuilding career, Arnold Schwarzenegger won the Mr. Olympia competition with a BMI of 31; the model on p. 261 also has a BMI greater than 30. Yet neither would be considered obese. Striking differences in body composition are also apparent among people of various ethnic and racial groups. For example, blacks tend to have a greater bone density and protein content than whites; consequently, using BMI as the standard may overestimate the prevalence of obesity among blacks.[19]

body mass index (BMI): an index of a person's weight in relation to height; determined by dividing the weight (in kilograms) by the square of the height (in meters).

underweight: body weight below some standard of acceptable weight that is usually defined in relation to height (such as BMI).

overweight: body weight above some standard of acceptable weight that is usually defined in relation to height (such as BMI).

FIGURE 8-6 BMI Values Used to Assess Weight

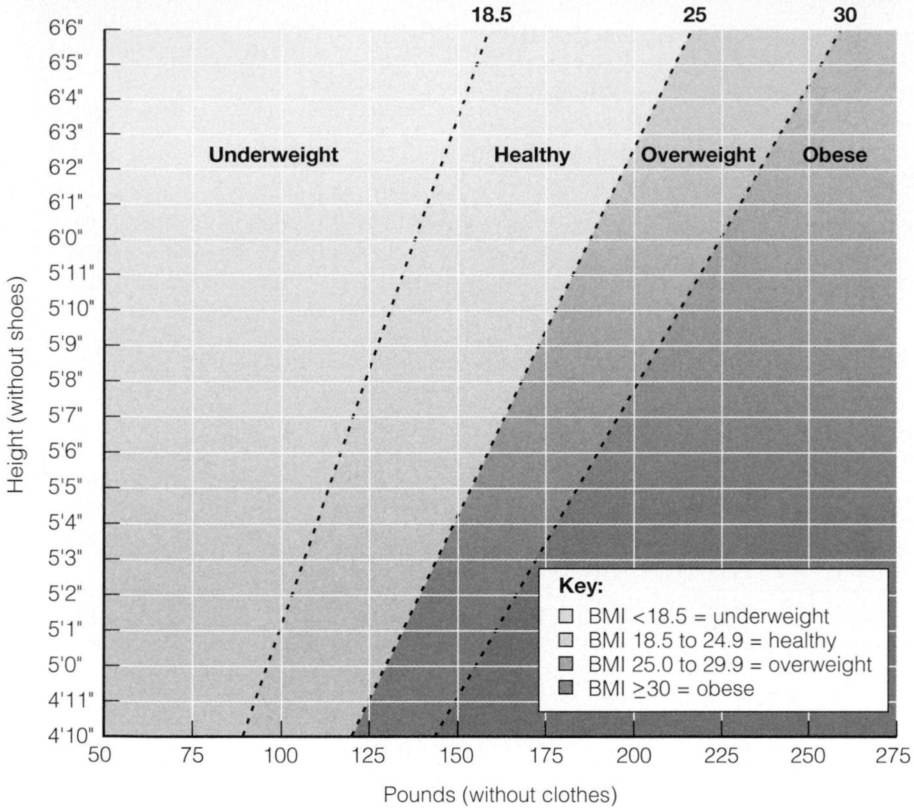
18.5
25
30
Underweight
Healthy
Overweight
Obese
Height (without shoes)
6'6"
6'5"
6'4"
6'3"
6'2"
6'1"
6'0"
5'11"
5'10"
5'9"
5'8"
5'7"
5'6"
5'5"
5'4"
5'3"
5'2"
5'1"
5'0"
4'11"
4'10"
50
75
100
125
150
175
200
225
250
275
Pounds (without clothes)
Key:
BMI <18.5 = underweight
BMI 18.5 to 24.9 = healthy
BMI 25.0 to 29.9 = overweight
BMI ≥30 = obese

NOTE: Chapter 15 presents BMI values for children and adolescents age 2 to 20.
SOURCE: U.S. Department of Agriculture and U.S. Department of Health and Human Services, *Nutrition and Your Health: Dietary Guidelines for Americans* (Washington, D.C.: 2000), p. 7.

FIGURE 8-7 Distribution of Body Weights in U.S. Adults

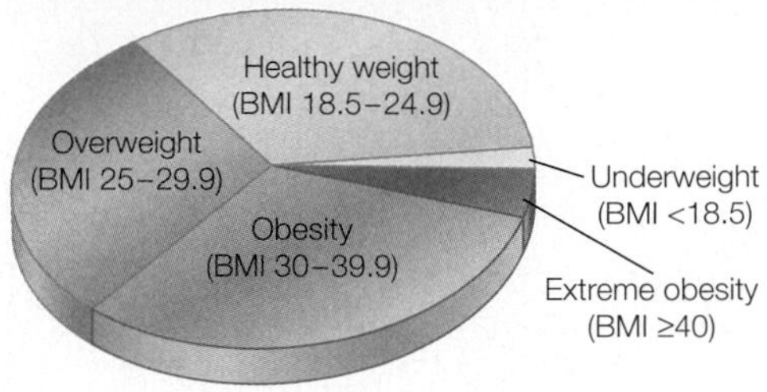
Healthy weight
(BMI 18.5–24.9)
Overweight
(BMI 25–29.9)
Obesity
(BMI 30–39.9)
Underweight
(BMI <18.5)
Extreme obesity
(BMI ≥40)

IN SUMMARY Current standards for body weight are based on a person's weight in relation to height, called the body mass index (BMI), and reflect disease risks. To its disadvantage, BMI does not reflect body fat, and it may misclassify very muscular people as overweight.

Body Fat and Its Distribution

Although weight measures are inexpensive, easy to take, and highly accurate, they fail to reveal two valuable pieces of information in assessing disease risk: how much of the weight is fat and where the fat is located. The ideal amount of body fat depends partly on the person. A normal-weight man may have from 13 to 21 percent body fat; a woman, because of her greater quantity of essential fat, 23 to 31 percent. In general, health problems typically develop when body fat exceeds 22 percent in young men, 25 percent in men over age 40, 32 percent in young women, and 35 percent in women over age 40. Body fat may contribute as much as 70 percent in excessively obese adults. Figure 8-8 (on p. 265) compares the body composition of healthy weight men and women.

Some People Need Less Body Fat For many athletes, a lower percentage of body fat may be ideal—just enough fat to provide fuel, insulate and protect the body, assist in nerve impulse transmissions, and support normal hormone activity, but not so much as to burden the body with excess bulk. For some athletes, then, ideal body fat might be 5 to 10 percent for men and 15 to 20 percent for women.

HOW TO Determine Body Weight Based on BMI

A person whose BMI reflects an unacceptable health risk can choose a desired BMI and then calculate an appropriate body weight. For example, a woman who is 5 feet 5 inches (1.65 meters) tall and weighs 180 pounds (82 kilograms) has a BMI of 30:

$$\text{BMI} = \frac{82 \text{ kg}}{1.65 \text{ m}^2} = 30$$

or

$$\text{BMI} = \frac{180 \text{ lb} \times 703}{65 \text{ in}^2} = 30.$$

A reasonable target for most overweight people is a BMI 2 units below their current one. To determine a desired goal weight based on a BMI of 28, for example, the woman could divide the desired BMI by the factor appropriate for her height from the table below:

$$\text{Desired BMI} \div \text{factor} = \text{goal weight.}$$

$$28 \div 0.166 = 169 \text{ lb.}$$

To reach a BMI of 28, this woman would need to lose 11 pounds. Such a calculation can help a person to determine realistic weight goals using health risk as a guide. Alternatively, a person could search the table on the inside back cover for the weight that corresponds to his or her height and the desired BMI.

Height	Factor	Height	Factor	Height	Factor
4′7″	0.232	5′3″	0.177	5′11″	0.139
4′8″	0.224	5′4″	0.172	6′0″	0.136
4′9″	0.216	5′5″	0.166	6′1″	0.132
4′10″	0.209	5′6″	0.161	6′2″	0.128
4′11″	0.202	5′7″	0.157	6′3″	0.125
5′0″	0.195	5′8″	0.152	6′4″	0.122
5′1″	0.189	5′9″	0.148	6′5″	0.119
5′2″	0.183	5′10″	0.143	6′6″	0.116

SOURCE: R. P. Abernathy, Body mass index: Determination and use. Copyright the American Dietetic Association. Reprinted by permission from *Journal of the American Dietetic Association* 91 (1991): 843.

(You may want to review the photo on p. 261 to appreciate what 8 percent body fat looks like.)

Some People Need More Body Fat For an Alaska fisherman, a higher percentage of body fat is probably beneficial because fat provides an insulating blanket to prevent excessive loss of body heat in cold climates. A woman starting a pregnancy needs sufficient body fat to support conception and fetal growth. Below a certain threshold for body fat, hormone synthesis falters, and individuals may become infertile, develop depression, experience abnormal hunger regulation, or become unable to keep warm. These thresholds differ for each function and for each individual; much remains to be learned about them.

Fat Distribution The distribution of fat on the body may be more critical than the total amount of fat alone. **Intra-abdominal fat** that is stored around the organs of the abdomen is referred to as **central obesity** or upper-body fat and, independently of total body fat, is associated with increased risks of heart disease, stroke, diabetes, hypertension, and some types of cancer.[20]

Abdominal fat is most common in men and to a lesser extent in women past menopause. Even when total body fat is similar, men have more abdominal fat than women. Regardless of gender, the risks of cardiovascular disease, diabetes, and mortality are increased for those with excessive abdominal fat.

Fat around the hips and thighs, sometimes referred to as lower-body fat, is most common in women during their reproductive years and seems relatively harmless. In fact, overweight people who do not have abdominal fat are less susceptible to health problems than overweight people with abdominal fat. Figure 8-9 compares the body shapes of people with upper-body fat and lower-body fat.

intra-abdominal fat: fat stored within the abdominal cavity in association with the internal abdominal organs, as opposed to the fat stored directly under the skin (subcutaneous fat).

central obesity: excess fat around the trunk of the body; also called **abdominal fat** or **upper-body fat.**

FIGURE 8-8 Male and Female Body Compositions Compared

The differences between male and female body compositions become apparent during adolescence. Lean body mass (primarily muscle) increases more in males than in females. Fat assumes a larger percentage of female body composition as essential body fat is deposited in the mammary glands and pelvic region in preparation for childbearing. Both men and women have essential fat associated with the bone marrow, the central nervous system, and the internal organs.

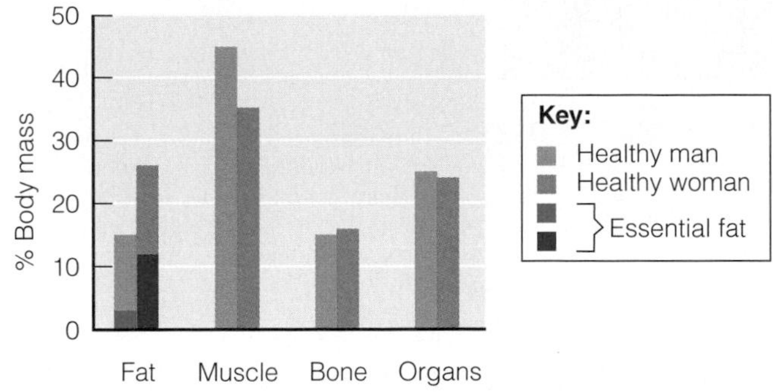
50
40
30
20
10
0
% Body mass
Fat
Muscle
Bone
Organs
Key:
Healthy man
Healthy woman
Essential fat

SOURCE: R. E. C. Wildman and D. M. Medeiros, *Advanced Human Nutrition* (Boca Raton, Fla.: CRC Press, 2000), pp. 321–323. Used with permission.

FIGURE 8-9 "Apple" and "Pear" Body Shapes Compared

Upper-body fat is more common in men than in women and is closely associated with heart disease, stroke, diabetes, hypertension, and some types of cancer. In contrast, lower-body fat is more common in women than in men and is not usually associated with chronic diseases. Popular articles sometimes call bodies with upper-body fat "apples" and those with lower-body fat, "pears." Researchers sometimes refer to upper-body fat as "android" (manlike) obesity and to lower-body fat as "gynoid" (womanlike) obesity.

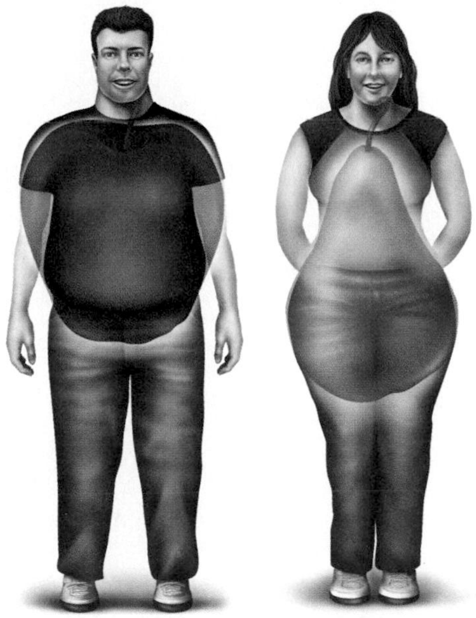

Waist Circumference A person's **waist circumference** is the most practical indicator of fat distribution and abdominal fat.*[21] In general, women with a waist circumference of greater than 35 inches (88 centimeters) and men with a waist circumference of greater than 40 inches (102 centimeters) have a high risk of central obesity–related health problems, such as diabetes and cardiovascular disease.[22] Appendix E includes instructions for measuring waist circumference and assessing abdominal fat.

Other Measures of Body Composition Health care professionals commonly use BMI and waist circumference to access a person's body weight and to monitor changes over time because these measures are relatively easy to determine and inexpensive.[23] Researchers needing more precise measures of body composition may choose any of several other techniques to estimate body fat and its distribution (see Figure 8-10 on p. 266). Mastering these techniques requires proper instruction and practice to ensure reliability. Appendix E provides additional details and includes many of the tables and charts routinely used in assessment procedures.†

IN SUMMARY The ideal amount of body fat varies from person to person, but researchers have found that body fat in excess of 22 percent for young men and 32 percent for young women (the levels rise slightly with age) poses health risks. Central obesity in which excess fat is distributed around the trunk of the body presents greater health risks than excess fat distributed on the lower body.

Health Risks Associated with Body Weight and Body Fat

Body weight and fat distribution correlate with disease risks and life expectancy.[24] These risks indicate a greater *likelihood* of developing a chronic disease and shortening life expectancy. Not all overweight and underweight people will get sick and

waist circumference: an anthropometric measurement used to assess a person's abdominal fat.

*The National Heart, Lung, and Blood Institute has replaced waist-hip ratio with waist circumference for assessment of obesity health risks.

†In addition to the methods shown in Figure 8-10, researchers sometimes estimate body composition using these methods: total body water, radioactive potassium count, near-infrared spectrophotometry, ultrasound, computed tomography, and magnetic resonance imaging. Each has advantages and disadvantages with respect to cost, technical difficulty, and precision of estimating body fat (see Appendix E for a comparison).

FIGURE 8-10 Methods Used to Assess Body Fat

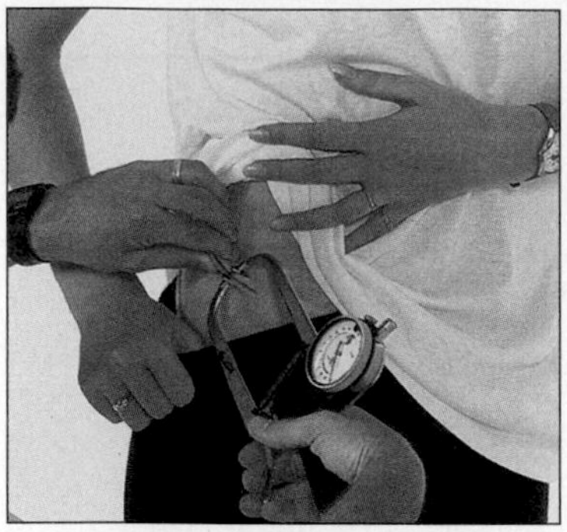

© Fitness & Wellness, Boise, Idaho

Fatfold measures estimate body fat by using a caliper to gauge the thickness of a fold of skin on the back of the arm (over the triceps), below the shoulder blade (subscapular), and in other places (including lower-body sites) and then comparing these measurements with standards.

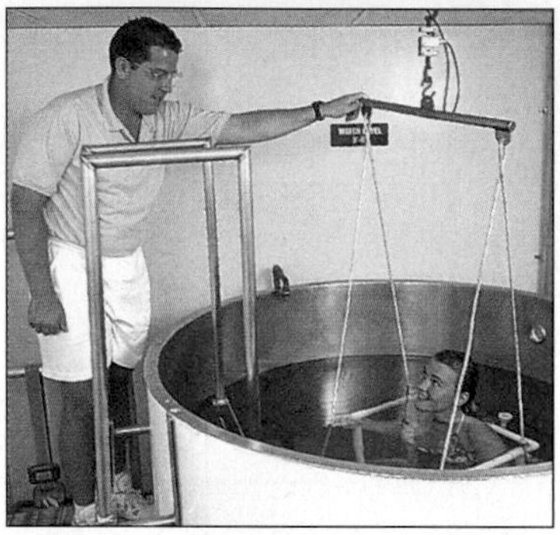

© David Young-Wolff/PhotoEdit

Hydrodensitometry measures body density by weighing the person first on land and then again while submerged in water. The difference between the person's actual weight and underwater weight provides a measure of the body's volume. A mathematical equation using the two measurements (volume and actual weight) determines body density, from which the percentage of body fat can be estimated.

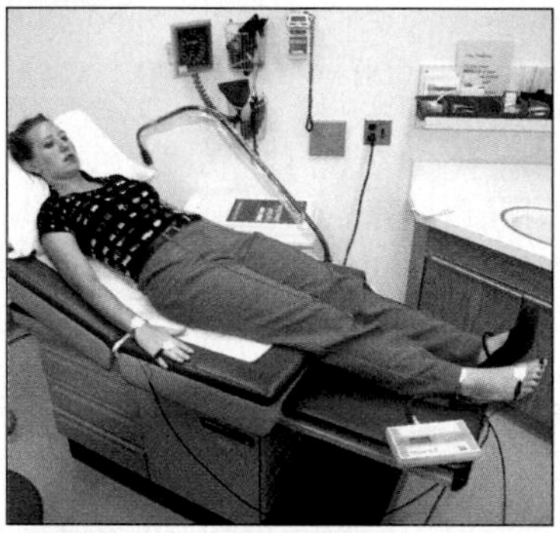

© Geri Engberg

Bioelectrical impedance measures body fat by using a low-intensity electrical current. Because electrolyte-containing fluids, which readily conduct an electrical current, are found primarily in lean body tissues, the leaner the person, the less resistance to the current. The measurement of electrical resistance is then used in a mathematical equation to estimate the percentage of body fat.

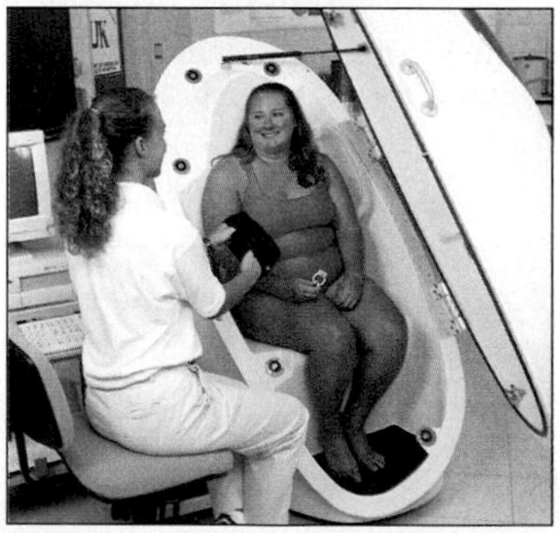

Photo Courtesy of Life Measurement, Inc.

Air displacement plethysmography estimates body composition by having a person sit inside a chamber while computerized sensors determine the amount of air displaced by the person's body.

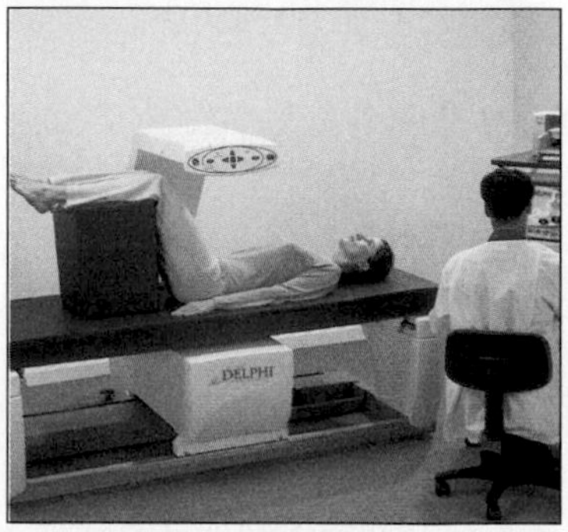
DELPHI

© Photo Courtesy of Hologic, Inc.

Dual energy X-ray absorptiometry (DEXA) uses two low-dose X-rays that differentiate among fat-free soft tissue (lean body mass), fat tissue, and bone tissue, providing a precise measurement of total fat and its distribution in all but extremely obese subjects.

die before their time nor will all normal-weight people live long healthy lives. These are *correlations,* not *causes.* For the most part, people with a BMI between 18.5 and 24.9 have relatively few health risks; risks increase as BMI falls below or rises above this range, indicating that both too little and too much body fat impair health.[25] Epidemiological data show a J- or U-shaped relationship between body weights and mortality (see Figure 8-11).[26] People who are extremely underweight or extremely obese carry higher risks of early deaths than those whose weights fall within the acceptable range. These mortality risks decline with age.[27]

Independently of BMI, factors such as smoking habits raise health risks, and physical fitness lowers them.[28] A man with a BMI of 22 who smokes two packs of cigarettes a day is jeopardizing his health, whereas a woman with a BMI of 32 who walks briskly for an hour a day is improving her health.

Health Risks of Underweight Some underweight people enjoy an active, healthy life, but others are underweight because of malnutrition, smoking habits, substance abuse, or illnesses. Weight and fat measures alone would not reveal these underlying causes, but a complete assessment that includes a diet and medical history, physical examination, and biochemical analysis would.

An underweight person, especially an older adult, may be unable to preserve lean tissue during the fight against a wasting disease such as cancer or a digestive disorder, especially when the disease is accompanied by malnutrition. Without adequate nutrient and energy reserves, an underweight person will have a particularly tough battle against such medical stresses. In fact, many people with cancer die, not from the cancer itself, but from malnutrition. Underweight women develop menstrual irregularities and become infertile. Exactly how infertility develops is unclear, but contributing factors include not only body weight but also restricted energy and fat intake and depleted body fat stores. Those who do conceive may give birth to unhealthy infants. An underweight woman can improve her chances of having a healthy infant by gaining weight prior to conception, during pregnancy, or both. Underweight and significant weight loss are also associated with osteoporosis and bone fractures.[29] For all these reasons, underweight people may benefit from enough of a weight gain to provide an energy reserve and protective amounts of all the nutrients that can be stored.

Health Risks of Overweight As for excessive body fat, the health risks are so many that it has been designated a disease: obesity. Among the health risks associated with obesity are diabetes, hypertension, cardiovascular disease, sleep apnea (abnormal ceasing of breathing during sleep), osteoarthritis, some cancers, gallbladder disease, respiratory problems (including Pickwickian syndrome, a breathing blockage linked with sudden death), and complications in pregnancy and surgery. Each year, these obesity-related illnesses cost our nation billions of dollars—in fact, as much as the medical costs of smoking.[30]

The cost in terms of lives is also great: an estimated 300,000 people die each year from obesity-related diseases.[31] In fact, obesity is second only to tobacco in causing preventable illnesses and premature deaths. Mortality increases as excess weight increases; people with a BMI greater than 35 are twice as likely to die prematurely as others. The risks associated with a high BMI appear to be greater for whites than for blacks.[32] In fact, the health risks associated with obesity do not become apparent in black women until a BMI of 37.[33]

Equally important, both central obesity and weight gains of more than 20 pounds between early and middle adulthood correlate with increased mortality. Fluctuations in body weight, as typically occur with "yo-yo" dieting, also increase the risks of chronic diseases and premature death.[34] In contrast, sustained weight loss improves physical well-being, reduces disease risks, and increases life expectancy.[35]

Cardiovascular Disease The relationship between obesity and cardiovascular disease risk is strong, with links to both elevated blood cholesterol and hypertension. Central obesity may raise the risk of heart attack and stroke as much as the

FIGURE 8-11 BMI and Mortality

This J-shaped curve describes the relationship between body mass index (BMI) and mortality and shows that both underweight and overweight present risks of a premature death.

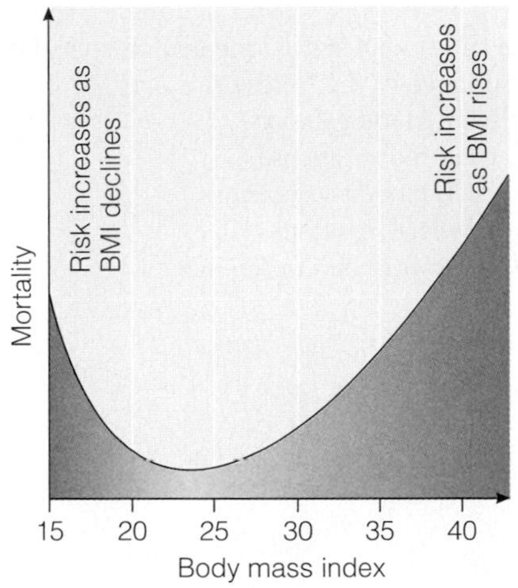
Mortality
Risk increases as BMI declines
Risk increases as BMI rises
15
20
25
30
35
40
Body mass index

- Cardiovascular disease risk factors associated with obesity:
  - High LDL cholesterol.
  - Low HDL cholesterol.
  - High blood pressure (hypertension).
  - Diabetes.

  Chapter 27 provides many more details.

- The metabolic syndrome is a cluster of at least three of the following:
  - High blood pressure.
  - High blood glucose.
  - High blood triglycerides.
  - Low HDL cholesterol.
  - High waist circumference.

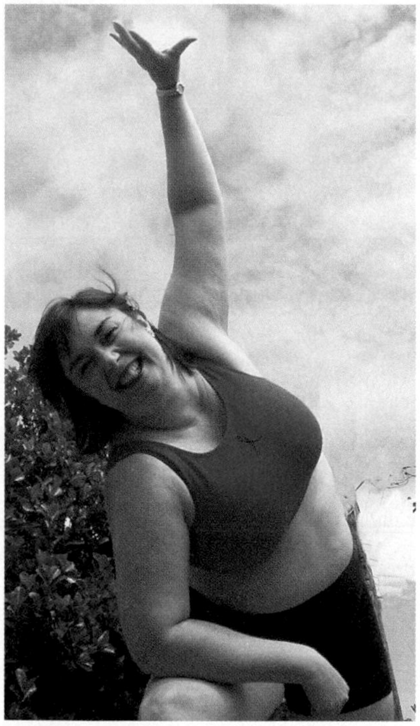

© Joe Sampson, Courtesy of Jennifer Portnick

Being active—even if overweight—is healthier than being sedentary. With a BMI of 36, aerobics instructor Jennifer Portnick is considered obese, but her daily workout routine helps to keep her in good health.

three leading risk factors (high LDL cholesterol, hypertension, and smoking) do.■ In addition to body fat and its distribution, weight gain also increases the risk of cardiovascular disease. Weight loss, on the other hand, can effectively lower both blood cholesterol and blood pressure in obese people. Of course, lean and normal-weight people may also have high blood cholesterol and blood pressure, and these factors are just as dangerous in lean people as in obese people.

Diabetes Diabetes (type 2) is three times more likely to develop in an obese person than in a nonobese person. Furthermore, the person with type 2 diabetes often has central obesity. Central-body fat cells appear to be larger and more insulin-resistant than lower-body fat cells. The association between **insulin resistance** and obesity is strong.[36] Both are major risk factors for the development of type 2 diabetes. Highlight 26 describes the central role obesity plays, together with other risk factors■—collectively known as the metabolic syndrome—in raising health risks dramatically.[37]

Diabetes appears to be influenced by weight gains as well as by body weight. A weight gain of more than 10 pounds since age 18 doubles the risk of developing diabetes, even in women of average weight. In contrast, weight loss is effective in improving glucose tolerance and insulin resistance.[38]

Cancer The risk of some cancers increases with both body weight and weight gain, but researchers do not fully understand the relationships.[39] One possible explanation may be that obese people have elevated levels of hormones that could influence cancer development.[40] For example, adipose tissue is the major site of estrogen synthesis in women, obese women have elevated levels of estrogen, and estrogen has been implicated in the development of cancers of the female reproductive system—cancers that account for half of all cancers in women.

Fit and Fat versus Sedentary and Slim Importantly, BMI and weight gains and losses do not tell all of the story. Cardiorespiratory fitness also plays a major role in health and longevity, independently of BMI.[41] Normal-weight people who are fit have a lower risk of mortality than normal-weight people who are unfit. Furthermore, overweight but fit people have lower risks than normal-weight, unfit ones. Clearly, a healthy body weight is good, but it may not be good enough. Fitness, in and of itself, offers many health benefits. The next chapter explores weight management and the benefits of achieving and maintaining a healthy weight.

IN SUMMARY The weight appropriate for an individual depends largely on factors specific to that individual, including body fat distribution, family health history, and current health status. At the extremes, both overweight and underweight carry clear risks to health.

Nutrition in Your Life

When combined with fitness, a healthy body weight will help you to defend against chronic diseases.

- **Do you balance your food intake with physical activity?**
- **Is your BMI between 18.5 and 24.9?**
- **Is your waist circumference less than 35 inches for a woman or 40 inches for a man?**

insulin resistance: the reduced ability of insulin to regulate glucose metabolism.

NUTRITION ON THE NET

Access these websites for further study of topics covered in this chapter.

- Find updates and quick links to these and other nutrition-related sites at our website: **www.wadsworth.com/nutrition**
- Obtain food composition data from the USDA Nutrient Data Laboratory: **www.nal.usda.gov/fnic/foodcomp**
- Learn about the 10,000 Steps Program at Shape Up America: **www.shapeup.org**
- Visit the special web pages and interactive applications for Healthy Weight: **www.nhlbi.nih.gov/subsites/index.htm**

NUTRITION CALCULATIONS

These problems give you practice in estimating energy needs. Once you have mastered these examples, you will be prepared to examine your own energy intakes and energy expenditures. Be sure to show your calculations for each problem and check p. 271 for answers.

1. Compare the energy a person might spend on various physical activities. Refer to Table 8-2 on p. 258, and compute how much energy a person who weighs 142 pounds would spend doing each of the following. You may want to compare various activities based on your weight.

   30 min vigorous aerobic dance:

   $$0.062 \text{ kcal/lb/min} \times 142 \text{ lb} = 8.8 \text{ kcal/min.}$$

   $$8.8 \text{ kcal/min} \times 30 \text{ min} = 264 \text{ kcal.}$$

   a. 2 hours golf, carrying clubs.
   b. 20 minutes running at 9 mph.
   c. 45 minutes swimming at 20 yd/min.
   d. 1 hour walking at 3.5 mph.
2. Consider the effect of age on BMR. An infant who weighs 20 pounds has a BMR of 500 kcalories/day; an adult who weighs 170 pounds has a BMR of about 1500. Based on body weight, who has the faster BMR?
3. Compute daily energy needs for a woman, age 20, who is 5 feet 6 inches tall, weighs 130 pounds, and is lightly active.
4. Discover what weight is needed to achieve a desired BMI. Refer to the table on p. 264 and consider a person who is 5 feet 4 inches tall. Suppose this person wants to have a BMI of 21. What should this person weigh? Does this agree with the table on the inside back cover?

STUDY QUESTIONS

These questions will help you review the chapter. You will find the answers in the discussions on the pages provided.

1. What are the consequences of an unbalanced energy budget? (p. 252)
2. Define hunger, appetite, satiation, and satiety and describe how each influences food intake. (pp. 253–255)
3. Describe each component of energy expenditure. What factors influence each? How can energy expenditure be estimated? (pp. 256–260)
4. Distinguish between body weight and body composition. What assessment techniques are used to measure each? (pp. 260–266)
5. What problems are involved in defining "ideal" body weight? (pp. 261–262)
6. What is central obesity, and what is its relationship to disease? (pp. 264–265)
7. What risks are associated with excess body weight and excess body fat? (pp. 265–268)

These multiple choice questions will help you prepare for an exam. Answers can be found on p. 271.

1. A person who consistently consumes 1700 kcalories a day and spends 2200 kcalories a day for a month would be expected to:
   a. lose ½ to 1 pound.
   b. gain ½ to 1 pound.
   c. lose 4 to 5 pounds.
   d. gain 4 to 5 pounds.
2. A bomb calorimeter measures:
   a. physiological fuel.
   b. energy available from foods.
   c. kcalories a person derives from foods.
   d. heat a person releases in basal metabolism.
3. The psychological desire to eat that accompanies the sight, smell, or thought of food is known as:
   a. hunger.
   b. satiety.
   c. appetite.
   d. palatability.

4. A person watching television after dinner reaches for a snack during a commercial in response to:
   a. external cues.
   b. hunger signals.
   c. stress arousal.
   d. satiety factors.
5. The largest component of energy expenditure is:
   a. basal metabolism.
   b. physical activity.
   c. indirect calorimetry.
   d. thermic effect of food.
6. A major factor influencing BMR is:
   a. hunger.
   b. food intake.
   c. body composition.
   d. physical activity.
7. The thermic effect of an 800-kcalorie meal is about:
   a. 8 kcalories.
   b. 80 kcalories.
   c. 160 kcalories.
   d. 200 kcalories.
8. For health's sake, a person with a BMI of 21 might want to:
   a. lose weight.
   b. maintain weight.
   c. gain weight.
9. Which of the following reflects height and weight?
   a. body mass index
   b. central obesity
   c. waist circumference
   d. body composition
10. Which of the following increases disease risks?
   a. BMI 19–21
   b. BMI 22–25
   c. lower-body fat
   d. central obesity

REFERENCES

1. A. Del Parigi and coauthors, Sex differences in the human brain's response to hunger and satiation, *American Journal of Clinical Nutrition* 75 (2002): 1017–1022.
2. B. J. Rolls, E. L. Morris, and L. S. Roe, Portion size of food affects energy intake in normal-weight and overweight men and women, *American Journal of Clinical Nutrition* 76 (2002): 1207–1213; R. J. Stubbs and coauthors, Effect of altering the variety of sensorially distinct foods, of the same macronutrient content, on food intake and body weight in men, *European Journal of Clinical Nutrition* 55 (2001): 19–28.
3. C. Marmonier, D. Chapelot, and J. Louis-Sylvestre, Effects of macronutrient content and energy density of snacks consumed in a satiety state on the onset of the next meal, *Appetite* 34 (2000): 161–168; M. S. Westerterp-Plantenga and coauthors, Satiety related to 24 h diet-induced thermogenesis during high protein/carbohydrate vs high fat diets measured in a respiration chamber, *European Journal of Clinical Nutrition* 53 (1999): 495–502.
4. B. Burton-Freeman, P. A. Davis, and B. O. Schneeman, Plasma cholecystokinin is associated with subjective measures of satiety in women, *American Journal of Clinical Nutrition* 76 (2002): 659–667; C. Feinle, D. O'Donovan, and M. Horowitz, Carbohydrate and satiety, *Nutrition Reviews* 60 (2002): 155–169; G. A. Bray, Afferent signals regulating food intake, *Proceedings of the Nutrition Society* 59 (2000): 373–384; T. H. Moran, Cholecystokinin and satiety: Current perspectives, *Nutrition* 16 (2000): 858–865.
5. S. H. A. Holt, J. C. Brand-Miller, and P. A. Stitt, The effects of equal-energy portions of different breads on blood glucose levels, feelings of fullness and subsequent food intake, *Journal of the American Dietetic Association* 101 (2001): 767–773.
6. M. W. Schwartz and coauthors, Model for the regulation of energy balance and adiposity, *American Journal of Clinical Nutrition* 69 (1999): 584–596.
7. J. T. Lemmer and coauthors, Effect of strength training on resting metabolic rate and physical activity: Age and gender comparisons, *Medicine and Science in Sports and Exercise* 33 (2001): 532–541.
8. G. P. Granata and L. J. Brandon, The thermic effect of food and obesity: Discrepant results and methodological variations, *Nutrition Reviews* 60 (2002): 223–233; L. Jonge and G. A. Bray, The thermic effect of food is reduced in obesity, *Nutrition Reviews* 60 (2002): 295–297.
9. F. X. Pi-Sunyer, Overnutrition and undernutrition as modifiers of metabolic processes in disease states, *American Journal of Clinical Nutrition* 72 (2000): 533S–537S.
10. S. Rubinstein and B. Caballero, Is Miss America an undernourished role model? *Journal of the American Medical Association* 283 (2000): 1569.
11. J. Wardle, J. Waller, and E. Fox, Age of onset and body dissatisfaction in obesity, *Addictive Behaviors* 27 (2002): 561–573; A. E. Field and coauthors, Peer, parent, and media influences on the development of weight concerns and frequent dieting among preadolescent and adolescent girls and boys, *Pediatrics* 107 (2001): 54–60.
12. K. K. Davison and L. L. Birch, Weight status, parent reaction, and self-concept in five-year-old girls, *Pediatrics* 107 (2001): 46–53.
13. H. Truby and S. J. Paxton, Development of the Children's Body Image Scale, *British Journal of Clinical Psychology* 41 (2002): 185–203; H. A. Hausenblas and coauthors, Body image in middle school children, *Eating and Weight Disorders* 7 (2002): 244–248.
14. C. A. Drury and M. Louis, Exploring the association between body weight, stigma of obesity, and health care avoidance, *Journal of the American Academy of Nurse Practitioners* 14 (2002): 554–561.
15. R. J. Kuczmarski and K. M. Flegal, Criteria for definition of overweight in transition: Background and recommendations for the United States, *American Journal of Clinical Nutrition* 72 (2000): 1074–1081.
16. K. M. Flegal and coauthors, Prevalence and trends in obesity among US adults, *Journal of the American Medical Association* 288 (2002): 1723–1727.
17. J. Stevens and coauthors, Evaluation of WHO and NHANES II standards for overweight using mortality rates, *Journal of the American Dietetic Association* 100 (2000): 825–827; A. Must and coauthors, The disease burden associated with overweight and obesity, *Journal of the American Medical Association* 282 (1999): 1523–1529.
18. L. J. Hoffer, Metabolic consequences of starvation, in M. E. Shils and coeditors, *Modern Nutrition in Health and Disease* (Baltimore: Williams & Wilkins, 1999), pp. 645–665.
19. D. R. Wagner and V. H. Heyward, Measures of body composition in blacks and whites: A comparative review, *American Journal of Clinical Nutrition* 71 (2000): 1392–1402.
20. T. B. Nguyen-Duy and coauthors, Visceral fat and liver fat are independent predictors of metabolic risk factors in men, *American Journal of Physiology. Endocrinology and Metabolism* (2003); G. Davì and coauthors, Platelet activation in obese women—Role of inflammation and oxidant stress, *Journal of the American Medical Association* 288 (2002): 2008–2014; J. M. Oppert and coauthors, Anthropometric estimates of muscle and fat mass in relation to cardiac and cancer mortality in men: The Paris Prospective Study, *American Journal of Clinical Nutrition* 75 (2002): 1107–1113.
21. I. Janssen and coauthors, Body mass index and waist circumference independently contribute to the prediction of nonabdominal, abdominal subcutaneous, and visceral fat, *American Journal of Clinical Nutrition* 75 (2002): 683–688.
22. S. K. Zhu and coauthors, Waist circumference and obesity-associated risk factors among whites in the third National Health and Nutrition Examination Survey: Clinical action thresholds, *American Journal of Clinical Nutrition* 76 (2002): 743–749.

23. J. C. Seidell and coauthors, Report from a Centers for Disease Control and Prevention workshop on use of adult anthropometry for public health and primary health care, *American Journal of Clinical Nutrition* 73 (2001): 123–126.
24. A. H. Mokdad and coauthors, Prevalence of obesity, diabetes, and obesity-related health risk factors, 2001, *Journal of the American Medical Association* 289 (2003): 76–79; K. R. Fontaine and coauthors, Years of life lost due to obesity, *Journal of the American Medical Association* 289 (2003): 187–193; Must and coauthors, 1999.
25. A. Thorogood and coauthors, Relation between body mass index and mortality in an unusually slim cohort, *Journal of Epidemiology and Community Health* 57 (2003) 130–133; P. T. Katzmarzyk, C. L. Craig, and C. Bouchard, Original article underweight, overweight and obesity: Relationships with mortality in the 13-year follow-up of the Canada Fitness Study, *Journal of Clinical Epidemiology* 54 (2001): 916–920; R. Bender and coauthors, Effect of age on excess mortality in obesity, *Journal of the American Medical Association* 281 (1999): 1498–1504.
26. R. G. Rogers, R. A. Hummer, and P. M. Krueger, The effect of obesity on overall, circulatory disease- and diabetes-specific mortality, *Journal of Biosocial Science* 35 (2003): 107–129; D. B. Allison and coauthors, Differential associations of body mass index and adiposity with all-cause mortality among men in the first and second National Health and Nutrition Examination Surveys (NHANES I and NHANES II) follow-up studies, *International Journal of Obesity and Related Metabolic Disorders* 26 (2002): 410–416; H. E. Meyer and coauthors, Body mass index and mortality: The influence of physical activity and smoking, *Medicine and Science in Sports and Exercise* 34 (2002): 1065–1070; P. N. Singh, K. D. Lindsted, and G. E. Fraser, Body weight and mortality among adults who never smoked, *American Journal of Epidemiology* 150 (1999): 1152–1164; E. E. Calle and coauthors, Body-mass index and mortality in a prospective cohort of U.S. adults, *New England Journal of Medicine* 341 (1999): 1097–1105.
27. I. Baik and coauthors, Adiposity and mortality in men, *American Journal of Epidemiology* 152 (2000): 264–271; J. Stevens, Impact of age on associations between weight and mortality, *Nutrition Reviews* 58 (2000): 129–137; Bender and coauthors, 1999.
28. A. Peeters and coauthors, Obesity in adulthood and its consequences for life expectancy: A life-table analysis, *Annals of Internal Medicine* 138 (2003): 24–32; Meyer and coauthors, 2002; M. Wei and coauthors, Relationship between low cardiorespiratory fitness and mortality in normal-weight, overweight, and obese men, *Journal of the American Medical Association* 282 (1999): 1547–1553.
29. L. M. Salamone and coauthors, Effect of a lifestyle intervention on bone mineral density in premenopausal women: A randomized trial, *American Journal of Clinical Nutrition* 70 (1999): 97–103.
30. E. A. Finkelstein, I. C. Fiebelkorn, and G. Wang, National medical expenditures attributable to overweight and obesity: How much, and who's paying? 2003, available at **www.healthaffairs.org/WebExclusives/Finkelstein_Web_Excl_051403.htm**.
31. D. B. Allison and coauthors, Annual deaths attributable to obesity in the United States, *Journal of the American Medical Association* 282 (1999): 1530–1538.
32. J. Stevens and coauthors, The effect of decision rules on the choice of a body mass index cutoff for obesity: Examples from African American and white women, *American Journal of Clinical Nutrition* 75 (2002): 986–992; J. Stevens, Obesity and mortality in African-Americans, *Nutrition Reviews* 58 (2000): 346–353; Calle and coauthors, 1999.
33. J. E. Manson and S. S. Bassuk, Obesity in the United States: A fresh look at its high toll, *Journal of the American Medical Association* 289 (2003): 229–230.
34. K. A. Petersmark and coauthors, The effect of weight cycling on blood lipids and blood pressure in the Multiple Risk Factor Intervention Trial special intervention group, *International Journal of Obesity and Related Metabolic Disorders* 23 (1999): 1246–1255.
35. Davì, 2002; D. F. Williamson and coauthors, Intentional weight loss and mortality among overweight individuals with diabetes, *Diabetes Care* 23 (2000): 1499–1504; J. T. Fine and coauthors, A prospective study of weight change and health-related quality of life in women, *Journal of the American Medical Association* 282 (1999): 2136–2142; K. Karason and coauthors, Weight loss and progression of early atherosclerosis in the carotid artery: A four-year controlled study of obese subjects, *International Journal of Obesity and Related Metabolic Disorders* 23 (1999): 948–956; G. Oster and coauthors, Lifetime health and economic benefits of weight loss among obese persons, *American Journal of Public Health* 89 (1999): 1536–1542.
36. J. L. Sievenpiper and coauthors, Simple skinfold-thickness measurements complement conventional anthropometric assessments in predicting glucose tolerance, *American Journal of Clinical Nutrition* 73 (2001): 567–573; D. H. Bessesen, Obesity as a factor, *Nutrition Reviews* 58 (2000): S12–S15; M. Rosenbaum and coauthors, Effects of changes in body weight on carbohydrate metabolism, catecholamine excretion, and thyroid function, *American Journal of Clinical Nutrition* 71 (2000): 1421–1432.
37. P. Maison and coauthors, Do different dimensions of the metabolic syndrome change together over time? Evidence supporting obesity as the central feature, *Diabetes Care* 24 (2001): 1758–1763.
38. B. A. Gower and coauthors, Effects of weight loss on changes in insulin sensitivity and lipid concentrations in premenopausal African American and white women, *American Journal of Clinical Nutrition* 76 (2002): 923–927.
39. D. S. Michaud and coauthors, Physical activity, obesity, height, and the risk of pancreatic cancer, *Journal of the American Medical Association* 286 (2001): 921–929; G. H. Rauscher, S. T. Mayne, and D. T. Janerich, Relation between body mass index and lung cancer risk in men and women never and former smokers, *American Journal of Epidemiology* 152 (2000): 506–513; W. H. Chow and coauthors, Obesity, hypertension, and the risk of kidney cancer in men, *New England Journal of Medicine* 343 (2000): 1305–1311; S. D. Li and S. Mobarhan, Association between body mass index and adenocarcinoma of the esophagus and gastric cardia, *Nutrition Reviews* 58 (2000): 54–56; J. Kermström and E. Barrett-Connor, Obesity, weight change, fasting insulin, proinsulin, C-peptide, and insulin-like growth factor-1 levels in women with and without breast cancer: The Rancho Bernardo Study, *Journal of Women's Health and Gender-based Medicine* 8 (1999): 1265–1272.
40. G. A. Bray, The underlying basis for obesity: Relationship to cancer, *Journal of Nutrition* 132 (2002): 3451S–3455S.
41. S. W. Farrell and coauthors, The relation of body mass index, cardiorespiratory fitness, and all-cause mortality in women, *Obesity Research* 10 (2002): 417–423; C. D. Lee and S. N. Blair, Cardiorespiratory fitness and smoking-related and total cancer mortality in men, *Medicine and Science in Sports and Exercise* 34 (2002): 735–739; C. D. Lee and S. N. Blair, Cardiorespiratory fitness and stroke mortality in men, *Medicine and Science in Sports and Exercise* 34 (2002): 592–595; M. Wei and coauthors, Relationship between low cardiorespiratory fitness and mortality in normal-weight, overweight, and obese men, *Journal of the American Medical Association* 282 (1999): 1547–1553.

ANSWERS

Nutrition Calculations

1. a. 0.045 kcal/lb/min × 142 lb = 6.4 kcal/min.
   6.4 kcal/min × 120 min = 768 kcal.
   b. 0.103 kcal/lb/min × 142 lb = 14.6 kcal/min.
   14.6 kcal/min × 20 min = 292 kcal.
   c. 0.032 kcal/lb/min × 142 lb = 4.5 kcal/min.
   4.5 kcal/min × 45 min = 202.5 kcal.
   d. 0.035 kcal/lb/min × 142 lb = 5 kcal/min.
   5 kcal/min × 60 min = 300 kcal.
2. The infant has the faster BMR (500 kcal/day ÷ 20 lb = 25 kcal/lb/day and 1500 kcal/day ÷ 170 lb = 8.8 kcal/lb/day).
   Because the infant has a BMR of 25 kcal/lb, whereas the adult has a BMR of 8.8 kcal/lb, the infant's BMR is almost 3 times faster than the adult's based on body weight.
3. EER = 354 − 6.91 × 20 + 1.12 × [(9.36 × 59) + (726 × 1.68)].
   EER = 354 − 138.2 + 1.12 (552.24 + 1219.68).
   EER = 354 − 138.2 + 1984.6 = 2200 kcal/day.
4. 21 ÷ 0.172 = 122 lb. Yes.

Study Questions (multiple choice)

1. c 2. b 3. c 4. a 5. a 6. c 7. b 8. b
9. a 10. d

HIGHLIGHT

The Latest and Greatest Weight-Loss Diet—Again

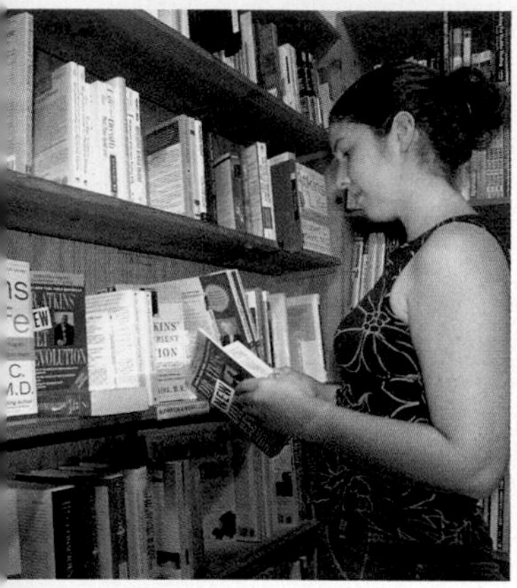

© Geri Engberg

To paraphrase William Shakespeare, "a fad diet by any other name would still be a fad diet." And the names are legion: the Atkins New Diet Revolution, the Calories Don't Count diet, the Protein Power diet, the Carbohydrate Addict's diet, the Lo-Carbo diet, the Healthy for Life diet, the Zone diet.* Year after year, "new and improved" diets appear on bookstore shelves and circulate among friends. People of all sizes eagerly try the best diet on the market ever, hoping that this one will really work. Sometimes fad diets seem to work for a while, but more often than not, their success is short-lived. Then another fad diet takes the spotlight. Here's how Dr. K. Brownell, an obesity researcher at Yale University, describes this phenomenon: "When I get calls about the latest diet fad, I imagine a trick birthday cake candle that keeps lighting up and we have to keep blowing it out."

Realizing that fad diets do not offer a safe and effective plan for weight loss, health professionals speak out, but they never get the candle blown out permanently. New fad diets can keep making outrageous claims because no one requires their advocates to prove what they say. Fad diet gurus do not have to conduct credible research on the benefits or dangers of their diets. They can simply make recommendations and then later, if questioned, search for bits and pieces of research that support the conclusions they have already reached. That's backwards. Diet and health recommendations should *follow* years of sound research that has been reviewed by panels of scientists *before* being offered to the public.

Because anyone can publish anything—in books or on the Internet—peddlers of fad diets can make unsubstantiated statements that fall far short of the truth, but sound impressive to the uninformed. They often offer distorted bits of legitimate research. They may start with one or more actual facts, but then leap from one erroneous conclusion to the next. Anyone who wants to believe them is forced to wonder how the thousands of scientists working on obesity research over the past century could possibly have missed such obvious connections. Table H8-1 presents some of the claims and truths of fad diets.

*The following sources offer comparisons and evaluations of various fad diets for your review: S. T. St. Jeor and coauthors, Dietary protein and weight reduction: A statement for healthcare professionals from the nutrition committee of the Council on Nutrition, Physical Activity, and Metabolism of the American Heart Association, *Circulation* 104 (2001): 1869–1874; G. L. Blackburn and V. H. He, The changing nature of obesity in the U.S.: How serious is the problem? *Nutrition & the M.D.*, June 1999, pp. 3–7.

TABLE H8-1 The Claims and Truths of Fad Diets

The Claim:	You can lose weight with "exceptionally easy rules."
The Truth:	Most fad diet plans have complicated rules that require you to calculate protein requirements, count carbohydrate grams, combine certain foods, time meal intervals, purchase special products, plan daily menus, and measure serving sizes.
The Claim:	You can lose weight by eating a specific ratio of carbohydrates, protein, and fat.
The Truth:	Weight loss depends on spending more energy than you take in.
The Claim:	This "revolutionary diet" can "reset your genetic code."
The Truth:	You inherited your genes and cannot alter your genetic code.
The Claim:	High-protein diets are popular, selling more than 20 million books, because they work.
The Truth:	Weight-loss books are popular because people grasp for quick fixes and simple solutions to their weight problems. If book sales were an indication of weight-loss success, we would be a lean nation—but they're not, and neither are we.
The Claim:	People gain weight on low-fat diets.
The Truth:	People can gain weight on low-fat diets if they overindulge in carbohydrates and proteins while cutting fat; low-fat diets are not necessarily low-kcalorie diets. But people can also lose weight on low-fat diets if they cut kcalories as well as fat.
The Claim:	High-protein diets energize the brain.
The Truth:	The brain depends on glucose for its energy; the primary dietary source of glucose is carbohydrate, not protein.
The Claim:	Thousands of people have been successful with this plan.
The Truth:	Authors of fad diets have not published their research findings in scientific journals. Success stories are anecdotal and failures are not reported.
The Claim:	Carbohydrates raise blood glucose levels, triggering insulin production and fat storage.
The Truth:	Insulin promotes fat storage when energy intake exceeds energy needs. Furthermore, insulin is only one hormone involved in the complex processes of maintaining the body's energy balance and health.
The Claim:	Eat protein and lose weight.
The Truth:	For every complicated problem, there is a simple—and wrong—solution.

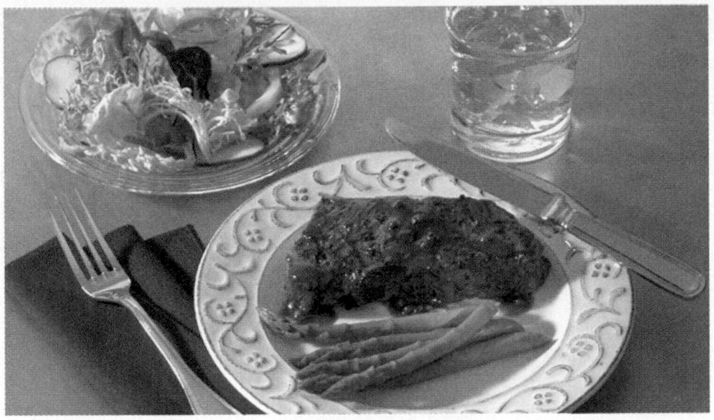

Matthew Farruggio

High-protein, low-carbohydrate meals overemphasize meat, fish, poultry, eggs, and cheeses, and shun breads, pastas, fruits, and vegetables.

No matter what their names are, most fad diets espouse essentially the same high-protein, low-carbohydrate diet. After all, diets may come in all flavors, but only in three proportions: high fat, high carbohydrate, or high protein. Few consumers would believe that high-fat diets could lead to weight loss; contrary to such a claim, dietary fat does not promote fat oxidation. Consumers already hear from many free sources that high-carbohydrate diets support good health, so peddling that idea would not be a profitable venture. That leaves high-protein diets, and they surface regularly in various guises as the best way to lose weight. High-protein diets are by design relatively low in carbohydrate. This highlight examines some of the science and the science fiction behind high-protein, low-carbohydrate fad diets.

The Diet's Appeal

Perhaps the greatest appeal of a high-protein, low-carbohydrate diet is that it turns current diet recommendations upside down. Foods such as meats and milk products that need to be selected carefully to limit saturated fat can now be eaten with abandon. Grains, legumes, vegetables, and fruits that we are told to eat in abundance can now be ignored. For some people, this is a dream come true: steaks without the potatoes, ribs without the coleslaw, and meatballs without the pasta. Who can resist the promise of weight loss while eating freely from a list of favorite foods?

To lure dieters in, proponents of high-protein diets often blame the currently recommended high-carbohydrate, low-fat diet for our obesity troubles. They claim that the incidence of obesity is rising because we are eating less fat. Such a claim may impress the naive, but it sends skeptical people running for the facts. True, the incidence of obesity has risen dramatically over the past two decades.[1] True, our intake of fat has dropped from 35 to 33 percent of daily energy intake.[2] Such facts might seem to imply that lowering fat intake leads to obesity, but this is an erroneous conclusion. The *percentage* declined only because average energy intakes increased by almost 200 kcalories a day (from 1878 kcalories a day to 2056). Actual fat intake *increased* by 3 grams a day (from 73 grams to 76). Furthermore, fewer than half of us engage in regular physical activity.[3] Obesity experts blame our high energy intakes and low energy outputs for the increase in obesity. Weight loss, after all, depends on a negative energy balance. To their credit, some of these diet plans recommend exercise—and regular physical activity is an integral component of successful weight loss.[4]

Dieters are also lured into fad diets by sophisticated—yet often erroneous—explanations of the metabolic consequences of eating certain foods. Terms such as *eicosanoids* and *de novo lipogenesis* are scattered about, intimidating readers into believing that the authors must be right given their brilliance in understanding the body.

One common misconception currently circulating amongst fad diets focuses on insulin. High-protein diet proponents claim that carbohydrates are bad. Some go so far as to equate carbohydrates with toxic poisons or addictive drugs. Starches and sugars are considered evil because they are absorbed easily and raise blood glucose. The pancreas then responds by secreting insulin—and insulin is touted as the real villain responsible for our nation's epidemic of obesity.

What does insulin do? Among its roles, insulin facilitates the transport of glucose into the cells, the storage of fatty acids as fat, and the synthesis of cholesterol. It is an anabolic hormone that builds and stores. True—but not the whole truth and nothing but the truth. Insulin is only one of many factors involved in the body's metabolism of nutrients and regulation of body weight.[5] Furthermore, as Chapter 4's discussion of the glycemic index pointed out, blood glucose and insulin do not always respond to foods as might be expected. Many carbohydrates—fruits, vegetables, legumes, and whole grains—are rich in fibers that slow glucose absorption and moderate insulin response. Most importantly, insulin is critical to maintaining health, as any person with type 1 diabetes can attest. Insulin causes problems only when a person develops insulin resistance—that is, when the body's cells do not respond to the large quantities of insulin that the pancreas continues to pump out in an effort to get a response. Insulin resistance is a major health problem—but it is not caused by carbohydrate, or by protein, or by fat. It results from being overweight. When a person loses weight, insulin response improves.

Another crazy distortion of the facts is the claim that high-protein foods expend more energy. As Chapter 8 mentioned, the thermic effect of food for protein is higher than for carbohydrate or fat, but the increase is still insignificant—perhaps the equivalent of two pounds per year.

If high-protein diets were as successful as some people claim, then consumers who tried them would lose lots of weight, and our obesity problems would be solved. Obviously, this is not the case. Similarly, if high-protein diets were as worthless as others claim, then consumers would eventually stop pursuing them. Clearly, this is not happening either. These diets have enough going for them that they work for some people at least for a short time, but they fail to produce long-lasting results for most people. Studies report that people following high-protein, low-carbohydrate diets do lose weight.[6] In fact, they lose more than people following conventional high-carbohydrate, low-fat diets—but only for the first six months. Their later gains make up the difference, so total weight loss is no different after one year.[7] The following sections examine some of the apparent achievements and shortcomings of high-protein diets.[8]

The Diet's Achievements

With over half of our nation's adults overweight and many more concerned about their weight, the market for a weight-loss book, product, or program is huge (no pun intended). Americans spend an estimated $33 billion a year on weight-loss books and products. Even a plan that offers only minimal weight-loss success easily attracts a following. High-protein diet plans offer a little success to some people for a short time. Here's why.

Don't Count kCalories

Who wants to count kcalories? Even experienced dieters find counting kcalories burdensome, not to mention timeworn. They want a new, easy way to lose weight, and high-protein diet plans seem to offer this boon. But while these diets often claim to disregard kcalories, their design typically ensures a low energy intake. They advise dieters to stop counting kcalories, but then recommend three meals "not to exceed 500 kcalories each and two snacks of less than 100 kcalories each." Most of the sample menu plans provided by these diets are designed to deliver 800 to 1200 kcalories a day.

Even when counting kcalories is truly not necessary, the total tends to be low simply because food intake is so limited. Without its refried beans, tortilla wrapping, and chopped vegetables, a burrito is reduced to a pile of ground beef. Without the baked potato, there's no need for butter and sour cream. Weight loss occurs because of the low energy intake—not the proportion of energy nutrients.[9] Success, then, depends on the restricted intake, not on protein's magical powers or carbohydrate's evil forces. This is an important point. Any diet can produce weight loss, at least temporarily, if intake is restricted. The real value of a diet is determined by its ability to maintain weight loss and support good health over the long term. The goal is not simply weight loss, but health gains—and whether high-protein, low-carbohydrate diets can support optimal health over time remains unknown.

Satisfy Hunger

As Chapter 8 mentioned, of the three energy-yielding nutrients, protein is the most satiating. Consequently, high-protein meals may suppress hunger and delay the start of the next meal. Furthermore, studies have reported that people tend to eat less after a high-protein meal than after a low-protein one.[10] In real-life situations, though, there is a strong association between a person's protein intake and BMI—the higher the intake, the higher the BMI.[11] This association remains apparent even after adjusting for energy intake and physical activity. All meals—whether designed for weight loss or not—should include enough protein to satisfy hunger, but not so much as to contribute to weight gain.

Follow a Plan

Most people need specific instructions and examples to make dietary changes. Fad diets offer dieters a plan. The user doesn't have to decide what foods to eat, how to prepare them, or how much to eat. Unfortunately, these instructions serve short-term weight-loss needs only. They do not provide for long-term changes in lifestyle that will support weight maintenance or health goals.

The success of any weight-loss diet depends on the person adopting the plan and sticking with it. People who prefer the high-protein, low-carbohydrate diet over the high-carbohydrate, low-fat diet may have more success at sticking with it. Again, weight loss occurs because of the duration of a low-kcalorie plan—not the proportion of energy nutrients.[12]

Limit Choices

Diets that omit hundreds of foods and several food groups limit a person's options and lack variety. Chapter 2 praised variety as a valuable way to ensure an adequate intake of nutrients, but variety also entices people to eat more food and gain more weight.[13] Without variety, some people lose interest in eating, which further reduces energy intake. Even if the allowed foods are favorites, eating the same foods week after week can become monotonous.

The Diet's Shortcomings

People who have followed high-protein diet plans for several months have lost weight. But can these diets also be harmful?

Too Much Fat

Some fad diets focus so intently on promoting protein and curbing carbohydrate that they fail to account for the fat that accompanies many high-protein foods. A breakfast of bacon and eggs, lunch of ham and cheese, and dinner of barbecued short ribs would provide 100 grams of protein—and 121 grams of fat! Yet this day's meals, even with a snack of peanuts, provide only 1600 kcalories. Without careful selection, protein-rich diets can be extraordinarily high in saturated fat and cholesterol—dietary factors that raise LDL cholesterol and the risks for heart disease.

Overall, studies report that people following high-protein, low-carbohydrate diets have little or no change in blood pressure or blood lipids—risk factors for heart disease.[14] Some researchers speculate that the weight loss that occurs on these diets offsets the adverse effects of a diet high in saturated fat and low in fruits and vegetables.[15]

Too Much Protein

Moderation has been a recurring theme throughout this text, with recommendations to get enough, but not too much, and cautions that too much can be as harmful as too little. The DRI Committee did not establish an upper limit for protein, but it does recognize that high-protein diets have been implicated in chronic diseases such as osteoporosis, kidney stones and kidney disease, some cancers, heart disease, and obesity.[16] One four-month study reports no adverse effects on bone metabolism.[17] Health recommendations typically advise a protein intake of 50 to 100 grams per day and within the range of 10 to 35 percent of energy intake.[18] Popular high-protein diets suggest a protein intake of 70 to 160 grams per day, representing 25 to 65 percent of energy intake.[19]

Too Little Everything Else

The quality of the diet suffers when carbohydrates are restricted.[20] Without fruits, vegetables, and whole grains, high-protein diets lack not only carbohydrate, but fiber, vitamins, minerals, and phytochemicals as well—all dietary factors protective against disease. To help shore up some of these inadequacies, fad diets often recommend a daily supplement. Conveniently, many of the companies selling fad diets also peddle these supplements. But as Highlights 10 and 11 explain, foods offer many more health benefits than any supplement can provide. Quite simply, if the diet is inadequate, it needs to be improved, not supplemented.

The Body's Perspective

When a person consumes a low-carbohydrate diet, a metabolism similar to that of fasting prevails (see Chapter 7 for a review of fasting). With little dietary carbohydrate coming in, the body uses its glycogen stores to provide glucose for the cells of the brain, nerves, and blood. Once the body depletes its glycogen reserves, it begins making glucose from the amino acids of protein (gluconeogenesis). A low-carbohydrate diet may provide abundant protein from food, but the body still uses some protein from body tissues.

Dieters can know glycogen depletion has occurred and gluconeogenesis has begun by monitoring their urine. Whenever glycogen or protein is broken down, water is released and urine production increases. Low-carbohydrate diets also induce ketosis, and ketones can be detected in the urine. Ketones form whenever glucose is lacking and fat breakdown is incomplete.

Many fad diets regard ketosis as the key to losing weight, but a study comparing weight-loss diets found no relation between ketosis and weight loss.[21] People in ketosis may experience a loss of appetite and a dramatic weight loss within the first few days. They would be disillusioned if they were aware that much of this weight loss reflects the loss of glycogen and protein together with large quantities of body fluids and important minerals.[22] They need to learn to appreciate the difference between loss of *fat* and loss of *weight.* Fat losses on ketogenic diets are no greater than on other diets providing the same number of kcalories. Once the dieter returns to well-balanced meals that provide adequate energy, carbohydrate, fat, protein, vitamins, and minerals, the body avidly retains these needed nutrients. The weight will return, quite often to a level higher than the starting point. Table H8-2 lists other consequences of a ketogenic diet.

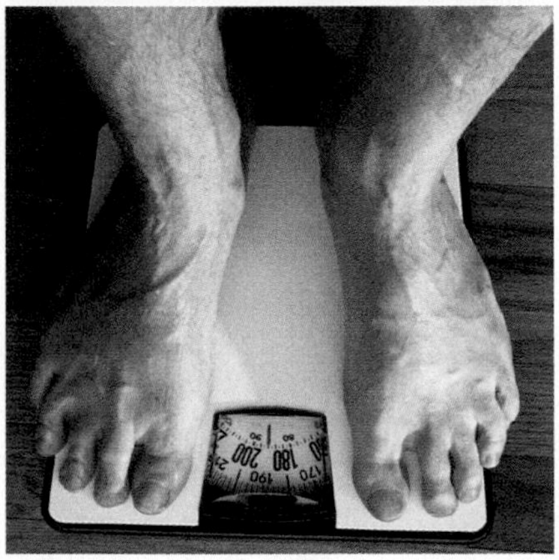

The wise consumer distinguishes between loss of fat and loss of weight.

Table H8-3 offers guidelines for identifying fad diets and other weight-loss scams; it includes the hallmarks of a reasonable weight-loss program as well. Diets that overemphasize protein and fall short on carbohydrate may not harm healthy people if used for only a little while, but they cannot support optimal health for long. Chapter 9 includes reasonable approaches to weight management and concludes that the ideal diet is one you can live with for the rest of your life. Keep that criterion in mind when you evaluate the next "latest and greatest weight-loss diet" that comes along.

TABLE H8-2 Adverse Side Effects of Low-Carbohydrate, Ketogenic Diets

- Nausea
- Fatigue (especially if physically active)
- Constipation
- Low blood pressure
- Elevated uric acid (which may exacerbate kidney disease and cause inflammation of the joints in those predisposed to gout)
- Stale, foul taste in the mouth (bad breath)
- In pregnant women, fetal harm and stillbirth

TABLE H8-3 Guidelines for Identifying Fad Diets and Other Weight-Loss Scams

1. They promise dramatic, rapid weight loss. Weight loss should be gradual and not exceed 2 pounds per week.
2. They promote diets that are nutritionally unbalanced or extremely low in kcalories. Diets should provide:
   - A reasonable number of kcalories (not fewer than 1200 kcalories per day for women and 1500 kcalories per day for men).
   - Enough, but not too much, protein (between the RDA and twice the RDA).
   - Enough, but not too much fat (between 20 and 35 percent of daily energy intake from fat).
   - Enough carbohydrate to spare protein and prevent ketosis (at least 100 grams per day) and 20 to 30 grams of fiber from food sources.
   - A balanced assortment of vitamins and minerals from a variety of foods from each of the food groups.
   - At least 1 liter (about 1 quart) of water daily or 1 milliliter per kcalorie daily—whichever is more.
3. They use liquid formulas rather than foods. Foods should accommodate a person's ethnic background, taste preferences, and financial means.
4. They attempt to make clients dependent upon special foods or devices. Programs should teach clients how to make good choices from the conventional food supply.
5. They fail to encourage permanent, realistic lifestyle changes. Programs should provide physical activity plans that involve spending at least 300 kcalories a day and behavior-modification strategies that help to correct poor eating habits.
6. They misrepresent salespeople as "counselors" supposedly qualified to give guidance in nutrition and/or general health. Even if adequately trained, such "counselors" would still be objectionable because of the obvious conflict of interest that exists when providers profit directly from products they recommend and sell.
7. They collect large sums of money at the start or require that clients sign contracts for expensive, long-term programs. Programs should be reasonably priced and run on a pay-as-you-go basis.
8. They fail to inform clients of the risks associated with weight loss in general or the specific program being promoted. They should provide information about dropout rates, the long-term success of their clients, and possible side effects.
9. They promote unproven or spurious weight-loss aids such as human chorionic gonadotropin hormone (HCG), starch blockers, diuretics, sauna belts, body wraps, passive exercise, ear stapling, acupuncture, electric muscle-stimulating (EMS) devices, spirulina, amino acid supplements (e.g., arginine, ornithine), glucomannan, methylcellulose (a "bulking agent"), "unique" ingredients, and so forth.
10. They fail to provide for weight maintenance after the program ends.

SOURCES: Adapted from American College of Sports Medicine, *ACSM's Guidelines for Exercise Testing and Prescription* (Baltimore: Williams & Wilkins, 1995), pp. 218–219; J. T. Dwyer, Treatment of obesity: Conventional programs and fad diets, in *Obesity*, ed. P. Björntorp and B. N. Brodoff (Philadelphia: J. B. Lippincott, 1992), p. 668; *National Council Against Health Fraud Newsletter*, March/April 1987, National Council Against Health Fraud, Inc.

NUTRITION ON THE NET

Access these websites for further study of topics covered in this highlight.

- Find updates and quick links to these and other nutrition-related sites at our website: **www.wadsworth.com/nutrition**
- Search for the Great Nutrition Debate at the USDA's site: **www.usda.gov**

REFERENCES

1. A. H. Mokdad and coauthors, The spread of the obesity epidemic in the United States, 1991–1998, *Journal of the American Medical Association* 282 (1999): 1519–1522.
2. P. Chanmugam and coauthors, Did fat intake in the United States really decline between 1989–1991 and 1994–1996? *Journal of the American Dietetic Association* 103 (2003): 867–872.
3. P. M. Barnes and C. A. Schoenborn, *Physical Activity among Adults: United States, 2000*, 2003, available at **www.cdc.gov/nchs/about/major/nhis/released200306.htm#7**.
4. M. Jakicic and coauthors, Appropriate intervention strategies for weight loss and prevention of weight regain for adults, *Medicine and Science in Sports and Exercise* 33 (2001): 2145–2156.
5. J. C. Brüning and coauthors, Role of brain insulin receptor in control of body weight and reproduction, *Science* 289 (2000): 2122–2125.
6. E. C. Westman and coauthors, Effect of 6-month adherence to a very low carbohydrate diet program, *American Journal of Medicine* 113 (2002): 30–36.
7. G. D. Foster and coauthors, A randomized trial of a low-carbohydrate diet for obesity, *New England Journal of Medicine* 348 (2003): 2082–2090.
8. J. Eisenstein and coauthors, High-protein weight-loss diets: Are they safe and do they work? A review of the experimental and epidemiologic data, *Nutrition Reviews* 60 (2002): 189–200.
9. D. K. Layman and coauthors, A reduced ratio of dietary carbohydrate to protein improves body composition and blood lipid profiles during weight loss in adult women, *Journal of Nutrition* 133 (2003): 411–417; D. M. Bravata and coauthors, Efficacy and safety of low-carbohydrate diets, *Journal of the American Medical Association* 289 (2003): 1837–1850; M. R. Freedman, J. King, and E. Kennedy, Popular

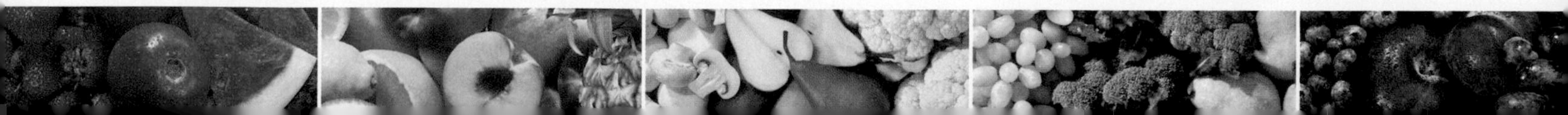

diets: A scientific review, *Obesity Research* 9 (2001): 1S–5S; A. Golay and coauthors, Similar weight loss with low-energy food combining or balanced diets, *International Journal of Obesity and Related Metabolic Disorders* 24 (2000): 492–496; N. H. Baba and coauthors, High protein vs high carbohydrate hypoenergetic diet for the treatment of obese hyperinsulinemic subjects, *International Journal of Obesity and Related Metabolic Disorders* 23 (1999): 1202–1206.
10. A. R. Skov and coauthors, Randomized trial on protein vs carbohydrate in ad libitum fat reduced diet for the treatment of obesity, *International Journal of Obesity and Related Metabolic Disorders* 23 (1999): 528–536.
11. A. Trichopoulou and coauthors, Lipid, protein and carbohydrate intake in relation to body mass index, *European Journal of Clinical Nutrition* 56 (2002): 37-43.
12. Bravata and coauthors, 2003.
13. M. A. McCrory and coauthors, Dietary variety within food groups: Association with energy and body fatness in men and women, *American Journal of Clinical Nutrition* 69 (1999): 440–447.
14. Bravata and coauthors, 2003.
15. Foster and coauthors, 2003.
16. Committee on Dietary Reference Intakes, *Dietary Reference Intakes for Energy, Carbohydrate, Fiber, Fat, Fatty Acids, Cholesterol, Protein, and Amino Acids* (Washington, D.C.: National Academies Press, 2002).
17. E. Farnsworth and coauthors, Effect of a high-protein, energy-restricted diet on body composition, glycemic control, and lipid concentrations in overweight and obese hyperinsulinemic men and women, *American Journal of Clinical Nutrition* 78 (2003): 31–39.
18. Committee on Dietary Reference Intakes, 2002; S. T. St. Jeor and coauthors, Dietary protein and weight reduction: A statement for healthcare professionals from the nutrition committee of the Council on Nutrition, Physical Activity, and Metabolism of the American Heart Association, *Circulation* 104 (2001): 1869–1874.
19. St. Jeor and coauthors, 2001.
20. E. T. Kennedy and coauthors, Popular diets: Correlation to health, nutrition, and obesity, *Journal of the American Dietetic Association* 101 (2001): 411–420.
21. Foster and coauthors, 2003.
22. St. Jeor and coauthors, 2001.

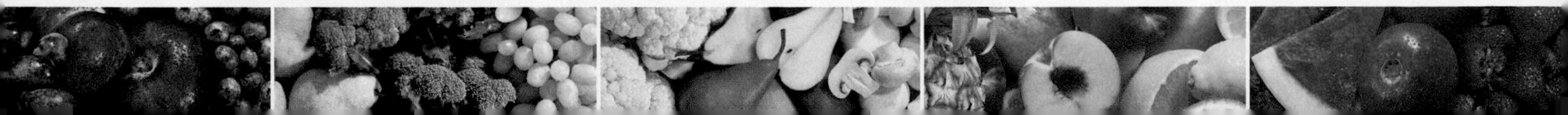

Chapter 9

Weight Management: Overweight and Underweight

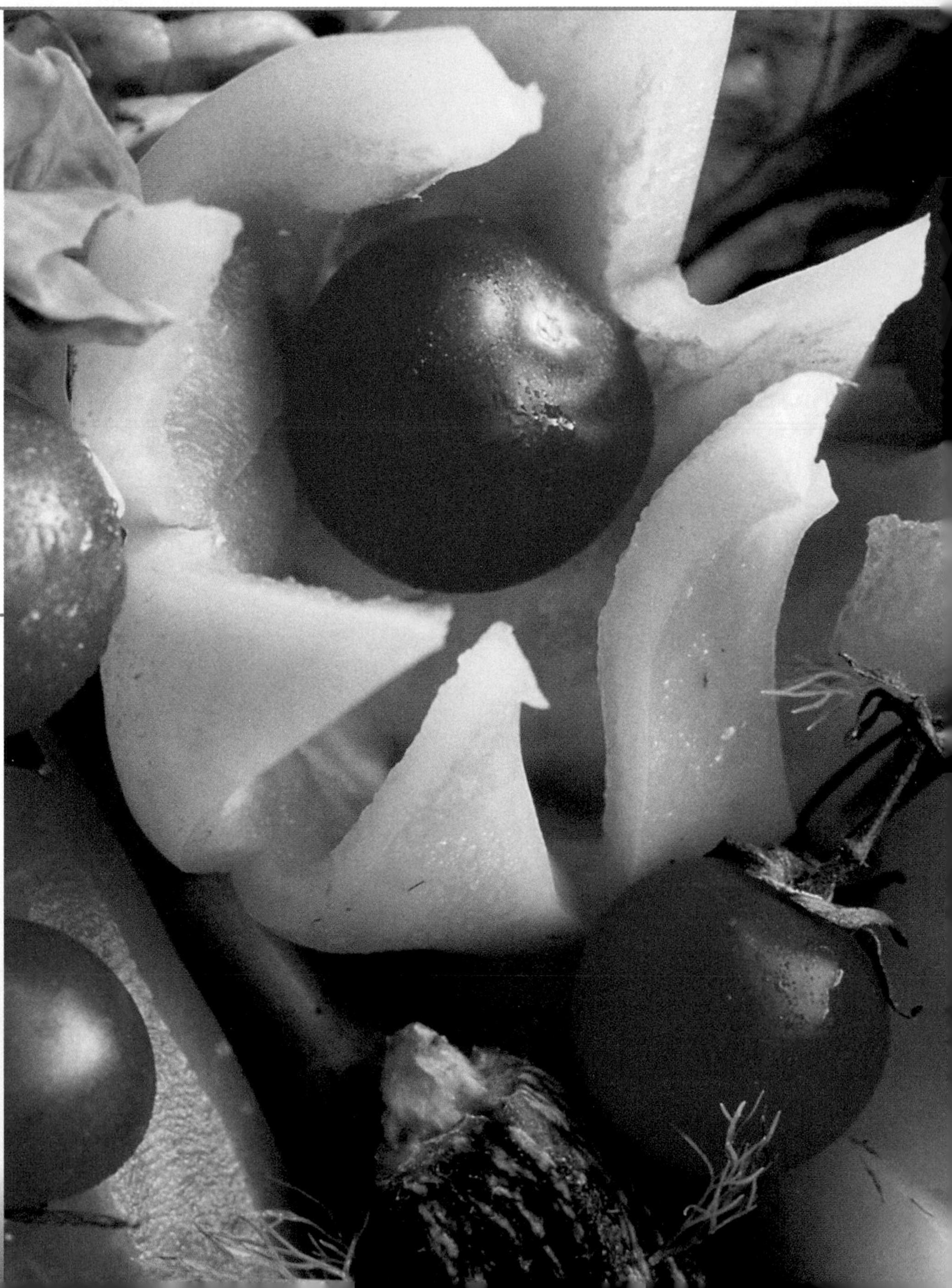

© Ken Scott/Stone/Getty Images

Chapter Outline

Available Online

http://nutrition.wadsworth.com/uncn7

Nutrition Animation: *Balancing Energy In and Energy Out*

Student Practice Test

Glossary Terms

Nutrition on the Net

Nutrition in Your Life

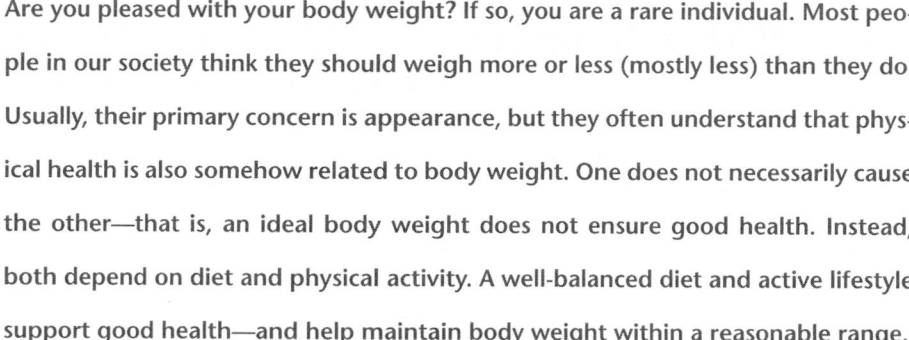

Are you pleased with your body weight? If so, you are a rare individual. Most people in our society think they should weigh more or less (mostly less) than they do. Usually, their primary concern is appearance, but they often understand that physical health is also somehow related to body weight. One does not necessarily cause the other—that is, an ideal body weight does not ensure good health. Instead, both depend on diet and physical activity. A well-balanced diet and active lifestyle support good health—and help maintain body weight within a reasonable range.

The previous chapter described how body weight is stable when energy in equals energy out. Weight gains occur when energy intake exceeds energy expended, and conversely, weight losses occur when energy expended exceeds energy intake. At the extremes, both overweight and underweight present health risks. This chapter emphasizes overweight, partly because it has been more intensively studied and partly because it is a widespread health problem in developed countries and a growing concern in developing countries. Information on underweight is presented wherever appropriate. The highlight that follows this chapter delves into the eating disorders anorexia nervosa and bulimia nervosa.

Overweight

Despite our preoccupation with body image and weight loss, the prevalence of overweight and obesity in the United States continues to rise dramatically.[1] In the past decade, obesity increased in every state, in both genders, and across all ages, races, and educational levels (see Figure 9-1). Over half of the adults in the United States are now considered overweight or obese, as defined by a BMI of 25 or

■ BMI:
- Healthy weight: 18.5–24.9.
- Overweight: 25.0–29.9.
- Obese: ≥30.

FIGURE 9-1 Increasing Prevalence of Obesity (BMI ≥30) among U.S. Adults

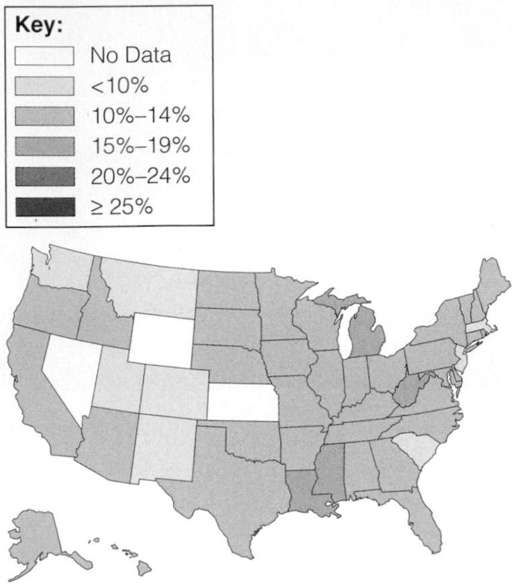
Key:
No Data
<10%
10%–14%
15%–19%
20%–24%
≥ 25%

1991: Only four states had obesity rates greater than 15 percent.

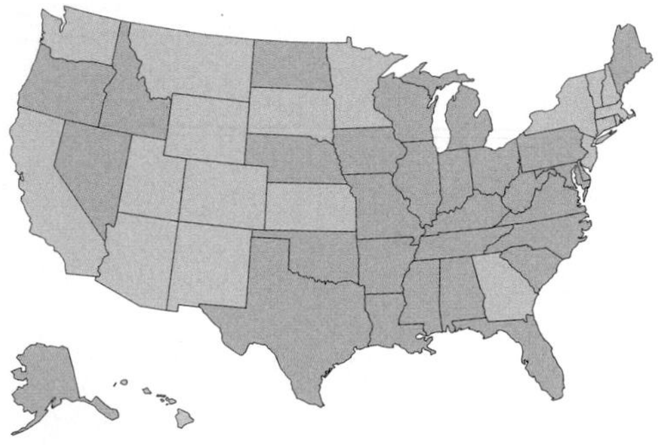

1996: Over half of the states had obesity rates greater than 15 percent.

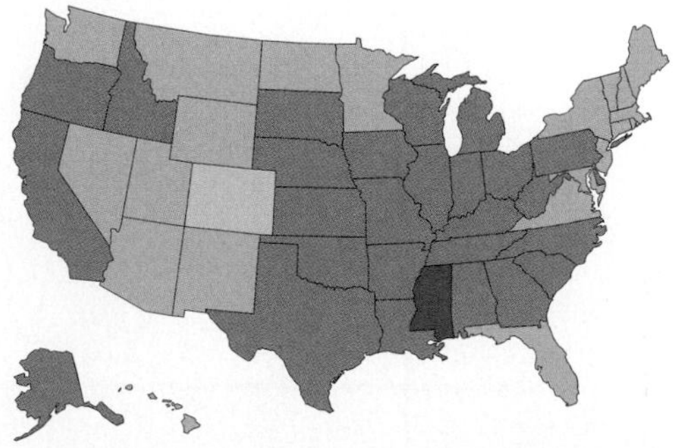

2001: Only one state had an obesity rate below 15 percent, most had obesity rates greater than 20 percent, and one had an obesity rate greater than 25 percent.

SOURCE: Mokdad A. H., et al. *Journal of the American Medical Association* 1999, 282:16; 2001, 286:10.

greater.■ The prevalence of overweight is especially high among women, the poor, blacks, and Hispanics.

The prevalence of overweight among children in the United States is also rising at an alarming rate. An estimated 15 percent of children and adolescents ages 6 to 19 years are overweight. Chapter 15 presents information on overweight during childhood and adolescence.

Obesity is so widespread and its prevalence is rising so rapidly that many refer to it as an **epidemic.**[2] According to the World Health Organization, this epidemic of obesity has spread worldwide, affecting over 300 million adults. Contrary to popular opinion, obesity is not limited to industrialized nations; over 115 million people in developing countries suffer from obesity-related problems. Before examining the suspected causes of obesity and the various strategies used to treat it, it may be helpful to understand the development and metabolism of body fat.

HEALTHY PEOPLE 2010

Increase the proportion of adults who are at healthy weight. Reduce the proportion of adults who are obese.

Fat Cell Development

When more energy is consumed than is spent, much of the excess energy is stored in the fat cells of adipose tissue. The amount of fat in a person's body reflects both the *number* and the *size* of the fat cells. The number of fat cells increases most rapidly during the growing years of late childhood and early puberty. After growth ceases, fat cell number may continue to increase whenever energy balance is positive. Obese people have more fat cells than healthy-weight people; their fat cells are also larger.

When energy intake exceeds expenditure, the fat cells accumulate triglycerides and expand in size (review Figure 5-20 on p. 157). When the cells enlarge, they stimulate cell proliferation so that their numbers increase again.[3] Thus obesity develops■ when a person's fat cells increase in number, in size, or quite often both. Figure 9-2 illustrates fat cell development.

When energy out exceeds energy in, the size of fat cells dwindles, but not their number. People with extra fat cells tend to regain lost weight rapidly; with weight gain, their many fat cells readily fill. In contrast, people with an average number of enlarged fat cells may be more successful in maintaining weight losses; when their cells shrink, both cell size and number are normal. Prevention of obesity is most critical, then, during the growing years when fat cells increase in number.

As mentioned, excess fat is typically stored in adipose tissue. This stored fat may be well tolerated, but fat accumulation in organs such as the heart or liver clearly plays a key role in the development of diseases such as heart failure or fatty liver.[4]■

Fat Cell Metabolism

The enzyme lipoprotein lipase (LPL)■ promotes fat storage in both adipose and muscle cells. Obese people generally have much more LPL activity in their fat cells than lean people do (their muscle cell LPL activity is similar, though). This high LPL activity makes fat storage especially efficient. Consequently, even modest excesses in energy intake have a more dramatic impact on obese people than on lean people.

The activity of LPL is partially regulated by gender-specific hormones—estrogen in women and testosterone in men. In women, fat cells in the breasts, hips, and thighs produce abundant LPL, putting fat away in those body sites; in men, fat

FIGURE 9-2 Fat Cell Development

Fat cells are capable of increasing their size by 20-fold and their number by several thousandfold.

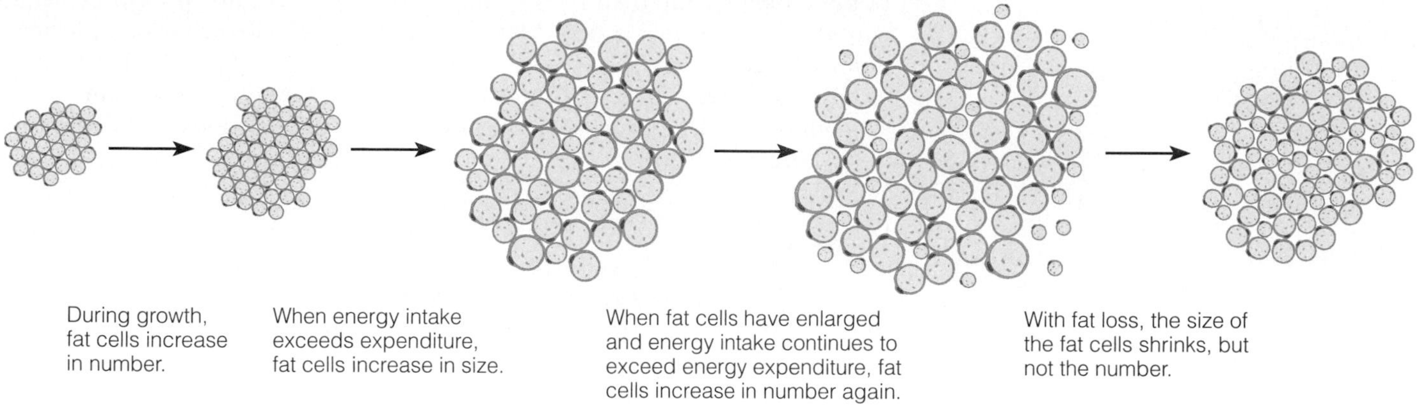
During growth, fat cells increase in number.
When energy intake exceeds expenditure, fat cells increase in size.
When fat cells have enlarged and energy intake continues to exceed energy expenditure, fat cells increase in number again.
With fat loss, the size of the fat cells shrinks, but not the number.

cells in the abdomen produce abundant LPL. This enzyme activity explains why men tend to develop central obesity around the abdomen whereas women more readily develop lower-body fat around the hips and thighs.

Gender differences are also apparent in the activity of the enzymes controlling the release and breakdown of fat in various parts of the body.[5] The release of lower-body fat is less active in women than in men, whereas the release of upper-body fat is similar. Furthermore, basal fat oxidation is lower in women than in men. Consequently, women may have a more difficult time losing fat in general, and from the hips and thighs in particular.

Enzyme activity may also explain why some people who lose weight regain it so easily. After weight loss, LPL activity increases, and it does so most dramatically in people who were fattest prior to weight loss. Apparently, weight loss serves as a signal to the gene that produces the LPL enzyme, saying "Make more enzyme to store fat." People easily regain weight after having lost it because they are battling against enzymes that want to store fat. The activities of these and other proteins provide an explanation for the observation that some inner mechanism seems to set a person's weight or body composition at a fixed point; the body will adjust to restore that **set point** if the person tries to change it.

- Obesity due to an increase in the *number* of fat cells is **hyperplastic obesity**. Obesity due to an increase in the *size* of fat cells is **hypertrophic obesity.**

- The adverse effects of fat in nonadipose tissues are known as **lipotoxicity.**

- Reminder: *Lipoprotein lipase (LPL)* is an enzyme that hydrolyzes triglycerides passing by in the bloodstream and directs their parts into the cells, where they can be metabolized or reassembled for storage.

Set-Point Theory

Many internal physiological variables, such as blood glucose, blood pH, and body temperature, remain fairly stable under a variety of conditions. The hypothalamus and other regulatory centers constantly monitor and delicately adjust conditions so as to maintain homeostasis.[6] The stability of such complex systems may depend on set-point regulators that maintain variables within specified limits.

Researchers have confirmed that after weight gains or losses, the body adjusts its metabolism so as to restore the original weight. Energy expenditure increases after weight gain and decreases after weight loss. These changes in energy expenditure differ from those expected based on body composition and help to explain why it is so difficult for an underweight person to maintain weight gains and an overweight person to maintain weight losses.

IN SUMMARY Fat cells develop by increasing in number and size. Prevention of excess weight gain depends on maintaining a reasonable number of fat cells. With gains or losses, the body adjusts to return to its previous status.

epidemic (EP-ee-DEM-ick): the appearance of a disease (usually infectious) or condition that attacks many people at the same time in the same region.
- **epi** = upon
- **demos** = people

set point: the point at which controls are set (for example, on a thermostat). The set-point theory that relates to body weight proposes that the body tends to maintain a certain weight by means of its own internal controls.

Causes of Obesity

Why do people accumulate excess body fat? The obvious answer is that they take in more food energy than they spend. But that answer falls short of explaining why they do this. Is it genetic? Environmental? Cultural? Behavioral? Socioeconomic? Psychological? Metabolic? All of these? Most likely, obesity has many interrelated causes. Why an imbalance between energy intake and energy expenditure occurs remains a bit of a mystery; the next sections summarize possible explanations.

Genetics

Genetics plays a true causative role in relatively few cases of obesity, for example, in Prader-Willi syndrome—a genetic disorder characterized by excessive appetite, massive obesity, short stature, and often mental retardation. Most cases of obesity, however, do not stem from a genetic mutation, yet genetic influences do seem to be involved.

Researchers have found that adopted children tend to be similar in weight to their biological parents, not to their adoptive parents. Studies of twins yield similar findings: identical twins are twice as likely to weigh the same as fraternal twins—even when reared apart. These findings suggest an important role for genetics in determining a person's *susceptibility* to obesity.[7] In other words, even if genes do not *cause* obesity, genetic factors may influence the food intake and activity patterns that lead to it and the metabolic pathways that maintain it.[8]

Clearly, something genetic makes a person more or less likely to gain or lose weight when overeating or undereating. Some people gain more weight than others on comparable energy intakes. Given an extra 1000 kcalories a day for 100 days, some pairs of identical twins gain less than 10 pounds while others gain up to 30 pounds. Within each pair, the amounts of weight gained, percentages of body fat, and locations of fat deposits are similar. Similarly, some people lose more weight than others following comparable exercise routines.

Researchers have been examining several genes in search of answers to obesity questions. As Chapter 6's section on protein synthesis described, each cell expresses only the genes for the proteins it needs, and each protein performs a unique function. The following paragraphs describe some recent research involving proteins that might help explain energy regulation and obesity development.[9]

Leptin Researchers have identified an obesity gene, called *ob,* that is expressed in the fat cells and codes for the protein **leptin.** Leptin acts as a hormone, primarily in the hypothalamus. Research suggests that leptin signals sufficient energy stores and promotes a negative energy balance by suppressing appetite and increasing energy expenditure.[10] Changes in energy expenditure primarily reflect changes in basal metabolism, but may also include changes in physical activity patterns.

Mice with a defective *ob* gene do not produce leptin and can weigh up to three times as much as normal mice and have five times as much body fat (see Figure 9-3). When injected with a synthetic form of leptin, the mice rapidly lose body fat. (Because leptin is a protein, it would be destroyed during digestion if given orally; consequently, it must be given by injection.) The fat cells not only lose fat, but they self-destruct (reducing cell number), which may explain why weight gains are delayed when the mice are fed again.

Although extremely rare, a genetic deficiency of leptin has been identified in human beings as well. An error in the gene that codes for leptin was discovered in three extremely obese children with barely detectable blood levels of leptin. Without leptin, the children have little appetite control; they are constantly hungry and eat considerably more than their siblings or peers. Given daily injections of leptin, these children lost a substantial amount of weight, confirming leptin's role in regulating appetite and body weight.[11]

leptin: a protein produced by fat cells under direction of the *ob* gene that decreases appetite and increases energy expenditure; sometimes called the ***ob* protein.**
- **leptos** = thin

FIGURE 9-3 Mice with and without Leptin Compared

Both of these mice have a defective *ob* gene. Consequently, they do not produce leptin. They both became obese, but the one on the right received daily injections of leptin, which suppressed food intake and increased energy expenditure, resulting in weight loss.

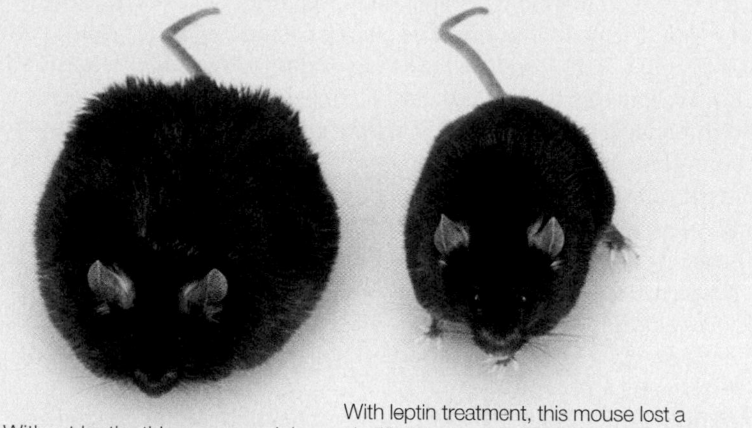

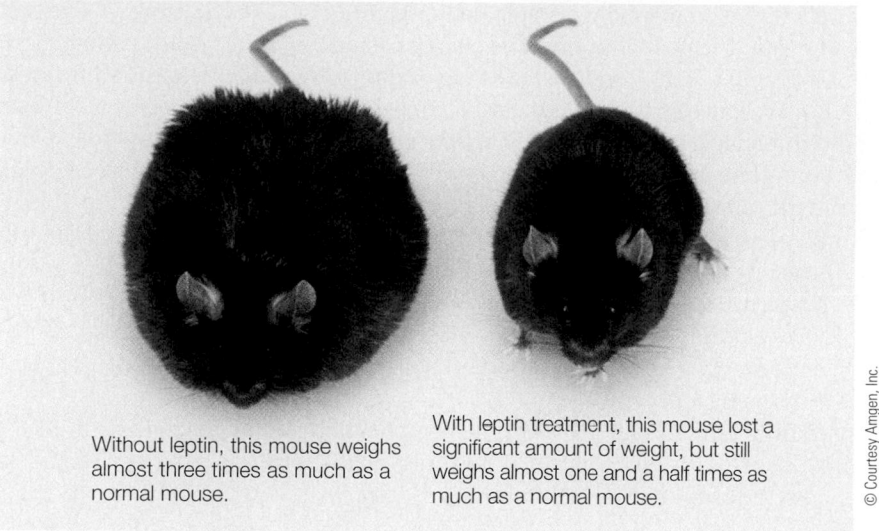

Without leptin, this mouse weighs almost three times as much as a normal mouse.

With leptin treatment, this mouse lost a significant amount of weight, but still weighs almost one and a half times as much as a normal mouse.

Not too surprisingly, leptin injections are only effective in suppressing appetite and supporting weight loss when overeating and obesity are the result of a leptin deficiency. Very few obese people have a leptin deficiency, however. In fact, blood levels of leptin usually correlate directly with body fat: the more body fat, the more leptin.[12] Obese people generally have high leptin levels, and weight gain increases leptin concentrations.[13] Researchers speculate that in obesity, leptin rises in an effort to overcome an insensitivity or resistance to leptin.[14]

Some researchers have reexamined the evidence on leptin from another point of view—one of undernutrition.[15] Instead of focusing on leptin's role as a satiety signal that might help prevent obesity by regulating food intake, they view leptin as a starvation hormone that signals energy deficits.[16] When energy intake is low, as occurs during starvation or undernutrition, leptin levels decline, and metabolism slows in an effort to reduce energy demands. Clearly, leptin plays a major role in energy regulation, but additional research is needed to clarify its actions when intake is either excessive or deficient.

In addition to serving as a satiety signal, leptin plays several other roles in the body.[17] For example, leptin may inform the female reproductive system about body fat reserves; stimulate growth of new blood vessels, especially in the cornea of the eye; enhance the maturation of bone marrow cells; promote formation of red blood cells; and help support a normal immune response.[18]

Ghrelin Researchers have recently discovered another protein that also acts as a hormone primarily in the hypothalamus, but it works in the opposite direction of leptin. Known as **ghrelin,** this protein is secreted primarily by the stomach cells and promotes a positive energy balance by stimulating appetite and promoting efficient energy storage.[19] The role ghrelin plays in regulating food intake and body weight is the subject of much intense research.[20]

Ghrelin triggers the desire to eat. Blood levels of ghrelin typically rise before and fall rapidly after a meal—reflecting the hunger and satiety that precede and follow eating.[21] In general, fasting blood levels correlate inversely with body weight: lean people have high ghrelin levels and obese people have low levels.[22] Interestingly, while ghrelin levels are high in underweight people, they are exceptionally high in anorexia nervosa and return to normal with nutrition intervention—indicating

ghrelin (GRELL-in): a protein produced by the stomach cells that enhances appetite and decreases energy expenditure.
- **ghre** = growth

that both body weight and nutrition status influence ghrelin levels.[23] Also noteworthy, ghrelin levels in Prader-Willi syndrome are markedly high and remain elevated even after a meal, which helps to explain the excessive appetite commonly seen in this disorder.[24] Similarly, ghrelin levels do not seem to decline after a meal in obese people, as they do for lean people.[25]

Ghrelin fights to maintain a stable body weight.[26] On average, ghrelin levels are high whenever the body is in negative energy balance, as occurs during low-kcalorie diets, for example. This response may help explain why weight loss is so difficult to maintain. Weight loss is more successful following gastric bypass surgery, in part, because ghrelin levels are abnormally low (why this is so remains unknown).[27] Ghrelin levels decline again whenever the body is in positive energy balance, as occurs with weight gains.[28]

Ghrelin levels also decline in response to high levels of PYY, a peptide that the GI cells secrete after a meal in proportion to the kcalories ingested.[29] In a recent study, people who were given PYY and then offered buffet meals consumed 30 percent fewer kcalories in a day than the control group.[30] Like the hormone leptin, PYY signals satiety and decreases food intake, but unlike leptin, PYY may be an effective treatment for obesity.

Like leptin, ghrelin plays roles in the body beyond energy regulation. In fact, it was first recognized for its participation in growth hormone activity.[31] Some research also indicates that ghrelin promotes sleep.[32]

Uncoupling Proteins Other genes code for proteins involved in energy metabolism. These proteins may influence the storing or expending of energy with different efficiencies or in different types of fat. The body has two types of fat: white and **brown adipose tissue.** White adipose tissue stores fat for other cells to use for energy; brown adipose tissue releases stored energy as heat. Recall from Chapter 7 that when fat is oxidized, some of the energy is released in heat and some is captured in ATP. In brown adipose tissue, oxidation may be uncoupled■ from ATP formation; it produces heat only. Radiating energy away as heat enables the body to spend, rather than store, energy. Heat production is particularly important in newborns, in adults who live in extremely cold climates, and in animals that hibernate; they have plenty of brown adipose tissue. In contrast, most human adults have small amounts of brown fat, and its role in body weight regulation, though probably minimal, is only just beginning to be understood.

■ Reminder: In *coupled reactions*, the energy released from the breakdown of one compound is used to create a bond in the formation of another compound. In *uncoupled reactions,* the energy is released as heat.

Uncoupling proteins are active not only in brown fat, but in white fat and many other tissues as well.[33] Their actions seem to influence the basal metabolic rate (BMR) and oppose the development of obesity.[34] Animals with abundant amounts of these uncoupling proteins resist weight gain, whereas those with minimal amounts gain weight easily. Similarly, people with a genetic variant of an uncoupling protein have lower metabolic rates and are more overweight than others.[35] Whether the body dissipates the energy from an ice cream sundae as heat or stores it in body fat has major consequences for a person's body weight.

Environment

Although genetic studies indicate that body weight may be at least partially heritable, they do not fully explain obesity. In contrast to the studies mentioned earlier that found similar weights between identical twins, some identical twins have dramatically different body weights.[36] With obesity rates rising over the past three decades and the **gene pool** remaining relatively unchanged, environment must play a role as well. The environment includes all of the circumstances that we encounter daily that push us toward fatness or thinness. Keep in mind that genetic and environmental factors are not mutually exclusive; genes can influence eating behaviors, for example.

Overeating One explanation for obesity is that overweight people overeat, although diet histories may not always reflect high intakes. Diet histories are not always accurate records of actual intakes; both normal-weight and obese people commonly

brown adipose tissue: masses of specialized fat cells packed with pigmented mitochondria that produce heat instead of ATP.

gene pool: all the genetic information of a population at a given time.

underreport their dietary intakes.[37] Most importantly, current dietary intakes may not reflect the eating habits that lead to obesity. Obese people who had a positive energy balance for years and accumulated excess body fat may not currently have a positive energy balance. This reality highlights an important point: the energy-balance equation must consider time. Both present *and* past eating and activity patterns influence current body weight.

We live in an environment that exposes us to an abundance of high-kcalorie, high-fat foods that are readily available, relatively inexpensive, heavily advertised, ■ and reasonably tasty.[38] Food is available everywhere, all the time—thanks largely to fast food. Our highways are lined with fast-food restaurants, and convenience stores and service stations offer fast food as well. Fast food is available in our schools, malls, and airports. It's convenient and it's available morning, noon, and night—and all times in between. Most alarming are the extraordinarily large serving sizes and ready-to-go meals that offer supersize■ combinations. People buy the large sizes and combinations, perceiving them to be a good value, but then they eat more than they need—a bad deal. Simply put, large portion sizes deliver more kcalories.[39] And portion sizes of virtually all foods and beverages have increased markedly in the past several decades, most notably at fast-food restaurants.[40] Not only have portion sizes increased over time, but they are now two to eight times larger than standard serving sizes.[41] The trend toward large portion sizes parallels the prevalence of overweight and obesity in the United States, beginning in the 1970s, increasing sharply in the 1980s, and continuing today.[42]

■ The food industry spends $30 billion a year on advertising. The message? "Eat more."

■ Want fries with that? A supersize portion delivers over 600 kcalories.

Restaurant food, especially fast food, is a major player in the development of obesity.[43] Fast food is often high in fat. Fat's 9 kcalories per gram quickly add up, amplifying people's energy intakes and enlarging their body fat stores. The combination of large portions and energy-dense foods is a double whammy. Reducing portion sizes is somewhat helpful, but the real kcalorie savings come from lowering the energy density.[44] After all, large portions of foods with low energy density such as fruits and vegetables can help with weight loss.

Physical Inactivity Our environment fosters physical inactivity as well. Life requires little exertion—escalators carry us up stairs, automobiles take us across town, buttons roll down windows, and remote controls change television channels. Modern technology has replaced physical activity at home, at work, and in transportation. Inactivity contributes to weight gain and poor health.[45] In turn, watching television, playing video games, and using the computer may contribute most to physical inactivity. The more time people spend in these sedentary activities, the more likely they are to be overweight.[46]

These sedentary activities contribute to weight gain in several ways. First, they require little energy beyond the resting metabolic rate. Second, they replace time spent in more vigorous activities. Watching television also influences food purchases and correlates with between-meal snacking on the high-kcalorie, high-fat foods most heavily advertised.

People may be obese, then, not because they eat too much, but because they move too little. Some obese people are so extraordinarily inactive that even when they eat less than lean people, they still have an energy surplus. Reducing their food intake further would jeopardize health and incur nutrient deficiencies. Physical activity is a necessary component of nutritional health. People must be physically active if they are to eat enough food to deliver all the nutrients they need without unhealthy weight gain. In fact, to prevent weight gain, the DRI■ suggests an accumulation of 60 minutes of moderately intense physical activities every day in addition to less intense activities of daily living.

■ DRI for physical activity: 60 min/day (moderate intensity).

IN SUMMARY Obesity has many causes and different combinations of causes in different people. Some causes, such as overeating and physical inactivity, may be within a person's control, and some, such as genetics, may be beyond it.

Problems of Obesity

An estimated 35 to 45 percent of all U.S. women (and 20 to 30 percent of U.S. men) are trying to lose weight at any given time, spending up to $40 billion each year to do so.[47] Some of these people do not even need to lose weight. Others may benefit from weight loss, but they are not successful; relatively few succeed, and even fewer succeed permanently. Whether an overweight person needs to lose weight is a question of health.

Health Risks

Chapter 8 described some of the health problems that commonly accompany obesity. In evaluating the risks to health from obesity, health care professionals use three indicators:[48]

- Body mass index■ (BMI, as described in Chapter 8).
- Waist circumference■ (also described in Chapter 8).
- Disease risk profile, taking into account family history, life-threatening diseases, and common risk factors for chronic diseases.[49]

■ BMI 25.0–29.9 = overweight.
BMI ≥30 = obese.

■ Men: >102 cm (>40 in).
Women: >88 cm (>35 in).

The higher the BMI, the greater the waist circumference, and the more risk factors, the greater the urgency to treat obesity.

People can best decide whether weight loss might be beneficial by considering their health status and motivation. People who are overweight by BMI standards, but otherwise in good health, might not benefit from losing weight; they might focus on preventing further weight gains instead. In contrast, those who are obese and suffering from a life-threatening disease such as diabetes might improve their health substantially by adopting a diet and exercise plan that supports weight loss. Regarding motivation, a person needs to be ready and willing to make lifestyle changes.

Overweight in Good Health Often a person's motivations for weight loss have nothing to do with health. A healthy young woman with a BMI of 26■ might want to lose a few pounds for spring break, but doing so might not improve her health. In fact, if she opts for a starvation diet or diet pills, she would be healthier *not* trying to lose weight.

■ For reference, a woman with a BMI of 26 might be:
- 5 ft 3 in, 146 lb.
- 5 ft 5 in, 156 lb.
- 5 ft 7 in, 166 lb.

Obese or Overweight with Risk Factors Weight loss is recommended for people who are obese and those who are overweight (or who have a high waist circumference) with two or more risk factors for chronic diseases.■ A 50-year-old man with a BMI of 28■ who has high blood pressure and a family history of heart disease can improve his health by adopting a diet low in saturated fat and a regular exercise plan.

■ Obese people and overweight people with two or more of these risk factors require aggressive treatment:
- Hypertension.
- Cigarette smoking.
- High LDL.
- Low HDL.
- Impaired glucose tolerance.
- Family history of heart disease.
- Men ≥45 yr; women ≥55 yr.

■ For reference, a man with a BMI of 28 might be:
- 5 ft 8 in, 184 lb.
- 5 ft 10 in, 195 lb.
- 6 ft, 206 lb.

Obese or Overweight with Life-Threatening Condition Weight loss is also recommended for a person who is either overweight or obese and suffering from a life-threatening condition such as heart disease, diabetes, or sleep apnea.■ The health benefits of weight loss are clear. For example, a 30-year-old man with a BMI of 40■ might be able to prevent or control the diabetes that runs in his family by losing 75 pounds. The effort required to do so may be great, but it is far less than the effort and consequences of living with diabetes.

■ Obese people and overweight people with any of these diseases require aggressive treatment:
- Heart disease.
- Diabetes (type 2).
- Sleep apnea, a disturbance of breathing during sleep, including temporarily stopping.

■ For reference, a man with a BMI of 40 might be:
- 5 ft 8 in, 265 lb.
- 5 ft 10 in, 280 lb.
- 6 ft, 295 lb.

Perceptions and Prejudices

Many people assume that every obese person can achieve slenderness and should pursue that goal. First consider that most obese people cannot—for whatever reason—successfully lose weight and maintain their losses.[50] Then consider the prejudice involved in that assumption. People come with varying weight tendencies, just as they come with varying potentials for height and degrees of health, yet we do not expect tall people to shrink or healthy people to get sick in an effort to become "normal."

Social Consequences Large segments of our society place such enormous value on thinness that obese people face prejudice and discrimination on the job, at school, and in social situations: they are judged on their appearance more than on their character.[51] Socially, obese people are stereotyped as lazy and lacking in self-control. Such a critical view of overweight is not prevalent in many other cultures, including segments of our society. Instead, overweight is simply accepted or even embraced as a sign of robust health and beauty. Many overweight people today are tired of our obsession with weight control and simply want to be accepted as they are. To free our society of its obsession with body weight and prejudice against obesity, we must first learn to judge others for who they are and not for what they weigh.

Psychological Problems Psychologically, obese people may suffer embarrassment when others treat them with hostility and contempt, and some have even come to view their own bodies as grotesque and loathsome. Parents and friends may scold them for lacking the discipline to resolve their weight problems. Health care professionals, including dietitians, are among the chief offenders. Criticism from others hurts self-esteem. Feelings of rejection, shame, or depression are common among obese people.

Most weight-loss programs assume that the problem can be solved simply by applying willpower and hard work. If determination were the only factor involved, though, the success rate would be far greater than it is. Overweight people may readily assume the blame for their failures to lose weight and maintain the losses when, in fact, the programs have failed. Ineffective treatment and its associated sense of failure add to a person's psychological burden. Figure 9-4 illustrates how the devastating psychological effects of obesity and dieting perpetuate themselves.

FIGURE 9-4 The Psychology of Weight Cycling

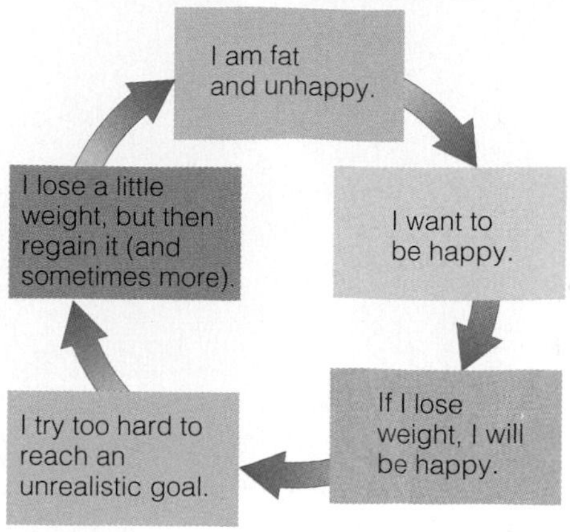
I am fat
and unhappy.
I want to
be happy.
If I lose
weight, I will
be happy.
I try too hard to
reach an
unrealistic goal.
I lose a little
weight, but then
regain it (and
sometimes more).

SOURCE: Adapted with permission from J. P. Foreyt and G. K. Goodrick, *Living Without Dieting* (Houston: Harrison Publishing, 1992).

Dangerous Interventions

People attach so many dreams of happiness to weight loss that they willingly risk huge sums of money for the slightest chance of success. As a result, weight-loss schemes flourish. Of the tens of thousands of claims, treatments, and theories for losing weight, few are effective—and many are downright dangerous. The negative effects must be carefully considered before embarking on any weight-loss program. Some interventions■ entail greater dangers than the risk of being overweight. Physical problems may arise from fad diets, "yo-yo" dieting, and drug use, and psychological problems may emerge from repeated "failures."

■ Scrutinize fad diets, magic potions, and wonder gizmos with a healthy dose of skepticism.

Some of the nation's most popular diet books and weight-loss programs have misled consumers with unsubstantiated claims and deceptive testimonials. Furthermore, they fail to provide an assessment of the short- and long-term results of their treatment plans, even though such evaluations are possible and would permit consumers to make informed decisions. Of course, some weight-loss programs are better than others in terms of cost, approach, and customer satisfaction, but few are particularly successful in helping people keep lost weight off. Clients can expect reputable programs to abide by a consumer bill of rights that explains the risks associated with weight-loss programs and provides honest predictions of success (see Table 9-1).

Fad Diets **Fad diets** often sound good, but typically fall short of delivering on their promises. They espouse exaggerated or false theories of weight loss and advise consumers to follow inadequate diets. Some fad diets are hazardous to health. Adverse reactions can be as minor as headaches, nausea, and dizziness or as serious as death. Table H8-3 in Highlight 8 (on p. 276) offers guidelines for identifying unsound weight-loss schemes and diets.

Over-the-Counter Drugs Millions of people in the United States use nonprescription weight-loss products. Most of them are women, especially young obese women, but almost 10 percent are of normal weight.[52] Only one over-the-counter

fad diets: popular eating plans that promise quick weight loss. Most fad diets severely limit certain foods or overemphasize others (for example, never eat potatoes or pasta or eat cabbage soup daily).

TABLE 9-1 Weight-Loss Consumer Bill of Rights (An Example)

1. *WARNING:* Rapid weight loss may cause serious health problems. Rapid weight loss is weight loss of more than 1½ to 2 pounds per week or weight loss of more than 1 percent of body weight per week after the second week of participation in a weight-loss program.
2. Consult your personal physician before starting any weight-loss program.
3. Only permanent lifestyle changes, such as making healthful food choices and increasing physical activity, promote long-term weight loss and successful maintenance.
4. Qualifications of this provider are available upon request.
5. *YOU HAVE A RIGHT TO:*
• Ask questions about the potential health risks of this program and its nutritional content, psychological support, and educational components.
• Receive an itemized statement of the actual or estimated price of the weight-loss program, including extra products, services, supplements, examinations, and laboratory tests.
• Know the actual or estimated duration of the program.
• Know the name, address, and qualifications of the dietitian or nutritionist who has reviewed and approved the weight-loss program.

■ **Benzocaine** is marketed under the trade names:
- Diet Ayds (candy).
- Slim Mint (gum).

■ Read labels of over-the-counter products to determine if they contain **phenylpropanolamine** (fen-ill-pro-pa-NOLE-a-mean).

■ Ephedrine is an amphetamine-like substance extracted from the Chinese ephedra herb *ma huang*.

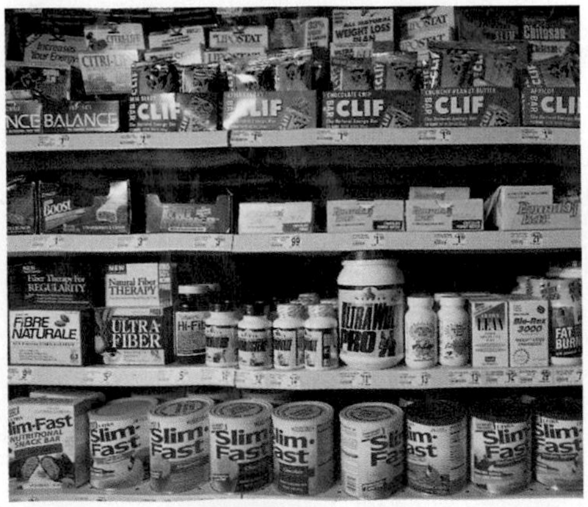
CLIF
Slim-Fast
© Anne Dowie

So many promises, so little success.

serotonin (SER-oh-tone-in): a neurotransmitter important in sleep regulation, appetite control, and sensory perception, among other roles. Serotonin is synthesized in the body from the amino acid tryptophan with the help of vitamin B_6.

medication to help with weight loss has been approved by the Food and Drug Administration (FDA). It contains benzocaine■ (in a candy or gum form), which anesthetizes the tongue, reducing taste sensations.

In 2000, the FDA recommended that manufacturers voluntarily discontinue marketing over-the-counter products containing phenylpropanolamine,■ an ingredient commonly used in products to suppress appetite.* Reported side effects include dry mouth, rapid pulse, nervousness, sleeplessness, hypertension, irregular heartbeats, kidney failure, seizures, and strokes.

Herbal Products and Dietary Supplements In their search for weight-loss magic, some consumers turn to "natural" herbal products and dietary supplements, even though few have proved to be effective.[53] St. John's wort, for example, contains substances that inhibit the uptake of **serotonin** and thus suppress appetite. In addition to the many cautions that accompany the use of any herbal remedies, consumers should be aware that St. John's wort is often prepared in combination with the herbal stimulant ephedrine.■ Ephedrine-containing supplements promote modest short-term weight loss (about 2 pounds a month), but the associated risks are high.[54] These supplements have been implicated in several cases of heart attacks and seizures and have been linked to about 100 deaths. For this reason, the FDA has banned the sale of dietary supplements containing ephedra.† Table 9-2 presents the claims and the dangers behind ephedrine and several other weight-loss supplements.[55]

Herbal laxatives containing senna, aloe, rhubarb root, cascara, castor oil, and buckthorn (or various combinations) are commonly sold as "dieter's tea." Such concoctions commonly cause nausea, vomiting, diarrhea, cramping, and fainting and may have contributed to the deaths of four women who had drastically reduced their food intakes. Consumers mistakenly believe that laxatives will diminish nutrient absorption and reduce kcalorie intake, but remember that absorption occurs primarily in the upper small intestine and these laxatives act on the lower large intestine. Chapter and Highlight 19 explore the possible benefits and potential dangers of herbal products and other alternative therapies. As it explains, current laws do not require manufacturers of dietary supplements to test the safety or effectiveness of any product. Consumers cannot assume that an herb or supplement of any kind is safe or effective just because it is available on the market. Supplements may contain contaminants and may not contain the amounts of active ingredients listed on the labels.[56] Anyone using dietary supplements for weight loss should first consult with a physician.

*Phenylpropanolamine is not commercially available in Canada.
†Ma huang (ephedrine) is illegal in Canada.

TABLE 9-2 Selected Herbal and Other Dietary Supplements Marketed for Weight Loss

Product	Manufacturers' Claims	Research Findings	Adverse Effects
Chitosan[a] (pronounced KITE-oh-san; derived from chitin, the substance that forms the hard shells of lobsters, crabs, and other crustaceans)	Binds to dietary fat, preventing digestion and absorption	Ineffective	Impaired absorption of fat-soluble vitamins
Chromium (trace mineral)	Eliminates body fat	Ineffective; weight gain reported when not accompanied by exercise	Headaches, sleep disturbances, and mood swings; hexavalent form is toxic and carcinogenic
Conjugated linoleic acid (CLA; a group of fatty acids related to linoleic acid, but with different *cis-* and *trans-*configurations)	Reduces body fat and suppresses appetite	Some evidence in animal studies, but ineffective in human studies	None known
Ephedrine[b] (amphetamine-like substance derived from the Chinese ephedra herb ma huang)	Speeds body's metabolism	Weight loss and dangerous side effects	Insomnia, tremors, heart attacks, strokes, and death; FDA has banned the sale of these products
Hydroxycitric acid[c] (active ingredient derived from the rind of the tropical fruit *garcinia cambogia*)	Inhibits the enzyme that converts citric acid to fat; suppresses appetite	Ineffective	Toxicity symptoms reported in animal studies
Pyruvate[d] (3-carbon compound produced during glycolysis)	Speeds body's metabolism	Modest weight loss with high doses	GI distress
Triiodothyroacetic acid[e] (TRIAC, a potent thyroid hormone)	Speeds up body's metaboiosm	Weight loss and dangerous side effects	Diarrhea, fatigue, drowsiness, insomnia, nervousness, sweating, heart attacks, and strokes; FDA warning issued
Yohimbine (derived from the bark of a West African tree)	Promotes weight loss	Ineffective	Nervousness, insomnia, anxiety, dizziness, tremors, headaches, nausea, vomiting, hypertension

NOTE: The FDA has not approved the use of any of these products; most products are used in conjunction with a 1000- to 1800-kcalorie diet.
[a]Marketed under the trade names Chitorich, Exofat, Fat Breaker, Fat Blocker, Fat Magnet, Fat Trapper, and Fatsorb.
[b]Marketed under the trade names Diet Fuel, Metabolife, and Nature's Nutrition Formula One.
[c]Marketed under the trade names Ultra Burn, Citralean, CitriMax, Citrin, Slim Life, Brindleslim, Medislim, and Beer Belly Busters.
[d]Marketed under the trade names Exercise in a Bottle, Pyruvate Punch, Pyruvate-c, and Provate.
[e]Marketed under the trade name Triax Metabolic Accelerator.

Other Gimmicks Other gimmicks don't help with weight loss either. Hot baths do not speed up metabolism so that pounds can be lost in hours. Steam and sauna baths do not melt the fat off the body, although they may dehydrate people so that they lose water weight. Brushes, sponges, wraps, creams, and massages intended to move, burn, or break up **"cellulite"** do nothing of the kind, because there is no such thing as cellulite.

IN SUMMARY The question whether a person should lose weight depends on many factors: the extent of overweight, age, health, and genetic makeup among them. Not all obesity will cause disease or shorten life expectancy. Just as there are unhealthy, normal-weight people, there are healthy, obese people. Some people may risk more in the process of losing weight than in remaining overweight. Weight-loss diets and supplements can be physically and psychologically damaging.

Aggressive Treatments of Obesity

The degree of obesity and the risk of disease guide the selection of appropriate strategies for weight reduction. An overweight person in good health may need to improve eating habits and increase physical activity, but someone with **clinically severe obesity** may need more aggressive treatment■ options—drugs or surgery.[57]

■ The field of medicine that specializes in treating obesity is called **bariatrics.**
- **bar** = weight

cellulite (SELL-you-light or SELL-you-leet): supposedly, a lumpy form of fat; actually, a fraud. Fatty areas of the body may appear lumpy when the strands of connective tissue that attach the skin to underlying muscles pull tight where the fat is thick. The fat itself is the same as fat anywhere else in the body. If the fat in these areas is lost, the lumpy appearance disappears.

clinically severe obesity: a BMI of 40 or greater or a BMI of 35 or greater with additional risk factors. A less preferred term used to describe the same condition is *morbid obesity.*

Drugs

Based on new understandings of obesity's genetic basis and its classification as a chronic disease, much research effort has focused on drug treatments for obesity. Experts reason that if obesity is a chronic disease, it should be treated as such—and the treatment of most chronic diseases includes drugs. The challenge, then, is to develop an effective drug that can be used over time without adverse side effects or the potential for abuse. No such drug currently exists.[58]

Several drugs for weight loss have been tried over the years. When used as part of a long-term, comprehensive weight-loss program, drugs can help obese people to lose up to 10 percent of their initial weight and maintain that loss for at least a year.[59] Because weight regain commonly occurs with the discontinuation of drug therapy, treatment must be long term. Yet the long-term use of drugs poses risks. We don't yet know whether a person would benefit more from maintaining a 20-pound excess or from taking a drug for a decade to keep the 20 pounds off. Physicians must prescribe drugs appropriately, inform consumers of the potential risks, and monitor side effects carefully. Two prescription drugs are currently on the market: sibutramine and orlistat. One reduces food intake; the other reduces nutrient absorption.[60]

Sibutramine **Sibutramine** suppresses appetite.* The drug is most effective when used in combination with a reduced-kcalorie diet and increased physical activity. Side effects include dry mouth, headache, constipation, rapid heart rate, and high blood pressure. The FDA advises those with high blood pressure not to use sibutramine and others to monitor their blood pressure.

Orlistat **Orlistat** takes a different approach to weight control.† It inhibits pancreatic lipase activity in the GI tract, thus blocking dietary fat digestion and absorption by about 30 percent. The drug is taken with meals and is most effective when accompanied by a reduced-kcalorie, low-fat diet. Side effects include gas, frequent bowel movements, and reduced absorption of fat-soluble vitamins.

Other Drugs Several other drugs are currently under study, including combinations that both decrease appetite and increase metabolism. Another approach being tested uses anticancer drugs to deprive the body's fat stores of needed blood vessels.[61]

Surgery

Surgery as an approach to weight loss is justified in some specific cases of clinically severe obesity. Surgical procedures effectively limit food intake by reducing the capacity of the stomach and suppress hunger by reducing production of the hormone ghrelin.[62] They reduce the size of the outlet as well, so they delay the passage of food from the stomach into the intestine for digestion and absorption (see Figure 9-5). The results are dramatic: most people achieve a lasting weight loss of more than 50 percent of their excess body weight.[63]

The long-term safety and effectiveness of gastric surgery depend, in large part, on compliance with dietary instructions. Common immediate postsurgical complications include infections, nausea, vomiting, and dehydration; in the long term, vitamin and mineral deficiencies and psychological problems are common. Lifelong medical supervision is necessary for those who choose the surgical route, but in suitable candidates, the health benefits of weight loss may prove worth the risks.[64]

Another surgical procedure is used, not to treat obesity, but to remove the evidence. Plastic surgeons can extract some fat deposits by suction lipectomy, or "liposuction." This cosmetic procedure has little effect on body weight, but can alter body shape slightly in specific areas. Liposuction is a popular procedure in part be-

sibutramine (sigh-BYOO-tra-mean): a drug used in the treatment of obesity that slows the reabsorption of serotonin in the brain, thus suppressing appetite and creating a feeling of fullness.

orlistat (OR-leh-stat): a drug used in the treatment of obesity that inhibits the absorption of fat in the GI tract, thus limiting kcaloric intake.

*Sibutramine is marketed under the trade name Meridia.
†Orlistat is marketed under the trade name Xenical.

FIGURE 9-5 Surgical Procedures Used in the Treatment of Severe Obesity

Both of these surgical procedures reduce the size of the stomach. Notice that the first procedure maintains a relatively normal flow, whereas the second one bypasses most of the stomach, all of the duodenum, and some of the jejunum. The dark pink areas highlight the flow of food through the GI tract. The pale pink areas indicate the sections that have been bypassed.

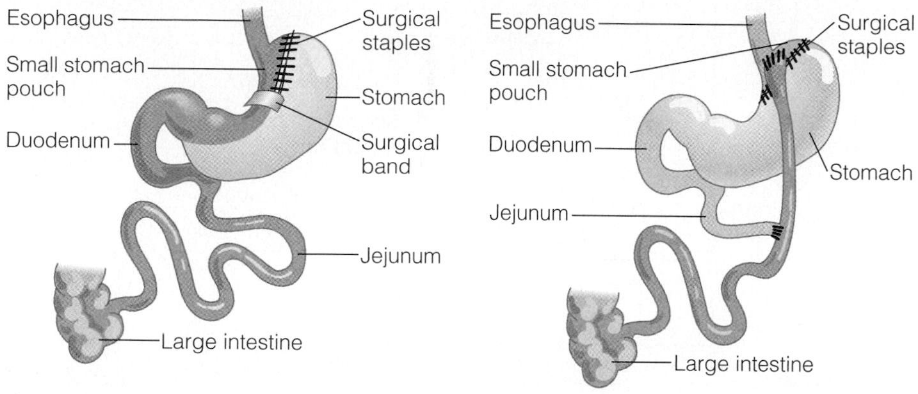
Esophagus
Small stomach pouch
Duodenum
Surgical staples
Stomach
Surgical band
Jejunum
Large intestine
Esophagus
Small stomach pouch
Duodenum
Jejunum
Surgical staples
Stomach
Large intestine

In vertical banded gastroplasty, the surgeon constructs a small stomach pouch and restricts the outlet from the stomach to the intestine.

In gastric bypass, the surgeon constructs a small stomach pouch and creates an outlet directly to the jejunum.

cause of its perceived safety, but, in fact, there can be serious complications that occasionally result in death.[65]

IN SUMMARY Obese people with high risks of medical problems may need aggressive treatment, including drugs or surgery. Others may benefit most from improving eating and exercise habits.

Weight-Loss Strategies

Successful weight-loss strategies embrace small changes, moderate losses, and reasonable goals. A person who loses 10 to 20 pounds in a year by consistently choosing nutrient-dense foods and engaging in regular physical activity is much more likely to maintain those losses and reap health benefits than if more weight were lost in less time by adopting a radical fad diet. In keeping with this philosophy, the 2005 *Dietary Guidelines* advise those who need to lose weight to "aim for a slow, steady weight loss by decreasing kcalorie intake while maintaining an adequate nutrient intake and increasing physical activity." Even modest weight loss brings health benefits.

Modest weight loss, even when a person is still overweight, can improve control of diabetes and reduce the risks of heart disease by lowering blood pressure and blood cholesterol, especially for those with central obesity. Improvements in physical capabilities and bodily pain become evident with even a 5-pound weight loss.[66] For these reasons, parameters such as blood pressure, blood cholesterol, or even vitality are more useful than body weight in marking success. People less concerned with disease risks may prefer to set goals for personal fitness, such as being able to play with children or climb stairs without becoming short of breath. Importantly, they can enjoy living a healthy life instead of focusing on the elusive goal of losing weight.

Whether the goal is health or fitness, expectations need to be reasonable. Unreachable targets ensure frustration and failure. If goals are achieved or exceeded, there will be rewards instead of disappointments.

FIGURE 9-6 Reasonable Weight Goals and Expectations Compared

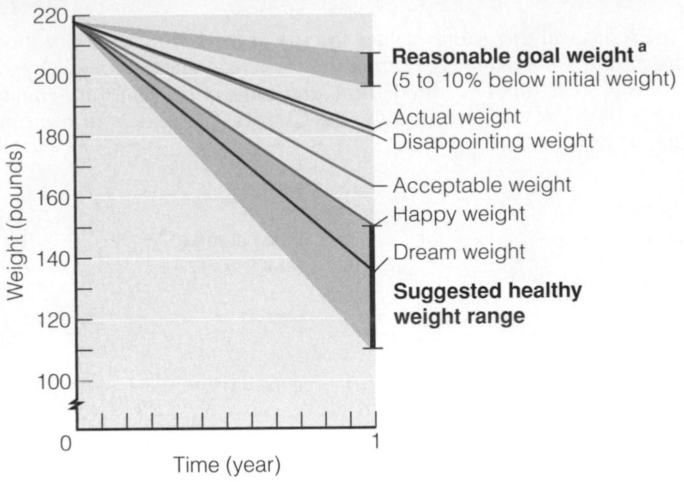
220
200
180
160
140
120
100
Weight (pounds)
0
1
Time (year)
Reasonable goal weight[a]
(5 to 10% below initial weight)
Actual weight
Disappointing weight
Acceptable weight
Happy weight
Dream weight
Suggested healthy weight range

[a]Reasonable goal weights reflect pounds lost over time. Given more time, reasonable goals may eventually fall within the suggested healthy-weight range.
SOURCE: Adapted from G. D. Foster and coauthors, What is a reasonable weight loss? Patients' expectations and evaluations of obesity treatment outcomes, *Journal of Consulting and Clinical Psychology* 65 (1997): 79–85.

Research findings highlight the great disparity between lofty expectations and reasonable success.[67] Before beginning a weight-loss program, obese women identified the weights they would describe as "dream," "happy," "acceptable," and "disappointing" (see Figure 9-6). All of these weights were below their starting weight. Their goal weights far exceeded the 5 to 10 percent recommended by experts, or even the 15 percent reported by the most successful weight-loss studies. Even their "disappointing" weights exceeded recommended goals. Close to a year later, and after an average loss of 35 pounds, almost half of the women did not achieve even their "disappointing" weights. They did, however, experience more physical, social, and psychological benefits than they had predicted for that weight. Still, in a culture that overvalues thinness, these women were not satisfied with a 16 percent reduction in weight—not because their efforts were unsuccessful, but because their expectations were unrealistic.

■ Safe rate for weight loss:
- ½ to 2 lb/week.
- 10% body weight/6 mo.

Depending on initial body weight, a reasonable rate of weight loss for overweight people is ½ to 2 pounds a week,■ or 10 percent of body weight over six months.[68] For a person weighing 250 pounds, a 10 percent loss is 25 pounds, or about 1 pound a week for six months. Such gradual weight losses are more likely to be maintained than rapid losses. Keep in mind that pursuing good health is a lifelong journey. Most adults are keenly aware of their body weights and shapes and realize that what they eat and what they do can make a difference to some extent. Those who are most successful at weight management seem to have fully incorporated healthful eating and physical activity into their daily lives.[69] Such advice—to reduce kcalorie intake and increase physical activity—would hardly surprise anyone, yet only one in five people trying to control their weight follows these recommendations.[70]

Eating Plans

Contrary to the claims of fad diets, no one food plan is magical, and no specific food must be included or avoided in a weight-management program. In designing a plan, people need only consider foods that they like or can learn to like, that are available, and that are within their means.

TABLE 9-3 Recommendations for a Weight-Loss Diet

Nutrient	Recommended Intake
kCalories	
For people with BMI ≥ 35	Approximately 500 to 1000 kcalories per day reduction from usual intake
For people with BMI between 27 and 35	Approximately 300 to 500 kcalories per day reduction from usual intake
Total fat	30% or less of total kcalories
Saturated fatty acids[a]	8 to 10% of total kcalories
Monounsaturated fatty acids	Up to 15% of total kcalories
Polyunsaturated fatty acids	Up to 10% of total kcalories
Cholesterol[a]	300 mg or less per day
Protein[b]	Approximately 15% of total kcalories
Carbohydrate[c]	55% or more of total kcalories
Sodium chloride	No more than 2400 mg of sodium or approximately 6 g of sodium chloride (salt) per day
Calcium	1000 to 1500 mg per day
Fiber[c]	20 to 30 g per day

[a]People with high blood cholesterol should aim for less than 7 percent kcalories from saturated fat and 200 milligrams of cholesterol per day.
[b]Protein should be derived from plant sources and lean sources of animal protein.
[c]Carbohydrates and fiber should be derived from vegetables, fruits, and whole grains.
SOURCE: National Institutes of Health Obesity Education Initiative, *The Practical Guide: Identification, Evaluation, and Treatment of Overweight and Obesity in Adults* (Washington, D.C.: U.S. Department of Health and Human Services, 2000), p. 27.

Be Realistic about Energy Intake The main characteristic of a weight-loss diet is that it provides less energy than the person needs to maintain present body weight. If food energy is restricted too severely, dieters may not receive sufficient nutrients and may lose lean tissue. Rapid weight loss usually means excessive loss of lean tissue, a lower BMR, and a rapid weight gain to follow. In addition, restrictive eating may set in motion the unhealthy behaviors of eating disorders (described in Highlight 9).

Table 9-3 outlines the recommendations of a weight-loss diet. Energy intake should provide nutritional adequacy without excess—that is, somewhere between deprivation and complete freedom to eat whatever, whenever. A reasonable suggestion is that an adult needs to increase activity and reduce food intake enough to create a deficit of 500 kcalories per day.[71] Such a deficit produces a weight loss of about 1 pound per week—a rate that supports the loss of fat efficiently while retaining lean tissue. In general, weight-loss diets provide 1200 to 1600 kcalories a day.[72]

Emphasize Nutritional Adequacy Nutritional adequacy is difficult to achieve on fewer than 1200 kcalories a day, and most healthy adults need never consume any less than that. A plan that provides an adequate intake supports a healthier and more successful weight loss than a restrictive plan that creates feelings of starvation and deprivation, which can lead to an irresistible urge to binge.

Table 2-3 (on p. 46) includes the recommended amounts for diets providing 1200 to 1600 kcalories. Such an intake would allow most people to lose weight and still meet their nutrient needs with careful, nutrient-dense food selections. (Women might need iron or calcium supplements.) Keep in mind, too, that well-balanced diets that emphasize fruits, vegetables, whole grains, lean meats or meat alternates, and low-fat milk products offer many health rewards even when they don't result in weight loss.[73]

Eat Small Portions As mentioned earlier, portion sizes at markets, at restaurants, and even at home have increased dramatically over the years.[74] We have come to expect large portions, and we have learned to clean our plates. Many of us pay more attention to these outside cues defining how much to eat than to our internal cues

FIGURE 9-7 Energy Density

Decreasing the energy density (kcal/g) of foods allows a person to eat satisfying portions while still reducing energy intake. To lower energy density, select foods high in water or fiber and low in fat.

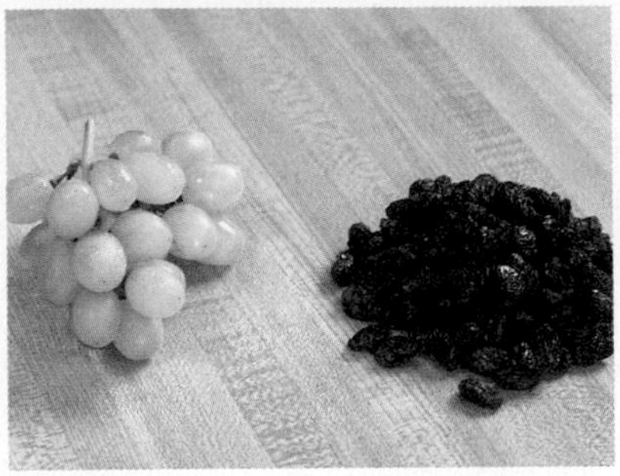

Selecting grapes with their high water content instead of raisins increases the volume and cuts the energy intake in half.

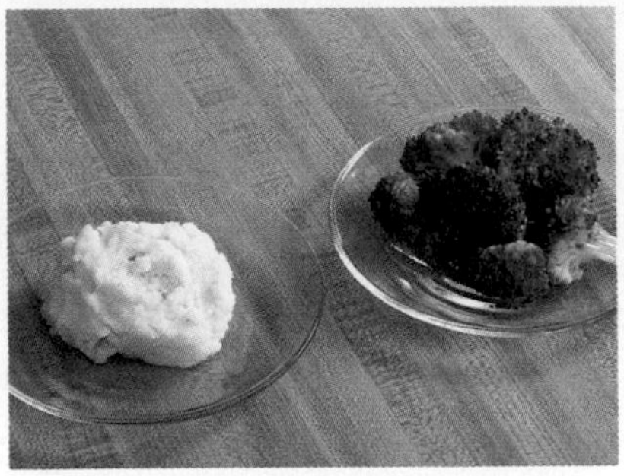

Even at the same weight and similar serving sizes, the fiber-rich broccoli delivers twice the fiber of the potatoes for about one-fourth the energy.

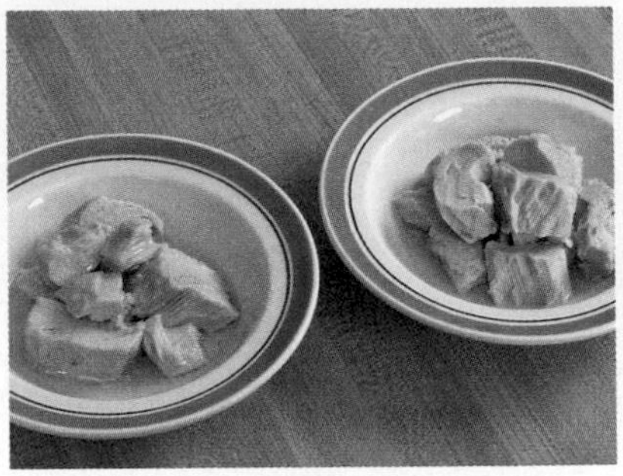

Matthew Farruggio (all)

By selecting the water-packed tuna (on the right), a person can enjoy the same amount for fewer kcalories.

of hunger and satiety. For health's sake, we may need to learn to eat less food at each meal—one piece of chicken for dinner instead of two, a teaspoon of butter on vegetables instead of a tablespoon, and one cookie for dessert instead of six. The goal is to eat enough food for energy, nutrients, and pleasure, but not more. This amount should leave a person feeling satisfied—not stuffed.

Keep in mind that even fat-free and low-fat foods can deliver a lot of kcalories when a person eats large quantities. A low-fat cookie or two can be a sweet treat even on a weight-loss diet, but larger portions defeat the savings.

Lower Energy Density Most people take their cues about how much to eat based on portion sizes and typically choose similar amounts from day to day.[75] To lower energy intake, a person can either reduce the portion size or reduce the energy density.[76] Figure 9-7 illustrates how water, fiber, and fat influence energy density, and the accompanying "How to" feature compares foods based on their energy density. Foods containing water, those rich in fiber, and those low in fat help to lower energy density, providing more satiety for fewer kcalories.

Remember Water Water helps with weight management in several ways. For one, foods with a high water content (such as broth-based soups) increase fullness, reduce hunger, and consequently reduce energy intake.[77] For another, drinking water fills the stomach between meals and satisfies the thirst that was formerly met by eating extra food (remember that foods provide water). Water also helps the GI tract adapt to a high-fiber diet.

Focus on Complex Carbohydrates Healthy meals and snacks center on complex carbohydrate foods. Fresh

HOW TO Compare Foods Based on Energy Density

Chapter 2 described how to evaluate foods based on their nutrient density—their nutrient contribution per kcalorie. Another way to evaluate foods is to consider their energy density—their energy contribution per gram. This example compares carrot sticks with french fries. The conclusion is no surprise, but understanding the mathematics may offer valuable insight into the concept of energy density. A carrot weighing 72 grams delivers 31 kcalories. To calculate the energy density, divide kcalories by grams:

$$\frac{31 \text{ kcal}}{72 \text{ g}} = 0.43 \text{ kcal/g}.$$

Do the same for french fries weighing 50 grams and contributing 167 kcalories:

$$\frac{167 \text{ kcal}}{50 \text{ g}} = 3.34 \text{ kcal/g}.$$

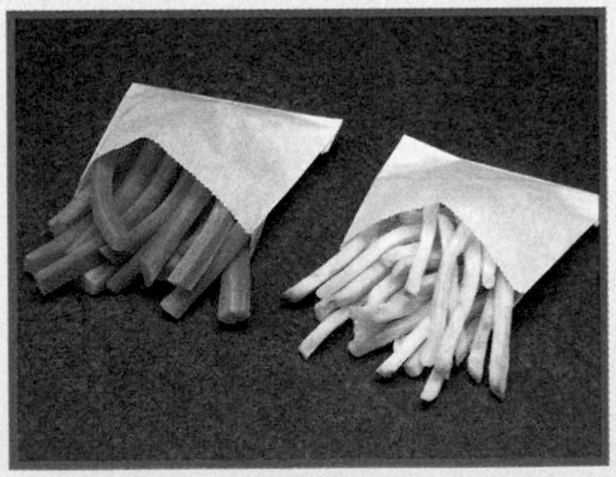

Matthew Farruggio

The more kcalories per gram, the greater the energy density. French fries are more energy dense than carrots. They provide more energy per gram—and per bite. Considering a food's energy density is especially useful in planning diets for weight management. Foods with a high energy density help with weight gain, whereas foods with a low energy density help with weight loss.

fruits, vegetables, legumes, and whole grains offer abundant vitamins, minerals, and fiber but little fat. Consequently, high-carbohydrate diets tend to be relatively low in energy and high in nutrients.[78]

High-fiber foods also require effort to eat—an added bonus. People who eat these foods in abundance spontaneously eat for longer times and take in fewer kcalories than when eating foods of high energy density. The satiety signal indicating fullness is sent after a 20-minute lag, so a person who slows down and savors each bite eats less before the signal reaches the brain. Of course, much depends on whether the person pays attention to internal satiety signals and stops eating or responds to external cognitive influences and continues.

Choose Fats Sensibly Ideally, a weight-loss diet will be both high in fiber and low in fat.[79] Lowering the fat content of a food lowers its energy density—for example, selecting fat-free milk instead of whole milk. That way, a person can consume the usual amount (say, a cup of milk) at a lower energy intake (85 instead of 150 kcalories).

Fat has a weak satiating effect, and satiation plays a key role in determining food intake during a meal. Consequently, a person eating a high-fat meal raises energy intake by adding both more food and more fat kcalories. For these reasons, measure fat with extra caution. Less fat in the diet means less fat in the body (review p. 165 for strategies to lower fat in the diet). Be careful not to take this advice to extremes, however; too little fat in the diet or in the body carries health risks as well, as Chapter 5 explained.

Whether a low-fat diet is the best option for weight loss is the subject of some controversy and much debate. An important point to notice in any discussion on weight-loss diets is total energy intake. *Low fat* simply means the energy derived from fat is relatively low compared with the total energy intake; it does not mean total energy intake is low. And reducing energy intake to less than expended is essential for weight loss. One way to lower energy intake is to lower fat intake. In these cases, adopting a low-fat diet can help with weight loss.[80]

Another currently popular way to lower energy intake is to lower carbohydrate intake. Highlight 8 discusses these diets fully, but findings from a recent study are worth mentioning here as well.[81] In this study, people were randomly assigned to one of two diets—either a low-carbohydrate diet or a low-fat diet. They were given descriptions of the diets and then fed themselves, as would be typical of many dieters. Both groups lost weight, but those on the low-carbohydrate diet lost more weight during the first six months; their diets produced a greater energy deficit. Interestingly, the differences in weight loss between the two groups disappeared by the end of one year. Between six months and one year, weight remained fairly stable in the low-fat group, but regains were evident in the low-carbohydrate group. These findings highlight an important point: weight loss requires a commitment to long-term changes in food choices. They also confirm another critical point: weight loss depends on a low energy intake—not the proportion of energy nutrients.[82]

Watch for Other Empty kCalories A person trying to achieve or maintain a healthy weight needs to pay attention not only to fat, but to sugar and alcohol, too.[83] Using them for pleasure on occasion is compatible with health as long as most daily choices are of nutrient-dense foods. Not only does alcohol add kcalories, but accompanying mixers can also add both kcalories and fat, especially in creamy drinks such as piña coladas (review Table H7-3 on p. 246). Furthermore, drinking alcohol reduces a person's inhibitions, which can sabotage weight-control efforts—at least temporarily.

IN SUMMARY A person who adopts a lifelong "eating plan for good health" rather than a "diet for weight loss" will be more likely to keep the lost weight off. Table 9-4 provides several tips for successful weight management.

TABLE 9-4 Weight-Management Strategies

In General

- Focus on healthy eating and activity habits, not on weight losses or gains.
- Adopt reasonable expectations about health and fitness goals and about how long it will take to achieve them.
- Make nutritional adequacy a high priority.
- Learn, practice, and follow a healthful eating plan for the rest of your life.
- Participate in some form of physical activity regularly.
- Adopt permanent lifestyle changes to achieve and maintain a healthy weight.

For Weight Loss

- Energy out should exceed energy in by about 500 kcalories/day. Increase your physical activity enough to spend more energy than you consume from foods.
- Emphasize foods with a low energy density and a high nutrient density.
- Eat small portions. Share a restaurant meal with a friend or take home half for lunch tomorrow.
- Eat slowly.
- Limit high-fat foods. Make legumes, whole grains, vegetables, and fruits central to your diet plan.
- Limit low-fat treats to the serving size on the label.
- Limit concentrated sweets and alcoholic beverages.
- Drink a glass of water before you begin to eat and another while you eat. Drink plenty of water throughout the day (8 glasses or more a day).
- Keep a record of diet and exercise habits; it reveals problem areas, the first step toward improving behaviors.
- Learn alternative ways to deal with emotions and stresses.
- Attend support groups regularly or develop supportive relationships with others.

For Weight Gain

- Energy in should exceed energy out by at least 500 kcalories/day. Increase your food intake enough to store more energy than you spend in exercise. Exercise and eat to build muscles.
- Expect weight gain to take time (1 pound per month would be reasonable).
- Emphasize energy-dense foods.
- Eat at least three meals a day.
- Eat large portions of foods and expect to feel full.
- Eat snacks between meals.
- Drink plenty of juice and milk.

Physical Activity

The best approach to weight management combines diet and physical activity. To prevent weight gains and support weight losses, current recommendations advise 60 minutes of moderately intense physical activity a day in addition to activities of daily life.[84] People who combine diet and exercise typically lose more fat, retain more muscle, and regain less weight than those who only diet. Even when people who include physical activity in their weight-management program do not lose more weight, they seem to follow their diet plans more closely and maintain their losses better than those who do not exercise.[85] Consequently, they benefit both from taking in a little less energy and from expending a little more energy in physical activity. Importantly, those who exercise reduce abdominal obesity and improve their blood pressure, insulin resistance, and cardiorespiratory fitness, regardless of weight loss.[86] The focus here is on the role of physical activity in weight management.

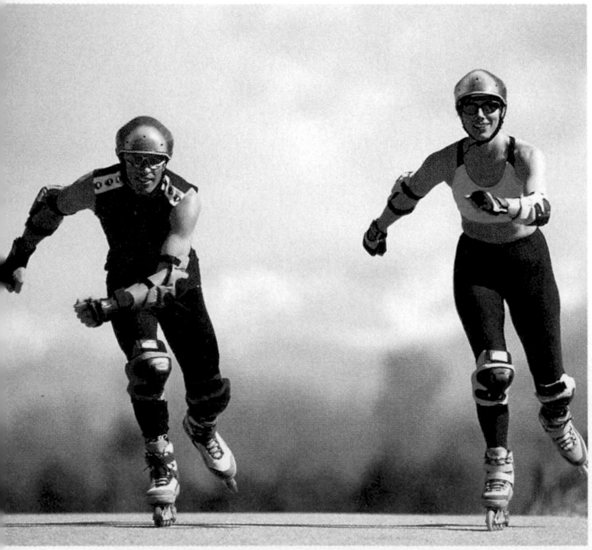

© Mike Chew/CORBIS

The key to good health is to combine sensible eating with regular exercise.

Activity and Energy Expenditure Table 8-2 (on p. 258) shows how much energy each of several activities uses. The number of kcalories spent in an activity depends on body weight, intensity, and duration. For example, a person who weighs 150 pounds and walks 3½ miles in 60 minutes expends about 315 kcalories. That same person running 3 miles in 30 minutes uses a similar amount. By comparison, a 200-pound person running 3 miles in 30 minutes expends an additional 100 kcalories or so. The goal is to expend as much energy as your time allows. The greater the energy deficit created by exercise, the greater the fat loss. And be careful not to compensate for the energy spent in exercise by eating more food. Otherwise, energy balance won't shift and fat loss will be less significant.

Available Online

http://nutrition.wadsworth.com/uncn7
Examine how much activity is needed to expend the energy contained in some commonly eaten foods.

Activity and Metabolism Activity also contributes to energy expenditure in an indirect way—by speeding up metabolism. It does this both immediately and over the long term. On any given day, metabolism remains slightly elevated for several hours after intense and prolonged exercise.■ Over the long term, a person who engages in daily vigorous activity gradually develops more lean tissue. Metabolic rate rises accordingly, and this supports continued weight loss or maintenance.

■ This postexercise effect raises the energy expenditure of exercise by about 15 percent.

Activity and Body Composition Physically active people have less body fat than sedentary people do—even if they have the same BMI.[87] Physical activity, even without weight loss, changes body composition: body fat decreases and lean body mass increases.[88] Furthermore, exercise specifically decreases abdominal fat.[89]

Activity and Appetite Control Physical activity also helps to control appetite. Many people think that exercising will make them eat more, but this is not entirely true. Active people do have healthy appetites, but immediately after an intense workout, most people do not feel like eating. They may be thirsty and want to shower, but they are not hungry. The reason is that the body has released fuels from storage to support the exercise, so glucose and fatty acids are abundant in the blood. At the same time, the body has suppressed its digestive functions. Hard physical work and eating are not compatible. A person must calm down, put energy fuels back in storage, and relax before eating. Thus exercise may actually help curb appetite, especially the inappropriate appetite that accompanies boredom, anxiety, or depression. Weight-management programs encourage people who feel the urge to eat when not hungry to go out and exercise instead. The activity passes time, relieves anxiety, and prevents inappropriate eating.

Activity and Psychological Benefits Activity also helps reduce stress. Since stress itself cues inappropriate eating for many people, activity can help here, too. In addition, the fit person looks and feels healthy and, as a result, gains self-esteem. High self-esteem motivates a person to persist in seeking good health and fitness, which keeps the beneficial■ cycle going.

■ Benefits of physical activity in a weight-management program:

- Short-term increase in energy expenditure (from exercise and from a slight rise in metabolism).
- Long-term increase in BMR (from an increase in lean tissue).
- Improved body composition.
- Appetite control.
- Stress reduction and control of stress eating.
- Physical, and therefore psychological, well-being.
- Improved self-esteem.

Choosing Activities Clearly, physical activity■ is a plus in a weight-management program. What kind of physical activity is best? People should choose activities that they enjoy and are willing to do regularly. What schedule of physical activity is best? It doesn't matter; whether a person chooses several short bouts of exercise or one continuous workout, the fitness and weight-loss benefits are the same—and any activity is better than being sedentary.[90]

■ For an active life, limit sedentary activities, engage in strength and flexibility activities and enjoy leisure activities often, engage in vigorous activities regularly, and be as active as possible every day.

Health care professionals frequently advise people to engage in activities of low-to-moderate intensity for a long duration, such as an hour-long fast-paced walk. The reasoning behind such advice is that people exercising at low-to-moderate intensity are more likely to stick with their activity for longer times and are less likely to injure themselves. A person who stays with an activity routine long enough to enjoy the rewards will be less inclined to give it up and will, over the long term, reap many health benefits. Activity of low-to-moderate intensity■ that expends at least 2000 kcalories per week is especially helpful for weight management.[91]

■ Estimated energy expended when walking at a moderate pace = 1 kcal/mi/kg body wt.

In addition to exercise, a person can incorporate hundreds of energy-spending activities into daily routines: take the stairs instead of the elevator, walk to the neighbor's apartment instead of making a phone call, and rake the leaves instead of using a blower. Remember that sitting uses more kcalories than lying down, standing uses more kcalories than sitting, and moving uses more kcalories than standing. A 175-pound person who replaces a 30-minute television program with a 2-mile walk a day can spend enough energy to lose (or at least not gain) 18 pounds in a year. One program recommends an activity goal of 10,000 steps a day. By wearing a pedometer, a person can easily track a day's activities without measuring miles or watching the clock. The point is: be active. Walk. Run. Swim. Dance. Cycle. Climb. Skip. Do whatever you enjoy doing—and do it often.

Spot Reducing People sometimes ask about "spot reducing." Unfortunately, muscles do not "own" the fat that surrounds them. Fat cells all over the body release fat in response to the demand of physical activity for use by whatever muscles are active. No exercise can remove the fat from any one particular area.

Exercise can help with trouble spots in another way, though. The "trouble spot" for most men is the abdomen, their primary site of fat storage. During aerobic exercise, abdominal fat readily releases its stores, providing fuel to the physically active body. With regular exercise and weight loss, men will deplete these abdominal fat stores before those in the lower body. Women may also deplete abdominal fat with exercise, but their "trouble spots" are more likely to be their hips and thighs.

In addition to aerobic activity, strength training can help to improve the tone of muscles in a trouble area, and stretching to gain flexibility can help with associated posture problems. A combination of aerobic, strength, and flexibility workouts best improves fitness and physical appearance.

IN SUMMARY Physical activity should be an integral part of a weight-control program. Physical activity can increase energy expenditure, improve body composition, help control appetite, reduce stress and stress eating, and enhance physical and psychological well-being.

Behavior and Attitude

Behavior modification once held a key position in weight-loss programs, but its status has diminished in recent years. Still, behavior and attitude play an important role in supporting efforts to achieve and maintain appropriate body weight and composition. Changing the hundreds of small behaviors of overeating and underexercising that lead to, and perpetuate, obesity requires time and effort. A person must commit to take action.

Adopting a positive, matter-of-fact attitude helps to ensure success. Healthy eating and activity choices are an essential part of healthy living and should simply be incorporated into the day—much like brushing one's teeth or wearing a safety belt.

Become Aware of Behaviors To solve a problem, a person must first identify all the behaviors that created the problem. Keeping a record will help to identify eating and exercise behaviors that may need changing (see Figure 9-8). It will also establish a baseline against which to measure future progress.

Change Behaviors Strategies■ focus on learning desired eating and exercise behaviors and eliminating unwanted behaviors. With so many possible behavior changes, a person can choose where to begin. Start simply and don't try to master them all at once. Attempting too many changes at one time can be overwhelming. Pick one trouble area that is manageable and start there. Practice a desired behavior until it becomes routine. Then select another trouble area to work on, and so on. Another bit of advice along the same lines: don't try to tackle major changes during a particularly stressful time of life.

■ Examples of behavioral strategies to support weight change:
- Do not grocery shop when hungry.
- Eat slowly (pause during meals, chew thoroughly, put down utensils between bites).
- Exercise when watching television.

behavior modification: the changing of behavior by the manipulation of antecedents (cues or environmental factors that trigger behavior), the behavior itself, and consequences (the penalties or rewards attached to behavior).

Personal Attitude For many people, overeating and being overweight have become an integral part of their identity. Those who fully understand their personal relationships with food are best prepared to make healthful changes in eating and exercise behaviors.

Sometimes habitual behaviors that are hazardous to health, such as smoking or drinking alcohol, contribute positively by helping people adapt to stressful situa-

FIGURE 9-8 Food Record

The entries in a food record should include the times and places of meals and snacks, the types and amounts of foods eaten, and a description of the individual's feelings when eating. The diary should also record physical activities: the kind, the intensity level, the duration, and the person's feelings about them.

Time	Place	Activity or food eaten	People present	Mood
10:30–10:40	School vending machine	6 peanut butter crackers and 12 oz. cola	by myself	starved
12:15–12:30	Restaurant	Sub sandwich and 12 oz. cola	friends	relaxed & friendly
3:00–3:45	Gym	Weight training	work out partner	tired
4:00–4:10	Snack bar	Small frozen yogurt	by myself	OK

tions. Similarly, many people overeat to cope with the stresses of life. To break out of that pattern, they must first identify the particular stressors that trigger the urge to overeat. Then, when faced with these situations, they must learn and practice problem-solving skills that will help them to respond appropriately.[92]

All this is not to imply that psychological therapy holds the magic answer to a weight problem. Still, efforts to improve one's general well-being may result in healthy eating and activity habits even when weight loss is not the primary goal. When the problems that trigger the urge to overeat are resolved in alternative ways, people may find they eat less. They may begin to respond appropriately to internal cues of hunger rather than inappropriately to external cues of stress. Sound emotional health supports a person's ability to take care of physical health in all ways—including nutrition, weight management, and fitness.

Support Groups Group support can prove helpful when making life changes. Some people find it useful to join a group such as Take Off Pounds Sensibly (TOPS), Weight Watchers (WW), Overeaters Anonymous (OA), or others. Some dieters prefer to form their own self-help groups or find support online. The Internet offers numerous opportunities for weight-loss education and counseling that may be effective alternatives to face-to-face programs.[93] As always, consumers need to choose wisely and avoid rip-offs.

HEALTHY PEOPLE 2010

Increase the proportion of worksites that offer nutrition or weight management classes or counseling.

IN SUMMARY A surefire remedy for obesity has yet to be found, although many people find a combination of the approaches just described to be most effective. Diet and exercise shift energy balance so that more energy is being spent than is taken in. Physical activity increases energy expenditure, builds lean tissue, and improves health. Energy intake should be reduced by 500 to 1000 kcalories per day. Behavior modification retrains habits to support a healthy eating and exercise plan. This treatment package requires time, individualization, and sometimes the assistance of a registered dietitian.

Weight Maintenance

People who are successful often experience much of their weight loss within half a year and then reach a plateau. This slowdown can be disappointing, but should be recognized as an opportunity for the body to adjust to its new weight. Reaching a plateau provides a little relief from the distraction of weight-loss dieting. An appropriate goal at this point is to continue eating and activity behaviors that will maintain weight. Attempting to lose additional weight at this point would require heroic efforts and would almost certainly meet with failure.

The prevalence of **successful weight-loss maintenance** is difficult to determine, in part because researchers have used different criteria.[94] Some look at success after one year and others after five years; some quantify success as 10 or more pounds lost and others as 5 or 10 percent of initial body weight lost. Furthermore, most research studies examine the success of one episode of weight loss in a structured program, but this scenario does not necessarily reflect the experiences of the general population. In reality, most people have lost weight several times in their lifetimes and did so on their own, not in a formal program. One survey reports that almost 50 percent of the overweight people who intentionally lost at least 10 percent of their initial body weight maintained the loss for at least a year and 25 percent maintained it for at least five years.[95] Using the same criteria, a review of research studies suggests a success rate of approximately 20 percent.[96]

Those who are successful in maintaining their weight loss have established vigorous exercise regimens and careful eating patterns, taking in less energy and a lower percentage of kcalories from fat than the national average.[97] Because these people are more efficient at storing fat, they do not have the same flexibility in their food and activity habits as their friends who have never been overweight.[98] With weight loss, metabolism shifts downward so that formerly overweight people require less energy than might be expected given their current body weight and body composition.[99] Consequently, to keep weight off, they must either eat less or exercise more than people the same size who have never been obese.

Physical activity plays a key role in maintaining weight.[100] Those who exercise vigorously are far more successful than those who are inactive.[101] On average, weight maintenance requires a person to expend about 2000 kcalories in physical activity per week.[102] To accomplish this, a person might exercise either moderately (such as brisk walking) for 60 minutes a day or vigorously (such as fast bicycling) for 35 minutes a day, for example.

In addition to limiting energy intake and exercising regularly, one other strategy may help with weight maintenance: frequent self-monitoring.[103] People who weigh themselves periodically and monitor their eating and exercise habits regularly can detect weight gains in the early stages and promptly initiate changes to prevent relapse.

Losing weight and maintaining the loss may not be as easy as gaining the weight in the first place, but it is possible. Those who have been successful find that it gets easier with time—the changes in diet and activity patterns become permanent.

successful weight-loss maintenance: achieving a weight loss of at least 10 percent of initial body weight and maintaining the loss for at least one year.

Prevention

Given the information presented up to this point in the chapter, the adage "An ounce of prevention is worth a pound of cure" seems particularly apropos. Obesity is a major risk factor for numerous diseases, and losing weight is challenging and

TABLE 9-5 Suggested Public Health Strategies

Strategies	Examples of Suggested Nutritional Strategies	Examples of Successful Nonnutritional Strategies
Impose safety standards to reduce the potential for harm.	• Regulate the kcalorie or fat density of foods. • Regulate the size of packages of high-fat foods.	• Mandate safety glass in automobiles. • Regulate the lead content of paint.
Control commercial advertising to limit the influence of harmful products.	• Improve nutrition labeling and product packaging. • Restrict the promotion of high-fat foods (especially when directed at children).	• Restrict cigarette advertising (especially when directed at children). • Add health warnings to alcoholic beverages.
Control the conditions under which products are sold to limit exposure to hazardous substances.	• Remove high-fat, low–nutrient density foods from school vending machines. • Restrict the number of vendors licensed to sell high-fat foods.	• Mandate minimum-age laws for the use of tobacco, alcohol, and automobiles. • Restrict the number of vendors licensed to sell alcohol.
Control prices to reduce consumption.	• Tax soft drinks and other foods high in kcalories, fat, or sugar.	• Tax alcohol and tobacco.

SOURCES: Adapted from M. Nestle and M. F. Jacobson, Halting the obesity epidemic: A public health policy approach, *Public Health Reports* 115 (2000): 12–24; R. W. Jeffery, Public health approaches to the management of obesity, in K. B. Brownell and C. G. Fairburn, eds., *Eating Disorder and Obesity—A Comprehensive Handbook* (New York: Guilford Press, 1995), pp. 558–563.

often temporary. Strategies for preventing weight gain■ are very similar to those for losing weight, with one exception: they begin early and continue throughout life. Over the years, they become an integral part of a person's life. It is much easier for a person to resist doughnuts for breakfast if he rarely eats them. Similarly, a person will have little trouble walking each morning if she has always been active.

■ To prevent excessive weight gain:
- Eat regular meals and limit snacking.
- Drink water instead of high-kcalorie beverages.
- Select sensible portion sizes and limit daily energy intake to no more than energy expended.
- Become physically active and limit sedentary activities.

Public Health Programs

Is there anyone in the United States who hasn't heard the message that obesity raises the risks of chronic diseases and that overweight people should aim for a healthy weight by eating sensibly and becoming physically active? Not likely. Yet implementing such advice is difficult in an environment of abundant food and physical inactivity. To successfully treat obesity, we may have to change the environment in which we live.[104] Table 9-5 provides examples of public health strategies that have been suggested to improve our nation's nutrition environment. Some of these strategies may seem radical, but dramatic measures may be needed if we are to curb the obesity epidemic that is sweeping across the nation.[105]

IN SUMMARY Preventing weight gains and maintaining weight losses require vigilant attention to diet and physical activity. Taking care of oneself is a lifelong responsibility.

Underweight

Underweight■ is a far less prevalent problem than overweight, affecting no more than 5 percent of U.S. adults (review Figure 8-7 on p. 263). Whether the underweight person needs to gain weight is a question of health and, like weight loss, a highly individual matter. People who are healthy at their present weights may stay there; there are no compelling reasons to try to gain weight. Those who are thin because of malnourishment or illness, however, might benefit from a diet that supports weight gain. Medical advice can help make the distinction.

■ Reminder: *Underweight* is a body weight so low as to have adverse health effects; it is generally defined as BMI <18.5.

Thin people may find gaining weight difficult.[106] Those who wish to gain weight for appearance's sake or to improve their athletic performance need to be aware that healthful weight gains can be achieved only by physical conditioning combined with high energy intakes. On a high-kcalorie diet alone, a person may gain weight, but it will be mostly fat. Even if the gain improves appearance, it can be detrimental to health and might impair athletic performance. Therefore, in weight gain, as in weight loss, physical activity and energy intake are essential components of a sound plan.

Problems of Underweight

The causes of underweight may be as diverse as those of overweight—hunger, appetite, and satiety irregularities; psychological traits; metabolic factors; and hereditary tendencies. Habits learned early in childhood, especially food aversions, may perpetuate themselves.

The demand for energy to support physical activity and growth often contributes to underweight. An active, growing boy may need more than 4000 kcalories a day to maintain his weight and may be too busy to take time to eat. Underweight people find it hard to gain weight due, in part, to their expenditure of energy in adaptive thermogenesis. So much energy may be spent adapting to a higher food intake that at first as many as 750 to 800 extra kcalories a day may be needed to gain a pound a week. Like those who want to lose weight, people who want to gain must learn new habits and learn to like new foods. They are also similarly vulnerable to potentially harmful schemes and would be wise to review the consumer bill of rights on p. 288, using "weight gain" instead of "weight loss" where appropriate.

An underweight condition known as anorexia nervosa sometimes develops in people who employ self-denial to control their weight. They go to such extremes that they become severely undernourished, achieving final body weights of 70 pounds or even less. The distinguishing feature of a person with anorexia nervosa, as opposed to other underweight people, is that the starvation is intentional. Anorexia nervosa and other eating disorders are the subject of the highlight that follows this chapter.

Weight-Gain Strategies

Weight-gain strategies center on eating foods that provide many kcalories in a small volume and exercising to build muscle. By using the USDA Food Guide recommendations for the higher kcalorie levels (see Table 2-3 on p. 46), a person can gain weight while meeting nutrient needs.

Energy-Dense Foods Energy-dense foods (the very ones eliminated from a successful weight-loss diet) hold the key to weight gain. Pick the highest-kcalorie items from each food group—that is, milk shakes instead of fat-free milk, salmon instead of snapper, avocados instead of cucumbers, a cup of grape juice instead of a small apple, and whole-wheat muffins instead of whole-wheat bread. Because fat provides more than twice as many kcalories per teaspoon as sugar does, fat adds kcalories without adding much bulk.

Be aware that health experts routinely recommend a low-fat diet because the biggest health problems in the United States involve obesity and heart disease. Eating high-kcalorie, high-fat foods is not healthy for most people, but may be essential for an underweight individual who needs to gain weight. An underweight person who is physically active and eating a nutritionally adequate diet can afford a few extra kcalories from fat. For health's sake, it would be wise to select foods with monounsaturated and polyunsaturated fats instead of those with saturated or *trans* fats: for example, sautéing vegetables in olive oil instead of butter or hydrogenated margarine.

Regular Meals Daily People who are underweight need to make meals a priority and take the time to plan, prepare, and eat each meal. They should eat at least three healthy meals every day and learn to eat more food within the first 20 minutes of a meal. Another suggestion is to eat meaty appetizers or the main course first and leave the soup or salad until later.

Large Portions Underweight people need to learn to eat more food at each meal. Put extra slices of ham and cheese on the sandwich for lunch, drink milk from a larger glass, and eat cereal from a larger bowl.

The person should expect to feel full. Most underweight individuals are accustomed to small quantities of food. When they begin eating significantly more, they feel uncomfortable. This is normal and passes over time.

Extra Snacks Since a substantially higher energy intake is needed each day, in addition to eating more food at each meal, it is necessary to eat more frequently. Between-meal snacks do not interfere with later meals; they can readily lead to weight gains.[107] For example, a student might make three sandwiches in the morning and eat them between classes in addition to the day's three regular meals. Snacking on dried fruit, nuts, and seeds is also an easy way to add kcalories.

Juice and Milk Beverages provide an easy way to increase energy intake. Consider that 6 cups of cranberry juice add almost 1000 kcalories to the day's intake. kCalories can be added to milk by mixing in powdered milk or packets of instant breakfast.

For people who are underweight due to illness, concentrated liquid formulas are often recommended because a weak person can swallow them easily. A physician or registered dietitian can recommend high-protein, high-kcalorie formulas to help an underweight person maintain or gain. Used in addition to regular meals, these can help considerably.

Exercising to Build Muscles To gain weight, use strength training primarily and increase energy intake to support that exercise. Eating extra food will then support a gain of both muscle and fat. About 700 to 1000 kcalories a day above normal energy needs is enough to support both the exercise and the building of muscle.

IN SUMMARY Both the incidence of underweight and the health problems associated with it are less prevalent than overweight and its associated problems. To gain weight, a person must train physically and increase energy intake by selecting energy-dense foods, eating regular meals, taking larger portions, and consuming extra snacks and beverages. Table 9-4 (on p. 296) includes a summary of weight-gain strategies.

Nutrition in Your Life

To enjoy good health and maintain a reasonable body weight, combine sensible eating habits and regular physical activity.

- **Do you try to lose or gain weight even though your BMI falls between 18.5 and 24.9?**
- **Does your weight fluctuate up and down dramatically over time?**
- **Do you follow fad diets or take over-the-counter drugs or herbal supplements?**

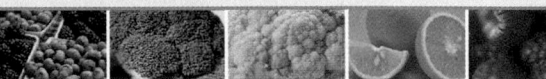

NUTRITION ON THE NET

Access these websites for further study of topics covered in this chapter.

- Find updates and quick links to these and other nutrition-related sites at our website: **www.wadsworth.com/nutrition**
- Search for "obesity" and "weight control" at the U.S. Government health information site: **www.healthfinder.gov**
- Review the Clinical Guidelines on the Identification, Evaluation, and Treatment of Overweight and Obesity in Adults: **www.nhlbi.nih.gov/guidelines/obesity/ob_home.htm**
- Learn about the drugs used for weight loss from the Center for Drug Evaluation and Research: **www.fda.gov/cder**
- Learn about weight control and the WIN program from the Weight-control Information Network: **www.niddk.nih.gov/health/nutrit/win.htm**
- Visit weight-loss support groups, such as Take Off Pounds Sensibly (TOPS), Overeaters Anonymous (OA), and Weight Watchers: **www.tops.org**, **www.oa.org**, and **www.weightwatchers.com**
- See what the obesity professionals think at the North American Association for the Study of Obesity and the American Society for Bariatric Surgery: **www.naaso.org** and **www.asbs.org**
- Consider the nondietary approaches of HUGS International: **www.hugs.com**
- Learn about the 10,000 Step Program from Shape Up America!: **www.shapeup.org/10000steps.html**
- Find helpful information on achieving and maintaining a healthy weight from the Calorie Control Council: **www.caloriecontrol.org**
- Learn how to end size discrimination and improve the quality of life for fat people from the National Association to Advance Fat Acceptance: **www.naafa.org**
- Find good advice on starting a weight-loss program from the Partnership for Healthy Weight Management: **www.consumer.gov/weightloss**
- Consider ways to live a healthy life at any weight: **www.bodypositive.com**

NUTRITION CALCULATIONS

These problems give you practice in doing simple energy-balance calculations (see p. 309 for answers). Once you have mastered these examples, you will be prepared to examine your own food choices. Be sure to show your calculations for each problem.

1. Critique a commercial weight-loss plan. Consumers spend billions of dollars a year on weight-loss programs such as Slim-Fast, Sweet Success, Weight Watchers, Nutri/System, Jenny Craig, Optifast, Medifast, and Formula One. One such plan calls for a milk shake in the morning, at noon, and as an afternoon snack and "a sensible, balanced, low-fat dinner" in the evening. One shake mixed in 8 ounces of vitamin A– and D–fortified fat-free milk offers 190 kcalories; 32 grams of carbohydrate, 13 grams of protein, and 1 gram of fat; at least one-third of the Daily Value for all vitamins and minerals; plus 2 grams of fiber.
   a. Calculate the kcalories and grams of carbohydrate, protein, and fat that three shakes provide.
   b. How do these values compare with the criteria listed in item 2 in Table H8-3 on p. 276?
   c. Plan "a sensible, balanced, low-fat dinner" that will help make this weight-loss plan adequate and balanced. Now, how do the day's totals compare with the criteria in item 2 in Table H8-3 on p. 276?
   d. Critique this plan using the other criteria described in Table H8-3 on p. 276 as a guide.
2. Evaluate a weight-gain attempt. People attempting to gain weight sometimes have a hard time because they choose low-kcalorie, high-bulk foods that make it hard to consume enough energy. Consider the following lunch: a chef's salad consisting of 2 cups iceberg lettuce, 1 whole tomato, 1 ounce swiss cheese, 1 ounce roasted ham (lean and fat), 1 hard-boiled egg, ½ cucumber, and ¼ cup mayonnaise-type salad dressing. If you weighed these foods, you'd find that they totaled 552 grams. This is a pretty filling meal.
   a. How much does this meal weigh in pounds?
   b. The meal provides 541 kcalories. What is the energy density of this meal, expressed in kcalories per gram?
   c. To gain weight, this person is advised to eat an additional 500 kcalories at this meal. Using foods with this same energy density, how much more chef's salad will this person have to eat?
   d. Suppose a person simply can't do this. Try to reduce the bulk of this meal by replacing some of the lettuce with more energy-dense foods. Delete 1 cup lettuce from the salad and add 1 ounce roast beef and 1 ounce cheddar cheese. Show how these

changes influence the weight and kcalories of this meal. (Use Appendix H.)

Item No./Food	Weight (g)	Energy (kcal)
Original totals:	552	541
Minus:		
#867 Lettuce, 1 c	–_______	–_______
Plus:		
#603 Roast beef, 1 oz	+_______	+_______
#37 Cheddar cheese, 1 oz	+_______	+_______
Totals:	_______	_______

e. How many kcalories did the changes add?
f. How much more *weight* of food did these changes add?

This exercise should reveal why people attempting to gain weight are advised to add high-fat items, within reason, to their daily meals.

STUDY QUESTIONS

These questions will help you review the chapter. You will find the answers in the discussions on the pages provided.

1. Describe how body fat develops, and suggest some reasons why it is difficult for an obese person to maintain weight loss. (pp. 280–281)
2. What factors contribute to obesity? (pp. 282–285)
3. List several aggressive ways to treat obesity, and explain why such methods are not recommended for every overweight person. (pp. 289–291)
4. Discuss reasonable dietary strategies for achieving and maintaining a healthy body weight. (pp. 291–295)
5. What are the benefits of increased physical activity in a weight-loss program? (pp. 296–298)
6. Describe the behavioral strategies for changing an individual's dietary habits. What role does personal attitude play? (pp. 298–299)
7. Describe strategies for successful weight gain. (pp. 302–303)

These multiple choice questions will help you prepare for an exam. Answers can be found on p. 309.

1. With weight loss, fat cells:
   a. decrease in size only.
   b. decrease in number only.
   c. decrease in both number and size.
   d. decrease in number, but increase in size.
2. Obesity is caused by:
   a. overeating.
   b. inactivity.
   c. defective genes.
   d. multiple factors.
3. The protein produced by the fat cells under the direction of the *ob* gene is called:
   a. leptin.
   b. serotonin.
   c. sibutramine.
   d. phentermine.
4. The biggest problem associated with the use of drugs in the treatment of obesity is:
   a. cost.
   b. chronic dosage.
   c. ineffectiveness.
   d. adverse side effects.
5. A realistic goal for weight loss is to reduce body weight:
   a. down to the weight a person was at age 25.
   b. down to the ideal weight in the weight-for-height tables.
   c. by 10 percent over six months.
   d. by 15 percent over three months.
6. A nutritionally sound weight-loss diet might restrict daily energy intake to create a:
   a. 1000-kcalorie-per-month deficit.
   b. 500-kcalorie-per-month deficit.
   c. 500-kcalorie-per-day deficit.
   d. 1000-kcalorie-per-day deficit.
7. Successful weight loss depends on:
   a. avoiding fats and limiting water.
   b. taking supplements and drinking water.
   c. increasing proteins and restricting carbohydrates.
   d. reducing energy intake and increasing physical activity.
8. Physical activity does not help a person to:
   a. lose weight.
   b. retain muscle.
   c. maintain weight loss.
   d. lose fat in trouble spots.
9. Which strategy would *not* help an overweight person to lose weight?
   a. Exercise.
   b. Eat slowly.
   c. Limit high-fat foods.
   d. Eat energy-dense foods regularly.
10. Which strategy would *not* help an underweight person to gain weight?
    a. Exercise.
    b. Drink plenty of water.
    c. Eat snacks between meals.
    d. Eat large portions of foods.

REFERENCES

1. K. M. Flegal and coauthors, Prevalence and trends in obesity among US adults, *Journal of the American Medical Association* 288 (2002): 1723–1727; C. E. Lewis, Weight gain continues in the 1990s: 10-year trends in weight and overweight from the CARDIA study, *American Journal of Epidemiology* 151 (2000): 1172–1181; A. H. Mokdad and coauthors, The spread of the obesity epidemic in the United States, 1991–1998, *Journal of the American Medical Association* 282 (1999): 1519–1522.
2. T. E. Kottke, L. A. Wu, and R. S. Hoffman, Economic and psychological implications of the obesity epidemic, *Mayo Clinic Proceedings* 78 (2003): 92–94; M. Kohn and M. Booth, The worldwide epidemic of obesity in adolescents, *Adolescent Medicine* 14 (2003): 1–9; G. du Toit and M. T. van der Merwe, The epidemic of childhood obesity, *South African Medical Journal* 93 (2003): 49–50; C. J. Schrodt, The obesity epidemic and physician responsibility, *Journal of the Kentucky Medical Association* 101 (2003): 27–28; W. H. Dietz and coauthors, Policy tools for the childhood obesity epidemic, *Journal of Law, Medicine, and Ethics* 30 (2002): 83–87; M. Chopra, S. Galbraith, and I. Darnton-Hill, A global response to a global problem: The epidemic of overnutrition, *Bulletin of the World Health Organization* 80 (2002): 952–958; J. P. Koplan and W. H. Dietz, Caloric imbalance and public health policy, *Journal of the American Medical Association* 282 (1999): 1579; Mokdad and coauthors, 1999.
3. E. D. Rosen, The molecular control of adipogenesis with special reference to lymphatic pathology, *Annals of the New York Academy of Sciences* 979 (2002): 143–158; D. B. Hausman and coauthors, The biology of white adipocyte proliferation, *Obesity Reviews* 2 (2001): 239–254.
4. J. E. Schaffer, Lipotoxicity: When tissues overeat, *Current Opinion in Lipidology* 14 (2003): 281–287.
5. E. Blaak, Gender differences in fat metabolism, *Current Opinion in Clinical Nutrition and Metabolic Care* 4 (2001): 499–502.
6. J. Webber and I. A. Macdonald, Signalling in body-weight homeostasis: Neuroendocrine efferent signals, *Proceedings of the Nutrition Society* 59 (2000): 397–404.
7. L. Pérusse and C. Bouchard, Gene-diet interactions in obesity, *American Journal of Clinical Nutrition* 72 (2000): 1285S–1290S.
8. P. Froguel and P. Boutin, Genetics of pathways regulating body weight in the development of obesity in humans, *Experimental Biology and Medicine* 226 (2001): 991–996.
9. D. E. Cummings and M. W. Schwartz, Genetics and pathophysiology of human obesity, *Annual Reviews of Medicine* 54 (2003): 453–471; J. Altman, Weight in the balance, *Neuroendocrinology* 76 (2002): 131–136; B. M. Spiegelman and J. S. Flier, Obesity and the regulation of energy balance, *Cell* 104 (2001): 531–543; M. W. Schwartz and coauthors, Central nervous system control of food intake, *Nature* 404 (2000): 661–671.
10. R. B. Ceddia, W. N. William Jr., and R. Curi, The response of skeletal muscle to leptin, *Frontiers in Bioscience* 6 (2001): D90–D97; C A. Baile, M. A. Della-Fera, and R. J. Martin, Regulation of metabolism and body fat mass by leptin, *Annual Review of Nutrition* 20 (2000): 105–127.
11. I. S. Farooqi and coauthors, Effects of recombinant leptin therapy in a child with congenital leptin deficiency, *New England Journal of Medicine* 341 (1999): 879–884.
12. C. E. Ruhl and J. E. Everhart, Leptin concentrations in the United States: Relations with demographic and anthropometric measures, *American Journal of Clinical Nutrition* 74 (2001): 295–301; B. Lönnerdal and P. J. Havel, Serum leptin concentrations in infants: Effects of diet, sex, and adiposity, *American Journal of Clinical Nutrition* 72 (2000): 484–489; H. Fors and coauthors, Serum leptin levels correlate with growth hormone secretion and body fat in children, *Journal of Clinical Endocrinology and Metabolism* 84 (1999): 3586–3590.
13. A. Polito and coauthors, Basal metabolic rate in anorexia nervosa: Relation to body composition and leptin concentrations, *American Journal of Clinical Nutrition* 71 (2000): 1495–1502.
14. J. Proietto and A. W. Thorburn, The therapeutic potential of leptin, *Expert Opinion on Investigational Drugs* 12 (2003): 373–378; W. A. Banks, Leptin transport across the blood-brain barrier: Implications for the cause and treatment of obesity, *Current Pharmaceutical Design* 7 (2001): 125–133; N. F. Chu and coauthors, Plasma leptin concentrations and four-year weight gain among US men, *International Journal of Obesity and Related Metabolic Disorders* 25 (2001): 346–353; Ceddia, William, and Curi, 2001.
15. R. H. Unger, Leptin physiology: A second look, *Regulatory Peptides* 92 (2000): 87–95.
16. A. M. Prentice and coauthors, Leptin and undernutrition, *Nutrition Reviews* 60 (2002): S56–S67.
17. J. Harvey and M. L. Ashford, *Neuropharmacology* 44 (2003): 845–854.
18. S. Takeda, F. Elefteriou, and G. Karsenty, Common endocrine control of body weight, reproduction, and bone mass, *Annual Review of Nutrition* 23 (2003): 403–411; Leptin: A key regulator in nutrition, *Nutrition Reviews* 60 (2002): entire issue; S. Moschos, J. L. Chan, and C. S. Mantzoros, Leptin and reproduction: A review, *Fertility and Sterility* 77 (2002): 433–444; R. B. S. Harris, Leptin—Much more than a satiety signal, *Annual Review of Nutrition* 20 (2000): 45–75; J. C. Fleet, Leptin and bone: Does the brain control bone biology? *Nutrition Reviews* 58 (2000): 209–211.
19. M. Kojima and K. Kangawa, Ghrelin, an orexigenic signaling molecule from the gastrointestinal tract, *Current Opinion in Pharmacology* 2 (2002): 665–668.
20. J. Eisenstein and A. Greenberg, Ghrelin: Update 2003, *Nutrition Reviews* 61 (2003): 101–104; O. Ukkola and S. Poykko, Ghrelin, growth and obesity, *Annals of Medicine* 34 (2002): 102–108.
21. G. Schaller and coauthors, Plasma ghrelin concentrations are not regulated by glucose or insulin: A double-blind, placebo-controlled crossover clamp study, *Diabetes* 52 (2003): 16–20; G. Iniguez and coauthors, Fasting and post-glucose ghrelin levels in SGA infants: Relationships with size and weight gain at one year of age, *Journal of Clinical Endocrinology and Metabolism* 87 (2002): 5830–5833.
22. M. Tanaka and coauthors, Habitual binge/purge behavior influences circulating ghrelin levels in eating disorders, *Journal of Psychiatric Research* 37 (2003): 17–22; J. H. Lindeman and coauthors, Ghrelin and the hyposomatotropism of obesity, *Obesity Research* 10 (2002): 1161–1166.
23. V. Tolle and coauthors, Balance in ghrelin and leptin plasma levels in anorexia nervosa patients and constitutionally thin women, *Journal of Clinical Endocrinology and Metabolism* 88 (2003): 109–116; M. F. Saad and coauthors, Insulin regulates plasma ghrelin concentration, *Journal of Clinical Endocrinology and Metabolism* 87 (2002): 3997–4000.
24. A. M. Haqq and coauthors, Serum ghrelin levels are inversely correlated with body mass index, age, and insulin concentrations in normal children and are markedly increased in Prader-Willi syndrome, *Journal of Clinical Endocrinology and Metabolism* 88 (2003): 174–178; A. DelParigi and coauthors, High circulating ghrelin: A potential cause for hyperphagia and obesity in Prader-Willi syndrome, *Journal of Clinical Endocrinology and Metabolism* 87 (2002): 5461–5464.
25. P. J. English and coauthors, Food fails to suppress ghrelin levels in obese humans, *Journal of Clinical Endocrinology and Metabolism* 87 (2002): 2984.
26. D. E. Cummings and coauthors, Plasma ghrelin levels after diet-induced weight loss or gastric bypass surgery, *New England Journal of Medicine* 346 (2002): 1623–1630.
27. Cummings and coauthors, 2002.
28. Iniguez and coauthors, 2002.
29. J. Korner and R. L. Leibel, To eat or not to eat—How the gut talks to the brain, *New England Journal of Medicine* 349 (2003): 926–930.
30. R. L. Batterham and coauthors, Inhibition of food intake in obese subjects by peptide YY_{3-36}, *New England Journal of Medicine* 349 (2003): 941–948.
31. F. Broglio and coauthors, Ghrelin: Endocrine and non-endocrine actions, *Journal of Pediatric Endocrinology and Metabolism* 15 (2002): 1219–1227.
32. J. C. Weikel and coauthors, Ghrelin promotes slow-wave sleep in humans, *American Journal of Physiology: Endocrinology and Metabolism* 284 (2003): E407–E415.
33. G. Wolf, The uncoupling proteins UCP2 and UCP3 in skeletal muscle, *Nutrition Reviews* 59 (2001): 56–57.
34. L. P. Kozak and M. E. Harper, Mitochondrial uncoupling proteins in energy expenditure, *Annual Review of Nutrition* 20 (2000): 339–363.
35. S. Y. S. Kimm and coauthors, Racial differences in the relation between uncoupling protein genes and resting energy expenditure, *American Journal of Clinical Nutrition* 75 (2002): 714–719; J. A. Yanovski and coauthors, Associations between uncoupling protein 2, body composition, and resting energy expenditure in lean and obese African American, white, and Asian children, *American Journal of Clinical Nutrition* 71 (2000): 1405–1412.
36. P. Hakala and coauthors, Environmental factors in the development of obesity in identical twins, *American Journal of Obesity and Related Metabolic Disorders* 23 (1999): 746–753.
37. A. H. C. Goris, M. S. Westerterp-Plantenga, and K. R. Westerterp, Undereating and underrecording of habitual food intake in obese men: Selective underreporting of fat intake, *American Journal of Clinical Nutrition* 71 (2000): 130–134.
38. J. C. Peters, The challenge of managing body weight in the modern world, *Asia Pacific Journal of Clinical Nutrition* 11 (2002): S714–S717.
39. B. J. Rolls, E. L. Morris, and L. S. Roe, Portion size of food affects energy intake

in normal-weight and overweight men and women, *American Journal of Clinical Nutrition* 76 (2002): 1207–1213.
40. S. J. Nielsen and B. M. Popkin, Patterns and trends in food portion sizes, 1977–1998, *Journal of the American Medical Association* 289 (2003): 450–453; H. Smiciklas-Wright and coauthors, Foods commonly eaten in the United States, 1989–1991 and 1994–1996: Are portion sizes changing? *Journal of the American Dietetic Association* 103 (2003): 41–47.
41. L. R. Young and M. Nestle, Expanding portion sizes in the US marketplace: Implications for nutrition counseling, *Journal of the American Dietetic Association* 103 (2003): 231–234.
42. L. R. Young and M. Nestle, The contribution of expanding portion sizes to the US obesity epidemic, *American Journal of Public Health* 92 (2002): 246–249.
43. J. K. Binkley, J. Eales, and M. Jekanowski, The relation between dietary change and rising US obesity, *International Journal of Obesity and Related Metabolic Disorders* 24 (2000): 1032–1039.
44. B. J. Rolls, The supersizing of America: Portion size and the obesity epidemic, *Nutrition Today* 38 (2003): 42–53.
45. M. Lahti-Koski and coauthors, Associations of body mass index and obesity with physical activity, food choices, alcohol intake, and smoking in the 1982–1997 FINRISK Studies, *American Journal of Clinical Nutrition* 75 (2002): 809–817; M. Wei and coauthors, The association between cardiorespiratory fitness and impaired glucose and type 2 diabetes mellitus in men, *Annals of Internal Medicine* 130 (1999): 89–96; U.S. Department of Health and Human Services, *Physical Activity and Health—A Report of the Surgeon General Executive Summary,* 1996.
46. F. B. Hu and coauthors, Television watching and other sedentary behaviors in relation to risk of obesity and type 2 diabetes mellitus in women, *Journal of the American Medical Association* 289 (2003): 1785–1791; J. Salmon and coauthors, The association between television viewing and overweight among Australian adults participating in varying levels of leisure-time physical activity, *International Journal of Obesity and Related Metabolic Disorders* 24 (2000): 600–606.
47. *U.S. News and World Report,* June 16, 2003, p. 36; **www.niddk.nih.gov/healthnutrit/pubs/statobes.htm**.
48. National Institutes of Health Obesity Education Initiative, *The Practical Guide: Identification, Evaluation, and Treatment of Overweight and Obesity in Adults* (Washington, D.C.: U.S. Department of Health and Human Services, 2000).
49. National Institutes of Health Obesity Education Initiative, 2000.
50. S. Sarlio-Lähteenkorva, A. Rissanen, and J. Kaprio, A descriptive study of weight loss maintenance: 6 and 15 year follow-up of initially overweight adults, *International Journal of Obesity and Related Metabolic Disorders* 24 (2000): 116–125.
51. N. S. Wellman and B. Friedberg, Causes and consequences of adult obesity: Health, social and economic impacts in the United States, *Asia Pacific Journal of Clinical Nutrition* 11 (2002): S705–S709.
52. H. M. Blanck, L. K. Khan, and M. K. Serdula, Use of nonprescription weight loss products: Results from a multistate survey, *Journal of the American Medical Association* 286 (2001): 930–935.
53. D. J. Dyck, Dietary fat intake, supplements, and weight loss, *Canadian Journal of Applied Physiology* 25 (2000): 495–523.
54. P. G. Shekelle and coauthors, Efficacy and safety of ephedra and ephedrine for weight loss and athletic performance: A meta-analysis, *Journal of the American Medical Association* 289 (2003): 1537–1545.
55. G. Egger, D. Cameron-Smith, and R. Stanton, The effectiveness of popular, non-prescription weight loss supplements, *Medical Journal of Australia* 171 (1999): 604–608; A. Sarubin, *The Health Professional's Guide to Popular Dietary Supplements* (Chicago: The American Dietetic Association, 1999); S. Foster and V. E. Tyler, *Tyler's Honest Herbal—A Sensible Guide to the Use of Herbs and Related Remedies* (New York: Haworth Herbal Press, 1999).
56. S. P. Dolan and coauthors, Analysis of dietary supplements for arsenic, cadmium, mercury, and lead using inductively coupled plasma mass spectrometry, *Journal of Agricultural and Food Chemistry* 51 (2003): 1307–1312; A. H. Feifer, N. E. Fleshner, and L. Klotz, Analytical accuracy and reliability of commonly used nutritional supplements in prostate disease, *Journal of Urology* 168 (2002): 150–154.
57. S. Z. Yanovski and J. A. Yanovski, Obesity, *New England Journal of Medicine* 346 (2002): 591–602.
58. C. H. Halsted, Is blockade of pancreatic lipase the answer? *American Journal of Clinical Nutrition* 69 (1999): 1059–1060.
59. G. Glazer, Long-term pharmacotherapy of obesity 2000: A review of efficacy and safety, *Archives of Internal Medicine* 161 (2001): 1814–1824.
60. S. Schurgin and R. D. Siegel, Pharmacotherapy of obesity: An update, *Nutrition in Clinical Care* 6 (2003): 27–37.
61. M. A. Rupnick and coauthors, Adipose tissue mass can be regulated through the vasculature, *Proceedings of the National Academy of Science* 99 (2002): 10730–10735.
62. Cummings and coauthors, 2002.
63. E. C. Mun, G. L. Blackburn, and J. B. Matthews, Current status of medical and surgical therapy for obesity, *Gastroenterology* 120 (2001): 669–681; H. J. Sugarman, The epidemic of severe obesity: The value of surgical treatment, *Mayo Clinic Proceedings* 75 (2000): 669–672.
64. R. E. Brolin, Bariatric surgery and long-term control of morbid obesity, *Journal of the American Medical Association* 288 (2002): 2793–2796.
65. J. G. Bruner and R. H. de Jong, Lipoplasty claims experience of U.S. insurance companies, *Plastic and Reconstructive Surgery* 107 (2001): 1285–1291; R. B. Rao, S. F. Ely, and R. S. Hoffman, Deaths related to liposuction, *New England Journal of Medicine* 340 (1999): 1471–1475.
66. J. T. Fine and coauthors, A prospective study of weight change and health-related quality of life in women, *Journal of the American Medical Association* 282 (1999): 2136–2142.
67. G. D. Foster and coauthors, Obese patients' perceptions of treatment outcomes and the factors that influence them, *Archives of Internal Medicine* 161 (2001): 2133–2139.
68. National Institutes of Health Obesity Education Initiative, 2000, p. 2.
69. Position of the American Dietetic Association: Weight management, *Journal of the American Dietetic Association* 102 (2002): 1145–1155.
70. M. K. Serdula and coauthors, Prevalence of attempting weight loss and strategies for controlling weight, *Journal of the American Medical Association* 282 (1999): 1353–1358.
71. National Institutes of Health Obesity Education Initiative, *Clinical Guidelines on the Identification, Evaluation, and Treatment of Overweight and Obesity in Adults* (Washington, D.C.: U.S. Department of Health and Human Services, 1998).
72. National Institutes of Health Obesity Education Initiative, 2000, pp. 26–27.
73. A. K. Kant and coauthors, A prospective study of diet quality and mortality in women, *Journal of the American Medical Association* 283 (2000): 2109–2115.
74. Nielsen and Popkin, 2003; Smiciklas-Wright and coauthors, 2003; Young and Nestle, 2002.
75. E. A. Bell and B. J. Rolls, Energy density of foods affects energy intake across multiple levels of fat content in lean and obese women, *American Journal of Clinical Nutrition* 73 (2001): 1010–1018.
76. T. V. Kral, L. S. Roe, and B. J. Rolls, Does nutrition information about the energy density of meals affect food intake in normal-weight women? *Appetite* 39 (2002): 137–145; B. J. Rolls and E. A. Bell, Dietary approaches to the treatment of obesity, *Medical Clinics of North America* 84 (2000): 401–418, vi.
77. B. J. Rolls, E. A. Bell, and M. L. Thorwart, Water incorporated into a food but not served with a food decreases energy intake in lean women, *American Journal of Clinical Nutrition* 70 (1999): 448–455.
78. S. A. Bowman and J. T. Spence, A comparison of low-carbohydrate vs. high-carbohydrate diets: Energy restriction, nutrient quality and correlation to body mass index, *Journal of the American College of Nutrition* 21 (2002): 268–274.
79. M. Yao and S. B. Roberts, Dietary energy density and weight regulation, *Nutrition Reviews* 59 (2001): 247–258.
80. A. Astrup and coauthors, Low-fat diets and energy balance: How does the evidence stand in 2002? *Proceedings of the Nutrition Society* 61 (2002): 299–309; S. D. Poppitt and coauthors, Long-term effects of ad libitum low-fat, high-carbohydrate diets on weight and serum lipids in overweight subjects with metabolic syndrome, *American Journal of Clinical Nutrition* 75 (2002): 11–20; S. E. Kasim-Karakas and coauthors, Changes in plasma lipoproteins during low-fat, high-carbohydrate diets: Effects of energy intake, *American Journal of Clinical Nutrition* 71 (2000): 1439–1447.
81. G. D. Foster and coauthors, A randomized trial of a low-carbohydrate diet for obesity, *New England Journal of Medicine* 348 (2003): 2082–2090.
82. D. K. Layman and coauthors, A reduced ratio of dietary carbohydrate to protein improves body composition and blood lipid profiles during weight loss in adult women, *Journal of Nutrition* 133 (2003): 411–417; D. M. Bravata and coauthors, Efficacy and safety of low-carbohydrate diets, *Journal of the American Medical Association* 289 (2003): 1837–1850; S. Pirozzo and coauthors, Advice on low-fat diets for obesity, *Cochrane Database of Systematic Review* (2002), available at **www.update-software.com/abstracts/ab003640.htm**; M. R. Freedman, J. King, and E. Kennedy, Popular diets: A scientific review, *Obesity Research* 9 (2001): 1S–5S; A. Golay and coauthors, Similar weight loss with low-energy food combining or balanced diets, *International Journal of Obesity and Related Metabolic Disorders* 24 (2000): 492–496; N. H. Baba and coauthors, High protein vs high carbohydrate hypoenergetic diet for the treatment of obese hyperinsulinemic subjects, *International Journal of Obesity and Related Metabolic Disorders* 23 (1999): 1202–1206.
83. Astrup and coauthors, 2002.
84. Committee on Dietary Reference Intakes, *Dietary Reference Intakes for Energy, Carbohydrate, Fiber, Fat, Fatty Acids, Cholesterol, Protein, and Amino Acids* (Washington, D.C.: National Academies Press, 2002).
85. J. W. Anderson and coauthors, Long-term weight-loss maintenance: A meta-analysis

of US studies, *American Journal of Clinical Nutrition* 74 (2001): 579–584.
86. J. F. Carroll and C. K. Kyser, Exercise training in obesity lowers blood pressure independent of weight change, *Medicine and Science in Sports and Exercise* 34 (2002): 596–601; B. Gutin and coauthors, Effects of exercise intensity on cardiovascular fitness, total body composition, and visceral adiposity of obese adolescents, *American Journal of Clinical Nutrition* 75 (2002): 818–826; R. Ross and coauathors, Reduction in obesity and related comorbid conditions after diet-induced weight loss and exercise induced weight loss in men, *Annals of Internal Medicine* 133 (2000): 92–103; A. L. Dunn and coauthors, Comparison of lifestyle and structured interventions to increase physical activity and cardiorespiratory fitness: A randomized trial, *Journal of the American Medical Association* 281 (1999): 327–334; J. M. Jakicic and coauthors, Effects of intermittent exercise and use of home exercise equipment on adherence, weight loss, and fitness in overweight women—A randomized trial, *Journal of the American Medical Association* 282 (1999): 1554–1560.
87. U. G. Kyle and coauthors, Physical activity and fat-free and fat mass by bioelectrical impedance in 3853 adults, *Medicine and Science in Sports and Exercise* 33 (2001): 576–584.
88. Gutin and coauthors, 2002; R. Ross and coauthors, Reduction in obesity and related comorbid conditions after diet-induced weight loss or exercise-induced weight loss in men: A randomized, controlled trial, *Annals of Internal Medicine* 133 (2000): 92–103; G. Benedetti and coauthors, Body composition and energy expenditure after weight loss following bariatric surgery, *Journal of the American College of Nutrition* 19 (2000): 270–274.
89. Gutin and coauthors, 2002; Ross and coauthors, 2000.
90. W. D. Schmidt, C. J. Biwer, and L. K. Kalscheuer, Effects of long *versus* short bout exercise on fitness and weight loss in overweight females, *Journal of the American College of Nutrition* 20 (2001): 494–501.
91. American College of Sports Medicine, Position stand: Appropriate intervention strategies for weight loss and prevention of weight regain for adults, *Medicine and Science in Sports and Exercise* 33 (2001): 2145–2156.
92. S. M. Byrne, Psychological aspects of weight maintenance and relapse in obesity, *Journal of Psychosomatic Research* 53 (2002): 1029–1036.
93. D. F. Tate, E. H. Jackvony, and R. R. Wing, Effects of Internet behavioral counseling on weight loss in adults at risk for type 2 diabetes: A randomized trial, *Journal of the American Medical Association* 289 (2003): 1833–1836.
94. R. R. Wing and J. O. Hill, Successful weight loss maintenance, *Annual Review of Nutrition* 21 (2001): 323–341.
95. M. T. Mcguire, R. R. Wing, and J. O. Hill, The prevalence of weight loss maintenance among American adults, *International Journal of Obesity and Related Metabolic Disorders* 23 (1999): 1314–1319.
96. Wing and Hill, 2001; M. R. Lowe, K. Miller-Kovach, and S. Phelan, Weight-loss maintenance in overweight individuals one to five years following successful completion of a commercial weight loss program, *International Journal of Obesity and Related Metabolic Disorders* 25 (2001): 325–331.
97. M. S. Leser, S. Z. Yanovski, and J. A. Yanovski, A low-fat intake and greater activity level are associated with lower weight regain 3 years after completing a very-low-calorie diet, *Journal of the American Dietetic Association* 102 (2002): 1252–1256.
98. A. Raben and coauthors, Diurnal metabolic profiles after 14d of an ad libitum high-starch, high-sucrose, or high-fat diet in normal-weight, never-obese and postobese women, *American Journal of Clinical Nutrition* 73 (2001): 177–189.
99. A. Astrup and coauthors, Meta-analysis of resting metabolic rate in formerly obese subjects, *American Journal of Clinical Nutrition* 69 (1999): 1117–1122.
100. R. L. Weinsier and coauthors, Free-living activity energy expenditure in women successful and unsuccessful at maintaining a normal body weight, *American Journal of Clinical Nutrition* 75 (2002): 499–504.
101. D. A. Schoeller, K. Shay, and R. F. Kushner, How much physical activity is needed to minimize weight gain in previously obese women? *American Journal of Clinical Nutrition* 66 (1997): 551–556.
102. American College of Sports Medicine, 2001.
103. Wing and Hill, 2001.
104. R. E. Killingsworth, Health promoting community design: A new paradigm to promote healthy and active communities, *American Journal of Health Promotion* 17 (2003): 169–170; M. Nestle and M. F. Jacobson, Halting the obesity epidemic: A public health policy approach, *Public Health Reports* 115 (2000): 12–24.
105. S. L. Mercer and coauthors, Possible lessons from the tobacco experience for obesity control, *American Journal of Clinical Nutrition* 77 (2003): 1073S–1082S.
106. T. B. VanItallie, Resistance to weight gain during overfeeding: A NEAT explanation, *Nutrition Reviews* 59 (2001): 48–51.
107. C. Marmonier and coauthors, Snacks consumed in a nonhungry state have poor satiating efficiency: Influence of snack composition on substrate utilization and hunger, *American Journal of Clinical Nutrition* 76 (2002): 518–528.

ANSWERS

Nutrition Calculations

1. a. Three milk shakes provide: 3 × 190 kcal = 570 kcal; 3 × 32 g carbohydrate = 96 g carbohydrate; 3 × 13 g protein = 39 g protein; and 3 × 1 g fat = 3 g fat.

   b. To meet this criteria, the plan needs *at least* an additional 630 kcalories (1200 kcal − 570 kcal = 630 kcal); an additional 5 to 24 grams of protein, depending on the person's RDA based on gender and age (63 g − 39 g = 24 g and 44 g − 39 g = 5 g); an additional 4 grams of carbohydrate (100 g − 96 g = 4 g); and some additional fat.

   c. Of course, there are many possible dinners that you could plan. One might be:

      Salad made with 1 c lettuce, 1 c chopped tomatoes and onions, ¼ c garbanzo beans, and 2 tbs low-fat dressing
      4 oz grilled chicken
      1 medium baked potato
      1 c summer squash and zucchini
      1 c melon cubes

   This meal brings the day's totals to 1215 kcalories, 90 g of protein, 192 g of carbohydrate, and 13 g of fat, which meets the goals for kcalories, protein, and carbohydrate. Because the milk shake has been fortified, all vitamin and mineral needs are covered as well. The only possible dietary shortcoming is that the day's percent kcalories from fat is low (only 10%), but because energy and nutrient recommendations have been met and the goal is weight loss, this may be acceptable.

   d. This weight-loss plan uses a liquid formula rather than foods, making clients dependent on a special device (the formula) rather than teaching them how to make good choices from the conventional food supply. It provides no information about dropout rates, the long-term success of clients, or weight maintenance after the program ends.

2. a. More than a pound (552 g ÷ 454 g/lb = 1.2 lb).

   b. 541 kcal ÷ 552 g = 0.98 kcal/g.

   c. More than another whole pound (0.98 kcal/g × 500 kcal = 490 g; 490 g ÷ 454 g/lb = 1.1 lb).

   d.

Item No./Food	Weight (g)	Energy (kcal)
Original totals:	552	541
Minus:		
#867 Lettuce, 1 c	−55	−7
Plus:		
#603 Roast beef, 1 oz	+28	+68
#37 Cheddar cheese, 1 oz	+28	+113
Totals:	553 g	715 kcal

   e. 715 kcal − 541 kcal = 174 kcal added.

   f. 553 g − 552 g = 1 g added.

Study Questions (multiple choice)

1. a 2. d 3. a 4. d 5. c 6. c 7. d 8. d 9. d 10. b

HIGHLIGHT

Eating Disorders

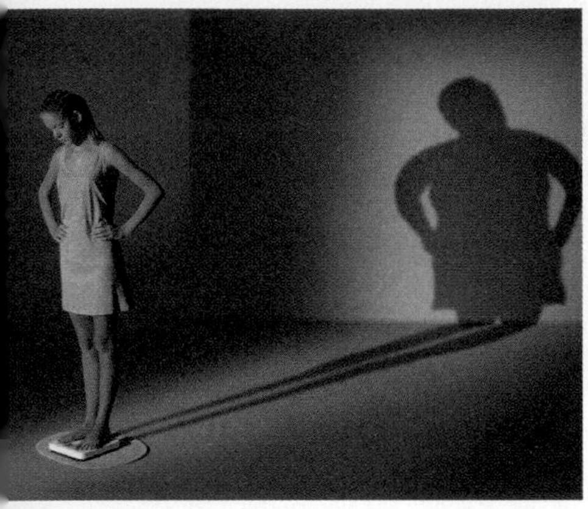
© Steve Niedorf Photography/The Image Bank/Getty Images

For some people, dieting to lose weight progresses to a dangerous and obsessive point. An estimated 5 million people in the United States, primarily girls and young women, suffer from the **eating disorders** anorexia nervosa and bulimia nervosa (the accompanying glossary defines these and related terms).[1] Many more suffer from binge-eating disorders or other unspecified conditions that do not meet the strict criteria for anorexia nervosa or bulimia nervosa, but still imperil a person's well-being.

Why do so many people in our society suffer from eating disorders? Most experts agree that the causes are multifactorial: sociocultural, psychological, and perhaps neurochemical. Excessive pressure to be thin is at least partly to blame. When low body weight becomes an important goal, people begin to view normal healthy body weight as being too fat, and they take unhealthy actions to lose weight.

Young people who attempt extreme weight loss may have learned to identify discomforts such as anger, jealousy, or disappointment with "feeling fat." They may also be depressed or suffer social anxiety. As weight loss becomes more of a focus, psychological problems worsen, and the likelihood of developing eating disorders intensifies. Athletes are among those most likely to develop eating disorders.[2]

The Female Athlete Triad

At age 14, Suzanne was a top contender for a spot on the state gymnastics team. Each day her coach reminded team members that they must weigh no more than their assigned weights in order to qualify for competition. The coach chastised gymnasts who gained weight, and Suzanne was terrified of being singled out. Convinced that the less she weighed the better she would perform, Suzanne weighed herself several times a day to confirm that she had not exceeded her 80-pound limit. Driven to excel in her sport, Suzanne kept her weight down by eating very little and training very hard. Unlike many of her friends, Suzanne never began to menstruate. A few months before her fifteenth birthday, Suzanne's coach dropped her back to the second-level team. Suzanne blamed her poor performance on a slow-healing stress fracture. Mentally stressed and physically exhausted, she quit gymnastics and began overeating between periods of self-starvation. Suzanne had developed the dangerous combination of problems that characterize the **female athlete triad**—disordered eating, amenorrhea, and osteoporosis (see Figure H9-1).

Disordered Eating

Part of the reason many athletes engage in **disordered eating** behaviors may be that they and their coaches have embraced unsuitable weight standards. An athlete's body must be heavier for a given height than a nonathlete's body because the athlete's body is dense, containing more healthy bone and muscle and less fat. When athletes rely on scales, they may mistakenly be-

GLOSSARY

amenorrhea (ay-MEN-oh-REE-ah): the absence of or cessation of menstruation. **Primary amenorrhea** is menarche delayed beyond 16 years of age. **Secondary amenorrhea** is the absence of three to six consecutive menstrual cycles.

anorexia (an-oh-RECK-see-ah) **nervosa:** an eating disorder characterized by a refusal to maintain a minimally normal body weight and a distortion in perception of body shape and weight.
- **an** = without
- **orex** = mouth
- **nervos** = of nervous origin

binge-eating disorder: an eating disorder whose criteria are similar to those of bulimia nervosa, excluding purging or other compensatory behaviors.

bulimia (byoo-LEEM-ee-ah) **nervosa:** an eating disorder characterized by repeated episodes of binge eating usually followed by self-induced vomiting, misuse of laxatives or diuretics, fasting, or excessive exercise.
- **buli** = ox

cathartic (ka-THAR-tik): a strong laxative.

disordered eating: eating behaviors that are neither normal nor healthy, including restrained eating, fasting, binge eating, and purging.

eating disorders: disturbances in eating behavior that jeopardize a person's physical or psychological health.

emetic (em-ETT-ic): an agent that causes vomiting.

female athlete triad: a potentially fatal combination of three medical problems: disordered eating, amenorrhea, and osteoporosis.

muscle dysmorphia (dis-MORE-fee-ah): a newly coined psychiatric disorder characterized by a preoccupation with building body mass.

stress fractures: bone damage or breaks caused by stress on bone surfaces during exercise.

unspecified eating disorders: eating disorders that do not meet the defined criteria for specific eating disorders.

FIGURE H9-1 The Female Athlete Triad

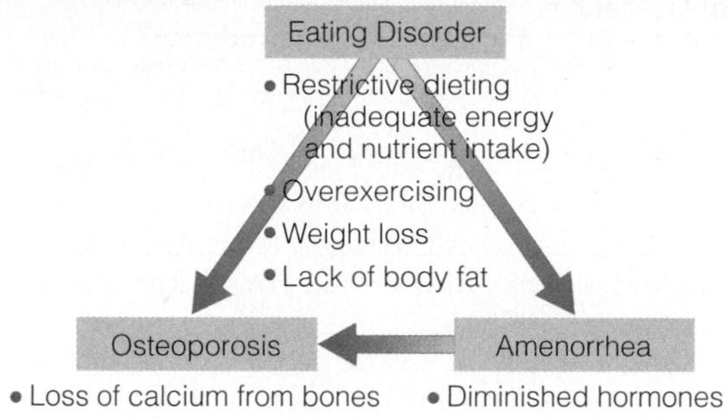
Eating Disorder
• Restrictive dieting (inadequate energy and nutrient intake)
• Overexercising
• Weight loss
• Lack of body fat
Osteoporosis
• Loss of calcium from bones
Amenorrhea
• Diminished hormones

lieve they are too fat because weight standards, such as the BMI, do not provide adequate information about body composition.

Many young athletes severely restrict energy intakes to improve performance, enhance the aesthetic appeal of their performance, or meet the weight guidelines of their specific sports. They fail to realize that the loss of lean tissue that accompanies energy restriction actually impairs their physical performance. The increasing incidence of abnormal eating habits among athletes is cause for concern. Male athletes, especially wrestlers and gymnasts, are affected by these disorders as well, but females are most vulnerable. Risk factors for eating disorders among athletes include:

- Young age (adolescence).
- Pressure to excel at a chosen sport.
- Focus on achieving or maintaining an "ideal" body weight or body fat percentage.
- Participation in endurance sports or competitions that emphasize a lean appearance or judge performance on aesthetic appeal such as gymnastics, wrestling, figure skating, or dance.
- Weight-loss dieting at an early age.
- Unsupervised dieting.

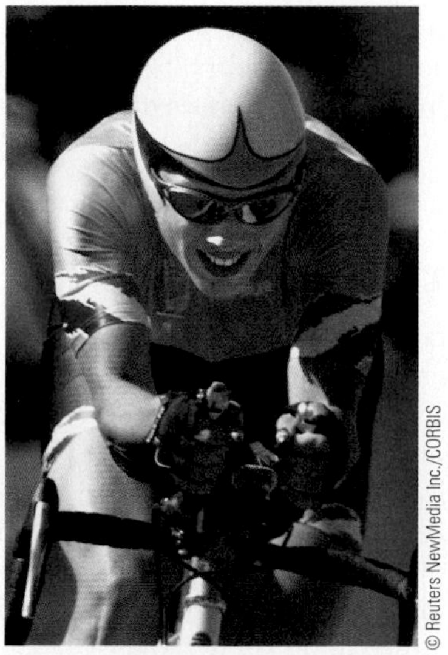

© Reuters NewMedia Inc./CORBIS

A few years earlier, this Olympic gold medalist would have been too weak and malnourished from anorexia nervosa to have set a world record in the cycling road race.

Amenorrhea

The prevalence of **amenorrhea** among premenopausal women in the United States is about 2 to 5 percent overall, but among female athletes, it may be as high as 66 percent. Contrary to previous notions, amenorrhea is *not* a normal adaptation to strenuous physical training: it is a symptom of something going wrong.[4] Amenorrhea is characterized by low blood estrogen, infertility, and often bone mineral losses. Excessive training, depleted body fat, low body weight, and inadequate nutrition all contribute to amenorrhea.[5] However amenorrhea develops, it threatens the integrity of the bones. Bone losses remain significant even after recovery.[6] (Women with bulimia frequently have menstrual irregularities, but they rarely cease menstruating, and so may be spared this loss of bone integrity.[7])

Osteoporosis

For most people, weight-bearing physical activity, dietary calcium, and the hormone estrogen protect against the bone loss of osteoporosis. For young women with disordered eating and amenorrhea, strenuous activity can impair bone health. Vigorous training combined with inadequate food intake raises stress hormones.[8] These stress hormones compromise bone health, greatly increasing the risks of **stress fractures** today and of osteoporosis in later life. Stress fractures, a serious form of bone injury, commonly occur among dancers and other athletes with amenorrhea, low calcium intakes, and disordered eating.[9] Many underweight young athletes have bones like those of postmenopausal women, and they may never recover their lost bone even after diagnosis and treatment—which makes prevention critical.[10] Athletes should be encouraged to consume at least 1300 milligrams of calcium each day, to eat nutrient-dense foods, and to obtain enough energy to support both weight gain and the energy expended in physical activity.

Other Dangerous Practices of Athletes

Only females face the threats of the female athlete triad, of course, but many male athletes face pressure to achieve a certain body weight and may develop eating disorders. Each week throughout the season, David drastically restricts his food and fluid intake before a wrestling match in an effort to "make weight." For at least three wrestlers in 1997, the consequences were deadly. Wrestlers and their coaches believe that competing in a lower weight class will give them a competitive advantage over smaller opponents. To that end, David practices in rubber suits, sits in saunas, and takes diuretics to lose 4 to 6 pounds.[11] He hopes to replenish the lost fluids, glycogen, and lean tissue during the hours between his weigh-in and competition, but the body needs days to correct this metabolic mayhem. Reestablishing fluid and electrolyte balances may take a day or two, replenishing glycogen stores may take two to three days, and replacing lean tissue may take even longer.

Ironically, the combination of food deprivation and dehydration impairs physical performance by reducing muscle strength, decreasing anaerobic power, reducing endurance capacity, and lowering oxygen consumption. For optimal performance, wrestlers need to first achieve their competitive weight during the off-season and then eat well-balanced meals and drink plenty of fluids during the competitive season.

Some athletes go to extreme measures to bulk up and *gain* weight. People afflicted with **muscle dysmorphia** eat high-protein diets, take dietary supplements, weight train for hours at a time, and often abuse steroids in an attempt to bulk up. Their bodies are large and muscular, yet they see themselves as puny 90-pound weaklings. They are preoccupied with the idea that their bodies are too small or inadequately muscular. Like others with distorted body images, people with muscle dysmorphia weigh themselves frequently and center their lives on diet and exercise. Paying attention to diet and pumping iron for fitness is admirable, but obsessing over it can cause serious social, occupational, and physical problems.

Preventing Eating Disorders in Athletes

To prevent eating disorders in athletes and dancers, the performers, their coaches, and their parents must learn about inappropriate body weight ideals, improper weight-loss techniques, eating disorder development, proper nutrition, and safe weight-control methods. Young people naturally search for identity and will often follow the advice of a person in authority without question. Therefore, coaches and dance instructors should never encourage unhealthy weight loss to qualify for competition or to conform with distorted artistic ideals. Athletes who truly need to lose weight should try to do so during the off-season and under the supervision of a health care professional. Frequent weighings can push young people who are striving to lose weight into a cycle of starving to confront the scale, then bingeing uncontrollably afterward. The erosion of self-esteem that accompanies these events can interfere with normal psychological development and set the stage for serious problems later on.

Table H9-1 includes suggestions to help athletes and dancers protect themselves against developing eating disorders. The remaining sections describe eating disorders that anyone, athlete or nonathlete, may experience.

TABLE H9-1 Tips for Combating Eating Disorders

General Guidelines
• Never restrict kcalories to below 1200 kcalories or food amounts to below those suggested for adequacy by the USDA Food Guide (see Table 2-3 on p. 46).
• Eat frequently. Include healthy snacks between meals. The person who eats frequently never gets so hungry as to allow hunger to dictate food choices.
• If not at a healthy weight, establish a reasonable weight goal based on a healthy body composition.
• Allow a reasonable time to achieve the goal. A reasonable loss of excess fat can be achieved at the rate of about 10 percent of body weight in six months.
• Establish a weight-maintenance support group with people who share interests.
Specific Guidelines for Athletes and Dancers
• Replace weight-based goals with performance-based goals.
• Restrict weight-loss activities to the off-season.
• Remember that eating disorders impair physical performance. Seek confidential help in obtaining treatment if needed.
• Focus on proper nutrition as an important facet of your training, as important as proper technique.

Anorexia Nervosa

Julie is 18 years old and a superachiever in school. She watches her diet with great care, and she exercises daily, maintaining a rigorous schedule of self-discipline. She is thin, but she is determined to lose more weight. She is 5 feet 6 inches tall and weighs 85 pounds. She has **anorexia nervosa.**

Characteristics of Anorexia Nervosa

Julie is unaware that she is undernourished, and she sees no need to obtain treatment. She developed amenorrhea several months ago and has become moody and chronically depressed. She insists that she is too fat, although her eyes are sunk in deep hollows in her face. Julie denies that she is ever tired, although she is close to physical exhaustion and no longer sleeps easily. Her family is concerned, and though reluctant to push her, they have finally insisted that she see a psychiatrist. Julie's psychiatrist has diagnosed anorexia nervosa (see Table H9-2) and prescribed group therapy as a start. If she does not begin to gain weight soon, she may need to be hospitalized.

As mentioned in the introduction, most anorexia nervosa victims are females; males account for only about 1 in 20 reported cases. Central to the diagnosis of anorexia nervosa is a

TABLE H9-2 Criteria for Diagnosis of Anorexia Nervosa

A person with anorexia nervosa demonstrates the following:

A. Refusal to maintain body weight at or above a minimal normal weight for age and height (e.g., weight loss leading to maintenance of body weight less than 85 percent of that expected; or failure to make expected weight gain during period of growth, leading to body weight less than 85 percent of that expected).

B. Intense fear of gaining weight or becoming fat, even though underweight.

C. Disturbance in the way in which one's body weight or shape is experienced, undue influence of body weight or shape on self-evaluation, or denial of the seriousness of the current low body weight.

D. In females past puberty, amenorrhea, i.e., the absence of at least three consecutive menstrual cycles. (A woman is considered to have amenorrhea if her periods occur only following hormone, e.g., estrogen, administration.)

Two types:

Restricting type: During the episode of anorexia nervosa, the person does not regularly engage in binge eating or purging behavior (i.e., self-induced vomiting or the misuse of laxatives, diuretics, or enemas).

Binge eating/purging type: During the episode of anorexia nervosa, the person regularly engages in binge eating or purging behavior (i.e., self-induced vomiting or the misuse of laxatives, diuretics, or enemas).

SOURCE: Reprinted with permission from American Psychiatric Association, *Diagnostic and Statistical Manual of Mental Disorders,* 4th ed. Text Revision. (Washington, D.C.: American Psychiatric Association, 2000).

distorted body image that overestimates personal body fatness. When Julie looks at herself in the mirror, she sees a "fat" 85-pound body. The more Julie overestimates her body size, the more resistant she is to treatment, and the more unwilling to examine her faulty values and misconceptions. Malnutrition is known to affect brain functioning and judgment in this way, causing lethargy, confusion, and delirium.

Anorexia nervosa cannot be self-diagnosed. Nearly everyone in our society is engaged in the pursuit of thinness, and denial runs high among people with anorexia nervosa. Some women have all the attitudes and behaviors associated with the condition, but without the dramatic weight loss.

Self-Starvation How can a person as thin as Julie continue to starve herself? Julie uses tremendous discipline against her hunger to strictly limit her portions of low-kcalorie foods. She will deny her hunger, and having adapted to so little food, she feels full after eating only a half-dozen carrot sticks. She knows the kcalorie contents of dozens of foods and the kcalorie costs of as many exercises. If she feels that she has gained an ounce of weight, she runs or jumps rope until she is sure she has exercised it off. If she fears that the food she has eaten outweighs the exercise, she may take laxatives to hasten the passage of food from her system. She drinks water incessantly to fill her stomach, risking dangerous mineral imbalances. She is desperately hungry. In fact, she is starving, but she doesn't eat because her need for self-control dominates.

Many people, on learning of this disorder, say they wish they had "a touch" of it to get thin. They mistakenly think that people with anorexia nervosa feel no hunger. They also fail to recognize the pain of the associated psychological and physical trauma.

Physical Consequences The starvation of anorexia nervosa damages the body just as the starvation of war and poverty does. In fact, after a few months, most people with anorexia nervosa have protein-energy malnutrition (PEM) that is similar to marasmus (described in Chapter 6). Their bodies have been depleted of both body fat and protein.[13] Victims are dying to be thin—quite literally. In young people, growth ceases and normal development falters. They lose so much lean tissue that basal metabolic rate slows. In addition, the heart pumps inefficiently and irregularly, the heart muscle becomes weak and thin, the chambers diminish in size, and the blood pressure falls.[14] Minerals that help to regulate heartbeat become unbalanced. Many deaths occur due to multiple organ system failure: the heart, kidneys, and liver cease to function.

Starvation brings other physical consequences as well: loss of brain tissue, impaired immune response, anemia, and a loss of digestive functions that worsens malnutrition. Peristalsis becomes sluggish, the stomach empties slowly, and the lining of the intestinal tract atrophies. The deteriorated GI tract fails to provide sufficient digestive enzymes and absorptive surfaces for handling any food that is eaten. The pancreas slows its production of digestive enzymes. The person may suffer from diarrhea, further worsening malnutrition.

Other effects of starvation include altered blood lipids, high blood vitamin A and vitamin E, low blood proteins, dry thin skin, abnormal nerve functioning, reduced bone density, low body temperature, low blood pressure, and the development of fine body hair (the body's attempt to keep warm). The electrical activity of the brain becomes abnormal, and insomnia is common. Both women and men lose their sex drives.

Women with anorexia nervosa develop amenorrhea (it is one of the diagnostic criteria). In young girls, the onset of menstruation is delayed. Menstrual periods typically resume with recovery, although some women never restart even after they have gained weight. Should an underweight woman with anorexia nervosa become pregnant, she is likely to give birth to an underweight baby—and low-birthweight babies face many health problems (as Chapter 14 explains). Mothers with anorexia nervosa may underfeed their children who then fail to grow and suffer the other consequences of starvation.

Treatment of Anorexia Nervosa

Treatment of anorexia nervosa requires a multidisciplinary approach.[15] Teams of physicians, nurses, psychiatrists, family therapists, and dietitians work together to resolve two sets of issues and behaviors: those relating to food and weight, and those involving relationships with oneself and others. The first dietary objective is to stop weight loss while establishing regular eating patterns. Appropriate diet is crucial to recovery and must be tailored individually to each client's needs.[16] Because body weight is low and fear of weight gain is high, initial food intake may be small. As eating becomes more comfortable, energy intake should increase gradually. Initially, clients may be unwilling to eat for themselves; they may need to be fed by tube. Those who will eat have a good chance of recovering without other interventions. Even after recovery, energy intakes may not fully return to normal.[17]

Because anorexia nervosa is like starvation physically, health care professionals classify clients based on indicators of PEM.* Low-risk clients need nutrition counseling. Intermediate-risk clients may need supplements such as high-kcalorie, high-protein formulas in addition to regular meals. High-risk clients may require hospitalization and may need to be fed by tube at first to prevent death. This step may cause psychological trauma. Drugs are commonly prescribed, but play a limited role in treatment.

Denial runs high among those with anorexia nervosa. Few seek treatment on their own. About half of the women who are treated can maintain their body weight at 85 percent or more of a healthy weight; at that weight, many of them begin menstruating again.[18] The other half have poor to fair treatment outcomes, relapse into abnormal eating behaviors, or die. Anorexia nervosa has one of the highest mortality rates among psychiatric disorders.[19] An estimated 1000 women die each year of anorexia nervosa—most commonly from cardiac complications due to malnutrition or suicide.[20]

Before drawing conclusions about someone who is extremely thin or who eats very little, remember that diagnosis requires professional assessment. Several national organizations offer information for people who are seeking help with anorexia nervosa, either for themselves or for others.†

TABLE H9-3 Criteria for Diagnosis of Bulimia Nervosa

A person with bulimia nervosa demonstrates the following:	
A.	Recurrent episodes of binge eating. An episode of binge eating is characterized by both of the following:
	1. Eating, in a discrete period of time (e.g., within any two-hour period), an amount of food that is definitely larger than most people would eat during a similar period of time and under similar circumstances.
	2. A sense of lack of control over eating during the episode (e.g., a feeling that one cannot stop eating or control what or how much one is eating).
B.	Recurrent inappropriate compensatory behavior in order to prevent weight gain, such as self-induced vomiting; misuse of laxatives, diuretics, enemas, or other medications; fasting; or excessive exercise.
C.	Binge eating and inappropriate compensatory behaviors both occur, on average, at least twice a week for three months.
D.	Self-evaluation unduly influenced by body shape and weight.
E.	The disturbance does not occur exclusively during episodes of anorexia nervosa.
Two types:	
	Purging type: The person regularly engages in self-induced vomiting or the misuse of laxatives, diuretics, or enemas.
	Nonpurging type: The person uses other inappropriate compensatory behaviors, such as fasting or excessive exercise, but does not regularly engage in self-induced vomiting or the misuse of laxatives, diuretics, or enemas.

SOURCE: Reprinted with permission from American Psychiatric Association, *Diagnostic and Statistical Manual of Mental Disorders,* 4th ed. Text Revision. (Washington, D.C.: American Psychiatric Association, 2000).

Bulimia Nervosa

Kelly is a charming, intelligent, 30-year-old flight attendant of normal weight who thinks constantly about food. She alternatively starves herself and secretly binges; when she has eaten too much, she makes herself vomit. Most readers recognize these symptoms as those of **bulimia nervosa.**

Characteristics of Bulimia Nervosa

Bulimia nervosa is distinct from anorexia nervosa and is more prevalent, although the true incidence is difficult to establish because bulimia nervosa is not as physically apparent. More men suffer from bulimia nervosa than from anorexia nervosa, but bulimia nervosa is still more common in women than in men. The secretive nature of bulimic behaviors makes recognition of the problem difficult, but once it is recognized, diagnosis is based on the criteria listed in Table H9-3.

Like the typical person with bulimia nervosa, Kelly is single, female, and white. She is well educated and close to her ideal body weight, although her weight fluctuates over a range of 10 pounds or so every few weeks. She prefers to weigh less than the weight that her body maintains naturally.

Kelly seldom lets her eating disorder interfere with work or other activities, although a third of all bulimics do. From early childhood she has been a high achiever and emotionally dependent on her parents. As a young teen, Kelly frequently followed severely restricted diets, but could never maintain the weight loss.[21] Kelly feels anxious at social events and cannot easily establish close personal relationships. She is usually depressed, is often impulsive, and has low self-esteem. When crisis hits, Kelly responds by replaying events, worrying excessively, and blaming herself but never asking for help— behaviors that interfere with effective coping.

Binge Eating Like the person with anorexia nervosa, the person with bulimia nervosa spends much time thinking

*Indicators of protein-energy malnutrition: a low percentage of body fat, low serum albumin, low serum transferrin, and impaired immune reactions.
†Internet sites are listed at the end of this highlight.

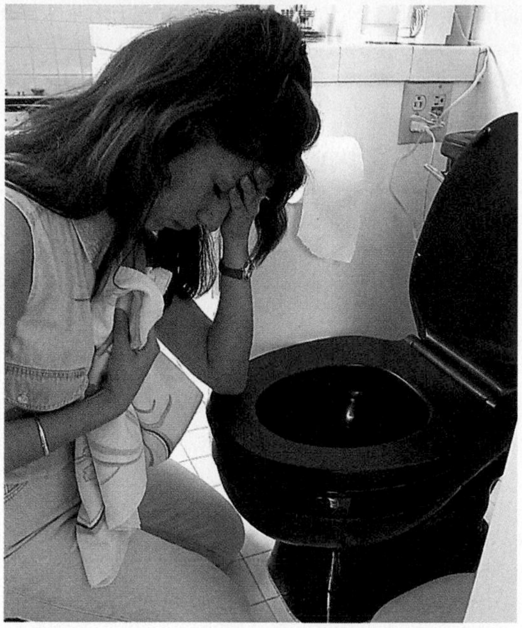

© Michael Newman/PhotoEdit

Bulimic binges are often followed by self-induced vomiting and feelings of shame or disgust.

about her body weight and food. Her preoccupation with food manifests itself in secret binge-eating episodes, which usually progress through several emotional stages: anticipation and planning, anxiety, urgency to begin, rapid and uncontrollable consumption of food, relief and relaxation, disappointment, and finally shame or disgust.

A bulimic binge is characterized by a sense of lacking control over eating. During a binge, the person consumes food for its emotional comfort and cannot stop eating or control what or how much is eaten. A typical binge occurs periodically, in secret, usually at night, and lasts an hour or more. Because a binge frequently follows a period of rigid dieting, eating is accelerated by intense hunger. Energy restriction followed by bingeing can set in motion a pattern of weight cycling, which may make weight loss and maintenance more difficult over time.

During a binge, Kelly consumes thousands of kcalories of easy-to-eat, low-fiber, high-fat, and, especially, high-carbohydrate foods. Typically, she chooses cookies, cakes, and ice cream—and she eats the entire bag of cookies, the whole cake, and every last spoonful in a carton of ice cream. After the binge, Kelly pays the price with swollen hands and feet, bloating, fatigue, headache, nausea, and pain.

Purging To purge the food from her body, Kelly may use a **cathartic**—a strong laxative that can injure the lower intestinal tract. Or she may induce vomiting, with or without the use of an **emetic**—a drug intended as first aid for poisoning. These purging behaviors are often accompanied by feelings of shame or guilt. Hence a vicious cycle develops: negative self-perceptions followed by dieting, bingeing, and purging, which in turn lead to negative self-perceptions (see Figure H9-2).

FIGURE H9-2 The Vicious Cycle of Restrictive Dieting and Binge Eating

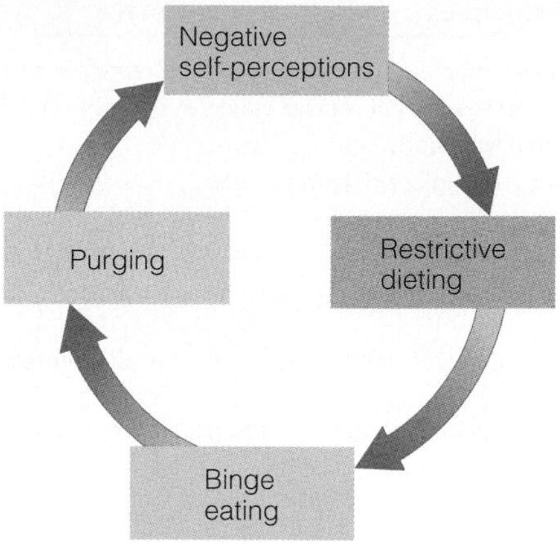
Negative self-perceptions
Restrictive dieting
Binge eating
Purging

On first glance, purging seems to offer a quick and easy solution to the problems of unwanted kcalories and body weight. Many people perceive such behavior as neutral or even positive, when, in fact, binge eating and purging have serious physical consequences. Signs of subclinical malnutrition are evident in a compromised immune system. Fluid and mineral imbalances caused by vomiting or diarrhea can lead to abnormal heart rhythms and injury to the kidneys. Urinary tract infections can lead to kidney failure. Vomiting causes irritation and infection of the pharynx, esophagus, and salivary glands; erosion of the teeth; and dental caries. The esophagus may rupture or tear, as may the stomach. Sometimes the eyes become red from pressure during vomiting. The hands may be calloused or cut by the teeth while inducing vomiting. Overuse of emetics depletes potassium concentrations and can lead to death by heart failure.

Unlike Julie, Kelly is aware that her behavior is abnormal, and she is deeply ashamed of it. She wants to recover, and this makes recovery more likely for her than for Julie, who clings to denial. Feeling inadequate ("I can't even control my eating"), Kelly tends to be passive and to look to others for confirmation of her sense of worth. When she experiences rejection, either in reality or in her imagination, her bulimia nervosa becomes worse. If Kelly's depression deepens, she may seek solace in drug or alcohol abuse or other addictive behaviors. Clinical depression is common in people with bulimia nervosa, and the rates of substance abuse are high.

Treatment of Bulimia Nervosa

Kelly needs to establish regular eating patterns. She may also benefit from a regular exercise program.[22] Weight maintenance, rather than cyclic weight gains and losses, is the treatment goal. Major steps toward recovery include discontinuing

TABLE H9-4 Diet Strategies for Combating Bulimia Nervosa

Planning Principles

- Plan meals and snacks; record plans in a food diary prior to eating.
- Plan meals and snacks that require eating at the table and using utensils.
- Refrain from finger foods.
- Refrain from "dieting" or skipping meals.

Nutrition Principles

- Eat a well-balanced diet and regularly timed meals consisting of a variety of foods.
- Include raw vegetables, salad, or raw fruit at meals to prolong eating times.
- Choose whole-grain, high-fiber breads, pasta, rice, and cereals to increase bulk.
- Consume adequate fluid, particularly water.

Other Tips

- Choose foods that provide protein and fat for satiety and bulky, fiber-rich carbohydrates for immediate feelings of fullness.
- Try including soups and other water-rich foods for satiety.
- Choose portions that meet the recommendations of the USDA Food Guide (pp. 44–45).
- For convenience (and to reduce temptation) select foods that naturally divide into portions. Select one potato, rather than rice or pasta that can be overloaded onto the plate; purchase yogurt and cottage cheese in individual containers; look for small packages of precut steak or chicken; choose frozen dinners with measured portions.
- Include 30 minutes of physical activity every day—exercise may be an important tool in defeating bulimia.

purging and restrictive dieting habits and learning to eat three meals a day plus snacks.[23] Initially, energy intake should provide enough food to satisfy hunger and maintain body weight. Table H9-4 offers diet strategies to correct the eating problems of bulimia nervosa. About half of the women diagnosed with bulimia nervosa recover completely after five to ten years, with or without treatment, but treatment probably speeds the recovery process.

A mental health professional should be on the treatment team to help clients with their depression and addictive behaviors. Some physicians prescribe the antidepressant drug fluoxetine in the treatment of bulimia nervosa.* Another drug that may be useful in the management of bulimia nervosa is naloxone, an opiate antagonist that suppresses the consumption of sweet and high-fat foods in binge-eaters.

Anorexia nervosa and bulimia nervosa are distinct eating disorders, yet they sometimes overlap in important ways. Anorexia victims may purge, and victims of both disorders share an overconcern with body weight and a tendency to drastically undereat. Many perceive foods as "forbidden" and "give in" to an eating binge. The two disorders can also appear in the same person, or one can lead to the other. Treatment is challenging and relapses are not unusual. Other people have **unspecified eating disorders** that fall short of the criteria for anorexia nervosa or bulimia nervosa, but share some of their features. One such condition is binge-eating disorder.

*Fluoxetine is marketed under the trade name Prozac.

HEALTHY PEOPLE 2010 Reduce the relapse rates for persons with eating disorders including anorexia nervosa and bulimia nervosa.

Binge-Eating Disorder

Charlie is a 40-year-old schoolteacher who has been overweight all his life. His friends and family are forever encouraging him to lose weight, and he has come to believe that if he only had more willpower, dieting would work. He periodically gives dieting his best shot—restricting energy intake for a day or two only to succumb to uncontrollable cravings, especially for high-fat foods. Like Charlie, up to half of the obese people who try to lose weight periodically binge; unlike people with bulimia nervosa, however, they typically do not purge. Such an eating disorder does not meet the criteria for either anorexia nervosa or bulimia nervosa—yet such compulsive overeating is a problem and occurs in people of normal weight as well as those who are severely overweight. Table H9-5 lists criteria for unspecified eating disorders, including binge eating. Obesity alone is not an eating disorder.

Clinicians note differences between people with bulimia nervosa and those with binge-eating disorder.[24] People with **binge-eating disorder** consume less during a binge, rarely purge, and exert less restraint during times of dieting. Similarities also exist, including feeling out of control, disgusted, depressed, embarrassed, guilty, or distressed because of their self-perceived gluttony.[25]

There are also differences between obese binge-eaters and obese people who do not binge. Those with the binge-eating disorder report higher rates of self-loathing, disgust about body size, depression, and anxiety. Their eating habits differ as well. Obese binge-eaters tend to consume more kcalories and more dessert and snack-type foods during regular meals and binges than obese people who do not binge.

Binge eating is a behavioral disorder that can be resolved with treatment. Resolving such behavior may not bring weight loss, but it may make participation in weight-control programs easier. It also improves physical health, mental health, and the chances of success in breaking the cycle of rapid weight losses and gains.

Eating Disorders in Society

Proof that society plays a role in eating disorders is found in their demographic distribution—they are known only in developed nations, and they become more prevalent as wealth increases

TABLE H9-5 Unspecified Eating Disorders,including Binge-Eating Disorder

Criteria for Diagnosis of Unspecified Eating Disorders, in General

Many people have eating disorders but do not meet all the criteria to be classified as having anorexia nervosa or bulimia nervosa. Some examples include those who:

A. Meet all of the criteria for anorexia nervosa, except irregular menses.
B. Meet all of the criteria for anorexia nervosa, except that their current weights fall within the normal ranges.
C. Meet all of the criteria for bulimia nervosa, except that binges occur less frequently than stated in the criteria.
D. Are of normal body weight and who compensate inappropriately for eating small amounts of food (example: self-induced vomiting after eating two cookies).
E. Repeatedly chew food, but spit it out without swallowing.
F. Have recurrent episodes of binge eating but who do not compensate as do those with bulimia nervosa.

Criteria for Diagnosis of Binge-Eating Disorder, Specifically

A person with a binge-eating disorder demonstrates the following:

A. Recurrent episodes of binge eating. An episode of binge eating is characterized by both of the following:
   1. Eating, in a discrete period of time (e.g., within any two-hour period) an amount of food that is definitely larger than most people would eat in a similar period of time under similar circumstances.
   2. A sense of lack of control over eating during the episode (e.g., a feeling that one cannot stop eating or control what or how much one is eating).
B. Binge-eating episodes are associated with at least three of the following:
   1. Eating much more rapidly than normal.
   2. Eating until feeling uncomfortably full.
   3. Eating large amounts of food when not feeling physically hungry.
   4. Eating alone because of being embarrassed by how much one is eating.
   5. Feeling disgusted with oneself, depressed, or very guilty after overeating.
C. The binge eating causes marked distress.
D. The binge eating occurs, on average, at least twice a week for six months.
E. The binge eating is not associated with the regular use of inappropriate compensatory behaviors (e.g., purging, fasting, excessive exercise) and does not occur exclusively during the course of anorexia nervosa or bulimia nervosa.

SOURCE: Reprinted with permission from American Psychiatric Association, *Diagnostic and Statistical Manual of Mental Disorders,* 4th ed. Text Revision. (Washington, D.C.: American Psychiatric Association, 2000).

and food becomes plentiful. Some people point to the vomitoriums of ancient times and claim that bulimia nervosa is not new, but the two are actually distinct. Ancient people were eating for pleasure, without guilt, and in the company of others; they vomited so that they could rejoin the feast. Bulimia nervosa is a disorder of isolation and is often accompanied by low self-esteem.

Chapter 8 described how our society sets unrealistic ideals for body weight, especially in women, and devalues those who do not conform to them. Anorexia nervosa and bulimia nervosa are not a form of rebellion against these unreasonable expectations, but rather an exaggerated acceptance of them. In fact, body dissatisfaction is a primary factor in the development of eating disorders.[26] Not that everyone who is dissatisfied will develop an eating disorder, but everyone with an eating disorder is dissatisfied. Characteristics of disordered eating such as restrained eating, fasting, binge eating, purging, fear of fatness, and distortion of body image are extraordinarily common among young girls. Most are "on diets," and many are poorly nourished.[27] Some eat too little food to support normal growth; thus they miss out on their adolescent growth spurts and may never catch up. Many eat so little that hunger propels them into binge-purge cycles.

Perhaps a person's best defense against these disorders is to learn to appreciate his or her own uniqueness. When people discover and honor the body's real physical needs, they become unwilling to sacrifice health for conformity. To respect and value oneself may be lifesaving.

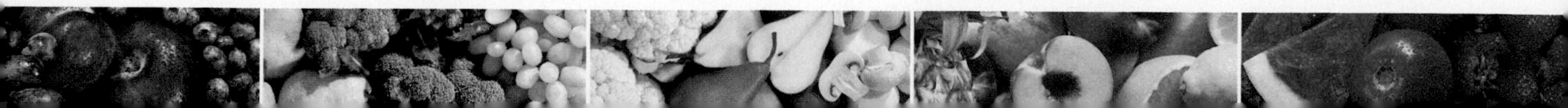

NUTRITION ON THE NET

Access these websites for further study of topics covered in this highlight.

- Find updates and quick links to these and other nutrition-related sites at our website: **www.wadsworth.com/nutrition**
- Search for "anorexia," "bulimia," and "eating disorders" at the U.S. Government health information site: **www.healthfinder.gov**
- Learn more about anorexia nervosa and related eating disorders from Anorexia Nervosa and Related Eating Disorders: **www.anred.com**
- Find out about help-lines, referral networks, support groups, and prevention programs from the American Anorexia Bulimia Association: **www.aabainc.org**
- Get facts about eating disorders from the National Institute of Mental Health: **www.nimh.nih.gov/publicat/eatingdisorder.cfm**

REFERENCES

1. Position of the American Dietetic Association: Nutrition intervention in the treatment of anorexia nervosa, bulimia nervosa, and eating disorders not otherwise specified (EDNOS), *Journal of the American Dietetic Association* 101 (2001): 810–819.
2. Position of the American Dietetic Association, 2001.
3. K. Kazis and E. Iglesias, The female athlete triad, *Adolescent Medicine* 14 (2003): 87–95; S. Sabatini, The female athlete triad, *American Journal of the Medical Sciences* 322 (2001): 193–195; Committee on Sports Medicine and Fitness, Medical concerns in the female athlete, *Pediatrics* 106 (2000): 610–613.
4. N. H. Golden, A review of the female athlete triad (amenorrhea, osteoporosis and disordered eating), *International Journal of Adolescent Medicine and Health* 14 (2002): 9–17.
5. M. Bass, L. Turner, and S. Hunt, Counseling female athletes: Application of the stages of change model to avoid disordered eating, amenorrhea, and osteoporosis, *Psychological Reports* 88 (2001): 1153–1160; M. P. Warren and A. L. Stiehl, Exercise and female adolescents: Effects on the reproductive and skeletal systems, *Journal of the American Medical Women's Association* 54 (1999): 115–120, 138.
6. D. Hartman and coauthors, Bone density of women who have recovered from anorexia nervosa, *International Journal of Eating Disorders* 28 (2000): 107–112.
7. S. J. Crow and coauthors, Long-term menstrual and reproductive function in patients with bulimia nervosa, *American Journal of Psychiatry* 159 (2002): 1048–1050; J. R. Newton and coauthors, Osteoporosis and normal weight bulimia nervosa—Which patients are at risk? *Journal of Psychosomatic Research* 37 (1993): 239–247.
8. J. A. McLean, S. I. Barr, and J. C. Prior, Cognitive dietary restraint is associated with higher urinary cortisol excretion in healthy premenopausal women, *American Journal of Clinical Nutrition* 73 (2001): 7–12.
9. A. I. Zeni and coauthors, Stress injury to the bone among women athletes, *Physical Medicine and Rehabilitation Clinics of North America* 11 (2000): 929–947; A. Nattiv, Stress fractures and bone health in track and field athletes, *Journal of Science and Medicine in Sport* 3 (2000): 268–279.
10. J. A. Hobart and D. R. Smucker, The female athlete triad, *American Family Physician* 61 (2000): 3357–3364, 3367.
11. R. B. Kiningham and D. W. Gorenflo, Weight loss methods of high school wrestlers, *Medicine and Science in Sports and Exercise* 33 (2001): 810–813.
12. D. Neumark-Sztainer and coauthors, Disordered eating among adolescents: Associations with sexual/physical abuse and other familial/psychosocial factors, *International Journal of Eating Disorders* 28 (2000): 249–258.
13. K. P. Kerruish and coauthors, Body composition in adolescents with anorexia nervosa, *American Journal of Clinical Nutrition* 75 (2002): 31–37.
14. C. Romano and coauthors, Reduced hemodynamic load and cardiac hypotrophy in patients with anorexia nervosa, *American Journal of Clinical Nutrition* 77 (2003): 308–312; C. Panagiotopoulos and coauthors, Electrocardiographic findings in adolescents with eating disorders, *Pediatrics* 105 (2000): 1100–1105.
15. Committee on Adolescence, Identifying and treating eating disorders, *Pediatrics* 111 (2003): 204–211.
16. A. E. Becker and coauthors, Eating disorders, *New England Journal of Medicine* 340 (1999): 1092–1098.
17. B. R. Carruth and J. D. Skinner, Dietary and physical activity patterns of young females with histories of eating disorders, *Topics in Clinical Nutrition* 16 (2000): 13–23.
18. H. C. Steinhausen, The outcome of anorexia nervosa in the 20th century, *American Journal of Psychiatry* 159 (2002): 1284–1293; B. Lowe and coauthors, Long-term outcome of anorexia nervosa in a prospective 21-year follow-up study, *Psychological Medicine* 31 (2001): 881–890.
19. P. K. Keel and coauthors, Predictors of mortality in eating disorders, *Archives of General Psychiatry* 60 (2003): 179–183.
20. M. B. Tamburrino and R. A. McGinnis, Anorexia nervosa: A review, *Panminerva Medica* 44 (2002): 301–311.
21. G. C. Patton and coauthors, Onset of adolescent eating disorders: Population based cohort study over 3 years, *British Medical Journal* 318 (1999): 765–768.
22. J. Sundgot-Borgen and coauthors, The effect of exercise, cognitive therapy, and nutritional counseling in treating bulimia nervosa, *Medicine and Science in Sports and Exercise* 34 (2002): 190–195.
23. Position of the American Dietetic Association, 2001.
24. A. E. Dingemans, M. J. Bruna, and E. F. van Furth, Binge eating disorder: A review, *International Journal of Obesity and Related Metabolic Disorders* 26 (2002): 299–307.
25. D. M. Ackard and coauthors, Overeating among adolescents: Prevalence and associations with weight-related characteristics and psychological health, *Pediatrics* 111 (2003): 67–74.
26. J. Polivy and C. P. Herman, Causes of eating disorders, *Annual Review of Psychology* 53 (2002): 187–213.
27. Federal Interagency Forum on Child and Family Statistics, *America's Children: Key National Indicators of Well-Being,* 1999, a report from the National Institutes of Health, available from National Maternal and Child Health Clearinghouse, 2070 Chain Bridge Road, Suite 450, Vienna, VA 22182 or on the Internet at **http://childstats.gov**.

Chapter 10

The Water-Soluble Vitamins: B Vitamins and Vitamin C

Available Online

http://nutrition.wadsworth.com/uncn7

Nutrition Animation: *Protecting the Vitamins in Foods*

Student Practice Test

Glossary Terms

Nutrition on the Net

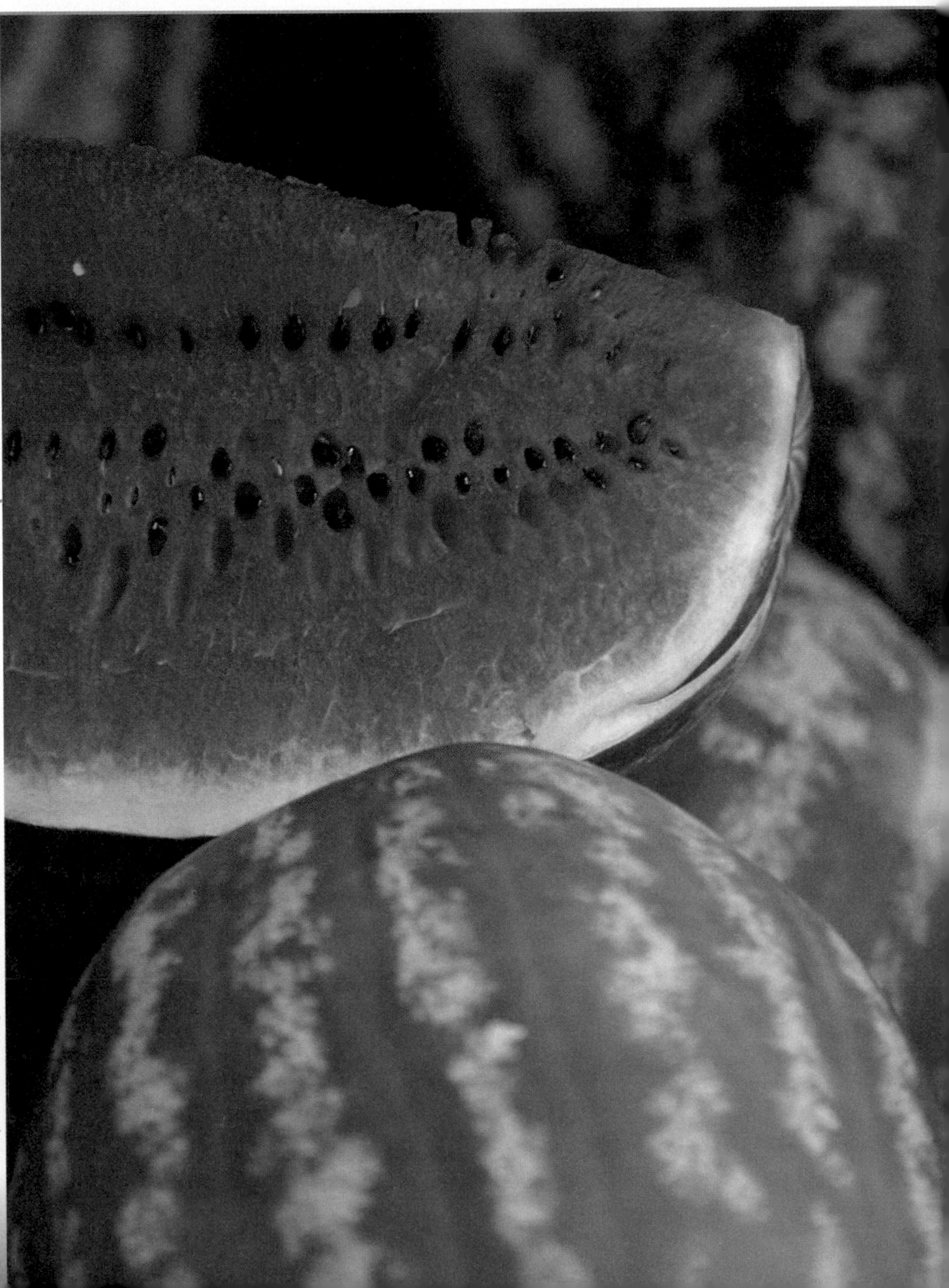

Nutrition in Your Life

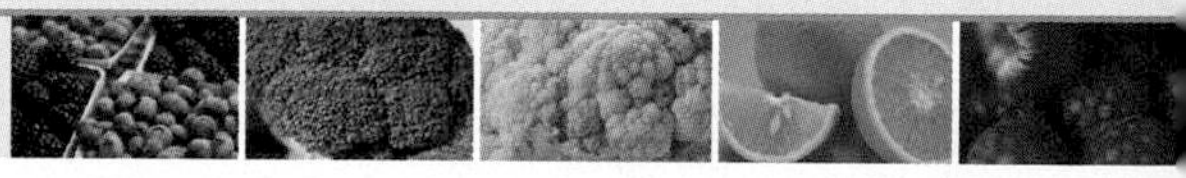

If you were playing a word game and your partner said "vitamins," how would you respond? If "pills" and "supplements" immediately come to mind, you may be missing the main message of the vitamin story—that hundreds of foods deliver over a dozen vitamins that participate in thousands of activities throughout your body. Quite simply, foods supply vitamins to support all that you are and all that you do—and supplements of any one of them, or even a combination of them, can't compete with foods in keeping you healthy.

Earlier chapters focused on the energy-yielding nutrients, which play leading roles in the body. The vitamins and minerals are their supporting cast. This chapter begins with an overview of the vitamins and then examines each of the water-soluble vitamins and a nonvitamin relative named choline; the next chapter features the fat-soluble vitamins. Chapters 12 and 13 present the minerals.

The Vitamins—An Overview

Researchers first recognized that there were substances in foods that were "vital to life" in the early 1900s. Since then, the world of vitamins has opened up dramatically. The vitamins■ are powerful substances, as their *absence* attests. Vitamin A deficiency can cause blindness; a lack of the B vitamin niacin can cause dementia; and a lack of vitamin D can retard bone growth. The consequences of deficiencies are so dire, and the effects of restoring the needed vitamins so dramatic, that people spend billions of dollars every year in the belief that vitamin pills will cure a host of ailments (see Highlight 10). Vitamins certainly support sound nutritional health, but they do not cure all ills. Furthermore, vitamin supplements do not offer the many benefits that come from vitamin-rich foods.

■ Reminder: The *vitamins* are organic, essential nutrients required in tiny amounts to perform specific functions that promote growth, reproduction, or the maintenance of health and life.
- **vita** = life
- **amine** = containing nitrogen (the first vitamins discovered contained nitrogen)

The *presence* of the vitamins also attests to their power. Vitamin C not only prevents the deficiency disease scurvy, but also seems to protect against certain types of cancer. Similarly, vitamin E seems to help protect against some facets of cardiovascular disease. The B vitamin folate helps to prevent birth defects. As you will see, the vitamins' roles in supporting optimal health extend far beyond preventing deficiency diseases. In fact, some of the credit given to low-fat diets in preventing disease actually belongs to the vitamins that diets rich in vegetables, fruits, and whole grains deliver (see Highlight 11 for more on vitamins in disease prevention).

The vitamins differ from carbohydrates, fats, and proteins in the following ways:

- *Structure.* Vitamins are individual units; they are not linked together (as are molecules of glucose or amino acids). Appendix C presents the chemical structure for each of the vitamins.
- *Function.* Vitamins do not yield usable energy when broken down; they assist the enzymes that release energy from carbohydrates, fats, and proteins.
- *Food contents.* The amounts of vitamins people ingest daily from foods and the amounts they require are measured in *micrograms* (µg) or *milligrams* (mg), rather than grams (g).■

■ 1 g = 1000 mg.
1 mg = 1000 µg.
For perspective, a dollar bill weighs about 1 g.

The vitamins are similar to the energy-yielding nutrients, though, in that they are vital to life, organic, and available from foods.

Bioavailability The amount of vitamins available from foods depends not only on the quantity provided by a food but also on the amount absorbed and used by the body—referred to as the vitamins' **bioavailability.** The quantity of vitamins in a food can be determined in a rather straightforward manner. Researchers analyze foods to determine their vitamin contents and publish the results in tables of food composition such as Appendix H. Determining the bioavailability of a vitamin is a more complex task because it depends on many factors, including:

- Efficiency of digestion and time of transit through the GI tract.
- Previous nutrient intake and nutrition status.
- Other foods consumed at the same time. (Chapters 10–13 describe factors that inhibit or enhance the absorption of individual vitamins and minerals.)
- Method of food preparation (raw, cooked, or processed).
- Source of the nutrient (synthetic, fortified, or naturally occurring).

Experts consider these factors when estimating recommended intakes.

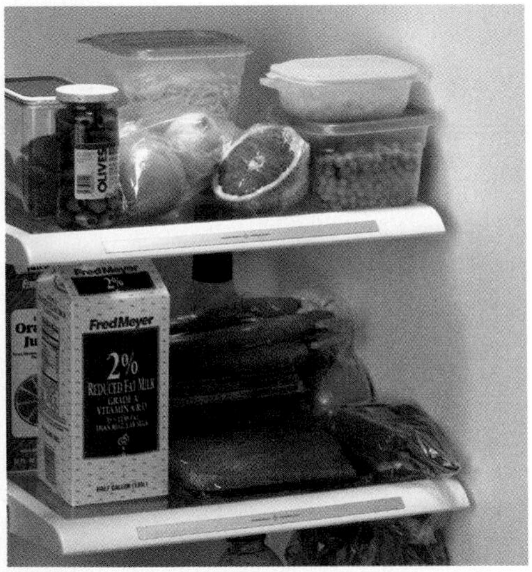
OLIVES
Fred Meyer
2%
REDUCED FAT MILK
Polara Studios, Inc.

To minimize vitamin losses, wrap cut fruits and vegetables or store them in airtight containers.

Precursors Some of the vitamins are available from foods in inactive forms known as **precursors,** or provitamins. Once inside the body, the precursor is converted to an active form of the vitamin. Thus, in measuring a person's vitamin intake, it is important to count both the amount of the active vitamin and the potential amount available from its precursors. The summary tables throughout this chapter and the next indicate which vitamins have precursors.

Organic Nature Being organic, vitamins can be destroyed and left unable to perform their duties. Therefore, they must be handled with care during storage and in cooking. Prolonged heating may destroy much of the thiamin in food. Because riboflavin can be destroyed by the ultraviolet rays of the sun or by fluorescent light, foods stored in transparent glass containers are most likely to lose riboflavin. Oxygen destroys vitamin C, so losses occur when foods are cut or broken and thereby exposed to air. Table 10-1 summarizes ways to minimize nutrient losses in the kitchen.

bioavailability: the rate at and the extent to which a nutrient is abosrbed and used.

precursors: substances that precede others; with regard to vitamins, compounds that can be converted into active vitamins; also known as **provitamins.**

Solubility As you may recall, carbohydrates and proteins are hydrophilic and lipids are hydrophobic. The vitamins divide along the same lines—the hy-

TABLE 10-1 Minimizing Nutrient Losses

- To slow the degradation of vitamins, refrigerate (most) fruits and vegetables.
- To minimize the oxidation of vitamins, store fruits and vegetables that have been cut in airtight wrappers and juices that have been opened in closed containers (and refrigerate them).
- To prevent losses during washing, rinse fruits and vegetables before cutting.
- To minimize losses during cooking, use a microwave oven or steam vegetables in a small amount of water. Add vegetables after water has come to a boil. Use the cooking water in mixed dishes such as casseroles and soups. Avoid high temperatures and long cooking times.

drophilic, water-soluble ones are the eight B vitamins and vitamin C; the hydrophobic, fat-soluble ones are vitamins A, D, E, and K. As each vitamin was discovered, it was given a name and sometimes a letter and number as well. Many of the water-soluble vitamins have multiple names, which has led to some confusion. The margin■ lists the standard names; summary tables throughout this chapter provide the common alternative names.

Solubility is apparent in the food sources of the different vitamins, and it affects their absorption, transport, storage, and excretion by the body. The water-soluble vitamins are found in the watery compartments of foods; the fat-soluble vitamins usually occur together in the fats and oils of foods. On being absorbed, the water-soluble vitamins move directly into the blood; like fats, the fat-soluble vitamins must first enter the lymph, then the blood. Once in the blood, many of the water-soluble vitamins travel freely; many of the fat-soluble vitamins require protein carriers for transport. Upon reaching the cells, water-soluble vitamins freely circulate in the water-filled compartments of the body; fat-soluble vitamins are held in fatty tissues and the liver until needed. The kidneys, monitoring the blood that flows through them, detect and remove small excesses of water-soluble vitamins (large excesses, however, may overwhelm the system, creating adverse effects); fat-soluble vitamins tend to remain in fat-storage sites in the body rather than being excreted, and so are more likely to reach toxic levels when consumed in excess.

Because the body stores fat-soluble vitamins, they can be eaten in large amounts once in a while and still meet the body's needs over time. Water-soluble vitamins are retained for varying periods in the body; a single day's omission from the diet does not bring on a deficiency, but still, the water-soluble vitamins must be eaten more regularly than the fat-soluble vitamins.

■ **Water-soluble vitamins:**
- B vitamins:
  - Thiamin.
  - Riboflavin.
  - Niacin.
  - Biotin.
  - Pantothenic acid.
  - Vitamin B_6.
  - Folate.
  - Vitamin B_{12}.
- Vitamin C.

Fat-soluble vitamins:
- Vitamin A.
- Vitamin D.
- Vitamin E.
- Vitamin K.

Toxicity Knowledge about some of the amazing roles of vitamins has prompted many people to begin taking supplements, assuming that more is better. But just as an inadequate intake can cause harm, so can an excessive intake. As mentioned, even some of the water-soluble vitamins have adverse effects when taken in large doses.

That a vitamin can be both essential and harmful may seem surprising, but the same is true of most nutrients. The effects of every substance depend on its dose, and this is one reason consumers should not self-prescribe supplements for their ailments. See the "How to" on the next page for a perspective on doses.

The Committee on Dietary Reference Intakes (DRI) addresses the possibility of adverse effects from high doses of nutrients by establishing Tolerable Upper Intake Levels. An Upper Level defines the highest amount of a nutrient that is likely not to cause harm for most healthy people when consumed daily. The risk of harm increases as intakes rise above the Upper Level. Of the nutrients discussed in this chapter, niacin, vitamin B_6, folate, choline, and vitamin C have had Upper Levels set, and these values are presented in their respective summary tables. Data are lacking to establish Upper Levels for the remaining B vitamins, but this does not mean that excessively high intakes would be without risk. (The inside front cover presents Upper Levels for the vitamins and minerals.)

HOW TO Understand Dose Levels and Effects

A substance may have a beneficial or harmful effect, but a critical thinker would not conclude that the substance itself was beneficial or harmful without first asking what dose was used. The accompanying figure shows three possible relationships between dose levels and effects. The third diagram represents the situation with nutrients—more is better up to a point, but beyond that point, still more is harmful.

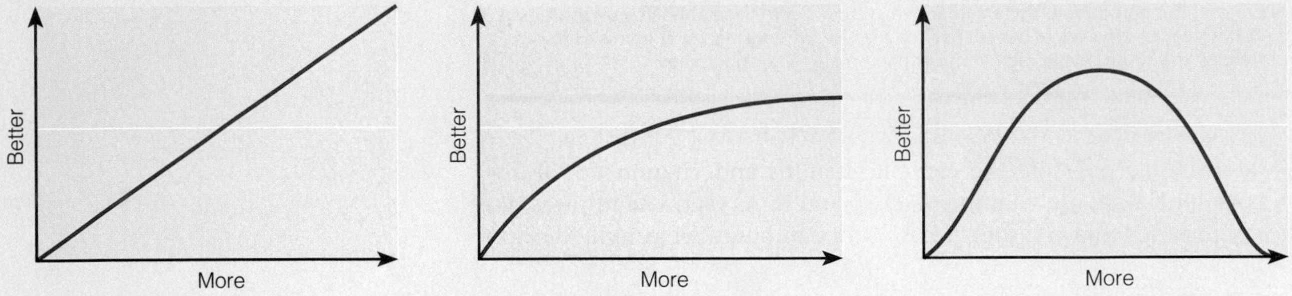
Better
More
Better
More
Better
More

As you progress in the direction of more, the effect gets better and better, with no end in sight (real life is seldom, if ever, like this).

As you progress in the direction of more, the effect reaches a maximum and then a plateau, becoming no better with higher doses.

As you progress in the direction of more, the effect reaches an optimum at some intermediate dose and then declines, showing that more is better up to a point and then harmful. That too much is as harmful as too little represents the situation with nutrients.

IN SUMMARY The vitamins are essential nutrients needed in tiny amounts in the diet both to prevent deficiency diseases and to support optimal health. The water-soluble vitamins are the B vitamins and vitamin C; the fat-soluble vitamins are vitamins A, D, E, and K. The accompanying table summarizes the differences between the water-soluble and fat-soluble vitamins.

	Water-Soluble Vitamins: B Vitamins and Vitamin C	Fat-Soluble Vitamins: Vitamins A, D, E, and K
Absorption	Directly into the blood.	First into the lymph, then the blood.
Transport	Travel freely.	Many require protein carriers.
Storage	Circulate freely in water-filled parts of the body.	Stored in the cells associated with fat.
Excretion	Kidneys detect and remove excess in urine.	Less readily excreted; tend to remain in fat-storage sites.
Toxicity	Possible to reach toxic levels when consumed from supplements.	Likely to reach toxic levels when consumed from supplements.
Requirements	Needed in frequent doses (perhaps 1 to 3 days).	Needed in periodic doses (perhaps weeks or even months).

NOTE: Exceptions occur, but these differences between the water-soluble and fat-soluble vitamins are valid generalizations.

The discussion of B vitamins that follows begins with a brief description of each of them, then offers a look at the ways they work together. Thus a preview of the individuals is followed by a survey of them all together, in concert.

The B Vitamins—As Individuals

Despite supplement advertisements that claim otherwise, the vitamins do not provide the body with fuel for energy. It is true, though, that without B vitamins the body would lack energy. The energy-yielding nutrients—carbohydrate, fat, and

FIGURE 10-1 Coenzyme Action

Some vitamins form part of the coenzymes that enable enzymes either to synthesize compounds (as illustrated by the lower enzymes in this figure) or to dismantle compounds (as illustrated by the upper enzymes).

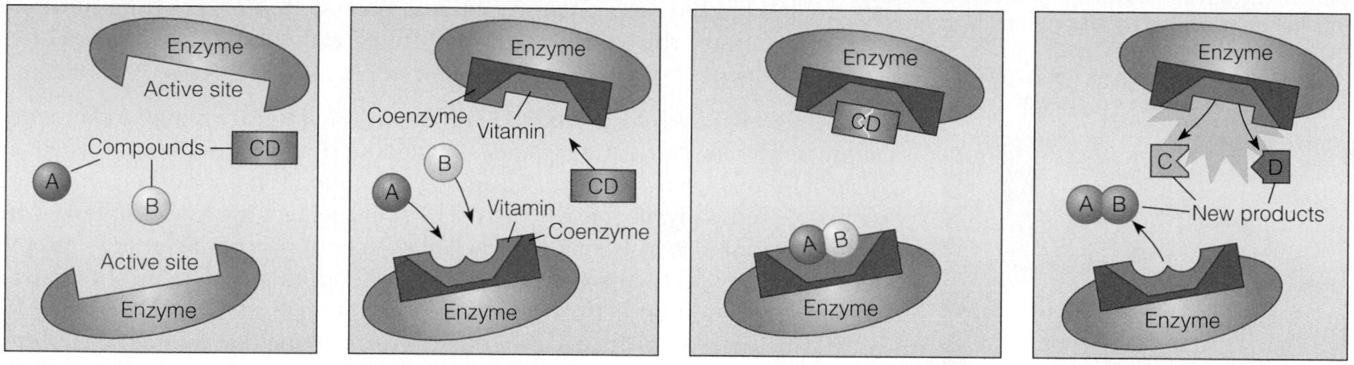
Enzyme
Active site
Compounds
CD
A
B
Active site
Enzyme
Enzyme
Coenzyme
Vitamin
B
A
CD
Vitamin
Coenzyme
Enzyme
Enzyme
CD
A B
Enzyme
Enzyme
C
D
A B
New products
Enzyme

Without coenzymes, compounds A, B, and CD don't respond to their enzymes.

With the coenzymes in place, compounds are attracted to their sites on the enzymes . . .

. . . and the reactions proceed instantaneously. The coenzymes often donate or accept electrons, atoms, or groups of atoms.

The reactions are completed with either the formation of a new product, AB, or the breaking apart of a compound into two new products, C and D, and the release of energy.

protein—are used for fuel; the B vitamins help the body to use that fuel. Several of the B vitamins—thiamin, riboflavin, niacin, pantothenic acid, and biotin—form part of the coenzymes■ that assist certain enzymes in the release of energy from carbohydrate, fat, and protein. Other B vitamins play other indispensable roles in metabolism. Vitamin B_6 assists enzymes that metabolize amino acids; folate and vitamin B_{12} help cells to multiply. Among these cells are the red blood cells and the cells lining the GI tract—cells that deliver energy to all the others.

■ Reminder: A *coenzyme* is a small organic molecule that associates closely with certain enzymes; many B vitamins form an integral part of coenzymes.

The vitamin portion of a coenzyme allows a chemical reaction to occur; the remaining portion of the coenzyme binds to the enzyme. Without its coenzyme, an enzyme cannot function. Thus symptoms of B vitamin deficiencies directly reflect the disturbances of metabolism incurred by a lack of coenzymes. Figure 10-1 illustrates coenzyme action.

The following sections describe individual B vitamins and note many coenzymes and metabolic pathways. Keep in mind that a later section will assemble these pieces of information into a whole picture.

The following sections also present the recommendations, deficiency and toxicity symptoms, and food sources for each vitamin. The recommendations for the B vitamins and vitamin C reflect the 1998 and 2000 DRI, respectively.[1] For thiamin, riboflavin, niacin, vitamin B_6, folate, vitamin B_{12}, and vitamin C, sufficient data were available to establish an RDA; for biotin, pantothenic acid, and choline, an Adequate Intake (AI) was set; only niacin, vitamin B_6, folate, choline, and vitamin C have Tolerable Upper Intake Levels. These values appear in the summary tables and figures that follow, as well as on the inside front covers.

Thiamin

Thiamin is the vitamin part of the coenzyme TPP (thiamin pyrophosphate), which assists in energy metabolism. The TPP coenzyme participates in the conversion of pyruvate to acetyl CoA (described in Chapter 7). The reaction removes one carbon from the 3-carbon pyruvate to make the 2-carbon acetyl CoA and carbon dioxide (CO_2). Later TPP participates in a similar step in the TCA cycle where it helps convert a 5-carbon compound to a 4-carbon compound. Besides playing these pivotal roles in the energy metabolism of all cells, thiamin occupies a special site on the

thiamin (THIGH-ah-min): a B vitamin. The coenzyme form is **TPP (thiamin pyrophosphate).**

FIGURE 10-2 Thiamin-Deficiency Symptom—The Edema of Beriberi

Beriberi may be characterized as "wet" (referring to edema) or "dry" (with muscle wasting, but no edema). Physical examination confirms that this person has wet beriberi. Notice how the impression of the physician's thumb remains on the leg.

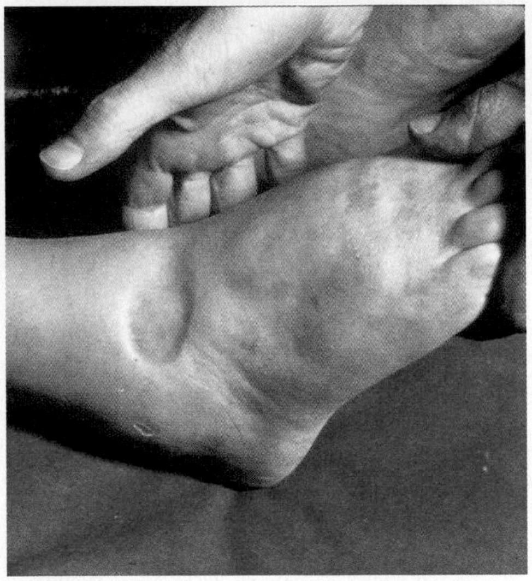

© NMSB/Custom Medical Stock Photo

■ Severe thiamin deficiency in alcohol abusers is called the **Wernicke-Korsakoff** (VER-nee-key KORE-sah-kof) **syndrome.** Symptoms include disorientation, loss of short-term memory, jerky eye movements, and staggering gait.

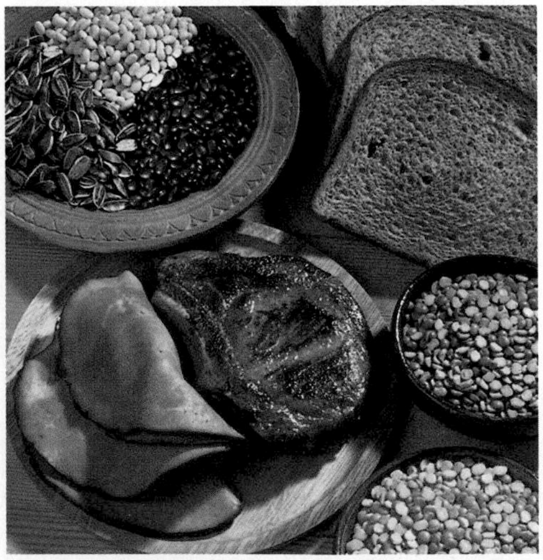

© Polara Studios Inc.

Pork is the richest source of thiamin, but enriched or whole-grain products typically make the greatest contribution to a day's intake because of the quantities eaten. Legumes such as split peas are also valuable sources of thiamin.

beriberi: the thiamin-deficiency disease.
- **beri** = weakness
- **beriberi** = "I can't, I can't"

membranes of nerve cells. Consequently, processes in nerves and in their responding tissues, the muscles, depend heavily on thiamin.

Thiamin Recommendations Dietary recommendations are based primarily on thiamin's role in enzyme activity. Generally, thiamin needs will be met if a person eats enough food to meet energy needs and obtains that energy from nutritious foods. The average thiamin intake in the United States and Canada meets or exceeds recommendations.

Thiamin Deficiency and Toxicity People who fail to eat enough food to meet energy needs risk nutrient deficiencies, including thiamin deficiency. Inadequate thiamin intakes have been reported among the nation's malnourished and homeless people. Similarly, people who derive most of their energy from empty-kcalorie items, like alcohol,■ risk thiamin deficiency. Alcohol contributes energy, but provides few, if any, nutrients and often displaces food. In addition, alcohol impairs thiamin absorption and enhances thiamin excretion in the urine, doubling the risk of deficiency. An estimated four out of five alcoholics are thiamin deficient.

Prolonged thiamin deficiency can result in the disease **beriberi,** which was first observed in Indonesia when the custom of polishing rice became widespread.[2] Rice provided 80 percent of the energy intake of the people of that area, and the germ and bran of the rice grain was their principal source of thiamin. When the germ and bran were removed in the preparation of white rice, beriberi spread like wildfire. The symptoms of beriberi include damage to the nervous system as well as to the heart and other muscles. Figure 10-2 presents one of the symptoms of beriberi. No adverse effects have been associated with excesses of thiamin; no Upper Level has been determined.

Thiamin Food Sources Before examining Figure 10-3, you may want to read the accompanying "How to," which describes the many features found in this and similar figures in this chapter and the next three chapters. When you look at Figure 10-3, notice that thiamin occurs in small quantities in many nutritious foods; highly refined foods contain almost no thiamin. The long red bar near the bottom of the graph shows that meats in the pork family are exceptionally rich in thiamin.

As mentioned earlier, prolonged cooking can destroy thiamin. Also, like other water-soluble vitamins, thiamin leaches into water when foods are boiled or blanched. Cooking methods that require little or no water such as steaming and microwave heating conserve thiamin and other water-soluble vitamins. The accompanying table summarizes thiamin's main functions, food sources, and deficiency symptoms.

IN SUMMARY Thiamin

Other Names

Vitamin B_1

1998 RDA

Men: 1.2 mg/day

Women: 1.1 mg/day

Chief Functions in the Body

Part of coenzyme TPP (thiamin pyrophosphate) used in energy metabolism

Significant Sources

Whole-grain, fortified, or enriched grain products; moderate amounts in all nutritious food; pork

Easily destroyed by heat

Deficiency Disease

Beriberi (wet, with edema; dry, with muscle wasting)

Deficiency Symptoms*

Enlarged heart, cardiac failure; muscular weakness; apathy, poor short-term memory, confusion, irritability; anorexia, weight loss

Toxicity Symptoms

None reported

*Severe thiamin deficiency is often related to heavy alcohol consumption.

FIGURE 10-3 Thiamin in Selected Foods

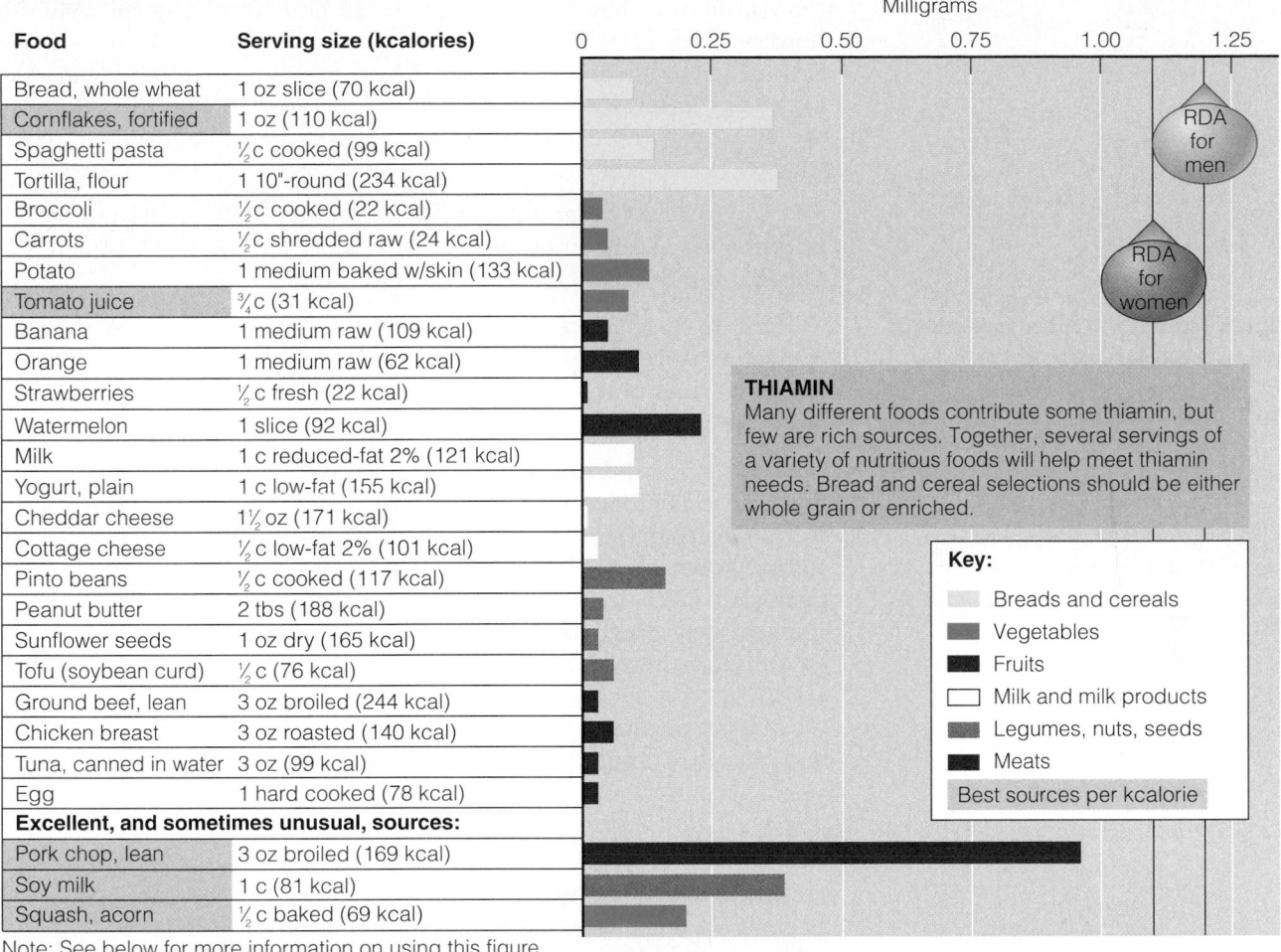

Food	Serving size (kcalories)
Bread, whole wheat	1 oz slice (70 kcal)
Cornflakes, fortified	1 oz (110 kcal)
Spaghetti pasta	½ c cooked (99 kcal)
Tortilla, flour	1 10"-round (234 kcal)
Broccoli	½ c cooked (22 kcal)
Carrots	½ c shredded raw (24 kcal)
Potato	1 medium baked w/skin (133 kcal)
Tomato juice	¾ c (31 kcal)
Banana	1 medium raw (109 kcal)
Orange	1 medium raw (62 kcal)
Strawberries	½ c fresh (22 kcal)
Watermelon	1 slice (92 kcal)
Milk	1 c reduced-fat 2% (121 kcal)
Yogurt, plain	1 c low-fat (155 kcal)
Cheddar cheese	1½ oz (171 kcal)
Cottage cheese	½ c low-fat 2% (101 kcal)
Pinto beans	½ c cooked (117 kcal)
Peanut butter	2 tbs (188 kcal)
Sunflower seeds	1 oz dry (165 kcal)
Tofu (soybean curd)	½ c (76 kcal)
Ground beef, lean	3 oz broiled (244 kcal)
Chicken breast	3 oz roasted (140 kcal)
Tuna, canned in water	3 oz (99 kcal)
Egg	1 hard cooked (78 kcal)
Excellent, and sometimes unusual, sources:	
Pork chop, lean	3 oz broiled (169 kcal)
Soy milk	1 c (81 kcal)
Squash, acorn	½ c baked (69 kcal)

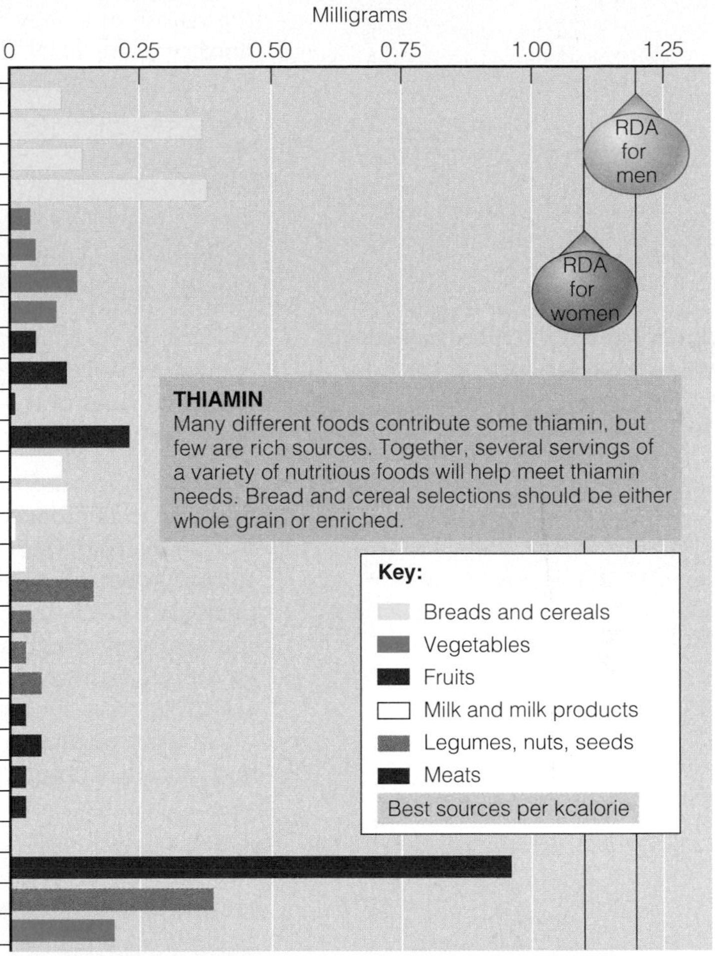
Milligrams
0
0.25
0.50
0.75
1.00
1.25
RDA for men
RDA for women
THIAMIN
Many different foods contribute some thiamin, but few are rich sources. Together, several servings of a variety of nutritious foods will help meet thiamin needs. Bread and cereal selections should be either whole grain or enriched.
Key:
Breads and cereals
Vegetables
Fruits
Milk and milk products
Legumes, nuts, seeds
Meats
Best sources per kcalorie

Note: See below for more information on using this figure.

HOW TO Evaluate Foods for Their Nutrient Contributions

Figure 10-3 is the first of a series of figures in this and the next three chapters that present the vitamins and minerals in foods. Each figure presents the same 24 foods, which were selected to ensure a variety of choices representative of each of the food groups as suggested by the USDA Food Guide. From the grains, for example, a bread, a cereal, and a pasta were chosen. The suggestion to include a variety of vegetables was also considered: dark green, leafy vegetables (broccoli); orange and deep yellow vegetables (carrots); starchy vegetables (potatoes); legumes (pinto beans); and other vegetables (tomato juice). The selection of fruits followed suggestions to use whole fruits (bananas); citrus fruits (oranges); melons (watermelon); and berries (strawberries). Items were selected from the milk and meat groups in a similar way. In addition to the 24 foods that appear in all of the figures, three different foods were selected for each of the nutrients to add variety and often reflect excellent, and sometimes unusual, sources.

Notice that the figures list the food, the serving size, and the food energy (kcalories) on the left. The amount of the nutrient per serving is presented in the graph on the right along with the RDA (or AI) for adults, so you can see how many servings would be needed to meet recommendations.

The colored bars show at a glance which food groups best provide a nutrient: yellow for breads and cereals; green for vegetables; purple for fruits; white for milk and milk products; brown for legumes; and red for meat, fish, and poultry. Because the USDA Food Guide mentions legumes with both the meat group and the vegetable group and because legumes are especially rich in many vitamins and minerals, they have been given their own color to highlight their nutrient contributions.

Notice how the bar graphs shift in the various figures. Careful study of all of the figures taken together will confirm that variety is the key to nutrient adequacy.

Another way to evaluate foods for their nutrient contributions is to consider their nutrient density (their thiamin *per 100 kcalories,* for example). Quite often, vegetables rank higher on a nutrient-per-kcalorie list than they do on a nutrient-per-serving list (see p. 41 to review how to evaluate foods based on nutrient density). The left column in the figure highlights five or so foods that offer the best deal for your energy "dollar" (the kcalorie). Notice how many of them are vegetables.

Realistically, people cannot eat for single nutrients. Fortunately, most foods deliver more than one nutrient, allowing people to combine foods into nourishing meals.

Riboflavin

Like thiamin, **riboflavin** serves as a coenzyme in many reactions, most notably in the release of energy from nutrients in all body cells. The coenzyme forms of riboflavin are FMN (flavin mononucleotide) and FAD (flavin adenine dinucleotide); both can accept and then donate two hydrogens (see Figure 10-4). During energy metabolism, FAD picks up two hydrogens (with their electrons) from the TCA cycle and delivers them to the electron transport chain (described in Chapter 7).

Riboflavin Recommendations Like thiamin's RDA, riboflavin's RDA is based primarily on its role in enzyme activity. Most people in the United States and Canada meet or exceed riboflavin recommendations.

■ Riboflavin deficiency is called **ariboflavinosis** (ay-RYE-boh-FLAY-vin-oh-sis).
- **a** = not
- **osis** = condition

Riboflavin Deficiency and Toxicity Riboflavin deficiency■ most often accompanies other nutrient deficiencies. Lack of the vitamin causes inflammation of the membranes of the mouth, skin, eyes, and GI tract. Excesses of riboflavin appear to cause no harm; no Upper Level has been established.

■ Turn to p. 41 for a review of how to evaluate foods based on nutrient density (per kcalorie).

Riboflavin Food Sources The greatest contributions of riboflavin come from milk and milk products (see Figure 10-5). Whole-grain or enriched bread and cereal products are also valuable sources because of the quantities typically consumed. When riboflavin sources are ranked by nutrient density (per kcalorie),■ many dark green, leafy vegetables (such as broccoli, turnip greens, asparagus, and spinach) appear high on the list. Vegans and others who don't use milk must rely on ample servings of dark greens and enriched grains for riboflavin. Nutritional yeast is another good source.

Ultraviolet light and irradiation destroy riboflavin. For these reasons, milk is sold in cardboard or opaque plastic containers, and precautions are taken when vitamin D

FIGURE 10-4 Riboflavin Coenzyme, Accepting and Donating Hydrogens

This figure shows the chemical structure of the riboflavin portion of the coenzyme only; the remainder of the coenzyme structure is represented by dotted lines (see Appendix C for the complete chemical structures of FAD and FMN). The reactive sites that accept and donate hydrogens are highlighted in white.

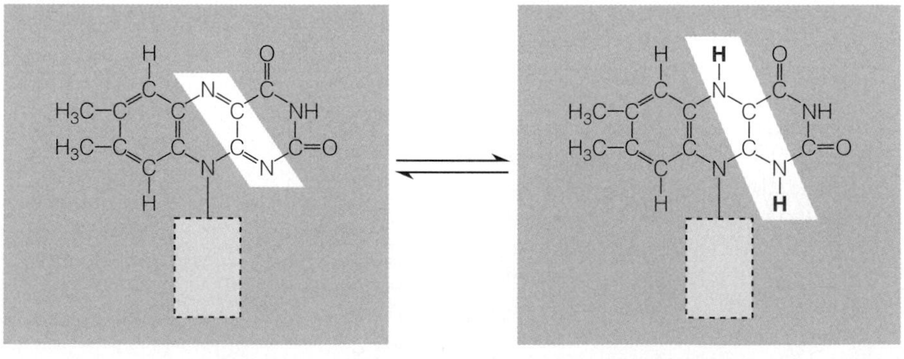

FAD ⇌ $FADH_2$

During the TCA cycle, compounds release hydrogens, and the riboflavin coenzyme FAD picks up two of them. As it accepts two hydrogens, FAD becomes $FADH_2$.

$FADH_2$ carries the hydrogens to the electron transport chain. At the end of the electron transport chain, the hydrogens are accepted by oxygen, creating water, and $FADH_2$ becomes FAD again. For every $FADH_2$ that passes through the electron transport chain, 2 ATP are generated.

riboflavin (RYE-boh-flay-vin): a B vitamin. The coenzyme forms are **FMN (flavin mononucleotide)** and **FAD (flavin adenine dinucleotide).**

FIGURE 10-5 Riboflavin in Selected Foods

Food	Serving size (kcalories)
Bread, whole wheat	1 oz slice (70 kcal)
Cornflakes, fortified	1 oz (110 kcal)
Spaghetti pasta	½ c cooked (99 kcal)
Tortilla, flour	1 10"-round (234 kcal)
Broccoli	½ c cooked (22 kcal)
Carrots	½ c shredded raw (24 kcal)
Potato	1 medium baked w/skin (133 kcal)
Tomato juice	¾ c (31 kcal)
Banana	1 medium raw (109 kcal)
Orange	1 medium raw (62 kcal)
Strawberries	½ c fresh (22 kcal)
Watermelon	1 slice (92 kcal)
Milk	1 c reduced-fat 2% (121 kcal)
Yogurt, plain	1 c low-fat (155 kcal)
Cheddar cheese	1½ oz (171 kcal)
Cottage cheese	½ c low-fat 2% (101 kcal)
Pinto beans	½ c cooked (117 kcal)
Peanut butter	2 tbs (188 kcal)
Sunflower seeds	1 oz dry (165 kcal)
Tofu (soybean curd)	½ c (76 kcal)
Ground beef, lean	3 oz broiled (244 kcal)
Chicken breast	3 oz roasted (140 kcal)
Tuna, canned in water	3 oz (99 kcal)
Egg	1 hard cooked (78 kcal)
Excellent, and sometimes unusual, sources:	
Liver	3 oz fried (184 kcal)
Clams, canned	3 oz (126 kcal)
Mushrooms	½ c cooked (21 kcal)

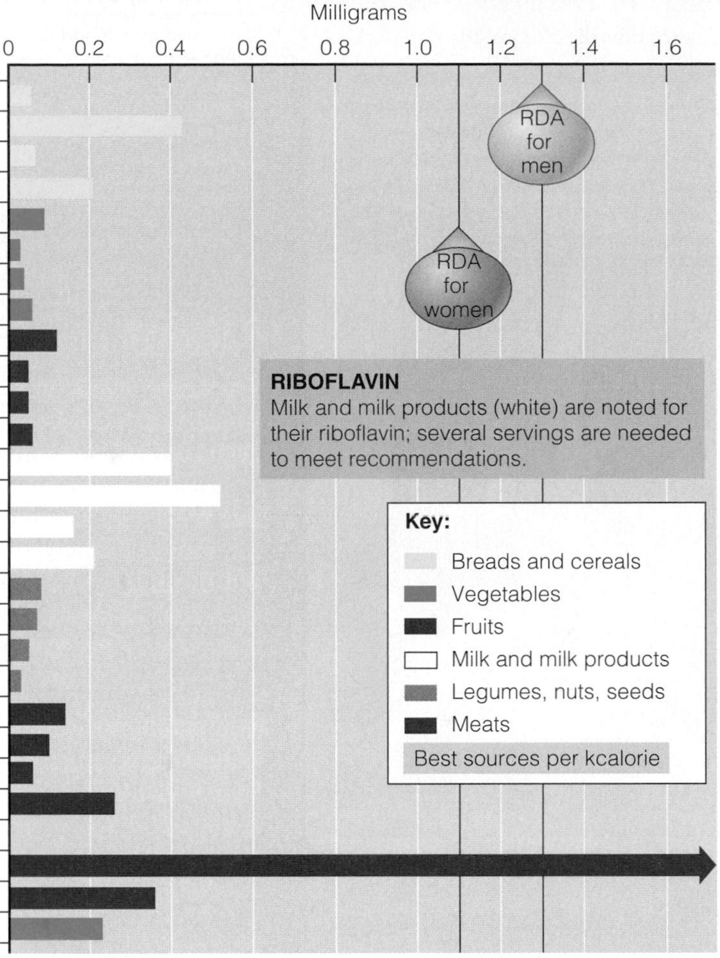
Milligrams
0
0.2
0.4
0.6
0.8
1.0
1.2
1.4
1.6
RDA for men
RDA for women
RIBOFLAVIN
Milk and milk products (white) are noted for their riboflavin; several servings are needed to meet recommendations.
Key:
Breads and cereals
Vegetables
Fruits
Milk and milk products
Legumes, nuts, seeds
Meats
Best sources per kcalorie

Note: See p. 327 for more information on using this figure.

is added to milk by irradiation.* In contrast, riboflavin is stable to heat, so cooking does not destroy it. The following summary table lists riboflavin's chief functions, food sources, and deficiency symptoms.

IN SUMMARY Riboflavin

Other Names

Vitamin B_2

1998 RDA

Men: 1.3 mg/day

Women: 1.1 mg/day

Chief Functions in the Body

Part of coenzymes FMN (flavin mononucleotide) and FAD (flavin adenine dinucleotide) used in energy metabolism

Significant Sources

Milk products (yogurt, cheese); enriched or whole grains; liver

Easily destroyed by ultraviolet light and irradiation

Deficiency Disease

Ariboflavinosis (ay-RYE-boh-FLAY-vin-oh-sis)

(continued)

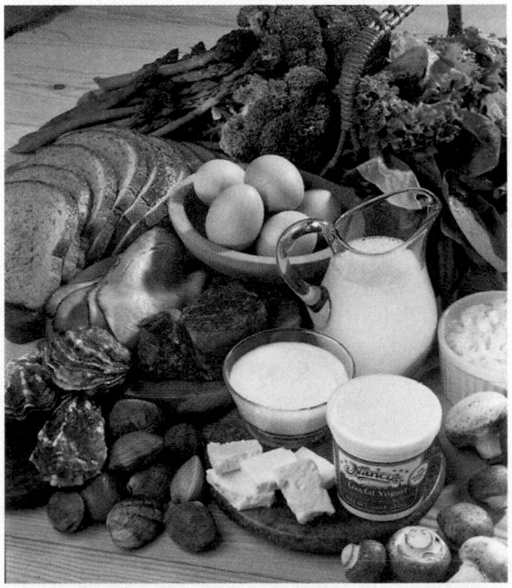

All of these foods are rich in riboflavin, but milk and milk products provide much of the riboflavin in the diets of most people.

*Vitamin D can be added to milk by feeding cows irradiated yeast or by irradiating the milk itself.

FIGURE 10-6 Niacin-Deficiency Symptom—The Dermatitis of Pellagra

In the dermatitis of pellagra, the skin darkens and flakes away as if it were sunburned. The protein-deficiency disease kwashiorkor also produces a "flaky paint" dermatitis, but the two are easily distinguished. The dermatitis of pellagra is bilateral and symmetrical and occurs only on those parts of the body exposed to the sun.

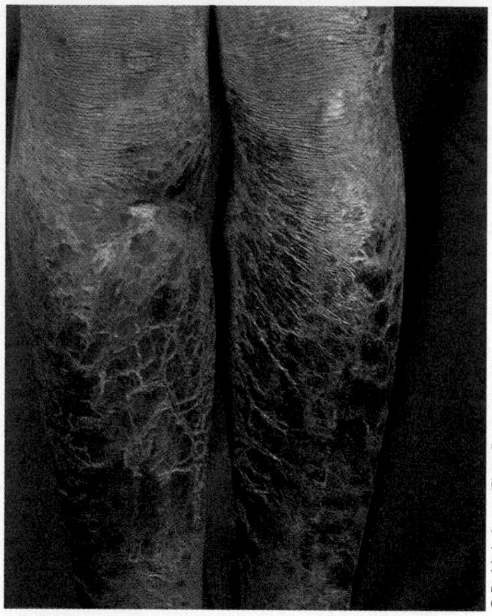

Riboflavin (continued)

Deficiency Symptoms	Toxicity Symptoms
Inflamed eyelids and sensitivity to light,[a] reddening of cornea; sore throat; cracks and redness at corners of mouth;[b] painful, smooth, purplish red tongue;[c] inflammation characterized by skin lesions covered with greasy scales	None reported

[a]Hypersensitivity to light is *photophobia* (FOE-toe-FOE-bee-ah).
[b]Cracks at the corners of the mouth are termed *cheilosis* (kye-LOH-sis or kee-LOH-sis).
[c]Smoothness of the tongue is caused by loss of its surface structures and is termed *glossitis* (gloss-EYE-tis).

Niacin

The name **niacin** describes two chemical structures: nicotinic acid and nicotinamide (also known as niacinamide). The body can easily convert nicotinic acid to nicotinamide, which is the major form of niacin in the blood.

The two coenzyme forms of niacin, NAD (nicotinamide adenine dinucleotide) and NADP (the phosphate form), participate in numerous metabolic reactions. They are central in energy-transfer reactions, especially the metabolism of glucose, fat, and alcohol. NAD is similar to the riboflavin coenzymes in that it carries hydrogens (and their electrons) during metabolic reactions, including the pathway from the TCA cycle to the electron transport chain.

Niacin Recommendations Niacin is unique among the B vitamins in that the body can make it from the amino acid tryptophan. To make 1 milligram of niacin requires approximately 60 milligrams of dietary tryptophan. For this reason, recommended intakes are stated in **niacin equivalents (NE).**■ A food containing 1 milligram of niacin and 60 milligrams of tryptophan provides the equivalent of 2 milligrams of niacin, or 2 niacin equivalents. The RDA for niacin allows for this conversion and is stated in niacin equivalents.

Niacin Deficiency The niacin-deficiency disease, **pellagra,** produces the symptoms of diarrhea, dermatitis, dementia, and eventually death (often called "the four Ds"). In the early 1900s, pellagra caused widespread misery and some 87,000 deaths in the U.S. South, where many people subsisted on a low-protein diet centered on corn. This diet supplied neither enough niacin nor enough tryptophan. At least 70 percent of the niacin in corn is bound to complex carbohydrates and small peptides, making it unavailable for absorption. Furthermore, corn is high in the amino acid leucine, which interferes with the tryptophan-to-niacin conversion, thus further contributing to the development of pellagra. Figure 10-6 illustrates the dermatitis of pellagra.

Pellagra was first believed to be caused by an infection. Medical researchers spent many years and much effort searching for infectious microbes until they realized that the problem was not what was present in the food, but what was *absent* from it. That a disease such as pellagra could be caused by diet—and not by germs—was a groundbreaking discovery. It contradicted commonly held medical opinions that diseases were caused only by infectious agents and advanced the science of nutrition dramatically.*

Niacin Toxicity Naturally occurring niacin from foods■ causes no harm, but large doses from supplements or drugs produce a variety of adverse effects, most notably **"niacin flush."** Niacin flush occurs when nicotinic acid is taken in doses only three to four times the RDA. It dilates the capillaries and causes a tingling sensation that can be painful. The nicotinamide form does not produce this effect—nor does it lower blood cholesterol.

■ 1 NE = 1 mg niacin or 60 mg tryptophan.

■ When a normal dose of a nutrient (levels commonly found in foods) provides a normal blood concentration, the nutrient is having a *physiological* effect. When a large dose (levels commonly available only from supplements) overwhelms some body system and acts like a drug, the nutrient is having a *pharmacological* effect.
- **physio** = natural
- **pharma** = drug

niacin (NIGH-a-sin): a B vitamin. The coenzyme forms are **NAD (nicotinamide adenine dinucleotide)** and **NADP (the phosphate form of NAD).** Niacin can be eaten preformed or made in the body from its precursor, tryptophan, one of the amino acids.

niacin equivalents (NE): the amount of niacin present in food, including the niacin that can theoretically be made from its precursor, tryptophan, present in the food.

pellagra (pell-AY-gra): the niacin-deficiency disease.
- **pellis** = skin
- **agra** = rough

niacin flush: a temporary burning, tingling, and itching sensation that occurs when a person takes a large dose of nicotinic acid; often accompanied by a headache and reddened face, arms, and chest.

*Dr. Joseph Goldberger, a physician for the U.S. government, headed the investigations that determined that pellagra was a dietary disorder, not an infectious disease. He died several years before Conrad Elevjhem discovered that a deficiency of niacin caused pellagra.

Large doses of nicotinic acid have been used to help lower blood cholesterol and prevent heart disease.[3] Such therapy must be closely monitored because of its adverse side effects (causes liver damage and aggravates peptic ulcers, among others). People with the following conditions may be particularly susceptible to the toxic effects of niacin: liver disease, diabetes, peptic ulcers, gout, irregular heartbeats, inflammatory bowel disease, migraine headaches, and alcoholism.

Niacin Food Sources Tables of food composition typically list preformed niacin only, but as mentioned, niacin can also be made in the body from the amino acid tryptophan. Hence diets that are high in protein are never lacking niacin. The "How to" on p. 332 shows how to estimate the total amount of niacin available from the diet. Dietary tryptophan could meet about half the daily need for most people, but the average diet easily supplies enough preformed niacin.

The predominance of the red bars in Figure 10-7 (on p. 332) explains why meat, poultry, and fish contribute about half the niacin most people need. An additional fourth of most people's niacin comes from enriched and whole grains. Mushrooms, asparagus, and leafy green vegetables are among the richest vegetable sources (per kcalorie) and can provide abundant niacin when eaten in generous amounts.

Niacin is less vulnerable to losses during food preparation and storage than other water-soluble vitamins. Being fairly heat-resistant, niacin can withstand reasonable cooking times, but like other water-soluble vitamins, it will leach into cooking water. The summary table includes food sources as well as niacin's various names, functions, and deficiency and toxicity symptoms.

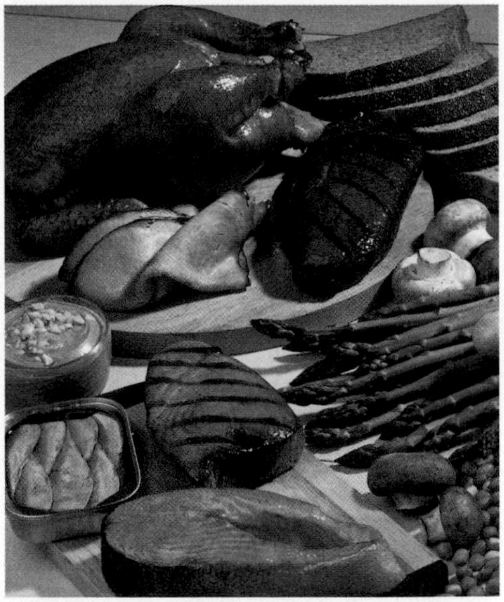

Protein-rich foods such as meat, fish, poultry, and peanut butter contribute much of the niacin in people's diets. Enriched breads and cereals and a few vegetables are also rich in niacin.

IN SUMMARY **Niacin**

Other Names

Nicotinic acid, nicotinamide, niacinamide, vitamin B_3; precursor is dietary tryptophan (an amino acid)

1998 RDA

Men: 16 mg NE/day

Women: 14 mg NE/day

Upper Level

Adults: 35 mg/day

Chief Functions in the Body

Part of coenzymes NAD (nicotinamide adenine dinucleotide) and NADP (its phosphate form) used in energy metabolism

Significant Sources

Milk, eggs, meat, poultry, fish, whole-grain and enriched breads and cereals, nuts, and all protein-containing foods

Deficiency Disease

Pellagra

Deficiency Symptoms

Diarrhea, abdominal pain, vomiting; inflamed, swollen, smooth, bright red tongue;[a] depression, apathy, fatigue, loss of memory, headache; bilateral symmetrical rash on areas exposed to sunlight

Toxicity Symptoms

Painful flush, hives, and rash ("niacin flush"); excessive sweating; blurred vision; liver damage, impaired glucose tolerance

[a]Smoothness of the tongue is caused by loss of its surface structures and is termed *glossitis* (gloss-EYE-tis).

Biotin

Biotin plays an important role in metabolism as a coenzyme that carries activated carbon dioxide. This role is critical in the TCA cycle: biotin delivers a carbon to 3-carbon pyruvate, thus replenishing oxaloacetate, the 4-carbon compound needed to combine with acetyl CoA to keep the TCA cycle turning. The biotin coenzyme also serves crucial roles in gluconeogenesis,■ fatty acid synthesis, and the breakdown of certain fatty acids and amino acids.

■ Reminder: The synthesis of glucose from noncarbohydrate sources such as amino acids or glycerol is called *gluconeogenesis*.

biotin (BY-oh-tin): a B vitamin that functions as a coenzyme in metabolism.

HOW TO Estimate Niacin Equivalents

To obtain a rough approximation of niacin equivalents:

- Calculate total protein consumed (grams).
- Assuming that the RDA amount of protein will be used first to make body protein, subtract the RDA to obtain "leftover" protein available to make niacin (grams). (Actually, the RDA provides a generous protein allowance, so "leftover" protein may be even greater than this.)
- About 1 gram of every 100 grams of high-quality protein is tryptophan, so divide by 100 to obtain the tryptophan in this leftover protein (grams).
- Multiply by 1000 to express this amount of tryptophan in milligrams.
- Divide by 60 to get niacin equivalents (milligrams).
- Finally, add the amount of preformed niacin obtained in the diet (milligrams).

For example, suppose that a 19-year-old woman who weighs 130 pounds consumes 75 grams of protein in a day. To calculate her protein RDA, first convert pounds to kilograms if necessary, and then multiply by 0.8 g/kg:

$$130 \text{ lb} \div 2.2 \text{ lb/kg} = 59 \text{ kg}$$
$$59 \text{ kg} \times 0.8 \text{ g/kg} = 47 \text{ g}.$$

Then determine her leftover protein by subtracting her RDA from her intake:

$$75 \text{ g protein intake} - 47 \text{ g protein RDA} = 28 \text{ g protein leftover}.$$

Next calculate the amount of tryptophan in this leftover protein:

$$28 \text{ g protein} \div 100 = 0.28 \text{ g tryptophan}.$$
$$0.28 \text{ g tryptophan} \times 1000 = 280 \text{ mg tryptophan}.$$

Then convert milligrams of tryptophan to niacin equivalents:

$$280 \text{ mg tryptophan} \div 60 = 4.7 \text{ mg NE}.$$

To determine the total amount of niacin available from the diet, add the amount available from tryptophan (4.7 mg NE) to the amount of preformed niacin obtained from the diet.

FIGURE 10-7 Niacin in Selected Foods

Food	Serving size (kcalories)
Bread, whole wheat	1 oz slice (70 kcal)
Cornflakes, fortified	1 oz (110 kcal)
Spaghetti pasta	½ c cooked (99 kcal)
Tortilla, flour	1 10"-round (234 kcal)
Broccoli	½ c cooked (22 kcal)
Carrots	½ c shredded raw (24 kcal)
Potato	1 medium baked w/skin (133 kcal)
Tomato juice	¾ c (31 kcal)
Banana	1 medium raw (109 kcal)
Orange	1 medium raw (62 kcal)
Strawberries	½ c fresh (22 kcal)
Watermelon	1 slice (92 kcal)
Milk	1 c reduced-fat 2% (121 kcal)
Yogurt, plain	1 c low-fat (155 kcal)
Cheddar cheese	1½ oz (171 kcal)
Cottage cheese	½ c low-fat 2% (101 kcal)
Pinto beans	½ c cooked (117 kcal)
Peanut butter	2 tbs (188 kcal)
Sunflower seeds	1 oz dry (165 kcal)
Tofu (soybean curd)	½ c (76 kcal)
Ground beef, lean	3 oz broiled (244 kcal)
Chicken breast	3 oz roasted (140 kcal)
Tuna, canned in water	3 oz (99 kcal)
Egg	1 hard cooked (78 kcal)
Excellent, and sometimes unusual, sources:	
Liver	3 oz fried (184 kcal)
Peanuts	1 oz roasted (165 kcal)
Mushrooms	½ c cooked (21 kcal)

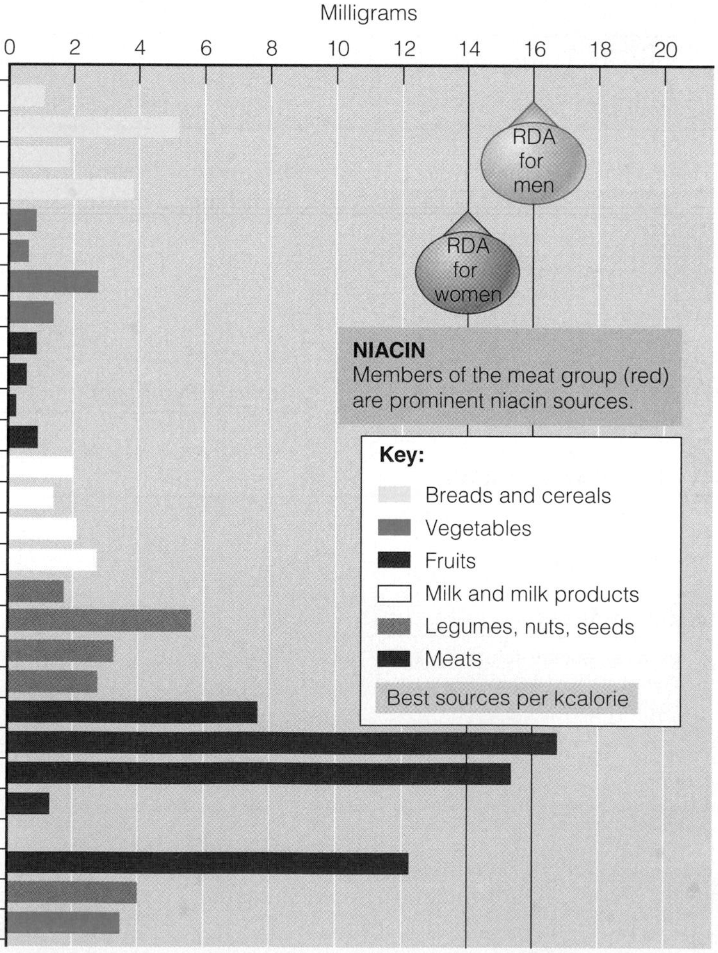

Milligrams
0 2 4 6 8 10 12 14 16 18 20
RDA for men
RDA for women
NIACIN
Members of the meat group (red) are prominent niacin sources.
Key:
Breads and cereals
Vegetables
Fruits
Milk and milk products
Legumes, nuts, seeds
Meats
Best sources per kcalorie

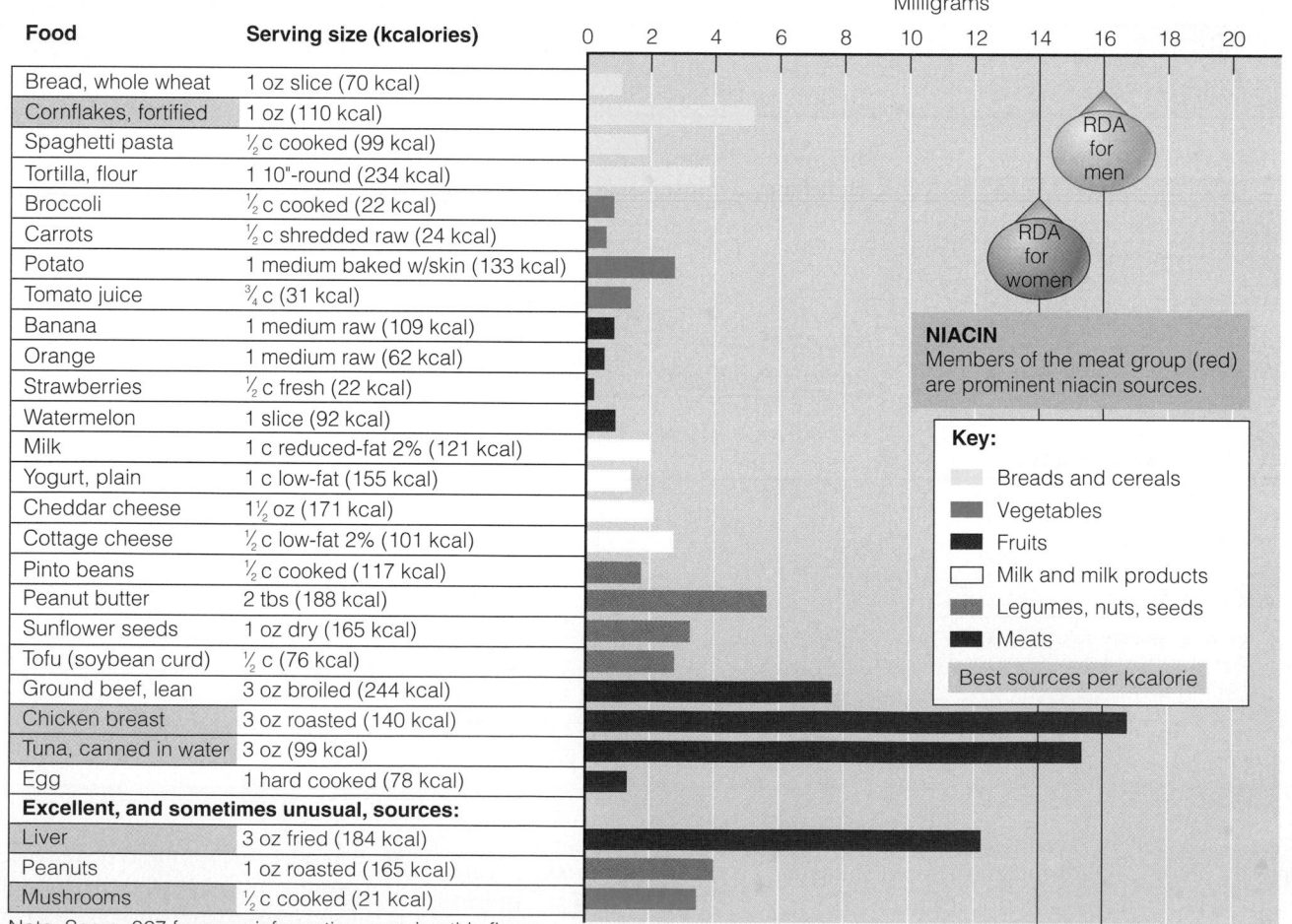

Note: See p. 327 for more information on using this figure.

Biotin Recommendations Biotin is needed in very small amounts. Instead of an RDA, an Adequate Intake (AI) has been determined.

Biotin Deficiency and Toxicity Biotin deficiencies rarely occur. Researchers can induce a biotin deficiency in animals or human beings by feeding them raw egg whites, which contain a protein■ that binds biotin and thus prevents its absorption. Biotin-deficiency symptoms include skin rash, hair loss, and neurological impairment. More than two dozen egg whites must be consumed daily for several months to produce these effects, however, and the eggs have to be raw; cooking denatures the binding protein. No adverse effects from high biotin intakes have been reported; it does not have an Upper Level.

■ The protein **avidin** (AV-eh-din) in egg whites binds biotin.
- **avid** = greedy

Biotin Food Sources Biotin is widespread in foods (including egg yolks), so eating a variety of foods protects against deficiencies. Some biotin is also synthesized by GI tract bacteria, but this amount may not contribute much to the biotin absorbed. A review of biotin facts is provided in the summary table.

IN SUMMARY Biotin

1998 Adequate Intake (AI)

Adults: 30 μg/day

Chief Functions in the Body

Part of a coenzyme used in energy metabolism, fat synthesis, amino acid metabolism, and glycogen synthesis

Significant Sources

Widespread in foods; organ meats, egg yolks, soybeans, fish, whole grains; also produced by GI bacteria

Deficiency Symptoms

Depression, lethargy, hallucinations, numb or tingling sensation in the arms and legs; red, scaly rash around the eyes, nose, and mouth; hair loss

Toxicity Symptoms

None reported

Pantothenic Acid

Pantothenic acid is involved in more than 100 different steps in the synthesis of lipids, neurotransmitters, steroid hormones, and hemoglobin as part of the chemical structure of coenzyme A—the same CoA that forms acetyl CoA, the "crossroads" compound in several metabolic pathways, including the TCA cycle. (Appendix C presents the chemical structures of these two molecules and shows that coenzyme A is made up in part of pantothenic acid.)

Pantothenic Acid Recommendations An Adequate Intake (AI) for pantothenic acid has been set. It reflects the amount needed to replace daily losses.

Pantothenic Acid Deficiency and Toxicity Pantothenic acid deficiency is rare. Its symptoms involve a general failure of all the body's systems and include fatigue, GI distress, and neurological disturbances. The "burning feet" syndrome that affected prisoners of war in Asia during World War II is thought to have been caused by pantothenic acid deficiency. No toxic effects have been reported, and no Upper Level has been established.

Pantothenic Acid Food Sources Pantothenic acid is widespread in foods, and typical diets seem to provide adequate intakes. Beef, poultry, whole grains, potatoes, tomatoes, and broccoli are particularly good sources. Losses of pantothenic acid during food production can be substantial because it is readily destroyed by the freezing, canning, and refining processes. The following summary table presents pantothenic acid facts.

pantothenic (PAN-toe-THEN-ick) **acid:** a B vitamin. The principal active form is part of coenzyme A, called "CoA" throughout Chapter 7.
- **pantos** = everywhere

IN SUMMARY Pantothenic Acid

1998 Adequate Intake (AI)

Adults: 5 mg/day

Chief Functions in the Body

Part of coenzyme A, used in energy metabolism

Significant Sources

Widespread in foods; organ meats, mushrooms, avocados, broccoli, whole grains

Easily destroyed by food processing

Deficiency Symptoms

Vomiting, nausea, stomach cramps; insomnia, fatigue, depression, irritability, restlessness, apathy; hypoglycemia, increased sensitivity to insulin

Toxicity Symptoms

None reported

Vitamin B_6

Vitamin B_6 occurs in three forms—pyridoxal, pyridoxine, and pyridoxamine. All three can be converted to the coenzyme PLP (pyridoxal phosphate), which is active in amino acid metabolism. Because PLP can transfer amino groups (NH_2) from an amino acid to a keto acid, the body can make nonessential amino acids (review Figure 7-15 on p. 228). The ability to add and remove amino groups makes PLP valuable in protein and urea metabolism as well. The conversions of the amino acid tryptophan to niacin or to the neurotransmitter serotonin■ also depend on PLP as does the synthesis of heme (the nonprotein portion of hemoglobin), nucleic acids (such as DNA and RNA), and lecithin.

■ Reminder: *Serotonin* is a neurotransmitter important in appetite control, sleep regulation, and sensory perception, among other roles; it is synthesized in the body from the amino acid tryptophan with the help of vitamin B_6.

A surge of research in the last decade has revealed that vitamin B_6 influences cognitive performance, immune function, and steroid hormone activity. Unlike other water-soluble vitamins, vitamin B_6 is stored extensively in muscle tissue.

Vitamin B_6 Recommendations Because the vitamin B_6 coenzymes play many roles in amino acid metabolism, previous RDA were expressed in terms of protein intakes; the current RDA for vitamin B_6, however, is not. Research does not support claims that large doses of vitamin B_6 enhance muscle strength or physical endurance. Vitamin supplements cannot compete with a nutritious diet and physical training.

Vitamin B_6 Deficiency Without adequate vitamin B_6, synthesis of key neurotransmitters diminishes, and abnormal compounds produced during tryptophan metabolism accumulate in the brain. Early symptoms of vitamin B_6 deficiency include depression and confusion; advanced symptoms include abnormal brain wave patterns and convulsions.

Alcohol contributes to the destruction and loss of vitamin B_6 from the body. As Highlight 7 described, when the body breaks down alcohol, it produces acetaldehyde. If allowed to accumulate, acetaldehyde dislodges the PLP coenzyme from its enzymes; once loose, PLP breaks down and is excreted.

Another drug that acts as a vitamin B_6 **antagonist** is INH, a medication that inhibits the growth of the tuberculosis bacterium.* This drug has saved countless lives, but as a vitamin B_6 antagonist, INH binds and inactivates the vitamin, inducing a deficiency. Whenever INH is used to treat tuberculosis, vitamin B_6 supplements must be given to protect against deficiency.

Oral contraceptives have raised concerns, but they may be unwarranted. Early studies reported signs of vitamin B_6 deficiency in oral contraceptive users, but that was when the pills contained estrogen at three to five times the quantities used today. Estrogen creates a shortage of vitamin B_6 by stimulating the breakdown of tryptophan, a process that requires the vitamin.

Vitamin B_6 Toxicity The first major report of vitamin B_6 toxicity appeared in 1983. Until that time, everyone (including researchers and dietitians) believed

vitamin B_6: a family of compounds—pyridoxal, pyridoxine, and pyridoxamine. The primary active coenzyme form is **PLP (pyridoxal phosphate).**

antagonist: a competing factor that counteracts the action of another factor. When a drug displaces a vitamin from its site of action, the drug renders the vitamin ineffective and thus acts as a vitamin antagonist.

*INH stands for isonicotinic acid hydrazide.

that, like the other water-soluble vitamins, vitamin B_6 could not reach toxic concentrations in the body. The report described neurological damage in people who had been taking more than 2 grams of vitamin B_6 daily (20 times the current Upper Level) for two months or more.

Some women use vitamin B_6 supplements in an attempt to treat premenstrual syndrome (PMS), the cluster of physical, emotional, and psychological symptoms that some women experience seven to ten days prior to menstruation. The cause of PMS remains undefined, although researchers generally agree that the hormonal changes of the menstrual cycle must be responsible. Without a full understanding of PMS causes, medical treatments flounder, and quack treatments abound. Among nutritional approaches, the taking of vitamin B_6 has received much attention, but seems to have done more harm than good.

Some people have taken vitamin B_6 supplements in an attempt to cure **carpal tunnel syndrome** and sleep disorders even though such treatment seems to be ineffective.[4] Self-prescribing is ill-advised because large doses of vitamin B_6 taken for months or years may cause irreversible nerve degeneration.

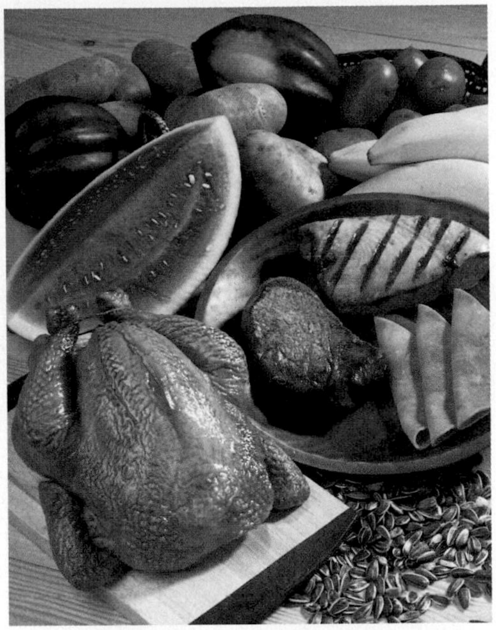

© Polara Studios Inc.

Most protein-rich foods such as meat, fish, and poultry provide ample vitamin B_6; some vegetables and fruits are good sources, too.

Vitamin B_6 Food Sources As you can see from the colored bars in Figure 10-8 (on p. 336), meats, fish, and poultry (red), potatoes and a few other vegetables (green), and fruits (purple) offer vitamin B_6. As is true of most of the other vitamins, fruits and vegetables would rank considerably higher if foods were ranked by nutrient density (vitamin B_6 per kcalorie). Several servings of vitamin B_6–rich foods are needed to meet recommended intakes.

Foods lose vitamin B_6 when heated. Information is limited, but vitamin B_6 bioavailability from plant-derived foods seems to be lower than from animal-derived foods; fiber does not appear to interfere with absorption. The summary table lists food sources of vitamin B_6 as well as its chief functions in the body and common symptoms of both deficiency and toxicity.

IN SUMMARY Vitamin B_6

Other Names

Pyridoxine, pyridoxal, pyridoxamine

1998 RDA

Adults (19–50 yr): 1.3 mg/day

Upper Level

Adults: 100 mg/day

Chief Functions in the Body

Part of coenzymes PLP (pyridoxal phosphate) and PMP (pyridoxamine phosphate) used in amino acid and fatty acid metabolism; helps to convert tryptophan to niacin and to serotonin; helps to make red blood cells

Significant Sources

Meats, fish, poultry, potatoes, legumes, noncitrus fruits, fortified cereals, liver, soy products

Easily destroyed by heat

Deficiency Symptoms

Scaly dermatitis; anemia (small-cell type);[a] depression, confusion, abnormal brain wave pattern, convulsions

Toxicity Symptoms

Depression, fatigue, irritability, headaches, nerve damage causing numbness and muscle weakness leading to an inability to walk and convulsions; skin lesions

[a]Small-cell–type anemia is *microcytic anemia.*

Folate

Folate, also known as folacin or folic acid, has a chemical name that would fit a flying dinosaur: pteroylglutamic acid (PGA for short). Its primary coenzyme form, THF (tetrahydrofolate), serves as part of an enzyme complex that transfers one-carbon compounds that arise during metabolism. This action helps convert vitamin B_{12} to one of its coenzyme forms and helps synthesize the DNA required for all rapidly growing cells.

carpal tunnel syndrome: a pinched nerve at the wrist, causing pain or numbness in the hand. It is often caused by repetitive motion of the wrist.

folate (FOLE-ate): a B vitamin; also known as folic acid, folacin, or pteroylglutamic (tare-o-EEL-glue-TAM-ick) acid (PGA). The coenzyme forms are **DHF (dihydrofolate)** and **THF (tetrahydrofolate).**

FIGURE 10-8 Vitamin B_6 in Selected Foods

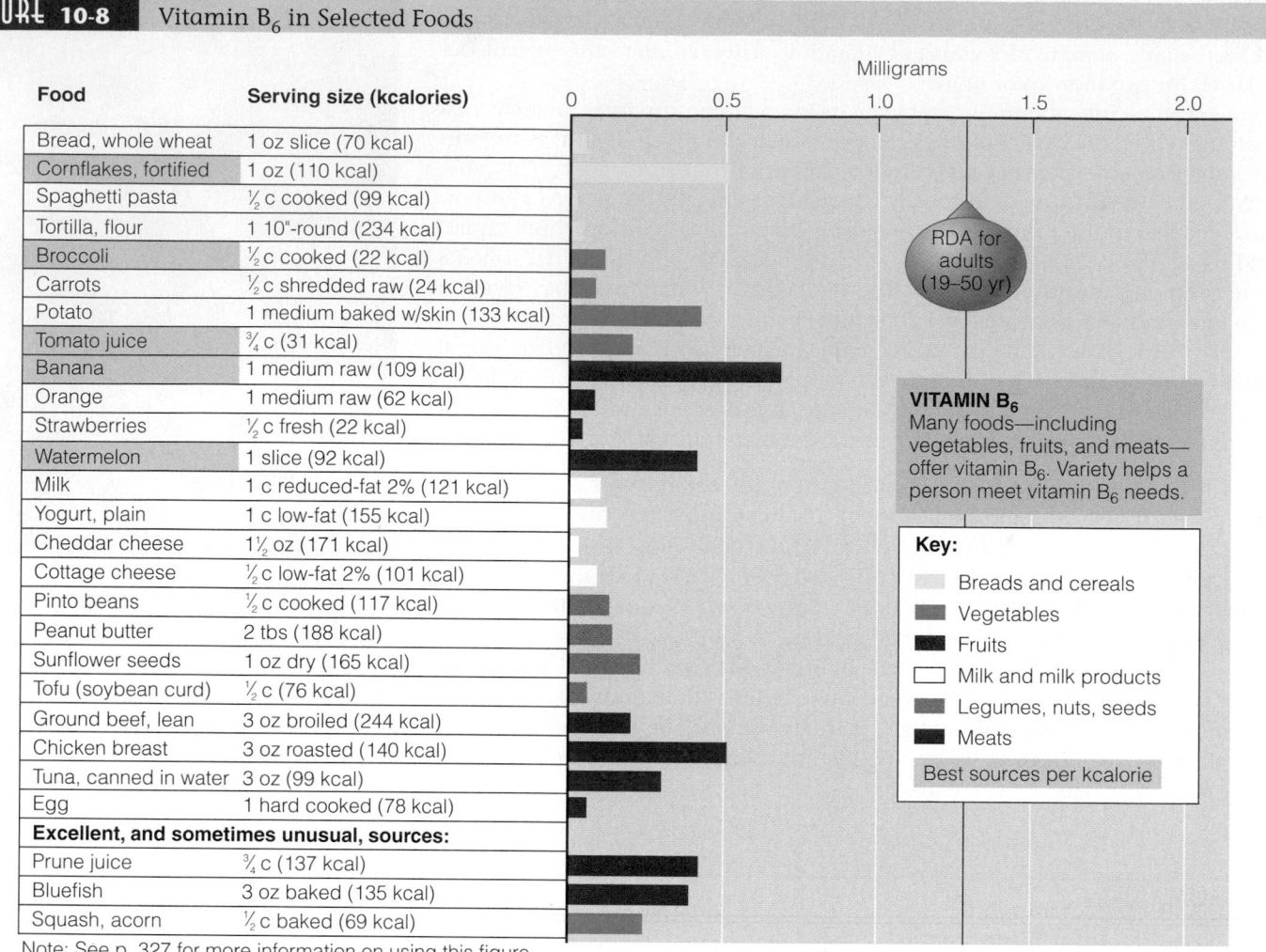

Food	Serving size (kcalories)
Bread, whole wheat	1 oz slice (70 kcal)
Cornflakes, fortified	1 oz (110 kcal)
Spaghetti pasta	½ c cooked (99 kcal)
Tortilla, flour	1 10"-round (234 kcal)
Broccoli	½ c cooked (22 kcal)
Carrots	½ c shredded raw (24 kcal)
Potato	1 medium baked w/skin (133 kcal)
Tomato juice	¾ c (31 kcal)
Banana	1 medium raw (109 kcal)
Orange	1 medium raw (62 kcal)
Strawberries	½ c fresh (22 kcal)
Watermelon	1 slice (92 kcal)
Milk	1 c reduced-fat 2% (121 kcal)
Yogurt, plain	1 c low-fat (155 kcal)
Cheddar cheese	1½ oz (171 kcal)
Cottage cheese	½ c low-fat 2% (101 kcal)
Pinto beans	½ c cooked (117 kcal)
Peanut butter	2 tbs (188 kcal)
Sunflower seeds	1 oz dry (165 kcal)
Tofu (soybean curd)	½ c (76 kcal)
Ground beef, lean	3 oz broiled (244 kcal)
Chicken breast	3 oz roasted (140 kcal)
Tuna, canned in water	3 oz (99 kcal)
Egg	1 hard cooked (78 kcal)
Excellent, and sometimes unusual, sources:	
Prune juice	¾ c (137 kcal)
Bluefish	3 oz baked (135 kcal)
Squash, acorn	½ c baked (69 kcal)

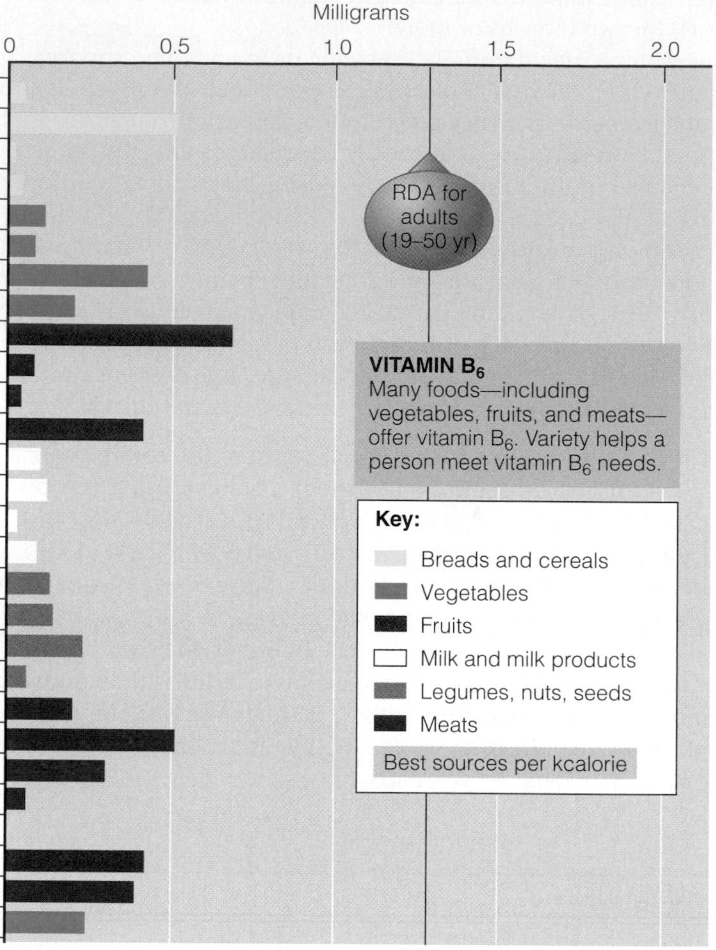

Milligrams
0
0.5
1.0
1.5
2.0
RDA for adults (19–50 yr)
VITAMIN B6
Many foods—including vegetables, fruits, and meats—offer vitamin B6. Variety helps a person meet vitamin B6 needs.
Key:
Breads and cereals
Vegetables
Fruits
Milk and milk products
Legumes, nuts, seeds
Meats
Best sources per kcalorie

Note: See p. 327 for more information on using this figure.

dietary folate equivalents (DFE): the amount of folate available to the body from naturally occurring sources, fortified foods, and supplements, accounting for differences in the bioavailability from each source.

neural tube defects: malformations of the brain, spinal cord, or both during embryonic development. The two main types of neural tube defects are **spina bifida** (literally, "split spine") and **anencephaly** ("no brain").

Foods deliver folate mostly in the "bound" form—that is, combined with a string of amino acids (glutamate), known as polyglutamate (see Appendix C for the chemical structure). The intestine prefers to absorb the "free" folate form—folate with only one glutamate attached (the monoglutamate form). Enzymes on the intestinal cell surfaces hydrolyze the polyglutamate to monoglutamate and several glutamates. Then the monoglutamate is attached to a methyl group (CH_3). Special transport systems deliver the monoglutamate with its methyl group to the liver and other body cells.

In order for the folate coenzyme to function, the methyl group must be removed by an enzyme that requires the help of vitamin B_{12}. Without that help, folate becomes trapped inside cells in its methyl form, unavailable to support DNA synthesis and cell growth. Figure 10-9 summarizes folate's absorption and activation.

To dispose of excess folate, the liver secretes most of it into bile and ships it to the gallbladder. Thus folate returns to the intestine in an enterohepatic circulation route like that of bile itself (review Figure 5-16 on p. 153).

This complicated system for handling folate is vulnerable to GI tract injuries. Since folate is actively secreted back into the GI tract with bile, it has to be reabsorbed repeatedly. If the GI tract cells are damaged, then folate is rapidly lost from the body. Such is the case in alcohol abuse; folate deficiency rapidly develops and, ironically, damages the GI tract further. The folate coenzymes, remember, are active in cell multiplication—and the cells lining the GI tract are among the most rapidly renewed cells in the body. Unable to make new cells, the GI tract deteriorates and not only loses folate, but also fails to absorb other nutrients.

FIGURE 10-9 Folate's Absorption and Activation

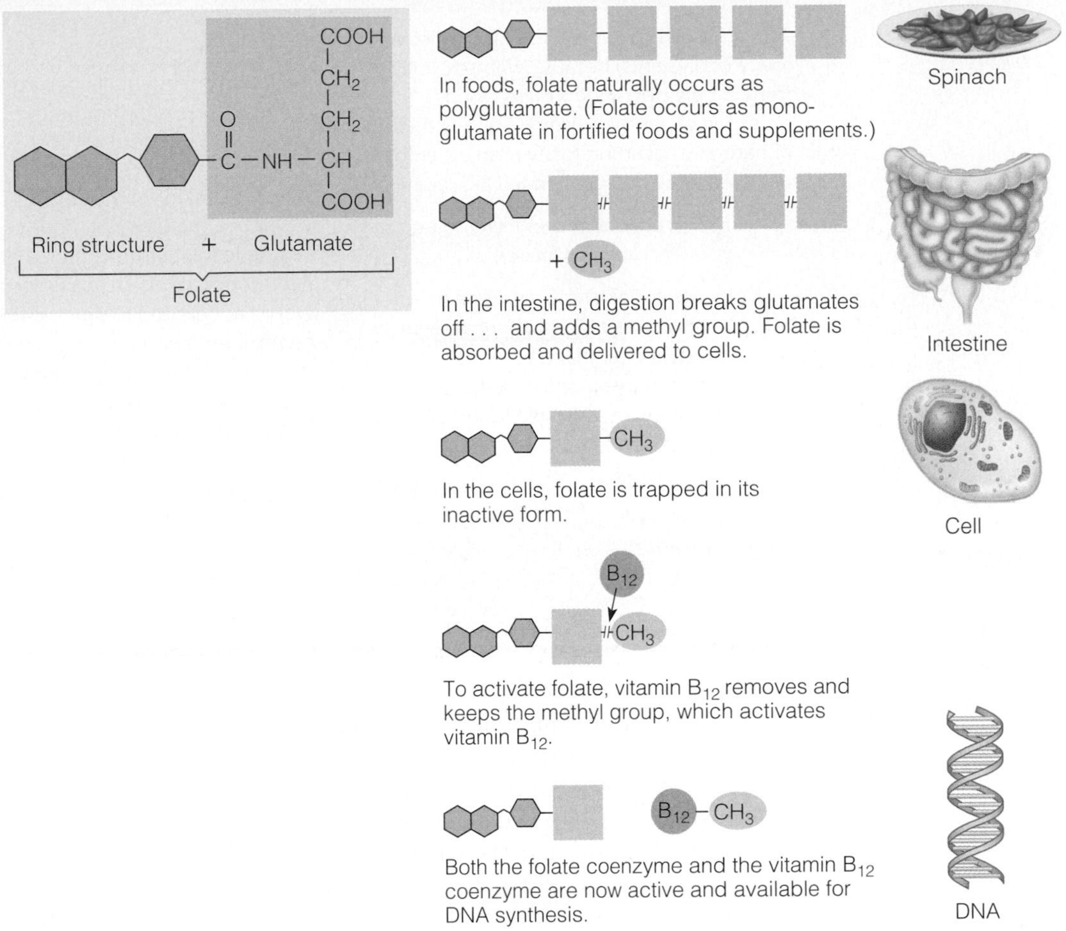
COOH
CH_2
CH_2
O
C—NH—CH
COOH
Ring structure + Glutamate
Folate
In foods, folate naturally occurs as polyglutamate. (Folate occurs as mono-glutamate in fortified foods and supplements.)
Spinach
+ CH_3
In the intestine, digestion breaks glutamates off . . . and adds a methyl group. Folate is absorbed and delivered to cells.
Intestine
CH_3
In the cells, folate is trapped in its inactive form.
Cell
B_{12}
CH_3
To activate folate, vitamin B_{12} removes and keeps the methyl group, which activates vitamin B_{12}.
B_{12}—CH_3
Both the folate coenzyme and the vitamin B_{12} coenzyme are now active and available for DNA synthesis.
DNA

Folate Recommendations The bioavailability of folate ranges from 50 percent for foods to 100 percent for supplements taken on an empty stomach. These differences in bioavailability were considered in establishing the folate RDA. Naturally occurring folate from foods is given full credit. Synthetic folate from fortified foods and supplements is given extra credit because, on average, it is 1.7 times more available than naturally occurring food folate. Thus a person consuming 100 micrograms of folate from foods and 100 micrograms from a supplement receives 270 **dietary folate equivalents (DFE).**■ (The "How to" on p. 338 describes how to estimate dietary folate equivalents.) The need for folate rises considerably during pregnancy and whenever cells are multiplying, so the recommendations for pregnant women are considerably higher than for other adults.

Folate and Neural Tube Defects Several research studies have confirmed the importance of folate in reducing the risks of **neural tube defects.**[5] The brain and spinal cord develop from the neural tube, and defects in its orderly formation during the early weeks of pregnancy may result in various central nervous system disorders and death. (Chapter 14 provides photos of neural tube development and a figure showing a neural tube defect.)

Folate supplements taken one month before conception and continued throughout the first trimester of pregnancy can help prevent neural tube defects.[6] For this reason, all women of childbearing age■ who are capable of becoming pregnant should consume 0.4 milligram (400 micrograms) of folate daily,■ although only one-third of them actually do.[7] This recommendation can be met through a diet that includes at least five servings of fruits and vegetables daily, but many

■ To calculate DFE:
DFE = µg food folate + (1.7 × µg synthetic folate).
Using the example in the text:
100 µg food
+ 170 µg supplement (1.7 × 100 µg)
270 µg DFE

■ Women of childbearing age (15 to 45 yr) should:
- Eat folate-rich foods.
- Eat folate-fortified foods.
- Take a multivitamin daily (most provide 400 µg folate).

■ Reminder: A milligram (mg) is one-thousandth of a gram. A microgram (µg) is one-thousandth of a milligram (or one-millionth of a gram).
- 0.4 mg = 400 µg.

HOW TO Estimate Dietary Folate Equivalents

Folate is expressed in terms of DFE (dietary folate equivalents) because synthetic folate from supplements and fortified foods is absorbed at almost twice (1.7 times) the rate of naturally occurring folate from other foods. Use the following equation to calculate:

$$\text{DFE} = \mu\text{g food folate} + (1.7 \times \mu\text{g synthetic folate}).$$

Consider, for example, a pregnant woman who takes a supplement and eats a bowl of fortified cornflakes, 2 slices of fortified bread, and a cup of fortified pasta. From the supplement and fortified foods, she obtains synthetic folate:

Supplement	100 μg folate
Fortified cornflakes	100 μg folate
Fortified bread	40 μg folate
Fortified pasta	60 μg folate
	300 μg folate

To calculate the DFE, multiply the amount of synthetic folate by 1.7:

$$300\ \mu\text{g} \times 1.7 = 510\ \mu\text{g DFE}.$$

Now add the naturally occurring folate from the other foods in her diet—in this example, another 90 μg of folate.

$$510\ \mu\text{g DFE} + 90\ \mu\text{g} = 600\ \mu\text{g DFE}.$$

Notice that if we had not converted synthetic folate from supplements and fortified foods to DFE, then this woman's intake would appear to fall short of the 600 μg recommendation for pregnancy (300 μg + 90 μg = 390 μg). But as our example shows, her intake does meet the recommendation. At this time, supplement and fortified food labels list folate in μg only, not μg DFE, making such calculations necessary.

women typically fail to do so and receive only half this amount from foods. Furthermore, because of the enhanced bioavailability of synthetic folate, supplementation or fortification improves folate status significantly. Women who have given birth to infants with neural tube defects previously should consume 4 milligrams of folate daily before conception and throughout the first trimester of pregnancy.

Because half of the pregnancies each year are unplanned and because neural tube defects occur early in development before most women realize they are pregnant, the Food and Drug Administration (FDA) has mandated that grain products be fortified to deliver folate to the U.S. population.* Labels on fortified products may claim that "adequate intake of folate has been shown to reduce the risk of neural tube defects." Fortification has improved folate status in women of childbearing age and lowered the number of neural tube defects that occur each year, as Figure 10-10 shows.[8]

Folate fortification raises safety concerns as well, especially since folate intakes from fortified foods are more than twice as high as originally predicted.[9] Because high intakes of folate complicate the diagnosis of a vitamin B_{12} deficiency, folate consumption should not exceed 1 milligram daily without close medical supervision.[10]

Recent research has uncovered relationships between folate deficiency and non–neural tube birth defects such as Down syndrome.[11] Folate's exact role in preventing these birth defects, however, remains unclear. Some women whose infants develop these defects are *not* deficient in folate, and others with severe folate deficiencies do *not* give birth to infants with birth defects. Researchers continue to look for other factors that must also be involved.

Folate and Heart Disease The FDA's decision to fortify grain products with folate was strengthened by research indicating an important role for folate in defending against heart disease. As Chapter 6 mentioned, research indicates that high levels of the amino acid homocysteine and low levels of folate increase the risk of fatal heart disease.[12] One of folate's key roles in the body is to break down homocysteine. Without folate, homocysteine accumulates, which seems to en-

*Bread products, flour, corn grits, cornmeal, farina, rice, macaroni, and noodles must be fortified with 140 micrograms of folate per 100 grams of grain. For perspective, 100 grams is roughly 3 slices of bread; 1 cup of flour, ½ cup of corn grits, cornmeal, farina, or rice; or ¾ cup of macaroni or noodles.

FIGURE 10-10 Decreasing Spina Bifida Rates since Folate Fortification

Neural tube defects have declined since folate fortification began in 1996.

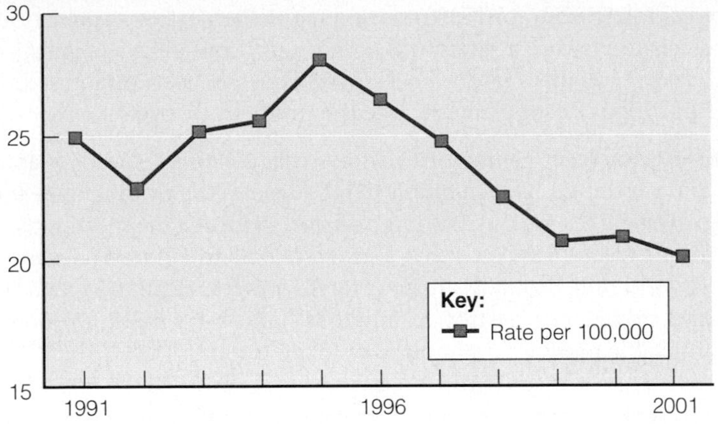
30
25
20
15
1991
1996
2001
Key:
Rate per 100,000

SOURCE: National Vital Statistics System, National Center for Health Statistics, Centers for Disease Control.

hance blood clot formation and arterial wall deterioration. Fortified foods and folate supplements raise blood folate and reduce blood homocysteine levels to an extent that may help to prevent heart disease.[13]

Folate and Cancer Folate may also play a role in preventing cancer.[14] Notably, folate may be most effective in protecting those most likely to develop cancers: men who smoke (against pancreatic cancer) and women who drink alcohol (against breast cancer).[15]

Folate Deficiency Folate deficiency impairs cell division and protein synthesis—processes critical to growing tissues. In a folate deficiency, the replacement of red blood cells and GI tract cells falters. Not surprisingly, then, two of the first symptoms of a folate deficiency are **anemia** and GI tract deterioration.

The anemia of folate deficiency is characterized by large,■ immature red blood cells. Without folate, DNA synthesis slows and the cells lose their ability to divide. The nucleus of the cell is not released as normally occurs during development. As a result, the immature blood cells are enlarged and oval-shaped. They cannot carry oxygen or travel through the capillaries as efficiently as normal red blood cells.

Folate deficiencies may develop from inadequate intake and have been reported in infants fed goat's milk, which is notoriously low in folate. Folate deficiency may also result from impaired absorption or an unusual metabolic need for the vitamin. Metabolic needs increase wherever cell multiplication must speed up: in pregnancies involving twins and triplets; in cancer; in skin-destroying diseases such as chicken pox and measles; and in burns, blood loss, GI tract damage, and the like.

Of all the vitamins, folate appears to be most vulnerable to interactions with drugs, which can lead to a secondary deficiency. Some medications, notably anticancer drugs, have a chemical structure similar to folate's structure and can displace the vitamin from enzymes and interfere with normal metabolism. Cancer cells, like all cells, need the real vitamin to multiply; without it, they die. Unfortunately, these drugs affect both cancerous cells and healthy cells and create a folate deficiency for all cells. (Chapter 19 discusses nutrient-drug interactions and includes a figure illustrating the similarities between the vitamin folate and the anticancer drug methotrexate.)

Aspirin and antacids also interfere with the body's handling of folate. Healthy adults who use these drugs to relieve an occasional headache or upset stomach need not be concerned, but people who rely heavily on aspirin or antacids should

■ Large-cell anemia is known as **macrocytic** or **megaloblastic anemia.**
- **macro** = large
- **cyte** = cell
- **mega** = large

anemia (ah-NEE-me-ah): literally, "too little blood." Anemia is any condition in which too few red blood cells are present, or the red blood cells are immature (and therefore large) or too small or contain too little hemoglobin to carry the normal amount of oxygen to the tissues. It is not a disease itself but can be a symptom of many different disease conditions, including many nutrient deficiencies, bleeding, excessive red blood cell destruction, and defective red blood cell formation.
- **an** = without
- **emia** = blood

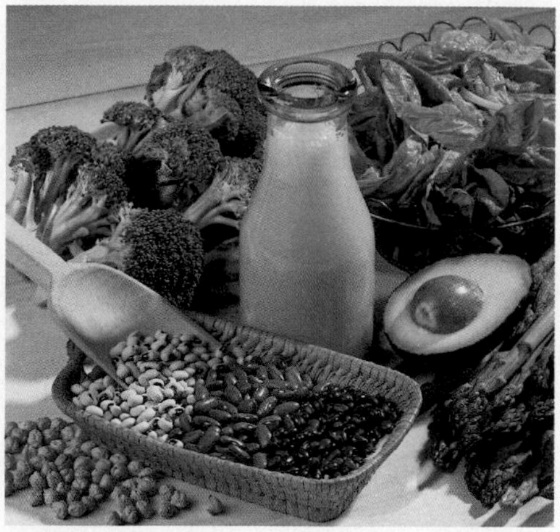
© Polara Studios Inc.

Leafy dark green vegetables (such as spinach and broccoli), legumes (such as black beans, kidney beans, and black-eyed peas), liver, and some fruits (notably citrus fruits and juices) are naturally rich in folate.

be aware of the nutrition consequences. Oral contraceptives may also impair folate status, as may smoking.

Folate Toxicity Naturally occurring folate from foods alone appears to cause no harm. Excess folate from fortified foods or supplements, however, can reach high enough levels to obscure a vitamin B_{12} deficiency and delay diagnosis of neurological damage. For this reason, an Upper Level has been established for folate from fortified foods or supplements (see the inside front cover).

Folate Food Sources Figure 10-11 shows that folate is especially abundant in legumes and vegetables. The vitamin's name suggests the word *foliage,* and indeed, leafy green vegetables are outstanding sources. With fortification, grain products also contribute folate. The small red and white bars in Figure 10-11 indicate that meats, milk, and milk products are poor folate sources. Heat and oxidation during cooking and storage can destroy as much as half of the folate in foods. The accompanying table provides a summary of folate information.

IN SUMMARY Folate

Other Names

Folic acid, folacin, pteroylglutamic acid (PGA)

1998 RDA

Adults: 400 µg/day

Upper Level

Adults: 1000 µg/day

Chief Functions in the Body

Part of coenzymes THF (tetrahydrofolate) and DHF (dihydrofolate) used in DNA synthesis and therefore important in new cell formation

Significant Sources

Fortified grains, leafy green vegetables, legumes, seeds, liver

Easily destroyed by heat and oxygen

Deficiency Symptoms

Anemia (large-cell type);[a] smooth, red tongue;[b] mental confusion, weakness, fatigue, irritability, headache

Toxicity Symptoms

Masks vitamin B_{12}–deficiency symptoms

[a] Large-cell–type anemia is known as either *macrocytic* or *megaloblastic anemia.*
[b] Smoothness of the tongue is caused by loss of its surface structures and is termed *glossitis* (gloss-EYE-tis).

Vitamin B_{12}

Vitamin B_{12} and folate are closely related: each depends on the other for activation. Recall that vitamin B_{12} removes a methyl group to activate the folate coenzyme; when folate gives up its methyl group, the vitamin B_{12} coenzyme becomes activated (review Figure 10-9 on p. 337).

The regeneration of the amino acid methionine and the synthesis of DNA and RNA depend on both folate and vitamin B_{12}.* In addition, without any help from folate, vitamin B_{12} maintains the sheath that surrounds and protects nerve fibers and promotes their normal growth. Bone cell activity and metabolism also depend on vitamin B_{12}.

In the stomach, hydrochloric acid and the digestive enzyme pepsin release vitamin B_{12} from the proteins to which it is attached in foods. As the vitamin passes to the small intestine, it binds with a molecule called **intrinsic factor.** Bound together, intrinsic factor and vitamin B_{12} travel to the end of the small intestine, where receptors recognize the complex. Importantly, the receptors do not recognize vitamin B_{12} alone without intrinsic factor. There the intrinsic factor is degraded, and the vitamin is gradually absorbed into the bloodstream. Transport of vitamin B_{12} in the blood depends on specific binding proteins.

vitamin B_{12}: a B vitamin characterized by the presence of cobalt (see Figure 13-12 in Chapter 13). The active forms of coenzyme B_{12} are **methylcobalamin** and **deoxyadenosylcobalamin.**

intrinsic factor: a glycoprotein (a protein with short polysaccharide chains attached) manufactured in the stomach that aids in the absorption of vitamin B_{12}.
• **intrinsic** = on the inside

*In the body, methionine serves as a methyl (CH_3) donor. In doing so, methionine can be converted to other amino acids. Some of these amino acids can regenerate methionine, but methionine is still considered an essential amino acid that is needed in the diet.

FIGURE 10-11 Folate in Selected Foods

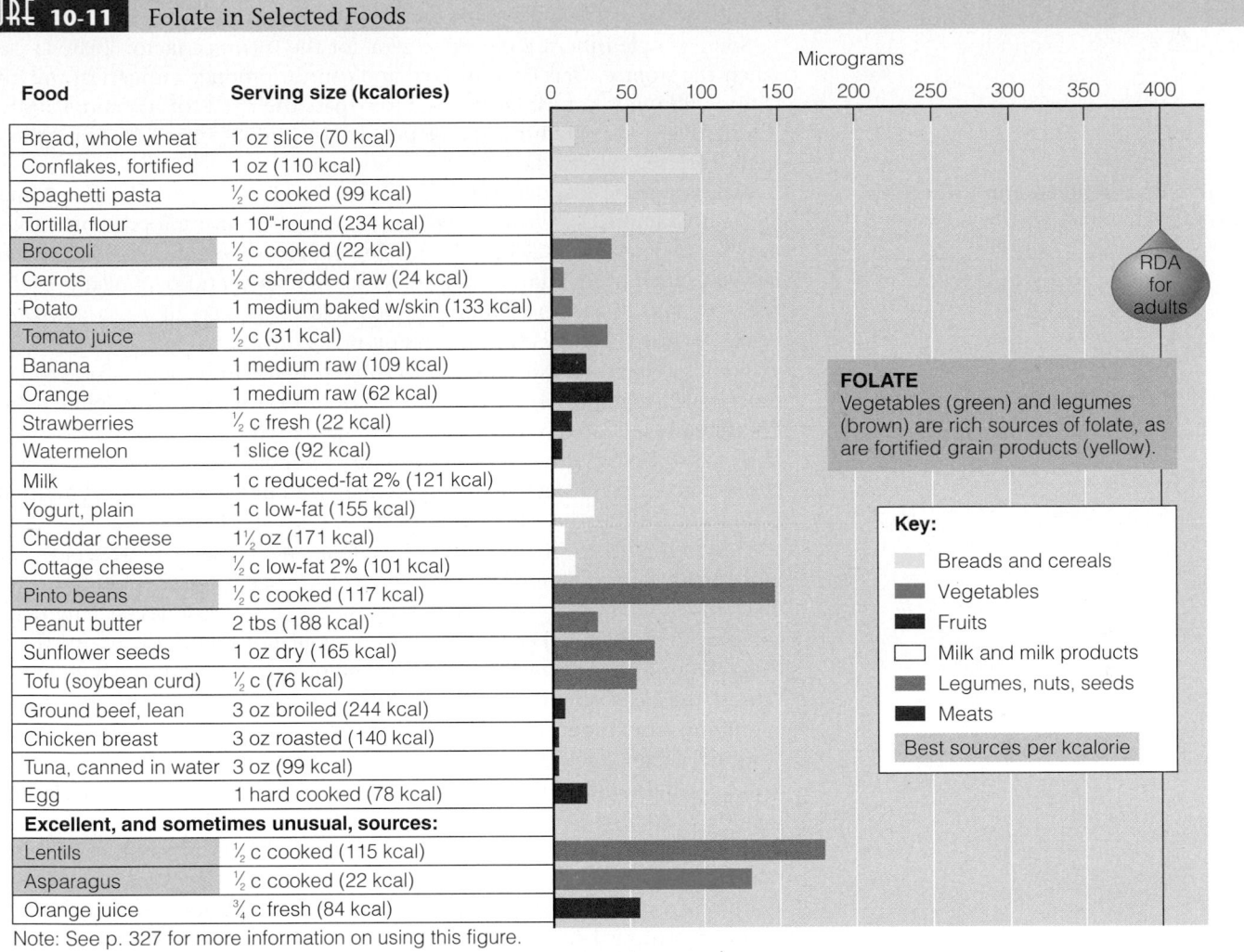

Food	Serving size (kcalories)
Bread, whole wheat	1 oz slice (70 kcal)
Cornflakes, fortified	1 oz (110 kcal)
Spaghetti pasta	½ c cooked (99 kcal)
Tortilla, flour	1 10"-round (234 kcal)
Broccoli	½ c cooked (22 kcal)
Carrots	½ c shredded raw (24 kcal)
Potato	1 medium baked w/skin (133 kcal)
Tomato juice	½ c (31 kcal)
Banana	1 medium raw (109 kcal)
Orange	1 medium raw (62 kcal)
Strawberries	½ c fresh (22 kcal)
Watermelon	1 slice (92 kcal)
Milk	1 c reduced-fat 2% (121 kcal)
Yogurt, plain	1 c low-fat (155 kcal)
Cheddar cheese	1½ oz (171 kcal)
Cottage cheese	½ c low-fat 2% (101 kcal)
Pinto beans	½ c cooked (117 kcal)
Peanut butter	2 tbs (188 kcal)
Sunflower seeds	1 oz dry (165 kcal)
Tofu (soybean curd)	½ c (76 kcal)
Ground beef, lean	3 oz broiled (244 kcal)
Chicken breast	3 oz roasted (140 kcal)
Tuna, canned in water	3 oz (99 kcal)
Egg	1 hard cooked (78 kcal)
Excellent, and sometimes unusual, sources:	
Lentils	½ c cooked (115 kcal)
Asparagus	½ c cooked (22 kcal)
Orange juice	¾ c fresh (84 kcal)

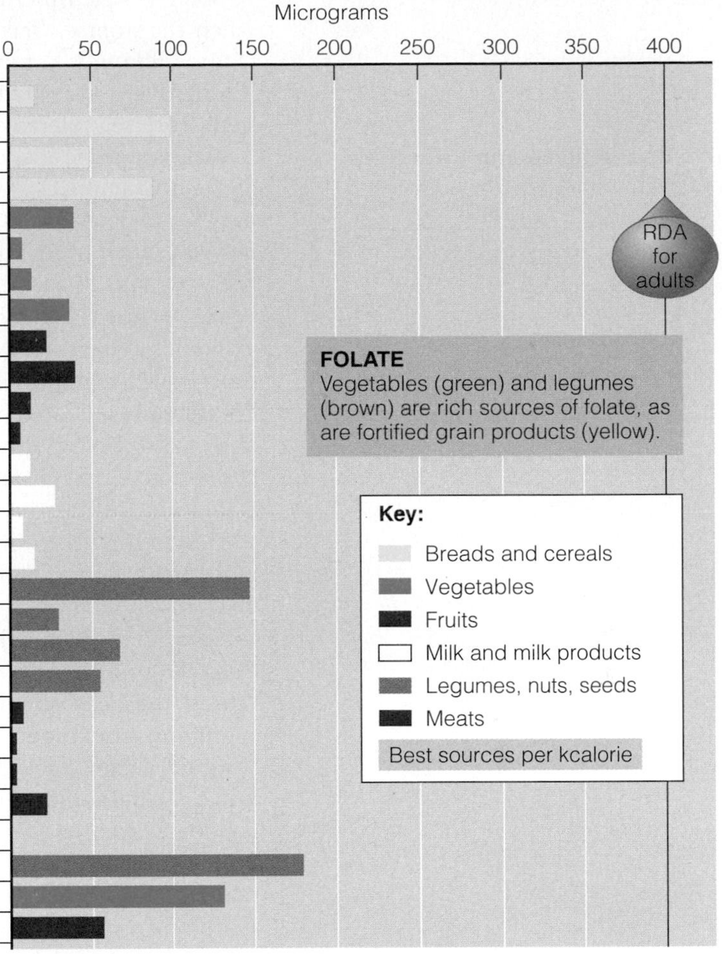
Micrograms
0
50
100
150
200
250
300
350
400
RDA for adults
FOLATE
Vegetables (green) and legumes (brown) are rich sources of folate, as are fortified grain products (yellow).
Key:
Breads and cereals
Vegetables
Fruits
Milk and milk products
Legumes, nuts, seeds
Meats
Best sources per kcalorie

Note: See p. 327 for more information on using this figure.

Like folate, vitamin B_{12} follows the enterohepatic circulation route. It is continually secreted into bile and delivered to the intestine, where it is reabsorbed. Because most vitamin B_{12} is reabsorbed, healthy people rarely develop a deficiency even when their intake is minimal.

Vitamin B_{12} Recommendations The RDA for adults is only 2.4 micrograms of vitamin B_{12} a day—just over two-millionths of a gram. The ink in the period at the end of this sentence may weigh about 2.4 micrograms. But tiny though this amount appears to the human eye, it contains billions of molecules of vitamin B_{12}, enough to provide coenzymes for all the enzymes that need its help.

Vitamin B_{12} Deficiency and Toxicity Most vitamin B_{12} deficiencies reflect inadequate absorption, not poor intake. Inadequate absorption typically occurs for one of two reasons: a lack of hydrochloric acid or a lack of intrinsic factor. Without hydrochloric acid, the vitamin is not released from the dietary proteins and so is not available for binding with the intrinsic factor. Without the intrinsic factor, the vitamin cannot be absorbed.

Many people, especially those over 50, develop **atrophic gastritis,** a common condition in older people that damages the cells of the stomach. Atrophic gastritis may also develop in response to iron deficiency or infection with *Helicobacter pylori,* the bacterium implicated in ulcer formation. Without healthy stomach cells, production of hydrochloric acid and intrinsic factor diminishes. Even with an adequate intake

atrophic (a-TRO-fik) **gastritis** (gas-TRY-tis): chronic inflammation of the stomach accompanied by a diminished size and functioning of the mucous membrane and glands.
- **atrophy** = wasting
- **gastro** = stomach
- **itis** = inflammation

from foods, vitamin B_{12} status suffers. The vitamin B_{12} deficiency caused by atrophic gastritis and a lack of intrinsic factor is known as **pernicious anemia.**

Some people inherit a defective gene for the intrinsic factor. In such cases, or when the stomach has been injured and cannot produce enough of the intrinsic factor, vitamin B_{12} must be injected to bypass the need for intestinal absorption. Alternatively, the vitamin may be delivered by nasal spray; absorption is rapid, high, and well tolerated.

■ Vitamin B_{12} is found primarily in foods derived from animals.

A prolonged inadequate intake, as can occur with a vegetarian diet,■ may also create a vitamin B_{12} deficiency.[16] People who stop eating foods containing vitamin B_{12} may take several years to develop deficiency symptoms because the body recycles much of its vitamin B_{12}, reabsorbing it over and over again. Even when the body fails to absorb vitamin B_{12}, deficiency may take up to three years to develop because the body conserves its supply.

Because vitamin B_{12} is required to convert folate to its active form, one of the most obvious vitamin B_{12}–deficiency symptoms is the anemia of folate deficiency. This anemia is characterized by large, immature red blood cells, which are indicative of slow DNA synthesis and an inability to divide (see Figure 10-12). When folate is trapped in its inactive (methyl folate) form due to vitamin B_{12} deficiency, or is unavailable due to folate deficiency itself, DNA synthesis slows.

First to be affected in a vitamin B_{12} or folate deficiency are the rapidly growing blood cells. Either vitamin B_{12} or folate will clear up the anemia, but if folate is given when vitamin B_{12} is needed, the result is disastrous: devastating neurological symptoms. Remember that vitamin B_{12}, but not folate, maintains the sheath that surrounds and protects nerve fibers and promotes their normal growth. Folate "cures" the *blood* symptoms of a vitamin B_{12} deficiency, but cannot stop the *nerve* symptoms from progressing. By doing so, folate "masks" a vitamin B_{12} deficiency. Marginal vitamin B_{12} deficiency impairs performance on tests measuring intelligence, spatial ability, and short-term memory.[17] Advanced neurological symptoms include a creeping paralysis that begins at the extremities and works inward and up the spine. Early detection and correction are necessary to prevent permanent nerve damage and paralysis. With sufficient folate in the diet, the neurological symptoms of vitamin B_{12} deficiency can develop without evidence of anemia. Such interactions between folate and vitamin B_{12} highlight some of the safety is-

FIGURE 10-12 Normal and Anemic Blood Cells

The anemia of folate deficiency is indistinguishable from that of vitamin B_{12} deficiency. Appendix E describes the biochemical tests used to differentiate the two conditions.

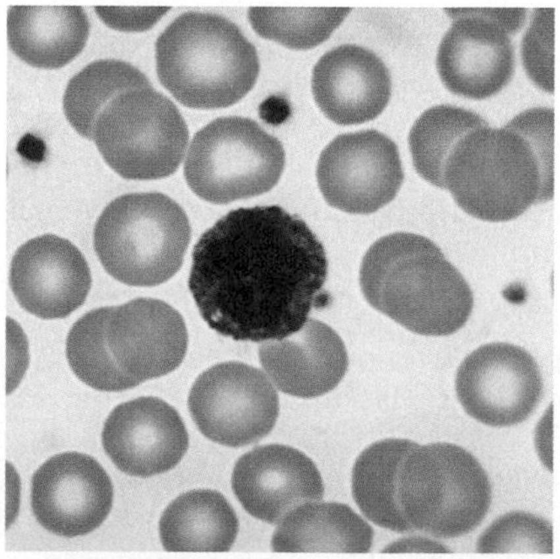

Normal blood cells. The size, shape, and color of the red blood cells show that they are normal.

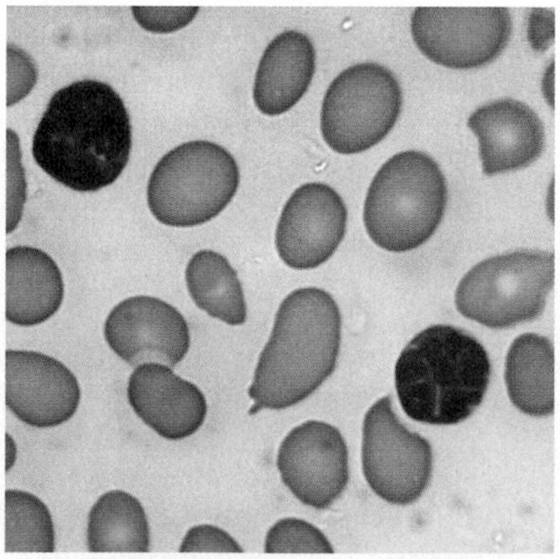

Blood cells in pernicious anemia (megaloblastic). Megaloblastic blood cells are slightly larger than normal red blood cells, and their shapes are irregular.

pernicious (per-NISH-us) **anemia:** a blood disorder that reflects a vitamin B_{12} deficiency caused by lack of intrinsic factor and characterized by abnormally large and immature red blood cells. Other symptoms include muscle weakness and irreversible neurological damage.
- **pernicious** = destructive

sues surrounding the use of supplements and the fortification of foods. No adverse effects have been reported for excess vitamin B_{12}, and no Upper Level has been set.

Vitamin B_{12} Food Sources Vitamin B_{12} is unique among the vitamins in being found almost exclusively in foods derived from animals. Anyone who eats reasonable amounts of meat is guaranteed an adequate intake, and vegetarians who use milk products or eggs are also protected from deficiency. Vegans, who restrict all foods derived from animals, need a reliable source, such as vitamin B_{12}–fortified soy milk or vitamin B_{12} supplements. Yeast grown on a vitamin B_{12}–enriched medium and mixed with that medium provides some vitamin B_{12}, but yeast itself does not contain active vitamin B_{12}. Fermented soy products such as miso (a soybean paste) and sea algae such as spirulina also do *not* provide active vitamin B_{12}. Extensive research shows that the amounts listed on the labels of these plant products are inaccurate and misleading because the vitamin B_{12} is in an inactive, unavailable form.

As mentioned earlier, the water-soluble vitamins are particularly vulnerable to losses in cooking. For most of these nutrients, microwave heating minimizes losses as well as, or better than, traditional cooking methods. Such is not the case for vitamin B_{12}, however. Microwave heating inactivates vitamin B_{12}. To preserve this vitamin, use the oven or stovetop instead of a microwave to cook meats and milk products (major sources of vitamin B_{12}). The accompanying table provides a summary of information about vitamin B_{12}.

IN SUMMARY **Vitamin B_{12}**

Other Names

Cobalamin (and related forms)

1998 RDA

Adults: 2.4 μg/day

Chief Functions in the Body

Part of coenzymes methylcobalamin and deoxyadenosylcobalamin used in new cell synthesis; helps to maintain nerve cells; reforms folate coenzyme; helps to break down some fatty acids and amino acids

Significant Sources

Animal products (meat, fish, poultry, shellfish, milk, cheese, eggs), fortified cereals

Easily destroyed by microwave cooking

Deficiency Disease

Pernicious anemia[a]

Deficiency Symptoms

Anemia (large-cell type);[b] fatigue, degeneration of peripheral nerves progressing to paralysis

Toxicity Symptoms

None reported

[a]The name *pernicious anemia* refers to the vitamin B_{12} deficiency caused by atrophic gastritis and a lack of intrinsic factor, but not to that caused by inadequate dietary intake.
[b]Large-cell–type anemia is known as either *macrocytic* or *megaloblastic anemia.*

Non-B Vitamins

Nutrition scientists debate whether other dietary compounds might also be considered vitamins. In some cases, the compounds may be conditionally essential—that is, needed by the body from foods when synthesis becomes insufficient to support normal growth and metabolism. In other cases, the compounds may be vitamin impostors—not needed under any circumstances.

Choline The essentiality of **choline** has been blurry for decades, in part because the body can make choline from the amino acid methionine. Furthermore, choline is commonly found in many foods as part of the lecithin molecule (review Figure 5-9 on p. 148). Consequently, choline deficiencies are rare. Without any

choline (KOH-leen): a nitrogen-containing compound found in foods and made in the body from the amino acid methionine. Choline is used to make the phospholipid lecithin and the neurotransmitter acetylcholine.

dietary choline, however, synthesis alone appears to be insufficient to meet the body's needs, making choline a conditionally essential nutrient. For this reason, the 1998 DRI report established an Adequate Intake (AI) for choline. The body uses choline to make the neurotransmitter acetylcholine and the phospholipid lecithin. The accompanying table summarizes key choline facts.

IN SUMMARY **Choline**

1998 Adequate Intake (AI)

Men: 550 mg/day

Women: 425 mg/day

Upper Level

Adults: 3500 mg/day

Chief Functions in the Body

Needed for the synthesis of the neurotransmitter acetylcholine and the phospholipid lecithin

Deficiency Symptoms

Liver damage

Toxicity Symptoms

Body odor, sweating, salivation, reduced growth rate, low blood pressure, liver damage

Significant Sources

Milk, liver, eggs, peanuts

Inositol and Carnitine **Inositol** is a part of cell membrane structures, and **carnitine** transports long-chain fatty acids from the cytosol to the mitochondria for oxidation. Like choline, these two substances can be made by the body, but unlike choline, no recommendations have been established. Researchers continue to explore the possibility that these substances may be essential. Even if they are essential, though, supplements are unnecessary because these compounds are widespread in foods.

Some vitamin companies include choline, inositol, and carnitine in their formulations to make their vitamin pills look more "complete" than others, but this strategy offers no real advantage. For a rational way to compare vitamin-mineral supplements, read Highlight 10.

Vitamin Impostors Other substances have been mistaken for essential nutrients for human beings because they are needed for growth by bacteria or other forms of life. Among them are PABA (para-aminobenzoic acid, a component of folate's ring structure), the bioflavonoids (vitamin P or hesperidin), pyrroloquinoline quinone (methoxatin), orotic acid, lipoic acid, and ubiquinone (coenzyme Q_{10}). Other names erroneously associated with vitamins are "vitamin O" (oxygenated salt water), "vitamin B_5" (another name for pantothenic acid), "vitamin B_{15}" (also called "pangamic acid," a hoax), and "vitamin B_{17}" (laetrile, an alleged "cancer cure" and not a vitamin or a cure by any stretch of the imagination—in fact, laetrile is a potentially dangerous substance).

IN SUMMARY The B vitamins serve as coenzymes that facilitate the work of every cell. They are active in carbohydrate, fat, and protein metabolism and in the making of DNA and thus new cells. Historically famous B vitamin–deficiency diseases are beriberi (thiamin), pellagra (niacin), and pernicious anemia (vitamin B_{12}). Pellagra can be prevented by adequate protein because the amino acid tryptophan can be converted to niacin in the body. A high intake of folate can mask the blood symptom of a vitamin B_{12} deficiency, but it will not prevent the associated nerve damage. Vitamin B_6 participates in amino acid metabolism and can be harmful in excess. Biotin and pantothenic acid serve important roles in energy metabolism and are common in a variety of foods. Many substances that people claim as B vitamins are not.

inositol (in-OSS-ih-tall): a nonessential nutrient that can be made in the body from glucose. Inositol is a part of cell membrane structures.

carnitine (CAR-neh-teen): a nonessential nutrient made in the body from the amino acid lysine. Carnitine transports long-chain fatty acids from the cytosol to the mitochondria for oxidation.

The B Vitamins—In Concert

This chapter has described some of the impressive ways that vitamins work individually, as if their many actions in the body could easily be disentangled. In fact, oftentimes it is difficult to tell which vitamin is truly responsible for a given effect because the nutrients are interdependent; the presence or absence of one affects another's absorption, metabolism, and excretion. You have already seen this interdependence with folate and vitamin B_{12}.

Riboflavin and vitamin B_6 provide another example. One of the riboflavin coenzymes, FMN, assists the enzyme that converts vitamin B_6 to its coenzyme form PLP. Consequently, a severe riboflavin deficiency can impair vitamin B_6 activity.[18] Thus a deficiency of one nutrient may alter the action of another. Furthermore, a deficiency of one nutrient may create a deficiency of another. For example, both riboflavin and vitamin B_6 (as well as iron) are required for the conversion of tryptophan to niacin. Consequently, an inadequate intake of either riboflavin or vitamin B_6 can diminish the body's niacin supply. These interdependent relationships are evident in many of the roles B vitamins play in the body.

B Vitamin Roles

Figure 10-13 (on p. 346) is intended to convey an *impression* of the many ways B vitamins busily work in metabolic pathways all over the body. Metabolism is the body's work, and the B vitamin coenzymes are indispensable to every step. In scanning the pathways of metabolism depicted in the figure, note the many abbreviations for the coenzymes that keep the processes going.

Look at the first step in the now-familiar pathway of glucose breakdown. To break down glucose to pyruvate, the cells must have certain enzymes. For the enzymes to work, they must have the niacin coenzyme NAD. To make NAD, the cells must be supplied with niacin (or enough of the amino acid tryptophan to make niacin). They can make the rest of the coenzyme without dietary help.

The next step is the breakdown of pyruvate to acetyl CoA. The enzymes involved in this step require both NAD and the thiamin and riboflavin coenzymes TPP and FAD, respectively. The cells can manufacture the enzymes they need from the vitamins, if the vitamins are in the diet.

Another coenzyme needed for this step is CoA. Predictably, the cells can make CoA except for an essential part that must be obtained in the diet—pantothenic acid. Another coenzyme requiring biotin serves the enzyme complex involved in converting pyruvate to oxaloacetate, the compound that combines with acetyl CoA to start the TCA cycle.

These and other coenzymes participate throughout all the metabolic pathways. When the diet provides riboflavin, the body synthesizes FAD—a needed coenzyme in the TCA cycle. Vitamin B_6 is an indispensable part of PLP—a coenzyme required for many amino acid conversions, for a crucial step in the making of the iron-containing portion of hemoglobin for red blood cells, and for many other reactions. Folate becomes THF—the coenzyme required for the synthesis of new genetic material and therefore new cells. The vitamin B_{12} coenzyme, in turn, regenerates THF to its active form; thus vitamin B_{12} is also necessary for the formation of new cells.

Thus each of the B vitamin coenzymes is involved, directly or indirectly, in energy metabolism. Some facilitate the energy-releasing reactions themselves; others help build new cells to deliver the oxygen and nutrients that allow the energy reactions to occur.

B Vitamin Deficiencies

Now suppose the body's cells lack one of these B vitamins—niacin, for example. Without niacin, the cells cannot make NAD. Without NAD, the enzymes involved in every step of the glucose-to-energy pathway cannot function. Then, because all

FIGURE 10-13 Metabolic Pathways Involving B Vitamins

These metabolic pathways were introduced in Chapter 7 and are presented here to highlight the many coenzymes that facilitate the reactions. These coenzymes depend on the following vitamins:

- NAD and NADP: niacin.
- TPP: thiamin.
- CoA: pantothenic acid.
- B_{12}: vitamin B_{12}.
- FMN and FAD: riboflavin.
- THF: folate.
- PLP: vitamin B_6.
- Biotin.

Pathways leading toward acetyl CoA and the TCA cycle are catabolic, and those leading toward amino acids, glycogen, and fat are anabolic. For further details, see Appendix C.

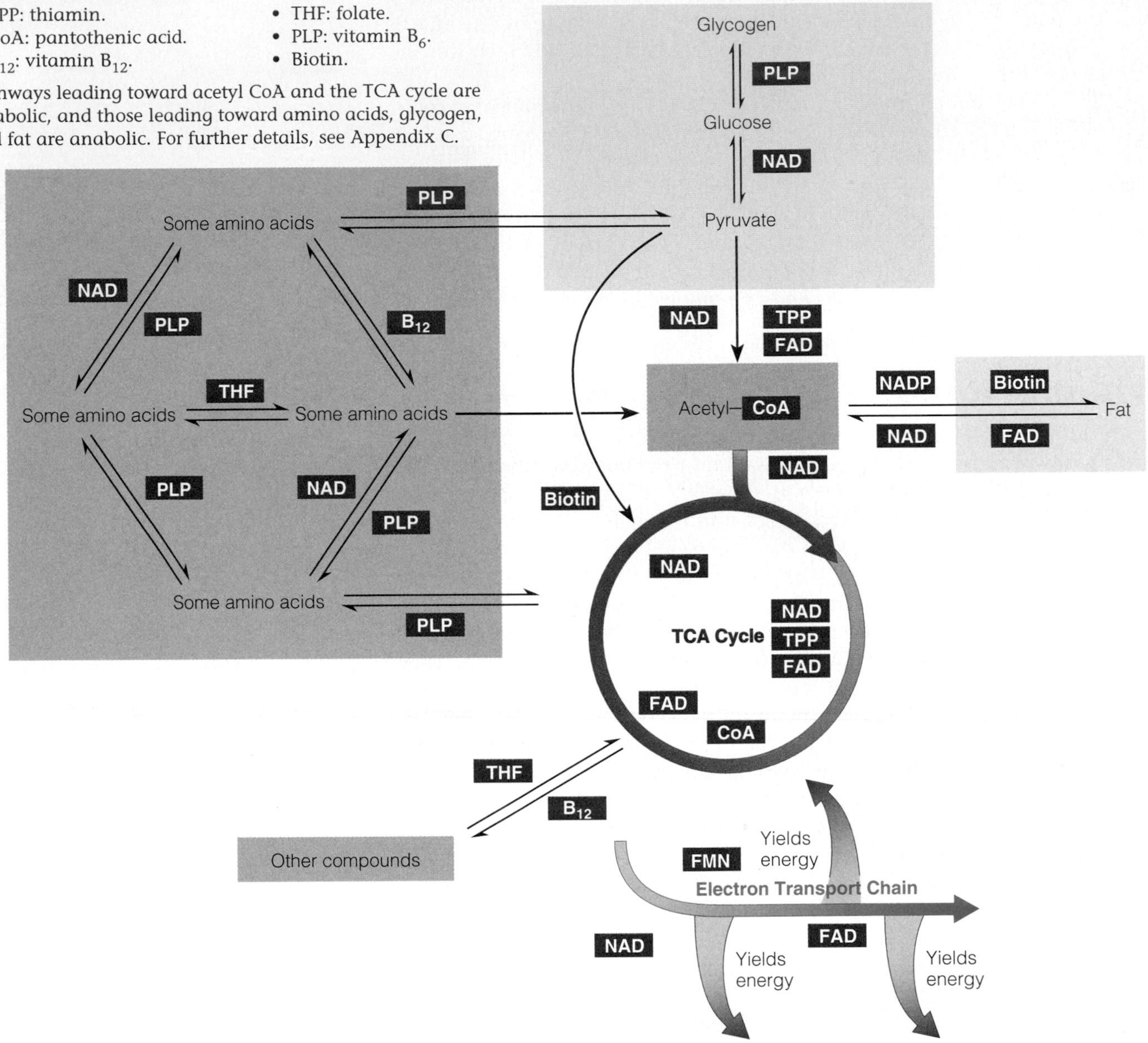
Glycogen
PLP
Glucose
NAD
Pyruvate
PLP
Some amino acids
NAD
PLP
B12
THF
Some amino acids
Some amino acids
PLP
NAD
PLP
Some amino acids
PLP
NAD
TPP
FAD
Acetyl–CoA
NADP
Biotin
Fat
NAD
FAD
NAD
Biotin
NAD
NAD
TCA Cycle
TPP
FAD
FAD
CoA
THF
B12
Other compounds
FMN
Yields energy
Electron Transport Chain
NAD
FAD
Yields energy
Yields energy

■ For want of a nail, a horseshoe was lost.
For want of a horseshoe, a horse was lost.
For want of a horse, a soldier was lost.
For want of a soldier, a battle was lost.
For want of a battle, the war was lost,
And all for the want of a horseshoe nail!
—Mother Goose

the body's activities require energy, literally everything begins to grind to a halt. This is no exaggeration. The deadly disease pellagra, caused by niacin deficiency, produces the "devastating four *Ds*": dermatitis, which reflects a failure of the skin; dementia, a failure of the nervous system; diarrhea, a failure of digestion and absorption; and eventually, as would be the case for any severe nutrient deficiency, death. These symptoms are the obvious ones, but a niacin deficiency affects all other organs, too, because all are dependent on the energy pathways. In short, niacin is like the horseshoe nail■ for want of which a war was lost.

All the vitamins are like horseshoe nails. With any B vitamin deficiency, many body systems become deranged, and similar symptoms may appear. A lack of "horseshoe nails" can have disastrous and far-reaching effects.

Deficiencies of single B vitamins seldom show up in isolation, however. After all, people do not eat nutrients singly; they eat foods, which contain mixtures of nutrients. Only in two cases described earlier—beriberi and pellagra—have dietary deficiencies associated with single B vitamins been observed on a large scale in human populations. Even in these cases, the deficiencies were not pure. Both diseases were attributed to deficiencies of single vitamins, but both were deficiencies of several vitamins in which one vitamin stood out above the rest. When foods containing the vitamin known to be needed were provided, the other vitamins that were in short supply came as part of the package.

Major deficiency diseases of epidemic proportions such as pellagra and beriberi are no longer seen in the United States and Canada, but lesser deficiencies of nutrients, including the B vitamins, sometimes occur in people whose food choices are poor because of poverty, ignorance, illness, or poor health habits like alcohol abuse. (Review Highlight 7 to fully appreciate how alcohol induces vitamin deficiencies and interferes with energy metabolism.) Remember from Chapter 1 that deficiencies can arise not only from deficient intakes (primary causes), but also for other (secondary) reasons.

In identifying nutrient deficiencies, it is important to realize that a particular symptom may not always have the same cause. The skin and the tongue (shown in Figure 10-14) appear to be especially sensitive to B vitamin deficiencies, but isolating these body parts in the summary tables earlier in this chapter gives them undue emphasis. Both the skin and the tongue■ are readily visible in a physical examination. The physician sees and reports the deficiency's outward symptoms, but the full impact of a vitamin deficiency occurs inside the cells of the body. If the skin develops a rash or lesions, other tissues beneath it may be degenerating, too. Similarly, the mouth and tongue are the visible part of the digestive system; if they are abnormal, most likely the rest of the GI tract is, too. The "How to" on the next page offers other insights into symptoms and their causes.

FIGURE 10-14 B Vitamin–Deficiency Symptom—The Smooth Tongue of Glossitis

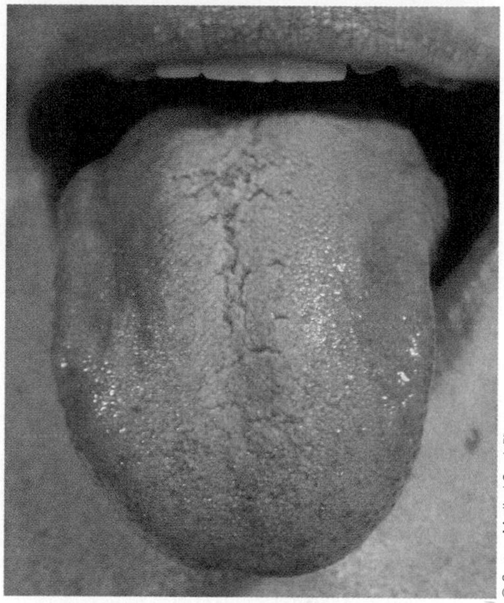

© Custom Medical Stock Photo

A healthy tongue has a rough and somewhat bumpy surface.

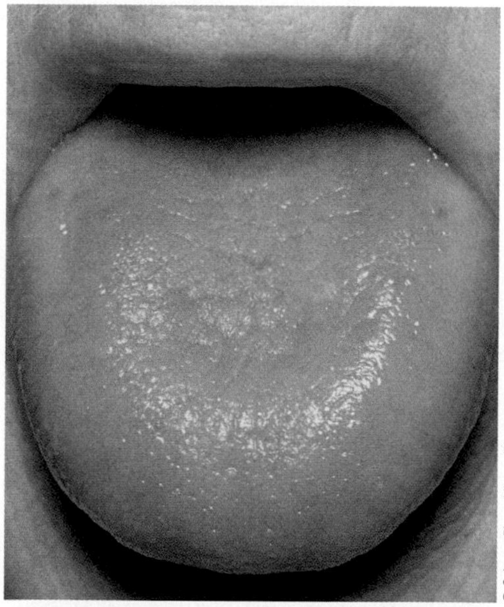

© Science Photo Library/Photo Researchers, Inc.

In a B vitamin deficiency, the tongue becomes smooth and swollen due to atrophy of the tissue (glossitis).

■ Two symptoms commonly seen in B vitamin deficiencies are **glossitis** (gloss-EYE-tis), an inflammation of the tongue, and **cheilosis** (kye-LOH-sis or kee-LOH-sis), a condition of reddened lips with cracks at the corners of the mouth.

- **glossa** = tongue
- **cheilos** = lip

B Vitamin Toxicities

Toxicities of the B vitamins from foods alone are unknown, but they can occur when people overuse supplements. With supplements, the quantities can quickly overwhelm the cells. Consider that one small capsule can easily deliver 2 milligrams of vitamin B_6, but it would take more than 3000 bananas, 6600 cups of rice, or 3600 chicken breasts to supply an equivalent amount. When the cells become oversaturated with a vitamin, they must work to eliminate the excess. The cells dispatch water-soluble vitamins to the urine for excretion, but sometimes they cannot keep pace with the onslaught. Homeostasis becomes disturbed and symptoms of toxicity develop.

B Vitamin Food Sources

Significantly, the deficiency diseases of beriberi and pellagra were eliminated by supplying foods—not pills. Vitamin pill advertisements make much of the fact that vitamins are indispensable to life, but human beings obtained their nourishment from foods for centuries before vitamin pills existed. If the diet lacks a vitamin, the first solution is to adjust food intake to obtain that vitamin.

Manufacturers of so-called *natural* vitamins boast that their pills are purified from real foods rather than synthesized in a laboratory. Think back on the course of human evolution; it is not *natural* to take any kind of pill. In reality, the finest, most natural vitamin "supplements" available are whole grains, vegetables, fruits, meat, fish, poultry, eggs, legumes, nuts, and milk and milk products.

The food figures presented in this chapter, taken together, sing the praises of a balanced diet. The cereal and bread group delivers thiamin, riboflavin, niacin, and folate. The fruit and vegetable groups excel in folate. The meat group serves thiamin, niacin, vitamin B_6, and vitamin B_{12} well. The milk group stands out for riboflavin and vitamin B_{12}. A diet that offers a variety of foods from each group, prepared with reasonable care, serves up ample B vitamins.

HOW TO Distinguish Symptoms and Causes

The cause of a symptom is not always apparent. The summary tables in this chapter show that deficiencies of riboflavin, niacin, biotin, and vitamin B_6 can all cause skin rashes. But so can a deficiency of protein, linoleic acid, or vitamin A. Because skin is on the outside and easy to see, it is a useful indicator of things-going-wrong-inside-cells. But, by itself, a skin symptom says nothing about its possible cause.

The same is true of anemia. Anemia is often caused by iron deficiency, but it can also be caused by a folate or vitamin B_{12} deficiency; by digestive tract failure to absorb any of these nutrients; or by such nonnutritional causes as infections, parasites, cancer, or loss of blood. No one specific nutrient will always cure a given symptom.

A person who feels chronically tired may be tempted to self-diagnose iron-deficiency anemia and self-prescribe an iron supplement. But this will relieve tiredness only if the cause is indeed iron-deficiency anemia. If the cause is a folate deficiency, taking iron will only prolong the fatigue. A person who is better informed may decide to take a vitamin supplement with iron, covering the possibility of a vitamin deficiency. But the symptom may have a nonnutritional cause. If the cause of the tiredness is actually hidden blood loss due to cancer, the postponement of a diagnosis may be fatal. When fatigue is caused by a lack of sleep, of course, no nutrient or combination of nutrients can replace a good night's rest. A person who is chronically tired should see a physician rather than self-prescribe. If the condition is nutrition related, a registered dietitian should be consulted as well.

IN SUMMARY The B vitamin coenzymes work together in energy metabolism. Some facilitate the energy-releasing reactions themselves; others help build cells to deliver the oxygen and nutrients that permit the energy pathways to run. These vitamins depend on each other to function optimally; a deficiency of any of them creates multiple problems. Fortunately, a variety of foods from each of the food groups will provide an adequate supply of all of the B vitamins.

Vitamin C

Two hundred and fifty years ago, any man who joined the crew of a seagoing ship knew he had at best a 50–50 chance of returning alive—not because he might be slain by pirates or die in a storm, but because he might contract the dread disease **scurvy.** As many as two-thirds of a ship's crew might die of scurvy on a long voyage. Only men on short voyages, especially around the Mediterranean Sea, were free of scurvy. No one knew the reason: that on long ocean voyages, the ship's cook used up the fresh fruits and vegetables early and then served cereals and meats until the return to port.

The first nutrition experiment ever performed on human beings was devised in the mid-1700s to find a cure for scurvy. James Lind, a British physician, divided 12 sailors with scurvy into six pairs. Each pair received a different supplemental ration: cider, vinegar, sulfuric acid, seawater, oranges and lemons, or a strong laxative mixed with spices. Those receiving the citrus fruits quickly recovered, but sadly, it was 50 years before the British navy required all vessels to provide every sailor■ with lime juice daily.

The antiscurvy "something" in limes and other foods was dubbed the **antiscorbutic factor.** Nearly 200 years later, the factor was isolated and found to be a six-carbon compound similar to glucose; it was named **ascorbic acid.** Shortly thereafter, it was synthesized, and today hundreds of millions of vitamin C pills are produced in pharmaceutical laboratories each year.

■ The tradition of providing British sailors with citrus juice daily to prevent scurvy gave them the nickname "limeys."

scurvy: the vitamin C–deficiency disease.

antiscorbutic (AN-tee-skor-BUE-tik) **factor:** the original name for vitamin C.
- **anti** = against
- **scorbutic** = causing scurvy

ascorbic acid: one of the two active forms of vitamin C (see Figure 10-15). Many people refer to vitamin C by this name.
- **a** = without
- **scorbic** = having scurvy

FIGURE 10-15 Active Forms of Vitamin C

The two hydrogens highlighted in yellow give vitamin C its acidity and its ability to act as an antioxidant.

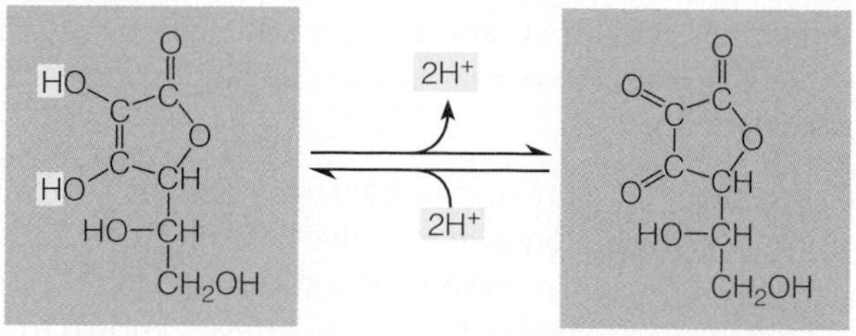
HO
HO
HO—CH
CH2OH
2H+
2H+
HO—CH
CH2OH

Ascorbic acid protects against oxidative damage by donating its two hydrogens with their electrons to free radicals (molecules with unpaired electrons). In doing so, ascorbic acid becomes dehydroascorbic acid.

Dehydroascorbic acid can readily accept hydrogens to become ascorbic acid. The reversibility of this reaction is key to vitamin C's role as an antioxidant.

Vitamin C Roles

Vitamin C parts company with the B vitamins in its mode of action. In some settings, vitamin C serves as a cofactor■ helping a specific enzyme perform its job, but in others, it acts as an antioxidant participating in more general ways.

■ Reminder: A *cofactor* is a small, inorganic or organic substance that facilitates the action of an enzyme.

As an Antioxidant Vitamin C loses electrons easily, a characteristic that allows it to perform as an **antioxidant.** In the body, antioxidants defend against **free radicals.** Free radicals are discussed in Highlight 11, but for now, a simple definition will suffice. A free radical is a molecule with one or more unpaired electrons, making it unstable and highly reactive. By donating an electron or two, antioxidants neutralize free radicals and protect other substances from their damage. Figure 10-15 illustrates how vitamin C can give up electrons to stop free-radical damage and then receive them again to become reactivated. This recycling of vitamin C is key to limiting losses and maintaining a reserve of antioxidants in the body.

Vitamin C is like a bodyguard for water-soluble substances; it stands ready to sacrifice its own life to save theirs. In the cells and body fluids, vitamin C protects tissues from **oxidative stress** and thus may play an important role in preventing diseases. In the intestines, vitamin C enhances iron absorption by protecting iron from oxidation. (Chapter 13 provides more details on the relationship between vitamin C and iron.)

As a Cofactor in Collagen Formation Vitamin C helps to form the fibrous structural protein of connective tissues known as collagen.■ Collagen serves as the matrix on which bones and teeth are formed. When a person is wounded, collagen glues the separated tissues together, forming scars. Cells are held together largely by collagen; this is especially important in the artery walls, which must expand and contract with each beat of the heart, and in the thin capillary walls, which must withstand a pulse of blood every second or so without giving way.

■ Reminder: *Collagen* is the structural protein from which connective tissues such as scars, tendons, ligaments, and the foundations of bones and teeth are made.

Chapter 6 described how the body makes proteins by stringing together chains of amino acids. During the synthesis of collagen, each time a proline or lysine is added to the growing protein chain, an enzyme hydroxylates it (adds an OH group to it), making the amino acid hydroxyproline or hydroxylysine, respectively. These two special amino acids facilitate the binding together of collagen fibers to make strong, ropelike structures. The conversion of proline to hydroxyproline requires both vitamin C and iron. Iron works as a cofactor in the reaction, and vitamin C protects iron from oxidation, thereby allowing iron to perform its duty. Without vitamin C and iron, the hydroxylation step does not occur.

antioxidant: a substance in foods that significantly decreases the adverse effects of free radicals on normal physiological functions in the human body.

free radicals: unstable molecules with one or more unpaired electrons.

oxidative stress: an imbalance between the production of free radicals and the body's ability to handle them and prevent damage.

FIGURE 10-16 Vitamin C Intake (mg/day)

Recommendations are generously above the minimum requirement and below the toxicity level.

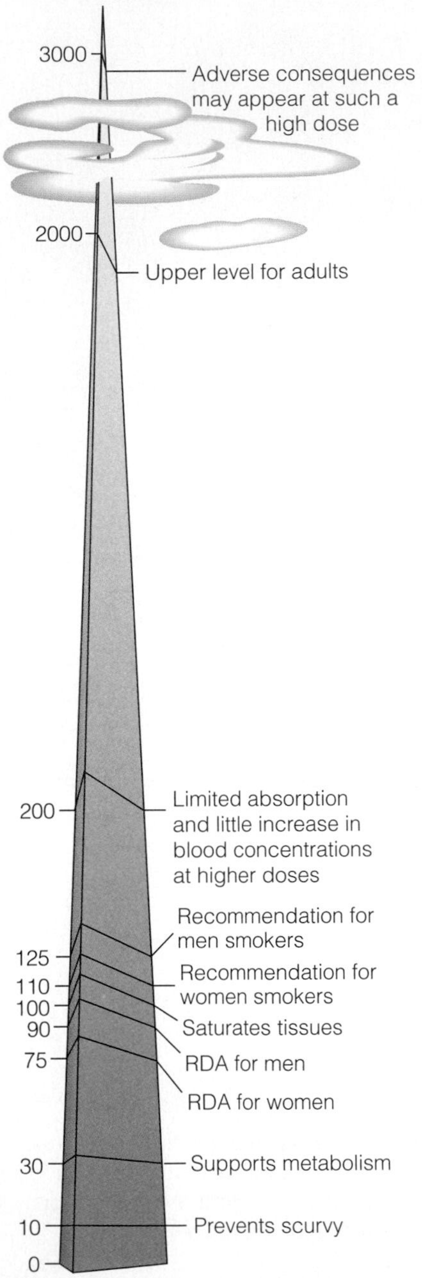
3000
Adverse consequences may appear at such a high dose
2000
Upper level for adults
200
Limited absorption and little increase in blood concentrations at higher doses
Recommendation for men smokers
125
Recommendation for women smokers
110
100
Saturates tissues
90
RDA for men
75
RDA for women
30
Supports metabolism
10
Prevents scurvy
0

■ For perspective, 1 c orange juice provides >100 mg vitamin C.

histamine (HISS-tah-mean or HISS-tah-men): a substance produced by cells of the immune system as part of a local immune reaction to an antigen; participates in causing inflammation.

As a Cofactor in Other Reactions Vitamin C also serves as a cofactor in the synthesis of several other compounds. As in collagen formation, vitamin C helps in the hydroxylation of carnitine, a compound that transports long-chain fatty acids into the mitochondria of a cell for energy metabolism. It participates in the conversions of the amino acids tryptophan and tyrosine to the neurotransmitters serotonin and norepinephrine, respectively. Vitamin C also assists in the making of hormones, including thyroxin, which regulates the metabolic rate; metabolism speeds up under times of extreme physical stress.

In Stress The adrenal glands contain more vitamin C than any other organ in the body, and during stress, these glands release the vitamin, together with hormones, into the blood. The vitamin's exact role in the stress reaction remains unclear, but physical stresses raise vitamin C needs. Among the stresses known to increase vitamin C needs are infections; burns; extremely high or low temperatures; intakes of toxic heavy metals such as lead, mercury, and cadmium; the chronic use of certain medications, including aspirin, barbiturates, and oral contraceptives; and cigarette smoking. When immune system cells are called into action, they use a lot of oxygen and produce free radicals. In this case, free radicals are helpful. They act as ammunition in an "oxidative burst" that demolishes the offending viruses and bacteria and destroys the damaged cells. Vitamin C steps in as an antioxidant to control this oxidative activity.

As a Cure for the Common Cold Newspaper headlines touting vitamin C as a cure for colds have appeared frequently over the years, but research supporting such claims has been conflicting and controversial. Some studies find no relationship between vitamin C and the occurrence of the common cold, whereas others report fewer colds, fewer days, and shorter duration of severe symptoms.[19] A review of the research on vitamin C in the treatment and prevention of the common cold reveals a modest benefit—a significant difference in duration of less than a day per cold in favor of those taking a daily dose of at least 1 gram of vitamin C.[20] The term *significant* means that *statistical* analysis suggests that the findings probably didn't arise by chance, but from the experimental treatment being tested. Is a day enough savings to warrant routine daily supplementation? Supplement users seem to think so.

Interestingly, those who received the placebo *but thought they were receiving vitamin C* had fewer colds than the group who received vitamin C *but thought they were receiving the placebo.* (Never underestimate the healing power of faith!)

Discoveries of the ways vitamin C works in the body provide possible links between the vitamin and the common cold. Anyone who has ever had a cold knows the discomfort of a runny or stuffed-up nose. Nasal congestion develops in response to elevated blood **histamine,** and people commonly take antihistamines for relief. Like an antihistamine, vitamin C comes to the rescue and deactivates histamine.

In Disease Prevention Whether vitamin C may help in preventing or treating cancer, heart disease, cataracts, and other diseases is still being studied, and findings are presented in Highlight 11. Conducting research in the United States and Canada can be difficult, however, because diets typically contribute enough vitamin C to provide optimal health benefits.

Vitamin C Recommendations

How much vitamin C does a person need? As Figure 10-16 illustrates, recommendations are set generously above the minimum requirement to prevent scurvy and well below the toxicity level.[21] Current recommendations are higher than the previous RDA, but not as high as some experts had proposed.[22]

The requirement—the amount needed to prevent the overt symptoms of scurvy—is only 10 milligrams daily. However, 10 milligrams a day does not saturate all the body tissues; higher intakes will increase the body's total vitamin C. At about 100 milligrams■ per day, 95 percent of the population probably reaches tis-

FIGURE 10-17 Vitamin C–Deficiency Symptoms—Scorbutic Gums and Pinpoint Hemmorhages

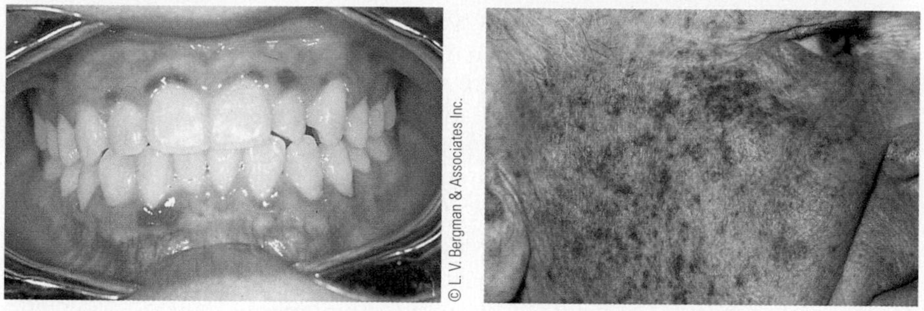

© L. V. Bergman & Associates Inc.

Scorbutic gums. Unlike other lesions of the mouth, scurvy presents a symmetrical appearance without infection.

© Dr. P. Marazzi/Photo Researchers, Inc.

Pinpoint hemorrhages. Small red spots appear in the skin, indicating spontaneous bleeding internally.

sue saturation. At about 200 milligrams, absorption reaches a maximum, and there is little, if any, increase in blood concentrations at higher doses. Excess vitamin C is readily excreted.

As mentioned earlier, cigarette smoking increases the need for vitamin C. Cigarette smoke contains oxidants, which greedily deplete this potent antioxidant. Exposure to cigarette smoke, especially when accompanied by low intakes of vitamin C, depletes the body's pool in both active and passive smokers; similarly, people who chew tobacco have low levels of vitamin C as well.[23] Because people who smoke cigarettes regularly suffer significant oxidative stress, their requirement for vitamin C is increased an additional 35 milligrams; nonsmokers regularly exposed to cigarette smoke should be sure to meet their RDA for vitamin C.

After oral surgery, dentists may prescribe supplemental vitamin C to hasten healing. After major operations or extensive burns, when scar tissue is forming, a physician may prescribe 1000 milligrams (1 gram) a day or even more. Self-medication is not recommended.

Vitamin C Deficiency

Two of the most notable signs of a vitamin C deficiency reflect its role in maintaining the integrity of blood vessels. The gums bleed easily around the teeth, and capillaries under the skin break spontaneously, producing pinpoint hemorrhages (see Figure 10-17).

When the vitamin C pool falls to about a fifth of its optimal size (this may take more than a month on a diet lacking vitamin C), scurvy symptoms begin to appear. Inadequate collagen synthesis causes further hemorrhaging. Muscles, including the heart muscle, degenerate. The skin becomes rough, brown, scaly, and dry. Wounds fail to heal because scar tissue will not form. Bone rebuilding falters; the ends of the long bones become softened, malformed, and painful, and fractures develop. The teeth become loose as the cartilage around them weakens. Anemia and infections are common. There are also characteristic psychological signs, including hysteria and depression. Sudden death is likely, caused by massive internal bleeding.

Once diagnosed, scurvy is readily resolved by vitamin C.[24] Moderate doses in the neighborhood of 100 milligrams per day are sufficient, curing the scurvy within about five days. Such an intake is easily achieved by including vitamin C–rich foods in the diet.

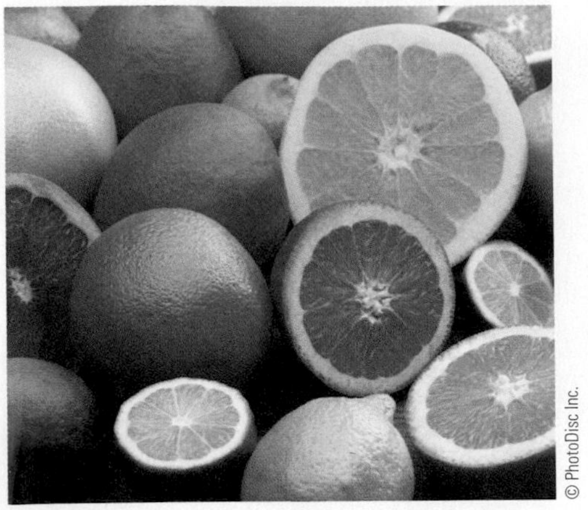

When dietitians say "vitamin C," people think "citrus fruits."

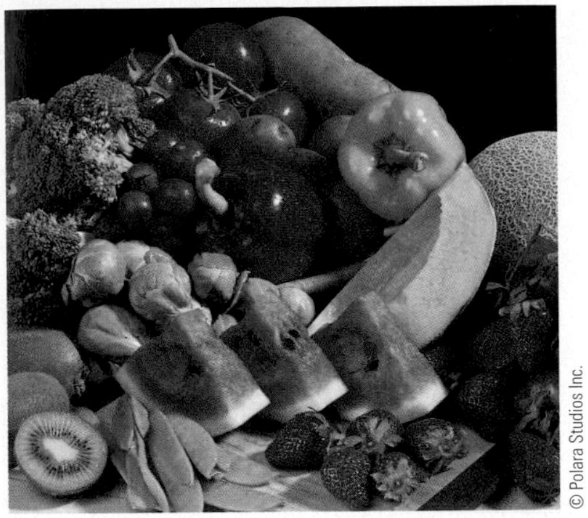

But these foods are also rich in vitamin C.

■ Reminder: *Gout* is a metabolic disease in which uric acid crystals precipitate in the joints.

false positive: a test result indicating that a condition is present (positive) when in fact it is not (therefore false).

false negative: a test result indicating that a condition is not present (negative) when in fact it is present (therefore false).

Vitamin C Toxicity

The easy availability of vitamin C supplements and the publication of books recommending vitamin C to prevent colds and cancer have led thousands of people to take large doses of vitamin C. Not surprisingly, toxic effects such as nausea, abdominal cramps, and diarrhea are often reported.

Several instances of interference with medical regimens are also known. Large amounts of vitamin C excreted in the urine obscure the results of tests used to detect diabetes, giving a **false positive** result in some instances and a **false negative** in others. People taking anticlotting medications may unwittingly counteract the effect if they also take massive doses of vitamin C.* Those with kidney disease, a tendency toward gout,■ or a genetic abnormality that alters vitamin C's breakdown to its excretion products are prone to forming kidney stones if they take large doses of vitamin C.† Vitamin C supplements may adversely affect people with iron overload. (Chapter 13 describes the damaging effects of too much iron.) Vitamin C enhances iron absorption and releases iron from body stores; free iron causes the kind of cellular damage typical of free radicals. These events illustrate how vitamin C can act as a *pro*oxidant when quantities exceed the body's needs.

The estimated average intake from both diet and supplements is 187 milligrams of vitamin C a day. Few instances warrant consuming more than 200 milligrams a day. For adults who dose themselves with up to 2 grams a day (and relatively few do), the risks may not be great; those taking more should be aware of the distinct possibility of adverse effects.

Vitamin C Food Sources

Fruits and vegetables can easily provide a generous amount of vitamin C. A cup of orange juice at breakfast, a salad for lunch, and a stalk of broccoli and a potato for dinner alone provide more than 300 milligrams. Clearly, a person making such food choices needs no vitamin C pills.

Figure 10-18 shows the amounts of vitamin C in various common foods. The overwhelming abundance of purple and green bars reveals not only that the citrus fruits are justly famous for being rich in vitamin C, but that other fruits and vegetables are in the same league. A half cup of broccoli, bell pepper, or strawberries provides more than 50 milligrams of the vitamin (and an array of other nutrients). Because vitamin C is vulnerable to heat, raw fruits and vegetables usually have a higher nutrient density than their cooked counterparts. Similarly, because vitamin C is readily destroyed by oxygen, foods and juices should be stored properly and consumed within a week of opening.[25]

The potato is an important source of vitamin C, not because one potato by itself meets the daily need, but because potatoes are such a common staple that they make significant contributions. In fact, scurvy was unknown in Ireland until the potato blight of the mid-1840s when some two million people died of malnutrition and infection.

The lack of yellow, white, brown, and red bars in Figure 10-18 confirms that grains, milk (except breast milk), legumes, and meats are notoriously poor sources of vitamin C. Organ meats (liver, kidneys, and others) and raw meats contain some vitamin C, but most people don't eat large quantities of these. Raw meats and fish contribute enough vitamin C to be significant in parts of Alaska, Canada, and Japan, but elsewhere fruits and vegetables are necessary to supply sufficient vitamin C.

*Vitamin C interferes with such anticoagulant drugs as warfarin, dicumarol, heparin, and coumadin. It is unclear whether vitamin C inhibits the absorption or the action of these drugs.

†Vitamin C is inactivated and degraded by several routes, and sometimes oxalate, which can form kidney stones, is produced along the way. People may also develop oxalate crystals in their kidneys regardless of vitamin C status.

FIGURE 10-18 Vitamin C in Selected Foods

Food	Serving size (kcalories)
Bread, whole wheat	1 oz slice (70 kcal)
Cornflakes, fortified	1 oz (110 kcal)
Spaghetti pasta	½ c cooked (99 kcal)
Tortilla, flour	1 10"-round (234 kcal)
Broccoli	½ c cooked (22 kcal)
Carrots	½ c shredded raw (24 kcal)
Potato	1 medium baked w/skin (133 kcal)
Tomato juice	¾ c (31 kcal)
Banana	1 medium raw (109 kcal)
Orange	1 medium raw (62 kcal)
Strawberries	½ c fresh (22 kcal)
Watermelon	1 slice (92 kcal)
Milk	1 c reduced-fat 2% (121 kcal)
Yogurt, plain	1 c low fat (155 kcal)
Cheddar cheese	1½ oz (171 kcal)
Cottage cheese	½ c low-fat 2% (101 kcal)
Pinto beans	½ c cooked (117 kcal)
Peanut butter	2 tbs (188 kcal)
Sunflower seeds	1 oz dry (165 kcal)
Tofu (soybean curd)	½ c (76 kcal)
Ground beef, lean	3 oz broiled (244 kcal)
Chicken breast	3 oz roasted (140 kcal)
Tuna, canned in water	3 oz (99 kcal)
Egg	1 hard cooked (78 kcal)
Excellent, and sometimes unusual, sources:	
Red bell pepper	½ c raw chopped (20 kcal)
Kiwi	1 (46 kcal)
Brussels sprouts	½ c cooked (30 kcal)

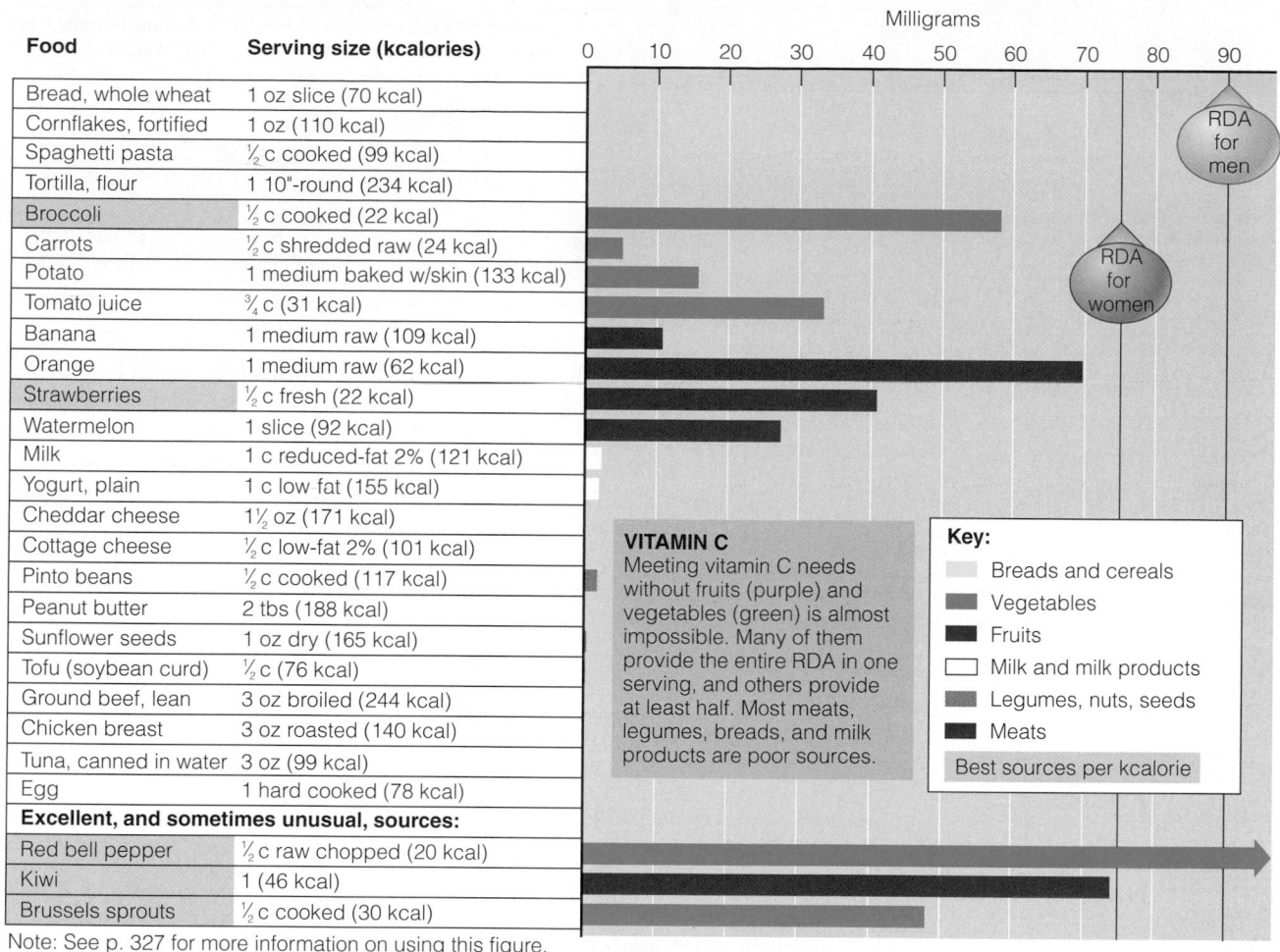

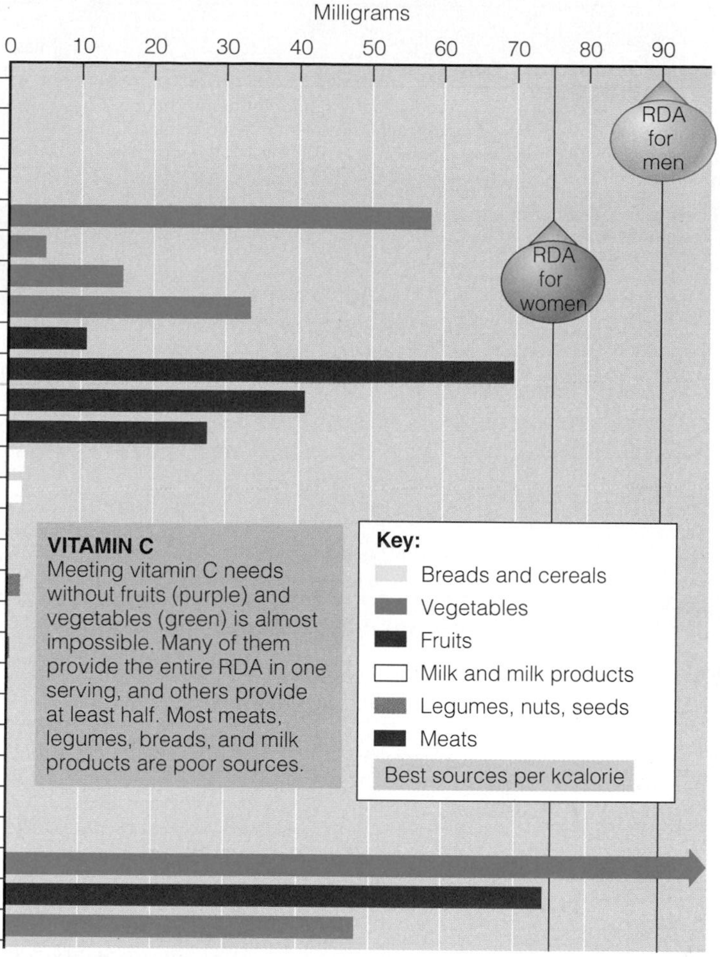
Milligrams
0
10
20
30
40
50
60
70
80
90
RDA for men
RDA for women
VITAMIN C
Meeting vitamin C needs without fruits (purple) and vegetables (green) is almost impossible. Many of them provide the entire RDA in one serving, and others provide at least half. Most meats, legumes, breads, and milk products are poor sources.
Key:
Breads and cereals
Vegetables
Fruits
Milk and milk products
Legumes, nuts, seeds
Meats
Best sources per kcalorie

Note: See p. 327 for more information on using this figure.

Because of vitamin C's antioxidant property, food manufacturers sometimes add a variation of vitamin C to some beverages and most cured meats, such as luncheon meats, to prevent oxidation and spoilage. This compound safely preserves these foods, but it does not have vitamin C activity in the body. Simply put, "ham and bacon cannot replace fruits and vegetables." See the accompanying table for a summary of vitamin C.

IN SUMMARY Vitamin C

Other Names

Ascorbic acid

2000 RDA

Men: 90 mg/day

Women: 75 mg/day

Smokers: +35 mg/day

Upper Level

Adults: 2000 mg/day

Chief Functions in the Body

Collagen synthesis (strengthens blood vessel walls, forms scar tissue, provides matrix for bone growth), antioxidant, thyroxin synthesis, amino acid metabolism, strengthens resistance to infection, helps in absorption of iron

Significant Sources

Citrus fruits, cabbage-type vegetables, dark green vegetables (such as bell peppers and broccoli), cantaloupe, strawberries, lettuce, tomatoes, potatoes, papayas, mangoes

Easily destroyed by heat and oxygen

(continued)

Vitamin C (continued)

Deficiency Disease

Scurvy

Deficiency Symptoms

Anemia (small-cell type),[a] atherosclerotic plaques, pinpoint hemorrhages; bone fragility, joint pain; poor wound healing, frequent infections; bleeding gums, loosened teeth; muscle degeneration and pain, hysteria, depression; rough skin, blotchy bruises

Toxicity Symptoms

Nausea, abdominal cramps, diarrhea; headache, fatigue, insomnia; hot flashes, rashes; interference with medical tests, aggravation of gout symptoms, urinary tract problems, kidney stones[b]

[a] Small-cell–type anemia is *microcytic anemia.*
[b] People with kidney disease, a tendency toward gout, or a genetic abnormality that alters the breakdown of vitamin C are prone to forming kidney stones. Vitamin C is inactivated and degraded by several routes, sometimes producing oxalate, which can form stones in the kidneys.

Vita means life. After this discourse on the vitamins, who could dispute that they deserve their name? Their regulation of metabolic processes makes them vital to the normal growth, development, and maintenance of the body. The accompanying summary table condenses the information provided in this chapter for a quick review. The remarkable roles of the vitamins continue in the next chapter.

IN SUMMARY The Water-Soluble Vitamins

Vitamin and Chief Functions	Deficiency Symptoms	Toxicity Symptoms	Food Sources
Thiamin Part of coenzyme TPP in energy metabolism	Beriberi (edema or muscle wasting), anorexia and weight loss, neurological disturbances, muscular weakness, heart enlargement and failure	None reported	Enriched, fortified, or whole-grain products; pork
Riboflavin Part of coenzymes FAD and FMN in energy metabolism	Inflammation of the mouth, skin, and eyelids; sensitivity to light	None reported	Milk products; enriched, fortified, or whole-grain products; liver
Niacin Part of coenzymes NAD and NADP in energy metabolism	Pellagra (diarrhea, dermatitis, and dementia)	Niacin flush, liver damage, impaired glucose tolerance	Protein-rich foods
Biotin Part of coenzyme in energy metabolism	Skin rash, hair loss, neurological disturbances	None reported	Widespread in foods; GI bacteria synthesis
Pantothenic acid Part of coenzyme A in energy metabolism	Digestive and neurological disturbances	None reported	Widespread in foods
Vitamin B_6 Part of coenzymes used in amino acid and fatty acid metabolism	Scaly dermatitis, depression, confusion, convulsions, anemia	Nerve degeneration, skin lesions	Protein-rich foods
Folate Activates vitamin B_{12}; helps synthesize DNA for new cell growth	Anemia, glossitis, neurological disturbances, elevated homocysteine	Masks vitamin B_{12} deficiency	Legumes, vegetables, fortified grain products
Vitamin B_{12} Activates folate; helps synthesize DNA for new cell growth; protects nerve cells	Anemia; nerve damage and paralysis	None reported	Foods derived from animals
Vitamin C Synthesis of collagen, carnitine, hormones, neurotransmitters; antioxidant	Scurvy (bleeding gums, pinpoint hemorrhages, abnormal bone growth, and joint pain)	Diarrhea, GI distress	Fruits and vegetables

Nutrition in Your Life

To obtain all the vitamins you need each day, be sure to select from a variety of foods.

- Do you often choose whole or enriched grains, dark green leafy vegetables, citrus fruits, and legumes?
- If you are a woman of childbearing age, do you eat folate-rich foods or take supplements regularly?
- Do you take supplements that provide more than the upper limit of the vitamins?

Available Online

http://nutrition.wadsworth.com/uncn7
Practice planning several lunch menus with varying energy needs while simultaneously meeting the recommended intakes of several vitamins.

NUTRITION ON THE NET

Access these websites for further study of topics covered in this chapter. Be aware that many websites on the Internet are peddling vitamin supplements, not accurate information.

- Find updates and quick links to these and other nutrition-related sites at our website: **www.wadsworth.com/nutrition**
- Search for "vitamins" at the American Dietetic Association: **www.eatright.org**
- Review the Dietary Reference Intakes for the water-soluble vitamins: **www.nap.edu/readingroom**
- Visit the World Health Organization to learn about "vitamin deficiencies" around the world: **www.who.int**
- Learn more about neural tube defects from the Spina Bifida Association of America: **www.sbaa.org**
- Read about Dr. Joseph Goldberger and his groundbreaking discovery linking pellagra to diet by searching for his name at: **www.nih.gov** or **www.pbs.org**
- Learn how fruits and vegetables support a healthy diet rich in vitamins from the National Cancer Institute or the 5 A Day for Better Health program: **www.5aday.gov** or **5aday.org**

NUTRITION CALCULATIONS

These problems give you practice in doing simple vitamin-related calculations (answers are provided on p. 358). Be sure to show your calculations for each problem.

1. Review the units in which vitamins are measured (a spot check).
   a. For each of these vitamins, note the unit of measure:

Thiamin	Folate
Riboflavin	Vitamin B_{12}
Niacin	Vitamin C
Vitamin B_6	

   b. Recall from the chapter's description of people's self-dosing with vitamin B_6 that people who suffer toxicity symptoms may be taking more than 2 grams a day, whereas the RDA is less than 2 *milligrams*. How much higher than 2 milligrams is 2 grams?
   c. Vitamin B_{12} is measured in micrograms. How many micrograms are in a gram? How many grams are in a teaspoon of a granular powder? How many micrograms does that represent? What is your RDA for vitamin B_{12}?

   This exercise should convince you that the amount of vitamins a person needs is indeed quite small—yet still essential.

2. Be aware of how niacin intakes are affected by dietary protein availability.
   a. Refer to the "How to" on p. 332, and calculate how much niacin a woman receives from a diet that

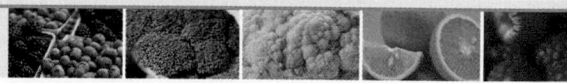

delivers 90 grams protein and 9 milligrams niacin. (Assume her RDA for protein is 46 grams/day.)

b. Is this woman getting her RDA of niacin (14 milligrams NE)?

This exercise should demonstrate that protein helps meet niacin needs.

STUDY QUESTIONS

These questions will help you review the chapter. You will find the answers in the discussions on the pages provided.

1. How do the vitamins differ from the energy nutrients? (p. 322)
2. Describe some general differences between fat-soluble and water-soluble vitamins. (pp. 322–324)
3. Which B vitamins are involved in energy metabolism? Protein metabolism? Cell division? (pp. 324–325)
4. For thiamin, riboflavin, niacin, biotin, pantothenic acid, vitamin B_6, folate, vitamin B_{12}, and vitamin C, state:
   - Its chief function in the body.
   - Its characteristic deficiency symptoms.
   - Its significant food sources. (See respective summary tables.)
5. What is the relationship of tryptophan to niacin? (p. 330)
6. Describe the relationship between folate and vitamin B_{12}. (pp. 336, 337, 340, 342)
7. What risks are associated with high doses of niacin? Vitamin B_6? Vitamin C? (pp. 330, 334–335, 352)

These questions will help you prepare for an exam. Answers can be found on p. 358.

1. Vitamins:
   a. are inorganic compounds.
   b. yield energy when broken down.
   c. are soluble in either water or fat.
   d. perform best when linked in long chains.
2. The rate at and the extent to which a vitamin is absorbed and used in the body is known as its:
   a. bioavailability.
   b. intrinsic factor.
   c. physiological effect.
   d. pharmacological effect.
3. Many of the B vitamins serve as:
   a. coenzymes.
   b. antagonists.
   c. antioxidants.
   d. serotonin precursors.
4. With respect to thiamin, which of the following is the most nutrient dense?
   a. 1 slice whole-wheat bread (69 kcalories and 0.1 milligram thiamin)
   b. 1 cup yogurt (144 kcalories and 0.1 milligram thiamin)
   c. 1 cup snow peas (69 kcalories and 0.22 milligram thiamin)
   d. 1 chicken breast (141 kcalories and 0.06 milligram thiamin)
5. The body can make niacin from:
   a. tyrosine.
   b. serotonin.
   c. carnitine.
   d. tryptophan.
6. The vitamin that protects against neural tube defects is:
   a. niacin.
   b. folate.
   c. riboflavin.
   d. vitamin B_{12}.
7. A lack of intrinsic factor may lead to:
   a. beriberi.
   b. pellagra.
   c. pernicious anemia.
   d. atrophic gastritis.
8. Which of the following is a B vitamin?
   a. inositol
   b. carnitine
   c. vitamin B_{15}
   d. pantothenic acid
9. Vitamin C serves as a(n):
   a. coenzyme.
   b. antagonist.
   c. antioxidant.
   d. intrinsic factor.
10. The requirement for vitamin C is highest for:
    a. smokers.
    b. athletes.
    c. alcoholics.
    d. the elderly.

REFERENCES

1. Committee on Dietary Reference Intakes, *Dietary Reference Intakes for Vitamin C, Vitamin E, Selenium, and Carotenoids* (Washington, D.C.: National Academy Press, 2000); Committee on Dietary Reference Intakes, *Dietary Reference Intakes for Thiamin, Riboflavin, Niacin, Vitamin B_6, Folate, Vitamin B_{12}, Pantothenic Acid, Biotin, and Choline* (Washington, D.C.: National Academy Press, 1998).
2. K. J. Carpenter, *Beriberi, White Rice, and Vitamin B: A Disease, a Cause, and a Cure* (Berkeley: University of California Press, 2000).
3. B. G. Brown and coauthors, Simvastatin and niacin, antioxidant vitamins, or the combination for the prevention of coronary disease, *New England Journal of Medicine* 345 (2001): 1583–1592; T. A. Jacobson, Combination lipid-altering therapy: An emerging treatment paradigm for the 21st century, *Current Atherosclerosis Reports* 3 (2001): 373–382.
4. A. A. Gerritsen and coauthors, Conservative treatment options for carpal tunnel syndrome: A systematic review of randomized controlled trials, *Journal of Neurology* 249 (2002): 272–280; R. Luboshitzky and coauthors, The effect of pyridoxine administration on melatonin secretion in normal men, *Neuroendocrinology Letters* 23 (2002): 213–217.
5. A. Fleming, The role of folate in the prevention of neural tube defects: Human and animal studies, *Nutrition Reviews* 59 (2001): S13–S20; S. M. Gross and coauthors, Inadequate folic acid intakes are prevalent among young women with neural tube defects, *Journal of the American Dietetic Association* 101 (2001): 342–345; Committee on Genetics, Folic acid for the prevention of neural tube defects, *Pediatrics* 104 (1999): 325–327; L. D. Botto and coauthors, Neural-tube defects, *New England Journal of Medicine* 341 (1999): 1509–1519.
6. R. J. Berry and coauthors, Prevention of neural-tube defects with folic acid in China, *New England Journal of Medicine* 341 (1999): 1485–1490; Committee on Genetics, 1999.
7. Knowledge and use of folic acid by women of childbearing age—United States, 1995 and 1998, *Morbidity and Mortality Weekly Report* 48 (1999): 327–328; C. J. Lewis and coauthors, Estimated folate intakes: Data updated to reflect food fortification, increased bioavailability, and dietary supplement use, *American Journal of Clinical Nutrition* 70 (1999): 198–207.
8. J. Erickson, Folic acid and prevention of spina bifida and anencephaly, *Morbidity and Mortality Weekly Report* 51 (2002): 1–3; M. A. Honein and coauthors, Impact of folic acid fortification of the US food supply on the occurrence of neural tube defects, *Journal of the American Medical Association* 285 (2001): 2981–2986; R. E. Stevenson and coauthors, Decline in prevalence of neural tube defects in a high-risk region of the United States, *Pediatrics* 106 (2000): 677–683.
9. E. P. Quinlivan and J. F. Gregory III, Effect of food fortification on folic acid intake in the United States, *American Journal of Clinical Nutrition* 77 (2003): 221–225; G. J. Cuskelly, H. McNulty, and J. M. Scott, Fortification with low amounts of folic acid makes a significant difference in folate status in young women: Implications for the prevention of neural tube defects, *American Journal of Clinical Nutrition* 70 (1999): 234–239; P. F. Jacques and coauthors, The effect of folic acid fortification on plasma folate and total homocysteine concentrations, *New England Journal of Medicine* 340 (1999): 1449–1454.
10. Committee on Dietary Reference Intakes, 1998.
11. S. Moyers and L. B. Bailey, Fetal malformations and folate metabolism: Review of recent evidence, *Nutrition Reviews* 59 (2001): 215–224; S. J. James and coauthors, Abnormal folate metabolism and mutation in the methylenetetrahydrofolate reductase gene may be maternal risk factors for Down syndrome, *American Journal of Clinical Nutrition* 70 (1999): 495–501; D. S. Rosenblatt, Folate and homocysteine metabolism and gene polymorphisms in the etiology of Down syndrome, *American Journal of Clinical Nutrition* 70 (1999): 429–430.
12. D. S. Wald, M. Law, and J. K. Morris, Homocysteine and cardiovascular disease: Evidence on causality from a meta-analysis, *British Medical Journal* 325 (2002): 1202; M. L. Bots and coauthors, Homocysteine and short-term risk of myocardial infarction and stroke in the elderly: The Rotterdam Study, *Archives of Internal Medicine* 159 (1999): 38–44.
13. F. V. van Oort and coauthors, Folic acid and reduction of plasma homocysteine concentrations in older adults: A dose-response study, *American Journal of Clinical Nutrition* 77 (2003): 1318–1323; B. J. Venn and coauthors, Dietary counseling to increase natural folate intake: A randomized placebo-controlled trial in free-living subjects to assess effects on serum folate and plasma total homocysteine, *American Journal of Clinical Nutrition* 76 (2002): 758–765; G. Schnyder and coauthors, Decreased rate of coronary restenosis after lowering of plasma homocysteine levels, *New England Journal of Medicine* 345 (2001): 1539–1600; L. J. Riddell and coauthors, Dietary strategies for lowering homocysteine concentrations, *American Journal of Clinical Nutrition* 71 (2000): 448–454; Jacques and coauthors, 1999; I. A. Brouwer and coauthors, Low-dose folic acid supplementation decreases plasma homocysteine concentrations: A randomized trial, *American Journal of Clinical Nutrition* 69 (1999): 99–104.
14. G. C. Rampersaud, L. B. Bailey, and G. P. A. Kauwell, Relationship of folate to colorectal and cervical cancer: Review and recommendations for practitioners, *Journal of the American Dietetic Association* 102 (2002): 1273–1282; S. W. Choi and J. B. Mason, Folate and carcinogenesis: An integrated scheme, *Journal of Nutrition* 130 (2000): 129–132; Y. I. Kim, Methylenetetrahydrofolate reductase polymorphisms, folate, and cancer risk: A paradigm of gene-nutrient interactions in carcinogenesis, *Nutrition Reviews* 58 (2000): 205–209.
15. Y. Kim, Folate and cancer prevention: A new medical application of folate beyond hyperhomocysteinemia and neural tube defects, *Nutrition Reviews* 57 (1999): 314–321; S. Zhang and coauthors, A prospective study of folate intake and the risk of breast cancer, *Journal of the American Medical Association* 281 (1999): 1632–1637.
16. B. D. Hokin and T. Butler, Cyanocobalamin (vitamin B-12) status in Seventh-day Adventist ministers in Australia, *American Journal of Clinical Nutrition* 70 (1999): 576S–578S.
17. M. W. J. Louwman and coauthors, Signs of impaired cognitive function in adolescents with marginal cobalamin status, *American Journal of Clinical Nutrition* 72 (2000): 762–769.
18. H. J. Powers, Riboflavin (vitamin B-2) and health, *American Journal of Clinical Nutrition* 77 (2003): 1352–1360.
19. H. Hemilä and coauthors, Vitamin C, vitamin E, and beta-carotene in relation to common cold incidence in male smokers, *Epidemiology* 13 (2002): 32–37; B. Takkouche and coauthors, Intake of vitamin C and zinc and risk of common cold: A cohort study, *Epidemiology* 13 (2002): 38–44; M. van Straten and P. Josling, Preventing the common cold with a vitamin C supplement: A double-blind, placebo-controlled survey, *Advances in Therapy* 19 (2002): 151–159; H. C. Gorton and K. Jarvis, The effectiveness of vitamin C in preventing and relieving the symptoms of virus-induced respiratory infections, *Journal of Manipulative and Physiological Therapeutics* 22 (1999): 530–533.
20. R. M. Douglas, E. B. Chalker, and B. Treacy, Vitamin C for preventing and treating the common cold (Cochrane Review), *Cochrane Database of Systematic Reviews* 2 (2000): CD000980; H. Hemilä and Z. S. Herman, Vitamin C and the common cold: A retrospective analysis of Chalmer's review, *Journal of the American College of Nutrition* 14 (1995): 116–123.
21. Committee on Dietary Reference Intakes, 2000.
22. Researchers proposed 120 mg/day. M. Levine and coauthors, Criteria and recommendations for vitamin C intake, *Journal of the American Medical Association* 281 (1999): 1415–1423; A. C. Carr and B. Frei, Toward a new recommended dietary allowance for vitamin C based on antioxidant and health effects in humans, *American Journal of Clinical Nutrition* 69 (1999): 1086–1107.
23. A. M. Preston and coauthors, Influence of environmental tobacco smoke on vitamin C status in children, *American Journal of Clinical Nutrition* 77 (2003): 167–172; R. S. Strauss, Environmental tobacco smoke and serum vitamin C levels in children, *Pediatrics* 107 (2001): 540–542; J. Lykkesfeldt and coauthors, Ascorbate is depleted by smoking and repleted by moderate supplementation: A study in male smokers and nonsmokers with matched dietary antioxidant intakes, *American Journal of Clinical Nutrition* 71 (2000): 530–536.
24. M. Weinstein, P. Babyn, and S. Zlotkin, An orange a day keeps the doctor away: Scurvy in the year 2000, **http://www.pediatrics.org/cgi/content/full/108/3/e55**.
25. C. S. Johnston and D. L. Bowling, Stability of ascorbic acid in commercially available orange juices, *Journal of the American Dietetic Association* 102 (2002): 525–529.

ANSWERS

Nutrition Calculations

1. a. Thiamin: mg.
   Riboflavin: mg.
   Niacin: mg NE.
   Vitamin B_6: mg.
   Folate: μg DFE.
   Vitamin B_{12}: μg.
   Vitamin C: mg.

   b. A thousand times higher (2 g × 1000 mg/g = 2000 mg; 2000 mg ÷ 2 mg = 1000).

   c. 1 g = 1000 mg; 1 mg = 1000 μg (1000 × 1000 = 1,000,000); 1 million μg = 1 g.
   1 tsp = 5 g.
   5 × 1,000,000 μg = 5,000,000 μg/tsp.
   See inside front cover for your RDA based on age and gender.

2. a. She eats 90 g protein. Assume she uses 46 g as protein. This leaves 90 g − 46 g = 44 g protein "leftover."
   44 g protein ÷ 100 = 0.44 g tryptophan.
   0.44 g tryptophan × 1000 = 440 mg tryptophan.
   440 mg tryptophan ÷ 60 = 7.3 mg NE.
   7.3 mg NE + 9 mg niacin = 16.3 mg NE.

   b. Yes.

Study Questions (multiple choice)

1. c 2. a 3. a 4. c 5. d 6. b 7. c 8. d
9. c 10. a

HIGHLIGHT

Vitamin and Mineral Supplements

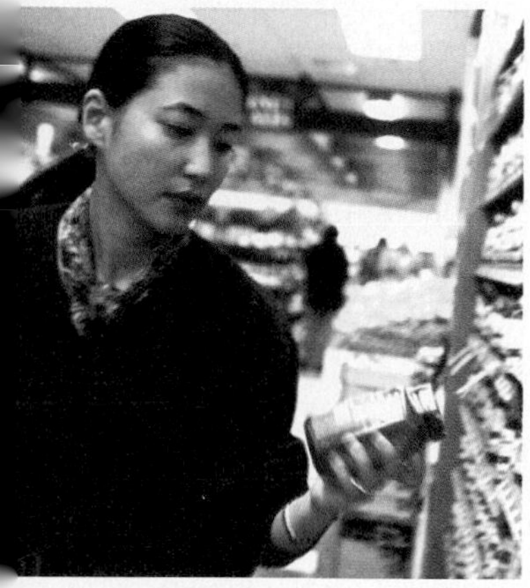

© J. Share/Stone/Getty Images

Almost half of the population in the United States takes vitamin and mineral supplements regularly, spending billions of dollars on them each year.[1] Many people take supplements as dietary insurance—in case they are not meeting their nutrient needs from foods alone. Others take supplements as health insurance—to protect against certain diseases.

One out of every five people takes multinutrient pills daily. Others take large doses of single nutrients, most commonly, vitamin C, vitamin E, beta-carotene, iron, and calcium. In many cases, taking supplements is a costly but harmless practice; sometimes, it is both costly and harmful to health.

For the most part, people self-prescribe supplements, taking them on the advice of friends, television, websites, or books that may or may not be reliable. Sometimes, they take supplements on the recommendation of a physician. When such advice follows a valid nutrition assessment, supplementation may be warranted, but even then the preferred course of action is to improve food choices and eating habits.[2] Without an assessment, the advice to take supplements may be inappropriate. A registered dietitian can help with the decision.[3]

When people think of supplements, they often think of vitamins, but minerals are important, too, of course. People whose diets lack vitamins, for whatever reason, probably lack several minerals as well. This highlight asks several questions related to vitamin-mineral **supplements** (the accompanying glossary defines supplements and related terms). What are the arguments *for* taking supplements? What are the arguments *against* taking them? Finally, if people do take supplements, how can they choose the appropriate ones? (In addition to vitamins and minerals, supplements may also provide amino acids or herbs, which are discussed in Chapters 6 and 19, respectively.)

Arguments for Supplements

Vitamin-mineral supplements may be appropriate in some circumstances. In some cases, they can correct deficiencies; in others, they can reduce the risk of diseases.

Correct Overt Deficiencies

In the United States and Canada, adults rarely suffer nutrient deficiency diseases such as scurvy, pellagra, and beriberi, but they do still occur. To correct an overt deficiency disease, a physician may prescribe therapeutic doses two to ten times the RDA (or AI) of a nutrient. At such high doses, the supplement is acting as a drug.

Improve Nutrition Status

In contrast to the classical deficiencies, which present a multitude of symptoms and are relatively easy to recognize, subclinical deficiencies are subtle and easy to overlook—and they are also more likely to occur. People who do not eat enough food to deliver the needed amounts of nutrients, such as habitual dieters and the elderly, risk developing subclinical deficiencies. Similarly, vegetarians who restrict their use of entire food groups without appropriate substitutions may fail to fully meet their nutrient needs. If there is no way for these people to eat enough nutritious foods to meet their needs, then vitamin-mineral supplements may be appropriate to help prevent nutrient deficiencies.

GLOSSARY

FDA (Food and Drug Administration): a federal agency that is responsible for, among other things, supplement safety, manufacturing, and information, including product labeling, package inserts, and accompanying literature. Another federal agency, the **FTC (Federal Trade Commission),** is responsible for, among other things, supplement advertising.

high potency: 100% or more of the Daily Value for the nutrient in a single supplement and for at least two-thirds of the nutrients in a multinutrient supplement.

supplements: pills, capsules, tablets, liquids, or powders that contain vitamins, minerals, herbs, or amino acids; intended to increase dietary intake of these substances.

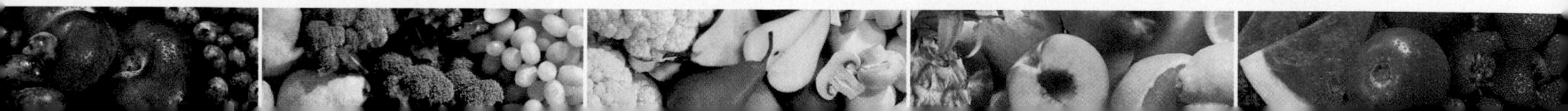

Reduce Disease Risks

Few people consume the optimal amounts of all the vitamins and minerals by diet alone. Inadequate intakes have been linked to chronic diseases such as heart disease, some cancers, and osteoporosis.[4] For this reason, some physicians recommend that all adults take vitamin-mineral supplements.[5] Others recognize the lack of conclusive evidence and the potential harm of supplementation and advise against such a recommendation.[6]

Highlight 11 reviews the relationships between supplement use and disease prevention. It describes some of the accumulating evidence suggesting that intakes of certain nutrients at levels much higher than can be attained from foods alone may be beneficial in reducing disease risks. It also presents research confirming the associated risks. Clearly, consumers must be cautious in taking supplements to prevent disease.

Many people, especially postmenopausal women and those who are intolerant to lactose or allergic to milk, may not receive enough calcium to forestall the bone degeneration of old age, osteoporosis. For them, nonmilk calcium-rich foods are especially valuable, but calcium supplements may also be appropriate (Highlight 12 provides more details).

Support Increased Nutrient Needs

As Chapters 14–16 explain, nutrient needs increase during certain stages of life, making it difficult to meet some of those needs without supplementation. For example, women who lose a lot of blood and therefore a lot of iron during menstruation each month may need an iron supplement. Women of childbearing age need folate supplements to reduce the risks of neural tube defects. Similarly, pregnant women and women who are breastfeeding their infants have exceptionally high nutrient needs and so usually need special supplements. Newborns routinely receive a single dose of vitamin K at birth to prevent abnormal bleeding. Infants may need other supplements as well, depending on whether they are breastfed or receiving formula, and on whether their water contains fluoride.

Improve the Body's Defenses

Health care professionals may provide special supplementation to people being treated for addictions to alcohol or other drugs and to people with prolonged illnesses, extensive injuries, or other severe stresses such as surgery. Illnesses that interfere with appetite, eating, or nutrient absorption limit nutrient intakes, yet nutrient needs are often heightened by diseases or medications. In all these cases, supplements are appropriate.

Who Needs Supplements?

In summary, the following list acknowledges that in these specific conditions, these people may need to take supplements:

- People with nutrient deficiencies.
- People with low food energy intakes (fewer than 1200 kcalories per day) need a multivitamin and mineral supplement.
- People who eat all-plant diets (vegans) and those with atrophic gastritis need vitamin B_{12}.
- Women who bleed excessively during menstruation need iron.
- People with lactose intolerance or milk allergies, or who otherwise do not consume enough dairy products to forestall extensive bone loss, need calcium.
- People in certain stages of the life cycle who have increased nutrient needs (for example, infants need iron and fluoride, women of childbearing age need folate, pregnant women need iron, and the elderly need vitamins B_{12} and D).
- People with limited milk intake and sun exposure need vitamin D.
- People who have diseases, infections, or injuries or who have undergone surgery that interferes with the intake, absorption, metabolism, or excretion of nutrients.
- People taking medications that interfere with the body's use of specific nutrients.

Except for people in these circumstances, most adults can normally get all the nutrients they need by eating a varied diet of nutrient-dense foods. Even athletes can meet their nutrient needs without the help of supplements.

Arguments against Supplements

Foods rarely cause nutrient imbalances or toxicities, but supplements can. The higher the dose, the greater the risk of harm. People's tolerances for high doses of nutrients vary, just as their risks of deficiencies do. Amounts that some can tolerate may be harmful for others, and no one knows who falls where along the spectrum. It is difficult to determine just how much of a nutrient is enough—or too much. The Tolerable Upper Intake Levels of the DRI answer the question how much is too much by defining the highest amount that appears safe for most healthy people. Table H10-1 presents these suggested Upper Levels and Daily Values for selected vitamins and minerals and the quantities typically found in supplements.

Toxicity

The extent and severity of supplement toxicity remain unclear. Only a few alert health care professionals can recognize toxicity, even when it is acute. When it is chronic, with the effects developing subtly and progressing slowly, it often goes unrecognized. In view of the potential hazards, some authori-

TABLE H10-1 Vitamin and Mineral Intakes for Adults

Nutrient	Tolerable Upper Intake Levels[a]	Daily Values	Typical Multivitamin-Mineral Supplement	Average Single-Nutrient Supplement
Vitamins				
Vitamin A	3000 μg (10,000 IU)	5000 IU	5000 IU	8000 to 10,000 IU
Vitamin D	50 μg (2000 IU)	400 IU	400 IU	400 IU
Vitamin E	1000 mg (1500 to 2200 IU)[b]	30 IU	30 IU	100 to 1000 IU
Vitamin K	—[c]	80 μg	40 μg	—[e]
Thiamin	—[c]	1.5 mg	1.5 mg	50 mg
Riboflavin	—[c]	1.7 mg	1.7 mg	25 mg
Niacin (as niacinamide)	35 mg[b]	20 mg	20 mg	100 to 500 mg
Vitamin B_6	100 mg	2 mg	2 mg	100 to 200 mg
Folate	1000 μg[b]	400 μg	400 μg	400 μg
Vitamin B_{12}	—[c]	6 μg	6 μg	100 to 1000 μg
Pantothenic acid	—[c]	10 mg	10 mg	100 to 500 mg
Biotin	—[c]	300 μg	30 μg	300 to 600 μg
Vitamin C	2000 mg	60 mg	10 mg	500 to 2000 mg
Choline	3500 mg	—	10 mg	250 mg
Minerals				
Calcium	2500 mg	1000 mg	160 mg	250 to 600 mg
Phosphorus	4000 mg	1000 mg	110 mg	—[e]
Magnesium	350 mg[d]	400 mg	100 mg	250 mg
Iron	45 mg	18 mg	18 mg	18 to 30 mg
Zinc	40 mg	15 mg	15 mg	10 to 100 mg
Iodine	1100 μg	150 μg	150 μg	—[e]
Selenium	400 μg	70 μg	10 μg	50 to 200 μg
Fluoride	10 mg	—	—	—[e]
Copper	10 mg	2 mg	0.5 mg	—[e]
Manganese	11 mg	2 mg	5 mg	—[e]
Chromium	—[c]	120 μg	25 μg	200 to 400 μg
Molybdenum	2000 μg	75 μg	25 μg	—[e]

[a] Unless otherwise noted, Upper Levels represent total intakes from food, water, and supplements.
[b] Upper Levels represent intakes from supplements, fortified foods, or both.
[c] These nutrients have been evaluated by the DRI Committee for Tolerable Upper Intake Levels, but none were established because of insufficient data. No adverse effects have been reported with intakes of these nutrients at levels typical of supplements, but caution is still advised, given the potential for harm that accompanies excessive intakes.
[d] Upper Levels represent intakes from supplements only.
[e] Available as a single supplement by prescription.

ties believe supplements should bear warning labels, advising consumers that large doses may be toxic.

Toxic overdoses of vitamins and minerals in children are more readily recognized and, unfortunately, fairly common. Fruit-flavored, chewable vitamins shaped like cartoon characters entice young children to eat them like candy in amounts that can cause poisoning. High-potency iron supplements (30 milligrams of iron or more per tablet) are especially toxic and are the leading cause of accidental ingestion fatalities among children. Even mild overdoses cause GI distress, nausea, and black diarrhea that reflects gastric bleeding. Severe overdoses result in bloody diarrhea, shock, liver damage, coma, and death.

Life-Threatening Misinformation

Another problem arises when people who are ill come to believe that high doses of vitamins or minerals can be therapeutic. Not only can high doses be toxic, but the person may take them instead of seeking medical help. Furthermore, there are no guarantees that the supplements will be effective.

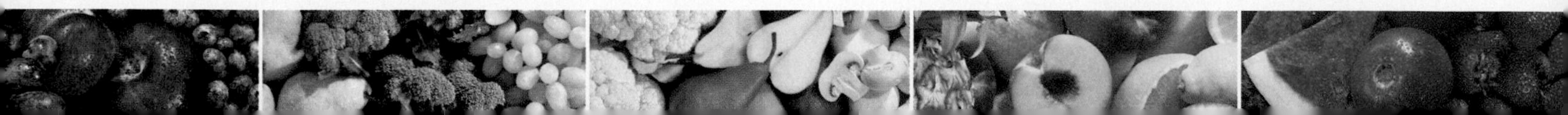

Marketing materials for supplements often make health statements that are required to be "truthful and not misleading," but often fall far short of both. Chapter and Highlight 19 revisit this topic and include discussions of herbal preparations and other alternative therapies.

Unknown Needs

Another argument against the use of supplements is that no one knows exactly how to formulate the "ideal" supplement. What nutrients should be included? Which, if any, of the phytochemicals should be included? How much of each? On whose needs should the choices be based? Surveys have repeatedly shown little relationship between the supplements people take and the nutrients they actually need.

False Sense of Security

Another argument against supplement use is that it may lull people into a false sense of security. A person might eat irresponsibly, thinking, "My supplement will cover my needs." Or, experiencing a warning symptom of a disease, a person might postpone seeking a diagnosis, thinking, "I probably just need a supplement to make this go away." Such self-diagnosis is potentially dangerous.

Other Invalid Reasons

Other invalid reasons why people might take supplements include:

- The belief that the food supply or soil contains inadequate nutrients.
- The belief that supplements can provide energy.
- The belief that supplements can enhance athletic performance or build lean body tissues without physical work or faster than work alone.
- The belief that supplements will help a person cope with stress.
- The belief that supplements can prevent, treat, or cure conditions ranging from the common cold to cancer.

Ironically, people with health problems are more likely to take supplements than other people, yet today's health problems are more likely to be due to overnutrition and poor lifestyle choices than to nutrient deficiencies. The truth—that most people would benefit from improving their eating and exercise habits—is harder to swallow than a supplement pill.

Bioavailability and Antagonistic Actions

In general, the body absorbs nutrients best from foods in which the nutrients are diluted and dispersed among other substances that may facilitate their absorption. Taken in pure, concentrated form, nutrients are likely to interfere with one another's absorption or with the absorption of nutrients in foods eaten at the same time. Documentation of these effects is particularly extensive for minerals: zinc hinders copper and calcium absorption, iron hinders zinc absorption, calcium hinders magnesium and iron absorption, and magnesium hinders the absorption of calcium and iron. Similarly, binding agents in supplements limit mineral absorption.

Although minerals provide the most familiar and best-documented examples, interference among vitamins is now being seen as supplement use increases. The vitamin A precursor beta-carotene, long thought to be nontoxic, interferes with vitamin E metabolism when taken over the long term as a dietary supplement. Vitamin E, on the other hand, antagonizes vitamin K activity and so should not be used by people being treated for blood-clotting disorders. Consumers who want the benefits of optimal absorption of nutrients should eat ordinary foods, selected for nutrient density and variety.

Whenever the diet is inadequate, the person should first attempt to improve it so as to obtain the needed nutrients from foods. If that is truly impossible, then the person needs a multivitamin-mineral supplement that supplies between 50 and 150 percent of the Daily Value for each of the nutrients. These amounts reflect the ranges commonly found in foods and therefore are compatible with the body's normal handling of nutrients (its physiologic tolerance). The next section provides some pointers to assist in the selection of an appropriate supplement.

Selection of Supplements

Whenever a physician or registered dietitian recommends a supplement, follow the directions carefully. When selecting a supplement yourself, look for a single, balanced vitamin-mineral supplement.

If you decide to take a vitamin-mineral supplement, ignore the eye-catching art and meaningless claims. Pay attention to the form the supplements are in, the list of ingredients, and the price. Here's where the truth lies, and from it you can make a rational decision based on facts. You have two basic questions to answer.

Form

The first question: What form do you want—chewable, liquid, or pills? If you'd rather drink your supplements than chew them, fine. (If you choose a chewable form, though, be aware that chewable vitamin C can dissolve tooth enamel.) If you choose pills, look for statements about the disintegration time. The U.S. Pharmacopeia (USP) suggests that supplements should completely disintegrate within 30 to 45 minutes.* Obviously, supplements that don't dissolve have little chance of

*The USP establishes standards for quality, strength, and purity of supplements.

entering the bloodstream, so look for a brand that claims to meet USP disintegration standards.

Contents

The second question: What vitamins and minerals do *you* need? Generally, an appropriate supplement provides vitamins and minerals in amounts that do not exceed recommended intakes.[7] Avoid supplements that, in a daily dose, provide more than the Tolerable Upper Intake Level for *any* nutrient. Avoid preparations with more than 10 milligrams of iron per dose, except as prescribed by a physician. Iron is hard to get rid of once it's in the body, and an excess of iron can cause problems, just as a deficiency can (see Chapter 13).

Misleading Claims

Ignore "organic" or "natural" claims. Such supplements are no better than others and often cost more. The word *synthetic* may sound like "fake," but to synthesize just means to put together. Whether vitamins are synthesized in a laboratory or synthesized by plants and animals, your body uses them similarly. Only your wallet can tell the difference.

Avoid products that make **"high potency"** claims. More is not better (review the "How to" on p. 324). Remember that foods are also providing these nutrients. Nutrients can build up and cause unexpected problems. For example, a man who takes vitamins and begins to lose his hair may think his hair loss means he needs *more* vitamins, when in fact it may be the early sign of a vitamin A overdose. (Of course, it may be completely unrelated to nutrition as well.)

Be wise to fake vitamins and preparations that contain items not needed in human nutrition, such as carnitine and inositol. Such ingredients reveal a marketing strategy aimed at your pocket, not at your health. The manufacturer wants you to believe that its pills contain the latest "new" nutrient that other brands omit, but in reality, these substances are not known to be needed by human beings.

Realize that the claim that supplements "relieve stress" is another marketing ploy. If you give even passing thought to what people mean by "stress," you'll realize manufacturers could never design a supplement to meet everyone's needs. Is it stressful to take an exam? Well, yes. Is it stressful to survive a major car wreck with third-degree burns and multiple bone fractures? Definitely yes. The body's responses to these stresses are different. The body does use vitamins and minerals in mounting a stress response, but a body fed a well-balanced diet can meet the needs of most minor stresses. As for the major ones, medical intervention is needed. In any case, taking a vitamin supplement won't make life any less stressful.

Other marketing tricks to sidestep are "green" pills that contain dehydrated, crushed parsley, alfalfa, and other fruit and vegetable extracts. The nutrients and phytochemicals advertised can be obtained from a serving of vegetables more easily and for less money. Such pills may also provide enzymes, but these are inactivated in the stomach during protein digestion.

Be aware that some geriatric "tonics" are low in vitamins and minerals, yet so high in alcohol as to threaten inebriation. The liquids designed for infants are more complete.

Recognize the latest nutrition buzzwords. Manufacturers were marketing "antioxidant" supplements before the print had time to dry on the first scientific reports of antioxidant vitamins' action in preventing cancer and cardiovascular disease. Remember, too, that high doses can alter a nutrient's action in the body. An antioxidant in physiological quantities may be beneficial, but in pharmacological quantities, it may act as a prooxidant and produce harmful by-products. Highlight 11 explores antioxidants and supplement use in more detail.

Finally, be aware that advertising on the Internet is cheap and not closely regulated. Promotional e-mails can be sent to millions of people in an instant. Internet messages can easily cite references and provide links to other sites, implying an endorsement when in fact none has been given.[8] Be cautious when examining unsolicited information and search for a balanced perspective.

Cost

When shopping for supplements, remember that local or store brands may be just as good as nationally advertised brands. If they are less expensive, it may be because the price does not have to cover the cost of national advertising.

Regulation of Supplements

The Dietary Supplement Health and Education Act of 1994 was intended to enable consumers to make informed choices about nutrient supplements. The act subjects supplements to the same general labeling requirements that apply to foods. Specifically:

- Nutrition labeling for dietary supplements is required.
- Labels may make nutrient claims (as "high" or "low") according to specific criteria (for example, "an excellent source of vitamin C").
- Labels may claim that the lack of a nutrient can cause a deficiency disease, but if they do, they must also include the prevalence of that deficiency disease in the United States.
- Labels may make health claims that are supported by significant scientific agreement and are not brand specific (for example, "folate protects against neural tube defects"). To date, the following health claims have been approved for supplements: folate and neural tube defects, calcium and osteoporosis, soluble fiber from

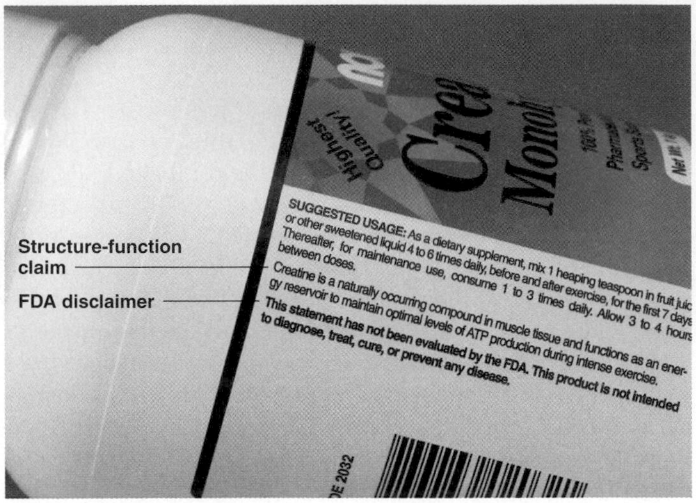
Structure-function claim
FDA disclaimer
This statement has not been evaluated by the FDA. This product is not intended to diagnose, treat, cure, or prevent any disease.

© Anne Dowie

Structure-function claims do not need FDA authorization, but they must be accompanied by a disclaimer.

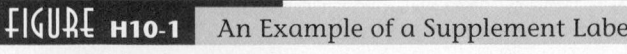

FIGURE H10-1 An Example of a Supplement Label

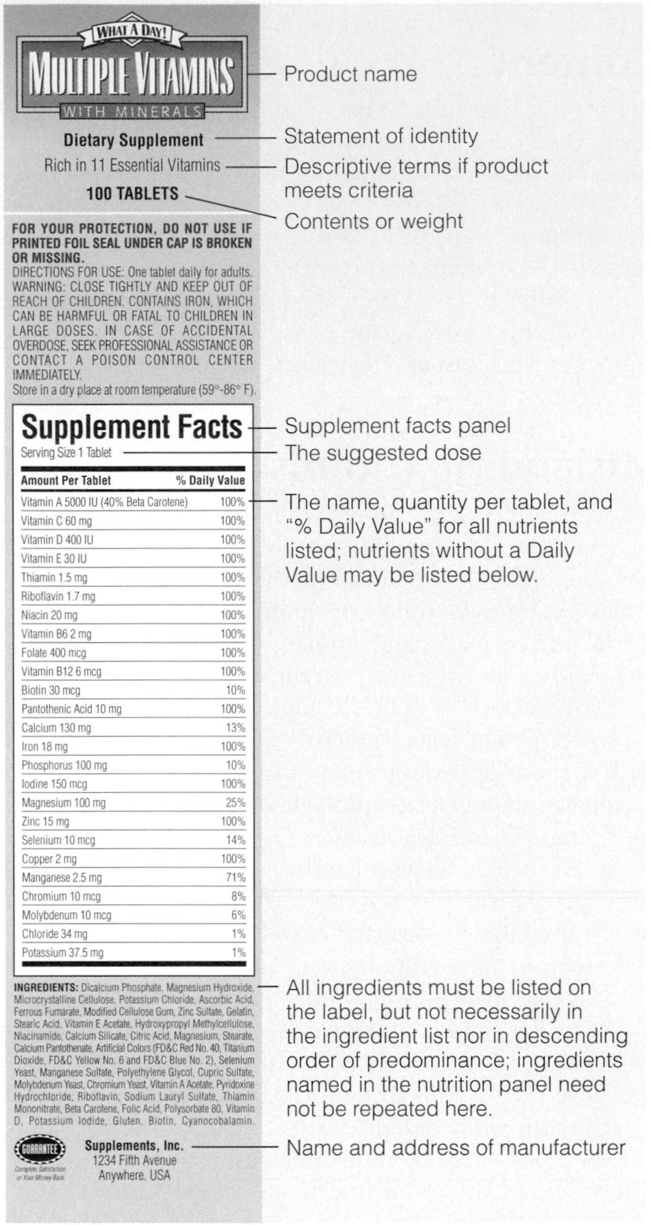
WHAT A DAY!
MULTIPLE VITAMINS
WITH MINERALS
Dietary Supplement
Rich in 11 Essential Vitamins
100 TABLETS
FOR YOUR PROTECTION, DO NOT USE IF PRINTED FOIL SEAL UNDER CAP IS BROKEN OR MISSING.
DIRECTIONS FOR USE: One tablet daily for adults.
WARNING: CLOSE TIGHTLY AND KEEP OUT OF REACH OF CHILDREN. CONTAINS IRON, WHICH CAN BE HARMFUL OR FATAL TO CHILDREN IN LARGE DOSES. IN CASE OF ACCIDENTAL OVERDOSE, SEEK PROFESSIONAL ASSISTANCE OR CONTACT A POISON CONTROL CENTER IMMEDIATELY.
Store in a dry place at room temperature (59°-86° F).
Supplement Facts
Serving Size 1 Tablet
Amount Per Tablet % Daily Value
Vitamin A 5000 IU (40% Beta Carotene) 100%
Vitamin C 60 mg 100%
Vitamin D 400 IU 100%
Vitamin E 30 IU 100%
Thiamin 1.5 mg 100%
Riboflavin 1.7 mg 100%
Niacin 20 mg 100%
Vitamin B6 2 mg 100%
Folate 400 mcg 100%
Vitamin B12 6 mcg 100%
Biotin 30 mcg 10%
Pantothenic Acid 10 mg 100%
Calcium 130 mg 13%
Iron 18 mg 100%
Phosphorus 100 mg 10%
Iodine 150 mcg 100%
Magnesium 100 mg 25%
Zinc 15 mg 100%
Selenium 10 mcg 14%
Copper 2 mg 100%
Manganese 2.5 mg 71%
Chromium 10 mcg 8%
Molybdenum 10 mcg 6%
Chloride 34 mg 1%
Potassium 37.5 mg 1%
INGREDIENTS: Dicalcium Phosphate, Magnesium Hydroxide, Microcrystalline Cellulose, Potassium Chloride, Ascorbic Acid, Ferrous Fumarate, Modified Cellulose Gum, Zinc Sulfate, Gelatin, Stearic Acid, Vitamin E Acetate, Hydroxypropyl Methylcellulose, Niacinamide, Calcium Silicate, Citric Acid, Magnesium, Stearate, Calcium Pantothenate, Artificial Colors (FD&C Red No. 40, Titanium Dioxide, FD&C Yellow No. 6 and FD&C Blue No. 2), Selenium Yeast, Manganese Sulfate, Polyethylene Glycol, Cupric Sulfate, Molybdenum Yeast, Chromium Yeast, Vitamin A Acetate, Pyridoxine Hydrochloride, Riboflavin, Sodium Lauryl Sulfate, Thiamin Mononitrate, Beta Carotene, Folic Acid, Polysorbate 80, Vitamin D, Potassium Iodide, Gluten, Biotin, Cyanocobalamin.
GUARANTEE
Complete Satisfaction or Your Money Back
Supplements, Inc.
1234 Fifth Avenue
Anywhere, USA
Product name
Statement of identity
Descriptive terms if product meets criteria
Contents or weight
Supplement facts panel
The suggested dose
The name, quantity per tablet, and "% Daily Value" for all nutrients listed; nutrients without a Daily Value may be listed below.
All ingredients must be listed on the label, but not necessarily in the ingredient list nor in descending order of predominance; ingredients named in the nutrition panel need not be repeated here.
Name and address of manufacturer

oat bran and from psyllium husks and cardiovascular disease, and omega-3 fatty acids and cardiovascular disease.

- Labels may claim to diagnose, treat, cure, or relieve common complaints such as menstrual cramps or memory loss, but may *not* make claims about specific diseases (except as noted above).
- Labels may make structure-function claims about the role a nutrient plays in the body, how the nutrient performs its function, and how consuming the nutrient is associated with general well-being. These claims must be accompanied by an **FDA** disclaimer statement: "This statement has not been evaluated by the Food and Drug Administration. This product is not intended to diagnose, treat, cure or prevent any disease." Figure H10-1 provides an example of a supplement label that complies with the requirements.

The multibillion-dollar-a-year supplement industry spends much money and effort influencing these regulations. The net effect of the Dietary Supplement Health and Education Act was a deregulation of the supplement industry. Unlike food additives or drugs, supplements do not need to be proved safe and effective, nor do they need the FDA's approval before being marketed. Furthermore, there are no standards for potency or dosage. Should a problem arise, the burden falls to the FDA to prove that the supplement poses an unreasonable risk and should be removed from the market. When asked, most Americans express support for greater regulation of dietary supplements.[9] Health professionals agree.[10]

If all the nutrients we need can come from food, why not just eat food? Foods have so much more to offer than supplements do. Nutrients in foods come in an infinite variety of combinations with a multitude of different carriers and absorption enhancers. They come with water, fiber, and an array of beneficial phytochemicals. Foods stimulate the GI tract to keep it healthy. They provide energy, and since you need energy each day, why not have nutritious foods deliver it? Foods offer pleasure, satiety, and opportunities for socializing while eating. In no way can nutrient supplements hold a candle to foods as a means of meeting human health needs. For further proof, read Highlight 11.

NUTRITION ON THE NET

Access these websites for further study of topics covered in this highlight.

- Find updates and quick links to these and other nutrition-related sites at our website: **www.wadsworth.com/nutrition**
- Gather information from the Office of Dietary Supplements or Health Canada: **dietary-supplements.info.nih.gov** or **www.hc-sc.gc.ca**
- Report adverse reactions associated with dietary supplements to the FDA's MedWatch program: **www.fda.gov/medwatch**
- Search for "supplements" at the American Dietetic Association: **www.eatright.org**
- Learn more about supplements from the FDA Center for Food Safety and Applied Nutrition: **www.cfsan.fda.gov/~dms/supplmnt.html**
- Obtain consumer information on dietary supplements from the U.S. Pharmacopeia: **www.usp.org**
- Review the Federal Trade Commission policies for dietary supplement advertising: **www.ftc.gov/bcp/conline/pubs/buspubs/dietsupp.htm**

REFERENCES

1. L. S. Balluz and coauthors, Vitamin and mineral supplement use in the United States: Results from the third National Health and Nutrition Examination Survey, *Archives of Family Medicine* 9 (2000): 258–262.
2. Position of the American Dietetic Association: Food fortification and dietary supplements, *Journal of the American Dietetic Association* 101 (2001): 115–125.
3. J. R. Hunt, Tailoring advice on dietary supplements: An opportunity for dietetics professionals, *Journal of the American Dietetic Association* 102 (2002): 1754–1755; C. Thomson and coauthors, Guidelines regarding the recommendation and sale of dietary supplements, *Journal of the American Dietetic Association* 102 (2002): 1158–1164.
4. K. M. Fairfield and R. H. Fletcher, Vitamins for chronic disease prevention in adults: Scientific review, *Journal of the American Medical Association* 287 (2002): 3116–3126.
5. R. H. Fletcher and K. M. Fairfield, Vitamins for chronic disease prevention in adults: Clinical applications, *Journal of the American Medical Association* 287 (2002): 3127–3129.
6. C. D. Morris and S. Carson, Routine vitamin supplementation to prevent cardiovascular disease: A summary of the evidence for the U.S. Preventive Services Task Force, *Annals of Internal Medicine* 139 (2003): 56–70; B. Hasanain and A. D. Mooradian, Antioxidant vitamins and their influence in diabetes mellitus, *Current Diabetes Reports* 2 (2002): 448–456.
7. W. C. Willett and M. J. Stampfer, What vitamins should I be taking, doctor? *New England Journal of Medicine* 345 (2001): 1819–1824.
8. J. M. Drazen, Inappropriate advertising of dietary supplements, *New England Journal of Medicine* 348 (2003): 777–778.
9. R. J. Blendon and coauthors, Americans' views on the use and regulation of dietary supplements, *Archives of Internal Medicine* 161 (2001): 805–810.
10. P. B. Fontanarosa, D. Rennie, and C. D. DeAngelis, The need for regulation of dietary supplements—Lessons from ephedra, *Journal of the American Medical Association* 289 (2003): 1568–1570.

Chapter 11

The Fat-Soluble Vitamins: A, D, E, and K

Chapter Outline

Available Online

http://nutrition.wadsworth.com/uncn7

Nutrition Animation: *Free-Radical Action in the Body*

Student Practice Test

Glossary Terms

Nutrition on the Net

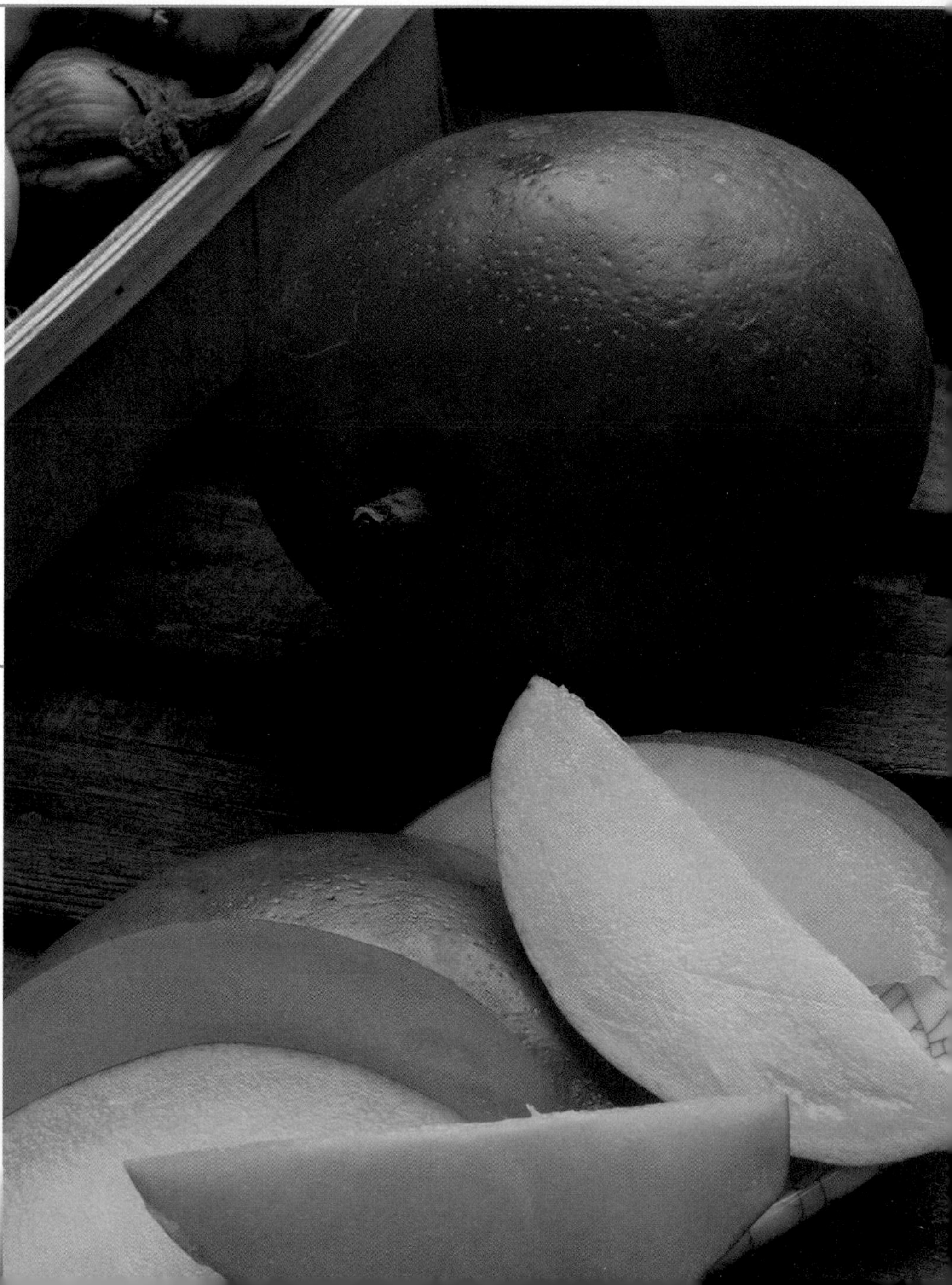

Nutrition in Your Life

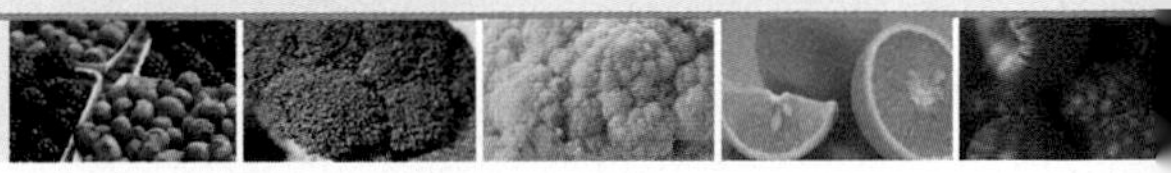

Realizing that vitamin A from vegetables participates in vision, a mom encourages her children to "eat your carrots" because "they're good for your eyes." A dad takes his children outside to "enjoy the fresh air and sunshine" because they need the vitamin D that is made with the help of the sun. A physician recommends that a patient use vitamin E to slow the progression of heart disease. Another physician gives a newborn a dose of vitamin K to protect against life-threatening blood loss. These common daily occurrences highlight some of the heroic work of the fat-soluble vitamins.

The fat-soluble vitamins A, D, E, and K■ differ from the water-soluble vitamins in several significant ways (review the table on p. 324). Being insoluble in water, the fat-soluble vitamins require bile for their absorption. Upon absorption, fat-soluble vitamins travel through the lymphatic system within chylomicrons before entering the bloodstream, where many of them require protein carriers for transport. The fat-soluble vitamins participate in numerous activities all over the body, but excesses are stored primarily in the liver and adipose tissue. The body maintains blood concentrations by retrieving these vitamins from storage as needed; thus people can eat less than their daily need for days, weeks, or even months or years without ill effects. They need only ensure that over time *average* daily intakes approximate recommendations. By the same token, because fat-soluble vitamins are not readily excreted, the risk of toxicity is greater than it is for the water-soluble vitamins.

■ The fat-soluble vitamins:
- Vitamin A.
- Vitamin D.
- Vitamin E.
- Vitamin K.

Vitamin A and Beta-Carotene

Vitamin A was the first fat-soluble vitamin to be recognized. Almost a century later, vitamin A and its precursor, **beta-carotene,** continue to intrigue researchers with their diverse roles and profound effects on health.

vitamin A: all naturally occurring compounds with the biological activity of retinol (RET-ih-nol), the alcohol form of vitamin A.

beta-carotene (BAY-tah KARE-oh-teen): one of the carotenoids; an orange pigment and vitamin A precursor found in plants. A **precursor** is a compound that can be converted into an active vitamin.

FIGURE 11-1 Forms of Vitamin A

In this diagram, corners represent carbon atoms, as in all previous diagrams in this book. A further simplification here is that methyl groups (CH_3) are understood to be at the ends of the lines extending from corners. (See Appendix C for complete structures.)

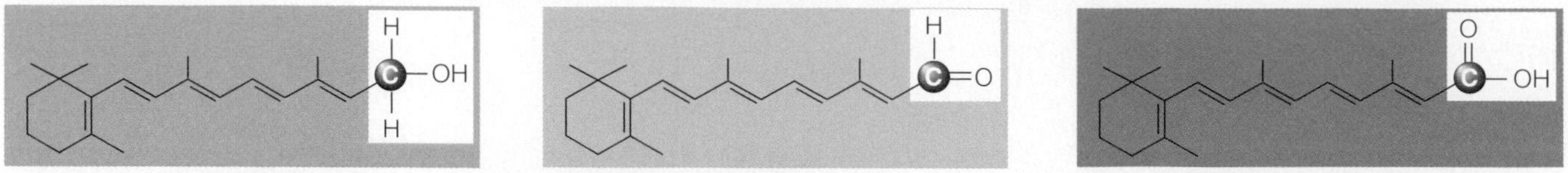
H
C
OH
H
H
C
O
O
C
OH

Retinol, the alcohol form

Retinal, the aldehyde form

Retinoic acid, the acid form

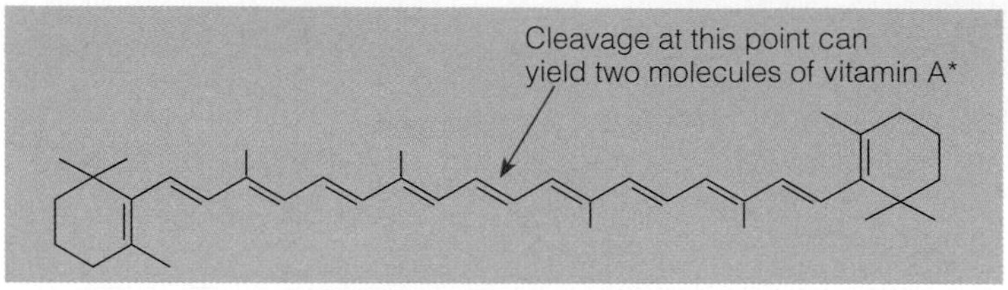
Cleavage at this point can yield two molecules of vitamin A*

Beta-carotene, a precursor

*Sometimes cleavage occurs at other points as well, so that one molecule of beta-carotene may yield only one molecule of vitamin A. Furthermore, not all beta-carotene is converted to vitamin A, and absorption of beta-carotene is not as efficient as that of vitamin A. For these reasons, 12 µg of beta-carotene are equivalent to 1 µg of vitamin A. Conversion of other carotenoids to vitamin A is even less efficient.

■ Carotenoids are among the best-known phytochemicals.

Three different forms of vitamin A are active in the body: retinol, retinal, and retinoic acid. Collectively, these compounds are known as **retinoids.** Foods derived from animals provide compounds (retinyl esters) that are easily converted to retinol in the intestine. Foods derived from plants provide **carotenoids,**■ some of which have **vitamin A activity.*** The most studied of the carotenoids is beta-carotene, which can be split to form retinol in the intestine and liver. Beta-carotene's absorption and conversion are significantly less efficient than those of the retinoids.[1] Figure 11-1 illustrates the structural similarities and differences of these vitamin A compounds and the cleavage of beta-carotene.[2]

The cells can convert retinol and retinal to the other active forms of vitamin A as needed. The conversion of retinol to retinal is reversible, but the further conversion of retinal to retinoic acid is irreversible (see Figure 11-2). This irreversibility is significant because each form of vitamin A performs a function that the others cannot.

A special transport protein, **retinol-binding protein (RBP),** picks up vitamin A from the liver, where it is stored, and carries it in the blood. Cells that use vitamin A have special protein receptors for it, as if the vitamin were fragile and had to be passed carefully from hand to hand without being dropped.[3] Each form of vitamin A has its own receptor protein (retinol has several) within the cells.

*Carotenoids with vitamin A activity include alpha-carotene, beta-carotene, and beta-cryptoxanthin; carotenoids with no vitamin A activity include lycopene, lutein, and zeaxanthin.

retinoids (RET-ih-noyds): chemically related compounds with biological activity similar to that of retinol; metabolites of retinol.

carotenoids (kah-ROT-eh-noyds): pigments commonly found in plants and animals, some of which have vitamin A activity. The carotenoid with the greatest vitamin A activity is beta-carotene.

vitamin A activity: a term referring to both the active forms of vitamin A and the precursor forms in foods without distinguishing between them.

retinol-binding protein (RBP): the specific protein responsible for transporting retinol.

FIGURE 11-2 Conversion of Vitamin A Compounds

Notice that the conversion from retinol to retinal is reversible, whereas the pathway from retinal to retinoic acid is not.

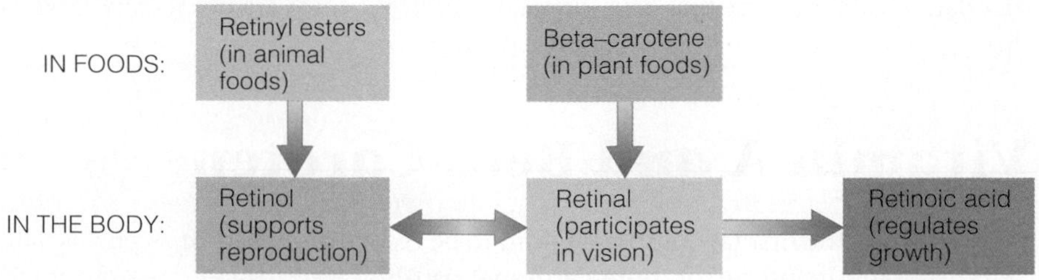
IN FOODS:
Retinyl esters (in animal foods)
Beta–carotene (in plant foods)
IN THE BODY:
Retinol (supports reproduction)
Retinal (participates in vision)
Retinoic acid (regulates growth)

Roles in the Body

Vitamin A is a versatile vitamin. Its major roles include:

- Promoting vision.
- Participating in protein synthesis and cell differentiation (and thereby maintaining the health of epithelial tissues and skin).
- Supporting reproduction and growth.

As mentioned, each form of vitamin A performs specific tasks. Retinol supports reproduction and is the major transport and storage form of the vitamin. Retinal is active in vision and is also an intermediate in the conversion of retinol to retinoic acid (review Figure 11-2). Retinoic acid acts like a hormone, regulating cell differentiation, growth, and embryonic development.[4] Animals raised on retinoic acid as their sole source of vitamin A can grow normally, but they become blind because retinoic acid cannot be converted to retinal (review Figure 11-2).

Vitamin A in Vision Vitamin A plays two indispensable roles in the eye: it helps maintain a crystal-clear outer window, the **cornea,** and it participates in the conversion of light energy into nerve impulses at the **retina** (see Figure 11-3 for details). The cells of the retina contain **pigment** molecules called **rhodopsin;** each rhodopsin molecule is composed of a protein called **opsin** bonded to a molecule of retinal.■ When light passes through the cornea of the eye and strikes the cells of the retina, rhodopsin responds by changing shape and becoming bleached. As it does, the retinal shifts from a *cis* to a *trans* configuration, just as fatty acids do during hydrogenation (see pp. 146–147). The *trans*-retinal cannot remain bonded to opsin. When retinal is released, opsin changes shape, thereby disturbing the membrane of the cell and generating an electrical impulse that travels along the cell's length. At the other end of the cell, the impulse is transmitted to a nerve cell, which conveys the message to the brain. Much of the retinal is then converted back to its active *cis* form and combined with the opsin protein to regenerate the pigment rhodopsin. Some retinal, however, may be oxidized to retinoic acid, a biochemical dead end for the visual process.

Visual activity leads to repeated small losses of retinal, necessitating its constant replenishment either directly from foods or indirectly from retinol stores. Ultimately, foods supply all the retinal in the pigments of the eye.

Vitamin A in Protein Synthesis and Cell Differentiation Despite its important role in vision, only one-thousandth of the body's vitamin A is in the retina. Much more is in the cells lining the body's surfaces. There the vitamin participates

■ Over 100 million cells reside in the retina, and each contains about 30 million molecules of vitamin A–containing visual pigments.

cornea (KOR-nee-uh): the transparent membrane covering the outside of the eye.

retina (RET-in-uh): the layer of light-sensitive nerve cells lining the back of the inside of the eye; consists of rods and cones.

pigment: a molecule capable of absorbing certain wavelengths of light so that it reflects only those that we perceive as a certain color.

rhodopsin (ro-DOP-sin): a light-sensitive pigment of the retina; contains the retinal form of vitamin A and the protein opsin.
- **rhod** = red (pigment)
- **opsin** = visual protein

opsin (OP-sin): the protein portion of the visual pigment molecule.

FIGURE 11-3 Vitamin A's Role in Vision

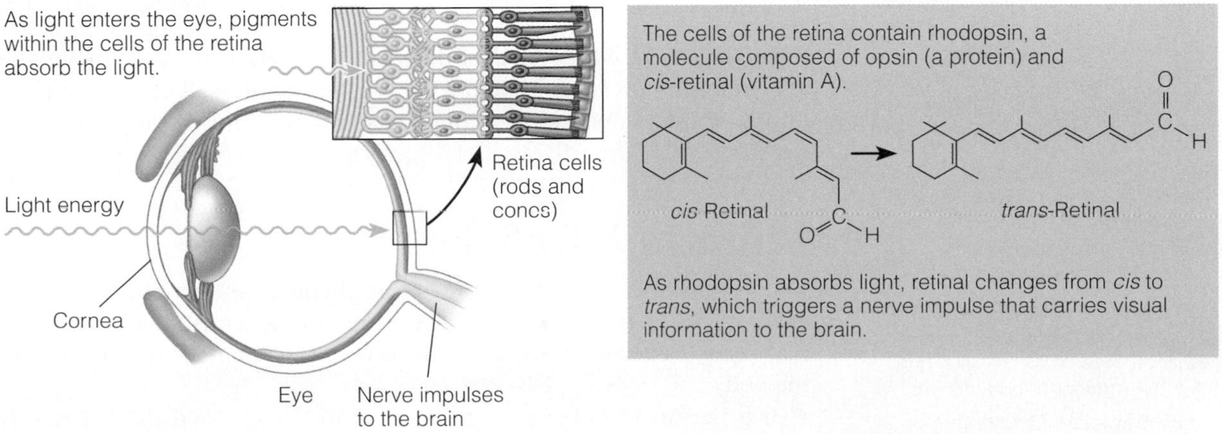
As light enters the eye, pigments within the cells of the retina absorb the light.
Retina cells (rods and cones)
Light energy
Cornea
Eye
Nerve impulses to the brain
The cells of the retina contain rhodopsin, a molecule composed of opsin (a protein) and cis-retinal (vitamin A).
cis Retinal
trans-Retinal
As rhodopsin absorbs light, retinal changes from cis to trans, which triggers a nerve impulse that carries visual information to the brain.

FIGURE 11-4 Mucous Membrane Integrity

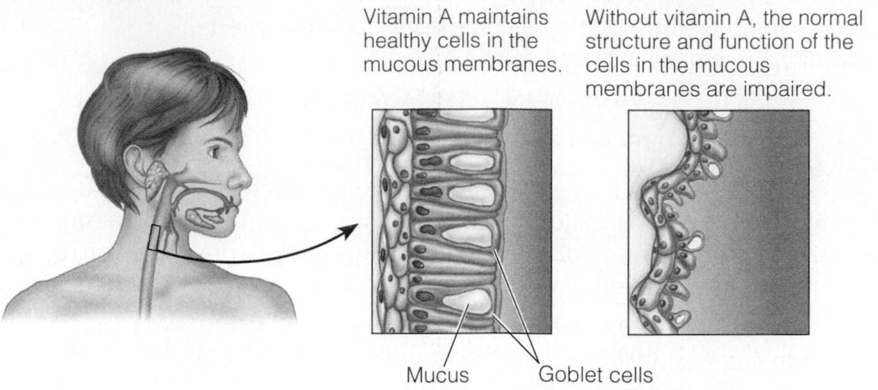
Vitamin A maintains healthy cells in the mucous membranes.
Without vitamin A, the normal structure and function of the cells in the mucous membranes are impaired.
Mucus
Goblet cells

in protein synthesis and **cell differentiation,** a process by which each type of cell develops to perform a specific function.

All body surfaces, both inside and out, are covered by layers of cells known as **epithelial cells.** The **epithelial tissue** on the outside of the body is, of course, the skin. The epithelial tissues that line the inside of the body are the **mucous membranes:** the linings of the mouth, stomach, and intestines; the linings of the lungs and the passages leading to them; the linings of the urinary bladder and urethra; the linings of the uterus and vagina; and the linings of the eyelids and sinus passageways. Within the body, the mucous membranes of the GI tract alone line an area larger than a quarter of a football field, and vitamin A helps to maintain their integrity (see Figure 11-4).

Vitamin A promotes differentiation of both epithelial cells and goblet cells, one-celled glands that synthesize and secrete mucus. Mucus coats and protects the epithelial cells from invasive microorganisms and other harmful substances, such as gastric juices.

Vitamin A in Reproduction and Growth As mentioned, vitamin A also supports reproduction and growth. In men, retinol participates in sperm development, and in women, vitamin A supports normal fetal development during pregnancy. Children lacking vitamin A fail to grow. When given vitamin A supplements, these children gain weight and grow taller.[5]

The growth of bones illustrates that growth is a complex phenomenon of **remodeling.** To convert a small bone into a large bone, the bone-remodeling cells must "undo" some parts of the bone as they go,■ and vitamin A participates in the dismantling. The cells that break down bone contain sacs of degradative enzymes.■ With the help of vitamin A, these enzymes eat away at selected sites in the bone, removing the parts that are not needed.

Beta-Carotene as an Antioxidant In the body, beta-carotene serves primarily as a vitamin A precursor.[6] Not all dietary beta-carotene is converted to active vitamin A, however. Some beta-carotene may act as an antioxidant capable of protecting the body against disease (see Highlight 11 for details).

Vitamin A Deficiency

Vitamin A status depends mostly on the adequacy of vitamin A stores, 90 percent of which are in the liver. Vitamin A status also depends on a person's protein status because retinol-binding proteins serve as the vitamin's transport carriers inside the body.

If a person were to stop eating vitamin A–rich foods, deficiency symptoms would not begin to appear until after stores were depleted—one to two years for a

■ The cells that destroy bone during growth are **osteoclasts**; those that build bone are **osteoblasts.**
- **osteo** = bone
- **clast** = break
- **blast** = build

■ The sacs of degradative enzymes are **lysosomes** (LYE-so-zomes).

cell differentiation (DIF-er-EN-she-AY-shun): the process by which immature cells develop specific functions different from those of the original that are characteristic of their mature cell type.

epithelial (ep-i-THEE-lee-ul) **cells:** cells on the surface of the skin and mucous membranes.

epithelial tissue: the layer of the body that serves as a selective barrier between the body's interior and the environment (examples are the cornea, the skin, the respiratory lining, and the lining of the digestive tract).

mucous (MYOO-kus) **membranes:** the membranes, composed of mucus-secreting cells, that line the surfaces of body tissues.

remodeling: the dismantling and re-formation of a structure, in this case, bone.

healthy adult but much sooner for a growing child. Then the consequences would be profound and severe. Vitamin A deficiency is uncommon in the United States, but it is one of the developing world's major nutrition problems.[7] More than 100 million children worldwide have some degree of vitamin A deficiency, and so are vulnerable to infectious diseases and blindness.

Infectious Diseases In developing countries around the world, measles is a devastating infectious disease, killing as many as 2 million children each year. The severity of the illness often correlates with the degree of vitamin A deficiency; deaths are usually due to related infections such as pneumonia and severe diarrhea.[8] Providing large doses of vitamin A reduces the risk of dying from these infections.

The World Health Organization (WHO) and UNICEF (the United Nations International Children's Emergency Fund) have made the control of vitamin A deficiency a major goal in their quest to improve child health and survival throughout the developing world. They recommend routine vitamin A supplementation for all children with measles in areas where vitamin A deficiency is a problem or where the measles death rate is high. In the United States, the American Academy of Pediatrics recommends vitamin A supplementation for certain groups of measles-infected infants and children. Vitamin A supplementation also protects against the complications of other life-threatening infections, including malaria, lung diseases, and HIV (human immunodeficiency virus, the virus that causes AIDS).[9]

Night Blindness **Night blindness** is one of the first detectable signs of vitamin A deficiency and permits early diagnosis.[10] In night blindness, the retina does not receive enough retinal to regenerate the visual pigments bleached by light. The person loses the ability to recover promptly from the temporary blinding that follows a flash of bright light at night or to see after the lights go out. In many parts of the world, after the sun goes down, vitamin A–deficient people become night-blind: children cannot find their shoes or toys, and women cannot fetch water or wash dishes.[11] They often cling to others or sit still, afraid that they may trip and fall or lose their way if they try to walk alone. In many developing countries, night blindness due to vitamin A deficiency is so common that the people have special words to describe it. In Indonesia, the term is *buta ayam,* which means "chicken eyes" or "chicken blindness." (Chickens do not have the cells of the retina that respond to dim light and therefore cannot see at night.) Figure 11-5 shows the eyes' slow recovery in response to a flash of bright light in night blindness.

Blindness (Xerophthalmia) Beyond night blindness is total blindness—failure to see at all. Night blindness is caused by a lack of vitamin A at the back of the eye, the retina; total blindness is caused by a lack at the front of the eye, the cornea.

night blindness: slow recovery of vision after flashes of bright light at night or an inability to see in dim light; an early symptom of vitamin A deficiency.

FIGURE 11-5 Vitamin A–Deficiency Symptom—Night Blindness

These photographs illustrate the eyes' slow recovery in response to a flash of bright light at night. In animal research studies, the response rate is measured with electrodes.

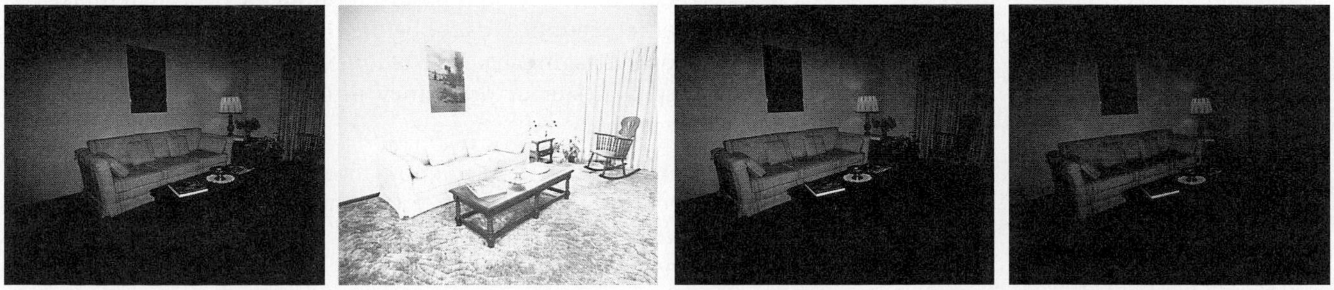

In dim light, you can make out the details in this room. You are using your rods for vision.

A flash of bright light momentarily blinds you as the pigment in the rods is bleached.

You quickly recover and can see the details again in a few seconds.

With inadequate vitamin A, you do not recover but remain blinded for many seconds.

FIGURE 11-6 Vitamin A–Deficiency Symptom—The Rough Skin of Keratinization

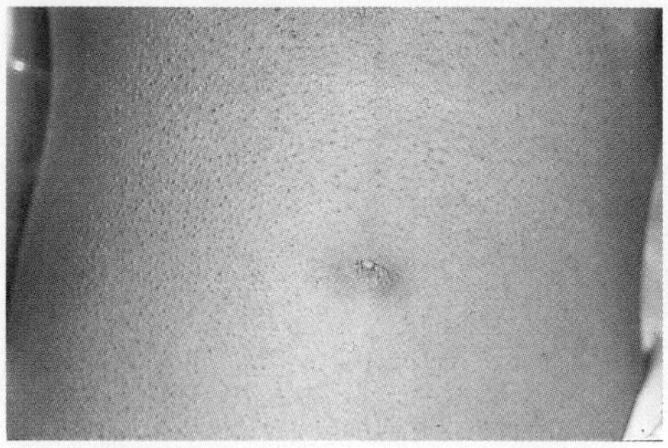

Ken Greer/Visuals Unlimited

In vitamin A deficiency, the epithelial cells secrete the protein keratin in a process known as *keratinization.* (Keratinization doesn't occur in the GI tract, but mucus-producing cells dwindle, and mucus production declines.) The progression of this condition to the extreme is *hyperkeratinization* or *hyperkeratosis.* When keratin accumulates around each hair follicle, the condition is known as *follicular hyperkeratosis.*

Severe vitamin A deficiency is the major cause of childhood blindness in the world, causing more than half a million preschool children to lose their sight each year.[12] Blindness due to vitamin A deficiency, known as **xerophthalmia,** develops in stages. First, the cornea becomes dry and hard, a condition known as **xerosis.** Corneal xerosis can quickly progress to **keratomalacia,** the softening of the cornea that leads to irreversible blindness.

Keratinization Elsewhere in the body, vitamin A deficiency affects other surfaces. Without vitamin A, the goblet cells in the GI tract diminish in number and activity, limiting the secretion of mucus. With less mucus, normal digestion and absorption of nutrients falter, and this, in turn, worsens malnutrition by limiting the absorption of whatever nutrients the diet may deliver. Similar changes in the cells of other epithelial tissues weaken defenses, making infections of the respiratory tract, the GI tract, the urinary tract, the vagina, and possibly the inner ear likely. On the body's outer surface, the epithelial cells change shape and begin to secrete the protein **keratin**—the hard, inflexible protein of hair and nails. As Figure 11-6 shows, the skin becomes dry, rough, and scaly as lumps of keratin accumulate **(keratinization).**

Vitamin A Toxicity

Just as a deficiency of vitamin A affects all body systems, so does a toxicity. Symptoms of toxicity begin to develop when all the binding proteins are swamped, and free vitamin A damages the cells. Such effects are unlikely when a person depends on a balanced diet for nutrients, but with concentrated amounts of **preformed vitamin A** from foods derived from animals, fortified foods, or supplements, toxicity is a real possibility. Children are most vulnerable to toxicity because they need less and are more sensitive to overdoses. An Upper Level has been set for preformed vitamin A (see inside front cover).

Beta-carotene, which is found in a wide variety of fruits and vegetables, is not converted efficiently enough in the body to cause vitamin A toxicity; instead, it is stored in the fat just under the skin. Overconsumption of beta-carotene from foods may turn the skin yellow, but this is not harmful (see Figure 11-7).[13] In contrast, overconsumption of beta-carotene from supplements may be quite harmful. In excess, this antioxidant may act as a prooxidant, promoting cell division and destroying vitamin A.[14] Furthermore, the adverse effects of beta-carotene supplements are most evident in people who drink alcohol and smoke cigarettes.[15]

Bone Defects Excessive amounts of vitamin A over the years may weaken the bones and contribute to osteoporosis.[16] People consuming large amounts of vitamin A either from supplements or from foods containing retinol have a significantly greater risk of hip fractures.[17] Such findings suggest that most people should not take vitamin A supplements. Even multivitamin supplements■ provide more vitamin A than most people need.[18]

Birth Defects Excessive vitamin A poses a **teratogenic** risk. High intakes (10,000 IU■ of supplemental vitamin A daily) before the seventh week of pregnancy appear to be the most damaging. For this reason, vitamin A is not given as a supplement in the first trimester of pregnancy unless there is specific evidence of deficiency, which is rare.

Not for Acne Adolescents need to know that massive doses of vitamin A have no beneficial effect on **acne.** The prescription medicine Accutane is made from vitamin A but is chemically different. Taken orally, Accutane is effective against the deep lesions of cystic acne. It is highly toxic, however, especially during growth, and has caused birth defects in infants when women have taken it during their pregnancies. For this reason, women taking Accutane must begin using an effective form of contraception at least one month before taking the drug and continue using contraception at least one month after discontinuing its use.

■ Multivitamin supplements typically provide:
- 750 µg (2500 IU).
- 1500 µg (5000 IU).

For perspective, the RDA for vitamin A is 700 µg for women and 900 µg for men.

■ For perspective, 10,000 IU ≈ 3000 µg vitamin A, roughly four times the RDA for women.

xerophthalmia (zer-off-THAL-mee-uh): progressive blindness caused by severe vitamin A deficiency.
- **xero** = dry
- **ophthalm** = eye

xerosis (zee-ROW-sis): abnormal drying of the skin and mucous membranes; a sign of vitamin A deficiency.

keratomalacia (KARE-ah-toe-ma-LAY-shuh): softening of the cornea that leads to irreversible blindness; seen in severe vitamin A deficiency.

keratin (KARE-uh-tin): a water-insoluble protein; the normal protein of hair and nails. Keratin-producing cells may replace mucus-producing cells in vitamin A deficiency.

keratinization: accumulation of keratin in a tissue; a sign of vitamin A deficiency.

preformed vitamin A: dietary vitamin A in its active form.

teratogenic (ter-AT-oh-jen-ik): causing abnormal fetal development and birth defects.
- **terato** = monster
- **genic** = to produce

Another vitamin A relative, Retin-A, fights acne, the wrinkles of aging, and other skin disorders. Applied topically, this ointment smooths and softens skin; it also lightens skin that has become darkly pigmented after inflammation. During treatment, the skin becomes red and tender and peels.

Vitamin A Recommendations

Because the body can derive vitamin A from various retinoids and carotenoids, its contents in foods and its recommendations are expressed as **retinol activity equivalents (RAE).** A microgram of retinol counts as 1 RAE,■ as does 12 micrograms of dietary beta-carotene. Most food and supplement labels report their vitamin A contents using international units (IU),■ an old measure of vitamin activity used before direct chemical analysis was possible.

Vitamin A in Foods

The richest sources of the retinoids are foods derived from animals—liver, fish liver oils, milk and milk products, butter, and eggs. Since vitamin A is fat soluble, it is lost when milk is skimmed. To compensate, reduced-fat and fat-free milks are often fortified so as to supply 6 to 10 percent of the Daily Value per cup.* Margarine is usually fortified so as to provide the same amount of vitamin A as butter.

Plants contain no retinoids, but many vegetables and some fruits contain vitamin A precursors—the carotenoids, red and yellow pigments of plants. Only a few carotenoids have vitamin A activity; the carotenoid with the greatest vitamin A activity is beta-carotene.

The Colors of Vitamin A Foods The dark leafy greens (like spinach—not celery or cabbage) and the rich yellow or deep orange vegetables and fruits (such as winter squash, cantaloupe, carrots, and sweet potatoes—not corn or bananas) help people meet their vitamin A needs (see Figure 11-8 on p. 374). A diet including several servings of such carotene-rich sources helps to ensure a sufficient intake.

An attractive meal that includes foods of different colors most likely supplies vitamin A as well. Most foods with vitamin A activity are brightly colored—green, yellow, orange, and red. Any plant food with significant vitamin A activity must have some color, since beta-carotene is a rich, deep yellow, almost orange compound. The beta-carotene in dark green, leafy vegetables is abundant but masked by large amounts of the green pigment **chlorophyll.**

Bright color is not always a sign of vitamin A activity, however. Beets and corn, for example, derive their colors from the red and yellow **xanthophylls,** which have no vitamin A activity. As for white plant foods such as potatoes, cauliflower, pasta, and rice, they also offer little or no vitamin A.

Vitamin A–Poor Fast Foods Fast foods often lack vitamin A. Anyone who dines frequently on hamburgers, french fries, and colas would be wise to emphasize colorful vegetables and fruits at other meals.

Vitamin A–Rich Liver People sometimes wonder if eating liver too frequently can cause vitamin A toxicity. Liver is a rich source because vitamin A is stored there in animals, just as in humans.† Arctic explorers who have eaten large quantities of polar bear liver have become ill with symptoms suggesting vitamin A toxicity, as have young children who regularly ate a chicken liver spread that provided three times their daily recommended intake. Liver offers many nutrients, and eating it periodically may improve a person's nutrition status, but caution is warranted not to eat too

*Vitamin A fortification of milk in the United States is required to a level found in whole milk (1200 IU per quart), but many manufacturers commonly fortify to a higher level (2000 IU per quart). Similarly, in Canada all milk that has had fat removed must be fortified with vitamin A.

†The liver is not the only organ that stores vitamin A. The kidneys, adrenals, and other organs do, too, but the liver stores the most and is the one most commonly eaten.

FIGURE 11-7 Symptom of Beta-Carotene Excess—Discoloration of the Skin

The hand on the right shows the skin discoloration that occurs when blood levels of beta-carotene rise in response to a low-kcalorie diet that features carrots, pumpkins, and orange juice. (The hand on the left belongs to someone else and is shown for comparison.)

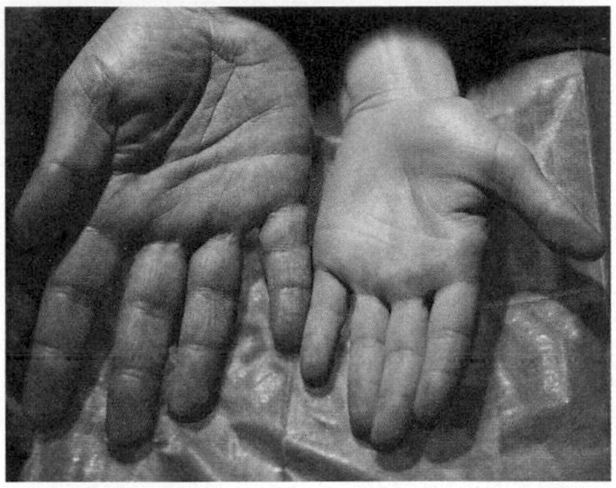

■ 1 μg RAE = 1 μg retinol.
= 2 μg beta-carotene (supplement).
= 12 μg beta-carotene (dietary).
= 24 μg of other vitamin A precursor carotenoids.

■ 1 IU retinol = 0.3 μg retinol or 0.3 μg RAE.
1 IU beta-carotene (supplement) = 0.5 IU retinol or 0.15 μg RAE.
1 IU beta-carotene (dietary) = 0.165 IU retinol or 0.05 μg RAE.
1 IU other vitamin A precursor carotenoids = 0.025 μg RAE.

acne: a chronic inflammation of the skin's follicles and oil-producing glands, which leads to an accumulation of oils inside the ducts that surround hairs; usually associated with the maturation of young adults.

retinol activity equivalents (RAE): a measure of vitamin A activity; the amount of retinol that the body will derive from a food containing preformed retinol or its precursor beta-carotene.

chlorophyll (KLO-row-fil): the green pigment of plants, which absorbs light and transfers the energy to other molecules, thereby initiating photosynthesis.

xanthophylls (ZAN-tho-fills): pigments found in plants; responsible for the color changes seen in autumn leaves.

FIGURE 11-8 Vitamin A in Selected Foods

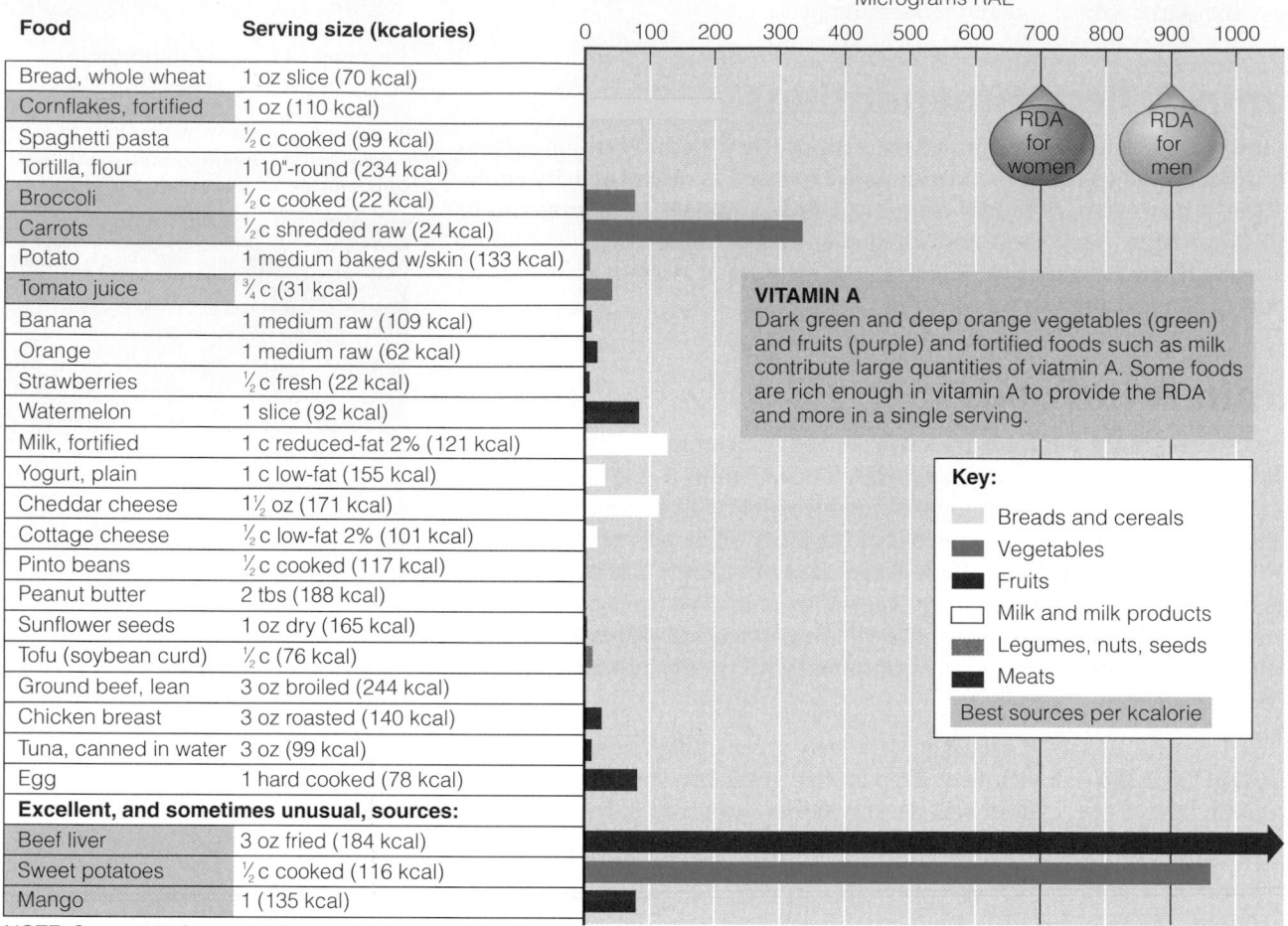

Food	Serving size (kcalories)
Bread, whole wheat	1 oz slice (70 kcal)
Cornflakes, fortified	1 oz (110 kcal)
Spaghetti pasta	½ c cooked (99 kcal)
Tortilla, flour	1 10"-round (234 kcal)
Broccoli	½ c cooked (22 kcal)
Carrots	½ c shredded raw (24 kcal)
Potato	1 medium baked w/skin (133 kcal)
Tomato juice	¾ c (31 kcal)
Banana	1 medium raw (109 kcal)
Orange	1 medium raw (62 kcal)
Strawberries	½ c fresh (22 kcal)
Watermelon	1 slice (92 kcal)
Milk, fortified	1 c reduced-fat 2% (121 kcal)
Yogurt, plain	1 c low-fat (155 kcal)
Cheddar cheese	1½ oz (171 kcal)
Cottage cheese	½ c low-fat 2% (101 kcal)
Pinto beans	½ c cooked (117 kcal)
Peanut butter	2 tbs (188 kcal)
Sunflower seeds	1 oz dry (165 kcal)
Tofu (soybean curd)	½ c (76 kcal)
Ground beef, lean	3 oz broiled (244 kcal)
Chicken breast	3 oz roasted (140 kcal)
Tuna, canned in water	3 oz (99 kcal)
Egg	1 hard cooked (78 kcal)
Excellent, and sometimes unusual, sources:	
Beef liver	3 oz fried (184 kcal)
Sweet potatoes	½ c cooked (116 kcal)
Mango	1 (135 kcal)

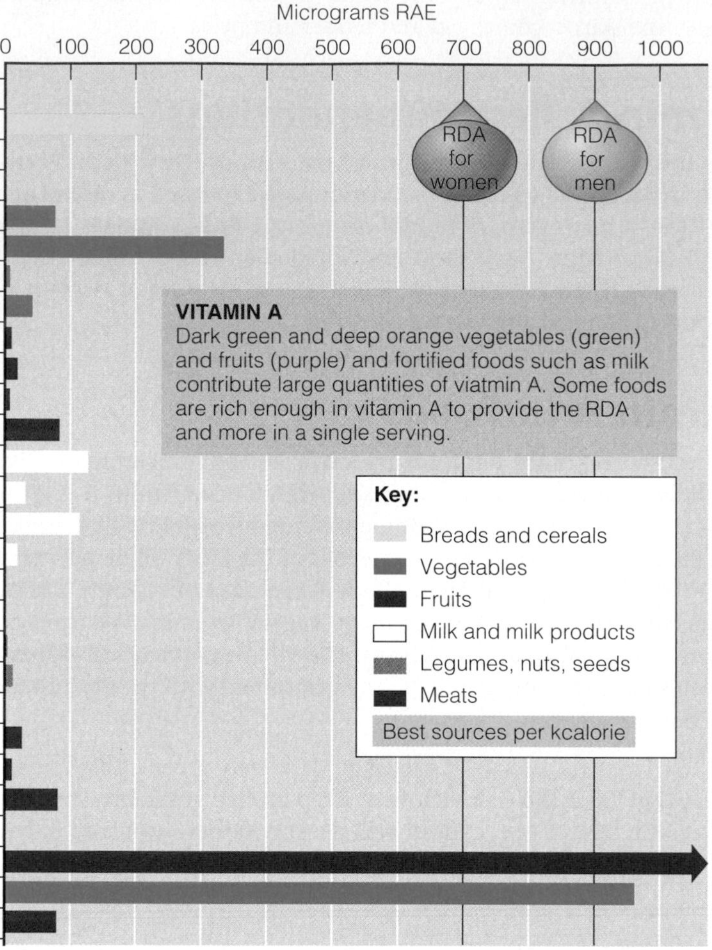
Micrograms RAE
0 100 200 300 400 500 600 700 800 900 1000
RDA for women
RDA for men
VITAMIN A
Dark green and deep orange vegetables (green) and fruits (purple) and fortified foods such as milk contribute large quantities of viatmin A. Some foods are rich enough in vitamin A to provide the RDA and more in a single serving.
Key:
Breads and cereals
Vegetables
Fruits
Milk and milk products
Legumes, nuts, seeds
Meats
Best sources per kcalorie

NOTE: See p. 327 for more information on using this figure.

much too often, especially for pregnant women. With one ounce of beef liver providing more than three times the RDA for vitamin A, intakes can rise quickly.

IN SUMMARY Vitamin A is found in the body in three forms: retinol, retinal, and retinoic acid. Together, they are essential to vision, healthy epithelial tissues, and growth. Vitamin A deficiency is a major health problem worldwide, leading to infections, blindness, and keratinization. Toxicity can also cause problems and is most often associated with supplement abuse. Animal-derived foods such as liver and milk provide retinoids, whereas brightly colored plant-derived foods such as spinach, carrots, and pumpkins provide beta-carotene and other carotenoids. In addition to serving as a precursor for vitamin A, beta-carotene may act as an antioxidant in the body. The accompanying table summarizes vitamin A's functions in the body, deficiency symptoms, toxicity symptoms, and food sources.

Vitamin A

Other Names	2001 RDA
Retinol, retinal, retinoic acid; precursors are carotenoids such as beta-carotene	Men: 900 μg RAE/day Women: 700 μg RAE/day

(continued)

Vitamin A (continued)

Upper Level

Adults: 3000 µg/day

Chief Functions in the Body

Vision; maintenance of cornea, epithelial cells, mucous membranes, skin; bone and tooth growth; reproduction; immunity

Significant Sources

Retinol: fortified milk, cheese, cream, butter, fortified margarine, eggs, liver

Beta-carotene: spinach and other dark leafy greens; broccoli, deep orange fruits (apricots, cantaloupe) and vegetables (squash, carrots, sweet potatoes, pumpkin)

Deficiency Disease

Hypovitaminosis A

Deficiency Symptoms

Night blindness, corneal drying (xerosis), triangular gray spots on eye (Bitot's spots), softening of the cornea (keratomalacia), and corneal degeneration and blindness (xerophthalmia); impaired immunity (infectious diseases); plugging of hair follicles with keratin, forming white lumps (hyperkeratosis)

Toxicity Disease

Hypervitaminosis A[a]

Chronic Toxicity Symptoms

Increased activity of osteoclasts[b] causing reduced bone density; liver abnormalities; birth defects

Acute Toxicity Symptoms

Blurred vision, nausea, vomiting, vertigo; increase of pressure inside skull, mimicking brain tumor; headaches

[a] A related condition, *hypercarotenemia,* is caused by the accumulation of too much of the vitamin A precursor beta-carotene in the blood, which turns the skin noticeably yellow. Hypercarotenemia is not, strictly speaking, a toxicity symptom.
[b] *Osteoclasts* are the cells that destroy bone during its growth. Those that build bone are *osteoblasts.*

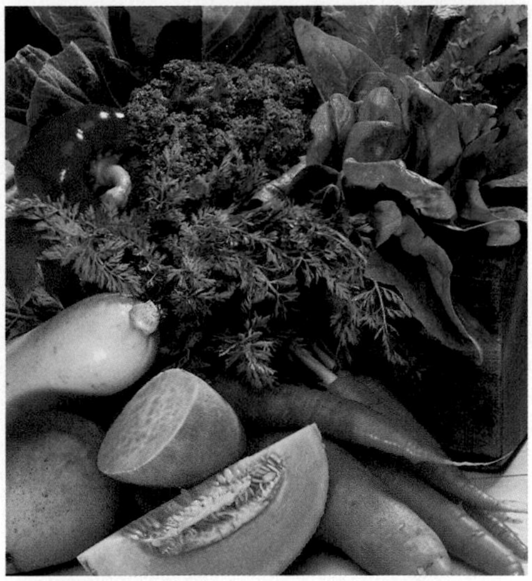

The carotenoids in foods bring colors to meals; the retinoids in our eyes allow us to see them.

Vitamin D

Vitamin D (calciferol)■ is different from all the other nutrients in that the body can synthesize it, with the help of sunlight, from a precursor that the body makes from cholesterol. Therefore, vitamin D is not an essential nutrient: given enough time in the sun, people need no vitamin D from foods.[19]

■ Vitamin D comes in many forms, the two most important being a plant version called **vitamin D_2** or **ergocalciferol** (ER-go-kal-SIF-er-ol) and an animal version called **vitamin D_3** or **cholecalciferol** (KO-lee-kal-SIF-er-ol).

Figure 11-9 (on p. 376) diagrams the pathway for making and activating vitamin D. Ultraviolet rays from the sun hit the precursor in the skin and convert it to previtamin D_3. This compound works its way into the body and slowly, over the next 36 hours, is converted to its active form with the help of the body's heat. The biological activity of the active vitamin is 500- to 1000-fold greater than that of its precursor.

Regardless of whether the body manufactures vitamin D_3 or obtains it directly from foods, two hydroxylation reactions must occur before the vitamin becomes fully active. First, the liver adds an OH group, and then the kidneys add another OH group to produce the active vitamin. A review of Figure 11-9 reveals how diseases affecting either the liver or the kidneys can interfere with the activation of vitamin D and produce symptoms of deficiency.

Roles in the Body

Though called a vitamin, vitamin D is actually a hormone—a compound manufactured by one part of the body that causes another part to respond. Like vitamin A, vitamin D has a binding protein that carries it to the target organs—most notably, the intestines, the kidneys, and the bones. All respond to vitamin D by making the bone minerals available.

Vitamin D in Bone Growth Vitamin D is a member of a large and cooperative bone-making and maintenance team composed of nutrients and other compounds, including vitamins A, C, and K; the hormones parathormone and calcitonin; the protein collagen; and the minerals calcium, phosphorus, magnesium,

FIGURE 11-9 Vitamin D Synthesis and Activation

The precursor of vitamin D is made in the liver from cholesterol (see Figure 5-11 on p. 150 and Appendix C). The activation of vitamin D is a closely regulated process. The final product, active vitamin D, is also known as1,25-dihydroxycholecalciferol (or calcitriol).

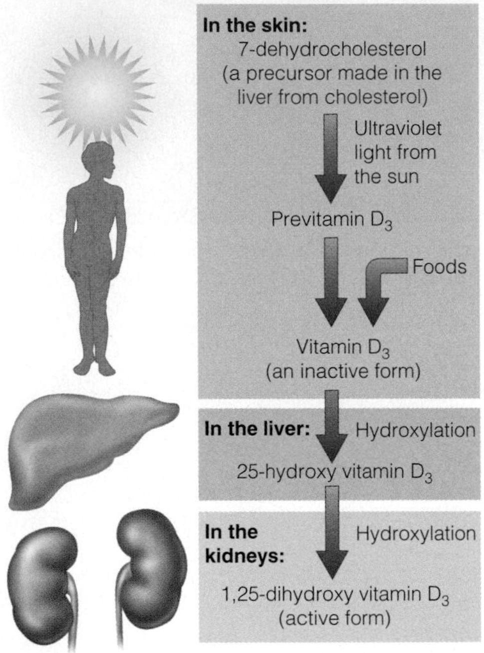
In the skin:
7-dehydrocholesterol (a precursor made in the liver from cholesterol)
Ultraviolet light from the sun
Previtamin D3
Foods
Vitamin D3 (an inactive form)
In the liver:
Hydroxylation
25-hydroxy vitamin D3
In the kidneys:
Hydroxylation
1,25-dihydroxy vitamin D3 (active form)

■ Because the poorly formed rib attachments resemble rosary beads, this symptom is commonly known as **rachitic** (ra-KIT-it) **rosary** ("the rosary of rickets").

rickets: the vitamin D–deficiency disease in children characterized by inadequate mineralization of bone (manifested in bowed legs or knock-knees, outward-bowed chest, and knobs on ribs). A rare type of rickets, not caused by vitamin D deficiency, is known as *vitamin D–refractory rickets.*

osteomalacia (OS-tee-oh-ma-LAY-shuh): a bone disease characterized by softening of the bones. Symptoms include bending of the spine and bowing of the legs. The disease occurs most often in adult women.
- **osteo** = bone
- **malacia** = softening

and fluoride. Vitamin D's special role in bone growth is to maintain blood concentrations of calcium and phosphorus. The bones grow denser and stronger as they absorb and deposit these minerals.

Vitamin D raises blood concentrations of these minerals in three ways. It enhances their absorption from the GI tract, their reabsorption by the kidneys, and their mobilization from the bones into the blood. The vitamin may work alone, as it does in the GI tract, or in combination with parathormone, as it does in the bones and kidneys. Vitamin D is the director, but the star of the show is calcium. Details of calcium balance appear in Chapter 12.

Vitamin D in Other Roles Scientists have discovered many other vitamin D target tissues, including cells of the immune system, brain and nervous system, pancreas, skin, muscles and cartilage, and reproductive organs. Because vitamin D has numerous functions, it may be valuable in treating a number of disorders. Recent evidence suggests that vitamin D may protect against multiple sclerosis.[20]

Vitamin D Deficiency

Factors that contribute to vitamin D deficiency include dark skin, breastfeeding without supplementation, lack of sunlight, and use of nonfortified milk.[21] In vitamin D deficiency, production of the protein that binds calcium in the intestinal cells slows. Thus, even when calcium in the diet is adequate, it passes through the GI tract unabsorbed, leaving the bones undersupplied. Consequently, a vitamin D deficiency creates a calcium deficiency. Adolescents may not reach their peak bone mass.[22]

Rickets Worldwide, the vitamin D–deficiency disease **rickets** still afflicts many children.[23] The bones fail to calcify normally, causing growth retardation and skeletal abnormalities. The bones become so weak that they bend when they have to support the body's weight (see Figure 11-10). A child with rickets who is old enough to walk characteristically develops bowed legs, often the most obvious sign of the disease. Another sign is the beaded ribs■ that result from the poorly formed attachments of the bones to the cartilage.

Osteomalacia The adult form of rickets, **osteomalacia,** occurs most often in women who have low calcium intakes and little exposure to sun and who go through repeated pregnancies and periods of lactation. Given this combination of risk factors, the leg bones may soften to such an extent that a young woman who is tall and straight at 20 may become bent, bowlegged, and stooped before she is 30.

Osteoporosis Any failure to synthesize adequate vitamin D or obtain enough from foods sets the stage for a loss of calcium from the bones, which can result in fractures. In a group of women with osteoporosis hospitalized for hip fractures, half had an undetected vitamin D deficiency.[24] Highlight 12 describes the many factors that lead to osteoporosis, a condition of reduced bone density.

The Elderly Vitamin D deficiency is especially likely in older adults for several reasons. For one, the skin, liver, and kidneys lose their capacity to make and activate vitamin D with advancing age. For another, older adults typically drink little or no milk—the main dietary source of vitamin D. And finally, older adults typically spend much of the day indoors, and when they do venture outside, many of them cautiously wear protective clothing or apply sunscreen to all sun-exposed areas of their skin. Dark-skinned people living in northern regions are particularly vulnerable.[25] All of these factors increase the likelihood of vitamin D deficiency and its consequences: bone losses and fractures.

Vitamin D Toxicity

Vitamin D clearly illustrates how nutrients in optimal amounts support health, but both inadequacies and excesses cause trouble. Vitamin D is the most likely of the vitamins to have toxic effects when consumed in excessive amounts. The

FIGURE 11-10 Vitamin D–Deficiency Symptoms—Bowed Legs and Beaded Ribs of Rickets

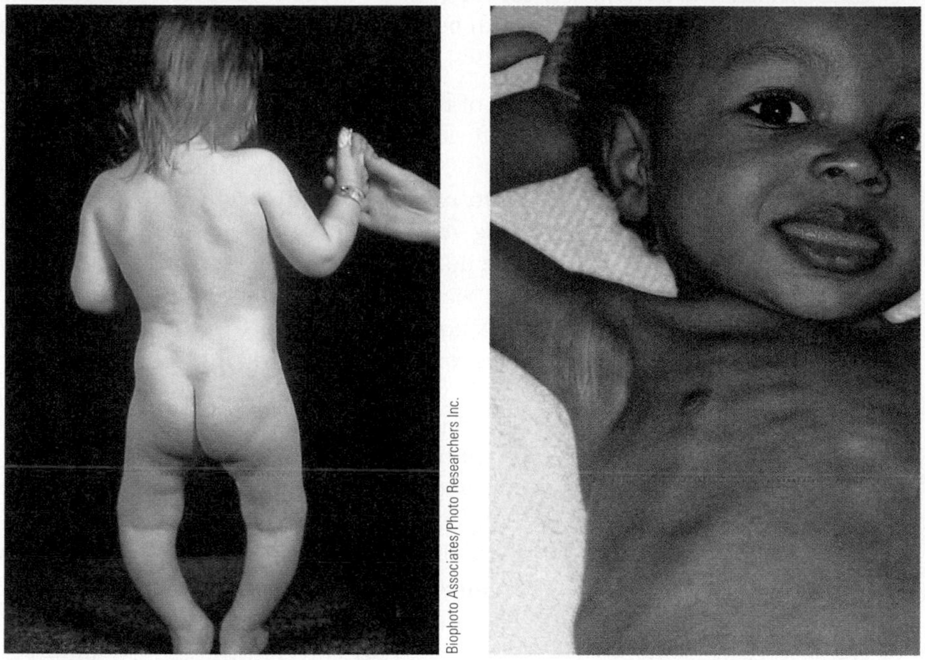

Biophoto Associates/Photo Researchers Inc.

Bowed legs. In rickets, the poorly formed long bones of the legs bend outward as weight-bearing activities such as walking begin.

© Photo Courtesy of Dr. Normal Carvalho at Children's Healthcare of Atlanta

Beaded ribs. In rickets, a series of "beads" develop where the cartilages and bones attach.

amounts of vitamin D made by the skin and found in foods are well within the safe limits set by the Upper Level, but supplements containing the vitamin in concentrated form should be kept out of the reach of children and used cautiously, if at all, by adults.

An excess of vitamin D raises the concentration of blood calcium.■ Excess blood calcium tends to precipitate in the soft tissue, forming stones, especially in the kidneys where calcium is concentrated in the effort to excrete it. Calcification may also harden the blood vessels and is especially dangerous in the major arteries of the heart and lungs, where it can cause death.

■ High blood calcium is known as **hypercalcemia** and may develop from a variety of disorders, including vitamin D toxicity. It does *not* develop from a high calcium intake.

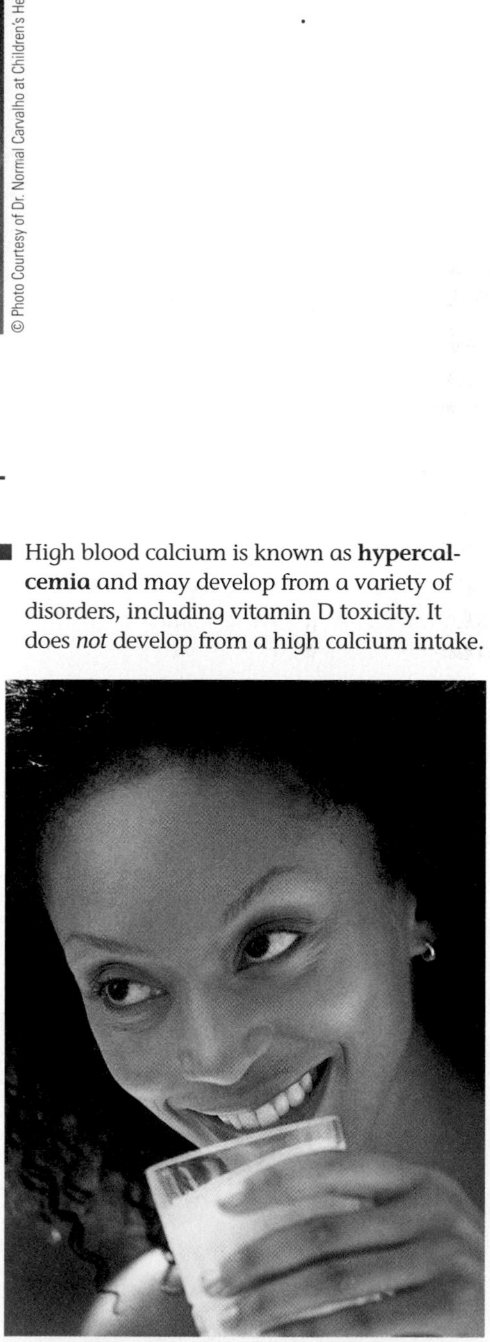

© Francisco Cruz/Super Stock

A cool glass of milk refreshes as it replenishes vitamin D and other bone-building nutrients.

Vitamin D Recommendations and Sources

Only a few foods contain vitamin D naturally. Fortunately, the body can make all the vitamin D it needs with the help of a little sunshine. In setting dietary recommendations, however, the DRI Committee assumed that no vitamin D was available from this source.

Vitamin D in Foods Most adults, especially in sunny regions, need not make special efforts to obtain vitamin D from food. People who are not outdoors much or who live in northern or predominantly cloudy or smoggy areas are advised to drink at least 2 cups of vitamin D–fortified milk a day. The fortification of milk with vitamin D is the best guarantee that people will meet their needs and underscores the importance of milk in a well-balanced diet.* For those who use margarine in place of butter, fortified margarine is also a significant source. A plant

*Vitamin D fortification of milk in the United States is 10 micrograms cholecalciferol (400 IU) per quart; in Canada, 9.6 micrograms (385 IU) per liter.

version of vitamin D may yield an active compound on irradiation, but its contribution is minor. Without adequate sunshine, fortification, or supplementation, a vegan diet cannot meet vitamin D needs. Vegetarians who do not include milk in their diets may use vitamin D–fortified soy milk. Importantly, feeding infants and young children nonfortified "health beverages" instead of milk or infant formula can create severe nutrient deficiencies, including rickets.[26]

Vitamin D from the Sun Most of the world's population relies on natural exposure to sunlight to maintain adequate vitamin D nutrition. The sun imposes no risk of vitamin D toxicity; prolonged exposure to sunlight degrades the vitamin D precursor in the skin, preventing its conversion to the active vitamin. Even lifeguards on southern beaches are safe from vitamin D toxicity from the sun.

Prolonged exposure to sunlight does, however, prematurely wrinkle the skin and present the risk of skin cancer. Sunscreens help reduce these risks, but unfortunately, sunscreens with sun protection factors (SPF) of 8 and higher also prevent vitamin D synthesis. A strategy to avoid this dilemma is to apply sunscreen after enough time has elapsed to provide sufficient vitamin D synthesis. For most people, exposing hands, face, and arms on a clear summer day for 10 to 15 minutes a few times a week should be sufficient to maintain vitamin D nutrition.

The pigments of dark skin provide some protection from the sun's damage, but they also reduce vitamin D synthesis. Dark-skinned people require longer sunlight exposure than light-skinned people: heavily pigmented skin achieves the same amount of vitamin D synthesis in three hours as fair skin in 30 minutes. Latitude, season, and time of day■ also have dramatic effects on vitamin D synthesis (see Figure 11-11). The ultraviolet (UV) rays of the sun that promote vitamin D synthesis are blocked by heavy clouds, smoke, or smog. Differences in skin pigmentation, latitude, and smog may account for the finding that African American people, especially those in northern, smoggy cities, are most likely to develop rickets.[27] For these people, and for those who are unable to go outdoors frequently, dietary vitamin D is essential. Vitamin D stores from summer synthesis alone are insufficient to meet winter needs.[28]

■ Factors that may limit sun exposure and, therefore, vitamin D synthesis:
- Geographic location.
- Season of the year.
- Time of day.
- Air pollution.
- Clothing.
- Tall buildings.
- Indoor living.
- Sunscreens.

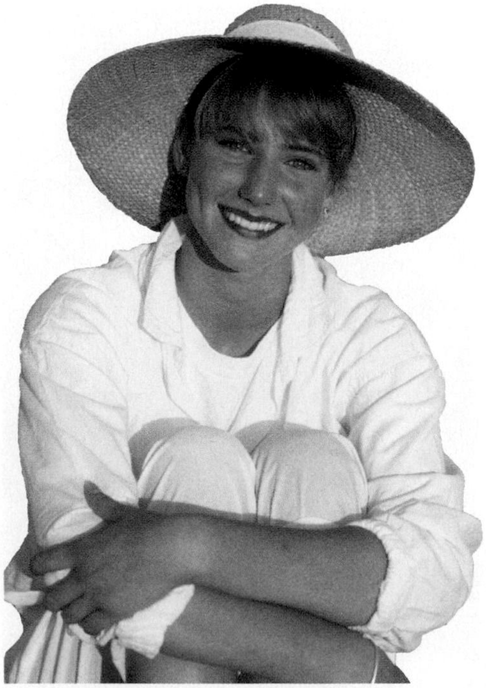

The sunshine vitamin: vitamin D.

FIGURE 11-11 Vitamin D Synthesis and Latitude

Above 40° north latitude (and below 40° south latitude in the southern hemisphere), vitamin D synthesis essentially ceases for the four months of winter. Synthesis increases as spring approaches, peaks in summer, and declines again in the fall. People living in regions of extreme northern (or extreme southern) latitudes may miss as much as six months of vitamin D production.

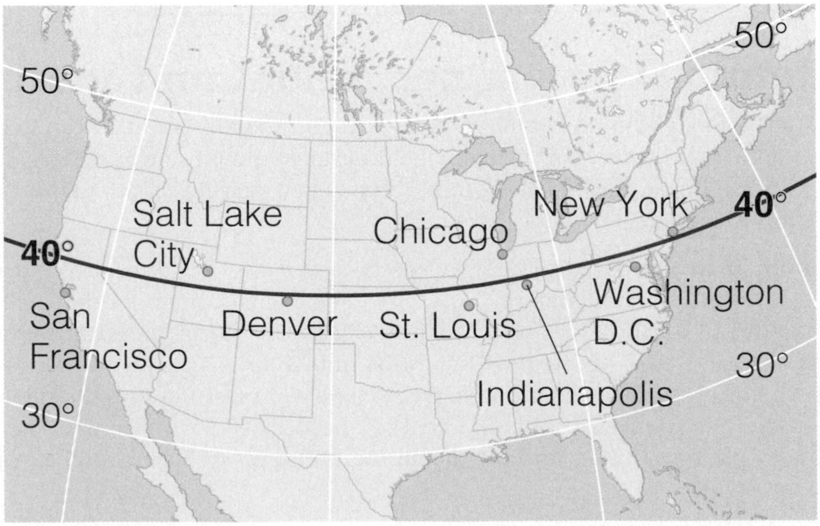
50°
50°
Salt Lake City
Chicago
New York
40°
40°
San Francisco
Denver
St. Louis
Washington D.C.
Indianapolis
30°
30°

Depending on the radiation used, the UV rays from tanning lamps and tanning booths may also stimulate vitamin D synthesis, but the hazards outweigh any possible benefits.* The Food and Drug Administration (FDA) warns that if the lamps are not properly filtered, people using tanning booths risk burns, damage to the eyes and blood vessels, and skin cancer.

IN SUMMARY Vitamin D can be synthesized in the body with the help of sunlight or obtained from foods derived from animals. It sends signals to three primary target sites: the GI tract to absorb more calcium and phosphorus, the bones to release more, and the kidneys to retain more. These actions maintain blood calcium concentrations and support bone formation. A deficiency causes rickets in childhood and osteomalacia in later life. Fortified milk is an important food source. The accompanying table summarizes vitamin D facts.

Vitamin D

Other Names

Calciferol (kal-SIF-er-ol), 1,25-dihydroxy vitamin D (calcitriol); the animal version is vitamin D_3 or cholecalciferol; the plant version is vitamin D_2 or ergocalciferol; precursor is the body's own cholesterol

1997 Adequate Intake (AI)■

Adults: 5 μg/day (19–50 yr)
10 μg/day (51 –70 yr)
15 μg/day (>70 yr)

Upper Level

Adults: 50 μg/day

Chief Functions in the Body

Mineralization of bones (raises blood calcium and phosphorus by increasing absorption from digestive tract, withdrawing calcium from bones, stimulating retention by kidneys)

Significant Sources

Synthesized in the body with the help of sunlight; fortified milk, margarine, butter, cereals, and chocolate mixes; veal, beef, egg yolks, liver, fatty fish (herring, salmon, sardines) and their oils

Deficiency Diseases

Rickets, osteomalacia

Deficiency Symptoms

Rickets in Children

Inadequate calcification, resulting in misshapen bones (bowing of legs); enlargement of ends of long bones (knees, wrists); deformities of ribs (bowed, with beads or knobs);[a] delayed closing of fontanel, resulting in rapid enlargement of head (see figure below); lax muscles resulting in protrusion of abdomen; muscle spasms

Osteomalacia in Adults

Loss of calcium, resulting in soft, flexible, brittle, and deformed bones; progressive weakness; pain in pelvis, lower back, and legs

Toxicity Disease

Hypervitaminosis D

Toxicity Symptoms

Elevated blood calcium; calcification of soft tissues (blood vessels, kidneys, heart, lungs, tisues around joints), frequent urination

Fontanel
A fontanel is an open space in the top of a baby's skull before the bones have grown together. In rickets, closing of the fontanel is delayed.

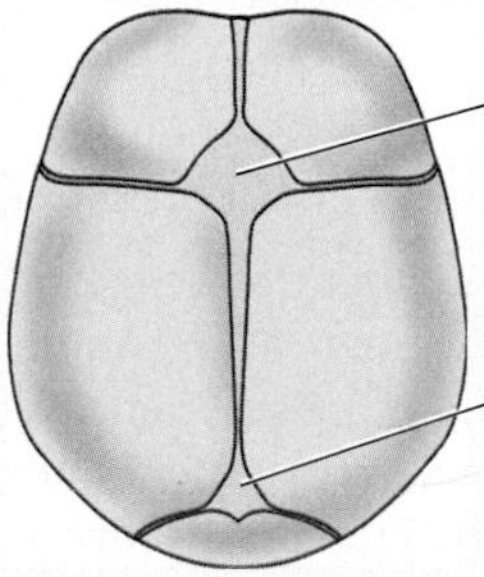
Anterior fontanel normally closes by the end of the second year
Posterior fontanel normally closes by the end of the first year

[a]Bowing of the ribs causes the symptoms known as *pigeon breast*. The beads that form on the ribs resemble rosary beads; thus this symptom is known as *rachitic* (ra-KIT-ik) *rosary* ("the rosary of rickets").

■ Vitamin D activity was previously expressed in international units (IU), but is now expressed in micrograms of cholecalciferol. To convert, use the following factor:
1 IU = 0.025 μg cholecalciferol.

For example:
- 100 IU = 2.5 μg (100 IU × 0.025 μg).
- 400 (IU) = 10 μg (400 IU × 0.025 μg).

*The best wavelengths for vitamin D synthesis are UV-B rays between 290 and 310 nanometers. Some tanning parlors advertise "UV-A rays only, for a tan without the burn," but in fact, UV-A rays can damage the skin.

FIGURE 11-12 Free-Radical Formation and Antioxidant Protection

Free-radical formation and damage

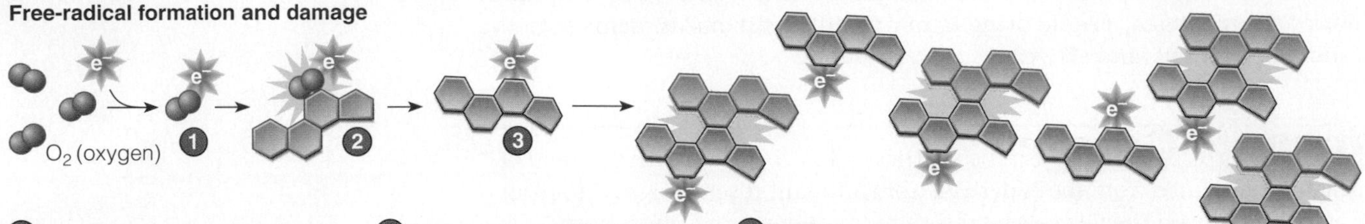
e
O_2 (oxygen)
1
2
3

1 Occasionally, oxygen gains an extra electron from the electron transport chain, thereby generating a free radical.

2 To regain its stability, the free radical attacks a nearby molecule (such as a lipid or protein) and steals an electron.

3 Left with an unpaired electron, this molecule becomes a free radical itself and attacks another nearby molecule. The chain reaction continues, causing widespread damage.

Antioxidant protection

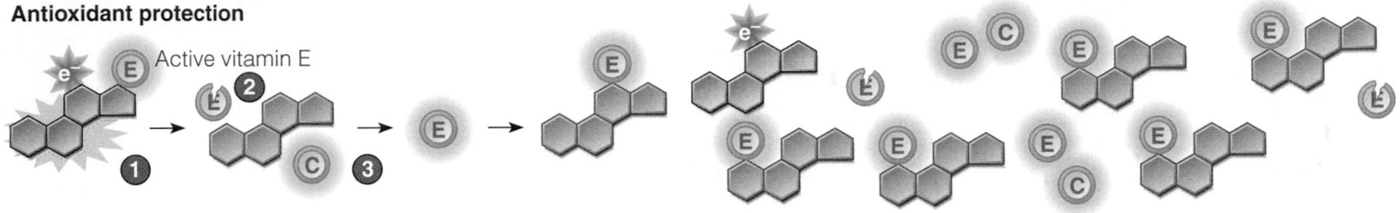
Active vitamin E
E
C
1
2
3

1 Antioxidants, such as vitamin E, neutralize free radicals by donating one of their own electrons.

2 The destructive chain reaction is stopped, but vitamin E is no longer active.

3 Like vitamin E, vitamin C acts as an antioxidant; it also restores vitamin E to its active form. An abundance of dietary antioxidants minimizes free-radical damage.

Available Online

Watch how free radicals damage macromolecules such as proteins, lipids, and DNA in a self-perpetuating chain reaction. Observe how antioxidants stabilize these highly reactive compounds and interrupt this destructive cycle.

Vitamin E

Researchers discovered a component of vegetable oils necessary for reproduction in rats and named this antisterility factor **tocopherol,** which means "to bring forth offspring." When chemists isolated four different tocopherol compounds, they designated them by the first four letters of the Greek alphabet: alpha, beta, gamma, and delta. The tocopherols consist of a complex ring structure and a long saturated side chain (Appendix C provides the chemical structures). The positions of methyl groups (CH_3) on the side chain and their chemical rotations distinguish one tocopherol from another. **Alpha-tocopherol** is the only one with vitamin E activity in the human body.[29] The other tocopherols are not readily converted to alpha-tocopherol in the body, nor do they perform the same roles. Whether these other tocopherols might be beneficial in other ways is the subject of current research.[30]

Vitamin E as an Antioxidant

Vitamin E is a fat-soluble antioxidant and one of the body's primary defenders against the adverse effects of free radicals. Its main action is to stop the chain reaction of free radicals producing more free radicals (see Figure 11-12). In doing so, vitamin E protects the vulnerable components of the cells and their membranes from destruction. Most notably, vitamin E prevents the oxidation of the polyunsaturated fatty acids, but it protects other lipids and related compounds (for example, vitamin A) as well.

Accumulating evidence suggests that vitamin E may reduce the risk of heart disease by protecting low-density lipoproteins (LDL) against oxidation. The oxidation of LDL has been implicated as a key factor in the development of heart disease. Highlight 11 provides many more details on how vitamin E and other antioxidants protect against chronic diseases, such as heart disease and cancer.

tocopherol (tuh-KOFF-er-ol): a general term for several chemically related compounds, one of which has vitamin E activity (see Appendix C for chemical structures).

alpha-tocopherol: the active vitamin E compound.

While research continues to reveal possible roles for vitamin E, it also has clearly discredited claims that vitamin E improves physical performance, enhances sexual performance, or cures sexual dysfunction in males. Vitamin E does not slow or prevent the processes of aging such as hair turning gray or skin wrinkling. Nor does it slow the progression of Parkinson's disease.

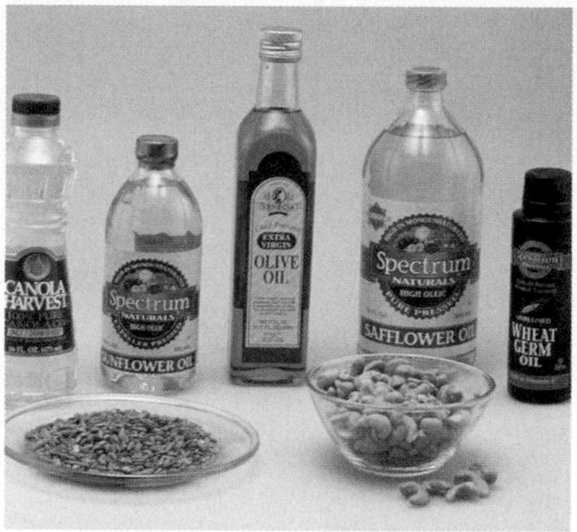
CANOLA HARVEST
Spectrum
OLIVE OIL
Spectrum
SAFFLOWER OIL
WHEAT GERM OIL

© Craig M. Moore

Fat-soluble vitamin E is found predominantly in vegetable oils, seeds, and nuts.

Vitamin E Deficiency

In human beings, a primary deficiency of vitamin E (from a poor intake) is rare; deficiency is usually associated with diseases of fat malabsorption such as cystic fibrosis. Without vitamin E, the red blood cells break open and spill their contents, probably due to oxidation of the polyunsaturated fatty acids in their membranes. This classic sign of vitamin E deficiency, known as **erythrocyte hemolysis,** is seen in premature infants, born before the transfer of vitamin E from the mother to the infant that takes place in the last weeks of pregnancy. Vitamin E treatment corrects **hemolytic anemia.**

Prolonged vitamin E deficiency also causes neuromuscular dysfunction involving the spinal cord and retina of the eye. Common symptoms include loss of muscle coordination and reflexes and impaired vision and speech. Vitamin E treatment corrects these neurological symptoms of vitamin E deficiency, but it does *not* prevent or cure the hereditary **muscular dystrophy** that afflicts children. Children with this condition do not benefit from vitamin E treatment and usually die at an early age when their respiratory muscles deteriorate.

Two other conditions seem to respond to vitamin E treatment, although results are inconsistent. One is a nonmalignant breast disease **(fibrocystic breast disease),** and the other is an abnormality of blood flow that causes cramping in the legs **(intermittent claudication).**

Vitamin E Toxicity

Vitamin E supplement use has risen in recent years as its protective actions against chronic diseases have been recognized. Still, toxicity is rare, and its effects are not as detrimental as with vitamins A and D. The Upper Level for vitamin E (1000 milligrams) is more than 65 times greater than the recommended intake for adults (15 milligrams). Extremely high doses of vitamin E may interfere with the blood-clotting action of vitamin K and enhance the effects of drugs used to oppose blood clotting, causing hemorrhage.

Vitamin E Recommendations

The current RDA for vitamin E differs from previous recommendations in being based on the alpha-tocopherol form only. As mentioned earlier, the other tocopherols cannot be converted to alpha-tocopherol, nor can they perform the same metabolic roles in the body. A person who consumes large quantities of polyunsaturated fatty acids needs more vitamin E. Fortunately, vitamin E and polyunsaturated fatty acids tend to occur together in the same foods.

Vitamin E in Foods

Vitamin E is widespread in foods. Much of the vitamin E in the diet comes from vegetable oils and products made from them, such as margarine and salad dressings. Wheat germ oil is especially rich in vitamin E.

Vitamin E is readily destroyed by heat processing (such as deep-fat frying) and oxidation, so fresh or lightly processed foods are preferable sources. Most processed and convenience foods do not contribute enough vitamin E to ensure an adequate intake.

erythrocyte (eh-RITH-ro-cite) **hemolysis** (he-MOLL-uh-sis): the breaking open of red blood cells (erythrocytes); a symptom of vitamin E–deficiency disease in human beings.
- **erythro** = red
- **cyte** = cell
- **hemo** = blood
- **lysis** = breaking

hemolytic (HE-moh-LIT-ick) **anemia:** the condition of having too few red blood cells as a result of erythrocyte hemolysis.

muscular dystrophy (DIS-tro-fee): a hereditary disease in which the muscles gradually weaken. Its most debilitating effects arise in the lungs.

fibrocystic (FYE-bro-SIS-tik) **breast disease:** a harmless condition in which the breasts develop lumps, sometimes associated with caffeine consumption. In some, it responds to abstinence from caffeine; in others, it can be treated with vitamin E.
- **fibro** = fibrous tissue
- **cyst** = closed sac

intermittent claudication (klaw-dih-KAY-shun): severe calf pain caused by inadequate blood supply. It occurs when walking and subsides during rest.
- **intermittent** = at intervals
- **claudicare** = to limp

■ Appendix H accurately presents vitamin E data in milligrams of alpha-tocopherol.

Prior to 2000, values of the vitamin E in foods reflected all of the various tocopherols and were expressed in "milligrams of tocopherol equivalents."■ These measures overestimated the amount of alpha-tocopherol. To estimate the alpha-tocopherol content of foods stated in tocopherol equivalents, multiply by 0.8.[31]

IN SUMMARY Vitamin E acts as an antioxidant, defending lipids and other components of the cells against oxidative damage. Deficiencies are rare, but do occur in premature infants, the primary symptom being erythrocyte hemolysis. Vitamin E is found predominantly in vegetable oils and appears to be one of the least toxic of the fat-soluble vitamins. The summary table reviews vitamin E's functions, deficiency symptoms, toxicity symptoms, and food sources.

Vitamin E

Other Names

Alpha-tocopherol

2000 RDA

Adults: 15 mg/day

Upper Level

Adults: 1000 mg/day

Chief Functions in the Body

Antioxidant (stabilization of cell membranes, regulation of oxidation reactions, protection of polyunsaturated fatty acids [PUFA] and vitamin A)

Significant Sources

Polyunsaturated plant oils (margarine, salad dressings, shortenings), leafy green vegetables, wheat germ, whole grains, liver, egg yolks, nuts, seeds

Easily destroyed by heat and oxygen

Deficiency Symptoms

Red blood cell breakage,[a] nerve damage

Toxicity Symptoms

Augments the effects of anticlotting medication

[a]The breaking of red blood cells is called *erythrocyte hemolysis*.

Vitamin K

■ *K* stands for the Danish word *koagulation* ("coagulation" or "clotting").

Like vitamin D, vitamin K can be obtained from a nonfood source. Bacteria in the GI tract synthesize vitamin K that the body can absorb. Vitamin K■ acts primarily in blood clotting, where its presence can make the difference between life and death. Blood has a remarkable ability to remain a liquid, but can turn solid within seconds when the integrity of that system is disturbed. (If blood did not clot, a single pinprick could drain the entire body of all its blood, just as a tiny hole in a bucket makes the bucket forever useless for holding water.)

Roles in the Body

More than a dozen different proteins and the mineral calcium are involved in making a blood clot. Vitamin K is essential for the activation of several of these proteins, among them prothrombin, made by the liver as a precursor of the protein thrombin (see Figure 11-13). When any of the blood-clotting factors is lacking, **hemorrhagic disease** results. If an artery or vein is cut or broken, bleeding goes unchecked. (Of course, this is not to say that hemorrhaging is always caused by vitamin K deficiency. Another cause is the hereditary disorder **hemophilia,** which is not curable with vitamin K.)

Vitamin K also participates in the synthesis of bone proteins. Without vitamin K, the bones produce an abnormal protein that cannot bind to the minerals that normally form bones; bone density is low.[32] An adequate intake of vitamin K helps to make the bone protein correctly and protect against hip fractures.[33]

hemorrhagic (hem-oh-RAJ-ik) **disease:** a disease characterized by excessive bleeding.

hemophilia (HE-moh-FEEL-ee-ah): a hereditary disease that is caused by a genetic defect and has no relation to vitamin K. The blood is unable to clot because it lacks the ability to synthesize certain clotting factors.

FIGURE 11-13 Blood-Clotting Process

When blood is exposed to air, foreign substances, or secretions from injured tissues, platelets (small, cell-like structures in the blood) release a phospholipid known as thromboplastin. Thromboplastin catalyzes the conversion of the inactive protein prothrombin to the active enzyme thrombin. Thrombin then catalyzes the conversion of the precursor protein fibrinogen to the active protein fibrin that forms the clot.

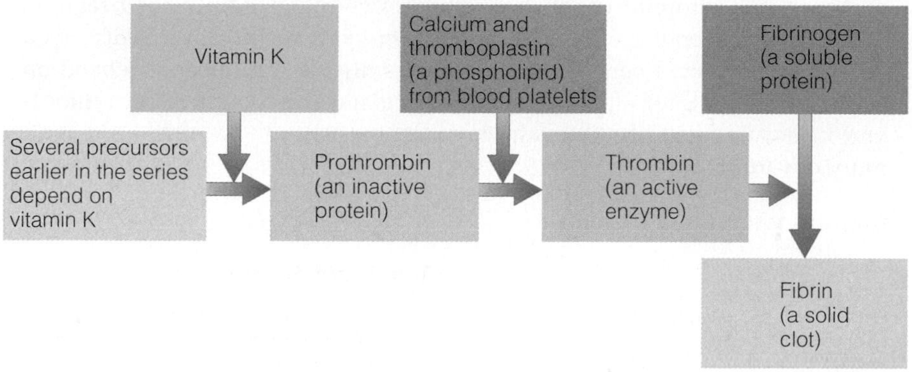
Vitamin K
Calcium and thromboplastin (a phospholipid) from blood platelets
Fibrinogen (a soluble protein)
Several precursors earlier in the series depend on vitamin K
Prothrombin (an inactive protein)
Thrombin (an active enzyme)
Fibrin (a solid clot)

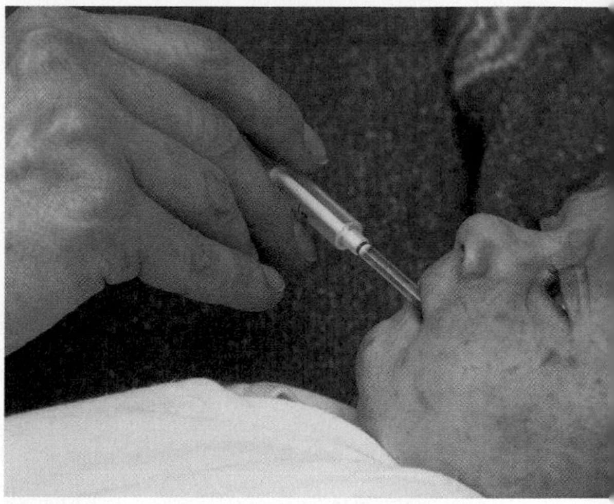

Soon after birth, newborn infants receive a dose of vitamin K to prevent hemorrhagic disease.

Vitamin K is historically known for its role in blood clotting, and more recently for its participation in bone building, but researchers continue to discover proteins needing vitamin K's assistance. These proteins have been identified in the plaques of atherosclerosis, the kidneys, and the nervous system.

Vitamin K Deficiency

A primary deficiency■ of vitamin K is rare, but a secondary deficiency may occur in two circumstances. First, whenever fat absorption falters, as occurs when bile production fails, vitamin K absorption diminishes. Second, some drugs disrupt vitamin K's synthesis and action in the body: antibiotics kill the vitamin K–producing bacteria in the intestine, and anticoagulant drugs interfere with vitamin K metabolism and activity. When vitamin K deficiency does occur, it can be fatal.

Newborn infants present a unique case of vitamin K nutrition because they are born with a **sterile** intestinal tract, and the vitamin K–producing bacteria take weeks to establish themselves. At the same time, plasma prothrombin concentrations are low (this reduces the likelihood of fatal blood clotting during the stress of birth). To prevent hemorrhagic disease in the newborn, a single dose of vitamin K■ (usually as the naturally occurring form, phylloquinone) is given at birth either orally or by intramuscular injection. Concerns that vitamin K given at birth raises the risks of childhood cancer are unproved and unlikely.

■ Reminder: A *primary deficiency* develops in response to an inadequate dietary intake whereas a *secondary deficiency* occurs for other reasons.

■ The natural form of vitamin K is **phylloquinone** (FILL-oh-KWIN-own); the synthetic form is **menadione** (men-uh-DYE-own). See Appendix C for the chemistry of these structures.

Vitamin K Toxicity

Toxicity is not common, and no adverse effects have been reported with high intakes of vitamin K. Therefore, an Upper Level has not been established. High doses of vitamin K can reduce the effectiveness of anticoagulant drugs used to prevent blood clotting. People taking these drugs should eat vitamin K–rich foods in moderation and keep their intakes consistent from day to day.

Vitamin K Recommendations and Sources

As mentioned earlier, vitamin K is made in the GI tract by the billions of bacteria that normally reside there. Once synthesized, vitamin K is absorbed and stored in the liver. This source provides only about half of a person's needs. Vitamin K–rich

sterile: free of microorganisms, such as bacteria.

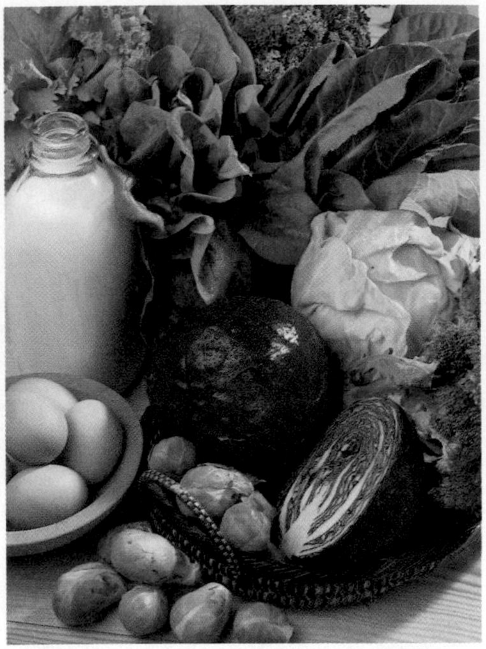
© Polara Studios Inc.

Notable food sources of vitamin K include milk, eggs, brussels sprouts, collards, liver, cabbage, spinach, and broccoli.

foods such as liver, leafy green vegetables, and members of the cabbage family can easily supply the rest. Milk, meats, eggs, cereals, fruits, and vegetables provide smaller, but still significant, amounts.

IN SUMMARY Vitamin K helps with blood clotting, and its deficiency causes hemorrhagic disease (uncontrolled bleeding). Bacteria in the GI tract can make the vitamin; people typically receive about half of their requirements from bacterial synthesis and half from foods such as liver, leafy green vegetables, and members of the cabbage family. Because people depend on bacterial synthesis for vitamin K, deficiency is most likely in newborn infants and in people taking antibiotics. The accompanying table provides a summary of vitamin K facts.

Vitamin K

Other Names

Phylloquinone, menaquinone, menadione, naphthoquinone

2001 AI

Men: 120 μg/day

Women: 90 μg/day

Chief Functions in the Body

Synthesis of blood-clotting proteins and bone proteins

Significant Sources

Bacterial synthesis in the digestive tract;[a] liver; leafy green vegetables, cabbage-type vegetables; milk

Deficiency Symptoms

Hemorrhaging

Toxicity Symptoms

None known

[a]Vitamin K needs cannot be met from bacterial synthesis alone; however, it is a potentially important source in the small intestine, where absorption efficiency ranges from 40 to 70 percent.

The Fat-Soluble Vitamins—In Summary

The four fat-soluble vitamins play many specific roles in the growth and maintenance of the body. Their presence affects the health and function of the eyes, skin, GI tract, lungs, bones, teeth, nervous system, and blood; their deficiencies become apparent in these same areas. Toxicities of the fat-soluble vitamins are possible, especially when people use supplements, because the body stores excesses.

As with the water-soluble vitamins, the function of one fat-soluble vitamin often depends on the presence of another. Recall that vitamin E protects vitamin A from oxidation. In vitamin E deficiency, vitamin A absorption and storage are impaired. Three of the four fat-soluble vitamins—A, D, and K—play important roles in bone growth and remodeling. As mentioned, vitamin K helps synthesize a specific bone protein, and vitamin D regulates that synthesis. Vitamin A, in turn, may control which bone-building genes respond to vitamin D.

Fat-soluble vitamins also interact with minerals: vitamin D and calcium cooperate in bone formation; and zinc is required for the synthesis of vitamin A's transport protein, retinol-binding protein. Zinc also assists the enzyme that regenerates retinal from retinol in the eye.

The roles of the fat-soluble vitamins differ from those of the water-soluble vitamins, and they appear in different foods, yet they are just as essential to life. The need for them underlines the importance of eating a wide variety of nourishing foods daily. The following table condenses the information on fat-soluble vitamins into a short summary.

IN SUMMARY The Fat-Soluble Vitamins

Vitamin and Chief Functions	Deficiency Symptoms	Toxicity Symptoms	Significant Sources
Vitamin A Vision; maintenance of cornea, epithelial cells, mucous membranes, skin; bone and tooth growth; reproduction; immunity	Infectious diseases, night blindness, blindness (xerophthalmia), keratinization	Reduced bone mineral density, liver abnormalities, birth defects	Retinol: milk and milk products Beta-carotene: dark green leafy and deep yellow/orange vegetables
Vitamin D Mineralization of bones (raises blood calcium and phosphorus by increasing absorption from digestive tract, withdrawing calcium from bones, stimulating retention by kidneys)	Rickets, osteomalacia	Calcium imbalance (calcification of soft tisues and formation of stones)	Synthesized in the body with the help of sunshine; fortified milk
Vitamin E Antioxidant (stabilization of cell membranes, regulation of oxidation reactions, protection of polyunsaturated fatty acids [PUFA] and vitamin A)	Erythrocyte hemolysis, nerve damage	Hemorrhagic effects	Vegetable oils
Vitamin K Synthesis of blood-clotting proteins and bone proteins	Hemorrhage	None known	Synthesized in the body by GI bacteria; green leafy vegetables

Nutrition in Your Life

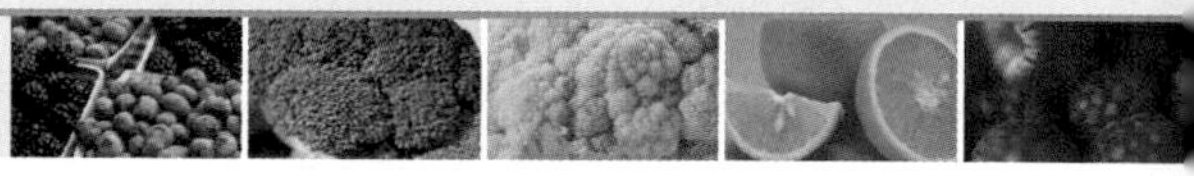

For the fat-soluble vitamins, select colorful fruits and vegetables, fortified milk or soy products, and vegetable oils; use supplements with caution, if at all.

- **Do you eat dark green, leafy or deep yellow vegetables daily?**
- **Do you drink vitamin D–fortified milk or go outside in the sunshine regularly?**
- **Do you use vegetable oils when you cook?**

NUTRITION ON THE NET

Access these websites for further study of topics covered in this chapter. Be aware that many websites on the Internet are peddling vitamin supplements, not accurate information.

- Find updates and quick links to these and other nutrition-related sites at our website: **www.wadsworth.com/nutrition**
- Search for "vitamins" at the American Dietetic Association: **www.eatright.org**
- Review the Dietary Reference Intakes for vitamins A, D, E, and K and the carotenoids by searching for "DRI": **www.nap.edu**
- Visit the World Health Organization to learn about "vitamin deficiencies" around the world: **www.who.int**
- Search for "vitamins" at the U.S. Government health information site: **www.healthfinder.gov**
- Learn how fruits and vegetables support a healthy diet rich in vitamins from the 5 A Day for Better Health program: **www.5aday.com** or **www.5aday.gov**

NUTRITION CALCULATIONS

These exercises will help you learn the best food sources for the vitamins and prepare you to examine your own food choices. See p. 388 for answers.

1. Review the units in which vitamins are measured (a spot check). For each of these vitamins, note the unit of measure:

Vitamin A	Vitamin D
Vitamin E	Vitamin K

2. Analyze the vitamin contents of foods. Review the figures, photos, and food sources sections in Chapters 10 and 11 and list the food group(s) that contributed the most of each vitamin. Which food groups offer the most thiamin? The most riboflavin? The most niacin? The most vitamin B_6? The most folate? The most vitamin B_{12}? The most vitamin C? The most vitamin A? The most vitamin D? The most vitamin E?

   List the groups that provided "the most" and compare them with the USDA Food Guide in Chapter 2.

This exercise should convince you that each of the food groups provides some, but not all, of the vitamins needed daily. For a full array, a person needs to eat a variety of foods from each of the food groups regularly.

STUDY QUESTIONS

These questions will help you review the chapter. You will find the answers in the discussions on the pages provided.

1. List the fat-soluble vitamins. What characteristics do they have in common? How do they differ from the water-soluble vitamins? (p. 367)
2. Summarize the roles of vitamin A and the symptoms of its deficiency. (pp. 369–372)
3. What is meant by vitamin precursors? Name the precursors of vitamin A, and tell in what classes of foods they are located. Give examples of foods with high vitamin A activity. (pp. 367, 373–374)
4. How is vitamin D unique among the vitamins? What is its chief function? What are the richest sources of this vitamin? (pp. 375–376, 377–379)
5. Describe vitamin E's role as an antioxidant. What are the chief symptoms of vitamin E deficiency? (pp. 380–381)
6. What is vitamin K's primary role in the body? What conditions may lead to vitamin K deficiency? (pp. 382–383)

These multiple choice questions will help you prepare for an exam. Answers can be found on p. 388.

1. Fat-soluble vitamins:
   a. are easily excreted.
   b. seldom reach toxic levels.
   c. require bile for absorption.
   d. are not stored in the body's tissues.
2. The form of vitamin A active in vision is:
   a. retinal.
   b. retinol.
   c. rhodopsin.
   d. retinoic acid.
3. Vitamin A–deficiency symptoms include:
   a. rickets and osteomalacia.
   b. hemorrhaging and jaundice.
   c. night blindness and keratomalacia.
   d. fibrocystic breast disease and erythrocyte hemolysis.
4. Good sources of vitamin A include:
   a. oatmeal, pinto beans, and ham.
   b. apricots, turnip greens, and liver.
   c. whole-wheat bread, green peas, and tuna.
   d. corn, grapefruit juice, and sunflower seeds.
5. To keep minerals available in the blood, vitamin D targets:
   a. the skin, the muscles, and the bones.
   b. the kidneys, the liver, and the bones.
   c. the intestines, the kidneys, and the bones.
   d. the intestines, the pancreas, and the liver.
6. Vitamin D can be synthesized from a precursor that the body makes from:
   a. bilirubin.
   b. tocopherol.
   c. cholesterol.
   d. beta-carotene.
7. Vitamin E's most notable role is to:
   a. protect lipids against oxidation.
   b. activate blood-clotting proteins.
   c. support protein and DNA synthesis.
   d. enhance calcium deposits in the bones.
8. The classic sign of vitamin E deficiency is:
   a. rickets.
   b. xeropthalmia.
   c. muscular dystrophy.
   d. erythrocyte hemolysis.
9. Without vitamin K:
   a. muscles atrophy.
   b. bones become soft.
   c. skin rashes develop.
   d. blood fails to clot.
10. A significant amount of vitamin K comes from:
    a. vegetable oils.
    b. sunlight exposure.
    c. bacterial synthesis.
    d. fortified grain products.

REFERENCES

1. S. J. Hickenbottom and coauthors, Variability in conversion of ß-carotene to vitamin A in men as measured by using a double-tracer study design, *American Journal of Clinical Nutrition* 75 (2002): 900–907; K. J. Yeum and R. M. Russell, Carotenoid bioavailability and bioconversion, *Annual Review of Nutrition* 22 (2002): 483–504.
2. G. Wolf, The enzymatic cleavage of ß-carotene: End of a controversy, *Nutrition Reviews* 59 (2001): 116–118.
3. J. L. Napoli, A gene knockout corroborates the integral function of cellular retinol-binding protein in retinoic metabolism, *Nutrition Reviews* 58 (2000): 230–236.
4. M. Clagett-Dame and H. F. DeLuca, The role of vitamin A in mammalian reproduction and embryonic development, *Annual Review of Nutrition* 22 (2002): 347–381.
5. H. Hadi and coauthors, Vitamin A supplementation selectively improves the linear growth of Indonesian preschool children: Results from a randomized controlled trial, *American Journal of Clinical Nutrition* 71 (2000): 507–513.
6. Committee on Dietary Reference Intakes, *Dietary Reference Intakes for Vitamin C, Vitamin E, Selenium, and Carotenoids* (Washington, D.C.: National Academy Press, 2000).
7. C. Ballew and coauthors, Serum retinol distributions in residents of the United States: Third National Health and Nutrition Examination Survey, 1988–1994, *American Journal of Clinical Nutrition* 73 (2001): 586–593.
8. C. E. West, Vitamin A and measles, *Nutrition Reviews* 58 (2000): S46–S54.
9. E. Villamor and coauthors, Vitamin A supplements ameliorate the adverse effect of HIV-1, malaria, and diarrheal infections on child growth, *Pediatrics* 109 (2002): e6; C. Duggan and W. Fawzi, Micronutrients and child health: Studies in international nutrition and HIV infection, *Nutrition Reviews* 59 (2001): 358–369; A. H. Shankar and coauthors, Effect of vitamin A supplementation on morbidity due to *Plasmodium falciparum* in young children in Papua New Guinea randomised trial, *Lancet* 354 (1999): 203–209; J. E. Tyson and coauthors, Vitamin A supplementation for extremely-low-birth-weight infants, *New England Journal of Medicine* 340 (1999): 1962–1968; F. Sempértegui and coauthors, The beneficial effects of weekly low-dose vitamin A supplementation on acute lower respiratory infections and diarrhea in Ecuadorian children, *Pediatrics* 104 (1999): e6.
10. R. M. Russell, The vitamin A spectrum: From deficiency to toxicity, *American Journal of Clinical Nutrition* 71 (2000): 878–884.
11. P. Christian and coauthors, Working after the sun goes down: Exploring how night blindness impairs women's work activities in rural Nepal, *European Journal of Clinical Nutrition* 52 (1998): 519–524.
12. A. Sommer, Xerophthalmia and vitamin A status, *Progress in Retinal and Eye Research* 17 (1998): 9–31.
13. A. Mazzone and A. dal Canton, Images in clinical medicine—Hypercarotenemia, *New England Journal of Medicine* 346 (2002): 821.
14. X.-D. Wang and coauthors, Retinoid signaling and activator protein-1 expression in ferrets given ß-carotene supplements and exposed to tobacco smoke, *Journal of the National Cancer Institute* 91 (1999): 60–66.
15. M. A. Leo and C. S. Lieber, Alcohol, vitamin A, and ß-carotene: Adverse interactions, including hepatotoxicity and carcinogenicity, *American Journal of Clinical Nutrition* 69 (1999): 1071–1085.
16. S. Johansson and coauthors, Subclinical hypervitaminosis A causes fragile bones in rats, *Bone* 31 (2002): 685–689; N. Binkley and D. Krueger, Hypervitaminosis A and bone, *Nutrition Reviews* 58 (2000): 138–144.
17. K. Michaelsson and coauthors, Serum retinol levels and the risk of fractures, *New England Journal of Medicine* 348 (2003): 287–294; D. Feskanich and coauthors, Vitamin A intake and hip fractures among postmenopausal women, *Journal of the American Medical Association* 287 (2002): 47–54; S. J. Whiting and B. Lemke, Excess retinol intake may explain the high incidence of osteoporosis in northern Europe, *Nutrition Reviews* 57 (1999): 192–195.
18. L. M. Voyles and coauthors, High levels of retinol intake during the first trimester of pregnancy result from use of over-the-counter vitamin/mineral supplements, *Journal of the American Dietetic Association* 100 (2000): 1068–1070.
19. R. P. Heaney, Lessons for nutritional science from vitamin D, *American Journal of Clinical Nutrition* 69 (1999): 825–826.
20. I. A. van der Mei and coauthors, Past exposure to sun, skin phenotype, and risk of multiple sclerosis: Case-control study, *British Medical Journal* 327 (2003): 316–321.
21. I. N. Sills, Nutritional rickets: A preventable disease, *Topics in Clinical Nutrition* 17 (2001): 36–43.
22. M. K. M. Lehtonen-Veromaa and coauthors, Vitamin D and attainment of peak bone mass among peripubertal Finnish girls: A 3-y prospective study, *American Journal of Clinical Nutrition* 76 (2002): 1446–1453; T. A. Outila, M. U. M. Kärkkäinen, and C. J. E. Lamberg-Allardt, Vitamin D status affects serum parathyroid hormone concentrations during winter in female adolescents: Associations with forearm bone mineral density, *American Journal of Clinical Nutrition* 74 (2001): 206–210.
23. S. A. Abrams, Nutritional rickets: An old disease returns, *Nutrition Reviews* 60 (2002): 111–115.
24. M. S. LeBoff and coauthors, Occult vitamin D deficiency in postmenopausal US women with acute hip fracture, *Journal of the American Medical Association* 281 (1999): 1505–1511.
25. M. S. Calvo and S. J. Whiting, Prevalence of vitamin D insufficiency in Canada and the United States: Importance to health status and efficacy of current food fortification and dietary supplement use, *Nutrition Reviews* 61 (2003): 107–113.
26. N. F. Carvalho and coauthors, Severe nutritional deficiencies in toddlers resulting from health food milk alternatives, *Pediatrics* 107 (2001): e46.
27. T. A. Sentongo and coauthors, Vitamin D status in children, adolescents, and young adults with Crohn disease, *American Journal of Clinical Nutrition* 76 (2002): 1077–1081; S. Nesby-O'Dell and coauthors, Hypovitaminosis D prevalence and determinants among African American and white women of reproductive age: Third National Health and Nutrition Examination Survey, 1988–1994, *American Journal of Clinical Nutrition* 76 (2002): 187–192; S. R. Kreiter and coauthors, Nutritional rickets in African American breast-fed infants, *Journal of Pediatrics* 137 (2000): 153–157.
28. R. P. Heaney and coauthors, Human serum 25-hydroxycholecalciferol response to extended oral dosing with cholecalciferol, *American Journal of Clinical Nutrition* 77 (2003): 204–210.
29. Committee on Dietary Reference Intakes, 2000.
30. A. M. Papas, Beyond α-tocopherol: The role of the other tocopherols and tocotrienols, in M. S. Meskin and coeditors, *Phytochemicals in Nutrition and Health* (Boca Raton, Fla.: CRC Press, 2002), pp. 61–77; Q. Jiang and coauthors, γTocopherol, the major form of vitamin E in the US diet, deserves more attention, *American Journal of Clinical Nutrition* 74 (2001): 714–722.
31. Committee on Dietary Reference Intakes, 2000.
32. S. L. Booth and coauthors, Vitamin K intake and bone mineral density in women and men, *American Journal of Clinical Nutrition* 77 (2003): 512–516.
33. N. C. Binkley and coauthors, A high phylloquinone intake is required to achieve maximal osteocalcin γ-carboxylation, *American Journal of Clinical Nutrition* 76 (2002): 1055–1060; N. C. Binkley and coauthors, Vitamin K supplementation reduces serum concentrations of under-γ-carboxylated osteocalcin in healthy young and elderly adults, *American Journal of Clinical Nutrition* 72 (2000): 1523–1528; S. L. Booth and coauthors, Dietary vitamin K intakes are associated with hip fracture but not with bone mineral density in elderly men and women, *American Journal of Clinical Nutrition* 71 (2000): 1201–1208; D. Feskanich and coauthors, Vitamin K intake and hip fractures in women: A prospective study, *American Journal of Clinical Nutrition* 69 (1999): 74–79.

ANSWERS

Nutrition Calculations

1. Vitamin A: µg RAE. Vitamin D: µg.
   Vitamin E: mg. Vitamin K: µg.
2. Thiamin: Legumes and grains
   Riboflavin: Milks, grains, and meats
   Niacin: Meats and grains
   Vitamin B_6: Meats
   Folate: Legumes and vegetables
   Vitamin B_{12}: Meats and milks
   Vitamin C: Vegetables and fruits
   Vitamin A: Vegetables, fruits, and milks
   Vitamin D: Milks
   Vitamin E: Legumes and oils

Taken together, "the most" groups form the USDA Food Guide—grains, vegetables, legumes, fruits, milks, meats, and oils.

Study Questions (multiple choice)

1. c 2. a 3. c 4. b 5. c 6. c 7. a 8. d 9. d 10. c

HIGHLIGHT

Antioxidant Nutrients in Disease Prevention

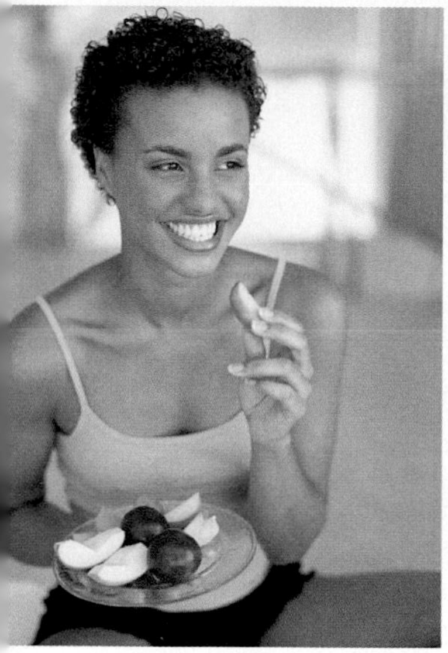

Count on supplement manufacturers to exploit the day's hot topics in nutrition. The moment bits of research news surface, new supplements appear—and terms like "antioxidants" and "lycopene" become household words. Friendly faces in TV commercials try to persuade us that these supplements hold the magic in the fight against aging and disease. New supplements hit the market and cash registers ring. Vitamin C, for years the leading single nutrient supplement, gains new popularity, and sales of lutein, beta-carotene, and vitamin E supplements soar as well.

In the meantime, scientists and medical experts around the world continue their work to clarify and confirm the roles of antioxidants in preventing chronic diseases.[1] This highlight summarizes some of the accumulating evidence. It also revisits the advantages of foods over supplements. But first it is important to introduce the troublemakers—the **free radicals** (the accompanying glossary defines free radicals and related terms).

Free Radicals and Disease

Chapter 7 described how the body's cells use oxygen in metabolic reactions. In the process, oxygen sometimes reacts with body compounds and produces highly unstable molecules known as free radicals. In addition to normal body processes, environmental factors such as ultraviolet radiation, air pollution, and tobacco smoke generate free radicals.

A free radical is a molecule with one or more unpaired electrons.* An electron without a partner is unstable and highly reactive. To regain its stability, the free radical quickly finds a stable but vulnerable compound from which to steal an electron (see Figure H11-1 on p. 390).

With the loss of an electron, the formerly stable molecule becomes a free radical itself and steals an electron from another nearby molecule. Thus an electron-snatching chain reaction is under way with free radicals producing more free radicals. Antioxidants neutralize free radicals by donating one of their own electrons, thus ending the chain reaction. When they lose electrons, antioxidants do not become free radicals because they are stable in either form. (Review Figure 10-15 on p. 349 to see how ascorbic acid can give up two hydrogens with their electrons and become dehydroascorbic acid.)

Once formed, free radicals attack. Occasionally, these free-radical attacks are helpful. For example, cells of the immune system use free radicals as ammunition in an "oxidative burst" that demolishes disease-causing viruses and bacteria. Most often, however, free-radical attacks cause widespread damage. They commonly damage the polyunsaturated fatty acids in lipoproteins and in cell membranes, disrupting the transport of substances into and out of cells. Free radicals also damage

*Many free radicals exist, but the oxygen-derived ones are most common in the human body. Examples of oxygen-derived free radicals include superoxide radical ($O_2\cdot^-$), hydroxyl radical ($OH\cdot$), and nitric oxide ($NO\cdot$). (The dots in the symbols represent the unpaired electrons.) Technically, hydrogen peroxide (H_2O_2) and singlet oxygen are not free radicals because they contain paired electrons, but the unstable conformation of their electrons makes radical-producing reactions likely. Scientists sometimes use the term *reactive oxygen species (ROS)* to describe all of these compounds.

GLOSSARY

free radicals: unstable and highly reactive atoms or molecules that have one or more unpaired electrons in the outer orbital (see Appendix B for a review of basic chemistry concepts).

oxidants (OK-see-dants): compounds (such as oxygen itself) that oxidize other compounds. Compounds that prevent oxidation are called *anti*oxidants, whereas those that promote it are called *pro*oxidants.
- **anti** = against
- **pro** = for

oxidative stress: a condition in which the production of oxidants and free radicals exceeds the body's ability to defend itself.

prooxidants: substances that significantly induce oxidative stress.

Reminder: *Dietary antioxidants* are substances typically found in foods that significantly decrease the adverse effects of free radicals on normal functions in the body. *Nonnutrients* are compounds in foods that do not fit into the six classes of nutrients. *Phytochemicals* are nonnutrient compounds found in plant-derived foods that have biological activity in the body.

FIGURE H11-1 The Actions of Free Radicals and Antioxidants

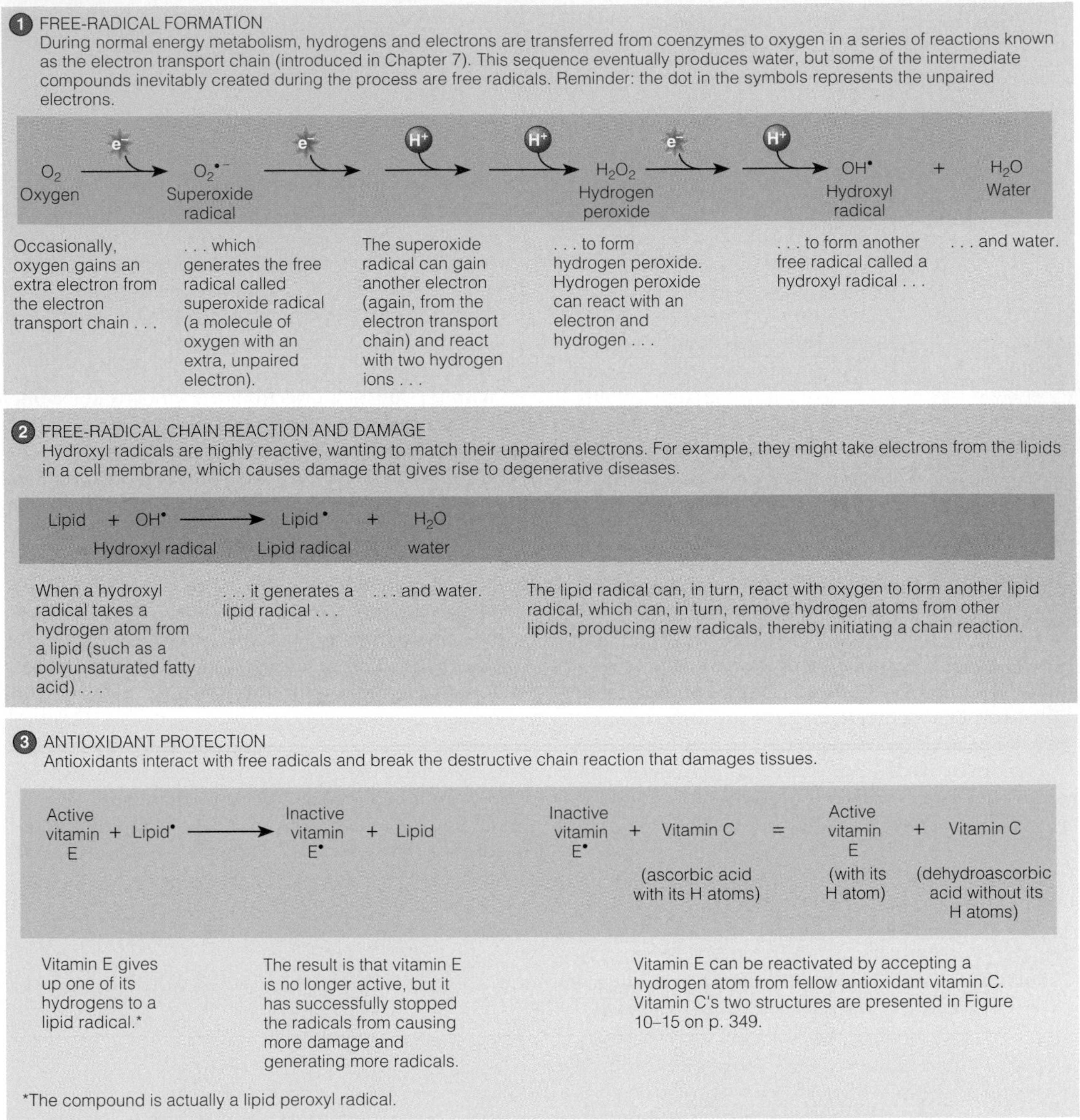
1 FREE-RADICAL FORMATION
During normal energy metabolism, hydrogens and electrons are transferred from coenzymes to oxygen in a series of reactions known as the electron transport chain (introduced in Chapter 7). This sequence eventually produces water, but some of the intermediate compounds inevitably created during the process are free radicals. Reminder: the dot in the symbols represents the unpaired electrons.
e⁻
e⁻
H+
H+
e⁻
H+
O_2
Oxygen
$O_2^{\bullet -}$
Superoxide radical
H_2O_2
Hydrogen peroxide
$OH^{\bullet}$
Hydroxyl radical
+
H_2O
Water
Occasionally, oxygen gains an extra electron from the electron transport chain . . .
. . . which generates the free radical called superoxide radical (a molecule of oxygen with an extra, unpaired electron).
The superoxide radical can gain another electron (again, from the electron transport chain) and react with two hydrogen ions . . .
. . . to form hydrogen peroxide. Hydrogen peroxide can react with an electron and hydrogen . . .
. . . to form another free radical called a hydroxyl radical . . .
. . . and water.
2 FREE-RADICAL CHAIN REACTION AND DAMAGE
Hydroxyl radicals are highly reactive, wanting to match their unpaired electrons. For example, they might take electrons from the lipids in a cell membrane, which causes damage that gives rise to degenerative diseases.
Lipid + $OH^{\bullet}$ → $Lipid^{\bullet}$ + H_2O
Hydroxyl radical
Lipid radical
water
When a hydroxyl radical takes a hydrogen atom from a lipid (such as a polyunsaturated fatty acid) . . .
. . . it generates a lipid radical . . .
. . . and water.
The lipid radical can, in turn, react with oxygen to form another lipid radical, which can, in turn, remove hydrogen atoms from other lipids, producing new radicals, thereby initiating a chain reaction.
3 ANTIOXIDANT PROTECTION
Antioxidants interact with free radicals and break the destructive chain reaction that damages tissues.
Active vitamin E + $Lipid^{\bullet}$ → Inactive vitamin $E^{\bullet}$ + Lipid
Inactive vitamin $E^{\bullet}$ + Vitamin C = Active vitamin E + Vitamin C
(ascorbic acid with its H atoms)
(with its H atom)
(dehydroascorbic acid without its H atoms)
Vitamin E gives up one of its hydrogens to a lipid radical.*
The result is that vitamin E is no longer active, but it has successfully stopped the radicals from causing more damage and generating more radicals.
Vitamin E can be reactivated by accepting a hydrogen atom from fellow antioxidant vitamin C. Vitamin C's two structures are presented in Figure 10–15 on p. 349.
*The compound is actually a lipid peroxyl radical.

cell proteins (altering their functions) and DNA (creating mutations).

The body's natural defenses and repair systems try to control the destruction caused by free radicals, but these systems are not 100 percent effective. In fact, they become less effective with age, and the unrepaired damage accumulates. To some extent, dietary antioxidants defend the body against **oxidative stress,** but if antioxidants are unavailable, or if free-radical production becomes excessive, health problems may develop. Oxygen-derived free radicals may cause diseases not only by indiscriminately destroying the valuable components of cells, but also by serving as signals for specific activities within the cells. Scientists have identified oxidative stress as a causative factor and antioxidants as a protective factor in cognitive performance and the aging process and in the development of diseases such as cancer, arthritis, cataracts, and heart disease.[2]

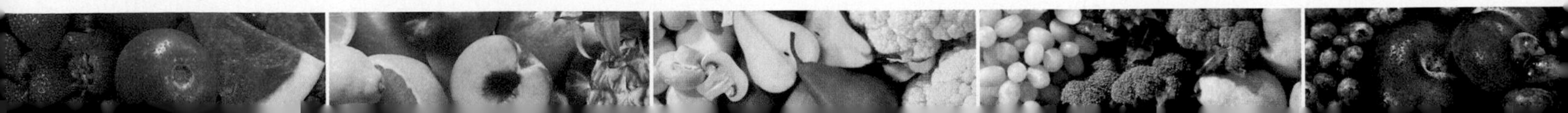

Defending against Free Radicals

The body maintains a couple lines of defense against free-radical damage. A system of enzymes disarms the most harmful **oxidants.*** The action of these enzymes depends on the minerals selenium, copper, manganese, and zinc. If the diet fails to provide adequate supplies of these minerals, this line of defense weakens. The body also uses the antioxidant vitamins: vitamin E and vitamin C. Vitamin E defends the body's lipids (cell membranes and lipoproteins, for example) by efficiently stopping the free-radical chain reaction. Vitamin C protects the body's watery components, such as the fluid of the blood, against free-radical attacks. Vitamin C seems especially adept at neutralizing free radicals from polluted air and cigarette smoke; it may also restore oxidized vitamin E to its active state.

Dietary antioxidants may also include *non*nutrients—some of the phytochemicals (featured in Highlight 13). Together, nutrients and phytochemicals with antioxidant activity minimize damage by:

- Limiting free-radical formation.
- Destroying free radicals or their precursors.
- Stimulating antioxidant enzyme activity.
- Repairing oxidative damage.
- Stimulating repair enzyme activity.

These actions play key roles in defending the body against cancer and heart disease.

Defending against Cancer

Cancers arise when cellular DNA is damaged—sometimes by free-radical attacks. Antioxidants may reduce cancer risks by protecting DNA from this damage. Many researchers have reported low rates of cancer in people whose diets include abundant vegetables and fruits, rich in antioxidants.[3] Preliminary reports suggest an inverse relationship between DNA damage and vegetable intake and a positive relationship with beef and pork intake. Laboratory studies with animals and with cells in tissue culture also seem to support such findings.

Foods rich in vitamin C seem to protect against certain types of cancers, especially those of the mouth, larynx, esophagus, and stomach. Such a correlation may reflect the benefits of a diet rich in fruits and vegetables and low in fat; it does not necessarily support taking vitamin C supplements to treat or prevent cancer.

*These enzymes include glutathione peroxidase, thioredoxin reductase, superoxide dismutase, and catalase.

Evidence that vitamin E helps guard against cancer is less consistent than for vitamin C. Still, people with low blood levels of vitamin E have high rates of some cancers. Several studies report a cancer-preventing benefit of vegetables and fruits rich in beta-carotene and the other carotenoids as well.[4]

Defending against Heart Disease

High blood cholesterol carried in LDL is a major risk factor for cardiovascular disease, but how do LDL exert their damage? One scenario is that free radicals within the arterial walls oxidize LDL, changing their structure and function. The oxidized LDL then accelerate the formation of artery-clogging plaques. These free radicals also oxidize the polyunsaturated fatty acids of the cell membranes, sparking additional changes in the arterial walls, which impede the flow of blood. Susceptibility to such oxidative damage within the arterial walls is heightened by a diet high in saturated fat or cigarette smoke. In contrast, diets that include plenty of fruits and vegetables, especially when combined with little saturated fat, strengthen antioxidant defenses against LDL oxidation.[5] Antioxidant nutrients taken as supplements also seem to slow the early progression of atherosclerosis.[6]

Antioxidants, especially vitamin E, may protect against cardiovascular disease.[7] Epidemiological studies suggest that people who eat foods rich in vitamin E have low rates of death from heart disease.[8] Similarly, large doses of vitamin E supplements may slow the progression of heart disease. Among its many protective roles, vitamin E defends against LDL oxidation, inflammation, arterial injuries, and blood clotting.[9] Less clear is whether vitamin E supplements benefit people who already have heart disease or multiple risk factors for it.[10] Antioxidant supplements may not be beneficial and, in fact, may even be harmful for these people.[11]

Some studies suggest that vitamin C protects against LDL oxidation, raises HDL, lowers total cholesterol, and improves blood pressure. Vitamin C may also minimize the free-radical action within the arterial wall that typically follows a high-fat meal.[12] In fact, blood flow through the arteries is similar to that seen after a low-fat meal.

Foods, Supplements, or Both?

In the process of scavenging and quenching free radicals, antioxidants themselves become oxidized. To some extent, they can be regenerated, but still, losses occur and free radicals attack continuously. To maintain defenses, a person must replenish dietary antioxidants regularly. But should antioxidants be replenished from foods or from supplements?

Foods—especially fruits and vegetables—offer not only antioxidants, but an array of other valuable vitamins and minerals as well. Importantly, deficiencies of these nutrients can damage DNA as readily as free radicals can.[13] Eating fruits and vegetables in abundance protects against both deficiencies and diseases. A major review of the evidence gathered from metabolic studies, epidemiologic studies, and dietary intervention trials identified three dietary strategies most effective in preventing heart disease:[14]

- Use unsaturated fats (that have not been hydrogenated) instead of saturated or *trans* fats (see Highlight 5).
- Select foods rich in omega-3 fatty acids (see Chapter 5).
- Consume a diet high in fruits, vegetables, nuts, and whole grains and low in refined grain products.

Such a diet combined with exercise, weight control, and not smoking serves as the best prescription for health. Notably, taking supplements is not among these disease-prevention recommendations.

Some research suggests a protective effect from as little as a daily glass of orange juice or carrot juice (rich sources of vitamin C and beta-carotene, respectively). Other intervention studies, however, have used levels of nutrients that far exceed current recommendations and can be achieved only by taking supplements. In making their recommendations for the antioxidant nutrients, members of the DRI Committee considered whether these studies support substantially higher intakes to help protect against chronic diseases. They did raise the recommendations for vitamins C and E, but do not support taking vitamin pills over eating a healthy diet.

While awaiting additional research, should people anticipate the go-ahead and start taking antioxidant supplements now? Most scientists agree that it is too early to make such a recommendation. Though fruits and vegetables containing many antioxidant nutrients and phytochemicals have been associated with a diminished risk of many cancers, supplements have not always proved beneficial. In fact, sometimes the benefits are more apparent when the vitamins come from foods rather than from supplements. Without data to confirm the benefits of supplements, we cannot accept the potential risks. And the risks are real.

Consider the findings from a study to determine whether daily supplements of vitamin E, beta-carotene, or both would reduce the incidence of lung cancer among smokers. After five to eight years of supplementation, there was no reduction in the incidence of lung cancer; in fact, the researchers found a *higher* incidence of lung cancer among smokers receiving the beta-carotene. Another group of researchers reported similar findings: smokers and asbestos workers receiving beta-carotene and vitamin A supplements for four years had a higher incidence of lung cancer and risk of death than those taking a placebo. These findings brought the study to an end much earlier than planned. Given the association between high intakes of *foods* rich in beta-carotene and low rates of lung cancer reported in earlier epidemiological studies, findings of increased risk were surprising, to say the least.[15] As is often true of most nutrients, the action of beta-carotene differs dramatically at various levels of intake.[16] Amounts commonly found in foods may be beneficial, but high doses trigger the production of keratin in the delicate cells of the lungs, and this effect is magnified with smoking.[17]

Clearly, remedies to life-threatening diseases such as lung cancer are not as simple as taking supplements. Smokers are much wiser to stop smoking than to rely on pills to protect them from lung cancer.

Even if research clearly proves that a particular nutrient is the ultimate protective ingredient in foods, supplements would not be the answer because their contents are limited. Vitamin E supplements, for example, usually contain alpha-tocopherol, but foods provide an assortment of tocopherols among other nutrients, many of which provide valuable protection against free-radical damage. Supplements shortchange users.

Furthermore, much more research is needed to define optimal and dangerous levels of intake. This much we know: antioxidants behave differently under various conditions. At physiological levels typical of a healthy diet, they act as antioxidants, but at pharmacological doses typical of supplements, they may act as **prooxidants,** stimulating the production of free radicals.[18] This is especially likely in the presence of other antioxidants or minerals such as iron. Until the optimum intake of these nutrients can be determined, the risks of supplement use remain unclear. The best way to add antioxidants to the diet is to eat generous servings of fruits and vegetables daily.

It should be clear by now that we cannot know the identity and action of every chemical in every food. Even if we did, why create a supplement to replicate a food? Why not eat foods and enjoy the pleasure, nourishment, and health benefits they provide? The beneficial constituents in foods are widespread among plants. Among the fruits, pomegranates,

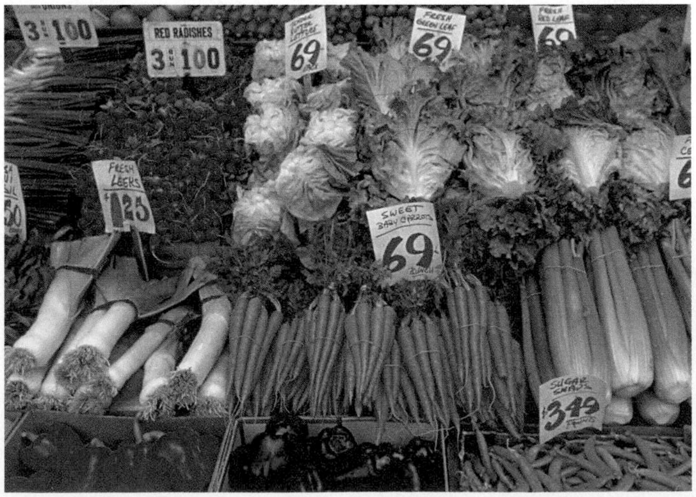
RED RADISHES
3 100
FRESH LEEKS
SWEET BABY CARROTS
69
© Jeffry Myers/Stock, Boston/PictureQuest

Many cancer-fighting products are available now at your local produce counter.

berries, and citrus rank high in antioxidants; top antioxidant vegetables include kale, spinach, and brussels sprouts; millet and oats contain the most antioxidants among the grains; pinto beans and soybeans are the outstanding legumes; and walnuts outshine the other nuts.[19] But don't try to single out one particular food for its magic nutrient, antioxidant, or phytochemical. Instead, eat a wide variety of fruits and vegetables in generous quantities every day—and get *all* the magic compounds these foods have to offer.

REFERENCES

1. P. Møller and S. Loft, Oxidative DNA damage in human white blood cells in dietary antioxidant intervention studies, *American Journal of Clinical Nutrition* 76 (2002): 303–310; B. Halliwell, Why and how should we measure oxidative DNA damage in nutritional studies? How far have we come? *American Journal of Clinical Nutrition* 72 (2000): 1082–1087.
2. F. Grodstein, J. Chen, and W. C. Willett, High-dose antioxidant supplements and cognitive function in community-dwelling elderly women, *American Journal of Clinical Nutrition* 77 (2003): 975–984; M. J. Engelhart and coauthors, Dietary intake of antioxidants and risk of Alzheimer disease, *Journal of the American Medical Association* 287 (2002): 3223–3229; H. L. Hu and coauthors, Mechanisms of ageing and development, *Science Direct* 121 (2001): 217–230; M. Meydani, Antioxidants and cognitive function, *Nutrition Reviews* 59 (2001): S75–S80; J. W. Miller, Vitamin E and memory: Is it vascular protection? *Nutrition Reviews* 58 (2000): 109–111.
3. A. Martin and coauthors, Roles of vitamins E and C on neurodegenerative diseases and cognitive performance, *Nutrition Reviews* 60 (2002): 308–326; H. Chen and coauthors, Dietary patterns and adenocarcinoma of the esophagus and distal stomach, *American Journal of Clinical Nutrition* 75 (2002): 137–144; B. Halliwell, Establishing the significance and optimal intake of dietary antioxidants: The biomarker concept, *Nutrition Reviews* 57 (1999): 104–113.
4. E. R. Berton and coauthors, A population-based case-control study of carotenoid and vitamin A intake and ovarian cancer (United States), *Cancer Causes Control* 12 (2001): 83–90; D. S. Michaud and coauthors, Intake of specific carotenoids and risk of lung cancer in 2 prospective US cohorts, *American Journal of Clinical Nutrition* 72 (2000): 990–997; M. L. Slattery and coauthors, Carotenoids and colon cancer, *American Journal of Clinical Nutrition* 71 (2000): 575–582; N. McKeown and coauthors, Antioxidants and breast cancer, *Nutrition Reviews* 57 (1999): 321–324; D. A. Cooper, A. L. Eldridge, and J. C. Peters, Dietary carotenoids and lung cancer: A review of recent research, *Nutrition Reviews* 57 (1999): 133–134; P. Riso and coauthors, Does tomato consumption effectively increase the resistance of lymphocyte DNA to oxidative damage? *American Journal of Clinical Nutrition* 69 (1999): 712–718; E. Giovannucci, Tomatoes, tomato-based products, lycopene, and cancer: Review of the epidemiologic literature, *Journal of the National Cancer Institute* 91 (1999): 317–331.
5. R. A. Jacob, Evidence that diet modification reduces in vivo oxidant damage, *Nutrition Reviews* 57 (1999): 255–258.
6. L. Liu and M. Meydani, Combined vitamin C and E supplementation retards early progression of arteriosclerosis in heart transplant patients, *Nutrition Reviews* 60 (2002): 368–371; H. Y. Huang and coauthors, Effects of vitamin C and vitamin E on in vivo lipid peroxidation: Results of a randomized controlled trial, *American Journal of Clinical Nutrition* 76 (2002): 549–555; C. R. Gale, H. E. Ashurst, and H. J. Powers, Antioxidant vitamin status and carotid atherosclerosis in the elderly, *American Journal of Clinical Nutrition* 74 (2001): 402–408; F. Nappo, Impairment of endothelial functions by acute hyperhomocysteinemia and reversal by antioxidant vitamins, *Journal of the American Medical Association* 281 (1999): 2113–2118.
7. A. Iannuzzi and coauthors, Dietary and circulating antioxidant vitamins in relation to carotid plaques in middle-aged women, *American Journal of Clinical Nutrition* 76 (2002): 582–587; M. Meydani, Effect of functional food ingredients: Vitamin E modulation of cardiovascular diseases and immune status in the elderly, *American Journal of Clinical Nutrition* 71 (2000): 1665S–1668S.
8. L. A. Yochum, A. R. Folsom, and L. H. Kushi, Intake of antioxidant vitamins and risk of death from stroke in postmenopausal women, *American Journal of Clinical Nutrition* 72 (2000): 476–483.
9. S. Devaraj, A. Harris, and I. Jialal, Modulation of monocyte-macrophage function with α-tocopherol: Implications for atherosclerosis, *Nutrition Reviews* 60 (2002): 8–14; L. J. van Tits and coauthors, α-Tocopherol supplementation decreases production of superoxide and cytokines by leukocytes ex vivo in both normolipidemic and hypertriglyceridemic individuals, *American Journal of Clinical Nutrition* 71 (2000): 458–464; M. Meydani, Vitamin E and prevention of heart disease in high-risk patients, *Nutrition Reviews* 58 (2000): 278–281.
10. B. G. Brown and coauthors, Simvastatin and niacin, antioxidant vitamins, or the combination for the prevention of coronary disease, *New England Journal of Medicine* 345 (2001): 1583–1592.
11. D. D. Waters and coauthors, Effects of hormone replacement therapy and antioxidant vitamin supplements on coronary atherosclerosis in postmenopausal women: A randomized controlled trial, *Journal of the American Medical Association* 288 (2002): 2432–2440; Collaborative Group of the Primary Prevention Project (PPP), Low-dose aspirin and vitamin E in people at cardiovascular risk: A randomized trial in general practice, *Lancet* 357 (2001): 89–95.
12. L. Liu and coauthors, Vitamin C preserves endothelial function in patients with coronary heart disease after a high-fat meal, *Clinical Cardiology* 25 (2002): 219–224.
13. B. N. Ames, Micronutrient deficiencies: A major cause of DNA damage, *Annals of the New York Academy of Sciences* 889 (1999): 87–106.
14. F. B. Hu and W. C. Willett, Optimal diets for prevention of coronary heart disease, *Journal of the American Medical Association* 288 (2002): 2569–2578.
15. W. A. Pryor, W. Stahl, and C. L. Rock, Beta carotene: From biochemistry to clinical trials, *Nutrition Reviews* 58 (2000): 39–53.
16. J. S. Bertram, Carotenoids and gene regulation, *Nutrition Reviews* 57 (1999): 182–191.
17. G. Wolf, The effect of low and high doses of ß-carotene and exposure to cigarette smoke on the lungs of ferrets, *Nutrition Reviews* 60 (2002): 88–90.
18. X. D. Wang and R. M. Russell, Procarcinogenic and anticarcinogenic effects of ß-carotene, *Nutrition Reviews* 57 (1999): 263–272.
19. B. L. Halvorsen and coauthors, A systematic screening of total antioxidants in dietary plants, *Journal of Nutrition* 132 (2002): 461–471.

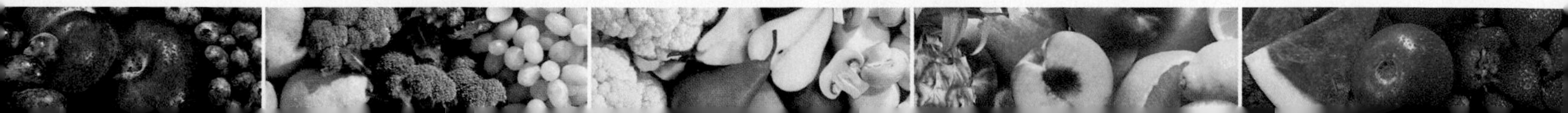

Chapter 12

Water and the Major Minerals

Chapter Outline

Available Online

http://nutrition.wadsworth.com/uncn7

Nutrition Animation: *Maintaining Water Balance in the Body*

Student Practice Test

Glossary Terms

Nutrition on the Net

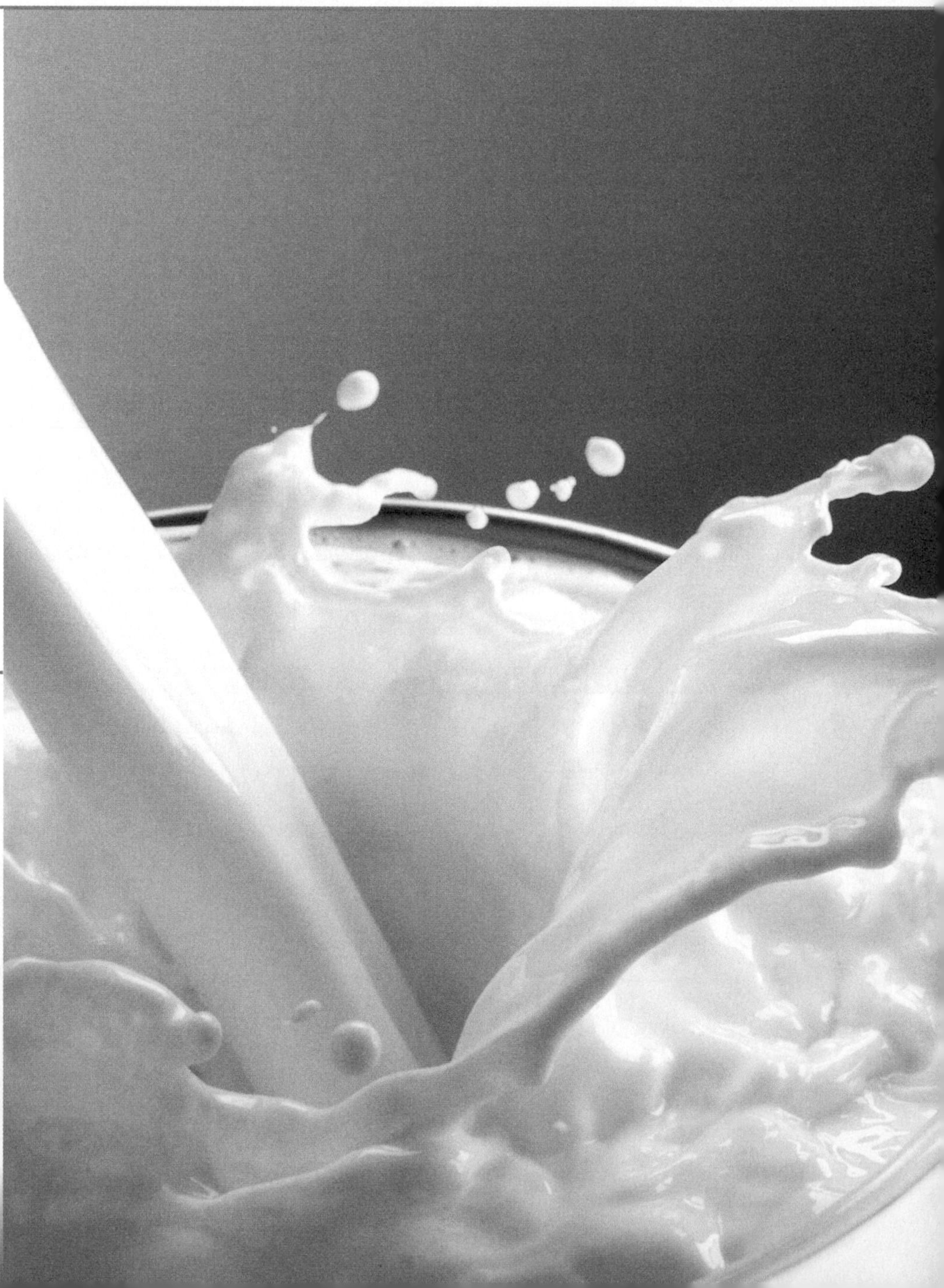

Nutrition in Your Life

What's your beverage of choice? If you said water, then congratulate yourself for recognizing its importance in maintaining your body's fluid balance. If you answered milk, then pat yourself on the back for taking good care of your bones. Faced with a lack of water, you would realize within days how vital it is to your very survival. The consequences of a lack of milk (or other calcium-rich foods) are also dramatic, but may not become apparent for decades. Water, calcium, and all the other major minerals support fluid balance and bone health. Before getting too comfortable reading this chapter, you might want to get yourself a glass of water or milk. Your body will thank you.

Water is an essential nutrient, more important to life than any of the others. The body needs more water each day than any other nutrient. Furthermore, you can survive only a few days without water, whereas a deficiency of the other nutrients may take weeks, months, or even years to develop.

This chapter begins with a look at water and the body's fluids. The body maintains an appropriate balance and distribution of water with the help of another class of nutrients—the minerals. In addition to introducing the minerals that help regulate body fluids, the chapter describes many of the other important functions minerals perform in the body.

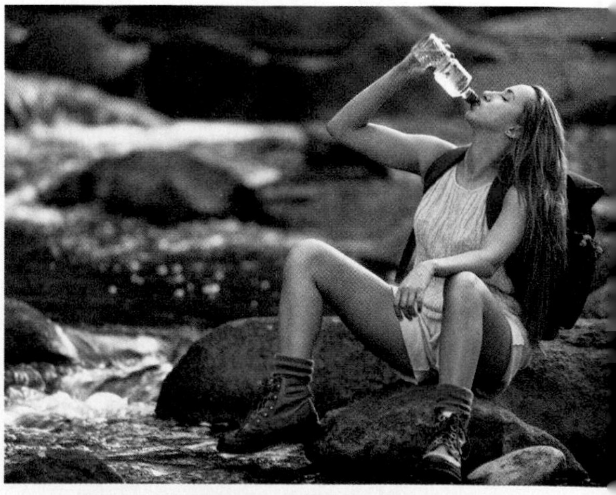

Water is the most indispensable nutrient.

Water and the Body Fluids

Water constitutes about 60 percent of an adult's body weight and a higher percentage of a child's. Because water makes up about three-fourths of the weight of lean tissue and less than one-fourth of the weight of fat, a person's body composition influences how much of the body's weight is water. The proportion of water is generally smaller in females, obese people, and the elderly because of their smaller proportion of lean tissue.

In the body, water becomes the fluid in which all life processes occur. The water in the body fluids:

temp regulation
blood volume
transport

- Carries nutrients and waste products throughout the body.
- Maintains the structure of large molecules such as proteins and glycogen.
- Participates in metabolic reactions.
- Serves as the solvent for minerals, vitamins, amino acids, glucose, and many other small molecules so that they can participate in metabolic activities.
- Acts as a lubricant and cushion around joints and inside the eyes, the spinal cord, and, in pregnancy, the amniotic sac surrounding the fetus in the womb.
- Aids in the regulation of normal body temperature; evaporation of sweat from the skin removes excess heat from the body.
- Maintains blood volume.

To support these and other vital functions, the body actively maintains an appropriate **water balance.**■

■ Water balance: intake = output.

Water Balance and Recommended Intakes

Every cell contains fluid of the exact composition that is best for that cell **(intracellular fluid)** and is bathed externally in another such fluid **(interstitial fluid).** Interstitial fluid is the largest component of **extracellular fluid.** Figure 12-1 illustrates a cell and its associated fluids. These fluids continually lose and replace their components, yet the composition in each compartment remains remarkably constant under normal conditions. Because imbalances can be devastating, the body quickly responds by adjusting both water intake and excretion as needed. Consequently, the entire system of cells and fluids remains in a delicate but controlled state of homeostasis.

Available Online

Watch how water balance is maintained in the body through equalization of water sources and water losses.

Water Intake **Thirst** and satiety influence water intake, apparently in response to changes sensed by the mouth, hypothalamus,■ and nerves. When the blood becomes concentrated (having lost water, but not the dissolved substances within it), the mouth becomes dry, and the hypothalamus initiates drinking behavior. Stretch receptors in the stomach send signals to stop drinking as do receptors in the heart that monitor blood volume.

■ Reminder: The *hypothalamus* is a brain center that controls activities such as maintenance of water balance, regulation of body temperature, and control of appetite.

Thirst drives a person to seek water, but it lags behind the body's need. When too much water is lost from the body and not replaced, **dehydration** develops. A first sign of dehydration is thirst, the signal that the body has already lost some of its fluid. If a person is unable to obtain fluid or, as in many elderly people, fails to perceive the thirst message, the symptoms of dehydration may progress rapidly from thirst to weakness, exhaustion, and delirium and end in death if not corrected (see Table 12-1). Dehydration may easily develop with either water deprivation or excessive water losses.

Water intoxication, on the other hand, is rare but can occur with excessive water ingestion and kidney disorders that reduce urine production. The symptoms may include confusion, convulsions, and even death in extreme cases. Excessive water ingestion contributes to the dangerous condition known as hyponatremia, sometimes seen in endurance athletes.

Water Sources The obvious dietary sources of water are water itself and other beverages, but nearly all foods also contain water. Most fruits and vegetables contain up to 90 percent water; many meats and cheeses contain at least 50 percent (see Table 12-2 for selected foods and Appendix H for many more). Water is also generated during metabolism. Recall that when the energy-yielding nutrients break down, their carbons and hydrogens combine with oxygen to yield carbon

water balance: the balance between water intake and output (losses).

intracellular fluid: fluid within the cells, usually high in potassium and phosphate. Intracellular fluid accounts for approximately two-thirds of the body's water.
- **intra** = within

interstitial (IN-ter-STISH-al) **fluid:** fluid between the cells (intercellular), usually high in sodium and chloride. Interstitial fluid is a large component of extracellular fluid.
- **inter** = in the midst, between

extracellular fluid: fluid outside the cells. Extracellular fluid includes two main components—the interstitial fluid and plasma. Extracellular fluid accounts for approximately one-third of the body's water.
- **extra** = outside

thirst: a conscious desire to drink.

dehydration: the condition in which body water output exceeds water input. Symptoms include thirst, dry skin and mucous membranes, rapid heartbeat, low blood pressure, and weakness.

water intoxication: the rare condition in which body water contents are too high in all body fluid compartments.

TABLE 12-1 Signs of Dehydration

Body Weight Lost (%)	Symptoms
1–2	Thirst, fatigue, weakness, vague discomfort, loss of appetite
3–4	Impaired physical performance, dry mouth, reduction in urine, flushed skin, impatience, apathy
5–6	Difficulty in concentrating, headache, irritability, sleepiness, impaired temperature regulation, increased respiratory rate
7–10	Dizziness, spastic muscles, loss of balance, delirium, exhaustion, collapse

NOTE: The onset and severity of symptoms at various percentages of body weight lost depend on the activity, fitness level, degree of acclimation, temperature, and humidity. If not corrected, dehydration can lead to death.

dioxide (CO_2)—and water (H_2O). As Table 12-3 (on p. 398) shows, the water derived daily from these three sources averages about 2½ liters (roughly 2½ quarts).

Water Losses The body must excrete a minimum of about 500 milliliters of water each day■ as urine—enough to carry away the waste products generated by a day's metabolic activities. Above this amount, excretion adjusts to balance intake. If a person drinks more water, the kidneys excrete more urine, and the urine becomes more dilute. In addition to urine, water is lost from the lungs as vapor and from the skin as sweat; some is also lost in feces.* The amount of fluid lost from each source varies, depending on the environment (such as heat or humidity) and physical conditions (such as exercise or fever). On average, daily losses total about 2½ liters. Table 12-3 (on p. 398) shows how water excretion balances intake; maintaining this balance requires healthy kidneys and an adequate intake of fluids.

Water Recommendations Because water needs vary depending on diet, activity, environmental temperature, and humidity, a general water requirement is difficult to establish. In the past, recommendations■ were expressed in proportion to the amount of energy expended under average environmental conditions. The recommended water intake for a person who expends 2000 kcalories a day, for example, would be about 2 to 3 liters of water (about 7 to 11 cups). This recommendation is in line with the Adequate Intake (AI) for *total* water set by the DRI Committee.■ Total water includes not only drinking water, but water in other beverages and in foods as well.[1]

*Water lost from the lungs and skin accounts for almost one-half of the daily losses even when a person is not visibly perspiring; these losses are commonly referred to as *insensible water losses*.

TABLE 12-2 Percentage of Water in Selected Foods

100%	Water, diet sodas
90–99%	Fat-free milk, strawberries, watermelon, lettuce, cabbage, celery, spinach, broccoli
80–89%	Fruit juice, yogurt, apples, grapes, oranges, carrots
70–79%	Shrimp, bananas, corn, potatoes, avocados, cottage cheese, ricotta cheese
60–69%	Pasta, legumes, salmon, ice cream, chicken breast
50–59%	Ground beef, hot dogs, feta cheese
40–49%	Pizza
30–39%	Cheddar cheese, bagels, bread
20–29%	Pepperoni sausage, cake, biscuits
10–19%	Butter, margarine, raisins
1–9%	Crackers, cereals, pretzels, taco shells, peanut butter, nuts
0%	Oils

FIGURE 12-1 One Cell and Its Associated Fluids

Fluids are found within the cells (intracellular) or outside the cells (extracellular). Extracellular fluids include plasma (the fluid portion of blood in the intravascular spaces of blood vessels) and interstitial fluids (the tissue fluid that fills the intercellular spaces between the cells).

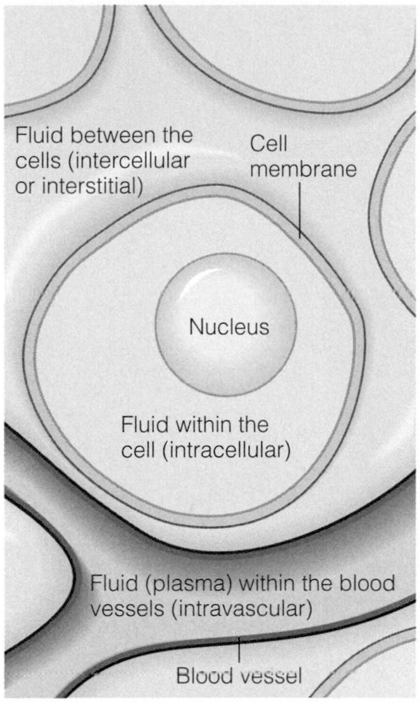
Fluid between the cells (intercellular or interstitial)
Cell membrane
Nucleus
Fluid within the cell (intracellular)
Fluid (plasma) within the blood vessels (intravascular)
Blood vessel

■ The amount of water the body has to excrete each day to dispose of its wastes is the **obligatory** (ah-BLIG-ah-TORE-ee) **water excretion**—about 500 mL (about 2 c, or a pint).

■ Water recommendation:
- 1.0 to 1.5 mL/kcal expended (adults).†
- 1.5 mL/kcal expended (infants and athletes).

Conversion factors:
- 1 mL = 0.03 fluid ounce.
- 125 mL ≈ ½ c.

Easy estimation: ½ c per 100 kcal expended.

†For those using kilojoules: 4.2 to 6.3 mL/kJ expended.

■ AI for *total* water:
- Men: 3.7 L/day.
- Women: 2.7 L/day.

Conversion factors:
- 1 L = 33.8 fluid oz.
- 1 L = 1.06 qt.
- 1 c = 8 fluid oz.

TABLE 12-3 Water Balance

Water Sources	Amount (mL)	Water Losses	Amount (mL)
Liquids	550 to 1500	Kidneys (urine)	500 to 1400
Foods	700 to 1000	Skin (sweat)	450 to 900
Metabolic water	200 to 300	Lungs (breath)	350
		GI tract (feces)	150
Total	1450 to 2800	Total	1450 to 2800

Because a wide range of water intakes will prevent dehydration and its harmful consequences, the AI is based on average intakes. People who are physically active or who live in hot environments may need more. Survey data show that people are drinking more water, juice, soft drinks, coffee, tea, and alcoholic beverages than previously.[2] Regardless of which beverages people drink, they lose some fluid within a few hours, which is why they have to replenish daily.

Some research indicates that people who drink caffeinated beverages lose a little more fluid than when drinking water because caffeine acts as a diuretic.[3] The DRI Committee considered such findings in their recommendations for water intake and concluded that "caffeinated beverages contribute to the daily total water intake similar to that contributed by non-caffeinated beverages."[4] In other words, it doesn't seem to matter whether people rely on caffeine-containing beverages or other beverages to meet their fluid needs.

As Highlight 7 explains, alcohol acts as a diuretic, and it has many adverse effects on health and nutrition status. Alcohol should not be used to meet fluid needs.

Health Effects of Water In addition to meeting the body's fluid needs, drinking plenty of water may protect the bladder against cancer by diluting the urine and reducing its holding time. The risk of bladder cancer in men decreases when fluid intake is high.[5] An adequate water intake may also protect against kidney stones, prostate cancer, and breast cancer.[6]

The kind of water you drink may also make a difference to health. Water is usually either hard or soft. **Hard water** has high concentrations of calcium and magnesium; sodium or potassium is the principal mineral of **soft water** (see the accompanying glossary for these and other common terms used to describe water). In practical terms, soft water makes more bubbles with less soap; hard water leaves

GLOSSARY OF WATER TERMS

artesian water: water drawn from a well that taps a confined aquifer in which the water is under pressure.

bottled water: drinking water sold in bottles.

carbonated water: water that contains carbon dioxide gas, either naturally occurring or added, that causes bubbles to form in it; also called *bubbling* or *sparkling water.* Seltzer, soda, and tonic waters are legally soft drinks and are not regulated as water.

distilled water: water that has been vaporized and recondensed, leaving it free of dissolved minerals.

filtered water: water treated by filtration, usually through *activated carbon filters* that reduce the lead in tap water, or by *reverse osmosis* units that force pressurized water across a membrane removing lead, arsenic, and some microorganisms from tap water.

hard water: water with a high calcium and magnesium content.

mineral water: water from a spring or well that typically contains 250 to 500 parts per million (ppm) of minerals. Minerals give water a distinctive flavor. Many mineral waters are high in sodium.

natural water: water obtained from a spring or well that is certified to be safe and sanitary. The mineral content may not be changed, but the water may be treated in other ways such as with ozone or by filtration.

public water: water from a municipal or county water system that has been treated and disinfected.

purified water: water that has been treated by distillation or other physical or chemical processes that remove dissolved solids. Because purified water contains no minerals or contaminants, it is useful for medical and research purposes.

soft water: water with a high sodium or potassium content.

spring water: water originating from an underground spring or well. It may be bubbly (carbonated), or "flat" or "still," meaning not carbonated. Brand names such as "Spring Pure" do not necessarily mean that the water comes from a spring.

well water: water drawn from ground water by tapping into an aquifer.

a ring on the tub, a crust of rocklike crystals in the teakettle, and a gray residue in the laundry.

Soft water may seem more desirable around the house, and some homeowners purchase water softeners that replace magnesium and calcium with sodium. In the body, however, soft water with sodium may aggravate hypertension and heart disease.[7] In contrast, hard water may benefit these conditions by virtue of its calcium content.[8]

Soft water also more easily dissolves certain contaminant minerals, such as cadmium and lead, from old plumbing pipes. As Chapter 13 explains, these contaminant minerals harm the body by displacing the nutrient minerals from their normal sites of action. People who live in old buildings should run the cold water tap a minute to flush out harmful minerals whenever the water faucet has been off for more than six hours. Many people turn to **bottled water** as an alternative to tap water, believing it to be safer than tap water and therefore worth its substantial cost.

IN SUMMARY Water makes up about 60 percent of the adult body's weight. It assists with the transport of nutrients and waste products throughout the body, participates in chemical reactions, acts as a solvent, serves as a shock absorber, and regulates body temperature. To maintain water balance, intake from liquids, foods, and metabolism must equal losses from the kidneys, skin, lungs, and GI tract. The amount and type of water a person drinks may have positive or negative health effects.

Blood Volume and Blood Pressure

Fluids maintain the blood volume, which in turn influences blood pressure. Central to the regulation of blood volume and blood pressure are the kidneys. All day, every day, the kidneys reabsorb needed substances and water and excrete wastes with some water in the urine (see Figure 12-2 on p. 400). The kidneys meticulously adjust the volume and the concentration of the urine to accommodate changes in the body, including variations in the day's food and beverage intakes. Instructions on whether to retain or release substances or water come from ADH, renin, angiotensin, and aldosterone.

ADH and Water Retention Whenever blood volume or blood pressure falls too low, or whenever the extracellular fluid becomes too concentrated, the hypothalamus signals the pituitary gland to release **antidiuretic hormone (ADH).** ADH is a water-conserving hormone■ that stimulates the kidneys to reabsorb water. Consequently, the more water you need, the less your kidneys excrete. These events also trigger thirst. Drinking water and retaining fluids raise the blood volume and dilute the concentrated fluids, thus helping to restore homeostasis.

■ Recall from Highlight 7 that alcohol depresses ADH activity, thus promoting fluid losses and dehydration. In addition to its antidiuretic effect, ADH elevates blood pressure and so is also called **vasopressin** (VAS-oh-PRES-in).
- **vaso** = vessel
- **press** = pressure

Renin and Sodium Retention Cells in the kidneys respond to low blood pressure by releasing an enzyme called **renin.** Through a complex series of events, renin causes the kidneys to reabsorb sodium. Sodium reabsorption, in turn, is always accompanied by water retention, which helps to restore blood volume and blood pressure.

Angiotensin and Blood Vessel Constriction Renin also activates the blood protein angiotensinogen to **angiotensin.** Angiotensin is a powerful **vasoconstrictor**: it narrows the diameters of blood vessels, thereby raising the blood pressure.

Aldosterone and Sodium Retention Angiotensin also mediates the release of the hormone **aldosterone** from the **adrenal glands.** Aldosterone signals the kidneys to retain more sodium and therefore water because when sodium moves, fluids follow. Again, the effect is that when more water is needed, less is excreted.

antidiuretic hormone (ADH): a hormone released by the pituitary gland in response to highly concentrated blood. The kidneys respond by reabsorbing water, thus preventing water loss.
- **anti** = against
- **dia** = through
- **ure** = urine

renin (REN-in): an enzyme from the kidneys that activates angiotensin.

angiotensin (AN-gee-oh-TEN-sin): a hormone involved in blood pressure regulation. Its precursor protein is called **angiotensinogen.**

vasoconstrictor (VAS-oh-kon-STRIK-tor): a substance that constricts or narrows the blood vessels.

aldosterone (al-DOS-ter-own): a hormone secreted by the adrenal glands that stimulates the reabsorption of sodium by the kidneys. Aldosterone also regulates chloride and potassium concentrations.

adrenal glands: glands adjacent to, and just above, each kidney.

FIGURE 12-2 A Nephron, One of the Kidney's Many Functioning Units

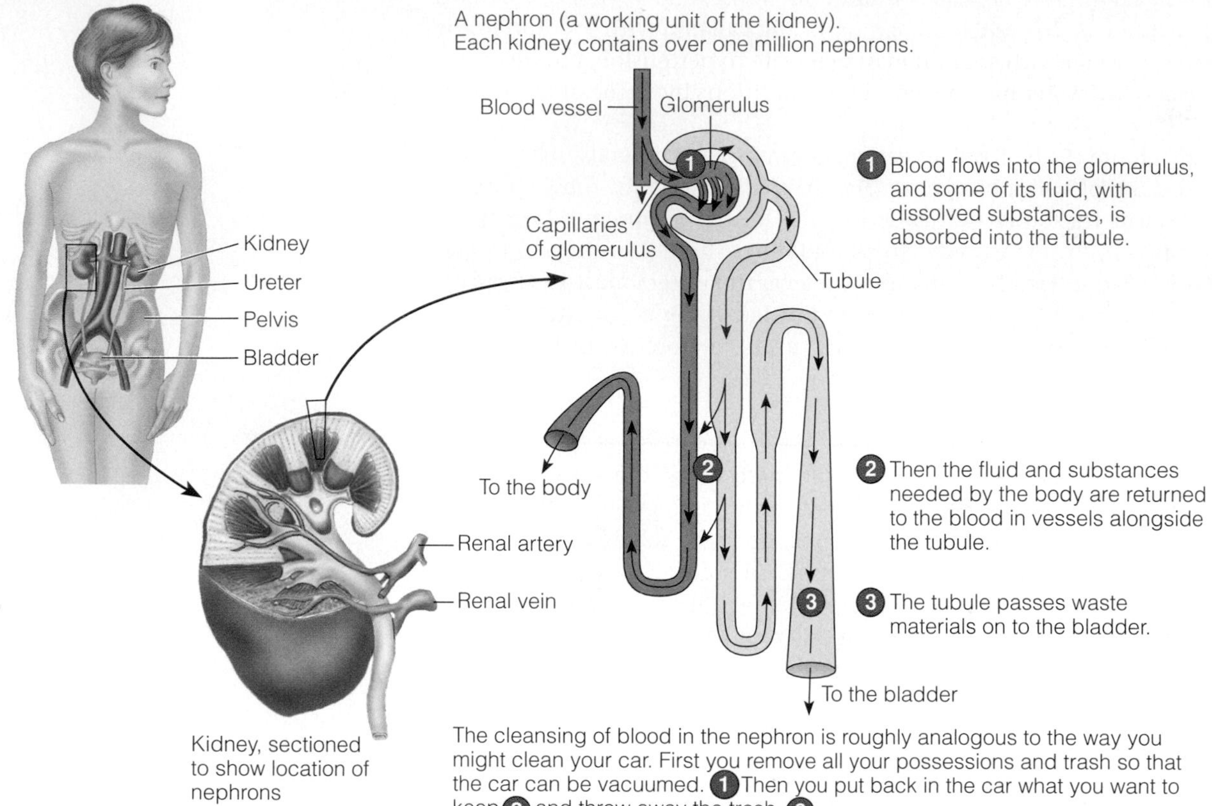
A nephron (a working unit of the kidney).
Each kidney contains over one million nephrons.
Blood vessel
Glomerulus
Capillaries of glomerulus
Tubule
Kidney
Ureter
Pelvis
Bladder
To the body
Renal artery
Renal vein
Kidney, sectioned to show location of nephrons
To the bladder
1 Blood flows into the glomerulus, and some of its fluid, with dissolved substances, is absorbed into the tubule.
2 Then the fluid and substances needed by the body are returned to the blood in vessels alongside the tubule.
3 The tubule passes waste materials on to the bladder.

The cleansing of blood in the nephron is roughly analogous to the way you might clean your car. First you remove all your possessions and trash so that the car can be vacuumed. (1) Then you put back in the car what you want to keep (2) and throw away the trash. (3)

All of these actions are presented in Figure 12-3 and help to explain why high-sodium diets aggravate conditions such as hypertension or edema. Too much sodium causes water retention and an accompanying rise in blood pressure or swelling in the interstitial spaces. Chapter 27 discusses hypertension in detail.

IN SUMMARY In response to low blood volume, low blood pressure, or highly concentrated body fluids, these actions combine to effectively restore homeostasis:

- ADH retains water.
- Renin retains sodium.
- Angiotensin constricts blood vessels.
- Aldosterone retains sodium.

These actions can maintain water balance only if a person drinks enough water.

■ The major minerals:
- Sodium.
- Chloride.
- Potassium.
- Calcium.
- Phosphorus.
- Magnesium.
- Sulfur.

salt: a compound composed of a positive ion other than H^+ and a negative ion other than OH^-. An example is sodium chloride ($Na^+ Cl^-$).
- **Na** = sodium.
- **Cl** = chloride.

dissociates (dis-SO-see-ates): physically separates.

ions (EYE-uns): atoms or molecules that have gained or lost electrons and therefore have electrical charges. Examples include the positively charged sodium ion (Na^+) and the negatively charged chloride ion (Cl^-). For a closer look at ions, see Appendix B.

Fluid and Electrolyte Balance

Maintaining a balance of about two-thirds of the body fluids inside the cells and one-third outside is vital to the life of the cells. If too much water were to enter the cells, it might rupture them; if too much water were to leave, they would collapse. To control the movement of water, the cells direct the movement of the major minerals.■

Dissociation of Salt in Water When a mineral **salt** such as sodium chloride (NaCl) dissolves in water, it separates **(dissociates)** into **ions**—positively and neg-

FIGURE 12-3 How the Body Regulates Blood Volume

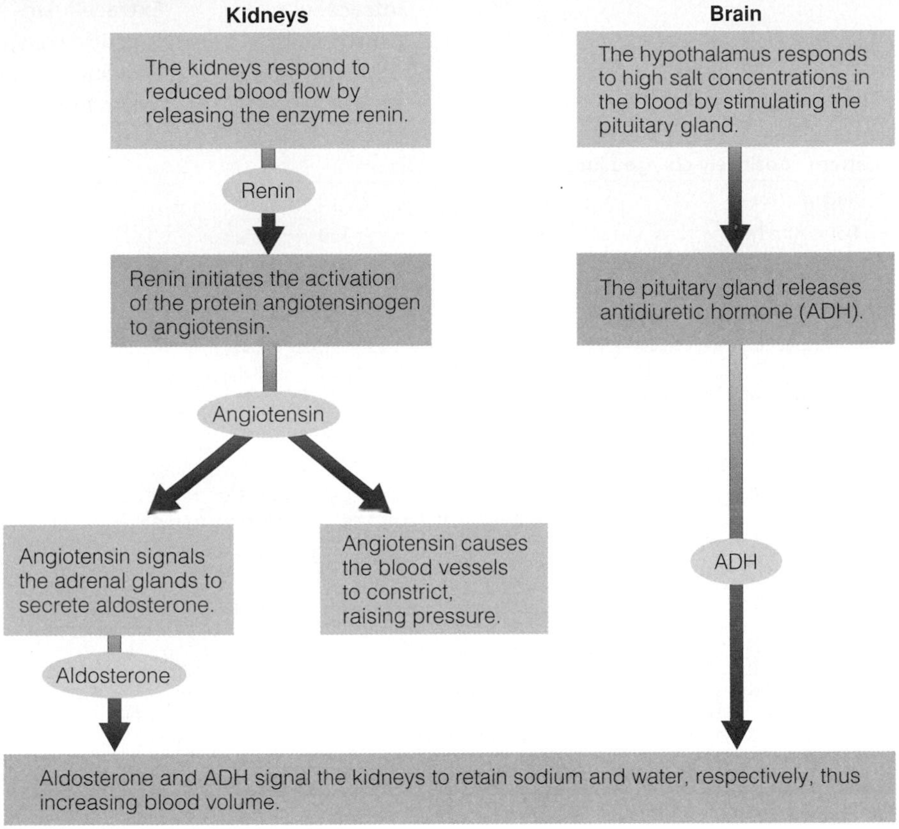
Kidneys
Brain
The kidneys respond to reduced blood flow by releasing the enzyme renin.
The hypothalamus responds to high salt concentrations in the blood by stimulating the pituitary gland.
Renin
Renin initiates the activation of the protein angiotensinogen to angiotensin.
The pituitary gland releases antidiuretic hormone (ADH).
Angiotensin
Angiotensin signals the adrenal glands to secrete aldosterone.
Angiotensin causes the blood vessels to constrict, raising pressure.
ADH
Aldosterone
Aldosterone and ADH signal the kidneys to retain sodium and water, respectively, thus increasing blood volume.

atively charged particles (Na^+ and Cl^-). The positive ions are **cations;** the negative ones are **anions.**■ Unlike pure water, which conducts electricity poorly, ions dissolved in water carry electrical current. For this reason, salts that dissociate into ions are called **electrolytes,** and fluids that contain them are **electrolyte solutions.**

In all electrolyte solutions, anion and cation concentrations balance (the number of negative and positive charges are equal). If a fluid contains 1000 negative charges, it must contain 1000 positive charges, too. If an anion enters the fluid, a cation must accompany it or another anion must leave so that electrical neutrality will be maintained. Whenever Na^+ ions leave a cell, other positive ions enter: potassium (K^+) ions, for example. In fact, it's a good bet that whenever Na^+ and K^+ ions are moving, they are going in opposite directions.

Table 12-4 (on p. 402) shows that, indeed, the positive and negative charges inside and outside cells are perfectly balanced even though the numbers of each kind of ion differ over a wide range. Inside the cells, the positive charges total 202 and the negative charges balance these perfectly. Outside the cells, the amounts and proportions of the ions differ from those inside, but again the positive and negative charges balance. (Scientists count these charges in **milliequivalents, mEq.**)

Electrolytes Attract Water Electrolytes attract water. Each water molecule has a net charge of zero,■ but the oxygen side of the molecule is slightly negatively charged, and the hydrogens are slightly positively charged. Figure 12-4 shows the result in an electrolyte solution: both positive and negative ions attract clusters of water molecules around them. This attraction dissolves salts in water and enables the body to move fluids into appropriate compartments.

■ To help you remember the difference, think of the "t" in cations as a "plus" (+) sign and the "n" in anions as "negative."

■ A neutral molecule, such as water, that has opposite charges spatially separated within the molecule is **polar;** see Appendix B for more details.

cations (CAT-eye-uns): positively charged ions.

anions (AN-eye-uns): negatively charged ions.

electrolytes: salts that dissolve in water and dissociate into charged particles called ions.

electrolyte solutions: solutions that can conduct electricity.

milliequivalents (mEq): the concentration of electrolytes in a volume of solution. Milliequivalents are a useful measure when considering ions because the number of charges reveals characteristics about the solution that are not evident when the concentration is expressed in terms of weight.

TABLE 12-4 Important Body Electrolytes

Electrolytes	Intracellular (inside cells) Concentration (mEq/L)	Extracellular (outside cells) Concentration (mEq/L)
Cations (positively charged ions)		
Sodium (Na^+)	10	142
Potassium (K^+)	150	5
Calcium (Ca^{++})	2	5
Magnesium (Mg^{++})	40	3
	202	155
Anions (negatively charged ions)		
Chloride (Cl^-)	2	103
Bicarbonate (HCO_3^-)	10	27
Phosphate ($HPO_4^=$)	103	2
Sulfate ($SO_4^=$)	20	1
Organic acids (lactate, pyruvate)	10	6
Proteins	57	16
	202	155

NOTE: The numbers of positive and negative charges in a given fluid are the same. For example, in extracellular fluid, the cations and anions both equal 155 milliequivalents per liter (mEq/L). Of the cations, sodium ions make up 142 mEq/L; and potassium, calcium, and magnesium ions make up the remainder. Of the anions, chloride ions number 103 mEq/L; bicarbonate ions number 27; and the rest are provided by phosphate ions, sulfate ions, organic acids, and protein.

■ The word ending *-ate* denotes a salt of the mineral. Thus phosphate is the salt form of the mineral phosphorus, and sulfate is the salt form of sulfur.

Water Follows Electrolytes Some electrolytes reside primarily outside the cells (notably, sodium and chloride), while others are predominantly inside the cells (notably, potassium, magnesium, phosphate,■ and sulfate). Cell membranes are selectively permeable, meaning that they allow the passage of some molecules, but not of others. Whenever electrolytes move across the membrane, water follows.

FIGURE 12-4 Water Dissolves Salts and Follows Electrolytes

The structural arrangement of the two hydrogen atoms and one oxygen atom enables water to dissolve salts. Water's role as a solvent is one of its most valuable characteristics.

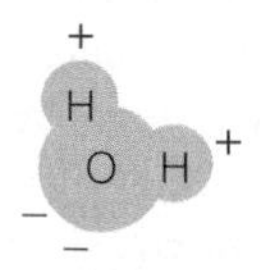
+
H
O H
+
–
–

The negatively charged electrons that bond the hydrogens to the oxygen spend most of their time near the oxygen atom. As a result, the oxygen is slightly negative, and the hydrogens are slightly positive (see Appendix B).

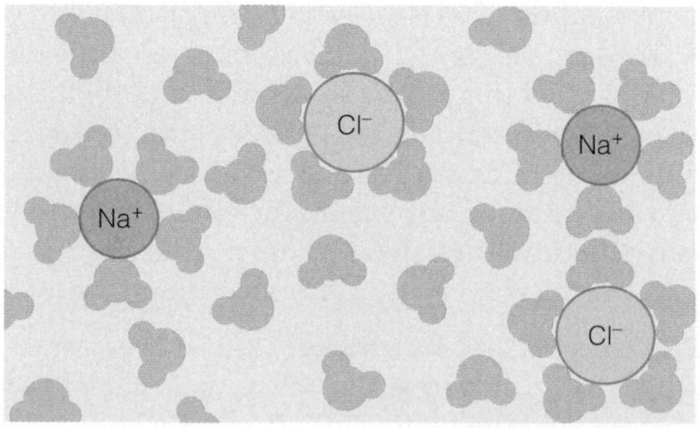
Cl⁻
Na⁺
Na⁺
Cl⁻

In an electrolyte solution, water molecules are attracted to both anions and cations. Notice that the negative oxygen atoms of the water molecules are drawn to the sodium cation (Na^+), while the positive hydrogen atoms of the water molecules are drawn to the chloride ions (Cl^-).

FIGURE 12-5 Osmosis

Water flows in the direction of the more highly concentrated solution.

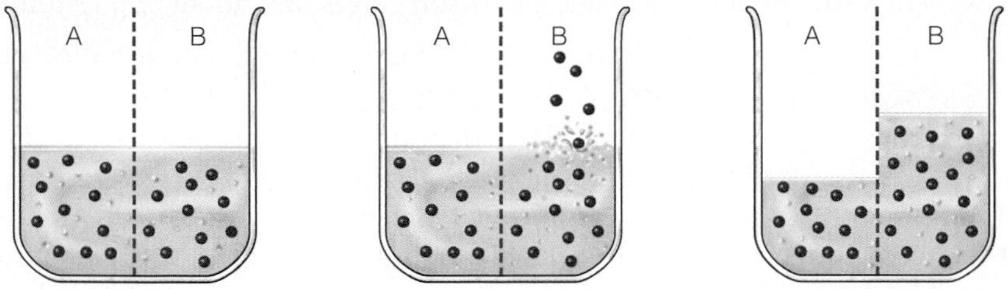
A
B
A
B
A
B

1 With equal numbers of solute particles on both sides, the concentrations are equal, and the tendency of water to move in either direction is about the same.

2 Now additional solute is added to side B. Solute cannot flow across the divider (in the case of a cell, its membrane).

3 Water can flow both ways across the divider, but has a greater tendency to move from side A to side B, where there is a greater concentration of solute. The volume of water becomes greater on side B, and the concentrations on side A and B become equal.

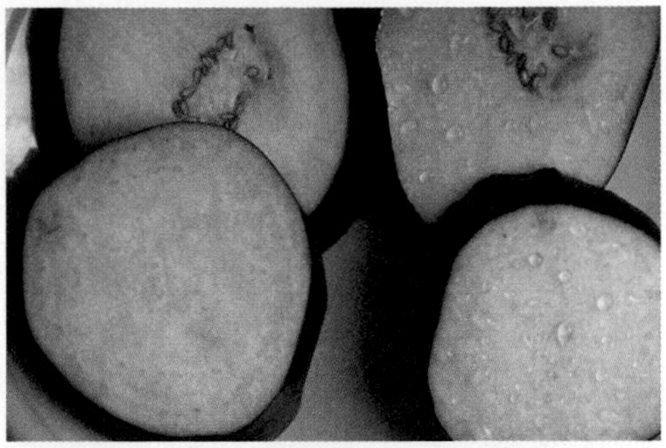

© Craig M. Moore

When sprinkled with salt, vegetables "sweat" because water moves toward the higher concentration of salt outside the eggplant.

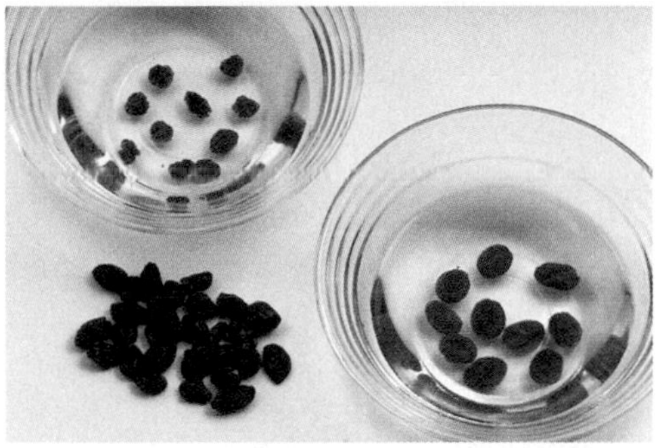

© Craig M. Moore

When immersed in water, raisins get plump because water moves toward the higher concentration of sugar inside the raisins.

The movement of water across a membrane toward the more concentrated **solutes** is called **osmosis.** The amount of pressure needed to prevent the movement of water across a membrane is called the **osmotic pressure.** Figure 12-5 presents osmosis and the photos of salted eggplant and rehydrated raisins provide familiar examples.

Proteins Regulate Flow of Fluids and Ions Chapter 6 described how proteins attract water and help to regulate fluid movement. In addition, transport proteins in the cell membranes regulate the passage of positive ions and other substances from one side of the membrane to the other. Negative ions follow positive ions, and water flows toward the more concentrated solution.

A well-understood protein that regulates the flow of fluids and ions in and out of cells is the sodium-potassium pump. The pump actively exchanges sodium for potassium across the cell membrane, using ATP as an energy source. Figure 6-10 on p. 191 illustrates this action.

Regulation of Fluid and Electrolyte Balance The amounts of various minerals in the body must remain nearly constant. Regulation occurs chiefly at two sites: the GI tract and the kidneys.

The digestive juices of the GI tract contain minerals. These minerals and those from foods are reabsorbed in the large intestine as needed. Each day, 8 liters of fluids and associated minerals are recycled this way, providing ample opportunity for the regulation of electrolyte balance.

The kidneys' control of the body's *water* content by way of the hormone ADH has already been described (see p. 399). To regulate the *electrolyte* contents, the kidneys depend on the adrenal glands, which send out messages by way of the hormone aldosterone (also explained on p. 399). If the body's sodium is low, aldosterone stimulates sodium reabsorption from the kidneys. As sodium is reabsorbed, potassium (another positive ion) is excreted in accordance with the rule that total positive charges must remain in balance with total negative charges.

Fluid and Electrolyte Imbalance

Normally, the body defends itself successfully against fluid and electrolyte imbalances. Certain situations and some medications, however, may overwhelm the body's ability to compensate. Severe and prolonged vomiting and diarrhea and heavy sweating, burns, and traumatic wounds may incur such great fluid and electrolyte losses as to precipitate a medical emergency.

solutes (SOLL-yutes): the substances that are dissolved in a solution. The number of molecules in a given volume of fluid is the **solute concentration.**

osmosis: the movement of water across a membrane *toward* the side where the solutes are more concentrated.

osmotic pressure: the amount of pressure needed to prevent the movement of water across a membrane.

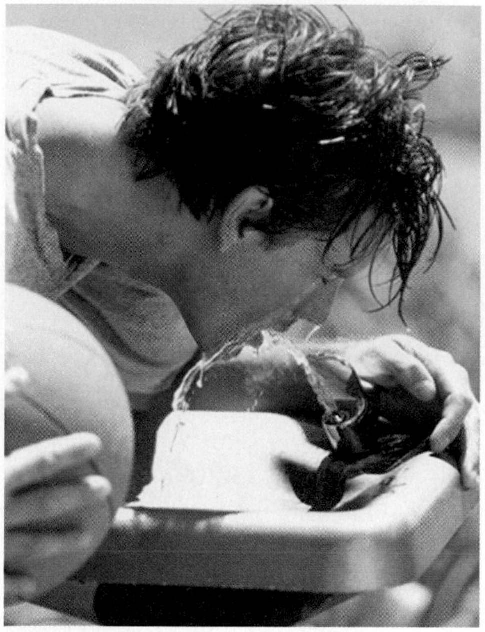
© Norbert Schaefer/CORBIS
Physically active people must remember to replace their body fluids.

Sodium and Chloride Most Easily Lost Because sodium and chloride are the body's principal extracellular cation and anion, they are first to be lost when fluid is lost by sweating, bleeding, or excretion. It is no coincidence that after sweating excessively or losing fluid in other ways, a person craves salty foods and refreshing drinks.

Different Solutes Lost by Different Routes If fluid is lost by vomiting or diarrhea, sodium is lost indiscriminately. If the adrenal glands oversecrete aldosterone, as occurs when a tumor develops, the kidneys may excrete too much potassium. And the person with uncontrolled diabetes may lose a solute not normally excreted: glucose, and with it, large amounts of fluid. All three situations bring on dehydration, but drinking water alone cannot restore electrolyte balance. In each case, medical intervention is required.

Replacing Lost Fluids and Electrolytes In many cases, people can replace the fluids and minerals lost in sweat or in a temporary bout of diarrhea by drinking plain cool water and eating regular foods. Some cases, however, demand rapid replacement of fluids and electrolytes—for example, when diarrhea threatens the life of a malnourished child. Caregivers around the world have learned to use simple formulas■ to treat mild-to-moderate cases of diarrhea at home. These lifesaving formulas do not require hospitalization and can be prepared from ingredients available locally. Caregivers need only learn to measure ingredients carefully and use sanitary water. Once rehydrated, a person can begin eating foods.

■ Health care workers use **oral rehydration therapy (ORT)**—a simple solution of sugar, salt, and water, taken by mouth—to treat dehydration caused by diarrhea. A simple ORT recipe (cool before giving):
- ½ L boiling water.
- A small handful of sugar (4 tsp).
- 3 pinches of salt (½ tsp).

Chapter 24 provides a more exact recipe.

Acid-Base Balance

The body uses its ions not only to help maintain fluid and electrolyte balance, but also to regulate the acidity **(pH)** of its fluids. The pH scale of Chapter 3 is repeated here, in Figure 12-6, with the normal and abnormal pH ranges of the blood added. As you can see, the body must maintain the pH within a narrow range to avoid life-threatening consequences. Slight deviations in either direction can damage proteins, causing metabolic mayhem. Enzymes couldn't catalyze reactions and hemoglobin couldn't carry oxygen—to name just two examples.

The acidity of the body's fluids is determined by the concentration of hydrogen ions (H^+). A high concentration of hydrogen ions would be very acidic. Normal energy metabolism generates hydrogen ions, as well as many other acids, that must be neutralized. Three systems defend the body against fluctuations in pH—buffers in the blood, respiration in the lungs, and excretion in the kidneys.

Regulation by the Buffers **Bicarbonate** (a base) and **carbonic acid** (an acid) in the body fluids, as well as some proteins, protect the body against changes in acidity by acting as buffers—substances that can neutralize acids or bases. These buffer systems serve as a first line of defense against changes in the fluids' acid-base balance.

Regulation by the Lungs Respiration provides another defense. Carbon dioxide, which is formed all the time during cellular metabolism, forms carbonic acid in the blood, which then dissociates to form hydrogen ions and bicarbonate ions. The appropriate balance between carbonic acid and bicarbonate is essential to maintaining optimal blood pH. If too much carbonic acid builds up, the respiration rate speeds up; this hyperventilation increases the amount of carbon dioxide exhaled, thereby lowering the carbonic acid concentration and restoring homeostasis. Conversely, if bicarbonate builds up, the respiration rate slows; carbon dioxide is retained and forms more carbonic acid. Again, homeostasis is restored.

Regulation by the Kidneys The kidneys play the primary role in maintaining long-term control of acid-base balance. By selecting which ions to retain and which to excrete, the kidneys adjust the body's acid-base balance. Their work is complex, but its net effect is easy to sum up. The *body's* total acid burden remains nearly constant; *urine's* acidity fluctuates to accommodate that balance.

pH: a measure of the concentration of H^+ ions (see Appendix B). The lower the pH, the higher the H^+ ion concentration and the stronger the acid. A pH above 7 is alkaline, or base (a solution in which OH^- ions predominate).

bicarbonate: a compound with the formula HCO_3 that results from the dissociation of carbonic acid; of particular importance in maintaining the body's acid-base balance. (Bicarbonate is also an alkaline secretion of the pancreas, part of the pancreatic juice.)

carbonic acid: a compound with the formula H_2CO_3 that results from the combination of carbon dioxide (CO_2) and water (H_2O); of particular importance in maintaining the body's acid-base balance.

FIGURE 12-6 The pH Scale

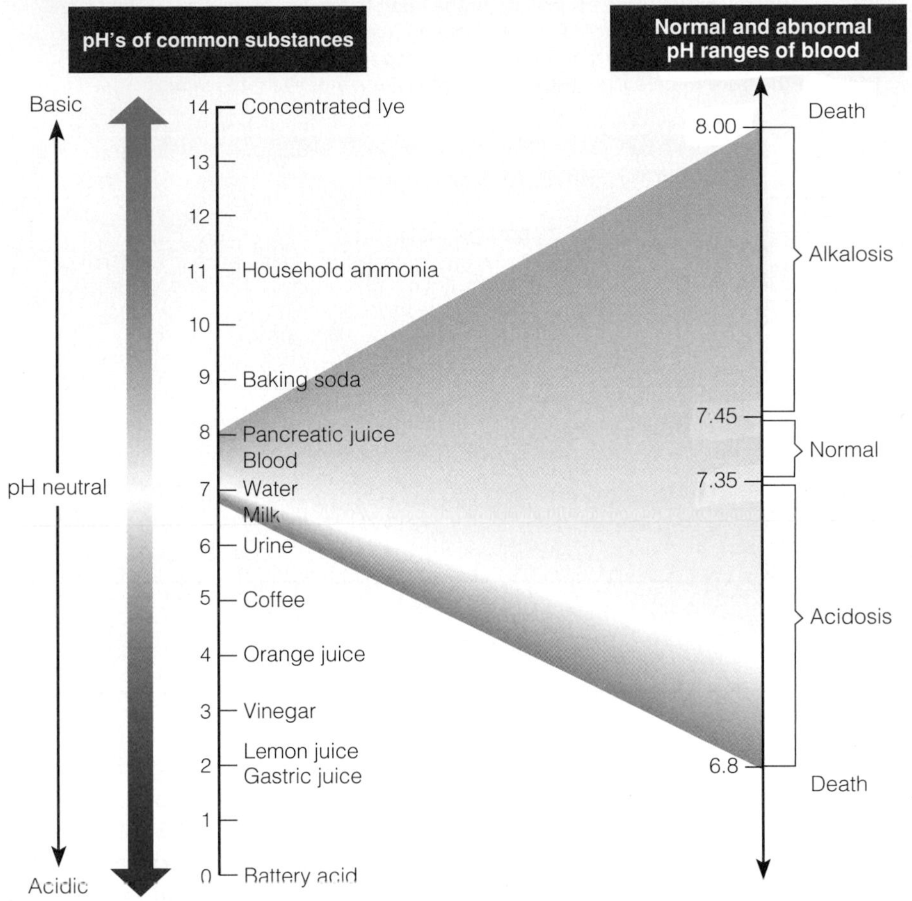
pH's of common substances
Normal and abnormal pH ranges of blood
Basic
pH neutral
Acidic
14 Concentrated lye
13
12
11 Household ammonia
10
9 Baking soda
8 Pancreatic juice
Blood
7 Water
Milk
6 Urine
5 Coffee
4 Orange juice
3 Vinegar
2 Lemon juice
Gastric juice
1
0 Battery acid
Death
8.00
Alkalosis
7.45
Normal
7.35
Acidosis
6.8
Death

NOTE: Each step is ten times as concentrated in base (1/10 as much acid, or H^+) as the one below it.

IN SUMMARY Electrolytes (charged minerals) in the fluids help distribute the fluids inside and outside the cells, thus ensuring the appropriate water balance and acid-base balance to support all life processes. Excessive losses of fluids and electrolytes upset these balances; the kidneys play a key role in restoring homeostasis.

The Minerals—An Overview

Figure 12-7 shows the amounts of the **major minerals** found in the body and, for comparison, some of the trace minerals. The distinction between the major and trace minerals does not mean that one group is more important than the other—all minerals are vital. The major minerals are so named because they are present, and needed, in larger amounts in the body. They are shown at the top of the figure and are discussed in this chapter. The trace minerals (shown at the bottom) are discussed in Chapter 13. A few generalizations pertain to all of the minerals and distinguish them from the vitamins. Especially notable is their chemical nature.

Inorganic Elements Unlike the organic vitamins, which are easily destroyed, minerals are inorganic elements that always retain their chemical identity. Once minerals enter the body proper, they remain there until excreted; they cannot be

major minerals: essential mineral nutrients found in the human body in amounts larger than 5 g; sometimes called **macrominerals.**

FIGURE 12-7 Minerals in a 60-kilogram (132-pound) Human Body

Not only are the major minerals present in the body in larger amounts than the trace minerals, but they are also needed by the body in larger amounts. Recommended intakes for the major minerals are stated in *hundreds of milligrams* or *grams,* whereas those for the trace minerals are listed in *tens of milligrams* or even *micrograms.*

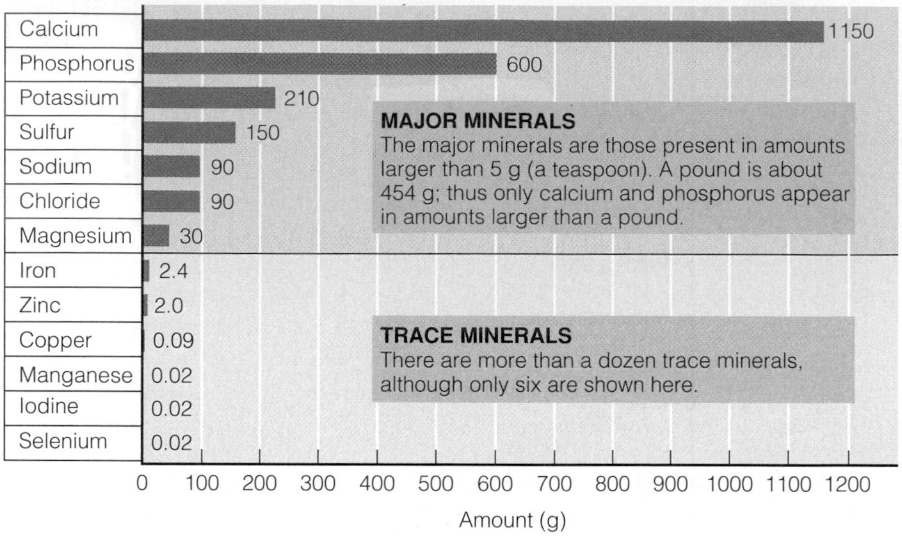

Calcium
1150
Phosphorus
600
Potassium
210
Sulfur
150
Sodium
90
Chloride
90
Magnesium
30
Iron
2.4
Zinc
2.0
Copper
0.09
Manganese
0.02
Iodine
0.02
Selenium
0.02
MAJOR MINERALS
The major minerals are those present in amounts larger than 5 g (a teaspoon). A pound is about 454 g; thus only calcium and phosphorus appear in amounts larger than a pound.
TRACE MINERALS
There are more than a dozen trace minerals, although only six are shown here.
0 100 200 300 400 500 600 700 800 900 1000 1100 1200
Amount (g)

changed into anything else. Iron, for example, may temporarily combine with other charged elements in salts, but it is always iron. Neither can minerals be destroyed by heat, air, acid, or mixing; consequently, little care is needed to preserve minerals during food preparation. In fact, the ash that remains when a food is burned contains all the minerals that were in the food originally. Minerals can be lost from food only when they leach into water that is then poured down the drain.

The Body's Handling of Minerals The minerals also differ from the vitamins in the amounts the body can absorb and in the extent to which they must be specially handled. Some minerals, such as potassium, are easily absorbed into the blood, transported freely, and readily excreted by the kidneys, much like the water-soluble vitamins. Other minerals, such as calcium, are more like fat-soluble vitamins in that they must have carriers to be absorbed and transported. And, like some of the fat-soluble vitamins, minerals taken in excess can be toxic.

Variable Bioavailability The bioavailability■ of minerals varies. Some foods contain **binders** that combine chemically with minerals, preventing their absorption and carrying them out of the body with other wastes. Examples of binders include phytates, which are found primarily in legumes and grains, and oxalates, which are present in rhubarb and spinach, among other foods. These foods contain more minerals than the body actually receives for use.

■ Reminder: *Bioavailability* refers to the rate at and the extent to which a nutrient is absorbed and used.

Nutrient Interactions Chapter 10 described how the presence or absence of one vitamin can affect another's absorption, metabolism, and excretion. The same is true of the minerals. The interactions between sodium and calcium, for example, cause both to be excreted when sodium intakes are high. Phosphorus binds with magnesium in the GI tract, so magnesium absorption is limited when phosphorus intakes are high. These are just two examples of the interactions involving minerals featured in this chapter. Discussions in both this chapter and the next point out additional problems that arise from such interactions. Notice how often they reflect an excess of one mineral creating an inadequacy of another and how supplements—not foods—are most often to blame.

binders: chemical compounds in foods that combine with nutrients (especially minerals) to form complexes the body cannot absorb. Examples include **phytates** (FYE-tates) and **oxalates** (OCK-sa-lates).

Varied Roles While all the major minerals help to maintain the body's fluid balance described earlier, sodium, chloride, and potassium are most noted for that role. For this reason, these three minerals are discussed first here. Later sections describe the minerals most noted for their roles in bone growth and health—calcium, phosphorus, and magnesium.

IN SUMMARY The major minerals are found in larger quantities in the body, whereas the trace minerals occur in smaller amounts. Minerals are inorganic elements that retain their chemical identities; they usually receive special handling and regulation in the body; and they may bind with other substances or interact with other minerals, thus limiting their absorption.

Sodium

People have held salt (sodium chloride) in high regard throughout recorded history. We say "you are the salt of the earth" to someone we admire and "you are not worth your salt" to someone we consider worthless. Even the word *salary* comes from the Latin word for salt.

Cultures vary in their use of salt, but most people find its taste innately appealing. Salt brings its own tangy taste and enhances other flavors, most likely by suppressing the bitter flavors. You can taste this effect for yourself: tonic water with its bitter quinine tastes sweeter with a little salt added.

Sodium Roles in the Body **Sodium** is the principal cation of the extracellular fluid and the primary regulator of its volume. Sodium also helps maintain acid-base balance and is essential to nerve impulse transmission and muscle contraction.*

Foods usually provide more sodium than the body needs. Sodium is readily absorbed by the intestinal tract and travels freely in the blood until it reaches the kidneys, which filter all the sodium out of the blood; then, with great precision, they return to the bloodstream the exact amount the body needs. Normally, the amount excreted is approximately equal to the amount ingested on a given day. When blood sodium rises, as when a person eats salted foods, thirst signals the person to drink until the appropriate sodium-to-water ratio is restored. Then the kidneys excrete both the excess water and the excess sodium together.

Sodium Recommendations Diets rarely lack sodium and even when intakes are low, the body adapts by reducing sodium losses in urine and sweat, thus making deficiencies unlikely. Sodium recommendations■ are set low enough to protect against high blood pressure, but high enough to allow an adequate intake of other nutrients. Because high sodium intakes correlate with high blood pressure, the Upper Level for adults is set at 2300 milligrams per day, slightly lower than the Daily Value used on food labels (2400 milligrams).

■ AI for sodium:
- 1500 mg/day (19–50 yr).
- 1300 mg/day (51–70 yr).
- 1200 mg/day (>70 yr).

HEALTHY PEOPLE 2010

Increase the proportion of persons aged 2 years and older who consume 2400 mg or less of sodium daily.

Sodium and Hypertension For years, a high *sodium* intake was considered the primary factor responsible for high blood pressure. Then research pointed to *salt* (sodium chloride) as the dietary culprit. Salt has a greater effect on blood pressure than either sodium or chloride alone or in combination with other ions.

sodium: the principal cation in the extracellular fluids of the body; critical to the maintenance of fluid balance, nerve impulse transmissions, and muscle contractions.

*One of the ways the kidneys regulate acid-base balance is by excreting hydrogen ions (H^+) in exchange for sodium ions (Na^+).

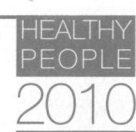

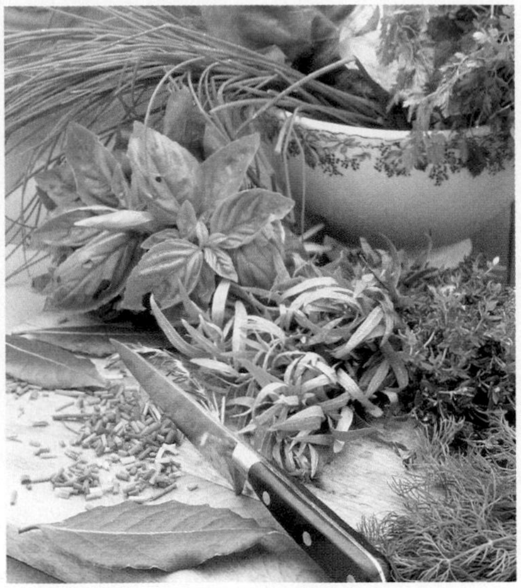
© BSIP Agency/Index Stock Imagery

Fresh herbs add flavor to a recipe without adding salt.

■ 2005 *Dietary Guidelines:*
- Consume less than 2300 mg (approximately 1 tsp of salt) of sodium per day.

■ Salt (sodium chloride) is about 40% sodium.
1 g salt contributes 400 mg sodium.
5 g salt = 1 tsp.
1 tsp salt contributes 2000 mg sodium.

salt sensitivity: a characteristic of individuals who respond to a high salt intake with an increase in blood pressure or to a low salt intake with a decrease in bloood pressure.

Some individuals respond sensitively to excesses in salt intake and experience high blood pressure. People most likely to have a **salt sensitivity** include those whose parents had high blood pressure; those with chronic kidney disease or diabetes; African Americans; and people over 50 years of age.* Overweight people also appear to be particularly sensitive to the effect of salt on blood pressure. For them, a high salt intake correlates strongly with heart disease, and salt restriction helps to lower their blood pressure.[9]

In fact, a salt-restricted diet lowers blood pressure in people without hypertension as well.[10] Because reducing salt intake causes no harm and diminishes the risk of hypertension and heart disease, the 2005 *Dietary Guidelines*■ advise limiting daily salt intake to about 1 teaspoon (the equivalent of 2.3 grams or 2300 milligrams of *sodium*).■ Higher intakes seem to be well tolerated in most healthy people, however. The accompanying "How to" offers strategies for cutting salt (and therefore sodium) intake.

One diet plan, known as the DASH (Dietary Approaches to Stop Hypertension) diet, also lowers blood pressure.[11] The DASH approach emphasizes fruits, vegetables, and low-fat dairy products; includes whole grains, nuts, poultry, and fish; and calls for reduced intakes of red meat, butter, and other high-fat foods. The DASH diet in combination with a reduced sodium intake is even more effective in lowering blood pressure than either strategy alone. Chapter 27 offers a complete discussion of hypertension and the dietary recommendations for its prevention and treatment.

Sodium and Osteoporosis A high sodium intake is also associated with calcium excretion, but whether it influences bone loss is less clear.[12] One review of the research concludes that evidence is insufficient to recommend reducing sodium intakes to prevent osteoporosis.[13] Other researchers disagree, acknowledging that while no long-term evidence shows that a reduced sodium intake prevents osteoporosis, less convincing evidence, together with the absence of harm, supports such a recommendation.[14] In other words, reducing sodium intake can't hurt and it may help. Some research shows that potassium may counteract the effects of sodium on calcium excretion.[15] Dietary advice to prevent osteoporosis might therefore suggest selecting foods that are high in calcium and potassium and low in sodium.

Sodium in Foods In general, processed foods have the most sodium, while unprocessed foods such as fresh fruits, vegetables, milk, and meats have the least. In fact, as much as 75 percent of the sodium in people's diets comes from salt added to foods by manufacturers; about 15 percent comes from salt added during cooking and at the table; and only 10 percent comes from the natural content in foods.

Because processed foods may contain sodium without chloride, as in additives such as sodium bicarbonate or sodium saccharin, they do not always taste salty. Most people are surprised to learn that 1 ounce of cornflakes contains more sodium than 1 ounce of salted peanuts—and that ½ cup of instant chocolate pudding contains still more. (The peanuts taste saltier because the salt is all on the surface, where the tongue's sensors immediately pick it up.)

HOW TO Cut Salt Intake

Most people eat more salt (and therefore sodium) than they need, and some people can lower their blood pressure by avoiding highly salted foods and removing the saltshaker from the table. Foods eaten without salt may seem less tasty at first, but with repetition, people can learn to enjoy the natural flavors of many unsalted foods. Strategies to cut salt intake include:

- Cook with little or no added salt.
- Prepare foods with sodium-free spices such as basil, bay leaves, curry, garlic, ginger, mint, oregano, pepper, rosemary, and thyme; lemon juice; vinegar; or wine.
- Add little or no salt at the table; taste foods before adding salt.
- Read labels with an eye open for salt. (See the glossary on p. 59 for terms used to describe the sodium contents of foods on labels.)
- Select low-salt or salt-free products when available.

Use these foods sparingly:

- Foods prepared in brine, such as pickles, olives, and sauerkraut.
- Salty or smoked meats, such as bologna, corned or chipped beef, bacon, frankfurters, ham, lunch meats, salt pork, sausage, and smoked tongue.
- Salty or smoked fish, such as anchovies, caviar, salted and dried cod, herring, sardines, and smoked salmon.
- Snack items such as potato chips, pretzels, salted popcorn, salted nuts, and crackers.
- Condiments such as bouillon cubes; seasoned salts; MSG; soy, teriyaki, Worcestershire, and barbeque sauces; prepared horseradish, catsup, and mustard.
- Cheeses, especially processed types.
- Canned and instant soups.

*Compared with others, salt-sensitive individuals have elevated concentrations of renin in their blood.

FIGURE 12-8 What Processing Does to the Sodium and Potassium Contents of Foods

People who eat foods high in salt often happen to be eating fewer potassium-containing foods at the same time. Note how potassium is lost and sodium is gained as foods become more processed, causing the potassium-to-sodium ratio to fall dramatically. Even when potassium isn't lost, the addition of sodium still lowers the potassium-to-sodium ratio. Limiting sodium intake may help in two ways, then—by lowering blood pressure in salt-sensitive individuals and by indirectly raising potassium intakes in all individuals.

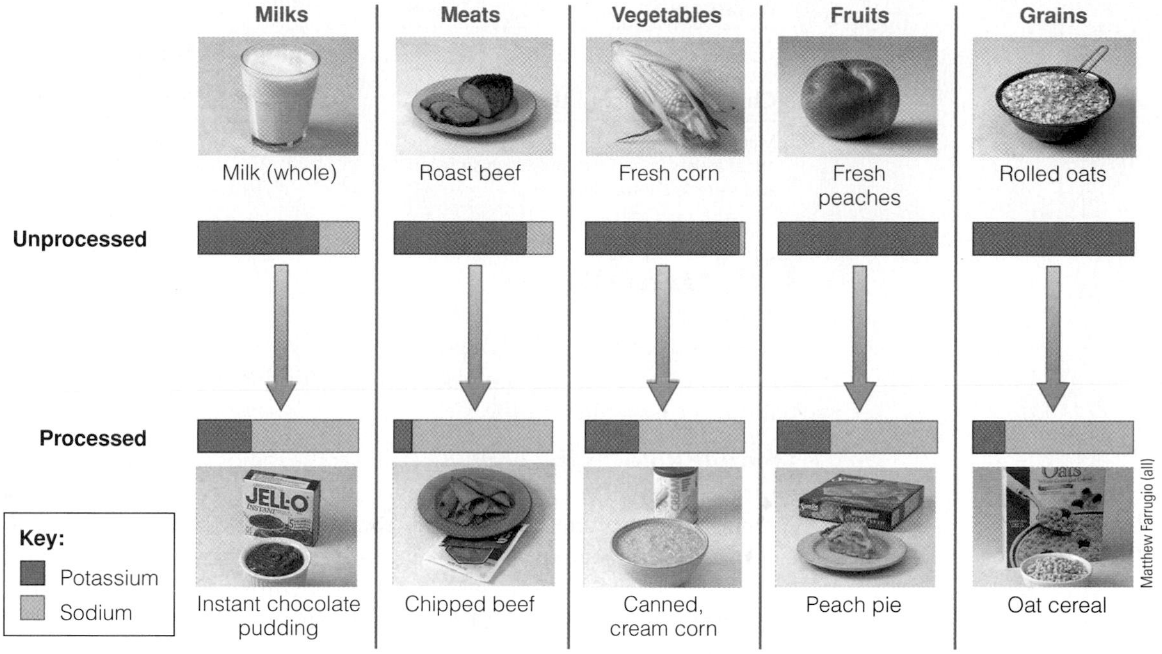
Milks
Meats
Vegetables
Fruits
Grains
Milk (whole)
Roast beef
Fresh corn
Fresh peaches
Rolled oats
Unprocessed
Processed
JELL-O
Key:
Potassium
Sodium
Instant chocolate pudding
Chipped beef
Canned, cream corn
Peach pie
Oat cereal
Matthew Farrugio (all)

Figure 12-8 shows that processed foods not only contain more sodium than their less processed counterparts, but also have less potassium.■ Low potassium may be as significant as high sodium when it comes to blood pressure regulation, so processed foods have two strikes against them.

■ 2005 *Dietary Guidelines:*
- Choose and prepare foods with little salt. At the same time, consume potassium-rich foods, such as fruits and vegetables.

Sodium Deficiency If blood sodium drops, as may occur with vomiting, diarrhea, or heavy sweating, both sodium and water must be replenished. Under normal conditions of sweating due to exercise, salt losses can easily be replaced later in the day with ordinary foods. Salt tablets are not recommended because too much salt, especially if taken with too little water, can induce dehydration. During intense activities, such as ultra-endurance events, athletes can lose so much sodium and drink so much water that they develop hyponatremia—too little sodium in the blood.

Sodium Toxicity and Excessive Intakes The immediate symptoms of acute sodium toxicity are edema and hypertension, but such toxicity poses no problem as long as water needs are met. Prolonged excessive sodium intake■ may contribute to hypertension in some people, as explained earlier.

■ UL for sodium: 2300 mg/day.

IN SUMMARY Sodium is the main cation outside cells and one of the primary electrolytes responsible for maintaining fluid balance. Dietary deficiency is rare, and excesses may aggravate hypertension in some people. For this reason, health professionals advise a diet moderate in salt and sodium. The table on the next page summarizes information about sodium.

Sodium

2004 Adequate Intake (AI)	Deficiency Symptoms
Adults: 1500 mg/day (19–50 yr) 1300 mg/day (51–70 yr) 1200 mg/day (>70 yr)	Muscle cramps, mental apathy, loss of appetite
Upper Level	**Toxicity Symptoms**
Adults: 2300 mg/day	Edema, acute hypertension
Chief Functions in the Body	**Significant Sources**
Maintains normal fluid and electrolyte balance; assists in nerve impulse transmission and muscle contraction	Table salt, soy sauce; moderate amounts in meats, milks, breads, and vegetables; large amounts in processed foods

Chloride

The element *chlorine* (Cl_2) is a poisonous gas. When chlorine reacts with sodium or hydrogen, however, it forms the negative chloride ion (Cl^-). *Chloride* is an essential nutrient, required in the diet.

Chloride Roles in the Body **Chloride** is the major anion of the extracellular fluids (outside the cells), where it occurs mostly in association with sodium. Chloride can move freely across membranes and so also associates with potassium inside cells. Like sodium and potassium, chloride maintains fluid and electrolyte balance.

In the stomach, the chloride ion is part of hydrochloric acid, which maintains the strong acidity of the gastric juice. One of the most serious consequences of vomiting is the loss of this acid■ from the stomach, which upsets the acid-base balance.* Such imbalances are commonly seen in bulimia nervosa, as Highlight 9 describes.

■ Reminder: The loss of acid can lead to *alkalosis,* an above-normal alkalinity in the blood and body fluids.

Chloride Recommendations and Intakes Chloride is abundant in foods (especially processed foods) as part of sodium chloride and other salts. Because the proportion of chloride in salt is greater than sodium,■ chloride recommendations are slightly higher than, but still equivalent to, those of sodium. In other words, ¾ teaspoon of salt will deliver some sodium, more chloride, and still meet the AI for both.

■ Salt (sodium chloride) is about 60% chloride.
1 g salt contributes 600 mg chloride.
5 g salt = 1 tsp.
1 tsp salt contributes 3000 mg chloride.

Chloride Deficiency and Toxicity Diets rarely lack chloride. Chloride losses may occur in conditions such as heavy sweating, chronic diarrhea, and vomiting. The only known cause of high blood chloride concentrations is dehydration due to water deficiency. In both cases, consuming ordinary foods and beverages can restore chloride balance.

IN SUMMARY Chloride is the major anion outside cells, and it associates closely with sodium. In addition to its role in fluid balance, chloride is part of the stomach's hydrochloric acid. The accompanying table summarizes information on chloride.

Chloride

2004 Adequate Intake (AI)	Upper Level
Adults: 2300 mg/day (19–50 yr) 2000 mg/day (51—70 yr) 1800 mg/day (>70 yr)	Adults: 3600 mg/day

(continued)

chloride (KLO-ride): the major anion in the extracellular fluids of the body. Chloride is the ionic form of chlorine, Cl^-; see Appendix B for a description of the chlorine-to-chloride conversion.

*Hydrochloric acid secretion into the stomach involves the addition of bicarbonate ions (base) to the plasma. These bicarbonate ions (HCO_3^-) are neutralized by hydrogen ions (H^+) from the gastric secretions that are reabsorbed into the plasma. When hydrochloric acid is lost during vomiting, these hydrogen ions are no longer available for reabsorption, and so, in effect, the concentrations of bicarbonate ions in the plasma are increased. In this way, excessive vomiting of acidic gastric juices leads to *metabolic alkalosis.*

Chloride (continued)

Chief Functions in the Body	Toxicity Symptoms
Maintains normal fluid and electrolyte balance; part of hydrochloric acid found in the stomach, necessary for proper digestion	Vomiting

Deficiency Symptoms	Significant Sources
Do not occur under normal circumstances	Table salt, soy sauce; moderate amounts in meats, milks, eggs; large amounts in processed foods

Potassium

Like sodium, **potassium** is a positively charged ion. In contrast to sodium, potassium is the body's principal cation *inside* the body cells.

Potassium Roles in the Body Potassium plays a major role in maintaining fluid and electrolyte balance and cell integrity. During nerve impulse transmission and muscle contraction, potassium and sodium briefly trade places across the cell membrane. The cell then quickly pumps them back into place. Controlling potassium distribution is a high priority for the body because it affects many aspects of homeostasis, including a steady heartbeat.

Potassium Recommendations and Intakes Potassium is abundant in all living cells, both plant and animal. Because cells remain intact unless foods are processed, the richest sources of potassium are *fresh* foods of all kinds—as Figure 12-9 (p. 412) shows. Most processed foods such as canned vegetables, ready-to-eat cereals, and luncheon meats contain less potassium—and more sodium (recall Figure 12-8). To meet the AI for potassium, most people need to increase their intake of fruits and vegetables to the amounts recommended by the USDA Food Guide.

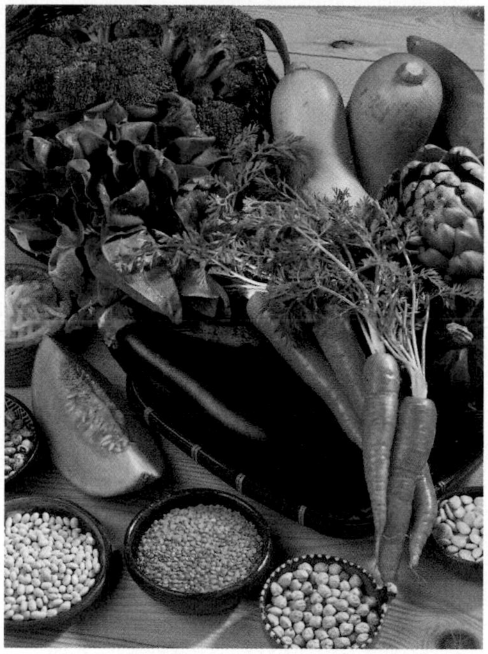

© Polara Studios Inc.

Fresh foods, especially fruits and vegetables, provide potassium in abundance.

Potassium and Hypertension Diets low in potassium seem to play an important role in the development of high blood pressure. Low potassium intakes raise blood pressure, whereas high potassium intakes appear to both prevent and correct hypertension.[16] ■ Potassium-rich fruits and vegetables also appear to reduce the risk of stroke—more so than can be explained by the reduction in blood pressure alone.

■ Reminder: The DASH diet, used to lower blood pressure, emphasizes potassium-rich foods such as fruits and vegetables.

Potassium Deficiency Potassium deficiency is the most common electrolyte imbalance. It is more often caused by excessive losses than by deficient intakes. Conditions such as diabetic acidosis, dehydration, or prolonged vomiting or diarrhea can create a potassium deficiency, as can the regular use of certain drugs, including diuretics, steroids, and strong laxatives.* For this reason, many physicians prescribe potassium supplements along with these potassium-wasting drugs. One of the earliest symptoms of deficiency is muscle weakness.

Potassium Toxicity Potassium toxicity does not result from overeating foods high in potassium; therefore an Upper Level was not set. It can result from overconsumption of potassium salts or supplements (including some "energy fitness shakes") and from certain diseases or treatments.[17] Given more potassium than the body needs, the kidneys accelerate their excretion. If the GI tract is bypassed, however, and potassium is injected directly into a vein, it can stop the heart.

IN SUMMARY Potassium, like sodium and chloride, is an electrolyte that plays an important role in maintaining fluid balance. Potassium is the primary cation inside cells; fresh foods, notably fruits and vegetables, are its best sources. The table on the next page summarizes facts about potassium.

potassium: the principal cation within the body's cells; critical to the maintenance of fluid balance, nerve impulse transmissions, and muscle contractions.

*People using diuretics to control hypertension should know that some cause potassium excretion and can induce a deficiency. Those using these drugs must be particularly careful to include rich sources of potassium in their daily diets. (Some diuretics are designed to spare potassium.)

FIGURE 12-9 Potassium in Selected Foods

Food	Serving size (kcalories)
Bread, whole wheat	1 oz slice (70 kcal)
Cornflakes, fortified	1 oz (110 kcal)
Spaghetti pasta	½ c cooked (99 kcal)
Tortilla, flour	1 10"-round (234 kcal)
Broccoli	½ c cooked (22 kcal)
Carrots	½ c shredded raw (24 kcal)
Potato	1 medium baked w/skin (133 kcal)
Tomato juice	¾ c (31 kcal)
Banana	1 medium raw (109 kcal)
Orange	1 medium raw (62 kcal)
Strawberries	½ c fresh (22 kcal)
Watermelon	1 slice (92 kcal)
Milk	1 c reduced-fat 2% (121 kcal)
Yogurt, plain	1 c low-fat (155 kcal)
Cheddar cheese	1½ oz (171 kcal)
Cottage cheese	½ c low-fat 2% (101 kcal)
Pinto beans	½ c cooked (117 kcal)
Peanut butter	2 tbs (188 kcal)
Sunflower seeds	1 oz dry (165 kcal)
Tofu (soybean curd)	½ c (76 kcal)
Ground beef, lean	3 oz broiled (244 kcal)
Chicken breast	3 oz roasted (140 kcal)
Tuna, canned in water	3 oz (99 kcal)
Egg	1 hard cooked (78 kcal)
Excellent, and sometimes unusual, sources:	
Squash, acorn	½ c baked (69 kcal)
Soybeans	½ c cooked (149 kcal)
Artichoke	1 (60 kcal)

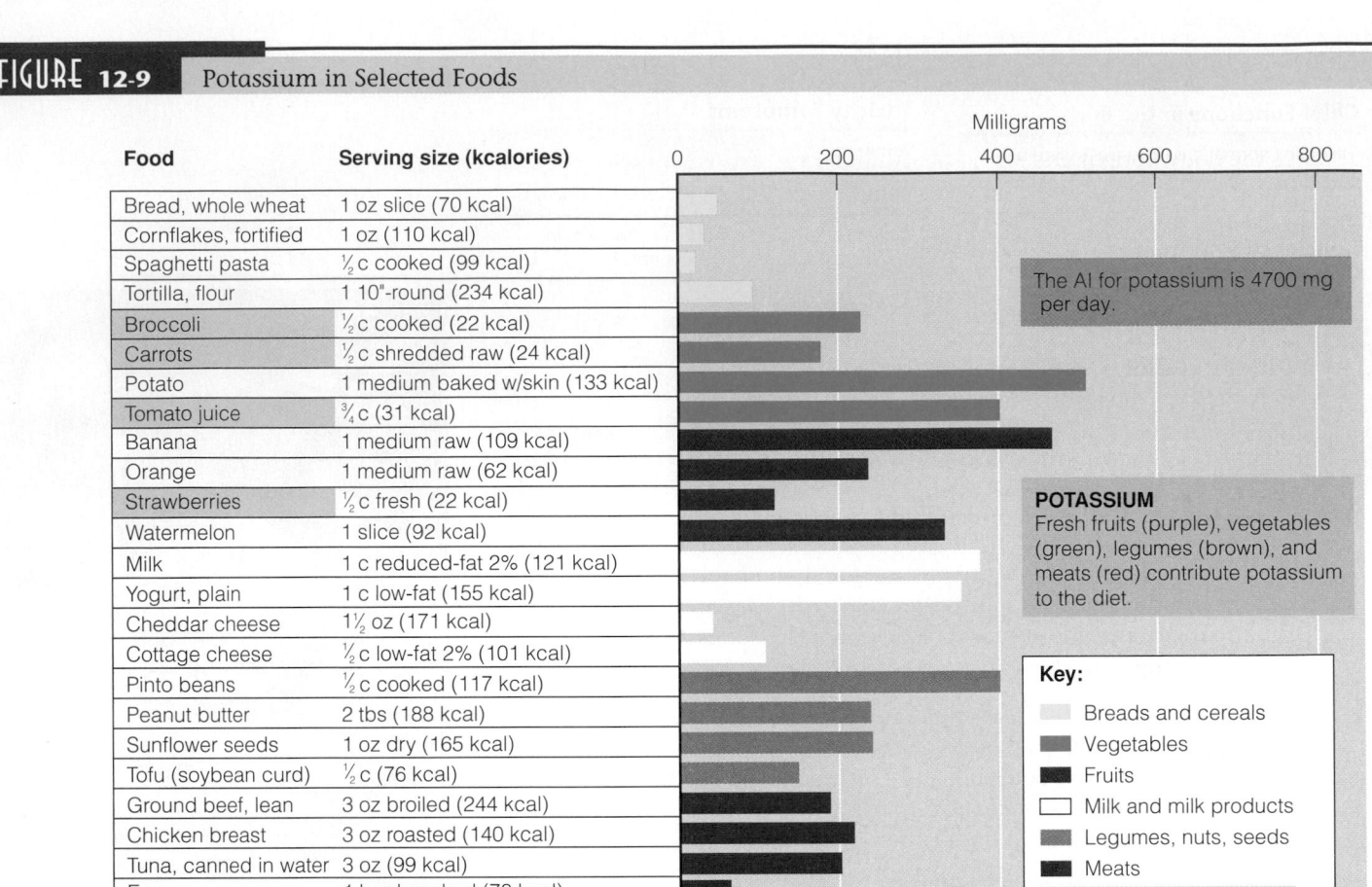

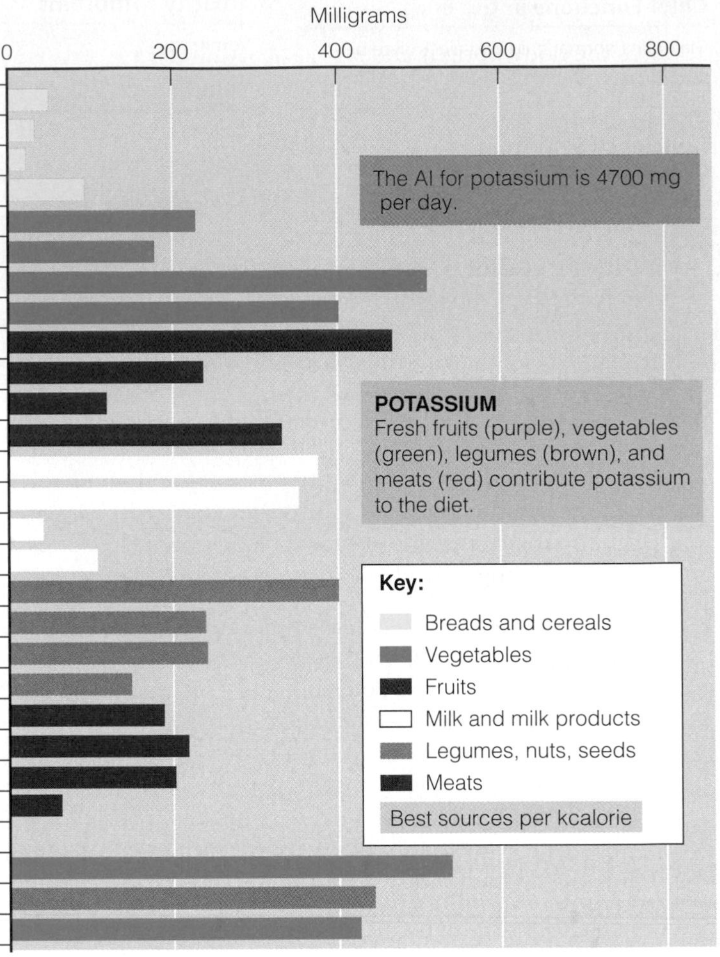
Milligrams
0
200
400
600
800
The AI for potassium is 4700 mg per day.
POTASSIUM
Fresh fruits (purple), vegetables (green), legumes (brown), and meats (red) contribute potassium to the diet.
Key:
Breads and cereals
Vegetables
Fruits
Milk and milk products
Legumes, nuts, seeds
Meats
Best sources per kcalorie

NOTE: See p. 327 for more information on using this figure.

Potassium

2004 Adequate Intake (AI)

Adults: 4700 mg/day

Chief Functions in the Body

Maintains normal fluid and electrolyte balance; facilitates many reactions; supports cell integrity; assists in nerve impulse transmission and muscle contractions

Deficiency Symptoms[a]

Muscular weakness, paralysis, confusion

Toxicity Symptoms

Muscular weakness; vomiting; if given into a vein, can stop the heart

Significant Sources

All whole foods: meats, milks, fruits, vegetables, grains, legumes

[a]Deficiency accompanies dehydration.

Calcium

Calcium is the most abundant mineral in the body. It receives much emphasis in this chapter and in the highlight that follows because an adequate intake helps grow a healthy skeleton in early life and minimize bone loss in later life.

calcium: the most abundant mineral in the body; found primarily in the body's bones and teeth.

Calcium Roles in the Body

Ninety-nine percent of the body's calcium is in the bones (and teeth), where it plays two roles. First, it is an integral part of bone structure, providing a rigid frame that holds the body upright and serves as attachment points for muscles, making motion possible. Second, it serves as a calcium bank, offering a readily available source of the mineral to the body fluids should a drop in blood calcium occur.

Calcium in Bones As bones begin to form, calcium salts form crystals, called **hydroxyapatite,** on a matrix of the protein collagen. During **mineralization,** as the crystals become denser, they give strength and rigidity to the maturing bones. As a result, the long leg bones of children can support their weight by the time they have learned to walk.

Many people have the idea that once a bone is built, it is inert like a rock. Actually, the bones are gaining and losing minerals continuously in an ongoing process of remodeling. Growing children gain more bone than they lose, and healthy adults maintain a reasonable balance. When withdrawals substantially exceed deposits, problems such as osteoporosis develop (as described in Highlight 12).

The formation of teeth follows a pattern similar to that of bones. The turnover of minerals in teeth is not as rapid as in bone, however; fluoride hardens and stabilizes the crystals of teeth, opposing the withdrawal of minerals from them.

Calcium in Body Fluids The 1 percent of the body's calcium that circulates in the fluids as ionized calcium is vital to life. The calcium ion participates in the regulation of muscle contractions, the clotting of blood, the transmission of nerve impulses, the secretion of hormones, and the activation of some enzyme reactions.

Calcium also activates a protein called **calmodulin.** This protein relays messages from the cell surface to the inside of the cell. Several of these messages help to maintain normal blood pressure.

Calcium and Disease Prevention Calcium may protect against hypertension.[18] For this reason, restricting sodium to treat hypertension is narrow advice, especially considering the success of the DASH diet in lowering blood pressure. The DASH diet is not particularly low in sodium, but it is rich in calcium, as well as in magnesium and potassium. As mentioned earlier, the DASH diet, together with a reduced sodium intake, is more effective in lowering blood pressure than either strategy alone. Some research also suggests protective relationships between dietary calcium and blood cholesterol, diabetes, and colon cancer.[19] Highlight 12 explores calcium's role in preventing osteoporosis.

Calcium and Obesity Calcium may also play a role in maintaining a healthy body weight.[20] Analyses of national survey data as well as small clinical studies show an inverse relationship between calcium intake and body fatness: the higher the calcium intake, the lower the body fatness.[21] In particular, calcium from dairy foods seems to exert greater effects on body weight than calcium in supplement form.[22] Notably, calcium intake does not simply reflect a healthy lifestyle; the relationship remains strong even when factors such as energy intake and exercise are considered. An adequate dietary calcium intake may help prevent excessive fat accumulation by stimulating hormonal action that targets the breakdown of stored fat.[23] Large, well-designed clinical studies are needed to confirm the effects of dietary calcium intake on body weight.

Calcium Balance Calcium homeostasis is one of the body's highest priorities and involves a system of hormones and vitamin D. Whenever blood calcium falls too low or rises too high, three organ systems respond: the intestines, bones, and kidneys. Figure 12-10 illustrates how vitamin D and the hormones **parathormone** and **calcitonin** return blood calcium to normal.

The calcium in bone provides a nearly inexhaustible bank of calcium for the blood. The blood borrows and returns calcium as needed so that even with a dietary deficiency, *blood* calcium remains normal—even as *bone* calcium diminishes

hydroxyapatite (high-drox-ee-APP-ah-tite): crystals made of calcium and phosphorus.

mineralization: the process in which calcium, phosphorus, and other minerals crystallize on the collagen matrix of a growing bone, hardening the bone.

calmodulin (cal-MOD-you-lin): an inactive protein that becomes active when bound to calcium. Once activated, it becomes a messenger that tells other proteins what to do. The system serves as an interpreter for hormone- and nerve-mediated messages arriving at cells.

parathormone (PAIR-ah-THOR-moan): a hormone from the parathyroid glands that regulates blood calcium by raising it when levels fall too low; also known as **parathyroid hormone.**

calcitonin (KAL-see-TOE-nin): a hormone from the thyroid gland that regulates blood calcium by lowering it when levels rise too high.

FIGURE 12-10 Calcium Balance

Blood calcium is regulated in part by vitamin D and two hormones—calcitonin and parathormone. Bone serves as a reservoir when blood calcium is high and as a source of calcium when blood calcium is low. Osteoclasts break down bone and release calcium into the blood; osteoblasts build new bone using calcium from the blood.

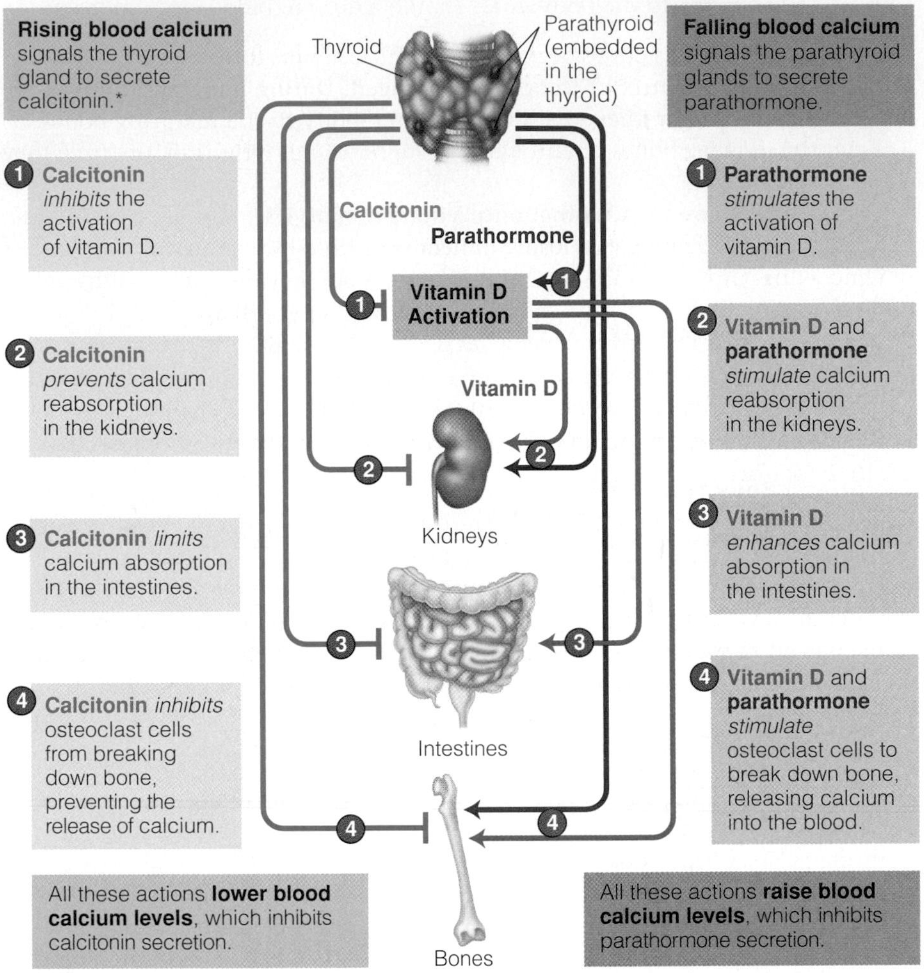

Rising blood calcium signals the thyroid gland to secrete calcitonin.*
Thyroid
Parathyroid (embedded in the thyroid)
Falling blood calcium signals the parathyroid glands to secrete parathormone.
1 **Calcitonin** *inhibits* the activation of vitamin D.
Calcitonin
Parathormone
Vitamin D Activation
1 **Parathormone** *stimulates* the activation of vitamin D.
2 **Calcitonin** *prevents* calcium reabsorption in the kidneys.
Vitamin D
2 **Vitamin D** and **parathormone** *stimulate* calcium reabsorption in the kidneys.
Kidneys
3 **Calcitonin** *limits* calcium absorption in the intestines.
3 **Vitamin D** *enhances* calcium absorption in the intestines.
Intestines
4 **Calcitonin** *inhibits* osteoclast cells from breaking down bone, preventing the release of calcium.
4 **Vitamin D** and **parathormone** *stimulate* osteoclast cells to break down bone, releasing calcium into the blood.
Bones
All these actions **lower blood calcium levels**, which inhibits calcitonin secretion.
All these actions **raise blood calcium levels**, which inhibits parathormone secretion.

*Calcitonin plays a major role in defending infants and young children against the dangers of rising blood calcium that can occur when regular feedings of milk deliver large quanities of calcium to a small body. In contrast, calcitonin plays a relatively minor role in adults because their absorption of calcium is less efficient and their bodies are larger, making elevated blood calcium unlikely.

(see Figure 12-11). Blood calcium changes only in response to abnormal regulatory control, not to diet. A person can have an inadequate calcium intake for years and suffer no noticeable symptoms. Only late in life does it become apparent that the integrity of the bones has been compromised.

Blood calcium above normal results in **calcium rigor:** the muscles contract and cannot relax. Similarly, blood calcium below normal causes **calcium tetany**—also characterized by uncontrolled muscle contraction. These conditions do *not* reflect a *dietary* excess or lack of calcium; they are caused by a lack of vitamin D or by abnormal secretion of the regulatory hormones. A chronic *dietary* deficiency of calcium, or a chronic deficiency due to poor absorption over the years, depletes the savings account in the bones. Again: the *bones,* not the blood, are robbed by a calcium deficiency.

Calcium Absorption Many factors affect calcium absorption, but on average, adults absorb about 25 percent of the calcium they ingest. The stomach's acidity helps to keep calcium soluble, and vitamin D helps to make the **calcium-binding protein** needed for absorption. (This explains why calcium-rich milk is the best food for vitamin D fortification.)

calcium rigor: hardness or stiffness of the muscles caused by high blood calcium concentrations.

calcium tetany (TET-ah-nee): intermittent spasm of the extremities due to nervous and muscular excitability caused by low blood calcium concentrations.

calcium-binding protein: a protein in the intestinal cells, made with the help of vitamin D, that facilitates calcium absorption.

Whenever calcium is needed, the body increases its production of the calcium-binding protein to improve calcium absorption. The result is obvious in the case of a pregnant woman, who absorbs 50 percent of the calcium from the milk she drinks. Similarly, growing children absorb 50 to 60 percent of the calcium they consume. Then, when bone growth slows or stops, absorption falls to the adult level of about 25 percent. In addition, absorption becomes more efficient during times of inadequate intakes.[24]

Many of the conditions that enhance calcium absorption inhibit its absorption when they are absent. For example, sufficient vitamin D supports absorption, while a deficiency impairs it. In addition, fiber, in general, and the binders phytate and oxalate, in particular, interfere with calcium absorption, but their effects are relatively minor at intakes typical of U.S. diets. Vegetables with oxalates and whole grains with phytates are nutritious foods, of course, but they are not useful calcium sources. The margin■ presents factors that influence calcium balance.

FIGURE 12-11 Maintaining Blood Calcium from the Diet and from the Bones

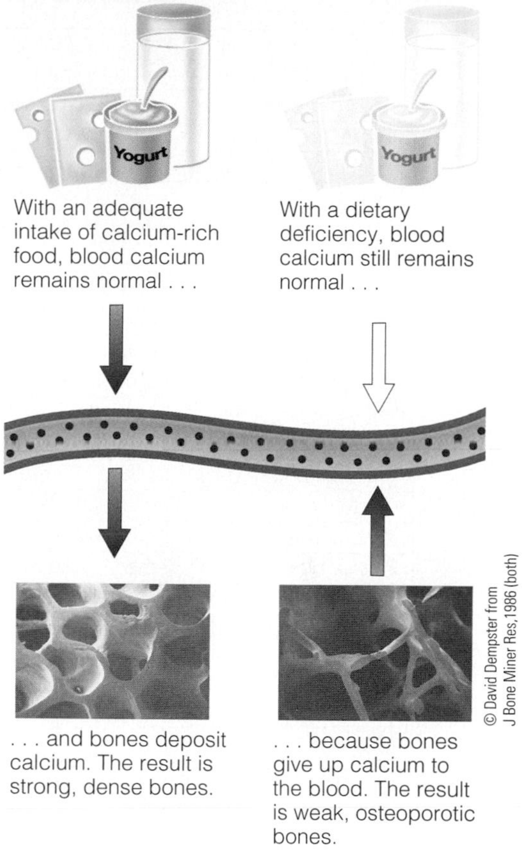
Yogurt
Yogurt
With an adequate intake of calcium-rich food, blood calcium remains normal . . .
With a dietary deficiency, blood calcium still remains normal . . .
. . . and bones deposit calcium. The result is strong, dense bones.
. . . because bones give up calcium to the blood. The result is weak, osteoporotic bones.
© David Dempster from J Bone Miner Res, 1986 (both)

Calcium Recommendations and Sources

Calcium is unlike most other nutrients, in that hormones maintain its *blood* concentration regardless of dietary intake. As Figure 12-11 shows, when intake is high, the *bones* benefit; when intake is low, the *bones* suffer. Calcium recommendations are therefore based on the amount needed to retain the most calcium in bones. By retaining the most calcium possible, the bones can develop to their fullest potential in size and density—their **peak bone mass**—within genetic limits.

Calcium Recommendations Because obtaining enough calcium during growth helps to ensure that the skeleton will be strong and dense, recommendations have been set high at 1300 milligrams daily for adolescents up to the age of 18 years. Between the ages of 19 and 50, recommendations are lowered to 1000 milligrams a day; for later life, recommendations are raised again to 1200 milligrams a day to minimize the bone loss that tends to occur later in life. Some authorities advocate as much as 1500 milligrams a day for women over 50. Many people in the United States and Canada, particularly women, have calcium intakes far below current recommendations. High intakes of calcium from supplements may have adverse effects such as kidney stone formation; for this reason, an Upper Level has been established (see inside front cover).

Increase the proportion of persons aged 2 years and older who meet dietary recommendations for calcium. HEALTHY PEOPLE 2010

High intakes of both dietary protein and sodium increase calcium losses, but whether these losses impair bone development remains unclear.[25] In establishing an Adequate Intake (AI) for calcium, the DRI Committee considered these nutrient interactions, but did not adjust dietary recommendations based on this information.

Calcium in Milk Products Figure 12-12 on p. 416 shows that calcium is found most abundantly in a single class of foods—milk and milk products. Unfortunately, many people, for a variety of reasons, cannot or do not drink milk. For example, some people are lactose intolerant, while others simply do not enjoy the taste of milk.

The person who doesn't like to drink milk may prefer to eat cheese or yogurt. Alternatively, milk and milk products can be concealed in foods. Powdered fat-free milk can be added to casseroles, soups, and other mixed dishes during preparation; 5 heaping tablespoons offer the equivalent of a cup of milk. This simple step is an excellent way for older women to obtain not only extra calcium, but more protein, vitamins, and minerals as well.

It is especially difficult for children who don't drink milk to meet their calcium needs. Children who don't drink milk have lower calcium intakes and poorer bone

■ Factors that *enhance* calcium absorption:

- Stomach acid.
- Vitamin D.
- Lactose.
- Growth hormones.

Factors that *inhibit* calcium absorption:

- Lack of stomach acid.
- Vitamin D deficiency.
- High phosphorus intake.
- High-fiber diet.
- Phytates (in seeds, nuts, grains).
- Oxalates (in beet greens, rhubarb, spinach).

peak bone mass: the highest attainable bone size and density for an individual, developed during the first three decades of life.

FIGURE 12-12 Calcium in Selected Foods

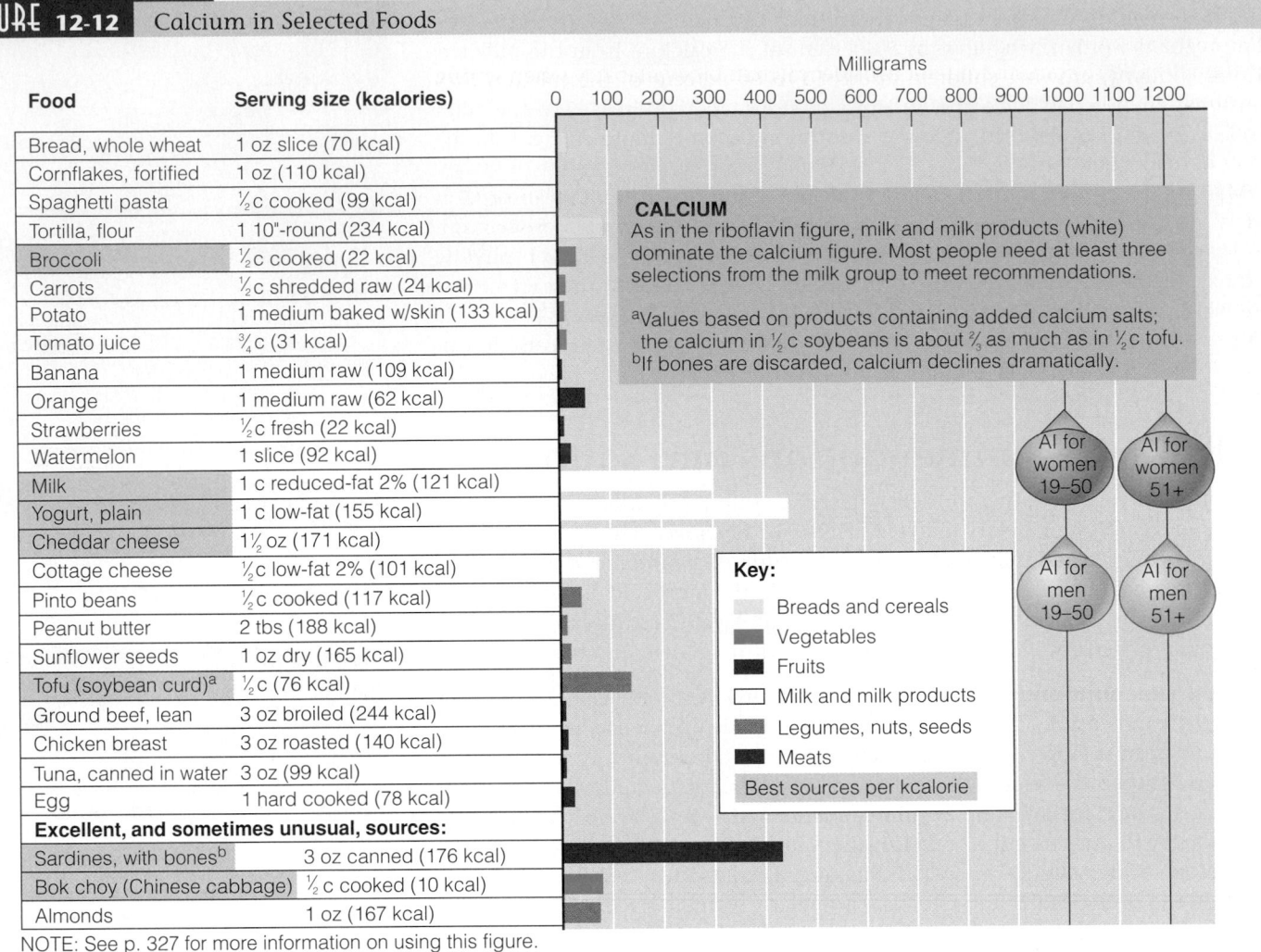

Food	Serving size (kcalories)
Bread, whole wheat	1 oz slice (70 kcal)
Cornflakes, fortified	1 oz (110 kcal)
Spaghetti pasta	½ c cooked (99 kcal)
Tortilla, flour	1 10"-round (234 kcal)
Broccoli	½ c cooked (22 kcal)
Carrots	½ c shredded raw (24 kcal)
Potato	1 medium baked w/skin (133 kcal)
Tomato juice	¾ c (31 kcal)
Banana	1 medium raw (109 kcal)
Orange	1 medium raw (62 kcal)
Strawberries	½ c fresh (22 kcal)
Watermelon	1 slice (92 kcal)
Milk	1 c reduced-fat 2% (121 kcal)
Yogurt, plain	1 c low-fat (155 kcal)
Cheddar cheese	1½ oz (171 kcal)
Cottage cheese	½ c low-fat 2% (101 kcal)
Pinto beans	½ c cooked (117 kcal)
Peanut butter	2 tbs (188 kcal)
Sunflower seeds	1 oz dry (165 kcal)
Tofu (soybean curd)[a]	½ c (76 kcal)
Ground beef, lean	3 oz broiled (244 kcal)
Chicken breast	3 oz roasted (140 kcal)
Tuna, canned in water	3 oz (99 kcal)
Egg	1 hard cooked (78 kcal)
Excellent, and sometimes unusual, sources:	
Sardines, with bones[b]	3 oz canned (176 kcal)
Bok choy (Chinese cabbage)	½ c cooked (10 kcal)
Almonds	1 oz (167 kcal)

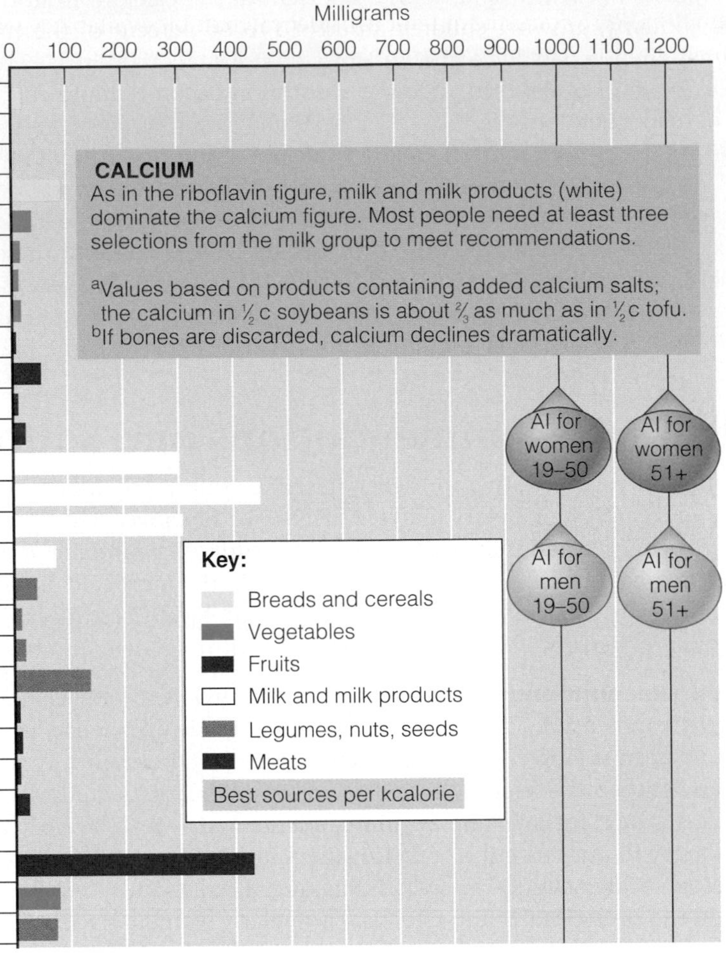
Milligrams
0 100 200 300 400 500 600 700 800 900 1000 1100 1200
CALCIUM
As in the riboflavin figure, milk and milk products (white) dominate the calcium figure. Most people need at least three selections from the milk group to meet recommendations.
[a]Values based on products containing added calcium salts; the calcium in ½ c soybeans is about 2/3 as much as in ½ c tofu.
[b]If bones are discarded, calcium declines dramatically.
AI for women 19–50
AI for women 51+
AI for men 19–50
AI for men 51+
Key:
Breads and cereals
Vegetables
Fruits
Milk and milk products
Legumes, nuts, seeds
Meats
Best sources per kcalorie

NOTE: See p. 327 for more information on using this figure.

health than those who drink milk regularly, and are shorter as well.[26] The consequences of drinking too little milk during childhood and adolescence persist into adulthood. Women who seldom drank milk as children or teenagers have lower bone density and greater risk of fractures than those who drank milk regularly.[27] It is possible for people who do not drink milk to obtain adequate calcium, but only if they carefully select other calcium-rich foods.

■ People with lactose intolerance may be able to consume small quantities of milk, as Chapter 4 explains.

Calcium in Other Foods Some cultures do not use milk in their cuisines; some vegetarians exclude milk as well as meat; and some people are allergic to milk protein or are lactose intolerant.■ These people need to find nonmilk sources of calcium to help meet their calcium needs. Some brands of tofu, corn tortillas, some nuts (such as almonds), and some seeds (such as sesame seeds) can supply calcium for the person who doesn't use milk products. A slice of most breads contains only about 5 to 10 percent of the calcium found in milk, but can be a major source for people who eat many slices because the calcium is well absorbed.

Among the vegetables, mustard and turnip greens, bok choy, kale, parsley, watercress, and broccoli are good sources of available calcium. So are some seaweeds such as the nori popular in Japanese cooking. Some dark green, leafy vegetables—notably spinach and Swiss chard—appear to be calcium-rich but actually provide little, if any, calcium to the body because of the binders they contain. It would take 8 cups of spinach—containing six times as much calcium as 1 cup of milk—to deliver the equivalent in *absorbable* calcium.[28]

With the exception of foods such as spinach that contain calcium binders, however, the calcium content of foods is usually more important than bioavailability.[29] Consequently, recognizing that people eat a variety of foods containing calcium, the DRI Committee did not consider calcium bioavailability when setting recommendations. The margin drawing■ ranks selected foods according to their calcium bioavailability.

Oysters are also a rich source of calcium, as are small fish eaten with their bones, such as canned sardines. Many Asians prepare a stock from bones that helps account for their adequate calcium intake without the use of milk. They soak the cracked bones from chicken, turkey, pork, or fish in vinegar and then slowly boil the bones until they become soft. The bones release calcium into the acidic broth, and most of the vinegar boils off. Cooks then use the stock, which contains more than 100 milligrams of calcium per tablespoon, in place of water to prepare soups, vegetables, and rice. Similarly, cooks in the Navajo tribe use an ash prepared from the branches and needles of the juniper tree in their recipes. One teaspoon of juniper ash provides about as much calcium as a cup of milk.

Some mineral waters provide as much as 500 milligrams of calcium per liter, offering a convenient way to meet both calcium and water needs.[30] Similarly, calcium-fortified orange juice and other fruit and vegetable juices allow a person to meet both calcium and vitamin needs easily. Other examples of calcium-fortified foods include high-calcium milk (milk with extra calcium added) and calcium-fortified cereals. The "How to" on p. 418 describes a shortcut method for estimating your calcium intake. Highlight 12 discusses calcium supplements.

A generalization that has been gaining strength throughout this book is supported by the information given here about calcium. A balanced diet that supplies a variety of foods is the best plan to ensure adequacy for all essential nutrients. All food groups should be included, and none should be overemphasized. In our culture, calcium intake is usually inadequate wherever milk is lacking in the diet—whether through ignorance, poverty, simple dislike, fad dieting, lactose intolerance, or allergy. By contrast, iron is usually lacking whenever milk is overemphasized, as Chapter 13 explains.

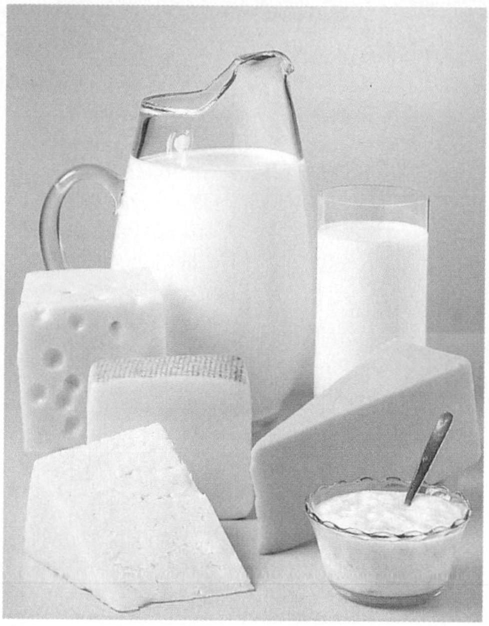

Milk and milk products are rightly famous for their calcium contents.

■ Bioavailability of Calcium from Selected Foods

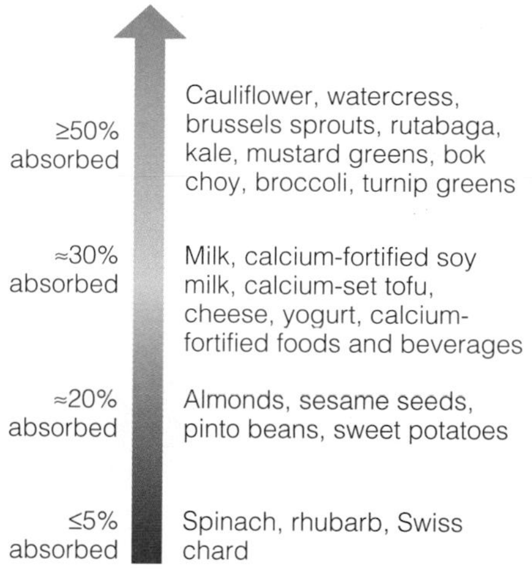
≥50% absorbed
Cauliflower, watercress, brussels sprouts, rutabaga, kale, mustard greens, bok choy, broccoli, turnip greens
≈30% absorbed
Milk, calcium-fortified soy milk, calcium-set tofu, cheese, yogurt, calcium-fortified foods and beverages
≈20% absorbed
Almonds, sesame seeds, pinto beans, sweet potatoes
≤5% absorbed
Spinach, rhubarb, Swiss chard

Calcium Deficiency

A low calcium intake during the growing years limits the bones' ability to reach their optimal mass and density. Most people achieve a peak bone mass by their late 20s, and dense bones best protect against age-related bone loss and fractures (see Figure 12-13). All adults lose bone as they grow older, beginning between the ages of 30 and 40. Should bone losses reach the point of causing fractures under common, everyday stresses, the condition is known as **osteoporosis.** Osteoporosis afflicts more than 25 million people in the United States, mostly older women.

FIGURE 12-13 Phases of Bone Development throughout Life

The active growth phase occurs from birth to approximately age 20. The next phase of peak bone mass development occurs between the ages of 12 and 30. The final phase, when bone resorption exceeds formation, begins between the ages of 30 and 40 and continues through the remainder of life.

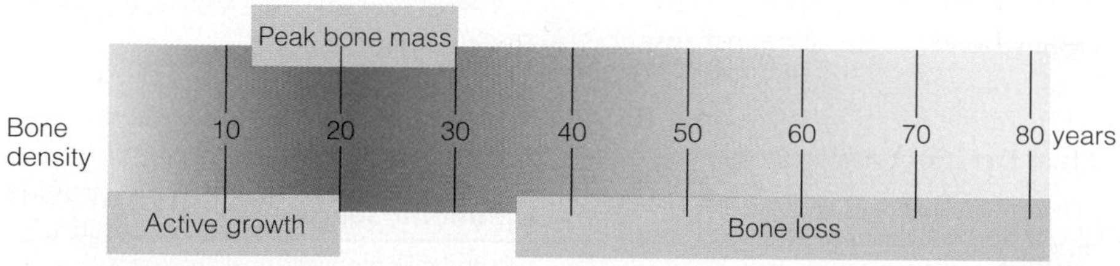
Peak bone mass
Bone density
10
20
30
40
50
60
70
80 years
Active growth
Bone loss

osteoporosis (OS-tee-oh-pore-OH-sis): a disease in which the bones become porous and fragile due to a loss of minerals; also called **adult bone loss.**
- **osteo** = bone
- **porosis** = porous

HOW TO Estimate Your Calcium Intake

Most dietitians have developed useful shortcuts to help them estimate nutrient intakes and "see" inadequacies in the diet. They can tell at a glance whether a day's meals fall short of calcium recommendations, for example.

To estimate calcium intakes, keep two bits of information in mind:

- A cup of milk provides about 300 milligrams of calcium.
- Adults need between 1000 and 1200 milligrams of calcium per day, which represents 3 to 4 cups of milk—or the equivalent:

$$1000 \text{ mg} \div 300 \text{ mg/c} = 3\tfrac{1}{3} \text{ c.}$$
$$1200 \text{ mg} \div 300 \text{ mg/c} = 4 \text{ c.}$$

If a person drinks 3 to 4 cups of milk a day, it's easy to see that calcium needs are being met. If not, it takes some detective work to identify the other sources and estimate total calcium intake.

To estimate a person's daily calcium intake, use this shortcut, which compares the calcium in calcium-rich foods to the calcium content of milk. The calcium in a cup of milk is assigned 1 point, and the goal is to attain 3 to 4 points per day. Foods are given points as follows:

- 1 c milk, yogurt, or fortified soy milk or 1½ oz cheese = 1 point.
- 4 oz canned fish with bones (sardines) = 1 point.
- 1 c ice cream, cottage cheese, or calcium-rich vegetable (see the text) = ½ point.

Then, because other foods also contribute small amounts of calcium, together they are given a point.

- Well-balanced diet containing a variety of foods = 1 point.

Now consider a day's meals with calcium in mind. Cereal with 1 cup of milk for breakfast (1 point for milk), a ham and cheese sub sandwich for lunch (1 point for cheese), and a cup of broccoli and lasagna for dinner (½ point for calcium-rich vegetable and 1 point for cheese in lasagna)—plus 1 point for all other foods eaten that day—adds up to 4½ points. This shortcut estimate indicates that calcium recommendations have been met, and a diet analysis of these few foods reveals a calcium intake of over 1000 milligrams. By knowing the best sources of each nutrient, you can learn to scan the day's meals and quickly see if you are meeting your daily goals.

HEALTHY PEOPLE 2010

Reduce the prevalence of osteoporosis, among people aged 50 and over.

Unlike many diseases that make themselves known through symptoms such as pain, shortness of breath, skin lesions, tiredness, and the like, osteoporosis is silent. The body sends no signals saying bones are losing their calcium and, as a result, their integrity. Blood samples offer no clues because blood calcium remains normal regardless of bone content, and measures of bone density are not routinely taken. Highlight 12 suggests strategies to protect against bone loss, of which eating calcium-rich foods is only one. Even during adulthood, however, high calcium intakes may promote bone strength, prevent further deterioration, and reverse bone loss.[31]

IN SUMMARY Most of the body's calcium is in the bones where it provides a rigid structure and a reservoir of calcium for the blood. Blood calcium participates in muscle contraction, blood clotting, and nerve impulses and is closely regulated by a system of hormones and vitamin D. Calcium is found predominantly in milk and milk products, but some other foods including certain vegetables and tofu also provide calcium. Even when calcium intake is inadequate, blood calcium remains normal, but at the expense of bone loss, which can lead to osteoporosis. Calcium's roles, deficiency symptoms, and food sources are summarized below.

Calcium

1997 Adequate Intake (AI)

Adults: 1000 mg/day (19–50 yr)
1200 mg/day (>51 yr)

Upper Level

Adults: 2500 mg/day

Chief Functions in the Body

Mineralization of bones and teeth; also involved in muscle contraction and relaxation, nerve functioning, blood clotting, blood pressure, and immune defenses

Deficiency Symptoms

Stunted growth in children; bone loss (osteoporosis) in adults

Toxicity Symptoms

Constipation; increased risk of urinary stone formation and kidney dysfunction; interference with absorption of other minerals

Significant Sources

Milk and milk products, small fish (with bones), tofu (bean curd), greens (broccoli, chard), legumes

Phosphorus

Phosphorus is the second most abundant mineral in the body. About 85 percent of it is found combined with calcium in the hydroxyapatite crystals of bones and teeth.

Phosphorus Roles in the Body Phosphorus salts (phosphates) are found not only in bones and teeth, but in all body cells as part of a major buffer system (phosphoric acid and its salts). Phosphorus is also part of DNA and RNA and is therefore necessary for all growth.

Phosphorus assists in energy metabolism. Many enzymes and the B vitamins become active only when a phosphate group is attached. ATP itself, the energy currency of the cells, uses three phosphate groups to do its work.

Lipids containing phosphorus as part of their structures (phospholipids) help to transport other lipids in the blood. Phospholipids are also the major structural components of cell membranes, where they control the transport of nutrients into and out of the cells. Some proteins, such as the casein in milk, contain phosphorus as part of their structures (phosphoproteins).

Phosphorus Recommendations and Intakes Diets that provide adequate energy and protein also supply adequate phosphorus. Dietary deficiencies of phosphorus are unknown. As Figure 12-14 shows, foods rich in proteins are the best sources of phosphorus. In addition to legumes and foods from the milk and meat groups, processed foods (including soft drinks) are usually high in phosphorus (from the additives).

phosphorus: a major mineral found mostly in the body's bones and teeth.

FIGURE 12-14 Phosphorus in Selected Foods

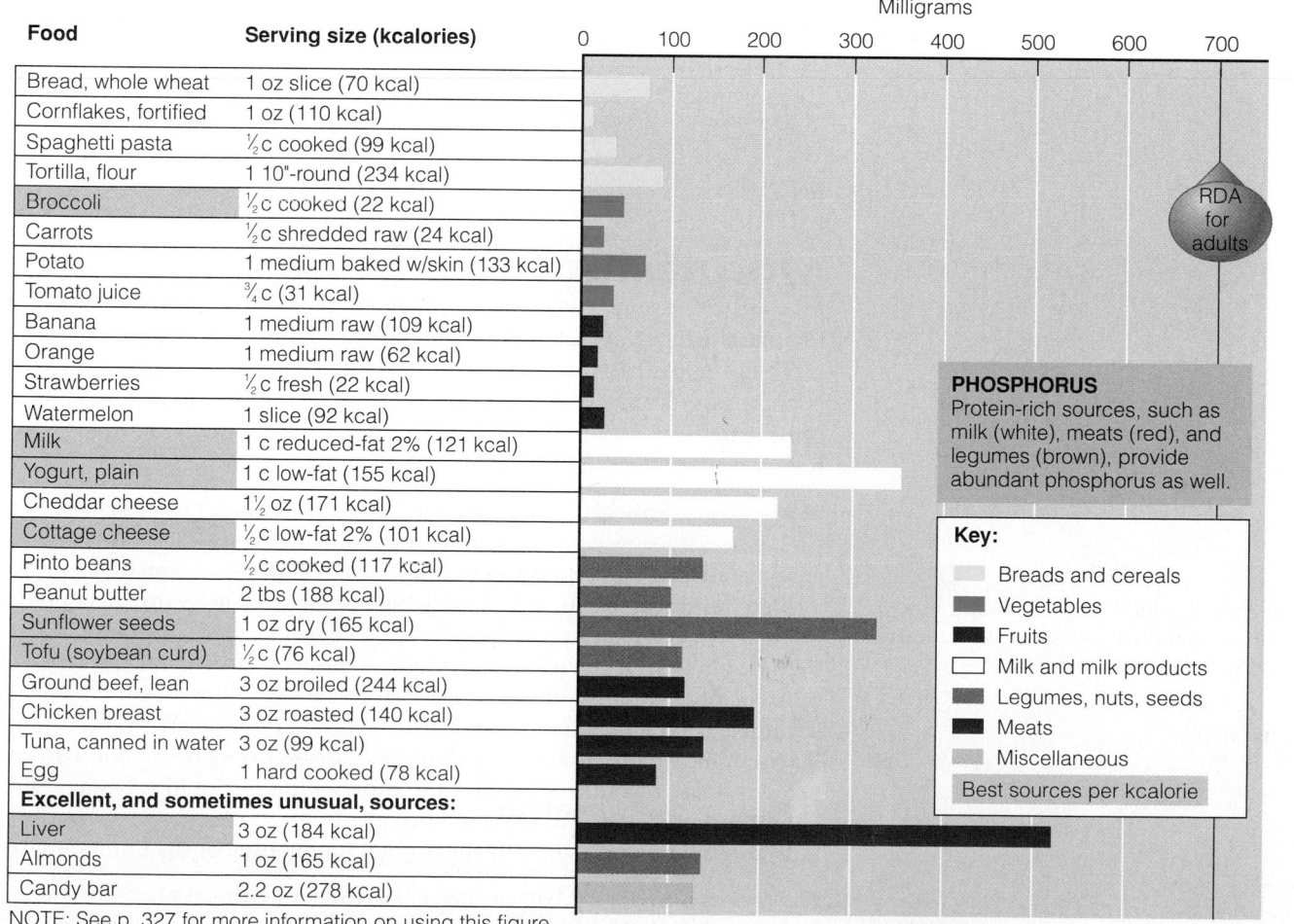

Food	Serving size (kcalories)
Bread, whole wheat	1 oz slice (70 kcal)
Cornflakes, fortified	1 oz (110 kcal)
Spaghetti pasta	½ c cooked (99 kcal)
Tortilla, flour	1 10"-round (234 kcal)
Broccoli	½ c cooked (22 kcal)
Carrots	½ c shredded raw (24 kcal)
Potato	1 medium baked w/skin (133 kcal)
Tomato juice	¾ c (31 kcal)
Banana	1 medium raw (109 kcal)
Orange	1 medium raw (62 kcal)
Strawberries	½ c fresh (22 kcal)
Watermelon	1 slice (92 kcal)
Milk	1 c reduced-fat 2% (121 kcal)
Yogurt, plain	1 c low-fat (155 kcal)
Cheddar cheese	1½ oz (171 kcal)
Cottage cheese	½ c low-fat 2% (101 kcal)
Pinto beans	½ c cooked (117 kcal)
Peanut butter	2 tbs (188 kcal)
Sunflower seeds	1 oz dry (165 kcal)
Tofu (soybean curd)	½ c (76 kcal)
Ground beef, lean	3 oz broiled (244 kcal)
Chicken breast	3 oz roasted (140 kcal)
Tuna, canned in water	3 oz (99 kcal)
Egg	1 hard cooked (78 kcal)
Excellent, and sometimes unusual, sources:	
Liver	3 oz (184 kcal)
Almonds	1 oz (165 kcal)
Candy bar	2.2 oz (278 kcal)

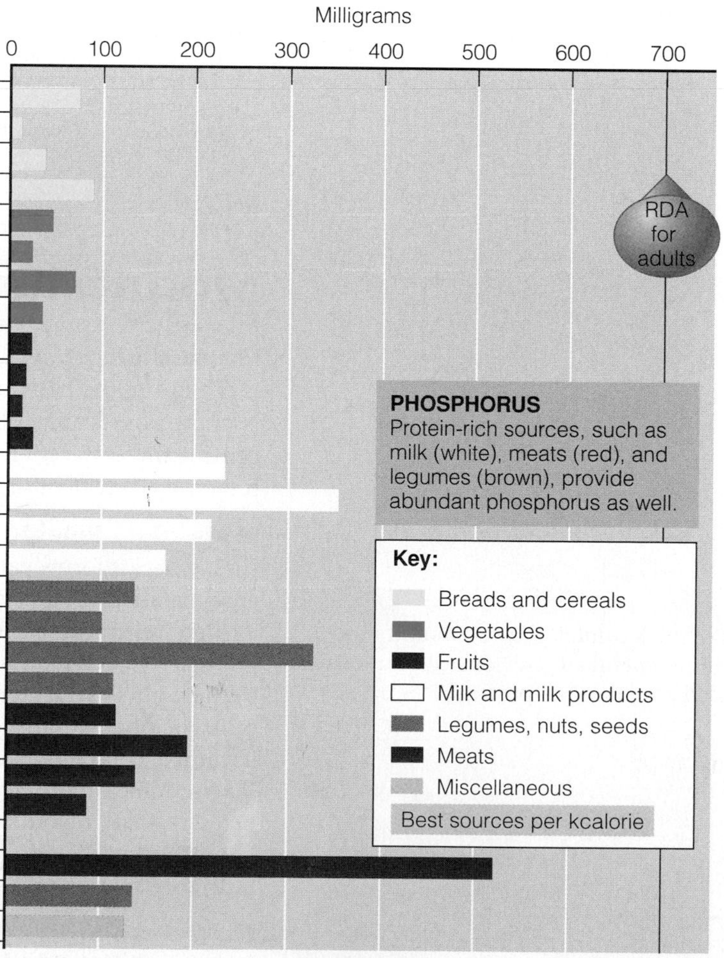
Milligrams
0
100
200
300
400
500
600
700
RDA for adults
PHOSPHORUS
Protein-rich sources, such as milk (white), meats (red), and legumes (brown), provide abundant phosphorus as well.
Key:
Breads and cereals
Vegetables
Fruits
Milk and milk products
Legumes, nuts, seeds
Meats
Miscellaneous
Best sources per kcalorie

NOTE: See p. 327 for more information on using this figure.

In the past, researchers emphasized the importance of an ideal calcium-to-phosphorus ratio from the diet to support calcium metabolism, but there is little or no evidence to support this concept.[32] The quantities of calcium and phosphorus in the diet are far more important than their ratio to each other. A high phosphorus intake has been blamed for bone loss when, in fact, a low calcium intake—not a phosphorus toxicity or an improper ratio—is responsible.[33] Research shows that the displacement of milk in the diet by cola drinks, not the phosphoric acid content of the beverages, has adverse effects on bone.[34] No adverse effects of high dietary phosphorus intakes have been reported; still, an Upper Level has been established (see inside front cover).

IN SUMMARY Phosphorus accompanies calcium both in the crystals of bone and in many foods such as milk. Phosphorus is also important in energy metabolism, as part of phospholipids, and as part of the genetic materials DNA and RNA. The summary table below lists functions of, and other information about, phosphorus.

Phosphorus

1997 RDA

Adults: 700 mg/day

Upper Level

Adults (19–70 yr): 4000 mg/day

Chief Functions in the Body

Mineralization of bones and teeth; part of every cell; important in genetic material, part of phospholipids, used in energy transfer and in buffer systems that maintain acid-base balance

Deficiency Symptoms

Muscular weakness, bone pain[a]

Toxicity Symptoms

Calcification of nonskeletal tissues, particularly the kidneys

Significant Sources

All animal tissues (meat, fish, poultry, eggs, milk)

[a]Dietary deficiency rarely occurs, but some drugs can bind with phosphorus making it unavailable and resulting in bone loss that is characterized by weakness and pain.

Magnesium

Magnesium barely qualifies as a major mineral: only about 1 ounce of magnesium is present in the body of a 130-pound person. Over half of the body's magnesium is in the bones. Most of the rest is in the muscles and soft tissues, with only 1 percent in the extracellular fluid. As with calcium, bone magnesium may serve as a reservoir to ensure normal blood concentrations.

Magnesium Roles in the Body Magnesium acts in all the cells of the soft tissues, where it forms part of the protein-making machinery and is necessary for energy metabolism. It participates in hundreds of enzyme systems. A major role is as a catalyst■ in the reaction that adds the last phosphate to the high-energy compound ATP. As a required component for ATP metabolism, magnesium is essential to the body's use of glucose; the synthesis of protein, fat, and nucleic acids; and the cells' membrane transport systems. Together with calcium, magnesium is involved in muscle contraction and blood clotting: calcium promotes the processes, whereas magnesium inhibits them. This dynamic interaction between the two minerals helps regulate blood pressure and the functioning of the lungs. Magnesium also helps prevent dental caries by holding calcium in tooth enamel. Like many other nutrients, magnesium supports the normal functioning of the immune system.

■ Reminder: A *catalyst* is a compound that facilitates chemical reactions without itself being changed in the process.

magnesium: a cation within the body's cells, active in many enzyme systems.

Magnesium Intakes Average dietary magnesium estimates for U.S. adults fall below recommendations. Dietary intake data, however, do not include the contribution made by water. In areas with hard water, the water contributes both calcium and magnesium to daily intakes. Mineral waters noted earlier for their calcium content may also be magnesium-rich and can be important sources of this mineral for those who drink them.[35] Bioavailability of magnesium from mineral water is about 50 percent, but improves when the water is consumed with a meal.[36]

The brown bars in Figure 12-15 indicate that legumes, seeds, and nuts make significant magnesium contributions. Magnesium is part of the chlorophyll molecule, so leafy green vegetables are also good sources.

Magnesium Deficiency Even with average magnesium intakes below recommendations, deficiency symptoms rarely appear except with diseases. Magnesium deficiency may develop in cases of alcohol abuse, protein malnutrition, kidney disorders, and prolonged vomiting or diarrhea. People using diuretics may also show symptoms. A severe magnesium deficiency causes a tetany similar to the calcium tetany described earlier. Magnesium deficiencies also impair central nervous system activity and may be responsible for the hallucinations experienced during alcohol withdrawal.

Magnesium and Hypertension Magnesium is critical to heart function and seems to protect against hypertension and heart disease. Interestingly, people living in areas of the country with hard water, which contains high concentrations of calcium and magnesium, tend to have low rates of heart disease. With magnesium deficiency, the walls of the arteries and capillaries tend to constrict, a possible explanation for the hypertensive effect.

FIGURE 12-15 Magnesium in Selected Foods

Food	Serving size (kcalories)
Bread, whole wheat	1 oz slice (70 kcal)
Cornflakes, fortified	1 oz (110 kcal)
Spaghetti pasta	½ c cooked (99 kcal)
Tortilla, flour	1 10"-round (234 kcal)
Broccoli	½ c cooked (22 kcal)
Carrots	½ c shredded raw (24 kcal)
Potato	1 medium baked w/skin (133 kcal)
Tomato juice	¾ c (31 kcal)
Banana	1 medium raw (109 kcal)
Orange	1 medium raw (62 kcal)
Strawberries	½ c fresh (22 kcal)
Watermelon	1 slice (92 kcal)
Milk	1 c reduced-fat 2% (121 kcal)
Yogurt, plain	1 c low-fat (155 kcal)
Cheddar cheese	1½ oz (171 kcal)
Cottage cheese	½ c low-fat 2% (101 kcal)
Pinto beans	½ c cooked (117 kcal)
Peanut butter	2 tbs (188 kcal)
Sunflower seeds	1 oz dry (165 kcal)
Tofu (soybean curd)	½ c (76 kcal)
Ground beef, lean	3 oz broiled (244 kcal)
Chicken breast	3 oz roasted (140 kcal)
Tuna, canned in water	3 oz (99 kcal)
Egg	1 hard cooked (78 kcal)
Excellent, and sometimes unusual, sources:	
Halibut	3 oz baked (199 kcal)
Cashews	1 oz (161 kcal)
Artichoke	1 (60 kcal)

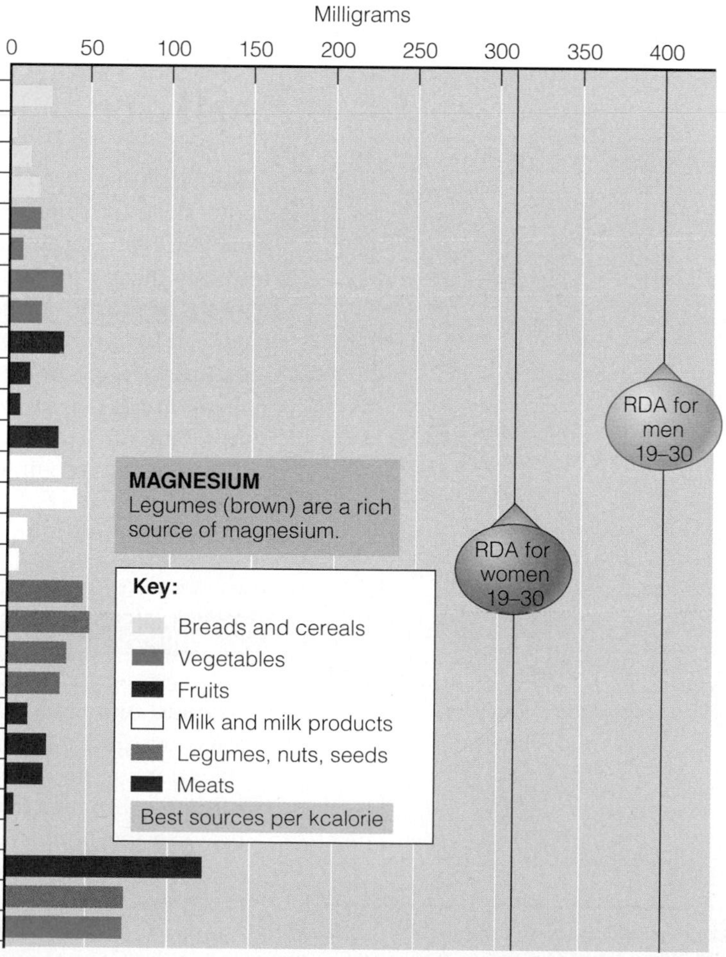
Milligrams
0
50
100
150
200
250
300
350
400
RDA for men 19–30
RDA for women 19–30
MAGNESIUM
Legumes (brown) are a rich source of magnesium.
Key:
Breads and cereals
Vegetables
Fruits
Milk and milk products
Legumes, nuts, seeds
Meats
Best sources per kcalorie

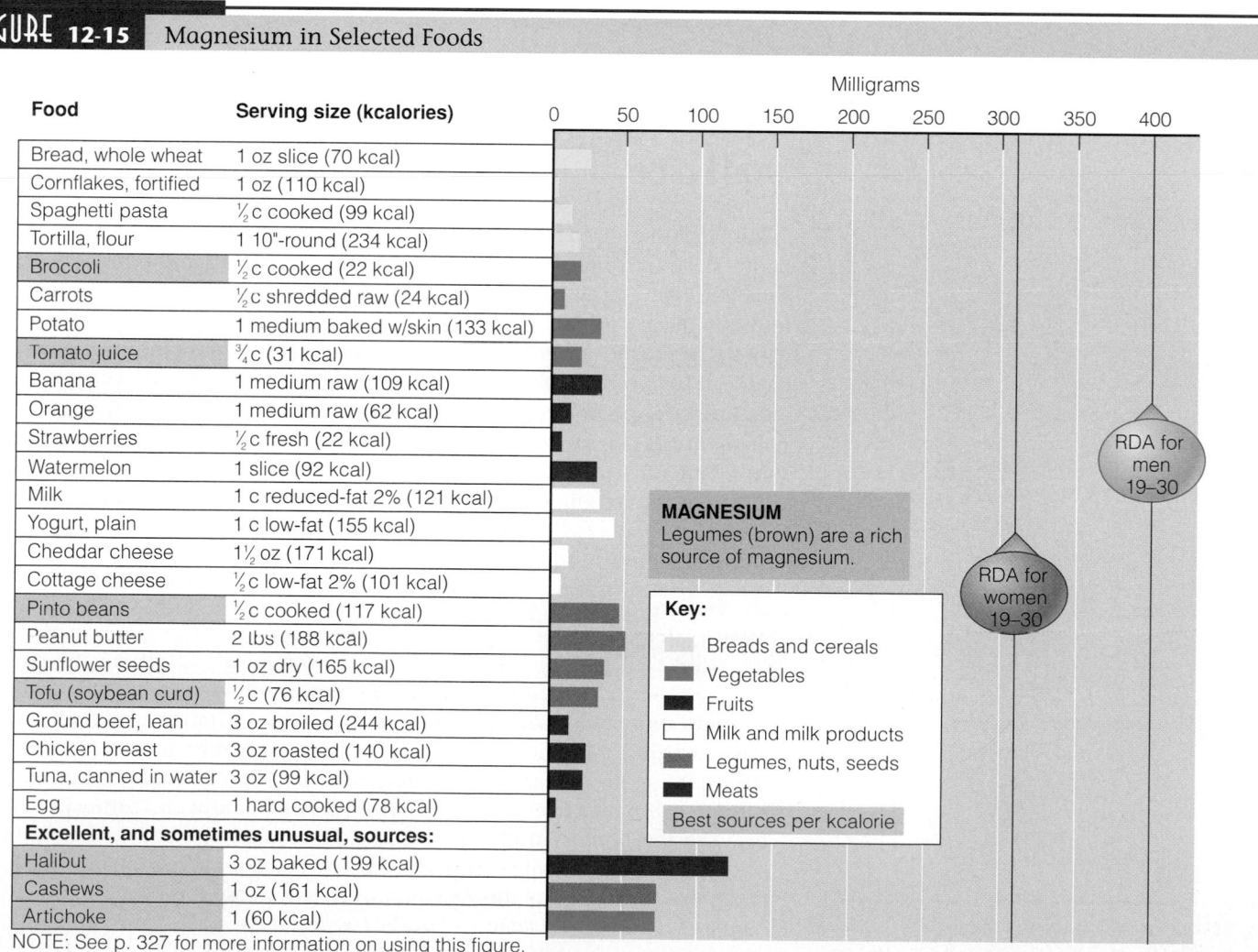

NOTE: See p. 327 for more information on using this figure.

Magnesium Toxicity Magnesium toxicity is rare, but it can be fatal.[37] The Upper Level for magnesium applies only to nonfood sources such as supplements or magnesium salts.

IN SUMMARY Like calcium and phosphorus, magnesium supports bone mineralization. Magnesium is also involved in numerous enzyme systems and in heart function. It is found abundantly in legumes and leafy green vegetables and, in some areas, in water. The table below offers a summary.

Magnesium

1997 RDA

Men (19–30 yr): 400 mg/day

Women (19–30 yr): 310 mg/day

Upper Level

Adults: 350 mg nonfood magnesium/day

Chief Functions in the Body

Bone mineralization, building of protein, enzyme action, normal muscle contraction, nerve impulse transmission, maintenance of teeth, and functioning of immune system

Deficiency Symptoms

Weakness; confusion; if extreme, convulsions, bizarre muscle movements (especially of eye and face muscles), hallucinations, and difficulty in swallowing; in children, growth failure[a]

Toxicity Symptoms

From nonfood sources only; diarrhea, alkalosis, dehydration

Significant Sources

Nuts, legumes, whole grains, dark green vegetables, seafood, chocolate, cocoa

[a]A still more severe deficiency causes tetany, an extreme, prolonged contraction of the muscles similar to that caused by low blood calcium.

Sulfate

Sulfate is the oxidized form of the mineral **sulfur** as it exists in food and water. The body's need for sulfate is easily met by a variety of foods and beverages. In addition, the body receives sulfate from the amino acids methionine and cysteine found in dietary protein. These sulfur-containing amino acids help determine the contour of protein molecules. The sulfur-containing side chains in cysteine molecules can link to each other, forming disulfide bridges, which stabilize the protein structure (see the drawing of insulin with its disulfide bridges on p. 184). Skin, hair, and nails contain some of the body's more rigid proteins, which have a high sulfur content.

There is no recommended intake for sulfate, and no deficiencies are known. Only when people lack protein to the point of severe deficiency will they lack the sulfur-containing amino acids.

IN SUMMARY Like the other nutrients, the minerals' actions are coordinated to get the body's work done. The major minerals, especially sodium, chloride, and potassium, influence the body's fluid balance; whenever an anion moves, a cation moves—always maintaining homeostasis. Sodium, chloride, potassium, calcium, and magnesium are key members of the team of nutrients that direct nerve impulse transmission and muscle contraction; they are also the primary nutrients involved in regulating blood pressure. Phosphorus and magnesium participate in many reactions involving glucose, fatty acids, amino acids, and the vitamins. Calcium, phosphorus, and magnesium combine to form the structure of the bones and teeth. Each major mineral also plays other specific roles in the body. (See the summary table on p. 423.)

sulfate: the oxidized form of sulfur.

sulfur: a mineral present in the body as part of some proteins.

The Major Minerals

Mineral and Chief Functions	Deficiency Symptoms	Toxicity Symptoms	Significant Sources
Sodium Maintains normal fluid and electrolyte balance; assists in nerve impulse transmission and muscle contraction	Muscle cramps, mental apathy, loss of appetite	Edema, acute hypertension	Table salt, soy sauce; moderate amounts in meats, milks, breads, and vegetables; large amounts in processed foods
Chloride Maintains normal fluid and electrolyte balance; part of hydrochloric acid found in the stomach, necessary for proper digestion	Do not occur under normal circumstances	Vomiting	Table salt, soy sauce; moderate amounts in meats, milks, eggs; large amounts in processed foods
Potassium Maintains normal fluid and electrolyte balance; facilitates many reactions; supports cell integrity; assists in nerve impulse transmission and muscle contractions	Muscular weakness, paralysis, confusion	Muscular weakness; vomiting; if given into a vein, can stop the heart	All whole foods; meats, milks, fruits, vegetables, grains, legumes
Calcium Mineralization of bones and teeth; also involved in muscle contraction and relaxation, nerve functioning, blood clotting, blood pressure, and immune defenses	Stunted growth in children; bone loss (osteoporosis) in adults	Constipation; increased risk of urinary stone formation and kidney dysfunction; interference with absorption of other minerals	Milk and milk products, small fish (with bones), tofu, greens (broccoli, chard), legumes
Phosphorus Mineralization of bones and teeth; part of every cell; important in genetic material, part of phospholipids, used in energy transfer and in buffer systems that maintain acid-base balance	Muscular weakness, bone pain[a]	Calcification of nonskeletal tissues, particularly the kidneys	All animal tissues (meat, fish, poultry, eggs, milk)
Magnesium Bone mineralization, building of protein, enzyme action, normal muscle contraction, nerve impulse transmission, maintenance of teeth, and functioning of immune system	Weakness; confusion; if extreme, convulsions, bizarre muscle movements (especially of eye and face muscles), hallucinations, and difficulty in swallowing; in children, growth failure[b]	From nonfood sources only; diarrhea, alkalosis, dehydration	Nuts, legumes, whole grains, dark green vegetables, seafood, chocolate, cocoa
Sulfate As part of proteins, stabilizes their shape by forming disulfide bridges; part of the vitamins biotin and thiamin and the hormone insulin	None known; protein deficiency would occur first	Toxicity would occur only if sulfur-containing amino acids were eaten in excess; this (in animals) depresses growth	All protein-containing foods (meats, fish, poultry, eggs, milk, legumes, nuts)

[a]Dietary deficiency rarely occurs, but some drugs can bind with phosphorus making it unavailable and resulting in bone loss that is characterized by weakness and pain.
[b]A still more severe deficiency causes tetany, an extreme, prolonged contraction of the muscles similar to that caused by low blood calcium.

With all of the tasks these minerals perform, they are of great importance to life. Consuming enough of each of them every day is easy, given a variety of foods from each of the food groups. Whole-grain breads supply magnesium; fruits, vegetables, and legumes also provide magnesium and potassium, too; milks offer calcium and phosphorus; meats also offer phosphorus and sulfate as well; all foods provide sodium and chloride, excesses being more problematic than inadequacies. The message is quite simple and has been repeated throughout this text: for an adequate intake of all the nutrients, including the major minerals, choose different foods from each of the five food groups. And drink plenty of water.

Nutrition in Your Life

Many people may miss the mark when it comes to drinking enough water to keep their bodies well hydrated or obtaining enough calcium to promote strong bones; in contrast, sodium intakes often exceed those recommended for health.

- **Do you drink plenty of water—about 8 glasses—every day?**
- **Do you select and prepare foods with less salt?**
- **Do you drink at least 3 glasses of milk—or get the equivalent in calcium—every day?**

NUTRITION ON THE NET

Access these websites for further study of topics covered in this chapter.

- Find updates and quick links to these and other nutrition-related sites at our website: **www.wadsworth.com/nutrition**
- Search for "minerals" at the American Dietetic Association site: **www.eatright.org**
- Learn about sodium in foods and on food labels from the Food and Drug Administration: **www.fda.gov/fdac/foodlabel/sodium.html**
- Find tips and recipes for including more milk in the diet: **www.whymilk.com**
- Learn about the benefits of calcium from the National Dairy Council: **www.nationaldairycouncil.org**

NUTRITION CALCULATIONS

These problems give you an appreciation for the minerals in foods. Be sure to show your calculations (see p. 427 for answers).

1. For each of these minerals, note the unit of measure:
   Calcium Magnesium Phosphorus
   Potassium Sodium
2. Learn to appreciate calcium-dense foods. The foods in the accompanying table are ranked in order of their calcium contents per serving.
   a. Which foods offer the most calcium per kcalorie? To calculate calcium density, divide calcium (mg) by energy (kcal). Record your answer in the table (round your answers); the first one is done for you.
   b. The top five items ranked in order of calcium contents per serving are sardines > milk > cheese > salmon > broccoli. What are the top five items in order of calcium contents per kcalorie?

Food	Calcium (mg)	Energy (kcal)	Calcium Density (mg/kcal)
Sardines, 3 oz canned	325	176	1.85
Milk, fat-free, 1 c	301	85	
Cheddar cheese, 1 oz	204	114	
Salmon, 3 oz canned	182	118	
Broccoli, cooked from fresh, chopped, ½ c	36	22	
Sweet potato, baked in skin, 1 ea	32	140	
Cantaloupe melon, ½	29	93	
Whole-wheat bread, 1 slice	21	64	
Apple, 1 medium	15	125	
Sirloin steak, lean, 3 oz	9	171	

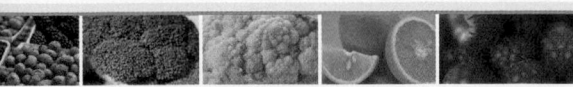

This information should convince you that milk, milk products, fish eaten with their bones, and dark green vegetables are the best choices for calcium.

3. a. Consider how the rate of absorption influences the amount of calcium available for the body's use. Use the drawing on p. 417 to determine how much calcium the body actually receives from the foods listed in the accompanying table by multiplying the milligrams of calcium in the food by the percentage absorbed. The first one is done for you.
   b. To appreciate how the absorption rate influences the amount of calcium available to the body, compare broccoli with almonds. Which provides more calcium in foods and to the body?
   c. To appreciate how the calcium content of foods influences the amount of calcium available to the body, compare cauliflower with milk. How much cauliflower would a person have to eat to receive an equivalent amount of calcium as from 1 cup of milk? How does your answer change when you account for differences in their absorption rates?

Food	Calcium in the Food (mg)	Absorption Rate (%)	Calcium in the Body (mg)
Cauliflower, ½ c cooked, fresh	10	≥50	≥5
Broccoli, ½ c cooked, fresh	36		
Milk, 1 c 1% low-fat	300		
Almonds, 1 oz	75		
Spinach, 1 c raw	55		

STUDY QUESTIONS

These questions will help you review the chapter. You will find the answers in the discussions on the pages provided.

1. List the roles of water in the body. (p. 396)
2. List the sources of water intake and routes of water excretion. (pp. 396–397)
3. What is ADH? Where does it exert its action? What is aldosterone? How does it work? (p. 399)
4. How does the body use electrolytes to regulate fluid balance? (pp. 400–403)
5. What do the terms *major* and *trace* mean when describing the minerals in the body? (p. 405)
6. Describe some characteristics of minerals that distinguish them from vitamins. (pp. 405–407)
7. What is the major function of sodium in the body? Describe how the kidneys regulate blood sodium. Is a dietary deficiency of sodium likely? Why or why not? (pp. 407–409)
8. List calcium's roles in the body. How does the body keep blood calcium constant regardless of intake? (pp. 413–414)
9. Name significant food sources of calcium. What are the consequences of inadequate intakes? (pp. 415–418)
10. List the roles of phosphorus in the body. Discuss the relationships between calcium and phosphorus. Is a dietary deficiency of phosphorus likely? Why or why not? (pp. 419–420)
11. State the major functions of chloride, potassium, magnesium, and sulfur in the body. Are deficiencies of these nutrients likely to occur in your own diet? Why or why not? (pp. 410, 411, 420–421, 422)

These multiple choice questions will help you prepare for an exam. Answers can be found on p. 427.

1. The body generates water during the:
   a. buffering of acids.
   b. dismantling of bone.
   c. metabolism of minerals.
   d. breakdown of energy nutrients.
2. Regulation of fluid and electrolyte balance and acid-base balance depends primarily on the:
   a. kidneys.
   b. intestines.
   c. sweat glands.
   d. specialized tear ducts.
3. The distinction between the major and trace minerals reflects the:
   a. ability of their ions to form salts.
   b. amounts of their contents in the body.
   c. importance of their functions in the body.
   d. capacity to retain their identity after absorption.
4. The principal cation in extracellular fluids is:
   a. sodium.
   b. chloride.
   c. potassium.
   d. phosphorus.
5. The role of chloride in the stomach is to help:
   a. support nerve impulses.
   b. convey hormonal messages.
   c. maintain a strong acidity.
   d. assist in muscular contractions.

6. Which would provide the most potassium?
   a. bologna
   b. potatoes
   c. pickles
   d. whole-wheat bread
7. Calcium homeostasis depends on:
   a. vitamin K, aldosterone, and renin.
   b. vitamin K, parathormone, and renin.
   c. vitamin D, aldosterone, and calcitonin.
   d. vitamin D, calcitonin, and parathormone.
8. Calcium absorption is hindered by:
   a. lactose.
   b. oxalates.
   c. vitamin D.
   d. stomach acid.
9. Phosphorus assists in many activities in the body, but *not:*
   a. energy metabolism.
   b. the clotting of blood.
   c. the transport of lipids.
   d. bone and teeth formation.
10. Most of the body's magnesium can be found in the:
   a. bones.
   b. nerves.
   c. muscles.
   d. extracellular fluids.

REFERENCES

1. Committee on Dietary Reference Intakes, *Dietary Reference Intakes for Water, Potassium, Sodium, Chloride, and Sulfate* (Washington, D.C.: National Academies Press, 2004), p. 67.
2. U.S. Department of Agriculture, *1994–1996, 1998 Continuing Survey of Food Intakes by Individuals (CSFII) 1994–1996, and Diet and Health Knowledge Survey, 2000.* (Available from the National Technical Information Service, Springfield, VA: tel 1-800-553-6847; CD-ROM accession number PB2000-500027).
3. M. Neuhäuser-Berthold and coauthors, Coffee consumption and total body water homeostasis as measured by fluid balance and bioelectrical impedance analysis, *Annals of Nutrition and Metabolism* 41 (1997): 29–36.
4. Committee on Dietary Reference Intakes, 2004, pp. 120–121.
5. D. S. Michaud and coauthors, Fluid intake and the risk of bladder cancer in men, *New England Journal of Medicine* 340 (1999): 1390–1397.
6. S. M. Kleiner, Water: An essential but overlooked nutrient, *Journal of the American Dietetic Association* 99 (1999): 200–206.
7. M. P. Sauvant and D. Pepin, Geographic variation of the mortality from cardiovascular disease and drinking water in a French small area (Puy de Dome), *Environmental Research* 84 (2000): 219–227.
8. H. Bohmer, H. Muller, and K. L. Resch, Calcium supplementation with calcium-rich mineral waters: A systematic review and meta-analysis of its bioavailability, *Osteoporosis International* 11 (2000): 938–943; R. Maheswaran and coauthors, Magnesium in drinking water supplies and mortality from acute myocardial infarction in north west England, *Heart* 82 (1999): 455–460.
9. J. He and coauthors, Dietary sodium intake and subsequent risk of cardiovascular disease in overweight adults, *Journal of the American Medical Association* 282 (1999): 2027–2034.
10. F. M. Sacks and coauthors, Effects on blood pressure of reduced dietary sodium and the Dietary Approaches to Stop Hypertension (DASH) diet, *New England Journal of Medicine* 344 (2001): 3–10.
11. Sacks and coauthors, 2001.
12. M. Harrington and K. D. Cashman, High salt intake appears to increase bone resorption in postmenopausal women but high potassium intake ameliorates this adverse effect, *Nutrition Reviews* 61 (2003): 179–183.
13. A. J. Cohen and F. J. Roe, Review of risk factors for osteoporosis with particular reference to a possible aetiological role of dietary salt, *Food and Chemical Toxicology* 38 (2000): 237–253.
14. F. P. Cappuccio and coauthors, Unravelling the links between calcium excretion, salt intake, hypertension, kidney stones and bone metabolism, *Journal of Nephrology* 13 (2000): 169–177.
15. D. E. Sellmeyer, M. Schloetter, and A. Sebastin, Potassium citrate prevents increased urine calcium excretion and bone resorption induced by a high sodium chloride diet, *Journal of Clinical Endocrinology and Metabolism* 87 (2002): 2008–2012.
16. F. J. He and G. A. MacGregor, Beneficial effects of potassium, *British Medical Journal* 323 (2001): 497–501.
17. K. Kathleen, Hyperkalemia, *American Journal of Nursing* 100 (2000): 55–56.
18. R. Jorde and K. H. Bønaa, Calcium from dairy products, vitamin D intake, and blood pressure: The Tromsø study, *American Journal of Clinical Nutrition* 71 (2000): 1530–1535.
19. M. Jacqmain and coauthors, Calcium intake, body composition, and lipoprotein-lipid concentrations, *American Journal of Clinical Nutrition* 77 (2003): 1448–1452; E. Kampman and coauthors, Calcium, vitamin D, sunshine exposure, dairy products and colon cancer risk (United States), *Cancer Causes and Control* 5 (2000): 459–466; E. Kallay and coauthors, Dietary calcium and growth modulation of human colon cancer cells: Role of the extracellular calcium-sensing receptor, *Cancer Detection and Prevention* 24 (2000): 127–136.
20. S. J. Parikh and J. A. Yanovski, Calcium and adiposity, *American Journal of Clinical Nutrition* 77 (2003): 281–287; D. Teegarden, Calcium intake and reduction in weight or fat mass, *Journal of Nutrition* 133 (2003): 249S–251S; R. P. Heaney, K. M. Davies, and M. J. Barger-Lux, Calcium and weight: Clinical studies, *Journal of the American College of Nutrition* 21 (2002): 152–155.
21. Jacqmain and coauthors, 2003; Teegarden, 2003; Heaney, Davies, and Barger-Lux, 2002; M. B. Zemel and coauthors, Regulation of adiposity by dietary calcium, *FASEB Journal* 14 (2000): 1132–1138.
22. M. B. Zemel and coauthors, Dietary calcium and dairy products accelerate weight and fat loss during energy restriction in obese adults, *American Journal of Clinical Nutrition* 75 (2002): 342S.
23. M. B. Zemel, Mechanisms of dairy modulation of adiposity, *Journal of Nutrition* 133 (2003): 252S–256S.
24. R. L. Wolf and coauthors, Factors associated with calcium absorption efficiency in pre- and perimenopausal women, *American Journal of Clinical Nutrition* 72 (2000): 466–471; Committee on Dietary Reference Intakes, *Dietary Reference Intakes for Calcium, Phosphorus, Magnesium, Vitamin D, and Fluoride* (Washington, D.C.: National Academy Press, 1997), pp. 72–73.
25. Committee on Dietary Reference Intakes, 1997, pp. 75–76.
26. R. E. Black and coauthors, Children who avoid drinking cow milk have low dietary calcium intakes and poor bone health, *American Journal of Clinical Nutrition* 76 (2002): 675–680.
27. H. J. Kalkwarf, J. C. Khoury, and B. P. Lanphear, Milk intake during childhood and adolescence, adult bone density, and osteoporotic fractures in US women, *American Journal of Clinical Nutrition* 77 (2003): 257–265.
28. C. M. Weaver, W. R. Proulx, and R. Heaney, Choices for achieving adequate dietary calcium with a vegetarian diet, *American Journal of Clinical Nutrition* 70 (1999): 543S–548S.
29. Committee on Dietary Reference Intakes, 1997, pp. 73–74.
30. P. Galan and coauthors, Contribution of mineral waters to dietary calcium and magnesium intake in a French adult population, *Journal of the American Dietetic Association* 102 (2002): 1658–1662; J. Guillemant and coauthors, Mineral water as a source of dietary calcium: Acute effects on parathyroid function and bone resorption in young men, *American Journal of Clinical Nutrition* 71 (2000): 999–1002.
31. R. P. Heaney and coauthors, Dietary changes favorably affect bone remodeling in older adults, *Journal of the American Dietetic Association* 99 (1999): 1228–1233.

32. Committee on Dietary Reference Intakes, 1997, pp. 152–154.
33. Committee on Dietary Reference Intakes, 1997, p. 182.
34. R. P. Heaney and K. Rafferty, Carbonated beverages and urinary calcium excretion, *American Journal of Clinical Nutrition* 74 (2001): 343–347.
35. Galan and coauthors, 2002.
36. M. Sabatier and coauthors, Meal effect on magnesium bioavailability from mineral water in healthy women, *American Journal of Clinical Nutrition* 75 (2002): 65–71.
37. J. K. McGuire, M. S. Kulkarni, and H. P. Baden, Fatal hypermagnesemia in a child treated with megavitamin/megamineral therapy, *Pediatrics* 105 (2000): e18.

ANSWERS

Nutrition Calculations

1. Calcium: mg. Magnesium: mg. Phosphorus: mg. Potassium: mg. Sodium: mg.

2. a.

Food	Calcium Density (mg/kcal)
Sardines, 3 oz canned	325 mg ÷ 176 kcal = 1.85 mg/kcal
Milk, fat-free, 1 c	301 mg ÷ 85 kcal = 3.54 mg/kcal
Cheddar cheese, 1 oz	204 mg ÷ 114 kcal = 1.79 mg/kcal
Salmon, 3 oz canned	182 mg ÷ 118 kcal = 1.54 mg/kcal
Broccoli, cooked from fresh, chopped, ½ c	36 mg ÷ 22 kcal = 1.64 mg/kcal
Sweet potato, baked in skin, 1 ea	32 mg ÷ 140 kcal = 0.23 mg/kcal
Cantaloupe melon, ½	29 mg ÷ 93 kcal = 0.31 mg/kcal
Whole-wheat bread, 1 slice	21 mg ÷ 64 kcal = 0.33 mg/kcal
Apple, 1 medium	15 mg ÷ 125 kcal = 0.12 mg/kcal
Sirloin steak, lean, 3 oz	9 mg ÷ 171 kcal = 0.05 mg/kcal

b. Milk > sardines > cheese > broccoli > salmon.

3. a.

Food	Calcium in Food (mg) × Absorption rate (%) = Calcium in the Body (mg)
Cauliflower, ½ c cooked, fresh	10 mg × 0.50 = 5 mg (or more)
Broccoli, ½ c cooked, fresh	36 mg × 0.50 = 18 mg (or more)
Milk, 1 c 1% low-fat	300 mg × 0.30 = 90 mg
Almonds, 1 oz	75 mg × 0.20 = 15 mg
Spinach, 1 c raw	55 mg × 0.05 = 3 mg (or less)

b. The almonds offer more than twice as much calcium per serving, but an equivalent amount after absorption.

c. To equal the 300 milligrams provided by milk, a person would need to eat 15 cups of cauliflower (300 mg/c milk ÷ 10 mg/½ c cauliflower = 30 ½ c or 15 c). After considering the better absorption rate of cauliflower, a person would need to eat 9 cups of cauliflower (5 mg/½ c or 10 mg/c; 90 mg ÷ 10 mg/c = 9 c) to match the 90 milligrams available to the body from milk after absorption. The better absorption rate reduced the quantity of cauliflower significantly, but that's still a lot of cauliflower.

Study Questions (multiple choice)

1. d 2. a 3. b 4. a 5. c 6. b 7. d 8. b 9. b 10. a

HIGHLIGHT

Osteoporosis and Calcium

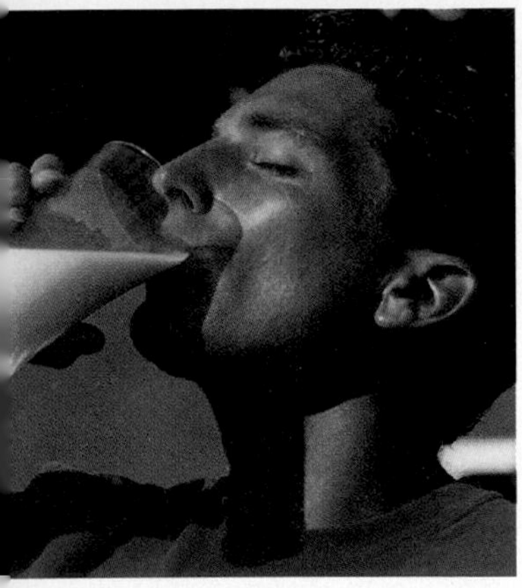

© Photo Disc Inc.

Osteoporosis becomes apparent during the later years, but it develops much earlier—and without warning. Few people are aware that their bones are being robbed of their strength. The problem often first becomes evident when someone's hip suddenly gives way. People say, "She fell and broke her hip," but in fact the hip may have been so fragile that it broke *before* she fell. Even bumping into a table may be enough to shatter a porous bone into fragments so numerous and scattered that they cannot be reassembled. Removing them and replacing them with an artificial joint requires major surgery. An estimated 300,000 people in the United States are hospitalized each year because of hip fractures related to osteoporosis. About a fourth die of complications within a year. A fourth of those who survive will never walk or live independently again. Their quality of life slips downward.

This highlight examines osteoporosis, one of the most prevalent diseases of aging, affecting more than 44 million people in the United States—most of them women over 50. It reviews the many factors that contribute to the 1.5 million breaks in the bones of the hips, vertebrae, wrists, arms, and ankles each year. And it presents strategies to reduce the risks, paying special attention to the role of dietary calcium.

Bone Development and Disintegration

Bone has two compartments: the outer, hard shell of **cortical bone,** and the inner, lacy matrix of **trabecular bone.** (The glossary defines these and other bone-related terms.) Both can lose minerals, but in different ways and at different rates. The photograph on p. 429 shows a human leg bone sliced lengthwise, exposing the lacy, calcium-containing crystals of trabecular bone. These crystals give up calcium to the blood when the diet runs short, and they take up calcium again when the supply is plentiful (review Figure 12-11 on p. 415). For people who have eaten calcium-rich foods throughout the bone-forming years of their youth, these deposits make bones dense and provide a rich reservoir of calcium.

Surrounding and protecting the trabecular bone is a dense, ivorylike exterior shell—the cortical bone. Cortical bone composes the shafts of the long bones, and a thin cortical shell caps the end of the bone, too. Both compartments confer strength on bone: cortical bone provides the sturdy outer wall, while trabecular bone provides support along the lines of stress.

The two types of bone play different roles in calcium balance and osteoporosis. Supplied with blood vessels and metabolically active, trabecular bone is sensitive to hormones that govern day-to-day deposits and withdrawals of calcium. It readily gives up minerals whenever blood calcium needs replenishing.

GLOSSARY

antacids: acid-buffering agents used to counter excess acidity in the stomach. Calcium-containing preparations (such as Tums) contain available calcium. Antacids with aluminum or magnesium hydroxides (such as Rolaids) can accelerate calcium losses.

bone meal or **powdered bone:** crushed or ground bone preparations intended to supply calcium to the diet. Calcium from bone is not well absorbed and is often contaminated with toxic minerals such as arsenic, mercury, lead, and cadmium.

bone density: a measure of bone strength. When minerals fill the bone matrix (making it dense), they give it strength.

cortical bone: the very dense bone tissue that forms the outer shell surrounding trabecular bone and comprises the shaft of a long bone.

dolomite: a compound of minerals (calcium magnesium carbonate) found in limestone and marble. Dolomite is powdered and is sold as a calcium-magnesium supplement, but may be contaminated with toxic minerals, is not well absorbed, and interacts adversely with absorption of other esssential minerals.

oyster shell: a product made from the powdered shells of oysters that is sold as a calcium supplement, but is not well absorbed by the digestive system.

trabecular (tra-BECK-you-lar) **bone:** the lacy inner structure of calcium crystals that supports the bone's structure and provides a calcium storage bank.

type I osteoporosis: osteoporosis characterized by rapid bone losses, primarily of trabecular bone.

type II osteoporosis: osteoporosis characterized by gradual losses of both trabecular and cortical bone.

Reminder: *Osteoporosis* is a disease characterized by porous and fragile bones.

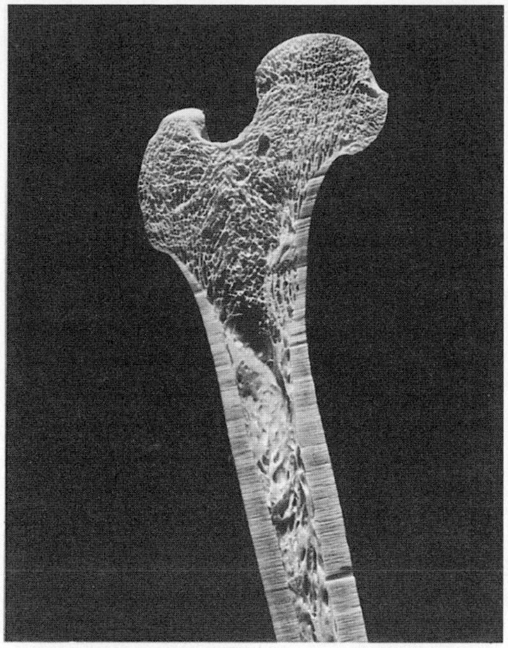
Courtesy of Gjon Mili

Trabecular bone is the lacy network of calcium-containing crystals that fills the interior. Cortical bone is the dense, ivorylike bone that forms the exterior shell.

Losses of trabecular bone start becoming significant for men and women in their 30s, although losses can occur whenever calcium withdrawals exceed deposits.

Cortical bone also gives up calcium, but slowly and at a steady pace. Cortical bone losses typically begin at about age 40 and continue slowly but surely thereafter.

Losses of trabecular and cortical bone reflect two types of osteoporosis, which cause two types of bone breaks. **Type I osteoporosis** involves losses of trabecular bone (see Figure H12-1). These losses sometimes exceed three times the expected rate, and bone breaks may occur suddenly. Trabecular bone becomes so fragile that even the body's own weight can overburden the spine—vertebrae may suddenly disintegrate and crush down, painfully pinching major nerves. Wrists may break as bone ends weaken, and teeth may loosen or fall out as the trabecular bone of the jaw recedes. Women are most often the victims of this type of osteoporosis, outnumbering men six to one.

In **type II osteoporosis,** the calcium of both cortical and trabecular bone is drawn out of storage, but slowly over the years. As old age approaches, the vertebrae may compress into wedge shapes, forming what is often called a "dowager's hump," the posture many older people assume as they "grow shorter." Figure H12-2 (on p. 430) shows the effect of compressed spinal bone on a woman's height and posture. Because both the cortical shell and the trabecular interior weaken, breaks most often occur in the hip, as mentioned in the introductory paragraph. A woman is twice as likely as a man to suffer type II osteoporosis.

Table H12-1 summarizes the differences between the two types of osteoporosis. Physicians can diagnose osteoporosis and assess the risk of bone fractures by measuring **bone density** using dual-energy X-ray absorptiometry (DEXA scan) or ultrasound. They also consider risk factors that predict bone fractures, including age, personal and family history of fracture, heritage, BMI, and physical inactivity.[1] Table H12-2 summarizes the major risk factors and protective factors for osteoporosis. The more risk factors that apply to a person, the greater the chances of bone loss. Notice that several risk factors that are influential in the development of osteoporosis—such as age, gender, and heritage—cannot be changed. Other risk factors—such as diet, physical activity, body weight, smoking, and alcohol use—are personal behaviors that can be changed. By eating a well-balanced diet rich in calcium, being physically active, abstaining from smoking, and drinking alcohol in moderation (if at all), people can defend themselves against osteoporosis. These decisions are particularly important for those with other risk factors that cannot be changed.

Whether a person develops osteoporosis seems to depend on the interactions of several factors, including nutrition. The strongest predictor of bone density is age: osteoporosis is responsible for 90 percent of the hip fractures in women and 80 percent in men over the age of 65.

FIGURE H12-1 Healthy and Osteoporotic Trabecular Bones

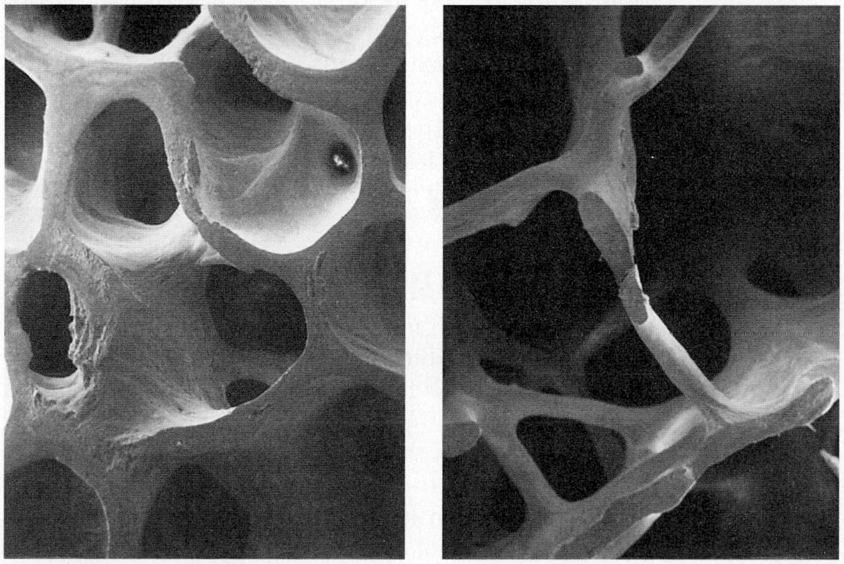
Permission by David Dempster from J Eone Miner Res, 1986 (both)

Electron micrograph of healthy trabecular bone.

Electron micrograph of trabecular bone affected by osteoporosis.

FIGURE H12-2 Loss of Height in a Woman Caused by Osteoporosis

The woman on the left is about 50 years old. On the right, she is 80 years old. Her legs have not grown shorter: only her back has lost length, due to collapse of her spinal bones (vertebrae). Collapsed vertebrae cannot protect the spinal nerves from pressure that causes excruciating pain.

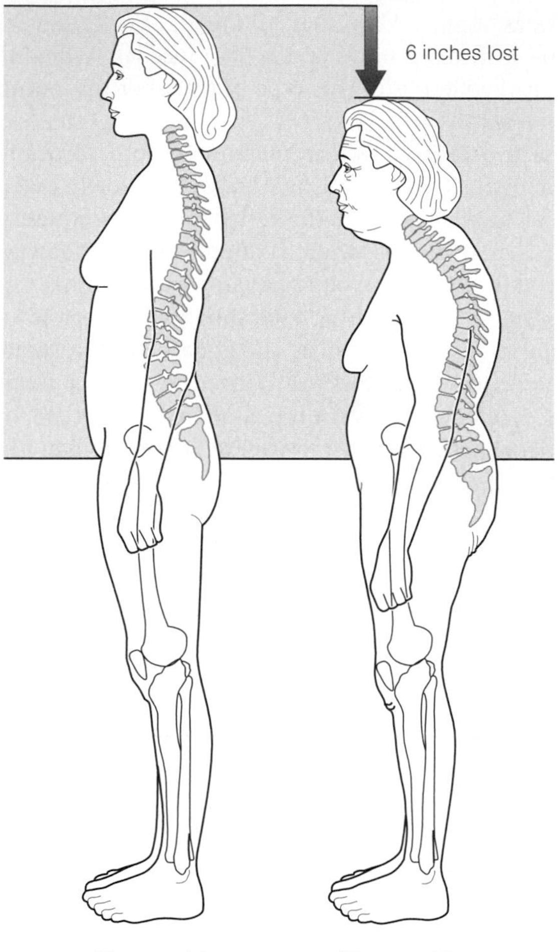
6 inches lost
50 years old
80 years old

TABLE H12-1 Types of Osteoporosis Compared

	Type I	Type II
Other name	Postmenopausal osteoporosis	Senile osteoporosis
Age of onset	50 to 70 years old	70 years and older
Bone loss	Trabecular bone	Both trabecular and cortical bone
Fracture sites	Wrist and spine	Hip
Gender incidence	6 women to 1 man	2 women to 1 man
Primary causes	Rapid loss of estrogen in women following menopause; loss of testosterone in men with advancing age	Reduced calcium absorption, increased bone mineral loss, increased propensity to fall

TABLE H12-2 Risk Factors and Protective Factors for Osteoporosis

Risk Factors	Protective Factors
• Older age	• Younger age
• Low BMI	• High BMI
• Caucasian, Asian, or Hispanic heritage	• African American heritage
• Cigarette smoking	• No smoking
• Alcohol consumption in excess	• Alcohol consumption in moderation
• Sedentary lifestyle	• Regular weight-bearing exercise
• Use of glucocorticoids or anticonvulsants	• Use of diuretics
• Female gender	• Male gender
• Maternal history of osteoporosis fracture or personal history of fracture	• Bone density assessment and treatment (if necessary)
• Estrogen deficiency in women (amenorrhea or menopause, especially early or surgically induced); testosterone deficiency in men	• Use of estrogen therapy
• Lifetime diet inadequate in calcium and vitamin D	• Lifetime diet rich in calcium and vitamin D

Age and Bone Calcium

Two major stages of life are critical in the development of osteoporosis. The first is the bone-acquiring stage of childhood and adolescence. The second is the bone-losing decades of late adulthood (especially in women after menopause). The bones gain strength and density all through the growing years and into young adulthood. As people age, the cells that build bone gradually become less active, but those that dismantle bone continue working. The result is that bone loss exceeds bone formation. Some bone loss is inevitable, but losses can be curtailed by maximizing bone mass.

Maximizing Bone Mass

To maximize bone mass, the diet must deliver an adequate supply of calcium during the first three decades of life. Children and teens who get enough calcium and vitamin D have denser bones than those with inadequate intakes. With little or no calcium from the diet, the body must depend on bone to supply calcium to the blood; bone mass diminishes, and bones lose their density and strength. When people reach the bone-losing years of middle age, those who formed dense bones during their youth have the advantage. They simply have more bone starting out and can lose more before suffering ill effects. Figure H12-3 demonstrates this effect.

FIGURE H12-3 Bone Losses over Time Compared

Peak bone mass is achieved by age 30. Women gradually lose bone mass until menopause, when losses accelerate dramatically and then gradually taper off.

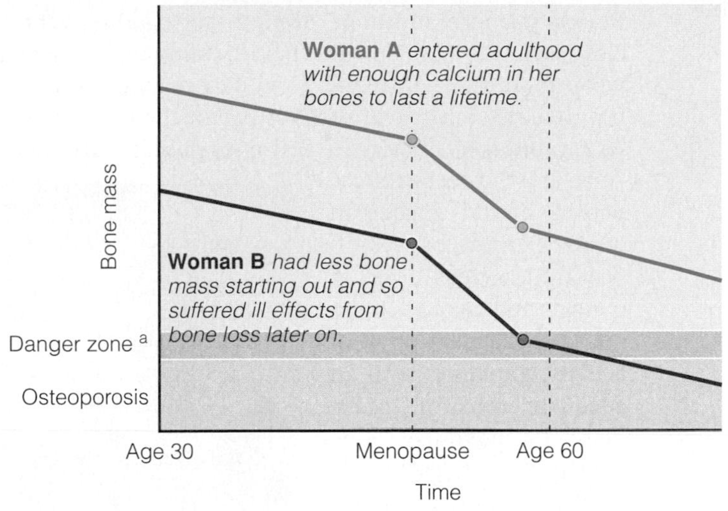
Woman A entered adulthood with enough calcium in her bones to last a lifetime.
Woman B had less bone mass starting out and so suffered ill effects from bone loss later on.
Bone mass
Danger zone a
Osteoporosis
Age 30
Menopause
Age 60
Time

[a]People with a moderate degree of bone mass reduction are said to have *osteopenia* and are at increased risk of fractures.
SOURCE: Data from Committee on Dietary Reference Intakes, *Dietary Reference Intakes for Calcium, Phosphorus, Magnesium, Vitamin D, and Fluoride* (Washington, D.C.: National Academy Press, 1997), pp. 71–145.

Minimizing Bone Loss

Not only does dietary calcium build strong bones in youth, but it remains important in protecting against losses in the later years.[2] Unfortunately, calcium intakes of older adults are typically low, and calcium absorption declines after about the age of 65 years. The kidneys do not activate vitamin D as well as they did earlier (recall that active vitamin D enhances calcium absorption). Also, sunlight is needed to form vitamin D, and many older people spend little or no time outdoors in the sunshine. For these reasons, and because intakes of vitamin D are typically low anyway, blood vitamin D declines.

Some of the hormones that regulate bone and calcium metabolism also change with age and accelerate bone mineral withdrawal.* Together, these age-related factors contribute to bone loss: inefficient bone remodeling, reduced calcium intakes, impaired calcium absorption, poor vitamin D status, and hormonal changes that favor bone mineral withdrawal.

Gender and Hormones

After age, gender is the next strongest predictor of osteoporosis: men have greater bone density than women at maturity, and women have greater losses than men in later life. Consequently, women account for four out of five cases of osteoporosis. Menopause imperils women's bones. Bone dwindles rapidly when the hormone estrogen diminishes and menstruation ceases. Women may lose up to 20 percent of their bone mass during the six to eight years following menopause. Eventually, losses taper off so that women again lose bone at the same rate as men their age. Losses of bone minerals continue throughout the remainder of a woman's lifetime, but not at the free-fall pace of the menopause years (review Figure H12-3).

Rapid bone losses also occur when *young* women's ovaries fail to produce enough estrogen, causing menstruation to cease. In some, diseased ovaries are to blame and must be removed; in others, the ovaries fail to produce sufficient estrogen because the women suffer from anorexia nervosa and have unreasonably restricted their body weight (see Highlight 9). The amenorrhea and low body weights explain much of the bone loss seen in these young women, even years after diagnosis and treatment.[3] Estrogen therapy can help nonmenstruating women prevent further bone loss and reduce the incidence of fractures.[4] Because estrogen therapy may increase the risks for heart disease and breast cancer, women must carefully weigh any potential benefits against the possible dangers.[5] Other drugs used to prevent or treat osteoporosis include raloxifene, alendronate, risedronate, and calcitonin.† A combination of hormone replacement and a drug may be an option for some women.[6]

Some women who choose not to use estrogen therapy turn to soy as an alternative treatment. Interestingly, the phytochemicals commonly found in soybeans mimic the actions of estrogen in the body. When natural estrogen is lacking, as after menopause, these phytochemicals may step in to stimulate estrogen-sensitive tissues. By way of this action, soy and its phytochemicals may help to prevent the rapid bone losses of the menopause years.[7] Research is far from conclusive, but some evidence suggests that soy may indeed offer some protection.[8]

If estrogen deficiency is a major cause of osteoporosis in women, what is the cause of bone loss in men? The male sex hormone testosterone appears to play a role. Men with low levels of testosterone, as occurs after removal of diseased testes or when testes lose function with aging, suffer more fractures. Treatment for men with osteoporosis includes

*Among the hormones suggested as influential are parathormone, calcitonin, and estrogen.

†Raloxifene (rah-LOX-ih-feen) is a selective estrogen-receptor modulator (SERM), marketed as Evista; alendronate (a-LEN-droe-nate) is a bisphosphonate, marketed as Fosamax; risedronate (rih-SEH-droe-nate) is a bisphosphonate, marketed as Actonel; and calcitonin is a hormone, marketed as Calcimar and Miacalcin.

testosterone replacement therapy. Thus both male and female sex hormones participate in the development and treatment of osteoporosis.

Most hormone and drug treatments for osteoporosis work by inhibiting the activities of the bone-dismantling cells, thus allowing the bone-building cells to slowly shore up bone tissue with new calcium deposits.* Research is also under way to develop drugs that will stimulate the bone-building cells to accelerate fracture healing and restore bone strength.[9] Leading contenders include parathormone, cholesterol-lowering drugs (statins), and leptin.

Genetics and Ethnicity

Osteoporosis may, in part, be hereditary; family history of osteoporosis or fracture is a risk factor. The exact role of genetics is unclear, but most likely it influences both the peak bone mass achieved during growth and the bone loss incurred during the later years. The extent to which a given genetic potential is realized, however, depends on many outside factors. Diet and physical activity, for example, can maximize peak bone density during growth, whereas alcohol and tobacco abuse can accelerate bone losses later in life.

Risks of osteoporosis appear to run along racial lines and reflect genetic differences in bone development. African Americans, for example, seem to use and conserve calcium more efficiently than Caucasians. Consequently, even though their calcium intakes are typically lower, black people have denser bones than white people do. Greater bone density expresses itself in a lower rate of osteoporosis among blacks. Fractures, for example, are about twice as likely in white women age 65 or older as in black women.

Other ethnic groups have a high risk of osteoporosis. Asians from China and Japan, Mexican Americans, Hispanic people from Central and South America, and Inuit people from St. Lawrence Island typically have lower bone density than Caucasians. One might expect that these groups would suffer more bone fractures, but this is not always the case. Again, genetic differences may explain why. Asians, for example, generally have small, compact hips, which makes them less susceptible to fractures.

Findings from around the world demonstrate that although a person's genes may lay the groundwork, environmental factors influence the genes' ultimate expression. Diet in general, and calcium in particular, are among those environmental factors. Others include physical activity, body weight, smoking, and alcohol. Importantly, all of these factors are within a person's control.

*The generic name of the drug is aldendronate, marketed as Fosamax. This drug belongs to a group of nonhormonal medicines called bisphosphonates.

Physical Activity and Body Weight

Muscle strength and bone strength go together. When muscles work, they pull on the bones, stimulating them to develop more trabeculae and grow denser. The hormones that promote new muscle growth also favor the building of bone. As a result, active bones are denser than sedentary bones.[10]

To keep bones healthy, a person should engage in weight-training or weight-bearing activities (such as dancing and vigorous walking) daily. Regular physical activity combined with an adequate calcium intake helps to maximize bone density in adolescence.[11] Adults can also maximize and maintain bone density with a regular program of weight training.[12] Even past menopause when most women are losing bone, weight training improves bone density.[13]

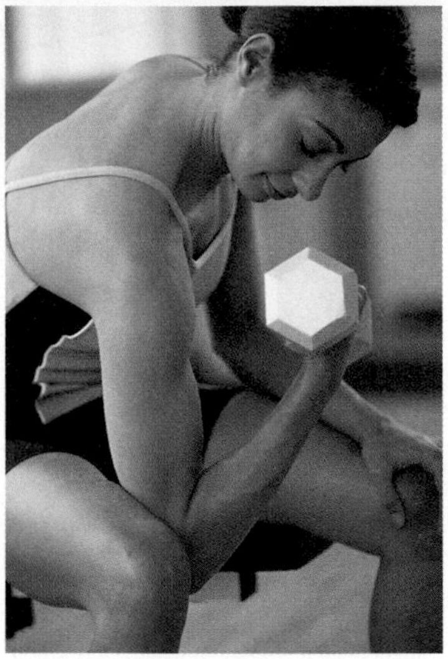
© Rob Lewine/CORBIS

Strength training helps to build strong bones.

Heavier body weights and weight gains place a similar stress on the bones and promote their density. In fact, underweight and weight losses are significant and consistent predictors of bone density losses and risk of fractures.[14] As mentioned in Highlight 9, the combination of underweight, severely restricted energy intake, extreme daily exercise, and amenorrhea reliably predicts bone loss. Interestingly, some evidence suggests that the bone density associated with overweight may be due not to body weight alone but to the lack of, or inability to respond to, leptin.[15]

Cells respond, with the help of the necessary regulators, to the demands put upon them. Then they select the nutrients they need from what is offered. To increase bone density, put a demand on the bones, make them work, and then provide the raw materials from which they can grow strong: calcium and all the other nutrients in the right balance.

Smoking and Alcohol

Add bone damage to the list of ill consequences associated with smoking. Bones of smokers are less dense than those of nonsmokers—even after controlling for differences in age, body weight, and physical activity habits.[16] Blood levels of vitamin D and bone-related hormones in smokers favor decreased calcium absorption and increased bone resorption.[17]

Fortunately, these damaging effects can be reversed with smoking cessation. Blood indicators of beneficial bone activity are apparent six weeks after a person stops smoking.[18] In time, bone density is similar for former smokers and nonsmokers.

People who abuse alcohol often suffer from osteoporosis and experience more bone breaks than others. Several factors appear to be involved: alcohol enhances fluid excretion, leading to excessive calcium losses in the urine; upsets the hormonal balance required for healthy bones; slows bone formation, leading to lower bone density; stimulates bone breakdown; and increases the risk of falling. Alcohol in moderate amounts, however, may protect bone density by decreasing remodeling activity.[19]

Dietary Calcium Is the Key to Prevention

Bone strength later in life depends most on how well the bones were built during childhood and adolescence. Adequate calcium nutrition during the growing years is essential to achieving optimal peak bone mass.[20] Simply put, growing children who do not get enough calcium do not have strong bones.[21] Neither do adults who did not get enough calcium during their childhood and adolescence.[22] To that end, the DRI Committee recommends 1300 milligrams of calcium per day for everyone 9 through 18 years of age. Unfortunately, few girls meet the recommendations for calcium during these bone-forming years. (Boys generally obtain intakes close to those recommended because they eat more food.) Consequently, most girls start their adult years with less-than-optimal bone density. As for adults, women rarely meet their recommended intakes of 1000 to 1200 milligrams from food. Some authorities suggest 1500 milligrams of calcium for postmenopausal women who are not receiving estrogen, but warn that intakes exceeding 2500 milligrams a day could cause health problems.

Other Nutrients Play Supporting Roles

Much research has focused on calcium, but other nutrients support bone health, too. Adequate protein protects bones and reduces the likelihood of hip fractures.[23] As mentioned earlier, vitamin D is needed for optimal bone health.[24] Supplementation with vitamin D reduces bone loss and the risk of fractures.[25] Vitamin K protects against hip fractures.[26] The minerals magnesium and potassium also help to maintain bone mineral density.[27] Vitamin A is needed in the bone-remodeling process, but too much may be associated with osteoporosis.[28] Additional research points to the bone benefits not of a specific nutrient, but of a diet rich in fruits and vegetables.[29] In contrast, diets containing too much salt, candy, or caffeine are associated with bone losses.[30] Clearly, a well-balanced diet that depends on all the food groups to supply a full array of nutrients is central to bone health.

A Perspective on Supplements

Bone health improves when people increase their intake of calcium-rich foods.[31] People who do not consume milk products or other calcium-rich foods in amounts that provide even half the recommended calcium should consider consulting a registered dietitian who can assess the diet and suggest food choices to correct any inadequacies. For those who are unable to consume enough calcium-rich foods to forestall osteoporosis, taking calcium supplements may be appropriate.

Selecting a calcium supplement requires a little investigative work to sort through the many options. Before examining calcium supplements, recognize that multivitamin-mineral pills contain little or no calcium. The label may list a few milligrams of calcium, but remember that the recommended intake is a gram or more for adults.

Calcium supplements are typically sold as compounds of calcium carbonate (common in **antacids** and fortified chocolate candies), citrate, gluconate, lactate, malate, or phosphate. These supplements often include magnesium, vitamin D, or both. In addition, there are calcium supplements made from **bone meal, oyster shell,** or **dolomite** (limestone). Many calcium supplements, especially those derived from these natural products, contain lead—which impairs health in numerous ways, as Chapter 13 points out.[32] Fortunately, calcium interferes with the absorption and action of lead in the body.

The first question to ask is how much calcium the supplement provides. Most calcium supplements provide between 250 and 1000 milligrams of calcium. To be safe, total calcium intake from both foods and supplements should not exceed 2500 milligrams a day. Read the label to find out how much a dose supplies. Be aware that a 1000-milligram tablet of calcium carbonate contains only 400 milligrams of calcium. Unless the label states otherwise, supplements of calcium carbonate are 40 percent calcium; those of calcium citrate are 21 percent; lactate, 13 percent; and gluconate, 9 percent. Select a low-dose supplement and take it several times a day rather than taking a large-dose supplement all at once. Taking supplements in doses of 500 milligrams or less improves absorption. Small doses also help ease the GI distress (constipation, intestinal bloating, and excessive gas) that sometimes accompanies calcium supplement use.

The next question to ask is how well the body absorbs and uses the calcium from various supplements. Most healthy people absorb calcium equally well—and as well as from milk—from any of these supplements: calcium carbonate, citrate, or phosphate. More important than supplement solubility is tablet disintegration. When manufacturers compress

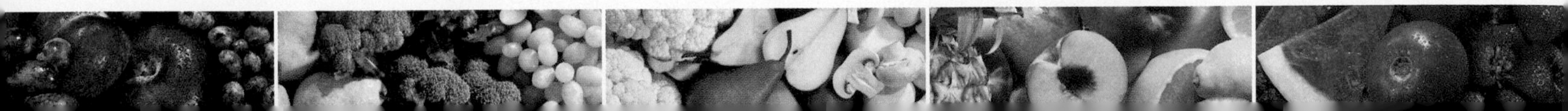

large quantities of calcium into small pills, the stomach acid has difficulty penetrating the pill. To test a supplement's ability to dissolve, drop it into a 6-ounce cup of vinegar, and stir occasionally. A high-quality formulation will dissolve within half an hour.

Finally, having chosen a supplement, a person must take it regularly, but when should you take it? To circumvent adverse nutrient interactions, take calcium supplements between, not with, meals. (Importantly, do not take calcium supplements with iron supplements or iron-rich meals; calcium inhibits iron absorption.) To enhance calcium absorption, take supplements with meals. If such contradictory advice drives you crazy, reconsider the benefits of food sources of calcium. Most experts agree that foods are the best source of calcium.

Some Closing Thoughts

Unfortunately, many of the strongest risk factors for osteoporosis are beyond people's control: age, gender, and genetics. But there are still several effective strategies for prevention.[33] First, ensure an optimal peak bone mass during childhood and adolescence by eating a balanced diet rich in calcium and engaging in regular physical activity. Then maintain that bone mass by continuing those healthy diet and activity habits, abstaining from cigarette smoking, and using alcohol moderately, if at all. Finally, minimize bone loss by maintaining an adequate nutrition and activity regimen and, for women, consult a physician about calcium supplements or other drug therapies that may be effective both in preventing bone loss and in restoring lost bone. The reward is the best possible chance of preserving bone health throughout life.

NUTRITION ON THE NET

Access these websites for further study of topics covered in this highlight.

- Find updates and quick links to these and other nutrition-related sites at our website: **www.wadsworth.com/nutrition**
- Search for "falls and fractures" at the National Institute on Aging: **www.nih.gov/nia**
- Visit the National Institutes of Health Osteoporosis and Related Bone Diseases' National Resource Center: **www.osteo.org**
- Obtain additional information from the National Osteoporosis Foundation: **www.nof.org**

REFERENCES

1. E. S. Siris and coauthors, Identification and fracture outcomes of undiagnosed low bone mineral density in postmenopausal women: Results from the National Osteoporosis Risk Assessment, *Journal of the American Medical Association* 286 (2001): 2815–2822; D. J. van der Voort and coauthors, Screening for osteoporosis using easily obtainable biometrical data: Diagnostic accuracy of measured, self-reported and recalled BMI, and related costs of bone mineral density measurements, *Osteoporosis International* 11 (2000): 233–239; L. W. Turner, P. A. Faile, and R. Tomlinson, Jr., Osteoporosis diagnosis and fracture, *Orthopaedic Nursing*, September/October 1999, pp. 21–27.
2. B. A. Peterson and coauthors, The effects of an educational intervention on calcium intake and bone mineral content in young women with low calcium intake, *American Journal of Health Promotion* 14 (2000): 149–156.
3. D. Hartman and coauthors, Bone density of women who have recovered from anorexia nervosa, *International Journal of Eating Disorders* 28 (2000): 107–112.
4. H. J. Kloosterboer and A. G. Ederveen, Pros and cons of existing treatment modalities in osteoporosis: A comparison between tibolone, SERMs and estrogen (+/− progestogen) treatments, *Journal of Steroid Biochemistry and Molecular Biology* 83 (2002): 157–165; R. A. Sayegh and P. G. Stubblefield, Bone metabolism and the perimenopause overview, risk factors, screening, and osteoporosis preventive measures, *Obstetrics and Gynecology Clinics of North America* 29 (2002): 495–510.
5. R. T. Chlebowski and coauthors, Influence of estrogen plus progestin on breast cancer and mammography in healthy post-menopausal women: The Women's Health Initiative Randomized Trial, *Journal of the American Medical Association* 289 (2003): 3243–3253; C. G. Solomon and R. G. Dluhy, Rethinking postmenopausal hormone therapy, *New England Journal of Medicine* 348 (2003): 579–580; Writing Group for the Women's Health Initiative Investigators, Risks and benefits of estrogen plus progestin in healthy postmenopausal women: Principal results from the Women's Health Initiative Randomized Controlled Trial, *Journal of the American Medical Association* 288 (2002): 321–333; O. Ylikorkala and M. Metsa-heikkila, Hormone replacement therapy in women with a history of breast cancer, *Gynecological Endocrinology* 16 (2002): 469–478.
6. S. L. Greenspan, N. M. Resnick, and R. A. Parker, Combination therapy with hormone replacement and alendronate for prevention of bone loss in elderly women: A randomized controlled trial, *Journal of the American Medical Association* 289 (2003): 2525–2533.

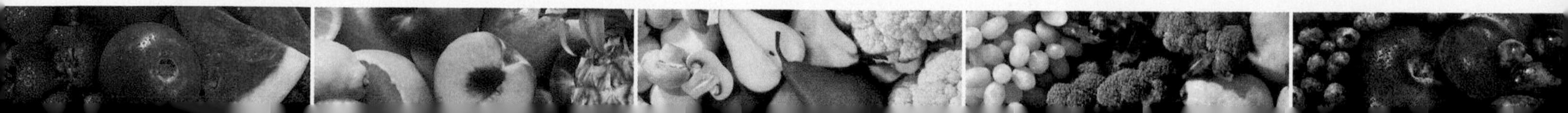

7. R. Brynin, Soy and its isoflavones: A review of their effects on bone density, *Alternative Medicine Review* 7 (2002): 317–327.
8. B. H. Arjmandi and coauthors, Soy protein has a greater effect on bone in postmenopausal women not on hormone replacement therapy, as evidenced by reducing bone resorption and urinary calcium excretion, *Journal of Clinical Endocrinology and Metabolism* 88 (2003): 1048–1054; T. Uesugi, Y. Fukui, and Y. Yamori, Beneficial effects of soybean isoflavone supplementation on bone metabolism and serum lipids in postmenopausal Japanese women: A four-week study, *Journal of the American College of Nutrition* 21 (2002): 97–102.
9. J. F. Whitfield, How to grow bone to treat osteoporosis and mend fractures, *Current Rheumatology Reports* 5 (2003): 45–56.
10. K. Delvaux and coauthors, Bone mass and lifetime physical activity in Flemish males: A 17-year follow-up study, *Medicine and Science in Sports and Exercise* 33 (2001): 1868–1875; L. Metcalfe and coauthors, Postmenopausal women and exercise for prevention of osteoporosis: The Bone, Estrogen, Strength Training (BEST) Study, *ACSM'S Health and Fitness Journal,* May/June 2001, pp. 6–14.
11. M. C. Wang and coauthors, Diet in midpuberty and sedentary activity in prepuberty predict peak bone mass, *American Journal of Clinical Nutrition* 77 (2003): 495–503; S. J. Stear and coauthors, Effect of a calcium and exercise intervention on the bone mineral status of 16-18-y-old adolescent girls, *American Journal of Clinical Nutrition* 77 (2003): 985–992; J. J. B. Anderson, Calcium requirements during adolescence to maximize bone health, *Journal of the American College of Nutrition* 20 (2001): 186S–191S.
12. J. E. Layne and M. E. Nelson, The effects of progressive resistance training on bone density: A review, *Medicine and Science in Sports and Exercise* 31 (1999): 25–30.
13. E. C. Cussler and coauthors, Weight lifted in strength training predicts bone change in postmenopausal women, *Medicine and Science in Sports and Exercise* 35 (2003): 10–17; Metcalfe and coauthors, 2001.
14. T. A. Ricci and coauthors, Moderate energy restriction increases bone resorption in obese postmenopausal women, *American Journal of Clinical Nutrition* 73 (2001): 347–352; D. Chao and coauthors, Effect of voluntary weight loss on bone mineral density in older overweight women, *Journal of the American Geriatrics Society* 48 (2000): 753–759; L. M. Salamone and coauthors, Effect of a lifestyle intervention on bone mineral density in premenopausal women: A randomized trial, *American Journal of Clinical Nutrition* 70 (1999): 97–103.
15. J. C. Fleet, Leptin and bone: Does the brain control bone biology? *Nutrition Reviews* 58 (2000): 209–211.
16. P. Gerdhem and K. J. Obrant, Effects of cigarette-smoking on bone mass as assessed by dual-energy X-ray absorptiometry and ultrasound, *Osteoporosis International* 13 (2002): 932–936; K. D. Ward and R. C. Klesges, A meta-analysis of the effects of cigarette smoking on bone mineral density, *Calcified Tissue International* 68 (2001): 259–270.
17. P. B. Rapuri and coauthors, Smoking and bone metabolism in elderly women, *Bone* 27 (2000): 429–436; A. P. Hermann and coauthors, Premenopausal smoking and bone density in 2015 perimenopausal women, *Journal of Bone and Mineral Research* 15 (2000): 780–787.
18. C. Oncken and coauthors, Effects of smoking cessation or reduction on hormone profiles and bone turnover in postmenopausal women, *Nicotine and Tobacco Research* 4 (2002): 451–458.
19. P. B. Rapuri and coauthors, Alcohol intake and bone metabolism in elderly women, *American Journal of Clinical Nutrition* 72 (2000): 1206–1213; O. Ganry, C. Baudoin, and P. Fardellone, for the EPIDOS, Effect of alcohol intake on bone mineral density in elderly women: The EPIDOS Study, *American Journal of Epidemiology* 151 (2000): 773–780.
20. D. Teegarden and coauthors, Previous milk consumption is associated with greater bone density in young women, *American Journal of Clinical Nutrition* 69 (1999): 1014–1017.
21. R. E. Black and coauthors, Children who avoid drinking cow milk have low dietary calcium intakes and poor bone health, *American Journal of Clinical Nutrition* 76 (2002): 675–680.
22. H. J. Kalkwarf, J. C. Khoury, and B. P. Lanphear, Milk intake during childhood and adolescence, adult bone density, and osteoporotic fractures in US women, *American Journal of Clinical Nutrition* 77 (2003): 257–265.
23. J. Bell, Elderly women need dietary protein to maintain bone mass, *Nutrition Reviews* 60 (2002): 337–341; B. Dawson-Hughes and S. S. Harris, Calcium intake influences the association of protein intake with rates of bone loss in elderly men and women, *American Journal of Clinical Nutrition* 75 (2002): 773–779; J. H. E. Promislow and coauthors, Protein consumption and bone mineral density in the elderly: The Rancho Bernardo Study, *American Journal of Epidemiology* 155 (2002): 636–644; R. G. Munger, J. R. Cerhan, and B. C. Chiu, Prospective study of dietary protein intake and risk of hip fracture in postmenopausal women, *American Journal of Clinical Nutrition* 69 (1999): 147–152.
24. A. G. Need and coauthors, Vitamin D status: Effects on parathyroid hormone and 1,25-dihydroxyvitamin D in postmenopausal women, *American Journal of Clinical Nutrition* 71 (2000): 1577–1581.
25. D. Feskanich, W. C. Willett, and G. A. Colditz, Calcium, vitamin D, milk consumption, and hip fractures: A prospective study among postmenopausal women, *American Journal of Clinical Nutrition* 77 (2003): 504–511.
26. N. C. Binkley and coauthors, A high phylloquinone intake is required to achieve maximal osteocalcin γ-carboxylation, *American Journal of Clinical Nutrition* 76 (2002): 1055–1060; S. L. Booth and coauthors, Dietary vitamin K intakes are associated with hip fracture but not with bone mineral density in elderly men and women, *American Journal of Clinical Nutrition* 71 (2000): 1201–1208; D. Feskanich and coauthors, Vitamin K intake and hip fractures in women: A prospective study, *American Journal of Clinical Nutrition* 69 (1999): 74–79.
27. K. L. Tucker and coauthors, Potassium, magnesium, and fruit and vegetable intakes are associated with greater bone mineral density in elderly men and women, *American Journal of Clinical Nutrition* 69 (1999): 727–736.
28. K. Michaelsson and coauthors, Serum retinol levels and the risk of fractures, *New England Journal of Medicine* 348 (2003): 287–294; D. Feskanich and coauthors, Vitamin A intake and hip fractures among postmenopausal women, *Journal of the American Medical Association* 287 (2002): 47–54; S. Johnasson and coauthors, Subclinical hypervitaminosis A causes fragile bones in rats, *Bone* 31 (2002): 685–689; N. Binkley and D. Krueger, Hypervitaminosis A and bone, *Nutrition Reviews* 58 (2000): 138–144; S. J. Whiting and B. Lemke, Excess retinol intake may explain the high incidence of osteoporosis in northern Europe, *Nutrition Reviews* 57 (1999): 192–195.
29. K. L. Tucker and coauthors, Bone mineral density and dietary patterns in older adults: The Framingham Osteoporosis Study, *American Journal of Clinical Nutrition* 76 (2002): 245–252; D. M. Hegsted, Fractures, calcium, and the modern diet, *American Journal of Clinical Nutrition* 74 (2001): 571–573; S. A. New and coauthors, Dietary influences on bone mass and bone metabolism: Further evidence of a positive link between fruit and vegetable consumption and bone health? *American Journal of Clinical Nutrition* 71 (2000): 142–151; J. J. B. Anderson, Plant-based diets and bone health: Nutritional implications, *American Journal of Clinical Nutrition* 70 (1999) 539S–542S; Tucker and coauthors, 1999.
30. M. Harrington and K. D. Cashman, High salt intake appears to increase bone resorption in postmenopausal women but high potassium intake ameliorates this adverse effect, *Nutrition Reveiws* 61 (2003): 179–183; Tucker and coauthors, 2002; P. B. Rapuri and coauthors, Caffeine intake increases the rate of bone loss in elderly women and interacts with vitamin D receptor genotypes, *American Journal of Clinical Nutrition* 74 (2001): 694–700.
31. R. P. Heaney and coauthors, Dietary changes favorably affect bone remodeling in older adults, *Journal of the American Dietetic Association* 99 (1999): 1228–1233.
32. E. A. Ross, N. J. Szabo, and I. R. Tebbett, Lead content of calcium supplements, *Journal of the American Medical Association* 284 (2000): 1425–1429.
33. NIH Consensus Development Panel on Osteoporosis Prevention, Diagnosis, and Therapy, Osteoporosis prevention, diagnosis, and therapy, *Journal of the American Medical Association* 285 (2001): 785–795.

Chapter 13

The Trace Minerals

Chapter Outline

Available Online

http://nutrition.wadsworth.com/uncn7

Nutrition Animation: *Meal Planning to Meet Recommended Intakes of Minerals*

Student Practice Test

Glossary Terms

Nutrition on the Net

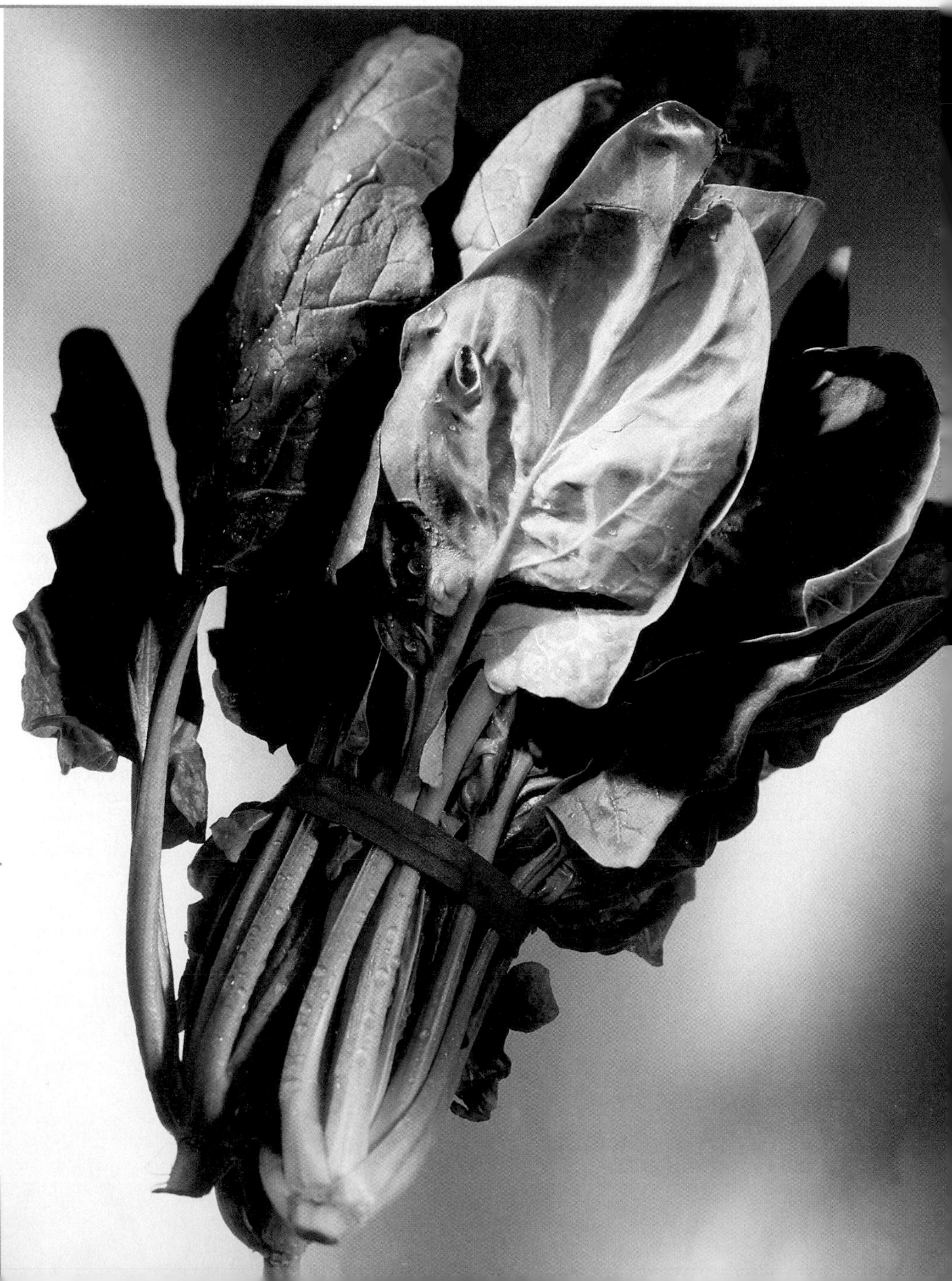

Nutrition in Your Life

Trace—barely a perceptible amount. But the trace minerals tackle big jobs. Your blood can't carry oxygen without iron, and insulin can't deliver glucose without chromium. Teeth become decayed without fluoride, and thyroid glands develop goiter without iodine. Together, the trace minerals—iron, zinc, iodine, selenium, copper, manganese, fluoride, chromium, and molybdenum—keep you healthy and strong. Where can you get these amazing minerals? A variety of foods, especially those from the meat and meat alternate group, sprinkled with a little iodized salt and complemented by a glass of fluoridated water will do the trick. It's remarkable what your body can do with only a few milligrams—or even micrograms—of the trace minerals.

Figure 12-7 in the last chapter (p. 406) showed the tiny quantities of **trace minerals** in the human body. The trace minerals are so named because they are present, and needed, in relatively small amounts in the body. All together, they would produce only a bit of dust, hardly enough to fill a teaspoon. Yet they are no less important than the major minerals or any of the other nutrients. Each of the trace minerals performs a vital role. A deficiency of any of them may be fatal, and an excess of many is equally deadly. Remarkably, people's diets normally supply just enough of these minerals to maintain health.

The Trace Minerals—An Overview

The body requires the trace minerals in minuscule quantities. They participate in diverse tasks all over the body, each having special duties that only it can perform.

Food Sources The trace mineral contents of foods depend on soil and water composition and on how foods are processed. Furthermore, many factors in the

trace minerals: essential mineral nutrients found in the human body in amounts smaller than 5 g; sometimes called **microminerals.**

■ Reminder: *Bioavailability* refers to the rate at and the extent to which a nutrient is absorbed and used.

diet and within the body affect the minerals' bioavailability.■ Still, outstanding food sources for each of the trace minerals, just like those for the other nutrients, include a wide variety of foods, especially unprocessed, whole foods.

Deficiencies Severe deficiencies of the better-known minerals are easy to recognize. Deficiencies of the others may be harder to diagnose, and for all minerals, mild deficiencies are easy to overlook. Because the minerals are active in all the body systems—the GI tract, cardiovascular system, blood, muscles, bones, and central nervous system—deficiencies can have wide-reaching effects and can affect people of all ages. The most common result of a deficiency in children is failure to grow and thrive.

Toxicities Some of the trace minerals are toxic at intakes not far above the estimated requirements. Thus it is important not to habitually exceed the Upper Level of recommended intakes. Many vitamin-mineral supplements contain trace minerals, making it easy for users to exceed their needs. The Food and Drug Administration (FDA) has no authority to limit the amounts of trace minerals in supplements; consumers have demanded the freedom to choose their own doses of nutrients.* Individuals who take supplements must therefore be aware of the possible dangers and select supplements that contain no more than 100 percent of the Daily Value. It would be easier and safer to meet nutrient needs by selecting a variety of foods than by combining an assortment of supplements (see Highlight 10).

Interactions Interactions among the trace minerals are common and often well coordinated to meet the body's needs. For example, several of the trace minerals support insulin's work, influencing its synthesis, storage, release, and action.[1]

At other times, interactions lead to nutrient imbalances. An excess of one may cause a deficiency of another. (A slight manganese overload, for example, may aggravate an iron deficiency.) A deficiency of one may interfere with the work of another. (A selenium deficiency halts the activation of the iodine-containing thyroid hormones.) A deficiency of a trace mineral may even open the way for a contaminant mineral to cause a toxic reaction. (Iron deficiency, for example, makes the body vulnerable to lead poisoning.) These examples reinforce the need to balance intakes and to use supplements wisely, if at all. A good food source of one nutrient may be a poor food source of another; and factors that enhance the action of some trace minerals may hinder others. (Meats are a good source of iron, but a poor source of calcium; vitamin C enhances the absorption of iron but hinders that of copper.) Research on the trace minerals is active, suggesting that we have much more to learn about them.

IN SUMMARY Although the body uses only tiny amounts of the trace minerals, they are vital to health. Because so little is required, the trace minerals can be toxic at levels not far above estimated requirements—a consideration for supplement users. Like the other nutrients, the trace minerals are best obtained by eating a variety of whole foods.

Iron

Iron is an essential nutrient, vital to many of the cells' activities, but it poses a problem for millions of people: some people simply don't eat enough iron-containing foods to support their health optimally, while others absorb so much iron that it threatens their health. Iron exemplifies the principle that both too little and too much of a nutrient in the body can be harmful.

*Canada limits the amounts of trace minerals in supplements.

Iron Roles in the Body

Iron has the knack of switching back and forth between two ionic states.■ In the reduced state, iron has lost two electrons and therefore has a net positive charge of two; it is known as *ferrous iron*. In the oxidized state, iron has lost a third electron, has a net positive charge of three, and is known as *ferric iron*. Because ferrous iron can be oxidized to ferric iron and ferric iron can be reduced to ferrous iron, iron can serve as a cofactor■ to enzymes involved in oxidation-reduction reactions—reactions so widespread in metabolism that they occur in all cells. Iron is also required by enzymes involved in the making of amino acids, collagen, hormones, and neurotransmitters. (For details about ions, oxidation, and reduction, see Appendix B.)

■ Iron's two ionic states:
- Ferrous iron (reduced): Fe^{++}.
- Ferric iron (oxidized): Fe^{+++}.

■ Reminder: A *cofactor* is a substance that works with an enzyme to facilitate a chemical reaction.

Iron forms a part of the electron carriers that participate in the electron transport chain (discussed in Chapter 7).* In this pathway, these carriers transfer hydrogens and electrons to oxygen, forming water, and in the process make ATP for the cells' energy use.

Most of the body's iron is found in two proteins: hemoglobin■ in the red blood cells and **myoglobin** in the muscle cells. In both, iron helps accept, carry, and then release oxygen.

■ Reminder: *Hemoglobin* is the oxygen-carrying protein of the red blood cells that transports oxygen from the lungs to tissues throughout the body; hemoglobin accounts for 80% of the body's iron.

Iron Absorption and Metabolism

The body conserves iron. Because it is difficult to excrete iron once it is in the body, balance is maintained primarily through absorption: more iron is absorbed when stores are empty, and less is absorbed when stores are full.[2]

Iron Absorption Special proteins help the body absorb iron from food (see Figure 13-1). One protein, called mucosal **ferritin,** receives iron from food and stores it in the mucosal cells■ of the small intestine. When the body needs iron, mucosal ferritin

■ A mucous membrane such as the one that lines the GI tract is sometimes called the **mucosa** (mu-KO-sa). The adjective of mucosa is **mucosal** (mu-KO-sal).

myoglobin: the oxygen-holding protein of the muscle cells.
- **myo** = muscle

ferritin (FAIR-ih-tin): the iron storage protein.

*The iron-containing electron carriers of the electron transport chain are known as *cytochromes*. See Appendix C for details of this pathway.

FIGURE 13-1 Iron Absorption

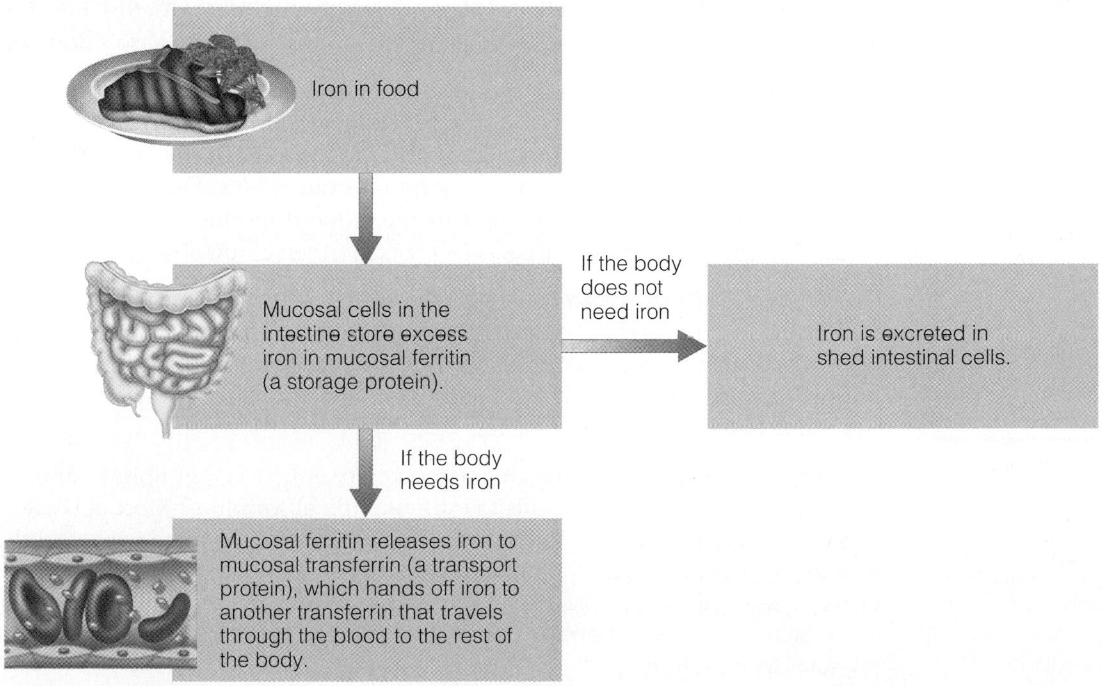
Iron in food
Mucosal cells in the intestine store excess iron in mucosal ferritin (a storage protein).
If the body does not need iron
Iron is excreted in shed intestinal cells.
If the body needs iron
Mucosal ferritin releases iron to mucosal transferrin (a transport protein), which hands off iron to another transferrin that travels through the blood to the rest of the body.

FIGURE 13-2 Heme and Nonheme Iron in Foods

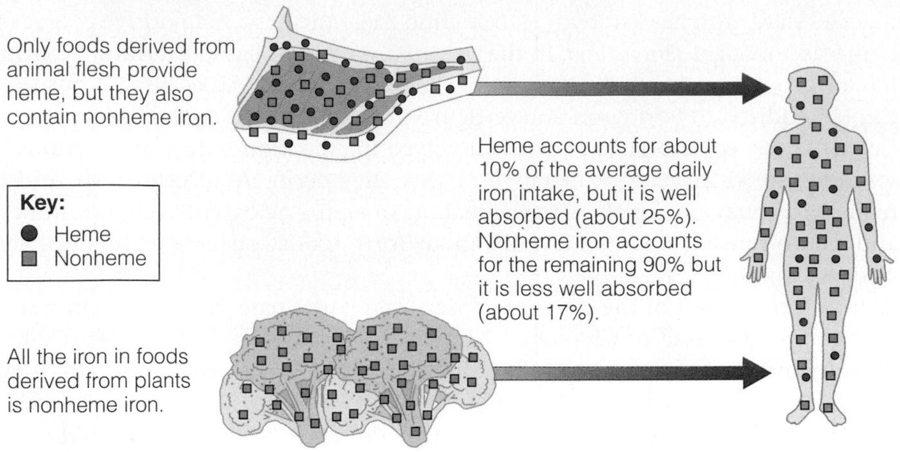
Only foods derived from animal flesh provide heme, but they also contain nonheme iron.
Key:
Heme
Nonheme
Heme accounts for about 10% of the average daily iron intake, but it is well absorbed (about 25%). Nonheme iron accounts for the remaining 90% but it is less well absorbed (about 17%).
All the iron in foods derived from plants is nonheme iron.

releases some iron to another protein, called mucosal **transferrin.** Mucosal transferrin transfers the iron to another protein, *blood transferrin,* which transports the iron to the rest of the body. If the body does not need iron, it is carried out when the intestinal cells are shed and excreted in the feces; intestinal cells are replaced about every three days. By holding iron temporarily, these cells can either deliver iron when the day's intake falls short or dispose of it when intakes exceed needs.

Heme and Nonheme Iron Iron absorption depends in part on its source. Iron occurs in two forms in foods: as **heme** iron, which is found only in foods derived from the flesh of animals, such as meats, poultry, and fish; and as nonheme iron, which is found in both plant-derived and animal-derived foods (see Figure 13-2). On average, heme iron represents about 10 percent of the iron a person consumes in a day. Even though heme iron accounts for only a small proportion of the intake, it is so well absorbed that it contributes significant iron: about 25 percent of heme iron is absorbed. By comparison, only 17 percent of nonheme iron is absorbed, depending on dietary factors and the body's iron stores.[3] In iron deficiency, absorption increases, and in iron overload, absorption declines.[4] Researchers disagree as to whether heme iron absorption responds to iron stores as sensitively as nonheme iron absorption does.

Absorption-Enhancing Factors Meat, fish, and poultry contain not only the well-absorbed heme iron, but also a factor (called the **MFP factor**) that promotes the absorption of nonheme iron■ from other foods eaten at the same meal. Vitamin C also enhances nonheme iron absorption from foods eaten in the same meal by capturing the iron and keeping it in the reduced ferrous form, ready for absorption. Some acids and sugars also enhance nonheme iron absorption.

■ Factors that *enhance* nonheme iron absorption:
- MFP factor.
- Vitamin C (ascorbic acid).
- Citric acid and lactic acid from foods and HCl acid from the stomach.
- Sugars (including the sugars in wine).

Absorption-Inhibiting Factors Some dietary factors bind with nonheme iron, inhibiting absorption.■ These factors include the phytates and fibers in soy products, whole grains, and nuts; oxalates in some vegetables; the calcium and phosphorus in milk; the EDTA in food additives;* and the tannic acid in tea, coffee, nuts, and some fruits and vegetables.

■ Factors that *inhibit* nonheme iron absorption:
- Phytates and fibers (grains and vegetables).
- Oxalates (spinach, beets, rhubarb).
- Calcium and phosphorus (milk).
- EDTA (food additives).
- Tannic acid (and other polyphenols in tea and coffee).

Dietary Factors Combined The many dietary enhancers, inhibitors, and their combined effects make it difficult to estimate iron absorption.[5] Most of these factors exert a strong influence individually, but not when combined with the others in a meal. Furthermore, the impact of the combined effects diminishes when a diet is evaluated over several days. When multiple meals are analyzed together, three factors appear to be most relevant: MFP and vitamin C as enhancers and phytates as inhibitors.[6]

transferrin (trans-FAIR-in): the iron transport protein.

heme (HEEM): the iron-holding part of the hemoglobin and myoglobin proteins. About 40% of the iron in meat, fish, and poultry is bound into heme; the other 60% is **nonheme** iron.

MFP factor: a factor associated with the digestion of **m**eat, **f**ish, and **p**oultry that enhances nonheme iron absorption.

*EDTA is ethylenediamine tetra acetate, a chelating agent that is used in food processing to retard crystal formation and promote color retention.

Individual Variation Overall, about 18 percent of dietary iron is absorbed from mixed diets and only about 10 percent from vegetarian diets.[7] As you might expect, vegetarian diets do not have the benefit of easy-to-absorb heme iron or the help of MFP in enhancing absorption, but even the absorption of nonheme iron is low.[8] In addition to dietary influences, iron absorption also depends on an individual's health, stage in the life cycle, and iron status. Absorption can be as low as 2 percent in a person with GI disease or as high as 35 percent in a rapidly growing, healthy child. The body adapts to absorb more iron when a person's iron stores fall short, or when the need increases for any reason (such as pregnancy). The body makes more mucosal transferrin to absorb more iron from the intestines and more blood transferrin to carry more iron around the body. Similarly, when iron stores are sufficient, the body adapts to absorb less iron.[9]

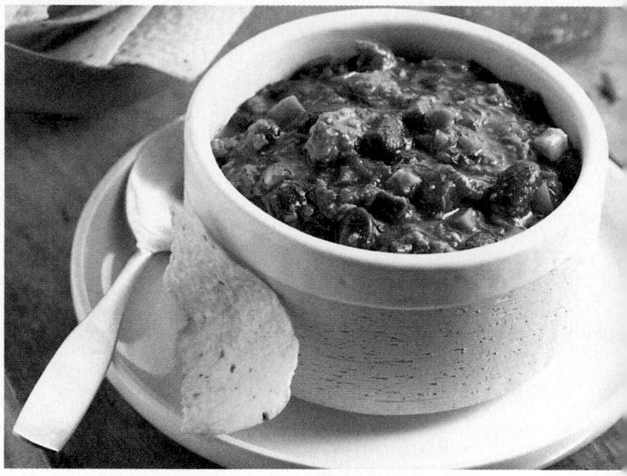

This chili dinner provides several factors that may enhance iron absorption: heme and nonheme iron and MFP from meat, nonheme iron from legumes, and vitamin C from tomatoes.

Iron Transport and Storage Blood transferrin delivers iron to the bone marrow and other tissues. The bone marrow uses large quantities to make new red blood cells, whereas other tissues use less. Surplus iron is stored in the protein ferritin, primarily in the liver, but also in the bone marrow and spleen. When dietary iron has been plentiful, ferritin is constantly and rapidly made and broken down, providing an ever-ready supply of iron. When iron concentrations become abnormally high, the liver converts some ferritin into another storage protein called **hemosiderin.** Hemosiderin releases iron more slowly than ferritin does. By storing excess iron, the body protects itself: free iron acts as a free radical, attacking cell lipids, DNA, and protein.[10] (See Highlight 11 for more information on free radicals and the damage they can cause.)

Iron Recycling The average red blood cell lives about four months; then the spleen and liver cells remove it from the blood, take it apart, and prepare the degradation products for excretion or recycling. The iron is salvaged: the liver attaches it to blood transferrin, which transports it back to the bone marrow to be reused in making new red blood cells. Thus, although red blood cells live for only about four months, the iron recycles through each new generation of cells (see Figure 13-3).

hemosiderin (heem-oh-SID-er-in): an iron storage protein primarily made in times of iron overload.

FIGURE 13-3 Iron Recycled in the Body

Once iron enters the body, most of it is recycled. Some is lost with body tissues and must be replaced by eating iron-containing food.

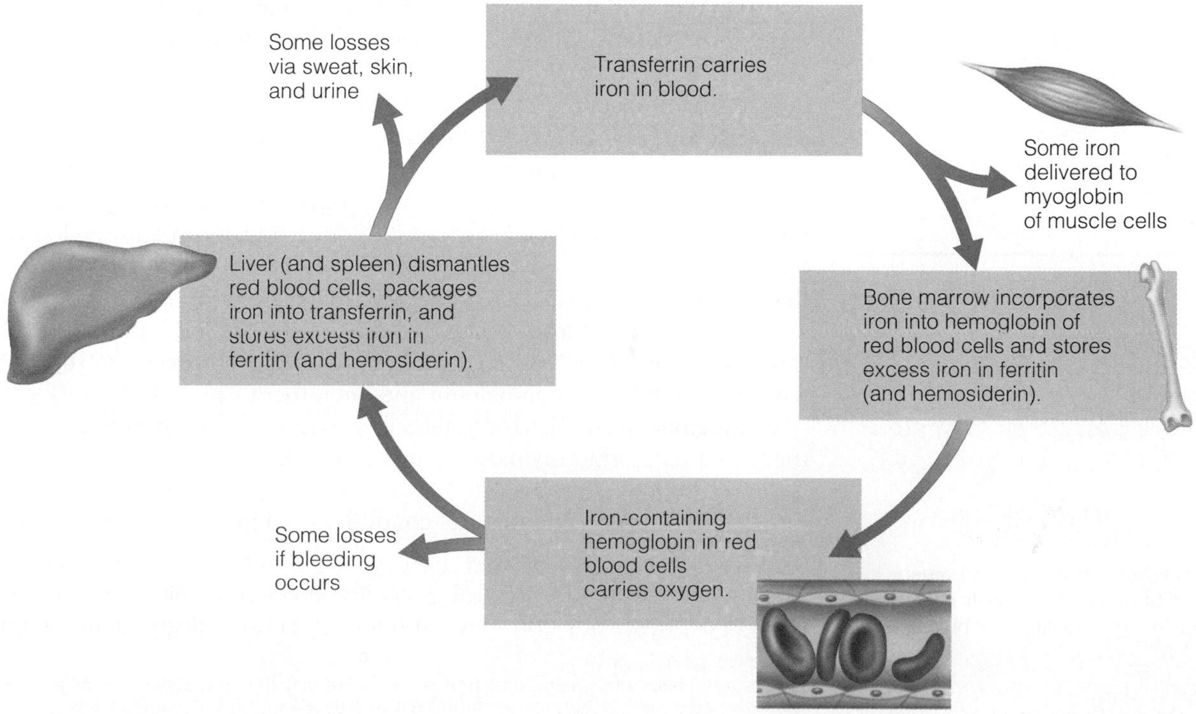
Some losses via sweat, skin, and urine
Transferrin carries iron in blood.
Some iron delivered to myoglobin of muscle cells
Liver (and spleen) dismantles red blood cells, packages iron into transferrin, and stores excess iron in ferritin (and hemosiderin).
Bone marrow incorporates iron into hemoglobin of red blood cells and stores excess iron in ferritin (and hemosiderin).
Some losses if bleeding occurs
Iron-containing hemoglobin in red blood cells carries oxygen.

The body loses some iron daily via the GI tract and, if bleeding occurs, in blood; only tiny amounts of iron are lost in urine, sweat, and shed skin.*

Iron Deficiency

Worldwide, **iron deficiency** is the most common nutrient deficiency, affecting more than 1.2 billion people.[11] In developing countries, almost half of the preschool children and pregnant women suffer from **iron-deficiency anemia.**[12] In the United States, iron deficiency is less prevalent, but still affects 10 percent of toddlers, adolescent girls, and women of childbearing age; preventing and correcting iron deficiency are high priorities.[13]

■ High risk for iron deficiency:
- Women in their reproductive years.
- Pregnant women.
- Infants and young children.
- Teenagers.

Vulnerable Stages of Life Some stages of life■ both demand more iron and provide less, making deficiency likely.[14] Women in their reproductive years are especially prone to iron deficiency because of repeated blood losses during menstruation. Pregnancy demands additional iron to support the added blood volume, growth of the fetus, and blood loss during childbirth. Infants and young children receive little iron from their high-milk diets, yet need extra iron to support their rapid growth. The rapid growth of adolescence, especially for males, and the menstrual losses of females also demand extra iron that a typical teen diet may not provide. An adequate iron intake is especially important during these stages of life.

HEALTHY PEOPLE 2010

Reduce iron deficiency among young children, females of childbearing age, and pregnant females.

■ The iron content of blood is about 0.5 mg/100 mL blood. A person donating a pint of blood (approximately 500 mL) loses about 2.5 mg of iron.

Blood Losses Bleeding■ from any site incurs iron losses. In some cases, as in an active ulcer, the bleeding may not be obvious, but even small chronic blood losses significantly deplete iron reserves; treating the ulcer resolves the iron deficiency.[15] In developing countries, blood loss is often brought on by malaria and parasitic infections of the GI tract. People who donate blood regularly also incur losses and may benefit from iron supplements. As mentioned, menstrual losses can be considerable as they tap women's iron stores regularly.

■ Stages of iron deficiency:
- Iron stores diminish.
- Transport iron decreases.
- Hemoglobin production declines.

Assessment of Iron Deficiency Iron deficiency develops in stages.■ This section provides a brief overview of how to detect these stages, and Appendix E provides more details. In the first stage of iron deficiency, iron stores diminish. Measures of serum ferritin (in the blood) reflect iron stores and are most valuable in assessing iron status at this earliest stage.

The second stage of iron deficiency is characterized by a decrease in transport iron: serum iron falls, and the iron-carrying protein transferrin *increases* (an adaptation that enhances iron absorption). Together, these two measures can determine the severity of the deficiency—the more transferrin and the less iron in the blood, the more advanced the deficiency is. Transferrin saturation—the percentage of transferrin that is saturated with iron—decreases as iron stores decline.

The third stage of iron deficiency occurs when the lack of iron limits hemoglobin production. Now the hemoglobin precursor, **erythrocyte protoporphyrin,** begins to accumulate as hemoglobin and **hematocrit** values decline.

Hemoglobin and hematocrit tests are easy, quick, and inexpensive, so they are the tests most commonly used in evaluating iron status; their usefulness is limited, however, because they are late indicators of iron deficiency. Furthermore, other nutrient deficiencies and medical conditions can influence their values.

Iron Deficiency and Anemia Iron deficiency and iron-deficiency anemia are not the same: people may be iron deficient without being anemic. The term *iron deficiency* refers to depleted body iron stores without regard to the degree of depletion or to the

iron deficiency: the state of having depleted iron stores.

iron-deficiency anemia: severe depletion of iron stores that results in low hemoglobin and small, pale red blood cells. Anemias that impair hemoglobin synthesis are **microcytic.**
- **micro** = small
- **cytic** = cell

erythrocyte protoporphyrin (PRO-toe-PORE-fe-rin): a precursor to hemoglobin.

hematocrit (hee-MAT-oh-krit): measurement of the volume of the red blood cells packed by centrifuge in a given volume of blood.

*Adults lose about 1.0 milligram of iron per day. Women lose additional iron in menses. Menstrual losses vary considerably, but over a month, they average about 0.5 milligram per day.

FIGURE 13-4 Normal and Anemic Blood Cells

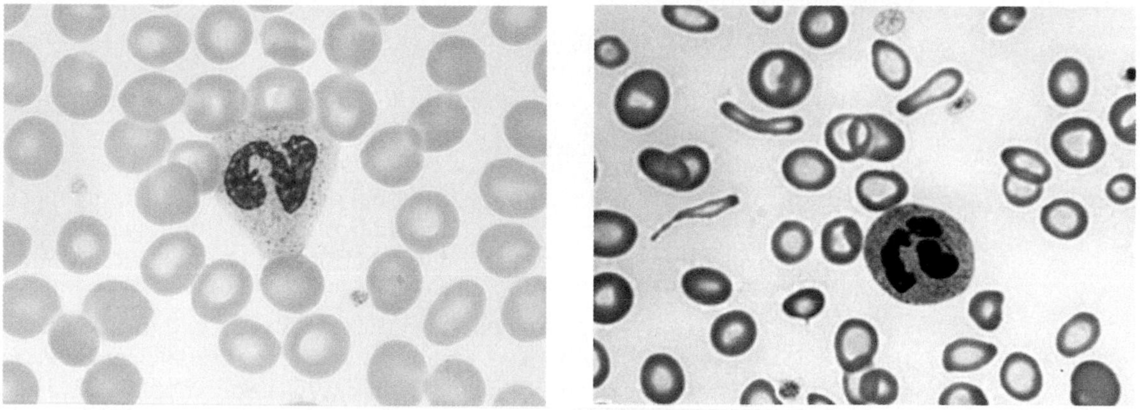

Both size and color are normal in these blood cells.

Blood cells in iron-deficiency anemia are small (microcytic) and pale (hypochromic) because they contain less hemoglobin.

presence of anemia. The term *iron-deficiency anemia* refers to the severe depletion of iron stores that results in a low hemoglobin concentration. In iron-deficiency anemia, red blood cells are pale and small■ (see Figure 13-4). They can't carry enough oxygen from the lungs to the tissues. Without adequate iron, energy metabolism in the cells falters. The result is fatigue, weakness, headaches, apathy, pallor, and poor resistance to cold temperatures. Since hemoglobin is the bright red pigment of the blood, the skin of a fair person who is anemic may become noticeably pale. In a dark-skinned person, the tongue and eye lining, normally pink, will be very pale.

■ Iron-deficiency anemia is a **microcytic** (my-cro-SIT-ic) **hypochromic** (high-po-KROME-ic) **anemia.**
- **micro** = small
- **cytic** = cell
- **hypo** = too little
- **chrom** = color

The fatigue that accompanies iron-deficiency anemia differs from the tiredness a person experiences from a simple lack of sleep. People with anemia feel fatigue only when they exert themselves. Iron supplementation can relieve the fatigue and improve the body's response to physical activity.[16] Whether iron deficiency without clinical signs of anemia impairs physical performance is less clear.

Iron Deficiency and Behavior Long before the red blood cells are affected and anemia is diagnosed, a developing iron deficiency affects behavior. Even at slightly lowered iron levels, energy metabolism is impaired and neurotransmitter synthesis is altered, reducing physical work capacity and mental productivity.[17] Without the physical energy and mental alertness to work, plan, think, play, sing, or learn, people simply do these things less. They have no obvious deficiency symptoms; they just appear unmotivated, apathetic, and less physically fit. Work productivity and voluntary activities decline.[18]

Many of the symptoms associated with iron deficiency are easily mistaken for behavioral or motivational problems. A restless child who fails to pay attention in class might be thought contrary. An apathetic homemaker who has let housework pile up might be thought lazy. No responsible dietitian would ever claim that all behavioral problems are caused by nutrient deficiencies, but poor nutrition is always a possible contributor to problems like these. When investigating a behavioral problem, check the adequacy of the diet and seek a routine physical examination before undertaking more expensive, and possibly harmful, treatment options. (The effects of iron deficiency on children's behavior are discussed further in Chapter 15.)

Iron Deficiency and Pica A curious behavior seen in some iron-deficient people, especially in women and children of low-income groups, is **pica**—an appetite for ice, clay, paste, and other nonfood substances. These substances contain no iron and cannot remedy a deficiency; in fact, clay actually inhibits iron absorption, which may explain the iron deficiency that accompanies such behavior.

pica (PIE-ka): a craving for nonfood substances. Also known as **geophagia** (gee-oh-FAY-gee-uh) when referring to clay eating and **pagophagia** (pag-oh-FAY-gee-uh) when referring to ice craving.

Iron Toxicity

In general, even a diet that includes fortified foods poses no special risk for iron toxicity.[19] The body normally absorbs less iron when its stores are full, but some individuals are poorly defended against excess iron. Once considered rare, **iron overload** has emerged as an important disorder of iron metabolism and regulation.

Iron Overload Iron overload is known as **hemochromatosis** and is usually caused by a genetic disorder that enhances iron absorption.[20] Hereditary hemochromatosis is the most common genetic disorder in the United States, affecting some 1.5 million people. Other causes of iron overload include repeated blood transfusions (which bypass the intestinal defense), massive doses of supplementary iron (which overwhelm the intestinal defense), and other rare metabolic disorders. Excess iron may cause **hemosiderosis,** a condition characterized by large deposits of the iron storage protein hemosiderin in the liver and other tissues.

Some of the signs and symptoms of iron overload are similar to those of iron deficiency: apathy, lethargy, and fatigue. Therefore, taking iron supplements before assessing iron status is clearly unwise; hemoglobin tests alone would fail to make the distinction because excess iron accumulates in storage. Iron overload assessment tests measure transferrin saturation and serum ferritin.

Iron overload is characterized by tissue damage, especially in iron-storing organs such as the liver. Infections are likely because bacteria thrive on iron-rich blood. Symptoms are most severe in alcohol abusers because alcohol damages the intestine, further impairing its defenses against absorbing excess iron. Untreated hemochromatosis aggravates the risks of diabetes, liver cancer, heart disease, and arthritis.

Iron overload is more common in men than in women and is twice as prevalent among men as iron deficiency. The widespread fortification of foods with iron makes it difficult for people with hemochromatosis to follow a low-iron diet, and greater dangers lie in the indiscriminate use of iron and vitamin C supplements. Vitamin C not only enhances iron absorption, but releases iron from ferritin, allowing free iron to wreak the damage typical of free radicals.[21] This example shows how vitamin C acts as a *pro*oxidant when taken in high doses. (See Highlight 11 for a discussion of free radicals and their effects on disease development.)

Iron and Heart Disease Some research suggests a link between heart disease and elevated iron stores, but the evidence is inconsistent and unconvincing.[22] As mentioned, free radicals can attack ferritin, causing it to release iron from storage. Free iron, in turn, acts as an oxidant that can generate more free radicals. Whether iron's oxidation of LDL plays a role in the development of heart disease has not been proved.[23]

Iron and Cancer There may be an association between iron and some cancers. Explanations for how iron might be involved in causing cancer focus on its free-radical activity, which can damage DNA (see Highlight 11). One of the benefits of a high-fiber diet may be that its phytates bind iron, making it less available for such reactions.

Iron Poisoning Large doses of iron supplements cause GI distress, including constipation, nausea, vomiting, and diarrhea. These effects may not be as serious as other consequences of iron toxicity, but they are consistent enough to establish an Upper Level of 45 milligrams per day for adults.

Ingestion of iron-containing supplements remains a leading cause of accidental poisoning in small children.[24] Symptoms of intoxication include nausea, vomiting, diarrhea, a rapid heartbeat, a weak pulse, dizziness, shock, and confusion. As few as five iron tablets containing as little as 200 milligrams of iron have caused the deaths of dozens of young children. The exact cause of death is uncertain, but excessive free-radical damage is thought to play a role in heart failure and respiratory distress; autopsy reports reveal iron deposits and cell death in the stomach, small intestine, liver, and blood vessels (which can cause internal bleeding).[25]

iron overload: toxicity from excess iron.

hemochromatosis (HE-moh-KRO-ma-toe-sis): a hereditary defect in iron absorption characterized by deposits of iron-containing pigment in many tissues, with tissue damage.

hemosiderosis (HE-moh-sid-er-OH-sis): a condition characterized by the deposition of hemosiderin in the liver and other tissues.

HOW TO Estimate the Recommended Daily Intake for Iron

To calculate the recommended daily iron intake, the DRI Committee considers a number of factors. For example, for a woman of childbearing age (19 to 50):

- Losses from feces, urine, sweat, and shed skin: 1.0 milligram.
- Losses through menstruation (about 14 milligrams total averaged over 28 days): 0.5 milligram.

These losses reflect an average daily need (total) of 1.5 milligrams of *absorbed* iron.

An estimated average requirement is determined based on the daily need and the assumption that an average of 18 percent of ingested iron is absorbed:

1.5 mg iron (needed) ÷ 0.18 (percent iron absorbed) = 8 mg iron (estimated average requirement).

Then a margin of safety is added to cover the needs of essentially all women of childbearing age, and the RDA is set at 18 milligrams.

Keep iron-containing tablets out of the reach of children. If you suspect iron poisoning, call the nearest poison control center or a physician immediately.

Iron Recommendations and Sources

To obtain enough iron, people must first select iron-rich foods and then eat so as to maximize iron absorption. This discussion begins by identifying iron-rich foods, then reviews factors affecting absorption.

Recommended Iron Intakes The usual diet in the United States provides about 6 to 7 milligrams of iron for every 1000 kcalories. The recommended daily intake for men is 8 milligrams, and most men eat more than 2000 kcalories a day, so they can meet their iron needs with little effort. Women in their reproductive years, however, need 18 milligrams a day. (The accompanying "How to" explains how to calculate the recommended intake.) Vegetarians need 1.8 times as much iron to make up for the low bioavailability typical of their diets.[26] ■

■ To calculate the RDA for vegetarians, multiply by 1.8:
- 8 mg × 1.8 = 14 mg/day (vegetarian men).
- 18 mg × 1.8 = 32 mg/day (vegetarian women, 19 to 50 yr).

Because women have higher iron needs and lower energy needs, they sometimes have trouble obtaining enough iron. On average, women receive only 12 to 13 milligrams of iron per day, not enough until after menopause. To meet their iron needs from foods, premenopausal women need to select iron-rich foods at every meal.

Iron in Foods Figure 13-5 (on p. 446) shows the amounts of iron in selected foods. Meats, fish, and poultry contribute the most iron; other protein-rich foods such as legumes and eggs are also good sources. Although an indispensable part of the diet, foods in the milk group are notoriously poor in iron. Grain foods vary, with whole-grain, enriched, and fortified breads and cereals providing the most iron. Finally, dark greens (such as broccoli) and dried fruits (such as raisins) contribute some iron.

Iron-Enriched Foods Iron is one of the enrichment nutrients for grain products. One serving of enriched bread or cereal provides only a little iron, but because people eat many servings of these foods, the contribution can be significant. Iron added to foods is not absorbed as well as naturally occurring iron, but when eaten with absorption-enhancing foods, enrichment iron can make a difference. In cases of iron overload, enrichment may exacerbate the problem.[27]

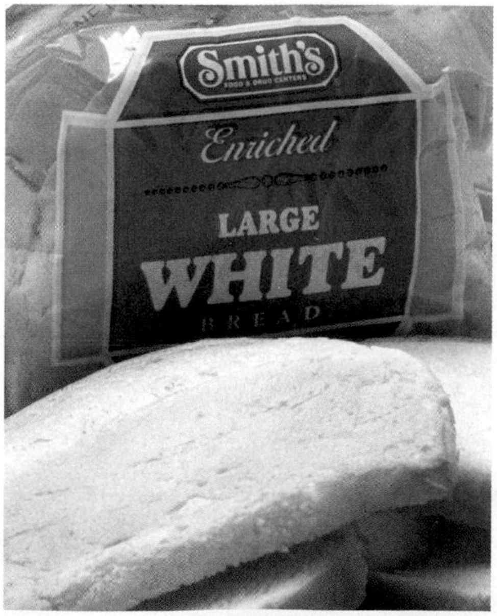
Smith's
Enriched
LARGE
WHITE
BREAD
© Craig M. Moore

When the label on a grain product says "enriched," it means iron and several B vitamins have been added.

Maximizing Iron Absorption In general, the bioavailability of iron in meats, fish, and poultry is high; in grains and legumes, intermediate; and in most vegetables, especially those high in oxalates such as spinach, low. As mentioned earlier, the amount of iron ultimately absorbed from a meal depends on the combined effects of several enhancing and inhibiting factors. For maximum absorption of nonheme iron, eat meat for MFP and fruits or vegetables for vitamin C. The iron of baked beans, for example, will be enhanced by the MFP in a piece of ham served with them; the iron of bread will be enhanced by vitamin C in a slice of tomato on a sandwich.

FIGURE 13-5 Iron in Selected Foods

Food	Serving size (kcalories)
Bread, whole wheat	1 oz slice (70 kcal)
Cornflakes, fortified	1 oz (110 kcal)
Spaghetti pasta	½ c cooked (99 kcal)
Tortilla, flour	1 10"-round (234 kcal)
Broccoli	½ c cooked (22 kcal)
Carrots	½ c shredded raw (24 kcal)
Potato	1 medium baked w/skin (133 kcal)
Tomato juice	½ c (31 kcal)
Banana	1 medium raw (109 kcal)
Orange	1 medium raw (62 kcal)
Strawberries	½ c fresh (22 kcal)
Watermelon	1 slice (92 kcal)
Milk	1 c reduced-fat 2% (121 kcal)
Yogurt, plain	1 c low-fat (155 kcal)
Cheddar cheese	1½ oz (171 kcal)
Cottage cheese	½ c low-fat 2% (101 kcal)
Pinto beans	½ c cooked (117 kcal)
Peanut butter	2 tbs (188 kcal)
Sunflower seeds	1 oz dry (165 kcal)
Tofu (soybean curd)	½ c (76 kcal)
Ground beef, lean	3 oz broiled (244 kcal)
Chicken breast	3 oz roasted (140 kcal)
Tuna, canned in water	3 oz (99 kcal)
Egg	1 hard cooked (78 kcal)
Excellent, and sometimes unusual, sources:	
Clams, canned	3 oz (126 kcal)
Beef liver	3 oz fried (184 kcal)
Parsley	1 c raw (22 kcal)

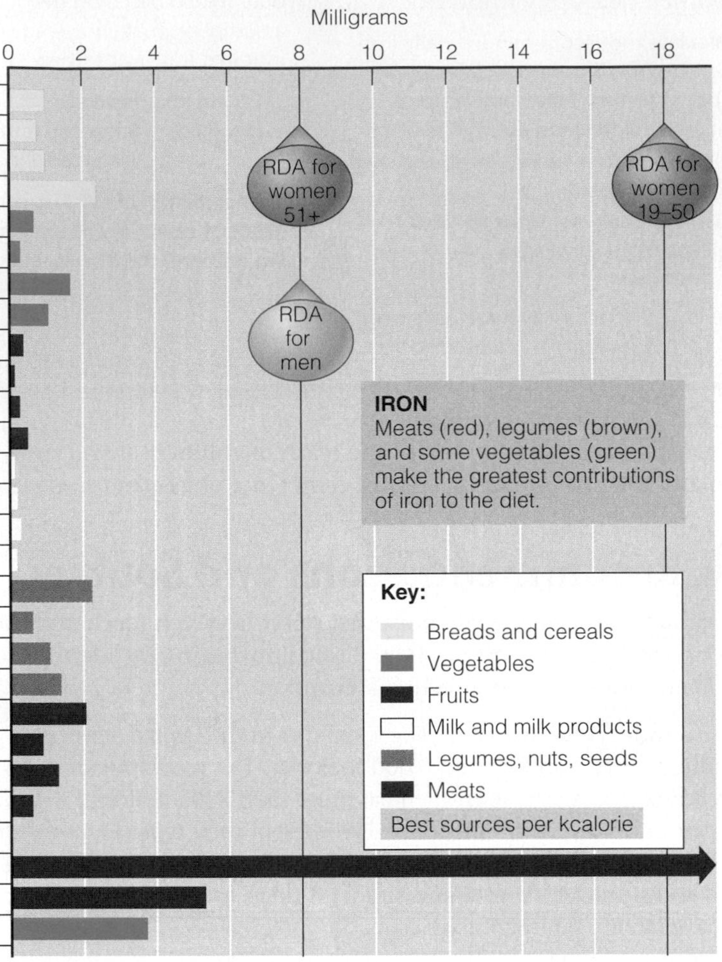
Milligrams
0 2 4 6 8 10 12 14 16 18
RDA for women 51+
RDA for women 19–50
RDA for men
IRON
Meats (red), legumes (brown), and some vegetables (green) make the greatest contributions of iron to the diet.
Key:
Breads and cereals
Vegetables
Fruits
Milk and milk products
Legumes, nuts, seeds
Meats
Best sources per kcalorie

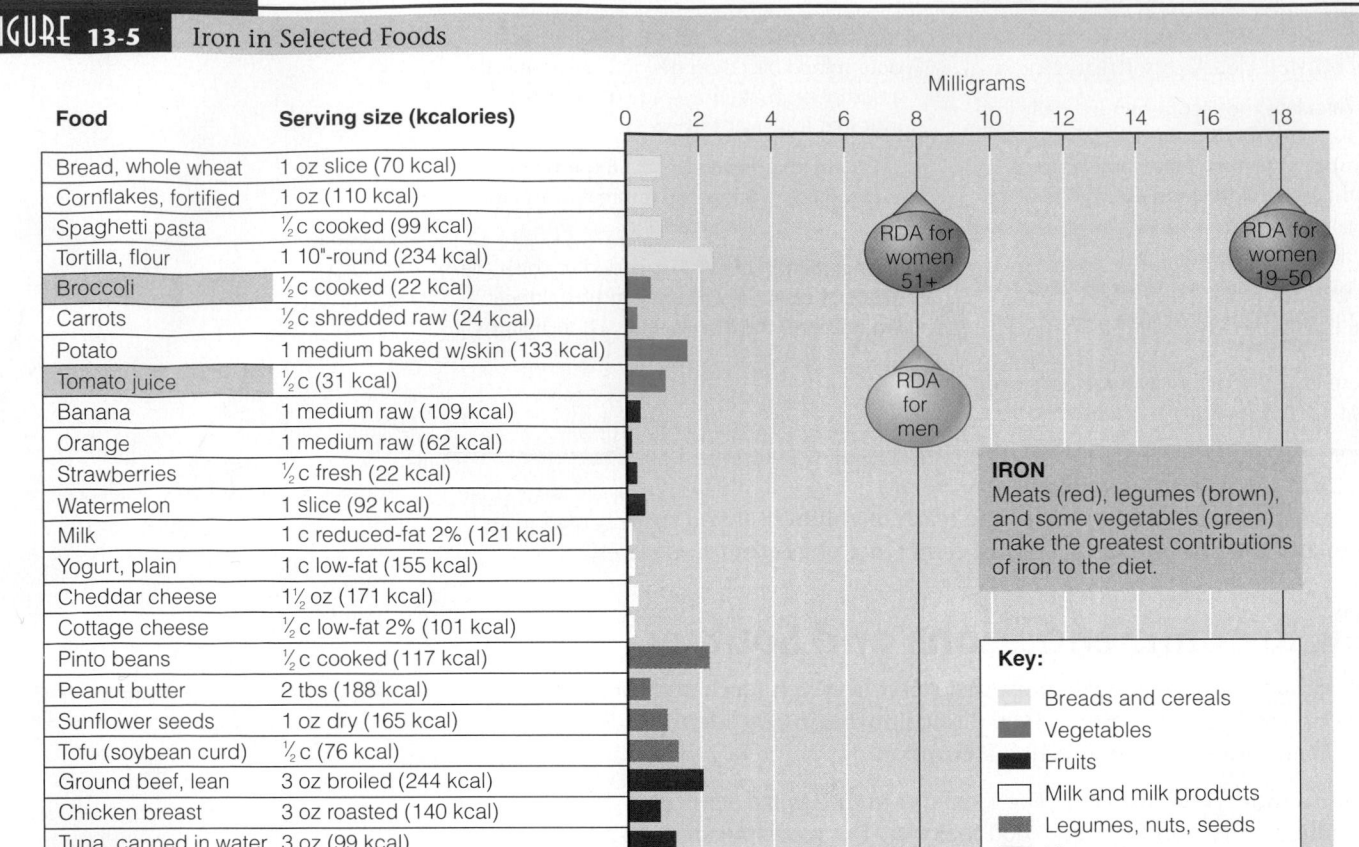

NOTE: See p. 327 for more information on using this figure.

Iron Contamination and Supplementation

In addition to the iron from foods, **contamination iron** from nonfood sources of inorganic iron salts can contribute to the day's intakes. People can also get iron from supplements.

Contamination Iron Foods cooked in iron cookware take up iron salts. The more acidic the food, and the longer it is cooked in iron cookware, the higher the iron content. The iron content of eggs can triple in the time it takes to scramble them in an iron pan. Admittedly, the absorption of this iron may be poor (perhaps only 1 to 2 percent), but every little bit helps a person who is trying to increase iron intake.

Iron Supplements People who are iron deficient may need supplements as well as an iron-rich, absorption-enhancing diet. Many physicians routinely recommend iron supplements to pregnant women, infants, and young children. Iron from supplements is less well absorbed than that from food, so the doses have to be high. The absorption of iron taken as ferrous sulfate or as an iron **chelate** is better than that from other iron supplements. Absorption also improves when supplements are taken between meals or at bedtime on an empty stomach, and with liquids other than milk, tea, or coffee, which inhibit absorption. Taking iron supplements in a single dose instead of several doses per day is equally effective and may improve a person's willingness to take it regularly.[28]

There is no benefit to taking iron supplements with orange juice because vitamin C does not enhance absorption from supplements as it does from foods. (Vitamin C

contamination iron: iron found in foods as the result of contamination by inorganic iron salts from iron cookware, iron-containing soils, and the like.

chelate (KEY-late): a substance that can grasp the positive ions of a metal.
- **chele** = claw

enhances iron absorption by converting insoluble ferric iron in foods to the more soluble ferrous iron, and supplemental iron is already in the ferrous form.) Constipation is a common side effect of iron supplementation; drinking plenty of water may help to relieve this problem.

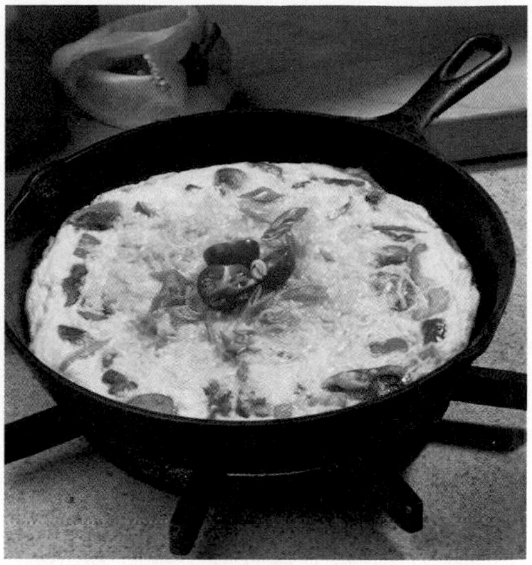

© Polara Studios Inc.

An old-fashioned iron skillet adds iron to foods.

IN SUMMARY Most of the body's iron is in hemoglobin and myoglobin where it carries oxygen for use in energy metabolism; some iron is also required for enzymes involved in a variety of reactions. Special proteins assist with iron absorption, transport, and storage—all helping to maintain an appropriate balance, because both too little and too much iron can be damaging. Iron deficiency is most common among infants and young children, teenagers, women of childbearing age, and pregnant women; symptoms include fatigue and anemia. Iron overload is most common in men. Heme iron, which is found only in meat, fish, and poultry, is better absorbed than nonheme iron, which occurs in most foods. Nonheme iron absorption is improved by eating iron-containing foods with foods containing the MFP factor and vitamin C; absorption is limited by phytates and oxalates. The summary table presents a few iron facts.

Iron

2001 RDA

Men: 8 mg/day

Women: 18 mg/day (19–50 yr)

8 mg/day (51+)

Upper Level

Adults: 45 mg/day

Chief Functions in the Body

Part of the protein hemoglobin, which carries oxygen in the blood; part of the protein myoglobin in muscles, which makes oxygen available for muscle contraction; necessary for the utilization of energy as part of the cells' metabolic machinery

Significant Sources

Red meats, fish, poultry, shellfish, eggs, legumes, dried fruits

Deficiency Symptoms

Anemia: weakness, fatigue, headaches; impaired work performance and cognitive function; impaired immunity; pale skin, nailbeds, mucous membranes, and palm creases; concave nails; inability to regulate body temperature; pica

Toxicity Symptoms

GI distress

Iron overload: infections, fatigue, joint pain, skin pigmentation, organ damage

Zinc

Zinc is a versatile trace element required as a cofactor■ by more than 100 enzymes. Virtually all cells contain zinc, but the highest concentrations are in muscle and bone.

■ Reminder: A *cofactor* is a substance that works with an enzyme to facilitate a chemical reaction.

Zinc Roles in the Body

Zinc supports the work of numerous proteins in the body, including the **metalloenzymes,**■ which are involved in a variety of metabolic processes.* In addition, zinc stabilizes cell membranes, helping to strengthen their defense against free-radical attacks. Zinc also assists in immune function and in growth and development. Zinc participates in the synthesis, storage, and release of the hormone insulin in the pancreas, although it does not appear to play a direct role in insulin's action. Zinc interacts with platelets in blood clotting, affects thyroid hormone function, and influences behavior and learning performance. It is needed to produce the active form of vitamin A (retinal) in visual pigments and the retinol-binding protein that transports vitamin A. It is essential to normal taste perception, wound healing, the making of sperm, and

■ Metalloenzymes that require zinc:
- Help make parts of the genetic materials DNA and RNA.
- Manufacture heme for hemoglobin.
- Participate in essential fatty acid metabolism.
- Release vitamin A from liver stores.
- Metabolize carbohydrates.
- Synthesize proteins.
- Metabolize alcohol in the liver.
- Dispose of damaging free radicals.

metalloenzymes (meh-TAL-oh-EN-zimes): enzymes that contain one or more minerals as part of their structures.

*Among the metalloenzymes requiring zinc are carbonic anhydrase, deoxythymidine kinase, DNA and RNA polymerase, and alkaline phosphatase.

fetal development. A zinc deficiency impairs all these and other functions, underlining the vast importance of zinc in supporting the body's proteins.

Zinc Absorption and Metabolism

The body's handling of zinc resembles that of iron in some ways and differs in others. A key difference is the circular passage of zinc from the intestine to the body and back again.

Zinc Absorption The rate of zinc absorption varies from about 15 to 40 percent, depending on a person's zinc status: if more is needed, more is absorbed. Also, dietary factors influence zinc absorption. For example, fiber and phytates bind zinc, thus limiting its bioavailability.[29]

Upon absorption into an intestinal cell, zinc has several options. It may become involved in the metabolic functions of the cell itself. Alternatively, it may be retained within the cell by **metallothionein,** a special binding protein similar to the iron storage protein, mucosal ferritin.

Metallothionein in the intestinal cells helps to regulate zinc absorption by holding it in reserve until the body needs zinc. Then metallothionein releases it into the blood where it can be transported around the body. Metallothionein in the liver performs a similar role, binding zinc until other body tissues signal a need for it.

Zinc Recycling Some zinc eventually reaches the pancreas, where it is incorporated into many of the digestive enzymes that the pancreas releases into the intestine at mealtimes. The intestine thus receives two doses of zinc with each meal—one from foods and the other from the zinc-rich pancreatic secretions. The recycling of zinc in the body from the pancreas to the intestine and back to the pancreas is referred to as the **enteropancreatic circulation** of zinc. As this zinc circulates through the intestine, it may be refused entry by the intestinal cells or retained in them on any of its times around (see Figure 13-6). The body loses zinc

metallothionein (meh-TAL-oh-THIGH-oh-neen): a sulfur-rich protein that avidly binds with and transports metals such as zinc.
- **metallo** = containing a metal
- **thio** = containing sulfur
- **ein** = a protein

enteropancreatic (EN-ter-oh-PAN-kree-AT-ik) **circulation:** the circulatory route from the pancreas to the intestine and back to the pancreas.

FIGURE 13-6 Enteropancreatic Circulation of Zinc

Some zinc from food is absorbed by the small intestine and sent to the pancreas to be incorporated into digestive enzymes that return to the small intestine. This cycle is called the enteropancreatic circulation of zinc.

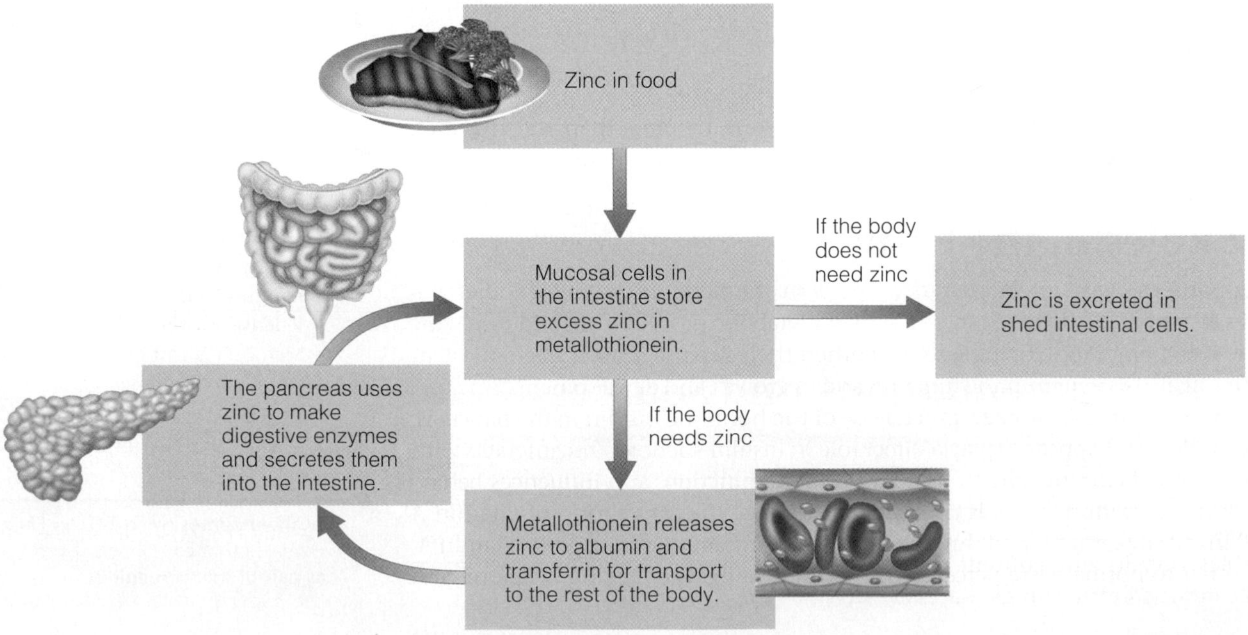
Zinc in food
Mucosal cells in the intestine store excess zinc in metallothionein.
If the body does not need zinc
Zinc is excreted in shed intestinal cells.
The pancreas uses zinc to make digestive enzymes and secretes them into the intestine.
If the body needs zinc
Metallothionein releases zinc to albumin and transferrin for transport to the rest of the body.

primarily in feces. Smaller losses occur in urine, shed skin, hair, sweat, menstrual fluids, and semen.

Zinc Transport Zinc's main transport vehicle in the blood is the protein albumin. Some zinc also binds to transferrin—the same transferrin that carries iron in the blood. In healthy individuals, transferrin is usually less than 50 percent saturated with iron, but in iron overload, it is more saturated. Diets that deliver more than twice as much iron as zinc leave too few transferrin sites available for zinc. The result: poor zinc absorption. The converse is also true: large doses of zinc inhibit iron absorption.

Large doses of zinc create a similar problem with another essential mineral, copper. These nutrient interactions highlight one of the many reasons why people should use supplements conservatively, if at all: supplementation can easily create imbalances.

Zinc Deficiency

Severe zinc deficiencies are not widespread in developed countries, but they do occur in vulnerable groups—pregnant women, young children, the elderly, and the poor. Human zinc deficiency was first reported in the 1960s in children and adolescent boys in Egypt, Iran, and Turkey. Children have especially high zinc needs because they are growing rapidly and synthesizing many zinc-containing proteins; the native diets among those populations were not meeting these needs. Middle Eastern diets are typically low in the richest zinc source, meats, and the staple foods are legumes, unleavened breads, and other whole-grain foods—all high in fiber and phytates, which inhibit zinc absorption.*

Figure 13-7 shows the severe growth retardation and mentions the arrested sexual maturation characteristic of zinc deficiency. In addition, zinc deficiency hinders digestion and absorption, causing diarrhea, which worsens malnutrition not only for zinc, but for all nutrients. It impairs the immune response, making infections likely—among them, infections of the GI tract, which worsen malnutrition, including zinc malnutrition (a classic downward spiral of events). Chronic zinc deficiency damages the central nervous system and brain and may lead to poor motor development and cognitive performance. Because zinc deficiency directly impairs vitamin A metabolism, vitamin A–deficiency symptoms often appear. Zinc deficiency also disturbs thyroid function and the metabolic rate. It alters taste, causes loss of appetite, and slows wound healing—in fact, its symptoms are so all-pervasive that generalized malnutrition and sickness are more likely to be the diagnosis than simple zinc deficiency.

Zinc Toxicity

High doses (50 to 450 milligrams) of zinc may cause vomiting, diarrhea, headaches, exhaustion, and other symptoms. An Upper Level for adults was set at 40 milligrams based on zinc's interference in copper metabolism—an effect that, in animals, leads to degeneration of the heart muscle.

Zinc Recommendations and Sources

Figure 13-8 shows zinc amounts in foods per serving. Zinc is highest in protein-rich foods such as shellfish (especially oysters), meats, poultry, and liver. Legumes and whole-grain products are good sources of zinc if eaten in large quantities; in typical U.S. diets, phytate intake from grains is not high enough to impair zinc absorption. Vegetables vary in zinc content depending on the soil in which they are grown. Average intakes in the United States are slightly higher than recommendations.

*Unleavened bread contains no yeast, which normally breaks down phytates during fermentation.

FIGURE 13-7 Zinc-Deficiency Symptoms—The Stunted Growth of Dwarfism

The Egyptian man on the right is an adult of average height. The Egyptian boy on the left is 17 years old but is only 4 feet tall, like a 7-year-old in the United States. His genitalia are like those of a 6-year-old. The growth retardation, known as dwarfism, is rightly ascribed to zinc deficiency because it is partially reversible when zinc is restored to the diet.

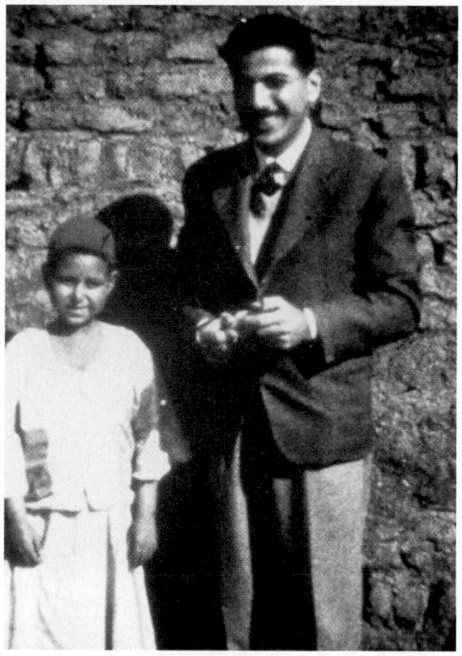

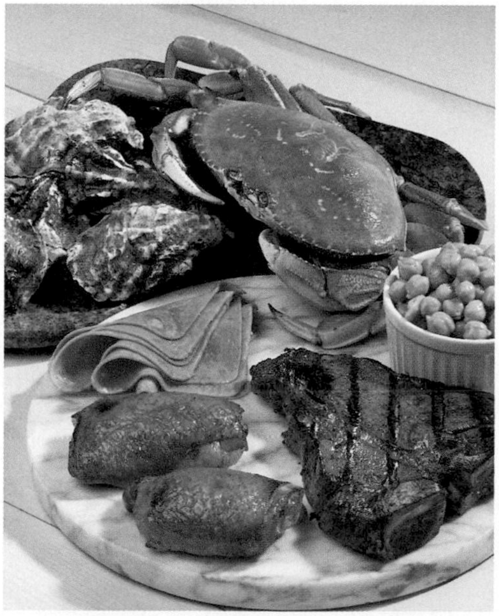

Zinc is highest in protein-rich foods such as oysters, beef, poultry, legumes, and nuts.

FIGURE 13-8 Zinc in Selected Foods

Food	Serving size (kcalories)
Bread, whole wheat	1 oz slice (70 kcal)
Cornflakes, fortified	1 oz (110 kcal)
Spaghetti pasta	1/2 c cooked (99 kcal)
Tortilla, flour	1 10"-round (234 kcal)
Broccoli	1/2 c cooked (22 kcal)
Carrots	1/2 c shredded raw (24 kcal)
Potato	1 medium baked w/skin (133 kcal)
Tomato juice	3/4 c (31 kcal)
Banana	1 medium raw (109 kcal)
Orange	1 medium raw (62 kcal)
Strawberries	1/2 c fresh (22 kcal)
Watermelon	1 slice (92 kcal)
Milk	1 c reduced-fat 2% (121 kcal)
Yogurt, plain	1 c low-fat (155 kcal)
Cheddar cheese	1 1/2 oz (171 kcal)
Cottage cheese	1/2 c low-fat 2% (101 kcal)
Pinto beans	1/2 c cooked (117 kcal)
Peanut butter	2 tbs (188 kcal)
Sunflower seeds	1 oz dry (165 kcal)
Tofu (soybean curd)	1/2 c (76 kcal)
Ground beef, lean	3 oz broiled (244 kcal)
Chicken breast	3 oz roasted (140 kcal)
Tuna, canned in water	3 oz (99 kcal)
Egg	1 hard cooked (78 kcal)
Excellent, and sometimes unusual, sources:	
Oysters	3 oz cooked (139 kcal)
Sirloin steak, lean	3 oz broiled (172 kcal)
Crab	3 oz cooked (94 kcal)

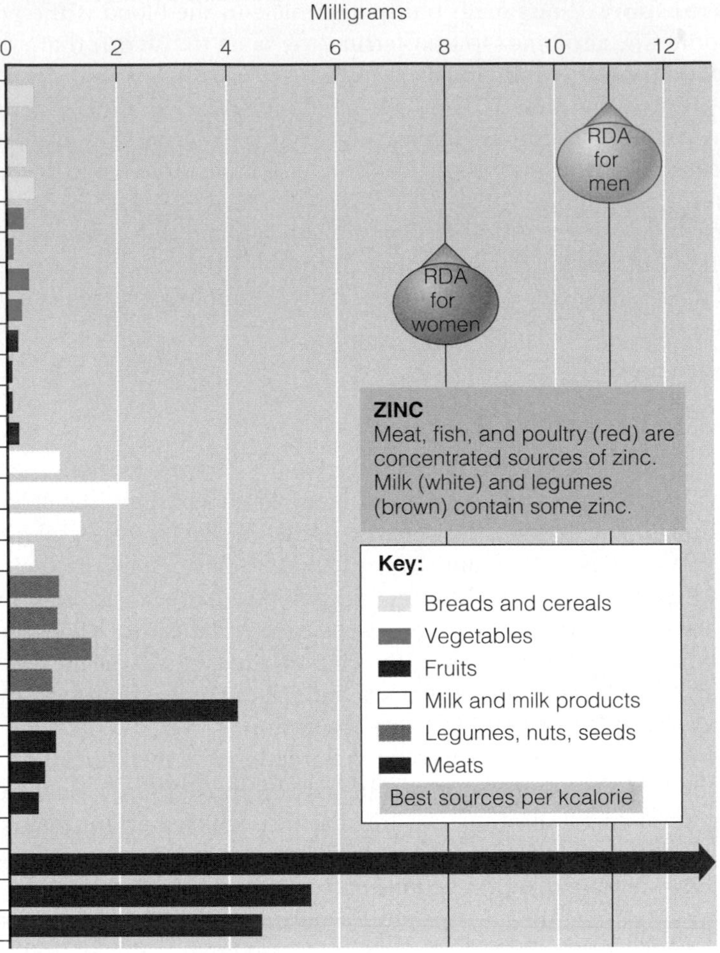
Milligrams
0
2
4
6
8
10
12
RDA for men
RDA for women
ZINC
Meat, fish, and poultry (red) are concentrated sources of zinc. Milk (white) and legumes (brown) contain some zinc.
Key:
Breads and cereals
Vegetables
Fruits
Milk and milk products
Legumes, nuts, seeds
Meats
Best sources per kcalorie

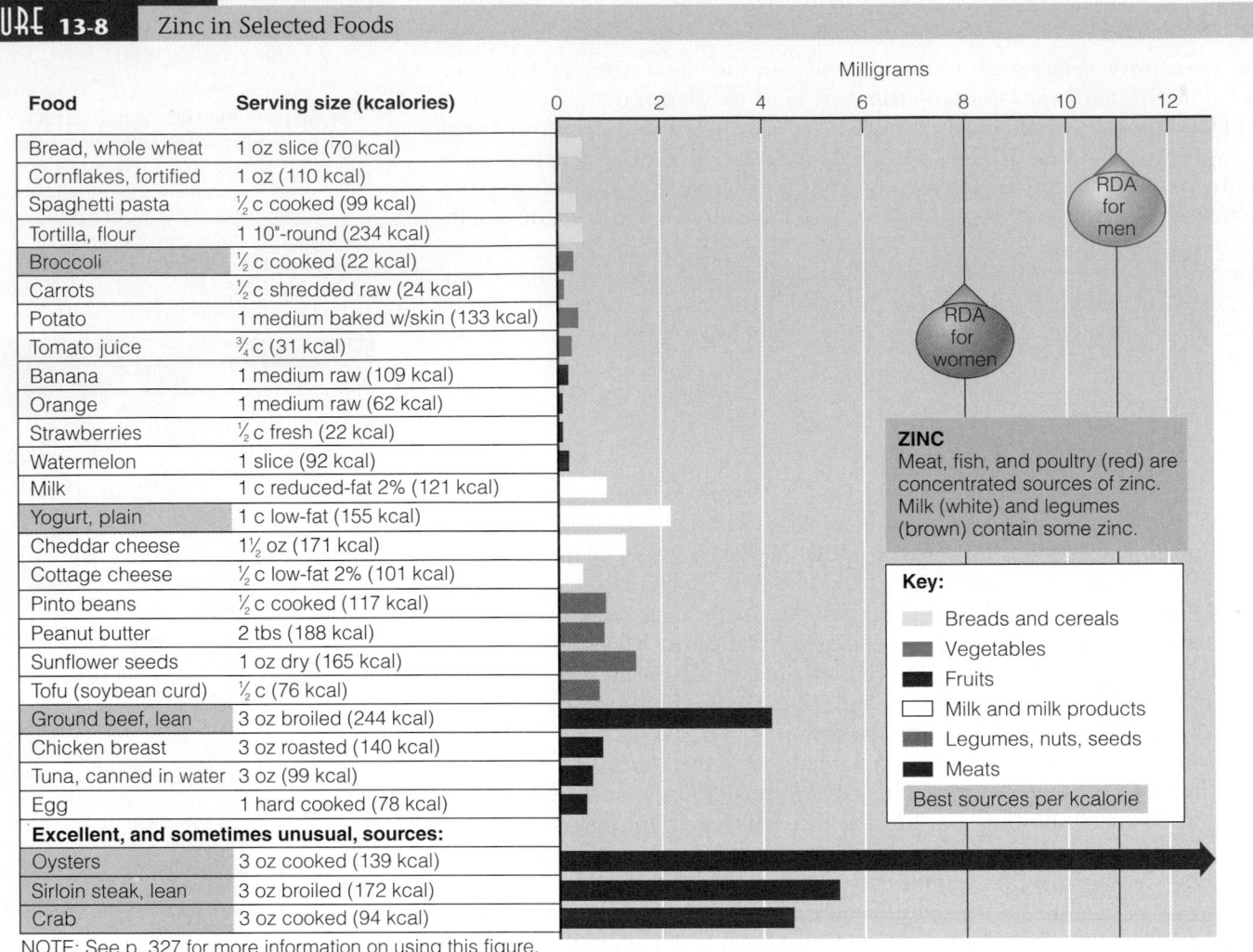

NOTE: See p. 327 for more information on using this figure.

Zinc Supplementation

In developed countries, most people can get enough zinc from the diet without resorting to supplements. In developing countries, zinc supplements play a major role in the treatment of childhood infectious diseases. Zinc supplements effectively reduce the incidence of disease and death associated with diarrhea.[30]

The use of zinc lozenges to treat the common cold has been controversial and inconclusive, with some studies finding them effective and others not.[31] The different study results may reflect the effectiveness of various zinc compounds. Some studies using zinc gluconate report shorter duration of cold symptoms, whereas most studies using other combinations of zinc report no effect. Common side effects of zinc lozenges include nausea and bad taste reactions.

IN SUMMARY Zinc-requiring enzymes participate in a multitude of reactions affecting growth, vitamin A activity, and pancreatic digestive enzyme synthesis, among others. Both dietary zinc and zinc-rich pancreatic secretions (via enteropancreatic circulation) are available for absorption. Absorption is monitored by a special binding protein (metallothionein) in the intestine. Protein-rich foods derived from animals are the best sources of bioavailable zinc. Fiber and phytates in cereals bind zinc, limiting absorption. Growth retardation and sexual immaturity are hallmark symptoms of zinc deficiency. These facts and others are included in the following table.

Zinc

2001 RDA

Men: 11 mg/day

Women: 8 mg/day

Upper Level

Adults: 40 mg/day

Chief Functions in the Body

Part of many enzymes; associated with the hormone insulin; involved in making genetic material and proteins, immune reactions, transport of vitamin A, taste perception, wound healing, the making of sperm, and the normal development of the fetus

Significant Sources

Protein-containing foods: red meats, shellfish, whole grains

Deficiency Symptoms[a]

Growth retardation, delayed sexual maturation, impaired immune function, hair loss, eye and skin lesions, loss of appetite

Toxicity Symptoms

Loss of appetite, impaired immunity, low HDL, copper and iron deficiencies

[a]A rare inherited disease of zinc malabsorption, *acrodermatitis* (AK-roh-der-ma-TIE-tis) *enteropathica* (EN-ter-oh-PATH-ick-ah), causes additional and more severe symptoms.

Iodine

Traces of the iodine ion (called iodide)■ are indispensable to life. In the GI tract, iodine from foods becomes iodide; this chapter uses *iodine* when referring to the nutrient in foods and iodide when referring to it in the body. Iodide occurs in the body in minuscule amounts, but its principal role in the body and its requirement are well established.

Iodide Roles in the Body Iodide is an integral part of the thyroid hormones■ that regulate body temperature, metabolic rate, reproduction, growth, blood cell production, nerve and muscle function, and more. By controlling the rate at which the cells use oxygen, these hormones influence the amount of energy released during basal metabolism.

Iodine Deficiency The hypothalamus regulates thyroid hormone production by controlling the release of the pituitary's thyroid-stimulating hormone (TSH).■ With iodine deficiency, thyroid hormone production declines, and the body responds by secreting more TSH in a futile attempt to accelerate iodide uptake by the thyroid gland. If a deficiency persists, the cells of the thyroid gland enlarge, so as to trap as much iodide as possible. Sometimes the gland enlarges until it makes a visible lump in the neck, a simple **goiter** (shown in Figure 13-9 on p. 452).

Goiter afflicts about 200 million people the world over, many of them in South America, Asia, and Africa. In all but 4 percent of these cases, the cause is iodine deficiency. As for the 4 percent (8 million), most have goiter because they regularly eat excessive amounts of foods■ that contain an antithyroid substance **(goitrogen)** whose effect is not counteracted by dietary iodine. The goitrogens present in plants remind us that even natural components of foods can cause harm when eaten in excess.

Goiter may be the earliest and most obvious sign of iodine deficiency, but the most tragic and prevalent damage occurs in the brain. Children with even a mild iodine deficiency typically have goiters and perform poorly in school; with treatment, mental performance in the classroom improves.[32]

A severe iodine deficiency during pregnancy causes the extreme and irreversible mental and physical retardation known as **cretinism.**■ Cretinism affects approximately 6 million people worldwide and can be averted by the early diagnosis and treatment of maternal iodine deficiency. A worldwide effort to provide iodized salt to people living in iodine-deficient areas has been dramatically successful.

■ The ion form of *iodine* is called *iodide.*

■ The thyroid gland releases tetraiodothyronine (T_4), commonly known as **thyroxine** (thigh-ROCKS-in), to its target tissues. Upon reaching the cells, T_4 is deiodinated to triiodothyronine (T_3), which is the active form of the hormone.

■ Thyroid-stimulating hormone is also called *thyrotropin.*

■ Examples of goitrogen-containing foods:
- Cabbage, spinach, radishes, rutabagas.
- Soybeans, peanuts.
- Peaches, strawberries.

■ The underactivity of the thyroid gland is known as *hypothyroidism* and may be caused by iodine deficiency or any number of other causes. Without treatment, an infant with *congenital hypothyroidism* will develop the physical and mental retardation of *cretinism.*

goiter (GOY-ter): an enlargement of the thyroid gland due to an iodine deficiency, malfunction of the gland, or overconsumption of a goitrogen. Goiter caused by iodine deficiency is **simple goiter.**

goitrogen (GOY-troh-jen): a substance that enlarges the thyroid gland and causes **toxic goiter**. Goitrogens occur naturally in such foods as cabbage, kale, brussels sprouts, cauliflower, broccoli, and kohlrabi.

cretinism (CREE-tin-ism): a congenital disease characterized by mental and physical retardation and commonly caused by maternal iodine deficiency during pregnancy.

FIGURE 13-9 Iodine-Deficiency Symptom—The Enlarged Thyroid of Goiter

In iodine deficiency, the thyroid gland enlarges—a condition known as simple goiter.

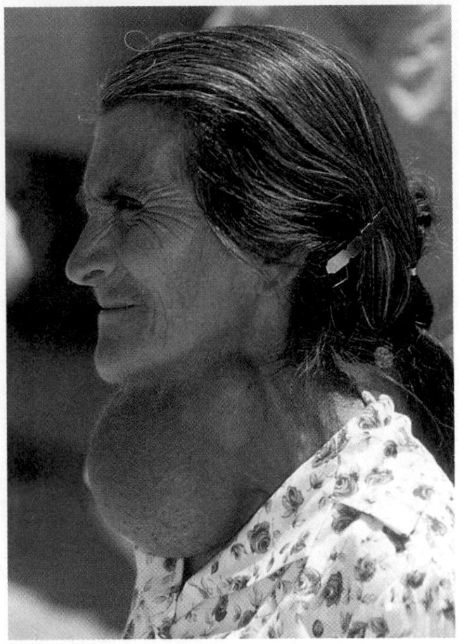

© Bob Daemmrich/The Image Works

Iodine Toxicity Excessive intakes of iodine can enlarge the thyroid gland, just as deficiency can. During pregnancy, exposure to excessive iodine from foods, prenatal supplements, or medications is especially damaging to the developing infant. An infant exposed to toxic amounts of iodine during gestation may develop a goiter so severe as to block the airways and cause suffocation. The Upper Level is over 1000 micrograms per day for an adult—several times higher than average intakes.

Iodine Recommendations and Sources The ocean is the world's major source of iodine. In coastal areas, seafood, water, and even iodine-containing sea mist are dependable iodine sources. Further inland, the amount of iodine in foods is variable and generally reflects the amount present in the soil in which plants are grown or on which animals graze. Landmasses that were once under the ocean have soils rich in iodine; those in flood-prone areas where water leaches iodine from the soil are poor in iodine. In the United States and Canada, the iodization of salt■ has eliminated the widespread misery caused by iodine deficiency during the 1930s, but iodized salt is not available in many parts of the world. Some countries add iodine to bread, fish paste, or drinking water instead.

- ■ Iodized salt contains about 60 µg iodine per gram salt.

Average consumption of iodine in the United States exceeds recommendations, but falls below toxic levels as well. Some of the excess iodine in the U.S. diet stems from fast foods, which use iodized salt liberally. Some iodine comes from bakery products and from milk. The baking industry uses iodates (iodine salts) as dough conditioners, and most dairies feed cows iodine-containing medications and use iodine to disinfect milking equipment. Now that these sources have been identified, food industries have reduced their use of these compounds, but the sudden emergence of this problem points to a need for continued surveillance of the food supply. Processed foods in the United States do not use iodized salt.

The recommended intake of iodine for adults is a minuscule amount. The need for iodine is easily met by consuming seafood, vegetables grown in iodine-rich soil, and iodized salt.■ In the United States, labels indicate whether salt is iodized; in Canada, all table salt is iodized.

- ■ On average, ½ tsp iodized salt provides the RDA for iodine.

IN SUMMARY Iodide, the ion of the mineral iodine, is an essential component of the thyroid hormone. An iodine deficiency can lead to simple goiter—enlargement of the thyroid gland—and can impair fetal development, causing cretinism. Iodization of salt has largely eliminated iodine deficiency in the United States and Canada. The table provides a summary of iodine.

Iodine

2001 RDA

Adults: 150 µg/day

Upper Level

1100 µg/day

Chief Functions in the Body

A component of two thyroid hormones that help to regulate growth, development, and metabolic rate

Significant Sources

Iodized salt, seafood, bread, dairy products, plants grown in iodine-rich soil and animals fed those plants

Deficiency Disease

Simple goiter, cretinism

Deficiency Symptoms

Underactive thyroid gland, goiter, mental and physical retardation in infants (cretinism)

Toxicity Symptoms

Underactive thyroid gland, elevated TSH, goiter

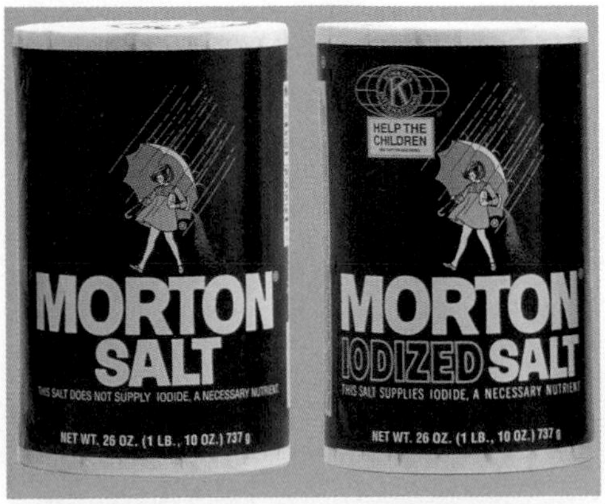
MORTON SALT
THIS SALT DOES NOT SUPPLY IODIDE, A NECESSARY NUTRIENT
NET WT. 26 OZ. (1 LB., 10 OZ.) 737 g
HELP THE CHILDREN
MORTON IODIZED SALT
THIS SALT SUPPLIES IODIDE, A NECESSARY NUTRIENT
NET WT. 26 OZ. (1 LB., 10 OZ.) 737 g

© Craig M. Moore

Only "iodized salt" has had iodine added.

Selenium

The essential mineral **selenium** shares some of the chemical characteristics of the mineral sulfur. This similarity allows selenium to substitute for sulfur in the amino acids methionine, cysteine, and cystine.[33]

Selenium Roles in the Body Selenium is one of the body's antioxidant nutrients, working primarily as a part of the enzyme glutathione peroxidase. Glutathione peroxidase and vitamin E work in concert. Glutathione peroxidase prevents free-radical formation, thus blocking the chain reaction before it begins; if free radicals do form and a chain reaction starts, vitamin E stops it. (Highlight 11 describes free-radical formation, chain reactions, and antioxidant action in detail.) Another enzyme that converts the thyroid hormone to its active form also contains selenium.

Selenium Deficiency Selenium deficiency is associated with a heart disease■ that is prevalent in regions of China where the soil and foods lack selenium. The primary cause of this heart disease is probably a virus, but selenium deficiency appears to predispose people to it, and adequate selenium seems to prevent it.

■ The heart disease associated with selenium deficiency is named **Keshan** (KESH-an or ka-SHAWN) **disease** for one of the provinces of China where it was studied. Keshan disease is characterized by heart enlargement and insufficiency; fibrous tissue replaces the muscle tissue that normally composes the middle layer of the walls of the heart.

Selenium and Cancer Some research suggests that selenium may protect against some types of cancers. Given the potential for harm and the lack of conclusive evidence, however, recommendations to take selenium supplements would be premature—and perhaps ineffective as well. Selenium from foods is far more effective in inhibiting cancer growth than selenium from supplements.[34] Such a finding reinforces a theme that has been repeated throughout this text—foods offer many more health benefits than supplements.

Selenium Recommendations and Sources The soil in many regions of the United States and Canada contains selenium. People living in regions with selenium-poor soil may still get enough selenium, partly because they eat vegetables and grains transported from other regions and partly because they eat meats and other animal products, which are reliable sources of selenium. Average intakes in the United States and Canada are above the RDA, which is based on the amount needed to maximize glutathione peroxidase activity.

Selenium Toxicity Because high doses of selenium are toxic, an Upper Level has been set. Selenium toxicity causes loss and brittleness of hair and nails, garlic breath odor, and nervous system abnormalities.

IN SUMMARY Selenium is an antioxidant nutrient that works closely with the glutathione peroxidase enzyme and vitamin E. Selenium is found in association with protein in foods. Deficiencies are associated with a predisposition to a type of heart disease and possibly with some kinds of cancer. See the table below for a summary of selenium.

Selenium

2000 RDA

Adults: 55 µg/day

Upper Level

Adults: 400 µg/day

Chief Functions in the Body

Defends against oxidation; regulates thyroid hormone

Significant Sources

Seafood, meat, whole grains, vegetables (depending on soil content)

Deficiency Symptoms

Predisposition to heart disease characterized by cardiac tissue becoming fibrous (Keshan disease)

Toxicity Symptoms

Loss and brittleness of hair and nails; skin rash, fatigue, irritability, and nervous system disorders; garlic breath odor

selenium (se-LEEN-ee-um): a trace element.

Copper

The body contains about 100 milligrams of copper. It is found in a variety of cells and tissues.

Copper Roles in the Body Copper serves as a constituent of several enzymes. The copper-containing enzymes have diverse metabolic roles with one common characteristic: all involve reactions that consume oxygen or oxygen radicals. For example, copper-containing enzymes catalyze the oxidation of ferrous iron to ferric iron.[*35] Copper's role in iron metabolism makes it a key factor in hemoglobin synthesis. Two copper- and zinc-containing enzymes participate in the body's natural defense against free radicals.[†] Still another copper enzyme helps to manufacture collagen and heal wounds.[‡] Copper, like iron, is needed in many of the metabolic reactions related to the release of energy.[§]

Copper Deficiency and Toxicity Copper deficiency is rare. In animals, copper deficiency raises blood cholesterol and damages blood vessels, raising questions about whether low dietary copper might contribute to cardiovascular disease in humans. Typical U.S. diets provide adequate amounts. Some genetic disorders create a copper toxicity, but excessive intakes from foods are unlikely. Excessive intakes from supplements may cause liver damage, and therefore an Upper Level has been set.

Two rare genetic disorders affect copper status in opposite directions. In Menkes disease, the intestinal cells absorb copper, but cannot release it into circulation, causing a life-threatening deficiency. In Wilson's disease, copper accumulates in the liver and brain, creating a life-threatening toxicity. Wilson's disease can be controlled by reducing copper intake, using chelating agents such as penicillamine, and taking zinc supplements, which interfere with copper absorption. (The use of chelation in health care is mentioned in Highlight 19's discussion of alternative therapies.)

Copper Recommendations and Sources The richest food sources of copper are legumes, whole grains, nuts, shellfish, and seeds. Over half of the copper from foods is absorbed, and the major route of elimination appears to be bile. Water may also provide copper, depending on the type of plumbing pipe and the hardness of the water.

IN SUMMARY Copper is a component of several enzymes, all of which are involved in some way with oxygen or oxidation. Some act as antioxidants; others are essential to iron metabolism. Legumes, whole grains, and shellfish are good sources of copper. See the table for a summary of copper facts.

Copper

2001 RDA	Significant Sources
Adults: 900 μg/day	Seafood, nuts, whole grains, seeds, legumes
Upper Level	**Deficiency Symptoms**
Adults: 10,000 μg/day (10 mg/day)	Anemia, bone abnormalities
Chief Functions in the Body	**Toxicity Symptoms**
Necessary for the absorption and use of iron in the formation of hemoglobin; part of several enzymes	Liver damage

*The copper-containing enzyme *ceruloplasmin* participates in the oxidation of ferrous iron to ferric iron.
†Two copper-containing *superoxide dismutase* enzymes defend against free radicals.
‡The copper-containing enzyme *lysyl oxidase* helps synthesize connective tissues.
§The copper-containing enzyme *cytochrome C oxidase* participates in the electron transport chain.

Manganese

The human body contains a tiny 20 milligrams of manganese. Most of it can be found in the bones and metabolically active organs such as the liver, kidneys, and pancreas.

Manganese Roles in the Body Manganese acts as a cofactor for many enzymes that facilitate the metabolism of carbohydrate, lipids, and amino acids. In addition, manganese-containing metalloenzymes assist in bone formation and the conversion of pyruvate to a TCA cycle compound.

Manganese Deficiency and Toxicity Manganese requirements are low, and many plant foods contain significant amounts of this trace mineral, so deficiencies are rare. As is true of other trace minerals, however, dietary factors such as phytates inhibit its absorption. In addition, high intakes of iron and calcium limit manganese absorption, so people who use supplements of these minerals regularly may impair their manganese status.

Toxicity is more likely to occur from an environment contaminated with manganese than from dietary intake. Miners who inhale large quantities of manganese dust on the job over prolonged periods show symptoms of a brain disease, along with abnormalities in appearance and behavior. Still, an Upper Level has been established based on intakes from food, water, and supplements.

Manganese Recommendations and Sources Grain products make the greatest contribution of manganese to the diet. With insufficient information to establish an RDA, an AI was set based on average intakes.

IN SUMMARY Manganese-dependent enzymes are involved in bone formation and various metabolic processes. Manganese is widespread in plant foods, so deficiencies are rare, although regular use of calcium and iron supplements may limit manganese absorption. A summary of manganese appears in the table below.

Manganese

2001 AI	Significant Sources
Men: 2.3 mg/day	Nuts, whole grains, leafy vegetables, tea
Women: 1.8 mg/day	
Upper Level	**Deficiency Symptoms**
Adults: 11 mg/day	Rare
Chief Functions in the Body	**Toxicity Symptoms**
Cofactor for several enzymes	Nervous system disorders

Fluoride

Fluoride is present in virtually all soils, water supplies, plants, and animals. Only a trace of fluoride occurs in the human body, but with this amount, the crystalline deposits in bones and teeth are larger and more perfectly formed.

Fluoride Roles in the Body During the mineralization of bones and teeth, calcium and phosphorus form crystals called hydroxyapatite. Then fluoride replaces the hydroxyl (OH) portions of the hydroxyapatite crystal, forming **fluorapatite,** which makes the bones stronger and the teeth more resistant to decay.

Fluoride and Dental Caries Dental caries ranks as the nation's most widespread health problem: an estimated 95 percent of the population have decayed,

fluorapatite (floor-APP-uh-tite): the stabilized form of bone and tooth crystal, in which fluoride has replaced the hydroxyl groups of hydroxyapatite.

FIGURE 13-10 U.S. Population with Access to Fluoridated Water through Public Water Systems

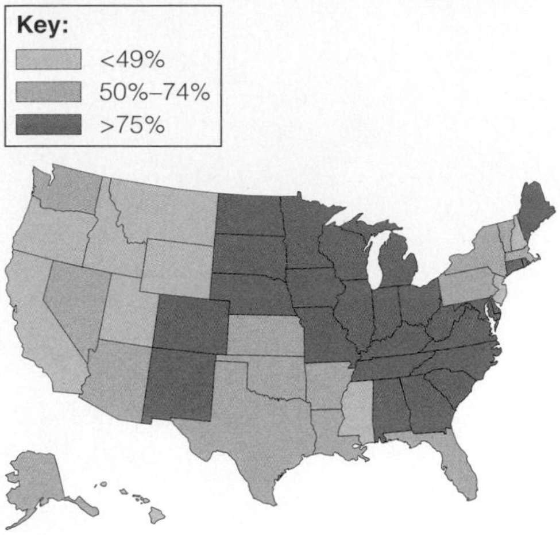
Key:
<49%
50%–74%
>75%

missing, or filled teeth. By interfering with a person's ability to chew and eat a wide variety of foods, these dental problems can quickly lead to a multitude of nutrition problems. Where fluoride is lacking, dental decay is common.

Drinking water is usually the best source of fluoride; over 65 percent of the U.S. population receives fluoride through the public water system (see Figure 13-10).[36] (Most bottled waters lack fluoride.) Fluoridation of drinking water to raise the concentration to 1 part fluoride per 1 million■ parts water offers the greatest protection against dental caries at virtually no risk of toxicity.[37] By fluoridating the drinking water, a community offers its residents, particularly the children, a safe, economical, practical, and effective way to defend against dental caries.[38]

Fluoride Toxicity Too much fluoride can damage the teeth, causing **fluorosis.** For this reason, an Upper Level has been established. In mild cases, the teeth develop small white specks; in severe cases, the enamel becomes pitted and permanently stained (as shown in Figure 13-11). Fluorosis occurs only during tooth development and cannot be reversed, making its prevention■ a high priority. To limit fluoride ingestion, take care not to swallow fluoride-containing dental products such as toothpaste and mouthwash.

Fluoride Recommendations and Sources As mentioned earlier, much of the U.S. population has access to water with an optimal fluoride concentration, which typically delivers about 1 milligram per person per day.[39] Fish and most teas contain appreciable amounts of natural fluoride.

■ For perspective, 1 part per million (1 ppm) is approximately 1 mg per liter.

■ To prevent fluorosis:
- Monitor the fluoride content of the local water supply.
- Supervise toddlers when they brush their teeth and use only a little toothpaste (pea-size amount).
- Use fluoride supplements only as prescribed by a physician.

HEALTHY PEOPLE 2010

Increase the proportion of the U.S. population served by community water systems with optimally fluoridated water.

IN SUMMARY Fluoride makes bones stronger and teeth more resistant to decay. Fluoridation of public water supplies can significantly reduce the incidence of dental caries, but an excess of fluoride during tooth development can cause fluorosis—discolored and pitted tooth enamel. The table below summarizes fluoride information.

Fluoride

1997 AI	Significant Sources
Men: 3.8 mg/day Women: 3.1 mg/day	Drinking water (if fluoride containing or fluoridated), tea, seafood
Upper Level	**Deficiency Symptoms**
Adults: 10 mg/day	Susceptibility to tooth decay
Chief Functions in the Body	**Toxicity Symptoms**
Involved in the formation of bones and teeth; helps to make teeth resistant to decay	Fluorosis (pitting and discoloration of teeth)

FIGURE 13-11 Fluoride-Toxicity Symptom—The Mottled Teeth of Fluorosis

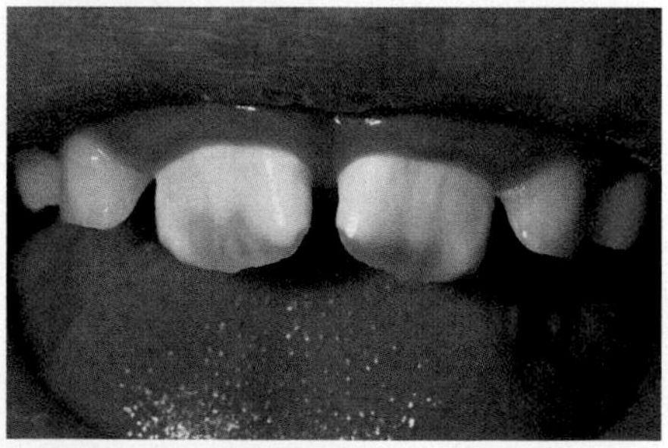

© Dr. P. Marrazi/Science Photo Library/ Photo Researchers Inc.

Chromium

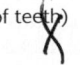

Chromium is an essential mineral that participates in carbohydrate and lipid metabolism. Like iron, chromium assumes different charges. In the case of chromium, the Cr^{+++} ion is the most stable and most commonly found in foods.

Chromium Roles in the Body Chromium helps maintain glucose homeostasis by enhancing the activity of the hormone insulin.■ When chromium is lacking, a diabeteslike condition may develop with elevated blood glucose and impaired

■ Small organic compounds that enhance insulin's action are called **glucose tolerance factors (GTF).** Some glucose tolerance factors contain chromium.

fluorosis (floor-OH-sis): discoloration and pitting of tooth enamel caused by excess fluoride during tooth development.

glucose tolerance, insulin response, and glucagon response. In spite of these relationships, research findings suggest that chromium supplements do not effectively improve glucose or insulin responses in diabetes.[40]

Chromium Recommendations and Sources Chromium is present in a variety of foods. The best sources are unrefined foods, particularly liver, brewer's yeast, and whole grains. The more refined foods people eat, the less chromium they ingest.

Chromium Supplements Supplement advertisements have succeeded in convincing consumers that they can lose fat and build muscle by taking chromium picolinate. Whether chromium—picolinate or plain—supplements reduce body fat or improve muscle strength remains controversial. Initial studies reported that chromium picolinate supplements increased lean body mass and reduced body fat in weight trainers, but later studies show no effects of supplementation on strength, lean body mass, or body fat.

IN SUMMARY Chromium enhances insulin's action. A deficiency can result in a diabeteslike condition. Chromium is widely available in unrefined foods including brewer's yeast, whole grains, and liver. The table below provides a summary of chromium.

Chromium

2001 AI	Deficiency Symptoms
Men: 35 μg/day	Diabeteslike condition
Women: 25 μg/day	
Chief Functions in the Body	**Toxicity Symptoms**
Enhances insulin action	None reported
Significant Sources	
Meats (especially liver), whole grains, brewer's yeast	

Molybdenum

Molybdenum acts as a working part of several metalloenzymes. Dietary deficiencies of molybdenum are unknown because the amounts needed are minuscule—as little as 0.1 part per million parts of body tissue. Legumes, breads and other grain products, leafy green vegetables, milk, and liver are molybdenum-rich foods. Average daily intakes fall within the suggested range of intakes.

Molybdenum toxicity is rare, but has been reported in animal studies, and an Upper Level has been established. Characteristics include kidney damage and reproductive abnormalities. For a summary of molybdenum facts, see the accompanying table.

Molybdenum

2001 RDA	Significant Sources
Adults: 45 μg/day	Legumes, cereals, organ meats
Upper Level	**Deficiency Symptoms**
Adults: 2 mg/day	Unknown
Chief Functions in the Body	**Toxicity Symptoms**
Cofactor for several enzymes	None reported; reproductive effects in animals

molybdenum (mo-LIB-duh-num): a trace element.

FIGURE 13-12 Cobalt with Vitamin B_{12}

The intricate vitamin B_{12} molecule contains one atom of the mineral cobalt. The alternative name for vitamin B_{12}, cobalamin, reflects the presence of cobalt in its structure.

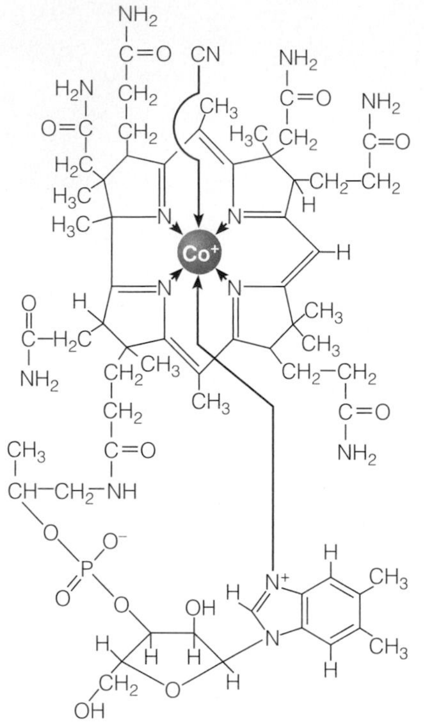

Other Trace Minerals

Research to determine whether other trace minerals are essential is difficult, both because their quantities in the body are so small and because human deficiencies are unknown. Guessing their functions in the body can be particularly problematic. Much of the available knowledge comes from research using animals.

Nickel may serve as a cofactor for certain enzymes. Silicon is involved in the formation of bones and collagen. Vanadium, too, is necessary for growth and bone development and also for normal reproduction. Cobalt is a key mineral in the large vitamin B_{12} molecule (see Figure 13-12), but it is not an essential nutrient and no recommendation has been established. Boron may play a key role in brain activities; in animals, boron strengthens bones.[41]

In the future many other trace minerals may turn out to play key nutritional roles. Even arsenic—famous as a poison used by murderers and known to be a carcinogen—may turn out to be essential for human beings in tiny quantities; it has already proved useful in the treatment of some types of leukemia.

Contaminant Minerals

Chapter 12 and this chapter have told of the many ways minerals serve the body—maintaining fluid and electrolyte balance, providing structural support to the bones, transporting oxygen, and assisting enzymes. In contrast to those minerals that the body requires, contaminant minerals impair the body's growth, work capacity, and general health. Contaminant minerals include the **heavy metals** lead, mercury, and cadmium that enter the food supply by way of soil, water, and air pollution. This section focuses on lead poisoning because it is the most serious environmental threat to young children, but all contaminant minerals disrupt body processes and impair nutrition status similarly.

Like other minerals, lead is indestructible; the body cannot change its chemistry. Chemically similar to nutrient minerals like iron, calcium, and zinc (cations with two positive charges), lead displaces them from some of the metabolic sites they normally occupy, but is then unable to perform their roles. For example, lead competes with iron in heme, but then cannot carry oxygen; similarly, lead competes with calcium in the brain, but then cannot signal messages from nerve cells. Excess lead in the blood also deranges the structure of red blood cell membranes, making them leaky and fragile. Lead interacts with white blood cells, too, impairing their ability to fight infection, and it binds to antibodies, thwarting their effort to resist disease.

In addition to its effects on the blood, lead damages many body systems, particularly the vulnerable nervous system, kidneys, and bone marrow. It impairs such normal activities as growth by interfering with hormone activity.[42] It interferes with tooth development and may contribute to dental caries as well.[43] Even at low levels, blood lead concentrations correlate with poor IQ scores.[44] In short, lead's interactions in the body have profound adverse effects. The greater the exposure, the more damaging the effects. The American Academy of Pediatrics recommends testing children who have been identified as having a high risk for lead poisoning. Those with high blood lead levels are treated with drugs that bind to lead and carry it out in the urine. Table 13-1 lists symptoms of lead toxicity.

Lead typifies the ways all heavy metals behave in the body: they interfere with nutrients that are trying to do their jobs. The "good guy" nutrients are shoved aside by the "bad guy" contaminants. Then the contaminants cannot perform

TABLE 13-1 Symptoms of Lead Toxicity

In Children

- Learning disabilities (reduced short-term memory; impaired concentration)
- Low IQ
- Behavior problems
- Slow growth
- Iron-deficiency anemia
- Dental caries
- Sleep disturbances (night waking, restlessness, head banging)
- Nervous system disorders; seizures
- Slow reaction time; poor coordination
- Impaired hearing

In Adults

- Hypertension
- Reproductive complications
- Kidney failure

the roles of the nutrients, and health diminishes. To safeguard our health, we must defend ourselves against contamination by eating nutrient-rich foods and preserving a clean environment.

Closing Thoughts on the Nutrients

This chapter completes the introductory lessons on the nutrients. Each nutrient from the amino acids to zinc has been described rather thoroughly—its chemistry, roles in the body, sources in the diet, symptoms of deficiency and toxicity, and influences on health and disease. Such a detailed examination is informative, but it can also be misleading. It is important to step back from the myopic study of the individual nutrients to look at them as a whole. After all, people eat foods, not nutrients, and most foods deliver dozens of nutrients. Furthermore, nutrients work cooperatively with each other in the body; their actions are most often *interactions*. This chapter alone mentioned how iron depends on vitamin C to keep it in its active form and copper to incorporate it into hemoglobin; how zinc is needed to activate and transport vitamin A; and how both iodine and selenium are needed for the synthesis of thyroid hormone. The accompanying table condenses the information on the trace minerals for your review.

heavy metals: any of a number of mineral ions such as mercury and lead, so called because they are of relatively high atomic weight. Many heavy metals are poisonous.

IN SUMMARY The Trace Minerals

Mineral and Chief Functions	Deficiency Symptoms	Toxicity Symptoms[a]	Significant Sources
Iron Part of the protein hemoglobin, which carries oxygen in the blood; part of the protein myoglobin in muscles, which makes oxygen available for muscle contraction; necessary for energy metabolism	Anemia: weakness, fatigue, headaches; impaired work performance; impaired immunity; pale skin, nail beds, mucous membranes, and palm creases; concave nails; inability to regulate body temperature; pica	GI distress; iron overload: infections, fatigue, joint pain, skin pigmentation, organ damage	Red meats, fish, poultry, shellfish, eggs, legumes, dried fruits
Zinc Part of insulin and many enzymes; involved in making genetic material and proteins, immune reactions, transport of vitamin A, taste perception, wound healing, the making of sperm, and normal fetal development	Growth retardation, delayed sexual maturation, impaired immune function, hair loss, eye and skin lesions, loss of appetite.	Loss of appetite, impaired immunity, low HDL, copper and iron deficiencies	Protein-containing foods: red meats, fish, shellfish, poultry, whole grains
Iodine A component of the thyroid hormones that help to regulate growth, development, and metabolic rate	Underactive thyroid gland, goiter, mental and physical retardation (cretinism)	Underactive thyroid gland, elevated TSH, goiter	Iodized salt; seafood; plants grown in iodine-rich soil and animals fed those plants
Selenium Part of an enzyme that defends against oxidation; regulates thyroid hormone	Associated with Keshan disease	Nail and hair brittleness and loss; fatigue, irritability, and nervous system disorders, skin rash, garlic breath odor	Seafoods, organ meats; other meats, whole grains, and vegetables (depending on soil content)
Copper Helps form hemoglobin; part of several enzymes	Anemia, bone abnormalities	Liver damage	Seafood, nuts, legumes, whole grains, seeds

[a]Acute toxicities of many minerals cause abdominal pain, nausea, vomiting, and diarrhea.

continued

The Trace Minerals—*continued*

Mineral and Chief Functions	Deficiency Symptoms	Toxicity Symptoms[a]	Significant Sources
Manganese Cofactor for several enzymes	Rare	Nervous symptom disorders	Nuts, whole grains, leafy vegetables, tea
Fluoride Helps form bones and teeth; confers decay resistance on teeth	Susceptibility to tooth decay	Fluorosis (pitting and discoloration) of teeth,	Drinking water if fluoride containing or fluoridated, tea, seafood
Chromium Enhances insulin action	Diabeteslike condition	None reported	Meats (liver), whole grains, brewer's yeast
Molybdenum Cofactor for several enzymes	Unknown	None reported	Legumes, cereals, organ meats

Estimates of how much of each particular nutrient the body needs fall between intakes that are inadequate and cause illness and intakes that are excessive and cause illness. Between deficiency and toxicity lies a wide range of intakes that support health—to varying degrees. In the past, nutrient needs were determined by how much was needed to prevent deficiency symptoms. If lack of a nutrient caused illness, it was defined as essential. Today, nutrient needs are based on how much is needed to support optimal health. The amount of vitamin C needed to prevent scurvy is much less than the amount correlated with reducing the risk of cancer, for example. Furthermore, nutrients are being examined within the context of the whole diet. Health benefits are not credited to vitamin C alone, but to the vitamin C–rich fruits and vegetables that also provide many other nutrients—and nonnutrients (phytochemicals)—important to health.

People can also improve their health with physical activity. Energy expenditure is unlike money expenditure: it is desirable to *spend* energy, not to save it (within reason, of course). The more energy people spend, the more food they can afford to eat—food that delivers both nutrients and pleasure.

Nutrition in Your Life

Trace minerals from a variety of foods, especially those in the meat and meat alternate group, support many of your body's activities.

- **Do you eat a variety of foods, including some meats, seafood, poultry, or legumes, daily?**
- **Do you use iodized salt?**
- **Do you drink fluoridated water?**

Available Online

http://nutrition.wadsworth.com/uncn7
Practice planning meals with varying energy needs to meet recommended intakes of several minerals.

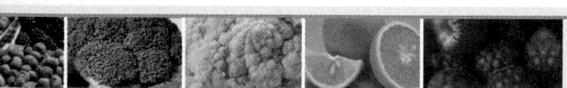

NUTRITION ON THE NET

Access these websites for further study of topics covered in this chapter.

- Find updates and quick links to these and other nutrition-related sites at our website: **www.wadsworth.com/nutrition**
- Search for "minerals" at the American Dietetic Association: **www.eatright.org**
- Search for the individual minerals by name at the U.S. Government health information site: **www.healthfinder.gov**
- Learn more about iron overload from the Iron Overload Diseases Association: **www.ironoverload.org**
- Learn more about iodine and thyroid disease from the American Thyroid Association: **www.thyroid.org**

NUTRITION CALCULATIONS

Once you have mastered these examples, you will understand minerals a little better and be prepared to examine your own food choices. Be sure to show your calculations for each problem. (see p. 464 for answers.)

1. For each of these minerals, note the unit of measure for recommendations:

Iron	Manganese
Zinc	Fluoride
Iodine	Chromium
Selenium	Molybdenum
Copper	

2. Appreciate foods for their iron density. Following is a list of foods with the energy amount and the iron content per serving.
   a. Rank these foods by iron per serving.
   b. Calculate the iron density (divide milligrams by kcalories) for these foods and rank them by their iron per kcalorie.
   c. Name three foods that are higher on the second list than they were on the first list.
   d. What do these foods have in common?

Food	Iron (mg)	Energy (kcal)	Iron Density (mg/kcal)
Milk, fat-free, 1 c	0.10	85	
Cheddar cheese, 1 oz	0.19	114	
Broccoli, cooked from fresh, chopped, 1 c	1.31	44	
Sweet potato, baked in skin, 1 ea	0.51	117	
Cantaloupe melon, ½	0.56	93	
Carrots, from fresh, ½ c	0.48	35	
Whole-wheat bread, 1 slice	0.87	64	
Green peas, cooked from frozen, ½ c	1.26	62	
Apple, medium	0.38	125	
Sirloin steak, lean, 4 oz	3.81	228	
Pork chop, lean, broiled, 1 ea	0.66	166	

STUDY QUESTIONS

These questions will help you review the chapter. You will find the answers in the discussions on the pages provided.

1. Distinguish between heme and nonheme iron. Discuss the factors that enhance iron absorption. (pp. 440–441)
2. Distinguish between iron deficiency and iron-deficiency anemia. What are the symptoms of iron-deficiency anemia? (pp. 442–443)
3. What causes iron overload? What are its symptoms? (p. 444)
4. Describe the similarities and differences in the absorption and regulation of iron and zinc. (pp. 440–441, 448–449)
5. Discuss possible reasons for a low intake of zinc. What factors affect the bioavailability of zinc? (p. 449)
6. Describe the principal functions of iodide, selenium, copper, manganese, fluoride, chromium, and molybdenum in the body. (pp. 451, 453, 454, 455, 456, 457)
7. What public health measure has been used in preventing simple goiter? What measure has been recommended for protection against tooth decay? (pp. 451, 456)
8. Discuss the importance of balanced and varied diets in obtaining the essential minerals and avoiding toxicities. (pp. 458–459)
9. Describe some of the ways trace minerals interact with each other and with other nutrients. (p. 459)

These multiple choice questions will help you prepare for an exam. Answers can be found on p. 464.

1. Iron absorption is impaired by:
   a. heme.
   b. phytates.

c. vitamin C.
d. MFP factor.

2. Which of these people is *least* likely to develop an iron deficiency?
   a. 3-year-old boy
   b. 52-year-old man
   c. 17-year-old girl
   d. 24-year-old woman
3. Which of the following would *not* describe the blood cells of a severe iron deficiency?
   a. anemic
   b. microcytic
   c. pernicious
   d. hypochromic
4. Which provides the most absorbable iron?
   a. 1 apple
   b. 1 c milk
   c. 3 oz steak
   d. ½ c spinach
5. The intestinal protein that helps to regulate zinc absorption is:
   a. albumin.
   b. ferritin.
   c. hemosiderin.
   d. metallothionein.
6. A classic sign of zinc deficiency is:
   a. anemia.
   b. goiter.
   c. mottled teeth.
   d. growth retardation.
7. Cretinism is caused by a deficiency of:
   a. iron.
   b. zinc.
   c. iodine.
   d. selenium.
8. The mineral best known for its role as an antioxidant is:
   a. copper.
   b. selenium.
   c. manganese.
   d. molybdenum.
9. Fluorosis occurs when fluoride:
   a. is excessive.
   b. is inadequate.
   c. binds with phosphorus.
   d. interacts with calcium.
10. Which mineral enhances insulin activity?
    a. zinc
    b. iodine
    c. chromium
    d. manganese

REFERENCES

1. R. A. Anderson, Role of dietary factors: Micronutrients, *Nutrition Reviews* 58 (2000): S10–S11.
2. M. Wessling-Resnick, Iron transport, *Annual Review of Nutrition* 20 (2000): 129–151; N. C. Andrews, Disorders of iron metabolism, *New England Journal of Medicine* 341 (1999): 1986–1995.
3. Committee on Dietary Reference Intakes, *Dietary Reference Intakes for Vitamin A, Vitamin K, Arsenic, Boron, Chromium, Copper, Iodine, Iron, Manganese, Molybdenum, Nickel, Silicon, Vanadium, and Zinc* (Washington, D.C.: National Academy Press, 2001), p. 315.
4. S. Miret, R. J. Simpson, and A. T. McKie, Physiology and molecular biology of dietary iron absorption, *Annual Review of Nutrition* 23 (2003): 283–301.
5. L. Hallberg and L. Hulthén, Prediction of dietary iron absorption: An algorithm for calculating absorption and bioavailability of dietary iron, *American Journal of Clinical Nutrition* 71 (2000): 1147–1160.
6. M. B. Reddy, R. F. Hurrell, and J. D. Cook, Estimation of nonheme-iron bioavailability from meal composition, *American Journal of Clinical Nutrition* 71 (2000): 937–943.
7. Committee on Dietary Reference Intakes, 2001, p. 351.
8. J. R. Hunt and Z. K. Roughead, Nonheme-iron absorption, fecal ferritin excretion, and blood indexes of iron status in women consuming controlled lactoovovegetarian diets for 8 wk, *American Journal of Clinical Nutrition* 69 (1999): 944–952.
9. J. R. Hunt and Z. K. Roughead, Adaptation of iron absorption in men consuming diets with high or low iron bioavailability, *American Journal of Clinical Nutrition* 71 (2000): 94–102.
10. R. S. Eisenstein, Iron regulatory proteins and the molecular control of mammalian iron metabolism, *Annual Review of Nutrition* 20 (2000): 627–662.
11. J. L. Beard and J. R. Connor, Iron status and neural functioning, *Annual Review of Nutrition* 23 (2003): 41–58.
12. World Health Organization, **http://www.who.int/nut/ida.htm**.
13. Iron deficiency—United States, 1999–2000, *Morbidity and Mortality Weekly Report* 51 (2002): 897–899.
14. L. Hallberg, Perspectives on nutritional iron deficiency, *Annual Review of Nutrition* 21 (2001): 1–21.
15. B. Annibale and coauthors, Reversal of iron deficiency anemia after *Helicobacter pylori* eradication in patients with asymptomatic gastritis, *Annals of Internal Medicine* 131 (1999): 668–672.
16. T. Brownlie and coauthors, Marginal iron deficiency without anemia impairs aerobic adaptation among previously untrained women, *American Journal of Clinical Nutrition* 75 (2002): 734–742.
17. J. Beard, Iron deficiency alters brain development and functioning, *Journal of Nutrition* 133 (2003): 1468S–1472S; E. M. Ross, Evaluation and treatment of iron deficiency in adults, *Nutrition in Clinical Care* 5 (2002): 220–224.
18. J. D. Haas and T. Brownlie, Iron deficiency and reduced work capacity: A critical review of the research to determine a causal relationship, *Journal of Nutrition* 131 (2001): 676S–690S.
19. A. L. M. Heath and S. J. Fairweather-Tait, Health implications of iron overload: The role of diet and genotype, *Nutrition Reviews* 61 (2003): 45–62.
20. R. E. Fleming and W. S. Sly, Mechanisms of iron accumulation in hereditary hemochromatosis, *Annual Review of Physiology* 64 (2002): 663–680; R. J. Wood, The "anemic" enterocyte in hereditary hemochromatosis: Molecular insights into the control of intestinal iron absorption, *Nutrition Reviews* 60 (2002): 144–148; M. J. Nowicki and B. R. Bacon, Hereditary hemochromatosis in siblings: Diagnosis by genotyping, *Pediatrics* 105 (2000): 426–429; A. S. Tavill, Clinical implications of the hemochromatosis gene, *New England Journal of Medicine* 341 (1999): 755–757.
21. B. Lachili and coauthors, Increased lipid peroxidation in pregnant women after iron and vitamin C supplementation, *Biological Trace Element Research* 83 (2001): 103–110; V. Herbert, S. Shaw, and E. Jayatilleke, Vitamin C–driven free radical generation from iron, *Journal of Nutrition* 126 (1996): 1213S–1220S.
22. U. Ramakrishnan, E. Kuklina, and A. D. Stein, Iron stores and cardiovascular disease risk factors in women of reproductive age in the United States, *American Journal of Clinical Nutrition* 76 (2002): 1256–1260;

C. T. Stempos and coauthors, Serum ferritin and death from all causes and cardiovascular disease: The NHANES II Mortality Study, National Health and Nutrition Examination Study, *Annals of Epidemiology* 10 (2000): 441–448; J. Danesh and P. Appleby, Coronary heart disease and iron status: Meta-analyses of prospective studies, *Circulation* 99 (1999): 852–854; B. de Valk and J. J. Marx, Iron, atherosclerosis, and ischemic heart disease, *Archives of Internal Medicine* 159 (1999): 1542–1548; K. Klipstein-Grobusch and coauthors, Serum ferritin and risk of myocardial infarction in the elderly: The Rotterdam Study, *American Journal of Clinical Nutrition* 69 (1999): 1231–1236.

23. J. L. Derstine and coauthors, Iron status in association with cardiovascular disease risk in 3 controlled feeding studies, *American Journal of Clinical Nutrition* 77 (2003): 56–62; K. Klipstein-Grobusch and coauthors, Dietary iron and risk of myocardial infarction in the Rotterdam Study, *American Journal of Epidemiology* 149 (1999): 421–428.
24. M. Shannon, Ingestion of toxic substances by children, *New England Journal of Medicine* 342 (2000): 186–191; C. C. Morris, Pediatric iron poisonings in the United States, *Southern Medicine Journal* 93 (2000): 352–358.
25. W. J. Bartfay and coauthors, Cytotoxic aldehyde generation in heart following acute iron-loading, *Journal of Trace Elements in Medicine and Biology* 14 (2000): 14–20; A. S. Ioannides and J. M. Panisello, Acute respiratory distress syndrome in children with acute iron poisoning: The role of intravenous desferrioxamine, *European Journal of Pediatrics* 159 (2000): 158–159; J. P. Pestaner and coauthors, Ferrous sulfate toxicity: A review of autopsy findings, *Biological Trace Element Research* 69 (1999): 191–198.
26. Committee on Dietary Reference Intakes, 2001, p. 351.
27. J. R. Backstrand, The history and future of food fortification in the United States: A public health perspective, *Nutrition Reviews* 60 (2002): 15–26.
28. S. Zlotkin and coauthors, Randomized, controlled trial of single versus 3-times-daily ferrous sulfate drops for treatment of anemia, *Pediatrics* 108 (2001): 613–616.
29. C. L. Adams and coauthors, Zinc absorption from a low-phytic acid maize, *American Journal of Clinical Nutrition* 76 (2002): 556–559.
30. T. A. Strand and coauthors, Effectiveness and efficacy of zinc for the treatment of acute diarrhea in young children, *Pediatrics* 109 (2002): 898–903; N. Bhandari and coauthors, Substantial reduction in severe diarrheal morbidity by daily zinc supplementation in young North Indian children, *Pediatrics* 109 (2002): e86; C. Duggan and W. Fawzi, Micronutrients and child health: Studies in international nutrition and HIV infection, *Nutrition Reviews* 59 (2001): 358–369; The Zinc Investigators' Collaborative Group, Therapeutic effects of oral zinc in acute and persistent diarrhea in children in developing countries: Pooled analysis of randomized controlled trials, *American Journal of Clinical Nutrition* 72 (2000): 1516–1522; R. B. Costello and J. Grumstrup-Scott, Zinc: What role might supplements play? *Journal of the American Dietetic Association* 100 (2000): 371–375.
31. B. H. McElroy and S. P. Miller, Effectiveness of zinc gluconate glycine lozenges (Cold-Eeze) against the common cold in school-aged subjects: A retrospective chart review, *American Journal of Therapeutics* 9 (2002): 472–475; I. Marshall, Zinc for the common cold, *Cochrane Database of Systematic Reviews* 2 (2000): CD001364; J. L. Jackson, E. Lesho, and C. Peterson, Zinc and the common cold: A meta-analysis revisited, *Journal of Nutrition* 130 (2000): 1512S–1515S; A. S. Prasad and coauthors, Duration of symptoms and plasma cytokine levels in patients with the common cold treated with zinc acetate: A randomized, double-blind, placebo-controlled trial, *Annals of Internal Medicine* 133 (2000): 245–252; R. B. Turner and W. E. Cetnarowski, Effect of treatment with zinc gluconate or zinc acetate on experimental and natural colds, *Clinical Infectious Diseases* 31 (2000): 1202–1208.
32. T. van den Briel and coauthors, Improved iodine status is associated with improved mental performance of schoolchildren in Benin, *American Journal of Clinical Nutrition* 72 (2000): 1179–1185.
33. D. M. Driscoll and P. R. Copeland, Mechanism and regulation of selenoprotein synthesis, *Annual Review of Nutrition* 23 (2003): 17–40.
34. J. W. Finley and C. D. Davis, Selenium (Se) from high-selenium broccoli is utilized differently than selenite, selanate and selenomethionine, but is more effective in inhibiting colon carcinogenesis, *Biofactors* 14 (2001): 191–196.
35. N. E. Hellman and J. D. Gitlin, Ceruloplasmin metabolism and function, *Annual Review of Nutrition* 22 (2002): 439–458.
36. Populations receiving optimally fluoridated public drinking water—United States, 2000, *Morbidity and Mortality Weekly Report* 51 (2002): 144–147.
37. Position of the American Dietetic Association: The impact of fluoride on health, *Journal of the American Dietetic Association* 101 (2001): 126–132.
38. Recommendations for using fluoride to prevent and control dental caries in the United States, *Morbidity and Mortality Weekly Report* 50 (2001): entire supplement.
39. Populations receiving optimally fluoridated public drinking water—United States, 2000, 2002.
40. M. D. Althuis and coauthors, Glucose and insulin responses to dietary chromium supplements: A meta-analysis, *American Journal of Clinical Nutrition* 76 (2002): 148–155; L. G. Trow and coauthors, Lack of effect of dietary chromium supplementation on glucose tolerance, plasma insulin and lipoprotein levels in patients with type 2 diabetes, *International Journal of Vitamin and Nutrition Research* 70 (2000): 14–18.
41. T. A. Devirian and S. L. Volpe, The physiological effects of dietary boron, *Critical Reviews in Food and Science Nutrition* 43 (2003): 219–231.
42. S. G. Selevan and coauthors, Blood lead concentration and delayed puberty in girls, *New England Journal of Medicine* 348 (2003): 1527–1536.
43. M. E. Moss, B. P. Lanphear, and P. A. Auinger, Association of dental caries and blood lead levels, *Journal of the American Medical Association* 281 (1999): 2294–2298.
44. R. L. Canfield and coauthors, Intellectual impairment in children with blood lead concentrations below 10 µg per deciliter, *New England Journal of Medicine* 348 (2003): 1517–1526.

ANSWERS

Nutrition Calculations

1. Iron: mg. Selenium: µg. Fluoride: mg.
   Zinc: mg. Copper: µg. Chromium: µg.
   Iodine: µg. Manganese: mg. Molybdenum: µg.
2. a. Sirloin steak > broccoli > green peas > bread > pork chop > cantaloupe > sweet potato > carrots > apple > cheese > milk.
   b.

Food	Iron Density (mg/kcal)
Milk, fat-free, 1 c	0.10 mg ÷ 85 kcal = 0.0012 mg/kcal
Cheddar cheese, 1 oz	0.19 mg ÷ 114 kcal = 0.0017 mg/kcal
Broccoli, cooked from fresh, chopped, 1 c	1.31 mg ÷ 44 kcal = 0.0298 mg/kcal
Sweet potato, baked in skin, 1 ea	0.51 mg ÷ 117 kcal = 0.0044 mg/kcal
Cantaloupe melon, ½	0.56 mg ÷ 93 kcal = 0.0060 mg/kcal
Carrots, from fresh, ½ c	0.48 mg ÷ 35 kcal = 0.0137 mg/kcal
Whole-wheat bread, 1 slice	0.87 mg ÷ 64 kcal = 0.0136 mg/kcal
Green peas, cooked from frozen, ½ c	1.26 mg ÷ 62 kcal = 0.0203 mg/kcal
Apple, medium	0.38 mg ÷ 125 kcal = 0.0030 mg/kcal
Sirloin steak, lean, 4 oz	3.81 mg ÷ 228 kcal = 0.0167 mg/kcal
Pork chop, lean broiled, 1 ea	0.66 mg ÷ 166 kcal = 0.0040 mg/kcal

   Broccoli > green peas > sirloin steak > carrots > bread > cantaloupe > sweet potato > pork chop > apple > cheese > milk.

   c. Broccoli, green peas, and carrots are all higher on the per-kcalorie list.

   d. They are all vegetables.

Study Questions (multiple choice)

1. b 2. b 3. c 4. c 5. d 6. d 7. c 8. b
9. a 10. c

HIGHLIGHT

Phytochemicals and Functional Foods

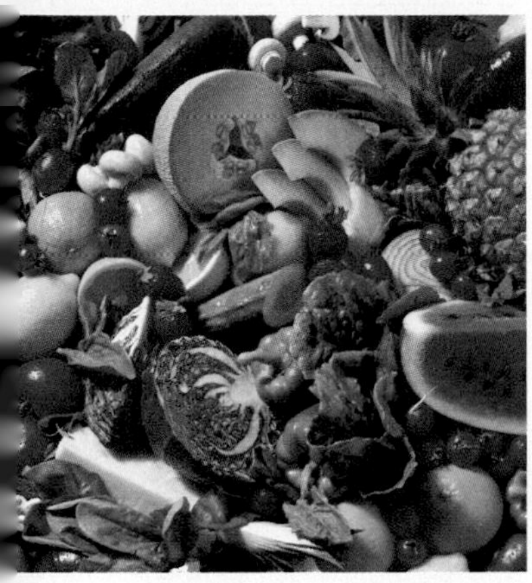

© John E. Kelly/FoodPix/Getty Images

Chapter 13 completes the introductory discussions on the six classes of nutrients—carbohydrates, lipids, proteins, vitamins, minerals, and water. In addition to these nutrients, foods contain thousands of nonnutrient compounds, including the phytochemicals. Chapter 1 introduced the phytochemicals as compounds found in plant-derived foods (*phyto* means plant) that have biological activity in the body. Research on phytochemicals is unfolding daily, adding to our knowledge of their roles in human health, but there are still many questions and only tentative answers. Just a few of the tens of thousands of phytochemicals have been researched at all, and only a sampling are mentioned in this highlight—enough to illustrate their wide variety of food sources and roles in supporting health.

The concept that foods provide health benefits beyond those of the nutrients emerged from numerous epidemiological studies showing the protective effects of plant-based diets on cancer and heart disease. People have been using foods to maintain health and prevent disease for years, but now these foods have been given a name—they are called **functional foods** (the accompanying glossary defines this and related terms). Much of this text touts the benefits of nature's functional foods—grains rich in dietary fibers, fish rich in omega-3 fatty acids, and fruits rich in phytochemicals, for example. This highlight begins with a look at some of these familiar functional foods, the phytochemicals they contain, and their roles in disease prevention. Then the discussion turns to examine the most controversial of functional foods—novel foods to which phytochemicals have been added to promote health.[1] How these foods fit into a healthy diet is still unclear.[2]

The Phytochemicals

In foods, phytochemicals impart tastes, aromas, colors, and other characteristics. They give hot peppers their burning sensation, garlic its pungent flavor, and tomatoes their dark red color. In the body, phytochemicals can have profound physiological effects, acting as antioxidants, mimicking hormones, and suppressing the development of diseases.[3] Table H13-1 (on p. 466) presents the names, possible effects, and food sources of some of the better-known phytochemicals.

Defending against Cancer

A variety of phytochemicals from a variety of foods appear to protect against DNA damage and defend the body against cancer.[4] A few examples follow.

GLOSSARY

flavonoids (FLAY-von-oyds): yellow pigments in foods; phytochemicals that may exert physiological effects on the body.

flaxseed: the small brown seed of the flax plant; used in baking, cereals, or other foods and valued by industry as a source of linseed oil and fiber.

functional foods: foods that contain physiologically active compounds that provide health benefits beyond basic nutrition; sometimes called *designer foods* or *nutraceuticals*.

lignans: phytochemicals present in flaxseed, but not in flax oil, that are converted to phytosterols by intestinal bacteria and are under study as possible anticancer agents.

lutein (LOO-teen): a plant pigment of yellow hue; a phytochemical believed to play roles in eye functioning and health.

lycopene (LYE-koh-peen): a pigment responsible for the red color of tomatoes and other red-hued vegetables; a phytochemical that may act as an antioxidant in the body.

phytoestrogens: plant-derived compounds that have structural and functional similarities to human estrogen. Phytoestrogens include genistein, daidzein, and glycitein.

phytosterols: plant-derived compounds that have structural similarities to cholesterol and lower blood cholesterol by competing with cholesterol for absorption. Phytosterols include sterol esters and stanol esters.

probiotics: microbial food ingredients that are beneficial to health. Nondigestible food ingredients that encourage the growth of favorable bacteria are called **prebiotics.**
- **pro** = for
- **bios** = life
- **pre** = before

yogurt: milk fermented by specific bacterial cultures.

Reminder: *Phytochemicals* are nonnutrient compounds found in plant-derived foods that have biological activity in the body.

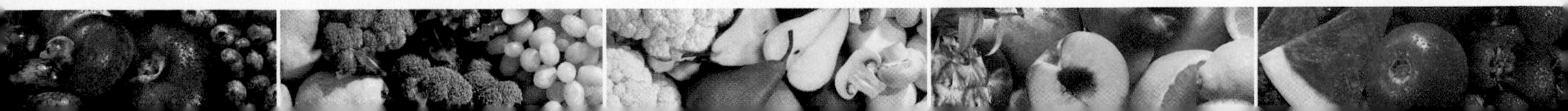

TABLE H13-1 Phytochemicals—Their Food Sources and Actions

Name	Possible Effects	Food Sources
Capsaicin	Modulates blood clotting, possibly reducing the risk of fatal clots in heart and artery disease.	Hot peppers
Carotenoids (include beta-carotene, lycopene, lutein, and hundreds of related compounds)[a]	Act as antioxidants, possibly reducing risks of cancer and other diseases.	Deeply pigmented fruits and vegetables (apricots, broccoli, cantaloupe, carrots, pumpkin, spinach, sweet potatoes, tomatoes)
Curcumin	May inhibit enzymes that activate carcinogens.	Tumeric, a yellow-colored spice
Flavonoids (include flavones, flavonols, isoflavones, catechins, and others)[b,c]	Act as antioxidants; scavenge carcinogens; bind to nitrates in the stomach, preventing conversion to nitrosamines; inhibit cell proliferation.	Berries, black tea, celery, citrus fruits, green tea, olives, onions, oregano, purple grapes, purple grape juice, soybeans and soy products, vegetables, whole wheat, wine
Indoles[d]	May trigger production of enzymes that block DNA damage from carcinogens; may inhibit estrogen action.	Broccoli and other cruciferous vegetables (brussels sprouts, cabbage, cauliflower), horseradish, mustard greens
Isothiocyanates (including sulforaphane)	Inhibit enzymes that activate carcinogens; trigger production of enzymes that detoxify carcinogens.	Broccoli and other cruciferous vegetables (brussels sprouts, cabbage, cauliflower), horseradish, mustard greens
Lignans[e]	Block estrogen activity in cells, possibly reducing the risk of cancer of the breast, colon, ovaries, and prostate.	Flaxseed and its oil, whole grains
Monoterpenes (include limonene)	May trigger enzyme production to detoxify carcinogens; inhibit cancer promotion and cell proliferation.	Citrus fruit peels and oils
Organosulfur compounds	May speed production of carcinogen-destroying enzymes; slow production of carcinogen-activating enzymes.	Chives, garlic, leeks, onions
Phenolic acids[c]	May trigger enzyme production to make carcinogens water soluble, facilitating excretion.	Coffee beans, fruits (apples, blueberries, cherries, grapes, oranges, pears, prunes), oats, potatoes, soybeans
Phytic acid	Binds to minerals, preventing free-radical formation, possibly reducing cancer risk.	Whole grains
Phytoestrogens (genistein and daidzein)	Estrogen inhibition may produce these actions: inhibit cell replication in GI tract; reduce risk of breast, colon, ovarian, prostate, and other estrogen-sensitive cancers; reduce cancer cell survival. Estrogen mimicking may reduce risk of osteoporosis.	Soybeans, soy flour, soy milk, tofu, textured vegetable protein, other legume products
Protease inhibitors	May suppress enzyme production in cancer cells, slowing tumor growth; inhibit hormone binding; inhibit malignant changes in cells.	Broccoli sprouts, potatoes, soybeans and other legumes, soy products
Resveratrol	Offsets artery-damaging effects of high-fat diets.	Red wine, peanuts
Saponins	May interfere with DNA replication, preventing cancer cells from multiplying; stimulate immune response.	Alfalfa sprouts, other sprouts, green vegetables, potatoes, tomatoes
Tannins[c]	May inhibit carcinogen activation and cancer promotion; act as antioxidants.	Black-eyed peas, grapes, lentils, red and white wine, tea

[a]Other carotenoids include alpha-carotene, beta-cryptoxanthin, and zeaxanthin.
[b]Other flavonoids of interest include ellagic acid and ferulic acid; see also *phytoestrogens*.
[c]A subset of the larger group *phenolic phytochemicals*.
[d]Indoles include dithiothiones, isothiocyantes, and others.
[e]Lignans act as phytosterols, but their food sources are limited.

Soybeans and products made from them correlate with low rates of cancer, especially cancers of the breast and prostate.[5] Soybeans—as well as **flaxseed** oil, whole grains, fruits, and vegetables—are a rich source of an array of phytochemicals, among them the **phytoestrogens.** Phytoestrogens are plant compounds that weakly mimic or modulate the effects of the steroid hormone estrogen in the body.[6] These phytoestrogens have antioxidant activity and appear to slow the growth of breast and prostate cancers.[7]

Tomatoes seem to offer protection against cancers of the esophagus, lung, prostate, and stomach. Among the phytochemicals responsible for this effect is **lycopene,** one of beta-carotene's many carotenoid relatives. Lycopene is the pigment that gives apricots, guava, papaya, pink grapefruits, and watermelon their red color—and it is especially abundant in tomatoes and cooked tomato products. Lycopene is a powerful antioxidant that seems to inhibit the growth of cancer cells.[8] Importantly, these benefits are seen when people eat *foods* containing lycopene-rich tomato products.[9]

Soybeans and tomatoes are only two of the many fruits and vegetables credited with providing anticancer activity. Researchers speculate that people might cut their risks of cancers

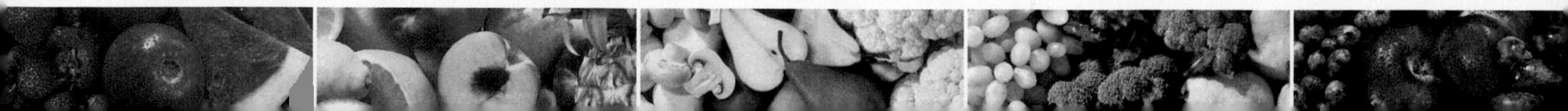

in half simply by eating the recommended amounts of fruits and vegetables each day.

Defending against Heart Disease

Diets based primarily on unprocessed foods appear to support heart health better than those founded on highly refined foods—perhaps because of the abundance of nutrients, fiber, or phytochemicals such as the **flavonoids.**[10] Flavonoids, a large group of phytochemicals known for their health-promoting qualities, are found in whole grains, legumes, soy, vegetables, fruits, herbs, spices, teas, chocolate, nuts, olive oil, and red wines.[11] Flavonoids are powerful antioxidants that may help to protect LDL cholesterol against oxidation and reduce blood platelet stickiness, making blood clots less likely.[12] An abundance of flavonoid-containing *foods* in the diet lowers the risks of chronic diseases.[13] Importantly, no claims can be made for flavonoids themselves as the protective factor, particularly when they are extracted from foods and sold as supplements.[14]

In addition to flavonoids, fruits and vegetables are rich in carotenoids. Studies suggest that a diet rich in carotenoids is also associated with a lower risk of heart disease.[15] Notable among the carotenoids that may defend against heart disease are **lutein** and lycopene.[16]

The **phytosterols** of soybeans and other vegetables may also protect against heart disease.[17] These cholesterol-like molecules are naturally found in all plants and inhibit cholesterol absorption in the body.[18] As a result, blood cholesterol levels decline. The phytoestrogens of soy may also protect against heart disease by acting as antioxidants and lowering blood pressure.[19]

The Phytochemicals in Perspective

Because foods deliver thousands of phytochemicals in addition to dozens of nutrients, researchers must be careful in giving credit for particular health benefits to any one compound. Diets rich in whole grains, legumes, vegetables, fruits, and nuts seem to be protective against heart disease and cancer, but identifying *the* specific foods or components of foods that are responsible is difficult.[20] Each food possesses a unique array of phytochemicals—citrus fruits provide monoterpenes; grapes, resveratrol; and flaxseed, **lignans.** Broccoli may contain as many as 10,000 different phytochemicals—each with the potential to influence some action in the body. Beverages such as wine, spices such as oregano, and oils such as olive oil contain phytochemicals that may explain, in part, why people who live in the Mediterranean region have reduced risks of heart disease.[21] Even identifying all of the phytochemicals and their effects doesn't answer all the questions because the actions of phytochemicals may be complementary or overlapping—which reinforces the principle of variety in diet planning.[22] For an appreciation of the array of phytochemicals offered by a variety of fruits and vegetables, see Figure H13-1 (on p. 468).

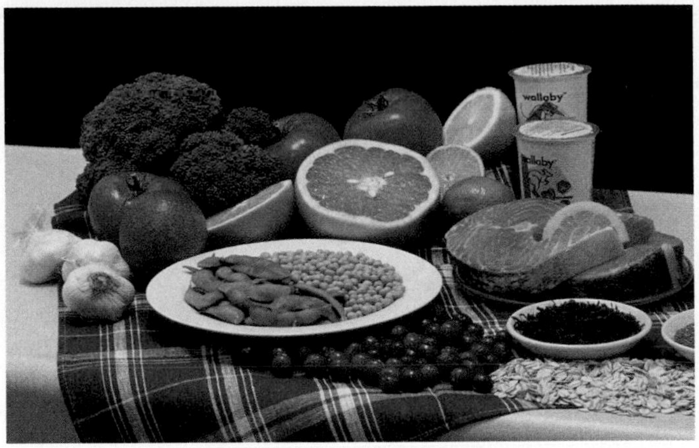
walaby

© Craig M. Moore

Nature offers a variety of functional foods that provide us with many health benefits.

Functional Foods

Because foods naturally contain thousands of phytochemicals that are biologically active in the body, virtually all of them have some special value in supporting health. In other words, even simple, whole foods, in reality, are functional foods. Cranberries may help protect against urinary tract infections; garlic may lower blood cholesterol; and tomatoes may protect against some cancers, just to name a few examples.[23] But that hasn't stopped food manufacturers from trying to create functional foods as well. The creation of more functional foods has become the fastest-growing trend and the greatest influence transforming the American food supply.[24]

Many processed foods become functional foods when they are fortified with nutrients or enhanced with phytochemicals or herbs (calcium-fortified orange juice, for example). Less frequently, an entirely new food is created, as in the case of a meat substitute made of mycoprotein—a protein derived from a fungus.*[25] This functional food not only provides dietary fiber, polyunsaturated fats, and high-quality protein, but it lowers LDL cholesterol, raises HDL cholesterol, improves glucose response, and prolongs satiety after a meal. Such a novel functional food raises the question—is it a food or a drug?

Foods as Pharmacy

Not too long ago, most of us could agree on what was a food and what was a drug. Today, functional foods blur the distinctions. They have characteristics similar to both foods and drugs, but do not fit neatly into either category.

*This mycoprotein product is marketed under the trade name Quorn (pronounced KWORN).

FIGURE H13-1 An Array of Phytochemicals in a Variety of Fruits and Vegetables

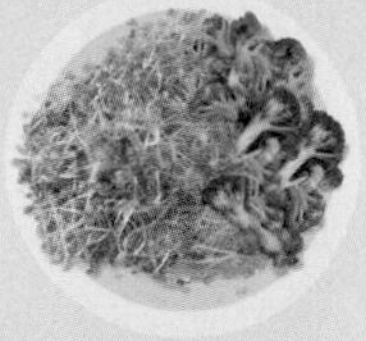

Broccoli and broccoli sprouts contain an abundance of the cancer-fighting phytochemical sulforaphane.

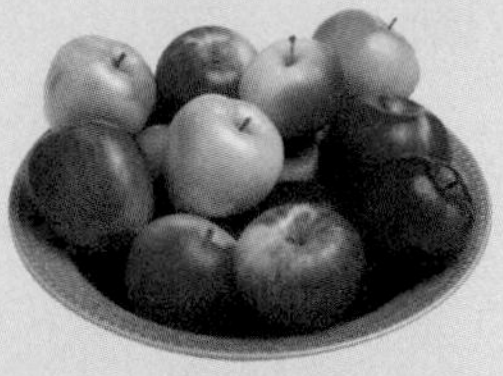

An apple a day—rich in flavonoids—may protect against lung cancer.

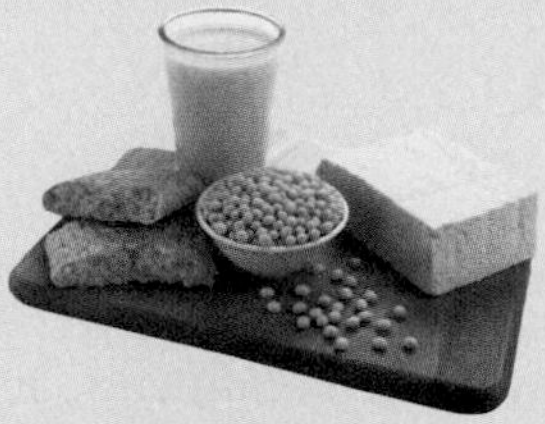

The phytoestrogens of soybeans seem to starve cancer cells and inhibit tumor growth; the phytosterols may lower blood cholesterol and protect cardiac arteries.

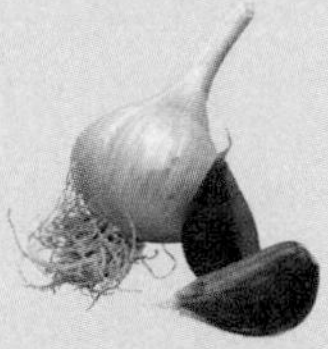

Garlic, with its abundant organosulfur compounds, may lower blood cholesterol and protect against stomach cancer.

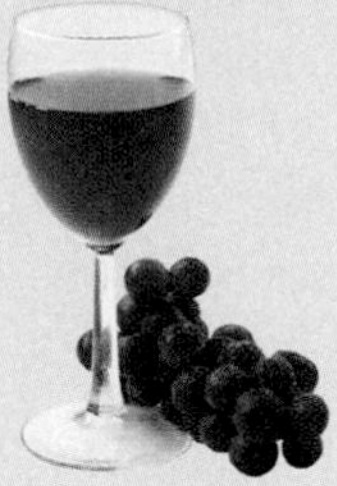

The phytochemical resveratrol found in grapes (and nuts) protects against cancer by inhibiting cell growth and against heart disease by limiting clot formation and inflammation.

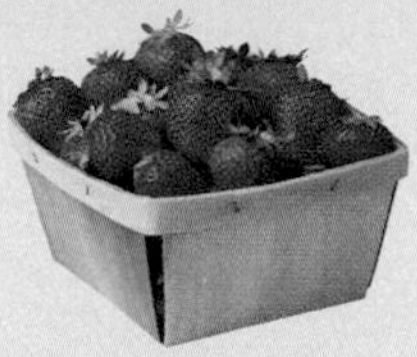

The ellagic acid of strawberries may inhibit certain types of cancer.

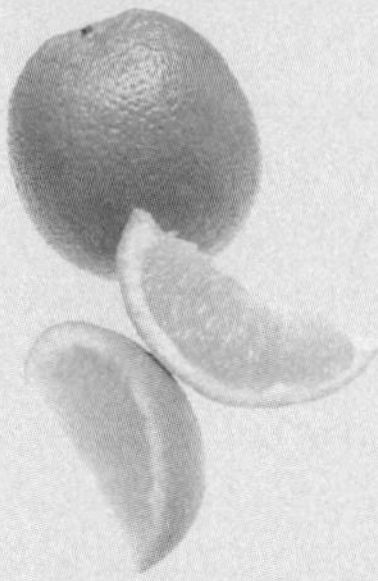

The monoterpenes of citrus fruits (and cherries) may inhibit cancer growth.

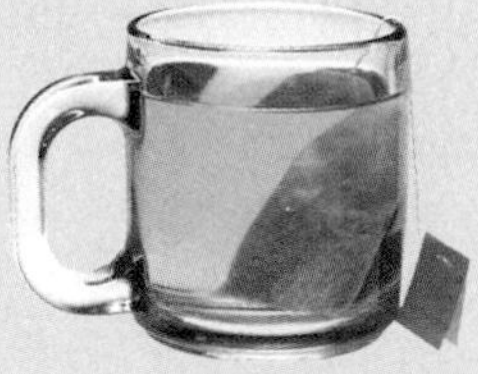

The flavonoids in black tea may protect against heart disease, whereas those in green tea may defend against cancer.

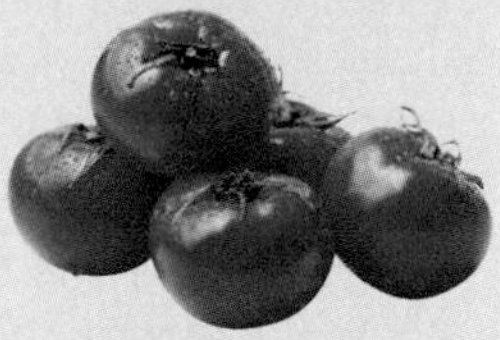

Tomatoes, with their abundant lycopene, may defend against cancer by protecting DNA from oxidative damage.

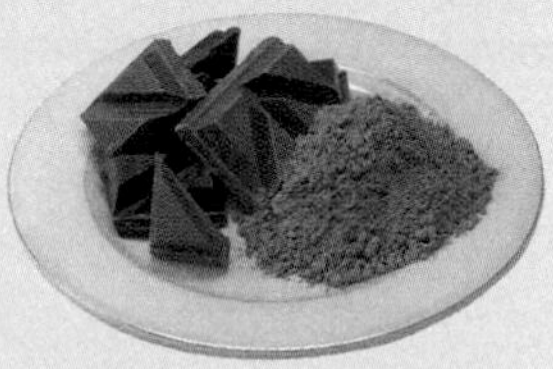

The flavonoids in cocoa and chocolate defend against oxidation and reduce the tendency of blood to clot.

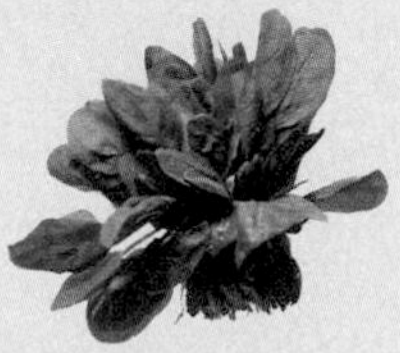

Spinach and other colorful vegetables contain the carotenoids lutein and zeaxanthin, which help protect the eyes against macular degeneration.

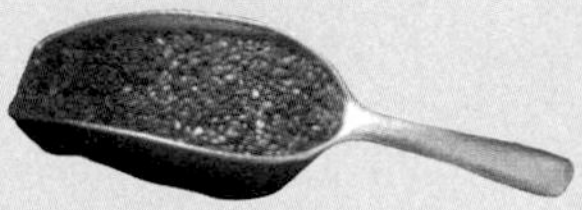

Flaxseed, the richest source of lignans, may prevent the spread of cancer.

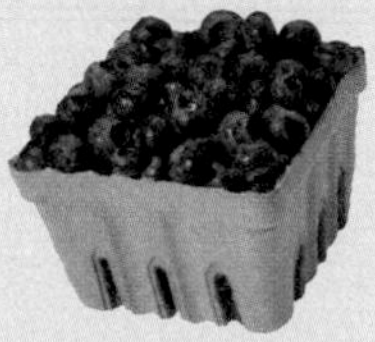

Blueberries, a rich source of flavonoids, improve memory in animals.

© Courtesy of Brassica Protection Products, © 2001 PhotoDisc, © EyeWire, Inc., Courtesy of Flax Council of Canada, Photodisc/Getty Images, Matthew Farruggio

Consider the healing powers of **yogurt,** for example. Yogurt contains *Lactobacillus* and other living bacteria that ferment milk into yogurt. These microorganisms, called **probiotics,** change the population of microbes in the GI tract, which improves defenses against GI disorders.[26] Research is under way to determine whether probiotics may help to alleviate diarrhea, inflammatory bowel disease, and lactose intolerance; enhance immune function; protect against GI cancer; and lower blood cholesterol.[27] As information on the potential benefits of probiotics unfolds, food manufacturers may begin to include these microorganisms in a variety of other foods. Food companies have already developed products with added phytochemicals. Consider margarine, for example.

Eating nonhydrogenated margarine sparingly instead of butter generously may lower blood cholesterol slightly over several months and clearly falls into the food category. Taking the drug Lipitor, on the other hand, lowers blood cholesterol significantly within weeks and clearly falls into the drug category. But margarine enhanced with a phytosterol that lowers blood cholesterol is in a gray area between the two. The margarine looks and tastes like a food, but it acts like a drug.

The use of functional foods as drugs creates a whole new set of diet-planning problems. Not only must foods provide an adequate intake of all the nutrients to support good health, but they must also deliver druglike ingredients to protect against disease. Like drugs used to treat chronic diseases, functional foods may need to be eaten several times a day for several months or years to have a beneficial effect. Sporadic users may be disappointed in the results. When used four times a day for four weeks, margarine enriched with phytosterols reduces cholesterol by 8 percent, much more than regular margarine does, but not nearly as much as the 32 percent reduction seen with cholesterol-lowering drugs.[28] For this reason, functional foods may be more useful for prevention and mild cases of disease than for intervention and more severe cases.

Foods and drugs differ dramatically in cost as well. Functional foods such as fruits and vegetables incur no added costs, of course, but foods that have been manufactured with added phytochemicals can be expensive, costing up to six times as much as their conventional counterparts. The price of functional foods typically falls between that of traditional foods and medicines.

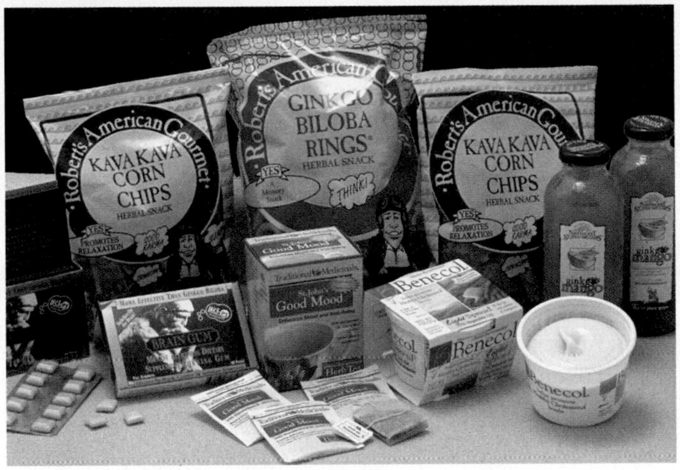
Robert's American Gourmet
KAVA KAVA CORN CHIPS
HERBAL SNACK
GINKGO BILOBA RINGS
Good Mood
Benecol

© Craig M. Moore

Functional foods currently on the market promise to "enhance mood," "promote relaxation and good karma," "increase alertness," and "improve memory," among other claims.

Unanswered Questions

To achieve a desired health effect, which is the better choice: to eat a food designed to affect some body function or simply to adjust the diet? Does it make more sense to use a margarine enhanced with a phytosterol that lowers blood cholesterol or simply to limit the amount of butter eaten?*[29] Is it smarter to eat eggs enriched with omega-3 fatty acids or to restrict egg consumption?[30] Might functional foods offer a sensible solution for improving our nation's health—if done correctly? Perhaps so—but there is a problem with functional foods: the food industry is moving too fast for either scientists or the Food and Drug Administration to keep up. Consumers were able to buy soup with St. John's wort that claimed to enhance mood and fruit juice with echinacea that was supposed to fight colds while scientists were still conducting their studies on these ingredients. Research to determine the safety and effectiveness of these substances is still in progress. Until this work is complete, consumers are on their own in finding the answers to the following questions:[31]

- *Does it work?* Research is generally lacking and findings are often inconclusive.
- *How much does it contain?* Food labels are not required to list the quantities of added phytochemicals. Even if they were, consumers have no standard for comparison and cannot deduce whether the amounts listed are a little or a lot. Most importantly, until research is complete, food manufacturers do not know what amounts (if any) are most effective—or most toxic.
- *Is it safe?* Functional foods can act like drugs. They contain ingredients that can alter body functions and cause allergies, drug interactions, drowsiness, and other side effects. Yet, unlike drug labels, food labels do not provide instructions for the dosage, frequency, or duration of treatment.
- *Is it healthy?* Adding phytochemicals to a food does not magically make it a healthy choice. A candy bar may be fortified with phytochemicals, but it is still made mostly of sugar and fat.

Critics suggest that the designation "functional foods" may be nothing more than a marketing tool. After all, even the most experienced researchers cannot yet identify the perfect combination of nutrients and phytochemicals to support optimal health. Yet manufacturers are freely experimenting with various concoctions as if they possessed that knowledge. Is it okay for them to sprinkle phytochemicals on fried snack foods and label them "functional," thus implying health benefits? Do we want our children receiving their nourishment from fortified caramel candies and chocolate cakes?

Future Foods

Nature has elegantly designed foods to provide us with a complex array of dozens of nutrients and thousands of additional compounds that may benefit health—most of which we have yet to identify or understand. Over the years, we have taken those foods and first deconstructed them and then reconstructed them in an effort to "improve" them. With new scientific understandings of how nutrients—and the myriad of other compounds in foods—interact with genes, we may someday be able to design foods to meet the *exact* health needs of *each* individual.[32] Indeed, our knowledge of the human

*Margarine products that lower blood cholesterol contain either sterol esters from vegetable oils, soybeans, and corn or stanol esters from wood pulp.

genome and of human nutrition may well merge to allow for specific recommendations for individuals based on their predisposition to diet-related diseases.[33]

If the present trend continues, then someday physicians may be able to prescribe the perfect foods to enhance your health, and farmers will be able to grow them. Scientists have already developed gene technology to alter the composition of food crops. They can grow rice enriched with vitamin A and tomatoes containing a hepatitis vaccine, for example. It seems quite likely that foods can be created to meet every possible human need. But then, in a sense, that was largely true 100 years ago when we relied on the bounty of nature.

NUTRITION ON THE NET

Access these websites for further study of topics covered in this highlight.

- Find updates and quick links to these and other nutrition-related sites at our website: **www.wadsworth.com/nutrition**
- Search for "functional foods" at the International Food Information Council: **www.ificinfo.org**
- Search for "functional foods" at the Center for Science in the Public Interest: **www.cspinet.org**
- Find out if warnings have been issued for any food ingredients at the FDA website: **www.fda.gov**

REFERENCES

1. J. A. Milner, Functional foods: The US perspective, *American Journal of Clinical Nutrition* 71 (2000): 1654S–1659S.
2. C. H. Halsted, Dietary supplements and functional foods: 2 sides of a coin? *American Journal of Clinical Nutrition* 77 (2003): 1001S–1007S.
3. P. M. Kris-Etherton and coauthors, Bioactive compounds in foods: Their role in the prevention of cardiovascular disease and cancer, *American Journal of Medicine* 113 (2002): 71S–88S.
4. C. S. Yang and coauthors, Inhibition of carcinogenesis by dietary polyphenolic compounds, *Annual Review of Nutrition* 21 (2001): 381–406; M. Abdulla and P. Gruber, Role of diet modification in cancer prevention, *Biofactors* 12 (2000): 45–51.
5. C. A. Lamartiniere, Protection against breast cancer with genistein: A component of soy, *American Journal of Clinical Nutrition* 71 (2000): 1705S–1707S.
6. I. C. Munro and coauthors, Soy isoflavones: A safety review, *Nutrition Reviews* 61 (2003): 1–33.
7. C. A. Lamartiniere and coauthors, Genistein chemoprevention: Timing and mechanisms of action in murine mammary and prostate, *Journal of Nutrition* 132 (2002): 552S–558S.
8. D. Heber and Q. Y. Lu, Overview of mechanisms of action of lycopene, *Experimental Biology and Medicine* 227 (2002): 920–923; T. M. Vogt and coauthors, Serum lycopene, other serum carotenoids, and risk of prostate cancer in US blacks and whites, *American Journal of Epidemiology* 155 (2002): 1023–1032; Q. Y. Lu and coauthors, Inverse associations between plasma lycopene and other carotenoids and prostate cancer, *Cancer Epidemiology, Biomarkers and Prevention* 10 (2001): 749–756.
9. E. Giovannucci and coauthors, A prospective study of tomato products, lycopene, and prostate cancer risk, *Journal of the National Cancer Institute* 94 (2002): 391–398; L. Chen and coauthors, Oxidative DNA damage in prostate cancer patients consuming tomato sauce–based entrees as a whole-food intervention, *Journal of the National Cancer Institute* 93 (2001): 1872–1879.
10. J. A. Ross and C. M. Kasum, Dietary flavonoids: Bioavailability, metabolic effects, and safety, *Annual Review of Nutrition* 22 (2002): 19–34.
11. F. M. Steinberg, M. M. Bearden, and C. L. Keen, Cocoa and chocolate flavonoids: Implications for cardiovascular health, *Journal of the American Dietetic Association* 103 (2003): 215–223; F. Visioli, and C. Galli, Biological properties of olive oil phytochemicals, *Critical Reviews in Food Science and Nutrition* 42 (2002): 209–221; Y. J. Surh, Anti-tumor promoting potential of selected spice ingredients with antioxidative and anti-inflammatory activities: A short review, *Food and Chemical Toxicology* 40 (2002): 1091–1097; J. M. Geleijnse and coauthors, Inverse association of tea and flavonoid intakes with incident myocardial infarction: The Rotterdam Study, *American Journal of Clinical Nutrition* 75 (2002): 880–886, C. L. Keen, Chocolate: Food as medicine/medicine as food, *Journal of the American College of Nutrition* 20 (2001): 436S–439S.
12. B. Fuhrman and M. Aviram, Flavonoids protect LDL from oxidation and attenuate atherosclerosis, *Current Opinion in Lipidology* 12 (2001): 41–48.
13. M. Messina, C. Gardner, and S. Barnes, Gaining insight into the health effects of soy but a long way still to go: Commentary on the Fourth International Symposium on the Role of Soy in Preventing and Treating Chronic Disease, *Journal of Nutrition* 132 (2002): 547S–551S; P. Knekt and coauthors, Flavonoid intake and risk of chronic diseases, *American Journal of Clinical Nutrition* 76 (2002): 560–568.
14. Ross and Kasum, 2002.
15. S. K. Osganian and coauthors, Dietary carotenoids and risk of coronary artery disease in women, *American Journal of Clinical Nutrition* 77 (2003): 1390–1399; S. Liu and coauthors, Intake of vegetables rich in carotenoids and risk of coronary heart disease in men: The Physicians' Heart Study, *International Journal of Epidemiology* 30 (2001): 130–135; S. B. Kritchevsky, beta-Carotene, carotenoids and the prevention of coronary heart disease, *Journal of Nutrition* 129 (1999): 5–8.
16. T. H. Rissanen and coauthors, Serum lycopene concentrations and carotid atherosclerosis: The Kuopio Ischaemic Heart Disease Risk Factor Study, *American Journal of Clinical Nutrition* 77 (2003): 133–138; Heber and Lu, 2002; J. H. Dwyer and coauthors, Oxygenated carotenoid lutein and progression of early atherosclerosis: The Los Angeles atherosclerosis study, *Circulation* 103 (2001): 2922–2927; L. Arab and S. Steck, Lycopene and cardiovascular disease, *American Journal of Clinical Nutrition* 71 (2000): 1691S–1695S.
17. R. E. Ostlund, Jr., Phytosterols in human nutrition, *Annual Review of Nutrition* 22 (2002): 533–549.
18. C. A. Vanstone and coauthors, Unesterified plant sterols and stanols lower LDL-cholesterol concentrations equivalently in hypercholesterolemic persons, *American Journal of Clinical Nutrition* 76 (2002): 1272–1278.
19. M. Rivas and coauthors, Soy milk lowers blood pressure in men and women with mild to moderate essential hypertension, *Journal of Nutrition* 132 (2002): 1900–1902.
20. Kris-Etherton and coauthors, 2002; C. M. Steinmaus, S. Nunez, and A. H. Smith, Diet and bladder cancer: A meta-analysis of six dietary variables, *American Journal of Epidemiology* 151 (2000): 693–702.
21. F. Visioli, A. Poli, and C. Gall, Antioxidant and other biological activities of phenols from olives and olive oil, *Medicinal Research Reviews* 22 (2002): 65–75; A. Trichopoulou, E. Vasilopoulou, and A. Lagiou, Mediterranean diet and coronary heart disease: Are antioxidants critical? *Nutrition Reviews* 57 (1999): 253–255.
22. J. W. Lampe, Health effects of vegetables and fruit: Assessing mechanism of action in human experimental studies, *American Journal of Clinical Nutrition* 70 (1999): 475S–490S.

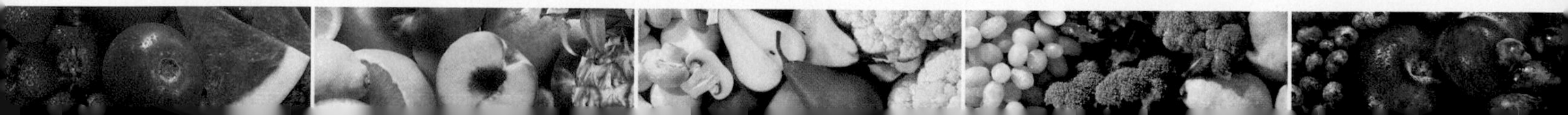

23. A. B. Howell and B. Foxman, Cranberry juice and adhesion of antibiotic resistant uropathogens, *Journal of the American Medical Association* 287 (2002): 3082–3083; C. W. Hadley and coauthors, Tomatoes, lycopene, and prostate cancer: Progress and promise, *Experimental Biology and Medicine* 227 (2002): 869–880; R. T. Ackermann and coauthors, Garlic shows promise for improving some cardiovascular risk factors, *Archives of Internal Medicine* 161 (2001): 813–824.
24. Position of the American Dietetic Association: Functional foods, *Journal of the American Dietetic Association* 99 (1999): 1278–1285.
25. T. Peregrin, Mycoprotein: Is America ready for a meat substitute derived from a fungus? *Journal of the American Dietetic Association* 102 (2002): 628.
26. M. E. Sanders, Probiotics: Considerations for human health, *Nutrition Reviews* 61 (2003): 91–99; M. H. Floch and J. Hong-Curtiss, Probiotics and functional foods in gastrointestinal disorders, *Current Gastroenterology Reports* 3 (2001): 343–350; Probiotics and prebiotics, *American Journal of Clinical Nutrition* (supplement) 73 (2001): entire issue.
27. J. M. Saavedra and A. Tschernia, Human studies with probiotics and prebiotics: Clinical implications, *British Journal of Nutrition* 87 (2002): S241–S246; P. Marteau and M. C. Boutron-Ruault, Nutritional advantages of probiotics and prebiotics, *British Journal of Nutrition* 87 (2002): S153–S157; G. T. Macfarlane and J. H. Cummings, Probiotics, infection and immunity, *Current Opinion in Infectious Diseases* 15 (2002): 501–506; L. Kopp-Hoolihan, Prophylactic and therapeutic uses of probiotics: A review, *Journal of the American Dietetic Association* 101 (2001): 229–238; M. B. Roberfroid, Prebiotics and probiotics: Are they functional foods? *American Journal of Clinical Nutrition* 71 (2000): 1682S–1687S.
28. L. A. Simons, Additive effect of plant sterol-ester margarine and cerivastatin in lowering low-density lipoprotein cholesterol in primary hypercholesterolemia, *American Journal of Cardiology* 90 (2002): 737–740.
29. P. Nestel and coauthors, Cholesterol-lowering effects of plant sterol esters and non-esterified stanols in margarine, butter and low-fat foods, *European Journal of Clinical Nutrition* 55 (2001): 1084–1090.
30. D. J. Farrell, Enrichment of hen eggs with n-3 long-chain fatty acids and evaluation of enriched eggs in humans, *American Journal of Clinical Nutrition* 68 (1998): 538–544.
31. C. Hasler and coauthors, How to evaluate the safety, efficacy, and quality of functional foods and their ingredients, *Journal of the American Dietetic Association* 101 (2001): 733–736; B. Brophy and D. Schardt, Functional foods, *Nutrition Action Healthletter,* April 1999, pp. 3–7.
32. J. A. Milner, Functional foods and health: A US perspective, *British Journal of Nutrition* 88 (2002): S151–S158.
33. C. M. Hasler, The changing face of functional foods, *Journal of the American College of Nutrition* 19 (2000): 499S–506S; I. H. Rosenberg, *What Is a Nutrient? Defining the Food-Drug Continuum* (Washington, D.C.: Center for Food and Nutrition Policy, 1999).

Chapter 14

Life Cycle Nutrition: Pregnancy and Lactation

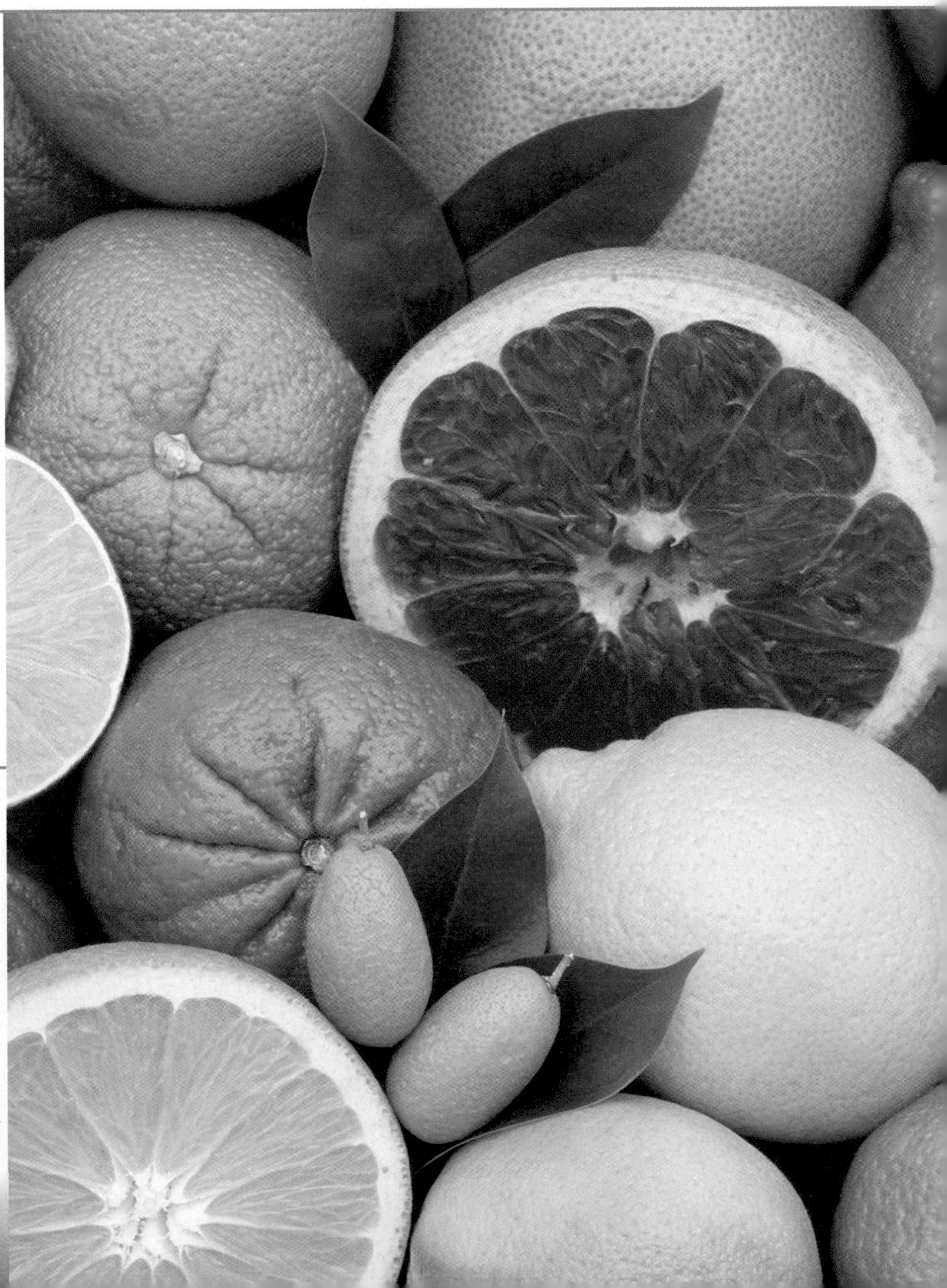

© Wally Eberhart/Botanica/Getty Images

Chapter Outline

Available Online

http://nutrition.wadsworth.com/uncn7

Nutrition Animation: *Nutrient Needs of Women and Infants*

Student Practice Test

Glossary Terms

Nutrition on the Net

Nutrition in Your Life

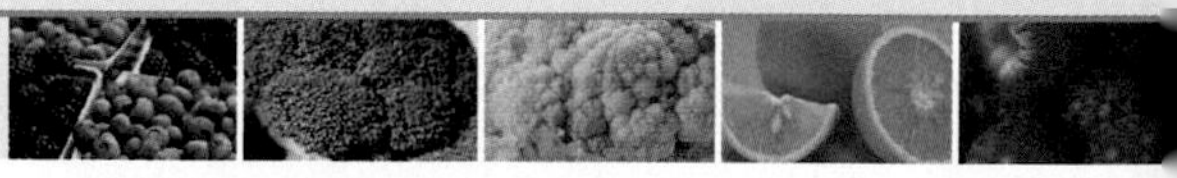

Food choices have consequences. Sometimes they happen immediately, as when you get heartburn after eating a pepperoni and jalapeño pizza. Other times they sneak up on you, as when you gain weight after indulging in double hot fudge sundaes. Quite often, they are temporary and easily resolved, as when hunger pangs strike after you drink only a diet cola for lunch. During pregnancy, however, the consequences of a woman's food choices are dramatic. They affect not only her health, but also the growth and development of another human being—not just for today, but for years to come. Making smart food choices is a huge responsibility, but fortunately, it's fairly simple.

All people—pregnant and lactating women, infants, children, adolescents, and adults—need the same nutrients, but the amounts they need vary depending on their stage of life. This chapter focuses on nutrition in preparation for, and support of, pregnancy and lactation. The next two chapters address the needs of infants, children, adolescents, and older adults.

Nutrition prior to Pregnancy

A section on nutrition prior to pregnancy must, by its nature, focus mainly on women. A man's nutrition may affect his **fertility** and possibly the genetic contributions he makes to his children, but nutrition exerts its primary influence through the woman. Her body provides the environment for the growth and development of a new human being. Prior to pregnancy, a woman has a unique opportunity to prepare herself physically, mentally, and emotionally for the many

fertility: the capacity of a woman to produce a normal ovum periodically and of a man to produce normal sperm; the ability to reproduce.

changes to come. In preparation for a healthy pregnancy, a woman can establish the following habits:

- *Achieve and maintain a healthy body weight.* Both underweight and overweight women, and their newborns, face increased risks of complications.
- *Choose an adequate and balanced diet.* Malnutrition reduces fertility and impairs the early development of an infant should a woman become pregnant.
- *Be physically active.* A women who wants to be physically active *when* she is pregnant needs to become physically active *beforehand.*
- *Avoid harmful influences.* Both maternal and paternal ingestion of harmful substances (such as cigarettes, alcohol, drugs, or environmental contaminants) can alter genes or their expression, interfering with fertility and causing abnormalities.

Young adults who nourish and protect their bodies do so not only for their own sakes, but also for future generations.

Growth and Development during Pregnancy

A whole new life begins at **conception.** Organ systems develop rapidly, and nutrition plays many supportive roles. This section describes placental development and fetal growth, paying close attention to times of intense developmental activity.

conception: the union of the male sperm and the female ovum; fertilization.

placenta (plah-SEN-tuh): the organ that develops inside the uterus early in pregnancy, through which the fetus receives nutrients and oxygen and returns carbon dioxide and other waste products to be excreted.

uterus (YOU-ter-us): the muscular organ within which the infant develops before birth.

amniotic (am-nee-OTT-ic) **sac:** the "bag of waters" in the uterus, in which the fetus floats.

umbilical (um-BILL-ih-cul) **cord:** the ropelike structure through which the fetus's veins and arteries reach the placenta; the route of nourishment and oxygen to the fetus and the route of waste disposal from the fetus. The scar in the middle of the abdomen that marks the former attachment of the umbilical cord is the **umbilicus** (um-BILL-ih-cus), commonly known as the "belly button."

ovum (OH-vum): the female reproductive cell, capable of developing into a new organism upon fertilization; commonly referred to as an egg.

sperm: the male reproductive cell, capable of fertilizing an ovum.

zygote (ZY-goat): the product of the union of ovum and sperm; so-called for the first two weeks after fertilization.

implantation: the stage of development in which the zygote embeds itself in the wall of the uterus and begins to develop; occurs during the first two weeks after conception.

Placental Development

In the early days of pregnancy, a spongy structure known as the **placenta** develops in the **uterus.** Two associated structures also form (see Figure 14-1). One is the **amniotic sac,** a fluid-filled balloonlike structure that houses the developing fetus. The other is the **umbilical cord,** a ropelike structure containing fetal blood vessels that extends through the fetus's "belly button" (the umbilicus) to the placenta. These three structures play crucial roles during pregnancy and then are expelled from the uterus during childbirth.

The placenta develops as an interweaving of fetal and maternal blood vessels embedded in the uterine wall. The maternal blood transfers oxygen and nutrients to the fetus's blood and picks up fetal waste products. By exchanging oxygen, nutrients, and waste products, the placenta performs the respiratory, absorptive, and excretory functions that the fetus's lungs, digestive system, and kidneys will provide after birth.

The placenta is a versatile, metabolically active organ. Like all body tissues, the placenta uses energy and nutrients to support its work. Like a gland, it produces an array of hormones that maintain pregnancy and prepare the mother's breasts for lactation (making milk). A healthy placenta is essential for the developing fetus to attain its full potential.

Fetal Growth and Development

Fetal development begins with the fertilization of an **ovum** by a **sperm.** Three stages follow: the zygote, the embryo, and the fetus (see Figure 14-2).

The Zygote The newly fertilized ovum, or **zygote,** begins as a single cell and divides to become many cells during the days after fertilization. Within two weeks, the zygote embeds itself in the uterine wall—a process known as **implantation.** Cell division continues—each set of cells divides into many other cells. As development proceeds, the zygote becomes an embryo.

FIGURE 14-1 The Placenta and Associated Structures

To understand how placental villi absorb nutrients without maternal and fetal blood interacting directly, think of how the intestinal villi work. The GI side of the intestinal villi is bathed in a nutrient-rich fluid (chyme). The intestinal villi absorb the nutrient molecules and release them into the body via capillaries. Similarly, the maternal side of the placental villi is bathed in nutrient-rich maternal blood. The placental villi absorb the nutrient molecules and release them to the fetus via fetal capillaries.

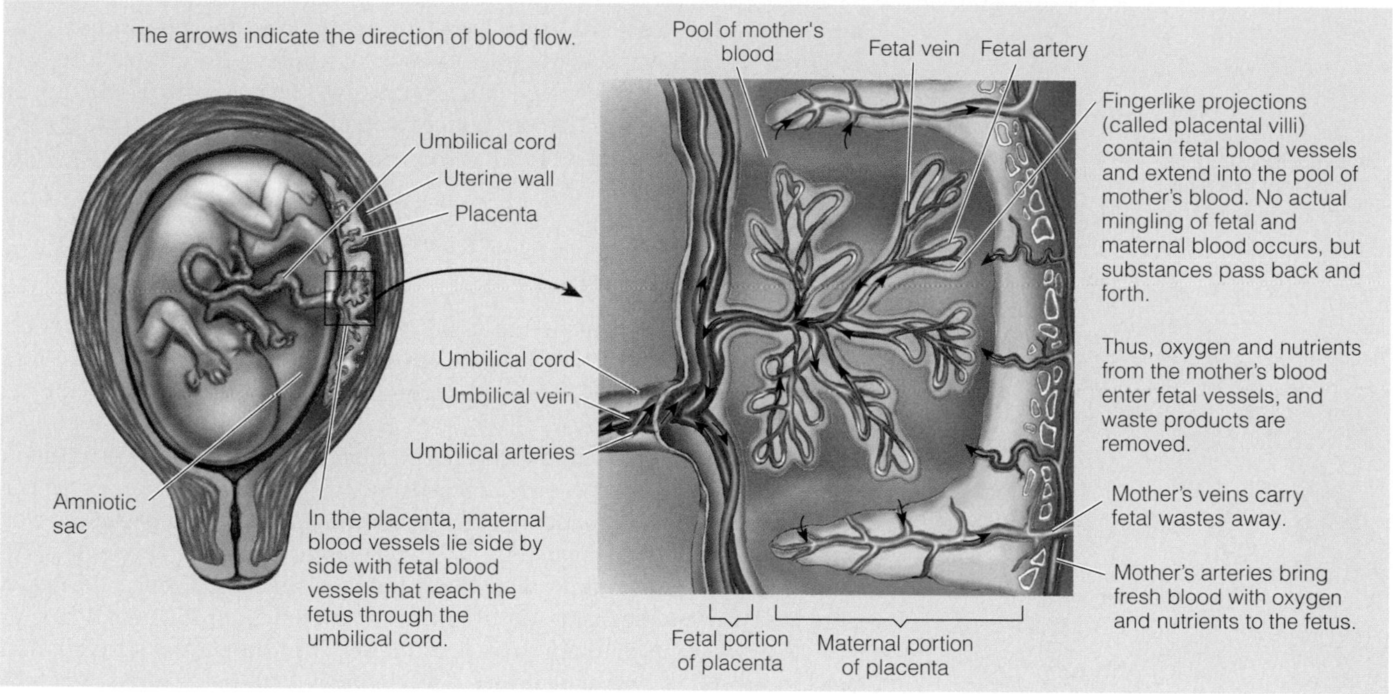
The arrows indicate the direction of blood flow.
Umbilical cord
Uterine wall
Placenta
Amniotic sac
In the placenta, maternal blood vessels lie side by side with fetal blood vessels that reach the fetus through the umbilical cord.
Pool of mother's blood
Fetal vein
Fetal artery
Umbilical cord
Umbilical vein
Umbilical arteries
Fingerlike projections (called placental villi) contain fetal blood vessels and extend into the pool of mother's blood. No actual mingling of fetal and maternal blood occurs, but substances pass back and forth.
Thus, oxygen and nutrients from the mother's blood enter fetal vessels, and waste products are removed.
Mother's veins carry fetal wastes away.
Mother's arteries bring fresh blood with oxygen and nutrients to the fetus.
Fetal portion of placenta
Maternal portion of placenta

FIGURE 14-2 Stages of Embryonic and Fetal Development

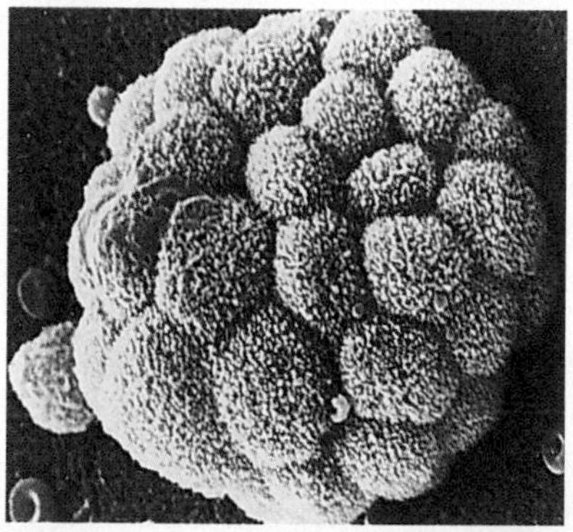

1 A newly fertilized ovum is about the size of a period at the end of this sentence. This **zygote** at less than one week after fertilization is not much bigger and is ready for implantation.

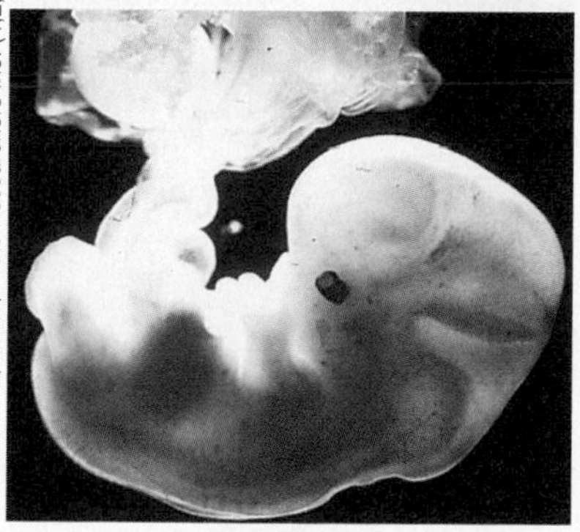

2 After implantation, the placenta develops and begins to provide nourishment to the developing embryo. An **embryo** five weeks after fertilization is about ½ inch long.

© Petit Format/Nestle/Photo Researchers Inc. (1,2,3)

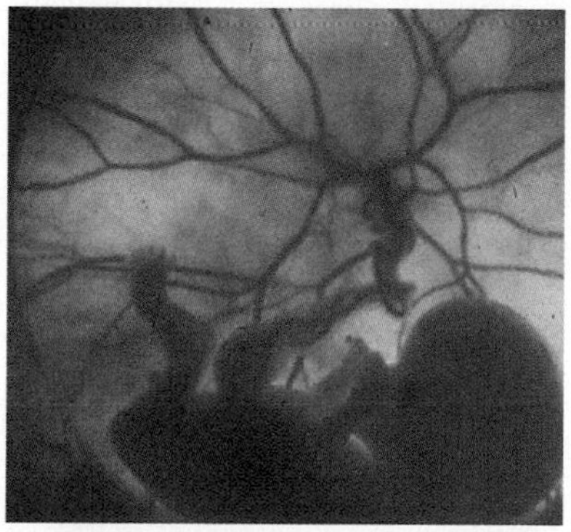

3 A **fetus** after 11 weeks of development is just over an inch long. Notice the umbilical cord and blood vessels connecting the fetus with the placenta.

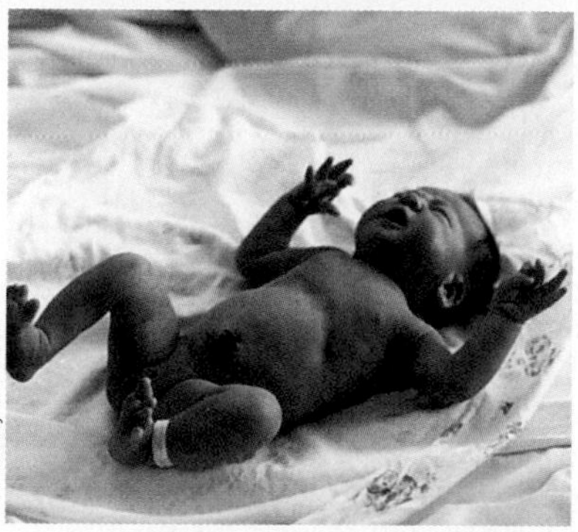

4 A **newborn infant** after nine months of development measures close to 20 inches in length. From eight weeks to term, this infant grew 20 times longer and 50 times heavier.

© Anthony M. Vanelli

FIGURE 14-3 The Concept of Critical Periods

Critical periods occur early in development. An adverse influence felt early can have a much more severe and prolonged impact than one felt later on.

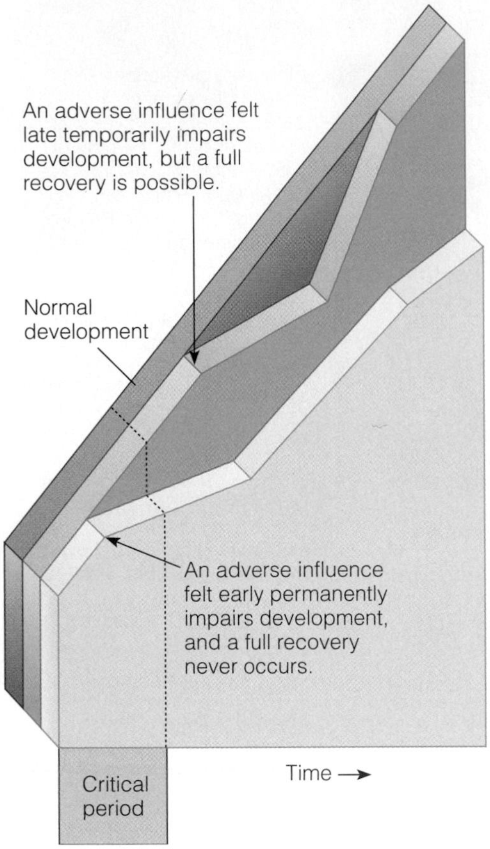
An adverse influence felt late temporarily impairs development, but a full recovery is possible.
Normal development
An adverse influence felt early permanently impairs development, and a full recovery never occurs.
Critical period
Time →

■ Reminder: The *neural tube* is the structure that eventually becomes the brain and spinal cord.

The Embryo The **embryo** develops at an amazing rate. At first, the number of cells in the embryo doubles approximately every 24 hours; later the rate slows, and only one doubling occurs during the final ten weeks of pregnancy. The embryo's size changes very little, but at eight weeks, the 1¼-inch embryo has a complete central nervous system, a beating heart, a digestive system, well-defined fingers and toes, and the beginnings of facial features.

The Fetus The **fetus** continues to grow during the next seven months. Each organ grows to maturity according to its own schedule, with greater intensity at some times than at others. As Figure 14-2 shows, fetal growth is phenomenal: weight increases from less than an ounce to about 7½ pounds (3500 grams). Most successful pregnancies last 39 to 41 weeks and produce a healthy infant weighing between 6½ and 9 pounds.

Critical Periods

Times of intense development and rapid cell division are called **critical periods**—critical in the sense that those cellular activities can occur only at those times. If cell division and number are limited during a critical period, full recovery is not possible (see Figure 14-3).

Each organ and tissue is most vulnerable to adverse influences (such as nutrient deficiencies or toxins) during its own critical period (see Figure 14-4). The critical period for neural tube■ development, for example, is from 17 to 30 days **gestation.** Consequently, neural tube development is most vulnerable to nutrient deficiencies, nutrient excesses, or toxins during this critical time—when most women do not even realize that they are pregnant. Any abnormal development of the neural tube or its failure to close completely can cause a major defect in the central nervous system. Figure 14-5 shows photos of neural tube development in the early weeks of gestation.

FIGURE 14-4 Critical Periods of Development

During embryonic development (from 2 to 8 weeks), many of the tissues are in their critical periods (purple area of the bars); events occur that will have irreversible effects on the development of those tissues. In the later stages of development (green area of the bars), the tissues continue to grow and change, but the events are less critical in that they are relatively minor or reversible.

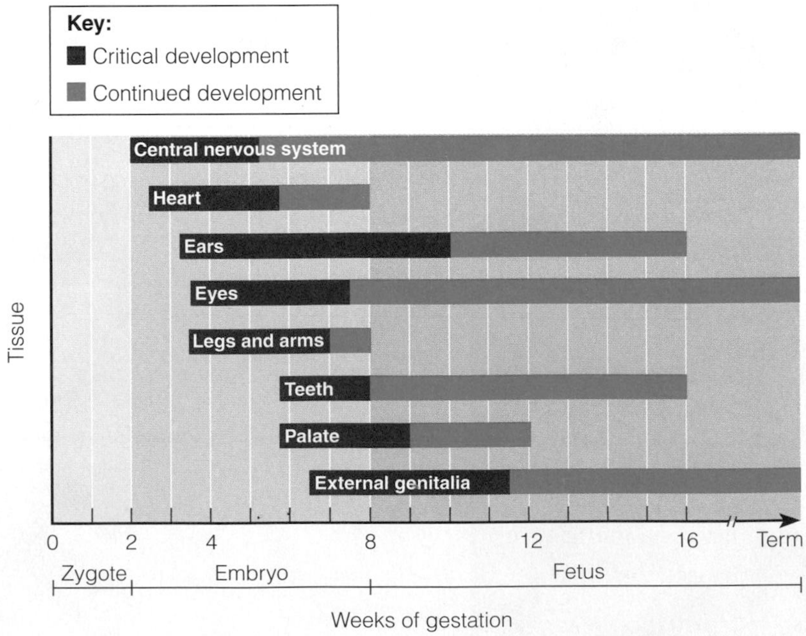
Key:
Critical development
Continued development
Central nervous system
Heart
Ears
Eyes
Legs and arms
Teeth
Palate
External genitalia
Tissue
0
2
4
8
12
16
Term
Zygote
Embryo
Fetus
Weeks of gestation

SOURCE: Adapted with permission from *Before We Were Born* by K. L. Moore. (Philadelphia: W. B. Saunders, 1974).

embryo (EM-bree-oh): the developing infant from two to eight weeks after conception.

fetus (FEET-us): the developing infant from eight weeks after conception until term.

critical periods: finite periods during development in which certain events occur that will have irreversible effects on later developmental stages; usually a period of rapid cell division.

gestation (jes-TAY-shun): the period from conception to birth. For human beings, the average length of a healthy gestation is 40 weeks. Pregnancy is often divided into thirds, called **trimesters.**

FIGURE 14-5 Neural Tube Development

The neural tube is the beginning structure of the brain and spinal cord. Any failure of the neural tube to close or to develop normally results in central nervous system disorders such as spina bifida and anencephaly. Successful development of the neural tube depends, in part, on the vitamin folate.

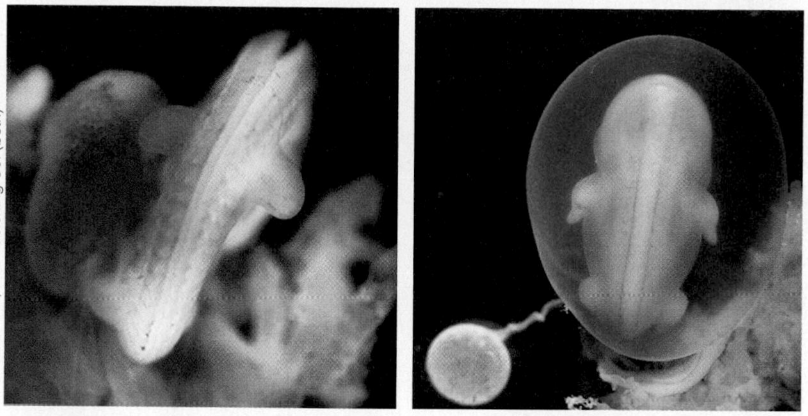

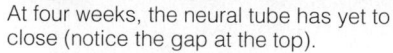

At four weeks, the neural tube has yet to close (notice the gap at the top).

At six weeks, the neural tube (outlined by the delicate red vertebral arteries) has successfully closed.

Neural Tube Defects In the United States, approximately 30 of every 100,000 infants are born with a **neural tube defect;** some 1000 or so infants are affected each year.* Many other pregnancies with neural tube defects end in abortions or stillbirths.

The two most common types of neural tube defects are anencephaly and spina bifida. In **anencephaly,** the upper end of the neural tube fails to close. Consequently, the brain is either missing or fails to develop. Pregnancies affected by anencephaly often end in miscarriage; infants born with anencephaly die shortly after birth.

Spina bifida is characterized by incomplete closure of the spinal cord and its bony encasement (see Figure 14-6 on p. 478). The meninges membranes covering the spinal cord often protrude as a sac, which may rupture and lead to meningitis, a life-threatening infection. Spina bifida is accompanied by varying degrees of paralysis, depending on the extent of the spinal cord damage. Mild cases may not even be noticed, but severe cases lead to death. Common problems include clubfoot, dislocated hip, kidney disorders, curvature of the spine, muscle weakness, mental handicaps, and motor and sensory losses.

A pregnancy affected by a neural tube defect can occur in any woman, but these factors make it more likely:

- A previous pregnancy affected by a neural tube defect.
- Maternal diabetes (type 1).
- Maternal use of antiseizure medications.
- Maternal obesity.
- Exposure to high temperatures early in pregnancy (prolonged fever or hot-tub use).
- Race/ethnicity (neural tube defects are more common among whites and Hispanics than among others).
- Low socioeconomic status.

Folate supplementation reduces the risk.

neural tube defect: a serious central nervous system birth defect that often results in lifelong disability or death.

anencephaly (AN-en-SEF-a-lee): an uncommon and always fatal type of neural tube defect; characterized by the absence of a brain.
- **an** = not (without)
- **encephalus** = brain

spina (SPY-nah) **bifida** (BIFF-ih-dah): one of the most common types of neural tube defects; characterized by the incomplete closure of the spinal cord and its bony encasement.
- **spina** = spine
- **bifida** = split

*Worldwide, some 300,000 to 400,000 infants are born with neural tube defects each year.

FIGURE 14-6 Spina Bifida

Spina bifida, a common neural tube defect, occurs when the vertebrae of the spine fail to close around the spinal cord, leaving it unprotected. The B vitamin folate helps prevent spina bifida and other neural tube defects.

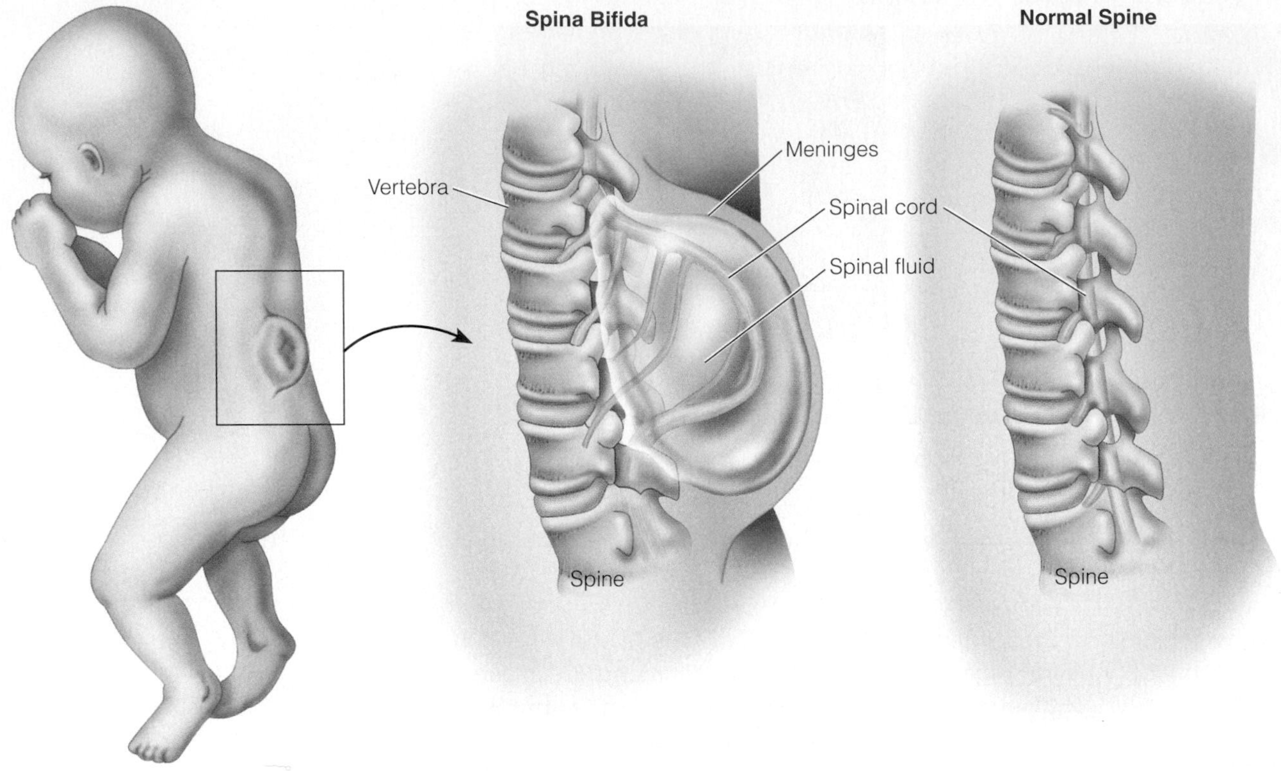
Spina Bifida
Normal Spine
Meninges
Vertebra
Spinal cord
Spinal fluid
Spine
Spine

SOURCE: From the *Journal of the American Medical Association,* June 20, 2001, Vol. 285, No. 23, p. 3050. Reprinted with permission of the American Medical Association.

Folate Supplementation Chapter 10 described how folate supplements taken one month before conception and continued throughout the first trimester can help prevent neural tube defects. For this reason, all women of childbearing age■ who are capable of becoming pregnant should consume 400 micrograms (0.4 milligram) of folate daily. Most over-the-counter multivitamin supplements contain 400 micrograms of folate; prenatal supplements usually contain at least 800 micrograms. A woman who has previously had an infant with a neural tube defect may be advised by her physician to take folate supplements in doses ten times larger—4 milligrams daily. Because high doses of folate can mask the pernicious anemia of a vitamin B_{12} deficiency, quantities of 1 milligram or more require a prescription.

Because half of the pregnancies each year are unplanned and because neural tube defects occur early in development before most women realize they are pregnant, grain products in the United States are fortified with folate to ensure an adequate intake. Labels on fortified products may claim that an "adequate intake of folate has been shown to reduce the risk of neural tube defects." Fortification has improved folate status in women of childbearing age and lowered the number of neural tube defects that occur each year, as Figure 10-10 on p. 339 shows.[1]

■ Folate RDA:
- For women: 400 μg (0.4 mg)/day.
- During pregnancy: 600 μg (0.6 mg)/day.

2005 *Dietary Guidelines:*
- Consume adequate synthetic folate from fortified foods and supplements in addition to naturally occurring folate from a variety of foods.

HEALTHY PEOPLE 2010

Reduce the occurrence of spina bifida and other neural tube defects. Increase the proportion of pregnancies begun with an optimum folate level.

Chronic Diseases Some research suggests that adverse influences at critical times set the stage for chronic diseases in adult life.[2] Poor maternal diet during critical periods may permanently alter body functions such as blood pressure, glucose tolerance, and immune functions that influence disease development.[3] For example, maternal malnutrition may alter blood vessel growth and program lipid metabolism and lean body mass development in such a way that the infant will develop risk factors for cardiovascular disease as an adult.[4]

Malnutrition during the critical period of pancreatic cell growth provides an example of how type 2 diabetes may develop in adulthood.[5] The pancreatic cells responsible for producing insulin (the beta cells) normally increase more than 130-fold between 12 weeks gestation and five months after birth. Nutrition is a primary determinant of beta cell growth, and infants who have suffered prenatal malnutrition have significantly fewer beta cells than well-nourished infants. They are also more likely to be low-birthweight infants—and low birthweight correlates with a high risk of type 2 diabetes during adulthood.[6] One hypothesis suggests that diabetes may develop from the interaction of inadequate nutrition early in life with abundant nutrition later in life: the small mass of beta cells developed in lean times during fetal development may be insufficient in times of overnutrition during adulthood when the body needs more insulin.

Hypertension may develop from a similar scenario of inadequate growth during placental and gestational development followed by accelerated growth during early childhood: the small mass of kidney cells developed in lean times may be insufficient to handle the excessive demands of later life.[7] Low-birthweight infants who gain weight rapidly as young children are likely to develop hypertension and heart disease as adults.[8]

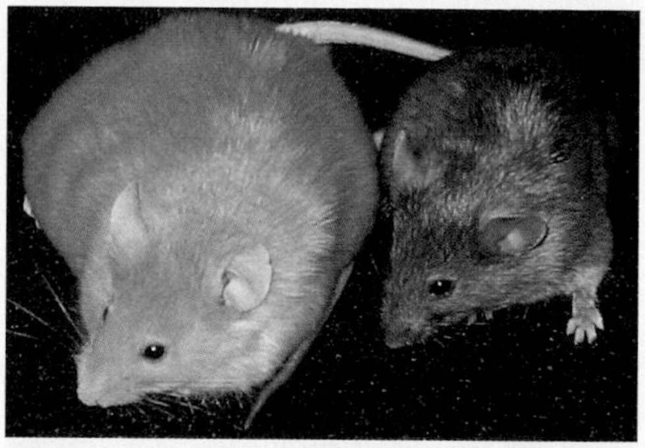
© Jirtle and Waterland

Both of these mice have the gene that tends to produce fat, yellow pups, but their mothers had different diets. The mother of the mouse on the right received a dietary supplement, which silenced the gene, resulting in brown pups with normal appetites.

Fetal Programming Recent genetic research may help to explain this phenomenon of substances such as nutrients influencing the development of diseases later on in adulthood—a process known as **fetal programming.** Researchers know that simply having a certain gene does not ensure that its associated trait will be expressed; the gene has to be activated.[9] (Similarly, owning lamps does not ensure you will have light in your home unless you turn them on.) Nutrients play key roles in activating or silencing genes. Switching genes on and off does not change the genetic sequence itself,■ but it can have dramatic consequences for a person's health. In the case of pregnancy, the mother's nutrition can permanently change gene expression in her fetus as well.[10]

■ The study of heritable changes in gene function that occur without a change in the DNA sequence is called **epigenetics.**

Whether silencing or activating a gene is good or bad depends on what the gene does. Silencing a gene that stimulates cancer growth, for example, would be good, but silencing a gene that suppresses cancer growth would be bad. Similarly, activating a gene that defends against obesity would be good, but activating a gene that promotes obesity would be bad. Much research is under way to determine which nutrients activate or silence which genes.

IN SUMMARY Maternal nutrition before and during pregnancy affects both the mother's health and the infant's growth. As the infant develops through its three stages—the zygote, embryo, and fetus—its organs and tissues grow, each on its own schedule. Times of intense development are critical periods that depend on nutrients to proceed smoothly. Without folate, for example, the neural tube fails to develop completely during the first month of pregnancy, prompting recommendations that all women of childbearing age take folate daily.

Because critical periods occur throughout pregnancy, a woman should continuously take good care of her health. That care should include achieving and maintaining a healthy body weight prior to pregnancy and gaining sufficient weight during pregnancy to support a healthy infant.

fetal programming: the influence of substances during fetal growth on the development of diseases in later life.

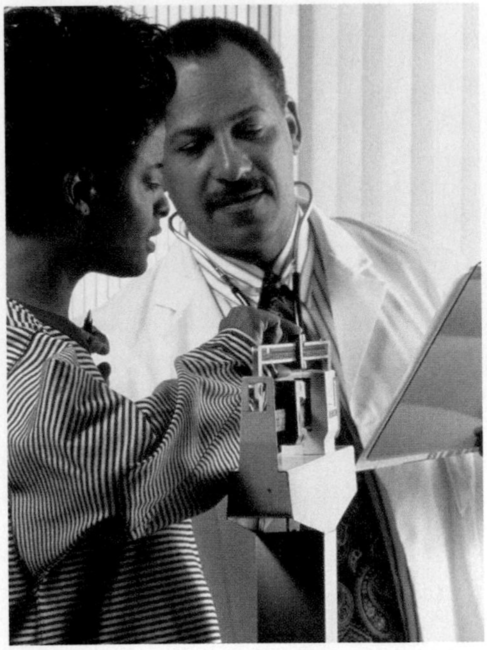

Fetal growth and maternal health depend on a sufficient weight gain during pregnancy.

Maternal Weight

Birthweight is the most reliable indicator of an infant's health. As a later section of this chapter explains, an underweight infant is more likely to have physical and mental defects, become ill, and die than a normal-weight infant. In general, higher birthweights present fewer risks for infants. Two characteristics of the mother's weight influence an infant's birthweight: her weight *prior* to conception and her weight gain *during* pregnancy.

Weight prior to Conception

A woman's weight prior to conception influences fetal growth. Even with the same weight gain during pregnancy, underweight women tend to have smaller babies than heavier women.

Underweight An underweight woman has a high risk of having a low-birthweight infant, especially if she is unable to gain sufficient weight during pregnancy. In addition, the rates of **preterm** births and infant deaths are higher for underweight women. An underweight woman improves her chances of having a healthy infant by gaining sufficient weight prior to conception or by gaining extra pounds during pregnancy. To gain weight, an underweight woman can follow the dietary recommendations for pregnant women (described in Figure 14-11 on p. 486).

Overweight and Obesity Overweight and obesity also create problems related to pregnancy and childbirth.[11] Obese women have an especially high risk of medical complications such as hypertension, gestational diabetes, and postpartum infections.[12] Compared with other women, obese women are also more likely to have other complications of labor and delivery.[13]

Overweight women have the lowest rate of low-birthweight infants. In fact, infants of overweight women are more likely to be born **post term** and to weigh more than 9 pounds.■ Large newborns increase the likelihood of a difficult labor and delivery, birth trauma, and **cesarean section.** Consequently, these infants have a greater risk of poor health and death than infants of normal weight.

■ The term **macrosomia** (mak-roh-SO-me-ah) describes high-birthweight infants (roughly 9 lb, or 4000 g, or more); macrosomia results from prepregnancy obesity, excessive weight gain during pregnancy, or uncontrolled diabetes.
- **macro** = large
- **soma** = body

Of greater concern than infant birthweight is the poor development of infants born to obese mothers. Obesity may double the risk for neural tube defects. In addition, both overweight and obese women have a greater risk of giving birth to infants with heart defects and other abnormalities.[14]

Weight-loss dieting during pregnancy is never advisable. Overweight women should try to achieve a healthy body weight before becoming pregnant, avoid excessive weight gain during pregnancy, and postpone weight loss until after childbirth. Weight loss is best achieved by eating moderate amounts of nutrient-dense foods and exercising to lose body fat.

Weight Gain during Pregnancy

All pregnant women must gain weight—fetal growth and maternal health depend on it. Maternal weight gain during pregnancy correlates closely with infant birthweight, which is a strong predictor of the health and subsequent development of the infant.

Recommended Weight Gains Table 14-1 presents recommended weight gains for various prepregnancy weights. The recommended gain for a woman who begins pregnancy at a healthy weight and is carrying a single fetus is 25 to 35 pounds. An underweight woman needs to gain between 28 and 40 pounds; and an overweight woman, between 15 and 25 pounds. Some women should strive for gains at the upper end of the target range, notably, adolescents who are still growing themselves and black women whose infants tend to be smaller than white infants even with the same maternal weight gain. Short women (5 feet 2 inches and under) should strive for gains at the lower end of the target range. Women who are

preterm (infant): an infant born prior to the 38th week of pregnancy; also called a **premature infant.** A **term** infant is born between the 38th and 42nd week of pregnancy.

post term (infant): an infant born after the 42nd week of pregnancy.

cesarean section: a surgically assisted birth involving removal of the fetus by an incision into the uterus, usually by way of the abdominal wall.

TABLE 14-1 Recommended Weight Gains Based on Prepregnancy Weight

Prepregnancy Weight	Recommended Weight Gain
Underweight (BMI <18.5)	28 to 40 lb (12.5 to 18.0 kg)
Healthy weight (BMI 18.5 to 24.9)	25 to 35 lb (11.5 to 16.0 kg)
Overweight (BMI 25.0 to 29.9)	15 to 25 lb (7.0 to 11.5 kg)
Obese (BMI ≥30)	15 lb minimum (6.8 kg minimum)

NOTE: These classifications for BMI are slightly different from those developed in 1990 by the Committee on Nutritional Status during Pregnancy and Lactation for the publication *Nutrition during Pregnancy* (Washington, D.C.: National Academy Press). That committee acknowledged that because such classifications had not been validated by research on pregnancy outcome, "any cut off points will be arbitrary for women of reproductive age." For these reasons, it seems appropriate to use the values developed for adults in 1998 by the National Institutes of Health (see Chapter 8).

carrying twins should aim for a weight gain of 35 to 45 pounds. If a woman gains more than is recommended early in pregnancy, she should not restrict her energy intake later in order to lose weight. A large weight gain over a short time, however, indicates excessive fluid retention and may be the first sign of the serious medical complication preeclampsia, discussed later.

Increase the proportion of mothers who achieve a recommended weight gain during their pregnancies.

HEALTHY PEOPLE 2010

Weight-Gain Patterns For the normal-weight woman, weight gain ideally follows a pattern of 3½ pounds during the first trimester and 1 pound per week thereafter. Health care professionals monitor weight gain using a prenatal weight-gain grid (see Figure 14-7).

Components of Weight Gain Women often express concern about the weight gain that accompanies a healthy pregnancy. They may find comfort in a reminder that most of the gain supports the growth and development of the placenta,

FIGURE 14-7 Recommended Prenatal Weight Gain Based on Prepregnancy Weight

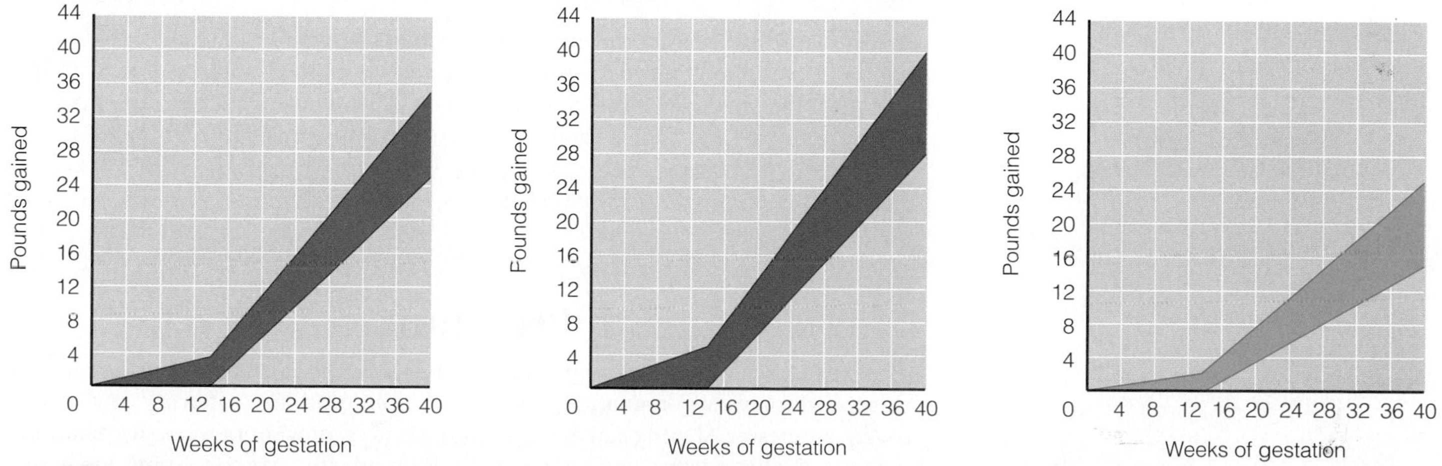
Pounds gained
44 40 36 32 28 24 20 16 12 8 4 0
4 8 12 16 20 24 28 32 36 40
Weeks of gestation
Founds gained
Weeks of gestation
Pounds gained
Weeks of gestation

Normal-weight women should gain about 3½ pounds in the first trimester and just under 1 pound/week thereafter, achieving a total gain of 25 to 35 pounds by term.

Underweight women should gain about 5 pounds in the first trimester and just over 1 pound/week thereafter, achieving a total gain of 28 to 40 pounds by term.

Overweight women should gain about 2 pounds in the first trimester and ⅔ pound/week thereafter, achieving a total gain of 15 to 25 pounds.

FIGURE 14-8 Components of Weight Gain during Pregnancy

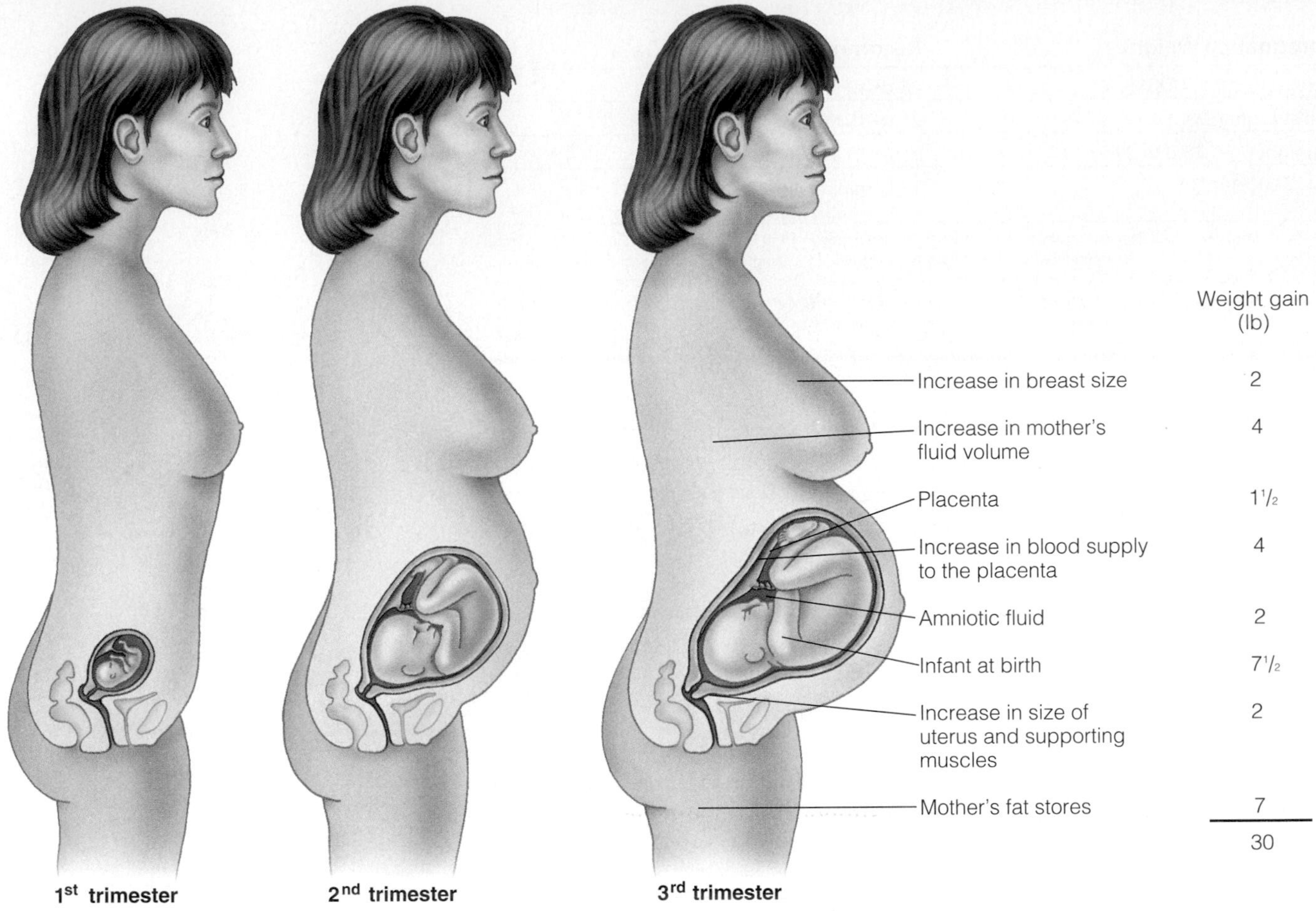
Weight gain (lb)
Increase in breast size 2
Increase in mother's fluid volume 4
Placenta 1½
Increase in blood supply to the placenta 4
Amniotic fluid 2
Infant at birth 7½
Increase in size of uterus and supporting muscles 2
Mother's fat stores 7
30
1st trimester
2nd trimester
3rd trimester

uterus, blood, and breasts, as well as an optimally healthy 7½-pound infant. A small amount goes into maternal fat stores, and even that fat is there for a special purpose: to provide energy for labor and lactation. Figure 14-8 shows the components of a typical 30-pound weight gain.

Weight Loss after Pregnancy The pregnant woman loses some weight at delivery. In the following weeks, she loses more as her blood volume returns to normal and she sheds accumulated fluids. The typical woman does not, however, return to her prepregnancy weight. In general, the more weight a woman gains beyond the needs of pregnancy, the more she will retain. Even with an average weight gain, though, most women tend to retain a couple of pounds with each pregnancy.

Exercise during Pregnancy

An active, physically fit woman experiencing a normal pregnancy can continue to exercise throughout pregnancy, adjusting the duration and intensity as the pregnancy progresses. Staying active can improve fitness, prevent or manage gestational diabetes, facilitate labor, and reduce stress. Women who exercise during pregnancy report fewer discomforts throughout their pregnancies. Regular exercise develops the strength and endurance a woman needs to carry the extra weight through pregnancy and to labor through an intense delivery. It also maintains the habits that help a woman lose excess weight and get back into shape after the birth.

FIGURE 14-9 Exercise Guidelines during Pregnancy

DO

Do exercise regularly (at least three times a week).

Do warm up with 5 to 10 minutes of light activity.

Do exercise for 20 to 30 minutes at your target heart rate.

Do cool down with 5 to 10 minutes of slow activity and gentle stretching.

Do drink water before, after, and during exercise.

Do eat enough to support the additional needs of pregnancy plus exercise.

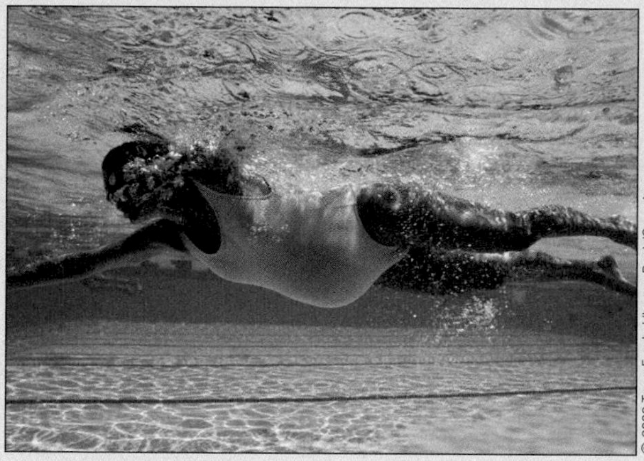

Pregnant women can enjoy the benefits of exercise.

DON'T

Don't exercise vigorously after long periods of inactivity.

Don't exercise in hot, humid weather.

Don't exercise when sick with fever.

Don't exercise while lying on your back after the first trimester of pregnancy or stand motionless for prolonged periods.

Don't exercise if you experience any pain or discomfort.

Don't participate in activities that may harm the abdomen or involve jerky, bouncy movements.

A pregnant woman should participate in "low-impact" activities■ and avoid sports in which she might fall or be hit by other people or objects. For example, playing singles tennis with one person on each side of the net is safer than a fast-moving game of racquetball in which the two competitors can collide. Swimming and water aerobics are particularly beneficial because they allow the body to remain cool and move freely with the water's support, thus reducing back pain.[15] Figure 14-9 provides some guidelines for exercise during pregnancy.[16] Several of the guidelines are aimed at preventing excessively high internal body temperature and dehydration, both of which can harm fetal development. To this end, pregnant women should also stay out of saunas, steam rooms, and hot whirlpools.

■ 2005 *Dietary Guidelines:*
- Healthy pregnant women should incorporate 30 minutes or more of moderately intense physical activity on most, if not all, days of the week and avoid activities with a high risk of falling or abdominal trauma.

IN SUMMARY A healthy pregnancy depends on a sufficient weight gain. Women who begin their pregnancies at a healthy weight need to gain about 30 pounds, which covers the growth and development of the placenta, uterus, blood, breasts, and infant. By remaining active throughout pregnancy, a woman can develop the strength she needs to carry the extra weight and maintain habits that will help her lose it after the birth.

Nutrition during Pregnancy

A woman's body changes dramatically during pregnancy. Her uterus and its supporting muscles increase in size and strength; her blood volume increases by half to carry the additional nutrients and other materials; her joints become more flexible in preparation for childbirth; her feet swell in response to high concentrations of the hormone estrogen, which promotes water retention and helps to ready the uterus for delivery; and her breasts enlarge in preparation for lactation. The hormones that mediate all these changes may influence her mood. She can best prepare to handle these changes given a nutritious diet, regular physical activity, plenty of rest, and caring companions. This section highlights the role of nutrition.

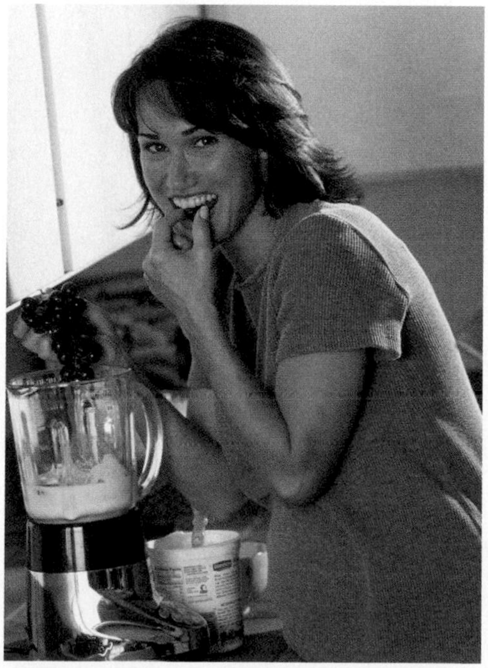

A pregnant woman's food choices support both her health and her infant's growth and development.

Energy and Nutrient Needs during Pregnancy

From conception to birth, all parts of the infant—bones, muscles, organs, blood cells, skin, and other tissues—are made from nutrients in the foods the mother eats. For most women, nutrient needs during pregnancy and lactation■ are higher than at any other time (see Figure 14-10). To meet the high nutrient demands of pregnancy, a woman will need to make careful food choices, but her body will also help by maximizing absorption and minimizing losses.[17]

■ The table on the inside front cover provides separate listings for women during pregnancy and lactation, reflecting their heightened nutrient needs.

Energy The energy needs of pregnant women are greater than those of nonpregnant women—an additional 340 kcalories during the second trimester and an extra 450 kcalories during the third.■ Underweight women and physically active women may require more. A woman can easily get these added kcalories with nutrient-dense selections from the five food groups. Table 2-3 (on p. 46) provides suggested dietary patterns for several kcalorie levels, and Figure 14-11 (on p. 486) presents a sample menu for pregnant and lactating women. Alternatively, a woman who has been neglecting her calcium needs may want to use her additional kcalories for milk and milk products. A variety of strategies are appropriate in meeting the energy demands of pregnancy.[18]

■ Energy requirement during pregnancy:
- 2nd trimester: +340 kcal/day.
- 3rd trimester: +450 kcal/day.

For a 2000-kcalorie daily intake, these added kcalories represent about 15 to 20 percent more food energy than before pregnancy. The increase in nutrient needs is often greater than this, so nutrient-dense foods should supply the extra kcalories: foods such as whole-grain breads and cereals, legumes, dark green vegetables, citrus fruits, low-fat milk and milk products, and lean meats, fish, poultry, and eggs. Ample carbohydrate (ideally, 175 grams or more per day and certainly no less than 135 grams) is necessary to fuel the fetal brain and spare the protein needed for growth.

Protein The protein RDA■ for pregnancy is an additional 25 grams per day higher than for nonpregnant women. Pregnant women can easily meet their protein needs by selecting meats, milk products, and protein-containing plant foods such as legumes, whole grains, nuts, and seeds. Use of high-protein supplements during pregnancy may be harmful and is discouraged.

■ Protein RDA during pregnancy:
- +25 g/day.

Essential Fatty Acids The high nutrient requirements of pregnancy leave little room in the diet for excess fat, but the essential long-chain polyunsaturated fatty acids are particularly important to the growth and development of the fetus.[19] The brain is largely made of lipid material, and it depends heavily on the long-chain omega-3 and omega-6 fatty acids for its growth, function, and structure. (See Table 5-2 on p. 161 for a list of good food sources of the omega fatty acids.)

Nutrients for Blood Production and Cell Growth New cells are laid down at a tremendous pace as the fetus grows and develops. At the same time, the mother's red blood cell mass expands. All nutrients are important in these processes, but for folate, vitamin B_{12}, iron, and zinc, the needs are especially great due to their key roles in the synthesis of DNA and new cells.

The requirement for folate increases dramatically during pregnancy.■ It is best to obtain sufficient folate from a combination of supplements, fortified foods, and a diet that includes fruits, juices, green vegetables, and whole grains.[20] The "How to" feature in Chapter 10 on p. 338 describes how folate from each of these sources contributes to a day's intake.

■ Folate RDA during pregnancy:
- 600 μg/day.

The pregnant woman also has a slightly greater need for the B vitamin that activates the folate enzyme—vitamin B_{12}.■ Generally, even modest amounts of meat, fish, eggs, or milk products together with body stores easily meet the need for vitamin B_{12}. Vegans who exclude all foods of animal origin, however, need daily supplements of vitamin B_{12} or vitamin B_{12}–fortified foods to prevent the neurological complications of a deficiency.

■ Vitamin B_{12} RDA during pregnancy:
- 2.6 μg/day.

Pregnant women need iron■ to support their enlarged blood volume and to provide for placental and fetal needs. The developing fetus draws on maternal iron stores to create stores of its own to last through the first four to six months after birth

■ Iron RDA during pregnancy:
- 27 mg/day.

FIGURE 14-10 Comparison of Nutrient Recommendations for Nonpregnant, Pregnant, and Lactating Women

For actual values, turn to the table on the inside front cover.

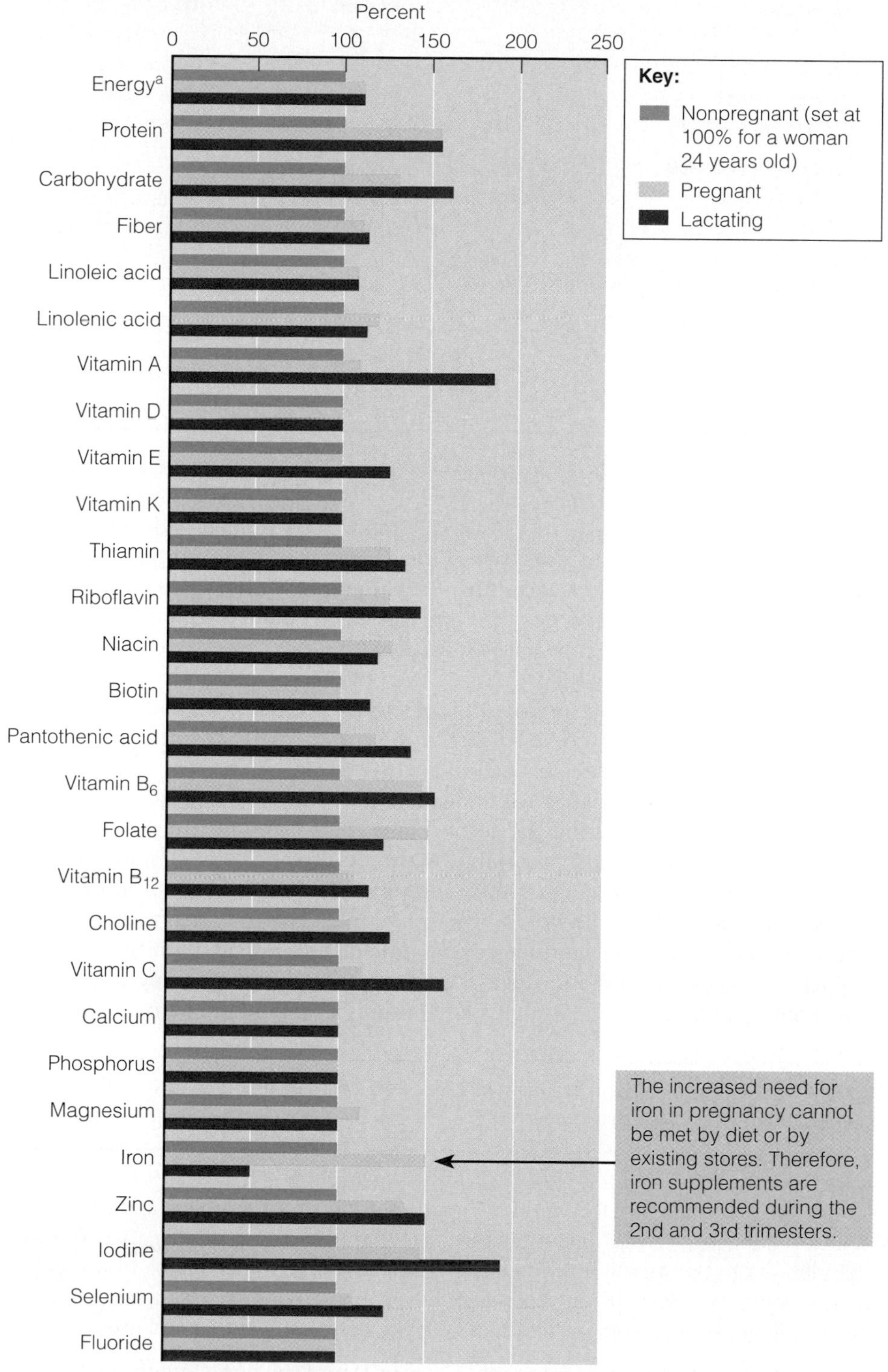

Percent
0
50
100
150
200
250
Energy[a]
Protein
Carbohydrate
Fiber
Linoleic acid
Linolenic acid
Vitamin A
Vitamin D
Vitamin E
Vitamin K
Thiamin
Riboflavin
Niacin
Biotin
Pantothenic acid
Vitamin B_6
Folate
Vitamin B_{12}
Choline
Vitamin C
Calcium
Phosphorus
Magnesium
Iron
Zinc
Iodine
Selenium
Fluoride
Key:
Nonpregnant (set at 100% for a woman 24 years old)
Pregnant
Lactating
The increased need for iron in pregnancy cannot be met by diet or by existing stores. Therefore, iron supplements are recommended during the 2nd and 3rd trimesters.

[a]Energy allowance during pregnancy is for 2nd trimester; energy allowance during the 3rd trimester is slightly higher; no additional allowance is provided during the 1st trimester. Energy allowance during lactation is for the first 6 months; energy allowance during the second 6 months is slightly higher.

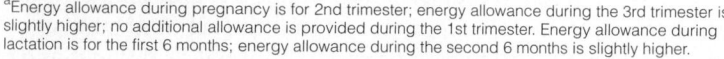

Available Online

Examine how pregnancy and lactation alter the nutrient needs of women, and examine the nutrient needs of infants.

FIGURE 14-11 Daily Food Choices for Pregnant and Lactating Women

SAMPLE MENU

Breakfast
1 whole-wheat English muffin
2 tbs peanut butter
1 c low-fat vanilla yogurt
1/2 c fresh strawberries
1 c orange juice

Midmorning snack
1/2 c cranberry juice
1 oz pretzels

Lunch
Sandwich (tuna salad on whole-wheat bread)
1/2 carrot (sticks)
1 c low-fat milk

Dinner
Chicken cacciatore
3 oz chicken
1/2 c stewed tomatoes
1 c rice
1/2 c summer squash
1 1/2 c salad (spinach, mushrooms, carrots)
1 tbs salad dressing
1 slice Italian bread
2 tsp soft margarine
1 c low-fat milk

NOTE: This sample meal plan provides about 2500 kcalories (55% from carbohydrate, 20% from protein, and 25% from fat) and meets most of the vitamin and mineral needs of pregnant and lactating women.

when milk, which lacks iron, will be its sole food. Even women with inadequate stores transfer significant amounts of iron, suggesting that the iron needs of the fetus have priority over those of the mother.[21] In addition, the blood losses inevitable at birth, especially during a cesarean section, can further drain the mother's supply.*

During pregnancy, the body makes several adaptations to help meet the exceptionally high need for iron. Menstruation, the major route of iron loss in women, ceases, and iron absorption improves thanks to an increase in blood transferrin, the body's iron-absorbing and iron-carrying protein. Without sufficient intake, though, iron stores would quickly dwindle.

Few women enter pregnancy with adequate iron stores, so a daily iron supplement is recommended during the second and third trimesters for all pregnant women. For this reason, most prenatal supplements provide 30 to 60 milligrams of iron a day. To enhance iron absorption, the supplement should be taken between meals or at bedtime and with liquids other than milk, coffee, or tea, which inhibit iron absorption. (Drinking orange juice does not enhance iron absorption from supplements as it does from foods; vitamin C enhances iron absorption by converting iron from ferric to ferrous, but supplemental iron is already in the ferrous form.)

HEALTHY PEOPLE 2010

Reduce iron deficiency among pregnant females. Reduce anemia among low-income pregnant females in their third trimester.

■ Zinc RDA during pregnancy:
- 12 mg/day (≤18 yr).
- 11 mg/day (19–50 yr).

Zinc■ is required for DNA and RNA synthesis and thus for protein synthesis and cell development. Typical zinc intakes for pregnant women are lower than recommendations, but routine supplementation is not advised. Women taking iron supplements (more than 30 milligrams per day), however, may need zinc supplementation because large doses of iron can interfere with the body's absorption and use of zinc.

Nutrients for Bone Development Vitamin D and the bone-building minerals calcium, phosphorus, magnesium, and fluoride are in great demand during pregnancy. Insufficient intakes may produce abnormal fetal bones and teeth.

■ The AI for Vitamin D does not increase during pregnancy.

Vitamin D■ plays a vital role in calcium absorption and utilization. Consequently, severe maternal vitamin D deficiency interferes with normal calcium metabolism, resulting in rickets in the fetus and osteomalacia in the mother. Regular

*On average almost twice as much blood is lost during a cesarean delivery as during the average vaginal delivery of a single fetus.

exposure to sunlight and consumption of vitamin D–fortified milk are usually sufficient to provide the recommended amount of vitamin D during pregnancy. Routine supplementation is not recommended because of the toxicity risk. Vegans who avoid milk, eggs, and fish may receive enough vitamin D from regular exposure to sunlight and from fortified soy milk.

Calcium absorption more than doubles early in pregnancy, helping the mother to meet the calcium needs of pregnancy.■ During the last trimester, as the fetal bones begin to calcify, over 300 milligrams a day are transferred to the fetus. Recommendations to ensure an adequate calcium intake during pregnancy are aimed at conserving maternal bone while supplying fetal needs.

■ The AI for calcium does not increase during pregnancy.

Calcium intakes for pregnant women■ typically fall below recommendations. Because bones are still actively depositing minerals until about age 25 or so, adequate calcium is especially important for young women. Pregnant women under age 25 who receive less than 600 milligrams of dietary calcium daily need to increase their intake of milk, cheese, yogurt, and other calcium-rich foods. Alternatively, and less preferably, they may need a daily supplement of 600 milligrams of calcium.

■ The USDA Food Guide suggests consuming 3 cups per day of fat-free or low-fat milk or the equivalent in milk products.

Other Nutrients The nutrients mentioned here are those most intensely involved in blood production, cell growth, and bone growth. Of course, other nutrients are also needed during pregnancy to support the growth and health of both fetus and mother. Even with adequate nutrition, repeated pregnancies less than a year apart deplete nutrient reserves: fetal growth may be compromised and maternal health may decline. The optimal interval between pregnancies is 18 to 23 months.[22]

Nutrient Supplements Physicians routinely recommend daily multivitamin-mineral supplements for pregnant women. Prenatal supplements typically contain greater amounts of folate, iron, and calcium than regular vitamin-mineral supplements. These supplements are particularly beneficial for women who do not eat adequately and for those in high-risk groups: women carrying multiple fetuses, cigarette smokers, and alcohol and drug abusers. The use of prenatal supplements may help reduce the risks of preterm delivery, low infant birthweights, and birth defects.[23] Figure 14-12 presents a label from a standard prenatal supplement.

FIGURE 14-12 Example of a Prenatal Supplement

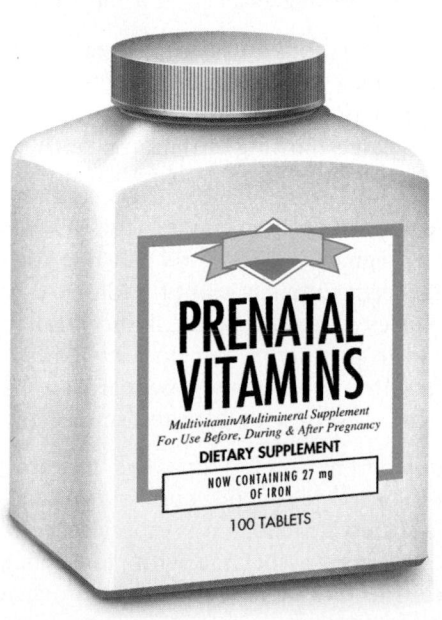
PRENATAL
VITAMINS
Multivitamin/Multimineral Supplement
For Use Before, During & After Pregnancy
DIETARY SUPPLEMENT
NOW CONTAINING 27 mg OF IRON
100 TABLETS

Supplement Facts
Serving Size 1 Tablet

Amount Per Tablet	% Daily Value for Pregnant/ Lactating Women
Vitamin A 4000 IU	50%
Vitamin C 100 mg	167%
Vitamin D 400 IU	100%
Vitamin E 11 IU	37%
Thiamin 1.84 mg	108%
Riboflavin 1.7 mg	85%
Niacin 18 mg	90%
Vitamin B6 2.6 mg	104%
Folate 800 mcg	100%
Vitamin B12 4 mcg	50%
Calcium 200 mg	15%
Iron 27 mg	150%
Zinc 25 mg	167%

INGREDIENTS: calcium carbonate, microcrystalline cellulose, dicalcium phosphate, ascorbic acid, ferrous fumarate, zinc oxide, acacia, sucrose ester, niacinamide, modified cellulose gum, di-alpha tocopheryl acetate, hydroxypropyl methylcellulose, hydroxypropyl cellulose, artificial colors (FD&C blue no. 1 lake, FD&C red no. 40 lake, FD&C yellow no. 6 lake, titanium dioxide), polyethylene glycol, starch, pyridoxine hydrochloride, vitamin A acetate, riboflavin, thiamin mononitrate, folic acid, beta carotene, cholecalciferol, maltodextrin, gluten, cyanocobalamin, sodium bisulfite.

TABLE 14-2 Strategies to Alleviate Maternal Discomforts

To Alleviate the Nausea of Pregnancy	To Prevent or Alleviate Constipation	To Prevent or Relieve Heartburn
• On waking, arise slowly. • Eat dry toast or crackers. • Chew gum or suck hard candies. • Eat small, frequent meals. • Avoid foods with offensive odors. • When nauseated, do not drink citrus juice, water, milk, coffee, or tea.	• Eat foods high in fiber (fruits, vegetables, and whole-grain cereals). • Exercise regularly. • Drink at least eight glasses of liquids a day. • Respond promptly to the urge to defecate. • Use laxatives only as prescribed by a physician; do not use mineral oil, because it interferes with absorption of fat-soluble vitamins.	• Relax and eat slowly. • Chew food thoroughly. • Eat small, frequent meals. • Drink liquids between meals. • Avoid spicy or greasy foods. • Sit up while eating; elevate the head while sleeping. • Wait an hour after eating before lying down. • Wait two hours after eating before exercising.

Common Nutrition-Related Concerns of Pregnancy

Nausea, constipation, heartburn, and food sensitivities are common nutrition-related concerns during pregnancy. A few simple strategies can help alleviate maternal discomforts (see Table 14-2).

Nausea Not all women have queasy stomachs in the early months of pregnancy, but many do. The nausea of "morning" (actually, anytime) sickness ranges from mild queasiness to debilitating nausea and vomiting. Severe and continued vomiting may require hospitalization if it results in acidosis, dehydration, or excessive weight loss. The hormonal changes of early pregnancy seem to be responsible for a woman's sensitivities to the appearance, texture, or smell of foods. Traditional strategies for quelling nausea are listed in Table 14-2, but some women benefit most from simply eating the foods they want when they feel like eating. They may also find comfort in a cleaner, quieter, and more temperate environment.

Constipation and Hemorrhoids As the hormones of pregnancy alter muscle tone and the growing fetus crowds intestinal organs, an expectant mother may experience constipation. She may also develop hemorrhoids (swollen veins of the rectum). These can be painful, and straining during bowel movements may cause bleeding. She can gain relief by following the strategies listed in Table 14-2.

Heartburn Heartburn is another common complaint during pregnancy. The hormones of pregnancy relax the digestive muscles, and the growing fetus puts increasing pressure on the mother's stomach. This combination allows stomach acid to back up into the lower esophagus and create a burning sensation near the heart. Tips to help relieve heartburn are included in Table 14-2.

Food Cravings and Aversions Some women develop cravings for, or aversions to, particular foods and beverages during pregnancy. These **food cravings** and **food aversions** are fairly common, but do not seem to reflect real physiological needs. In other words, a woman who craves pickles does not necessarily need salt. Similarly, cravings for ice cream are common in pregnancy, but do not signify a calcium deficiency. Cravings and aversions that arise during pregnancy are most likely due to hormone-induced changes in sensitivity to taste and smell.

Nonfood Cravings Some pregnant women develop cravings for nonfood items■ such as laundry starch, clay, soil, or ice—a practice known as pica.[24] Pica is a cultural phenomenon that reflects a society's folklore; it is especially common among African American women. Pica is often associated with iron-deficiency anemia, but whether iron deficiency leads to pica or pica leads to iron deficiency is unclear. Eating clay or soil may interfere with iron absorption and displace iron-rich foods from the diet.

■ Reminder: The general term for eating nonfood items is *pica*. The specific craving for nonfood items that come from the earth, such as clay or dirt, is known as *geophagia*.

food cravings: strong desires to eat particular foods.

food aversions: strong desires to avoid particular foods.

IN SUMMARY Energy and nutrient needs are high during pregnancy. A balanced diet that includes an extra serving from each of the five food groups can usually meet these needs, with the exception of iron and folate (supplements are recommended). The nausea, constipation, and heartburn that sometimes accompany pregnancy can usually be alleviated with a few simple strategies. Food cravings do not typically reflect physiological needs.

High-Risk Pregnancies

Some pregnancies jeopardize the life and health of the mother and infant. Table 14-3 identifies several characteristics of a **high-risk pregnancy.** A woman with none of these risk factors is said to have a **low-risk pregnancy.** The more factors that apply, the higher the risk. All pregnant women, especially those in high-risk categories, need prenatal care, including dietary■ advice.

■ Nutrition advice in prenatal care:
- Eat well-balanced meals.
- Gain enough weight to support fetal growth.
- Take prenatal supplements as prescribed.
- Stop drinking alcohol.

Increase the proportion of pregnant women who receive early and adequate prenatal care.

HEALTHY PEOPLE 2010

The Infant's Birthweight

A high-risk pregnancy is likely to produce an infant with **low birthweight.** Low-birthweight infants, defined as infants who weigh 5½ pounds or less, are classified according to their gestational age. Preterm infants are born before they are fully developed; they are often underweight and have trouble breathing because their lungs are immature. Preterm infants may be small, but if their size and weight are appropriate for their age,■ they can catch up in growth given adequate nutrition support. In contrast, small-for-gestational-age infants have

■ Some preterm infants are of a weight **appropriate for gestational age (AGA);** others are **small for gestational age (SGA),** often reflecting malnutrition.

TABLE 14-3 High-Risk Pregnancy Factors

Factor	Condition That Raises Risk
Maternal weight	
Prior to pregnancy	Prepregnancy BMI either <18.5 or >25
During pregnancy	Insufficient or excessive pregnancy weight gain
Maternal nutrition	Nutrient deficiencies or toxicities; eating disorders
Socioeconomic status	Poverty, lack of family support, low level of education, limited food available
Lifestyle habits	Smoking, alcohol or other drug use
Age	Teens, especially 15 years or younger; women 35 years or older
Previous pregnancies	
Number	Many previous pregnancies (3 or more to mothers under age 20; 4 or more to mothers age 20 or older)
Interval	Short intervals between pregnancies (<18 months)
Outcomes	Previous history of problems
Multiple births	Twins or triplets
Birthweight	Low- or high-birthweight infants
Maternal health	
High blood pressure	Development of pregnancy-related hypertension
Diabetes	Development of gestational diabetes
Chronic diseases	Diabetes; heart, respiratory, and kidney disease; certain genetic disorders; special diets and medications

high-risk pregnancy: a pregnancy characterized by indicators that make it likely the birth will be surrounded by problems such as premature delivery, difficult birth, retarded growth, birth defects, and early infant death.

low-risk pregnancy: a pregnancy characterized by indicators that make a normal outcome likely.

low birthweight (LBW): a birthweight of 5½ lb (2500 g) or less; indicates probable poor health in the newborn and poor nutrition status in the mother during pregnancy, before pregnancy, or both. Normal birthweight for a full-term baby is 6½ to 8¾ lb (about 3000 to 4000 g).

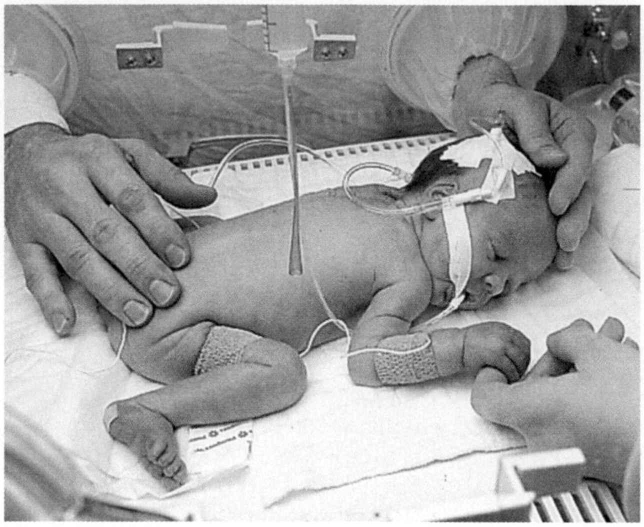
© Nik Kleinberg/Stock Boston

Low-birthweight babies need special care and nourishment.

suffered growth failure in the uterus and do not catch up as well. For the most part, survival improves with increased gestational age and birthweight.

Low-birthweight infants are more likely to experience complications during delivery than normal-weight babies. They also have a statistically greater chance of having physical and mental birth defects, contracting diseases, and dying early in life. Of infants who die before their first birthdays, about two-thirds were low-birthweight newborns. Very-low-birthweight infants (3½ pounds or less) struggle not only for their immediate physical health and survival, but for their future cognitive development and abilities as well.[25]

A strong relationship is evident between socioeconomic disadvantage and low birthweight. Low socioeconomic status impairs fetal development by causing stress and by limiting access to medical care and to nutritious foods. Low socioeconomic status often accompanies teen pregnancies, smoking, and alcohol and drug abuse—all predictors of low birthweight.

HEALTHY PEOPLE 2010

Reduce low birthweight (LBW) and very low birthweight (VLBW).

Malnutrition and Pregnancy

Good nutrition clearly supports a pregnancy. In contrast, malnutrition interferes with the ability to conceive, the likelihood of implantation, and the subsequent development of a fetus should conception and implantation occur.

Malnutrition and Fertility The nutrition habits and lifestyle choices people make can influence the course of a pregnancy they are not even planning at the time. Severe malnutrition and food deprivation can reduce fertility: women may develop amenorrhea,■ and men may lose their ability to produce viable sperm. Furthermore, both men and women lose sexual interest during times of starvation. Starvation arises predictably during famines, wars, and droughts, but can also occur amidst peace and plenty. Many young women who diet excessively are starving and suffering from malnutrition (see Highlight 9).

■ Reminder: *Amenorrhea* is the temporary or permanent absence of menstrual periods. Amenorrhea is normal before puberty, after menopause, during pregnancy, and during lactation; otherwise it is abnormal.

Malnutrition and Early Pregnancy If a malnourished woman does become pregnant, she faces the challenge of supporting both the growth of a baby and her own health with inadequate nutrient stores. Malnutrition prior to and around conception prevents the placenta from developing fully. A poorly developed placenta cannot deliver optimum nourishment to the fetus, and the infant will be born small and possibly with physical and cognitive abnormalities. If this small infant is a female, she may develop poorly and have an elevated risk of developing a chronic condition that could impair her ability to give birth to a healthy infant. Thus a woman's malnutrition can adversely affect not only her children but her *grandchildren.*

Malnutrition and Fetal Development Without adequate nutrition during pregnancy, fetal growth and infant health are compromised. In general, consequences of malnutrition during pregnancy include fetal growth retardation, congenital malformations (birth defects), spontaneous abortion and stillbirth, premature birth, and low infant birthweight. Malnutrition, coupled with low birthweight, is a factor in more than half of all deaths of children under four years of age worldwide.

Food Assistance Programs

Women in high-risk pregnancies can find assistance from the WIC program—a high-quality, cost-effective health care and nutrition services program for women, infants, and children in the United States.[26] Formally known as the Special Supplemental Nutrition Program for Women, Infants, and Children, WIC provides nutrition education and nutritious foods to infants, children up to age five, and pregnant and breastfeeding women who qualify financially and have a high risk of medical or nutritional problems. The program is both remedial and preventive: services include health care referrals, nutrition education, and food packages or vouchers for specific foods. These foods supply nutrients known to be lacking in the diets of the target population: most notably, protein, calcium, iron, vitamin A, and vitamin C. WIC-sponsored foods include tuna fish, carrots, eggs, milk, iron-fortified cereal, vitamin C–rich juice, cheese, legumes, peanut butter, and infant formula.

Over 7 million people—most of them young children—receive WIC benefits each month. Prenatal WIC participation can effectively reduce infant mortality, low birthweight, and maternal and newborn medical costs. In 2002, Congress appropriated over $4 billion for WIC. For every dollar spent on WIC, an estimated three dollars in medical costs are saved in the first two months after birth.

Maternal Health

Medical disorders can threaten the life and health of both mother and fetus. If diagnosed and treated early, many diseases can be managed to ensure a healthy outcome—another strong argument for early prenatal care.

Preexisting Diabetes Whether diabetes presents risks depends on how well it is controlled before and during pregnancy. Without proper management of maternal diabetes, women face high infertility rates, and those who do conceive may experience episodes of severe hypoglycemia or hyperglycemia, spontaneous abortions, and pregnancy-related hypertension. Infants may be large, suffer physical and mental abnormalities, and experience other complications such as severe hypoglycemia or respiratory distress, both of which can be fatal. Ideally, a woman with diabetes will receive the prenatal care needed to achieve glucose control before conception and continued glucose control throughout pregnancy.

Gestational Diabetes Approximately 1 in 14 women who does not have diabetes develops a condition known as **gestational diabetes** during pregnancy. Gestational diabetes usually develops during the second half of pregnancy, with subsequent return to normal after childbirth. Some women with gestational diabetes, however, develop diabetes (usually type 2) after pregnancy, especially if they are overweight. For this reason, health care professionals advise against excessive weight gain.

The most common consequences of gestational diabetes are complications during labor and delivery and a high infant birthweight.[27] Birth defects associated with gestational diabetes include heart damage, limb deformities, and neural tube defects. To ensure that the problems of gestational diabetes are dealt with promptly, physicians screen for the risk factors■ listed in the margin and test high-risk women for glucose intolerance immediately and average-risk women between 24 and 28 weeks gestation.[28] Dietary recommendations should meet the needs of pregnancy and maternal blood glucose goals.[29] To maintain normal blood glucose levels, carbohydrates should be restricted to 35 to 40 percent of energy intake. To limit excessive weight gain, obese women should limit energy intake to about 25 kcalories per kilogram body weight. Diet and moderate exercise may control gestational diabetes, but if blood glucose fails to normalize, insulin or other drugs may be required.[30]

Preexisting Hypertension Hypertension complicates pregnancy and affects its outcome in different ways, depending on when the hypertension first develops and on how severe it becomes. In addition to the threats hypertension always carries (such as heart attack and stroke), high blood pressure increases the risks of a low-birthweight infant or the separation of the placenta from the wall of the uterus before the birth, resulting in stillbirth. Ideally, before a woman with hypertension becomes pregnant, her blood pressure will be under control.

■ Risk factors for gestational diabetes:
- Age 35 or older.
- BMI >25 or excessive weight gain.
- Complications in previous pregnancies, including high-birthweight infant.
- Symptoms of diabetes.
- Family history of diabetes.
- Hispanic, black, Native American, South or East Asian, Pacific Islander, or indigenous Australian.

gestational diabetes: abnormal glucose tolerance during pregnancy.

Transient Hypertension of Pregnancy Some women develop hypertension during the second half of pregnancy.* Most often, the rise in blood pressure is mild and does not affect the pregnancy adversely. Blood pressure usually returns to normal during the first few weeks after childbirth. This **transient hypertension of pregnancy** differs from the life-threatening hypertensive diseases■ of pregnancy—preeclampsia and eclampsia.

■ The hypertensive diseases of pregnancy are sometimes called **toxemia.**

Preeclampsia and Eclampsia Hypertension may signal the onset of **preeclampsia,** a condition characterized not only by high blood pressure but also by protein in the urine and fluid retention (edema). The edema■ of preeclampsia is a whole-body edema, distinct from the localized fluid retention women normally experience late in pregnancy.

■ The normal edema of pregnancy responds to gravity; fluid pools in the ankles. The edema of preeclampsia is a generalized edema. The differences between these two types of edema help with the diagnosis of preeclampsia.

Preeclampsia usually occurs with first pregnancies■ and most often after 20 weeks gestation. Symptoms typically regress within two days of delivery. Both men and women who were born of pregnancies complicated by preeclampsia are more likely to have a child born of a pregnancy complicated by preeclampsia, suggesting a genetic predisposition.[31] Black women have a much greater risk of preeclampsia than white women.

■ Warning signs of preeclampsia:
- Hypertension.
- Protein in the urine.
- Upper abdominal pain.
- Severe and constant headaches.
- Swelling, especially of the face.
- Dizziness.
- Blurred vision.
- Sudden weight gain (1 lb/day).
- Fetal growth retardation.

Preeclampsia affects almost all of the mother's organs—the circulatory system, liver, kidneys, and brain. Blood flow through the vessels that supply oxygen and nutrients to the placenta diminishes. For this reason, preeclampsia often retards fetal growth. In some cases, the placenta separates from the uterus, resulting in premature birth or stillbirth.

Preeclampsia can progress rapidly to **eclampsia**—a condition characterized by convulsive seizures and coma. Maternal death during pregnancy and childbirth is extremely rare in developed countries, but when it does occur, eclampsia is a common cause. The rate of death for black women with eclampsia is over four times the rate for white women.[32]

Preeclampsia demands prompt medical attention. Treatment focuses on controlling blood pressure and preventing convulsions. If preeclampsia develops early and is severe, induced labor or cesarean section may be necessary, regardless of gestational age. The infant will be preterm, with all of the associated problems, including poor lung development and special care needs. Several dietary factors have been studied, but none have proved conclusive in preventing preeclampsia.[33] Calcium supplementation may be effective for some women.[34]

transient hypertension of pregnancy: high blood pressure that develops in the second half of pregnancy and resolves after childbirth, usually without affecting the outcome of the pregnancy.

preeclampsia (PRE-ee-KLAMP-see-ah): a condition characterized by hypertension, fluid retention, and protein in the urine; formerly known as *pregnancy-induced hypertension.**

eclampsia (eh-KLAMP-see-ah): a severe stage of preeclampsia characterized by convulsions.

*The Working Group on High Blood Pressure in Pregnancy, convened by the National High Blood Pressure Education Program of the National Heart, Lung, and Blood Institute, suggested abandoning the term *pregnancy-induced hypertension* because it failed to differentiate between the mild, transient hypertension of pregnancy and the life-threatening hypertension of preeclampsia.

The Mother's Age

Maternal age also influences the course of a pregnancy. Compared with women of the physically ideal childbearing age of 20 to 25, both younger and older women face more complications of pregnancy.

Pregnancy in Adolescents Many adolescents become sexually active before age 19, and over 800,000 adolescent girls face pregnancies each year in the United States; over half of them give birth.[35] Put another way, about 1 out of every 20 babies is born to a teenager. Nourishing a growing fetus adds to a teenage girl's nutrition burden, especially if her growth is still incomplete. Simply being young increases the risks of pregnancy complications independently of important socioeconomic factors.

Common complications among adolescent mothers include iron-deficiency anemia (which may reflect poor diet and inadequate prenatal care) and prolonged labor (which reflects the mother's physical immaturity). On a positive note, maternal death is lowest for mothers under age 20.

*Blood pressure of 140/90 millimeters mercury during the second half of pregnancy in a woman who has not previously exhibited hypertension indicates high blood pressure. So does a rise in systolic blood pressure of 30 millimeters or in diastolic blood pressure of 15 millimeters on at least two occasions more than six hours apart. By this rule, an apparently "normal" blood pressure of 120/85 would be high for a woman whose normal value was 90/70.

Pregnant teenagers have higher rates of stillbirths, preterm births, and low-birthweight infants than do adult women. Many of these infants suffer physical problems, require intensive care, and die within the first year. The care of infants born to teenagers costs our society an estimated $1 billion annually. Because teenagers have few financial resources, they cannot pay these costs. Furthermore, their low economic status contributes significantly to the complications surrounding their pregnancies. At a time when prenatal care is most important, it is less accessible. And the pattern of teenage pregnancies continues from generation to generation, with almost 40 percent of the daughters born to teenage mothers becoming teenage mothers themselves. Clearly, teenage pregnancy is a major public health problem.

HEALTHY PEOPLE 2010

Reduce pregnancies among adolescent females.

To support the needs of both mother and fetus, young teenagers (13 to 16 years old) are encouraged to strive for the highest weight gains recommended for pregnancy. For a teen who enters pregnancy at a healthy body weight, a weight gain of approximately 35 pounds is recommended; this amount minimizes the risk of delivering a low-birthweight infant. Gaining less weight may limit fetal growth. Pregnant and lactating teenagers can use the food guide presented in Figure 2-1 (on p. 44–45), making sure to select a high enough kcalorie level to support adequate weight gain.

Without the appropriate economic, social, and physical support, a young mother will not be able to care for herself during her pregnancy and for her child after the birth. To improve her chances for a successful pregnancy and a healthy infant, she must seek prenatal care. WIC helps pregnant teenagers obtain adequate food for themselves and their infants (WIC was introduced on p. 490).

Pregnancy in Older Women In the last several decades, many women have delayed childbearing while they pursue education and careers. As a result, the number of first births to women 35 and older has increased dramatically. Most of these women, even those over age 50, have healthy pregnancies.[36]

The few complications associated with later childbearing often reflect chronic conditions such as hypertension and diabetes, which can complicate an otherwise healthy pregnancy. These complications may result in a cesarean section, which is twice as common in women over 35 as among younger women. For all these reasons, maternal death rates are higher in women over 35 than in younger women.

The babies of older mothers face problems of their own including higher rates of premature births and low birthweight.[37] Their rates of birth defects are also high. Because 1 out of 50 pregnancies in older women produces an infant with genetic abnormalities, obstetricians routinely screen women older than 35. For a 40-year-old mother, the risk of having a child with **Down syndrome,** for example, is about 1 in 100 compared with 1 in 300 for a 35-year-old and 1 in 10,000 for a 20-year-old. In addition, fetal death is twice as high for women 35 years and older than for younger women. Why this is so remains a bit of a mystery. One possibility is that the uterine blood vessels of older women may not fully adapt to the increased demands of pregnancy.

Practices Incompatible with Pregnancy

Besides malnutrition, a variety of lifestyle factors can have adverse effects on pregnancy; and some may be teratogenic.■ People who are planning to have children can make the choice to practice healthy behaviors.

■ Reminder: The word *teratogenic* describes a factor that causes abnormal fetal development and birth defects.

Alcohol One out of eight pregnant women drinks alcohol at some time during her pregnancy; 1 out of 30 drinks frequently.[38] Alcohol consumption during pregnancy can cause irreversible mental and physical retardation of the fetus—fetal alcohol

Down syndrome: a genetic abnormality that causes mental retardation, short stature, and flattened facial features.

syndrome (FAS). Of the leading causes of mental retardation, FAS is the only one that is totally *preventable*. To that end, the surgeon general urges all pregnant women to refrain from drinking alcohol. Fetal alcohol syndrome is the topic of Highlight 14, which includes mention of how alcohol consumption by men may also affect fertility and fetal development.

HEALTHY PEOPLE 2010

Increase abstinence from alcohol among pregnant women. Reduce the occurrence of fetal alcohol syndrome (FAS).

Medicinal Drugs Drugs other than alcohol can also cause complications during pregnancy, problems in labor, and serious birth defects. For these reasons, pregnant women should not take any medicines without consulting their physicians, who must weigh the benefits against the risks.[39]

Herbal Supplements Similarly, pregnant women should seek a physician's advice before using herbal supplements as well. Women sometimes seek herbal preparations during their pregnancies to induce labor, aid digestion, promote water loss, support restful sleep, and fight depression. As Chapter 19 explains, some herbs may be safe, but many others are definitely harmful.

Illicit Drugs The recommendation to avoid drugs during pregnancy also includes illicit drugs, of course. Unfortunately, use of illicit drugs, such as cocaine and marijuana, is common among some pregnant women.*

Drugs of abuse, such as cocaine, easily cross the placenta and impair fetal growth and development.[40] Furthermore, they are responsible for preterm births, low-birthweight infants, perinatal deaths,■ and sudden infant deaths. If these newborns survive, central nervous system damage is evident: their cries, sleep, and behaviors early in life are abnormal, and their cognitive development later in life is impaired.[41] They may be hypersensitive or underaroused; those who test positive for drugs suffer the greatest effects of toxicity and withdrawal.[42]

■ The word *perinatal* refers to the time between the 28th week of gestation and one month after birth.

Smoking and Chewing Tobacco Smoking cigarettes or chewing tobacco at any time exerts harmful effects, and pregnancy dramatically magnifies the hazards of these practices. Smoking restricts the blood supply to the growing fetus and so limits oxygen and nutrient delivery and waste removal. A mother who smokes is more likely to have a complicated birth and a low-birthweight infant.[43] Indeed, of all preventable causes of low birthweight in the United States, smoking has the greatest impact. Although most infants born to cigarette smokers are low birthweight, some are not, suggesting that the effect of smoking on birthweight also depends, in part, on genes involved in the metabolism of smoking toxins.[44] Smokers also tend to eat less nutritious foods during their pregnancies than do nonsmokers, further impairing fetal development. Unfortunately, an estimated one out of eight pregnant women smokes, and rates are even higher for unmarried women and those who have not graduated from high school.[45]

In addition to contributing to low birthweight, smoking can cause death in an otherwise healthy fetus or newborn. A positive relationship exists between **sudden infant death syndrome (SIDS)** and both cigarette smoking during pregnancy and postnatal exposure to passive smoke. Smoking during pregnancy may even harm the intellectual and behavioral development of the child later in life. The margin■ lists other complications of smoking during pregnancy.

■ Complications associated with smoking during pregnancy:
- Fetal growth retardation.
- Low birthweight.
- Complications at birth (prolonged final stage of labor).
- Mislocation of the placenta.
- Premature separation of the placenta.
- Vaginal bleeding.
- Spontaneous abortion.
- Fetal death.
- Sudden infant death syndrome (SIDS).
- Middle ear diseases.
- Cardiac and respiratory diseases.

sudden infant death syndrome (SIDS): the unexpected and unexplained death of an apparently well infant; the most common cause of death of infants between the second week and the end of the first year of life; also called *crib death*.

HEALTHY PEOPLE 2010

Increase smoking cessation during pregnancy. Increase abstinence from cigarettes among pregnant women.

*It is estimated that 17 percent of pregnant women use marijuana and at least 6 percent use cocaine.

Infants of mothers who chew tobacco also have low birthweights and high rates of fetal deaths. Any woman who smokes cigarettes or chews tobacco and is considering pregnancy or who is already pregnant should try to quit.

Environmental Contaminants Infants and young children of pregnant women exposed to environmental contaminants such as lead show signs of delayed mental and psychomotor development. During pregnancy, lead readily moves across the placenta, inflicting severe damage on the developing fetal nervous system.[46] In addition, infants exposed to even low levels of lead during gestation weigh less at birth and consequently struggle to survive. For these reasons, it is particularly important that pregnant women receive foods and beverages grown and prepared in environments free of contamination. A diet high in calcium will also help to defend against lead contamination.[47] Breastfeeding the infant may also help to counterbalance the developmental damage incurred from contamination during pregnancy.[48]

Among the contaminants of concern is mercury. As Chapter 5 mentioned, fatty fish are a good source of omega-3 fatty acids, but some fish contain large amounts of the pollutant mercury, which can harm the developing brain and nervous system.[49] For this reason, pregnant (and lactating) women should:[50]

- Avoid shark, swordfish, king mackerel, and tilefish.
- Limit average weekly consumption to 12 ounces (cooked or canned) of ocean, coastal, and other commercial fish *or* to 6 ounces (cooked) of freshwater fish caught by family and friends.

Supplements of fish oil are not recommended both because they may contain concentrated toxins and because their effects on pregnancy remain unknown.

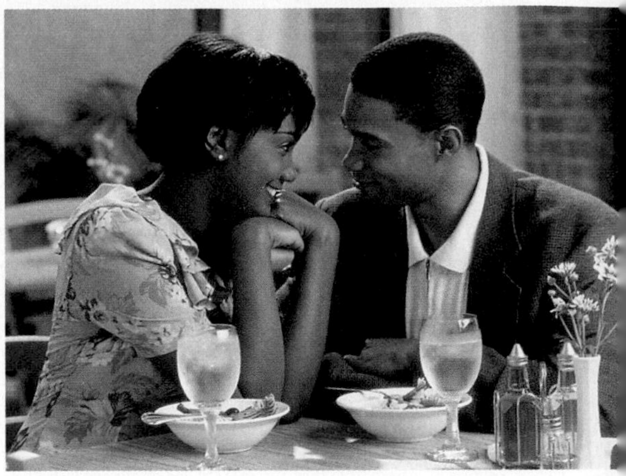

© Jose I. Pelaez, Inc./CORBIS

Young adults can prepare for a healthy pregnancy by taking care of themselves today.

Foodborne Illness Foodborne illnesses arise when people eat foods that contain infectious microbes or microbes that produce toxins. At best, the vomiting and diarrhea associated with these illnesses can leave a pregnant woman exhausted and dehydrated; at worse, foodborne illnesses can cause meningitis, pneumonia, or even fetal death. Pregnant women are about 20 times more likely than other healthy adults to get the foodborne illness **listeriosis.**■

■ To prevent listeriosis:

- Use only pasteurized juices and dairy products; avoid Mexican soft cheeses, feta cheese, brie, Camembert, and blue-veined cheeses such as Roquefort.
- Thoroughly cook meat, poultry, eggs, and seafood.
- Thoroughly reheat hot dogs, luncheon meats, and deli meats, including cured meats such as salami.
- Wash all fruits and vegetables.
- Avoid refrigerated pâté, meat spreads, smoked seafood such as salmon or trout, and any fish labeled "nova," "lox," or "kippered," unless prepared in a cooked dish.

Vitamin-Mineral Megadoses The pregnant woman who is trying to eat well may mistakenly assume that more is better when it comes to vitamin-mineral supplements. This is simply not true; many vitamins and minerals are toxic when taken in excess. Excessive vitamin A is particularly infamous for its role in malformations of the cranial nervous system. Intakes before the seventh week appeared to be the most damaging. (Review Figure 14-4 on p. 476 to see how many tissues are in their critical periods prior to the seventh week.) For this reason, vitamin A is not given as a supplement in the first trimester of pregnancy unless there is specific evidence of deficiency, which is rare. A pregnant woman can obtain all the vitamin A and most of the other vitamins and minerals she needs by making wise food choices. She should take supplements only on the advice of a registered dietitian or physician.

Caffeine Caffeine crosses the placenta, and the developing fetus has a limited ability to metabolize it. Research studies have not proved that caffeine (even in high doses) causes birth defects in human infants (as it does in animals), but some evidence suggests that moderate-to-heavy use may increase the risk of spontaneous abortion.[51](Heavy caffeine use was defined as the equivalent of 3 to 6 cups of coffee a day.) All things considered, it might be most sensible to limit caffeine consumption to the equivalent of a cup of coffee or two 12-ounce cola beverages a day. (The caffeine contents of selected beverages, foods, and drugs are listed at the beginning of Appendix H.)

Weight-Loss Dieting Weight-loss dieting, even for short periods, is hazardous during pregnancy. Low-carbohydrate diets or fasts that cause ketosis deprive the fetal brain of needed glucose and may impair cognitive development. Such diets are also likely to lack other nutrients vital to fetal growth. Regardless of prepregnancy weight, pregnant women should never intentionally lose weight.

listeriosis: an infection caused by eating food contaminated with the bacterium *Listeria monocytogenes,* which can be killed by pasteurization and cooking, but can survive at refrigerated temperatures; certain ready-to-eat foods, such as hot dogs and deli meats, may become contaminated after cooking or processing, but before packaging.

Sugar Substitutes Artificial sweeteners have been extensively investigated and found to be acceptable during pregnancy if used within the Food and Drug Administration's guidelines (presented in Highlight 4).[52] Still, it would be prudent for pregnant women to use sweeteners in moderation and within an otherwise nutritious and well-balanced diet. Women with phenylketonuria should not use aspartame, as Highlight 4 explains.

IN SUMMARY High-risk pregnancies, especially for teenagers, threaten the life and health of both mother and infant. Proper nutrition and abstinence from smoking, alcohol, and other drugs improve the outcome. In addition, prenatal care includes monitoring pregnant women for gestational diabetes and preeclampsia.

In general, most women can enjoy a healthy pregnancy if they:[53]

- Get prenatal care.
- Eat a balanced diet, safely prepared.
- Take prenatal supplements as prescribed.
- Gain a healthy amount of weight.
- Refrain from cigarettes, alcohol, and drugs (including herbs) unless prescribed by a physician.

Childbirth marks the end of pregnancy and the beginning of a new set of parental responsibilities—including feeding the newborn.

Nutrition during Lactation

Before the end of her pregnancy, a woman will need to consider whether to feed her infant breast milk,■ infant formula, or both. These options are the only recommended foods for an infant during the first four to six months of life. The rate of breastfeeding is close to the Healthy People 2010 goal of 75 percent at birth, but falls far short of goals at six months and a year.[54] This section focuses on how the mother's nutrition supports the making of breast milk; the next chapter describes how the infant benefits from drinking breast milk.

■ To learn about breastfeeding, a pregnant woman can read at least one of the many books available. Nutrition on the Net at the end of this chapter provides a list of other nutrition resources, including LaLeche League International.

HEALTHY PEOPLE 2010

Increase the proportion of mothers who breastfeed their babies.

In many countries around the world, a woman breastfeeds her newborn without considering the alternatives or consciously making a decision. In other parts of the world, a woman feeds her newborn formula simply because she knows so little about breastfeeding. She may have misconceptions or feel uncomfortable about a process she has never seen or experienced. Breastfeeding offers many health benefits to both mother and infant, and every pregnant woman should seriously consider it (see Table 14-4).[55] Still, there are valid reasons for not breastfeeding, and formula-fed infants grow and develop into healthy children.

Lactation: A Physiological Process

Lactation naturally follows pregnancy, as the mother's body continues to nourish the infant. The **mammary glands** secrete milk for this purpose. The mammary glands develop during puberty, but remain fairly inactive until pregnancy. During pregnancy, hormones promote the growth and branching of a duct system in the breasts and the development of the milk-producing cells.

lactation: production and secretion of breast milk for the purpose of nourishing an infant.

mammary glands: glands of the female breast that secrete milk.

TABLE 14-4 Benefits of Breastfeeding

For Infants:
• Provides the appropriate composition and balance of nutrients with high bioavailability.
• Provides hormones that promote physiological development.
• Improves cognitive development.
• Protects against a variety of infections.
• May protect against some chronic diseases, such as diabetes (type 1) and hypertension, later in life.
• Protects against food allergies.
For Mothers:
• Contracts the uterus.
• Delays the return of regular ovulation, thus lengthening birth intervals. (It is not, however, a dependable method of contraception.)
• Conserves iron stores (by prolonging amenorrhea).
• May protect against breast and ovarian cancer.
Other:
• Cost savings from not needing medical treatment for childhood illnesses or time off work to care for them.
• Cost savings from not needing to purchase formula (even after adjusting for added foods in the diet of a lactating mother).[a]
• Environmental savings to society from not needing to manufacture, package, and ship formula and dispose of the packaging.

[a]A nursing mother produces over 35 gallons of milk during the first six months, saving her roughly $450 in formula costs.

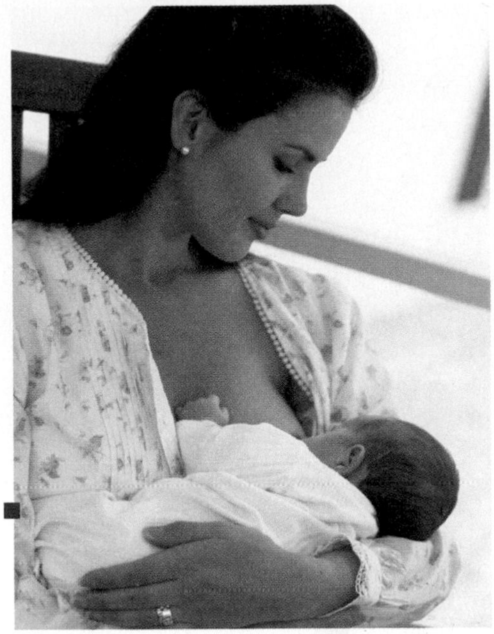

© Ariel Skelley/CORBIS

A woman who decides to breastfeed offers her infant a full array of nutrients and protective factors to support optimal health and development.

The hormones **prolactin** and **oxytocin** finely coordinate lactation. The infant's demand for milk stimulates the release of these hormones, which signal the mammary glands to supply milk. Prolactin is responsible for milk production. Prolactin concentrations remain high and milk production continues as long as the infant is nursing.

The hormone oxytocin causes the mammary glands to eject milk into the ducts, a response known as the **let-down reflex.** The mother feels this reflex as a contraction of the breast, followed by the flow of milk and the release of pressure. By relaxing and eating well, the nursing mother promotes easy let-down of milk and greatly enhances her chances of successful lactation.

Breastfeeding: A Learned Behavior

Lactation is an automatic physiological process that virtually all mothers are capable of doing. Breastfeeding, on the other hand, is a learned behavior that not all mothers decide to do. Of women who do breastfeed, those who receive early and repeated information and support breastfeed their infants longer than others. Health care professionals■ play an important role in providing encouragement and accurate information on breastfeeding.[56] Women who have been successful breastfeeding can offer advice and dispel misperceptions about lifestyle issues.[57] Table 14-5 (on p. 498) lists ten steps maternity facilities and health care professionals can take to promote successful breastfeeding among new mothers.[58]

The mother's partner also plays an important role in encouraging breastfeeding.[59] When partners support the decision, mothers are more likely to start and continue breastfeeding. Clearly, educating those closest to the mother could change attitudes and promote breastfeeding.

Most healthy women who want to breastfeed can do so with a little preparation. Physical obstacles to breastfeeding are rare, although most nursing mothers quit before the recommended six months because of perceived difficulties.[60] Successful

■ Some hospitals employ *certified lactation consultants* who specialize in helping new mothers establish a healthy breastfeeding relationship with their newborn. These consultants are often registered nurses with specialized training in breast and infant anatomy and physiology.

prolactin (pro-LAK-tin): a hormone secreted from the anterior pituitary gland that acts on the mammary glands to initiate and sustain milk production.
- **pro** = promote
- **lacto** = milk

oxytocin (OCK-see-TOH-sin): a hormone that stimulates the mammary glands to eject milk during lactation and the uterus to contract during childbirth.

let-down reflex: the reflex that forces milk to the front of the breast when the infant begins to nurse.

TABLE 14-5 Ten Steps to Successful Breastfeeding

To promote breastfeeding, every maternity facility should:

- Develop a written breastfeeding policy that is routinely communicated to all health care staff.
- Train all health care staff in the skills necessary to implement the breastfeeding policy.
- Inform all pregnant women about the benefits and management of breastfeeding.
- Help mothers initiate breastfeeding within ½ hour of birth.
- Show mothers how to breastfeed and how to maintain lactation, even if they need to be separated from their infants.
- Give newborn infants no food or drink other than breast milk, unless medically indicated.
- Practice rooming-in, allowing mothers and infants to remain together 24 hours a day.
- Encourage breastfeeding on demand.
- Give no artificial nipples or pacifiers to breastfeeding infants.[a]
- Foster the establishment of breastfeeding support groups and refer mothers to them at discharge from the facility.

[a]Compared with nonusers, infants who use pacifiers breastfeed less frequently and stop breastfeeding at a younger age. C. G. Victora and coauthors, Pacifier use and short breastfeeding duration: Cause, consequence, or coincidence? *Pediatrics* 99 (1997): 445–453.

SOURCE: United Nations Children's Fund and World Health Organization, *Protecting, Promoting and Supporting Breastfeeding: The Special Role of Maternity Services.*

breastfeeding requires adequate nutrition and rest. This, plus the support of all who care, will help to enhance the well-being of mother and infant.

The Mother's Nutrient Needs

Ideally, the mother who chooses to breastfeed her infant will continue to eat nutrient-dense foods throughout lactation. An adequate diet is needed to support the stamina, patience, and self-confidence that nursing an infant demands.

■ Energy requirement during lactation:
- 1st 6 mo: +330 kcal/day.
- 2nd 6 mo: +400 kcal/day.

Energy Intake and Exercise A nursing mother produces about 25 ounces of milk per day, with considerable variation from woman to woman and in the same woman from time to time, depending primarily on the infant's demand for milk. To produce an adequate supply of milk, a woman needs extra energy—almost 500 kcalories a day above her regular need during the first six months of lactation. To meet this energy need,■ she can eat an extra 330 kcalories of food each day and let the fat reserves she accumulated during pregnancy provide the rest. Most women need at least 1800 kcalories a day to receive all the nutrients required for successful lactation. Severe energy restriction may hinder milk production.

After the birth of the infant, many women are in a hurry to lose the extra body fat they accumulated during pregnancy. Opinions differ as to whether breastfeeding helps with postpartum weight loss. In general, most women lose 1 to 2 pounds a month during the first four to six months of lactation; some may lose more, and others may maintain or even gain weight. Neither the quality nor the quantity of breast milk is adversely affected by moderate weight loss, and infants grow normally.[61]

Women often exercise to lose weight and improve fitness, and this is compatible with breastfeeding and infant growth.[62] Intense physical activity can raise the lactic acid concentration of breast milk, which may influence the milk's taste. Some infants may prefer milk produced prior to exercise (which has a lower lactic acid content). In these cases, mothers can either breastfeed before exercise or express their milk before exercise for use afterward.

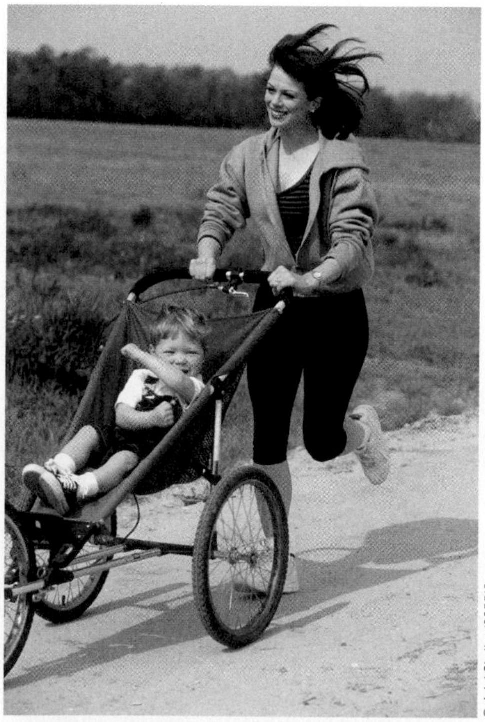
© Ariel Skelley/CORBIS

A jog through the park provides an opportunity for physical activity and fresh air.

Energy Nutrients Recommendations for protein and fatty acids remain about the same during lactation as during pregnancy, but increase for carbohydrates and fibers. Nursing mothers need additional carbohydrate to replace the glucose used to make the lactose in breast milk. The fiber recommendation is 1 gram higher simply because it is based on kcalorie intake, which increases during lactation.

Vitamins and Minerals A question often raised is whether a mother's milk may lack a nutrient if she fails to get enough in her diet. The answer differs from one nutrient to the next, but in general, nutritional inadequacies reduce the *quantity,* not the *quality,* of breast milk. Women can produce milk with adequate protein, carbohydrate, fat, and most minerals, even when their own supplies are limited. For these nutrients and for the vitamin folate as well, milk quality is maintained at the expense of maternal stores. This is most evident in the case of calcium: dietary calcium has no effect on the calcium concentration of breast milk, but maternal bones lose some of their density during lactation. Bone density increases again when lactation ends; breastfeeding has no long-term harmful effects on bones.[63] Nutrients in breast milk most likely to decline in response to prolonged inadequate intakes are the vitamins—especially vitamins B_6, B_{12}, A, and D. Review Figure 14-10 (on p. 485) to compare a lactating woman's nutrient needs with those of pregnant and nonpregnant women.

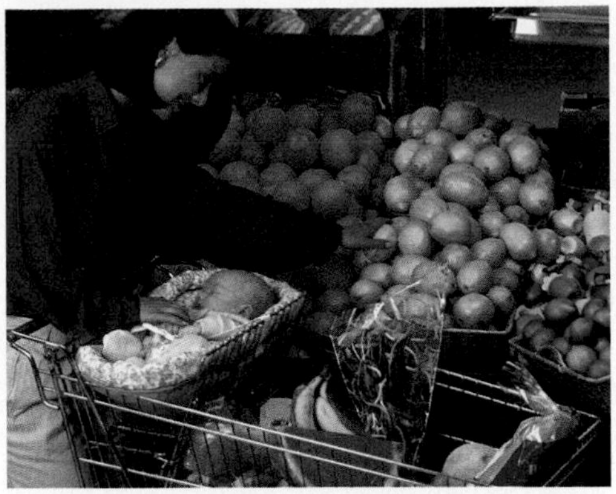

© Photo Disc Inc.

Nutritious foods support successful lactation.

Water Despite misconceptions, a mother who drinks more fluid does not produce more breast milk. To protect herself from dehydration, however, a lactating woman needs to drink plenty of fluids.■ A sensible guideline is to drink a glass of milk, juice, or water at each meal and each time the infant nurses.

■ AI for *total* water (including drinking water, other beverages, and foods) during lactation: 3.8 L/day.

Nutrient Supplements Most lactating women can obtain all the nutrients they need from a well-balanced diet without taking vitamin-mineral supplements. Nevertheless, some may need iron supplements, not to enhance the iron in their breast milk, but to refill their depleted iron stores. Maternal iron stores dwindle during pregnancy when the fetus takes iron to meet its own needs during the first four to six months after birth. In addition, childbirth may have incurred blood losses. Thus a woman may need iron supplements during lactation, even though, until menstruation resumes, her iron requirement is about half that of other nonpregnant women her age.

Particular Foods Foods with strong or spicy flavors (such as garlic) may alter the flavor of breast milk. A sudden change in the taste of the milk may annoy some infants. Familiar flavors may enhance enjoyment.[64]

Infants who develop symptoms of food allergy may be more comfortable if the mother's diet excludes the most common offenders—cow's milk, eggs, fish, peanuts, and tree nuts.[65] Generally, infants with a strong family history of food allergies benefit from breastfeeding.

A nursing mother can usually eat whatever nutritious foods she chooses. If she suspects a particular food is causing the infant discomfort, her physician may recommend a dietary challenge: eliminate the food from the diet to see if the infant's reactions subside; then return the food to the diet, and again monitor the infant's reactions. If a food must be eliminated for an extended time, appropriate substitutions must be made to ensure nutrient adequacy.

Practices Incompatible with Lactation

Some substances impair milk production or enter breast milk and interfere with infant development. This section discusses practices that a breastfeeding mother should avoid.

Alcohol Alcohol easily enters breast milk, and its concentration peaks within an hour of ingestion. Infants drink less breast milk when their mothers have consumed even small amounts of alcohol (equivalent to a can of beer). Three possible reasons, acting separately or together, may explain why. For one, the alcohol may have altered the flavor of the breast milk and thereby the infants' acceptance of it. For another, because infants metabolize alcohol inefficiently, even low doses may be potent enough to suppress their feeding and cause sleepiness. Third, the alcohol may have interfered with lactation by inhibiting the hormone oxytocin.

In the past, alcohol has been recommended to mothers to facilitate lactation despite a lack of scientific evidence that it does so. The research summarized here suggests that alcohol actually hinders breastfeeding. An occasional glass of wine or beer is considered within safe limits, but in general, lactating women should consume little or no alcohol.

Medicinal Drugs Most medicines are compatible with breastfeeding, but some are contraindicated, either because they suppress lactation or because they are secreted into breast milk and can harm the infant.[66] As a precaution, a nursing mother should consult with her physician prior to taking any drug, including herbal supplements.

Illicit Drugs Illicit drugs, of course, are harmful to the physical and emotional health of both the mother and the nursing infant. Breast milk can deliver such high doses of illicit drugs as to cause irritability, tremors, hallucinations, and even death in infants. Women whose infants have overdosed on illicit drugs contained in breast milk have been convicted of murder.

Smoking Cigarette smoking reduces milk volume, so smokers may produce too little milk to meet their infants' energy needs. The milk they do produce contains nicotine, which alters its smell and flavor. Consequently, infants of breastfeeding mothers who smoke gain less weight than infants of those who do not smoke. Furthermore, infant exposure to passive smoke negates the protective effect breastfeeding offers against SIDS and increases the risks dramatically.

Environmental Contaminants Some environmental contaminants, such as DDT, PCBs, and dioxin, can find their way into breast milk. Inuit mothers living in Arctic Québec who eat seal and beluga whale blubber have high concentrations of DDT and PCBs in their breast milk, but the impact on infant development is unclear. Preliminary studies indicate that the children of these Inuit mothers are developing normally. Researchers speculate that the abundant omega-3 fatty acids of the Inuit diet may protect against damage to the central nervous system. Breast milk tainted with dioxins interferes with tooth development during early infancy, producing soft, mottled teeth that are vulnerable to dental caries.[67] To limit mercury intake, lactating women should heed the fish restrictions mentioned earlier for pregnant women.

Caffeine Caffeine enters breast milk and may make an infant irritable and wakeful. As during pregnancy, caffeine consumption should be moderate—the equivalent of 1 to 2 cups of coffee a day. Larger doses of caffeine may interfere with the bioavailability of iron from breast milk and impair the infant's iron status.

Maternal Health

If a woman has an ordinary cold, she can continue nursing without worry. If susceptible, the infant will catch it from her anyway. (Thanks to the immunological protection of breast milk, the baby may be less susceptible than a formula-fed baby would be.) With appropriate treatment, a woman who has an infectious disease such as tuberculosis or hepatitis can breastfeed; transmission is rare.[68] Women with HIV (human immunodeficiency virus) infections, however, should consider other options.

HIV Infection and AIDS Mothers with HIV infections can transmit the virus (which causes AIDS) to their infants through breast milk, especially during the early months of breastfeeding.[69] Where safe alternatives are available, HIV-positive women should *not* breastfeed their infants. In developing countries, where the feeding of inappropriate or contaminated formulas causes 1.5 million infant deaths each year, the decision is less obvious.[70] To prevent the mother-to-child transmission of HIV, WHO and UNICEF urge mothers in developing countries *not* to breastfeed, but stress the importance of finding suitable feeding alternatives to prevent the malnutrition, disease, and death that commonly occur when women in these countries do not breastfeed.

Diabetes Women with diabetes (type 1) may need careful monitoring and counseling to ensure successful lactation. These women need to adjust their energy intakes and insulin doses to meet the heightened needs of lactation. Maintaining good glucose control helps to initiate lactation and support milk production.

Postpartum Amenorrhea Women who breastfeed experience prolonged **postpartum amenorrhea.** Absent menstrual periods, however, do not protect a woman from pregnancy. To prevent pregnancy, a couple must use some form of contraception—but not oral contraceptive agents. Standard oral contraceptives contain estrogen, which reduces milk volume and the protein content of breast milk.

Breast Health Some women fear that breastfeeding will cause their breasts to sag. The breasts do swell and become heavy and large immediately after the birth, but even when they are producing enough milk to nourish a thriving infant, they eventually shrink back to their prepregnant size. Given proper support, diet, and exercise, breasts often return to their former shape and size when lactation ends. Breasts change their shape as the body ages, but breastfeeding does not accelerate this process.

Whether the physical and hormonal events of lactation protect women from later breast cancer is an area of active research. Some research suggests no association between breastfeeding and breast cancer, whereas other research suggests a protective effect.[71] The reduction in breast cancer risk is most apparent for premenopausal women who were young when they breastfed and who breastfed for a long time.

IN SUMMARY The lactating woman needs extra fluid and enough energy and nutrients to produce about 25 ounces of milk a day. Alcohol, other drugs, smoking, and contaminants may reduce milk production or enter breast milk and impair infant development.

This chapter has focused on the nutrition needs of the mother during pregnancy and lactation. The next chapter explores the dietary needs of infants, children, and adolescents.

postpartum amenorrhea: the normal temporary absence of menstrual periods immediately following childbirth.

Nutrition in Your Life

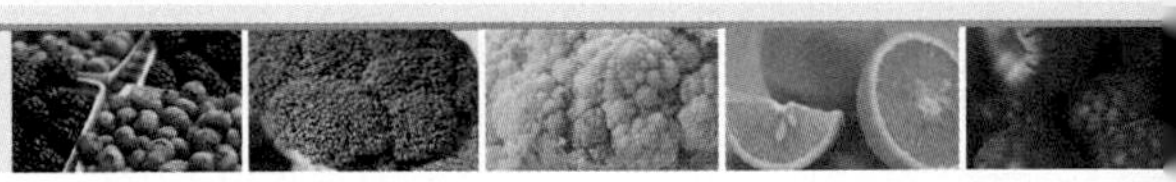

The choices a woman makes in preparation for, and in support of, pregnancy and lactation can influence both her health and her infant's development—today and for decades to come.

- **For women of childbearing age, do you consume at least 400 micrograms of folate daily?**
- **For women who are pregnant, are you paying attention to your nutrition needs and gaining the amount of weight recommended?**
- **For women who are about to give birth, have you carefully considered all the advantages of breastfeeding your infant and received the advice and support you need to be successful?**

NUTRITION ON THE NET

Access these websites for further study of topics covered in this chapter.

- Find updates and quick links to these and other nutrition-related sites at our website: **www.wadsworth.com/nutrition**
- Visit the pregnancy and child health center of the Mayo Clinic: **www.mayohealth.org**
- Learn more about having a healthy baby and about birth defects from the March of Dimes and the National Center on Birth Defects and Developmental Disabilities: **www.modimes.org** and **www.cdc.gov/ncbddd**
- Learn more about neural tube defects from the Spina Bifida Association of America: **www.sbaa.org**
- Search for "birth defects," "pregnancy," "adolescent pregnancy," "maternal and infant health," and "breastfeeding" at the U.S. Government health information site: **www.healthfinder.gov**
- Search for "pregnancy" at the American Dietetic Association site: **www.eatright.org**
- Learn more about the WIC program: **www.fns.usda.gov/fns**
- Visit the American College of Obstetricians and Gynecologists: **www.acog.org**
- Learn more about gestational diabetes from the American Diabetes Association: **www.diabetes.org**
- Learn more about breastfeeding from LaLeche League International: **www.lalecheleague.org**
- Obtain prenatal nutrition guidelines from Health Canada: **www.hc-sc.gc.ca**

STUDY QUESTIONS

These questions will help you review the chapter. You will find the answers in the discussions on the pages provided.

1. Describe the placenta and its function. (pp. 474–475)
2. Describe the normal events of fetal development. How does malnutrition impair fetal development? (pp. 474–476, 490)
3. Define the term *critical period*. How do adverse influences during critical periods affect later health? (pp. 476–479)
4. Explain why women of childbearing age need folate in their diets. How much is recommended, and how can women ensure that these needs are met? (pp. 477–478, 484)
5. What is the recommended pattern of weight gain during pregnancy for a woman at a healthy weight? For an underweight woman? For an overweight woman? (pp. 480–481)
6. What does a pregnant woman need to know about exercise? (pp. 482–483)
7. Which nutrients are needed in the greatest amounts during pregnancy? Why are they so important? Describe wise food choices for the pregnant woman. (pp. 484–487)
8. Define low-risk and high-risk pregnancies. What is the significance of infant birthweight in terms of the child's future health? (pp. 489–490)
9. Describe some of the special problems of the pregnant adolescent. Which nutrients are needed in increased amounts? (pp. 492–493)
10. What practices should be avoided during pregnancy? Why? (pp. 493–496)
11. How do nutrient needs during lactation differ from nutrient needs during pregnancy? (pp. 498–499)

These multiple choice questions will help you prepare for an exam. Answers can be found on (p. 504).

1. The spongy structure that delivers nutrients to the fetus and returns waste products to the mother is called the:
   a. embryo.
   b. uterus.
   c. placenta.
   d. amniotic sac.
2. Which of these strategies is *not* a healthy option for an overweight woman?
   a. Limit weight gain during pregnancy.
   b. Postpone weight loss until after pregnancy.
   c. Follow a weight-loss diet during pregnancy.
   d. Try to achieve a healthy weight before becoming pregnant.
3. A reasonable weight gain during pregnancy for a normal-weight woman is about:
   a. 10 pounds.
   b. 20 pounds.
   c. 30 pounds.
   d. 40 pounds.
4. Energy needs during pregnancy increase by about:
   a. 100 kcalories/day.
   b. 300 kcalories/day.
   c. 500 kcalories/day.
   d. 700 kcalories/day.
5. To help prevent neural tube defects, grain products are now fortified with:
   a. iron.
   b. folate.
   c. protein.
   d. vitamin C.

6. Pregnant women should *not* take supplements of:
   a. iron.
   b. folate.
   c. vitamin A.
   d. vitamin C.
7. The combination of high blood pressure, protein in the urine, and edema signals:
   a. jaundice.
   b. preeclampsia.
   c. gestational diabetes.
   d. gestational hypertension.
8. To facilitate lactation, a mother needs:
   a. about 5000 kcalories a day.
   b. adequate nutrition and rest.
   c. vitamin and mineral supplements.
   d. a glass of wine or beer before each feeding.
9. A breastfeeding woman should drink plenty of water to:
   a. produce more milk.
   b. suppress lactation.
   c. prevent dehydration.
   d. dilute nutrient concentration.
10. A woman may need iron supplements during lactation:
    a. to enhance the iron in her breast milk.
    b. to provide iron for the infant's growth.
    c. to replace the iron in her body's stores.
    d. to support the increase in her blood volume.

REFERENCES

1. J. Erickson, Folic acid and prevention of spina bifida and anencephaly, *Morbidity and Mortality Weekly Report* 51 (2002): 1–3; M. A. Honein and coauthors, Impact of folic acid fortification of the US food supply on the occurrence of neural tube defects, *Journal of the American Medical Association* 285 (2001): 2981–2986.
2. C. N. Hales and S. E. Ozanne, For debate: Fetal and early postnatal growth restriction lead to diabetes, the metabolic syndrome and renal failure, *Diabetologia* 46 (2003): 1013–1019; K. M. Rasmussen, The "fetal origins" hypothesis: Challenges and opportunities for maternal and child nutrition, *Annual Review of Nutrition* 21 (2001): 73–95; K. M. Godfrey and D. J. P. Barker, Fetal nutrition and adult disease, *American Journal of Clinical Nutrition* 71 (2000): 1344S–1352S; A. Lucas, M. S. Fewtrell, and J. Cole, Fetal origins of adult disease—The hypothesis revisited, *British Medical Journal* 319 (1999): 245–249.
3. B. E. Birgisdottir and coauthors, Size at birth and glucose intolerance in a relatively genetically homogeneous, high-birth weight population, *American Journal of Clinical Nutrition* 76 (2002): 399–403; T. W. McDade and coauthors, Prenatal undernutrition, postnatal environments, and antibody response to vaccination in adolescence, *American Journal of Clinical Nutrition* 74 (2001): 543–548.
4. P. Szitányi, J. Janda, and R. Poledne, Intrauterine undernutrition and programming as a new risk of cardiovascular disease in later life, *Physiological Research* 52 (2003): 389–395; A. Singhal and coauthors, Programming of lean body mass: A link between birth weight, obesity, and cardiovascular disease? *American Journal of Clinical Nutrition* 77 (2003): 726–730; T. J. Roseboom and coauthors, Plasma lipid profiles in adults after prenatal exposure to the Dutch famine, *American Journal of Clinical Nutrition* 72 (2000): 1101–1106.
5. G. Wolf, Adult type 2 diabetes induced by intrauterine growth retardation, *Nutrition Reviews* 61 (2003): 176–179.
6. J. W. Rich-Edwards and coauthors, Birthweight and the risk for type 2 diabetes mellitus in adult women, *Annals of Internal Medicine* 130 (1999): 278–284.
7. K. M. Moritz, M. Dodic, and E. M. Wintour, Kidney development and the fetal programming of adult disease, *Bioessays* 25 (2003): 212–220; M. Symonds and coauthors, Maternal nutrient restriction during placental growth, programming of fetal adiposity and juvenile blood pressure control, *Archives of Physiology and Biochemistry* 111 (2003): 45–52; J. Eriksson and coauthors, Fetal and childhood growth and hypertension in adult life, *Hypertension* 36 (2000): 790–794.
8. C. M. Law and coauthors, Fetal, infant, and childhood growth and adult blood pressure: A longitudinal study from birth to 22 years of age, *Circulation* 105 (2002): 1088–1092; J. G. Ericksson and coauthors, Early growth and coronary heart disease in later life: Longitudinal study, *British Medical Journal* 322 (2001): 949–953.
9. E. Pennisi, Behind the scenes of gene expression, *Science* 293 (2001): 1064–1067.
10. R. A. Waterland and R. L. Jirtle, Transposable elements: Targets for early nutritional effects on epigenetic gene regulation, *Molecular and Cellular Biology* 23 (2003): 5293–5300.
11. J. M. Baeten, E. A. Bukusi, and M. Lambe, Pregnancy complications and outcomes among overweight and obese nulliparous women, *American Journal of Public Health* 91 (2001): 436–440.
12. F. Galtier-Dereure, C. Boegner, and J. Bringer, Obesity and pregnancy: Complications and cost, *American Journal of Clinical Nutrition* 71 (2000): 1242S–1248S.
13. T. K. Young and B. Woodmansee, Factors that are associated with cesarean delivery in a large private practice: The importance of pregnancy body mass index and weight gain, *American Journal of Obstetrics and Gynecology* 187 (2002): 312–318.
14. M. L. Watkins and coauthors, Maternal obesity and risk for birth defects, *Pediatrics* 111 (2003): 1152–1158.
15. M. Kihlstrand and coauthors, Water gymnastics reduced the intensity of back/low back pain in pregnant women, *Acta Obstetrica Gynecologica Scandinavica* 78 (1999): 180–185.
16. R. Artal and M. O'Toole, Guidelines of the American College of Obstetricians and Gynecologists for exercise during pregnancy and the postpartum period, *British Journal of Sports Medicine* 37 (2003): 6–12; Committee on Obstetric Practice, Exercise during pregnancy and the postpartum period, *Obstetrics and Gynecology* 99 (2002): 171–173.
17. J. C. King, Physiology of pregnancy and nutrient metabolism, *American Journal of Clinical Nutrition* 71 (2000): 1218S–1225S.
18. D. L. Dufour, J. C. Reina, and G. B. Spurr, Energy intake and expenditure of free-living, pregnant Colombian women in an urban setting, *American Journal of Clinical Nutrition* 70 (1999): 269–276; L. E. Kopp-Hoolihan and coauthors, Longitudinal assessment of energy balance in well-nourished pregnant women, *American Journal of Clinical Nutrition* 69 (1999): 697–704.
19. M. Makrides and R. A. Gibson, Long-chain polyunsaturated fatty acid requirements during pregnancy and lactation, *American Journal of Clinical Nutrition* 71 (2000): 307S–311S; M. D. M. Al, A. C. van Houwelingen, and G. Hornstra, Long-chain polyunsaturated fatty acids, pregnancy, and pregnancy outcome, *American Journal of Clinical Nutrition* 71 (2000): 285S–291S; A. K. Dutta-Roy, Transport mechanisms for long-chain polyunsaturated fatty acids in the human placenta, *American Journal of Clinical Nutrition* 71 (2000): 315S–322S; S. M. Innis, Maternal diet, length of gestation, and long-chain polyunsaturated fatty acid status of infants at birth, *American Journal of Clinical Nutrition* 70 (1999): 181–182.
20. Committee on Dietary Reference Intakes, *Dietary Reference Intakes for Thiamin, Riboflavin, Niacin, Vitamin B_6, Folate, Vitamin B_{12}, Pantothenic Acid, Biotin, and Choline* (Washington, D.C.: National Academy Press, 1998), pp. 196–305.
21. K. O. O'Brien and coauthors, Maternal iron status influences iron transfer to the fetus during the third trimester of pregnancy, *American Journal of Clinical Nutrition* 77 (2003): 924–930.
22. B. P. Zhu and coauthors, Effect of the interval between pregnancies on perinatal outcomes, *New England Journal of Medicine* 340 (1999): 589–594.
23. M. M. Werler and coauthors, Multivitamin supplementation and risk of birth defects, *American Journal of Epidemiology* 150 (1999): 675–682.
24. E. A. Rose, J. H. Porcerelli, and A. V. Neale, Pica: Common but commonly missed, *Journal of the American Board of Family Practice* 13 (2000): 353–358.
25. S. Saigal and coauthors, School difficulties at adolescence in a regional cohort of children who were extremely low birth weight, *Pediatrics* 105 (2000): 325–331.
26. American Academy of Pediatrics, WIC program, *Pediatrics* 108 (2001): 1216–1217.
27. W. van Wootten and R. E. Turner, Macrosomia in neonates of mothers with gestational diabetes is associated with body mass index and previous gestational diabetes, *Journal of the American Dietetic Association* 102 (2002): 241–243.
28. Report of the Expert Committee on the Diagnosis and Classification of Diabetes Mellitus, *Diabetes Care* 26 (2003): S5–S20.
29. Position statement from the American Diabetes Association: Gestational diabetes mellitus, *Diabetes Care* 26 (2003): S103–S105.
30. O. Langer and coauthors, A comparison of glyburide and insulin women with

gestational diabetes mellitus, *New England Journal of Medicine* 343 (2000): 1134–1138.
31. M. S. Esplin and coauthors, Paternal and maternal components of the predisposition to preeclampsia, *New England Journal of Medicine* 344 (2001): 867–872.
32. *National Vital Statistics Reports* 47 (1999): 14.
33. D. Maine, Role of nutrition in the prevention of toxemia, *American Journal of Clinical Nutrition* 72 (2000): 298S–300S.
34. J. Villar and J. M. Belizan, Same nutrient, different hypotheses: Disparities in trials of calcium supplementation during pregnancy, *American Journal of Clinical Nutrition* 71 (2000): 1375S–1379S.
35. National Center for Health Statistics, Centers for Disease Control, **www. cdc.gov/nchs,** visited April 25, 2003; National and state-specific pregnancy rates among adolescents —United States, 1995–1997, *Morbidity and Mortality Weekly Report* 49 (2000): 605–611.
36. R. J. Paulson and coauthors, Pregnancy in the sixth decade of life—Obstetric outcomes in women of advanced reproductive age, *Journal of the American Medical Association* 288 (2002): 2320–2323.
37. S. C. Tough and coauthors, Delayed childbearing and its impact on population rate changes in lower birth weight, multiple birth, and preterm delivery, *Pediatrics* 109 (2002): 399–403.
38. Alcohol use among women of childbearing age—United States, 1991–1999, *Morbidity and Mortality Weekly Report* 51 (2002): 273–276.
39. Committee on Drugs, American Academy of Pediatrics, Use of psychoactive medication during pregnancy and possible effects on the fetus and newborn, *Pediatrics* 105 (2000): 880–887.
40. E. S. Bandstra and coauthors, Intrauterine growth of full-term infants: Impact of prenatal cocaine exposure, *Pediatrics* 108 (2001): 1309–1319; D. A. Frank and coauthors, Level of in utero cocaine exposure and neonatal ultrasound findings, *Pediatrics* 104 (1999): 1101–1105; G. A. Richardson and coauthors, Growth of infants prenatally exposed to cocaine/crack: Comparison of a prenatal care and a no prenatal care sample, *Pediatrics* 104 (1999): e8.
41. L. T. Singer and coauthors, Cognitive and motor outcomes of cocaine-exposed infants, *Journal of the American Medical Association* 287 (2002): 1952–1960; M. S. Scher, G. A. Richardson, and N. L. Day, Effects of prenatal cocaine/crack and other drug exposure on electroencephalographic sleep studies at birth and one year, *Pediatrics* 105 (2000): 39–48.
42. Committee on Drugs, American Academy of Pediatrics, Neonatal drug withdrawal, *Pediatrics* 101 (1998): 1079–1088.
43. J. M. Lightwood, C. S. Phibbs, and S. A. Glantz, Short-term health and economic benefits of smoking cessation: Low birth weight, *Pediatrics* 104 (1999): 1312–1320; S. Cnattingius and coauthors, The influence of gestational age and smoking habits on the risk of subsequent preterm deliveries, *New England Journal of Medicine* 341 (1999): 943–948.
44. X. Wang and coauthors, Maternal cigarette smoking, metabolic gene polymorphism, and infant birth weight, *Journal of the American Medical Association* 287 (2002): 195–202.
45. S. J. Ventura and coauthors, Trends and variations in smoking during pregnancy and low birth weight. Evidence from the birth certificate, 1990–2000, *Pediatrics* 111 (2003): 1176–1180; S. H. Ebrahim and coauthors, Trends in pregnancy-related smoking rates in the United States, 1987–1996, *Journal of the American Medical Association* 283 (2000): 361–366.
46. A. Gomaa and coauthors, Maternal bone lead as an independent risk factor for fetal neurotoxicity: A prospective study, *Pediatrics* 110 (2002): 110–118.
47. M. A. Johnson, High calcium intake blunts pregnancy-induced increases in maternal blood lead, *Nutrition Reviews* 59 (2001): 152–156.
48. N. Ribas-Fitó and coauthors, Breastfeeding, exposure to organochlorine compounds, and neurodevelopment in infants, *Pediatrics* 111 (2003): e580–e585.
49. S. E. Schober and coauthors, Blood mercury levels in US children and women of childbearing age, 1999–2000, *Journal of the American Medical Association* 289 (2003): 1667–1674.
50. Fish advisories, **www.epa.gov/ost/fish** visited April 23, 2003.
51. S. Cnattingius and coauthors, Caffeine intake and the risk of first-trimester spontaneous abortion, *New England Journal of Medicine* 343 (2000): 1839–1845; M. A. Klebanoff and coauthors, Maternal serum paraxanthine, a caffeine metabolite, and the risk of spontaneous abortion, *New England Journal of Medicine* 341 (1999): 1639–1644.
52. Position of the American Dietetic Association: Use of nutritive and nonnutritive sweetners, *Journal of the American Dietetic Association* 98 (1998): 580–587.
53. Position of the American Dietetic Association: Nutrition and lifestyle for a healthy pregnancy outcome, *Journal of the American Dietetic Association* 102 (2002): 1479–1490.
54. R. Li and coauthors, Prevalence of breastfeeding in the United States: The 2001 National Immunization Survey, *Pediatrics* 111 (2003): 1198–1201; A. S. Ryan, Z. Wenjun, and A. Acosta, Breastfeeding continues to increase into the new millennium, *Pediatrics* 110 (2002): 1103–1109.
55. Position of the American Dietetic Association: Breaking the barriers to breastfeeding, *Journal of the American Dietetic Association* 101 (2001): 1213–1220; Department of Health and Human Services, *Breastfeeding—HHS Blueprint for Action on Breastfeeding,* 2000.
56. Physicians and breastfeeding promotion in the United States: A call to action, *Pediatrics* 107 (2001): 584–588.
57. D. R. Zimmerman and N. Guttman, "Breast is best": Knowledge among low-income mothers is not enough, *Journal of Human Lactation* 17 (2001): 14–19.
58. B. L. Philipp and coauthors, Baby-friendly hospital initiative improves breastfeeding initiation rates in a US hospital setting, *Pediatrics* 108 (2001): 677–681.
59. C. L. Dennis, Breastfeeding initiation and duration: A 1990–2000 literature review, *Journal of Obstetric, Gynecologic and Neonatal Nursing* 31 (2002): 12–32; S. Arora and coauthors, Major factors influencing breastfeeding rates: Mother's perception of father's attitude and milk supply, *Pediatrics* 106 (2000): e67.
60. Dennis, 2002.
61. M. A. McCrory, Does dieting during lactation put infant growth at risk? *Nutrition Reviews* 59 (2001): 18–21.
62. C. A. Lovelady and coauthors, The effect of weight loss in overweight, lactating women on the growth of their infants, *New England Journal of Medicine* 342 (2000): 449–453; M. A. McCrory and coauthors, Randomized trial of the short-term effects of dieting compared with dieting plus aerobic exercise on lactation performance, *American Journal of Clinical Nutrition* 69 (1999): 959–967.
63. L. M. Paton and coauthors, Pregnancy and lactation have no long-term deleterious effect on measures of bone mineral in healthy women: A twin study, *American Journal of Clinical Nutrition* 77 (2003): 707–714.
64. J. A. Mennella, C. P. Jagnow, and G. K. Beauchamp, Prenatal and postnatal flavor learning by human infants, *Pediatrics* 107 (2001): e88.
65. Committee on Nutrition, American Academy of Pediatrics, Hypoallergenic infant formulas, *Pediatrics* 106 (2000): 346–349.
66. S. Ito and A. Lee, Drug excretion into breast milk—Overview, *Advanced Drug Delivery Reviews* 55 (2003): 617–627; Committee on Drugs, American Academy of Pediatrics, The transfer of drugs and other chemicals into human milk, *Pediatrics* 108 (2001): 776–789.
67. S. Alaluusua and coauthors, Developing teeth as biomarker of dioxin exposure, *Lancet* 353 (1999): 206.
68. J. S. Wang, Q. R. Zhu, and X. H. Wang, Breastfeeding does not pose any additional risk of immunoprophylaxis failure on infants of HBV carrier mothers, *International Journal of Clinical Practice* 57 (2003): 100–102; J. B. Hill and coauthors, Risk of hepatitis B transmission in breast-fed infants of chronic hepatitis B carriers, *Obstetrics and Gynecology* 99 (2002): 1049–1052; M. L. Newell and L. Pembrey, Mother-to-child transmission of hepatitis C virus infection, *Drugs of Today* 38 (2002): 321–337; E. R. Stiehm and M. A. Keller, Breast milk transmission of viral disease, *Advances in Nutritional Research* 10 (2001): 105–122.
69. J. S. Read and the Committee on Pediatric AIDS, human milk, breastfeeding, and transmission of human immunodeficiency virus type 1 in the United States, *Pediatrics* 112 (2003): 1196–1205; R. Nduati and coauthors, Effect of breastfeeding and formula feeding on transmission of HIV-1: A randomized clinical trial, *Journal of the American Medical Association* 283 (2000): 1167–1174.
70. J. Humphrey and P. Iliff, Is breast not best? Feeding babies born to HIV-positive mothers: Bringing balance to a complex issue, *Nutrition Reviews* 59 (2001): 119–127; E. Hormann, Breast-feeding and HIV: What choices does a mother really have? *Nutrition Today* 34 (1999): 189–196; M. G. Fowler, J. Bertolli, and P. Nieburg, When is breastfeeding not best? The dilemma facing HIV-infected women in resource poor settings, *Journal of the American Medical Association* 282 (1999): 781–783.
71. L. Lipworth, L. R. Bailey, and D. Trichopoulow, History of breast-feeding in relation to breast cancer risk: A review of the epidemiologic literature, *Journal of the National Cancer Institute* 92 (2000): 302–312.

ANSWERS

Study Questions (multiple choice)

1. c 2. c 3. c 4. b 5. b 6. c 7. b 8. b 9. c 10. c

HIGHLIGHT

Fetal Alcohol Syndrome

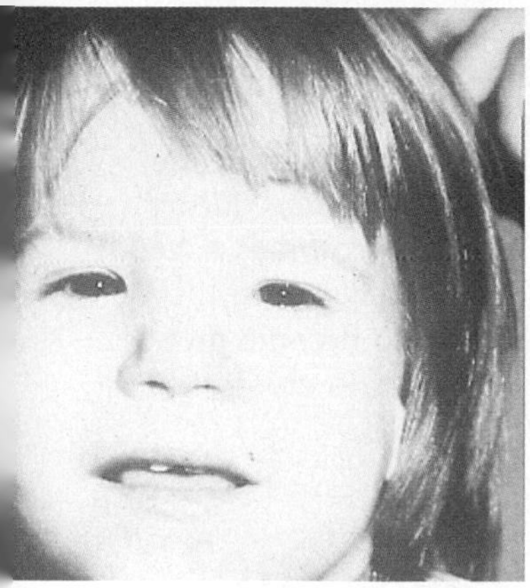

© Streissguth, A. P./Landesman-Dwyer, S., Martin, J. C., & Smith, D. W.

As Chapter 14 mentioned, drinking alcohol during pregnancy endangers the fetus. Alcohol crosses the placenta freely and deprives the developing fetus of both nutrients and oxygen. The result may be **fetal alcohol syndrome (FAS;** see the glossary on p. 506), a cluster of physical, mental, and neurobehavioral symptoms that includes:

- Prenatal and postnatal growth retardation.
- Impairment of the brain and central nervous system, with consequent mental retardation, poor motor skills and coordination, and hyperactivity.
- Abnormalities of the face and skull (see Figure H14-1).
- Increased frequency of major birth defects: cleft palate, heart defects, and defects in ears, eyes, genitals, and urinary system.

Tragically, the damage evident at birth persists: children with FAS never fully recover.[1]

Each year, as many as 12,000 infants are born with FAS because their mothers drank too much alcohol during pregnancy. In addition, three times as many infants are born with less serious, yet still significant, damage because their mothers drank alcohol—just not as much. These abnormalities fall short of FAS and were formerly known as **fetal alcohol effects (FAE).** This catchall term has been replaced by two terms that describe the mental and physical symptoms of **prenatal alcohol exposure.**[2] The cluster of mental problems associated with prenatal alcohol exposure is known as **alcohol-related neurodevelopmental disorder (ARND),** and the physical malformations are referred to as **alcohol-related birth defects (ARBD).** Some children with ARBD and ARND have no outward signs; others may be short or have only minor facial abnormalities. They often go undiagnosed even when they develop learning difficulties in the early school years. Mood disorders and problem behaviors, such as aggression, are common.[3]

The surgeon general states that pregnant women should drink absolutely no alcohol. Abstinence from alcohol is the best policy for pregnant women both because alcohol consumption during pregnancy has such severe consequences and because FAS can only be prevented—it cannot be treated. Further, because the most severe damage occurs around the time of conception—*before a woman may even realize that she is pregnant*—even a woman planning to conceive should abstain.

Drinking during Pregnancy

As mentioned in Chapter 14, one out of eight pregnant women drinks alcohol at some time during her pregnancy; 1 out of 30 uses alcohol frequently, and 1 out of 40 admits to binge drinking.[4] When a woman drinks during pregnancy, she causes damage in two ways: directly, by intoxication, and indirectly, by malnutrition. Prior to the complete formation of the placenta (approximately 12 weeks), alcohol diffuses

FIGURE H14-1 Typical Facial Characteristics of FAS

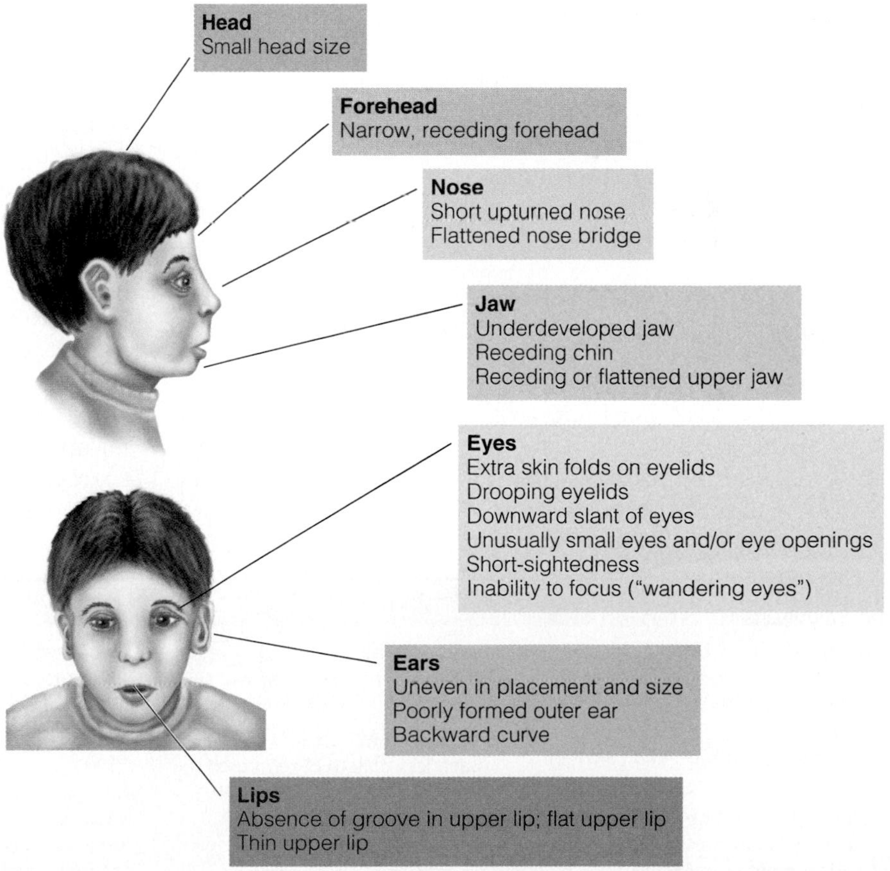
Head
Small head size
Forehead
Narrow, receding forehead
Nose
Short upturned nose
Flattened nose bridge
Jaw
Underdeveloped jaw
Receding chin
Receding or flattened upper jaw
Eyes
Extra skin folds on eyelids
Drooping eyelids
Downward slant of eyes
Unusually small eyes and/or eye openings
Short-sightedness
Inability to focus ("wandering eyes")
Ears
Uneven in placement and size
Poorly formed outer ear
Backward curve
Lips
Absence of groove in upper lip; flat upper lip
Thin upper lip

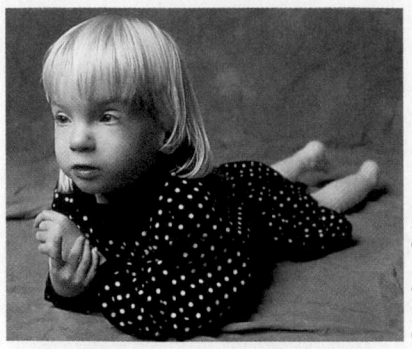

Characteristic facial features may diminish with time, but children with FAS typically continue to be short and underweight for their age.

directly into the tissues of the developing embryo, causing incredible damage. (Review Figure 14-4 on p. 476 and note that the critical periods for most tissues occur during embryonic development.) Alcohol interferes with the orderly development of tissues during their critical periods, reducing the number of cells and damaging those that are produced. The damage of alcohol toxicity during brain development is apparent in its reduced size and impaired function.[5]

When alcohol crosses the placenta, fetal blood alcohol rises until it reaches an equilibrium with maternal blood alcohol. The mother may not even appear drunk, but the fetus may be poisoned. The fetus's body is small, its detoxification system is immature, and alcohol remains in fetal blood long after it has disappeared from maternal blood.

A pregnant woman harms her unborn child not only by consuming alcohol but also by not consuming food. This combination enhances the likelihood of malnutrition and a poorly developed infant. It is important to realize, however, that malnutrition is not the cause of FAS. It is true that mothers of FAS children often have unbalanced diets and nutrient deficiencies. It is also true that malnutrition may augment the clinical signs seen in these children, but it is the *alcohol* that causes the damage. An adequate diet alone will not prevent FAS if alcohol abuse continues.

How Much Is Too Much?

A pregnant woman need not have an alcohol-abuse problem to give birth to a baby with FAS. She need only drink in excess of her liver's capacity to detoxify alcohol. Even one drink a day threatens neurological development and behaviors.[6] Four drinks a day dramatically worsens the risk of having an infant with physical malformations.

In addition to total alcohol intake, drinking patterns play an important role. Most FAS studies report their findings in terms of average intake per day, but people usually drink more heavily on some days than on others. For example, a woman who drinks an *average* of 1 ounce of alcohol (2 drinks) a day may not drink at all during the week, but then have 10 drinks on Saturday night, exposing the fetus to extremely toxic quantities of alcohol. Whether various drinking patterns incur damage depends on the frequency of consumption, the quantity consumed, and the stage of fetal development at the time of each drinking episode.

An occasional drink may be innocuous, but researchers are unable to say how much alcohol is safe to consume during pregnancy. For this reason, health care professionals urge women to stop drinking alcohol as soon as they realize they are pregnant or better, as soon as they *plan* to become pregnant. Why take any risk? Only the woman who abstains is sure of protecting her infant from FAS.

When Is the Damage Done?

The first month or two of pregnancy is a critical period of fetal development. Because pregnancy usually cannot be confirmed before five to six weeks, a woman may not even realize she is pregnant during that critical time. Therefore, it is advisable for women who are trying to conceive, or who suspect they might be pregnant, to abstain or curtail their alcohol intakes to ensure a healthy start.

The type of abnormality observed in an FAS infant depends on the developmental events occurring at the times of alcohol exposure. During the first trimester, developing organs such as the brain, heart, and kidneys may be malformed. During the second trimester, the risk of spontaneous abortion increases. During the third trimester, body and brain growth may be retarded.

Male alcohol ingestion may also affect fertility and fetal development.[7] Animal studies have found smaller litter sizes, lower birthweights, reduced survival rates, and impaired learning ability in the offspring of males consuming alcohol prior to conception. An association between paternal alcohol intake one month prior to conception and low infant birthweight is also

GLOSSARY

alcohol-related birth defects (ARBD): malformations in the skeletal and organ systems (heart, kidneys, eyes, ears) associated with prenatal alcohol exposure.

alcohol-related neurodevelopmental disorder (ARND): abnormalities in the central nervous system and cognitive development associated with prenatal alcohol exposure.

fetal alcohol effects (FAE): an older, less preferred, term used to describe both ARBD and ARND.

fetal alcohol syndrome (FAS): a cluster of physical, behavioral, and cognitive abnormalities associated with prenatal alcohol exposure, including facial malformations, growth retardation, and central nervous disorders.

prenatal alcohol exposure: subjecting a fetus to a pattern of excessive alcohol intake characterized by substantial regular use or heavy episodic drinking.

NOTE: See Highlight 7 for other alcohol-related terms and information.

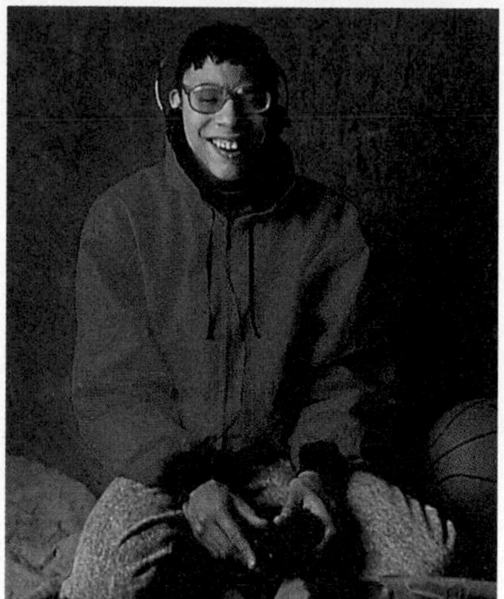

Children born with FAS must live with the long-term consequences of prenatal brain damage.

apparent in human beings. (Paternal alcohol intake was defined as an average of 2 or more drinks daily or at least 5 drinks on one occasion.) This relationship was independent of either parent's smoking and of the mother's use of alcohol, caffeine, or other drugs.

In view of the damage caused by FAS, prevention efforts focus on educating women not to drink during pregnancy.[8] Everyone should know of the potential dangers. Women who drink alcohol and who are sexually active may benefit from counseling and effective contraception to prevent pregnancy.[9] Almost half of all pregnancies are unintended, with many conceived during a binge drinking episode.[10]

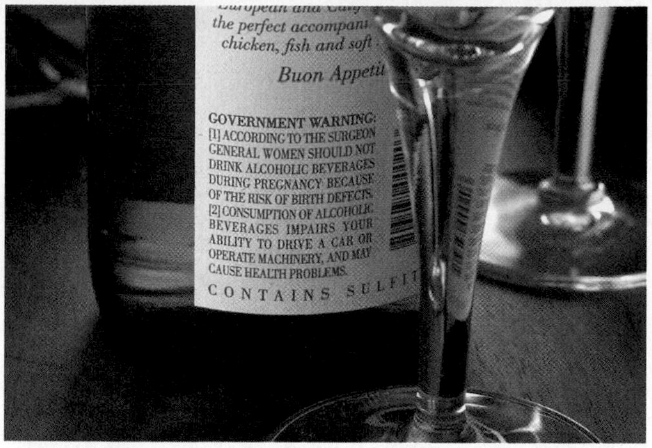
the perfect accompani
chicken, fish and soft
Buon Appetit
GOVERNMENT WARNING:
(1) ACCORDING TO THE SURGEON GENERAL WOMEN SHOULD NOT DRINK ALCOHOLIC BEVERAGES DURING PREGNANCY BECAUSE OF THE RISK OF BIRTH DEFECTS.
(2) CONSUMPTION OF ALCOHOLIC BEVERAGES IMPAIRS YOUR ABILITY TO DRIVE A CAR OR OPERATE MACHINERY, AND MAY CAUSE HEALTH PROBLEMS.
CONTAINS SULFIT

All containers of beer, wine, and liquor warn women not to drink alcoholic beverages during pregnancy because of the risk of birth defects.

Public service announcements and alcohol beverage warning labels help to raise awareness. Everyone should hear the message loud and clear: Don't drink alcohol prior to conception or during pregnancy.

NUTRITION ON THE NET

Access these websites for further study of topics covered in this highlight.

- Find updates and quick links to these and other nutrition-related sites at our website: **www.wadsworth.com/nutrition**
- Visit the National Organization on Fetal Alcohol Syndrome: **www.nofas.org**
- Search for "fetal alcohol syndrome" at the U.S. Government health information site: **www.healthfinder.gov**
- Request information on fetal alcohol syndrome from the National Clearinghouse for Alcohol and Drug Information: **www.health.org**
- Request information on drinking during pregnancy from the National Institute on Alcohol Abuse and Alcoholism: **www.niaaa.nih.gov**
- Gather facts on fetal alcohol syndrome from the March of Dimes: **www.modimes.org**

REFERENCES

1. N. L. Day and coauthors, Prenatal alcohol exposure predicts continued deficits in offspring size at 14 years of age, *Alcoholism: Clinical and Experimental Research* 26 (2002): 1584–1591; M. D. Cornelius and coauthors, Alcohol, tobacco and marijuana use among pregnant teenagers: 6-year follow-up of offspring growth effects, *Neurotoxicology and Teratology* 24 (2002): 703–710.
2. Committee on Substance Abuse and Committee on Children with Disabilities, American Academy of Pediatrics, Fetal alcohol syndrome and alcohol-related neurodevelopmental disorders, *Pediatrics* 106 (2000): 358–361.
3. M. J. O'Connor and coauthors, Psychiatric illness in a clinical sample of children with prenatal alcohol exposure, *American Journal of Drug and Alcohol Abuse* 28 (2002): 743–754; B. Sood and coauthors, Prenatal alcohol exposure and childhood behavior at age 6 to 7 years: Dose-response effect, *Pediatrics* 108 (2001): e34.
4. Alcohol use among women of childbearing age—United States 1991–1999, *Morbidity and Mortality Weekly Report* 51 (2002): 273–276.
5. J. W. Olney and coauthors, The enigma of fetal alcohol neurotoxicity, *Annals of Medicine* 34 (2002): 109–119.
6. S. W. Jacobson and coauthors, Validity of maternal report of prenatal alcohol, cocaine, and smoking in relation to neurobehavioral outcome, *Pediatrics* 109 (2002): 815–825.
7. H. Klonoff-Cohen, P. Lam-Kruglick, and C. Gonzalez, Effects of maternal and paternal alcohol consumption on the success rates of in vitro fertilization and gamete intrafallopian transfer, *Fertility and Sterility* 79 (2003): 330–339.
8. J. R. Hankin, Fetal alcohol syndrome prevention research, *Alcohol Research and Health* 26 (2002): 58–65.
9. The Project CHOICES Intervention Research Group, Reducing the risk of alcohol-exposed pregnancies: A study of a motivational intervention in community settings, *Pediatrics* 111 (2003): 1131–1135.
10. T. S. Naimi and coauthors, Binge drinking in the preconception period and the risk of unintended pregnancy: Implications for women and their children, *Pediatrics* 111 (2003): 1136–1141.

Chapter 15

Life Cycle Nutrition: Infancy, Childhood, and Adolescence

Chapter Outline

Nutrition during Infancy: *Energy and Nutrient Needs • Breast Milk • Infant Formula • Special Needs of Preterm Infants • Introducing Cow's Milk • Introducing Solid Foods • Mealtimes with Toddlers*

Nutrition during Childhood: *Energy and Nutrient Needs • Hunger and Malnutrition in Children • The Malnutrition-Lead Connection • Hyperactivity and "Hyper" Behavior • Food Allergy and Intolerance • Childhood Obesity • Mealtimes at Home • Nutrition at School*

Nutrition during Adolescence: *Growth and Development • Energy and Nutrient Needs • Food Choices and Health Habits • Problems Adolescents Face*

Highlight: *Childhood Obesity and the Early Development of Chronic Diseases*

Available Online

http://nutrition.wadsworth.com/uncn7

Nutrition Animation: *Nutrition in Childhood*

Student Practice Test

Glossary Terms

Nutrition on the Net

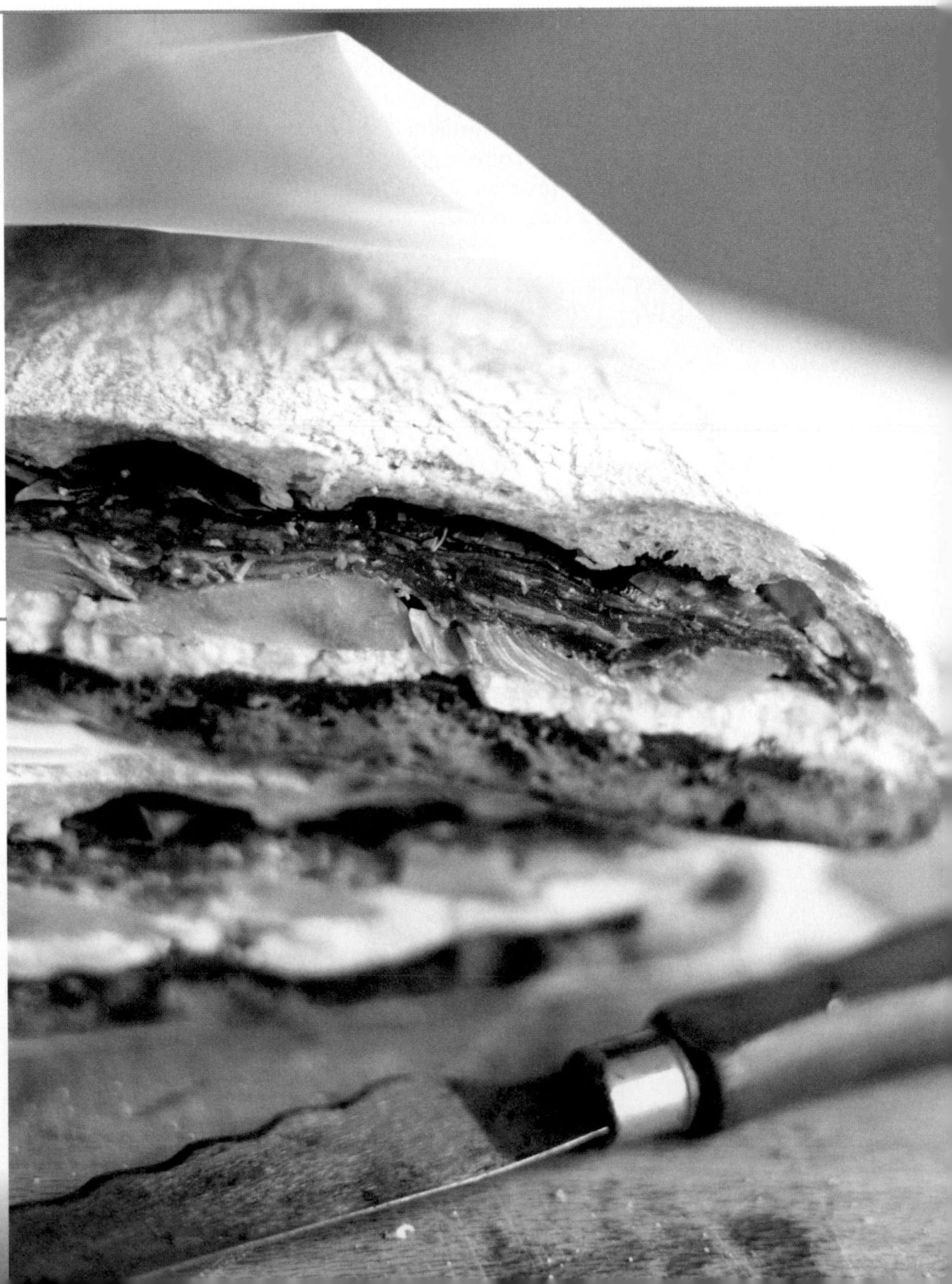

Nutrition in Your Life

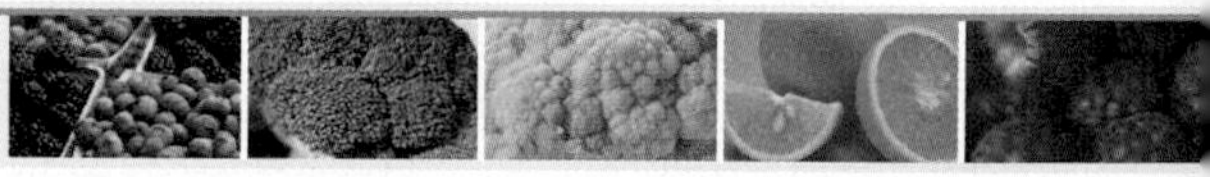

Much of this book has focused on you—your food choices and how they might affect your health. This chapter shifts the focus from you the recipient to you the caregiver. One day (if not already), children may depend on you to feed them well and teach them wisely. The responsibility of nourishing children can seem overwhelming at times, but the job is fairly simple: offer children a variety of nutritious foods to support their growth and teach them how to make healthy food and activity choices. Presenting foods in a relaxed and supportive environment nourishes both physical and emotional well-being.

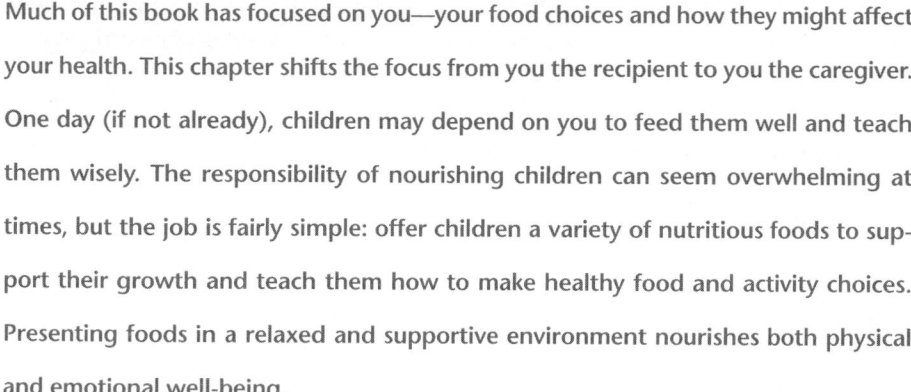

The first year of life is a time of phenomenal growth and development. After the first year, a child continues to grow and change, but more slowly. Still, the cumulative effects over the next decade are remarkable. Then, as the child enters the teen years, the pace toward adulthood accelerates dramatically. This chapter examines the special nutrient needs of infants, children, and adolescents.

Nutrition during Infancy

Initially, the infant drinks only breast milk or formula, but later begins to eat some foods, as appropriate. Common sense in the selection of infant foods and a nurturing, relaxed environment support an infant's health and well-being.

FIGURE 15-1 Weight Gain of Infants in Their First Five Years of Life

In the first year, an infant's birthweight may triple, but over the following several years, the rate of weight gain gradually diminishes.

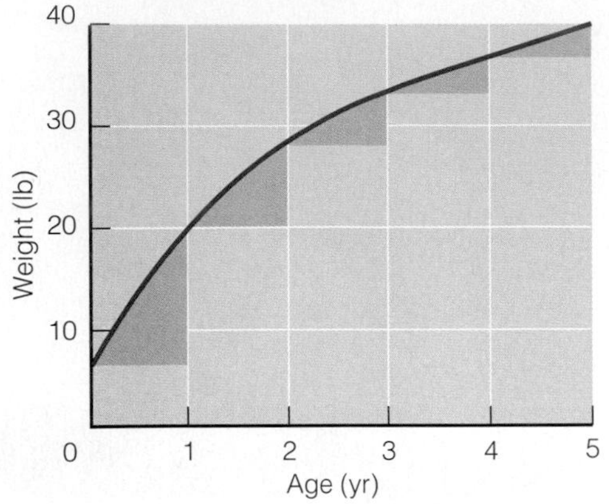
40
30
20
10
0
Weight (lb)
1
2
3
4
5
Age (yr)

	Infants	Adults
Heart rate (beats/minute)	120 to 140	70 to 80
Respiration rate (breaths/minute)	20 to 40	15 to 20
Energy needs (kcal/body weight)	45/lb (100/kg)	<18/lb (<40/kg)

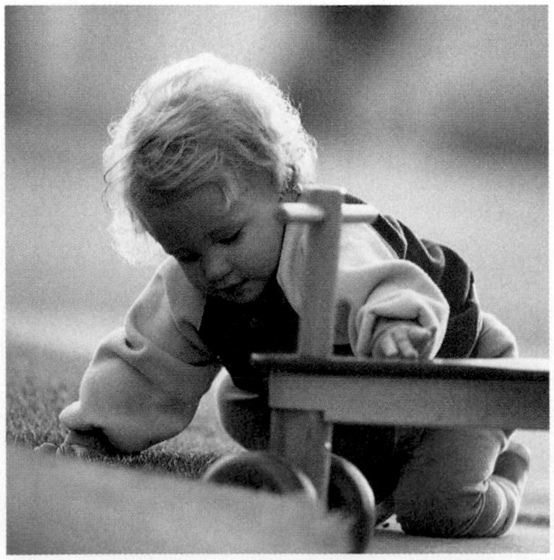

© Mark Scott/Taxi/Getty Images

After six months, energy saved by slower growth is spent in increased activity.

Energy and Nutrient Needs

An infant grows fast during the first year, as Figure 15-1 shows. Growth directly reflects nutrient intake and is an important parameter in assessing the nutrition status of infants and children. Health care professionals measure the heights and weights of infants and children at intervals and compare measures both with standard growth curves for gender and age and with previous measures of each child (see the "How to" on p. 512).[1]

Energy Intake and Activity A healthy infant's birthweight doubles by about five months of age and triples by one year, typically reaching 20 to 25 pounds. The infant's length changes more slowly than weight, increasing about 10 inches from birth to one year. By the end of the first year, infant growth slows considerably; an infant typically gains less than 10 pounds during the second year and grows about 5 inches in height.

Not only do infants grow rapidly, but their basal metabolic rate is remarkably high—about twice that of an adult, based on body weight. A newborn baby requires about 450 kcalories per day, whereas most adults require about 2000 kcalories per day. In terms of body weight, the difference is remarkable. Infants require about 100 kcalories per kilogram of body weight per day, whereas most adults need fewer than 40.■ If an infant's energy needs were superimposed on an adult, a 170-pound adult would require over 7000 kcalories a day. After six months, metabolic needs decline as the growth rate slows, but some of the energy saved by slower growth is spent in increased activity.

Energy Nutrients Recommendations for the energy nutrients—carbohydrate, fat, and protein—during the first six months of life are based on the average intakes of healthy, full-term infants fed breast milk.[2] During the second six months of life, recommendations reflect typical intakes from solid foods as well as breast milk.

As discussed in Chapter 4, carbohydrates provide energy to all the cells of the body, especially those in the brain, which depend primarily on glucose to fuel activities. Relative to the size of the body, an infant's brain is larger than an adult's and uses relatively more glucose—about 60 percent of the day's total energy intake.[3]

Fat provides most of the energy in breast milk and standard infant formula. Its high energy density supports the rapid growth of early infancy.

No single nutrient is more essential to growth than protein. All of the body's cells and most of its fluids contain protein; it is the basic building material of the body's tissues. Chapter 6 detailed the problems inadequate protein can cause. Excess dietary protein can cause problems, too, especially in a small infant. Too much protein stresses the liver and kidneys, which have to metabolize and excrete the excess nitrogen. Signs of protein overload include acidosis, dehydration, diarrhea, elevated blood ammonia, elevated blood urea, and fever. Such problems are not common, but have been observed in infants fed inappropriate foods, such as fat-free milk or concentrated formula.

Vitamins and Minerals Like the recommendations for the energy nutrients, those for the vitamins and minerals are based on the average amount of nutrients consumed by thriving infants breastfed by well-nourished mothers. An infant's needs for most of these nutrients, in proportion to body weight, are more than double those of an adult. Figure 15-2 illustrates this by comparing a five-month-old infant's needs per unit of body weight with those of an adult man. Some of the differences are extraordinary.

Water One of the most essential nutrients for infants, as for everyone, is water. The younger the infant, the greater the percentage of body weight is water. During early infancy, breast milk or infant formula normally provides enough water to replace fluid losses in a healthy infant. Even in hot, dry climates, neither breastfed nor bottle-fed infants need supplemental water.[4] Because much of the fluid in an infant's body is located *outside* the cells—between the cells and in the blood ves-

FIGURE 15-2 Recommended Intakes of an Infant and an Adult Compared on the Basis of Body Weight

Because infants are small, they need smaller total amounts of the nutrients than adults do, but when comparisons are based on body weight, infants need over twice as much of many nutrients. Infants use large amounts of energy and nutrients, in proportion to their body size, to keep all their metabolic processes going.

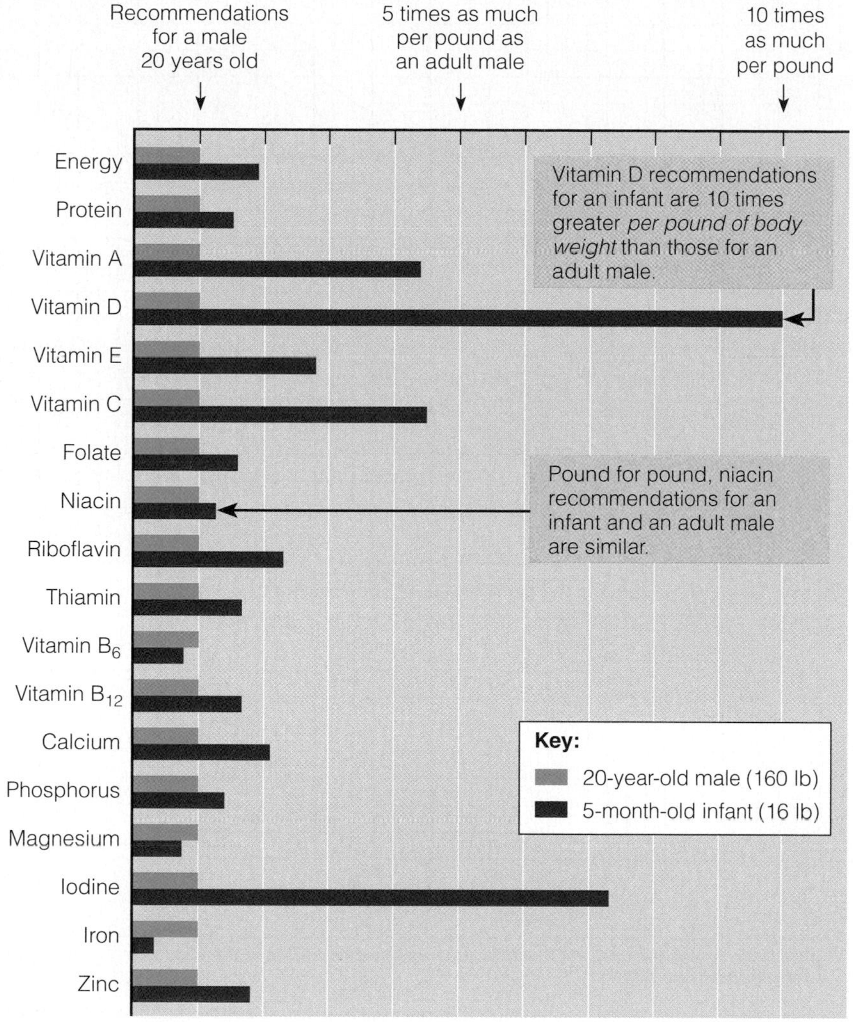

Recommendations for a male 20 years old
5 times as much per pound as an adult male
10 times as much per pound
Energy
Protein
Vitamin A
Vitamin D
Vitamin E
Vitamin C
Folate
Niacin
Riboflavin
Thiamin
Vitamin B6
Vitamin B12
Calcium
Phosphorus
Magnesium
Iodine
Iron
Zinc
Vitamin D recommendations for an infant are 10 times greater per pound of body weight than those for an adult male.
Pound for pound, niacin recommendations for an infant and an adult male are similar.
Key:
20-year-old male (160 lb)
5-month-old infant (16 lb)

sels—rapid fluid losses and the resulting dehydration can be life-threatening. Conditions that cause rapid fluid loss, such as diarrhea or vomiting, require an electrolyte solution designed for infants.

Breast Milk

In the United States and Canada, the two dietary practices that have the most effect on an infant's nutrition are the milk the infant receives and the age at which solid foods are introduced. A later section discusses the introduction of solid foods, but as to the milk, both the American Academy of Pediatrics (AAP) and the Canadian Paediatric Society strongly recommend breastfeeding for full-term infants, except where specific contraindications exist. The American Dietetic Association (ADA) also advocates breastfeeding for the nutritional health it confers on the infant as well as for the many other benefits it provides both infant and mother (review Table 14-4 on p. 497).[5]

HOW TO Plot Measures on a Growth Chart

You can assess the growth of infants and children by plotting their measurements on a percentile graph. Percentile graphs divide the measures of a population into 100 equal divisions so that half of the population falls at or above the 50th percentile, and half falls below. Using percentiles allows for comparisons among people of the same age and gender.

To plot measures on a growth chart, follow these steps:

- Select the appropriate chart based on age and gender. For this example, use the accompanying chart, which gives percentiles for weight for girls from birth to 36 months. (Appendix E provides other growth charts for both boys and girls of various ages.)
- Locate the infant's age along the horizontal axis at the bottom of the chart (in this example, 6 months).
- Locate the infant's weight in pounds or kilograms along the vertical axis of the chart (in this example, 17 pounds or 7.7 kilograms).
- Mark the chart where the age and weight lines intersect (shown here with a red dot), and read off the percentile.

This six-month-old infant is at the 75th percentile. Her pediatrician will weigh her again over the next few months and expect the growth curve to follow the same percentile throughout the first year. In general, dramatic changes or measures much above the 80th percentile or much below the 10th percentile may be cause for concern.

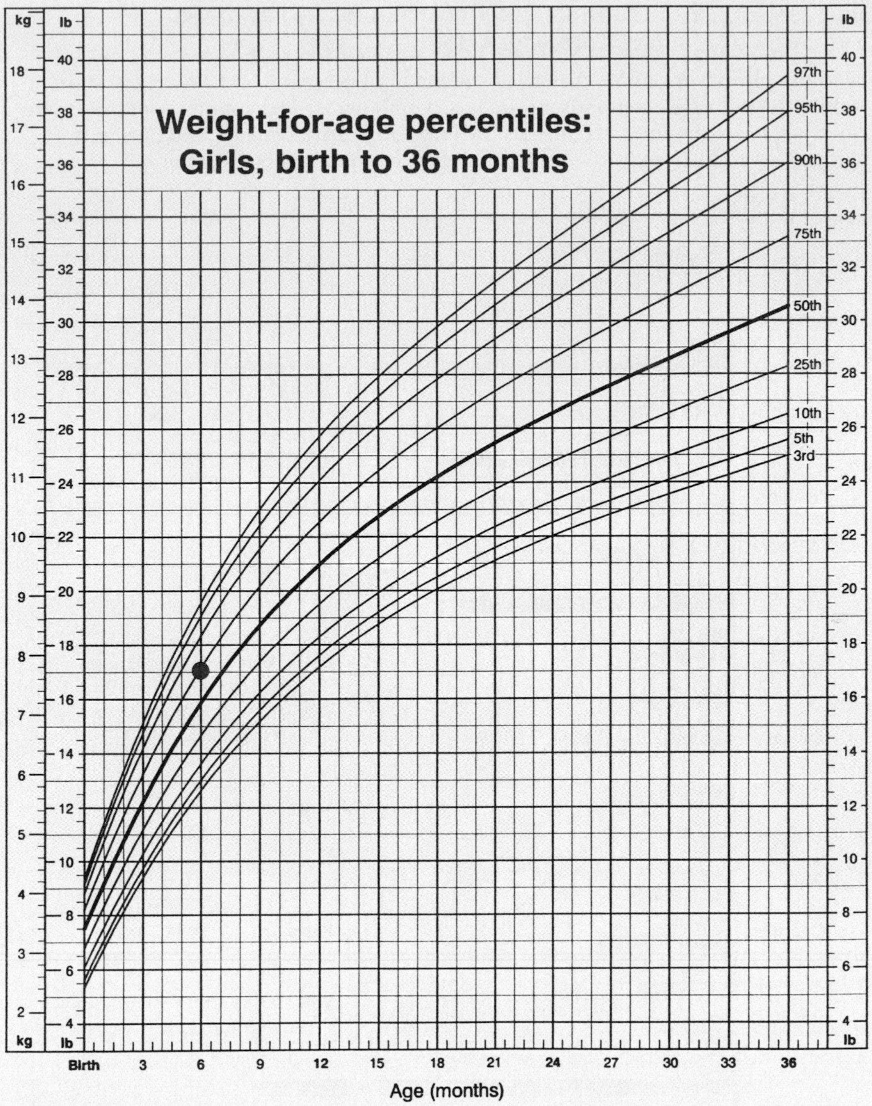
Weight-for-age percentiles:
Girls, birth to 36 months
kg
lb
97th
95th
90th
75th
50th
25th
10th
5th
3rd
Birth
3
6
9
12
15
18
21
24
27
30
33
36
Age (months)

SOURCE: Developed by the National Center for Health Statistics in collaboration with the National Center for Chronic Disease Prevention and Health Promotion (2000).

■ Reminder: Chapter 14 discusses breastfeeding, breastfeeding support, reasons why some women choose not to breastfeed, and contraindications to breastfeeding.

Breast milk excels as a source of nutrients for infants. Its unique nutrient composition and protective factors promote optimal infant health and development throughout the first year of life. Both the AAP and the ADA recognize exclusive breastfeeding for 6 months, and breastfeeding with complementary foods for at least 12 months, as the best feeding pattern for infants.[6] Experts add, though, that iron-fortified formula, which imitates the nutrient composition of breast milk, is an acceptable alternative. After all, the primary goal is to provide the infant nourishment in a relaxed and loving environment.■

Frequency and Duration of Breastfeeding Breast milk is more easily and completely digested than formula, so breastfed infants usually need to eat more frequently than formula-fed infants do. During the first few weeks, approximately 8 to 12 feedings a day, on demand, or whenever the infant cries with hunger, promote optimal milk production and infant growth. An infant who nurses every two to three hours and sleeps contentedly between feedings is adequately nourished.

Other Potential Benefits Breastfeeding may also help protect against excessive weight gain later on. A well-controlled survey of more than 15,000 adolescents and their mothers indicates that those who were mostly breastfed for the first six months of life were less likely to become overweight than those who were fed formula.[21] Another survey of more than 2000 children (ages nine to ten) had similar findings.[22] A study of much younger children (three to five years of age), however, found no clear evidence that breastfeeding influences body weight.[23] These researchers noted that other factors, especially the mother's weight, strongly predict overweight in children.

Breastfeeding may have a positive effect on later intelligence.[24] In one study, young adults who had been breastfed as long as nine months scored higher on two different intelligence tests than those who had been breastfed less than one month. Many other studies suggest a beneficial effect of breastfeeding on intelligence, but when subjected to strict standards of methodology (for example, large sample size and appropriate intelligence testing), the evidence is less convincing.[25] Nevertheless, the possibility that breastfeeding may positively affect later intelligence is intriguing. It may be that some specific component of breast milk, such as DHA, stimulates brain development or that certain factors associated with the feeding process itself promote intellect; most likely, a combination of factors contributes to the positive association. More large, well-controlled studies are needed to confirm the effects, if any, of breastfeeding on later intelligence.

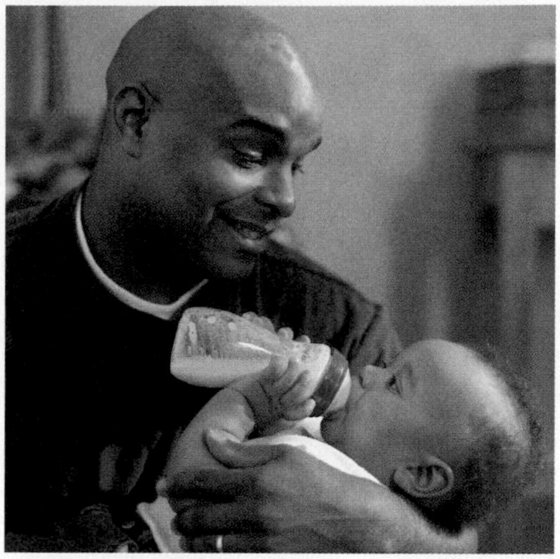

The infant thrives on infant formula offered with affection.

Infant Formula

A woman who breastfeeds for a year can **wean** her infant to cow's milk, bypassing the need for infant formula. However, a woman who decides to feed her infant formula from birth, to wean to formula after less than a year of breastfeeding, or to substitute formula for breastfeeding on occasion must select an appropriate infant formula and learn to prepare it.

Infant Formula Composition Formula manufacturers attempt to copy the nutrient composition of breast milk as closely as possible. Figure 15-4 illustrates the energy-nutrient balance of both. The AAP recommends that all formula-fed infants receive iron-fortified infant formulas. The increasing use of iron-fortified formulas during the past few decades is a major reason for the decline in iron-deficiency anemia among U.S. infants.

FIGURE 15-4 Percentages of Energy-Yielding Nutrients in Breast Milk and in Infant Formula

The average proportions of energy-yielding nutrients in human breast milk and formula differ slightly. In contrast, cow's milk provides too much protein and too little carbohydrate.

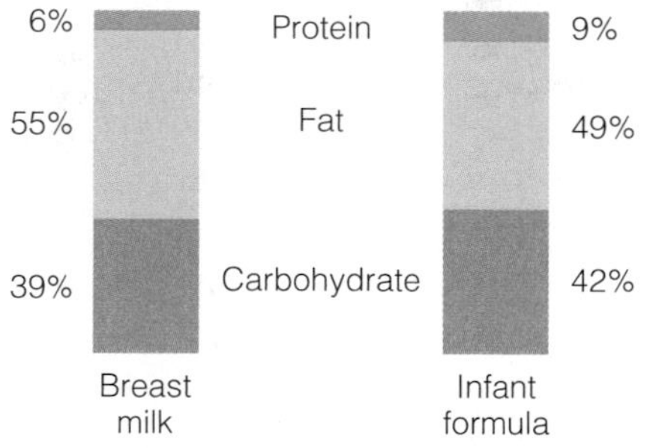
6%
Protein
9%
55%
Fat
49%
39%
Carbohydrate
42%
Breast milk
Infant formula

Risks of Formula Feeding Infant formulas contain no protective antibodies for infants, but in general, vaccinations, purified water, and clean environments in developed countries help protect infants from infections. Formulas can be prepared safely by following the rules of proper food handling and using water that is free of contamination. Of particular concern is lead-contaminated water, a major source of lead poisoning in infants. Because the first water drawn from the tap each day is highest in lead, a person living in a house with old, lead-soldered plumbing should let the water run a few minutes before drinking or using it to prepare formula or food.

In developing countries and in poor areas of the United States, formula may be unavailable, prepared with contaminated water, or overdiluted in an attempt to save money. More than 1.2 billion people in developing countries do not have access to safe drinking water. Contaminated formulas often cause infections, leading to diarrhea, dehydration, and malabsorption. Without sterilization and refrigeration, bottles of formula are an ideal breeding ground for bacteria. Whenever such risks are present, breastfeeding can be a life-saving option: breast milk is sterile, and its antibodies enhance an infant's resistance to infections.

Infant Formula Standards National and international standards have been set for the nutrient contents of infant formulas. In the United States, the standard developed by the AAP reflects "human milk taken from well-nourished mothers during the first or second month of lactation, when the infant's growth rate is high."

wean: gradually replacing breast milk with infant formula or other foods appropriate to an infant's diet.

FIGURE 15-5 Nursing Bottle Tooth Decay

This child was frequently put to bed sucking on a bottle filled with apple juice, so the teeth were bathed in carbohydrate for long periods of time—a perfect medium for bacterial growth. The upper teeth show signs of decay.

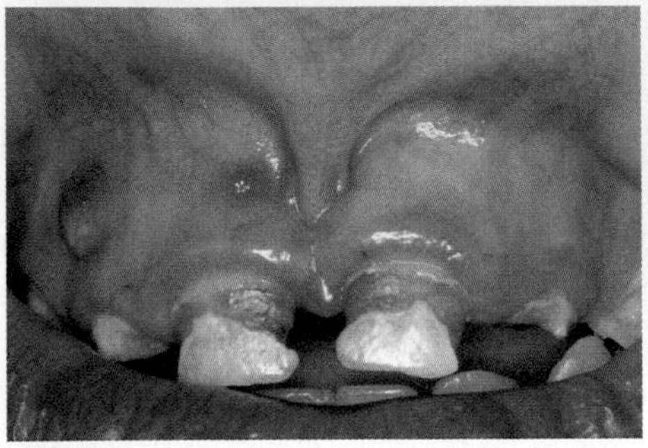

The Food and Drug Administration (FDA) mandates the safety and nutritional quality of infant formulas. Formulas meeting these standards have similar nutrient compositions; small differences are sometimes confusing, but usually unimportant.

Special Formulas Standard formulas are inappropriate for some infants. Special formulas have been designed to meet the dietary needs of infants with specific conditions such as prematurity or inherited diseases. Infants allergic to milk protein can drink special **hypoallergenic formulas** or formulas based on soy protein.[26] Soy formulas also use cornstarch and sucrose instead of lactose and so are recommended for infants with lactose intolerance as well. They are also useful as an alternative to milk-based formulas for vegan families. Despite these limited uses, soy formulas account for one-fourth of the infant formulas sold today. While soy formulas support the normal growth and development of infants, for infants who don't need them, they offer no advantage over milk formulas.

Inappropriate Formulas Caregivers must use only products designed for infants; soy *beverages,* for example, are nutritionally incomplete and inappropriate for infants. Goat's milk is also inappropriate for infants in part because of its low folate content. An infant receiving goat's milk is likely to develop "goat's milk anemia," an anemia characteristic of folate deficiency.

Nursing Bottle Tooth Decay An infant cannot be allowed to sleep with a bottle because of the potential damage to developing teeth. Salivary flow, which normally cleanses the mouth, diminishes as the infant falls asleep. Prolonged sucking on a bottle of formula, milk, or juice bathes the upper teeth in a carbohydrate-rich fluid that nourishes decay-producing bacteria. (The tongue covers and protects most of the lower teeth, but they, too, may be affected.) The result is extensive and rapid tooth decay (see Figure 15-5). To prevent **nursing bottle tooth decay,** no infant should be put to bed with a bottle of nourishing fluid.

Special Needs of Preterm Infants

An estimated one out of nine pregnancies in the United States results in a preterm birth.[27] The terms *preterm* and *premature* imply incomplete fetal development, or immaturity, of many body systems. As might be expected, preterm birth is a leading cause of infant deaths. Preterm infants face physical independence before some of their organs and body tissues are ready. The rate of weight gain in the fetus is greater during the last trimester of gestation than at any other time. Therefore, a preterm infant is most often a low-birthweight infant as well. With a premature birth, the infant is deprived of the nutritional support of the placenta during a time of maximal growth.

The last trimester of gestation is also a time of building nutrient stores. Being born with limited nutrient stores intensifies the precarious situation for the infant. Further compromising the nutrition status of preterm infants is their physical and metabolic immaturity. Nutrient absorption, especially of fat and calcium, from an immature GI tract is limited. Consequently, preterm, low-birthweight infants are candidates for nutrient imbalances. Deficiencies of the fat-soluble vitamins, calcium, iron, and zinc are common.

Preterm infants may miss out on the transfer of the long-chain fatty acids arachidonic acid and DHA, so critical to the healthy growth and development of the blood vessels and brain.[28] Supplementing breast milk or enriching infant formulas with these fatty acids may be beneficial for preterm infants.[29]

Preterm breast milk is well suited to meet a preterm infant's needs. During early lactation, preterm milk contains higher concentrations of protein and is lower in volume than term milk. The low milk volume is advantageous because preterm infants consume small quantities of milk per feeding, and the higher protein concentration allows for better growth. In many instances, supplements of nutrients specifically designed for preterm infants are added to the mother's expressed breast

hypoallergenic formulas: clinically tested infant formulas that do not provoke reactions in 90% of infants or children with confirmed cow's milk allergy. Like all infant formulas, hypoallergenic formulas must demonstrate nutritional suitability to support infant growth and development. Extensively hydrolyzed and free amino acid–based formulas are examples.

nursing bottle tooth decay: extensive tooth decay due to prolonged tooth contact with formula, milk, fruit juice, or other carbohydrate-rich liquid offered to an infant in a bottle.

milk and fed to the infant from a bottle. When fortified with a preterm supplement, preterm breast milk supports growth at a rate that approximates the growth rate that would have occurred within the uterus.

Introducing Cow's Milk

The age at which whole cow's milk should be introduced to the infant's diet has long been a source of controversy. The AAP advises that whole cow's milk is not appropriate during the first year.[30] Children one to two years of age should not be given reduced-fat, low-fat, or fat-free milk routinely; they need the fat of whole milk. Between the ages of two and five years, a gradual transition from whole milk to the lower-fat milks can take place, but care should be taken to avoid excessive restriction of dietary fat.

In some infants, particularly those younger than six months of age, whole cow's milk causes intestinal bleeding, which can lead to iron deficiency. Cow's milk is also a poor source of iron. Consequently, it both causes iron loss and fails to replace iron. Furthermore, the bioavailability of iron from infant cereal and other foods is reduced when cow's milk replaces breast milk or iron-fortified formula during the first year. Compared to breast milk or iron-fortified formula, cow's milk is higher in calcium and lower in vitamin C, characteristics that inhibit iron absorption. Furthermore, the higher protein concentration of cow's milk can stress the infant's kidneys. In short, cow's milk is a poor choice during the first year of life; infants need breast milk or iron-fortified infant formula.

Research examining the relationships between early exposure to cow's milk (or formula using cow's milk) and the development of type 1 diabetes (insulin-dependent) has been inconclusive and contradictory.[31] Families with a strong history of type 1 diabetes may want to breastfeed and avoid products containing cow's milk protein during the first year.

Introducing Solid Foods

The high nutrient needs of infancy are met first by breast milk or formula only and then by a limited diet to which foods■ are gradually added. Infants gradually develop the ability to chew, swallow, and digest the wide variety of foods available to adults. The caregiver's selection of appropriate foods at the appropriate stages of development is prerequisite to the infant's optimal growth and health.

■ The German word **beikost** (BYE-cost) describes any nonmilk foods given to an infant.

When to Begin In addition to breast milk or formula, an infant can begin eating solid foods between four and six months. The main purpose of introducing solid foods is to provide nutrients that are no longer supplied adequately by breast milk or formula alone. The foods chosen must be foods that the infant is developmentally capable of handling both physically and metabolically.■ The exact timing depends on the individual infant's needs and developmental readiness (see Table 15-2), which vary from infant to infant because of differences in growth rates, activities, and environmental conditions.

■ Digestive secretions gradually increase throughout the first year of life, making the digestion of solid foods more efficient.

Food Allergies To prevent allergy and to facilitate its prompt identification should it occur, experts recommend introducing single-ingredient foods, one at a time, in small portions, and waiting four to five days before introducing the next new food. For example, rice cereal is usually the first cereal introduced because it is least allergenic. When it is clear that rice cereal is not causing an allergy, another grain, perhaps barley or oats, is introduced. Wheat cereal is offered last because it is the most common offender. If a cereal causes an allergic reaction such as a skin rash, digestive upset, or respiratory discomfort, its use should be discontinued before introducing the next food. Highlight 24 and a later section in this chapter offer more on food allergies.

Choice of Infant Foods Infant foods should be selected to provide variety, balance, and moderation. Commercial baby foods offer a wide variety of palatable, nutritious

TABLE 15-2 Infant Development and Recommended Foods

NOTE: Because each stage of development builds on the previous stage, the foods from an earlier stage continue to be included in all later stages.

Age (mo)	Feeding Skill	Appropriate Foods Added to the Diet
0–4	Turns head toward any object that brushes cheek. Initially swallows using back of tongue; gradually begins to swallow using front of tongue as well. Strong reflex (extrusion) to push food out during first 2 to 3 months.	Feed breast milk or infant formula.
4–6	Extrusion reflex diminishes, and the ability to swallow nonliquid foods develops. Indicates desire for food by opening mouth and leaning forward. Indicates satiety or disinterest by turning away and leaning back. Sits erect with support at 6 months. Begins chewing action. Brings hand to mouth. Grasps objects with palm of hand.	Begin iron-fortified cereal mixed with breast milk, formula, or water. Begin pureed vegetables and fruits.
6–8	Able to feed self finger foods. Develops pincer (finger to thumb) grasp. Begins to drink from cup.	Begin textured vegetables and fruits. Begin unsweetened, diluted fruit juices from cup.
8–10	Begins to hold own bottle. Reaches for and grabs food and spoon. Sits unsupported.	Begin breads and cereals from table. Begin yogurt. Begin pieces of soft, cooked vegetables and fruit from table. Gradually begin finely cut meats, fish, casseroles, cheese, eggs, and mashed legumes.
10–12	Begins to master spoon, but still spills some.	Include breads and cereals from the table, in addition to infant cereal; fruits and soft or cooked vegetables; finely chopped or ground meat, fish or poultry; eggs, or mashed legumes.[a]

[a]Portion sizes for infants and young children are smaller than those for an adult. For example, a grain serving might be ½ slice of bread instead of 1 slice, or ¼ cup rice instead of ½ cup.

SOURCE: Adapted in part from Committee on Nutrition, American Academy of Pediatrics, *Pediatric Nutrition Handbook,* 5th ed., ed. R. E. Kleinman (Elk Grove Village, Ill.: American Academy of Pediatrics, 2004), pp. 103–115.

foods in a safe and convenient form. Homemade infant foods can be as nutritious as commercially prepared ones, as long as the cook minimizes nutrient losses during preparation. Ingredients for homemade foods should be fresh, whole foods without added salt, sugar, or seasonings. Pureed food can be frozen in ice cube trays, providing convenient-sized blocks of food that can be thawed, warmed, and fed to the infant. To guard against foodborne illnesses, hands and equipment must be kept clean.

Because recommendations to restrict fat do not apply to children under age two, labels on foods for children under two (such as infant meats and cereals) cannot carry information about fat. Fat information is omitted from infant food labels to prevent parents from restricting fat in infants' diets. Fearing that their infant will become overweight, parents may unintentionally malnourish the infant by limiting fat. In fact, infants and young children, because of their rapid growth, need more fat than older children and adults.

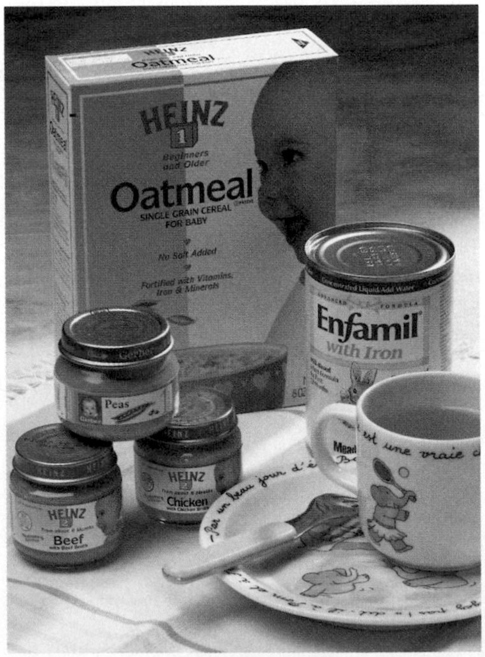
HEINZ
Oatmeal
Enfamil
with Iron
Peas
Chicken
Beef

Foods such as iron-fortified cereals and formulas, mashed legumes, and strained meats provide iron.

Foods to Provide Iron Rapid growth demands iron. At about four to six months, the infant begins to need more iron than stores plus breast milk or iron-fortified formula can provide. In addition to breast milk or iron-fortified formula, infants can receive iron from iron-fortified cereals and, once they readily accept solid foods, from meat or meat alternates such as legumes.[32] Iron-fortified cereals contribute a significant amount of iron to an infant's diet, but the iron's bioavailability is poor.[33] Caregivers can enhance iron absorption from iron-fortified cereals by serving vitamin C–rich foods and juices with meals.

Foods to Provide Vitamin C The best sources of vitamin C are fruits and vegetables. Some authorities suggest that an infant who is introduced to fruits before vegetables may develop a preference for sweets and find the vegetables less palatable. To prevent this, introduce vegetables first, fruits later.

Fruit juice may be a good source of vitamin C, but infants and young children may fail to grow and thrive when they drink so much juice each day that other, more energy- and nutrient-dense foods are displaced from their diets.[34] AAP recommendations set limits on juice consumption for infants and young children (one to six years of age): 4 to 6 ounces per day.[35] Fruit juices should be diluted and served in a cup, not a bottle, once the infant is six months of age or older.

Foods to Omit Concentrated sweets, including baby food "desserts," have no place in an infant's diet. They convey no nutrients to support growth, and the extra food energy can promote obesity. Products containing sugar alcohols such as sorbitol should also be limited, as they may cause diarrhea. Canned vegetables are also inappropriate for infants, as they often contain too much sodium. Honey and corn syrup should never be fed to infants because of the risk of **botulism.***

Infants and even young children cannot safely chew and swallow any of the foods listed in the margin;■ they can easily choke on these foods, a risk not worth taking. Nonfood items may present even greater choking hazards to infants and young children.[36] Parents and caregivers must pay careful attention to eliminate choking hazards in children's environments.

Foods at One Year At one year of age, whole cow's milk can become a primary source of most of the nutrients an infant needs; 2 to 3½ cups a day meets those needs sufficiently. More milk than this displaces iron-rich foods and can lead to **milk anemia.** If powdered milk is used, it should contain fat.

Other foods—meats, iron-fortified cereals, enriched or whole-grain breads, fruits, and vegetables—should be supplied in variety and in amounts sufficient to round out total energy needs. Ideally, a one-year-old will sit at the table, eat many of the same foods everyone else eats, and drink liquids from a cup, not a bottle. Figure 15-6 (on p. 520) shows a meal plan that meets a one-year-old's requirements.

Mealtimes with Toddlers

The nurturing of a young child involves more than nutrition. Those who care for young children are responsible for providing not only nutritious milk, foods, and water, but also a safe, loving, secure environment in which the children may grow and develop. In light of toddlers' developmental and nutrient needs and their often contrary and willful behavior, a few feeding guidelines may be helpful:

- Discourage unacceptable behavior, such as standing at the table or throwing food, by removing the young child from the table to wait until later to eat. Be consistent and firm, not punitive. The child will soon learn to sit and eat.
- Let toddlers explore and enjoy food, even if this means eating with fingers for a while. Use of the spoon will come in time.
- Don't force food on children. Rejecting new foods is normal; acceptance is more likely as children become familiar with new foods through repeated opportunities to taste them.
- Provide nutritious foods, and let children choose which ones, and how much, they will eat. Gradually, they will acquire a taste for different foods.
- Limit sweets. Infants and young children have little room for empty-kcaloric foods in their daily energy allowance. Do not use sweets as a reward for eating meals.
- Don't turn the dining table into a battleground. Make mealtimes enjoyable. Teach healthy food choices and eating habits in a pleasant environment.

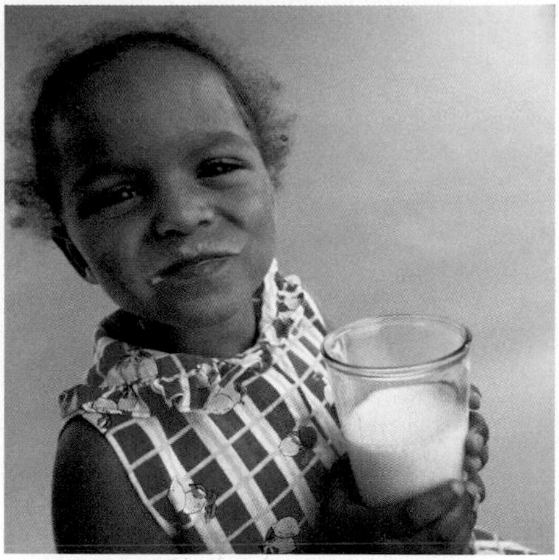

© Donna Day/Stone/Getty Images

Toddlers need vitamin A– and vitamin D–fortified whole milk.

■ To prevent choking, do not give infants or young children:

- Raw carrots.
- Cherries.
- Gum.
- Hard or gel-type candies.
- Hot dog slices.
- Marshmallows.
- Nuts.
- Peanut butter.
- Popcorn.
- Raw celery.
- Whole beans.
- Whole grapes.

Keep these nonfood items out of their reach:

- Balloons.
- Coins.
- Pen tops.
- Small balls.

botulism (BOT-chew-lism): an often fatal foodborne illness caused by the ingestion of foods containing a toxin produced by bacteria that grow without oxygen.

milk anemia: iron-deficiency anemia that develops when an excessive milk intake displaces iron-rich foods from the diet.

*In infants, but not older individuals, ingestion of *Clostridium botulinum* spores can cause illness when the spores germinate in the intestine and produce toxin, which is absorbed. Symptoms include poor feeding, constipation, loss of tension in the arteries and muscles, weakness, and respiratory compromise. Infant botulism has been implicated in 5 percent of cases of sudden infant death syndrome (SIDS).

FIGURE 15-6 Sample Meal Plan for a One-Year-Old

SAMPLE MENU	
Breakfast	½ c iron-fortified breakfast cereal
	¼ c whole milk (with cereal)
	½ c orange juice
Morning snack	1 to 2 oz cheese cubes
	Teething crackers
	½ c vitamin C–fortified fruit juice
Lunch	½ sandwich: 1 slice bread with 2 tbs tuna salad or egg salad
	½ c vegetables[a] (steamed carrots)
	1 c whole milk
Afternoon snack	1 slice toast
	1 to 2 tbs apple butter
	½ c whole milk
Dinner	2 to 3 oz chopped meat or well-cooked mashed legumes
	¼ c potato, rice, or pasta
	¼ c vegetables[a] (chopped broccoli)
	¼ c fruit[b] (sliced strawberries)
	1 c whole milk

[a]Include dark green, leafy and deep yellow vegetables.
[b]Include citrus fruits, melons, and berries.

IN SUMMARY The primary food for infants during the first 12 months is either breast milk or iron-fortified formula. In addition to nutrients, breast milk also offers immunological protection. At about four to six months, infants should gradually begin eating solid foods. By one year, they are drinking from a cup and eating many of the same foods as the rest of the family.

Nutrition during Childhood

Each year from age one to adolescence, a child typically grows taller by 2 to 3 inches and heavier by 5 to 6 pounds. Growth charts provide valuable clues to a child's health. Weight gains out of proportion to height gains may reflect overeating and inactivity, whereas measures significantly below the standard suggest malnutrition.

Increases in height and weight are only two of the many changes growing children experience (see Figure 15-7). At age one, children can stand alone and are beginning to toddle; by two, they can walk and are learning to run; by three, they can jump and are climbing with confidence. Bones and muscles increase in mass and density to make these accomplishments possible. Thereafter, further lengthening of the long bones and increases in musculature proceed unevenly and more slowly until adolescence.

Energy and Nutrient Needs

Children's appetites begin to diminish around one year, consistent with the slowing growth. Thereafter, children spontaneously vary their food intakes to coincide with their growth patterns; they demand more food during periods of rapid growth than during slow growth. Sometimes they seem insatiable; other times they seem to live on air and water.

Children's energy intakes also vary widely from meal to meal. Even so, their total daily intakes remain remarkably constant. If children eat less at one meal, they typically eat more at the next, and vice versa. Overweight children are an excep-

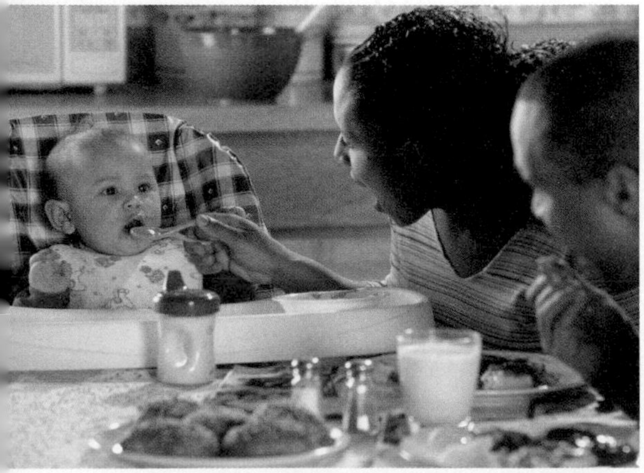

© SW Productions/Index Stock Imagery

Ideally, a one-year-old eats many of the same foods as the rest of the family.

FIGURE 15-7 Body Shape of One-Year-Old and Two-Year-Old Compared

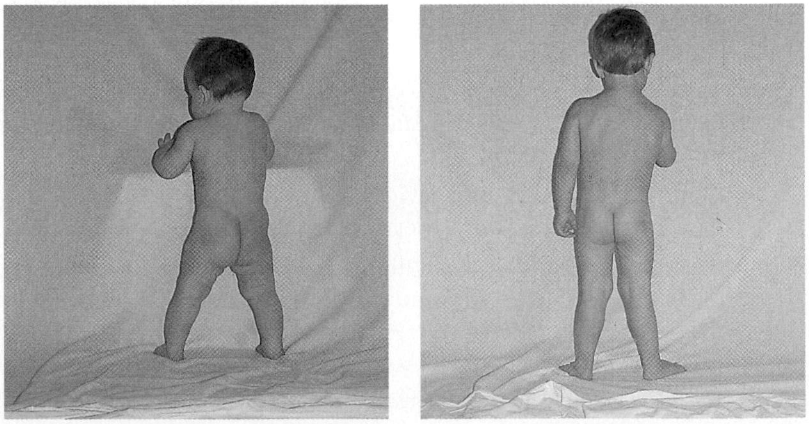

© Anthony M. Vanelli (both)

The body shape of a one-year-old (left) changes dramatically by age two (right). The two-year-old has lost much of the baby fat; the muscles (especially in the back, buttocks, and legs) have firmed and strengthened; and the leg bones have lengthened.

tion: they do not always adjust their energy intakes appropriately and may eat in response to external cues, disregarding hunger and satiety signals.

Energy Intake and Activity Individual children's energy needs vary widely, depending on their growth and physical activity. A one-year-old child needs about 800 kcalories a day; an active six-year-old needs twice as many kcalories a day. By age ten, an active child needs about 2000 kcalories a day. Total energy needs increase slightly with age, but energy needs per kilogram of body weight actually decline gradually.

Inactive children can become obese even when they eat less food than the average. Unfortunately, our nation's children are becoming less and less active, with young girls showing a marked reduction in their physical activity. Schools would serve our children well by offering activities to promote physical fitness.[37] Children who learn to enjoy physical play and exercise, both at home and at school, are best prepared to maintain active lifestyles as adults.

Some children, notably those adhering to a vegan diet, may have difficulty meeting their energy needs. Grains, vegetables, and fruits provide plenty of fiber, adding bulk, but may provide too few kcalories to support growth. Soy products, other legumes, and nut or seed butters offer more concentrated sources of energy to support optimal growth and development.[38]

Carbohydrate and Fiber Carbohydrate recommendations are based on glucose use by the brain. After a year of age, brain glucose use remains fairly constant and is within the adult range. Carbohydrate recommendations for children from the age of one year on are therefore the same as for adults (see inside front cover).[39]

Fiber recommendations derive from adult intakes shown to reduce the risk of coronary heart disease and are based on energy intakes. Consequently, children who have low energy intakes need less fiber than those with high intakes.[40] At a minimum, children's fiber intakes should at least equal their "age plus 5 grams."[41]

Fat and Fatty Acids As long as children's energy intakes are adequate, fat intakes below 30 percent of total energy do not impair growth.[42] Children who eat low-fat diets, however, have low intakes of some vitamins and minerals. The energy of dietary fat is important for young children who eat less food than older children and adults. No RDA for total fat has been established, but the DRI Committee recommends a fat intake of 30 to 40 percent of energy for children 1 to 3 years of age and 25 to 35 percent for children 4 to 18 years of age.[43] Recommended intakes of the essential fatty acids are based on average intakes (see inside front cover).

Protein Like energy needs, total protein needs increase slightly with age, but when the child's body weight is considered, the protein requirement actually declines slightly (see inside front cover). The estimation of protein needs considers the requirements for maintaining nitrogen balance, the quality of protein consumed, and the added needs of growth.

Vitamins and Minerals The vitamin and mineral needs of children increase with age (see inside front cover). A balanced diet of nutritious foods can meet children's needs for these nutrients, with the notable exception of iron. Iron-deficiency anemia is a major problem worldwide, as well as being the most prevalent nutrient deficiency among U.S. and Canadian children, especially toddlers one to two years of age.[44] During the second year of life, toddlers progress from a diet of iron-rich infant foods such as breast milk, iron-fortified formula, and iron-fortified infant cereal to a diet of adult foods and iron-poor cow's milk. In addition, their appetites often fluctuate; some become finicky about the foods they eat, and others prefer milk and juice to solid foods.[45] All of these situations can interfere with children eating iron-rich foods at a critical time for brain growth and development.

Reduce iron deficiency among young children.

HEALTHY PEOPLE 2010

To prevent iron deficiency, children's foods must deliver approximately 10 milligrams of iron per day. To achieve this goal, snacks and meals should include iron-rich foods, and milk intake should be reasonable so that it will not displace lean meats, fish, poultry, eggs, legumes, and whole-grain or enriched products. (Chapter 13 describes iron-rich foods and ways to maximize iron absorption.)

Supplements With the exception of specific recommendations for fluoride, iron, and vitamin D during infancy and childhood, the AAP and other professional groups agree that well-nourished children do not need vitamin and mineral supplements. Despite this, many children and adolescents take supplements.[46] Ironically, children with poor nutrient intakes do not receive supplements, and those who do take supplements receive extra nutrients they do not need. Furthermore, researchers are still studying the safety of supplement use by children.[47] In the meantime, parents and other caregivers need to rely on foods instead of supplements to nourish children.

The Federal Trade Commission has issued a consumer guidance warning parents about giving supplements advertised to prevent or cure childhood illnesses such as colds, ear infections, or asthma. The term *supplement* today includes many herbal products that have not been tested for safety and effectiveness in children.[48]

Available Online

Compare the nutrient density of several child-friendly meals and snacks, and evaluate how well they meet the dietary needs of children of several different ages.

Planning Children's Meals To provide all the needed nutrients, children's meals should include a variety of foods from each food group—in amounts suited to their appetites and needs. Figure 15-8 presents the Food Guide Pyramid for young children and provides examples of serving sizes for various foods. For two- to three-year-olds, serving sizes are smaller, about two-thirds the portion for a child over four years old.

Children whose diets follow the pattern presented in Figure 15-8 meet their nutrient needs fully, but few children eat according to these recommendations. Based on an analysis of the most recent national food intake data, the USDA found that most (81 percent) children between two and nine years of age have diets that need substantial improvement.[49] In another study, only 5 percent of the children consumed the suggested number of servings from even four of the five food groups. Consequently, intakes of several nutrients, notably calcium, iron, and zinc, typically fall below recommendations.[50]

Hunger and Malnutrition in Children

Most children in the United States and Canada have access to regular meals, but hunger and malnutrition do appear in certain circumstances. Low-income children, for example, may be hungry and malnourished. An estimated 12 million U.S. children are hungry at least some of the time and living in poverty.[51] Highlight 16 examines the causes and consequences of hunger in the United States.

When hunger is chronic, children become malnourished and suffer growth retardation. Worldwide, malnutrition takes a devastating toll on children, contributing to nearly half of the deaths of children under four years old. Vitamin A deficiency afflicts 3 to 10 million children worldwide, inducing blindness, stunted growth, and infections.[52] Zinc deficiency also retards growth and typically accompanies protein-energy malnutrition and vitamin A deficiency.

HEALTHY PEOPLE 2010

Reduce growth retardation among low-income children under age 5 years.

The United Nations Children's Fund, known as UNICEF, helps children living in poverty in developing countries get the nutrition and health care they need. UNICEF works with more than 160 countries through national governments, private-sector partners, and other international agencies to protect children and their rights, and to reduce childhood death and illness.

FIGURE 15-8 Food Guide Pyramid for Young Children

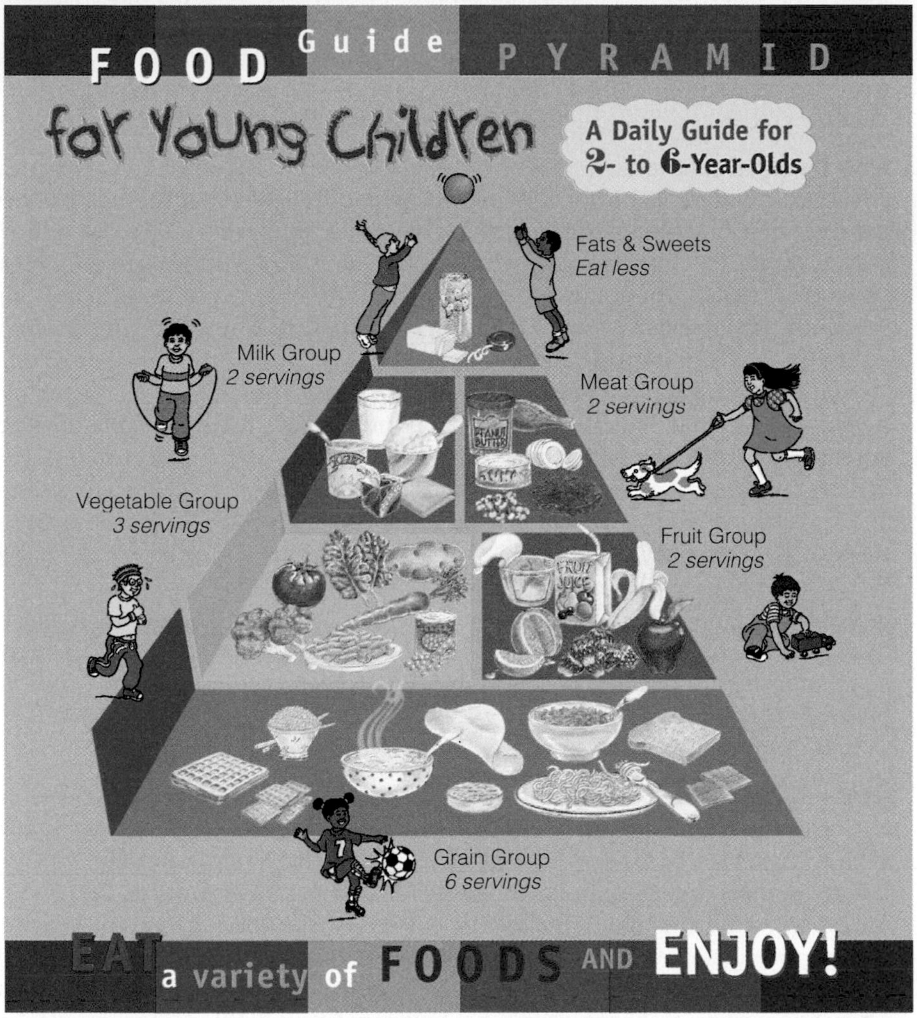
FOOD Guide PYRAMID
for Young Children
A Daily Guide for 2- to 6-Year-Olds
Fats & Sweets
Eat less
Milk Group
2 servings
Meat Group
2 servings
Vegetable Group
3 servings
Fruit Group
2 servings
Grain Group
6 servings
EAT a variety of FOODS AND ENJOY!

What counts as one serving?

GRAIN GROUP
1 slice bread
1/2 c cooked rice or pasta
1/2 c cooked cereal
1 oz ready-to-eat cereal

VEGETABLE GROUP
1/2 c chopped raw or cooked vegetables
1 c raw leafy vegetables

FRUIT GROUP
1 piece of fruit or melon wedge
3/4 c juice
1/2 c canned fruit
1/4 c dried fruit

MILK GROUP
1 c milk or yogurt
2 oz cheese

MEAT GROUP
2 to 3 oz cooked lean meat, poultry, or fish
1/2 c cooked dry beans, or 1 egg counts as 1 oz lean meat; 2 tbs of peanut butter count as 1 oz meat

FATS AND SWEETS
Limit kcalories from these.

Four- to six-year-olds can eat these serving sizes. Offer two- to three-year-olds less, except for milk. Two- to six-year-old children need a total of 2 servings from the milk group each day.

SOURCE: USDA Center for Nutrition and Policy Promotion, March 1999, Program AID 1649.

Hunger and Behavior Even when hunger is temporary, as when a child misses one meal, behavior and academic performance are affected. Children who eat nutritious breakfasts improve their school performance and are tardy or absent significantly less often than their peers who do not. Without breakfast, children perform poorly in tasks requiring concentration, their attention spans are shorter, and they even score lower on intelligence tests than their well-fed peers; malnourished children are particularly vulnerable. Unfortunately, an estimated 4 out of 30 students miss breakfast each day. Common sense dictates that it is unreasonable to expect anyone to learn and perform without fuel. For the child who hasn't had breakfast, the morning's lessons may be lost altogether. Even if a child has eaten breakfast, discomfort from hunger may become distracting by late morning.

The problem children face when attempting morning schoolwork on an empty stomach appears to be at least partly due to low blood glucose. The average child up to age ten or so needs to eat about every four hours to maintain a blood glucose concentration high enough to support the activity of the brain and the rest of the nervous system. A child's brain is as big as an adult's, and the brain is the body's chief glucose consumer, using about three times as much glucose per day as the rest of the body. A child's liver is much smaller than an adult's, however, and the liver is responsible for storing glucose as glycogen and releasing it into the blood

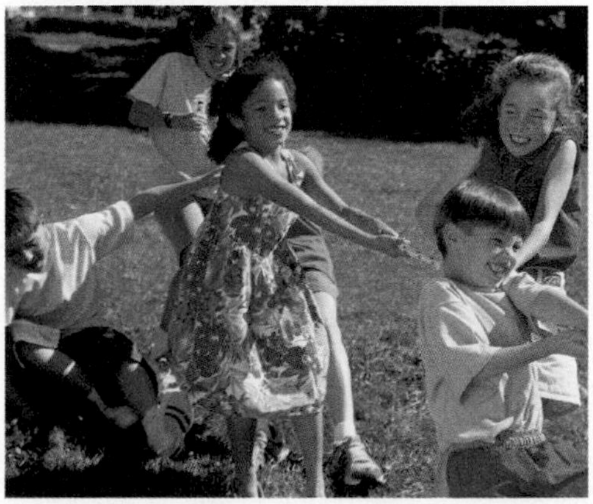

Healthy, well-nourished children are alert in the classroom and energetic at play.

as needed. A child's liver can store only about four hours' worth of glycogen—hence the need to eat fairly often. Teachers aware of the late-morning slump in their classrooms wisely request that midmorning snacks be provided; snacks improve classroom performance all the way to lunchtime.

Eating breakfast also helps children to meet their nutrient needs each day. Children who skip breakfast typically do not make up the deficits at later meals—they simply have lower intakes of energy, vitamins, and minerals than those who eat breakfast.

Iron Deficiency and Behavior Iron deficiency has well-known and widespread effects on children's behavior and intellectual performance.[53] In addition to carrying oxygen in the blood, iron transports oxygen within cells, which use it in energy metabolism. Iron is also used to make neurotransmitters—most notably, those that regulate the ability to pay attention, which is crucial to learning. Consequently, iron deficiency not only causes an energy crisis, but also directly affects attention span and learning ability.

Iron deficiency is often diagnosed by a quick, easy, inexpensive hemoglobin or hematocrit test that detects a deficit of iron in the *blood.* A child's *brain,* however, is sensitive to low iron concentrations long before the blood effects appear. Iron deficiency lowers the "motivation to persist in intellectually challenging tasks" and impairs overall intellectual performance. Anemic children perform less well on tests and are more disruptive than their nonanemic classmates; iron supplementation improves learning and memory. When combined with other nutrient deficiencies, iron-deficiency anemia has synergistic effects that are especially detrimental to learning. Furthermore, children who had iron-deficiency anemia *as infants* continue to perform poorly as they grow older, even if their iron status improves.[54] The long-term damaging effects on mental development make prevention of iron deficiency during infancy and early childhood a high priority.

Other Nutrient Deficiencies and Behavior A child with any of several nutrient deficiencies may be irritable, aggressive, disagreeable, or sad and withdrawn. Such a child may be labeled "hyperactive," "depressed," or "unlikable," when in fact these traits may arise from simple, even marginal, malnutrition. Parents and medical practitioners often overlook the possibility that malnutrition may account for abnormalities of appearance and behavior. Any departure from normal healthy appearance and behavior is a sign of possible poor nutrition (see Table 15-3). In any such case, inspection of the child's diet by a registered dietitian or other qualified health care professional is in order. Any suspicion of dietary inadequacies, no matter what other causes may be implicated, should prompt steps to correct those inadequacies immediately.

The Malnutrition-Lead Connection

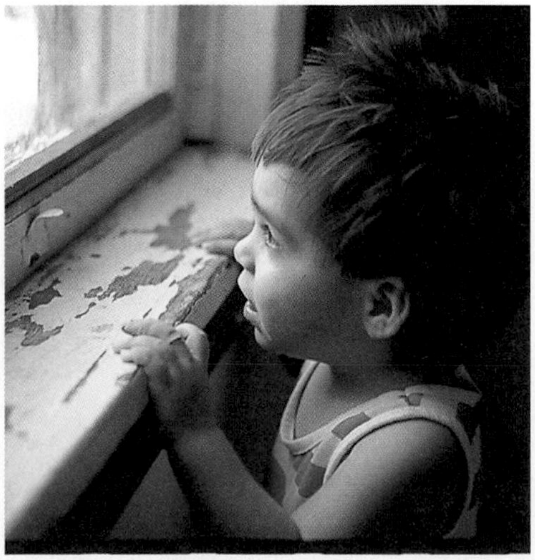
© Tony Freeman/PhotoEdit

Old, lead-based paint threatens the health of an exploring child.

Children who are malnourished are vulnerable to lead poisoning. They absorb more lead if their stomachs are empty; if they have low intakes of calcium, zinc, vitamin C, or vitamin D; and, of greatest concern because it is so common, if they have iron deficiencies.[55] Iron deficiency weakens the body's defenses against lead absorption, and lead poisoning can cause iron deficiency. Common to both iron deficiency and lead poisoning are a low socioeconomic background and a lack of immunizations against infectious diseases. Another common factor is pica—a craving for nonfood items. Many children with lead poisoning eat dirt or chips of old paint, two common sources of lead.

The anemia brought on by lead poisoning may be mistaken for a simple iron deficiency and therefore may be incorrectly treated. Like iron deficiency, mild lead toxicity has nonspecific symptoms, including diarrhea, irritability, and fatigue. The symptoms are not reversed by adding iron to the diet; exposure to lead must stop. With further exposure, the signs become more pronounced: children develop learning disabilities and behavioral problems. Still more severe lead toxicity can cause irreversible nerve damage, paralysis, mental retardation, and death.

TABLE 15-3 Physical Signs of Malnutrition in Children

	Well-Nourished	Malnourished	Possible Nutrient Deficiencies
Hair	Shiny, firm in the scalp	Dull, brittle, dry, loose; falls out	PEM
Eyes	Bright, clear pink membranes; adjust easily to light	Pale membranes; spots; redness; adjust slowly to darkness	Vitamin A, the B vitamins, zinc, and iron
Teeth and gums	No pain or caries, gums firm, teeth bright	Missing, discolored, decayed teeth; gums bleed easily and are swollen and spongy	Minerals and vitamin C
Face	Clear complexion without dryness or scaliness	Off-color, scaly, flaky, cracked skin	PEM, vitamin A, and iron
Glands	No lumps	Swollen at front of neck, cheeks	PEM and iodine
Tongue	Red, bumpy, rough	Sore, smooth, purplish, swollen	B vitamins
Skin	Smooth, firm, good color	Dry, rough, spotty; "sandpaper" feel or sores; lack of fat under skin	PEM, essential fatty acids, vitamin A, B vitamins, and vitamin C
Nails	Firm, pink	Spoon-shaped, brittle, ridged	Iron
Internal systems	Regular heart rhythm, heart rate, and blood pressure; no impairment of digestive function, reflexes, or mental status	Abnormal heart rate, heart rhythm, or blood pressure; enlarged liver, spleen; abnormal digestion; burning, tingling of hands, feet; loss of balance, coordination; mental confusion, irritability, fatigue	PEM and minerals
Muscles and bones	Muscle tone; posture, long bone development appropriate for age	"Wasted" appearance of muscles; swollen bumps on skull or ends of bones; small bumps on ribs; bowed legs or knock-knees	PEM, minerals, and vitamin D

More than 400,000 children—most of them under age six—have blood lead concentrations high enough to cause mental, behavioral, and other health problems.[56] Lead intoxication in young children comes from their own behaviors and activities—putting their hands in their mouths, playing in dirt and dust, and chewing on nonfood items. Unfortunately, the body readily absorbs lead during times of rapid growth and hoards it possessively thereafter. Lead is not easily excreted and accumulates mainly in the bones, but also in the brain, teeth, and kidneys. Tragically, a child's neuromuscular system is also maturing during these first few years of life. No wonder children with elevated lead levels experience impairment of balance, motor development, and the relaying of nerve messages to and from the brain. Unfortunately, deficits in intellectual development are only partially reversed when lead levels decline.[57]

HEALTHY PEOPLE 2010

Eliminate elevated blood lead levels in children. Increase the proportion of persons living in pre-1950s housing that has been tested for the presence of lead-based paint.

Federal laws mandating reductions in leaded gasolines, lead-based solder, and other products over the past three decades have helped to reduce the amounts of lead in food and in the environment in the United States. As a consequence, the prevalence of lead toxicity in children has declined dramatically for most of the United States, but lead exposure is still a threat in certain communities.[58] The "How to" on the next page presents strategies for defending children against lead toxicity.

Hyperactivity and "Hyper" Behavior

All children are naturally active, and many of them become overly active on occasion—for example, in anticipation of a birthday party. Such behavior is markedly different from true **hyperactivity.**

hyperactivity: inattentive and impulsive behavior that is more frequent and severe than is typical of others a similar age; professionally called **attention-deficit/hyperactivity disorder (ADHD).**

HOW TO Protect against Lead Toxicity

Researchers simultaneously made three major discoveries about lead toxicity: lead poisoning has *subtle* effects, the effects are *permanent,* and they occur at *low levels of exposure.* The amount of lead recognized to cause harm is only 10 micrograms per 100 milliliters of blood. Some research shows that blood lead concentrations *below* this amount may adversely affect children's scores on intelligence tests.[a] Consequently, consumers should take ultraconservative measures to protect themselves, and especially their infants and young children, from lead poisoning. The American Academy of Pediatrics and the Centers for Disease Control recommend screening in communities with a substantial number of houses built before 1950 and in those with a substantial number of children with elevated lead levels. In addition to screening children most likely to be exposed, pediatricians should alert all parents to the possible dangers of lead exposure and explain prevention strategies.

Preventive strategies include:

- In contaminated environments, keep small children from putting dirty or old painted objects in their mouths, and make sure children wash their hands before eating. Similarly, keep small children from eating any nonfood items. Lead poisoning has been reported in young children who have eaten crayons or pool cue chalk.
- Wet-mop floors and damp-sponge walls regularly. Children's blood lead levels decline when the homes they live in are cleaned regularly.
- Be aware that other countries do not have the same regulations protecting consumers against lead. Children have been poisoned by eating crayons made in China and drinking fruit juice canned in Mexico.
- Do not use lead-contaminated water to make infant formula.
- Once you have opened canned food, store it in a lead-free container to prevent lead migration into the food.
- Do not store acidic foods or beverages (such as vinegar or orange juice) in ceramic dishware or alcoholic beverages in pewter or crystal decanters.
- Many manufacturers are now making lead-safe products.[b] Old, handmade, or imported ceramic cups and bowls may contain lead and should not be used to heat coffee or tea or acidic foods such as tomato soup.
- U.S. wineries have stopped using lead in their foil seals, but older bottles may still be around and other countries may still use lead; to be safe, wipe the foil-sealed rim of a wine bottle with a clean wet cloth before removing the cork.
- Feed children nutritious meals regularly.
- Before using your newspaper to wrap food, mulch garden plants, or add to your compost, confirm with the publisher that the paper uses no lead in its ink.

The Environmental Protection Agency (EPA) also publishes a booklet, *Lead and Your Drinking Water,* in which the following cautions appear:

- Have the water in your home tested by a competent laboratory.
- Use only cold water for drinking, cooking, and making formula (cold water absorbs less lead).
- When water has been standing in pipes for more than two hours, flush the cold-water pipes by running water through them for 30 seconds before using it for drinking, cooking, or mixing formulas.
- If lead contamination of your water supply seems probable, obtain additional information and advice from the EPA and your local public health agency.

By taking these steps, parents can protect themselves and their children from this preventable danger.[c]

[a] R. L. Canfield and coauthors, Intellectual impairment in children with blood lead concentrations below 10 µg per deciliter, *New England Journal of Medicine* 348 (2003): 1517–1526.

[b] *A Shopper's Guide to Low-Lead China* is available from the Environmental Defense Fund, 257 Park Avenue South, New York, NY 10010; telephone (800) 284-3322.

[c] The National Lead Information Center provides two hotlines; call (800) LEAD-FYI (532-3394) for general information or (800) 424-LEAD (424-5323) with specific questions.

Hyperactivity Hyperactive children have trouble sleeping, cannot sit still for more than a few minutes at a time, act impulsively, and have difficulty paying attention. These behaviors interfere with social development and academic progress. The cause of hyperactivity remains unknown, but it affects 3 to 5 percent of young school-age children. To resolve the problems surrounding hyperactivity, physicians often recommend specific behavioral strategies, special educational programs, and psychological counseling; in many cases, they prescribe medication.[59]

Parents of hyperactive children sometimes seek help from alternative therapies, including special diets. They mistakenly believe a solution may lie in manipulating the diet—most commonly, by excluding sugar or food additives. Adding carrots or eliminating candy is such a simple solution that many parents eagerly give dietary advice a try. These dietary changes will not solve the problem of true hyperactivity. Studies have consistently found no convincing evidence that sugar causes hyperactivity or worsens behavior; in fact, sugar may actually have a sedative effect. Recommendations to restrict sugar in children's diets to prevent or treat behavioral problems are groundless.

Misbehaving Even a child who is not truly hyperactive can be difficult to manage at times. Michael may act unruly out of a desire for attention, Jessica may be cranky because of a lack of sleep, Christopher may react violently after watching too much television, and Sheila may be unable to sit still in class due to a lack of exercise. All of these children may benefit from more consistent care—regular hours of sleep, regular mealtimes, and regular outdoor activity.

Food Allergy and Intolerance

Food allergy is frequently blamed for physical and behavioral abnormalities in children, but only about 3 to 5 percent of children are diagnosed with true food allergies.[60] Food allergies diminish with age, until in adulthood they affect about 1 or 2 percent of the population.[61]

A true food allergy occurs when fractions of a food protein or other large molecule are absorbed into the blood and elicit an immunologic response. (Recall that proteins are normally dismantled in the digestive tract to amino acids that are absorbed without such a reaction.) The body's immune system reacts to these large food molecules as it does to other antigens—by producing antibodies, histamines, or other defensive agents. (Highlight 24 presents many more details.)

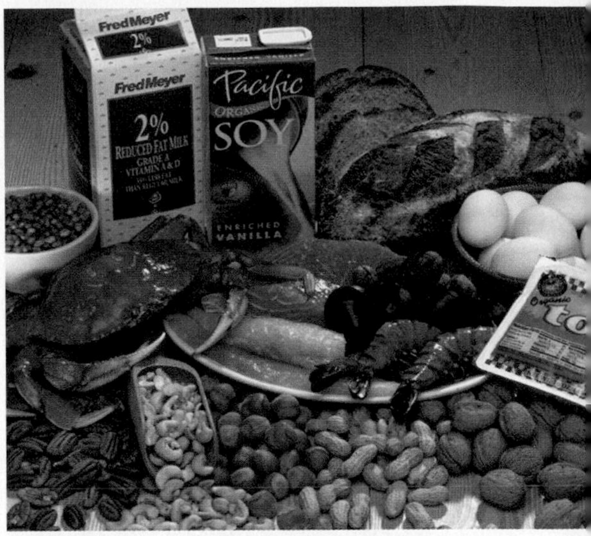

FredMeyer
2%
REDUCED FAT MILK
Pacific
SOY
ENRICHED VANILLA

Polara Studios, Inc.

These normally wholesome foods may cause life-threatening symptoms in people with allergies.

Detecting Food Allergy Allergies may have one or two components. They always involve antibodies; they may or may not involve symptoms.■ This means that allergies can be diagnosed only by testing for antibodies. Even symptoms exactly like those of an allergy may not be caused by one. Once a food allergy has been diagnosed, therapy requires strict elimination of the offending food. Children with allergies, like all children, need all their nutrients, so it is important to include other foods that offer the same nutrients as the omitted foods.[62]

■ A person who produces antibodies *without* having any symptoms has an **asymptomatic allergy;** a person who produces antibodies *and* has symptoms has a **symptomatic allergy.**

Allergic reactions to food may be immediate or delayed. In both cases, the antigen interacts immediately with the immune system, but the timing of symptoms varies from minutes to 24 hours after consumption of the antigen. Identifying the food that causes an immediate allergic reaction is fairly easy because the symptoms appear shortly after the food is eaten. Identifying the food that causes a delayed reaction is more difficult because the symptoms may not appear until much later. By this time, many other foods may have been eaten, complicating the picture.

Anaphylactic Shock The life-threatening food allergy reaction of **anaphylactic shock** is most often caused by peanuts, tree nuts, milk, eggs, wheat, soybeans, fish, or shellfish.[63] Among these foods, eggs, milk, soy, and peanuts most often cause problems in children. Children are more likely to outgrow allergies to eggs, milk, and soy than allergies to peanuts. Peanuts cause more life-threatening reactions than do all other food allergies combined. Research is currently under way to help those with peanut allergies tolerate small doses, thus saving lives and minimizing reactions.[64] One possible solution depends on finding a natural, hypoallergenic peanut among the 14,000 varieties of peanuts that grow. Families of children with a life-threatening food allergy and school personnel who supervise them must guard them against any exposure to the allergen.[65] The child must learn to identify which foods pose a problem and then learn and use refusal skills for all foods that may contain the allergen.

Reduce deaths from anaphylaxis caused by food allergies.

HEALTHY PEOPLE 2010

Parents of allergic children can pack safe foods for lunches and snacks and ask school officials to strictly enforce a "no swapping" policy in the lunchroom. The child must be able to recognize the symptoms of impending anaphylactic shock,■ such as a tingling of the tongue, throat, or skin, or difficulty breathing. Any person with food allergies severe enough to cause anaphylactic shock should wear a medical alert bracelet or necklace. Finally, the responsible child and the school staff should be prepared with injections of **epinephrine,** which prevents anaphylaxis after exposure to the allergen.[66] Many preventable deaths occur each year when people with food allergies accidentally ingest the allergen but have no epinephrine.[67]

■ Symptoms of impending anaphylactic shock:
- Tingling sensation in mouth.
- Swelling of the tongue and throat.
- Irritated, reddened eyes.
- Difficulty breathing, asthma.
- Hives, swelling, rashes.
- Vomiting, abdominal cramps, diarrhea.
- Drop in blood pressure.
- Loss of consciousness.
- Death.

food allergy: an adverse reaction to food that involves an immune response; also called **food-hypersensitivity reaction.**

anaphylactic (an-AFF-ill-LAC-tic) **shock:** a life-threatening whole-body allergic reaction.

epinephrine (EP-ih-NEFF-rin): a hormone of the adrenal gland administered by injection to counteract anaphylactic shock by opening the airways and maintaining heartbeat and blood pressure.

FIGURE 15-9 Trends in Childhood Obesity

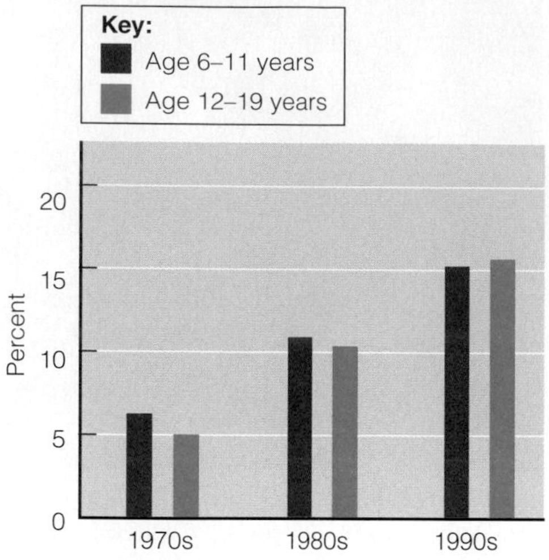
Key:
Age 6–11 years
Age 12–19 years
Percent
0
5
10
15
20
1970s
1980s
1990s

Allergens often sneak into foods in unexpected ways. To protect people with allergies, regulations require food manufacturers to declare common allergens, including food additives, on food labels.[68] Manufacturers must also prevent cross-contamination during production. Eliminating peanuts per se may not be too difficult, but avoiding peanut dust in a chocolate cookie can be a challenge. Equipment used for mixing peanut butter cookies must be disassembled and cleaned thoroughly before being used to make other products. When cross-contamination is likely, food labels must state that the product may contain an allergy-producing food. The FDA is currently working with the food industry to develop more clearly worded labels to alert consumers to the presence of food allergens.[69]

Food Intolerances Not all **adverse reactions** to foods are food allergies, although even physicians may describe them as such. Signs of adverse reactions to foods include stomachaches, headaches, rapid pulse rate, nausea, wheezing, hives, bronchial irritation, coughs, and other such discomforts. Among the causes may be reactions to chemicals in foods, such as the flavor enhancer monosodium glutamate (MSG), the natural laxative in prunes, or the mineral sulfur; digestive diseases, such as obstructions or injuries; enzyme deficiencies, such as lactose intolerance; and even psychological aversions. These reactions involve symptoms but no antibody production. Therefore, they are **food intolerances,** not allergies.

Pesticides on produce may also cause adverse reactions. Health risks from pesticide exposure may be small for healthy adults, but children are vulnerable. Therefore, government agencies set a **tolerance level** for each pesticide by first identifying foods that children commonly eat in large amounts and then considering the effects of pesticide exposure during each developmental stage.

Hunger, lead poisoning, hyperactivity, and allergic reactions can all adversely affect a child's nutrition status and health. Fortunately, each of these problems has solutions. They may not be easy solutions, but at least we have a reasonably good understanding of the problems and ways to correct them. Such is not the case with the most pervasive health problem for children in the United States—obesity.

Childhood Obesity

The number of overweight children has increased dramatically over the past three decades (see Figure 15-9). Like their parents, children in the United States are becoming fatter. An estimated 15 percent of U.S. children and adolescents 6 to 19 years of age are overweight.[70] Based on data from the BMI-for-age growth charts, children and adolescents are categorized as *at risk of overweight* above the 85th percentile and as *overweight* at the 95th percentile and above. Prevalence data reflect only children and adolescents in the overweight category; if those at risk of overweight were also included, the estimated 15 percent would likely double. Figure 15-10 presents the BMI for children and adolescents, indicating cutoff points for overweight and at risk of overweight.

HEALTHY PEOPLE 2010

Reduce the proportion of children and adolescents who are overweight or at risk of overweight.

The problem is especially troubling because overweight children have the potential of becoming obese adults with all the social, economic, and medical ramifications that often accompany obesity. They have additional problems, too, arising from differences in their growth, physical health, and psychological development. In trying to explain the rise in childhood obesity, researchers point to both genetic and environmental factors.

Genetic and Environmental Factors Parental obesity predicts an early increase in a young child's BMI, and it more than doubles the chances that a young

adverse reactions: unusual responses to food (including intolerances and allergies).

food intolerances: adverse reactions to foods that do not involve the immune system.

tolerance level: the maximum amount of a residue permitted in a food when a pesticide is used according to the label directions.

FIGURE 15-10 Body Mass Index-for-Age Percentiles: Boys and Girls, Age 2 to 20

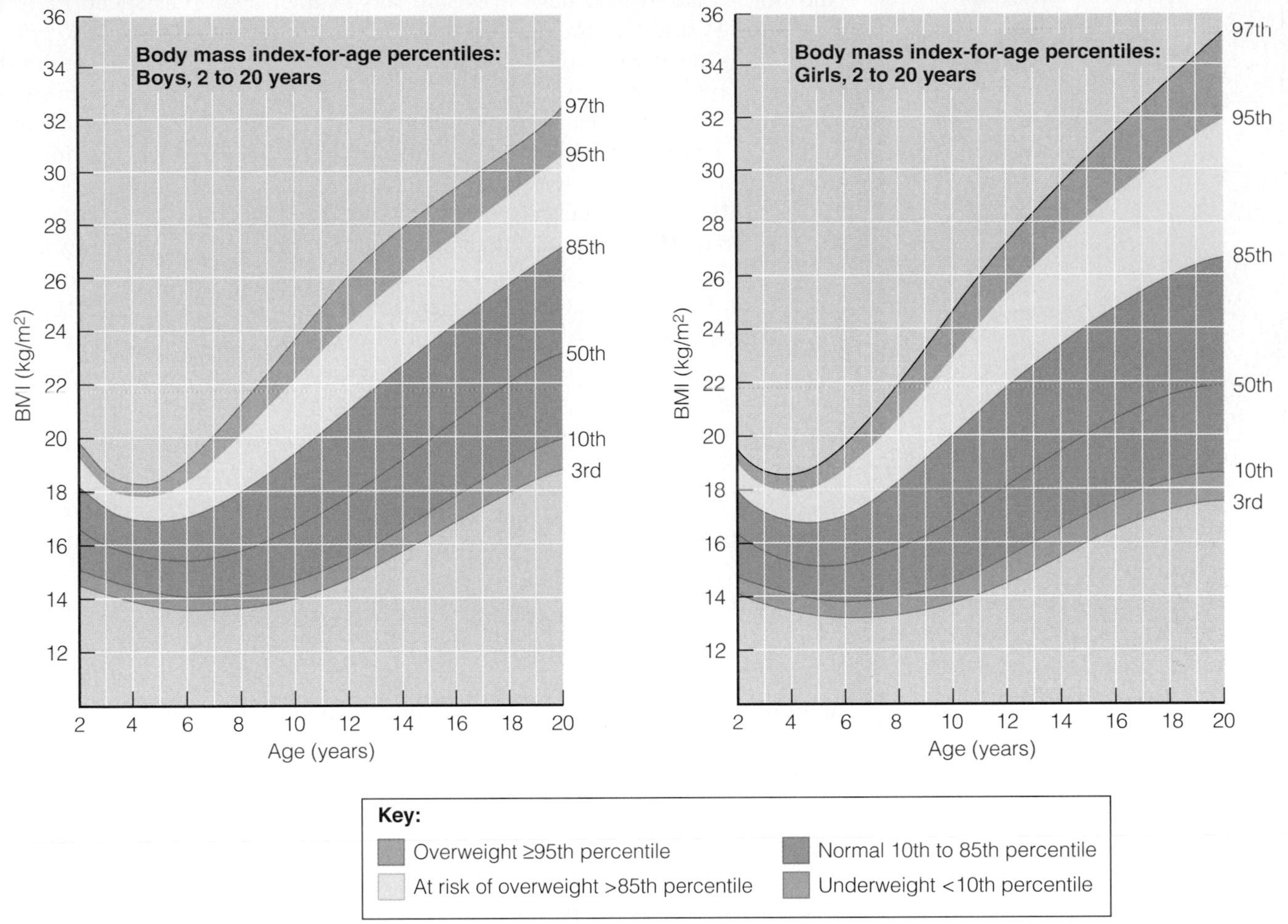
Body mass index-for-age percentiles:
Boys, 2 to 20 years
Body mass index-for-age percentiles:
Girls, 2 to 20 years
BMI (kg/m2)
Age (years)
97th
95th
85th
50th
10th
3rd
Key:
Overweight ≥95th percentile
At risk of overweight >85th percentile
Normal 10th to 85th percentile
Underweight <10th percentile

child will become an obese adult.[71] Nonobese children with neither parent obese have a less than 10 percent chance of becoming obese in adulthood, whereas obese teens with at least one obese parent have a greater than 80 percent chance of being obese adults. As children grow older, their own obesity also becomes an important factor in determining their obesity as adults.[72] The link between parental and child obesity reflects both genetic and environmental factors.

Diet and physical inactivity must also play a role in explaining why children are heavier today than they were 30 or so years ago. Children's dietary fat intakes vary, of course, but children who prefer high-fat foods tend to be more overweight than their peers.[73] Particularly noteworthy is that they also tend to have overweight parents. Such findings confirm the significant roles parents play in teaching children about healthy food choices, providing children with nutrient-dense foods, and serving as role models. When parents eat fruits and vegetables frequently, their children do, too.[74] The more fruits and vegetables children eat, the more vitamins and minerals and the less fat in their diets.

Most likely, children have grown more overweight because of their lack of physical activity.[75] An inactive child can become obese even while eating less food than an active child. Today's children are more sedentary and less physically fit than children were even 20 years ago.

Television watching■ may contribute most to physical inactivity. One study compared children who were experimentally set up with a stationary bicycle that they had to pedal in order to activate the television with children who did not

■ TV fosters obesity because it:
- Requires no energy beyond basal metabolism.
- Replaces vigorous activities.
- Encourages snacking.
- Promotes a sedentary lifestyle.

Playing video games influences children's activity patterns similarly.

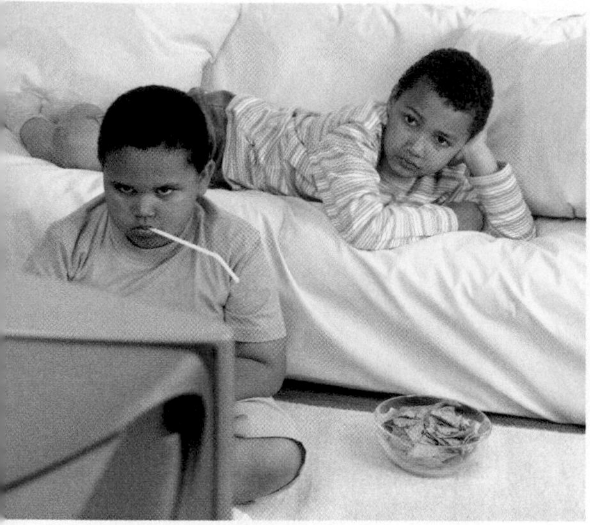
© Pat Doyle/CORBIS

Television watching influences children's eating habits and activity patterns.

have to pedal to watch TV, but could if they chose to.[76] The children who had to pedal were significantly more active, and watched much less TV, than those who did not. Children who have television sets in their bedrooms spend more time watching TV and are more likely to be overweight than children who do not have televisions in their rooms.[77] Children who watch a lot of television (four or more hours a day) are most likely to be obese and least likely to eat fruits and vegetables.[78] They often snack on the fattening foods that are advertised. The average child sees an estimated 30,000 TV commercials a year—many peddling foods high in sugar, fat, and salt such as sugar-coated breakfast cereals, candy bars, chips, fast foods, and carbonated beverages.

More than 25 percent of school-aged children in the United States watch four or more hours of television every day, and 67 percent watch two or more hours every day.[79] Time spent watching television is second only to sleep in time spent being physically inactive. Children also spend more time playing video games. These activities use no more energy than resting, displace participation in more vigorous activities, and foster snacking on high-fat foods.[80] Simply reducing the amount of time spent watching television (and playing video games) can improve a child's BMI.

Growth Overweight children develop a characteristic set of physical traits. They typically begin puberty earlier and so grow taller than their peers at first, but then stop growing at a shorter height. They develop greater bone and muscle mass in response to the demand of having to carry more weight—both fat and lean weight. Consequently, they appear "stocky" even when they lose their excess fat.

Physical Health Like overweight adults, overweight children display a blood lipid profile indicative that atherosclerosis is beginning to develop: high levels of total cholesterol, triglycerides, and LDL cholesterol. Overweight children also tend to have high blood pressure; in fact, obesity is the leading cause of pediatric hypertension. Their risks for developing type 2 diabetes and respiratory diseases (such as asthma) are also exceptionally high.[81] These relationships between childhood obesity and chronic diseases are discussed fully in Highlight 15.

Psychological Development In addition to the physical consequences, childhood obesity brings a host of emotional and social problems.[82] Because people frequently judge others on appearance more than on character, overweight children are often victims of prejudice. Many suffer discrimination by adults and rejection by their peers. They may have poor self-images, a sense of failure, and a passive approach to life. Television shows, which are a major influence in children's lives, often portray the fat person as the bumbling misfit. Overweight children themselves may come to accept this negative stereotype. Researchers investigating children's reactions to various body types find that both normal-weight and underweight children respond unfavorably to overweight bodies.

Prevention and Treatment of Obesity Medical science has worked wonders in preventing or curing many of even the most serious childhood diseases, but obesity remains a challenge.[83] Once excess fat has been stored, it is stubbornly difficult to remove. In light of all this, parents are encouraged to make major efforts to prevent childhood obesity or to begin treatment early—before adolescence.[84] Treatment must consider the many aspects of the problem and possible solutions. An integrated approach is recommended, involving diet, physical activity, psychological support, and behavioral changes.

Diet The initial goal for overweight children is to reduce the rate of weight gain; that is, to maintain weight while the child grows taller. Continued growth will then accomplish the desired change in weight for height. Weight loss is usually not recommended because diet restriction can interfere with growth and development.[85]

Whether the goal is to treat or prevent obesity, these strategies may be helpful:

- Serve family meals that reflect kcalorie control both in the foods offered and in the ways foods have been prepared.
- Involve children in shopping for, and preparing, meals.
- Encourage children to eat only when they are hungry, to eat slowly, to pause and enjoy their table companions, and to stop eating when they are full.
- Teach them how to select nutrient-dense foods that will meet their nutrient needs within their energy allowances and to serve themselves appropriate portions at meals; the amount of food offered influences the amount of food eaten.[86]
- Limit, but don't overly restrict, high-fat, high-sugar foods, including sugar-sweetened soft drinks.
- Never force children to clean their plates.
- Plan for snack times and provide a variety of nutritious snacks (see Table 15-5 later in this chapter).
- Discourage eating while watching TV.

Physical Activity The many benefits of physical activity are well known, but often are not incentive enough to motivate overweight people, especially children. Yet regular vigorous activity can improve a child's weight, body composition, and physical fitness.[87] Ideally, parents will limit sedentary activities and encourage daily physical activity to promote strong skeletal, muscular, and cardiovascular development and instill in their children the desire to be physically active throughout life. Most importantly, parents need to set a good example. Physical activity is a natural and lifelong behavior of healthy living. It can be as simple as riding a bike, playing tag, jumping rope, or doing chores. It need not be an organized sport; it just needs to be some activity on a regular basis. The AAP supports the efforts of schools to include more physical activity in the curriculum and encourages parents to support their children's participation.[88]

HEALTHY PEOPLE 2010

Increase the proportion of the nation's public and private schools that require daily school physical education for all students. Increase the proportion of adolescents who engage in moderate physical activity for at least 30 minutes on 5 or more days per week. Increase the proportion of adolescents who engage in vigorous physical activity that promotes cardiorespiratory fitness 3 or more days per week for 20 or more minutes per occasion. Increase the proportion of adolescents who spend physical education class time being physically active.

Psychological Support Weight-loss programs that involve parents and other caregivers in treatment report greater success than those without parental involvement. Because obesity in parents and their children tends to be positively correlated, both benefit from a weight-loss program. Parental attitudes about food greatly influence children's eating behavior, so it is important that the influence be positive. Otherwise, eating problems may become exacerbated. Unaware that they are teaching their children, parents pass on lessons at the dinner table, on television trays, and in drive-through restaurants. Overweight parents may model for their children the behaviors that have led to their weight gains—eating too much, dieting inappropriately, exercising too little. This pattern is especially evident between mothers and daughters.[89]

Behavioral Changes In contrast to traditional weight-loss programs that focus on *what* to eat, behavioral programs focus on *how* to eat. These techniques involve changing learned habits that lead a child to eat excessively.

Obesity is prevalent in our society. Its far-reaching effects lend urgency to the need to find a remedy. Because treatment of obesity is frequently unsuccessful, it is most important to prevent its onset. Above all, be sensible in teaching children how to

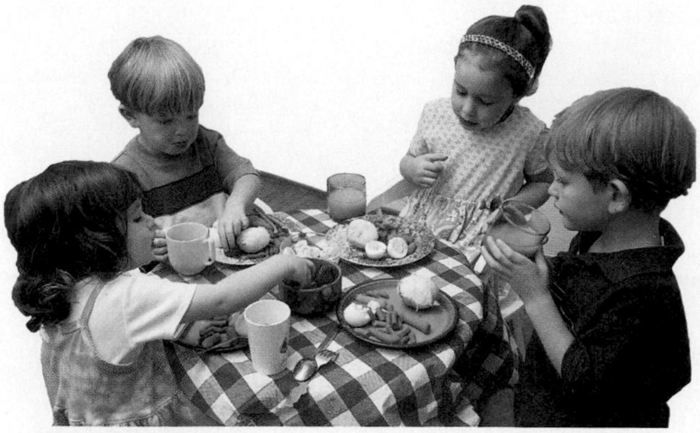
Mary Kate Denny/PhotoEdit

Eating is more fun for children when friends are there.

maintain appropriate body weight. Children can easily get the impression that their worth is tied to their body weight. Parents and the media are most influential in shaping self-concept, weight concerns, and dieting practices.[90] Some parents fail to realize that society's ideal of slimness can be perilously close to starvation and that a child encouraged to "diet" cannot obtain the energy and nutrients required for normal growth and development. Even healthy children without diagnosable eating disorders have been observed to limit their growth through "dieting." Weight gain in truly overweight children can be managed without compromising growth, but should be overseen by a health care professional.

Mealtimes at Home

Traditionally, parents served as **gatekeepers,** determining what foods and activities were available in their children's lives. Then the children made their own selections. Gatekeepers who wanted to promote nutritious choices and healthful habits provided access to nutrient-dense, delicious foods and opportunities for active play at home.

In today's consumer-oriented society, children have greater influence over family decisions concerning food—the fast-food restaurant the family chooses when eating out, the type of food the family eats at home, and the specific brands the family purchases at the grocery store. Parental guidance in food choices is still necessary, but equally important is teaching children consumer skills to help them make informed choices.

Honoring Children's Preferences Researchers attempting to explain children's food preferences encounter contradictions. Children say they like colorful foods, yet most often reject green and yellow vegetables while favoring brown peanut butter and white potatoes, apple wedges, and bread. They seem to like raw vegetables better than cooked ones, so it is wise to offer vegetables that are raw or slightly undercooked, served separately, and easy to eat. Foods should be warm, not hot, because a child's mouth is much more sensitive than an adult's. The flavor should be mild because a child has more taste buds, and smooth foods such as mashed potatoes or split-pea soup should contain no lumps (a child wonders, with some disgust, what the lumps might be). Children prefer foods that are familiar, so offer various foods regularly.

Make mealtimes fun for children. Young children like to eat at little tables and to be served small portions of food. They like sandwiches cut in different geometric shapes and common foods called silly names. They also like to eat with other children, and they tend to eat more when in the company of their friends. Children are also more likely to give up their prejudices against foods when they see their peers eating them.

Learning through Participation Allowing children to help plan and prepare the family's meals provides enjoyable learning experiences and encourages children to eat the foods they have prepared. Vegetables are pretty, especially when fresh, and provide opportunities for children to learn about color, growing vegetables and their seeds, and shapes and textures—all of which are fascinating to young children. Measuring, stirring, washing, and arranging foods are skills that even a young child can practice with enjoyment and pride (see Table 15-4).

Avoiding Power Struggles Problems over food often arise during the second or third year, when children begin asserting their independence. Many of these problems stem from the conflict between children's developmental stages and capabilities and parents who, in attempting to do what they think is best for their children, try to control every aspect of eating. Such conflicts can disrupt children's abilities to regulate their own food intakes or to determine their own likes and dis-

gatekeepers: with respect to nutrition, key people who control other people's access to foods and thereby exert profound impacts on their nutrition. Examples are the spouse who buys and cooks the food, the parent who feeds the children, and the caregiver in a day-care center.

likes. For example, many people share the misconception that children must be persuaded or coerced to try new foods. In fact, the opposite is true. When children are forced to try new foods, even by way of rewards, they are less likely to try those foods again than are children who are left to decide for themselves. Similarly, when children are restricted from eating their favorite foods, they are more likely to want those foods.[91] The parent is responsible for providing healthful foods, but the child is responsible for *how much* and even *whether* to eat.

When introducing new foods at the table, offer them one at a time and only in small amounts at first. The more often a food is presented to a young child, the more likely the child will accept that food. Offer the new food at the beginning of the meal, when the child is hungry, and allow the child to make the decision to accept or reject it. Never make an issue of food acceptance. A power struggle almost invariably sets a firm pattern of resistance and permanently closes the child's mind.

Choking Prevention Parents must always be alert to the dangers of choking. A choking child is silent, so an adult should be present whenever a child is eating. Make sure the child sits when eating; choking is more likely when a child is running or falling. (See p. 519 for a list of foods and nonfood items most likely to cause choking.)

Playing First Children may be more relaxed and attentive at mealtime if outdoor play or other fun activities are scheduled before, rather than immediately after, mealtime. Otherwise children "hurry up and eat" so that they can go play.

Snacking Parents may find that their children snack so much that they aren't hungry at mealtimes. Instead of teaching children *not* to snack, parents might be wise to teach them *how* to snack. Provide snacks that are as nutritious as the foods served at mealtime. Snacks can even be mealtime foods served individually over time, instead of all at once on one plate. When providing snacks to children, think of the five food groups and offer such snacks as pieces of cheese, tangerine slices, and peanut butter on whole-wheat crackers (see Table 15-5 on p. 534). Snacks that are easy to prepare should be readily available to children, especially if they arrive home from school before their parents.

To ensure that children have healthy appetites and plenty of room for nutritious foods when they are hungry, parents and teachers must limit access to candy, cola, and other concentrated sweets. Limiting access includes limiting the amount of pocket money children have to buy such foods themselves.[92] If these foods are permitted in large quantities, the only possible outcomes are nutrient deficiencies, obesity, or both. The preference for sweets is innate; most children do not naturally select nutritious foods on the basis of taste. When children are allowed to create meals freely from a variety of foods, they typically select foods that provide a lot of sugar. When their parents are watching, or even when they think their parents are watching, children improve their selections.[93]

Sweets need not be banned altogether. Children who are exceptionally active can enjoy high-kcalorie foods such as ice cream or pudding from the milk group or pancakes from the bread group. As for sedentary children, they need to become more active, so they can also enjoy some of these foods without unhealthy weight gain.

Preventing Dental Caries Children frequently snack on sticky, sugary foods that stay on the teeth and provide an ideal environment for the growth of bacteria that cause dental caries. Teach children to brush and floss after meals, to brush or rinse after eating snacks, to avoid sticky foods, and to select crisp or fibrous foods frequently.

Serving as Role Models In an effort to practice these many tips, parents may overlook perhaps the single most important influence on their children's food habits—themselves. Parents who don't eat carrots shouldn't be surprised when their children refuse to eat carrots. Likewise, parents who comment negatively on the smell of brussels sprouts may not be able to persuade children to try them. Children learn much through imitation. It is not surprising that children prefer the foods other family

TABLE 15-4 Food Skills of Preschool Children[a]

Age 1–2 years, when large muscles develop, the child:

- Uses short-shanked spoon.
- Helps feed self.
- Lifts and drinks from cup.
- Helps scrub, tear, break, or dip foods.

Age 3 years, when medium hand muscles develop, the child:

- Spears food with fork.
- Feeds self independently.
- Helps wrap, pour, mix, shake, or spread foods.
- Helps crack nuts with supervision.

Age 4 years, when small finger muscles develop, the child:

- Uses all utensils and napkin.
- Helps roll, juice, mash, or peel foods.
- Cracks egg shells.

Age 5 years, when fine coordination of fingers and hands develops, the child:

- Helps measure, grind, grate, and cut (soft foods with dull knife).
- Uses hand-cranked egg beater with supervision.

[a]These ages are approximate. Healthy, normal children develop at their own pace.

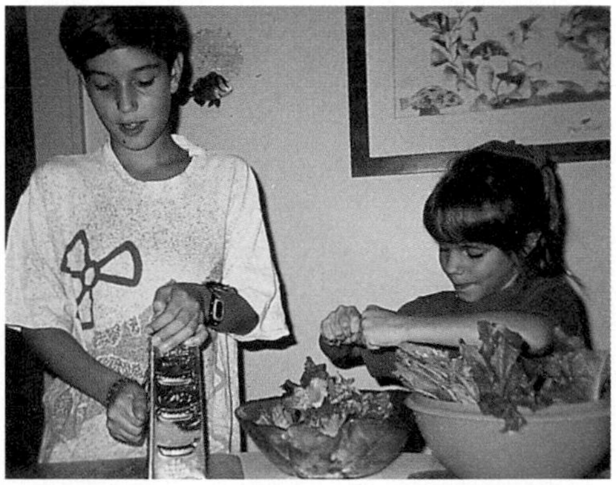

Children enjoy eating the foods they help to prepare.

TABLE 15-5 Healthful Snack Ideas—Think Food Groups, Alone and in Combination

Selecting two or more foods from different food groups adds variety and nutrient balance to snacks. The combinations are endless, so be creative.

Grains

Grain products are filling snacks, especially when combined with other foods:

- Cereal with fruit and milk
- Crackers and cheese
- Whole-grain toast with peanut butter
- Popcorn with grated cheese
- Oatmeal raisin cookies with milk

Vegetables

Cut-up fresh, raw vegetables make great snacks alone or in combination with foods from other food groups:

- Celery with peanut butter
- Broccoli, cauliflower, and carrot sticks with a flavored cottage cheese dip

Fruits

Fruits are delicious snacks and can be eaten alone—fresh, dried, or juiced—or combined with other foods:

- Apples and cheese
- Bananas and peanut butter
- Peaches with yogurt
- Raisins mixed with sunflower seeds or nuts

Meats and Legumes

Meat and legumes add protein to snacks:

- Refried beans with nachos and cheese
- Tuna on crackers
- Luncheon meat on whole-grain bread

Milk and Milk Products

Milk can be used as a beverage with any snack, and many other milk products, such as yogurt and cheese, can be eaten alone or with other foods as listed above.

members enjoy and dislike foods that are never offered to them.[94] Parents, older siblings, and other caregivers set an irresistible example by sitting with younger children, eating the same foods, and having pleasant conversations during mealtimes.

While serving and enjoying food, caregivers can promote both physical and emotional growth at every stage of a child's life. They can help their children to develop both a positive self-concept and a positive attitude toward food. If the beginnings are right, children will grow without the conflicts and confusions over food that can lead to nutrition and health problems.

Nutrition at School

While parents are doing what they can to establish good eating habits in their children at home, others are preparing and serving foods to their children at day-care centers and schools. In addition, children begin to learn about food and nutrition in the classroom. Meeting the nutrition and education needs of children is critical to supporting their healthy growth and development.[95]

Meals at School The U.S. government assists schools financially so that every student can receive nutritious meals at school. Both the School Breakfast Program and the National School Lunch Program provide meals at a reasonable cost to children from families with the financial means to pay. Meals are available free or at reduced cost to children from low-income families. In addition, schools can obtain food commodities. Nationally, the U.S. Department of Agriculture (USDA) administers the programs; on the state level, state departments of education operate them.* The programs usually cost local school districts little, but the educational rewards are great. Several studies have reported that children who participate in school food programs show improvements in learning.[96]

HEALTHY PEOPLE 2010

Increase the proportion of children and adolescents aged 6 to 19 years whose intakes of meals and snacks at school contribute to good overall dietary quality.

Approximately 27 million children receive lunches through the National School Lunch Program—half of them free or at a reduced price.[97] School lunches offer a variety of food choices and help children meet at least one-third of their recommended intakes for energy, protein, vitamin A, vitamin C, iron, and calcium. Table 15-6 shows school lunch patterns for children of different ages and specifies the numbers of servings of milk, protein-rich foods (meat, poultry, fish, cheese, eggs, legumes, or peanut butter), vegetables, fruits, and breads or other grain foods. Over a week's menus, these lunches are also required to meet the *Dietary Guidelines*. Schools making special efforts to lower fat in school lunches typically have trouble providing enough energy and nutrients, especially iron, to meet specifications. The American Dietetic Association (ADA) advocates the development of dietary guidelines specifically for children to ensure that school lunches will both provide adequate energy and nutrients and support health.[98] Other health professionals agree that there is a need for separate guidelines that address children's unique needs.[99]

*School lunches in Canada are administered locally and therefore vary from area to area.

TABLE 15-6 School Lunch Patterns for Different Ages[a]

Food Group	Preschool (Age)		Grade School through High School (Grade)		
	1 to 2	3 to 4	K to 3	4 to 6	7 to 12
Meat or meat alternate					
1 serving:					
Lean meat, poultry, or fish	1 oz	1½ oz	1½ oz	2 oz	3 oz
Cheese	1 oz	1½ oz	1½ oz	2 oz	3 oz
Large egg(s)	½	¾	¾	1	1½
Cooked dry beans or peas	¼ c	⅜ c	⅜ c	½ c	¾ c
Peanut butter	2 tbs	3 tbs	3 tbs	4 tbs	6 tbs
Yogurt	½ c	¾ c	¾ c	1 c	1½ c
Peanuts, soynuts, tree nuts, or seeds[b]	½ oz	¾ oz	¾ oz	1 oz	1½ oz
Vegetable and/or fruit					
2 or more servings, both to total	½ c	½ c	½ c	¾ c	¾ c
Bread or bread alternate[c]					
Servings	5 per week	8 per week	8 per week	8 per week	10 per week
Milk					
1 serving of fluid milk	¾ c	¾ c	1 c	1 c	1 c

[a]The quantities listed represent per-lunch minimums for each age and grade except those for the oldest group, which are recommendations. Schools unable to serve the recommended quantities for grades 7 to 12 must provide at least the amount shown for grades 4 to 6.
[b]These meat alternates may be used to meet no more than half of the meat or meat alternate requirement; therefore, they must be used in a meal with another meat or meat alternate.
[c]Schools must serve daily at least ½ serving of bread or bread alternate to the youngest age group and at least 1 serving to older children.
SOURCE: U.S. Department of Agriculture, National School Lunch Program Regulations, revised January 1, 1998.

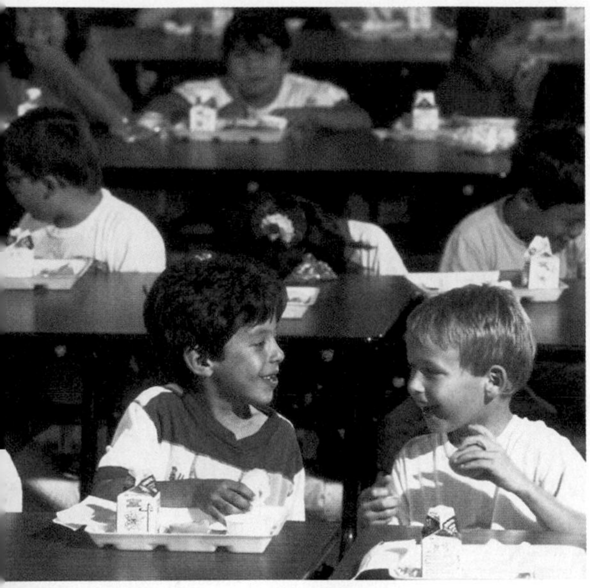

© Bob Daemmrich/Stock Boston/Picture Quest

School lunches provide children with nourishment at little or no charge.

The School Breakfast Program is available in slightly more than half of the nation's schools, and about 7 million children participate in it.[100] The school breakfast must provide at least a fourth of the RDA for each of many nutrients and contain at least one serving of milk; one serving of fruit, juice, or vegetable; and either two servings of bread (or bread alternates), two servings of meat (or meat alternates), or one serving of each.

Another federal program, the Child and Adult Care Food Program (CACFP), operates similarly and provides funds to organized child-care programs. All eligible children, centers, and family day-care homes may participate. Sponsors are reimbursed for most meal costs and may also receive USDA commodity foods.

Competing Influences at School Serving healthful lunches is only half the battle; students need to eat them, too. Short lunch periods and long waiting lines prevent some students from eating a school lunch and leave others with too little time to complete their meals.[101] Nutrition efforts at schools are also undermined when students can buy meals from fast-food restaurants or a la carte foods such as pizza or snack foods and carbonated beverages from snack bars, school stores, and vending machines.[102] These items compete with nutritious school lunches and are often high in fat and sugar.[103] Some states restrict the sale of competing foods and have higher rates of participation in school meal programs than the national average. Nutrition professionals advocate prohibiting sales of food and beverages from vending machines or school stores in middle and high schools until 30 minutes after the end of the last meal unless they are part of the school foodservice and meet *Dietary Guidelines* standards.[104]

Nutrition Education at School Coincident with the school breakfast and lunch programs is a program of nutrition education and training (NET) in all public schools. This program is minimally funded, but program administrators are ingenious and creative in accomplishing its highest-priority objectives. School health clinics offer another opportunity to provide nutrition education and intervention. Children need to be fed well *and* to learn enough about nutrition to make healthful food choices when the choices become theirs to make. Effective nutrition education programs involve children's families and focus on changing specific behaviors rather than teaching general nutrition facts.[105]

HEALTHY PEOPLE 2010

Increase the proportion of middle, junior high, and senior high schools that provide school health education to prevent health problems in several topics (including unhealthy dietary patterns and inadequate physical activity).

IN SUMMARY Children's appetites and nutrient needs reflect their stage of growth. Those who are chronically hungry and malnourished suffer growth retardation; when hunger is temporary and nutrient deficiencies are mild, the problems are usually more subtle—such as poor academic performance. Iron deficiency is widespread and has many physical and behavioral consequences. "Hyper" behavior is not caused by poor nutrition; misbehavior may reflect inconsistent care. Childhood obesity has become a major health problem. Adults at home and at school need to provide children with nutrient-dense foods and teach them how to make healthful diet and activity choices.

Nutrition during Adolescence

Teenagers make many more choices for themselves than they did as children. They are not fed, they eat; they are not sent out to play, they choose to go. At the same time, social pressures thrust choices at them: whether to drink alcoholic beverages and whether to develop their bodies to meet extreme ideals of slimness or athletic prowess. Their interest in nutrition—both valid information and misinformation—derives from personal, immediate experiences. They are concerned with how diet can improve their lives now—they engage in fad dieting in order to fit into a new bathing suit, avoid greasy foods in an effort to clear acne, or eat a pile of spaghetti to prepare for a big sporting event. In presenting information on the nutrition and health of adolescents, this section includes many topics of interest to teens.

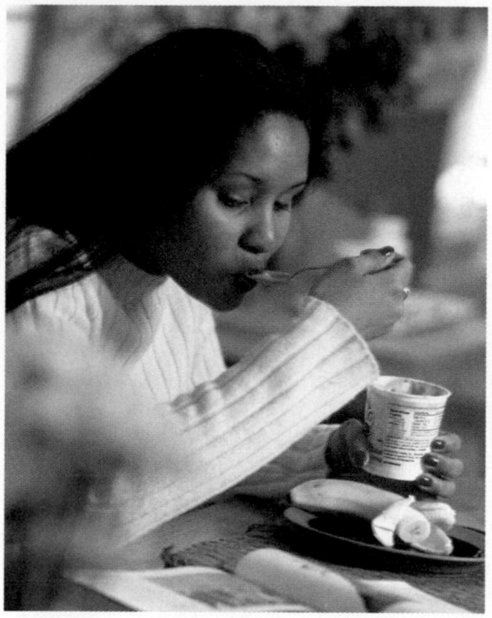

© Steve Dunwell/Index Stock Imagery

Nutritious snacks contribute valuable nutrients to an active teen's diet.

Growth and Development

With the onset of **adolescence,** the steady growth of childhood speeds up abruptly and dramatically, and the growth patterns of female and male become distinct. Hormones direct the intensity of the adolescent growth spurt, profoundly affecting every organ of the body, including the brain. After two to three years of intense growth and a few more at a slower pace, physically mature adults emerge.

In general, the adolescent growth spurt begins at age 10 or 11 for females and at 12 or 13 for males. It lasts about two and a half years. Before **puberty,** male and female body compositions differ only slightly, but during the adolescent spurt, differences between the genders become apparent in the skeletal system, lean body mass, and fat stores. In females, fat assumes a larger percentage of the total body weight, and in males, the lean body mass—principally muscle and bone—increases much more than in females (review Figure 8-8 on p. 265). On average, males grow 8 inches taller, and females, 6 inches taller. Males gain approximately 45 pounds, and females, about 35 pounds.

Energy and Nutrient Needs

Energy and nutrient needs are greater during adolescence than at any other time of life, except pregnancy and lactation. In general, nutrient needs rise throughout childhood, peak in adolescence, and then level off or even diminish as the teen becomes an adult.

Energy Intake and Activity The energy needs of adolescents vary greatly, depending on their current rate of growth, gender, body composition, and physical activity.[106] Boys' energy needs may be especially high; they typically grow faster than girls and, as mentioned, develop a greater proportion of lean body mass. An exceptionally active boy of 15 may need 3500 kcalories or more a day just to maintain his weight. Girls start growing earlier than boys and attain shorter heights and lower weights, so their energy needs peak sooner and decline earlier than those of their male peers. A sedentary girl of 15 whose growth is nearly at a standstill may need only 1700 kcalories a day if she is to avoid excessive weight gain. Thus adolescent girls need to pay special attention to being physically active and selecting foods of high nutrient density so as to meet their nutrient needs without exceeding their energy needs.

The insidious problem of obesity becomes ever more apparent in adolescence and often continues into adulthood. The problem is most evident in females, especially those of African American descent. Without intervention, overweight adolescents will face numerous physical and socioeconomic consequences for years to come. The consequences of obesity are so dramatic and our society's attitude toward obese people is so negative that even teens of normal or below-normal weight may perceive a need to lose weight. When taken to extremes, restrictive diets bring dramatic physical consequences of their own, as Highlight 9 explains.

Vitamins The RDA (or AI) for most vitamins increase during the adolescent years (see the table on the inside front cover). Several of the vitamin recommendations for adolescents are similar to those for adults, including the recommendation for vitamin D. During puberty, both the activation of vitamin D and the absorption of

adolescence: the period from the beginning of puberty until maturity.

puberty: the period in life in which a person becomes physically capable of reproduction.

calcium are enhanced, thus supporting the intense skeletal growth of the adolescent years without additional vitamin D.

Iron The need for iron increases during adolescence for both females and males, but for different reasons. Iron needs increase for females as they start to menstruate, and for males, as their lean body mass develops. Hence, the RDA increases at age 14 for both males and females. For females, the RDA remains high into late adulthood. For males, the RDA returns to preadolescent values in early adulthood.

In addition, iron needs increase when the adolescent growth spurt begins, whether that occurs before or after age 14. Therefore, boys in a growth spurt need an additional 2.9 milligrams of iron per day above the RDA for their age; girls need an additional 1.1 milligrams per day.[107]

Furthermore, iron recommendations for girls before age 14 do not reflect the iron losses of menstruation. The average age of menarche (first menstruation) in the United States is 12.5 years, however.[108] Therefore, for girls under the age of 14 who have started to menstruate, an additional 2.5 milligrams of iron per day is recommended.[109] Thus the RDA for iron depends not only on age and gender but also on whether the individual is in a growth spurt or has begun to menstruate, as listed in the margin.■

■ Iron RDA for males:
- 9–13 yr (8 mg/day).
- 9–13 yr in growth spurt (10.9 mg/day).
- 14–18 yr (11 mg/day).
- 14–18 yr in growth spurt (13.9 mg/day).

Iron RDA for females:
- 9–13 yr (8 mg/day).
- 9–13 yr in menarche (10.5 mg/day).
- 9–13 yr in menarche and growth spurt (11.6 mg/day).
- 14–18 yr (15 mg/day).
- 14–18 yr in growth spurt (16.1 mg/day).

Iron intakes often fail to keep pace with increasing needs, especially for females, who typically consume less iron-rich foods such as meat and fewer total kcalories than males. Not surprisingly, iron deficiency is most prevalent among adolescent girls. Iron-deficient children and teens score lower on standardized tests than those who are not iron deficient.[110]

Calcium Adolescence is a crucial time for bone development, and the requirement for calcium reaches its peak during these years. Unfortunately, many adolescents have calcium intakes below current recommendations. Low calcium intakes during times of active growth, especially if paired with physical inactivity, may compromise the development of peak bone mass, which is considered the best protection against adolescent fractures and adulthood osteoporosis.[111] Increasing milk products■ in the diet to meet calcium recommendations greatly increases bone density.[112] Once again, however, teenage girls are most vulnerable, for their milk—and therefore their calcium—intakes begin to decline at the time when their calcium needs are greatest.[113] Furthermore, women have much greater bone losses than men in later life. In addition to dietary calcium, sports activities during adolescence build strong bones.

■ To meet their calcium needs, teenagers should consume 3 cups of fat-free or low-fat milk or the equivalent in milk products each day. Chapter 12 presents other calcium-rich food choices.

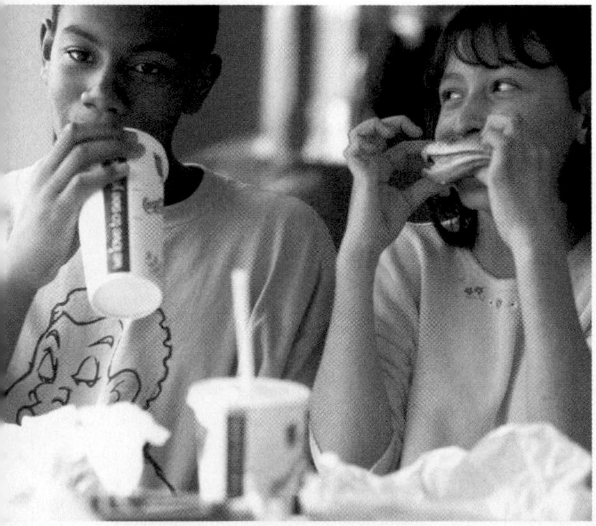

© Ariel Skelley/CORBIS

Because their lunches rarely include fruits, vegetables, or milk, many teens fail to get all the vitamins and minerals they need each day.

Food Choices and Health Habits

Teenagers like the freedom to come and go as they choose. They eat what they want if it is convenient and if they have the time.[114] With a multitude of afterschool, social, and job activities, they almost inevitably fall into irregular eating habits. At any given time on any given day, a teenager may be skipping a meal, eating a snack, preparing a meal, or consuming food prepared by a parent or restaurant. Adolescents who frequently eat meals with their families, however, eat more fruits, vegetables, grains, and calcium-rich foods, and drink fewer soft drinks, than those who seldom eat with their families.[115] Furthermore, they are less likely to smoke, drink alcohol, or use illegal drugs than adolescents who seldom eat meals with their families.[116]

Snacks Snacks typically provide at least a fourth of the average teenager's daily food energy intake. Most often, favorite snacks are high in fat and sodium and low in calcium, iron, vitamin A, vitamin C, folate, and fiber. Most adolescents need to eat a greater variety of foods to obtain these nutrients. Table 15-5 on p. 534 shows how to combine foods from different food groups to create healthy snacks. Vending machines rarely offer nutrient-dense options, and nutrition information alone does not convince people to make healthy choices.

Beverages Most frequently, adolescents drink soft drinks instead of fruit juice or milk with lunch, supper, and snacks. About the only time they select fruit juices is at breakfast. When they drink milk, they are more likely to consume it with a meal (especially breakfast) than as a snack. Because of their greater food intakes, boys are more likely than girls to drink enough milk to meet their calcium needs.

Over the past three decades, teens (especially girls) have been drinking more soft drinks and less milk, as Figure 15-11 shows.[117] Adolescents who drink soft drinks regularly have a higher energy intake and a lower calcium intake than those who do not; they are also more likely to be overweight.[118] The National Institutes of Health calls the low calcium intakes of America's teens "a crisis with long-term health effects." About 85 percent of girls and 64 percent of boys ages 12 to 19 years do not get enough calcium and are at serious risk for developing osteoporosis and other bone diseases in later life.[119]

For adolescents who can afford the kcalories and are meeting their calcium needs, soft drinks are an acceptable part of the diet. Soft drinks may present a different problem, however, when caffeine■ intake becomes excessive. Caffeine seems to be relatively harmless when used in moderate doses (the equivalent of fewer than four 12-ounce cola beverages a day). In greater amounts, it can cause the symptoms associated with anxiety—sweating, tenseness, and inability to concentrate.

FIGURE 15-11 Average Daily Intakes of Milk and Soft Drinks Compared

Over the years, adolescent milk intakes have decreased as soft drink intakes have increased.

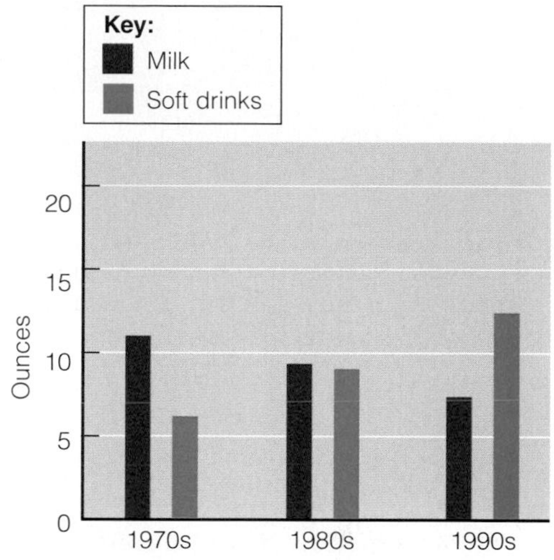
Key:
Milk
Soft drinks
Ounces
0
5
10
15
20
1970s
1980s
1990s

■ For perspective, caffeine-containing soft drinks typically deliver between 30 and 55 mg of caffeine per 12-ounce can. A pharmacologically active dose of caffeine is defined as 200 mg. Appendix H starts with a table listing the caffeine contents of selected foods, beverages, and drugs.

Eating Away from Home Adolescents eat about one-third of their meals away from home, and their nutritional welfare is enhanced or hindered by the choices they make. A lunch of a hamburger, a chocolate shake, and french fries supplies substantial quantities of many nutrients at a kcalorie cost of about 800, an energy intake some adolescents can afford. When they eat this sort of lunch, teens can adjust their breakfast and dinner choices to include fruits and vegetables for vitamin A, vitamin C, folate, and fiber and lean meats and legumes for iron and zinc. (See Appendix H for the nutrient contents of fast foods.) The more adolescents eat at fast-food restaurants, the fewer servings of fruits, vegetables, and milk they eat or drink.[120]

Peer Influence Many of the food and health choices adolescents make reflect the opinions and actions of their peers. When others perceive milk as "babyish," a teen will choose soft drinks instead; when others skip lunch and hang out in the parking lot, a teen may join in for the camaraderie, regardless of hunger. Adults need to remember that adolescents have the right to make their own decisions—even if they are contrary to the adults' views. Gatekeepers can set up the environment so that nutritious foods are available and can stand by with reliable nutrition information and advice, but the rest is up to the adolescents. Ultimately, they make the choices. (Highlight 9 examines the influence of social pressures on the development of eating disorders.)

Problems Adolescents Face

Physical maturity and growing independence present adolescents with new choices to make. The consequences of those choices will influence their nutritional health both today and throughout life. Some teenagers begin using drugs, alcohol, and tobacco; others wisely refrain. Information about the use of these substances is presented here because most people are first exposed to them during adolescence, but it actually applies to people of all ages.

Marijuana Almost half of the high school students in the United States report having at least tried marijuana.[121] Marijuana is unique among drugs in that it seems to enhance the enjoyment of eating, especially of sweets, a phenomenon commonly known as "the munchies." The active ingredient in marijuana is similar to chemicals that occur naturally in the brain. Known as endogenous cannabinoids, or endocannabinoids, these chemicals have receptors throughout the body and brain and may play roles in regulating appetite, pain, and memory. Research on how these chemicals work may shed light on why marijuana induces "the munchies." Whatever the mechanism, prolonged use of marijuana does not seem to bring about a weight gain.

Cocaine One in 11 high school seniors reports having used cocaine at least once.[122] Cocaine stimulates the nervous system and elicits the stress response—constricted blood vessels, raised blood pressure, widened pupils of the eyes, and increased body temperature. It also drives away feelings of fatigue. Cocaine occasionally causes immediate death—usually by heart attack, stroke, or seizure in an already damaged body system.

Weight loss is common, and cocaine abusers often develop eating disorders. Notably, the craving for cocaine replaces hunger; rats given unlimited cocaine will choose it over food until they starve to death. Thus, unlike marijuana use, cocaine use has major nutritional consequences.

Ecstasy The designer drug ecstasy has also lured 1 in 12 high school seniors at least once. Ecstasy signals the nerve cells to dump all their stored serotonin■ at once and then prevents its reabsorption. The rush of serotonin flooding the gap between the nerve cells (synapse) alters a person's mood, but may also damage nerve cells and impair memory. Because serotonin helps to regulate body temperature, overheating is a common and potentially dangerous side effect. People who use ecstasy regularly tend to lose weight.

■ Reminder: *Serotonin* is a neurotransmitter important in the regulation of appetite, sleep, and body temperature.

Drug Abuse, in General The nutrition problems associated with other drugs vary in degree, but drug abusers in general face multiple nutrition problems.■ During withdrawal from drugs, an important part of treatment is to identify and correct nutrient deficiencies.

■ Nutrition problems of drug abusers:
- They buy drugs with money that could be spent on food.
- They lose interest in food during "highs."
- They use drugs that depress appetite.
- Their lifestyle fails to promote good eating habits.
- If they use intravenous (IV) drugs, they may contract AIDS, hepatitis, or other infectious diseases, which increase their nutrient needs. Hepatitis also causes taste changes and loss of appetite.
- Medicines used to treat drug abuse may alter nutrition status.

Alcohol Abuse Sooner or later all teenagers face the decision of whether to drink alcohol. The law forbids the sale of alcohol to people under 21, but most adolescents who want it can get it. Four out of five high school students have had at least one alcoholic beverage; about half drink regularly; and one in three students drinks heavily (defined as five or more drinks on at least one occasion in the previous month).[123]

Highlight 7 describes how alcohol affects nutrition status. To sum it up, alcohol provides energy but no nutrients, and it can displace nutritious foods from the diet. Alcohol alters nutrient absorption and metabolism, so imbalances develop. People who cannot keep their alcohol use moderate must abstain to maintain their health. Highlight 7 lists resources for people with alcohol-related problems.

Smoking Slightly less than 30 percent of U.S. high school students report smoking a cigarette in the previous month.[124] This is the lowest rate of smoking among high schoolers since 1991. Cigarette smoking is a pervasive health problem causing thousands of people to suffer from cancer and diseases of the cardiovascular, digestive, and respiratory systems. These effects are beyond the scope of nutrition, but smoking cigarettes does influence hunger, body weight, and nutrient status.[125]

HEALTHY PEOPLE 2010

Reduce tobacco use by adolescents. Increase tobacco use cessation attempts by adolescent smokers.

Smoking a cigarette eases feelings of hunger. When smokers receive a hunger signal, they can quiet it with cigarettes instead of food. Such behavior ignores body signals and postpones energy and nutrient intake. Indeed, smokers tend to weigh less than nonsmokers and to gain weight when they stop smoking. People contemplating giving up cigarettes should know that the average weight gain is about 10 pounds in the first year. Smokers wanting to quit should prepare for the possibility of weight gain and adjust their diet and activity habits so as to maintain weight during and after quitting. Smoking cessation programs need to include strategies for weight management.[126]

Nutrient intakes of smokers and nonsmokers differ. Smokers tend to have lower intakes of dietary fiber, vitamin A, beta-carotene, folate, and vitamin C. The association between smoking and low intakes of fruits and vegetables rich in these nutrients may be noteworthy, considering their protective effect against lung cancer (see Highlight 11).

Compared to nonsmokers, smokers require more vitamin C■ to maintain steady body pools. Oxidants in cigarette smoke accelerate vitamin C metabolism and deplete smokers' body stores of this antioxidant.[127] This depletion is even evident to some degree in nonsmokers who are exposed to passive smoke.[128]

■ The vitamin C requirement for people who regularly smoke cigarettes is an additional 35 mg/day.

Beta-carotene enhances the immune response and protects against some cancer activity. Specifically, the risk of lung cancer is greatest for smokers who have the lowest intakes. Of course, such evidence should not be misinterpreted. It does not mean that as long as people eat their carrots, they can safely use tobacco. Nor does it mean that beta-carotene *supplements* would be beneficial; smokers taking beta-carotene supplements actually had a higher incidence of lung cancer and risk of death than those taking a placebo (see Highlight 11 for more details). Smokers are ten times more likely to get lung cancer than nonsmokers. Both smokers and nonsmokers, however, can reduce their cancer risks by eating fruits and vegetables rich in antioxidants (see Highlight 11 for details on antioxidant nutrients and disease prevention).

Smokeless Tobacco Nationwide, 1 in 15 high school students reports having used smokeless tobacco products.[129] Like cigarettes, smokeless tobacco use is linked to many health problems, from minor mouth sores to tumors in the nasal cavities, cheeks, gums, and throat. The risk of mouth and throat cancers is even greater than for smoking tobacco. Other drawbacks to tobacco chewing and snuff dipping include bad breath, stained teeth, and blunted senses of smell and taste. Tobacco chewing also damages the gums, tooth surfaces, and jawbones, making teeth loss later in life likely.

IN SUMMARY Nutrient needs rise dramatically as children enter the rapid growth spurt of the teen years. The busy lifestyles of adolescents add to the challenge of meeting their nutrient needs—especially for iron and calcium. In addition to making wise food choices, adolescents need to refrain from using substances that will impair their health—including illicit drugs, alcohol, and tobacco.

The nutrition and lifestyle choices people make as children and adolescents have long-term, as well as immediate, effects on their health. Highlight 15 describes how sound choices and good habits during childhood and adolescence can help prevent chronic diseases later in life.

Nutrition in Your Life

Encouraging children to eat nutritious foods today helps them learn how to make healthy food choices tomorrow.

- **If there are children in your life, do they receive enough food for healthy growth, but not so much as to lead to obesity?**
- **Are they physically active at home and at school?**
- **Do they get enough calcium and iron?**

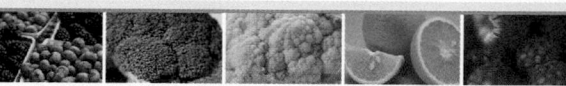

NUTRITION ON THE NET

Access these websites for further study of topics covered in this chapter.

- Find updates and quick links to these and other nutrition-related sites at our website: **www.wadsworth.com/nutrition**
- Search for "infants," "baby bottle tooth decay," "premature birth," "hyperactivity," "food allergies," and "adolescent health," at the U.S. Government health information site: **www.healthfinder.gov**
- Learn how to care for infants, children, and adolescents from the American Academy of Pediatrics and the Canadian Paediatric Society: **www.aap.org** and **www.cps.ca**
- Download the current growth charts and learn about their most recent revision: **www.cdc.gov/growthcharts**
- Get information on the Food Guide Pyramid for young children from the USDA: **www.usda.gov/cnpp**
- Get tips for feeding children from the American Dietetic Association and the Kids Food Cyber Club: **www.eatright.org** and **www.kidfood.org**
- Get tips for keeping children healthy from the Nemours Foundation: **www.kidshealth.org**
- Visit the National Center for Education in Maternal & Child Health and the National Institute of Child Health and Human Development: **www.ncemch.org** and **www.nichd.nih.gov**
- Learn about the Child Nutrition Programs: **www.fns.usda.gov/fns**
- Learn how UNICEF works to protect children: **www.unicef.org**
- Learn how to reduce lead exposure in your home from the U.S. Department of Housing and Urban Development Office of Lead Hazard Control: **www.hud.gov/lead**
- Learn more about food allergies from the American Academy of Allergy, Asthma, and Immunology; the Food Allergy Network; and the International Food Information Council: **www.aaaai.org**, **www.foodallergy.org**, and **www.ific.org**
- Learn more about hyperactivity from Children and Adults with Attention Deficit Disorders: **www.chadd.org**
- Visit the Milk Matters section of the National Institute of Child Health and Human Development (NICHD): **www.nichd.nih.gov**
- Learn more about caffeine from the International Food Information Council: **www.ific.org**
- To learn about healthy foods and to find recipes and ideas for physical activities, visit: **www.kidnetic.com**
- Get weight-loss tips for children and adolescents: **www.shapedown.com**
- Learn about nondietary approaches to weight loss from HUGS International: **www.hugs.com**
- Read the message for parents and teens on the risks of tobacco use from the American Academy of Pediatrics: **www.aap.org**
- Get help quitting smoking at QuitNet: **www.quitnet.com**
- Visit the Tobacco Information and Prevention Source (TIPS) of the Centers for Disease Control and Prevention: **www.cdc.gov/tobacco/sgr/sgr_2000**

STUDY QUESTIONS

These questions will help you review the chapter. You will find the answers in the discussions on the pages provided.

1. Describe some of the nutrient and immunological attributes of breast milk. (pp. 513–514)
2. What are the appropriate uses of formula feeding? What criteria would you use in selecting an infant formula? (pp. 515–516)
3. Why are solid foods not recommended for an infant during the first few months of life? When is an infant ready to start eating solid food? (pp. 517–519)
4. Identify foods that are inappropriate for infants and explain why they are inappropriate. (p. 519)
5. What nutrition problems are most common in children? What strategies can help prevent these problems? (pp. 521–522)
6. Describe the relationships between nutrition and behavior. How does television influence nutrition? (pp. 523–524, 529–530)
7. Describe a true food allergy. Which foods most often cause allergic reactions? How do food allergies influence nutrition status? (pp. 527–528)
8. Describe the problems associated with childhood obesity and the strategies for prevention and treatment. (pp. 528–532)
9. List strategies for introducing nutritious foods to children. (pp. 532–534)
10. What impact do school meal programs have on the nutrition status of children? (pp. 534–536)
11. Describe the changes in nutrient needs from childhood to adolescence. Why is an adolescent girl more likely to develop an iron deficiency than is a boy? (pp. 537–538)

12. How do adolescents' eating habits influence their nutrient intakes? (pp. 538–539)
13. How does the use of illicit drugs influence nutrition status? (pp. 539–540)
14. How do the nutrient intakes of smokers differ from those of nonsmokers? What impacts can those differences exert on health? (pp. 540–541)

These multiple choice questions will help you prepare for an exam. Answers can be found on p. 546.

1. A reasonable weight for a healthy five-month-old infant who weighed 8 pounds at birth might be:
   a. 12 pounds.
   b. 16 pounds.
   c. 20 pounds.
   d. 24 pounds.
2. Dehydration can develop quickly in infants because:
   a. much of their body water is extracellular.
   b. they lose a lot of water through urination and tears.
   c. only a small percentage of their body weight is water.
   d. they drink lots of breast milk or formula, but little water.
3. An infant should begin eating solid foods between:
   a. 2 and 4 weeks.
   b. 1 and 3 months.
   c. 4 and 6 months.
   d. 8 and 10 months.
4. Among U.S. and Canadian children, the most prevalent nutrient deficiency is of:
   a. iron.
   b. folate.
   c. protein.
   d. vitamin D.
5. A true food allergy always:
   a. elicits an immune response.
   b. causes an immediate reaction.
   c. creates an aversion to the offending food.
   d. involves symptoms such as headaches or hives.
6. Which of the following strategies is *not* effective?
   a. Play first, eat later.
   b. Provide small portions.
   c. Encourage children to help prepare meals.
   d. Use dessert as a reward for eating vegetables.
7. To help teenagers consume a balanced diet, parents can:
   a. monitor the teens' food intake.
   b. give up—parents can't influence teenagers.
   c. keep the pantry and refrigerator well stocked.
   d. forbid snacking and insist on regular, well-balanced meals.
8. During adolescence, energy and nutrient needs:
   a. reach a peak.
   b. fall dramatically.
   c. rise, but do not peak until adulthood.
   d. fluctuate so much that generalizations can't be made.
9. The nutrients most likely to fall short in the adolescent diet are:
   a. sodium and fat.
   b. folate and zinc.
   c. iron and calcium.
   d. protein and vitamin A.
10. To balance the day's intake, an adolescent who eats a hamburger, fries, and cola at lunch might benefit most from a dinner of:
    a. fried chicken, rice, and banana.
    b. ribeye steak, baked potato, and salad.
    c. pork chop, mashed potatoes, and apple juice.
    d. spaghetti with meat sauce, broccoli, and milk.

REFERENCES

1. R. J. Kuczmarski and coauthors, CDC Growth charts: United States, *Advanced Data* 314 (2000): 1–28.
2. Committee on Dietary Reference Intakes, *Dietary Reference Intakes for Energy, Carbohydrate, Fiber, Fat, Fatty Acids, Cholesterol, Protein, and Amino Acids* (Washington, D.C.: National Academies Press, 2002).
3. Committee on Dietary Reference Intakes, 2002, pp. 6-12–6-13.
4. Committee on Nutrition, American Academy of Pediatrics, *Pediatric Nutrition Handbook,* 5th ed., ed. R. E. Kleinman (Elk Grove Village, Ill.: American Academy of Pediatrics, 2004), pp. 103–115.
5. Position of the American Dietetic Association: Breaking the barriers to breastfeeding, *Journal of the American Dietetic Association* 101 (2001): 1213–1220.
6. Committee on Nutrition, American Academy of Pediatrics, 2004, pp. 55–85; Position of the American Dietetic Association, 2001.
7. J. D. Carver, Advances in nutritional modifications of infant formulas, *American Journal of Clinical Nutrition* 77 (2003): 1550S–1554S.
8. N. Auestad and coauthors, Growth and development in term infants fed long-chain polyunsaturate fatty acids: A double-masked, randomized, parallel, prospective, multivariate study, *Pediatrics* 108 (2001): 372–381; J. W. Anderson, B. M. Johnstone, and D. T. Remley, Breast-feeding and cognitive development: A meta-analysis, *American Journal of Clinical Nutrition* 70 (1999): 525–535.
9. Anderson, Johnstone, and Remley, 1999.
10. Auestad and coauthors, 2001.
11. E. E. Birch and coauthors, A randomized controlled trial of long-chain polyunsaturated fatty acid supplementation of formula in term infants after weaning at 6 wk of age, *American Journal of Clinical Nutrition* 75 (2002): 570–580.
12. C. Williams and coauthors, Stereoacuity at age 3.5 in children born fullterm is associated with prenatal and postnatal dietary factors: A report from a population-based cohort study, *American Journal of Clinical Nutrition* 73 (2001): 316–322.
13. D. L. O'Connor and coauthors, Growth and development in preterm infants fed long-chain polyunsaturated fatty acids: A prospective, randomized, controlled trial, *Pediatrics* 108 (2001): 359–371.
14. L. M. Gartner, F. R. Greer, and the Section on Breastfeeding and Committee on Nutrition, Prevention of rickets and vitamin D deficiency: New guidelines for vitamin D intake, *Pediatrics* 111 (2003): 908–910; S. Fitzpatrick and coauthors, Vitamin D-deficient rickets: A multifactorial disease, *Nutrition Reviews* 58 (2000): 218–222.
15. Gartner, Greer, and the Section on Breastfeeding and Committee on Nutrition, 2003.
16. Position of the American Dietetic Association, 2001: S. Arifeen and coauthors, Exclusive breastfeeding reduces acute respiratory infection and diarrhea deaths among infants in Dhaka slums, *Pediatrics* 108 (2001): e67.
17. B. Lönnerdal, Nutritional and physiologic significance of human milk proteins, *American Journal of Clinical Nutrition* 77 (2003): 1537S–1543S.
18. W. H. Oddy and coauthors, Association between breastfeeding and asthma in 6

year old children: Findings of a prospective birth cohort study, *British Medical Journal* 319 (1999): 815–819.
19. M. Gdalevich, D. Mimouni, and M. Mimouni, Breastfeeding and the risk of bronchial asthma in childhood: A systematic review with meta-analysis of prospective studies, *Journal of Pediatrics* 139 (2001): 261–266.
20. C. G. Owen and coauthors, Infant feeding and blood cholesterol: A study in adolescents and systematic review, *Pediatrics* 110 (2002): 597–608.
21. M. W. Gillman and coauthors, Risk of overweight among adolescents who were breastfed as infants, *Journal of the American Medical Association* 285 (2001): 2461–2467.
22. A. D. Liese and coauthors, Inverse association of overweight and breastfeeding in 9 to 10 year-old-children in Germany, *International Journal of Obesity and Related Metabolic Disorders* 25 (2001): 1644–1650.
23. M. L. Hediger and coauthors, Association between infant breastfeeding and overweight in young children, *Journal of the American Medical Association* 285 (2001): 2453–2460.
24. E. L. Mortensen and coauthors, The association between duration of breastfeeding and adult intelligence, *Journal of the American Medical Association* 287 (2002): 2365–2371.
25. A. Jain, J. Concato, and J. M. Leventhal, How good is the evidence linking breastfeeding and intelligence? *Pediatrics* 109 (2002): 1044–1053.
26. Committee on Nutrition, American Academy of Pediatrics, Hypoallergenic infant formulas, *Pediatrics* 106 (2000): 346–349.
27. M. F. MacDorman and coauthors, Annual summary of vital statistics—2001, *Pediatrics* 110 (2002): 1037–1052.
28. M. A. Crawford, Placental delivery of arachidonic and docosahexaenoic acids: Implications for the lipid nutrition of preterm infants, *American Journal of Clinical Nutrition* 71 (2000): 275S–284S.
29. O'Connor and coauthors, 2001; R. Uauy and D. R. Hoffman, Essential fat requirements of preterm infants, *American Journal of Clinical Nutrition* 71 (2000): 245S–250S.
30. Committee on Nutrition, American Academy of Pediatrics, 2004, p. 111.
31. L. Monetini and coauthors, Bovine beta-casein antibodies in breast- and bottle-fed infants: Their relevance in type 1 diabetes, *Diabetes/Metabolism Research and Reviews* 17 (2001): 51–54; C. D. Bernadier, Diabetes mellitus: Is there a connection with infant feeding practices? *Nutrition Today* 36 (2001): 241–248; M. Hummel and coauthors, No major association of breast-feeding, vaccinations, and child viral diseases with early islet autoimmunity in the German BABYDIAB study, *Diabetes Care* 23 (2000): 969–974.
32. S. J. Fomon, Feeding normal infants: Rationale for recommendations, *Journal of the American Dietetic Association* 101 (2001): 1002–1005.
33. L. Hallberg and coauthors, The role of meat to improve the critical iron balance during weaning, *Pediatrics* 111 (2003): 864–870; Fomon, 2001; L. Davidsson and coauthors, Iron bioavailability in infants from an infant cereal fortified with ferric pyrophosphate or ferrous fumarate, *American Journal of Clinical Nutrition* 71 (2000): 1597–1602.
34. B. A. Dennison and coauthors, Children's growth parameters vary by type of fruit juice consumed, *Journal of the American College of Nutrition* 18 (1999): 346–352.
35. Committee on Nutrition, American Academy of Pediatrics, The use and misuse of fruit juice in pediatrics, *Pediatrics* 107 (2001): 1210–1213.
36. Centers for Disease Control and Prevention, Nonfatal choking—related episodes among children—United States, 2001, *Morbidity and Mortality Weekly Report* 51 (2002): 945–948.
37. Committee on Sports Medicine and Fitness and Committee on School Health, Physical fitness and activity in schools, *Pediatrics* 105 (2000): 1156–1157.
38. V. Messina and A. R. Mangels, Considerations in planning vegan diets: Children, *Journal of the American Dietetic Association* 101 (2001): 661–669.
39. Committee on Dietary Reference Intakes, 2002, Chapter 6.
40. Committee on Dietary Reference Intakes, 2002, Chapter 7.
41. Position of the American Dietetic Association: Health implications of dietary fiber, *Journal of the American Dietetic Association* 102 (2002): 993–1000.
42. Committee on Dietary Reference Intakes, 2002, Chapter 8.
43. Committee on Dietary Reference Intakes, 2002, Chapter 11.
44. Centers for Disease Control and Prevention, Iron deficiency—United States, 1999–2000, *Morbidity and Mortality Weekly Report* 51 (2002): 897–899; M. F. Picciano and coauthors, Nutritional guidance is needed during dietary transition in early childhood, *Pediatrics* 106 (2000): 109–114.
45. S. L. Johnson, Children's food acceptance patterns: The interface of ontogeny and nutrition needs, *Nutrition Reviews* 60 (2002): S91–S94; Eden, 2001.
46. R. E. Kleinman, Current approaches to standards of care for children: How does the pediatric community currently approach this issue? *Nutrition Today* 37 (2002): 177–178.
47. D. J. Raiten, M. F. Picciano, and P. Coates, Dietary supplement use in children: Who, what, why, and where do we go from here: Executive summary, *Nutrition Today* 37 (2002): 167–169.
48. Federal Trade Commission, Consumer Features, Promotions for kids' dietary supplements leaves sour taste, **www.ftc.gov/bcp/conline/features/kidsupp.htm**. May 2000.
49. M. Lino, and coauthors, U.S. Department of Agriculture, Center for Nutrition Policy and Promotion, The quality of young children's diets, *Family Economics and Nutrition Review* 14 (2002): 52–59.
50. S. B. Roberts and M. B. Heyman, Micronutrient shortfalls in young children's diets: Common, and owing to inadequate intakes both at home and at child care centers, *Nutrition Reviews* 58 (2000): 27–29.
51. Federal Interagency Forum on Child and Family Statistics, *America's Children: Key National Indicators of Well-Being 2002*, available at **www.childstats.gov**.
52. Committee on Dietary Reference Intakes, *Dietary Reference Intakes for Vitamin A, Vitamin K, Arsenic, Boron, Chromium, Copper, Iodine, Iron, Manganese, Molybdenum, Nickel, Silicon, Vanadium, and Zinc* (Washington, D.C.: National Academy Press, 2001), pp. 82–161.
53. Committee on Dietary Reference Intakes, 2001, pp. 290–393; H. Saloojee and J. M. Pettifor, Iron deficiency and impaired child development, *British Medical Journal* 323 (2001): 1377–1378; J. S. Halterman and coauthors, Iron deficiency and cognitive achievement among school-aged children and adolescents in the United States, *Pediatrics* 107 (2001): 1381–1386; R. J. Stoltzfus, Iron-deficiency anemia: Reexamining the nature and magnitude of the public health problem. Summary: Implications for research and programs, *Journal of Nutrition* 131 (2001): 697S–700S.
54. B. Lozoff and coauthors, Poorer behavioral and developmental outcome more than 10 years after treatment for iron deficiency in infancy, *Pediatrics* 105 (2000): e51; E. K. Hurtado, A. H. Claussen, and K. G. Scott, Early childhood anemia and mild or moderate mental retardation, *American Journal of Clinical Nutrition* 69 (1999): 115–119.
55. J. A. Simon and E. S. Hudes, Relationship of ascorbic acid to blood lead levels, *Journal of the American Medical Association* 281 (1999): 2289–2293.
56. Centers for Disease Control and Prevention, Childhood lead poisoning, **www.cdc.gov/nceh/lead/factsheets/childhoodlead.htm**, site visited April 22, 2003.
57. X. Liu and coauthors, Do children with falling blood lead levels have improved cognition? *Pediatrics* 110 (2002): 787–791; W. J. Rogan and coauthors, The effect of chelation therapy with succimer on neuropsychological development in children exposed to lead, *New England Journal of Medicine* 344 (2001): 1421–1426; J. F. Rosen and P. Mushak, Primary prevention of childhood lead poisoning—The only solution, *New England Journal of Medicine* 344 (2001): 1470–1471.
58. Blood lead levels in young children—United States and selected states, 1996–1999, *Morbidity and Mortality Weekly Report* 49 (2000): 1133–1137.
59. S. Parmet, C. Lynm, and R. M. Glass, Attention-deficit/hyperactivity disorder, *Journal of the American Medical Association* 288 (2002): 1804; Subcommittee on Attention-Deficit/Hyperactivity Disorder, American Academy of Pediatrics, Clinical practice guideline: Treatment of the school-aged child with attention-deficit/hyperactivity disorder, *Pediatrics* 108 (2001): 1033–1044; The MTA Cooperative Group, A 14-month randomized clinical trial of treatment strategies for attention-deficit/hyperactivity disorder: Multimodal treatment study of children with ADHD, *Archives of General Psychiatry* 56 (1999): 1073–1086.
60. Food Allergy and Intolerances, National Institutes of Health Fact Sheet, **www.niaid.nih.gov/factsheets/food.htm**, site visited on April 23, 2003; R. Formanek, Food allergies: When food becomes the enemy, *FDA Consumer*, July/August 2001, pp. 10–16.
61. Formanek, 2001.
62. L. Christie and coauthors, Food allergies in children affect nutrient intake and growth, *Journal of the American Dietetic Association* 102 (2002): 1648–1651.
63. K. J. Falci, K. L. Gombas, and E. L. Elliot, Food allergen awareness: An FDA priority, *Food Safety Magazine*, February/March 2001, available at **www.cfsan.fda.gov/~dms/**.
64. H. Metzger, Two approaches to peanut allergy, *New England Journal of Medicine* 348 (2003): 1046–1048.
65. B. Wuthrich, Lethal or life-threatening allergic reactions to food, *Journal of Investigational Allergology and Clinical Immunology* 10 (2000): 59–65.
66. G. S. Rhim and M. S. McMorris, School readiness for children with food allergies, *Annals of Allergy, Asthma and Immunology* 86 (2001): 172–176.
67. S. A. Bock, A. Munoz-Furlong, and H. A. Sampson, Fatalities due to anaphylactic reactions to foods, *Journal of Allergy and Clinical Immunology* 107 (2001): 191–193.
68. J. M. Yeung, R. S. Applebaum, and R. Hildwine, Criteria to determine food

allergen priority, *Journal of Food Protection* 63 (2000): 982–986.
69. Formanek, 2001.
70. C. L. Ogden and coauthors, Prevalence and trends in overweight among US children and adolescents, 1999–2000, *Journal of the American Medical Association* 288 (2002): 1728–1732.
71. A. R. Dorosty and coauthors, Factors associated with early adiposity rebound, *Pediatrics* 105 (2000): 1115–1118.
72. A. Must, Does overweight in childhood have an impact on adult health? *Nutrition Reviews* 61 (2003): 139–142; S. S. Guo and coauthors, Predicting overweight and obesity in adulthood from body mass index values in childhood and adolescence, *American Journal of Clinical Nutrition* 76 (2002): 653–658; A. D. Salbe and coauthors, Assessing risk factors for obesity between childhood and adolescence: I. Birth weight, childhood adiposity, parental obesity, insulin, and leptin, *Pediatrics* 110 (2002): 299–306; M. Mijailovic, V. Mijailovic, and D. Micic, Childhood onset of obesity: Does an obese child become an obese adult? *Journal of Pediatric Endocrinology* 14 (2001): 1335S–1365S.
73. S. M. Robertson and coauthors, Factors related to adiposity among children aged 3 to 7 years, *Journal of the American Dietetic Association* 99 (1999): 938–943.
74. J. O. Fisher and coauthors, Parental influences on young girls' fruit and vegetable, micronutrient, and fat intakes, *Journal of the American Dietetic Association* 102 (2002): 58–64.
75. Centers for Disease Control and Prevention, Physical activity levels among children aged 9–13 years—United States, 2002, *Morbidity and Mortality Weekly Report* 52 (2003): 785–788; Committee on Nutrition, American Academy of Pediatrics, Prevention of pediatric overweight and obesity, *Pediatrics* 112 (2003): 424–430; R. Chatrath and coauthors, Physical fitness of urban American children, *Pediatric Cardiology* 23 (2002): 608–612; A. D. Salbe and coauthors, Assessing risk factors for obesity between childhood and adolescence: II. Energy metabolism and physical activity, *Pediatrics* 110 (2002): 307–314.
76. M. S. Faith and coauthors, Effects of contingent television on physical activity and television viewing in obese children, *Pediatrics* 107 (2001): 1043–1048.
77. B. A. Dennison, T. A. Erb, and P. L. Jenkins, Television viewing and television in bedroom associated with overweight risk among low-income preschool children, *Pediatrics* 109 (2002): 1028–1035.
78. C. J. Crespo and coauthors, Television watching, energy intake, and obesity in US children: Results from the third National Health and Nutrition Examination Survey, 1988–1994, *Archives of Pediatric and Adolescent Medicine* 155 (2001): 360–365; K. A. Coon and coauthors, Relationships between use of television during meals and children's food consumption patterns, *Pediatrics* 107 (2001): e71.
79. R. E. Andersen and coauthors, Relationship of physical activity and television watching with body weight and level of fatness among children, *Journal of the American Medical Association* 279 (1998): 938–942.
80. J. Utter and coauthors, Couch potatoes or french fries: Are sedentary behaviors associated with body mass index, physical activity, and dietary behaviors among adolescents? *Journal of the American Dietetic Association* 103 (2003): 1298–1305.
81. A. Must and S. E. Anderson, Effects of obesity on morbidity in children and adolescents, *Nutrition in Clinical Care* 6 (2003): 4–12; R. Sinha and coauthors, Prevalence of impaired glucose tolerance among children and adolescents with marked obesity, *New England Journal of Medicine* 346 (2002): 802–810.
82. J. B. Schwimmer, T. M. Burwinkle, and J. W. Varni, Health-related quality of life of severely obese children and adolescents, *Journal of the American Medical Association* 289 (2003): 1813–1819.
83. M. I. Goran, Metabolic precursors and effects of obesity in children: A decade of progress, 1990–1999, *American Journal of Clinical Nutrition* 73 (2001): 158–171.
84. American Heart Association's statement for health professionals on cardiovascular health in children, posted on July 1, 2002, **www.americanheart.org**.
85. Helping Your Overweight Child, **www.niddk.nih.gov/health/nutrit/pubs/helpchld.htm**, site visited on April 24, 2003.
86. B. J. Rolls, D. Engell, and L. L. Birch, Serving portion size influences 5-year-old but not 3-year-old children's food intakes, *Journal of the American Dietetic Association* 100 (2000): 232–234.
87. B. Gutin and coauthors, Effects of exercise intensity on cardiovascular fitness, total body composition, and visceral adiposity of obese adolescents, *American Journal of Clinical Nutrition* 75 (2002): 818–826; L. M. LeMura and M. T. Maziekas, Factors that alter body fat, body mass, and fat-free mass in pediatric obesity, *Medicine and Science in Sports and Exercise* 34 (2001): 487–496.
88. Committee on Sports Medicine and Fitness and Committee on School Health, American Academy of Pediatrics, Physical fitness and activity in schools, *Pediatrics* 105 (2000): 1156–1157.
89. T. M. Cutting and coauthors, Like mother, like daughter: Familiar patterns of overweight are mediated by mothers' dietary disinhibition, *American Journal of Clinical Nutrition* 69 (1999): 608–613.
90. D. Spruijt-Metz and coauthors, Relation between mothers' child-feeding practices and childrens' adiposity, *American Journal of Clinical Nutrition* 75 (2002): 581–586; A. E. Field and coauthors, Peer, parent, and media influences on the development of weight concerns and frequent dieting among preadolescent and adolescent girls and boys, *Pediatrics* 107 (2001): 54–60; K. K. Davison and L. L. Birch, Weight status, parent reaction, and self-concept in five-year-old girls, *Pediatrics* 107 (2001): 46–53.
91. J. O. Fisher and L. L. Birch, Restricting access to palatable foods affects children's behavioral response, food selection, and intake, *American Journal of Clinical Nutrition* 69 (1999): 1264–1272.
92. B. P. Roberts, A. S. Blinkhorn, and J. T. Duxbury, The power of children over adults when obtaining sweet snacks, *International Journal of Paediatric Dentistry* 13 (2003): 76–84.
93. R. E. Klesges and coauthors, Parental influence on food selection in young children and its relationships to childhood obesity, *American Journal of Clinical Nutrition* 53 (1991): 859–864.
94. J. D. Skinner and coauthors, Children's food preferences: A longitudinal analysis, *Journal of the American Dietetic Association* 102 (2002): 1638–1647.
95. Position of the American Dietetic Association, Society of Nutrition Education, and American School Food Service Association—Nutrition services: An essential component of comprehensive school health programs, *Journal of the American Dietetic Association* 103 (2003): 505–514; Position of the American Dietetic Association: Nutrition standards for child-care programs, *Journal of the American Dietetic Association* 99 (1999): 981–988.
96. Position of the American Dietetic Association, Society of Nutrition Education, and American School Food Service Association, 2003.
97. Position of the American Dietetic Association: Child and adolescent food and nutrition programs, *Journal of the American Dietetic Association* 103 (2003): 887–893.
98. Position of the American Dietetic Association: Dietary guidance for healthy children aged 2 to 11 years, *Journal of the American Dietetic Association* 99 (1999): 93–101.
99. M. F. Picciano, L. D. McBean, and V. A. Stallings, How to grow a healthy child: A conference report, *Nutrition Today* 34 (1999): 6–14.
100. Position of the American Dietetic Association, 2003.
101. E. A. Bergman and coauthors, Time spent by schoolchildren to eat lunch, *Journal of the American Dietetic Association* 100 (2000): 696–698.
102. J. L. Kramer-Atwood and coauthors, Fostering healthy food consumption in schools: Focusing on the challenges of competitive foods, *Journal of the American Dietetic Association* 102 (2002): 1228–1233; Position of the American Dietetic Association: Local support for nutrition integrity in schools, *Journal of the American Dietetic Association* 100 (2000): 108–111; K. W. Cullen and coauthors, Effect of a la carte and snack bar foods at school on children's lunchtime intake of fruits and vegetables, *Journal of the American Dietetic Association* 100 (2000): 1482–1486.
103. M. B. Wildey and coauthors, Fat and sugar levels are high in snacks purchased from student stores in middle schools, *Journal of the American Dietetic Association* 100 (2000): 319–322; L. Harnack and coauthors, Availability of a la carte food items in junior and senior high schools: A needs assessment, *Journal of the American Dietetic Association* 100 (2000): 701–703.
104. Position of the American Dietetic Association, Society for Nutrition Education, and American School Food Service Association, 2003.
105. Position of the American Dietetic Association, Society for Nutrition Education, and American School Food Service Association, 2003.
106. Committee on Dietary Reference Intakes, 2002, Chapter 5.
107. Committee on Dietary Reference Intakes, 2001, pp. 290–393.
108. W. C. Chumlea and coauthors, Age at menarche and racial comparisons in US girls, *Pediatrics* 111 (2003): 110–113.
109. Committee on Dietary Reference Intakes, 2001, pp. 290–393.
110. Halterman and coauthors, 2001.
111. Committee on Nutrition, American Academy of Pediatrics, Calcium requirements of infants, children, and adolescents, *Pediatrics* 104 (1999): 1152–1157.
112. H. J. Kalkwarf, J. C. Khoury, and B. P. Lanphear, Milk intake during childhood and adolescence, adult bone density, and osteoporotic fractures in US women, *American Journal of Clinical Nutrition* 77 (2003): 257–265.
113. S. A. Bowman, Beverage choices of young females: Changes and impact on nutrient intakes, *Journal of the American Dietetic Association* 102 (2002): 1234–1239.
114. M. Story, D. Neumark-Sztainer, and S. French, Individual and environmental influences on adolescent eating behaviors, *Journal of the American Dietetic Association* 102 (2002): S40–S51.

115. D. Neumark-Sztainer and coauthors, Family meal patterns: Associations with sociodemographic characteristics and improved dietary intake among adolescents, *Journal of the American Dietetic Association* 103 (2003): 317–322.
116. The National Center on Addiction and Substance Abuse of Columbia University (CASA), **www.casacolumbia.org**.
117. S. A. French, B. H. Lin, and J. F. Guthrie, National trends in soft drink consumption among children and adolescents age 6 to 17 years: Prevalence, amounts, and sources, 1977/1978 to 1994/1998, *Journal of the American Dietetic Association* 103 (2003): 1326–1331; Bowman, 2002.
118. D. S. Ludwig, K. E. Peterson, and S. L. Gortmaker, Relation between consumption of sugar-sweetened drinks and childhood obesity: A prospective, observational analysis, *Lancet* 357 (2001): 505–508; L. Harnack, J. Stang, and M. Story, Soft drink consumption among US children and adolescents: Nutritional consequences, *Journal of the American Dietetic Association* 99 (1999): 436–441.
119. Federal Update, Milk matters, *Journal of the American Dietetic Association* 102 (2002): 469.
120. S. A. French and coauthors, Fast food restaurant use among adolescents: Associations with nutrient intake, food choices, and behavioral and psychosocial variables, *International Journal of Obesity and Related Metabolic Disorders* 25 (2001): 1823–1833.
121. L. Kann and coauthors, Youth risk behavior surveillance—United States, 1999, *Morbidity and Mortality Weekly Report* 49 (2000): entire supplement.
122. Kann and coauthors, 2000.
123. Kann and coauthors, 2000.
124. Centers for Disease Control and Prevention, Trends in cigarette smoking among high school students—United States, 1991–2001, *Morbidity and Mortality Weekly Report* 51 (2002): 409–412.
125. J. S. Hampl and N. M. Betts, Cigarette use during adolescence: Effects on nutritional status, *Nutrition Reviews* 57 (1999): 215–221.
126. L. M. Varner, Impact of combined weight-control and smoking-cessation interventions on body weight: Review of the literature, *Journal of the American Dietetic Association* 99 (1999): 1272–1275.
127. J. Lykkesfeldt and coauthors, Ascorbate is depleted by smoking and repleted by moderate supplementation: A study in male smokers and nonsmokers with matched dietary antioxidant intakes, *American Journal of Clinical Nutrition* 71 (2000): 530–536.
128. A. M. Preston and coauthors, Influence of environmental tobacco smoke on vitamin C status in children, *American Journal of Clinical Nutrition* 77 (2003): 167–172.
129. Centers for Disease Control and Prevention, Youth tobacco surveillance—United States, 2000, *Morbidity and Mortality Weekly Report* (supplement) 50 (2001): 5–10.

ANSWERS

Study Questions (multiple choice)

1. b 2. a 3. c 4. a 5. a 6. d 7. c 8. a 9. c 10. d

HIGHLIGHT

Childhood Obesity and the Early Development of Chronic Diseases

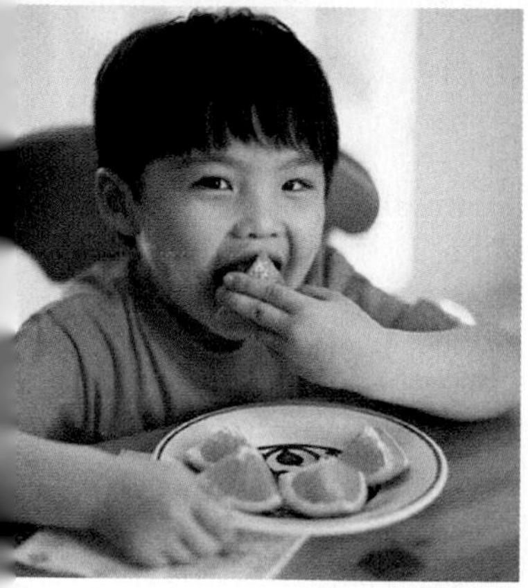

© Ross Whitaker/The Image Bank/Getty Images

When people think of the health problems of children and adolescents, they typically think of measles and acne, not heart disease or diabetes. They think of heart disease as the number one killer of adults in the United States and Canada, but it begins in childhood. Similarly, diabetes (type 2) has historically been called "adult onset," but it is now an epidemic among children and adolescents.[1] Risk factors for these two diseases develop early and are most evident in overweight youngsters.[2]

This highlight focuses on efforts to prevent childhood obesity and the development of heart disease and type 2 diabetes, but the benefits extend to other obesity-related diseases as well. The years of childhood (ages 2 to 18 years) are emphasized here, for the earlier in life health-promoting habits become established, the better they will stick. Later chapters fill in the rest of the story of nutrition's role in reducing chronic disease risk.

Invariably, questions arise as to what extent genetics is involved in disease development. For heart disease and type 2 diabetes, genetics does not appear to play a *determining* role; that is, a person is not simply destined at birth to develop these diseases. Instead, genetics appears to play a *permissive* role—the potential is inherited and then will develop, if given a push by poor health choices such as excessive weight gain, poor diet, sedentary lifestyle, and cigarette smoking.

Many experts agree that preventing or treating obesity in childhood will reduce the rate of chronic diseases in adulthood. Without intervention, most overweight children become overweight adolescents who become overweight adults, and being overweight exacerbates every chronic disease that adults face.[3]

Early Development of Type 2 Diabetes

Type 2 diabetes, a chronic disease closely linked with obesity, has been on the rise among children and adolescents as the prevalence of obesity in U.S. youth has increased in recent years.[4] An estimated 85 percent of the children diagnosed with type 2 diabetes are obese. Most are diagnosed during puberty, but as children become more obese and less active, the trend is shifting to younger children. Type 2 diabetes is most likely to occur in those who are obese and sedentary and have a family history of diabetes.

In type 2 diabetes, the cells become insulin-resistant—that is, insulin can no longer escort glucose from the blood into the cells. The combination of obesity and insulin resistance produces a cluster of symptoms, including high blood cholesterol and high blood pressure, which, in turn, promotes the development of atherosclerosis and the early development of heart disease.[5] Other common problems evident by early adulthood include kidney disease, blindness, and miscarriages. The complications of diabetes, especially when encountered at a young age, can shorten life expectancy.

Prevention and treatment of type 2 diabetes depend on weight management, which can be particularly difficult in a youngster's world of video games and candy bars. The activity and dietary suggestions to help defend against heart disease later in this highlight apply to type 2 diabetes as well.

Early Development of Heart Disease

Most people consider heart disease to be an adult disease because its incidence rises with advancing age, and symptoms rarely appear before age 30. In actuality, the disease process begins much earlier.

Atherosclerosis

Most **cardiovascular disease** involves **atherosclerosis** (see the glossary on p. 548 for these and related terms). Atherosclerosis develops when regions of an artery's walls become progressively thickened with **plaque**—an accumulation of fatty deposits, smooth muscle cells, and fibrous connective tissue. If it progresses, atherosclerosis may eventually block the flow of blood to the heart and cause a heart attack or cut off blood flow to the brain and cause a stroke. Infants are born with healthy, smooth, clear arteries, but within the first decade of life, **fatty streaks** may begin to appear (see Figure H15-1). During adolescence, these fatty streaks may begin to accumulate fibrous connective tissue. By early adulthood, the fibrous plaques may

GLOSSARY

atherosclerosis (ath-er-oh-scler-OH-sis): a type of artery disease characterized by accumulations of lipid-containing material on the inner walls of the arteries (see Chapter 27).
- **athero** = porridge or soft
- **scleros** = hard
- **osis** = condition

cardiovascular disease (CVD): a general term for all diseases of the heart and blood vessels. Atherosclerosis is the main cause of CVD. When the arteries that carry blood to the heart muscle become blocked, the heart suffers damage known as **coronary heart disease (CHD).**
- **cardio** = heart
- **vascular** = blood vessels

fatty streaks: accumulations of cholesterol and other lipids along the walls of the arteries.

plaque (PLACK): an accumulation of fatty deposits, smooth muscle cells, and fibrous connective tissue that develops in the artery walls in atherosclerosis.

begin to calcify and become raised lesions, especially in boys and young men. As the lesions grow more numerous and enlarge, the heart disease rate begins to rise, most dramatically at about age 45 in men and 55 in women. From this point on, arterial damage and blockage progress rapidly, and heart attacks and strokes threaten life. In short, the consequences of atherosclerosis, which become apparent only in adulthood, have their beginnings in the first decades of life.[6]

Atherosclerosis is not inevitable; people can grow old with relatively clear arteries. Early lesions may either progress or regress, depending on several factors, many of which reflect lifestyle behaviors. Smoking, for example, is strongly associated with the prevalence of fatty streaks and raised lesions, even in young adults.

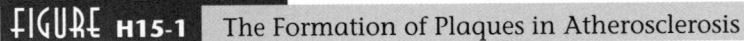

FIGURE H15-1 The Formation of Plaques in Atherosclerosis

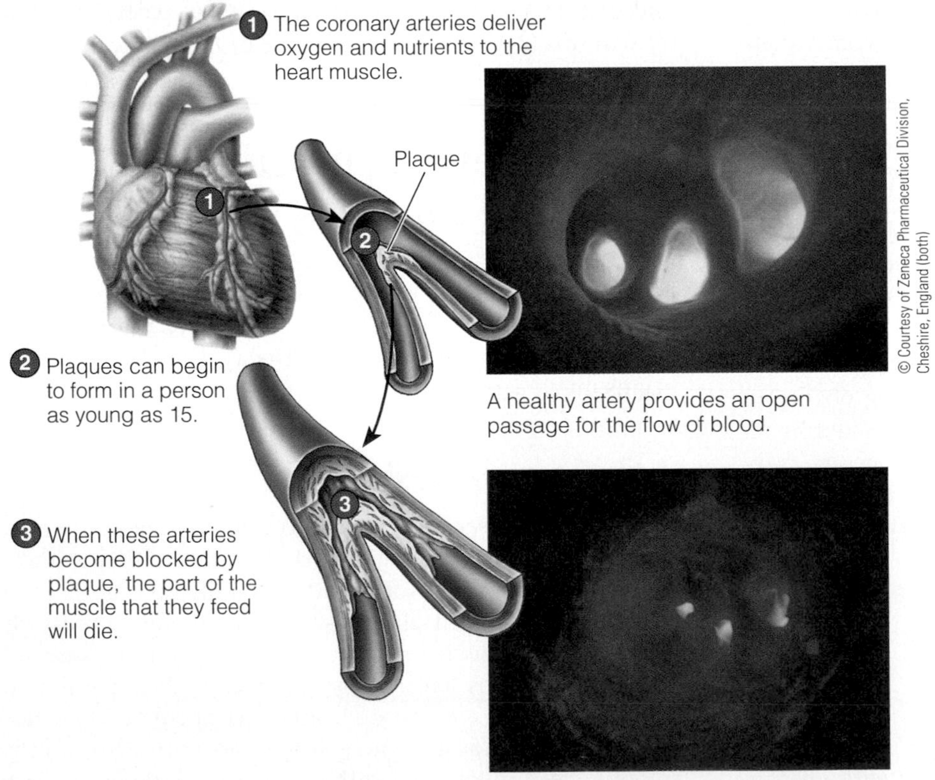
1 The coronary arteries deliver oxygen and nutrients to the heart muscle.
Plaque
2 Plaques can begin to form in a person as young as 15.
3 When these arteries become blocked by plaque, the part of the muscle that they feed will die.

A healthy artery provides an open passage for the flow of blood.

Plaques form along the artery's inner wall, reducing blood flow. Clots can form, aggravating the problem.

Blood Cholesterol

As blood cholesterol rises, atherosclerotic lesion coverage increases. Cholesterol values at birth are similar in all populations; differences emerge in early childhood. Standard values for cholesterol in children and adolescents (ages 2 to 18 years) are listed in Table H15-1.[7]

In general, blood cholesterol tends to rise as dietary saturated fat increases. In recent years, for example, Japanese children have adopted a diet more like that of the United States—higher in saturated fat—and as expected, their blood cholesterol has increased. Although their saturated fat intakes are still lower than intakes typical of U.S. children, their blood cholesterol has responded more dramatically, exceeding the levels seen in U.S. children.[8] Such findings suggest a genetic influence on the cholesterol response to dietary fat.[9]

Blood cholesterol also correlates with childhood obesity, especially central obesity.[10] LDL cholesterol rises with obesity, and HDL declines. These relationships are apparent throughout childhood, and their magnitude increases with age.

Children who are both overweight and have high blood cholesterol are quite likely to have parents who develop heart disease early.[11] For this reason, selective screening is recommended for children and adolescents whose parents (or grandparents) have heart disease; those whose parents have elevated blood cholesterol; and those

TABLE H15-1 Cholesterol Values for Children and Adolescents

Disease Risk	Total Cholesterol (mg/dL)	LDL Cholesterol (mg/dL)
Acceptable	<170	<110
Borderline	170–199	110–129
High	≥200	≥130

NOTE: Adult values appear in Chapter 27.

whose family history is unavailable, especially if other risk factors are evident.[12] Because blood cholesterol in children is a good predictor of adult values, some experts recommend universal screening to identify all children with high blood cholesterol. They note that many children who have high blood cholesterol would be missed under current screening criteria.

Among those children who may have high blood cholesterol, but may not meet screening criteria are those who are overweight. The incidence of high blood cholesterol in obese children with no other criteria is similar to that of nonobese children with family histories of heart disease. In addition to overweight, health care professionals should consider whether children smoke or consume a diet high in saturated fat.[13]

Early—but not advanced—atherosclerotic lesions are reversible, making screening and education a high priority. Both those with family histories of heart disease and those with multiple risk factors need intervention. Children with the highest risks of developing heart disease are sedentary and obese, with high blood pressure and high blood cholesterol.[14] In contrast, children with the lowest risks of heart disease are physically active and of normal weight, with low blood pressure and favorable lipid profiles. Routine pediatric care should identify these known risk factors and provide intervention when needed.

Blood Pressure

Pediatricians routinely monitor blood pressure in children and adolescents. High blood pressure may signal an underlying disease or the early onset of hypertension. Hypertension accelerates the development of atheroscerlosis. Standard values for hypertension in children and adolescents are given in Table H15-2.

Like atherosclerosis and high blood cholesterol, hypertension may develop in the first decades of life, especially among obese children.[15] Children can control their hypertension by participating in regular aerobic activity and by losing weight or maintaining their weight as they grow taller. No evidence

TABLE H15-2 Hypertension Standards for Children and Adolescents

	Systolic over Diastolic Pressure (mm Hg)			
	6 to 9 yr	10 to 12 yr	13 to 15 yr	16 to 18 yr
Mild hypertension	111–121 over 70–77	117–125 over 75–81	124–135 over 77–85	127–141 over 80–91
Moderate hypertension	122–129 over 70–85	126–133 over 82–89	136–143 over 86–91	142–149 over 92–97
Severe hypertension	>129 over >85	>133 over >89	>143 over >91	>149 over >97

NOTE: Adult values appear in Chapter 27.

suggests that restricting sodium lowers blood pressure in children and adolescents.

Physical Activity

Research has also confirmed an association between blood lipids and physical activity in children, similar to that seen in adults. Active children have a better lipid profile than physically inactive children.

Just as blood cholesterol and obesity track over the years, so does a youngster's level of physical activity. Those who are inactive now are likely to still be inactive years later. Similarly, those who are physically active now tend to remain so. Compared with inactive teens, those who are physically active weigh less, smoke less, eat a diet lower in saturated fats, and have better blood lipid profiles. Both obesity and blood cholesterol also correlate with the inactive pastime of watching television. The message is clear: physical activity offers numerous health benefits, and children who are active today are most likely to be active for years to come.

Dietary Recommendations for Children

Regardless of family history, experts agree that all children should eat a variety of foods and maintain desirable weight. There is less agreement, however, as to whether it is wise to restrict fat in children's diets.[16] Still, health experts recommend that children over age two receive at least 25 percent and no more than 35 percent of total energy from fat. Such a diet appears to improve blood lipids without compromising nutrient adequacy, physical growth, or neurological development.[17]

Moderation, Not Deprivation

Healthy children over age two can begin the transition to eating according to recommendations by eating fewer high-fat foods, replacing some high-fat foods with low-fat choices, and selecting more fruits and vegetables. All high-fat foods need not be eliminated, though. Healthy meals can still include moderate amounts of a child's favorite foods, even if they are high-fat selections such as french fries and ice cream. Without such additions, diets may be too low in fat, not to mention unappetizing and boring.

Parents and caregivers play a key role in helping children establish healthy eating habits.[18] Balanced meals need to provide lean meat, poultry, fish, and legumes; fruits and vegetables; whole grains; and low-fat milk products. Such meals can provide enough energy and nutrients to support growth and maintain blood cholesterol within a healthy range.

Pediatricians warn parents to avoid extremes; they caution that while intentions may be good, excessive food restriction may create nutrient deficiencies and impair growth. Furthermore, parental control over eating may instigate battles and foster attitudes about foods that can lead to inappropriate eating behaviors.

Diet First, Drugs Later

Experts agree that children with high blood cholesterol should first be treated with diet. If blood cholesterol remains high in children ten years and older after 6 to 12 months of dietary intervention, then drugs may be necessary to lower blood cholesterol. Drugs can effectively lower blood cholesterol without interfering with adolescent growth or development.[19]

Smoking

Even though the focus of this text is nutrition, another risk factor for heart disease that starts in childhood and carries over into adulthood must also be addressed—cigarette smoking. Each day 3000 children light up for the first time—typically in grade school. Among high school students, almost two out of three have tried smoking, and one in seven smokes regularly.[20] Approximately 80 percent of all adult smokers began smoking before the age of 18.[21]

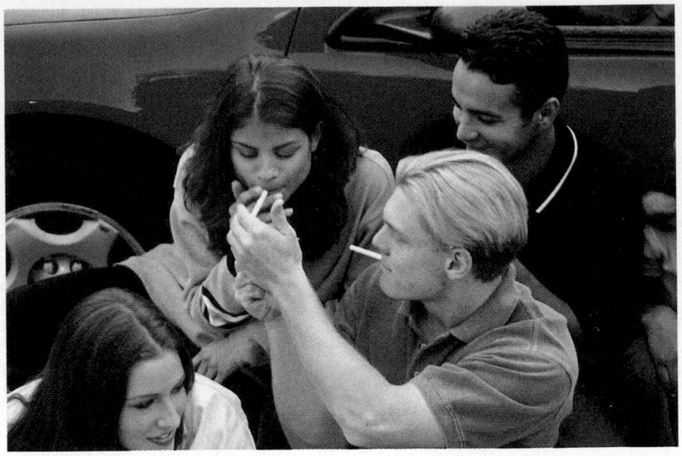

Cigarette smoking is the number one preventable cause of deaths.

Of those teenagers who continue smoking, half will eventually die of smoking-related causes. Efforts to teach children about the dangers of smoking need to be aggressive. Children are not likely to consider the long-term health consequences of tobacco use. They are more likely to be struck by the immediate health consequences, such as shortness of breath when playing sports, or social consequences, such as having bad breath. Whatever the context, the message to all children and teens should be clear: don't start smoking. If you've already started, quit.

In conclusion, *adult* heart disease is a major *pediatric* problem. Without intervention, some 60 million children are destined to suffer its consequences within the next 30 years. Optimal prevention efforts focus on children, especially on those who are overweight.[22]

Just as young children receive vaccinations against infectious diseases, they need screening for, and education about, chronic diseases. Many health education programs have been implemented in schools around the country. These programs are most effective when they include education in the classroom, heart-healthy meals in the lunchroom, fitness activities on the playground, and parental involvement at home.

NUTRITION ON THE NET

Access these websites for further study of topics covered in this highlight.

- Find updates and quick links to these and other nutrition-related sites at our website: **www.wadsworth.com/nutrition**
- Get weight-loss tips for children and adolescents: **www.shapedown.com**
- Learn about nondietary approaches to weight loss from HUGS International: **www.hugs.com**
- Visit the Nemours Foundation: **www.kidshealth.org**
- Find information on diabetes in children at the American Diabetes Association and Juvenile Diabetes Research Foundation: **www.diabetes.org** and **www.jdrf.org**

REFERENCES

1. T. Aye and L. L. Levitsky, Type 2 diabetes: An epidemic disease in childhood, *Current Opinion in Pediatrics* 15 (2003): 411–415.
2. G. D. Ball and L. J. McCargar, Childhood obesity in Canada: A review of prevalence estimates and risk factors for cardiovascular diseases and type 2 diabetes, *Canadian Journal of Applied Physiology* 28 (2003): 117–140.
3. A. Must, Does overweight in childhood have an impact on adult health? *Nutrition Reviews* 61 (2003): 139–142; D. S. Freedman, Clustering of coronary heart disease risk factors among obese children, *Journal of Pediatric Endocrinology and Metabolism* 15 (2002): 1099–1108.
4. D. S. Ludwig and C. B. Ebbeling, Type 2 diabetes mellitus in children: Primary care and public health considerations, *Journal of the American Medical Association* 286 (2001): 1427–1430; American Diabetes Association, Type 2 diabetes in children and adolescents, *Pediatrics* 105 (2000): 671–680.
5. R. Kohen-Avramoglu, A. Theriault, and K. Adeli, Emergence of the metabolic syndrome in childhood: An epidemiological overview and mechanistic link to dyslipidemia, *Clinical Biochemistry* 36 (2003): 413–420.
6. S. Li and coauthors, Childhood cardiovascular risk factors and carotid vascular changes in adulthood: The Bogalusa Heart Study, *Journal of the American Medical Association* 290 (2003): 2271–2276; K. B. Keller and L. Lemberg, Obesity and the metabolic syndrome, *American Journal of Clinical Care* 12 (2003): 167–170; H. C. McGill Jr. and coauthors, Origin of atherosclerosis in childhood and adolescence, *American Journal of Clinical Nutrition* 72 (2000): 1307S–1315S.
7. Committee on Nutrition, American Academy of Pediatrics, Cholesterol in childhood, *Pediatrics* 101 (1998): 141–147.
8. S. C. Couch and coauthors, Rapid westernization of children's blood cholesterol in 3 countries: Evidence for nutrient-gene interactions? *American Journal of Clinical Nutrition* 72 (2000): 1266S–1274S.
9. S. Q. Ye and P. O. Kwiterovich Jr., Influence of genetic polymorphisms on responsiveness to dietary fat and cholesterol, *American Journal of Clinical Nutrition* 72 (2000): 1275S–1284S.
10. O. Fiedland and coauthors, Obesity and lipid profiles in children and adolescents, *Journal of Pediatric Endocrinology and Metabolism* 15 (2002): 1011–1016; T. Dwyer and coauthors, Syndrome X in 8-y-old Australian children: Stronger associations with current body fatness than with infant size or growth, *International Journal of Obesity and Related Metabolic Disorders* 26 (2002): 1301–1309.
11. B. Glowinska, M. Urban, and A. Koput, Cardiovascular risk factors in children with obesity, hypertension and diabetes: Lipoprotein (a) levels and body mass index correlate with family history of cardiovascular disease, *European Journal of Pediatrics* 161 (2002): 511–518.
12. A. Wiegman and coauthors, Family history and cardiovascular risk in familial hypercholesterolemia: Data in more than 1000 children, *Circulation* 107 (2003): 1473–1478; Committee on Nutrition, American Academy of Pediatrics, 1998.
13. Committee on Nutrition, American Academy of Pediatrics, 1998.
14. V. N. Muratova and coauthors, The relation of obesity to cardiovascular risk factors among children: The CARDIAC project, *West Virginia Medical Journal* 98 (2002): 263–267.
15. Dwyer and coauthors, 2002.
16. R. E. Olson, Is it wise to restrict fat in the diets of children? *Journal of the American Dietetic Association* 100 (2000): 28–32; E. Satter, A moderate view on fat restriction, *Journal of the American Dietetic Association* 100 (2000): 32–36; L. A. Lytle, In defense of a low-fat diet for healthy children, *Journal of the American Dietetic Association* 100 (2000): 39–41.
17. E. Obarzanek and coauthors, Long-term safety and efficacy of a cholesterol-lowering diet in children with elevated low-density lipoprotein cholesterol: Seven-year results of the Dietary Intervention Study in Children (DISC), *Pediatrics* 107 (2001): 256–264; L. Rask-Nissilä and coauthors, Neurological development of 5-year-old children receiving a low-saturated fat, low-cholesterol diet since infancy: A randomized controlled study, *Journal of the American Medical Association* 284 (2000): 993–1000; R. M. Lauer and coauthors, Efficacy and safety of lowering dietary intake of total fat, saturated fat, and cholesterol in children with elevated LDL cholesterol: The Dietary Intervention Study in Children, *American Journal of Clinical Nutrition* 72 (2000): 1332S–1342S; N. F. Butte, Fat intake of children in relation to energy requirements, *American Journal of Clinical Nutrition* 72 (2000): 1246S–1252S.
18. T. A. Nicklas and coauthors, Family and child-care provider influences on preschool children's fruit, juice, and vegetable consumption, *Nutrition Reviews* 59 (2001): 224–235.
19. S. de Jongh and coauthors, Efficacy and safety of statin therapy in children with familial hypercholesterolemia: A randomized, double-blind, placebo-controlled trial with simvastatin, *Circulation* 106 (2002): 2231–2237.
20. Trends in cigarette smoking among high school students—United States, 1991–2001, *Morbidity and Mortality Weekly Report* 51 (2002): 409–412.
21. Youth tobacco surveillance—United States, 2000, *Morbidity and Mortality Weekly Report* 50 (2001): entire supplement.
22. Committee on Nutrition, American Academy of Pediatrics, Prevention of pediatric overweight and obesity, *Pediatrics* 112 (2003): 424–430.

Chapter 16

Life Cycle Nutrition: Adulthood and the Later Years

Chapter Outline

Nutrition and Longevity: *Observation of Older Adults • Manipulation of Diet*

The Aging Process: *Physiological Changes • Other Changes*

Energy and Nutrient Needs of Older Adults: *Water • Energy and Energy Nutrients • Vitamins and Minerals • Nutrient Supplements*

Nutrition-Related Concerns of Older Adults: *Cataracts and Macular Degeneration • Arthritis • The Aging Brain*

Food Choices and Eating Habits of Older Adults: *Food Assistance Programs • Meals for Singles*

Highlight: *Hunger and Community Nutrition*

Available Online

http://nutrition.wadsworth.com/uncn7

Nutrition Animation: *Nutrient Needs in Later Years*

Student Practice Test

Glossary Terms

Nutrition on the Net

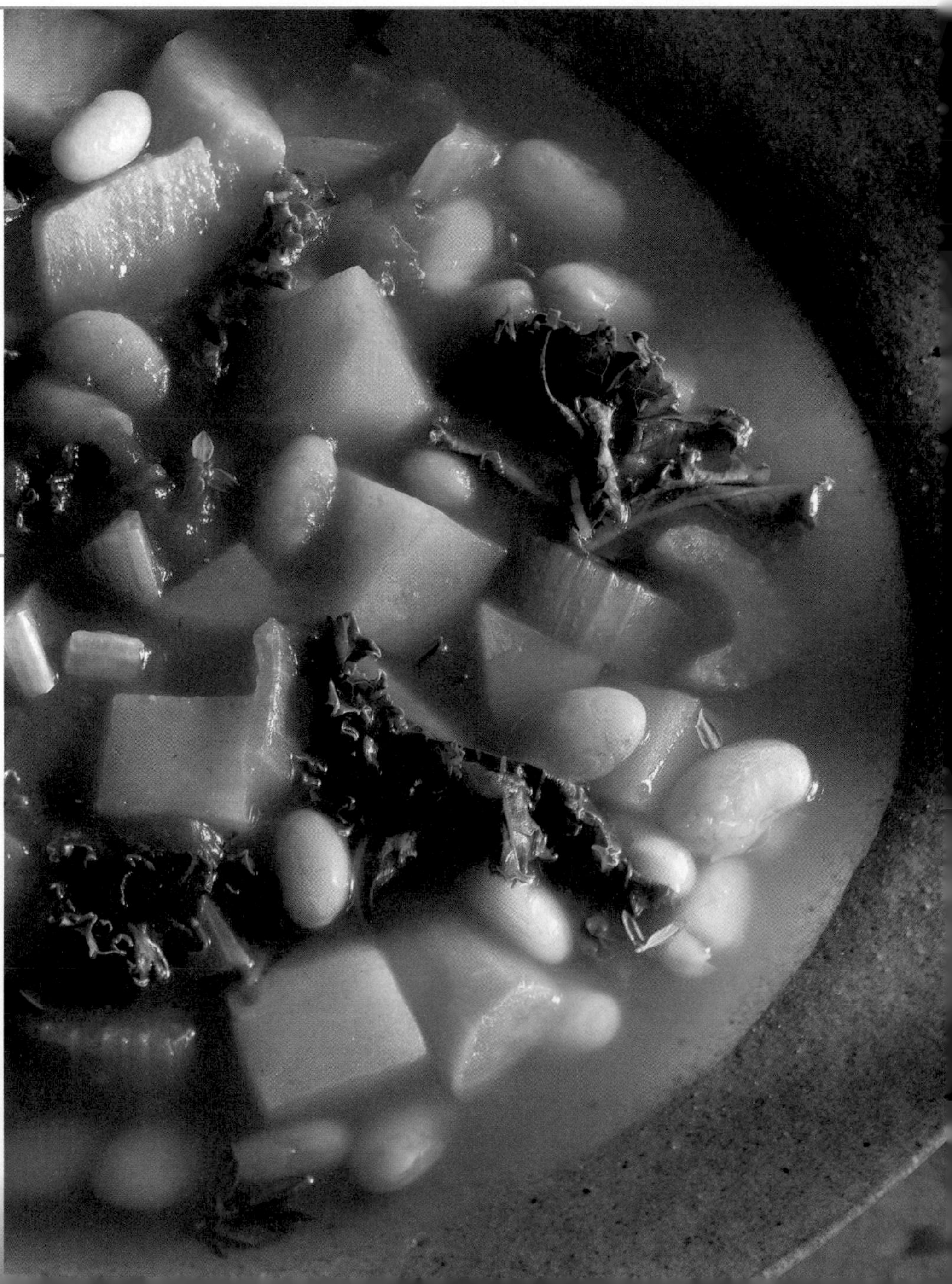

© Judd Pilossof/FoodPix/Getty Images

Nutrition in Your Life

Take a moment to envision yourself 20, 40, or even 60 years from now. Are you physically fit and healthy? Can you see yourself walking on the beach with friends or tossing a ball with children? Are you able to climb stairs and carry your own groceries? Importantly, are you enjoying life? If you're lucky, you will grow old with good health, but much of that depends on your actions today—and every day from now until then. Making nutritious foods and physical activities a priority in your life can help bring rewards of continued health and enjoyment in later life.

Wise food choices, made throughout adulthood, can support a person's ability to meet physical, emotional, and mental challenges and to enjoy freedom from disease. Two goals motivate adults to pay attention to their diets: promoting health and slowing aging. Much of this text has focused on nutrition to support health, and later chapters feature prevention and treatment of chronic diseases such as cancer and heart disease; this chapter focuses on aging and the nutrition needs of older adults.

The U.S. population is growing older. The majority is now middle-aged, and the ratio of old people to young is increasing, as Figure 16-1 (on p. 554) shows. In 1900, only 1 out of 25 people was 65 or older. In 2000, one out of eight had reached age 65. Projections for 2030 are one out of five.

Our society uses the arbitrary age of 65 years to define the transition point between middle age and old age, but growing "old" happens day by day, with changes occurring gradually over time. Since 1950 the population of those over 65 has almost tripled. Remarkably, the fastest-growing age group has been people over 85 years; since 1950 their numbers have increased sevenfold. The number of people in the United States age 100 or older doubled in the last decade. Similar trends are occurring in populations worldwide.[1]

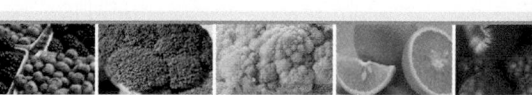

FIGURE 16-1 The Aging of the U.S. Population

In general the percentage of older people in the population has increased over the decades while the percentage of younger people has decreased.

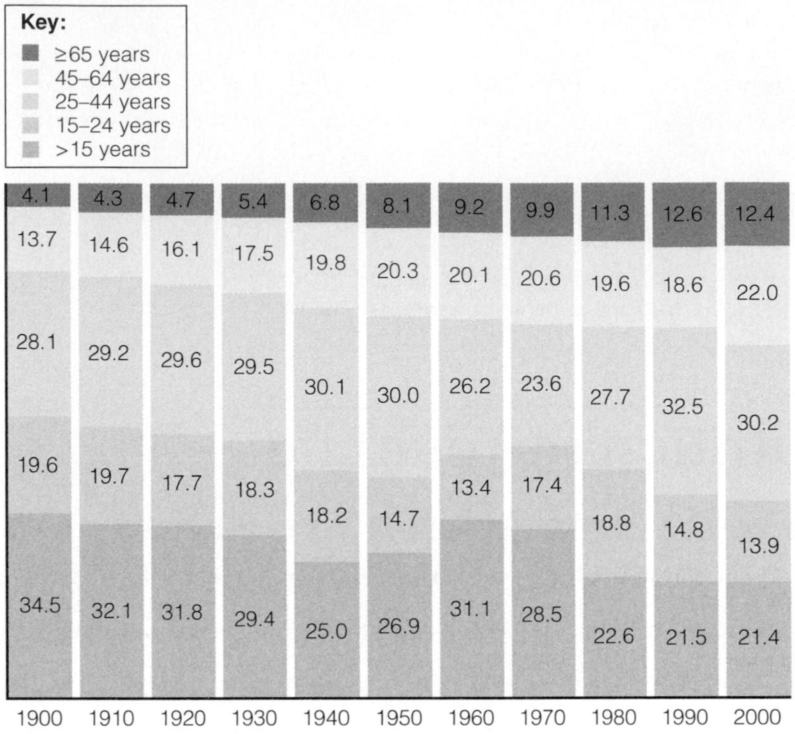
Key:
≥65 years
45–64 years
25–44 years
15–24 years
>15 years
4.1 13.7 28.1 19.6 34.5
4.3 14.6 29.2 19.7 32.1
4.7 16.1 29.6 17.7 31.8
5.4 17.5 29.5 18.3 29.4
6.8 19.8 30.1 18.2 25.0
8.1 20.3 30.0 14.7 26.9
9.2 20.1 26.2 13.4 31.1
9.9 20.6 23.6 17.4 28.5
11.3 19.6 27.7 18.8 22.6
12.6 18.6 32.5 14.8 21.5
12.4 22.0 30.2 13.9 21.4
1900 1910 1920 1930 1940 1950 1960 1970 1980 1990 2000

SOURCE: U.S. Census Bureau, Decennial census of population, 1900 to 2000.

Life expectancy in the United States for white women is 80 years and for black women, 75 years; for white men, it is 75 years and for black men, 68 years—all record highs and much higher than the average life expectancy of 47 years in 1900.[2] Women who live to 80 can expect to survive an additional nine years, on average; men, an additional seven. Advances in medical science—antibiotics and other treatments—are largely responsible for almost doubling the life expectancy in the twentieth century. Improved nutrition and an abundant supply of food have also contributed to lengthening life expectancy. The **life span** has not lengthened as dramatically; human **longevity** appears to have an upper limit. The potential human life span is currently 130 years. With recent advances in medical technology and genetic knowledge, however, researchers may one day be able to extend the life span even further by slowing, or perhaps preventing, aging and its accompanying diseases.

Nutrition and Longevity

Research in the field of aging is active—and difficult. Researchers are challenged by the diversity of older adults. When older adults experience health problems, it is hard to know whether to attribute these problems to genetics, aging, or other environmental factors such as nutrition. The idea that nutrition can influence the aging process is particularly appealing, because people can control and change their eating habits. The questions being asked include:

- To what extent is aging inevitable, and can it be slowed through changes in lifestyle and environment?

life expectancy: the average number of years lived by people in a given society.

life span: the maximum number of years of life attainable by a member of a species.

longevity: long duration of life.

- What role does nutrition play in the aging process, and what role can it play in slowing aging?

With respect to the first question, it seems that aging is an inevitable, natural process, programmed into the genes at conception. People can, however, slow the process within genetic limits by adopting healthy lifestyle habits such as eating nutritious food and engaging in physical activity. In fact, an estimated 70 to 80 percent of the average person's life expectancy may depend on individual health-related behaviors; genes determine the remaining 20 to 30 percent.[3]

With respect to the second question, good nutrition helps to maintain a healthy body and can therefore ease the aging process in many significant ways. Clearly, nutrition can improve the **quality of life** in the later years.

Observation of Older Adults

The strategies adults use to meet the two goals mentioned at the start of this chapter—promoting health and slowing aging—are actually very much the same. What to eat, when to sleep, how physically active to be, and other lifestyle choices greatly influence both physical health and the aging process.

Healthy Habits A person's **physiological age** reflects his or her health status and may or may not reflect the person's **chronological age.** Quite simply, some people seem younger, and others older, than their years. Six lifestyle behaviors seem to have the greatest influence on people's health and therefore on their physiological age:

- Sleeping regularly and adequately.
- Eating well-balanced meals, including breakfast, regularly.
- Engaging in physical activity regularly.
- Not smoking.
- Not using alcohol, or using it in moderation.
- Maintaining a healthy body weight.

Over the years, the effects of these lifestyle choices accumulate—that is, people who follow most of these practices live longer and have fewer disabilities as they age.[4] They are in better health, even when older in chronological age, than people who do not adopt these behaviors. Even though people cannot change their birth dates, they may be able to add years to, and enhance the quality of, their lives. Physical activity seems to be most influential in preventing or slowing the many changes that define a stereotypical "old" person. After all, many of the physical limitations that accompany aging occur because people become inactive, not because they become older.

Physical Activity The many remarkable benefits of regular physical activity■ are not limited to the young. Compared with those who are inactive, older adults who are active weigh less; have greater flexibility, more endurance, better balance, and better health; and live longer.[5] They reap additional benefits from various activities as well: aerobic activities improve cardiorespiratory endurance, blood pressure, and blood lipid concentrations; moderate endurance activities improve the quality of sleep; and strength training improves posture and mobility. In fact, regular physical activity is the most powerful predictor of a person's mobility in the later years. Physical activity also increases blood flow to the brain, thereby preserving mental ability, alleviating depression, and supporting independence.[6]

Muscle mass and muscle strength tend to decline with aging, making older people vulnerable to falls and immobility. Falls are a major cause of fear, injury, disability, and even death among older adults. Many lose their independence as a result of falls. Regular physical activity tones, firms, and strengthens muscles, helping to improve confidence, reduce the risk of falling, and lessen the risk of injury should a fall occur.

■ 2005 *Dietary Guidelines:*
- Older adults should participate in regular physical activity to reduce the functional declines associated with aging and to achieve the other benefits of physical activity identified for all adults.

quality of life: a person's perceived physical and mental well-being.

physiological age: a person's age as estimated from her or his body's health and probable life expectancy.

chronological age: a person's age in years from his or her date of birth.

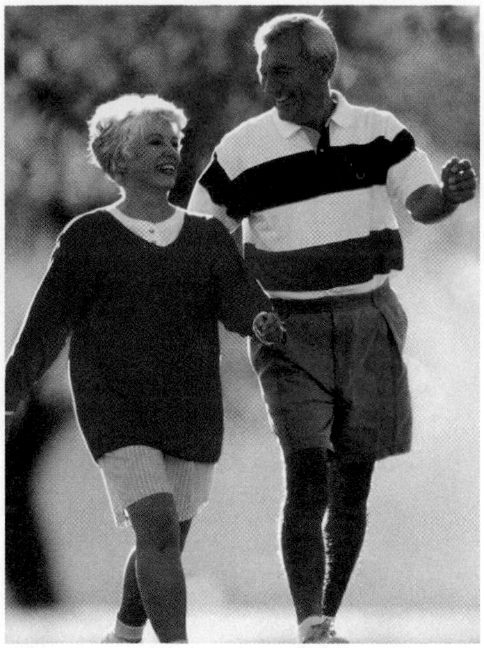
© R. W. Jones/Corbis

Regular physical activity promotes a healthy, independent lifestyle.

Even without a fall, older adults may become so weak that they can no longer perform life's daily tasks, such as climbing stairs, carrying packages, and opening jars. By improving muscle strength, which allows a person to perform these tasks, strength training helps to maintain independence. Even in frail, elderly people over 85 years of age, strength training not only improves balance, muscle strength, and mobility, but also increases energy expenditure and energy intake, thereby enhancing nutrient intakes. This finding highlights another reason to be physically active: a person spending energy can afford to eat more food and thus receives more nutrients as a result. People who are committed to an ongoing fitness program can benefit from higher energy and nutrient intakes and still maintain their body weights.

Ideally, physical activity should be part of each day's schedule and should be intense enough to prevent muscle atrophy and to speed up the heartbeat and respiration rate. Although aging reduces both speed and endurance to some degree, older adults can still train and achieve exceptional performances. Healthy older adults who have not been active can ease into a suitable routine. They can start by walking short distances until they are walking at least 10 minutes continuously, and then gradually increase their distance to a 30- to 45-minute workout at least five days a week. Table 16-1 provides exercise guidelines for seniors; people with medical conditions should check with a physician before beginning an exercise routine, as should sedentary men over 40 and women over 50 who want to participate in a vigorous program.

Manipulation of Diet

In their efforts to understand longevity, researchers have not only observed people, but have also manipulated influencing factors, such as diet, in animals. This research has given rise to some interesting and suggestive findings.

Energy Restriction in Animals Animals live longer and have fewer age-related diseases when their energy intakes are restricted.[7] These life-prolonging benefits become evident when the diet provides enough food to prevent malnutrition and an energy intake of about 70 percent of normal. Exactly how energy restriction

TABLE 16-1 Exercise Guidelines for Older Adults

	Endurance	Strength	Balance	Flexibility
Examples	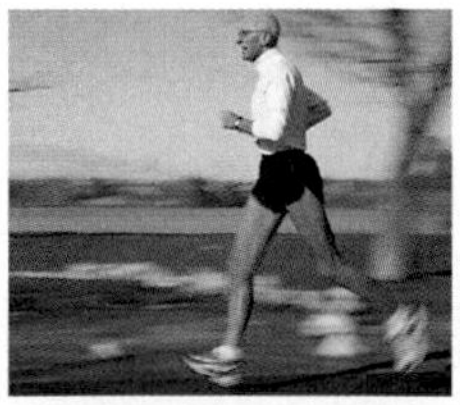 © Geoff Manasse/Photodisc/PictureQuest	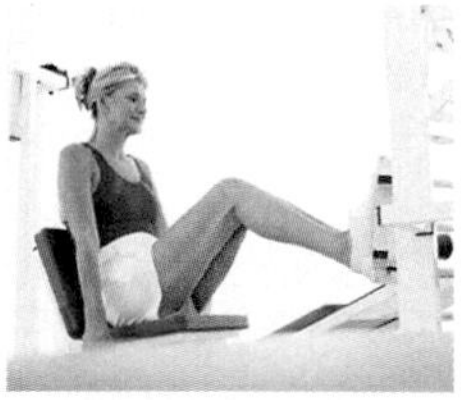 © IT Stock Free/PictureQuest	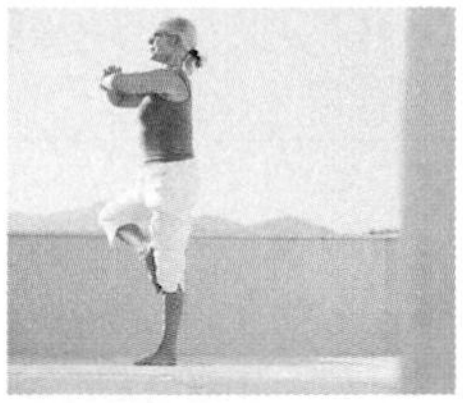 © IT Stock Free/PictureQuest	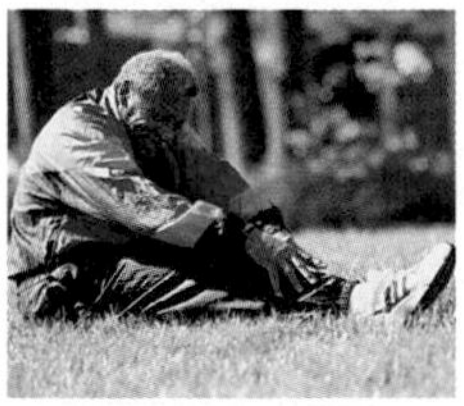 © Ron Chapple/Thinkstock/PictureQuest
Start easy	Be active 5 minutes on most or all days.	Using 0- to 2-pound weights, do 1 set of 8 repetitions twice a week.	Hold onto table or chair with one hand, then with one finger.	Hold stretch 10 seconds; do each stretch 3 times.
Progress gradually to goal	Be active 30 minutes (minimum) on most or all days.	Increase weight as able; do 2 sets of 8–15 repetitions twice a week.	Do not hold onto table or chair; then close eyes.	Hold stretch 30 seconds; do each stretch 5 times.
Cautions and comments	Stop if you are breathing so hard you can't talk or if you feel dizziness or chest pain.	Breathe out as you contract and in as you relax (do not hold breath); use smooth, steady movements.	Incorporate balance techniques with strength exercises as you progress.	Stretch after strength and endurance exercises for 20 minutes, 3 times a week; use slow, steady movements; bend joints slightly.

SOURCE: *Exercise: A Guide from the National Institute on Aging,* **www.nia.nih.gov**, accessed May 2003.

prolongs life remains largely unexplained, although gene activity appears to play a key role.[8] The genetic activity of old mice differs from that of young mice, with some genes becoming more active with age and others less active. With an energy-restricted diet, many of the genetic activities of older mice revert to those of younger mice. These "slow-aging" genetic changes are apparent in as little as one month on a restricted diet.[9]

The consequences of energy restriction include a delay in the onset, or prevention, of diseases such as atherosclerosis; prolonged growth and development; and improved blood glucose, insulin sensitivity, and blood lipids.[10] In addition, energy metabolism slows and body temperature drops—indications of a reduced rate of oxygen consumption.[11] As Highlight 11 explained, the use of oxygen during energy metabolism produces free radicals, which have been implicated in the aging process. Restricting energy intake not only produces fewer free radicals, but also increases antioxidant activity and enhances DNA repair. Reducing oxidative stress may at least partially explain how restricting energy intake lengthens life expectancy.[12]

Interestingly, longevity appears to depend on restricting energy intake and not on the amount of body fat. Genetically obese rats live longer when given a restricted diet even though their body fat is similar to that of other rats allowed to eat freely.

Energy Restriction in Human Beings Research on a variety of animals■ confirms the relationship between energy restriction and longevity. Applying the results of animal studies to human beings is problematic, however, and conducting studies on human beings raises numerous questions—beginning with how to define energy restriction.[13] Does it mean eating less or just weighing less? Is it less than you want or less than the average? Does eating less have to result in weight loss? Does it matter whether weight loss results from more exercise or from less food? Or whether weight loss is intentional or unintentional? Answers await research.

■ kCalorie-restricted research has been conducted on various species, including mice, rats, rhesus monkeys, cynomolgus monkeys, spiders, and fish.

Extreme starvation to extend life, like any extreme, is rarely, if ever, worth the price. Moderation, on the other hand, may be valuable. Many of the physiological responses to energy restriction seen in animals also occur in people whose intakes are *moderately* restricted. When people cut back on their usual energy intake by 10 to 20 percent,■ body weight, body fat, and blood pressure drop, and blood lipids and insulin response improve—favorable changes for preventing chronic diseases. The reduction in oxidative damage that occurs with energy restriction in animals also occurs in people whose diets include antioxidant nutrients and phytochemicals. As Highlights 11 and 13 explain, diets, such as the Mediterranean diet, that include an abundance of fruits, vegetables, olive oil, and red wine—with their array of antioxidants and phytochemicals—support good health and long life.[14]

■ For perspective, a person with a usual energy intake of 2000 kcalores might cut back to 1600 to 1800 kcalories.

IN SUMMARY Life expectancy in the United States increased dramatically in the twentieth century. Factors that enhance longevity include limited or no alcohol use, regular balanced meals, weight control, adequate sleep, abstinence from smoking, and regular physical activity. Energy restriction in animals seems to lengthen their lives. Whether such dietary intervention in human beings is beneficial remains unknown. At the very least, nutrition—especially when combined with regular physical activity—can influence aging and longevity in human beings by supporting good health and preventing disease.

The Aging Process

As people get older, each person becomes less and less like anyone else. The older people are, the more time has elapsed for such factors as nutrition, genetics, physical activity, and everyday **stress** to influence physical and psychological aging.

stress: any threat to a person's well-being; a demand placed on the body to adapt.

Both physical **stressors** (such as alcohol abuse, other drug abuse, smoking, pain, and illness) and psychological stressors (such as exams, divorce, moving, and the death of a loved one) elicit the body's **stress response.** The body responds to such stressors with an elaborate series of physiological steps, as the nervous and hormonal systems bring about defensive readiness in every body part. These effects favor physical action—the classic fight-or-flight response. Stress that is prolonged or severe can drain the body of its reserves and leave it weakened, aged, and vulnerable to illness, especially if physical action is not taken. As people age, they lose their ability to adapt to both external and internal disturbances. When disease strikes, the reduced ability to adapt makes the aging individual more vulnerable to death than a younger person.

Highlight 11 described the oxidative stresses that occur when free radicals exceed the body's ability to defend itself. Increased free-radical activity and decreased antioxidant protection are common, but not inevitable, features of aging—and antioxidants seem to help slow the aging process.[15] Healthy people over 100 years old who had higher intakes of vegetables showed less evidence of oxidative stress than people 70 to 99 years old. Such findings seem to suggest that the fountain of youth may actually be a cornucopia of fruits and vegetables rich in antioxidants. (Return to Highlight 11 for more details on the antioxidant action of fruits and vegetables in defending against oxidative stress.)

Physiological Changes

As aging progresses, inevitable changes in each of the body's organs contribute to the body's declining function. These physiological changes influence nutrition status, just as growth and development do in the earlier stages of the life cycle.

Body Weight Over half of the adults in the United States are now considered overweight or obese. Chapter 8 presented the many health problems that accompany obesity and the BMI guidelines for a healthy body weight (18.5 to 24.9). These guidelines apply to all adults, regardless of age, but they may be too restrictive for older adults. The importance of body weight in defending against chronic diseases differs for older adults. Being moderately overweight may not be harmful. For adults over 65, health risks do not become apparent until BMI reaches at least 27—and the relationship tends to diminish with age until it disappears by age 75.[16] Not all older adults are overweight, of course. In fact, the prevalence of overweight decreases with increasing age after age 55.[17]

For older adults, a low body weight may be more detrimental than a high one. Low body weight often reflects malnutrition and the trauma associated with a fall. Many older adults experience unintentional weight loss, in large part because of an inadequate food intake.[18] Without adequate nutrient reserves, an underweight person may be unprepared to fight against diseases. Even a slight weight loss (5 percent) increases the likelihood of disease and premature death, making every meal a life-saving event.[19]

Body Composition In general, older people tend to lose bone and muscle and gain body fat. Many of these changes occur because some hormones that regulate appetite and metabolism become less active with age, while others become more active.*

Loss of muscle, known as **sarcopenia,** can be significant in the later years, and its consequences can be quite dramatic (see Figure 16-2).[20] As muscles diminish and weaken, people lose their ability to move and maintain balance, making falls likely. The limitations that accompany the loss of muscle mass and strength play a key role in the diminishing health that often accompanies aging. Optimal nutri-

*Examples of hormones that change with age include growth hormone and androgens, which decline with advancing age, thus contributing to the decrease in lean body mass, and prolactin, which increases with age, helping to maintain body fat. Insulin sensitivity also diminishes as people grow older, most likely because of increases in body fat and decreases in physical activity.

stressors: environmental elements, physical or psychological, that cause stress.

stress response: the body's response to stress, mediated by both nerves and hormones.

sarcopenia (SAR-koh-PEE-nee-ah): loss of skeletal muscle mass, strength, and quality.
- **sarco** = flesh
- **penia** = loss or lack

FIGURE 16-2 Sarcopenia

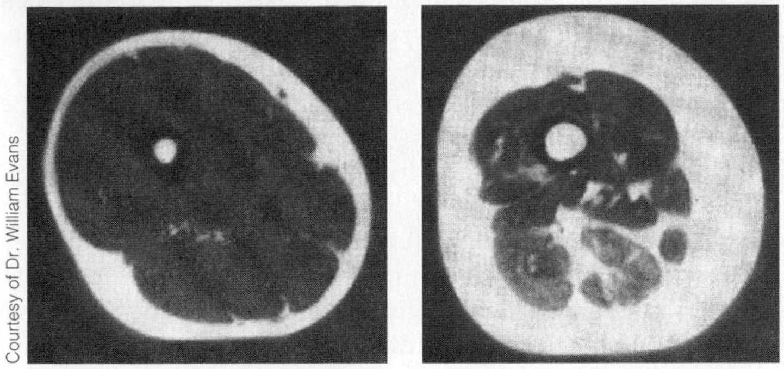
Courtesy of Dr. William Evans

These cross sections of two women's thighs may appear to be about the same size from the outside, but the 20-year-old woman's thigh (left) is dense with muscle tissue. The 64-year-old woman's thigh (right) has lost muscle and gained fat, changes that may be largely preventable with strength-building physical activities.

tion and regular physical activity can help maintain muscle mass and strength and minimize the changes in body composition associated with aging.[21]

Immune System Changes in the immune system also bring declining function with age. In addition, the immune system is compromised by nutrient deficiencies. Thus the combination of old age and malnutrition makes older people vulnerable to infectious diseases.[22] Adding insult to injury, antibiotics often are not effective against infections in people with compromised immune systems. Consequently, infectious diseases are a major cause of death in older adults. Older adults may improve their immune system responses by exercising regularly.[23]

GI Tract In the GI tract, the intestinal wall loses strength and elasticity with age, and GI hormone secretions change.[24] All of these actions slow motility. Constipation is much more common in the elderly than in the young.

Atrophic gastritis, a condition that affects almost one-third of those over 60, is characterized■ by an inflamed stomach, bacterial overgrowth, and a lack of hydrochloric acid and intrinsic factor. All of these can impair the digestion and absorption of nutrients, most notably, vitamin B_{12}, but also biotin, folate, calcium, iron, and zinc.

Difficulty in swallowing, medically known as **dysphagia,** occurs in all age groups, but especially in the elderly. Being unable to swallow a mouthful of food can be scary, painful, and dangerous. Even swallowing liquids can be a problem for some people. Consequently, the person may eat less food and drink fewer beverages, resulting in weight loss, malnutrition, and dehydration. Dietary intervention for dysphagia is highly individualized based on the person's abilities and tolerances. The diet typically provides moist, soft-textured, tender-cooked, or pureed foods and thickened liquids.

Tooth Loss Regular dental care over a lifetime protects against tooth loss and gum disease, which are common in old age. These conditions make chewing difficult or painful. Dentures, even when they fit properly, are less effective than natural teeth, and inefficient chewing can cause choking. People with tooth loss,■ gum disease, and ill-fitting dentures tend to limit their food selections to soft foods. If foods such as corn on the cob, apples, and hard rolls are replaced by creamed corn, applesauce, and rice, then nutrition status may not be greatly affected, but when food groups are eliminated and variety is limited, poor nutrition follows. People without teeth typically eat fewer fruits and vegetables and have less variety in their diets.[25] Consequently, they have low intakes of fiber and vitamins. To determine whether a visit to the dentist is needed, an older adult can check the conditions listed in the margin.■

■ Consequences of atrophic gastritis:
- Inflamed stomach.
- Increased bacterial growth.
- Reduced hydrochloric acid.
- Reduced intrinsic factor.
- Increased risk of nutrient deficiencies, notably of vitamin B_{12}.

■ The medical term for lack of teeth is **edentulous** (ee-DENT-you-lus).
- **e** = without
- **dens** = teeth

■ Conditions requiring dental care:
Dry mouth.
Eating difficulty.
No dental care within 2 years.
Tooth or mouth pain.
Altered food selections.
Lesions, sores, or lumps in mouth.

dysphagia (dis-FAY-gee-ah): difficulty in swallowing.

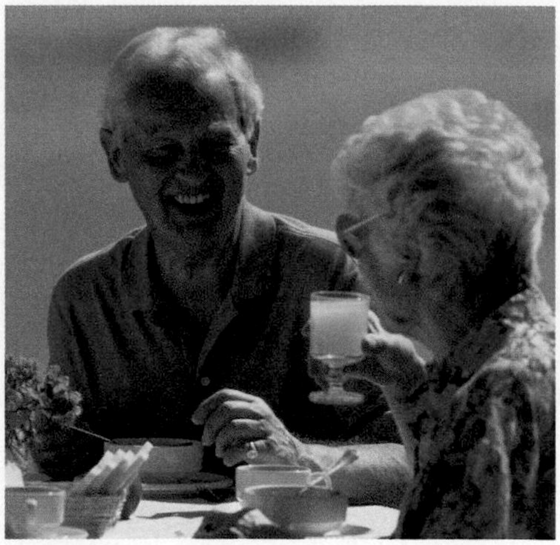

© Bob Thomas/Stone/Getty Images

Shared meals can brighten the day and enhance the appetite.

Sensory Losses and Other Physical Problems Sensory losses and other physical problems can also interfere with an older person's ability to obtain adequate nourishment. Failing eyesight, for example, can make driving to the grocery store impossible and shopping for food a frustrating experience. It may become so difficult to read food labels and count money that the person doesn't buy needed foods. Carrying bags of groceries may be an unmanageable task. Similarly, a person with limited mobility may find cooking and cleaning up too hard to do. Not too surprisingly, the prevalence of undernutrition is high among those who are homebound.

Sensory losses can also interfere with a person's ability or willingness to eat. Taste and smell sensitivities tend to diminish with age and may make eating less enjoyable. If a person eats less, then weight loss and nutrient deficiencies may follow. Loss of vision and hearing may contribute to social isolation, and eating alone may lead to poor intake.

Other Changes

In addition to the physiological changes that accompany aging, adults are changing in many other ways that influence their nutrition status.[26] Psychological, economic, and social factors play big roles in a person's ability and willingness to eat.

Psychological Changes Although not an inevitable component of aging, depression is common among older adults.[27] Depressed people, even those without disabilities, lose their ability to perform simple physical tasks. They frequently lose their appetite and the motivation to cook or even to eat. An overwhelming sense of grief and sadness at the death of a spouse, friend, or family member may leave a person, especially an elderly person, feeling powerless to overcome depression. When a person is suffering the heartache and loneliness of bereavement, cooking meals may not seem worthwhile. The support and companionship of family and friends, especially at mealtimes, can help overcome depression and enhance appetite.

Economic Changes Overall, older adults today have higher incomes than their cohorts of previous generations.[28] Still, poverty is a major problem for about 20 percent of the people over age 65. Factors such as living arrangements and income make significant differences in the food choices, eating habits, and nutrition status of older adults, especially those over age 80. People of low socioeconomic means are likely to have inadequate food and nutrient intakes. Only about one-third of the needy elderly receive assistance from federal programs.

Social Changes Malnutrition among older adults is most common in hospitals and nursing homes.[29] In the community, malnutrition is most likely to occur among those living alone, especially men; those with the least education; those living in federally funded housing (an indicator of low income); and those who have recently experienced a change in lifestyle. Adults who live alone do not necessarily make poor food choices, but they often consume too little food: loneliness is directly related to nutritional inadequacies, especially of energy intake.

IN SUMMARY Many changes that accompany aging can impair nutrition status. Among physiological changes, hormone activity alters body composition, immune system changes raise the risk of infections, atrophic gastritis interferes with digestion and absorption, and tooth loss limits food choices. Psychological changes such as depression, economic changes such as loss of income, and social changes such as loneliness contribute to poor food intake.

Energy and Nutrient Needs of Older Adults

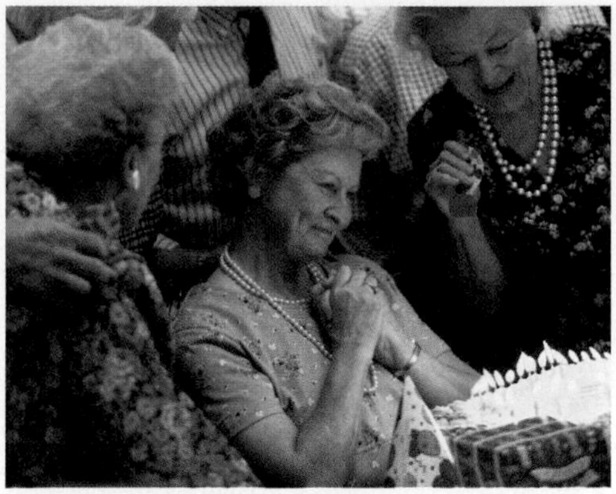
© Kwame Zikomo/Super Stock

Growing old can be enjoyable for people who take care of their health and live each day fully.

Knowledge about the nutrient needs and nutrition status of older adults has grown considerably in recent years. The Dietary Reference Intakes (DRI) cluster people over 50 into two age categories—one group of 51 to 70 years and one of 71 and older. Increasingly, research is showing that the nutrition needs of people 50 to 70 years old differ from those of people over 70.

Setting standards for older people is difficult because individual differences become more pronounced as people grow older. People start out with different genetic predispositions and ways of handling nutrients, and the effects of these differences become magnified with years of unique dietary habits. For example, one person may tend to omit fruits and vegetables from his diet, and by the time he is old, he may have a set of nutrition problems associated with a lack of fiber and antioxidants. Another person may have omitted milk and milk products all her life—her nutrition problems may be related to a lack of calcium. Also, as people age, they suffer different chronic diseases and take various medicines—both of which will affect nutrient needs. For all of these reasons, researchers have difficulty even defining "healthy aging," a prerequisite to developing recommendations to meet the "needs of practically all healthy persons." The following discussion gives special attention to the nutrients of greatest concern.

Water

Despite real fluid needs, many older people do not seem to feel thirsty or notice mouth dryness. Many nursing home employees say it is hard to persuade their elderly clients to drink enough water and fruit juices. Older adults may find it difficult and bothersome to get a drink or to get to a bathroom. Those who have lost bladder control may be afraid to drink too much water.

Dehydration is a risk for older adults. Total body water decreases as people age, so even mild stresses such as fever or hot weather can precipitate rapid dehydration in older adults. Dehydrated older adults seem to be more susceptible to urinary tract infections, pneumonia, **pressure ulcers,** and confusion and disorientation. To prevent dehydration, older adults need to drink at least 6 glasses of water a day.[30]

Energy and Energy Nutrients

On average, energy needs decline an estimated 5 percent per decade. One reason is that people usually reduce their physical activity as they age, although they need not do so. Another reason is that basal metabolic rate declines 1 to 2 percent per decade as lean body mass diminishes.

The lower energy expenditure of older adults means that they need to eat less food to maintain their weights. Accordingly, the estimated energy requirements■ for adults decrease steadily after age 19, as the "How to" on p. 562 explains.

On limited energy allowances, people must select mostly nutrient-dense foods. There is little leeway for added sugars, solid fats, or alcohol. The USDA Food Guide (on pp. 44–45) offers a dietary framework for adults of all ages.

Protein Because energy needs decrease, protein must be obtained from low-kcalorie sources of high-quality protein, such as lean meats, poultry, fish, and eggs; fat-free and low-fat milk products; and legumes. Protein is especially important for the elderly to support a healthy immune system and to prevent muscle wasting.

Available Online

http://nutrition.wadsworth.com/uncn7

Examine the various challenges elderly individuals face in meeting their nutrient needs.

■ Estimated energy requirements:
- Men: Subtract 10 kcal/day for each year of age above 19.
- Women: Subtract 7 kcal/day for each year of age above 19.

pressure ulcers: damage to the skin and underlying tissues as a result of compression and poor circulation; commonly seen in people who are bedridden or chairbound.

HOW TO Estimate Energy Requirements for Older Adults

The "How to" on p. 260 described how to estimate the energy requirements for adults using an equation that accounts for age, physical activity, weight, and height. Alternatively, energy requirements for older adults can be "guesstimated" by using the values listed in the tables in Appendix F for adults 30 years of age and subtracting 7 kcalories for women and 10 kcalories for men per day for each year over 30.

For example, Table F-4 lists 2556 kcalories per day for a woman who is 5 feet 5 inches tall, weighs 150 pounds, and has a low activity level. To estimate the energy requirements of a similar 50-year-old woman, subtract 7 kcalories per day for each year over 30:

$$50 - 30 = 20 \text{ yr.}$$
$$20 \text{ yr} \times 7 \text{ kcal/day} = 140 \text{ kcal/day.}$$
$$2556 \text{ kcal/day (at age 30)} - 140 \text{ kcal/day} = 2416 \text{ kcal/day (at age 50).}$$

Similarly, using Table F-5 to estimate the energy requirements of a sedentary 65-year-old man who is 5 feet 11 inches tall and weighs 250 pounds, subtract 10 kcalories per day for each year over 30:

$$65 - 30 = 35 \text{ yr.}$$
$$35 \text{ yr} \times 10 \text{ kcal/day} = 350 \text{ kcal/day.}$$
$$3088 \text{ kcal/day (at age 30)} - 350 \text{ kcal/day} = 2738 \text{ kcal/day (at age 65).}$$

(Adults between the ages of 19 and 30 can also use the values listed in the tables in Appendix F by adding 7 kcalories for women and 10 kcalories for men per day for each year below 30.)

Underweight or malnourished older adults need protein- and energy-dense snacks such as hard-boiled eggs, tuna fish and crackers, peanut butter on graham crackers, and hearty soups. Drinking liquid nutritional formulas between meals can also boost energy and nutrient intakes.[31] Importantly, the diet should provide enjoyment as well as nutrients.[32]

Carbohydrate and Fiber As always, abundant carbohydrate is needed to protect protein from being used as an energy source. Sources of complex carbohydrates such as legumes, vegetables, whole grains, and fruits are also rich in fiber and essential vitamins and minerals. Average fiber intakes among older adults are lower than current recommendations (14 grams per 1000 kcalories).[33] Eating high-fiber foods and drinking water can alleviate constipation—a condition common among older adults, especially nursing home residents. Physical inactivity and medications also contribute to the high incidence of constipation.

Fat As is true for people of all ages, fat intake needs to be moderate in the diets of most older adults—enough to enhance flavors and provide valuable nutrients, but not so much as to raise the risks of cancer, atherosclerosis, and other degenerative diseases. This recommendation should not be taken too far; limiting fat too severely may lead to nutrient deficiencies and weight loss—two problems that carry greater health risks in the elderly than overweight.

Vitamins and Minerals

Most people can achieve adequate vitamin and mineral intakes simply by including foods from all food groups in their diets, but older adults often omit fruits and vegetables. Similarly, few older adults consume the recommended amounts of milk or milk products.

Vitamin B_{12} An estimated 10 to 30 percent of adults over 50 have atrophic gastritis.■ As Chapter 10 explained, people with atrophic gastritis are particularly vulnerable to vitamin B_{12} deficiency: the bacterial overgrowth that accompanies this condition uses up the vitamin, and without hydrochloric acid and intrinsic factor, digestion and absorption of vitamin B_{12} are inefficient. Given the poor cognition, anemia, and devastating neurological effects associated with a vitamin B_{12} deficiency, an adequate intake is imperative.[34] The RDA for older adults is the same as for younger adults, but with the added suggestion to obtain most of a day's intake from vitamin B_{12}–fortified foods and supplements.[35]■ The bioavailability of vitamin B_{12} from these sources is better than from foods.

■ Reminder: *Atrophic gastritis* is a chronic inflammation of the stomach characterized by inadequate hydrochloric acid and intrinsic factor—two key players in vitamin B_{12} absorption.

■ 2005 *Dietary Guidelines:*
- People over age 50 should consume vitamin B_{12} from fortified foods or supplements.

Vitamin D Vitamin D deficiency is a problem among older adults. Only vitamin D–fortified milk provides significant vitamin D, and many older adults drink little or no milk.■ Further compromising the vitamin D status of many older people, especially those in nursing homes, is their limited exposure to sunlight. Finally, aging reduces the skin's capacity to make vitamin D and the kidneys' ability to convert it to its active form. Not only are older adults not getting enough vitamin D, but they may actually need more. To prevent bone loss and to maintain vitamin D status, especially in those who engage in minimal outdoor activity, adults 51 to 70 years old need 10 micrograms daily and those over 70 need 15 micrograms.[36]

■ 2005 *Dietary Guidelines:*
- Older adults should consume extra vitamin D from vitamin D–fortified foods and/or supplements.

Calcium Chapter and Highlight 12 emphasized the importance of abundant dietary calcium throughout life, and especially for women after menopause, to protect against osteoporosis. The DRI Committee recommends 1200 milligrams of calcium daily, but the calcium intakes of older people in the United States are well below recommendations.[37] Some older adults avoid milk and milk products because they dislike these foods or associate them with stomach discomfort. Simple solutions include using calcium-fortified juices, adding powdered milk to recipes, and taking supplements; Chapter 12 offers many other strategies for including nonmilk sources of calcium for those who do not drink milk.

Iron The iron needs of men remain unchanged throughout adulthood. For women, iron needs decrease substantially when blood loss through menstruation ceases. Consequently, iron-deficiency anemia is less common in older adults than in younger people. In fact, elevated iron stores are more likely than deficiency in older people, especially those who take iron supplements, eat red meat regularly, and include vitamin C–rich fruits in their daily diet.[38]

Nevertheless, iron deficiency may develop in older adults, especially when their food energy intakes are low. Aside from diet, two other factors may lead to iron deficiency in older people: chronic blood loss from diseases and medicines, and poor iron absorption due to reduced stomach acid secretion and antacid use. For older people with infectious diseases, the consequences of iron-deficiency anemia can be life-threatening.[39] Anyone concerned with older people's nutrition should keep these possibilities in mind.

Nutrient Supplements

People judge for themselves how to manage their nutrition, and some turn to supplements. Advertisers target older people with appeals to take supplements and eat "health" foods, claiming that these products prevent disease and promote longevity. About half of all women over 65 take some type of dietary supplement, while about one-fifth of older men do. When recommended by a physician or registered dietitian, vitamin D and calcium supplements for osteoporosis or vitamin B_{12} for pernicious anemia may be beneficial. Many health care professionals recommend a daily multivitamin-mineral supplement that provides 100 percent or less of the Daily Value for the listed nutrients.[40] They reason that such a supplement is more likely to be beneficial than to cause harm.

People with small energy allowances would do well to become more active so they can afford to eat more food. Food is the best source of nutrients for everybody. Supplements are just that—supplements to foods, not substitutes for them. For anyone who is motivated to obtain the best possible health, it is never too late to learn to eat well, drink water, exercise regularly, and adopt other lifestyle habits such as quitting smoking and moderating alcohol use.

IN SUMMARY The following table summarizes the nutrient concerns of aging. Although some nutrients need special attention in the diet, supplements are not routinely recommended. The ever-growing number of older people creates an urgent need to learn more about how their nutrient requirements differ from those of others and how such knowledge can enhance their health.

Nutrient	Effect of Aging	Comments
Water	Lack of thirst and decreased total body water make dehydration likely.	Mild dehydration is a common cause of confusion. Difficulty obtaining water or getting to the bathroom may compound the problem.
Energy	Need decreases as muscle mass decreases (sarcopenia).	Physical activity moderates the decline.
Fiber	Likelihood of constipation increases with low intakes and changes in the GI tract.	Inadequate water intakes and lack of physical activity, along with some medications, compound the problem.
Protein	Needs may stay the same or increase slightly.	Low-fat, high-fiber legumes and grains meet both protein and other nutrient needs.
Vitamin B_{12}	Atrophic gastritis is common.	Deficiency causes neurological damage; supplements may be needed.
Vitamin D	Increased likelihood of inadequate intake; skin synthesis declines.	Daily sunlight exposure in moderation or supplements may be beneficial.
Calcium	Intakes may be low; osteoporosis is common.	Stomach discomfort commonly limits milk intake; calcium substitutes or supplements may be needed.
Iron	In women, status improves after menopause; deficiencies are linked to chronic blood losses and low stomach acid output.	Adequate stomach acid is required for absorption; antacid or other medicine use may aggravate iron deficiency; vitamin C and meat increase absorption.

Nutrition-Related Concerns of Older Adults

Nutrition may play a greater role than has been realized in preventing many changes once thought to be inevitable consequences of growing older. The following discussions of cataracts and macular degeneration, arthritis, and the aging brain show that nutrition may provide at least some protection against some of the conditions associated with aging.

Cataracts and Macular Degeneration

Cataracts are age-related thickenings in the lenses of the eyes that impair vision. If not surgically removed, they ultimately lead to blindness. Cataracts occur even in well-nourished individuals as a result of ultraviolet light exposure, oxidative stress, injury, viral infections, toxic substances, and genetic disorders. Many cataracts, however, are vaguely called senile cataracts—meaning "caused by aging." In the United States, more than half of all adults 65 and older have a cataract.

Oxidative stress appears to play a significant role in the development of cataracts, and the antioxidant nutrients may help minimize the damage. Studies have reported an inverse relationship between cataracts and dietary intakes of vitamin C, vitamin E, and carotenoids; taking supplements of these antioxidant nutrients seems to slow the progression or reduce the risk of developing age-related cataracts.[41]

One other diet-related factor may play a role in the development of cataracts: overweight.[42] Overweight appears to be associated with cataracts, but its role has not been identified. Risk factors that typically accompany overweight, such as inactivity, diabetes, or hypertension, do not explain the association.

Another common cause of visual loss among older people is **macular degeneration,** a deterioration of the macular region of the retina.[43] Similarly to cataracts, risk factors for age-related macular degeneration include oxidative stress from sunlight, and preventive factors include supplements of antioxidant vitamins plus zinc and of the carotenoids lutein and zeaxanthin.[44] Total dietary fat may also be a risk factor for macular degeneration, but the omega-3 fatty acids of fish may be protective.[45]

cataracts (KAT-ah-rakts): thickenings of the eye lenses that impair vision and can lead to blindness.

macular (MACK-you-lar) **degeneration:** deterioration of the macular area of the eye that can lead to loss of central vision and eventual blindness. The **macula** is a small, oval, yellowish region in the center of the retina that provides the sharp, straight-ahead vision so critical to reading and driving.

arthritis: inflammation of a joint, usually accompanied by pain, swelling, and structural changes.

Arthritis

Over 40 million people in the United States have some form of **arthritis.**[46] As the population ages, it is expected that the prevalence will increase to 60 million by 2020.

Osteoarthritis The most common type of arthritis that disables older people is **osteoarthritis,** a painful deterioration of the cartilage in the joints. During movement, the ends of bones are normally protected from wear by cartilage and by small sacs of fluid that act as a lubricant. With age, bones sometimes disintegrate, and the joints become malformed and painful to move.

One known connection between osteoarthritis■ and nutrition is overweight. Weight loss may relieve some of the pain for overweight persons with osteoarthritis, partly because the joints affected are often weight-bearing joints that are stressed and irritated by having to carry excess poundage. Interestingly, though, weight loss often relieves the worst of the pain of arthritis in the hands as well, even though they are not weight-bearing joints. Jogging and other weight-bearing exercises do not worsen arthritis. In fact, both aerobic activity and strength training offer modest improvements in physical performance and pain relief.

■ Risk factors for osteoarthritis:
- Age.
- Smoking.
- BMI at age 40.
- Lack of hormone therapy (in women).

Rheumatoid Arthritis Another type of arthritis known as **rheumatoid arthritis** has possible links to diet through the immune system. In rheumatoid arthritis, the immune system mistakenly attacks the bone coverings as if they were made of foreign tissue. In some individuals, certain foods, notably vegetables and olive oil, may moderate the inflammatory responses and provide some relief.[47]

The omega-3 fatty acids commonly found in fish oil reduce joint tenderness and improve mobility in some people with rheumatoid arthritis.[48] The same diet recommended for heart health—one low in saturated fat from meats and milk products and high in omega-3 fats from fish—helps prevent or reduce the inflammation in the joints that makes arthritis so painful.

Another possible link between nutrition and rheumatoid arthritis involves the oxidative damage to the membranes within joints that causes inflammation and swelling. The antioxidant vitamins C and E defend against oxidation, and supplements of these nutrients may help prevent or relieve the pain of rheumatoid arthritis.[49]

Treatment Treatment for arthritis—dietary or otherwise—may help relieve discomfort and improve mobility, but it does not cure the condition. Traditional medical intervention for arthritis includes medication and surgery. Alternative therapies to treat arthritis abound, but none have proved safe and effective in scientific studies. Two currently popular supplements—glucosamine and chondroitin—may relieve pain and improve mobility as well as over-the-counter pain relievers, but stronger research studies are needed to confirm reports.[50] Drugs and supplements used to relieve arthritis can impose nutrition risks; many affect appetite and alter the body's use of nutrients, as Chapter 19 explains.

The Aging Brain

The brain, like all of the body's organs, responds to both genetic and environmental factors that can enhance or diminish its amazing capacities. One of the challenges researchers face when studying the human brain is to distinguish among normal age-related physiological changes, changes caused by diseases, and changes that result from cumulative, environmental factors such as diet.

The brain normally changes in some characteristic ways as it ages. For one thing, its blood supply decreases. For another, the number of **neurons,** the brain cells that specialize in transmitting information, diminishes as people age. When the number of nerve cells in one part of the cerebral cortex diminishes, hearing and speech are affected. Losses of neurons in other parts of the cortex can impair memory and cognitive function. When the number of neurons in the hindbrain diminishes, balance and posture are affected. Losses of neurons in other parts of the brain affect still other functions. Some of the cognitive loss and forgetfulness generally attributed to aging may be due in part to environmental, and therefore controllable, factors—including nutrient deficiencies.

Nutrient Deficiencies and Brain Function Nutrients influence the development and activities of the brain.[51] The ability of neurons to synthesize specific

osteoarthritis: a painful, degenerative disease of the joints that occurs when the cushioning cartilage in a joint deteriorates; joint structure is damaged, with loss of function; also called **degenerative arthritis.**

rheumatoid (ROO-ma-toyd) **arthritis:** a disease of the immune system involving painful inflammation of the joints and related structures.

neurons: nerve cells; the structural and functional units of the nervous system. Neurons initiate and conduct nerve transmissions.

TABLE 16-2 Summary of Nutrient-Brain Relationships

Brain Function	Depends on an Adequate Intake of:
Short-term memory	Vitamin B_{12}, vitamin C, vitamin E
Performance in problem-solving tests	Riboflavin, folate, vitamin B_{12}, vitamin C
Mental health	Thiamin, niacin, zinc, folate
Cognition	Folate, vitamin B_6, vitamin B_{12}, iron, vitamin E
Vision	Essential fatty acids, vitamin A
Neurotransmitter synthesis	Tyrosine, tryptophan, choline

neurotransmitters depends in part on the availability of precursor nutrients that are obtained from the diet.[52] The neurotransmitter serotonin, for example, derives from the amino acid tryptophan. To function properly, the enzymes involved in neurotransmitter synthesis require vitamins and minerals. Thus nutrient deficiencies may contribute to the loss of memory and cognition that some older adults experience.[53] Such losses may be preventable or at least diminished or delayed through diet. Table 16-2 summarizes some of the better-known connections between brain function and nutrients.

In some instances, the degree of cognitive loss is extensive. Such **senile dementia** may be attributable to a specific disorder such as a brain tumor or Alzheimer's disease.

Alzheimer's Disease Much attention has focused on the *abnormal* deterioration of the brain called **Alzheimer's disease,** which affects 10 percent of U.S. adults by age 65 and 30 percent of those over 85. Diagnosis of Alzheimer's disease depends on its characteristic symptoms: the victim gradually loses memory and reasoning, the ability to communicate, physical capabilities, and eventually life itself.[54] Nerve cells in the brain die, and communication between the cells breaks down.

Researchers are closing in on the exact cause of Alzheimer's disease.* Clearly, genetic factors are involved. Free radicals may also be involved.[55] Nerve cells in the brains of people with Alzheimer's disease show evidence of free-radical attack—damage to DNA, cell membranes, and proteins. They also show evidence of the minerals that trigger free-radical attacks—iron, copper, zinc, and aluminum.

In Alzheimer's disease, the brain is littered with clumps of a protein fragment called beta-amyloid. Free radicals and beta-amyloid have a sinister relationship: free radicals accelerate the clumping of beta-amyloid, and beta-amyloid produces more free radicals. Scientists believe beta-amyloid clogs the brain and damages or kills certain nerve cells, causing memory loss. Some research suggests that the antioxidant nutrients can limit free-radical damage and delay or prevent Alzheimer's disease.[56] Drug research is focusing on developing an immunization for beta-amyloid or an enzyme to block its production.[57]

Late in the course of the disease there is a decline in the activity of the enzyme that assists in the production of the neurotransmitter acetylcholine from choline and acetyl CoA.[58] Acetylcholine is essential to memory, but supplements of choline (or of lecithin, which contains choline) have no effect on memory or on the progression of the disease. Drugs that inhibit the breakdown of acetylcholine, on the other hand, have proved beneficial.

Research suggests that cardiovascular disease risk factors such as high blood pressure, diabetes, and elevated levels of homocysteine may be related to the development of Alzheimer's disease.[59] Diets designed to support a healthy heart may benefit a healthy brain as well.

Treatment for Alzheimer's disease involves providing care to clients and support to their families. Drugs are used to improve or at least to slow the loss of short-term memory and cognition, but they do not treat the disease.[60] Other drugs may be used to control depression, anxiety, and behavior problems.

Maintaining appropriate body weight may be the most important nutrition concern for the person with Alzheimer's disease.[61] Depression and forgetfulness can lead to changes in eating behaviors and poor food intake. Furthermore, changes in the body's weight-regulation system may contribute to weight loss. Perhaps the best that a caregiver can do nutritionally for a person with Alzheimer's disease is to supervise food planning and mealtimes. Providing well-liked and well-balanced meals and snacks in a cheerful atmosphere encourages food consumption. To minimize confusion, offer a few ready-to-eat foods, in bite-size pieces, with seasonings and sauces. To avoid mealtime disruptions, control distractions such as music, television, children, and the telephone.

senile dementia: the loss of brain function beyond the normal loss of physical adeptness and memory that occurs with aging.

Alzheimer's disease: a degenerative disease of the brain involving memory loss and major structural changes in neuron networks; also known as *senile dementia of the Alzheimer's type (SDAT), primary degenerative dementia of senile onset,* or *chronic brain syndrome.*

*A report on the genetic and other aspects of Alzheimer's is available from Alzheimer's Disease Education and Referral Center, P.O. Box 8250, Silver Springs, MD 20907-8250.

IN SUMMARY Senile dementia and other losses of brain function afflict millions of older adults, while others face loss of vision due to cataracts or macular degeneration, or cope with the pain of arthritis. As the number of people over age 65 continues to grow, the need for solutions to these problems becomes urgent. Some problems may be inevitable, but others are preventable and good nutrition may play a key role.

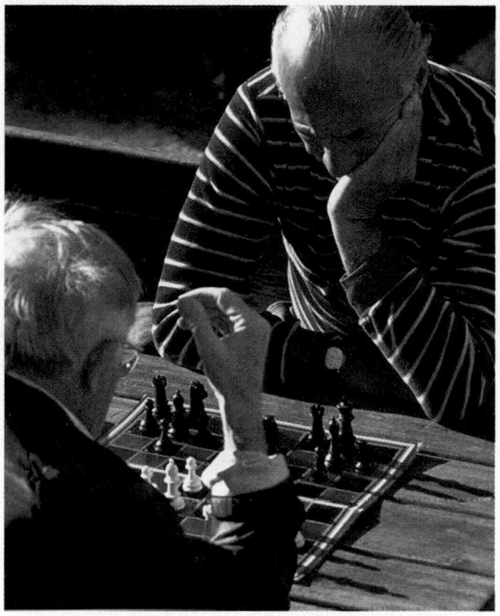
© Deborah Davis/PhotoEdit

Both foods and mental challenges nourish the brain.

Food Choices and Eating Habits of Older Adults

Older people are an incredibly diverse group, and for the most part they are independent, socially sophisticated, mentally lucid, fully participating members of society who report themselves to be happy and healthy. In fact, the quality of life among the elderly has improved, and their chronic disabilities have declined dramatically in recent years.[62] By practicing stress-management skills, maintaining physical fitness, participating in activities of interest, and cultivating spiritual health, as well as obtaining adequate nourishment, people can support a high quality of life into old age (see Table 16-3 for some strategies).

Older people spend more money per person on foods to eat at home than other age groups and less money on foods away from home. Manufacturers would be wise to cater to the preferences of older adults by providing good-tasting, nutritious foods in easy-to-open, single-serving packages with labels that are easy to read. Such services enable older adults to maintain their independence and to feel a sense of control and involvement in their own lives. Another way older adults can take care of themselves is by remaining or becoming physically active. As mentioned earlier, physical activity helps preserve one's ability to perform daily tasks and so promotes independence.

Familiarity, taste, and health beliefs are most influential on older people's food choices. Eating foods that are familiar, especially ethnic foods that recall family meals and pleasant times, can be comforting. People 65 and over are less likely to

TABLE 16-3 Strategies for Growing Old Healthfully

- Choose nutrient-dense foods.
- Be physically active. Walk, run, dance, swim, bike, or row for aerobic activity. Lift weights, do calisthenics, or pursue some other activity to tone, firm, and strengthen muscles. Practice balancing on one foot or doing simple movements with your eyes closed. Modify activities to suit changing abilities and tastes.
- Maintain appropriate body weight.
- Reduce stress (cultivate self-esteem, maintain a positive attitude, manage time wisely, know your limits, practice assertiveness, release tension, and take action).
- For women, discuss with a physician the risks and benefits of estrogen replacement therapy.
- For people who smoke, discuss with a physician strategies and programs to help you quit.
- Expect to enjoy sex, and learn new ways of enhancing it.
- Use alcohol only moderately, if at all; use drugs only as prescribed.
- Take care to prevent accidents.
- Expect good vision and hearing throughout life; obtain glasses and hearing aids if necessary.
- Take care of your teeth; obtain dentures if necessary.
- Be alert to confusion as a disease symptom, and seek diagnosis.
- Take medications as prescribed; see a physician before self-prescribing medicines or herbal remedies and a registered dietitian before self-prescribing supplements.
- Control depression through activities and friendships; seek professional help if necessary.
- Drink 6 to 8 glasses of water every day.
- Practice mental skills. Keep on solving math problems and crossword puzzles, playing cards or other games, reading, writing, imagining, and creating.
- Make financial plans early to ensure security.
- Accept change. Work at recovering from losses; make new friends.
- Cultivate spiritual health. Cherish personal values. Make life meaningful.
- Go outside for sunshine and fresh air as often as possible.
- Be socially active—play bridge, join an exercise or dance group, take a class, teach a class, eat with friends, volunteer time to help others.
- Stay interested in life—pursue a hobby, spend time with grandchildren, take a trip, read, grow a garden, or go to the movies.
- Enjoy life.

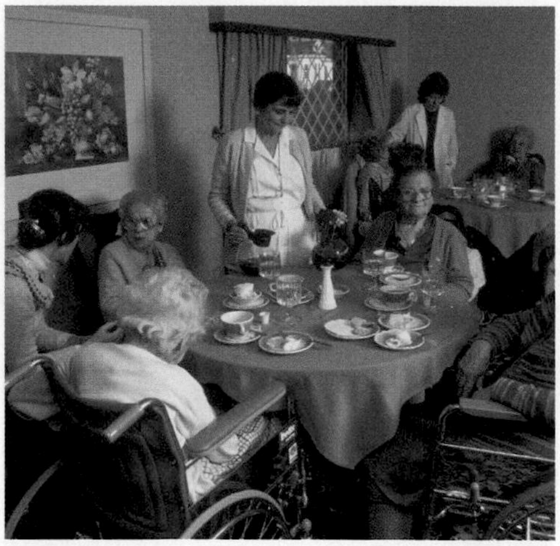

© Richard Pasley/Stock Boston/Picture Quest

Social interactions at a congregate meal site can be as nourishing as the foods served.

diet to lose weight than younger people are, but are more likely to diet in pursuit of medical goals such as controlling blood glucose and cholesterol.

Food Assistance Programs

The Nutrition Screening Initiative is part of a national effort to identify and treat nutrition problems in older persons; it uses a screening checklist. To *determine* the risk of malnutrition in older clients, health care professionals can keep in mind the characteristics and questions listed in Table 16-4.

The U.S. government funds the federal Elderly Nutrition Program to improve older people's nutrition status and enable them to avoid medical problems, continue living in communities of their own choice, and stay out of institutions. Its specific goals are to provide low-cost, nutritious meals; opportunities for social interaction; homemaker education and shopping assistance; counseling and referral to social services; and transportation. The program's mission has always been to provide "more than a meal."

The Elderly Nutrition Program provides for **congregate meals** at group settings such as community centers. Administrators try to select sites for congregate meals where as many eligible people as possible can participate. Volunteers may also deliver meals to those who are homebound either permanently or temporarily; these home-delivered meals are known as **Meals on Wheels.** The home-delivery program ensures nutrition, but its recipients miss out on the social benefits of the congregate meals; every effort is made to persuade older people to come to the shared meals, if they can. All persons aged 60 years and older and their spouses are eligible to receive meals from these programs, regardless of their income. Priority is given to those who are economically and socially needy. An estimated 3 million of our nation's older adults benefit from these meals.

These programs provide at least one meal a day that meets a third of the RDA for this age group; they must operate five or more days a week. Many programs voluntarily offer additional services designed to appeal to older adults: provisions for special diets (to meet medical needs or religious preferences), food pantries, ethnic meals, and delivery of meals to the homeless.

HEALTHY PEOPLE 2010

Increase the receipt of home foodservices by people aged 65 and older who have difficulty in preparing their own meals or are otherwise in need of home-delivered meals.

TABLE 16-4 Risk Factors for Malnutrition in Older Adults

	These questions help *determine* the risk of malnutrition in older adults:
Disease	• Do you have an illness or condition that changes the types or amounts of foods you eat?
Eating poorly	• Do you eat fewer than two meals a day? Do you eat fruits, vegetables, and milk products daily?
Tooth loss or mouth pain	• Is it difficult or painful to eat?
Economic hardship	• Do you have enough money to buy the food you need?
Reduced social contact	• Do you eat alone most of the time?
Multiple medications	• Do you take three or more different prescribed or over-the-counter medications daily?
Involuntary weight loss or gain	• Have you lost or gained 10 pounds or more in the last six months?
Needs assistance	• Are you physically able to shop, cook, and feed yourself?
Elderly person	• Are you older than 80?

congregate meals: nutrition programs that provide food for the elderly in conveniently located settings such as community centers.

Meals on Wheels: a nutrition program that delivers food for the elderly to their homes.

Older adults can learn about the available programs in their communities by looking in the Yellow Pages of the telephone book under "Social Services" or "Senior Citizens' Organizations."* In addition, the local senior center and hospital can usually direct people to programs providing nutrition and other health-related services.

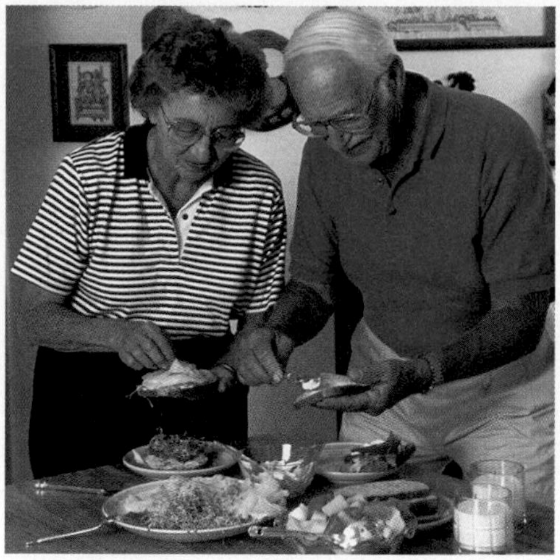

Myrleen Ferguson Cate/PhotoEdit

Taking time to nourish your body well is a gift you give yourself.

Meals for Singles

Many older adults live alone, and singles of all ages face challenges in purchasing, storing, and preparing food. Large packages of meat and vegetables are often intended for families of four or more, and even a head of lettuce can spoil before one person can use it all. Many singles live in small dwellings and have little storage space for foods. A limited income presents additional obstacles. This section offers suggestions that can help to solve some of the problems singles face.

Spend Wisely People who have the means to shop and cook for themselves can cut their food bills just by being wise shoppers. Large supermarkets are usually less expensive than convenience stores. A grocery list helps reduce impulse buying, and specials and coupons can save money when the items featured are those that the shopper needs and uses.

Buying the right amount so as not to waste any food is a challenge for people eating alone. They can buy fresh milk in the size best suited for personal needs. Pint-size and even cup-size boxes■ of milk are available and can be stored unopened on a shelf for up to three months without refrigeration.

■ Boxes of milk that can be stored at room temperature have been exposed to temperatures above those of pasteurization just long enough to sterilize the milk—a process called **ultrahigh temperature (UHT).**

Many foods that offer a variety of nutrients for practically pennies have a long shelf life; staples such as rice, pastas, dry powdered milk, and dried legumes can be purchased in bulk and stored for months at room temperature. Other foods that are usually a good buy include whole pieces of cheese rather than sliced or shredded cheese, fresh produce in season, variety meats such as chicken livers, and cereals that require cooking instead of ready-to-serve cereals.

A person who has ample freezing space can buy large packages of meat, such as pork chops, ground beef, or chicken, when they are on sale. Then the meat can be immediately wrapped into individual servings for the freezer. All the individual servings can be put in a bag marked appropriately with the contents and the date.

Frozen vegetables are more economical in large bags than in small boxes. The amount needed can be taken out, and the bag closed tightly with a twist tie or rubber band. If the package is returned quickly to the freezer each time, the vegetables will stay fresh for a long time.

Finally, breads and cereals usually must be purchased in larger quantities. Again the amount needed for a few days can be taken out and the rest stored in the freezer.

Grocers will break open a package of wrapped meat and rewrap the portion needed. Similarly, eggs can be purchased by the half-dozen. Eggs do keep for long periods, though, if stored properly in the refrigerator.

Fresh fruits and vegetables can be purchased individually. A person can buy fresh fruit at various stages of ripeness: a ripe one to eat right away, a semiripe one to eat soon after, and a green one to ripen on the windowsill. If vegetables are packaged in large quantities, the grocer can break open the package so that a smaller amount can be purchased. Small cans of fruits and vegetables, even though they are more expensive per unit, are a reasonable alternative, considering that it is expensive to buy a regular-size can and let the unused portion spoil.

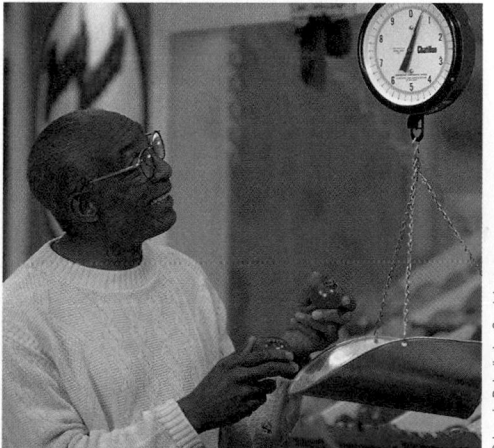

© Lonnie Duka/Index Stock Imagery

Buy only what you will use.

Be Creative Creative chefs think of various ways to use foods when only large amounts are available. For example, a head of cauliflower can be divided into thirds. Then one-third is cooked and eaten hot. Another third is put into a vinegar and oil marinade for use in a salad. And the last third can be used in a casserole or stew.

A variety of vegetables and meats can be enjoyed stir-fried; inexpensive vegetables such as cabbage, celery, and onion are delicious when crisp cooked in a little

*To find a local provider, call Eldercare Locator at (800) 677-1116.

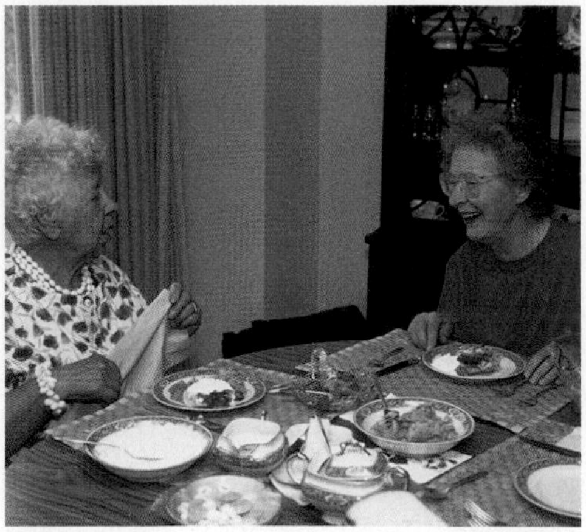
© Elena Rooraid/PhotoEdit

Invite guests to share a meal.

oil with herbs or lemon added. Interesting frozen vegetable mixtures are available in larger grocery stores. Cooked, leftover vegetables can be dropped in at the last minute. A bonus of a stir-fried meal is that there is only one pan to wash. Similarly, a microwave oven allows a chef to use fewer pots and pans. Meals and leftovers can also be frozen or refrigerated in microwavable containers to reheat as needed.

Many frozen dinners offer nutritious options. Adding a fresh salad, a whole-wheat roll, and a glass of milk can make a nutritionally balanced meal.

Also, single people shouldn't hesitate to invite someone to share meals with them whenever there is enough food. It's likely that the person will return the invitation, and both parties will get to enjoy companionship and a meal prepared by others.

IN SUMMARY Older people can benefit from both the nutrients provided and the social interaction available at congregate meals. Other government programs deliver meals to those who are homebound. With creativity and careful shopping, those living alone can prepare nutritious, inexpensive meals. Physical activity, mental challenges, stress management, and social activities can also help people grow old comfortably.

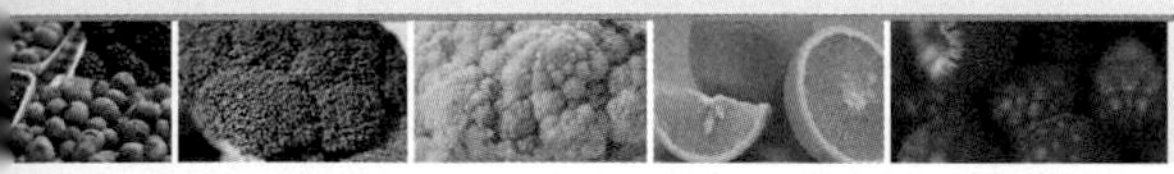

Nutrition in Your Life

By eating a balanced diet, maintaining a healthy body weight, and engaging in a variety of physical, social, and mental activities, you can enjoy good health in later life.

- **If there are older adults in your life, do they have the financial means, physical ability, and social support they need to eat adequately?**
- **Have they experienced an unintentional loss of weight recently?**
- **Are they active physically, socially, and mentally?**

NUTRITION ON THE NET

Access these websites for further study of topics covered in this chapter.

- Find updates and quick links to these and other nutrition-related sites at our website: **www.wadsworth.com/nutrition**
- Search for "aging," "arthritis," and "Alzheimer's" on the U.S. Government health information site: **www.healthfinder.gov**
- Visit the National Aging Information Center of the Administration on Aging: **www.aoa.gov**
- Visit the American Geriatrics Society: **www.americangeriatrics.org**
- Visit the National Institute on Aging: **www.nia.nih.gov**
- Visit the American Association of Retired Persons: **www.aarp.org**
- Get nutrition tips for growing older in good health from the American Dietetic Association: **www.eatright.org**
- Learn more about cataracts and macular degeneration from the National Eye Institute, the Macular Degeneration Partnership, and the American Society of Cataract and Refractive Surgery: **www.nei.nih.gov**, **www.macd.net**, and **www.ascrs.org**
- Learn more about arthritis from the Arthritis Society, the Arthritis Foundation, and the National Institute of Arthritis and Musculoskeletal and Skin Diseases: **www.arthritis.ca**, **www.arthritis.org**, and **www.niams.nih.gov**
- Learn more about Alzheimer's disease from the NIA Alzheimer's Disease Education and Referral Center and the Alzheimer's Association: **www.alzheimers.org** and **www.alz.org**
- Find out about federal government programs designed to help senior citizens maintain good health: **www.seniors.gov**

STUDY QUESTIONS

These questions will help you review the chapter. You will find the answers in the discussions on the pages provided.

1. What roles does nutrition play in aging, and what roles can it play in retarding aging? (pp. 554–557)
2. What are some of the physiological changes that occur in the body's systems with aging? To what extent can aging be prevented? (pp. 558–560)
3. Why does the risk of dehydration increase as people age? (p. 561)
4. Why do energy needs usually decline with advancing age? (p. 561)
5. Which vitamins and minerals need special consideration for the elderly? Explain why. Identify some factors that complicate the task of setting nutrient standards for older adults. (pp. 562–563)
6. Discuss the relationships between nutrition and cataracts and between nutrition and arthritis. (pp. 564–565)
7. What characteristics contribute to malnutrition in older people? (pp. 567–568)

These multiple choice questions will help you prepare for an exam. Answers can be found on p. 573.

1. Life expectancy in the United States is:
   a. 48 to 60 years.
   b. 58 to 70 years.
   c. 68 to 80 years.
   d. 78 to 90 years.
2. The human life span is about:
   a. 85 years.
   b. 100 years.
   c. 115 years.
   d. 130 years.
3. A 72-year-old person whose physical health is similar to that of people 10 years younger has a(n):
   a. chronological age of 62.
   b. physiological age of 72.
   c. physiological age of 62.
   d. absolute age of minus 10.
4. Rats live longest when given diets that:
   a. eliminate all fat.
   b. provide lots of protein.
   c. allow them to eat freely.
   d. restrict their energy intakes.
5. Which characteristic is *not* commonly associated with atrophic gastritis?
   a. inflamed stomach
   b. vitamin B_{12} toxicity
   c. bacterial overgrowth
   d. lack of intrinsic factor
6. On average, adult energy needs:
   a. decline 5 percent per year.
   b. decline 5 percent per decade.
   c. remain stable throughout life.
   d. rise gradually throughout life.
7. Which nutrients seem to protect against cataract development?
   a. minerals
   b. lecithins
   c. antioxidants
   d. amino acids
8. The best dietary advice for a person with osteoarthritis might be to:
   a. avoid milk products.
   b. take fish oil supplements.
   c. take vitamin E supplements.
   d. lose weight, if overweight.
9. Congregate meal programs are preferable to Meals on Wheels because they provide:
   a. nutritious meals.
   b. referral services.
   c. social interactions.
   d. financial assistance.
10. The Elderly Nutrition Program is available to:
    a. all people 65 years and older.
    b. all people 60 years and older.
    c. homebound people only, 60 years and older.
    d. low-income people only, 60 years and older.

REFERENCES

1. Trends in aging—United States and worldwide, *Morbidity and Mortality Weekly Report* 52 (2003): 101–106.
2. National vital statistics report, **www.cdc.gov/nchs**, site visited May 1, 2003.
3. T. Perls, Genetic and environmental influences on exceptional longevity and the AGE nomogram, *Annals of the New York Academy of Sciences* 959 (2002): 1–13.
4. G. E. Fraser and D. J. Shavlik, Ten years of life: Is it a matter of choice? *Archives of Internal Medicine* 161 (2001): 1645–1652.
5. E. W. Gregg and coauthors, Relationship of changes in physical activity and mortality among older women, *Journal of the American Medical Association* 289 (2003): 2379–2386; American College of Sports Medicine, Position stand: Exercise and physical activity for older adults, *Medicine and Science in Sports and Exercise* 30 (1998): 992–1008.
6. W. J. Strawbridge and coauthors, Physical activity reduces the risk of subsequent depression for older adults, *American Journal of Epidemiology* 156 (2002): 328–334; A. J. Schuit and coauthors, Physical activity and cognitive decline, the role of the apolipoprotein e4 allele, *Medicine and Science in Sports and Exercise* 33 (2001): 772–777.
7. I. M. Lee and coauthors, Epidemiologic data on the relationships of caloric intake, energy balance, and weight gain over the life span with longevity and morbidity, *Journals of Gerontology: Series A, Biological Sciences and Medical Sciences* 56 (2001): 7–19.
8. C. K. Lee and coauthors, Gene expression profile of aging and its retardation by calorie restriction, *Science* 285 (1999): 1390–1393.
9. S. X. Cao and coauthors, Genomic profiling of short- and long-term caloric restriction effects in the liver of aging mice, *Proceeding of the National Academy of Sciences of the United States of America* 98 (2001): 10630–10635.
10. J. M. Dhahbi and coauthors, Caloric restriction alters the feeding response of key metabolic enzyme genes, *Mechanisms of*

Ageing and Development 122 (2001): 1033–1048; J. J. Ramsey and coauthors, Dietary restriction and aging in rhesus monkeys: The University of Wisconsin study, *Experimental Gerontology* 35 (2000): 1131–1149; A. C. Gazdag and coauthors, Effect of long-term calorie restriction on GLUT4, phosphatidylinositol-3 kinase p85 subunit, and insulin receptor substrate-1 protein levels in rhesus monkey skeletal muscle, *Journals of Gerontology: Series A, Biological Sciences and Medical Sciences* 55 (2000): B44–B46; W. T. Cefalu and coauthors, Influence of caloric restriction on the development of atherosclerosis in nonhuman primates: Progress to date, *Toxicological Sciences* 52 (1999): 49–55.

11. J. P. DeLany and coauthors, Long-term calorie restriction reduces energy expenditure in aging monkeys, *Journals of Gerontology: Series A, Biological Sciences and Medical Sciences* 54 (1999): B5–B11.
12. G. Barja, Endogenous oxidative stress: Relationship to aging, longevity and caloric restriction, *Ageing Research and Reviews* 1 (2002): 397–411; B. J. Merry, Molecular mechanisms linking calorie restriction and longevity, *International Journal of Biochemistry and Cell Biology* 34 (2002): 1340–1354; J. Wanagat, D. B. Allison, and R. Weindruch, Calorie intake and aging: Mechanisms in rodents and a study in nonhuman primates, *Toxicological Sciences* 52 (1999): 35–40.
13. L. K. Heilbronn and E. Ravussin, Calorie restriction and aging: Review of the literature and implications for studies in humans, *American Journal of Clinical Nutrition* 78 (2003): 361–369; Lee and coauthors, 2001.
14. A. Trichopoulou and E. Vasilopoulou, Mediterranean diet and longevity, *British Journal of Nutrition* 84 (2000): S205–S209.
15. H. Hu and coauthors, Antioxidants may contribute in the fight against ageing: An in vitro model, *Mechanisms of Ageing and Development* 121 (2001): 217–230.
16. A. Heiat, V. Vaccarino, and H. M. Krumholz, An evidence-based assessment of federal guidelines for overweight and obesity as they apply to elderly persons, *Archives of Internal Medicine* 161 (2001): 1194–1203.
17. Surveillance for selected public health indicators affecting older adults—United States, *Morbidity and Mortality Weekly Report* 48 (1999): 94–95.
18. S. B. Roberts, Energy regulation and aging: Recent findings and their implications, *Nutrition Reviews* 58 (2000): 91–97; M. J. Toth and E. T. Poehlman, Energetic adaptation to chronic disease in the elderly, *Nutrition Reviews* 58 (2000): 61–66.
19. A. B. Newman and coauthors, Weight change in old age and its association with mortality, *Journal of the American Geriatrics Society* 49 (2001): 1309–1318; F. Landi and coauthors, Body mass index and mortality among older people living in the community, *Journal of the American Geriatrics Society* 47 (1999): 1072–1076.
20. H. K. Kamel, Sarcopenia and aging, *Nutrition Reviews* 61 (2003): 157–167; C. W. Bales and C. S. Ritchie, Sarcopenia, weight loss, and nutritional frailty in the elderly, *Annual Review of Nutrition* 22 (2002): 309–323; R. Roubenoff and C. Castaneda, Sarcopenia—Understanding the dynamics of aging muscle, *Journal of the American Medical Association* 286 (2001): 1230–1231.
21. R. D. Hansen and B. J. Allen, Habitual physical activity, anabolic hormones, and potassium content of fat-free mass in postmenopausal women, *American Journal of Clinical Nutrition* 75 (2002): 314–320; R. N. Baumgartner and coauthors, Predictors of skeletal muscle mass in elderly men and women, *Mechanisms of Ageing and Development* 107 (1999): 123–136.
22. G. Ravaglia and coauthors, Effect of micronutrient status on natural killer cell immune function in healthy free-living subjects aged ≥ 90 y, *American Journal of Clinical Nutrition* 71 (2000): 590–598.
23. M. J. M. Chin a Paw and coauthors, Immunity in frail elderly: A randomized controlled trial of exercise and enriched foods, *Medicine and Science in Sports and Exercise* 32 (2000): 2005–2011.
24. C. G. MacIntosh and coauthors, Effects of age on concentrations of plasma cholecystokinin, glucagon-like peptide 1, and peptide YY and their relation to appetite and pyloric motility, *American Journal of Clinical Nutrition* 69 (1999): 999–1006.
25. N. R. Sahyoun, C. L. Lin, and E. Krall, Nutritional status of the older adult is associated with dentition status, *Journal of the American Dietetic Association* 103 (2003): 61–66.
26. Position of the American Dietetic Association: Nutrition, aging, and the continuum of care, *Journal of the American Dietetic Association* 100 (2000): 580–595.
27. D. G. Blazer, Depression in late life: Review and commentary, *Journals of Gerontology: Series A, Biological Sciences and Medical Sciences* 58 (2003): 249–265; J. Unutzer, M. L. Bruce, and NIMH Affective Disorders Workgroup, The elderly, *Mental Health Services Research* 4 (2002): 245–247.
28. T. Hungerford and coauthors, Trends in the economic status of the elderly, 1976–2000, *Social Security Bulletin* 64 (2001): 12–22.
29. N. L. Crogan and A. Pasvogel, The influence of protein-calorie malnutrition on quality of life in nursing homes, *Journals of Gerontology: Series A, Biological Sciences and Medical Sciences* 58 (2003): 159–164; Y. Guigoz, S. Lauque, and B. J. Vellas, Identifying the elderly at risk for malnutrition: The Mini Nutritional Assessment, *Clinics in Geriatric Medicine* 18 (2002): 737–757; W. O. Seiler, Clinical pictures of malnutrition in ill elderly subjects, *Nutrition* 17 (2001): 496–498.
30. D. H. Holben and coauthors, Fluid intake compared with established standards and symptoms of dehydration among elderly residents of a long-term-care facility, *Journal of the American Dietetic Association* 99 (1999): 1447–1450.
31. M. M. G. Wilson, R. Purushothaman, and J. E. Morley, Effect of liquid dietary supplements on energy intake in the elderly, *American Journal of Clinical Nutrition* 75 (2002): 944–947.
32. Position of the American Dietetic Association: Liberalized diets for older adults in long-term care, *Journal of the American Dietetic Association* 102 (2002): 1316–1323.
33. Committee on Dietary Reference Intakes, *Dietary Reference Intakes for Energy, Carbohydrate, Fiber, Fat, Fatty Acids, Cholesterol, Protein, and Amino Acids* (Washington, D.C.: National Academies Press, 2002).
34. M. A. Johnson and coauthors, Hyperhomocysteinemia and vitamin B-12 deficiency in elderly using Title IIIc nutrition services, *American Journal of Clinical Nutrition* 77 (2003): 211–220; C. Ho, G. P. A. Kauwell, and L. B. Bailey, Practitioners' guide to meeting the vitamin B-12 Recommended Dietary Allowance for people aged 51 years and older, *Journal of the American Dietetic Association* 99 (1999): 725–727; H. W. Baik and R. M. Russell, Vitamin B_{12} deficiency in the elderly, *Annual Review of Nutrition* 19 (1999): 357–377.
35. Committee on Dietary Reference Intakes, *Dietary Reference Intakes for Thiamin, Riboflavin, Niacin, Vitamin B_6, Folate, Vitamin B_{12}, Pantothenic Acid, Biotin, and Choline* (Washington, D.C.: National Academy Press, 2000), p. 338.
36. Committee on Dietary Reference Intakes, *Dietary Reference Intakes for Calcium, Phosphorus, Magnesium, Vitamin D, and Fluoride* (Washington, D.C.: National Academy Press, 1997).
37. Committee on Dietary Reference Intakes, 1997.
38. D. J. Fleming and coauthors, Dietary factors associated with the risk of high iron stores in the elderly Framingham Heart Study cohort, *American Journal of Clinical Nutrition* 76 (2002): 1375–1384; D. J. Fleming and coauthors, Iron status of the free-living, elderly Framingham Heart Study cohort: An iron-replete population with a high prevalence of elevated iron stores, *American Journal of Clinical Nutrition* 73 (2001): 638–646.
39. G. J. Izaks, R. G. J. Westendorp, and D. L. Knook, The definition of anemia in older persons, *Journal of the American Medical Association* 281 (1999): 1714–1717.
40. R. H. Fletcher and K. M. Fairfield, Vitamins for chronic disease prevention in adults, *Journal of the American Medical Association* 287 (2002): 3127–3129; W. C. Willett and M. J. Stampfer, What vitamins should I be taking, doctor? *New England Journal of Medicine* 345 (2001): 1819–1824.
41. The REACT Group, The Roche European American Cataract Trial (REACT): A randomized clinical trial to investigate the efficacy of an oral antioxidant micronutrient mixture to slow progression of age-related cataract, *Ophthalmic Epidemiology* 9 (2002): 49–80; A. Taylor and coauthors, Long-term intake of vitamins and carotenoids and odds of early age-related cortical and posterior subcapsular lens opacities, *American Journal of Clinical Nutrition* 75 (2002): 540–549; L. Brown and coauthors, A prospective study of carotenoid intake and risk of cataract extraction in US men, *American Journal of Clinical Nutrition* 70 (1999): 517–524; L. Chason-Taber and coauthors, A prospective study of carotenoid and vitamin A intake and risk of cataract extraction in US women, *American Journal of Clinical Nutrition* 70 (1999): 509–516.
42. D. A. Schaumberg and coauthors, Relations of body fat distribution and height with cataract in men, *American Journal of Clinical Nutrition* 73 (2000): 1495–1502.
43. J. L. Gottlieb, Age-related macular degeneration, *Journal of the American Medical Association* 288 (2002): 2233–2236.
44. N. I. Krinsky, J. T. Landrum, and R. A. Bone, Biologic mechanisms of the protective role of lutein and zeaxanthin in the eye, *Annual Review of Nutrition* 23 (2003): 171–201; Age-Related Eye Disease Study Research Group, Antioxidants and zinc to prevent progression of age-related macular degeneration, *Journal of the American Medical Association* 286 (2001): 2466–2468.
45. E. Cho and coauthors, Prospective study of dietary fat and the risk of age-related macular degeneration, *American Journal of Clinical Nutrition* 73 (2001): 209–218.
46. Prevalence of arthritis—United States, 1997, *Morbidity and Mortality Weekly Report* 50 (2001): 334–336.
47. L. Skoldstam, L. Hagfors, and G. Johansson, An experimental study of a Mediterranean diet intervention for patients with rheumatoid arthritis, *Annals of the Rheumatic Diseases* 62 (2003): 208–214; A. Linos and coauthors, Dietary factors in relation to rheumatoid arthritis: A role for olive oil and cooked vegetables, *American Journal of Clinical Nutrition* 70 (1999): 1077–1082;

J. Kjeldsen-Kragh, Rheumatoid arthritis treated with vegetarian diets, *American Journal of Clinical Nutrition* 70 (1999): 594S–600S.

48. L. Cleland, M. James, and S. Proudman, The role of fish oils in the treatment of rheumatoid arthritis, *Drugs* 63 (2003): 845–853; J. M. Kremer, n-3 Fatty acid supplements in rheumatoid arthritis, *American Journal of Clinical Nutrition* 71 (2000): 349S–351S.
49. J. R. Cerhan and coauthors, Antioxidant micronutrients and risk of rheumatoid arthritis in a cohort of older women, *American Journal of Epidemiology* 157 (2003): 345–354; S. Tidow-Kebritchi and S. Mobarhan, Effects of diets containing fish oil and vitamin E on rheumatoid arthritis, *Nutrition Reviews* 59 (2001): 335–341.
50. T. E. McAlindon and coauthors, Glucosamine and chondroitin for treatment of osteoarthritis: A systematic quality assessment and meta-analysis, *Journal of the American Medical Association* 283 (2000): 1469–1475.
51. R. J. Kaplan and coauthors, Dietary protein, carbohydrate, and fat enhance memory performance in the healthy elderly, *American Journal of Clinical Nutrition* 74 (2001): 687–693; L. Dye, A. Lluch, and J. E. Blundell, Macronutrients and mental performance, *Nutrition* 16 (2000): 1021–1034; J. D. Fernstrom, Can nutrient supplements modify brain function? *American Journal of Clinical Nutrition* 71 (2000): 1669S–1673S.
52. R. J. Wurtman and coauthors, Effects of normal meals rich in carbohydrates or proteins on plasma tryptophan and tyrosine ratios, *American Journal of Clinical Nutrition* 77 (2003): 128–132.
53. S. J. Duthie and coauthors, Homocysteine, B vitamin status, and cognitive function in the elderly, *American Journal of Clinical Nutrition* 75 (2002): 908–913; J. Selhub and coauthors, B vitamins, homocysteine, and neurocognitive function in the elderly, *American Journal of Clinical Nutrition* 71 (2000): 614S–620S.
54. J. L. Cummings and G. Cole, Alzheimer disease, *Journal of the American Medical Association* 287 (2002): 2335–2338.
55. Y. Christen, Oxidative stress and Alzheimer disease, *American Journal of Clinical Nutrition* 71 (2000): 621S–629S.
56. M. J. Engelhart and coauthors, Dietary intake of antioxidants and risk of Alzheimer disease, *Journal of the American Medical Association* 287 (2002): 3223–3229; M. C. Morris, Dietary intake of antioxidant nutrients and the risk of incident Alzheimer disease in a biracial community study, *Journal of the American Medical Association* 287 (2002): 3230–3237; M. Grundman, Vitamin E and Alzheimer disease: The basis for additional clinical trials, *American Journal of Clinical Nutrition* 71 (2000): 630S–636S.
57. D. Schenk and coauthors, Immunization with amyloid-beta attenuates Alzheimer-disease-like pathology in the PDAPP mouse, *Nature* 400 (1999): 173–177; R. Vassar and coauthors, Beta-secretase cleavage of Alzheimer's amyloid precursor protein by the transmembrane aspartic protease BACE, *Science* 286 (1999): 735; I. Hussain and coauthors, Identification of novel aspartic protease (Asp 2) as beta-secretase, *Molecular and Cellular Neuroscience* 14 (1999): 419–427.
58. K. L. Davis and coauthors, Cholinergic markers in elderly patients with early signs of Alzheimer disease, *Journal of the American Medical Association* 281 (1999): 1401–1406.
59. S. Seshadri and coauthors, Plasma homocysteine as a risk factor for dementia and Alzheimer's disease, *New England Journal of Medicine* 346 (2002): 476–483; D. Snowdon and coauthors, Serum folate and the severity of atrophy of the neocortex in Alzheimer disease: Findings from the Nun Study, *American Journal of Clinical Nutrition* 71 (2000): 993–998; D. G. Weir and A. M. Molloy, Microvascular disease and dementia in the elderly: Are they related to hyperhomocysteinemia? *American Journal of Clinical Nutrition* 71 (2000): 859–860; J. W. Miller, Homocysteine and Alzheimer's disease, *Nutrition Reviews* 57 (1999): 126–129.
60. R. Mayeux and M. Sand, Treatment of Alzheimer's disease, *New England Journal of Medicine* 341 (1999): 1670–1679.
61. S. Gillette-Guyonnet and coauthors, Weight loss in Alzheimer disease, *American Journal of Clinical Nutrition* 71 (2000): 637S–642S; E. T. Poehlman and R. V. Dvorak, Energy expenditure, energy intake, and weight loss in Alzheimer disease, *American Journal of Clinical Nutrition* 71 (2000): 650S–655S; S. Rivière and coauthors, Nutrition and Alzheimer's disease, *Nutrition Reviews* 57 (1999): 363–367.
62. V. A. Freedman, L. G. Martin, and R. F. Schoeni, Recent trends in disability and functioning among older adults in the United States: A systematic review, *Journal of the American Medical Association* 288 (2002): 3137–3146; Y. Liao and coauthors, Quality of the last year of life of older adults: 1986 vs 1993, *Journal of the American Medical Association* 283 (2000): 512–518.

ANSWERS

Study Questions (multiple choice)

1. c 2. d 3. c 4. d 5. b 6. b 7. c 8. d 9. c 10. b

HIGHLIGHT

Hunger and Community Nutrition

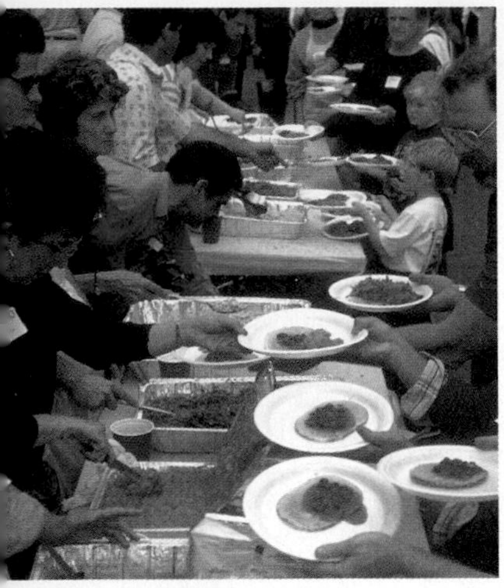

Joseph Sohm; ChromoSohm Inc./CORBIS

One person in every eight worldwide experiences persistent hunger—not the healthy appetite triggered by anticipation of a hearty meal, but the painful sensation caused by a lack of food. The physical feelings are the same, but in this highlight, hunger takes on greater meaning because the lack of food is recurrent and involuntary. Hunger deprives a person of the physical and mental energy needed to enjoy a full life and often leads to severe malnutrition and death. Tens of thousands of people die of starvation each day—one child every seven seconds.

Ideally, all people at all times would have access to enough food to support an active, healthy life; in other words, they would experience **food security.** Unfortunately, almost 34 million people in the United States, including 13 million children, live in poverty and cannot afford to buy enough food to maintain good health.[1] Said another way, one out of ten households experiences hunger or the threat of hunger. Given the agricultural bounty and enormous wealth in this country, do these numbers surprise you? The limited or uncertain availability of nutritionally adequate and safe foods is known as **food insecurity** and is a major social problem in our nation today. Inadequate diets lead to poor health in adults and impaired physical, psychological, and cognitive development in children.

The accompanying "How to" presents the questions used in national surveys to identify food insecurity in the United States, and Figure H16-1 shows the most recent findings. Responses to these questions provide crude, but necessary, data to estimate the degree of hunger in this country.[2]

Healthy People 2010: Increase food security among U.S. households and in so doing reduce hunger. HEALTHY PEOPLE 2010

Hunger in the United States

At its most extreme, people experience hunger because they have absolutely no food. More often, they have too little food **(food insufficiency)** and try to stretch their limited resources by eating small meals or skipping meals—often for days at a time. Sometimes hungry people obtain enough food to satisfy their hunger, perhaps by seeking food assistance or finding food through socially unacceptable ways—begging from strangers, stealing from markets, or scavenging through garbage cans, for example. Sometimes obtaining food raises concerns for food safety—for example, when rot, slime, mold, or insects have damaged foods or when people eat others' leftovers or meat from roadkill (an animal struck and killed by a motor vehicle).[3]

Hunger has many causes, but in developed countries, the primary cause is **food poverty.** People are hungry not because there is no food nearby to purchase, but because they lack money. An estimated one out of nine people in the United States lives in poverty. Even those above the poverty line may not have food security. Physical and mental illnesses

GLOSSARY

emergency kitchens: programs that provide prepared meals to be eaten on site; often called *soup kitchens.*

food bank: a facility that collects and distributes food donations to authorized organizations feeding the hungry.

food insecurity: limited or uncertain access to foods of sufficient quality or quantity to sustain a healthy and active life.

food insufficiency: an inadequate amount of food due to a lack of resources.

food pantries: programs that provide groceries to be prepared and eaten at home.

food poverty: hunger resulting from inadequate access to available food for various reasons, including inadequate resources, political obstacles, social disruptions, poor weather conditions, and lack of transportation.

food recovery: collecting wholesome food for distribution to low-income people who are hungry. Four common methods of food recovery are:

- *Field gleaning:* collecting crops from fields that either have already been harvested or are not profitable to harvest.
- *Perishable food rescue or salvage:* collecting perishable produce from wholesalers and markets.
- *Prepared food rescue:* collecting prepared foods from commercial kitchens.
- *Nonperishable food collection:* collecting processed foods from wholesalers and markets.

food security: certain access to enough food for all people at all times to sustain a healthy and active life.

HOW TO Identify Food Insecurity in a U.S. Household

To determine the extent of food insecurity in a household, surveys ask the following questions. These questions reflect stages people in a household experience as food insecurity becomes progressively worse. Positive responses to the first several questions identify those who have concerns about their food supplies and food budgets and make adjustments to meet their basic needs. As food insecurity worsens, the middle questions identify adults who experience hunger and eat less. Most often, adults tend to protect their children from this experience. In the most severe cases, children also suffer from hunger and eat less.

- We worried whether our food would run out before we got money to buy more.
- The food that we bought just didn't last, and we didn't have money to get more.
- We couldn't afford to eat balanced meals.
- We relied on only a few kinds of low-cost food to feed our children because we were running out of money to buy food.
- We couldn't feed our children a balanced meal because we couldn't afford that.
- Our children were not eating enough because we just couldn't afford enough food.
- In the last 12 months, did you or other adults in your household ever cut the size of your meals or skip meals because there wasn't enough money for food?
- How often did this happen? (Considered a positive response if it occurred in three or more months during the previous year.)
- In the last 12 months, did you ever eat less than you felt you should because there wasn't enough money for food?
- In the last 12 months, were you ever hungry but didn't eat because you couldn't afford enough food?
- In the last 12 months, did you lose weight because you didn't have enough money for food?
- In the last 12 months, did you or other adults in your household ever not eat for a whole day because there wasn't enough money for food?
- How often did this happen? (Considered a positive response if it occurred in three or more months during the previous year.)
- In the last 12 months, did you ever cut the size of your children's meals because there wasn't enough money for food?
- In the last 12 months, were the children ever hungry but you just couldn't afford more food?
- In the last 12 months, did your children ever skip a meal because there wasn't enough money for food?
- How often did this happen? (Considered a positive response if it occurred in three or more months during the previous year.)
- In the last 12 months, did your children ever not eat for a whole day because there wasn't enough money for food?

The more positive responses, the greater the food insecurity. Households with children answer all of the questions and are categorized as follows:

$\leq$2 positive responses = food secure.
3–7 positive responses = food insecure without hunger.
$\geq$8 positive responses = food insecure with hunger.

Households without children answer fewer questions and are categorized as follows:

$\leq$2 positive responses = food secure.
3–5 positive responses = food insecure without hunger.
$\geq$6 positive responses = food insecure with hunger.

Figure H16-1 (below) shows the results of the 2003 surveys.

FIGURE H16-1 Prevalence of Food Insecurity and Hunger in U.S. Households, 2003

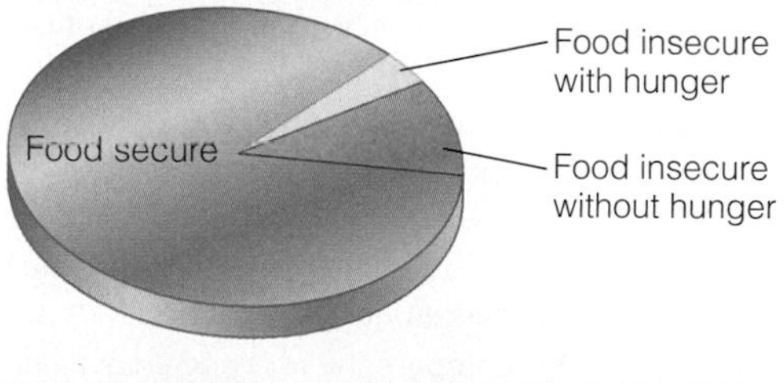
Food insecure
with hunger
Food secure
Food insecure
without hunger

SOURCE: Economic Research Service, U.S. Department of Agriculture, **www.ers.usda.gov/Briefing/FoodSecurity/** updated November 19, 2004 and visited on March 30, 2005.

and disabilities, unemployment, low-paying jobs, unexpected or ongoing medical expenses, and high living expenses threaten their financial stability. When money is tight, people are forced to choose between food and life's other necessities—utilities, housing, and medical care.[4] Food costs are more variable and flexible; a person can purchase fewer groceries to lower the monthly food bill, but usually can't pay only a portion of the bills for electricity, rent, or medication. Further contributing to food poverty are other problems such as abuse of alcohol and other drugs; lack of awareness of available food assistance programs; and the reluctance of people, particularly the elderly, to accept what they perceive as "welfare" or "charity." Lack of resources remains the major cause of food poverty, and solving this problem would do a lot to relieve hunger.

In the United States, poverty and hunger reach across various segments of society, touching single mothers living in households with their children; Hispanics, Native Americans, and African Americans; and those living in the inner cities more than others. People living in poverty are simply unable to buy sufficient amounts of nourishing foods, even if they are wise shoppers. For many of the children in these families, school lunch (and breakfast, where available) may be the only nourishment for the day. Otherwise they go hungry, waiting for an adult to find money for food. Not surprisingly, these children perform poorly in school and in social situations.[5]

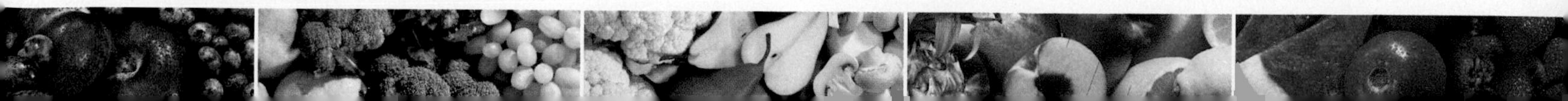

Relieving Hunger in the United States

The American Dietetic Association (ADA) calls for aggressive action to bring an end to domestic food insecurity and hunger and to achieve food and nutrition security for everybody living in the United States.[6] Many federal and local programs aim to prevent or relieve malnutrition and hunger in the United States.

Federal Food Assistance Programs

Adequate nutrition and food security are essential in supporting good health and achieving the public health goals of the United States.[7] To that end, an extensive network of federal assistance programs provides life-giving food daily to millions of U.S. citizens. One out of every six Americans receives food assistance of some kind, at a total cost of almost $40 billion per year. Even so, the programs are not fully successful in preventing hunger, but they do seem to improve the nutrient intakes of those who participate. Programs described in earlier chapters include the WIC program for low-income pregnant women, breastfeeding mothers, and their young children (Chapter 14); the school lunch, breakfast, and child-care food programs for children (Chapter 15); and the food assistance programs for older adults such as congregate meals and Meals on Wheels (Chapter 16).

The Food Stamp Program, administered by the U.S. Department of Agriculture (USDA), is the largest of the federal food assistance programs, both in amount of money spent and in number of people served. It provides assistance to almost 20 million people at a cost of over $20 billion per year; over half of the recipients are children.[8] The USDA issues food stamp coupons or debit cards through state agencies to households—people who buy and prepare food together. The amount a household receives depends on its size, resources, and income. The average monthly benefit is about $80 per person.[9] Recipients may use the coupons or cards like cash to purchase food and food-bearing plants and seeds, but not to buy tobacco, cleaning items, alcohol, or other nonfood items. The accompanying "How to" offers shopping tips for those on a limited budget.

The Food Stamp Program improves nutrient intakes significantly, but hunger continues to plague the United States. Of the estimated 2 million homeless people in the United States who are eligible for food assistance, only 15 percent of single adults and 50 percent of families receive food stamps.

National Food Recovery Programs

Efforts to resolve the problem of hunger in the United States do not depend solely on federal assistance programs. National **food recovery** programs have made a dramatic difference. The largest program, Second Harvest, coordinates the efforts of more than 250 **food pantries, emergency kitchens,** and homeless shelters in providing more than 1 billion pounds of food to 45,000 local agencies that feed over 23 million people a year.

Each year, an estimated one-fifth of our food supply is wasted in fields, commercial kitchens, grocery stores, and

HOW TO Plan Healthy, Thrifty Meals

Chapter 2 introduced the USDA Food Guide and principles for planning a healthy diet. Meeting that goal on a limited budget adds to the challenge. To save money and spend wisely, plan and shop for healthy meals with the following tips in mind:

Planning

- Make a grocery list before going to the store to avoid expensive "impulse" items. Do not shop when hungry.
- Use leftovers.
- Center meals on rice, noodles, and other grains.
- Use small quantities of meat, poultry, fish, or eggs.
- Use legumes instead of meat, poultry, fish, or eggs several times a week.
- Use cooked cereals such as oatmeal instead of ready-to-eat breakfast cereals.
- Cook large quantities when time and money allow.
- Check for sales and clip coupons for products you need; plan meals to take advantage of sale items.

Shopping

- Buy day-old bread and other products from the bakery outlet.
- Select whole foods instead of convenience foods (potatoes instead of instant mashed potatoes, for example).
- Try store brands.
- Buy fresh produce that is in season; buy canned or frozen items at other times.
- Buy only the amount of fresh food that you will eat before it spoils. Buy large bags of frozen items or dry goods; when cooking, take out the amount needed and store the remainder.
- Buy fat-free dry milk; mix and refrigerate quantities needed for a day or two. Buy fresh milk by the gallon or half-gallon.
- Buy less expensive cuts of meat. Chuck and bottom round roast are usually inexpensive; cover during cooking and cook long enough to make meat tender. Buy whole chickens instead of pieces.
- Compare the unit price (cost per ounce, for example) of similar foods so that you can select the least expensive brand or size.
- Buy nonfood items such as toilet paper and laundry detergent at discount stores instead of grocery stores.

For daily menus and recipes for healthy, thrifty meals, visit the USDA Center for Nutrition Policy and Promotion: **www.usda.gov/cnpp**

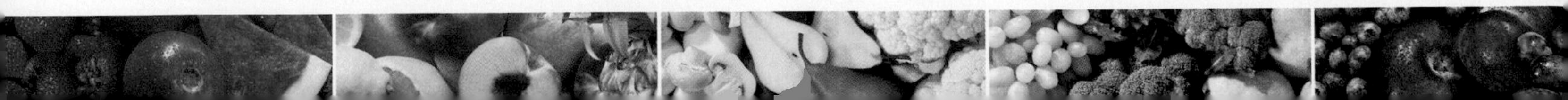

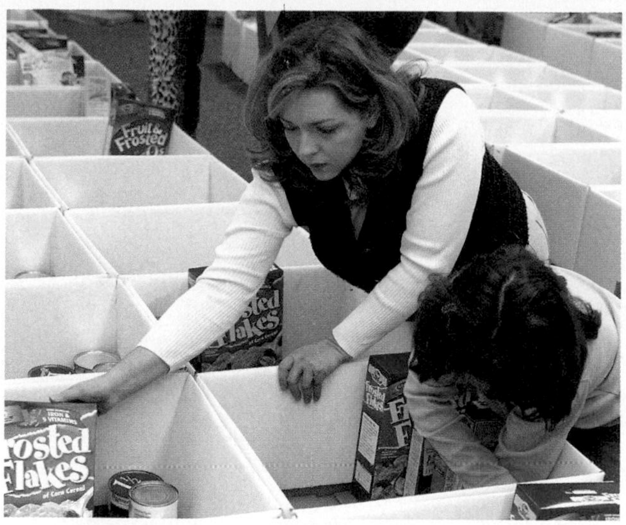
AP/Wide World Photos

Food banks depend on the helping hands of caring volunteers.

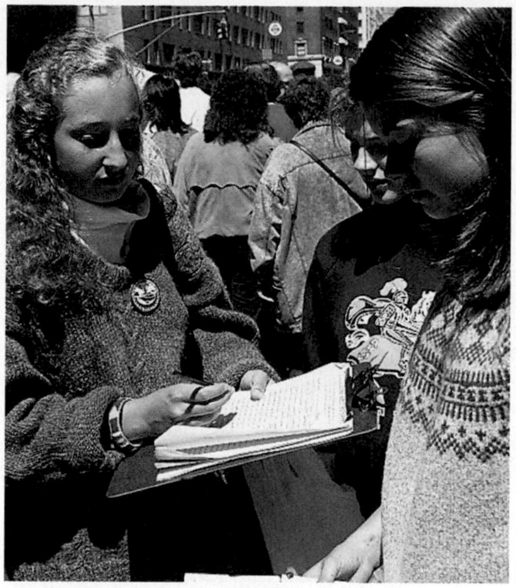
© Elsa Peterson-Stock Boston

Each person's choice to get involved and be heard can help lead to needed change.

restaurants—that's enough food to feed 49 million people. Food recovery programs collect and distribute good food that would otherwise go to waste. Volunteers might pick corn left in an already harvested field, a grocer might deliver ripe bananas to a local **food bank,** and a caterer might take leftover chicken salad to a community shelter, for example. All of these efforts help to feed the hungry in the United States.

Community Efforts

Food recovery programs depend on volunteers. Concerned citizens work through local agencies and churches to feed the hungry. Community-based food pantries provide groceries, and soup kitchens serve prepared meals. Meals often deliver adequate nourishment, but most homeless people receive fewer than one and a half meals a day, so many are still inadequately nourished.

Solutions

Every segment of our society can join in the fight against hunger and poverty. The federal government, the states, local communities, big business and small companies, educators, and all individuals, including dietitians and foodservice managers, have many opportunities to resolve these problems.

Government policies can direct tax dollars and other resources to develop energy conservation services and crop protection. Businesses can support antihunger programs. Many grocery stores and restaurants participate in food recovery programs by giving their leftover foods to community distribution centers.

Educators, including nutrition educators, can teach others about the underlying social and political causes of poverty, the root cause of hunger. At the college level, they can teach the relationships between hunger and population, hunger and environmental degradation, hunger and the status of women, and hunger and global economics. They can advocate legislation to address these problems. They can teach the poor to develop and run nutrition programs in their own communities and to fight on their own behalf for antipoverty, antihunger legislation.

Dietitians and foodservice managers have a special role to play, and their efforts can make an impressive difference. Their professional organization, the ADA, urges members to conserve resources and minimize waste in both their professional and their personal lives.[10] In addition, the ADA urges its members to educate themselves and others on hunger, its consequences, and programs to fight it; to conduct research on the effectiveness and benefits of programs; and to serve as advocates on the local, state, and national levels to help end hunger in the United States.[11] Globally, the ADA supports programs that combat malnutrition, provide food security, promote self-sufficiency, respect local cultures, protect the environment, and sustain the economy.[12]

Individuals can assist the global community in solving its poverty and hunger problems by joining and working for hunger-relief organizations (see Table H16-1 on p. 578). They can also support organizations that lobby for the needed changes in economic policies toward developing countries.

"Be part of the solution, not part of the problem," an adage says. In other words, don't waste time or energy moaning and groaning about how bad things are: do something to improve them. Your choice to get involved in the fight against hunger—whether in your community or across the globe—can make a big difference in the health and survival of others.

TABLE 16-1 Hunger-Relief Organizations

Action without Borders
79 Fifth Ave., 17th Floor
New York, NY 10118
(212) 843-3973
www.idealist.org

Bread for the World
50 F St. NW, Suite 500
Washington, DC 20001
(800) 82-BREAD or (800) 822-7323
(202) 639-9400; fax (202) 639-9401
www.bread.org

Center on Hunger and Poverty
Brandeis University
Mailstop 077
Waltham, MA 02454
(781) 736-8885
www.centeronhunger.org

Community Food Security Coalition
P.O. Box 909
Venice, CA 90294
(310) 822-5410
www.foodsecurity.org

Congressional Hunger Center
229½ Pennsylvania Ave.
Washington, DC 20003
(202) 547-7022
www.hungercenter.org

Oxfam America
26 West St.
Boston, MA 02111-1206
(800) 77-OXFAM or
(800) 776-9326
www.oxfamamerica.org

Pan American Health Organization
525 23rd St. NW
Washington, DC 20037
(202) 974-3000
www.paho.org

Second Harvest
35 E. Wacker Dr., #2000
Chicago, IL 60601
(800) 771-2303
www.secondharvest.org

Society of St. Andrew
3383 Sweet Hollow Rd.
Big Island, VA 24526
(800) 333-4597
www.endhunger.org

Food and Agriculture Organization (FAO) of the United Nations
2175 K St. NW, Suite 300
Washington, DC 20437
(202) 653-2400
www.fao.org

United Nations Children's Fund (UNICEF)
3 United Nations Plaza
New York, NY 10017-4414
(212) 326-7035
www.unicef.org

World Food Program
Via Vittorio Emanuele Orlando, 83
Rome, Italy 00148
www.wfp.org

World Health Organization (WHO)
525 23rd St. NW
Washington, DC 20037
(202) 974-3000
www.who.org

World Hunger Program
Brown University
Box 1831
Providence, RI 02912
(401) 863-1000

World Hunger Year (WHY)
505 Eighth Ave., 21st Floor
New York, NY 10018-6582
(800) GleanIt
www.worldhungeryear.org

HungerWeb
Tufts University
nutrition.tufts.edu/academic/hungerweb

REFERENCES

1. United States Department of Agriculture, *Household Food Security in the United States, 2001,* ERS Food Assistance and Nutrition Research Report no. FANRR-29, October 2002, available from www.ers.usda.gov/publications/fanrr29.
2. J. S. Hampl and R. Hill, Dietetic approaches to US hunger and food insecurity, *Journal of the American Dietetic Association* 102 (2002): 919–923.
3. K. M. Kempson and coauthors, Food management practices used by people with limited resources to maintain food sufficiency as reported by nutrition educators, *Journal of the American Dietetic Association* 102 (2002): 1795–1799.
4. M. Kim, J. Ohls, and R. Cohen, *Hunger in America, 2001—National Report Prepared for America's Second Harvest* (Princeton, N.J.: Mathematica Policy Research, Inc., 2001).
5. K. Alaimo, C. M. Olson, and E. A. Frongillo, Jr., Food insufficiency and American school-aged children's cognitive, academic, and psychosocial development, *Pediatrics* 108 (2001): 44–53.
6. Position of the American Dietetic Association: Domestic food and nutrition security, *Journal of the American Dietetic Association* 102 (2002): 1840–1847.
7. Position of the American Dietetic Association, 2002.
8. USDA Food and Nutrition Service, www.fns.usda.gov/, site visited June 3, 2003.
9. USDA Food and Nutrition Service, 2002 data, www.fns.usda.gov/pd/fsavgben.htm.
10. Position of the American Dietetic Association: Dietetic professionals can implement practices to conserve natural resources and protect the environment, *Journal of the American Dietetic Association* 101 (2001): 1221–1227.
11. Position of the American Dietetic Association, 2002.
12. Position of the American Dietetic Association: Addressing world hunger, malnutrition, and food insecurity, *Journal of the American Dietetic Association* 103 (2003): 1046–1057.

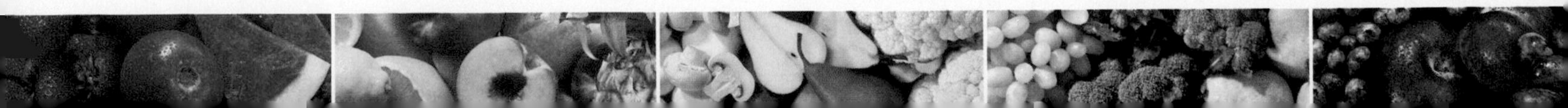

Chapter 17

Nutrition Care and Assessment

Chapter Outline

Available Online

http://nutrition.wadsworth.com/uncn7

Student Practice Test

Glossary Terms

Nutrition on the Net

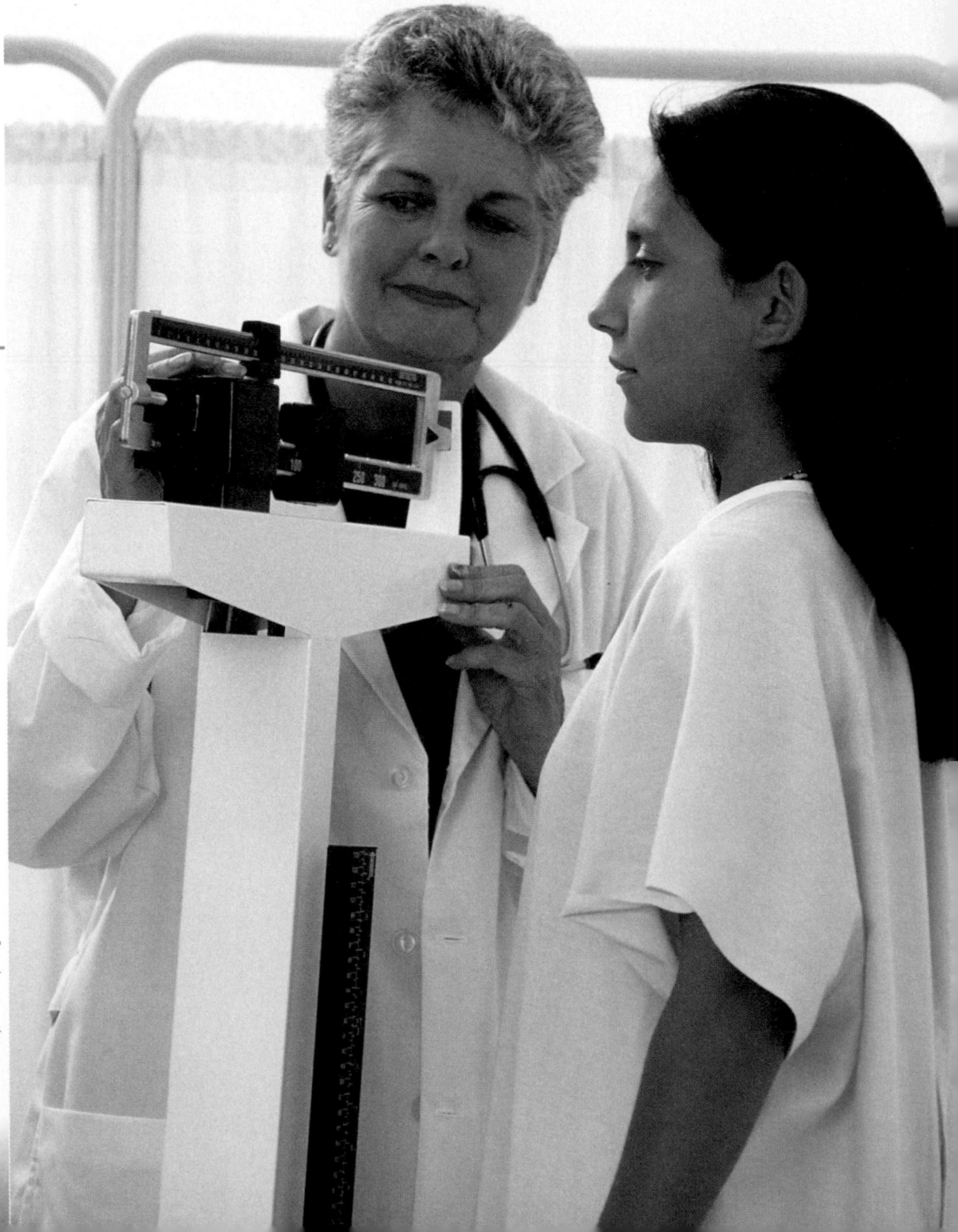

Nutrition in the Professional Setting

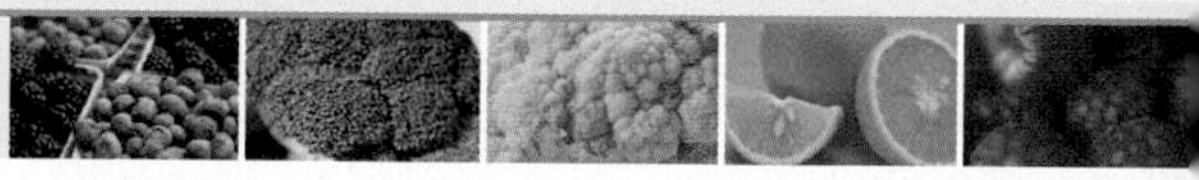

For a busy health practitioner, it can be easy to put a patient's nutrition needs on the back burner. After all, the benefits of diet therapy are not always as obvious or immediate as those of other medical treatments. Health practitioners who want to provide the best care for their patients, however, soon learn that an appropriate diet can improve both short-term and long-term outcomes of many disease treatments. Moreover, patients are often concerned about the impact their diet has on their disease condition. The remaining chapters of this book will show how dietary treatments can improve the quality of life for people who have become ill.

Earlier chapters of this book presented the nutrients and their roles in supporting health. Turning now to clinical nutrition, the remaining chapters describe how various medical conditions can affect nutrition status and nutrient needs. Health care professionals who include appropriate nutrition care in treatment decisions are best prepared to help patients recover from disease and maintain an optimal quality of life. This chapter focuses on the interrelationships between nutrition status and illness, the process used for providing nutrition care, and the components of nutrition assessment.

Nutrition in Health Care

Many medical conditions can alter nutrient needs and lead to malnutrition. Moreover, poor nutrition status can influence both the course of disease and the body's response to treatment. Malnutrition has been reported in 40 to 60 percent of patients hospitalized with acute illness, and patients with no nutrition problems often exhibit a decline in nutrition status within three weeks of admission.[1]

Recognizing and treating nutrition problems early in the disease process can improve the effectiveness of medical treatment and prevent complications. For this reason, a registered dietitian■ or similarly trained nutrition professional provides **medical nutrition therapy** services to assess, diagnose, and treat any nutrition problems that may arise during the course of disease management. These services may also include preventive nutrition programs and nutrition education services.[2]

■ Reminder: A *registered dietitian* is a nutrition professional who has met the minimum academic and professional requirements to qualify for the RD credential conferred by the American Dietetic Association. Minimum requirements include a bachelor's degree in nutrition or dietetics, a supervised internship, and the successful completion of a national examination.

Illness and Nutrition Status

An illness, its symptoms, and its treatments can lead to malnutrition by reducing food intake, impairing digestion and absorption, or altering nutrient metabolism and excretion (see Figure 17-1). For example, the nausea of foodborne illness or of cancer treatment may diminish appetite and reduce food intake; similarly, burns on the hands may make the physical act of eating uncomfortable, reducing food intake. Surgeries often require temporary dietary restrictions. The potential effects of medications (described in Chapter 19) are extensive and may include anorexia, gastrointestinal discomfort, or interference with the normal function and metabolism of nutrients. In many cases, the dietary changes required during illness are temporary and may be tailored to accommodate an individual's preferences and lifestyle. Other cases, notably chronic illnesses, may require long-term dietary modifications. For example, prevention of atherosclerosis■ may require lifelong changes in diet and lifestyle that some people may find difficult or unacceptable. The challenge for health professionals is to help these people appreciate the potential benefits and accept dietary changes that can improve their health.

■ Reminder: *Atherosclerosis* is a type of artery disease characterized by plaques along the inner walls of arteries.

In addition to the direct effects of illness on nutrition status, the cost of health care can drain financial resources and may limit ability to obtain high-quality foods. Some individuals may lack the space and equipment necessary to store and prepare special meals. Emotional health may also suffer as a result of chronic disease or terminal illness, and this can influence nutrition status as well (see Highlight 29).

medical nutrition therapy: nutrition care provided by a registered dietitian; includes diagnosing nutrition problems, prescribing diet plans, and providing dietary counseling.

FIGURE 17-1 Ways in Which Illness Can Affect Nutrition Status

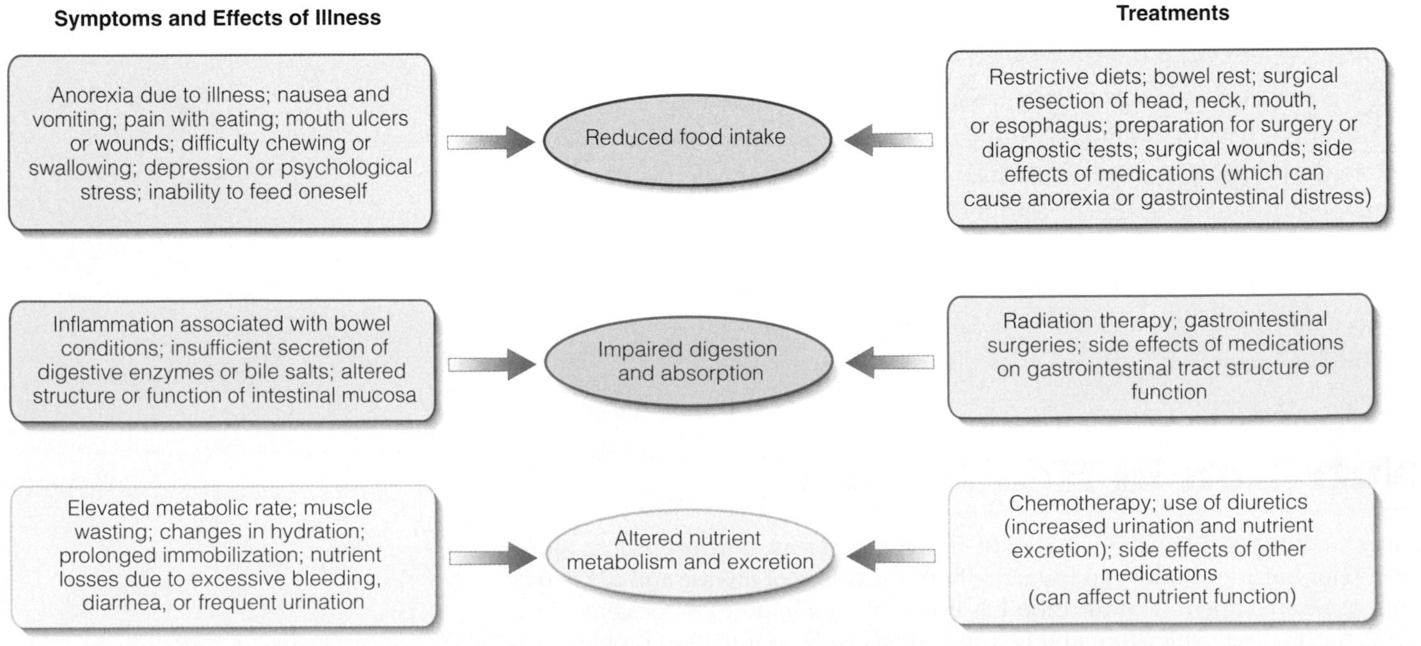
Symptoms and Effects of Illness
Treatments
Anorexia due to illness; nausea and vomiting; pain with eating; mouth ulcers or wounds; difficulty chewing or swallowing; depression or psychological stress; inability to feed oneself
Reduced food intake
Restrictive diets; bowel rest; surgical resection of head, neck, mouth, or esophagus; preparation for surgery or diagnostic tests; surgical wounds; side effects of medications (which can cause anorexia or gastrointestinal distress)
Inflammation associated with bowel conditions; insufficient secretion of digestive enzymes or bile salts; altered structure or function of intestinal mucosa
Impaired digestion and absorption
Radiation therapy; gastrointestinal surgeries; side effects of medications on gastrointestinal tract structure or function
Elevated metabolic rate; muscle wasting; changes in hydration; prolonged immobilization; nutrient losses due to excessive bleeding, diarrhea, or frequent urination
Altered nutrient metabolism and excretion
Chemotherapy; use of diuretics (increased urination and nutrient excretion); side effects of other medications (can affect nutrient function)

Health Professionals and Nutrition Care

The members of a health care team work together to ensure that the nutritional needs of an individual are met during illness. Their roles in nutrition care may overlap, and job descriptions in different institutions vary. In some cases, nutrition care is incorporated into the medical care plan developed by the entire health care team. Such plans, called **critical pathways** (or **clinical pathways**), outline coordinated plans of care for specific medical diagnoses, treatments, or procedures. This section describes the general roles of several different health care practitioners.

Physicians Physicians are responsible for all of a patient's medical needs, including nutrition. They may prescribe **diet orders** and other orders related to nutrition care, including those for nutrition assessment and diet counseling. Physicians rely on registered dietitians, nurses, and other health care professionals to alert them to nutrition problems, suggest strategies for handling nutrition problems, and provide nutrition services.

Registered Dietitians Registered dietitians have extensive knowledge about foods and human nutrition and are uniquely qualified to provide medical nutrition therapy. Dietitians conduct nutrition and dietary assessments; diagnose nutritional problems; develop, implement, and evaluate **nutrition care plans** (described in a later section); and plan and approve menus. They often work as managers of food and cafeteria services in health care institutions. Dietitians frequently depend on other health care professionals to alert them to patients who are having nutrition-related problems.

Registered dietitians stay abreast of the latest developments in clinical nutrition using publications and resources provided by the American Dietetic Association (ADA), the largest organization of nutrition professionals in the United States. Current dietary protocols for different medical conditions are available from clinical dietetics manuals compiled by the ADA, state dietetics organizations, or the dietetics staff at health care institutions.

Nurses Nurses interact frequently with patients and thus are in an ideal position to identify people who would benefit from nutrition services. Nurses often screen patients for nutrition problems and may participate in nutrition and dietary assessments. Certain nursing diagnoses may help to identify potential nutritional problems, as shown by the examples listed in Table 17-1. Nurses also provide direct nutrition care, such as encouraging patients to eat, finding practical solutions to food-related problems, recording a patient's food intake, and answering questions about special diets. **Nutrition support teams** (discussed in Chapter 21) rely on nurses to administer tube and intravenous feedings. In facilities that do not employ registered dietitians, nurses often assume responsibility for much of the nutrition care.

Registered Dietetic Technicians Registered dietetic technicians work in partnership with registered dietitians and assist in the implementation and monitoring of nutrition services. Depending on their background and experience, they may screen patients for nutrition problems, provide patient education and counseling, develop menus and recipes, ensure appropriate meal delivery, and monitor patients' food choices and intakes. Dietetic technicians often have supervisory positions in foodservice operations and may have roles in purchasing, inventory, quality control, sanitation, or safety.

Other Health Care Professionals Other heath care professionals may also assist with nutrition care. Pharmacists, physical therapists, occupational therapists, speech therapists, social workers, nursing assistants, and home health care aides can be instrumental in alerting dietitians or nurses to nutrition problems or may share relevant information about a patient's health status or personal needs.

TABLE 17-1 Examples of Nursing Diagnoses with Nutritional Implications

- Altered nutrition: more than body requirements
- Altered nutrition: less than body requirements
- Altered nutrition: risk for more than body requirements
- Chronic confusion
- Chronic pain
- Chronic sorrow
- Constipation
- Diarrhea
- Disturbed body image
- Feeding self-care deficit
- Impaired dentition
- Impaired oral mucous membrane
- Impaired physical mobility
- Impaired swallowing
- Nausea
- Risk for aspiration

SOURCE: North American Nursing Diagnoses Association (NANDA) Accepted Nursing Diagnoses.

critical pathways (or **clinical pathways**): interdisciplinary care plans for specific diagnoses, treatments, or procedures that merge the medical and nursing plans with those of other disciplines, such as physical therapy, nutrition, and mental health.

diet orders: specific instructions for dietary management; also called **diet prescriptions.**

nutrition care plans: strategies for meeting an individual's nutritional needs.

nutrition support teams: health care professionals responsible for the provision of nutrients by tube feedings or intravenous infusion.

TABLE 17-2 Useful Criteria for Identifying Nutritional Risks

- Age, medical diagnosis, severity of illness
- Height and weight, BMI, recent unintentional weight changes
- Recent changes in appetite or food intake
- Results of laboratory tests that indicate general health status (like albumin levels) or the presence of anemia or tissue wasting
- Use of medications and dietary supplements
- Dietary modifications prescribed for medical purposes
- Problems or symptoms that may make eating difficult (for example, problems with chewing or swallowing, nausea and vomiting, diarrhea, or constipation)
- Food allergies or intolerances
- History of diabetes, renal disease, or other chronic illness
- Presence of pressure sores or other skin conditions
- Depression or social isolation

Quality of Care

The **Joint Commission on Accreditation of Healthcare Organizations (JCAHO)** has developed an accreditation process that helps to ensure high-quality health care. This independent, nonprofit organization sets high standards for health care performance and safety and awards accreditation to health care organizations based on how well these standards are met. A team of JCAHO professionals conducts extensive on-site reviews at least once every three years to make accreditation decisions, which are available to the public on the organization's website (**www.jcaho.org**).

Nutrition Screening

The JCAHO has specified that **nutrition screening** be conducted within 24 hours of a patient's admission to a hospital (or other extended-care facility) to identify those who may need more extensive assessment and follow-up care. An effective screening process should be accurate enough to identify nutritional risk, yet simple enough to be completed within 5 to 15 minutes. Often a nurse, nursing assistant, registered dietitian, or dietetic technician performs and documents the screening, which varies according to the patient population, the type of care offered by the health care facility, and the patient's medical problem. The information used in screening includes the admitting diagnosis, information from the medical record, physical measurements and lab results collected during the admission process, and responses given by the patient or caregiver to an interview or questionnaire. Table 17-2 lists examples of information collected during screening that help to identify those who have a high risk of developing malnutrition.

Nutrition screening is often included in outpatient services and community health programs. The **Nutrition Screening Initiative** is a project sponsored by more than 25 national health and social services organizations to promote nutrition screening in the elderly. They have developed several screening tools, including the "DETERMINE Your Nutritional Health" checklist (see Figure 16-4 on p. 568) for use by individuals or community programs. The "determine" mnemonic aid for remembering the common warning signs of malnutrition is shown in the margin.■ Additional screening tools are more complex and need to be administered by trained health professionals.

■ Risk factors for malnutrition in older persons:
*D*isease.
*E*ating poorly.
*T*ooth loss or mouth pain.
*E*conomic hardship.
*R*educed social contact.
*M*ultiple medications.
*I*nvoluntary weight loss or gain.
*N*eed for assistance in self-care.
*E*lder years (above age 80).

A nutrition or health screening often leads to a referral for nutrition care. The following section describes the next step in the process: the method used by dietitians to address nutritional concerns.

The Nutrition Care Process

Registered dietitians use a systematic, logical approach to nutrition care called the **nutrition care process.** Figure 17-2 presents the four distinct, yet interrelated, steps of the nutrition care process:[3]

1. Nutrition assessment.
2. Nutrition diagnosis.
3. Nutrition intervention.
4. Nutrition monitoring and evaluation.

The nutrition care process is easiest to visualize as a series of steps, but in reality, the steps are frequently revisited in order to reassess and revise diagnoses and intervention strategies.[4] Follow-up visits are often required during nutrition care, so the cycle may be repeated until the desired outcomes have been accomplished. The discussion in this chapter focuses on individuals, but the nutrition care process can also be applied to groups or communities.

Joint Commission on Accreditation of Healthcare Organizations (JCAHO): a nonprofit organization that sets standards for health care performance and safety and awards accreditation to health care organizations that meet these standards.

nutrition screening: an examination process that identifies patients who require intervention for existing or potential nutritional problems.

Nutrition Screening Initiative: a collaboration by health, social service, and medical organizations that promotes nutrition screening in the elderly.

nutrition care process: an organized approach to nutrition care that consists of assessing, diagnosing, intervening, monitoring, and evaluating the patient's problems and progress.

Documentation at each step of the nutrition care process provides a record for future reference and facilitates communication among members of the health care team. The medical record is a legal document, and entries must follow the format specified by the hospital or health care facility that maintains the record. Documentation is discussed further in Chapter 18.

Nutrition Assessment Nutrition assessment, the first step of the nutrition care process, involves the collection of information needed to evaluate a patient's nutrition status and nutrient needs. The assessment data are used to develop a plan of action to prevent or correct any nutrient imbalances. Assessments are also done after nutrition care to help determine whether a care plan is working.

Remember that malnutrition can be caused by an illness or medical treatment and not just by inadequate dietary intake.■ To help determine the cause of a deficiency and therefore the best course of intervention, nutrition assessments draw on many sources of information including:

- Medical, social, and diet histories.
- Anthropometric data.
- Biochemical analyses.
- Physical examinations.

A meaningful assessment depends on both accurate information and a careful interpretation of findings. The second half of this chapter will describe each of the components of nutrition assessment in more detail.

Nutrition Diagnosis After completing a nutrition assessment, the dietitian can identify existing or potential nutrition problems and formulate specific nutrition diagnoses.[5] This step requires careful and objective analysis of the patterns and relationships among the data. Each problem receives a separate diagnosis, which is documented in the medical chart. Nutrition diagnoses, similar to nursing diagnoses, are stated in a format that includes the specific nutrition problem, the etiology or cause, and the signs and symptoms that provide evidence of the problem.■ For example, a nutrition diagnosis might state, "Unintentional weight loss *(the problem)* related to insufficient kcaloric intake *(the etiology or cause)* as evidenced by a 10-pound weight loss (representing 8 percent of body weight) in the past few months *(the sign or symptom)*." Note that unlike medical diagnoses, a nutrition diagnosis can change during the course of an illness.

Nutrition Intervention After nutrition problems have been identified, the appropriate treatments can be determined. The nutrition care plan typically includes behaviors and educational materials that can improve risk factors and correct nutrition problems.[6] For example, an intervention may include dietary modifications, nutrition handouts, or a change in medication. It should take into account an individual's food habits, lifestyle patterns, and other personal factors. To ensure cost-effective and high-quality implementation, the plan must be consistent with the care plans of other members of the health care team. Nutrition interventions used by dietitians are "evidence based"; that is, they are based on scientific rationale and supported by the results of high-quality research.

Goals of nutrition interventions are stated in terms of measurable outcomes, such as results of laboratory tests or anthropometric data. For example, the measurable outcomes for an overweight person with diabetes might include target ranges for blood glucose levels and body weight. Other important outcomes include positive changes in dietary behaviors and lifestyle: an interview with a heart disease patient may reveal that he or she has learned to use leaner cuts of meat and low-fat milk products and has started a regular walking program. Chapter 18 gives additional information about nutrition intervention.

Nutrition Monitoring and Evaluation After a nutrition intervention has begun, the effectiveness of the nutrition care plan must be evaluated. The original goals and outcome measures are typically reviewed at previously designated dates

FIGURE 17-2 The Nutrition Care Process

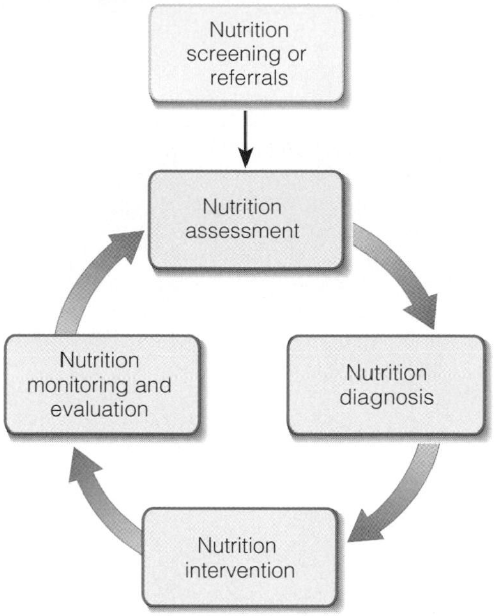
Nutrition screening or referrals
Nutrition assessment
Nutrition diagnosis
Nutrition intervention
Nutrition monitoring and evaluation

■ Reminder: A *primary* nutrient deficiency is caused by inadequate dietary intake, whereas a *secondary* nutrient deficiency may be caused by reduced nutrient absorption, changes in nutrient utilization within the body, increased losses of a nutrient, or increased nutrient needs.

■ This format is called the **PES Format** because it includes the **P**roblem, the **E**tiology, and the **S**igns and symptoms.

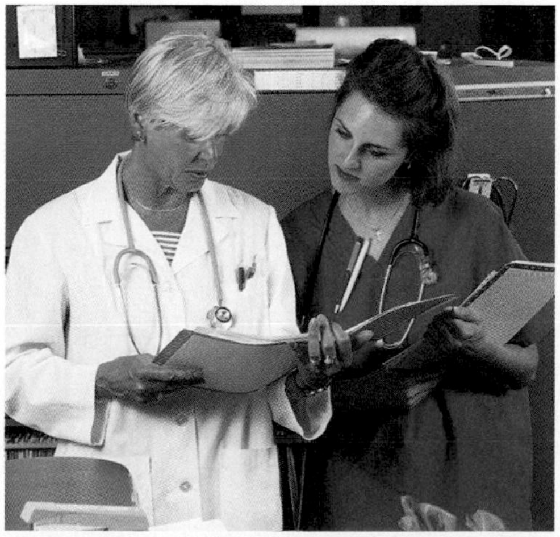

The medical record facilitates communication among members of the health care team.

and compared with earlier assessment data and diagnoses. Sometimes the patient's situation changes in a way that alters nutritional needs; for example, a change in medical treatment or medication may alter the ability to tolerate certain foods. A nutrition care plan needs to be flexible to adapt to the new situation.

If a patient is unable or unwilling to make the suggested changes, even the best plan will fall short of meeting goals. In this case, the care plan must be redesigned and should take into account why the previous plan was not successful. This new plan may need to include motivational techniques or additional patient education. When a patient is unwilling to modify behaviors despite the benefits that change might bring, little can be done except to try again at a later time when the patient may be more receptive.

IN SUMMARY Illness, its symptoms, and its treatments can affect food intake and nutrient metabolism, thereby leading to malnutrition. In turn, poor nutrition can reduce the effectiveness of medical treatment. The dietary treatment provided depends on a patient's medical condition and nutrition status and may require either short-term or long-term dietary and lifestyle changes. Nutrition screening identifies individuals who can benefit from nutrition assessment and follow-up care. A registered dietitian usually plays the primary role in developing a nutrition care plan, diagnosing nutrition problems, and counseling patients about dietary changes. A nutrition care plan includes four interrelated steps: nutrition assessment, nutrition diagnosis, nutrition intervention, and nutrition monitoring and evaluation.

Nutrition Assessment

As discussed earlier, a nutrition assessment provides the information needed to evaluate a person's nutrition status. With this information, a health care professional can diagnose problems and develop a nutrition care plan to prevent or correct imbalances. Follow-up assessments help to determine if the care plan is effective. Ideally, the assessment tools are sensitive enough to detect subtle nutrition problems and specific enough to identify problem nutrients. For most nutrient imbalances, no single test is adequate, and a variety of tests are needed to determine nutrition status. The remainder of this chapter discusses the types of information and measures that are most commonly used in a nutrition assessment.

Historical Information

Historical information reveals valuable clues about factors that influence nutrition status and nutrient requirements, as well as the personal preferences that need to be considered when developing a nutrition care plan. Table 17-3 summarizes the elements of medical, social, and diet histories that contribute to a comprehensive nutrition assessment.[7] Generally, this information can be obtained from the medical record or by an interview with the patient or caregiver.

TABLE 17-3 Historical Information Used in Nutrition Assessment

Medical History	Social History	Diet History
Current complaint(s)	Socioeconomic status	Dietary pattern
Past medical condition(s)	Cultural/ethnic identity	Dietary restrictions
Family history of illness	Educational level	Use of alcohol
Surgical history	Living situation	Food allergies and intolerances
Medication history	Shopping arrangements	Chewing and swallowing ability
Use of dietary/herbal supplements	Cooking facilities	Need for feeding assistance

Medical History Many medical conditions and their treatments have nutrition-related implications. Table 17-4 lists medical conditions that have been associated with a high risk of nutritional problems.[8] Many other conditions may also lead to malnutrition, especially if imbalances are not recognized and corrected. A review of the medical history can help to determine if specific dietary modifications are desirable or if food intake is likely to be affected by illness. Factors such as age, gender, and weight also need to be considered when assessing nutritional risk.

A medical history includes a survey of prescription drugs, over-the-counter medications, and dietary supplements that are used by the patient. As described in Chapter 19, some medications have deleterious effects on nutrition status, and some dietary components may alter the absorption and metabolism of drugs. For these reasons, the use of medications needs to be considered when planning nutrition care.

Social History Social factors influence food choices and an individual's ability to handle health and nutrition problems. For example, cultural heritage can affect food preferences. Financial concerns can limit a family's access to medical care or place a nutritious diet out of reach. If an individual depends on a family member to prepare food or make health care decisions, that person needs to participate in the nutrition care process. A person who lives alone or is depressed is less likely to eat well and may find it difficult or impossible to follow complex dietary instructions.

Diet History The **diet history** is a comprehensive record of past dietary practices. Information is collected about usual food intake, meal patterns, and lifestyle habits. Although different methods exist for obtaining data, the procedure often includes an interview about recent food intake (for example, a 24-hour recall) and a survey about usual food choices (such as a food frequency questionnaire). Because dietary intake is also influenced by an individual's health status, a diet history may include questions about food allergies and intolerances, physical disabilities, and the need for assistance during feeding. A good diet history can uncover current or potential nutrient imbalances and patterns of behavior that can contribute to health problems. The following section discusses the most common methods used for gathering food intake information.

TABLE 17-4 Medical Conditions Associated with High Risk for Nutritional Problems

- Acquired immune deficiency syndrome (AIDS)
- Alcoholic liver disease
- Anorexia nervosa
- Aspiration pneumonia
- Bulimia nervosa
- Burns, extensive or severe
- Celiac disease
- Dehydration
- Diabetes, newly diagnosed or uncontrolled
- Gestational diabetes
- Head trauma
- Hypoglycemia
- Inflammatory bowel disease
- Jaw fracture
- Multiple trauma
- Liver disease: hepatic encephalopathy
- Pregnancy-induced hypertension
- Renal disease, end-stage
- Skin ulcer
- Swallowing difficulty
- Vomiting, excessive

Dietary Assessment Methods

Knowledge of a person's usual diet can help a dietitian determine whether the person is likely to develop a nutrient deficiency. To assess nutrient adequacy, the diet's nutrient content is calculated using diet analysis software or a table of food composition (similar to that in Appendix H), and the results are compared with RDA and AI values. Another option is to compare the list of foods consumed with a diet-planning tool such as the USDA Food Guide. Knowing a person's food preferences can also be helpful for developing an appropriate nutrition care plan, planning menus, or providing dietary counseling.

Obtaining an accurate account of a person's usual food intake can be difficult. Results vary depending on both the patient's memory and honesty and the assessor's skill and training. In addition, each method has its own strengths and weaknesses, so the best results are obtained from a combination of several methods. Table 17-5 (p. 588) summarizes the different methods and indicates some advantages and disadvantages associated with their use.

The 24-Hour Recall The **24-hour recall** is a guided interview in which an individual recounts all the foods and beverages consumed in the past 24 hours or during the previous day. (A less precise alternative is to ask the person to recount the foods and beverages consumed in a "typical" day.) The interviewer includes questions about the times when meals or snacks were eaten, the amounts consumed, and the ways in which foods were prepared. The most accurate accounts are

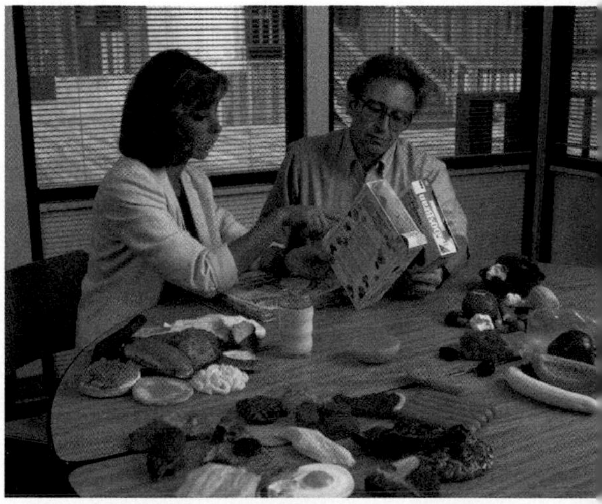

Food models and measuring utensils can help an individual visualize portion sizes.

diet history: a comprehensive record of a person's food intake and dietary practices.

24-hour recall: a record of foods consumed in the previous 24 hours; sometimes modified to include foods consumed in a typical day.

TABLE 17-5 Dietary Assessment Methods

Method	Description	Advantages	Disadvantages
24-hour recall	Guided interview in which the foods and beverages consumed in a 24-hour period are described in detail.	• Results are not dependent on literacy or educational level of respondent. • Interview occurs after food is consumed, so it does not interfere with food choices. • Relatively easy and quick assessment method.	• Reliant on memory. • Food items that cause embarrassment (alcohol, desserts) may be omitted. • Under- and overestimation of food intakes are common. • Skill of interviewer affects outcome. • Data from a single day cannot represent the respondent's usual intake accurately. • Seasonal variations may not be addressed.
Food frequency questionnaire	Written survey of food consumption during a specific period of time, often a one-year period.	• Examines long-term food intake, so day-to-day and seasonal variability should not affect results. • Completed after food is consumed, so does not interfere with food choices. • Low-cost method.	• Reliant on memory. • Not good for monitoring short-term changes in food intake. • Serving sizes are often difficult for respondents to evaluate without assistance. • Calculated nutrient intakes may not be accurate. • Food lists include common foods only. • Food lists for general population are of limited value in special populations.
Food record	Written account of food consumed during a specified period, usually several consecutive days. Accuracy is improved by including weights or measures of foods.	• Process does not rely on memory. • Recording foods as they are consumed improves likelihood of obtaining accurate food intake data. • Useful for controlling intake because keeping records can increase awareness of food choices.	• Recording process itself influences food intake. • Time-consuming and burdensome for respondent; requires high degree of motivation. • Underreporting is common. • Requires literacy and the physical ability to write. • Seasonal changes in diet are not taken into account.
Direct observation	Observation of meal trays or shelf inventories before and after eating; possible only in residential facilities.	• Process does not rely on memory. • Does not interfere with person's food intake. • Can be used to evaluate acceptability of prescribed diet.	• Possible only in residential situations. • Labor-intensive.

obtained when the respondent is repeatedly prompted to recall food items that are often forgotten, such as snack foods, beverages, and condiments.

To obtain food intake data using this method, the assessor may begin by asking, "What is the first thing you ate or drank yesterday morning?" (Or "What is the first thing you usually eat or drink during the day?") After the first food items are described, the follow-up questions might be, "What time was that?" and "How much did you eat?" Food models or measuring cups and spoons are usually used to help the individual visualize and describe the amounts consumed. Preparation methods are also ascertained with questions such as "How was your egg cooked?" The questioning continues (for example, "What was the *next* thing you ate?") until the intake record for the day is complete. After the day's intake is recounted, the interviewer asks whether the intake that day is fairly typical, and if not, how it varies from the person's usual intake. Sometimes a recall interview is conducted on several nonconsecutive days to get a better representation of a person's usual diet.

As mentioned previously, people often forget to mention beverages, condiments, and snack foods unless specifically prompted to do so. For example, a person may report eating two slices of toast but may not think to mention the four pats of butter and two tablespoons of jam on the toast. Or a cup of coffee may be mentioned, but not the spoonful of sugar or ounce of cream that was added. One researcher found that alcohol intake was rarely mentioned without prompting and that chocolate, take-out foods, butter, and red meat or pork frequently cause embarrassment during recall interviews.[9]

A recall interview can gather useful data for developing an acceptable nutrition care plan and for identifying food items that may need to be restricted due to illness. It is a poor technique, however, for determining the adequacy of a diet because it does not take into account fluctuations in food intake or seasonal variations. Furthermore, because the process relies on an individual's memory and reporting accuracy, food intakes are often underestimated. For these reasons, recall interviews are often followed up with a food frequency questionnaire, discussed next.

Food Frequency Questionnaire A **food frequency questionnaire** is a survey of foods and beverages routinely consumed over a certain time period. Some questionnaires are qualitative only: food lists contain commonly eaten foods, usually categorized by food group, with boxes to check to indicate frequency of consumption. Other types of questionnaires provide semiquantitative information by indicating the portion size consumed as well. Figure 17-3 shows a sample section of a semiquantitative questionnaire that surveys fruit intake over the previous year. Because the respondent is often asked to estimate food intakes over a one-year period, the results should not be affected by seasonal changes in diet. Conversely, a disadvantage of this method is its inability to determine recent changes in food intake.[10]

Long, detailed questionnaires can be cumbersome to complete, and simpler versions are available that focus on food categories relevant to a person's medical condition. For example, a questionnaire designed to evaluate calcium intake may include only milk products, fortified foods, certain fruits and vegetables, and dietary supplements that contain calcium. A computer analysis can then quickly estimate the individual's calcium intake and compare it to recommendations. Because food frequency questionnaires typically list only common foods, the calculated nutrient intakes are not as accurate as those obtained by dietary recall methods. In addition, some research has shown that short fruit and vegetable lists

food frequency questionnaire: a survey of foods routinely consumed. Some questionnaires ask about the types of food eaten and yield only qualitative information, whereas others include questions about portions consumed and yield semiquantitative data as well.

FIGURE 17-3 Sample Section of a Food Frequency Questionnaire

	HOW OFTEN								HOW MUCH			
FRUIT	Never or less than once per month	1 per mon.	2–3 per mon.	1 per week	2 per week	3–4 per week	5–6 per week	Every day	MEDIUM SERVING	YOUR SERVING SIZE S	M	L
EXAMPLE: Bananas	○	○	○	●	○	○	○	○	1 medium	○ 1/2	● 1	○ 2
Bananas	○	○	○	○	○	○	○	○	1 medium	○ 1/2	○ 1	○ 2
Apples, applesauce	○	○	○	○	○	○	○	○	1 medium or 1/2 cup	○ 1/2	○ 1	○ 2
Oranges (not including juice)	○	○	○	○	○	○	○	○	1 medium	○ 1/2	○ 1	○ 2
Grapefruit (not including juice)	○	○	○	○	○	○	○	○	1/2 medium	○ 1/4	○ 1/2	○ 1
Cantaloupe	○	○	○	○	○	○	○	○	1/4 medium	○ 1/8	○ 1/4	○ 1/2
Peaches, apricots (fresh, in season)	○	○	○	○	○	○	○	○	1 medium	○ 1/2	○ 1	○ 2
Peaches, apricots (canned or dried)	○	○	○	○	○	○	○	○	1 medium or 1/2 cup	○ 1/2	○ 1	○ 2
Prunes, or prune juice	○	○	○	○	○	○	○	○	1/2 cup	○ 1/4	○ 1/2	○ 1
Watermelon (in season)	○	○	○	○	○	○	○	○	1 slice	○ 1/2	○ 1	○ 2
Strawberries, other berries (in season)	○	○	○	○	○	○	○	○	1/2 cup	○ 1/4	○ 1/2	○ 1
Any other fruit, including kiwi, fruit cocktail, grapes, raisins, mangoes	○	○	○	○	○	○	○	○	1/2 cup	○ 1/4	○ 1/2	○ 1

may lead to underestimated intakes, whereas long lists may result in overestimated intakes.[11] Another weakness is that people often find it difficult and frustrating to estimate "average" portion sizes of foods irregularly consumed. In the clinical setting, food frequency questionnaires are best used when combined with 24-hour recalls to help verify the accuracy of the information obtained in an interview.

Food Record A **food record** is a written account of foods and beverages consumed during a specified time period, usually several consecutive days. Foods are recorded as they are consumed in order to obtain the most complete and accurate record possible; thus the process does not rely on memory. A detailed food record includes the types and amounts of foods and beverages consumed, times of consumption, and methods of preparation. For weight-management purposes, the food record may also include information about a person's mood (lonely, happy), the occasion (family meal, party), activities while eating (watching TV, driving a car), and daily physical activity. For establishing blood glucose control, the record may include information about medication schedule, physical activity, and the results of blood glucose monitoring.

The food record can provide valuable information about food intake as well as a person's response to and compliance with medical nutrition therapy. Food records may help pinpoint problem food patterns so that solutions can be implemented. Unfortunately, they require a great deal of time to complete, and people need to be highly motivated to keep accurate records. Another drawback is that the recording process itself may influence food intake. Furthermore, day-to-day and seasonal variations in food intake make it difficult to obtain accurate estimates of nutrient values in just a few days or even a week. It may be possible to obtain accurate intakes for some nutrients in a short time period (protein, total fat, calcium), but other nutrients may require weeks or months of accurate recording (vitamin A, vitamin B_{12}).[12]

Direct Observation For individuals in residential facilities, direct observation of meal trays or food inventories can identify problems with dietary intakes. During long-term care, this method can reveal a person's food preferences, changes in appetite, and any problems with a prescribed diet. Direct observation is labor-intensive, however, and requires regular and careful documentation. The amounts of foods and beverages provided must be recorded, as well as the amounts left over after the meal is finished. The differences are then used to calculate the amounts consumed and to estimate kcaloric and nutrient intakes.

Anthropometric Data

Nutrition assessments usually include some basic measures of body size. The most common anthropometric■ values used are height (or length) and weight, which help to assess growth in children and undernutrition and overnutrition in adults. Other helpful measurements include body composition tests (described in Chapter 8 and Appendix E) and circumferences of the head, waist, and limbs, which are discussed in the following sections.

Height (or Length) and Weight Poor growth in children is an indicator of malnutrition. In adults, height measurements alone do not reflect current nutrition status but can help to estimate healthy body weight and energy needs. Length is measured in infants and children up to age two or three, and height is measured in older children and adults. Length may also be measured in adults and children who are unable to stand for physical or medical reasons. The "How to" feature describes the proper techniques for measuring length and height.

In adults, height can be estimated from equations that include either knee height or the full arm span,■ both of which correlate well with height. The measure of knee height is frequently used in bedridden patients. Specific formulas have been developed for different age, gender, and ethnic groups.[13] For children

■ Reminder: *Anthropometric* refers to physical measurements of the human body.

■ Knee height is measured from the bottom of the heel to the top of the knee when the knee is bent at a 90° angle. Full arm span is measured from the longest fingertip of the right hand to the longest fingertip of the left hand when the arms are fully extended horizontally.

food record: a detailed log of food eaten during a specified time period, usually several days. A food record may also include information regarding disease symptoms, physical activity, emotions, or medication use; also called a **food diary.**

HOW TO Measure Length and Height

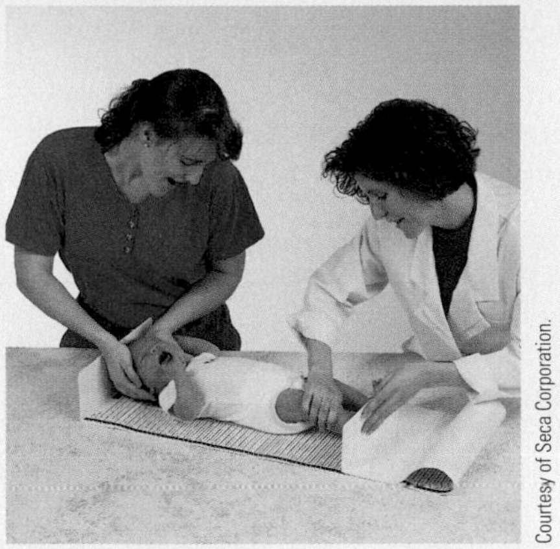

It often takes two people to measure the length of an infant.

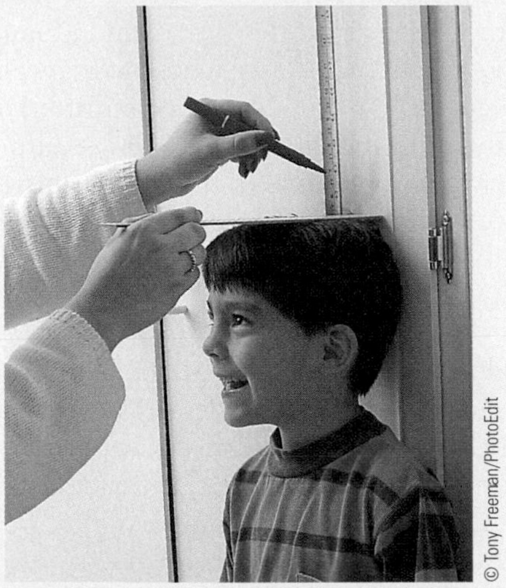

An accurate height measurement can be obtained by using a measuring tape fixed to a wall.

Tips for measuring length and height:

- Always measure—never ask! Self-reported heights are less accurate than measured heights. If height is not measured, document that the height is self-reported.
- Measure the length of infants and young children by using a measuring board with a fixed headboard and a movable footboard. It often takes two people to measure length. One person gently holds the infant's head against the headboard; the other straightens the infant's legs and moves the footboard to the bottom of the infant's feet.
- Using a measuring tape is a less accurate way to measure length in infants, but it is a useful alternative for measuring length in individuals who cannot stand erect. To use this method, straighten out the infant's or person's body, make a mark at the top of the head, make another mark at the bottom of the heel, and then measure the distance between the two marks.
- Measure height next to a wall to which a nonstretchable measuring tape or a board has been fixed. Ask the person to stand erect without shoes and with heels together. The person's eyes and head should be facing forward, with heels, buttocks, and shoulder blades touching the wall. Place a ruler or other flat, stiff object on the top of the head at a right angle to the wall and carefully note the height measurement. Although less accurate, the measuring rod of a scale can also be used to measure height.
- Higher values are obtained from supine measurements than from vertical height measurements due to gravity.

with disabilities that affect stature, alternative measures of linear growth include lower-leg lengths (knee to heel, which is similar to the adult's knee height measure) and upper-arm lengths (shoulder to elbow), which can be compared with reference percentiles.[14]

Body weights are usually monitored carefully during clinical care. Changes in body weight can reflect changes in hydration status, and an involuntary loss of body weight may signify protein-energy malnutrition (PEM). Body weights are often compared with healthy ranges, which can be obtained from height-weight tables and growth curves (see Appendix E) or calculated using a quick assessment tool■ based on empirical findings (see Table 17-6 on p. 592). The body mass index (BMI) is also widely used to assess weight for height; values outside the range of 18.5 to 25 suggest overweight or underweight (see Chapter 8).■ The suggested BMI range is not always appropriate for bodybuilders, older adults, and different ethnic groups.

Valid weight measurements require scales that have been carefully maintained, calibrated, and checked for accuracy at regular intervals. Beam balance and

■ This quick calculation of desirable body weight is sometimes called the **Hamwi method** after the researcher who developed it.

■ Reminder: $\text{BMI} = \dfrac{\text{weight (kg)}}{\text{height (m)}^2}$

FIGURE 17-4 Weight Measurement of an Infant

Infants sit or lie down on scales that are designed to hold them while they are being weighed.

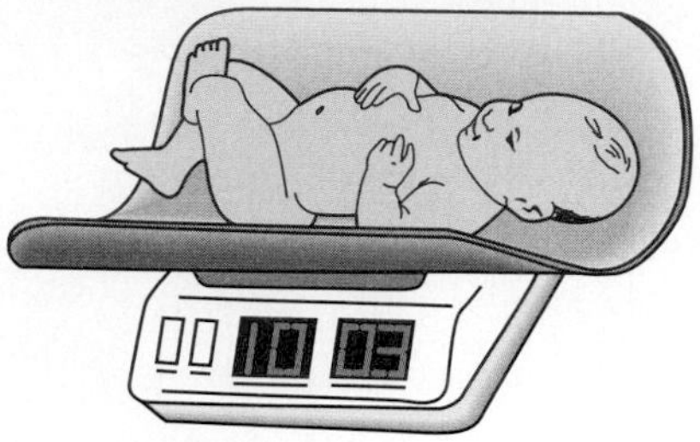

TABLE 17-6 Quick Estimate of Desirable Body Weight[a]

Men

- For first 5 feet, consider 106 pounds a reasonable weight. For each inch over 5 feet, add 6 pounds.
- For each inch under 5 feet, subtract 6 pounds.
- Add 10% for a large-framed individual; subtract 10% for a small-framed individual.
- *Example:* For a man 5 feet 8 inches tall (medium frame), a desirable weight would be 154 pounds (106 lb + 48 = 154 lb).

Women

- For first 5 feet, consider 100 pounds a reasonable weight. For each inch over 5 feet, add 5 pounds.
- For each inch under 5 feet, subtract 5 pounds.
- Add 10% for a large-framed individual; subtract 10% for a small-framed individual.
- *Example:* For a woman 5 feet 6 inches tall (medium frame), a desirable weight would be 130 pounds (100 lb + 30 = 130 lb).

[a]This method does not account for differences in age or race.

■ To calculate %IBW, use a person's current weight and a reasonable weight from height-weight tables or the Hamwi method:

$$\%IBW = \frac{\text{current weight}}{\text{ideal weight}} \times 100.$$

■ To calculate %UBW, use a person's current weight and usual weight:

$$\%UBW = \frac{\text{current weight}}{\text{usual weight}} \times 100.$$

FIGURE 17-5 Weight Measurement of an Older Child or Adult

Whenever possible, children and adults are measured on beam balance or electronic scales to ensure accuracy.

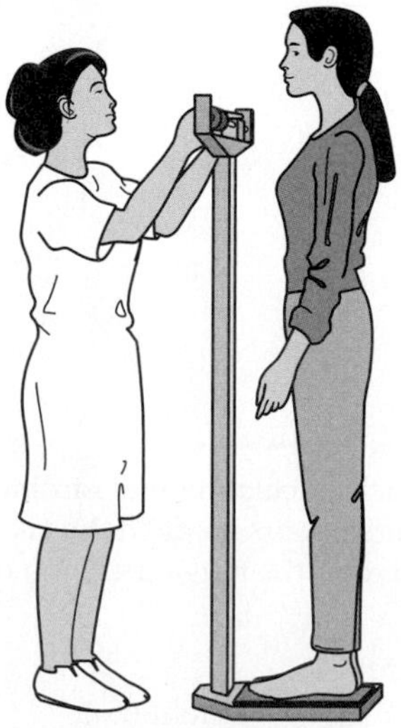

electronic scales are the most accurate. To measure an infant's weight, assessors use special scales that allow the infant to lie or sit (see Figure 17-4). Weighing infants naked and without diapers is standard procedure. Children who can stand are weighed in the same way as adults (see Figure 17-5). Standardized conditions are necessary when weighing so that repeated weight measurements give valid information: each weighing should take place at the same time of day (preferably before breakfast), in the same amount of clothing, after the person has voided, and on the same scale. Special scales and hospital beds with built-in scales are available for weighing people who are bedridden. Bathroom scales are inaccurate and inappropriate in the clinical setting.

Weight data are sometimes expressed as a percent of "ideal body weight" (%IBW)■ or a percent of "usual body weight" (%UBW)■ in order to assess the degree of nutritional risk associated with illness. The %UBW is more effective for interpreting weight changes that occur in overweight and obese individuals; %IBW fails to identify a significant weight loss. Conversely, in patients who have been underweight throughout life, a %IBW value could overstate the degree of weight loss due to illness. Table 17-7 shows how to evaluate %IBW and %UBW data.

Head Circumference Head circumference can help to assess brain growth and malnutrition in children up to three years of age, although this measure may not necessarily be reduced in a malnourished child.[15] Head circumference values are also used for tracking brain development in premature and small-for-gestational-age infants. To measure head circumference, the assessor encircles the largest circumference measure of a child's head with a nonstretchable measuring tape: the tape is placed just above the eyebrows and ears, and around the occipital prominence at the back of the head.

Circumferences of Waist and Limbs Circumferences of the waist and limbs help to evaluate body fat and muscle mass content, respectively.[16] Waist circumference correlates with visceral fat and can help evaluate overnutrition (see Appendix E). Circumferences of the mid-upper arm, mid-thigh, and mid-calf areas are used to assess the effects of illness, aging, and PEM on skeletal muscle content. Limb circumferences are more sensitive than body weight as indicators of muscle loss; for example, a study of mid-arm circumferences in elderly adults admitted to an acute care facility helped to identify 45 percent as being severely malnourished, even though only 28 percent were underweight.[17] For improved accuracy, circumference measurements are often used together with fatfold measurements to correct for the subcutaneous fat in limbs.

Anthropometric Assessment in Infants and Children To evaluate physical development, height, weight, and head circumference are monitored and compared with standard reference values, such as those depicted on growth charts (see the "How to" on p. 512 in Chapter 15). The most commonly used growth charts compare weight to age, height to age, BMI to age, and weight to height. Although individual growth patterns vary, a child's growth will generally stay at about the same percentile throughout childhood; a sudden drop in a previously steady growth pattern suggests malnutrition. Growth charts with BMI-for-age percentiles can be used to assess risk of underweight and overweight in children: the 10th and 85th percentiles have been used as cutoffs to identify children who may be malnourished or overweight, respectively.[18]

TABLE 17-7 Use of Body Weight for Assessing Nutritional Risk

%IBW	%UBW	Nutritional Risk
>120	—	Obesity
110–120	—	Overweight
90–109	—	Adequate weight—not at risk
80–89	85–95	Risk of mild malnutrition
70–79	75–84	Risk of moderate malnutrition
<70	<75	Risk of severe malnutrition

Anthropometric Assessment in Adults Weight and height are the primary anthropometric values recorded in medical charts and monitored during treatment.[19] Weight changes should be evaluated carefully because involuntary weight *loss* can indicate malnutrition and weight *gain* may suggest fluid retention. A 10 percent weight loss within a six-month period is considered significant, and greater losses signify a high risk of PEM. The weight gain that results from fluid accumulation can indicate worsening disease in patients with heart failure, liver cirrhosis, and kidney failure. Fluid retention itself can mask the weight loss associated with PEM. Weight changes may also be associated with the use of certain medications.

Changes in body composition often accompany illness and aging. Many of the illnesses discussed in later chapters are associated with lean tissue losses that resist nutrition intervention. Losses in both height and lean tissue are common with aging, whereas body weights may remain stable. Including anthropometric measures such as fatfold measurements and limb circumferences can help health care professionals identify body composition changes that need to be addressed in the treatment plan.

Biochemical Analyses

The approaches to nutrition assessment discussed previously examine only external attributes. Biochemical analyses help to determine what is happening to the body internally. Tests are usually based on analyses of blood■ and urine samples, which contain proteins, nutrients, and metabolites that reflect nutrition status. Table 17-8 (p. 594) lists and describes common blood tests with nutritional implications. Tests relevant to specific diseases will be discussed in the chapters that follow.

Interpreting laboratory values that fall outside normal ranges can be challenging because confounding variables can influence test results. For example, serum protein values are affected by hydration state,■ pregnancy, medications, and exercise.[20] Blood measurements of vitamins and minerals are often poor indicators of nutrient deficiency because the levels are affected by different physiological factors. Multiple tests are generally needed to diagnose a nutrition problem. Taken together with other assessment data, however, laboratory test results help to present a clearer picture than is possible otherwise.

■ Blood test results are often reported as either *plasma* or *serum* levels. *Plasma* is the yellow fluid that remains after cells are centrifuged; it contains clotting factors. *Serum* is the yellow fluid remaining after both cells and clotting factors have been removed.

■ Fluid retention can result in lab results that are deceptively low. Dehydration may cause lab results to be deceptively high.

Plasma Proteins Fluctuations in plasma proteins are not specific to only one illness or nutrition problem. For example, both PEM and liver disease■ can reduce plasma protein levels. Metabolic stress causes the release of hormones that alter plasma protein levels. Plasma protein values are also influenced by changes in hydration, pregnancy, kidney function, and some medications. Because plasma proteins are affected by so many factors, the values must be considered with other data to evaluate nutrition status. Blood plasma contains hundreds of proteins; the following paragraphs describe several of those commonly measured to assess nutrition status.

■ Most plasma proteins are synthesized in the liver.

Albumin Albumin is the most abundant plasma protein, and its levels are routinely measured. Albumin is influenced by many medical conditions but is slow to

TABLE 17-8 Routine Laboratory Tests with Nutritional Implications

This table presents a partial listing of some uses of commonly performed lab tests that have implications for nutritional problems.

Laboratory Test	Acceptable Range	Description
Hematology		
Red blood cell (RBC) count	Male: 4.3–5.7 million/μL Female: 3.8–5.1 million/μL	Number of RBC; aids anemia diagnosis.
Hemoglobin (Hb)	Male: 13.5–17.5 g/dL Female: 12.0–16.0 g/dL	Hemoglobin content of RBC; aids anemia diagnosis.
Hematocrit (Hct)	Male: 39–49% Female: 35–45%	Percentage RBC in total blood volume; aids anemia diagnosis.
Mean corpuscular volume (MCV)	81–99 fL	RBC size, helps to distinguish between microcytic and macrocytic anemias.
Mean corpuscular hemoglobin concentration (MCHC)	31–37% Hb/cell	Hb concentration within RBCs, helps to distinguish iron-deficiency anemia.
White blood cell (WBC) count	4500–11,000 cells/μL	Number of WBC; general assessment of immunity.
Blood Chemistry		
Serum Proteins		
• Total protein	6.4–8.3 g/dL	Protein levels are not specific to disease or highly sensitive; they can reflect poor protein intake, illness or infections, changes in hydration or metabolism, pregnancy, or medications.
• Albumin	3.4–4.8 g/dL	May reflect illness or PEM; slow to respond to improvement or worsening of disease.
• Transferrin	200–400 mg/dL >60 yr: 180–380 mg/dL	May reflect illness, PEM, or iron deficiency; slightly more sensitive to changes than albumin.
• Prealbumin (transthyretin)	10–40 mg/dL	May reflect illness or PEM; more responsive to health status changes than albumin or transferrin.
• C-reactive protein	68–8200 ng/mL	Indicator of inflammation or disease.
Serum Enzymes		
• Creatine kinase (CK)	Male: 38–174 U/L Female: 26–140 U/L	Different forms of CK are found in muscle, brain, and heart. High levels in blood may indicate heart attack, brain tissue damage, or skeletal muscle injury.
• Lactate dehydrogenase (LDH)	208–378 U/L	LDH is found in many tissues. Specific types may be elevated after heart attack, lung damage, or liver disease.
• Alkaline phosphatase	25–100 U/L	Found in many tissues; often measured to evaluate liver function.
• Aspartate aminotransferase (AST, formerly SGOT)	10–30 U/L	Usually monitored to assess liver damage; elevated in most liver diseases. Levels are somewhat increased after muscle injury.
• Alanine aminotransferase (ALT, formerly SGPT)	Male: 10–40 U/L Female: 7–35 U/L	Usually monitored to assess liver damage; elevated in most liver diseases. Levels are somewhat increased after muscle injury.
Serum Electrolytes		
• Sodium	136–146 mEq/L	Helps to evaluate hydration status or neuromuscular, kidney, and adrenal functions.
• Potassium	3.5–5.1 mEq/L	Helps to evaluate acid-base balance and kidney function; can detect potassium imbalances.
• Chloride	98–106 mEq/L	Helps to evaluate hydration status and detect acid-base and electrolyte imbalances.
Other		
• Glucose	74–106 mg/dL	Detects risk of glucose intolerance, diabetes mellitus, and hypoglycemia; helps to monitor diabetes treatment.
• Glycosylated hemoglobin (Hb A_{1c})	5.0–7.5% of Hb	Used to monitor long-term blood glucose control (approximately 1 to 3 months prior).
• Blood urea nitrogen (BUN)	6–20 mg/dL	Primarily used to monitor kidney function; value is altered by liver failure, dehydration, or shock.
• Uric acid	Male: 3.5–7.2 mg/dL Female: 2.6–6.0 mg/dL	Used for detecting gout or changes in kidney function; levels affected by age and diet; varies among different ethnic groups.
• Creatinine (serum or plasma)	Male: 0.7–1.3 mg/dL Female: 0.6–1.1 mg/dL	Used to monitor renal function.

NOTE: μL = microliter; dL = deciliter; fL = femtoliter; ng = nanogram; U/L = units per liter; mEq = milliequivalents.
SOURCE: L. Goldman and J. C. Bennett, eds. *Cecil Textbook of Medicine* (Philadelphia: Saunders, 2000).

reflect changes in nutrition status because of its large body pool and slow rate of degradation.■ In people with chronic PEM, albumin levels remain normal for long periods of time despite depletion of body proteins; levels fall only after prolonged malnutrition. Likewise, albumin concentrations increase slowly with appropriate nutrition support, so albumin is not a sensitive indicator of response to nutrition therapy.

■ The rate of degradation is defined by a substance's **half-life**—the time required by the body to metabolize or inactivate half of the amount of a substance. The albumin in plasma has a 3-week half-life, meaning that half of the amount circulating in plasma is degraded in a 3-week period.

Transferrin Transferrin transports iron, so its concentrations respond to both PEM and iron status. Transferrin breaks down in the body more rapidly than albumin,■ but it is relatively slow to respond to nutrition therapy. In addition, evaluating protein-energy status using transferrin is difficult if an iron deficiency is also present. Transferrin levels rise as iron deficiency worsens and fall as iron status improves.

■ Transferrin's half-life in plasma is approximately 8 to 10 days.

Prealbumin and Retinol-Binding Protein Levels of prealbumin (also called transthyretin) and retinol-binding protein decrease rapidly during PEM and respond quickly to changes in protein intake.■ Thus these proteins are more sensitive than albumin to changes in protein status. Like other plasma proteins, their usefulness in nutrition assessment is limited because they are affected by metabolic stress and various medical conditions. Also, their synthesis in the liver can be impaired by zinc deficiency. Prealbumin and retinol-binding protein are more expensive to measure than albumin, so they are not routinely included during nutrition assessment.

■ Half-lives of prealbumin and retinol-binding protein are 2 days and 12 hours, respectively.

Physical Examinations

As with other assessment methods, interpreting physical signs of malnutrition requires skill and clinical judgment. Most physical signs are nonspecific; they can reflect any of several nutrient deficiencies as well as conditions not related to nutrition. For example, cracked lips may be caused by one of several B vitamin deficiencies but may also be caused by sunburn, windburn, or dehydration. Dietary and laboratory data are needed as additional evidence to confirm suspected nutrient deficiencies.

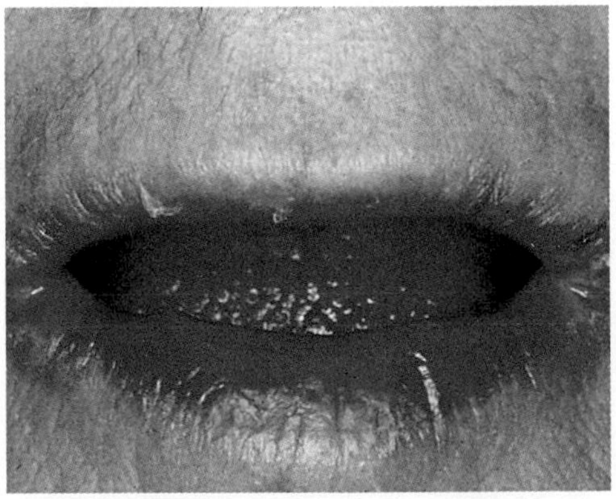

Physical signs of B vitamin deficiencies include dry, cracked lips and sores in the corners of the lips.

Clinical Signs of Malnutrition Signs of malnutrition appear most rapidly in parts of the body where cell replacement occurs at a rapid rate, such as the hair, skin, and digestive tract (including the mouth and tongue). Table 17-9 (p. 596) lists some clinical signs of nutrient deficiencies. Many of the symptoms listed occur only in advanced stages of nutrient deficiency. The summary tables in Chapters 10 through 13 also include signs and symptoms of specific vitamin and mineral imbalances.

Hydration State Various medical conditions and the use of some medications can upset fluid balance, causing either dehydration or fluid retention. Altered hydration is often evident during a physical exam and is important for interpreting the results of blood tests and the body weight measurement. The hydration state must also be considered when developing medical and nutrition care plans.

Dehydration Dehydration may result from fever, sweating, vomiting, diarrhea, excessive urination, and skin injury or burns (fluid can be lost through skin lesions). Symptoms include thirst, dry skin or mouth, and reduced skin tension. The urine may be dark yellow or amber colored, and urine volume may be unusually low. A dehydrated individual may have a headache or feel weak and confused. Early recognition of symptoms is critical because serious cases can cause coma or death. Dehydration risk is greatest in the elderly, who have reduced thirst responses to water deprivation.

Fluid Retention Fluid retention (edema)■ may accompany malnutrition, infection, or injury and is also a common side effect of some medications. It may be caused by impaired blood circulation and is often associated with diseases of the

■ Reminder: *Edema* is the abnormal accumulation of fluid in body tissues.

TABLE 17-9 Clinical Signs of Nutrient Deficiencies

Body System	Acceptable	Signs of Malnutrition	Other Possible Causes
Hair	Shiny, firm in scalp	Dull, brittle, dry, loose; falls out (PEM); corkscrew hair (copper)	Excessive hair bleaching; hair loss from aging, chemotherapy, or radiation therapy
Eyes	Bright, clear pink membranes; adjust easily to light	Pale membranes (iron); spots, dryness, nightblindness (vitamin A); redness at corners of eyes (B vitamins)	Anemia, unrelated to nutrition; eye disorders; allergies
Lips	Smooth	Dry, cracked, or with sores in the corner of the lips (B vitamins)	Sunburn, windburn, excessive salivation from ill-fitting dentures or other disorders
Mouth and gums	Red tongue without swelling, normal sense of taste; teeth without caries; gums without bleeding, swelling, or pain	Smooth or magenta tongue (B vitamins), decreased taste sensations (zinc); swollen, bleeding gums (vitamin C)	Medications, periodontal disease (poor oral hygiene)
Skin	Smooth, firm, good color	Poor wound healing (PEM, vitamin C, zinc); dry, rough, lack of fat under skin (essential fatty acids, PEM, B vitamins); bruising, bleeding under skin (vitamins C and K)	Poor skin care, diabetes mellitus, aging, medications
Nails	Smooth, firm, pink	Ridged (PEM); spoon shaped, pale (iron)	
Other		Dementia, peripheral neuropathy (B vitamins); swollen glands at front of neck (PEM, iodine); bowed legs (vitamin D)	Disorders of aging (dementia), diabetes mellitus (peripheral neuropathy)

heart, kidney, liver, and lungs. Fluid retention can be detected after 5 to 10 pounds of excess fluid accumulate in the body of an average-sized person.[21] Physical signs may include weight gain, facial puffiness, swelling of limbs, abdominal distention, and tight-fitting shoes. **Ascites,** a complication of liver cirrhosis, is the accumulation of fluid in the abdominal cavity. The pooling of fluids in one area can cause dehydration elsewhere in the body.

Functional Assessment Nutrient deficiencies can impair normal physiological functions; for example, zinc deficiency can depress immunity and slow wound healing. Protein-energy malnutrition and illness can cause **wasting,** the breakdown and loss of body tissues. A wide variety of functional tests help to evaluate the changes in physiological functions and losses in body strength that accompany malnutrition or disease. For example, exercise tolerance can be assessed using a treadmill or cycle ergometer. Handgrip strength can be tested with a hand dynamometer, a device that measures the strength and endurance of hand muscles. Respiratory muscle strength might be tested by holding a strip of paper 10 centimeters■ from the mouth and observing how the paper moves in response to respiration.[22] Assessment of immunity may include testing the skin's responses to antigens that typically cause redness and swelling if the immune system is functioning normally. The chapters that follow provide additional examples of functional assessment.

■ 10 cm = 4 inches.

Integrating Assessment Data

Several tools have been developed that combine the results from different assessment methods. One such technique is **Subjective Global Assessment (SGA),** which combines historical information with the results of a physical examination to predict the nutrition status of acute care patients (see Table 17-10). The elements typically included are weight and dietary changes, gastrointestinal symptoms, work capacity, level of metabolic stress, degree of muscle wasting and fat loss, and presence of edema or ascites. Subjective Global Assessment is widely used and has been found to be applicable to different patient populations.

ascites: an accumulation of fluid in the abdominal cavity.

wasting: the gradual atrophy (loss) of body tissues; associated with protein-energy malnutrition or chronic disease.

Subjective Global Assessment (SGA): a technique for assessing malnutrition that uses historical and physical information.

TABLE 17-10 Elements of Subjective Global Assessment

Medical and Diet Histories	• Body weight changes in past six months and past two weeks • Change in dietary intake and duration of change • Current diet: whether suboptimal, low-kcalorie, liquid, or starvation diet • Gastrointestinal symptoms: nausea, diarrhea, vomiting, or anorexia • Functional ability: full capacity or suboptimal, walking or bedridden • Current medical diagnosis • Degree of metabolic stress: low, moderate, or high
Physical Examination	• Loss of subcutaneous fat: in triceps or chest • Muscle wasting: in quadriceps or deltoids • Ankle edema • Sacral (lower spine) edema • Ascites
SGA Rating	• **Well-nourished** if recent weight gain, mild fat/muscle loss, improvement in histories • **Moderate malnutrition** suspected if >5% weight loss (not from hydration change), decreased food intake, mild fat/muscle wasting • **Severe malnutrition** if >10% weight loss (not from hydration change), severe fat/muscle wasting, some edema

SOURCE: A. S. Detsky and coauthors, What is subjective global assessment of nutritional status? *Journal of Parenteral and Enteral Nutrition* 11 (1987): 8–13.

IN SUMMARY Information from nutrition assessments is used to diagnose nutrition problems, plan nutrition care, and evaluate the success of nutrition care plans. Complete assessments include historical information, anthropometric data, biochemical analyses, and physical examinations. By combining the data from different assessment methods, health care professionals can better identify patients most likely to develop nutrition problems. The Case Study on p. 598 can help you review the different components of a nutrition assessment.

CASE STUDY

Nutrition Screening and Assessment

Mrs. Genova is an 85-year-old retired schoolteacher who lives alone. She uses a walker and has poorly fitting dentures. She was admitted to the hospital with pneumonia and also has congestive heart failure and diabetes. She routinely takes several medications to control blood glucose, hypertension, and heart function, and, in addition to these, the physician ordered antibiotics to treat the pneumonia. During an initial nutrition screening, Mrs. Genova stated that she had been eating very poorly over the past two weeks. She said that she usually weighs about 125 pounds (this fact was documented in her medical chart from a previous visit). Although she felt she was losing weight, she didn't know how much weight she may have lost or when she started losing weight. Upon admission to the hospital, Mrs. Genova weighed 115 pounds and was 5 feet, 2 inches tall. Her serum albumin level was 3.0 g/dL. A physical exam revealed edema, and a number of other laboratory tests confirmed that she was retaining fluid. As a result of the nutrition screening, Mrs. Genova was referred to the dietitian for a complete nutrition assessment.

1. From the brief description provided, which items in Mrs. Genova's medical, social, and diet histories might alert the nurse that she is at risk of malnutrition?

2. Identify a healthy body weight for Mrs. Genova and calculate her %IBW and %UBW. What do the results reveal? What effect does fluid retention have on Mrs. Genova's weight?

3. How can fluid retention alter Mrs. Genova's serum protein levels? What physical symptoms may have suggested that she was retaining excess fluid?

4. What tools can the dietitian use to estimate Mrs. Genova's usual food intake? What medical, physical, and social factors are likely to affect her dietary intake?

5. Describe some other types of assessment information the dietitian may need before developing a nutrition care plan.

STUDY QUESTIONS

These questions will help you review the chapter. You will find the answers in the discussions on the pages provided.

1. In what ways can illnesses affect nutrition status? (p. 582)
2. Contrast the roles of different health care practitioners in providing nutrition care. (p. 583)
3. What is the difference between nutrition screening and a complete nutrition assessment? (pp. 584–585)
4. Discuss the steps of the nutrition care process. (pp. 584–586)
5. Give examples of the types of information included in medical, social, and diet histories. (pp. 586–587)
6. Describe the methods of gathering food intake data, and indicate the advantages and disadvantages of each process. (pp. 587–590)
7. Which anthropometric measurements are often included in nutrition screenings and nutrition assessments? How do these measurements help in the evaluation of nutrition status? (pp. 590–593)
8. How can biochemical analyses help to assess nutrition status? Give examples. What confounding factors may influence the results of blood tests? (pp. 593–595)
9. Give examples of the information provided in a physical exam that can suggest malnutrition. (pp. 595–596)
10. What are some symptoms of dehydration and fluid retention? (pp. 595–596)

These multiple choice questions will help you prepare for an exam. Answers can be found on p. 600.

1. Mr. Smith experiences loss of appetite, difficulty swallowing, and mouth pain as a consequence of illness. Mr. Smith is at risk of malnutrition due to:
   a. altered metabolism.
   b. reduced food intake.
   c. altered excretion of nutrients.
   d. altered digestion and absorption.
2. The central role of nurses in health care makes them well positioned for:
   a. calculating patients' nutrient needs.
   b. providing medical nutrition therapy.
   c. conducting complete nutrition assessments.
   d. identifying patients at risk for malnutrition.
3. The nutrition care process is a systematic approach for:
   a. identifying the nutrient content of foods.
   b. ordering special diets.
   c. conducting nutrition screening.
   d. meeting the nutrition needs of patients.
4. To conduct complete nutrition assessments, dietitians rely on several sources of information, which include all of the following *except:*
   a. nutrition care plans.
   b. body measurements.
   c. medical, social, and diet histories.
   d. biochemical analyses.

5. All of the following factors place a person at risk for malnutrition *except:*
   a. health problems that are frequently associated with PEM.
   b. the use of prescription medications that affect nutrient needs.
   c. a social history that reveals that the individual lives with a spouse in a middle-income neighborhood.
   d. a significant reduction in food intake over the past five or more days.
6. After a nutrition screening revealed that Mrs. Jones had been eating very poorly during the past several weeks and had lost a considerable amount of weight, she was referred to the dietitian for a complete nutrition assessment. Which method(s) would the dietitian most likely use to get a clearer picture of Mrs. Jones's usual food intake?
   a. 24-hour recall interview
   b. food frequency questionnaire
   c. food record
   d. a and b
7. Height and weight measurements:
   a. are both affected by fluid status.
   b. cannot be performed on bedridden patients.
   c. are routine measurements in health care facilities.
   d. require equipment that is not readily available in most health care facilities.
8. The %IBW of a person who weighs 185 pounds and has a healthy body weight of 150 pounds is:
   a. 123 percent.
   b. 150 percent.
   c. 23 percent.
   d. 81 percent.
9. A malnourished patient has just begun to eat after days without significant amounts of food. Which of the following blood tests would change most quickly as the patient's nutrition status improves?
   a. albumin
   b. transferrin
   c. serum electrolytes
   d. retinol-binding protein
10. Physical signs of PEM might include all of the following *except:*
   a. low serum albumin.
   b. dull, brittle hair.
   c. poor grip strength.
   d. wasted appearance.

NUTRITION ON THE NET

Access these websites for further study of topics covered in this chapter.

- Find updates and quick links to these and other nutrition-related sites at our website: **www.wadsworth.com/nutrition**
- Obtain food composition data from the USDA Nutrient Data Laboratory: **www.nal.usda.gov/fnic/foodcomp/**
- Visit the Joint Commission on Accreditation of Healthcare Organizations (JCAHO) to learn more about the quality of health care and accreditation: **www.jcaho.org**
- Learn more about the Nutrition Screening Initiative from the American Academy of Family Physicians: **www.aafp.org**

REFERENCES

1. D. R. Thomas and coauthors, Malnutrition in subacute care, *American Journal of Clinical Nutrition* 75 (2002): 308–313.
2. K. Lacey and E. Pritchett, Nutrition care process and model: ADA adopts road map to quality care and outcomes management, *Journal of the American Dietetic Association* 103 (2003): 1061–1072.
3. Lacey and Pritchett, 2003.
4. Lacey and Pritchett, 2003.
5. Lacey and Pritchett, 2003; K. Lacey and N. Cross, A problem-based nutrition care model that is diagnostic driven and allows for monitoring and managing outcomes, *Journal of the American Dietetic Association* 102 (2002): 578–589.
6. Lacey and Pritchett, 2003.
7. American Dietetic Association, *Manual of Clinical Dietetics* (Chicago: American Dietetic Association, 2000).
8. D. B. Schwartz and D. Gudzin, Preadmission nutrition screening: Expanding hospital-based nutrition services by implementing earlier nutrition intervention, *Journal of the American Dietetic Association* 100 (2000): 81–87.
9. L. C. Tapsell, V. Brenninger, and J. Barnard, Applying conversation analysis to foster accurate reporting in the diet history interview, *Journal of the American Dietetic Association* 100 (2000): 818–824.
10. F. E. Thompson and A. F. Subar, Dietary assessment methodology, in A. M. Coulston, C. L. Rock, and E. R. Monsen, eds., *Nutrition in the Prevention and Treatment of Disease* (San Diego: Academic Press, 2001), pp. 3–30; J. Dwyer, Dietary assessment, in M. E. Shils and coeditors, *Modern Nutrition in Health and Disease* (Baltimore: Williams & Wilkins, 1999), pp. 937–959.
11. Thompson and Subar, 2001.
12. M. Nelson and coauthors, Between- and within-subject variation in nutrient intake from infancy to old age: Estimating the number of days required to rank dietary intakes with desired precision, *American Journal of Clinical Nutrition* 50 (1989): 155–167.
13. E. Saltzman and K. M. Mogensen, Physical assessment, in A. M. Coulston, C. L. Rock, and E. R. Monsen, eds., *Nutrition in the Prevention and Treatment of Disease* (San Diego: Academic Press, 2001), pp. 43–58; S. B. Heymsfield, R. N. Baumgartner, and S. F. Pan, Nutritional assessment of malnutrition by anthropometric methods, in M. E. Shils and coeditors, *Modern Nutrition in Health and Disease* (Baltimore: Williams & Wilkins, 1999), pp. 903–921.

14. V. A. Stallings and E. B. Fung, Clinical nutrition assessment of infants and children, in M. E. Shils and coeditors, *Modern Nutrition in Health and Disease* (Baltimore: Williams & Wilkins, 1999), pp. 885–893.
15. Stallings and Fung, 1999.
16. Saltzman and Mogensen, 2001; American Dietetic Association, 2000; Heymsfield, Baumgartner, and Pan, 1999.
17. Heymsfield, Baumgartner, and Pan, 1999.
18. K. M. Flegal, R. Wei, and C. Ogden, Weight-for-stature compared with body mass index-for-age growth charts for the United States from the Centers for Disease Control and Prevention, *American Journal of Clinical Nutrition* 75 (2002): 761–766.
19. Saltzman and Mogensen, 2001; Heymsfield, Baumgartner, and Pan, 1999.
20. American Dietetic Association, 2000.
21. G. A. Modest, Edema, in J. Noble and coeditors, *Textbook of Primary Care Medicine* (St. Louis: Mosby, 2001), pp. 178–182.
22. J. M. Newton and C. H. Halsted, Clinical and functional assessment of adults, in M. E. Shils and coeditors, *Modern Nutrition in Health and Disease* (Baltimore: Williams & Wilkins, 1999), pp. 895–902.

ANSWERS

Study Questions (multiple choice)

1. b 2. d 3. d 4. a 5. c 6. d 7. c 8. a 9. d 10. a

HIGHLIGHT

Nutrition and Immunity

The **immune system** protects the body by fighting infectious agents and eliminating abnormal or "worn-out" cells. Its elaborate network of interacting cells and molecules works to block invading organisms from entering the body and destroys those that do gain entry. Substances that elicit an immune response are called antigens; common examples include foreign proteins produced by bacteria, viruses, or fungi. Because the immune system can usually distinguish between the body's cells and proteins and those of invading organisms, the body's own tissues are protected.

This highlight introduces the immune system and its relationships to malnutrition and illness (the accompanying glossary defines relevant terms). Later chapters examine some of the relationships between specific illnesses and immune processes. Some diseases result from inadequate immune responses, as when infections spread, causing sepsis (Chapter 22), or when malignant cells develop into tumors (Chapter 29). Other conditions, such as inflammatory bowel diseases (Chapter 24) and atherosclerosis (Chapter 27), result from **inflammation** (Chapter 22). Most of the time, however, the immune system's carefully orchestrated actions are quietly working to preserve health.

Tissues of the Immune System

The immune system resides in no single organ, but depends on the physical and chemical interactions of a loosely organized network of cells and tissues scattered throughout the body. The tissues and organs involved in immunity are collectively

GLOSSARY

acute-phase proteins: plasma proteins released from the liver at the onset of acute infection. An example is **C-reactive protein,** which is considered one of the main indicators of severe infection and has antimicrobial effects.

adaptive immunity: immunity that is specific for particular antigens; adapts to antigens in an individual's environment and is characterized by "memory" for particular antigens. Also called **acquired immunity.**

allergy: an excessive and inappropriate immune reaction to a harmless substance.

allergen: any substance that triggers an inappropriate immune response.

autoimmune diseases: diseases characterized by an attack of immune defenses on the body's own cells.

B cells: lymphocytes that produce antibodies.

cell-mediated immunity: immunity conferred by T cells and macrophages.

complement: a group of plasma proteins that assist the activities of antibodies.

cytokines (SIGH-toe-kines): proteins produced by white blood cells that regulate immune cell development and immune responses.

humoral immunity: immunity conferred by B cells, which produce and release antibodies into body fluids.
- **humor** = fluid

hypersensitivity: immune responses that are excessive or inappropriate. One type of hypersensitivity is *allergy.*

immune system: the body's defense system against foreign substances.

immunoglobulins (IM-you-no-GLOB-you-linz): proteins produced by B cells that function as antibodies.

innate immunity: immunity that is present at birth, unchanging throughout life, and nonspecific for particular antigens; also called **natural immunity.**

inflammation: a nonspecific response to injury or infection; a type of innate immune response.

leukocytes: blood cells that function in immunity; also called **white blood cells.**

lymphoid tissues: tissues that contain lymphocytes.

lymphatic vessels: vessels through which lymph travels.

lymphocytes (LIM-foe-sites): white blood cells that recognize specific antigens and therefore function in adaptive immunity; include *T cells* and *B cells.*

lysozyme (LYE-so-zyme): enzyme with antibacterial properties found in immune cells and body secretions such as tears, saliva, and sweat.

macrophages (MAK-roe-fay-jez): monocytes that have left circulation and settled in a tissue, where they serve as scavengers and activate the immune response.

monocytes (MON-oh-sites): cells released from the bone marrow that move into tissues and mature into macrophages.

natural killer cells: lymphocytes that confer nonspecific immunity by destroying a wide array of viruses and tumor cells.

neutrophils (NEW-tro-fills): the most common type of white blood cell. Neutrophils destroy antigens by phagocytosis.

phagocytes (FAG-oh-sites): white blood cells (neutrophils and macrophages) that have the ability to engulf and destroy antigens.
- **phagein** = to eat

phagocytosis (FAG-oh-sigh-TOE-sis): the process by which phagocytes engulf and destroy antigens.

T cells: lymphocytes that attack antigens.

Reminder: *Antibodies* are large proteins produced by B cells in response to specific antigens; also called *immunoglobulins. Antigens* are substances that trigger an immune response. Examples include foreign proteins from bacteria, viruses, fungi, parasites, and proteins of other persons.

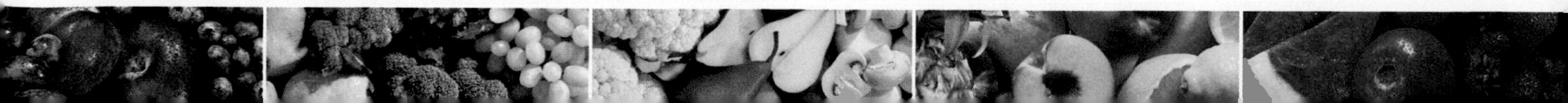

known as the lymphatic system (see Figure H17-1). **Lymphoid tissues** include the thymus gland and bone marrow, where **lymphocytes** are made, and the spleen, tonsils, adenoids, and lymph nodes, where foreign materials and debris are filtered out and discarded. Lymphoid tissue is also found within the body's mucosal linings where antigens are most likely to enter the body—in the gastrointestinal tract, the respiratory tract, and the genitourinary tract.

The cells active in immunity are the **leukocytes** (commonly known as **white blood cells**) and several types of accessory cells, as described in Table H17-1 and discussed in the following pages. These cells act by releasing chemicals such as enzymes, prostaglandins, histamine, and proteins called **cytokines** that bind to receptors on target cells. White blood cells travel between the tissues and blood in **lymphatic vessels** (see Chapter 3, p. 89).

FIGURE H17-1 The Lymphatic System

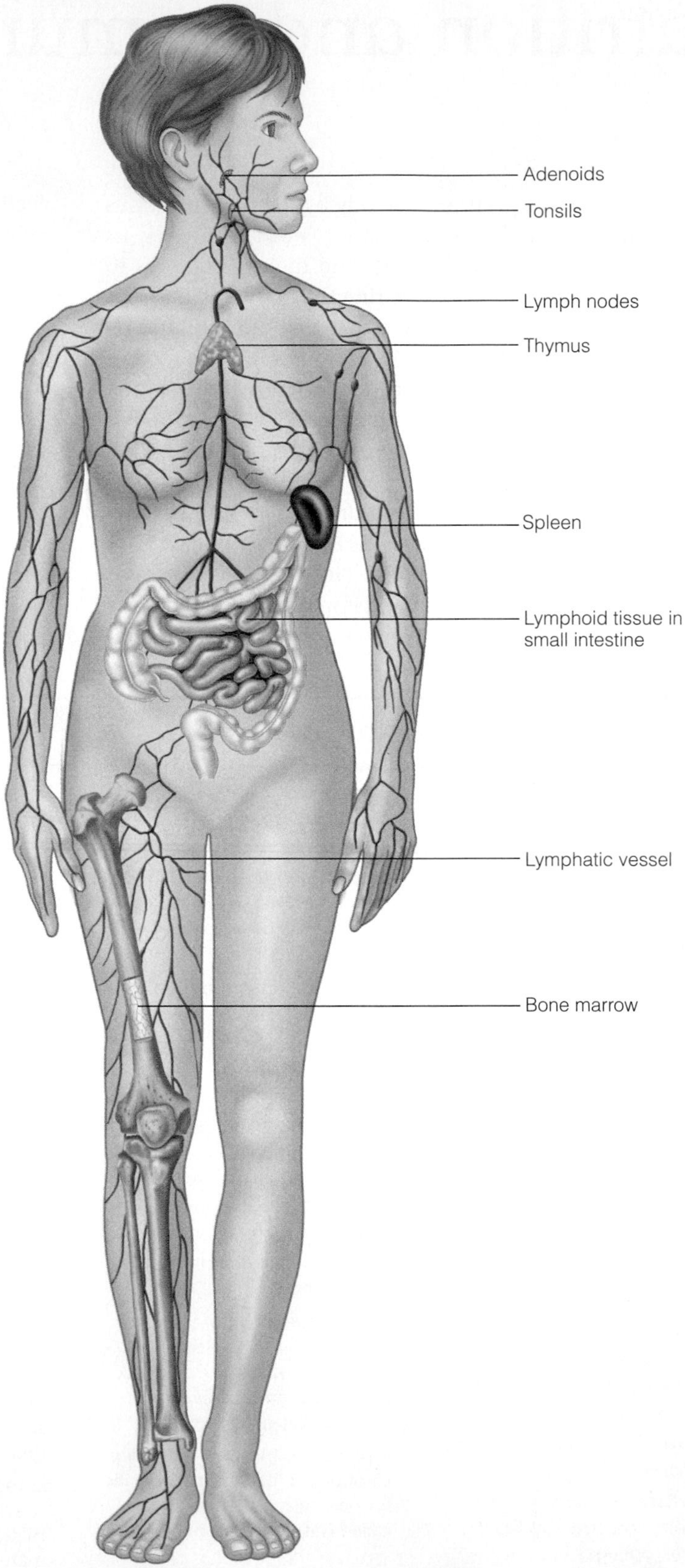
Adenoids
Tonsils
Lymph nodes
Thymus
Spleen
Lymphoid tissue in small intestine
Lymphatic vessel
Bone marrow

Examples of Innate Immunity

The immune protection present at birth is called **innate,** or **natural, immunity.** Innate immunity is nonspecific—it deters and destroys a wide range of pathogens. Nonspecific defenses include physical barriers to invading organisms, actions of defensive proteins, and activities of phagocytes and natural killer cells.

Physical Barriers to Infection

The body's first line of defense—the skin and mucous membranes—prevents the entry of infectious agents, which might otherwise gain easy access to tissues and blood. Skin not only provides an impenetrable physical barrier, but also contains its own lymphoid tissue and a variety of immune cells interspersed in its outer layers. Mucous membranes lining the gastrointestinal, respiratory, and genitourinary tracts also act as barriers to infection: mucus traps microorganisms and prevents them from attaching to tissue surfaces.[1]

Many microbes that arrive in the stomach face destruction from acidic gastric juices and enzymes. Those that survive enter the small in-

TABLE H17-1 Immune System Cells

White Blood Cells		
Lymphocytes	T cells	Activate macrophages Assist B cells Destroy virally infected cells
	B cells	Produce and secrete antibodies
	Natural killer cells	Destroy virally infected cells
Phagocytes	Monocytes/macrophages[a]	Present antigen fragments to T cells Engulf pathogens and cellular debris
	Neutrophils	Engulf pathogens and cellular debris
	Eosinophils	Release proteins that damage parasites Suppress inflammatory reactions
Accessory Cells		
Inflammatory mediators	Basophils	Release mediators that regulate inflammation
	Mast cells	Release mediators that regulate inflammation
	Platelets	Have primary role in blood clotting Release mediators that regulate inflammation

[a]Monocytes circulate in blood and become macrophages after they enter tissues.

testine, where digestive secretions and specialized cells, antibodies, and lymphoid tissue protect against infection. The large intestine also contains defensive cells and antibodies, as well as stable bacterial populations that actively maintain mucosal tissue and create a hostile environment for invasive bacteria.[2]

Defensive Proteins

Proteins contribute to nonspecific immune defenses by serving as enzymes or signaling molecules. The liver releases **acute-phase proteins** in response to trauma, infection, or inflammation. Some acute-phase proteins, such as **C-reactive protein,** have antimicrobial activities that destroy certain bacteria. C-reactive protein is considered a "marker" of acute inflammation and becomes elevated only when the body is fighting disease. Other acute-phase proteins include **complement,** a group of about 25 plasma proteins, so named because the proteins "complement" the activities of antibodies. When an antibody interacts with an antigen, a complex is formed that starts a series of reactions between the complement proteins. These actions may render microbes more susceptible to phagocytosis (described later), puncture a target cell's membrane, or help rid the body of antigen-antibody complexes. Another protein, **lysozyme,** attacks bacteria by breaking down carbohydrates on bacterial cell walls, causing the bacteria to burst.

Phagocytes

Upon entering the body, pathogens may encounter **phagocytes,** the scavenger cells of the immune system. Phagocytes engulf and digest bacteria, cellular debris (from damaged cells), and foreign particles in a process called **phagocytosis.** These cells are attracted to their targets by the presence of common microbial products, complement fragments, or chemical signals produced by cells. They pull in their prey by extending pseudopods ("false feet") and then douse it with a mix of potent chemicals that include hydrolytic enzymes, lysozyme, and free radicals.

The two main types of phagocytes are neutrophils and macrophages. **Neutrophils** are the most predominant leukocytes in blood, making up about 50 to 65 percent of the total. They also have the shortest life spans, surviving only a day or two after they are released from bone marrow. Neutophils migrate into tissues in response to injury or infection and accumulate in large numbers during the inflammatory process (discussed in Chapter 22). **Macrophages** are initially released from bone marrow as **monocytes;** after about a day in circulation, a monocyte migrates into one particular tissue where it develops into a macrophage and may survive for several months or longer. Each tissue has its own resident macrophages, and although their names may vary, they have similar functions in all tissues in which they reside. Examples of tissue macrophages include the Langerhans cells in the skin and the Kupffer cells in the liver.

Macrophages move and kill bacteria more slowly than neutrophils, but they are larger and can engulf larger targets, such as the body's dead and damaged cells. They also have the additional ability to display fragments of engulfed antigens on their cell surfaces for lymphocytes to recognize. This action triggers the immune responses of the lymphocytes (described in the later section "Examples of Adaptive Immunity").

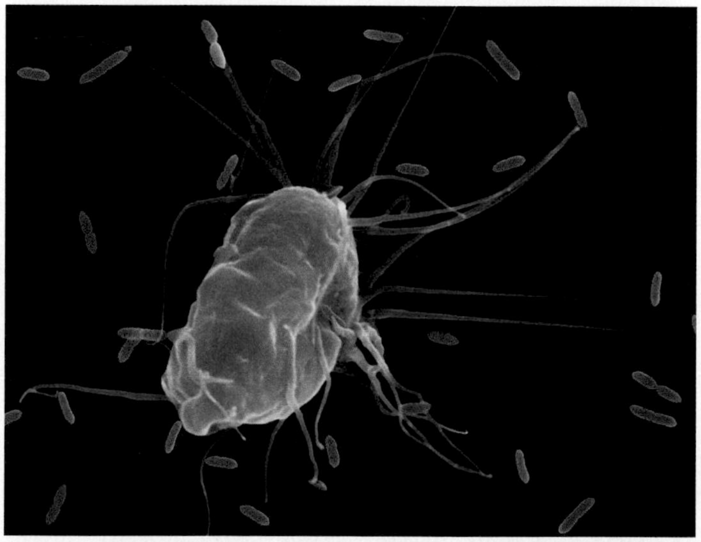

A macrophage extends pseudopods to pull in and engulf bacteria.

Natural Killer Cells

Natural killer cells are members of the lymphocyte family that recognize and destroy virus-infected cells and tumor cells. To destroy cells, these killer cells produce pore-forming proteins (called perforins) that can puncture the target cells' membranes. The killer cells then transfer destructive enzymes into the target cells that partially destroy their structures and encourage self-destruction. Phagocytes arrive at the scene to remove fragments left behind by the newly destroyed cell. The next section discusses the other members of the lymphocyte family, the B cells and T cells, which have critical roles in adaptive immunity.

Examples of Adaptive Immunity

In **adaptive,** or **acquired, immunity,** immune cells and proteins recognize *specific* pathogens as being foreign. Each **B cell** or **T cell** generates antibodies or receptors that can recognize only one specific type of antigen. Once activated, a lymphocyte produces other cells just like itself so that the newly formed army can attack the invading antigens and combat the infection. The lymphocytes are able to recognize a huge and diverse number of foreign molecules. Some of the lymphocytes serve as "memory cells," which survive for many years, enabling the immune system to respond rapidly if the same infection recurs.

B Cells

The B cells confer **humoral immunity,** so named because the cells' secretions, not the cells themselves, mount the defense within bodily fluids. B cells respond to antigens by producing antibodies that travel in the blood or tissue fluids to the site of infection. Antibodies, also known as **immunoglobulins,** are literally large globular proteins that provide immune protection. Each B cell expresses thousands of identical immunoglobulins on its cell surface. Once an antigen binds, the B cell multiplies. Its daughter cells produce large numbers of the same immunoglobulin and secrete them into the surrounding fluids. The free antibodies then attach to the surfaces of antigens to neutralize them or make them an easy target for attack by phagocytes. The antibodies can also bind to viral proteins to prevent viruses from entering cells.

T Cells

T cells participate in **cell-mediated immunity,** so named because the cells themselves direct an immune response. A T cell has thousands of identical receptors on its cell surface (called T-cell receptors) that can recognize one type of antigen. Antigens are displayed on the surfaces of antigen-presenting cells, specialized cells designed for this task (including macrophages and B cells). After a helper T cell binds to an antigen fragment on an antigen-presenting cell, it recruits a cytotoxic T cell to the region to attack and destroy the local antigens. The actions of cytotoxic T cells are similar to those of natural killer cells: they perforate cell membranes and deliver powerful chemicals that eventually lead to a cell's destruction. Helper T cells can also activate B cells to produce antibodies and can activate macrophages to destroy the pathogens they have engulfed.

Undesirable Effects of Immunity

Sometimes immune responses create problems. When excessive or inappropriate, immune reactions can lead to discomfort or illness—a condition referred to as **hypersensitivity. Allergy** is an example of an exaggerated response to an **allergen,** a harmless protein that may be eaten or inhaled. (Food allergy was introduced in Chapter 15 and is discussed further in Highlight 24.) Immune complexes formed from antigens and antibodies can also cause damage if not readily cleared by phagocytes. **Autoimmune diseases,** including such familiar diseases as type 1 diabetes mellitus and pernicious anemia, develop when immune responses are mounted against the body's own cells. Although the effects of the immune system are lifesaving when directed at harmful pathogens, they can be life-threatening when turned against the body.

Malnutrition, Immunity, and Infection

Malnutrition impairs immune function. Malnutrition is often accompanied by an increased risk of infection, and infection can reduce food intake and nutrient metabolism, further

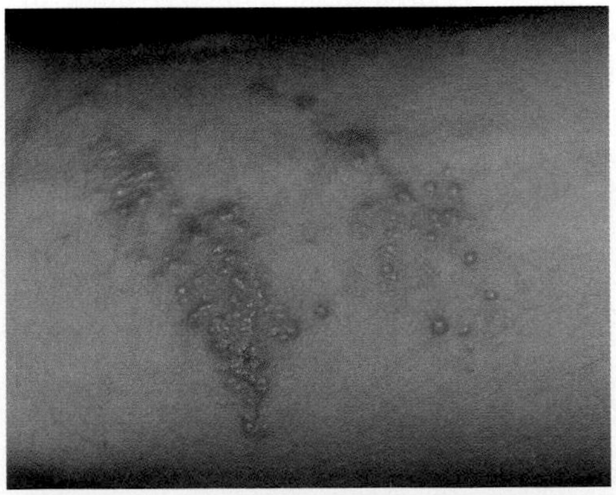

The rash that appears after contact with poison oak is an example of skin hypersensitivity.

worsening nutrition status. The result is a downward spiral in immunity and overall health. Although much of the discussion in this section centers on children in developing countries, malnutrition that is severe enough to impair immune function may occur in up to half of the adult hospital patients in the United States and is also common among the elderly.[3]

Malnutrition and Infection Risk

Protein-energy malnutrition (PEM), the most pervasive nutrition problem in the developing world, is frequently accompanied by serious infections. The risk of mortality from infection is much greater in children with PEM than in well-nourished children. Intervention studies have shown that infection rates can be dramatically improved by providing food supplements. In a five-year field trial among villages in rural Mexico, a program that provided food supplements to preschoolers was compared with another that vastly improved daily medical care. In the village that received medical care, preschoolers averaged 4.7 infections per year, whereas the children given food supplements averaged only 1.7 infections yearly.[4] The combination of malnutrition and infection severely affects growth rates in these children, and recovery periods are lengthy. One observational study that tracked whooping cough cases in a Guatemalan village found that a quarter of the children with the disease required about six months to regain the weight they had lost during illness.[5]

Malnutrition affects *all* aspects of immunity, including both innate and adaptive immune defenses. Both PEM and vitamin A deficiency can result in damage to skin and mucous membranes, which allows microorganisms easier entry into the body. Deficiencies of protein and some of the micronutrients can affect the synthesis of hydrolytic enzymes, complement, antibodies, and other proteins important for immune defenses. Cell-mediated immunity is impaired in numerous ways due to PEM and zinc deficiencies.[6]

Because PEM is usually associated with multiple micronutrient deficiencies, it has been difficult to separate out the individual effects of each nutrient. Zinc, iron, and vitamin A deficiencies are among the predominant micronutrient deficiencies worldwide, and a large body of research has demonstrated that each has a strong, independent influence on immunity. Supplementation of micronutrients (especially zinc and vitamin A) is frequently found to reduce the incidence or severity of illness.[7]

Effect of Infection on Nutrition Status

Recurrent infections are known to worsen nutrient deficiencies. Anorexia often results from infection and is worse when an infection is severe.[8] A study in Guatemala found that children with diarrhea consumed 18 percent fewer kcalories daily than healthy children. Another study found that Kenyan children reduced their kcaloric intake by 75 percent when they suffered from severe cases of measles. As mentioned earlier, body weights and growth are severely affected by infection. Some researchers found that negative nitrogen balance resulted from almost any infection, even when symptoms or fever were absent.[9]

Infection causes physical and metabolic changes that also worsen malnutrition.[10] For example, infections in the small intestine can disrupt its structure and function, frequently resulting in nutrient malabsorption. Damaged intestinal mucosa may increase fecal losses of nutrients: the breakdown of intestinal tissue can increase protein losses, and significant blood loss (as occurs in hookworm infection, for example) can cause iron status to deteriorate. Infections usually increase nutrient needs as well, due to the hypermetabolism that occurs during acute infection and the greater turnover rates of tissues that are more metabolically active during infection. Chapter 22 delves further into the consequences of severe infection and discusses the nutrient needs of individuals who suffer from these conditions.

REFERENCES

1. E. Isolauri and coauthors, Probiotics: Effects on immunity, *American Journal of Clinical Nutrition* 73 (2001): 444S–450S.
2. J. M. Saavedra and A. Tschernia, Human studies with probiotics and prebiotics: Clinical implications, *British Journal of Nutrition* 87 (2002): S241–S246; Isolauri and coauthors, 2001.
3. G. T. Keusch, The history of nutrition: Malnutrition, infection and immunity, *Journal of Nutrition* 133 (2003): 336S–340S.
4. N. S. Scrimshaw, Historical concepts of interactions, synergism and antagonism between nutrition and infection, *Journal of Nutrition* 133 (2003): 316S–321S.
5. Scrimshaw, 2003.
6. Scrimshaw, 2003.
7. Scrimshaw, 2003; K. H. Brown, Diarrhea and malnutrition, *Journal of Nutrition* 133 (2003): 328S–332S.
8. C. B. Stephensen, Vitamin A, infection, and immune function, *Annual Review of Nutrition* 21 (2001): 167–192.
9. Scrimshaw, 2003.
10. Keusch, 2003; Scrimshaw, 2003.

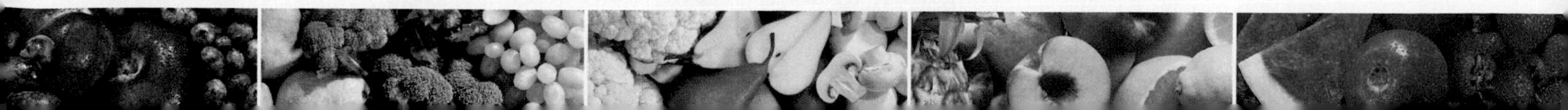

Chapter 18

Nutrition Intervention

Chapter Outline

Implementing Nutrition Care: *Approaches to Nutrition Care • The Medical Record • Reimbursement of Services*

Modified Diets: *Dietary Modifications • Alternative Feeding Routes • The Diet Order*

Foodservice: *Menu Planning • Food Selection • Food Preparation and Delivery • Improving Food Intake*

Highlight: *Nutritional Genomics*

Available Online

http://nutrition.wadsworth.com/uncn7

Student Practice Test

Glossary Terms

Nutrition on the Net

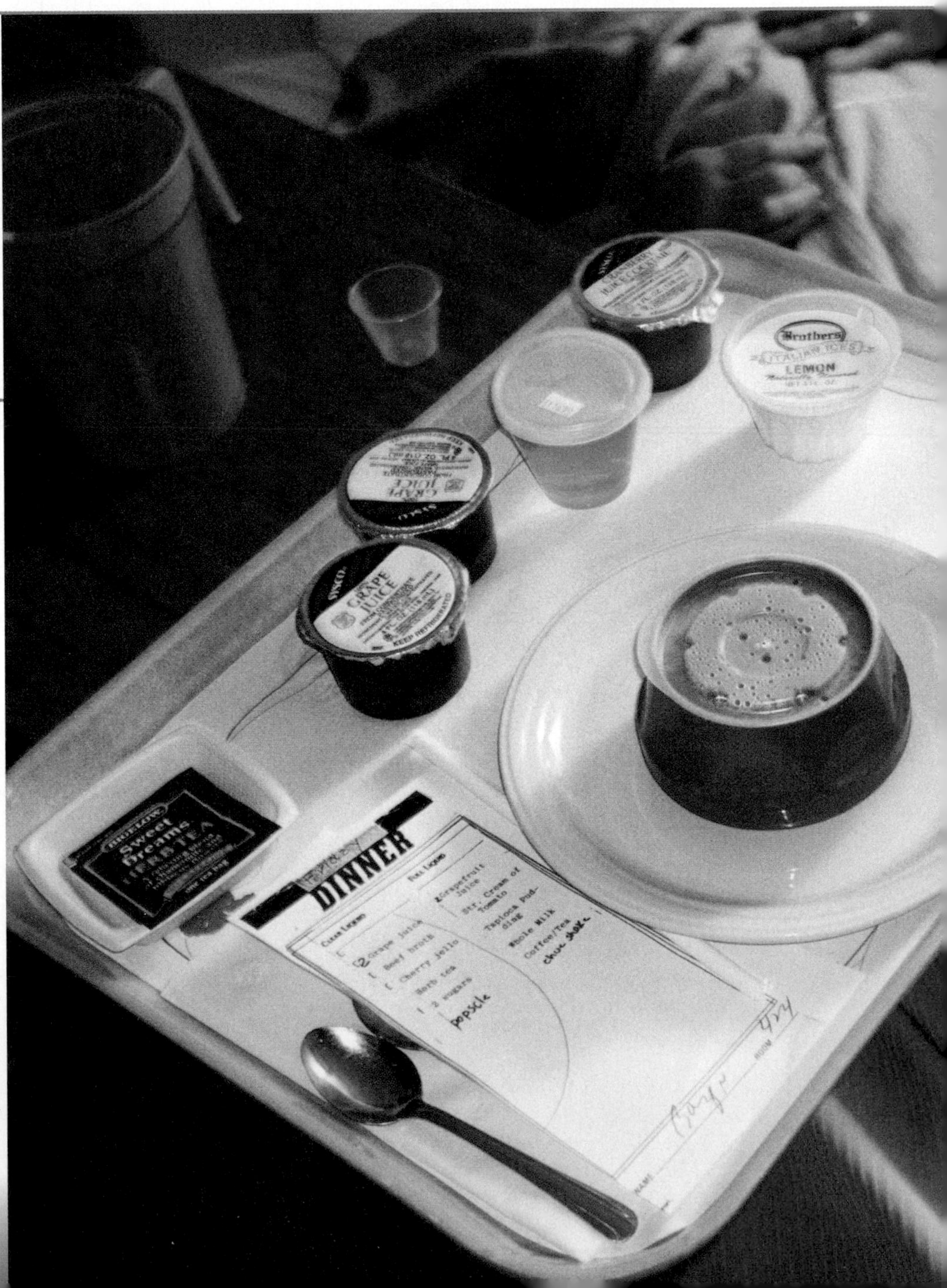

DINNER
GRAPE JUICE
LEMON

Nutrition in the Professional Setting

When working with patients, remember to establish a caring environment. Use familiar language, maintain eye contact, and be a good listener. Showing your interest can go a long way toward winning a patient's trust. Even an ideal dietary plan can sometimes be met with resentment and bitterness, for it may restrict a person's favorite foods and make it more difficult to cope with an illness. When interactions with health practitioners are positive and encouraging, an individual is more likely to make the dietary changes that benefit health.

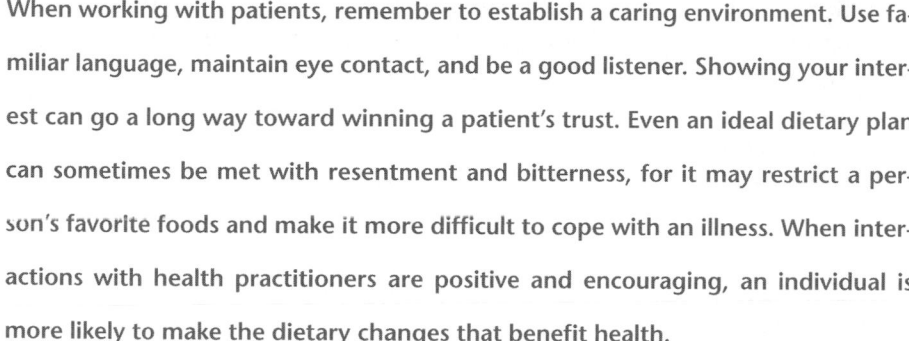

Chapter 17 discussed the interactions between illness and nutrition status and described the process of nutrition assessment. The results of a nutrition assessment help dietitians identify actual and potential nutrition problems. This chapter explains how health care professionals address such problems and provide nutrition care.

Implementing Nutrition Care

Nutrition interventions address and correct nutrition problems associated with acute disease or chronic illness and may play a role in the prevention of disease. A nutrition intervention requires two distinct, interrelated steps: the design of an appropriate nutrition care plan, and its implementation.[1] This section discusses several key components of these processes.

Approaches to Nutrition Care

As outlined in Chapter 17 (see pp. 584–586), a nutrition care plan consists of activities and educational materials that can help to resolve a person's immediate and long-term nutrition problems. The nutrition care plan should be compatible with the desires and abilities of the person it is designed to help. Because nutrition care often involves modifying eating habits, both education and behavior change techniques may be necessary.[2] The challenge is greater if dietary changes are required for extended periods.

Long-Term Dietary Intervention When long-term dietary changes are necessary, a nutrition care plan must take into account a person's current food habits, lifestyle, and degree of motivation. Because behavior change is a process that occurs in stages,[3] a single visit with a dietitian is rarely adequate. To ensure the success of long-term dietary modifications, follow-up visits are often necessary. The following approaches may be helpful in implementing long-term dietary changes:[4]

- *Determine the individual's readiness for change.* An effective nutrition care plan should be tailored to an individual's readiness to make dietary changes. Some people have no desire to change their dietary behaviors, and even those who are willing may not be fully prepared to take the necessary steps. A dietitian needs to consider a patient's readiness to adopt new dietary behaviors before attempting to implement an ambitious nutrition care plan.
- *Emphasize what to eat, rather than what not to eat.* Emphasizing foods that can be included in the diet, rather than those that should be restricted, can make dietary modifications more appealing. For example, suggesting additional fruits and vegetables is a more attractive message than telling the patient to restrict butter and cream sauces. In addition, an intervention will more likely be successful if the menus sound appetizing.
- *Encourage only one or two changes at a time.* People are more likely to try a dietary plan that does not deviate too much from their usual diet. If they are successful at adopting one or two changes, they are more likely to stick to the plan and be open to additional suggestions. Stricter plans may yield results more quickly, but are useful only for highly motivated people.

Nutrition Education Nutrition education is included in a nutrition care plan so that patients can learn about the dietary factors that affect a particular medical condition. Ideally, education also motivates individuals to make changes in diet and lifestyle that can measurably improve their health status.

A nutrition education program must be tailored to a person's age, level of literacy, and cultural background. Learning style should also be considered; some people learn best by lecture or discussion and are satisfied with written materials, whereas others prefer visual examples, such as food models, measuring devices, or food labels. Information can be provided in one-on-one counseling sessions or group discussions. A nutrition education session should also assess a person's understanding of the material and his or her commitment to making the necessary changes. Follow-up sessions can evaluate whether a person has adopted the desired behaviors.

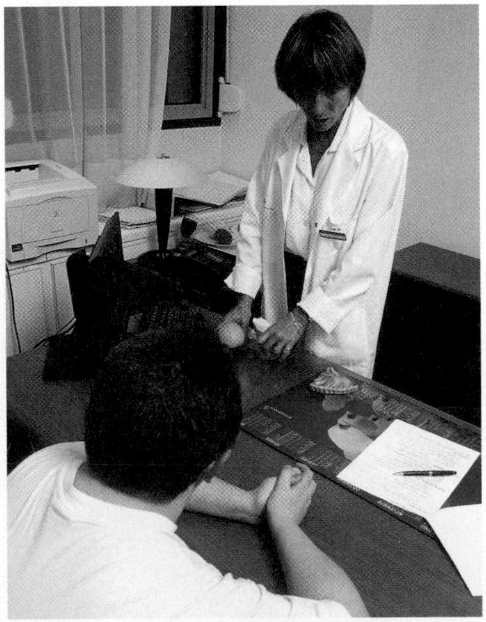

Dietary counseling requires sensitivity to cultural orientation, educational background, and motivation for change.

To provide nutrition education to a woman who is lactose intolerant and reluctant to use milk products, the dietitian might meet with the woman in a counseling session to teach her how to plan a nutritionally adequate diet that limits milk and milk products. Together they can design menus that take into account the woman's food preferences. Sample menus and food models can help to illustrate how altering food choices can change the calcium content of a meal. The Daily Value for calcium can be discussed using labels from foods such as calcium-fortified soy milk and supplements. The dietitian can also provide lists of foods that are good sources of calcium for the woman to take home to help with menu planning. In addition, the dietitian can assess the woman's understanding by having her identify nonmilk products that are high in calcium.

Follow-up Care Ideally, the dietitian monitors a patient's progress and regularly evaluates the effectiveness of a nutrition care plan. To achieve this, the dietitian usually compares relevant outcome measures (such as the results of blood tests) to initial values and meets with the patient to learn whether the plan has been satisfactory from the patient's point of view. Such follow-up efforts will reveal whether the care plan needs to be revised. A revised care plan may also be necessary if the person's situation changes. For example, after a pregnant woman delivers her baby, she may need instructions on how to feed her infant or how to modify her diet to support lactation (if she is breastfeeding) so that she can return to a healthy body weight. If a follow-up meeting with a dietitian is not possible, a dietetic technician or other qualified health practitioner will generally provide additional guidance and education.

The Medical Record

The medical record is a communication tool used by members of a health care team. It should accurately describe the health care provided to patients and identify the health care professional who provided the care. Medical records are legal documents and may be given to insurance carriers or to government and accrediting agencies to substantiate claims or determine the quality of care.

A medical record includes a patient's health history; the assessments, diagnoses, and prognoses of medical problems; the measures taken to treat those problems; and the results of tests and treatments. Entries by health care professionals document the care they have provided, the patient's condition and response to therapy, and the practitioner's recommendations for future care.

Medical Record Formats The format of medical documents varies among medical facilities, although there are a number of popular approaches. Problem-oriented medical records focus on a patient's medical problems and the strategies used to address those problems. This format is gradually being replaced by outcome- or goal-oriented records, which focus on quantifiable goals and the strategies for achieving them. For example, a problem-oriented medical record for a person with diabetes mellitus would list diabetes mellitus as a problem and then identify the strategies used to control the diabetes, such as diet planning, the use of medications to control blood sugar, and an exercise program. A goal-oriented medical record for the same patient would specify the patient's goal weight and desirable blood glucose levels and list the treatment plans for reaching these goals.

Documenting Nutrition Care Nutrition care is documented in various ways, but the most popular is the SOAP note.[5] The letters represent the types of information included: *S*ubjective, *O*bjective, *A*ssessment, and the *P*lan for care. *Subjective* information is obtained in an interview with the patient or patient's family and includes the main symptoms and complaints related to a particular medical problem. *Objective* information is available from the nutrition screening or assessment data; it includes results of biochemical analyses, anthropometric tests, and physical examinations. *Assessment* is a brief evaluation of the subjective and objective data and provides a concise diagnosis of the nutrition problem. The *Plan* describes recommendations, including dietary prescriptions, special equipment, nutrition education, and referrals that can help solve the problem. Figure 18-1 shows an example of a SOAP note, although there are many possible variations.

Other charting styles are also in use, but the content is more important than the particular format used. Health care professionals need to learn the charting procedures preferred by a medical facility before making entries in patients' medical records. Generally, entries in the medical record should be as succinct as possible so that they can be easily read and quickly understood by the other members of the health care team. The standardized templates used in electronic data systems also require concise language.

Reimbursement of Services

Managed care organizations■ often include outpatient nutrition services as a component of chronic disease management. Nevertheless, a survey of private health insurers in the United States found that only 52 percent covered the

■ Managed care is the provision of health care by a specified group of health care professionals and hospitals in order to manage costs or quality of care. Health maintenance organizations and preferred provider organizations are examples of managed care organizations.

FIGURE 18-1 Example of a SOAP Note

SOAP NOTE

Patient Name: Arthur Jones **Date:** Aug. 10, 2005

Age: 58 **Gender:** Male **Medical diagnosis:** Hypercholesterolemia

Subjective:

Patient recently learned of his hypercholesterolemia, has no obvious symptoms. Wants trial of dietary/lifestyle changes to reduce need for medication. Willing to attempt weight loss.

Objective:

Total cholesterol: 288 mg/dL
HDL-C: 48 mg/dL
LDL-C: 214 mg/dL
Triglycerides: 132 mg/dL

Glucose (fasting): 101 mg/dL
Hb_{A1c}: 5.7%
Weight: 268 lb
Height: 6'1"
Waist circumference: 45"
BMI: 35.4

Assessment:

Abdominal obesity; elevated LDL cholesterol. Weight loss and lifestyle changes may improve hypercholesterolemia; Mr. Jones is highly motivated to try these before resorting to meds.

Plan:

Goal: 15 lb weight loss over next 6 months; instruction about food portion sizes and lower-kcalorie food choices. Patient to start 30-minute walking program, evenings.

Follow-up visit: One month; patient will identify food portion sizes.

Referral: Heart-healthy workshop on August 17 (one week); patient to attend with wife.

Form completed by: Carmen Cordova, MPH, R.D. **Position:** Dietitian, Nutrition Services

medical nutrition therapy (MNT) provided by dietitians (an additional 12 percent were not sure).[6] Although MNT plays a critical role in disease management, reimbursement of services by insurers is quite limited.

Medicare benefits expanded in 1997 to cover MNT for outpatient diabetes management. In 2000, MNT was added for Medicare beneficiaries with diabetes and nondialysis kidney disease. Under additional provisions to take effect in 2005 and 2006, limited MNT services will be available to new beneficiaries of Medicare and to those with chronic diseases such as congestive heart failure and chronic obstructive pulmonary disease.[7] Private insurers often model their benefit packages after Medicare benefits, so it is anticipated that insurers may expand their coverage of nutrition services in the future.

IN SUMMARY Nutrition care plans are designed to correct the nutrition problems associated with illness. A care plan should be compatible with a person's food preferences and willingness to make dietary changes. Nutrition education may be provided in an individual counseling session or group workshop.

The evaluation of a care plan or nutrition education program ideally includes objective outcome measures of a person's health status. Nutrition care needs to be documented in the medical record and should be coordinated with overall medical care.

Modified Diets

During many illnesses, a person can meet energy and nutrient needs by following a **standard** or **regular diet.** In other cases, a **modified diet** is prescribed. Modified diets are usually altered in consistency or nutrient content or by including or eliminating certain foods. This section gives examples of common modified diets and explains their use during illness.

Dietary Modifications

Table 18-1 (on p. 612) lists examples of modified diets that are prescribed during illness. A diet's texture and consistency may be altered for people with chewing or swallowing impairments. Some dietary modifications relieve the symptoms of disease; for example, restricting dietary sodium can help to control fluid accumulation, and eliminating legumes and certain vegetables can reduce flatulence. Increasing the nutrient density of a diet may prevent or reverse malnutrition. Diets are also adjusted to improve nutrition-sensitive risk factors for chronic diseases, such as high blood cholesterol and hypertension. If a patient has more than one of these problems, several aspects of a diet may have to be modified.

Mechanically Altered Diets People who have difficulty chewing or swallowing may benefit from mechanically altered diets.[8] Swallowing impairment, or **dysphagia,** is a complication associated with certain diseases and disease treatments. Dysphagia may accompany neurological illnesses, surgical procedures that involve the head and neck, and a number of physiological and anatomical abnormalities that restrict the movement of food within the throat or esophagus. Diets for dysphagia are highly individualized because swallowing difficulties can vary greatly and because a person's swallowing ability can fluctuate over time. Diets used for dysphagia may also be prescribed for individuals with limited chewing abilities or dental problems.

Table 18-2 on p. 613 provides examples of foods that are included in mechanically altered diets.■ When soft, easy-to-chew foods such as breads, graham crackers, tender meats, soft fruits, and cooked vegetables are included, the diet is called a mechanical soft diet or simply a soft diet.

■ Mechanically altered diets include pureed diets and ground/minced diets.

Blenderized Liquid Diet Liquid diets are often prescribed following oral or facial surgeries (for example, jaw wiring) and may also be used by individuals with chewing problems.[9] The diet includes fluids and foods that have been blenderized to a liquid form. Soft or tender foods from all food groups can be blenderized (often with added liquid), including cereals and breads; cooked vegetables; fresh or cooked fruits without skins and seeds; cooked, tender meats and fish; and potatoes, rice, and pasta. Foods that do not blend well are excluded; examples include nuts and seeds, dried fruits, sausage and frankfurters, hard cheeses, raw vegetables, and corn. To prevent bacterial growth, blenderized foods should either be consumed immediately after preparation or be refrigerated for no more than 48 hours.[10]

Clear Liquid Diet Clear liquids require minimal digestion and are easily tolerated by the gastrointestinal (GI) tract. They are often the first foods offered to patients after acute gastrointestinal disturbances or intravenous feeding.[11] The **clear liquid diet** is also used before bowel surgeries and colonoscopy (a type of colon

standard or **regular diet:** a diet that includes all foods and meets the nutrient needs of healthy people.

modified diet: a diet that is adjusted to meet medical needs. Such diets may be adjusted in consistency, energy or nutrient content, or by the inclusion or elimination of certain foods.

dysphagia: difficulty swallowing.

clear liquid diet: a diet that consists of foods that are liquid at room temperature and leaves almost no residue (undigested material) in the intestines after digestion and absorption.

TABLE 18-1 Examples of Modified Diets

Type of Diet	Description of Diet	Appropriate Uses
Modified Texture and Consistency		
Mechanically altered diets	Contain foods that are modified in texture. Pureed diets include only pureed foods, ground/minced diets may include solid foods that are mashed, minced, ground, or soft.	Pureed diets are used for persons with swallowing difficulty, poor lip and tongue control, or oral hypersensitivity. Ground/minced diets are appropriate for persons with limited chewing ability or certain swallowing impairments.
Blenderized liquid diet	Contains fluids and foods that are blenderized to liquid form.	For persons who cannot chew, swallow, or tolerate solid foods.
Clear liquid diet	Contains clear fluids or foods that are liquid at room temperature and leave minimal residue in the colon.	For preparation for bowel surgery or colonoscopy, for acute gastrointestinal disturbances, or as a transition diet after intravenous feeding. For short-term use only.
Therapeutic Diets		
Fat-restricted diet	Restricts fat to low (<50 g/day) or very low (<25 g/day) levels in the diet.	For persons who have certain malabsorptive disorders or symptoms of diarrhea, flatulence, or steatorrhea (fecal fat) resulting from dietary fat intolerance.
Fiber-restricted diet	Restricts fiber to low levels in the diet (<10 g/day).	For acute phases of intestinal disorders or to reduce fecal output before surgery. Not recommended for long-term use.
High-kcalorie, high-protein diet	Contains foods that are kcalorie and protein dense.	Used for increased kcalorie and protein requirements (in cancer, AIDS, burns, trauma, and others); also used to reverse malnutrition, improve nutrition status, or promote weight gain.
Modified Mineral Diets		
Sodium-restricted diet	Restricts sodium; degree of restriction depends on symptoms and disease severity.	To prevent fluid retention or induce fluid loss; used in hypertension, congestive heart failure, renal disease, and liver disease.

SOURCE: American Dietetic Association, *Manual of Clinical Dietetics* (Chicago: American Dietetic Association, 2000).

examination). The diet consists of clear fluids and foods that are liquid at room temperature and leave little **residue** in the intestine (for this reason, milk products are not included in the diet). Permitted foods include clear or pulp-free fruit juices, clear broths, bouillon, consommé, fruit-flavored or unflavored gelatin, fruit ices made from clear juices, frozen juice bars, and plain hard candy.[12] Although the diet provides fluid and electrolytes, its nutrient and kcalorie contents are extremely limited. If used for longer than a day or two, it should be supplemented with commercially prepared low-residue formulas that can provide required nutrients. Figure 18-2 gives an example of a one-day clear liquid menu.

After a period without food, clear liquids are usually offered in small amounts at first to make sure the person can easily tolerate them. Most patients can then tolerate a rapid progression to solid foods, even after colon surgery.[13] Although preferences vary, a postoperative meal might include both liquids and solid foods, such as soup, sandwiches, pudding, juice, or milk. If a patient experiences gas or distention, smaller, more frequent meals may help. Small quantities of dry foods may be helpful if nausea or vomiting persists.

residue: material left in the intestine after digestion; includes mostly dietary fiber and undigested starches and proteins.

TABLE 18-2 Foods Included in Mechanically Altered Diets

Pureed Diets	Ground/Minced Diets
Milk products: Milk, smooth yogurt, pudding.	**Milk products:** Milk, yogurt with soft fruit, pudding, cottage cheese, processed cheeses, grated cheese.
Fruits: Pureed fruits without seeds or skins, juices, applesauce.	**Fruits:** Mashed or minced fruits without seeds or skins, mashed bananas, thickened juices and nectars, applesauce.
Vegetables: Pureed cooked vegetables without seeds or skins.	**Vegetables:** Mashed, minced, or soft (cooked) vegetables without seeds or skins, mashed winter squashes, moist mashed potatoes.
Meats and meat substitutes: Pureed meats (with gravy), pureed casseroles (with broth), pureed legumes.	**Meats and meat substitutes:** Ground meats, soft casseroles with gravy/broth.
Breads and cereals: Cream of wheat, cream of rice, slurried breads without crusts,[a] slurried pancakes, pureed rice and pasta	**Breads and cereals:** Smooth cooked cereals, pureed breads, pancakes with syrup, soft (bite-sized) pasta or rice (if tolerated).

[a]Slurried foods are mixed with liquid until the consistency is appropriate for the patient.
SOURCE: American Dietetic Association, *Manual of Clinical Dietetics* (Chicago: American Dietetic Association, 2000).

FIGURE 18-2 Menu—Clear Liquid Diet

SAMPLE MENU

Breakfast	Strained orange juice
	Flavored gelatin
	Ginger ale
	Coffee or tea, sugar
Lunch	Bouillon or consommé
	Flavored gelatin
	Frozen juice bars
	Apple or grape juice
	Coffee or tea, sugar
Supper	Bouillon or consommé
	Flavored gelatin
	Fruit ice
	Cranberry juice
	Coffee or tea, sugar
Snacks	Soft drinks
	Fruit ices
	Hard candy

Fat-Restricted Diet A fat-restricted diet may be recommended for reducing the symptoms of fat malabsorption that often accompany diseases of the liver, gallbladder, pancreas, lymphatic system, and intestines. Low-fat diets may also alleviate the symptoms of heartburn. Although fat intake is sometimes limited to as little as 25 grams daily, it should not be restricted more than necessary because fat is an important source of kcalories. Chapter 24 gives additional information about fat-restricted diets (pp. 744–746).

Most foods included in a fat-restricted diet provide less than 1 gram of fat per serving. The diet includes fat-free milk products, most breads and cooked grains, fat-free broths and soups, vegetables prepared without fats, most fruits, and fat-free candies and sweets (Table 24-4 on p. 746). Restricted foods include low-fat and whole-milk products, baked products with added fat (like muffins), and most prepared desserts. Lean meat and meat substitutes are permitted, but are restricted to 4 to 6 ounces per day, depending on the degree of restriction. Some patients with malabsorptive conditions do not tolerate large amounts of lactose or dietary fiber, so foods that include these substances may also need to be excluded from the diet.

Fiber-Restricted Diet A fiber-restricted diet is recommended during acute phases of intestinal disorders when the presence of fiber may exacerbate intestinal discomfort or cause diarrhea or blockages. Fiber-restricted diets are sometimes used before surgery to minimize fecal volume and after surgery during transition to a regular diet. Long-term fiber restriction is discouraged, however, because it is associated with constipation, diverticulosis, and other illnesses.

Fiber-restricted diets often eliminate whole-grain breads and cereals, nuts and seeds, raw and dried fruits, berries, dried beans and peas, chunky peanut butter, winter squash, and most raw vegetables. If required, even greater reductions in colonic residue can be achieved by excluding most fruits and vegetables and milk products. Additional guidance about the fiber content of foods can be found in Table 4-3 on p. 127 and in Appendix H.

High-kCalorie, High-Protein Diet The high-kcalorie, high-protein diet is used to increase kcalorie and protein intakes in patients who have unusually high requirements or in those who are eating poorly. High-fat foods are added to increase energy intakes; consequently, the diet may exceed 35 percent kcalories from fat. Consuming small, frequent meals and commercial liquid supplements also can help a patient meet increased energy, protein, and other nutrient needs.

TABLE 18-3 Foods Included in High-kCalorie, High-Protein Diets

Milk products	• Whole milk, half-and-half, cream • Cheese • Milk shakes, eggnog • Ice cream, whipped cream
Fruits	• Dried fruit • Canned fruit in heavy syrup • Avocado
Vegetables	• Vegetables prepared with butter, margarine, sour cream, mayonnaise, or salad dressing • Cream of vegetable soups
Meats and high-protein foods	• All meats, fish, and poultry, including bacon, frankfurters, and luncheon meats; eggs • All meats, prepared fried or covered in cream sauces and gravies • Nuts and seeds, peanut and other nut butters, coconut
Breads and cereals	• Granola and dry cereals prepared with whole milk or cream and dried fruit • Hot cereals with whole milk or cream, or added fat • Pasta, rice, and potatoes with added fat • Pancakes, waffles, French toast

Examples of foods included in high-kcalorie, high-protein diets are listed in Table 18-3. Some of these foods are high in saturated fat, which is restricted in heart-healthy diets. These foods are used liberally in malnourished patients to help correct their immediate nutrition problems—weight loss and muscle wasting. The "How to" offers additional suggestions for increasing the kcalorie and protein contents of meals.

Sodium-Restricted Diet A sodium-restricted diet is often used to prevent fluid retention and may be recommended for treatment of hypertension, congestive heart failure, kidney disease, or liver disease.[14] The degree of restriction depends on the illness, severity of symptoms, and the drug treatment prescribed. In most cases, sodium is restricted to 2000 or 3000 milligrams daily, although more severe restrictions may be used in the hospital setting.■ Sodium restriction is difficult to implement on a long-term basis because many patients find low-sodium diets unpalatable and fail to adhere to them.

■ Reminder: Although the Upper Level for sodium is 2300 mg, intakes in the United States generally exceed this amount.

Guidelines for sodium restriction usually include omitting the use of salt in cooking and at the table, eliminating most prepared foods and condiments, and limiting consumption of milk and milk products. Because so many processed foods are high in sodium, food labels should be checked and only low-sodium products consumed. Sodium restriction is discussed further in Chapters 27 and 28; see the "How to" on p. 838 and Table 28-1 on p. 855.

The modified diets discussed in this section can be adjusted to satisfy individual preferences and tolerances. They should also be altered as a patient's condition changes. Later chapters include other dietary modifications and strategies used in the treatment of the medical conditions discussed.

Alternative Feeding Routes

Patients most often meet their nutrient needs by consuming regular foods. If their nutrient needs are high or their appetites poor, liquid formulas can be added to their diets to supplement their intakes. Sometimes, however, a person's medical condition makes it difficult to meet nutrient needs orally. Two options remain: **tube feedings** or **intravenous feedings.**

tube feedings: liquid formulas delivered through a tube placed in the stomach or intestine.

intravenous feedings: the provision of nutrients through a vein, bypassing the intestine.

HOW TO Increase kCalories and Protein in Meals

To add kcalories to a meal, try these suggestions:

- *Butter or margarine.* Melt on pasta, potatoes, rice, and cooked vegetables. Add to hot cereals, casseroles, and soups. Spread liberally on bread, crackers, and rolls.
- *Mayonnaise.* Add to pasta, tuna, and potato salads. Use as a dressing for raw or cooked vegetables.
- *Cream cheese.* Mix into chopped fruits. Spread on raw vegetables, toast, and crackers. Use as a spread in sandwiches made with luncheon meats. Mix with yogurt for added flavor.
- *Half-and-half and cream.* Replace milk or water with half-and-half or cream in soups, sauces, hot chocolate, desserts, mashed potatoes, and cold and cooked cereals.
- *Nuts.* Add chopped nuts to pasta dishes, stir-fried vegetables, fruit salads, and green salads. Use nut meats in baked products.

These suggestions can help add protein to a meal:

- *Powdered milk (use full-fat milk powder if available).* Add to recipes that include milk. Dissolve extra milk powder into milk-containing beverages. Stir into hot cereals, potato dishes, casseroles, sauces, scrambled eggs, hamburger, and meat loaf.
- *Cheese.* Melt on burgers, meat loaf, cooked vegetables, scrambled eggs, casseroles, and potatoes. Add cottage cheese to casseroles, egg dishes, pasta recipes, and salad dressings. Grate hard cheeses and sprinkle on soups, salads, and cooked vegetable dishes.
- *Eggs.* Add raw eggs to casserole recipes, meatballs, and hamburgers. Add chopped hard-cooked eggs to salads, vegetable dishes, sandwich fillings, and pasta and potato salads.
- *Meats.* Add meat pieces to soups, egg dishes, casseroles, and pasta sauces. Add minced meats to vegetable dishes. Include meat in bean dishes.

- *Tube feedings.* Nutritionally complete formulas can be delivered through a tube placed directly into the stomach or intestine. Tube feedings are always preferred to intravenous feedings if the GI tract is functioning. A person in a coma, for example, is unable to eat but may be able to digest foods and absorb nutrients normally. In such a case, a tube feeding would be the most appropriate option (see Chapter 20).
- *Intravenous feedings.* In some cases, a person's medical condition prohibits the use of the GI tract to deliver nutrients. If the person is malnourished and the GI tract cannot be used for a long period of time, intravenous feedings can provide nutrients■ (see Chapter 21).

■ The intravenous provision of nutrients is called *parenteral nutrition.*

The Diet Order

As mentioned in Chapter 17, the physician has the primary responsibility for ordering an appropriate diet for a patient in a medical facility. The physician often relies on the dietitian to make recommendations when changes in the diet order appear warranted. If the dietitian recommends a change, it must be communicated clearly and quickly to the physician. In some medical facilities, dietitians may have some order-writing privileges so that optimal nutrition care can be provided as quickly and efficiently as possible.[15]

Diet Progression A diet order may read, "progress diet from clear liquids to a regular diet as tolerated." **Diet progression** changes the diet to adapt to a patient's increased tolerance to foods. There is little scientific evidence, however, to support a slow progression from clear liquids to solid foods after surgery, as was formerly believed.[16] Many patients tolerate a regular diet by the second postoperative meal. Symptoms such as nausea, vomiting, and flatulence can result from anesthesia and gut immobility, but dietary restrictions are not necessarily helpful.

Nothing by Mouth (NPO) An order to not give a patient anything at all—food, beverages, or medications—is abbreviated NPO for *non per os,* meaning "nothing by mouth." For example, an order may read "NPO for 24 hours" or "NPO

diet progression: a change in diet as a patient's tolerances permit.

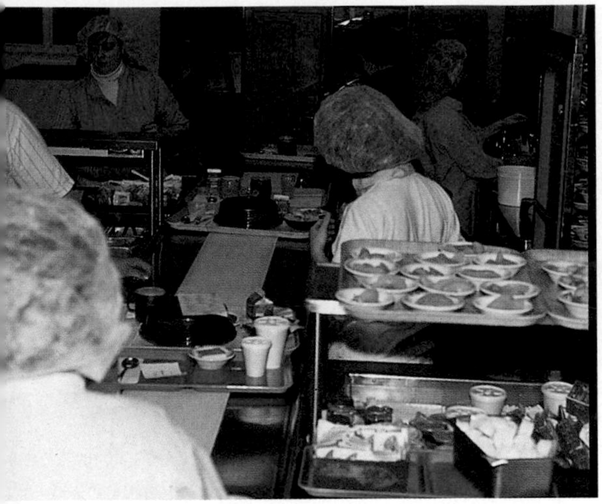

Foodservice departments strive to prepare appetizing and nutritious meals and may accommodate dozens of special diets.

until after X-ray." The NPO order is commonly used during certain acute illnesses and tests involving the GI tract.

IN SUMMARY A diet that is modified in consistency or nutrient content may be prescribed during illness. Diets modified in consistency can be used for people with swallowing and chewing difficulties and include the pureed, ground/minced, soft, and blenderized liquid diets. Clear liquid diets may be used briefly after acute gastrointestinal disturbances or intravenous feedings. Other medical conditions may require the restriction or supplementation of specific nutrients. In some cases, nutrients need to be delivered via tube feedings or intravenously. The physician has the primary responsibility for writing a diet order for a modified diet.

Foodservice

The work of a foodservice department can appear deceptively simple, with appropriate foods being delivered to patients who need specific types of diets. Behind the scenes, however, a complex system is at work. A foodservice department faces a daily challenge in planning, producing, and delivering hundreds of nutritious meals and accommodating dozens of special diets and food preferences.

Although this discussion focuses on the foodservice in hospitals, much of the information applies to foodservice in any health care facility, including nursing homes, assisted living centers, rehabilitation centers, and residential mental health care facilities. An important difference between hospitals and long-term health care facilities deserves mention, however. When patients in hospitals eat poorly, they can make up for nutrient deficits by eating well when they return home. Residents of a long-term care facility do not have this option. For this reason, foodservice departments in long-term care facilities must make even greater efforts to ensure that their patients receive and consume nutritious foods.

Menu Planning

In large facilities, the staff of dietitians may compile a **diet manual,** subject to approval by hospital administrators, several physicians, and representatives of the nursing service. Small facilities may adopt the diet manual of another hospital or an organization such as the state or national dietetic association. The diet manual describes the foods allowed and restricted for different modified diets, outlines the rationale and indications for use of the diets, and includes sample menus. The dietary department uses the diet manual to design menus for each diet. Registered dietitians and dietetic technicians may also assist in menu planning, especially for special diets.

Food Selection

Most hospitals provide **selective menus** from which patients can select their meals. A patient who must follow a modified diet receives menus that include only the foods specified in the hospital's diet manual for that particular diet (examples of menus are shown in Figure 18-3). By allowing a choice, this system ensures that patients will receive the foods they prefer and are most likely to eat. An added advantage is that patients can become familiar with the modified diets as they select foods from the appropriate menus.

Each menu identifies the patient and room number, the meal (breakfast, lunch, or supper), the type of diet, and the day the menu will be served. Often, patients need to make menu selections for a day or two in advance so that the foodservice

diet manual: a book that specifies the foods allowed and restricted on modified diets and provides sample menus.

selective menus: menus with two or more choices in some or all menu categories.

FIGURE 18-3 Sample Lunch Menus

LOW-FAT/LOW CHOLESTEROL/CARDIAC SUNDAY

Lunch

LF = Low Fat LSLF = Low Sodium, Low Fat

Meats

LSLF Baked chicken LSLF Baked fish (cod)

Starchy Vegetables

LSLF Rice LSLF Boiled potatoes

Vegetables

LSLF Baby carrots LSLF Green beans

Soup/Salad/Juice	Dressings
LSLF Coleslaw	Diet French
Gelatin	Diet Thousand Island
Tomato soup	Diet Italian
Tossed salad	

Desserts

Pears Fresh fruit

Breads

LF Dinner roll	Bran bread
White bread	LS Crackers
Wheat bread	

Beverages & Condiments

Coffee	Creamer
Decaf. coffee	Sugar
Hot tea	Sugar substitute
Decaf. hot tea	Herb seasoning
Iced tea	Lemon
Buttermilk	Margarine
Fat-free milk	Mustard
	Diet mayonnaise
	Catsup

Name ________________ Room _____

LOW SODIUM SUNDAY

Lunch

LF = Low Fat LSLF = Low Sodium, Low Fat

Meats

LSLF Baked chicken LSLF Baked fish (cod)

Starchy Vegetables

LSLF Rice LSLF Boiled potatoes

Vegetables

LSLF Baby carrots LSLF Green beans

Soup/Salad/Juice	Dressings
LSLF Coleslaw	Diet French
LS Chicken broth	Diet Thousand Island
Apple juice	Diet Italian
Tossed salad	

Desserts

Pears Fresh fruit

Breads

Dinner roll	Bran bread
White bread	LS Crackers
Wheat bread	

Beverages & Condiments

Coffee	Sugar
Decaf. coffee	Sugar substitute
Hot tea	Creamer
Decaf. hot tea	Lemon
Iced tea	Herb seasoning
Whole milk	Margarine
2% milk	Diet mustard
Fat-free milk	Diet mayonnaise
	Diet catsup

No salt

Name ________________ Room _____

RENAL SUNDAY

Lunch

LF = Low Fat LSLF = Low Sodium, Low Fat

Meats

LSLF Baked chicken LSLF Baked fish

Starchy Vegetables

LSLF Rice LSLF Dialyzed potatoes

Vegetables

LSLF Baby carrots LSLF Green beans

Soup/Salad/Juice	Dressings
Lemonade	Diet French
LSLF Coleslaw	Diet Thousand Island
Tossed salad (no tomato)	Diet Italian

Desserts

Pears Apple pie

Breads

Dinner roll	Bran bread
White bread	LS Crackers
Wheat bread	

Beverages & Condiments

Coffee	Sugar
Decaf. coffee	Sugar substitute
Hot tea	Creamer
Decaf. hot tea	Lemon
Iced tea	Margarine
	Diet mustard
	Mayonnaise

No salt

Name ________________ Room _____

department can estimate the amounts and types of food it needs to prepare. Menus are usually color-coded by diet, which helps to ensure that foodservice employees put the right foods on food trays. Color-coding also helps the person delivering the tray confirm that the right diet was delivered.

Patients typically select one or more items from each food category on a menu. If a menu is not marked correctly or is misplaced, the patient may receive a meal selected by the foodservice department. Potential problems that may arise when selective menus are used include:

- Patients may have difficulty seeing, reading, understanding, or physically marking menus.
- Patients may not understand that their selections will be for the next (or another) day.
- Patients may be out of their rooms (for tests, procedures, or physical activity) or asleep when the menus arrive and may miss the menu pick-up time.
- Patients may be too ill or too disinterested in food to make menu selections.

Problems with menu procedures can often be corrected by an explanation of the system or by taking the time to help patients mark menus.

Once food selections have been made and the menus collected, a member of the foodservice staff (usually, a dietetic technician or dietitian) may check them to ensure that the selections are appropriate. Completed menus can provide valuable clues about a person's usual eating habits or understanding of a modified diet.

Some hospitals do not offer selective menus. Instead, they may provide **nonselective menus** (menus with preselected food items) or menus that include

nonselective menus: menus that do not allow choices and list only preselected food items.

elements of both systems **(semiselective menus)**. Nonselective menus have been gaining popularity in hospital foodservice because they simplify operations and may help to cut costs.

Food Preparation and Delivery

The responsibility of budgeting, purchasing, planning, preparing, and serving appropriate meals rests with either a chief administrative dietitian or a foodservice director. Some facilities contract with outside foodservice companies to perform these duties. The logistics of preparing foods tailored to each modified diet can be overwhelming. For this reason, foodservice departments use systems designed to limit costs and minimize errors.

Meals may be produced in a central kitchen and delivered directly to patients' rooms, using serving equipment that keeps hot foods hot and cold foods cold. Another popular practice is to produce meals beforehand, deliver trays to the nursing unit, and then reheat hot food items in areas close to the patients' rooms. Generally, foodservice personnel deliver food carts directly to the nursing unit, and then either nursing or foodservice personnel take trays to patients.

The foodservice department needs to be contacted if a patient receives the wrong diet or consistently receives foods that differ from those requested. Foodservice departments often conduct periodic surveys to uncover problems patients may have with menu selections, food quality, or food service. Keep in mind that many foodservice employees do not have a nutrition background, and their ability to interpret diet orders and provide accurate information is limited.

Improving Food Intake

People in hospitals often lose their appetites as a result of their medical condition, treatment, or emotional distress. In addition, patients receive meals at specified times regardless of whether they are hungry and often must eat in bed without companionship; under these conditions, eating can be more of a chore than a pleasurable experience. Many medical conditions, medications, and treatments can dramatically alter taste perceptions. Meals may also be unwelcome if the person is in pain or has been sedated.

Dietitians, dietetic technicians, and nurses often play a central role in helping patients to eat. If either appetite or the sense of taste is affected by illness, the dietitian may be able to work with the patient to identify foods that can be enjoyed the most. Some problems can be handled directly by the person caring for the patient. For example, the nurse or assistant delivering trays can make sure that foods and utensils are arranged attractively when served and that the patient has had an opportunity to wash up before the meal. In some cases, the foodservice department must be contacted to solve food-related problems. The "How to" box lists additional suggestions to improve food intake at mealtimes.

The quality of foodservice strongly influences a patient's perception of the overall hospital stay.[17] Good communication between patients and the hospital staff about meals and food quality can improve a patient's satisfaction with foodservice.

IN SUMMARY Hospital foodservice departments often accommodate the special needs of hundreds of patients daily. Most hospitals provide selective menus from which patients can select meals that are appropriate for their specific medical conditions. Patients may need assistance with menu procedures and may need to be encouraged to consume adequate amounts of food.

semiselective menus: menus that combine aspects of both selective and nonselective menus.

HOW TO Help Hospital Patients Improve Their Food Intakes

1. Empathize with the patient. Show that you understand how difficult eating may be. Imagine feeling too sick to move or too tired to sit up.
2. Motivate. Be sure the patient understands how important nutrition is to recovery.
3. Help patients select the foods they like and mark menus appropriately. When appropriate and permissible, let friends or family members bring favorite foods from outside the hospital.
4. For patients who are weak, suggest foods that require little effort to eat. Eating a roast beef sandwich, for example, requires less effort than cutting and eating a steak. Drinking soup from a cup may be easier than eating it with a spoon.
5. Help patients prepare for meals. Help them get comfortable, either in bed or in a chair. Adjust the extension table to a comfortable distance and height, and make sure it is clean. Take these steps before the tray arrives, so the meal can be served promptly and at the right temperature.
6. When the food cart arrives, check the patient's tray. Confirm that the patient is receiving the right diet, that the foods on the tray are those selected from the menu, and that the foods look appealing. Order a new tray if foods are not appropriate.
7. Help with eating, if necessary. Help patients to open containers or cut foods, and help with feeding if patients cannot feed themselves.
8. Try to solve eating problems. Encourage patients with little appetite to eat the most nutritious foods first and to drink liquids between meals.
9. Take a positive attitude toward the hospital's food. Never say something like "I couldn't eat this either." Instead, say, "The foodservice department really tries to make foods appetizing. I'm sure we can find a solution."

CASE STUDY

Implementing Nutrition Care

Sam is a nine-year-old Native American who was admitted to the hospital after he passed out while playing with friends. Tests confirm a diagnosis of type 1 diabetes mellitus. Sam remains in the hospital for several days until his blood glucose and ketone levels are under control. During this time, he and his family learn about diabetes mellitus, the diet Sam needs to follow, the use of insulin, how to monitor blood glucose levels, and the required coordination of diet, insulin, and physical activity. The details of diabetes mellitus are reserved for Chapter 26, but for now you can consider the steps that are necessary for implementing a nutrition care plan.

1. Given the chronic nature of Sam's illness, what approach should be used when discussing the required dietary and medical treatments with Sam's family? What factors need consideration when designing a nutrition education program that includes Sam and his parents?
2. After a first visit with Sam and his family, what information should the dietitian include in Sam's medical record? Is enough information given above for designing a SOAP note? If not, what elements are missing?
3. Sam will need follow-up care to learn more about diabetes and to make the adjustments that will allow him to cope with his condition. Why is it important that plans for follow-up care be addressed before Sam leaves the hospital?

STUDY QUESTIONS

These questions will help you review the chapter. You will find the answers in the discussions on the pages provided.

1. Discuss the factors that should be considered when a patient is encouraged to make long-term dietary changes. What role can nutrition education play in this process? (pp. 607–609)
2. Describe how outcome measures can be used to monitor a patient's progress. (pp. 608–609)
3. Discuss the value and uses of the medical record, and identify the elements of a SOAP note. (pp. 609–610)
4. Compare the types of foods included in pureed diets, ground/minced diets, and blenderized diets. Give examples of patients who may benefit from these diets. (pp. 611–613)
5. Describe the uses of the clear liquid diet, and list permitted foods. (pp. 611–613)
6. Discuss the uses of the fat-restricted, fiber-restricted, and sodium-restricted diets. (pp. 612–614)
7. Give examples of menu changes that can improve the kcalorie and protein contents of meals. (pp. 613–615)
8. Discuss the advantages and potential problems associated with the use of selective menus by hospital foodservice departments. (pp. 616–617)
9. Describe how health care professionals can help hospital patients improve their food intakes. (pp. 618–619)

These multiple-choice questions will help you prepare for an exam. Answers can be found on p. 621.

1. Measurable goals for a person who must lose weight might include:
   a. the number of pounds the person is expected to lose each week.
   b. the type of diet the person is expected to follow.
   c. family members' attitudes toward the person's weight.
   d. the person's food intake record.
2. The most successful nutrition intervention would include a long list of:
   a. dietary changes that the person should consider making.
   b. foods that the person should avoid.
   c. appetizing meals and foods that the person can include in his or her diet.
   d. reasons why the person should make dietary changes.
3. The most important factor(s) that affect how nutrition education is presented is (are):
   a. the person's nutrient needs and nutrition status.
   b. the person's abilities and motivation.
   c. the person's medical history.
   d. the entries in the medical record.
4. A dietitian discusses a weight-reduction program with a patient, and together they set a goal for weight loss of 1 pound per week. The next step for the dietitian is to:
   a. assume the plan is working.
   b. formulate a new nutrition care plan.
   c. find a new strategy for meeting weight-loss goals.
   d. plan a follow-up meeting to weigh the patient and see how well the plan is working.
5. All of the following are true about medical records *except:*
   a. they are legal documents.
   b. they provide information about a patient's medical problems and the measures taken to address those problems.
   c. they all conform to the same format.

d. they are a communication tool used by the health care team.

6. Foods permitted on the clear liquid diet include all of the following *except:*
   a. milk.
   b. fruit ices.
   c. flavored gelatin.
   d. consommé.

7. The modified diet *least* likely to provide adequate nutrients and kcalories is the:
   a. pureed diet.
   b. clear liquid diet.
   c. ground/minced diet.
   d. high-kcalorie, high-protein diet.

8. Fiber restriction may be recommended:
   a. in patients with dysphagia.
   b. in patients who are unable to absorb fat normally.
   c. in patients with heartburn.
   d. during the acute phases of some intestinal disorders.

9. A hospital patient may occasionally be dissatisfied with selective menu procedures because:
   a. the system does not include food choices for individuals on modified diets.
   b. selective menus are difficult to understand and mark correctly.
   c. the opportunity to mark menus may be missed if patients are unavailable or asleep.
   d. foodservice operations cannot handle the food preferences of hundreds of patients.

10. A nurse notices a food on a patient's tray and is not sure if the food is allowed on the patient's diet. An appropriate action for the nurse to take would be to check the:
    a. care plan.
    b. diet order.
    c. diet manual.
    d. medical record.

NUTRITION ON THE NET

Access these websites for further study of topics covered in this chapter.

- Find updates and quick links to these and other nutrition-related sites at our website: **www.wadsworth.com/nutrition**
- Visit the website of the American Dietetic Association to find position papers on dietetics issues: **www.eatright.org**
- Design patient education materials with information from this government website: **http://medlineplus.gov/**
- Clinical issues are discussed at this Food and Drug Administration website, targeted to health professionals: **www.fda.gov/oc/oha/default.htm**

REFERENCES

1. K. Lacey and E. Pritchett, Nutrition care process and model: ADA adopts road map to quality care and outcomes management, *Journal of the American Dietetic Association* 103 (2003): 1061–1072.
2. J. M. Heins and L. Delahanty, Tools and techniques to facilitate eating behavior change, in A. M. Coulston, C. L. Rock, and E. R. Monsen, eds., *Nutrition in the Prevention and Treatment of Disease* (San Diego: Academic Press, 2001), pp. 105–122.
3. K. Glanz, Current theoretical bases for nutrition intervention and their uses, in A. M. Coulston, C. L. Rock, and E. R. Monsen, eds., *Nutrition in the Prevention and Treatment of Disease* (San Diego: Academic Press, 2001), pp. 83–93.
4. Glanz, 2001; M. C. Rosal and coauthors, Facilitating dietary change: The patient-centered counseling model, *Journal of the American Dietetic Association* 101 (2001): 332–338, 341.
5. C. Biesemeier and C. S. Chima, Computerized patient record: Are we prepared for our future practice? *Journal of the American Dietetic Association* 97 (1997): 1099–1104; P. Grace-Farfaglia and P. Rosow, Automating clinical dietetics documentation, *Journal of the American Dietetic Association* 95 (1995): 687–690.
6. C. S. Chima and H. A. Pollack, Position of the American Dietetic Association: Nutrition services in managed care, *Journal of the American Dietetic Association* 102 (2002): 1471–1478.
7. ADA Report on Medicare Conference Report, **www.eatright.org/Print/index_18143.cfm**, site visited October 5, 2004.
8. American Dietetic Association, *Manual of Clinical Dietetics* (Chicago: American Dietetic Association, 2000).
9. American Dietetic Association, 2000.
10. American Dietetic Association, 2000.
11. American Dietetic Association, 2000.
12. American Dietetic Association, 2000.
13. American Dietetic Association, 2000.
14. American Dietetic Association, 2000.
15. H. J. Silver and N. S. Wellman, Nutrition diagnosing and order writing: Value for practitioners, quality for clients, *Journal of the American Dietetic Association* 103 (2003): 1470–1472.
16. American Dietetic Association, 2000.
17. C. A. Watters and coauthors, Exploring patient satisfaction with foodservice through focus groups and meal rounds, *Journal of the American Dietetic Association* 103 (2003): 1347–1349.

ANSWERS

Study Questions (multiple choice)

1. a 2. c 3. b 4. d 5. c 6. a 7. b 8. d 9. c 10. c

Nutritional Genomics

Imagine this situation: a physician scrapes a sample of cells from inside your cheek and submits it to a **genomics** lab. Within an hour, you receive a report that reveals your disease susceptibilities and recommends dietary and lifestyle changes that can maintain health. You may even be given a prescription for a dietary supplement to prevent the diseases that you are most likely to develop. Improbable? Perhaps, but these possibilities are being explored by scientists involved with the new field of **nutritional genomics,** the study of dietary effects on **gene expression.**[1] Recent research suggests that some dietary factors may be more helpful (or more harmful) in people who have particular genetic variations. The promise of nutritional genomics is a custom-designed dietary prescription that fits each person's specific needs.

The recent surge of interest in genomics grew from the Human Genome Project, an international effort by industry and government scientists to sequence the human genome that was completed in April 2003. This project led to enormous advances in the research technologies needed to study genes and genetic variation. With recent knowledge about the general sequences of DNA within our chromosomes, researchers can now study how alterations in a person's diet and lifestyle can change the expression of a multitude of genes. The Herculean tasks ahead are to identify the individual genes in the genome and the roles of their respective protein products, the genes and protein products associated with diseases, and the dietary and lifestyle choices that most influence the expression of the genes involved in disease. The accompanying glossary defines genomics and related terms.

Defining Nutritional Genomics

Genetic differences among individuals have been studied for years, as have the specialized dietary therapies that are used to treat various **inherited disorders.** For example, an individual may inherit a genetic defect that inhibits the normal metabolism of an essential nutrient and may therefore need to con-

GLOSSARY

chromosomes: structures within the nucleus of a cell that contain the cell's DNA and associated proteins.

gene expression: the process by which a cell converts the genetic code into RNA and protein.

genes: segments of DNA that contain the information needed to make proteins.

genome: the full complement of genetic material in the chromosomes of a cell.

genomics: the study of genomes.

inherited disorders: medical conditions resulting from genetic defects.

microarray technology: research technology that monitors the expression of thousands of genes simultaneously.

multigene or **polygenic:** involving a number of genes, rather than a single gene.

noncoding sequences: regions of DNA that do not code for proteins. Some noncoding sequences may have regulatory or structural properties, but most have no known function.

nucleotides: the subunits of DNA and RNA molecules. These compounds—cytosine (C), thymine (T), uracil (U), guanine (G), and adenine (A)—are each composed of a phosphate group, a 5-carbon sugar (ribose), and a nitrogen-containing base. A DNA molecule is made up of two long chains of nucleotides held together by hydrogen bonding between nucleotide bases on opposing strands; each hydrogen-bonded nucleotide couple is called a **base pair.**

nutritional genomics: the study of dietary effects on genetic expression; also known as **nutrigenomics.**

polymorphisms: differences in the DNA sequences among individuals. A **single-nucleotide polymorphism** involves a single nucleotide at a particular area in the DNA strand.

- **poly** = many
- **morph** = form
- **ism** = condition

promoter: a region of DNA involved with gene activation.

transcription factors: proteins that bind DNA at specific sequences to regulate gene expression.

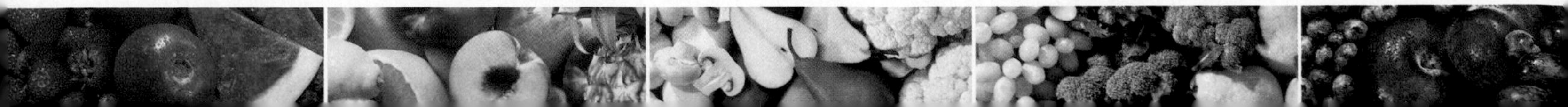

FIGURE H18-1 The Human Genome

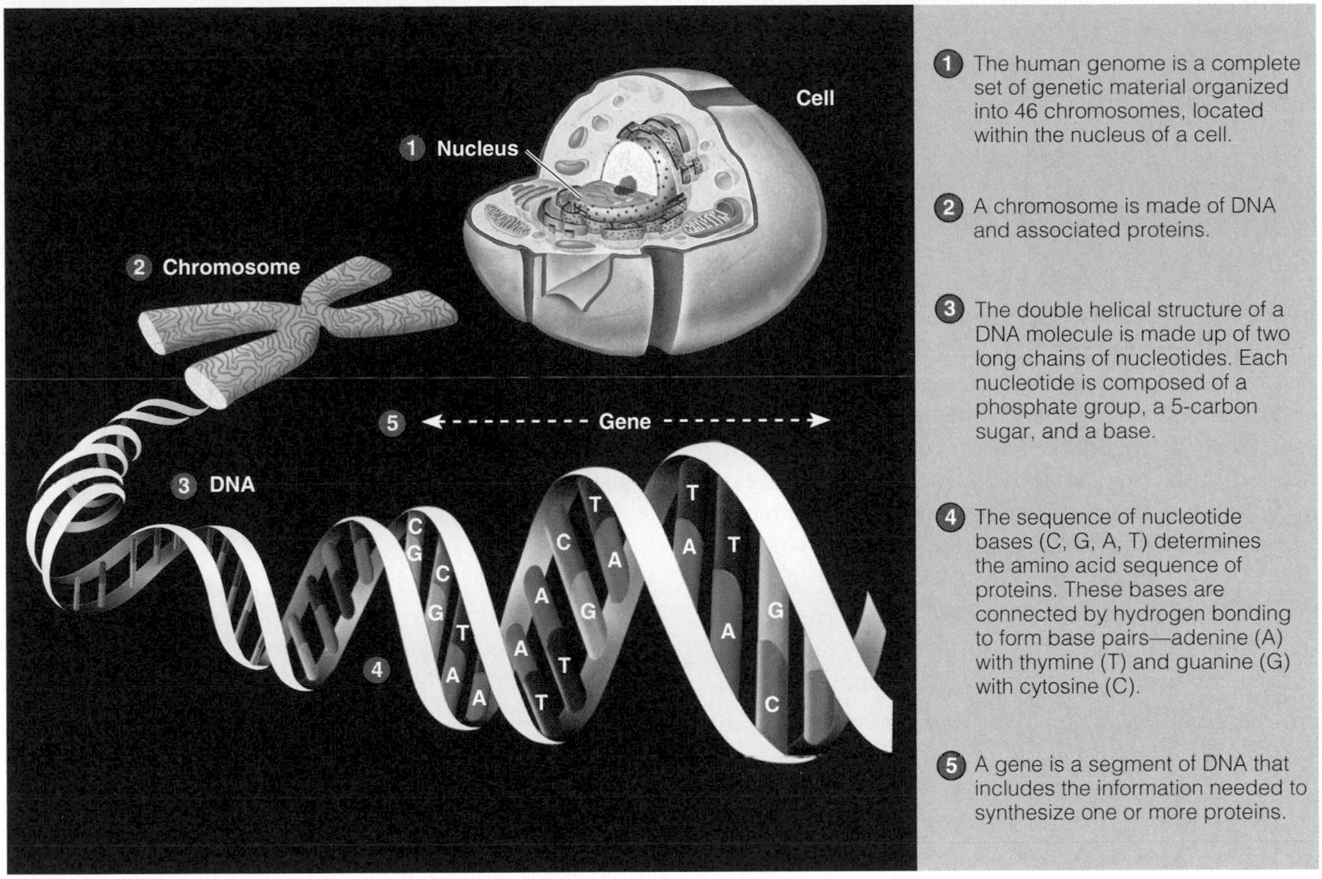
Cell
1 Nucleus
2 Chromosome
3 DNA
4
5 Gene
1 The human genome is a complete set of genetic material organized into 46 chromosomes, located within the nucleus of a cell.
2 A chromosome is made of DNA and associated proteins.
3 The double helical structure of a DNA molecule is made up of two long chains of nucleotides. Each nucleotide is composed of a phosphate group, a 5-carbon sugar, and a base.
4 The sequence of nucleotide bases (C, G, A, T) determines the amino acid sequence of proteins. These bases are connected by hydrogen bonding to form base pairs—adenine (A) with thymine (T) and guanine (G) with cytosine (C).
5 A gene is a segment of DNA that includes the information needed to synthesize one or more proteins.

Adapted from "A Primer: From DNA to Life," Human Genome Project, U.S. Department of Energy Office of Science; http://www.ornl.gov/sci/techresources/Human_Genome/primer_pic.shtml.

sume a diet that contains either more or less of this nutrient. An example of this type of condition is phenylketonuria (PKU), introduced on p. 135 and discussed further in Highlight 20. Genomic research takes this concept a few steps further: instead of focusing on alterations in one or two genes, researchers study the expression of *multiple* genes.

A Genomics Primer

As discussed in Chapter 6, our genetic information is encoded in DNA molecules within the nuclei of almost all of the cells in our bodies. Figure H18-1 shows how our genetic material is arranged to comprise the **genome,** which is the complete set of genetic information within our cells. The DNA molecules are tightly packed along with associated proteins within the 46 **chromosomes.** Segments of a DNA strand that can eventually be translated into proteins are called **genes.** The sequence of **nucleotides** within each gene encodes the amino acid sequence of a particular protein. Scientists currently estimate that there are between 20,000 and 25,000 genes in the human genome.[2] Only a small percentage of the genome codes for proteins, however: most DNA consists of **noncoding sequences** whose function, if any, is unclear.

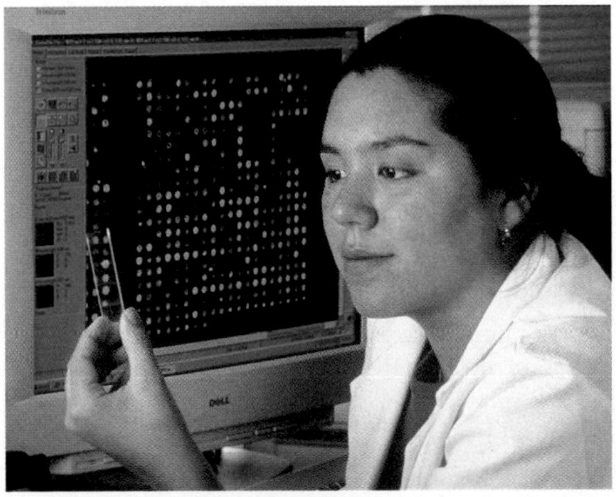

A DNA microarray allows researchers to monitor the expression of thousands of genes simultaneously.

When proteins are made, the information in the DNA sequence is first transcribed (copied) to messenger RNA molecules, which carry the genetic information out of the nucleus. Gene expression can be measured by determining the amounts of messenger RNA in a tissue sample. The expression of thousands of genes can be measured simultaneously using **microarray technology** (see the photo on p. 623).

How Nutrients Alter Gene Expression

Nutrients often function as signals that switch gene expression on or off.[3] The **promoter** region of a gene (a DNA region involved with gene activation) acts as the master switch. A large variety of proteins known as **transcription factors** recognize and bind to areas on the promoter and either enhance or inhibit gene expression. The number of transcription factors present in the nucleus and their tendency to bind to DNA are influenced by a combination of dietary factors and hormones. Examples of how nutrients can influence gene expression include:

- The transcription factor that enhances gene expression of enzymes required for cholesterol synthesis enters the nucleus only when the cellular cholesterol content is low.
- The transcription factor that inhibits expression of ferritin, an iron-storage protein, changes its affinity for DNA based on the iron content of the cell.

Genetic Variation and Disease

Except for identical twins, no two persons are genetically identical. The variation in the genomes of any two persons, however, is only about 0.1 percent, a difference of only one base in every 1000. The most common genetic differences, known as **polymorphisms,** are changes in single nucleotides **(single-nucleotide polymorphisms).** Such variations are significant only if they affect the amino acid sequence of a protein in such a way that protein function is altered.

Genetic variation gives rise to the diversity among human beings—it explains most of the differences in our physical appearances and metabolic characteristics. It also determines, along with environmental factors, our susceptibilities to diseases. Diseases characterized by a single-gene disorder tend to be relatively rare and usually exert their effects early in life. In contrast, the more common diseases, such as heart disease and cancer, are influenced by many genes and typically develop over several decades or even longer. In these more complex **multigene,** or **polygenic,** disorders, each of the genes can contribute to disease risk, but no single gene may be sufficient to cause the disease on its own.

Single-Gene Disorders

Single-gene disorders may seriously disrupt metabolism and may require significant dietary or medical intervention. Examples of single-gene disorders include PKU, sickle-cell anemia, and the iron-overload disease hemochromatosis. Not all single-gene disorders have life-threatening ramifications. For example, lactose intolerance can result from an alteration in the promoter of the lactase gene; it may cause gastrointestinal discomfort and is readily managed with dietary modification.

Multigene Disorders

Multigene diseases are often sensitive to environmental influences such as diet and lifestyle.[4] In many cases, these environmental risk factors directly influence the expression of the genes involved. Because multigene diseases tend to develop over many years, determining genetic susceptibility can allow a person to modify diet and lifestyle appropriately and reduce the risk of developing the disease.

Heart disease is an example of a disease with multiple gene influences. Its many risk factors represent the involvement of an assortment of genes that affect disparate aspects of physiology and metabolism. Consider that the major risk factors for heart disease include elevated blood cholesterol levels, obesity, diabetes, and hypertension. The underlying cause of any of these risk factors is rarely known; currently, clinicians screen for the presence of risk factors, but not the reasons why they occur. Should genomic research prove successful, a future assessment approach might be to identify specific genetic alterations and changes in metabolism that lead to the development of individual risk factors. For example, tests may determine whether blood cholesterol levels are high due to excessive cholesterol absorption, excessive liver production, or reduced cholesterol degradation.[5] This information could then guide clinicians to the most appropriate intervention. Similarly, dietitians would be better able to match their dietary recommendations to a person's genetic profile; for example, a high-carbohydrate, low-fat diet was long considered an appropriate intervention for heart disease patients, but it was later found to increase triglyceride levels in genetically susceptible individuals (see p. 824).

It is not yet possible to use our knowledge of the genome to screen patients for multigene disorders. Currently, the polymorphisms associated with disease are being documented, and procedures for multiple gene testing are being developed. How the current testing procedures will be integrated into future health care systems remains to be seen.

Micronutrient Status

Nutrient requirements of individuals are affected by genetic factors.[6] Although most people apparently can meet their nutrient needs by consuming nutrients at recommended levels, it would be useful to learn more about genetic variations within healthy populations. The techniques that have emerged from genomic research may provide a means for fine-tuning nutrient recommendations for individuals. Moreover, ideal indicators of nutrient status are still lacking for several of the minerals, such as zinc, magnesium, and chromium. Scientists hope to eventually produce genomic maps that will indicate how various nutrient deficiencies and combinations of deficiencies affect gene expression. These maps may eventually provide data that can help diagnose nutrient deficiencies.

Clinical Concerns and Ethical Issues

Enthusiasm surrounding genomic research needs to be put into perspective, in terms of both the status of clinical medicine at present and people's willingness to make difficult lifestyle choices. Critics have questioned whether genetic markers for disease would be more useful than simple and inexpensive clinical measurements, which reflect both genetic *and* environmental influences. In other words, knowing that a person is genetically predisposed toward high cholesterol levels is not necessarily more useful than knowing the person's actual blood cholesterol level.[7] Furthermore, if a disease has many genetic risk factors, each gene that contributes to susceptibility may have little influence on its own, so the benefits of identifying an individual genetic marker would be small. The long-range possibility is that many genetic markers will eventually be identified; the hope is that the combined information will be a more useful and accurate predictor of disease.

Additional knowledge about disease risk may not be useful unless people are motivated to make serious lifestyle changes. Despite the present abundance of disease prevention recommendations, many people seem unwilling to make the modifications known to improve health. For example, it has been estimated that heart disease and type 2 diabetes are 80 percent and 90 percent preventable, respectively, by changing one's lifestyle to include an appropriate diet, a healthy body weight, and regular exercise, among other factors.[8] Given the difficulty that people have with current recommendations, it is unlikely that they will enthusiastically adopt an even more detailed list of lifestyle modifications.

The ability to obtain detailed genetic information also raises important ethical concerns. A primary consideration is confidentiality: Should information about a person's susceptibility to disease be released to others without that person's consent? Because environmental factors play such an important role in disease risk, genetic predisposition usually cannot predict whether a person will develop a particular disease. Nevertheless, future insurers of medical services may attempt to charge higher rates or base their acceptance criteria on applicants' disease susceptibilities as evidenced by genetic testing. Another important concern is whether genetic testing is always in the best interest of children. Although early knowledge of a child's predisposition to illnesses may be useful for parents who want to provide optimal care, the release of this information could interfere with the child's privacy and increase the potential for "genetic discrimination" in the future.

Although genomic research has the potential to improve our ability to diagnose and treat disease, it is still unclear how knowledge of the genome will be translated into useful medical treatments. Still, health care professionals will need to keep informed of the ethical, legal, and social implications of genomics in the fields of medicine and nutrition as this remarkable research continues.

REFERENCES

1. J. B. German, M.-A. Roberts, and S. M. Watkins, Personal metabolomics as a next generation nutritional assessment, *Journal of Nutrition* 133 (2003): 4260–4266; S. M. Brown, *Essentials of Medical Genomics* (Hoboken, N.J.: Wiley-Liss, 2003).
2. International Human Genome Sequencing Consortium, Finishing the euchromatic sequence of the human genome, *Nature* 431 (2004): 931–945.
3. S. D. Clarke, The human genome and nutrition, in B. A. Bowman and R. M. Russell, eds., *Present Knowledge in Nutrition* (Washington, D.C.: ILSI Press, 2001), pp. 750–760.
4. W. C. Willett, Balancing life-style and genomics research for disease prevention, *Science* 296 (2002): 695–698.
5. German, Roberts, and Watkins, 2003.
6. R. A. Sunde, Research needs for human nutrition in the post-genome sequencing era, *Journal of Nutrition* 131 (2001): 3319–3323; B. N. Ames, H. Elson-Schwab, and E. A. Silver, High-dose vitamin therapy stimulates variant enzymes with decreased coenzyme binding affinity (increased K_m): Relevance to genetic disease and polymorphisms, *American Journal of Clinical Nutrition* 75 (2002): 616–658.
7. Willett, 2002.
8. Willett, 2002.

Chapter 19

Diet, Medications, and Dietary Supplements

Chapter Outline

Medications in Disease Treatment: *Risks versus Benefits of Medication Use • Patients at High Risk of Adverse Effects*

Dietary Supplements: *Effectiveness and Safety of Herbal Products • Use of Herbal Products for Illness*

Diet-Drug Interactions: *Medications and Food Intake • Diet-Drug Interactions and Absorption • Diet-Drug Interactions and Metabolism • Diet-Drug Interactions and Excretion • Diet-Drug Interactions and Toxicity*

Highlight: *Complementary and Alternative Medicine*

Available Online

http://nutrition.wadsworth.com/uncn7

Student Practice Test

Glossary Terms

Nutrition on the Net

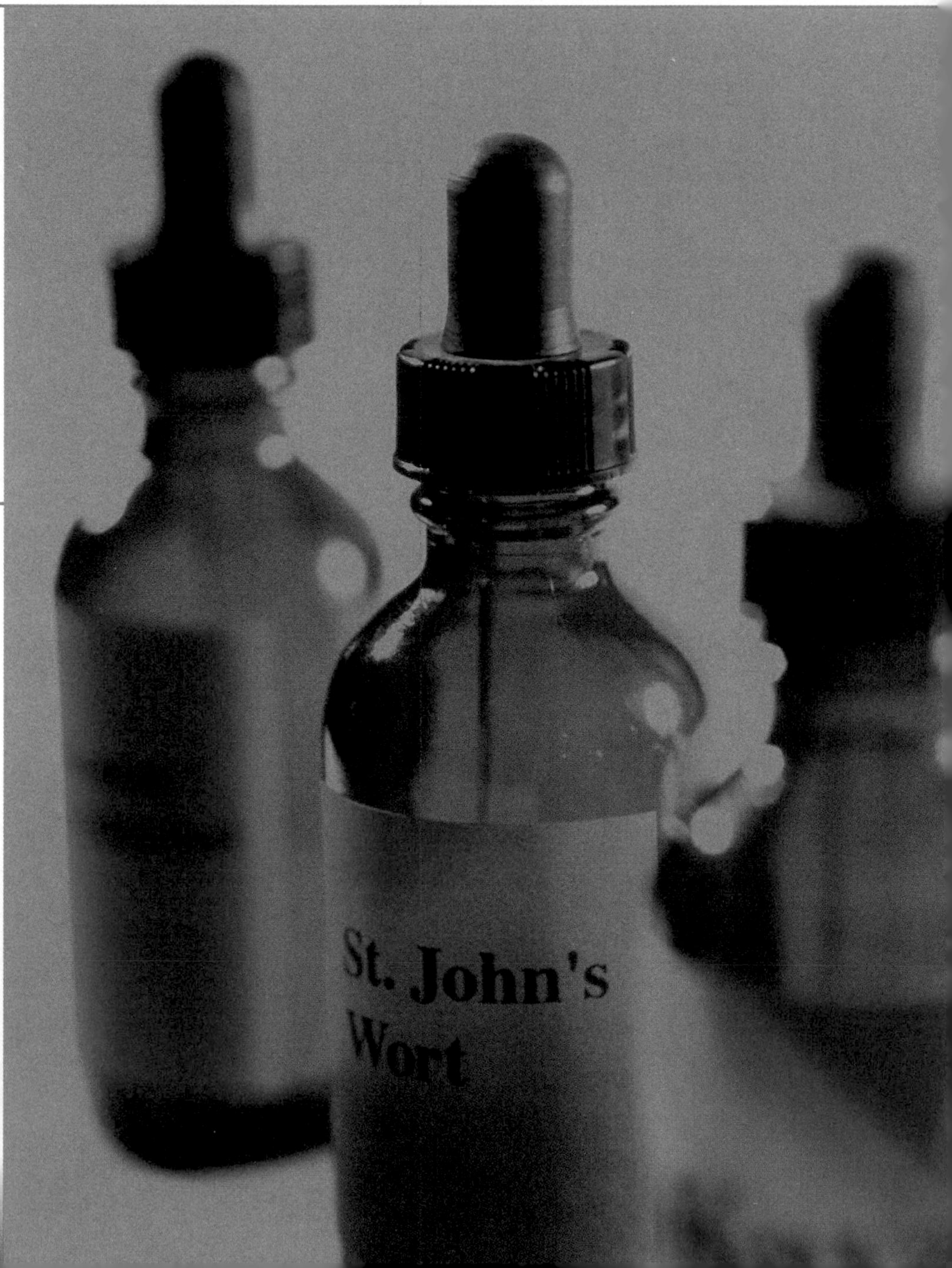
St. John's
Wort

© Ron Chapple/Taxi/Getty Images

Nutrition in the Professional Setting

After drugs are prescribed, follow-up is essential. Health practitioners should confirm that prescription directions are understood and that medications are taken carefully. Patients may feel uncomfortable admitting their uncertainty about directions, intolerance to side effects, or inability to purchase the drugs they need. Others may feel embarrassed discussing their use of dietary supplements. Patients are more likely to confide in health care providers who take the time to discuss these difficulties.

■ The term *drugs* includes not only medicines that are used to treat disease, but also products such as antiperspirants, sunscreens, dandruff shampoos, and fluoride toothpaste.

People frequently rely on medications to prevent and treat health problems. They may also use dietary supplements, which have become a popular alternative therapy. Because any ingested chemical can affect metabolism and potentially disrupt body processes, both medications and dietary supplements may produce adverse effects. Serious side effects may occur when medications interact with each other (drug-drug interactions) or with nutrients and other dietary components (diet-drug interactions). This chapter discusses the uses of medications and dietary supplements and describes the potential interactions among diet, drugs, and nutritional status. Highlight 19 describes the categories and common uses of complementary and alternative medicine.

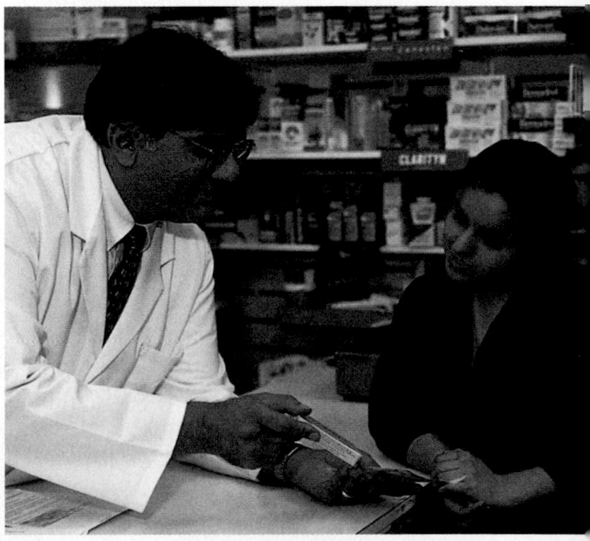
CLARITYN

Health care professionals can help recognize and prevent adverse effects associated with the use of medications and dietary supplements.

Medications in Disease Treatment

Drugs must be proved safe and effective before they can be marketed in the United States. The Food and Drug Administration (FDA) is responsible for approving sales of new medications and inspecting facilities where drugs are manufactured.[1] It also oversees the advertising of prescription drugs and the labeling of over-the-counter medications.■

Prescription Medications Prescription medications are usually given to treat serious conditions and may cause side effects. For these reasons, they are sold by prescription only, which ensures that a physician has evaluated the patient's medical condition and determined that the benefits of using the prescription medication outweigh the risks of incurring side effects.

Over-the-Counter Drugs Over-the-counter (OTC) drugs are those that can be used safely and effectively without medical supervision because, when used as directed, they ordinarily do not cause serious side effects. They are usually used to treat less serious illnesses that are easily self-diagnosed. Examples include aspirin to treat headaches or pain, decongestants to relieve stuffy noses, and antacids to combat indigestion. Prescription drugs considered safe enough for self-medication are frequently switched to OTC status, sometimes in smaller doses than are available by prescription. Labels on OTC drugs are regulated and provide information about their appropriate uses, dosages, and potential adverse effects.

Patients should be cautioned that adverse effects may occur if OTC drugs are used inappropriately. Under certain circumstances, the active ingredients in these drugs can worsen medical conditions, produce complications, and interact with other medications.[2] In addition, people using products with several active ingredients may inadvertently take toxic amounts of a substance when using several drugs simultaneously. For example, a person with a cold may take one medication to treat a cough and another medication for a headache without realizing that both contain an analgesic (pain medication).

Generic Drugs After the patent protection of brand-name drugs expires, generic versions of the drugs can be sold. Consumers can be confident that generic drugs are as safe and effective as the brand-name products they replace; they are chemically identical and reach the bloodstream in the same amount of time as the original drug. The advantage to the consumer is a substantial savings—generic drugs usually cost 20 to 75 percent less than their brand-name counterparts.

Risks versus Benefits of Medication Use

Some risk of an adverse reaction always accompanies the use of a medication. A drug is considered "safe" only when the benefits outweigh the risks associated with using it. Risks become greater when a drug is incorrectly prescribed or administered. This section discusses the types of risks associated with medication use and suggests some steps for managing risk.

Side Effects By the time a drug reaches the marketplace, large-scale clinical trials have revealed the majority of side effects associated with its use. Sometimes, however, rare side effects are detected only after a drug has been more widely used. In some instances, these effects occur because drugs are used for longer periods of time or in different circumstances than originally anticipated. The FDA monitors adverse events after drugs are marketed. Manufacturers are required to submit periodic reports, and individuals using the drugs are encouraged to report unexpected effects directly to the FDA.■ In some cases, the FDA may decide to change labeling information or even withdraw drugs from the marketplace due to their unacceptable risks to health.

■ The FDA's MedWatch program encourages health professionals and the public to report medication problems by mail, fax, telephone, or the Internet. The FDA also provides safety information about drugs and other medical products on the MedWatch website (**www.fda.gov/medwatch**).

Drug-Drug Interactions When multiple drugs are used, one drug may potentially alter the effects of another drug, and the risk of side effects increases. This problem is common in older adults, who are likely to use several medications daily over long periods. Primary care physicians often supervise the medications that patients use, but some individuals may use drugs prescribed by a number of different physicians. Others may use OTC medications and dietary supplements in addition to prescription drugs without being aware of the risks associated with certain combinations.

Diet-Drug Interactions Substances in the diet may alter the effectiveness of drugs, and drugs may affect food intake, digestion, absorption, metabolism or excretion of nutrients. The second half of this chapter describes these interactions and how they may affect nutritional status.

Medication Errors A medication error is any preventable action that causes inappropriate medication use or patient harm due to mistakes made by a health professional or patient. Medication errors are responsible for approximately 7000 deaths yearly.[3] An analysis of case reports submitted to the FDA from 1993 to 1998 found that errors involving improper dosages or incorrect drugs were the most common medication errors leading to patient death. Medication errors are often due to handwriting or transcription errors; for example, one patient died after receiving 10 milliliters of morphine solution instead of 10 milligrams—a 20-fold overdose. The wrong drug may be administered when two different drugs have names that look or sound alike or have similar packaging.

To help reduce the incidence of medication errors, several new recommendations and rulings have been proposed. In 2004, the Joint Committee on Accreditation of Healthcare Organizations (JCAHO)■ issued a new set of prohibited abbreviations, acronyms, and symbols to be included on the "Do Not Use" lists of accredited health care organizations (see the examples in Table 19-1). Because the terms are easily misread or misinterpreted, they can no longer be used on any clinical documentation related to patient care. Also in 2004, the FDA issued a regulation requiring bar code identifications on medications used in health care institutions. By 2006, most prescription drugs and some OTC drugs will have a bar

■ Reminder: The JCAHO is a nonprofit organization that sets standards for health care performance and safety (see p. 584).

TABLE 19-1 Terms Prohibited on Clinical Documentation

Prohibited Terms	Intended Meaning	Potential Problem	Correct Term for Documentation
U	Unit	Can be misread as the number 0 or 4; may cause 10-fold overdose or higher.	Write out "Unit."
IU	International Unit	Can be misread as IV (intravenous) or 10.	Write out "International Unit."
Trailing zero (1.0 mg) or lack of leading zero (.1 mg)	1 mg; 0.1 mg	Decimal point can be missed, leading to 10-fold error in dosages.	Never use zero by itself after a decimal. Always use zero before a decimal point.
HS, hs	*HS* means "half-strength"; *hs* means "bedtime" (abbreviation for "hours of sleep").	Can be mistaken for one another.	Write out "half-strength" or "bedtime."
μg	Microgram	Can be misread as mg (milligram).	Write "mcg."
A.S., A.D., A.U.	Abbreviations of the Latin for left ear, right ear, and both ears.	Can be misread as O.S., O.D., and O.U., meaning left eye, right eye, and both eyes.	Write out full words.
T.I.W.	Three times a week	Can be mistaken for "three times a day" or "twice weekly."	Write out "3 times weekly."
Q.D. (q.d.), Q.O.D (q.o.d.)	*Q.D.* means "every day"; Q.O.D. means "every other day."	Can be mistaken for one another or misread as "q.i.d." (four times daily).	Write out "daily" or "every other day."
q1d	Daily	Can be misread as q.i.d. (four times daily).	Write out "daily."

code identifying the drug. Hospital patients will wear bar-coded identification bracelets linked to computerized medical records with drug-dispensing information. Error messages will alert health care personnel if the drug, dosage, or timing of administration is not appropriate for the patient.

Patients at High Risk of Adverse Effects

Health care professionals should be aware that some patients are more likely than others to experience adverse effects from drugs. This is especially true of the populations that usually are not studied in the clinical trials that determine product safety: pregnant and lactating women, children, and people with diseases that are not the main focus of the study. In these groups, side effects may be discovered only after a drug has been marketed. Children may react in different ways to drugs than adults do, and the appropriate dosage for their age and size is often unknown. Also, only limited data are available on drug safety in older adults. Elderly people with chronic diseases that require multiple medications are most vulnerable. They are also more likely to have an impaired liver or kidneys—the two organs critical to metabolizing and eliminating drugs from the body.

To reduce the likelihood of adverse effects, health professionals should discuss with patients the potential benefits and risks of using medications before prescribing them. These suggestions may help:

- Advise patients that drugs should not be taken unless absolutely necessary. Discuss dietary or lifestyle alternatives that may have effects similar to those of drugs. For example, laxatives may not be needed if an individual increases consumption of foods high in fiber and begins exercising regularly.
- Request a complete list of prescription medications, OTC drugs, and dietary supplements that a patient is taking. Make sure that at least one physician is coordinating a patient's drug use. Encourage patients to purchase all medications at the same pharmacy so that the pharmacist can alert physicians and patients to potential problems.
- Encourage patients to keep track of side effects. Inform patients that new or unusual symptoms may be the result of a medication and may not be due to the medical condition itself. Other medications that treat the same symptoms may have fewer side effects.
- Make sure patients understand how to take medications properly and alert them to potential interactions between drugs and between drugs and dietary substances. Include information about drug safety when providing health education.

IN SUMMARY Both prescription and OTC drugs must be shown to be safe and effective before they are sold. The benefits of using a medication should be greater than the risks associated with its use. Potential risks include side effects, drug-drug and diet-drug interactions, and medication errors. The most common types of medication errors involve incorrect dosages or use of the wrong drug. Patients at highest risk of experiencing adverse effects include pregnant and nursing women, children, and the elderly. Health professionals should discuss the risks and benefits of medications with patients and alert them to potential dangers and possible solutions.

Dietary Supplements

Dietary supplements may contain vitamins, minerals, amino acids, herbs or other botanicals, and miscellaneous dietary constituents such as fish oils, enzymes, or shark cartilage. Many consumers use these products in the hope of improving their general health and preventing or treating specific diseases, but unlike drugs, dietary supplements do not need to be approved by the FDA before they are marketed. According to the Dietary Supplement Health and Education Act (DSHEA) of 1994, the companies that produce or distribute dietary supplements are responsible for determining their safety, but the companies are not required to provide any evidence. If a company receives reports of illness or injury related to use of its products, it is *not* required to submit this information to the FDA. The FDA must show that a supplement is unsafe before it can take action to remove the product from the marketplace.[4]

Although supplement labels may not make claims about preventing or treating specific diseases, suggestive statements are common. For example, a label on an herbal product may claim that it "promotes restful sleep" but cannot state that it cures insomnia. Stores often arrange supplements on the shelves by health condition; for example, posted signs may indicate the supplements suggested for "liver health" or "men's health." Reading materials positioned close to those shelves often suggest that the supplements can improve one's health. Because supplements have already been discussed in earlier sections of the text—fish oils (Chapter 5), protein and amino acids (Chapter 6), and vitamins and minerals (Highlight 10)—this discussion focuses on herbal and specialty products.

Effectiveness and Safety of Herbal Products

Use of herbal supplements has grown rapidly in the past decade. A 2004 study of 61,587 older adults (ages 50 to 76 years) found that one-third of the participants currently used herbal and other specialty supplements.[5]■ The top-selling herbal supplements include ginseng, echinacea, ginkgo biloba, garlic, and St. John's wort.[6] Table 19-2 lists popular herbs, their common uses, and potential risks associated with their use.

■ Technically speaking, an *herb* is a nonwoody, seed-producing plant that dies when the growing season ends. An *herbal supplement* may include other types of botanical products, such as garlic and ginkgo. *Specialty* supplements include nonplant products such as enzymes and shark cartilage.

The usefulness of herbal products sold in the United States is unclear. The marketplace is currently inundated with herbal "remedies" of dubious effectiveness. There is no question that many medicinal herbs contain naturally occurring compounds that can exert physiological effects. Few herbal products, however, have been rigorously tested, many make unfounded claims, and some contain contaminants or produce toxic effects.[7]

Efficacy Herbs have been used for centuries to treat medical conditions, and many have acquired reputations for being beneficial for specific diseases. Unfortunately, only a limited number of clinical studies support the traditional uses, and the results of studies that suggest little or no benefit are rarely publicized by the supplement industry. The National Center for Complementary and Alternative Medicine is currently funding large, controlled trials of several popular herbal treatments in an effort to obtain reliable efficacy and safety data. Several publications and websites provide reliable reviews of the research that has already been conducted (see the References and Nutrition on the Net at the end of this chapter).

Consistency of Herbal Ingredients Herbs contain numerous compounds, and it is often unclear which, if any, might produce the implied beneficial effect. Because the compounds in herbs vary among species and are affected by a plant's growing conditions, different samples of an herb can have different chemical compositions. The preparation method may also cause variations in the composition of an herbal product. Some manufacturers voluntarily standardize the herbal extracts they sell so that the compound believed to be beneficial can be reliably obtained from each dose.

Even when the active ingredients in a dietary supplement have been shown to be safe and effective, the dosage suggested on the label may not provide the amount of active ingredients found to be effective. For example, a consumer group (ConsumerLab.com) tested the compounds of nine ginkgo biloba products and found that seven of the products, when consumed at the recommended dose, lacked adequate levels of one or more compounds believed to be helpful.[8]

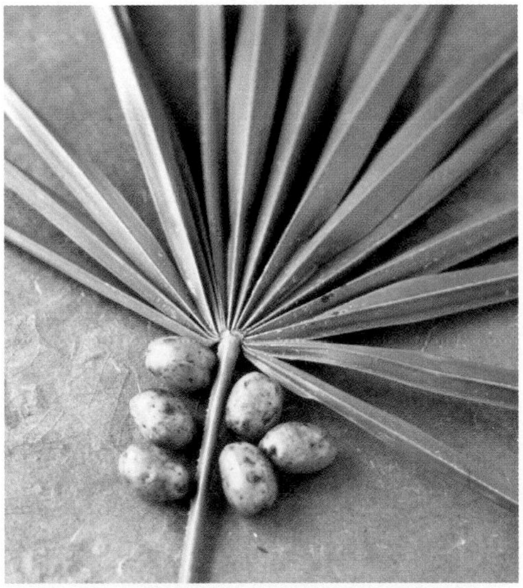

Some studies have shown that saw palmetto may improve the symptoms associated with an enlarged prostate.

TABLE 19-2 Popular Herbs, Their Common Uses, and Risks

Common Name	Scientific Source Name	Claims and Uses	Risks[a]
Aloe (gel)	*Aloe vera*	Promotes wound healing	Generally considered safe
Black cohosh	*Actaea racemos* (formerly *Cimicifuga racemosa*)	Eases menopause symptoms	May cause clotting in blood vessels of the eye, change the curvature of the cornea
Chamomile (flowers)	*Matricaria chamomilla*	Relieves indigestion	Generally considered safe
Chaparral (leaves and twigs)	*Larrea tridentata*	Slows aging, "cleanses" blood, heals wounds, cures cancer, treats acne	Acute, toxic hepatitis; liver damage
Comfrey (leafy plant)	*Symphytum officinale, S. asperum, S. x uplandicum*	Soothes nerves	Liver damage
Echinacea (roots)	*Enchinacea angustifolia, E. pallida, E. purpurea*	Alleviates symptoms of colds, flus, and infections; promotes wound healing; boosts immunity	Generally considered safe
Feverfew (leaves)	*Tanacetum parthenium*	Prevents migraine headaches	Generally considered safe; may cause mouth irritation, swelling, ulcers, and GI distress
Garlic (bulbs)	*Allium sativum*	Lowers blood lipids and blood pressure	Generally considered safe; may cause garlic breath, body odor, gas, and GI distress; inhibits blood clotting
Ginger	*Zingiber officinale*	Prevents motion sickness, nausea	Generally considered safe
Ginkgo (tree leaves)	*Ginkgo biloba*	Improves mental function in those with memory defects, relieves vertigo	Generally considered safe; may cause headache, GI distress, dizziness; may inhibit blood clotting
Ginseng (roots)	*Panax ginseng* (Asian), *P. quinquefolius* (American)	Boosts immunity, increases endurance, reduces blood glucose concentrations	Generally considered safe; may cause insomnia and high blood pressure
Goldenseal (roots)	*Hydrastis canadensis*	Relieves indigestion, treats urinary infections	Generally considered safe
Kava	*Piper methysticum*	Relieves anxiety, promotes relaxation	Liver failure
Saw palmetto (ripe fruits)	*Serenoa repens*	Relieves symptoms of enlarged prostate; diuretic; enhances sexual vigor; enlarges mammary glands	Generally considered safe
St. John's wort (leaves and tops)	*Hypericum perforatum*	Relieves depression and anxiety	Generally considered safe; may cause fatigue and GI distress
Valerian (roots)	*Valeriana officinalis*	Calms nerves, improves sleep	Generally considered safe
Yohimbe (tree bark)	*Pausinystalia yohimbe*	Enhances "male performance"	Kidney failure, seizures

[a]Allergies are always a possible risk; see Table 19-3 for drug interactions.

■ Nothing could be more natural—and deadly—than the poisonous herb hemlock.

Safety Issues Consumers of herbal supplements often assume that because plants are "natural," herbal products must be harmless.■ Many herbal remedies have toxic effects, however. The most common adverse effects of herbs include diarrhea, nausea, and vomiting.[9] The popular herbs kava, chaparral, and comfrey have caused liver damage. The use of yohimbe (promoted for bodybuilding) has been linked to renal failure, seizures, and heart palpitations. In 2004, the FDA removed the herb ephedra (also known as *ma huang*) from the market, advising that its side effects (which include elevated blood pressure and rapid heartbeat) could cause heart attack or stroke. The adverse effects of herbs are rarely listed on supplement labels.

Like drugs, herbs may either potentiate or interfere with the effects of other herbs and drugs. Information about herb-drug interactions is limited, and much of what is known was obtained from case studies rather than from controlled clinical trials. An herb may either increase or decrease the effects of medications, or it may raise the risk of toxicity. For example, garlic, ginkgo, and ginseng may increase the risk of bleeding when used with anticoagulant drugs. St. John's wort has been found to inhibit the actions of oral contraceptives, anticoagulants, and other drugs. Individuals may be more susceptible to the adverse effects of a drug if the

TABLE 19-3 Herb and Drug Interactions

Herb	Drug	Interaction
American ginseng	Estrogens, corticosteroids	Enhances hormonal response.
American ginseng	Breast cancer therapeutic agent	Synergistically inhibits cancer cell growth.
American ginseng, karela	Blood glucose regulators	Affect blood glucose levels.
Echinacea (possible immunostimulant)	Cyclosporine and corticosteroids (immunosuppressants)	May reduce drug effectiveness.
Evening primrose oil, borage	Anticonvulsants	Lower seizure threshold.
Feverfew	Aspirin, ibuprofen,and other nonsteroidal anti-inflammatory drugs	Negates the effect of the herb in treating migraine headaches.
Feverfew, garlic, ginkgo, ginger, and Asian ginseng	Warfarin, coumarin (anticlotting drugs, "blood thinners")	Prolong bleeding time; increase likelihood of hemorrhage.
Garlic	Protease inhibitor (HIV drug)	May reduce drug effectiveness.
Kava, valerian	Anesthetics	May enhance drug action.
Kelp (iodine source)	Synthroid or other thyroid hormone replacers	Interferes with drug action.
Kyushin, licorice, plantain, uzara root, hawthorn, Asian ginseng	Digoxin (cardiac antiarrhythmic drug derived from the herb foxglove)	Interfere with drug action and monitoring.
St. John's wort, saw palmetto, black tea	Iron	Tannins in herbs inhibit iron absorption.
Valerian	Barbiturates	Causes excessive sedation.

herb they are using has a similar effect; for example, ginger and ginseng contain compounds that raise blood pressure and may increase the toxicity of drugs that have a similar side effect.[10] Table 19-3 provides examples of herb and drug interactions.

Contamination of herbal products is another safety concern. In an analysis of 251 products imported from Asia, 10 percent were found to contain lead, 14 percent arsenic, and 14 percent mercury in excessive amounts.[11] Other contaminants occasionally found in herbal products include molds, bacteria, and pesticides that have been banned for use on food crops. Adulteration of imported products has been a serious concern: a Taiwanese study found that 24 percent of the 2609 herbal products tested contained synthetic drugs that were not declared on the label, and 53 percent of the adulterated products contained two or more added drugs.[12] There have also been reports of serious illnesses and fatalities occurring from the intentional or accidental substitutions of one plant species for another.[13]

Use of Herbal Products for Illness

When people self-medicate or ask the advice of store clerks instead of seeking effective medical treatments, the consequences can sometimes be serious and irreversible. A visit to the health food store for an herbal remedy may be less stressful than a visit to the doctor, but it may delay an appropriate treatment and allow an illness to progress. Consumers should inform their health care providers about the use of dietary supplements so that a comprehensive care plan can be developed and potential problems can be averted.

Many people are unaware that herbal products can interact with medications. Because research on herbs is often lacking, assessing potential interactions is difficult for health care professionals and patients alike. Some pharmacology textbooks and handbooks now contain information about herbal products and potential herb-drug interactions, and consumer websites and magazines regularly provide information about the safety of brand-name products. Several Internet resources for health practitioners and consumers are listed at the end of this chapter.

IN SUMMARY Although manufacturers and distributors of dietary supplements are responsible for determining product safety, the FDA takes action against unsafe supplements only after they reach the market. Herbal products are not reliable treatments for medical conditions; there is little evidence demonstrating their effectiveness and safety, and the concentrations of active ingredients may vary greatly. Safety concerns include adverse effects, herb-drug interactions, and contamination. Consumers using herbs may delay getting an appropriate treatment for their condition.

Diet-Drug Interactions

Clinicians often overlook or fail to recognize diet-drug interactions, yet such interactions can raise health care costs and result in serious, and sometimes fatal, complications. With hundreds of diet-drug interactions known and more to be identified in the future, health care professionals must learn to take steps to prevent them. This section discusses the main types of diet-drug interactions and their clinical importance.[14]

Diet-drug interactions generally fall into the following categories:

- Medications may alter food intake by affecting appetite or by causing complications that make food consumption difficult or unpleasant.
- Medications may alter the absorption, metabolism, and excretion of nutrients.
- Components of foods, including nutrients, may alter the absorption, metabolism, and excretion of medications.
- Acute toxicity may result from interactions between dietary components and medications.

Some specific examples of these types of diet-drug interactions are shown in Table 19-4. Examples of medications that may cause interactions are listed in Table 19-5, p. 636. The "How to" on p. 637 offers some practical recommendations that may help to prevent diet-drug interactions.

Medications and Food Intake

Although some medications have been developed to enhance or suppress food intake, an altered appetite is usually an undesirable side effect. This section discusses the various effects that medications may have that lead to changes in food intake.

Drug Complications That Alter Food Intake Some medications can make food intake difficult or unpleasant. Some induce nausea or vomiting, which reduces the desire to eat. Some cause inflammation or lesions in the mouth, stomach, or intestinal lining, resulting in pain or discomfort when food is eaten. Taste perceptions may change, leading to food aversions that may persist even after treatment has been discontinued. Sedatives can make a person too tired to eat. Table 19-6 (p. 636) lists other symptoms and complications associated with drug use that can lead to a poor appetite or make food consumption difficult.

Complications that limit food intake are significant only when they continue for a long period. For example, almost any drug may cause nausea in some individuals, but nausea often subsides after the first few doses of the medication. If nausea persists, however, weight loss and malnutrition may follow, which can impede recovery. Medications to treat certain complications of drug use may help improve food intake; for example, antinauseants and antiemetics may help to reduce nausea and vomiting.

TABLE 19-4 Examples of Diet-Drug Interactions

Drugs May Alter Food Intake by:

- Altering the appetite (amphetamines suppress appetite; corticosteroids increase appetite).
- Interfering with taste or smell (amphetamines change taste perceptions).
- Inducing nausea or vomiting (digitalis may do both).
- Interfering with oral function (some antidepressants may cause dry mouth).
- Causing sores or inflammation in the mouth (methotrexate may cause painful mouth ulcers).

Drugs May Alter Nutrient Absorption by:

- Changing the acidity of the digestive tract (antacids may interfere with iron and folate absorption).
- Damaging mucosal cells (cancer chemotherapy may damage mucosal cells).
- Binding to nutrients (bile acid binders bind to fat-soluble vitamins).

Foods and Nutrients May Alter Drug Absorption by:

- Stimulating secretion of gastric acid (the antifungal agent ketoconazole is absorbed better with meals due to increased acid secretion).
- Altering rate of gastric emptying (intestinal absorption of drugs may be delayed when they are taken with food).
- Binding to drugs (calcium binds to tetracycline, reducing drug and calcium absorption).
- Competing for absorption sites in the intestines (dietary amino acids interfere with levodopa absorption).

Drugs and Nutrients May Interact and Alter Metabolism by:

- Acting as structural analogs (as do warfarin and vitamin K).
- Using similar enzyme systems (phenobarbital induces liver enzymes that increase metabolism of folate, vitamin D, and vitamin K).
- Competing for transport on plasma proteins (fatty acids and drugs may compete for the same sites on the plasma protein albumin).

Drugs May Alter Nutrient Excretion by:

- Altering reabsorption in the kidneys (some diuretics increase the excretion of sodium and potassium).
- Causing diarrhea or vomiting (diarrhea and vomiting may cause electrolyte losses).

Foods May Alter Medication Excretion by:

- Inducing activities of liver enzymes that metabolize drugs to allow their excretion (components of charcoal-broiled meats increase metabolism of warfarin, theophylline, and acetominophen).

Toxicity May Occur from Combining Foods and Drugs by:

- Increasing side effects of the drug (caffeine in beverages can increase adverse effects of stimulants).
- Increasing drug action to excessive levels (grapefruit components may block metabolism of drugs and enhance drugs' actions and side effects).

Medications That Alter Appetite Medications are sometimes prescribed to stimulate food intake and encourage weight gain in patients with debilitating diseases such as cancer or AIDS. Examples include megestrol acetate, a progesterone analog, and dronabinol, which is derived from the active ingredient in marijuana. Unintentional weight gain may result from the use of some antipsychotics, antidepressants, and corticosteroids (for example, prednisone). People using these drugs may be unable to feel satiated and sometimes gain 40 to 60 pounds in just a few months.

Medications prescribed for obesity intentionally suppress the appetite and promote weight loss. Examples include sibutramine, amphetamines, and amphetamine-like compounds such as phentermine. When amphetamines are prescribed for other purposes, such as narcolepsy or attention-deficit hyperactivity disorder, appetite suppression and weight loss may be unwanted side effects.

TABLE 19-5 Classes of Medications That May Affect Nutrition Status

Classification	Possible Side Effects That May Affect Nutrition Status
Analgesics, narcotic	Sedation, nausea and vomiting, reduced motility of GI tract
Antacids	Constipation, diarrhea
Antibiotics	Nausea, vomiting, diarrhea
Anticonvulsants	Nausea, vomiting, GI distress
Antidepressants	Weight changes, dry mouth, nausea and vomiting, diarrhea, constipation
Antidiabetic agents	GI distress, diarrhea
Antidiarrheals	Nausea, constipation
Antifungal agents	Depressed appetite, nausea and vomiting, GI distress, diarrhea
Antihypertensives	Nausea, drowsiness, dry mouth, constipation, dizziness
Antilipemics	Nausea, GI distress, constipation
Antineoplastics	Depressed appetite, nausea and vomiting, dry mouth, taste alterations, mouth ulcers, mouth inflammation, fatigue, diarrhea, fever
Antiulcer agents	Reduced absorption of iron and vitamin B_{12}
Antiviral agents	Depressed appetite, nausea and vomiting, GI distress
Central nervous system stimulants	Depressed appetite, dry mouth, taste alterations
Corticosteroids	Nausea and vomiting, insulin resistance, altered calcium and vitamin D metabolism, negative nitrogen balance, sodium and fluid retention
Diuretics	Altered excretion of sodium, potassium, magnesium, phosphorus, calcium, and zinc
Hormonal agents	Appetite and weight changes; various other side effects depending on agent
Immunosuppressants	Nausea and vomiting, diarrhea, constipation, impaired renal function
Laxatives	Intestinal gas, laxative dependency

TABLE 19-6 Examples of Drug-Induced Side Effects That Can Limit Food Intake

- Altered tastes
- Anorexia
- Belching
- Bloating
- Blurred vision
- Chest pain
- Confusion
- Congestion, nasal
- Constipation
- Coughing
- Cramps, abdominal
- Diarrhea
- Dizziness
- Dry mouth
- Epigastric pain
- Fatigue
- GI distress
- Indigestion
- Inflammation of mouth tissue
- Intestinal gas
- Mouth ulcers or lesions
- Nausea
- Pain
- Sedation
- Shortness of breath
- Throat irritation

Diet-Drug Interactions and Absorption

As mentioned previously, some medications damage the lining of the gastrointestinal (GI) tract, resulting in pain or discomfort that can alter a person's appetite. These effects may also cause nutrient malabsorption and subsequent malnutrition. Conversely, the presence of food components in the GI tract may either enhance or reduce the absorption of medications and consequently alter the magnitude of a drug's effect in the body. Examples of these interactions are described in the following sections.

Medication Effects on Nutrient Absorption The medications most likely to cause widespread nutrient malabsorption are those that damage the intestinal mucosa. Antineoplastic and antiretroviral drugs are especially detrimental, however, nonsteroidal anti-inflammatory drugs (NSAIDS) and some antibiotics can have similar, though milder, effects. Other examples showing how medications may alter nutrient absorption include the following:

- *Drug-nutrient binding.* Some medications bind nutrients in the GI tract, preventing their absorption. For example, bile acid binders, used to reduce cholesterol levels, may also bind to the fat-soluble vitamins A, D, E, and K. Some antibiotics, notably tetracycline and ciprofloxacin, bind to the calcium in foods and supplements, which reduces the absorption of both the antibiotic and the calcium. Other minerals, such as iron, magnesium, and zinc, may also bind to the antibiotics. For this reason, consumers are advised to use dairy products and all mineral supplements at least 2 hours apart from these medications.
- *Altered acidity in the stomach.* Medications that reduce stomach acidity may potentially impair the absorption of vitamin B_{12}, folate, and iron. Several

HOW TO Prevent Diet-Drug Interactions

The JCAHO has advised that all patients be educated about potential diet-drug interactions. The physician, nurse, pharmacist, or dietitian should inform patients about precautions related to medications and dietary supplements and discuss signs of nutrition-related problems that may arise.

To prevent diet-drug interactions, first list the types and amounts of OTC and prescription medications and dietary supplements that the patient uses on a regular basis. Using a drug reference, look up each medication and make a note of:

- The appropriate method of administration (twice daily or at bedtime, for example).
- How the medication should be administered with respect to foods, beverages, and specific nutrients (for example, take on an empty stomach, take with food, do not take with milk, or do not drink alcoholic beverages with medication).
- How the medication should be used with respect to other medications.
- The side effects that may affect food intake (nausea and vomiting, constipation or diarrhea, or sedation, for example) or nutrient needs (may interfere with nutrient absorption or metabolism, for example).

A similar process can be used to review the dietary supplements that a person is taking. A reliable reference may provide information about their appropriate uses, possible side effects, and potential interactions with food and medications.

Patients who take multiple medications may need help learning when to take each medication to avoid drug-drug or diet-drug interactions. The health practitioner can use information from a patient's diet history (see Chapter 17) to help the patient coordinate meals and drugs so as to avoid interactions. Check with the pharmacist for additional information about a medication or potential interactions.

Some medications have well-known effects on nutritional status. The health practitioner should remain alert for signs of problems, especially when:

- Nutritional problems are a frequent result of using the medication.
- A patient uses multiple medications.
- The patient is in a high-risk group; for example, a child, a pregnant or lactating woman, an older adult, or a person who is malnourished, abuses alcohol, or has impaired liver or kidney function.
- The patient will need to use the medication for a long period of time.

Remember to alert the dietitian if you suspect a problem or think that the patient can benefit from nutrition counseling.

categories of antiulcer drugs reduce acidity by different mechanisms. For example, antacids neutralize stomach acidity by acting as weak bases. Proton pump inhibitors (like omeprazole) and H2 blockers (like cimetidine or ranitidine) interfere with acid secretion.

- *Direct inhibition.* Several drugs are known to directly impede the absorption of nutrients by interfering with their intestinal metabolism or transport into mucosal cells. For example, the antibiotics trimethoprim and pyrimethamine compete with folate for absorption into intestinal cells.

Dietary Effects on Medication Absorption Most drugs are absorbed in the upper small intestine. Major influences on drug absorption include the stomach emptying rate, level of acidity, and direct interactions with dietary components. The drug's formulation also influences its absorption, and instructions included with medications typically advise whether food should be included or avoided when using the medication. The following sections give examples of ways in which dietary factors can affect drug absorption.

Stomach Emptying Rate Drugs reach the small intestine more quickly when the stomach is empty. Therefore, taking a medication with meals may delay its absorption, although the total amount absorbed may not be affected. For example, aspirin works faster when taken on an empty stomach, but taking it with food is often encouraged to reduce stomach irritation.

If a drug has specific absorption sites in the intestine, slower stomach emptying may enhance absorption because the sites do not become saturated. A slow drug absorption rate, however, may be problematic if high blood concentrations are needed for effectiveness, as when a hypnotic drug is used to induce sleep.

Stomach Acidity Some drugs are better absorbed in an acid medium, so conditions that are too alkaline may reduce their absorption. Hence, acid-reducing therapies may reduce absorption of other drugs. Drugs that can be damaged by stomach acid are often available in coated forms that resist the acid environment.

Interactions with Food Components Both nutrients and nonnutrients may bind to drugs and inhibit their absorption. For example, high-fiber diets may decrease the absorption of some tricyclic antidepressants. Phytates■ in foods can bind to digoxin, a drug prescribed for heart disease. As mentioned earlier, calcium and other minerals may bind to some antibiotics, reducing absorption of both the minerals and the drug.

■ Reminder: *Phytates* are compounds found in many of the plant foods that contain fiber, such as whole grains and legumes. Phytates may bind to minerals and reduce their intestinal absorption.

Diet-Drug Interactions and Metabolism

Drugs and nutrients interact metabolically because they use the same enzyme systems in the small intestine and the liver. Drugs may enhance or inhibit the activities of enzymes that are needed for normal nutrient metabolism, and conversely, dietary components may enhance or inhibit the activities of enzymes that break down drugs prior to excretion. These alterations may affect the availability of nutrients, the actions of medications in the body, or various other physiological processes.

Medication Effects on Nutrient Metabolism Medications may interfere with the metabolism of only one or two nutrients or have broad effects that have many nutritional consequences. The drug methotrexate, used to treat cancer and inflammatory conditions, is an example of a medication that has dramatic effects on the metabolism of a single nutrient. Methotrexate resembles folate in structure (see Figure 19-1) and competes with the enzyme that converts folate to its active form. The adverse effects of using methotrexate therefore include symptoms of folate deficiency. These adverse effects can be reduced by using a pre-activated form of folate (called leucovorin) that is often prescribed along with methotrexate to "rescue" the rapidly dividing cells in the body that have high folate requirements. Corticosteroids, which are used as anti-inflammatory agents and immunosuppressants, provide an example of medications that have broad effects on nutritional health. Their long-term use may cause weight gain, muscle wasting, bone loss, and hyperglycemia, with eventual development of osteoporosis and diabetes.

Medications often alter the activities of liver enzymes that metabolize vitamins. For example, the anticonvulsants phenobarbital and phenytoin induce the liver enzymes that metabolize folate, vitamin D, and vitamin K; therefore, persons using these drugs require supplements of these vitamins. Phenobarbital and phenytoin interfere with metabolism of vitamins D and K in a number of other ways as well, causing increased risks of developing rickets in children and osteoporosis in adults.

Dietary Effects on Medication Metabolism Food components may affect the activities of enzymes that metabolize drugs or may counteract drug effects in other ways. For example, compounds in grapefruit juice (and whole grapefruit) have been found to inhibit or inactivate enzymes that metabolize a number of different drugs.[15] This lack of enzyme action increases blood concentrations of the drugs, leading to stronger physiological effects. The effect of the grapefruit juice lasts for a substantial period after the juice is consumed; in experiments with a drug prescribed for heart disease, the estimated half-life of its effect was 12 hours.■ Table 19-7 gives examples of drugs that have been found to interact with grapefruit juice, as well as some that are unaffected.

■ The term **half-life** is used here to define the time period of a chemical effect. If the grapefruit effect has a 12-hour half-life, this means that after 12 hours, its biological effect was half of the maximum effect that was measured.

FIGURE 19-1 Folate and Methotrexate

By competing for the enzyme that activates folate, methotrexate prevents cancer cells from obtaining the folate they need to multiply. In the process, normal cells are also deprived of the folate they need.

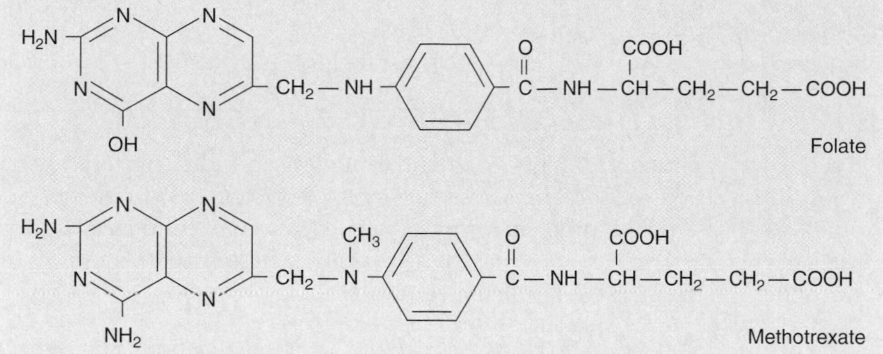
Folate
Methotrexate

A number of dietary factors affect the activity of the anticoagulant drug warfarin. The most important interaction is with vitamin K, which is structurally similar to warfarin. Warfarin acts by blocking the enzyme that activates vitamin K, thereby preventing the synthesis of blood-clotting factors. The amount of warfarin prescribed is dependent, in part, on how much vitamin K is in the diet. If vitamin K consumption from foods or supplements were to increase dramatically, it could

TABLE 19-7 Grapefruit Juice–Drug Interactions—Selected Examples

Drug Category	Drugs Affected by Grapefruit Juice	Drugs Unaffected by Grapefruit Juice
Cardiovascular drugs	Felodipine Nicardipine Nifedipine Verapamil	Amlodipine Diltiazem Propafenone Quinidine
Cholesterol-lowering drugs	Atorvastatin Lovastatin Simvastatin	Pravastatin
Central nervous system drugs	Buspirone Carbamazepine Diazepam Triazolam	Clomipramine Haloperidol
Anti-infective drugs	Saquinavir	Clarithromycin Itraconazole
Estrogens	Ethinylestradiol	17-ß-estradiol
Anticoagulants		Acenocoumarol Warfarin
Immunosuppressants	Cyclosporine Tacrolimus	Prednisone
Antiasthmatic drugs		Theophylline

SOURCE: D. G. Bailey, M. O. Arnold, and J. D. Spence, Inhibitors in the diet: Grapefruit juice–drug interactions, in R. H. Levy and coeditors, *Metabolic Drug Interactions* (Philadelphia: Lippincott Williams & Wilkins, 2000), pp. 661–669.

weaken the effect of the drug. Individuals using warfarin are advised to consume similar amounts of vitamin K daily to keep warfarin activity stable. The dietary sources highest in vitamin K are green leafy vegetables.

A number of popular herbs contain natural compounds that may enhance the activity of warfarin and therefore should be avoided during warfarin treatment. These herbs include St. John's wort, ginkgo, garlic, ginseng, dong quai, danshen, and others.[16]

Diet-Drug Interactions and Excretion

Diet-drug interactions may cause nutrient depletion and alter urinary losses of medications. When interactions cause nutrients to be excreted in greater-than-normal amounts, dietary supplements may be needed to prevent deficiency. Inadequate excretion of medications may cause toxicity, whereas excessive losses may reduce the amount available for therapeutic effect.

■ Reminder: *Reabsorption* of a substance *retains* it in the blood. Substances that are not reabsorbed are excreted in urine.

Medication Effects on Nutrient Excretion Some medications may interfere with the reabsorption of minerals by the kidneys,■ causing an increase in urinary losses. For example, some diuretics cause an accelerated excretion of calcium, potassium, and magnesium. Others may cause mineral retention instead. Risk of mineral depletion is highest if multiple drugs with the same effect are used, if kidney function is impaired, or if medications are used for a long time.

A number of drugs can increase excretion of vitamin B_6. An example is isoniazid (INH), an antituberculosis drug that is similar in structure to vitamin B_6. This drug induces excretion of vitamin B_6 and therefore has the potential to create a vitamin B_6 deficiency. Because the drug must be taken for at least six months to treat infection, vitamin B_6 supplements are routinely given to prevent deficiency.

■ Lithium is primarily used to prevent mood swings in patients with manic-depressive disorder.

Dietary Effects on Medication Excretion Food components may alter the reabsorption of drugs by the kidneys. For example, the amount of the medication lithium■ that is reabsorbed by the kidneys is generally similar to the amount of sodium reabsorbed. Consequently, dehydration or sodium depletion, which increase sodium reabsorption, may result in lithium retention. Similarly, a person with a high sodium intake will excrete more sodium in the urine and therefore more lithium. Individuals using lithium are advised to maintain a consistent sodium intake from day to day in order to maintain a stable blood level of lithium.

Urine acidity can affect medication excretion due to the effects of pH on a compound's ionic (chemical) form. The medication quinidine, used to treat arrhythmias, is excreted more readily in acidic urine. Foods or drugs that cause urine to become more alkaline (for example, sodium bicarbonate) may reduce quinidine excretion and raise blood levels.

Diet-Drug Interactions and Toxicity

Combinations of food components and drugs may sometimes cause toxicity or exacerbate a drug's side effects. The combination of tyramine, a compound in some foods, and monoamine oxidase (MAO) inhibitors, medications that treat depression, can be fatal. MAO inhibitors block an enzyme that normally inactivates tyramine and the hormones epinephrine and norepinephrine. When people who take MAO inhibitors consume excessive tyramine, the tyramine causes a sudden release of accumulated norepinephrine. This surge in norepinephrine results in severe headaches, rapid heartbeat, and a dangerous increase in blood pressure. For this reason, people taking MAO inhibitors are advised to restrict their intakes of foods rich in tyramine (see Table 19-8, p. 641).

TABLE 19-8 Foods Restricted in a Tyramine-Controlled Diet

Beverages	Red wines including chianti, sherry[a]
Cheeses	Aged cheeses, American, camembert, cheddar, gouda, gruyère, mozzarella, parmesan, provolone, romano, roquefort, stilton[b]
Meats	Liver; dried, salted, smoked, or pickled fish; sausage; pepperoni; salami; dried meats
Vegetables	Fava beans; Italian broad beans; sauerkraut; snow peas; fermented pickles and olives
Other	Brewer's yeast;[c] all aged and fermented products; soy sauce in large amounts; cheese-filled breads, crackers, and desserts; salad dressings containing cheese

NOTE: The tyramine contents of foods vary from product to product depending on the methods used to prepare, process, and store the food. In some cases, as little as 1 ounce of cheese can cause a severe hypertensive reaction in people taking monoamine oxidase inhibitors. In general, the following foods contain small enough amounts of tyramine that they can be consumed in small quantities: ripe avocado, banana, yogurt, sour cream, acidophilus milk, buttermilk, raspberries, and peanuts.

[a]Most wine and domestic beer can be consumed in small quantities.

[b]Unfermented cheeses, such as ricotta, cottage cheese, and cream cheese, are allowed.

[c]Products made with baker's yeast are allowed.

IN SUMMARY Medications may alter food intake and affect the absorption, metabolism, and excretion of nutrients. Components of foods can similarly affect the metabolism of medications. Some drugs may reduce appetite and cause damage to the GI tract. Binding between drugs and nutrients may inhibit their absorption. Drugs and nutrients may interfere with each other's metabolism because they use the same enzymes in the small intestine and liver. Diet-drug interactions may cause excessive losses of nutrients and alter the urinary excretion of medications.

Considering the many ways that medications and nutrients can interact and the number of medications and dietary supplements available, it is no wonder that serious side effects are increasingly recognized. Health care professionals are challenged to understand the mechanism of diet-drug interactions, identify them when they occur, and prevent them whenever possible.

NUTRITION ON THE NET

Access these websites for further study of topics covered in this chapter.

- Find updates and quick links to these and other nutrition-related sites at our website: **www.wadsworth.com/nutrition**
- Visit the Food and Drug Administration's home page for links to drug information: **www.fda.gov**
- To search for information about specific drugs, visit RxList: **www.rxlist.com**
- Report adverse effects associated with drugs to the FDA's MedWatch: **www.fda.gov/medwatch**
- Obtain information about herbal remedies from the Alternative Medicine Foundation or from the Integrative Medicine Service at Memorial Sloan-Kettering Cancer Center: **www.herbmed.org** or **www.mskcc.org/aboutherbs**
- Get dietary supplement information from the National Institutes of Health's Office of Dietary Supplements: **dietary-supplements.info.nih.gov**

STUDY QUESTIONS

These questions will help you review the chapter. You will find the answers in the discussions on the pages provided.

1. Describe similarities and differences among prescription medications, over-the-counter drugs, and generic versions of drugs. (p. 628)
2. Identify factors that frequently cause medication errors. What recommendations have been proposed to reduce incidences of these errors? (pp. 629–630)
3. Explain why some patient populations are at high risk for adverse effects from drugs. (p. 630)
4. Discuss why herbal remedies are not dependable treatments for medical conditions. Describe possible dangers associated with the use of these products. (pp. 631–633)
5. Discuss ways in which medications can affect food intake. (pp. 634–636)
6. Describe how medications can interfere with nutrient absorption and how dietary factors can affect drug absorption. (pp. 636–638)
7. Explain how drugs and nutrients may influence each other's metabolism. Provide some examples. (pp. 638–640)
8. Discuss diet-drug interactions that can alter the excretion of nutrients or medications. (p. 640)

These multiple choice questions will help you prepare for an exam. Answers can be found on p. 643.

1. Over-the-counter drugs are:
   a. unlikely to cause adverse effects.
   b. unlikely to interact with dietary components.
   c. generally used for longer periods of time than prescription medications.
   d. used to treat illnesses that are easily self-diagnosed and self-treated.
2. Recommendations for reducing incidences of medication errors include:
   a. physician supervision whenever drugs are administered.
   b. advising patients to take only one medication at a time.
   c. requiring that prescriptions be typed instead of handwritten.
   d. avoiding use of confusing terms on clinical documents.
3. Adverse drug effects are most likely when:
   a. multiple medications are used.
   b. generic drugs are substituted for brand-name drugs.
   c. patients are bedridden during an illness.
   d. medications are taken for just one or two days.
4. An important difference between medications and herbal products that reach the marketplace is that:
   a. medications that cause adverse effects cannot be sold.
   b. medications are subject to contamination with toxic metals, molds, and bacteria.
   c. herbal products are not required to prove safety and effectiveness.
   d. herbal products must provide standard amounts of active ingredients.
5. The most important step that health practitioners can take to limit risk of medication-related side effects is to:
   a. recommend use of over-the-counter drugs instead of prescription medications.
   b. encourage use of herbal remedies rather than prescription medications.
   c. advise patients to take medications separately from meals.
   d. ask patients to fully describe the types and amounts of medications and dietary supplements they are using.
6. Examples of medication-related symptoms that can significantly limit food intake include:
   a. skin rash and ringing in the ears.
   b. persistent nausea and vomiting.
   c. insomnia and sensitivity to sunlight.
   d. nasal congestion and hair loss.
7. Factors that typically interfere with drug absorption include:
   a. binding between drugs and food components.
   b. use of antacid therapies.
   c. rapid stomach emptying rate.
   d. all of the above.
8. Compounds in grapefruit juice:
   a. bind to antibiotics, reducing absorption.
   b. cause excessive drug excretion.
   c. strengthen effects of certain drugs.
   d. alter acidity in the stomach, impairing drug absorption.
9. Vitamin K consumption should be consistent in patients using:
   a. tetracycline.
   b. isoniazid.
   c. warfarin.
   d. lithium.
10. People who use MAO inhibiters must limit consumption of:
    a. whole milk and yogurt.
    b. aged cheeses.
    c. dark green leafy vegetables.
    d. grapefruit juice.

REFERENCES

1. Food and Drug Administration, *CDER 2002 Report to the Nation: Improving Public Health Through Human Drugs* (Rockville, Md.: Food and Drug Administration, 2002); Food and Drug Administration, *From Test Tube to Patient: New Drug Development in the United States* (Rockville, Md.: Food and Drug Administration, 1999).
2. R. L. Corelli and M. A. Koda-Kimble, Therapeutic and toxic potential of over-the-counter agents, in B. G. Katzung, ed., *Basic and Clinical Pharmacology* (New York: Lange Medical Books/McGraw-Hill, 2001), pp. 1077–1087.
3. J. Phillips and coauthors, Retrospective analysis of mortalities associated with medication errors, *American Journal of Health-System Pharmacy* 58 (2001): 1835–1841.
4. C. H. Halsted, Dietary supplements and functional foods: 2 sides of a coin? *American Journal of Clinical Nutrition* 77 (2003): 1001S–1007S; P. Mason, *Dietary Supplements* (Chicago: Pharmaceutical Press, 2001); K. L. Radimer, A. F. Subar, and F. E. Thompson, Nonvitamin, nonmineral dietary supplements: Issues and findings from NHANES III, *Journal of the American Dietetic Association* 100 (2000): 447–454.
5. S. Gunther and coauthors, Demographic and health-related correlates of herbal and specialty supplement use, *Journal of the American Dietetic Association* 104 (2004): 27–34.
6. Radimer, Subar, and Thompson, 2000.
7. Halsted, 2003; J. Barnes, L. A. Anderson, and J. D. Phillipson, *Herbal Medicines: A Guide for Healthcare Professionals* (Chicago: Pharmaceutical Press, 2002); M. Rotblatt and I. Ziment, eds., *Evidence-Based Herbal Medicine* (Philadelphia: Hanley & Belfus, 2002).
8. ConsumerLab.com, LLC, Product review: Ginkgo biloba and huperzine A—Memory enhancers, **www.consumerlab.com/results/ginkgobiloba.asp**, posted April 21, 2003 (site visited December 3, 2004).
9. Halsted, 2003.
10. Barnes, Anderson, and Phillipson, 2002.
11. Halsted, 2003.
12. W. F. Huang, K. C. Wen, and M. L. Hsiao, Adulteration by synthetic therapeutic substances of traditional Chinese medicines in Taiwan, *Journal of Clinical Pharmacology* 37 (1997): 344–350.
13. Barnes, Anderson, and Phillipson, 2002.
14. Z. M. Pronsky and J. P. Crowe, Food-drug interactions, in L. K. Mahan and S. Escott-Stump, eds., *Krause's Food, Nutrition, and Diet Therapy* (Philadelphia: Saunders, 2004); B. G. Katzung, ed., *Basic and Clinical Pharmacology* (New York: Lange Medical Books/McGraw-Hill, 2001); V. Utermohlen, Diet, nutrition, and drug interactions, in M. E. Shils and coeditors, *Modern Nutrition in Health and Disease* (Baltimore: Williams & Wilkins, 1999), pp. 1619–1641.
15. D. G. Bailey, Grapefruit juice–drug interaction issues, in J. I. Boullata and V. T. Armenti, eds., *Handbook of Drug-Nutrient Interactions* (Totowa, N.J.: Humana Press, 2004), pp. 175–194.
16. A. Fugh-Berman and E. Ernst, Herb-drug interactions: Review and assessment of report reliability, *British Journal of Clinical Pharmacology* 52 (2001): 587–596.

ANSWERS

Study Questions (multiple choice)

1. d 2. d 3. a 4. c 5. d 6. b 7. d 8. c 9. c 10. b

HIGHLIGHT

Complementary and Alternative Medicine

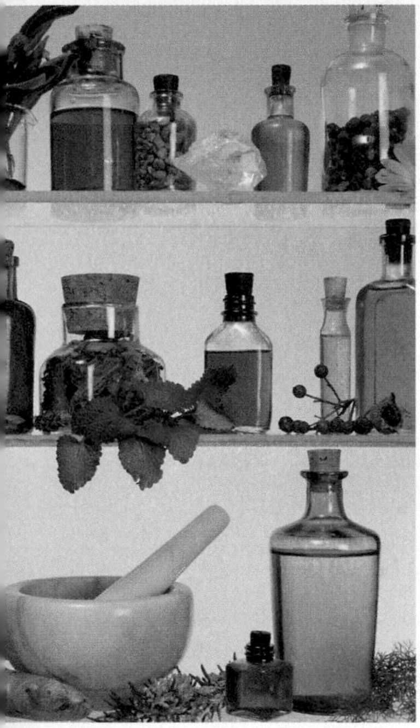

© Art Montes De Oca/Taxi/Getty Images

The medical treatments described in the clinical chapters are based upon current scientific understanding of human physiology and biochemistry and are generally supported by well-conducted clinical research. In **conventional medicine,** if a treatment is tested and found to be ineffective, it is eventually abandoned. If a novel therapy is demonstrated by clinical research to be effective and the benefits of using it outweigh its risks, it is incorporated into mainstream medical practice. This highlight examines therapies that have *not* been scientifically validated and are therefore not currently accepted by conventional medical professionals; they fall into a category called **complementary and alternative medicine (CAM)**. The accompanying glossary defines related terms.

In 1997, Americans spent an estimated $25 billion on CAM treatments. CAM is most prevalent among people with chronic, debilitating diseases; for example, 84 percent of AIDS patients reportedly use CAM.[1] CAM therapies remain popular despite the dearth of evidence demonstrating their effectiveness. Reasons for their popularity include consumers' growing interest in self-help measures, the noninvasive nature of many CAM therapies, and the positive interactions consumers have with CAM practitioners.[2]

In response to the enormous popularity of CAM in the United States, in 1998 Congress established the **National Center for Complementary and Alternative Medicine (NCCAM),** which is now one of the 27 institutes that make up the National Institutes of Health (NIH). NCCAM's missions are to investigate complementary and alternative therapies by funding well-designed scientific studies and to provide authoritative information for consumers and health professionals. If enough evidence is found to support the use of a complementary or alternative therapy, it may become a treatment regularly offered by conventional health practitioners.

Defining Complementary and Alternative Medicine

CAM includes a variety of approaches, philosophies, and treatments that have not been proved effective for treating disease; some of these are described in the glossary of alternative therapies (p. 646). When these therapies are used in place of conventional medicine, they are called *alternative;* when used together with conventional medicine, they are called *complementary.* The term *alternative* may be misleading in that it inappropriately implies that unproven methods of treatment are valid alternatives to conventional treatments.

Due to substantial consumer interest, health care professionals are finding it necessary to learn more about CAM therapies so that they can better communicate with patients regarding their medical care and advise them when an alternative approach conflicts with standard therapy or presents a danger to

GLOSSARY

alternative medicine: an approach that uses unconventional therapies *in place of* conventional medicine.

complementary and alternative medicine (CAM): diverse medical and health care systems, practices, and products that currently are not considered part of conventional medicine; also called *unconventional* or *unorthodox therapies.*

complementary medicine: an approach that uses unconventional therapies *in addition to,* and not simply as a replacement for, conventional medicine.

conventional medicine: diagnosis and treatment of diseases as practiced by medical doctors (M.D.) and doctors of osteopathy (D.O.) and assisted by allied health professionals such as registered nurses, pharmacists, and physical therapists; also called *Western, mainstream,* or *orthodox medicine.*

integrative medicine: an approach to medical care that combines mainstream medical therapies and CAM therapies for which there is some high-quality scientific evidence of safety and effectiveness.

National Center for Complementary and Alternative Medicine (NCCAM): a federal agency that researches and provides information about complementary and alternative therapies.

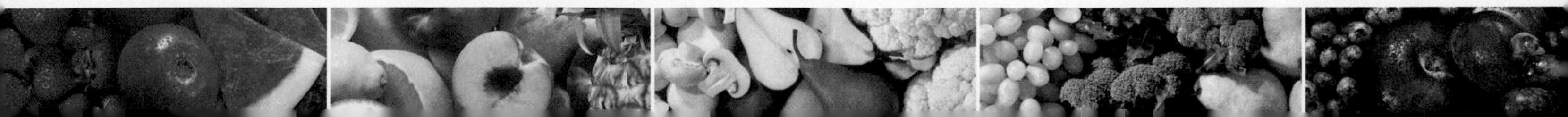

health. To provide medical students with objective information about CAM, half of U.S. medical schools now offer elective courses about alternative treatments.[3] Physicians who practice **integrative medicine** refer patients for complementary therapies while continuing to provide standard treatments.

Overview of CAM Therapies

CAM includes any and all therapies that are not part of conventional medicine. Consequently, the list of CAM approaches includes hundreds of advertised therapies purchased and used by consumers. Unfortunately, CAM has become a marketing buzzword and is used by unscrupulous sellers of worthless treatments.

NCCAM has classified CAM therapies as shown in Table H19-1 and defined in the glossary of alternative therapies on p. 646. Several popular examples are described in this highlight. Other examples are discussed on NCCAM's website (**http://nccam.nih.gov/health**).

TABLE H19-1 Examples of Complementary and Alternative Medicine

Alternative Medical Systems

- Naturopathic medicine
- Homeopathic medicine
- Traditional Chinese medicine
- Ayurveda

Mind-Body Interventions

- Meditation
- Faith healing (prayer)
- Mental healing (including hypnotherapy)
- Music, art, and dance therapy

Biologically Based Therapies

- Dietary supplements
- Foods and special diets
- Herbal products
- Hormones
- Aromatherapy

Manipulative and Body-Based Methods

- Chiropractic
- Massage therapy
- Osteopathic manipulation
- Reflexology

Energy Therapies

- Biofield therapies (including therapeutic touch, acupuncture, and qi gong)
- Bioelectrical fields (including electrical and magnetic fields)

Alternative Medical Systems

Alternative medical systems are based on theories other than the scientifically based theories underlying conventional medicine. Virtually all of these alternative systems were developed well over 100 years ago, before our bodies' biochemical and physiological processes were well understood. The alternative forms of diagnoses and treatments may appeal to consumers because the interventions are nontechnical and seem nonthreatening. In general, alternative theories and practices remain rooted in the past and have not been updated to include our current knowledge. Examples follow.

Naturopathic Medicine

Naturopathic medicine proposes that a person's natural "life force" can foster self-healing. This life force is allegedly stimulated by certain health-promoting factors and suppressed by excesses and deficiencies. Naturopaths believe that all ill health results from an internal disruption rather than from external disease-causing agents. Naturopathic therapies aim to enhance the natural healing powers of the body and may include special diets or fasting, herbal remedies and other dietary supplements, acupuncture, homeopathy, massage, and various other interventions.

Homeopathic Medicine

Homeopathic medicine is based on the dubious theory that "like cures like." Homeopaths believe that a substance that causes a particular set of symptoms can be used to cure a disease that has similar symptoms. Homeopathic remedies are usually substantially diluted in the belief that dilution increases potency; some remedies are so extremely diluted that the original substance is virtually no longer present. Homeopaths theorize that even though their remedies no longer contain a diluted substance, they still have powerful healing effects because the water structure is somehow altered during the dilution process used to prepare homeopathic medicines. This theory, however, conflicts with scientific understanding of water structure and properties.

Traditional Chinese Medicine

Traditional Chinese medicine (TCM) includes a large number of folk practices that originated in China. TCM is based on the theory that the body has pathways (called *meridians*) that conduct energy (called *qi;* pronounced *chee*). The interrupted flow of qi is believed to cause illness. TCM practices allegedly improve the flow of qi and include acupuncture, qi gong, herbal remedies, dietary practices, and massage. (Acupuncture and qi gong are described in a later section on energy therapies.) Ironically, TCM is used by relatively few in the Chinese population,

GLOSSARY OF ALTERNATIVE THERAPIES

acupuncture (AK-you-PUNK-cher): a therapy that involves inserting thin needles into the skin at specific anatomical points, allegedly to correct disruptions in the flow of energy within the body.

aromatherapy: inhalation of oil extracts from plants to cure illness or enhance health.

ayurveda: a traditional medical system from India that promotes the use of diet, herbs, meditation, massage, and yoga for preventing and treating illness.

bioelectrical or **bioelectromagnetic therapies:** therapies that involve the unconventional use of electric or magnetic fields to cure illness.

biofeedback: a technique in which individuals are trained to gain voluntary control of certain physiological processes, such as skin temperature or brain wave activity, to help reduce stress and anxiety.

biofield therapies: healing methods based on the belief that illnesses can be healed by manipulating energy fields that purportedly surround and penetrate the body. Examples include *acupuncture, qi gong,* and *therapeutic touch.*

chiropractic (KYE-roh-PRAK-tic): an alternative medical system based on the unproven theory that spinal manipulation can restore health.

- A *subluxation* is a misaligned vertebra or other spinal alteration that may cause illness.
- *Adjustment* describes the manipulative therapy practiced by chiropractors.

faith healing: the use of prayer or belief in divine intervention to promote healing.

homeopathic (HO-mee-oh-PATH-ic) **medicine:** a practice based on the theory that "like cures like"; that is, substances believed to cause certain symptoms are prescribed for curing the same symptoms, but are given in extremely diluted amounts.

- **homeo** = like
- **pathos** = suffering

hypnotherapy: a technique that uses hypnosis and the power of suggestion to improve health behaviors, relieve pain, and promote healing.

imagery: the use of mental images of things or events to aid relaxation or promote self-healing.

massage therapy: manual manipulation of muscles to reduce tension, increase blood circulation, improve joint mobility, and promote healing of injuries.

meditation: a self-directed technique of calming the mind and relaxing the body.

naturopathic (NAY-chur-oh-PATH-ic) **medicine:** an approach to medical care using practices alleged to enhance the body's natural healing abilities. Treatments may include a variety of alternative therapies including dietary supplements, herbal remedies, exercise, and homeopathy.

osteopathic (AHS-tee-oh-PATH-ic) **manipulation:** a manipulative technique performed by osteopaths that includes deep tissue massage and manipulation of joints, spine, and soft tissues. Doctors of Osteopathic Medicine (D.O.s) are fully trained and licensed medical physicians.

qi gong (chee GUNG): a Chinese system that combines movement, meditation, and breathing techniques and allegedly cures illness by enhancing the flow of "qi" energy within the body.

reflexology: a technique that applies pressure or massage on areas of the hands or feet to allegedly cure disease or relieve pain in other areas of the body; sometimes called **zone therapy.**

therapeutic touch: a technique of passing hands over a patient to purportedly identify energy imbalances and transfer healing power from therapist to patient; also called **laying on of hands.**

traditional Chinese medicine (TCM): an approach to medical care based on the concept that illness can be cured by enhancing the flow of "qi" energy within a person's body. Treatments may include herbal therapies, physical exercises, meditation, acupuncture, and remedial massage.

as Chinese physicians have largely adopted the Western approach to managing illness.[4]

Mind-Body Interventions

Mind-body therapies attempt to improve a person's sense of psychological or spiritual well-being despite the presence of illness. The treatments are also used in the hope of reducing stress, dealing with pain, or lowering blood pressure. Some of these therapies have been incorporated into mainstream medicine for stress reduction or relaxation. For example, **biofeedback** training, in which individuals learn to monitor skin temperature, muscle tension, or brain wave activity while practicing relaxation techniques, is frequently taught by behavioral medicine specialists to help patients reduce stress or anxiety. Other techniques to reduce stress and promote relaxation include **meditation,** art and music therapy, and prayer.

The clinical applications of other mind-body therapies are far more questionable. An example is guided **imagery,** in which a person tries to reverse the disease process (for example, shrink a tumor) by using mental pictures. Another example is the use of **faith healing** to cure disease in place of proven conventional treatments.

Biologically Based Therapies

Biological therapies include the use of natural products, such as vitamin supplements, herbal and plant extracts, and special foods. The most popular biological therapy is the use of herbal remedies, as discussed in Chapter 19. Other popular biologically based treatments follow.[5]

Hormones

Some hormones or hormonelike products that are derived from foods are considered dietary supplements and can be sold over the counter. Because the FDA does not regulate these products, there is no way of knowing whether they are

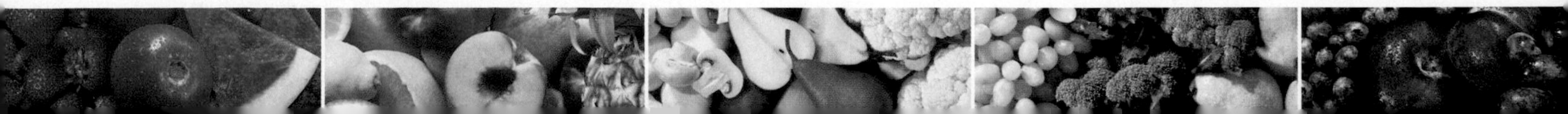

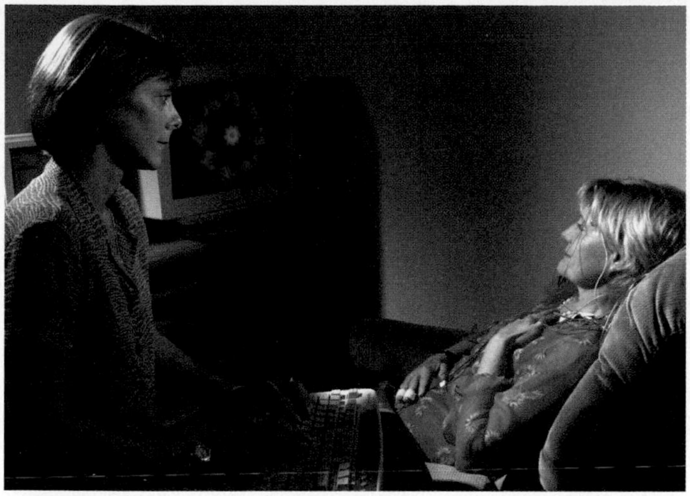

© Cindy Charles/PhotoEdit, Inc.

Biofeedback training is a stress reduction and relaxation technique.

safe or effective. Moreover, the dosages specified on the label may not be accurate, and the potential hazards of using them are not known. Examples include melatonin, a hormone made by the pineal gland and alleged to reverse sleep disorders and prevent jet lag. The adrenal hormone DHEA (dihydroepiandosterone) is promoted to enhance immunity, increase muscle mass, improve memory, and defend against aging.

Glucosamine-Chondroitin Supplements

The use of glucosamine and chondroitin supplements is an example of a CAM therapy in the process of moving to mainstream medicine. Glucosamine and chondroitin are produced in the body and help to maintain joint cartilage. Supplements containing either substance or a combination of the two may reduce pain and repair joint damage in people with osteoarthritis. Some high-quality studies have found that glucosamine and chondroitin reduce symptoms of arthritis better than a placebo, prompting some physicians to suggest using these supplements for pain relief. The overall benefits of using either or both of these substances are similar to those achieved using conventional anti-inflammatory drugs.[6]

Aromatherapy

Aromatherapy is the practice of inhaling aromatic substances derived from plants, called *essential oils*. Aromatherapy allegedly improves health and enhances natural healing processes. Popular examples of essential oils include those from eucalyptus, lavender, peppermint, rosemary, and lemon.

Manipulative and Body-Based Methods

Manipulative interventions include physical touch, forceful movement of different parts of the body, and the application of pressure. Some practitioners maintain that special energy fields are also manipulated during the physical treatment and that proper energy flow induces healing, as described in the later section on energy therapies.

Chiropractic

Chiropractic theory alleges that keeping the nervous system free from obstruction will allow the body to heal itself because the healing process stems from the brain and travels via the spinal cord and nerves to all parts of the body. Chiropractors claim to diagnose illnesses by detecting subluxations in the spine, which are variously described as misaligned vertebrae or pinched nerves that allegedly cause subtle interferences within the nervous system. The main treatment is the adjustment, a manual manipulation that is said to correct a subluxation and restore the body's natural healing ability. Although spinal manipulation has mainly been found to be helpful for improving back pain, most chiropractors still assert that chiropractic can cure disease rather than simply relieve symptoms.[7] For example, many still promote spinal manipulation to treat infectious diseases, prevent cancer, and regulate menstrual periods, even though the nervous system and spinal alignment do not play roles in the pathology of these conditions.

Massage Therapy

Massage therapy is the manipulation of muscle and connective tissue to improve muscle function, reduce pain, or promote relaxation. Massage therapists may also apply heat or cold and give advice about exercises that may improve muscle tone and range of motion. Although massage is often integrated into physical therapy treatment, some massage therapists may incorrectly suggest that massage is a valid treatment for a wide range of medical conditions.

"Energy" Therapies

Two categories of theories involve the alleged curative power of "energy." **Biofield therapies** are said to influence the energy that surrounds or pervades the human body, and their proponents claim that an energy therapy can strengthen or restore a person's "energy flow" and induce healing. Acupuncture, qi gong, and therapeutic touch are among the therapies that subscribe to these theories. It should be noted that CAM adherents often use the term *energy* unscientifically and that there is no objective evidence of this sort of energy flow. **Bioelectrical** or **bioelectromagnetic therapies** use electric or magnetic fields to allegedly promote healing; for example, magnets have been marketed with claims that they can improve circulation, reduce inflammation, and speed recovery from injuries.

Acupuncture

Acupuncture, a component of traditional Chinese medicine, is based on the theory that disease is caused by the disrupted flow of qi through the body. Acupuncture allegedly corrects such disruptions and restores health. The practice involves the shallow insertion of stainless steel needles into the skin at designated points on the body, sometimes accompanied by a low-frequency current to produce greater stimulation.

Qi Gong

Qi gong is another therapy originating in China that is said to improve the "flow of qi" within the body. A "qi gong master" allegedly cures disease by releasing energy from his or her body and passing it to the person being treated. Self-help practices include deep breathing, certain types of physical exercise, and concentration and relaxation techniques.

Therapeutic Touch

Therapeutic touch is based on the premise that the "healing force" of a practitioner can be used to cure disease. Practitioners claim to identify and correct energy imbalances by passing their hands above a patient's body and transferring "excess energy" to the patient.

Is CAM Safe and Effective?

As mentioned earlier, CAM treatments are generally excluded from mainstream medical practice because there is no evidence proving that they are effective for treating the diseases and medical conditions for which they are used. Many consumers think otherwise and seem satisfied that these treatments "work." How is this dichotomy to be explained?

Does CAM Work?

Consumers perceive their visits to CAM therapists as far more pleasant than visits to conventional health practitioners. CAM therapists spend more time with patients, are more attentive, and use less invasive interventions.[8] Self-help measures are encouraged, so the consumer has more control over the treatment. The therapies appear to be more "natural" and to have fewer side effects.

Possible explanations for "cures" include:[9]

- A person may seem "cured" because of misdiagnosis; that is, the condition diagnosed by the CAM practitioner may not have actually existed.
- The condition may have been self-limiting, or it may have gone into temporary remission after the treatment.
- Undue credit may be inappropriately assigned to the CAM therapy when the improvement was actually due to a previous or concurrent conventional treatment.
- The placebo effect may have had an influence on the course of disease.

The central question remains: Do the CAM therapies merely make people *feel* better, or do they really *get* better? This question can be answered only by well-controlled research studies.

Potential Hazards of CAM

One of the attractions of alternative therapies is the assumption that they are safe. Recall, however, the concerns associated with the use of herbal products discussed in Chapter 19, which include the potential toxicity of herbal ingredients, product contamination or adulteration, and interactions with conventional medications. The FDA recalled more than 100 dietary supplements between 1990 and 1999 due to hazards associated with their use.[10]

Another concern is that use of CAM therapies may delay the use of reliable treatments that have demonstrable benefits. Various reports have described how people with treatable medical conditions suffered permanent disability or death when they were misdiagnosed or improperly treated by CAM practitioners. For example, a rare but well-known risk of spinal cord injury or stroke is associated with a type of cervical manipulation performed by chiropractors.[11] Unfortunately, because most CAM therapies are not regulated or monitored, there are no accurate estimates of their adverse effects.

Working with Patients Who Use CAM

Health practitioners should be aware when their patients are using CAM therapies that may have consequences on the course of their disease and its treatment. It is important to routinely inquire about the use of CAM therapies and to educate patients about the hazards of postponing or stopping conventional treatment.[12] Patients should also be told about potential interactions between conventional treatments and CAM therapies. Some patients may want to learn about differences between evidence-based medical practices and untested CAM theories and may be interested in the integrative medicine options available.

Although alternative therapies come in a variety of shapes and sizes, they have one characteristic in common: their effectiveness is, for the most part, unproven. As mentioned previously, patients often choose alternative therapies because of their positive interactions with CAM practitioners. Empathizing with patients may go a long way toward winning their trust and improving their compliance with therapy. In addition, health practitioners need to regularly update their knowledge about unconventional practices, using reliable, objective resources, so that they can knowledgeably discuss these options with patients.

NUTRITION ON THE NET

Access these websites for further study of topics covered in this highlight.

- Find updates and quick links to these and other nutrition-related sites at our website: **www.wadsworth.com/nutrition**
- Learn about complementary and alternative medicine from the National Institutes of Health's National Center for Complementary and Alternative Medicine: **www.nccam.nih.gov**
- Search CAM or PubMed for a literature search of the complementary and alternative subset of PubMed: **www.nlm.nih.gov/nccam/camonpubmed.html**
- Review the backgrounds and practices of many popular practitioners of alternative treatments: **www.quackwatch.com**

REFERENCES

1. J. D. Berman and S. E. Straus, Implementing a research agenda for complementary and alternative medicine, *Annual Review of Medicine* 55 (2004): 239–254.
2. E. Ernst, The role of complementary and alternative medicine, *British Medical Journal* 321 (2000): 1133–1135.
3. B. Barzansky, H. S. Jonas, and S. I. Etzel, Educational programs in US medical schools, 1999–2000, *Journal of the American Medical Association* 284 (2000): 1114–1120.
4. D. Normile, The new face of Chinese medicine, *Science* 299 (2003): 188–190.
5. P. Mason, *Dietary Supplements* (Chicago: Pharmaceutical Press, 2001).
6. M. Rotblatt and I. Ziment, eds., *Evidence-Based Herbal Medicine* (Philadelphia: Hanley & Belfus, 2002).
7. American Medical Association, *Alternative Medicine (Report 12 of the Council on Scientific Affairs (A-97)* (American Medical Association, 1997), **www.ama-assn.org/ama/pub/category/13638.html**, site visited December 5, 2004.
8. American Medical Association, 1997.
9. American Medical Association, 1997.
10. Berman and Straus, 2004.
11. A. Vickers and C. Zollman, The manipulative therapies: Osteopathy and chiropractic, *British Medical Journal* 319 (1999): 1176–1179.
12. American Medical Association, 1997.

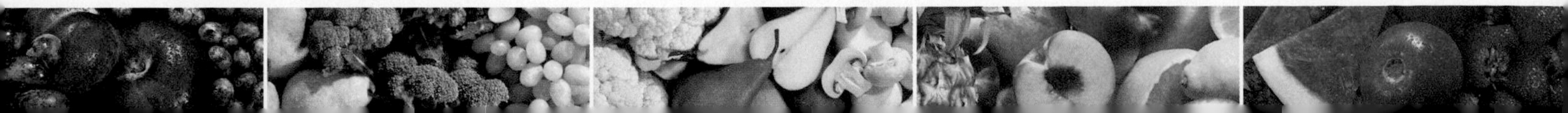

Chapter 20

Enteral Nutrition Support

Chapter Outline

Enteral Formulas: *Types of Formulas • Formula Characteristics*

Enteral Nutrition in Medical Care: *Oral Use of Enteral Formulas • Tube Feedings • Feeding Routes • Formula Selection*

Administration of Tube Feedings: *Safe Handling • Initiating and Progressing a Tube Feeding • Delivering Medications through Feeding Tubes • Complications of Tube Feeding • Documentation of Tube Feeding • Transition to Table Foods*

Highlight: *Enteral Nutrition and Inborn Errors of Metabolism*

Available Online

http://nutrition.wadsworth.com/uncn7

Student Practice Test

Glossary Terms

Nutrition on the Net

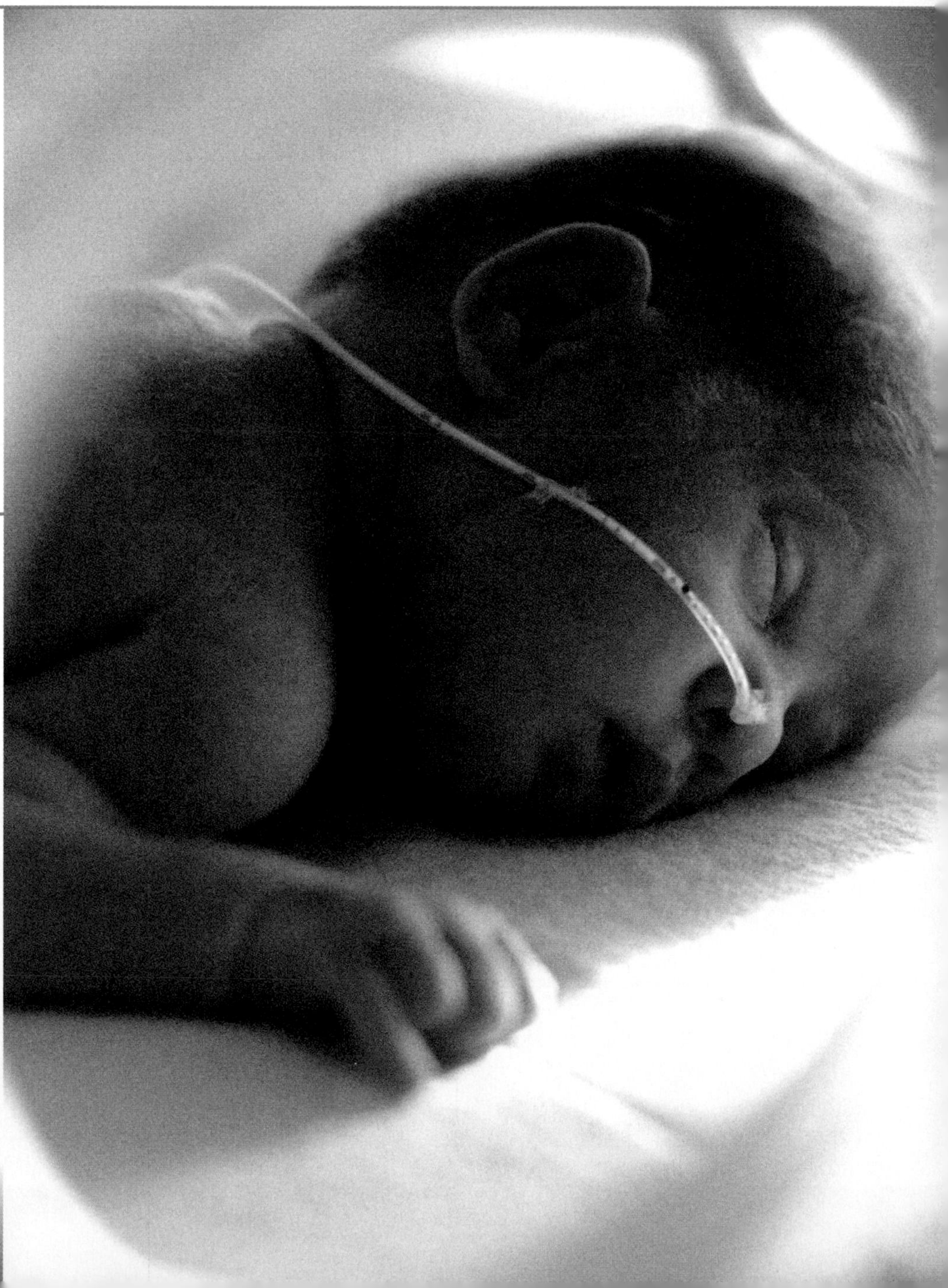

Nutrition in the Professional Setting

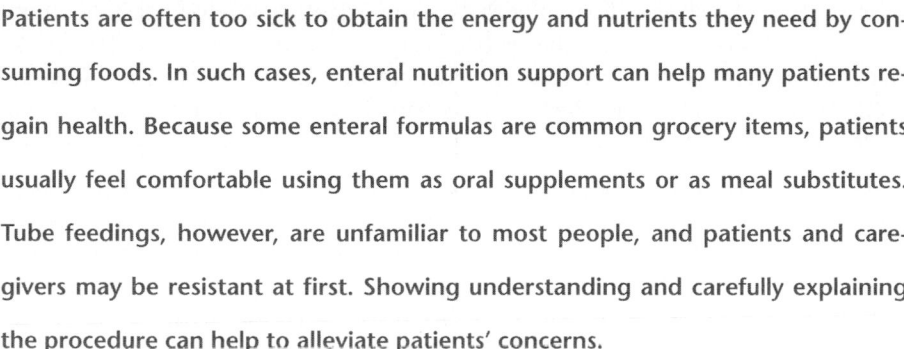

Patients are often too sick to obtain the energy and nutrients they need by consuming foods. In such cases, enteral nutrition support can help many patients regain health. Because some enteral formulas are common grocery items, patients usually feel comfortable using them as oral supplements or as meal substitutes. Tube feedings, however, are unfamiliar to most people, and patients and caregivers may be resistant at first. Showing understanding and carefully explaining the procedure can help to alleviate patients' concerns.

To meet nutritional needs using conventional foods, a person must be able to chew and swallow foods and digest and absorb nutrients in the amounts necessary to satisfy metabolic demands. As future chapters will show, illnesses may interfere with eating, digestion, and absorption to such a degree that conventional foods cannot supply the necessary nutrients. In such cases, **nutrition support**, the delivery of formulated nutrients, can meet a patient's nutritional needs. **Enteral nutrition** provides nutrients using the gastrointestinal (GI) tract. Enteral nutrition includes oral diets or supplements, but more commonly refers to the use of tube feedings,■ which supply nutrients directly to the stomach or intestine via a thin, flexible tube. **Parenteral nutrition** provides nutrients intravenously to patients who do not have adequate gastrointestinal function to handle enteral feedings (see Chapter 21).

If gastrointestinal function is normal and a poor appetite is the primary nutrition problem, enteral formulas can be provided as an oral supplement to the usual diet. If patients cannot consume enough food or drink enough formula to meet nutrient needs, it may be necessary to deliver nutrients using tube feedings, the main subject of this chapter.

■ Reminder: *Tube feedings* deliver liquid formulas through a tube placed in the stomach or intestine.

nutrition support: the delivery of formulated nutrients by feeding tube or intravenous infusion.

enteral (EN-ter-al) **nutrition:** provision of nutrients using the GI tract, including the use of tube feedings and oral diets.

parenteral (par-EN-ter-al) **nutrition:** intravenous provision of nutrients that bypasses the GI tract.
- **par** = beside
- **entero** = intestine

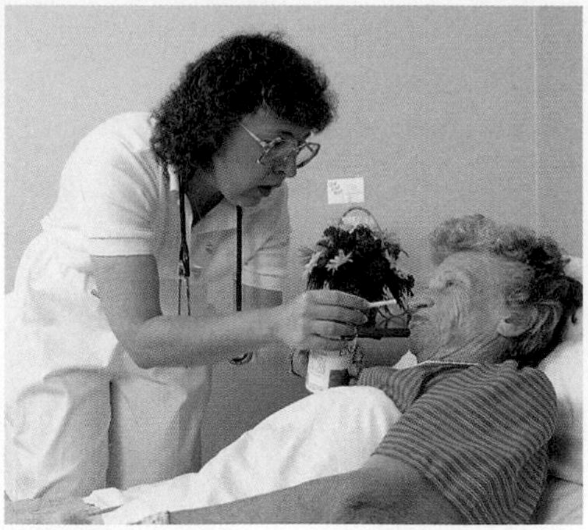

Enteral formulas can help to meet nutrient needs when patients cannot consume enough food from a conventional diet.

■ Reminder: The *macronutrients* are carbohydrates, fats, and proteins.

Enteral Formulas

The number of enteral formulas on the market is staggering (some examples are listed in Appendix J). Some products are available over-the-counter in pharmacies and grocery stores and are promoted in television and magazine advertisements. Most formulas are available in ready-to-use liquid form or in a powdered form that must be reconstituted with water. Designed to meet a variety of medical and nutrition needs, formulas can be used alone or given along with other foods. Thus a formula can be considered a liquid form of a standard or modified diet.

Many formulas are designed to supply all of an individual's nutrient requirements when consumed in sufficient volume. These nutritionally complete formulas are essential for a patient using a tube feeding or an oral liquid diet for more than a few days. They can also be, and often are, used in smaller quantities to supplement table foods.

Types of Formulas

Formulas are often categorized according to their macronutrient■ composition. Standard formulas usually contain intact proteins and polysaccharides, whereas hydrolyzed formulas contain broken down macronutrients that require less digestion. Some formulas contain only one or two macronutrients. Some formulas are designed to meet the specific nutrient needs of certain diseases. Because formulas are often used to replace meals, they typically contain vitamins and minerals as well. Table 20-1 lists examples of some macronutrient sources used in enteral formulas.

Standard Formulas **Standard formulas** are used for individuals who are able to digest and absorb nutrients without difficulty. They contain intact proteins isolated from milk or soybeans or a combination of **protein isolates** (purified proteins). The carbohydrate sources include modified starches, glucose polymers (such as maltodextrin), and sugars. A few formulas, called **blenderized formulas,** are made from whole foods and derive their protein primarily from pureed meat or poultry.

Hydrolyzed Formulas **Hydrolyzed formulas** are often provided to patients who have compromised digestive or absorptive functions. The formulas contain macronutrients that have been partially or fully broken down to fragments that require little (if any) digestion before absorption. Hydrolyzed formulas are often low in fat and may include medium-chain triglycerides (MCT) to ease digestion and absorption. These formulas are generally lactose-free and result in minimal fecal output.

Modular Formulas **Modular formulas** usually contain only one or two macronutrients and can be used to enhance other formulas. They may meet the needs of patients with specific nutritional problems; for example, a carbohydrate

standard formulas: general-purpose dietary formulas that contain intact proteins and polysaccharides; also called **polymeric** or **intact formulas.**

protein isolates: proteins that have been separated from foods. Examples include casein from milk and soy protein from soybeans.

blenderized formulas: dietary formulas that are made by blenderizing whole foods.

hydrolyzed formulas: dietary formulas that contain macronutrients that have been partially or fully hydrolyzed; also called **monomeric, defined,** or **elemental formulas.**

modular formulas: dietary formulas that contain only one or two macronutrients; used to enhance other formulas, meet specific nutrient needs, or create individualized formulas for people with unique needs.

TABLE 20-1 Examples of Protein, Carbohydrate, and Fat Sources in Enteral Formulas

Protein Sources	Carbohydrate Sources	Fat Sources
Casein	Cellulose	Canola oil
Egg white	Cornstarch	Corn oil
Free amino acids	Corn syrup	Fish oil
Hydrolyzed casein, whey, or soy protein	Maltodextrin	Medium-chain triglycerides (MCT)
Soy protein	Soy fiber	Soybean oil
Whey	Sucrose	Sunflower oil

formula may be used to increase the energy intake in a protein-restricted patient. Several modular formulas may be combined with liquid vitamin and mineral preparations to create individualized formulas for patients with unique nutrient needs. This process requires in-depth nutrition knowledge and skills.

Disease-Specific Formulas **Disease-specific formulas** contain nutrients that may meet the specific needs of patients with certain illnesses. For example, products have been developed for liver, kidney, and lung diseases; glucose intolerance; and metabolic stress. These disease-specific formulas are generally expensive, and their effectiveness is controversial.

Formula Characteristics

The varying energy and nutrient densities in enteral formulas enable them to meet the needs of patients while providing different volumes of fluid. The fiber content influences fecal bulk, colonic function, and blood glucose control. These properties affect the administration of tube feedings as well as the side effects that patients may experience.[1]

Energy Density The energy density of enteral formulas ranges between 0.5 and 2.0 kcalories per milliliter of fluid. Standard formulas generally provide 1.0 to 1.2 kcalories per milliliter and are appropriate for patients with average fluid requirements. Formulas that have greater energy density meet energy and nutrient needs in a smaller volume and therefore can benefit patients with high nutrient needs or those with fluid restrictions. Patients who have high fluid requirements can be given a formula that has low energy density, or they can be given a standard formula and provided with additional water via the feeding tube or intravenously.

Nutrient Density The percentages of protein, carbohydrate, and fat can vary greatly in enteral formulas. Protein content typically ranges between 8 and 29 percent of total kcalories. Protein requirements are high in patients with severe metabolic stress, but protein must be restricted in patients with renal failure. Carbohydrate and fat provide most of the energy in enteral formulas, and as with protein, the content of each varies among formulas. Standard formulas may provide 40 to 50 percent of kcalories from carbohydrate and 30 to 45 percent from fat.

Osmolality **Osmolality** refers to the osmotic property of a solution, that is, a solution's tendency to shift from one fluid compartment to another across a semipermeable membrane. The osmolality depends on a solution's concentrations of molecules and ionic particles. An enteral formula with an osmolality similar to that of blood serum (about 300 milliosmoles per kilogram) is an **isotonic formula,** whereas a **hypertonic formula** has an osmolality greater than that of blood serum. Generally, hydrolyzed formulas and nutrient-dense formulas have higher osmolalities than standard formulas.

Most enteral formulas have osmolalities between 300 and 700 milliosmoles per kilogram. Hypertonic formulas may reduce the nutrient absorption rate and cause diarrhea more often than isotonic formulas, but most people can tolerate both isotonic and hypertonic feedings without difficulty. When medications are infused along with enteral feedings, however, the osmotic load increases substantially and may contribute to the diarrhea experienced by many tube-fed patients.[2]

Fiber Content Fiber content influences the selection of an appropriate enteral formula. Fiber may be helpful for normalizing intestinal function, treating diarrhea and constipation, and maintaining blood glucose control. Fiber-containing formulas are avoided in patients with some intestinal conditions, those with pancreatitis, and patients undergoing examinations and procedures involving the intestines.

Cost Costs of enteral formulas vary greatly. As a general rule, hydrolyzed and disease-specific formulas are more expensive than standard formulas.

disease-specific formulas: dietary formulas designed to meet the nutrient needs of patients with specific illnesses.

osmolality (OZ-moh-LAL-eh-tee): the osmotic property of a solution, based on its concentrations of molecules and ionic particles. Osmolality is expressed as milliosmoles (mOsm) per kilogram.

isotonic formula: a formula with an osmolality similar to that of blood serum (300 mOsm/kg).
- **iso** = equal
- **tono** = pressure

hypertonic formula: a formula with an osmolality greater than that of blood serum.

IN SUMMARY Enteral formulas are liquid diets that meet a variety of nutrient and medical needs. Standard formulas that contain intact proteins and polysaccharides are used in patients who can digest and absorb nutrients without difficulty, whereas hydrolyzed formulas meet the nutrient needs of patients with limited digestive and absorptive functions. Modular formulas that contain single macronutrients can be used to modify other formulas. Specialized formulas are available for use in patients with specific diseases. Formulas differ in their macronutrient composition, energy density, osmolality, and fiber content. Most people tolerate isotonic and hypertonic formulas without difficulty.

Enteral Nutrition in Medical Care

A person with a functioning GI tract who cannot meet nutrition needs with conventional foods alone may benefit from enteral formulas. If GI function is severely impaired, parenteral nutrition, the subject of the next chapter, is an effective option. Enteral nutrition is always preferred, however, because it helps maintain normal gut function, causes fewer complications, and is less costly.[3] Enteral feedings also help to stimulate and improve intestinal function following intestinal surgeries or periods of GI tract disuse. Similarly, oral feedings are preferred to tube feedings if a person is able to drink an enteral formula. Drinking formulas prevents the stress, complications, and expense associated with tube feedings.

Oral Use of Enteral Formulas

Enteral formulas can fully meet the nutrient needs of individuals who can consume only liquids or who require hydrolyzed nutrients. More often, enteral formulas are used to supplement conventional diets when patients cannot consume the quantities of foods required to meet their needs. Enteral formulas provide a reliable source of nutrients and can add energy and protein to the diets of malnourished patients. Patients who are weak or debilitated may also find it easier to manage formulas than meals.

When a patient drinks a formula, taste becomes an important consideration. Allowing patients to sample different products and flavors and select the ones they prefer helps to promote acceptance. The "How to" offers additional suggestions for helping patients to accept oral formulas.

Tube Feedings

An individual with a functional GI tract who is unable to consume enough food or formula orally may need to be fed via a feeding tube. A tube feeding delivers a nutritionally complete formula directly to the stomach or intestine. Candidates for tube feedings include:

- People with physical problems that seriously interfere with chewing or swallowing.
- People who have little or no appetite for extended periods, especially if malnourished.
- People with gastrointestinal obstructions, some types of fistulas, or impaired motility in the upper GI tract.
- People who have impaired digestive function and who are unable to ingest hydrolyzed formulas orally.
- People who have undergone intestinal resections and are beginning enteral feedings.
- People who are mentally incapacitated due to confusion, dementia, or neurological difficulties.

HOW TO Help Patients Accept Oral Formulas

People using enteral formulas are often quite ill and have poor appetites. Even when a person enjoys a formula, the taste can eventually become monotonous. Hydrolyzed formulas are usually less palatable than standard formulas, and patients may find them difficult to drink. Health professionals can help by trying these suggestions:

- Allow the patient to sample different formulas that are appropriate for his or her needs; use only those the patient enjoys drinking.
- Serve formulas attractively and remind patients to drink them. Formulas that are offered in a glass on an attractive plate may be more appealing than those served from a can with an unfamiliar name.
- Some people may find the smell of formulas unappealing. Covering the top of the glass with plastic wrap or a lid, leaving just enough room for a straw, may help.
- Provide easy access. Keep the formula close to the patient's bed where little effort is required to reach it and within sight so that the patient is reminded to drink it. Patients who are very ill may lack the motivation even to reach for formula, let alone drink it. In such cases, offer the formula in smaller amounts that are easy to manage and serve it more frequently during the day.
- Try keeping the formula in an ice bath so that it will be cool and refreshing when the patient drinks it. Check with the patient to make sure the colder temperature is suitable.
- If the patient stops enjoying the formula, recommend different flavors or try other formulas.

- People in a coma.
- People with extremely high nutrient requirements.
- People on mechanical ventilators.

Feeding Routes

The tube feeding route chosen depends on a patient's medical condition, the expected duration of tube feeding, and the potential complications of a particular route. Figure 20-1 illustrates the main feeding routes, and the glossary on p. 656

FIGURE 20-1 Tube Feeding Routes

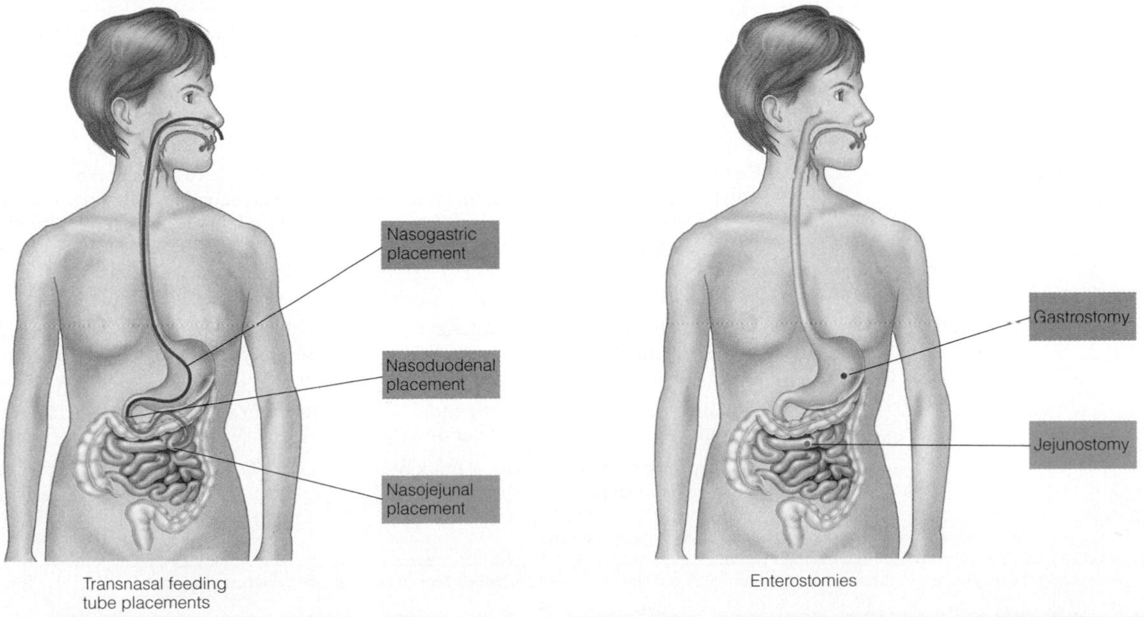
Nasogastric placement
Nasoduodenal placement
Nasojejunal placement
Transnasal feeding tube placements
Gastrostomy
Jejunostomy
Enterostomies

GLOSSARY OF TUBE FEEDING ROUTES

For each type of tube placement, the terms are listed in order from the upper to lower organs of the digestive system.

transnasal: through the nose. A **transnasal feeding tube** is one that is inserted through the nose.
- **naso** = nose

nasogastric (NG): tube is placed into the stomach via the nose.

nasoenteric: tube is placed into the GI tract via the nose. (*Nasoenteric feedings* usually refer to *nasoduodenal* and *nasojejunal* feedings.)

nasoduodenal (ND): tube is placed into the duodenum via the nose.

nasojejunal (NJ): tube is placed into the jejunum via the nose.

orogastric: tube is placed into the GI tract via the mouth. This method is often used to feed infants because a nasogastric tube can hinder the infant's breathing.

enterostomy (EN-ter-OSS-toe-mee): an opening into the GI tract through which a feeding tube can be passed.

gastrostomy (gas-TROSS-toe-mee): an opening into the stomach through which a feeding tube can be passed. A nonsurgical technique for creating a gastrostomy under local anesthesia is called **percutaneous endoscopic gastrostomy (PEG).**

jejunostomy (JE-ju-NOSS-toe-mee): an opening in the jejunum through which a feeding tube can be passed. A nonsurgical technique for creating a jejunostomy is called **percutaneous endoscopic jejunostomy (PEJ).** The tube can either be guided into the jejunum via a gastrostomy or passed directly into the jejunum **(direct PEJ).**

describes each route. Table 20-2 summarizes the advantages and disadvantages of each route. The following paragraphs provide details.

■ The final location of the feeding tube determines how the feeding route is classified.

When a patient is expected to be tube-fed for less than four weeks, a **nasoenteric** route is preferred; with this route, the feeding tube is passed into the GI tract via the nose. The patient is frequently awake during **transnasal** (through the nose) placement of a feeding tube. While the patient is in a slightly upright position with head tilted, the tube is inserted into a nostril and passed into the stomach **(nasogastric)**, duodenum **(nasoduodenal)**, or jejunum **(nasojejunal)**.■ If the patient is awake and alert, he or she can swallow water to ease the tube's passage. The final position of the feeding tube tip is often verified by abdominal X-ray or other means. In infants, **orogastric** placement, in which the feeding tube is passed into the stomach via the mouth, is preferred over transnasal routes. This placement allows the infant to breath more normally during feedings.

TABLE 20-2 Comparison of Tube Feeding Routes[a]

Insertion Method and Feeding Site	Advantages	Disadvantages
Transnasal	Does not require surgery or incisions for placement.	Easy to remove by disoriented patients; long-term use may irritate the nasal passages, throat, and esophagus.
Nasogastric	Easiest to insert and confirm placement; feedings can often be given intermittently and without an infusion pump.	Highest risk of aspiration in compromised patients.
Nasoduodenal and nasojejunal	Lower risk of aspiration in compromised patients; allow for enteral nutrition earlier than gastric feedings following severe stress; may allow for enteral feeding when obstructions, fistulas, or other medical conditions prevent gastric feeding.	More difficult to insert and confirm placement; feedings require an infusion pump for administration; may take longer to reach nutrition goals.
Tube enterostomies	Allow lower esophageal sphincter to remain closed, reducing the risk of aspiration; more comfortable than transnasal insertion for long-term use; site is not visible under clothing.	May require general anesthesia for insertion; require incisions; greater risk of complications from the insertion procedure; greater risk of infection; may cause skin irritation around the insertion site.
Gastrostomy	Feedings can often be given intermittently and without a pump; easier to insert than a jejunostomy.	Moderate risk of aspiration in high-risk patients.
Jejunostomy	Lowest risk of aspiration; allows for enteral nutrition earlier following severe stress; may allow for enteral feeding when obstructions, fistulas, or medical conditions prevent gastric feeding.	Most difficult to insert; feedings require an infusion pump for administration; may take longer to reach nutrition goals.

[a] Relative to other tube feeding routes. The actual advantages and disadvantages of different insertion procedures depend on the person's medical condition.

When a patient will be tube-fed for longer than four weeks or if the nasoenteric route is inaccessible due to an obstruction or other medical reasons, direct access to the stomach or intestine is made possible by passing the tube through an **enterostomy,** an opening in the stomach (**gastrostomy**) or jejunum (**jejunostomy**). An enterostomy may be made by surgical incision or nonsurgically using local anesthesia.

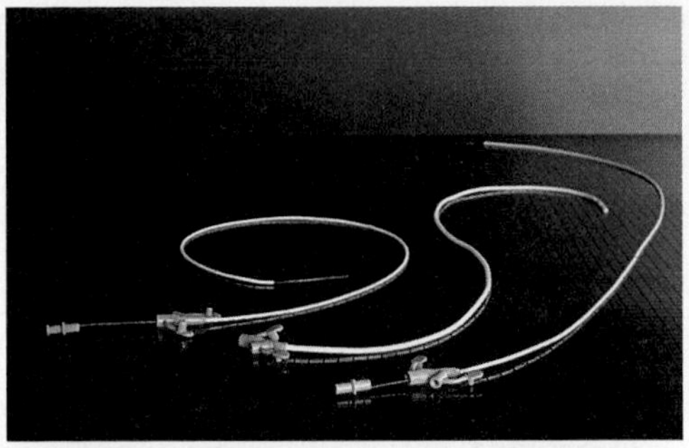

Feeding tubes come in many lengths and diameters. The thin wires protruding from the end of the feeding tubes are stylets, which stiffen the tube to ease insertion and are discarded thereafter. The Y-connector (shown here in orange) provides a port for administering water or medications without disrupting the feeding.

Selecting a Feeding Route When formulas are delivered into the stomach using a nasogastric tube or a gastrostomy, the digestive process begins in the stomach, just as it does when conventional foods are consumed. The stomach empties its contents at a controlled rate and delivers small volumes of nutrients into the intestine. For this reason, gastric feedings are often preferred whenever possible. Gastric feedings are not possible, however, for patients with gastric obstructions or conditions that significantly interfere with the stomach's ability to empty. For example, following a severe stress such as abdominal or intestinal surgery, GI motility may be temporarily impaired. Intestinal function often recovers within a few hours or a day, but the stomach may not empty normally for three or four days.[4] Thus the delivery of formulas into the small intestine can generally be initiated earlier than gastric feedings.

Gastric feedings may be a problem for patients at high risk of **aspiration,**■ a common complication in which formula or GI secretions enter the lungs, often from the backflow of stomach contents.[5] **Aspiration pneumonia,** a lung condition that is sometimes fatal, may result. To minimize the possibility of aspiration, clinicians may administer nasoduodenal or nasojejunal feedings. Avoiding gastric feedings to reduce aspiration is controversial, however, as studies have not consistently shown that they are associated with increased aspiration risk.[6] Some clinicians may prefer a jejunostomy because it allows the lower esophageal sphincter to remain tightly closed.

■ Aspiration risk is high in patients with esophageal disorders, neurological diseases, and conditions that reduce consciousness or cause dementia.

Feeding Tubes Feeding tubes are soft and flexible and come in a variety of lengths and diameters. The feeding tube selected depends on the patient's age and size, medical condition, the feeding route, and the viscosity of the formula. Once the appropriate length is determined, the tube selected is often the smallest tube through which the formula will flow without clogging.

The outer diameter of a tube is measured in **French sizes,** in which each unit is equal to one-third of a millimeter; thus a "12 French" feeding tube has a 4-millimeter diameter.■ The inner diameter depends on the thickness of the tubing material. Tubes are also available with double-lumen adapters so that one feeding tube can be used both for intestinal feedings and for **gastric decompression,** a procedure in which suction is used to remove the stomach contents of patients with motility disorders.

■ 1 French = $\frac{1}{3}$ mm.
12 French = $12 \times \frac{1}{3}$ mm = $\frac{12}{3}$ mm.
= 4 mm.

Formula Selection

Selecting an appropriate formula requires a logical approach, and some of the considerations involved are shown in Figure 20-2. Generally, the best formula is one that meets a patient's medical and nutrient needs with the lowest risk of complications and the lowest cost. If no available formulas can meet a patient's needs, modular formulas can be used to modify an existing formula.

The formula selected should meet nutrient needs as determined by a careful assessment of the patient's age, nutrition status, medical condition, and ability to digest and absorb nutrients. The vast majority of patients use standard formulas. A person with a functional, but impaired, GI tract may require a hydrolyzed formula. Other nutrition-related factors that affect the selection decision include:

- *A patient's energy, protein, and fluid requirements.* High nutrient needs must be met using the volume of formula a patient can tolerate. If fluids need to be restricted, the formula should be able to deliver the necessary nutrients in the volume prescribed.

aspiration: drawing in by suction or breathing; a common complication of enteral feedings in which foreign material enters the lungs, often from reflux of stomach contents.

aspiration pneumonia: a lung condition resulting from the abnormal entry of foreign material; caused by either bacterial infection or irritation of the lower airways.

French sizes: units of measure used for a feeding tube's outer diameter. One French unit is one-third of a millimeter.

gastric decompression: the use of suction to remove the stomach contents (including swallowed saliva, stomach secretions, and gas) of patients who have motility disorders or obstructions that prevent stomach emptying.

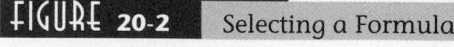

FIGURE 20-2 Selecting a Formula

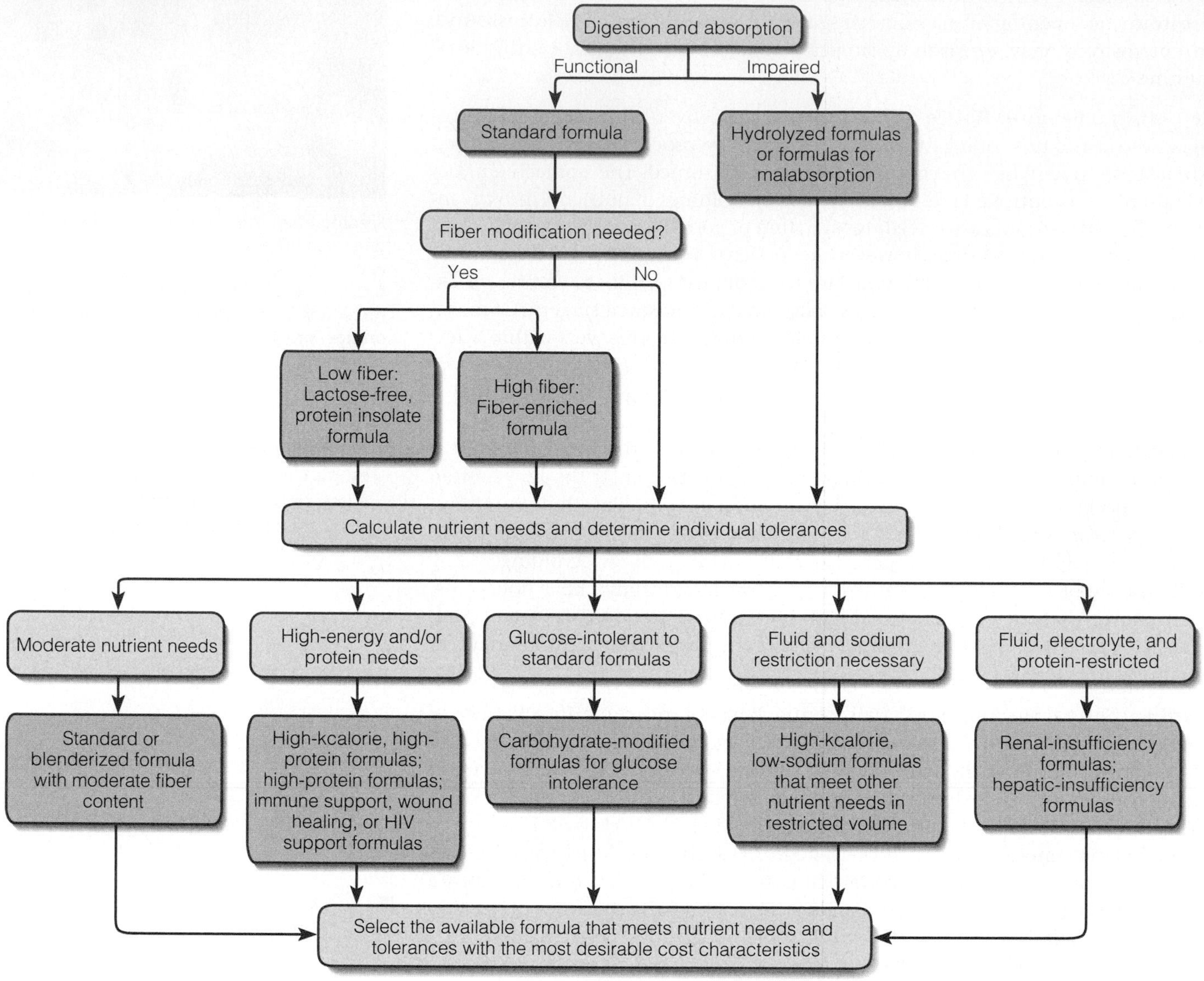
Digestion and absorption
Functional
Impaired
Standard formula
Hydrolyzed formulas or formulas for malabsorption
Fiber modification needed?
Yes
No
Low fiber: Lactose-free, protein insolate formula
High fiber: Fiber-enriched formula
Calculate nutrient needs and determine individual tolerances
Moderate nutrient needs
High-energy and/or protein needs
Glucose-intolerant to standard formulas
Fluid and sodium restriction necessary
Fluid, electrolyte, and protein-restricted
Standard or blenderized formula with moderate fiber content
High-kcalorie, high-protein formulas; high-protein formulas; immune support, wound healing, or HIV support formulas
Carbohydrate-modified formulas for glucose intolerance
High-kcalorie, low-sodium formulas that meet other nutrient needs in restricted volume
Renal-insufficiency formulas; hepatic-insufficiency formulas
Select the available formula that meets nutrient needs and tolerances with the most desirable cost characteristics

- *The need for fiber modifications.* The choice of formulas is narrowed if fiber intake needs to be low or high.
- *Individual tolerances (food allergies and sensitivities).* Most formulas are lactose-free because many patients who need enteral formulas are lactose intolerant. Many formulas are also gluten-free and can accommodate the needs of individuals with celiac disease (gluten sensitivity).
- *The size of the feeding tube lumen.* The formula selected must flow readily through the tube without clogging. Some fiber-containing or viscous formulas may require a tube with a wider lumen.

Health care facilities stock a limited number of formulas, so formula selection is usually limited by availability. Initially, the dietitian or physician may make an educated guess as to the best formula, based on the criteria previously mentioned. The decision can be reappraised as the patient's response to the formula is monitored.

IN SUMMARY Enteral formulas are used in patients who need to consume liquid or hydrolyzed diets or who require tube feedings. A nasoenteric feeding route is preferred for short-term tube feedings, whereas enterostomies are used for longer-term feedings. Because the stomach delivers nutrients into the intestine at a controlled rate, gastric feedings are often preferred, although they are usually avoided in patients at risk of aspiration. A chief concern in formula selection is the formula's ability to meet a patient's nutrient requirements.

Administration of Tube Feedings

Once a feeding route and formula have been selected, attention must be given to delivering the formula. The methods of tube feeding administration vary somewhat from one health care facility to the next. The procedures presented in the following sections are suggested guidelines.

Safe Handling

People who are ill or malnourished may have suppressed immune systems that make them vulnerable to infection from foodborne illness. To prevent contamination, all personnel involved in preparing or delivering formulas should work in clean environments, using clean equipment and clean hands. The foodservice department or pharmacy most often assumes responsibility for preparing formulas. Formulas are labeled with the patient's name, room number, date, and time of preparation (if necessary) and then sent to the nursing station.

Formulas are available as both **open feeding systems** and **closed feeding systems.** With an *open feeding system,* the formula must be transferred from its original packaging to a feeding container. The feeding container is connected to the feeding tube, and the formula is delivered to the patient. Examples of open feeding systems include formulas that are packaged in cans or bottles, concentrates that need to be diluted, and powders that require reconstitution. With a *closed feeding system,* the formula is prepackaged in a container that can be connected directly to a feeding tube. These closed systems reduce the risk of bacterial contamination, save nursing time, and can hang for longer periods of time than open systems. Although closed systems cost more initially, they may actually be less expensive in the long run by preventing bacterial contamination and thus avoiding the costs of treating infections.

Safety Guidelines Each institution has protocols for handling food products and formulas based on the identification of potential hazards and critical control points in food preparation, usually referred to as **HACCP (Hazard Analysis and Critical Control Point).** Personnel involved with preparing or delivering formula should be aware of the specific HACCP systems at their facility that are related to formula preparation and administration.

At the Nursing Station Once a formula reaches the nursing station, the nursing staff assumes responsibility for its safe handling. Hands should be carefully washed before handling formulas and feeding containers. In some facilities, nonsterile gloves are worn whenever formulas are handled. The following steps reduce the risk of formula contamination when open feeding systems are in use:

- Before opening a can of formula, carefully clean the can opener and the lid. If you do not use the entire can at one feeding, label the can with the time it was opened.
- Store opened cans or mixed formulas in clean, closed containers. Refrigerate the unused portion of formula promptly.

open feeding systems: delivery systems that require formula to be transferred from the original packaging to feeding containers before being administered through feeding tubes.

closed feeding systems: delivery systems in which formula comes prepackaged in containers that are ready to be attached to feeding tubes for administration.

HACCP (Hazard Analysis and Critical Control Point): systems of food or formula preparation that identify food safety hazards and critical control points during foodservice procedures; pronounced *hassip.*

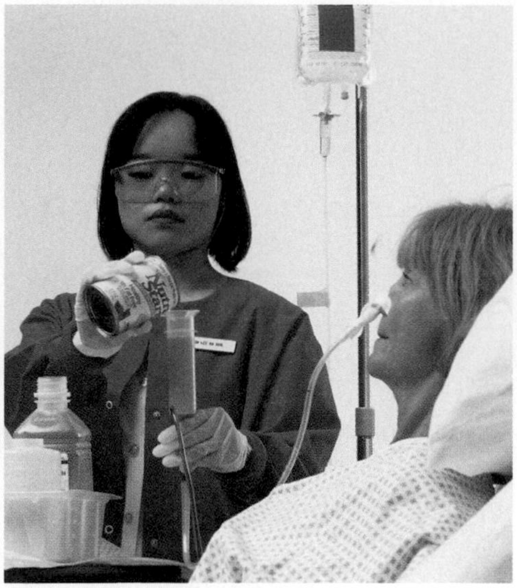
© Ed Eckstein/Phototake
With time, patients often adapt to larger amounts of formula administered over shorter periods of time.

- Discard unlabeled or improperly labeled containers and all opened containers of formula that are not used within 24 hours.

At Bedside These steps can help to reduce the risk of bacterial infections in tube-fed patients:

- Hang no more than an 8- to 12-hour supply of formula administered through an open system or no more than a 36- to 48-hour supply of formula administered through a closed system.
- For open systems, discard any formula that remains after 8 to 12 hours, rinse out the feeding bag and tubing, and add fresh formula to the feeding bag. Use a new feeding container and tubing (except for the feeding tube itself) every 24 hours.

Initiating and Progressing a Tube Feeding

Before beginning a tube feeding, health care professionals should discuss the procedure with the patient and family members, who may feel anxious about using a feeding tube. The discussion should address the reasons why tube feeding is appropriate and the benefits and risks of the procedure. The "How to" offers suggestions to help ease the concerns of patients who may benefit from tube feeding.

Minimizing the Risk of Incorrect Placement or Aspiration Serious complications may develop from tube feedings if the transnasal tube is accidentally placed into the respiratory tract or if formula or GI secretions are aspirated into the lungs. To minimize the risk of incorrect tube placement, clinicians usually use X-rays to verify the position of the feeding tube before a feeding is initiated. Nurses often monitor the feeding tube's position during the day by checking the position of the tubing after its placement has been confirmed. Another technique is to test the pH of a sample of bodily fluid drawn into the feeding tube, as the pH of stomach fluid is much lower than the pH of fluid obtained from the intestine or respiratory tract.

To reduce the risk of aspiration, the patient's upper body is elevated to at least a 30- to 45-degree angle during the feeding and for 30 minutes after the feeding whenever possible. The addition of blue food coloring to formula is sometimes suggested as a means of identifying aspirated formula in lung secretions; however, this practice is now discouraged because several deaths have been attributed to its use.[7]

Formula Delivery A day's nutrient needs can be met by delivering large amounts of formula several times a day **(intermittent feedings)** or smaller amounts continuously throughout the day **(continuous feedings).** A patient may also start on a continuous feeding and gradually transition to an intermittent feeding. Each method has specific uses, advantages, and disadvantages.

Intermittent feedings are best tolerated when they are delivered into the stomach (not the intestine). Generally, about 250 to 400 milliliters is delivered over 20 to 40 minutes using a gravity drip method or an infusion pump. The volume of formula required to meet a patient's nutrient needs is divided into several daily feedings. Because of the relatively high volume of formula delivered at a time, intermittent feedings may be difficult for some patients to tolerate, and the risk of aspiration may be higher than with continuous feedings. An advantage of intermittent feedings is that they mimic the usual pattern of eating and allow the patient freedom of movement between meals. They also require less time, making them less costly and easier to use at home.

Rapid delivery of a large volume of formula into the stomach (250 to 500 milliliters in less than 15 minutes) is called a **bolus feeding.** This type of feeding may be given every 3 to 4 hours using a syringe. Bolus feedings may cause abdominal discomfort, nausea, and cramping in some patients, especially when a feeding is initiated. The risk of aspiration is also greater than with other methods of feeding. For these reasons, bolus feedings are used only in patients who are not critically ill.

intermittent feedings: delivery of about 250 to 400 mL of formula over 20 to 40 minutes.

continuous feedings: slow delivery of formula at a constant rate over an 8- to 24-hour period.

bolus (BOH-lus) **feeding:** delivery of about 250 to 500 mL of formula in less than 15 minutes.

HOW TO Help Patients Cope with Tube Feedings

The thought of being "force-fed" is frightening to many people. Some may envision thick feeding tubes or fear that the procedure will be painful. Others may associate tube feedings only with irreversible illnesses. Patients may be less apprehensive once they understand the insertion procedure, the expected duration of the tube feeding, and the strategic role that nutrition plays in recovery from disease. The pointers that follow can help health care professionals prepare patients for transnasal tube feedings:

- Allow the patient to see and touch the feeding tube. Seeing firsthand that the tube is soft and narrow (only about half the diameter of a pencil) often alleviates anxiety.
- Show the patient how the feeding apparatus is attached to the feeding tube, and explain how the feeding will work. For young children, use dolls or stuffed toys to demonstrate tube insertion and feeding procedures.
- Explain that the patient remains fully alert during the procedure and helps pass the tube by swallowing. A numbing solution sprayed on the back of the throat minimizes discomfort and prevents gagging during the procedure.
- Tell the patient that once the tube has been inserted, most people become accustomed to its presence within a few hours. In most cases, the patient can easily swallow foods and liquids with the tube in place. If permitted, favorite foods or beverages can still be enjoyed.
- Assure the patient that the tube feeding will be temporary, if such assurance is appropriate.
- A tube feeding may be frightening for some patients, but others may feel relieved to know that they can receive sound nutrition without any effort. As they feel better and begin to eat again, the volume of the feeding can be reduced and then discontinued when oral intake is adequate.

Tube feedings may cause some patients to feel that they have lost control over an important aspect of their lives. They may also feel self-conscious about how the feeding tube looks or feel awkward when moving around with the equipment. A few simple measures can help:

- Involve patients in the decision-making and care process whenever possible. Patients can help to arrange their daily feeding schedules and can perform some of the feeding procedures themselves.
- Show patients how to manipulate the feeding equipment so that they can get out of bed and move around.
- Recommend that patients walk around and socialize with others, if permissible.
- Encourage patients to maintain contact with friends and keep busy with the hobbies and activities they enjoy. This measure is especially important for children, teens, and those on long-term feedings.
- When caring for infants and children, keep the developmental age of the child in mind and work with parents to ensure that appropriate feeding skills are mastered. Infants can be provided with a pacifier during feedings to help maintain the associations between sucking, swallowing, and fullness. When possible, the formula can be provided by bottle to an infant, or by spoon to a child, to further develop skills.

The more complex the procedure, the easier it becomes for health care professionals to focus on the procedure and disregard a patient's emotional reaction to the procedure. No matter how many technicalities you have to keep in mind, remember to stay focused on the person receiving your care.

Continuous feedings are delivered slowly and at a constant rate over a period of 8 to 24 hours. This type of feeding is recommended for critically ill patients because relatively small volumes are delivered at a time, which may reduce nausea, diarrhea, and the risk of aspiration. Continuous feedings are generally used in patients who receive intestinal feedings. An infusion pump is required to ensure accurate and steady flow rates; consequently, the feedings can limit the patient's freedom of movement and are more costly.

Formula Volume and Strength Formula administration schedules vary among institutions, so protocols should be reviewed carefully before working with patients. In general, almost all patients can receive undiluted formula (either isotonic or hypertonic) at the start of a feeding. Formulas, especially hypertonic formulas, are sometimes started slowly, and the volume gradually increased. In rare

HOW TO Plan a Tube Feeding Administration Schedule

After selecting a formula that meets the patient's medical and nutrient needs, the clinician determines the volume of formula that meets those needs. Consider a patient who needs 2000 kcalories daily using a standard formula that provides 1.0 kcalorie per milliliter. The total volume of formula required would be 2000 milliliters per day:

$$\chi \text{ mL} \times 1.0 \text{ kcal/mL} = 2000 \text{ kcal}.$$

$$\chi \text{ mL} = \frac{2000 \text{ kcal}}{1.0 \text{ kcal/mL}}.$$

$$\chi = 2000 \text{ mL}.$$

If the patient is to receive intermittent feedings six times a day, he will need about 330 milliliters of formula at each feeding:

$$2000 \text{ mL} \div 6 \text{ feedings} = 333 \text{ mL/feeding}.$$

Alternatively, if he is to receive intermittent feedings eight times a day, he will need 250 milliliters (or about one can of ready-to-feed formula) at each feeding:

$$2000 \text{ mL} \div 8 \text{ feedings} = 250 \text{ mL/feeding}.$$

He will probably tolerate this volume of formula best if it is delivered over a 30-minute period at each feeding. If the patient is to receive the formula continuously over 24 hours, he will need about 85 milliliters of formula each hour:

$$2000 \text{ mL} \div 24 \text{ hours} = 83 \text{ mL/hr}.$$

cases, formulas may be diluted until tolerated by the patient, although this practice is discouraged.

Intermittent feedings may start at about 120 to 150 milliliters at the initial feeding and be increased by 50 to 100 milliliters with every feeding until the goal volume is reached. Continuous feedings may start at about 30 to 40 milliliters per hour and be raised by 30 milliliters per hour every 6 to 8 hours. For both intermittent and continuous feedings, the rate and amount of increase depend on the patient's tolerance to the formula. If the new rate is not tolerated, the rate of delivery progresses more slowly to give the person additional time to adapt. If a patient on an intermittent feeding cannot tolerate the feeding, a continuous feeding may be a better choice. The "How to" describes several ways to plan tube feeding schedules.

Checking Gastric Residuals Nurses regularly measure the **gastric residual** (the volume of formula remaining in the stomach after a feeding) to ensure that the stomach is emptying properly. If formula accumulates in the stomach, the patient faces greater risks of nausea, vomiting, and aspiration of formula into the lungs. Gastric residuals are measured by gently withdrawing the gastric contents through the feeding tube using a syringe. The gastric residual is measured before each intermittent feeding and every 4 hours during continuous feedings. There is no consensus about the residual volume considered excessive, but it may be approximately 100 milliliters for a gastrostomy tube or 200 milliliters for a nasogastric tube.[8] If the residual volume is believed to be excessive, the feeding is held for an hour or two, and then the residual is rechecked. If the tendency to accumulate fluids persists, the physician may withhold the feeding, switch to an intestinal feeding, or begin drug therapy to stimulate gastric emptying.

Supplemental Water Formulas contain a considerable amount of water and therefore can meet a substantial portion of patients' water needs. Standard formulas are usually about 85 percent water and thus contain 850 milliliters of water per liter of formula. Nutrient-dense formulas may be 69 to 72 percent water (exact amounts can be obtained from a product label or manufacturer's information sheet). Many adults require about 2000 milliliters (approximately 2 quarts) of water daily.■ Fluids may be restricted in persons with kidney, liver, and heart diseases. Patients with fever, increased urine output, diarrhea, excessive sweating,

■ To estimate fluid requirements for adults and children:
- Allow 100 mL/kg for each of the first 10 kg of body weight.
- Allow 50 mL/kg for each of the next 10 kg of body weight.
- Allow 20 mL/kg for each kilogram of body weight above 20 kg.

gastric residual: the volume of formula that remains in the stomach from a previous feeding.

severe vomiting, fistula drainage, high-output ostomies, blood loss, or open wounds require additional water.

Additional water needs are usually met by flushes given via feeding tubes, or water can be given intravenously. To prevent clogging, feeding tubes are routinely flushed with water before and after each bolus or intermittent feeding and every 4 hours during continuous feedings.■ The water used for routine flushes should be included when estimating fluid intakes.

■ • For intermittent or bolus feedings, feeding tubes should be flushed before and after formula delivery with 20 to 60 mL of water.
• For continuous feedings, feeding tubes should be flushed with 20 to 60 mL of water every 4 hours.

In alert adults, thirst is often a good indicator of water needs. People who complain of thirst may receive more water, unless medical orders restrict fluids. In the elderly, thirst may be slow to develop in response to dehydration. Health care professionals can monitor patients' weight changes, record fluid intake and output, and measure urine specific gravity to evaluate hydration status. See Chapter 17 to review additional indicators of hydration status.

Delivering Medications through Feeding Tubes

Patients receiving tube feedings may require one or several medications that need to be delivered through feeding tubes. Proper administration is necessary to avoid complications. Medications may interact with enteral formulas in the same ways that they interact with foods, so the timing of administration must be considered. Feedings may need to be interrupted, and the feeding schedule altered, so that a medication can be given separately from formula. Some medications need to be exposed to the acidic stomach environment and cannot be given via an intestinal feeding tube. Medications can sometimes cause feeding tubes to clog. The following guidelines are recommended to prevent complications:

- Give medications by mouth instead of by tube whenever possible.
- If available, use liquid forms of medications. Dilute very viscous or hypertonic liquid medications with 10 to 30 milliliters of water before administering them through the feeding tube.
- If liquid forms are not available, use medications that can be given as injections or intravenously.
- Check with the pharmacist to learn whether drugs can be administered using intestinal feeding tubes, or if stomach acidity is required for proper absorption.
- Flush the feeding tube with 15 to 30 milliliters of warm (body temperature) water before and after administering a medication. Flush the tube with 5 milliliters of water between each medication given. Do not mix medications.
- If tablets must be used, check with the pharmacist to learn whether tablets are crushable. If so, crush tablets to a fine powder and mix with warm water before administering.
- Never crush enteric-coated or sustained-release medications due to the potential for adverse effects. In these cases, another form of medication must be given.
- Do not mix medications with enteral formulas, and avoid using medications known to be incompatible with formulas. Examples of medications that may be incompatible with some formulas are listed in Table 20-3.
- Check with the pharmacist about the proper timing of medication administration to avoid drug-nutrient interactions.

TABLE 20-3 Selected Medications That Are Incompatible with Formulas

Aluminum and magnesium hydroxide	MCT oil
Chlorpromazine concentrate	Mellaril concentrate
Cibalith-S syrup	Mellaril oral solution
Cimetidine	Paregoric elixir
Dimetane elixir	Potassium chloride
Dimetapp elixir	Reglan syrup
Feosol elixir	Riopan
Fleet's phosphosoda	Robitussin expectorant
Gevrabon liquid	Sudafed syrup
Klorvess syrup	Thorazine concentrate
Mandelamine Forte suspension	Zinc sulfate capsules

NOTE: These substances may be compatible with some formulas and not others.
SOURCES: Z. M. Pronsky, *Food-Medication Interactions*, 11th ed. (Pottstown, Pa.: Food-Medication Interactions, 2000); F. C. Thompson, M. R. Naysmith, and A. Lindsay, Managing drug therapy in patients receiving enteral and parenteral nutrition, *Hospital Pharmacist* 7 (2000): 155–164.

Diarrhea Medications are a major cause of the diarrhea that frequently accompanies tube feedings. Diarrhea is especially associated with the administration of some types of antibiotics and antacids, sorbitol-containing medications, and potassium supplements. The high osmolality of liquid medications can cause diarrhea, so dilution of hypertonic medications with 10 to 30 milliliters of water is often helpful.

Other Considerations Continuous feedings are ordinarily stopped during medication administration so that components of enteral formulas do not interfere with medication absorption. The feeding is typically halted for 15 minutes before and 15 minutes after medication delivery. Some medications may require a longer formula-free interval. For example, feedings need to be stopped for one to two hours before and after administering phenytoin, a medication that controls seizures.[9] In such cases, the delivery rate of formula needs to be increased so that the prescribed volume of formula can be delivered.

The feeding route also needs to be considered when medications are administered. A medication that is absorbed best in the duodenum may be poorly absorbed if a feeding tube is placed in the jejunum. In such cases, the medication may need to be injected or given intravenously.

Complications of Tube Feeding

Complications are a frequent occurrence during tube feedings. Common complications that may arise and some preventive and corrective measures are summarized in Table 20-4. The following paragraphs discuss some of the more common complications, which can be categorized as gastrointestinal problems, such as nausea and diarrhea; mechanical problems that are directly related to the tube feeding process; and metabolic problems, which include biochemical alterations and nutrient deficiencies.

Gastrointestinal Complications As mentioned earlier, diarrhea is frequently associated with tube feedings and may be caused by malabsorption problems, certain medications, bacterial overgrowth, malnutrition, or, more rarely, hypertonic formulas. Constipation sometimes occurs due to dehydration, motility impairments, obstructions, and low-fiber intakes. Impaired gastric motility or inadequate functioning of the lower esophageal sphincter may result in aspiration of GI secretions or formula. Other GI complications include abdominal discomfort, nausea, and vomiting.

Mechanical Complications Mechanical problems include clogged feeding tubes, malfunctioning feeding pumps, and dislodged feeding tubes after placement. The feeding tube itself may be a physical irritant and may warrant a change to a different type of tubing or a different feeding route. Nasoenteric tube placement may cause a number of side effects, such as dry mouth from increased mouth breathing and reduced salivary secretions; blocked eustachian tubes and resultant middle ear infections; and sinus infections due to blocking of the sinus tract. Sometimes ostomies are associated with leakage of gastrointestinal secretions at the site of tube insertion.

Metabolic Complications Common metabolic complications include fluid imbalances (either dehydration or overhydration), electrolyte imbalances, and glucose intolerance. Routine blood tests may be necessary to monitor levels of potassium, phosphorus, sodium, and glucose until a patient has stabilized. Some patients may need insulin or medications to reverse hyperglycemia. Vitamin K and essential fatty acid deficiencies may result if formulas lacking these nutrients are used for a prolonged period.

Many complications of tube feeding are preventable if the most appropriate feeding route, formula, and delivery method are chosen. Attention to a patient's primary medical condition and medication use is important as well. Table 20-5 on p. 666 provides a monitoring schedule that may help with the early detection of common tube feeding problems.

TABLE 20-4 Causes and Prevention or Correction of Tube Feeding Complications

Complications	Possible Causes	Preventive/Corrective Measures
Aspiration of formula	Compromised lower esophageal sphincter, delayed gastric emptying	Use nasoenteric, gastrostomy, or jejunostomy feedings in high-risk patients; check tube placement; elevate head of bed during and for 45 minutes after feeding; check gastric residuals.
Clogged feeding tube	Formula too thick for tube	Select appropriate tube size; flush tubing with water before and after giving formula; use infusion pump to deliver thick formulas. Remedies reported to help unclog feeding tubes include cola, cranberry juice, meat tenderizer, and pancreatic enzymes.
	Medications delivered through feeding tube	Use oral, liquid, or injectable medications whenever possible; dilute thick or sticky liquid medications with water before administering; crush tablets to a fine powder and mix with water; flush tubing with water before and after medications are given; give medications individually; do not add medications to the feeding container.
Constipation	Low-fiber formula	Provide additional fluids; use high-fiber formula.
	Lack of exercise	Encourage walking and other activities, if appropriate.
Dehydration and electrolyte imbalance	Excessive diarrhea	See items under *Diarrhea.*
	Inadequate fluid intake	Provide additional fluid.
	Carbohydrate intolerance	Use continuous drip administration of formula; monitor blood glucose; select a formula with a lower amount or different type of carbohydrate; provide a formula with a higher fat content.
	Excessive protein intake	Monitor blood electrolyte levels; reduce protein intake.
Diarrhea, cramps, abdominal distention	Bacterial contamination	Use fresh formula every 24 hours; store opened or mixed formula in a refrigerator; rinse feeding bag and tubing before adding fresh formula; change feeding apparatus every 24 hours; prepare formula with clean hands using clean equipment in a clean environment.
	Lactose intolerance	Use lactose-free formula in patients with current or potential lactose-intolerance.
	Hypertonic formula	Use small volume of formula and increase volume gradually.
	Rapid formula administration	Slow administration rate or use continuous drip feedings.
	Malnutrition/low serum albumin	Use small volume of dilute formula and increase volume and concentration gradually.
Hyperglycemia	Diabetes, hypermetabolism, drug therapy	Check blood glucose; slow administration rate; provide adequate fluids; select a formula with a lower amount or different type of carbohydrate; provide a formula with a higher fat content.
Nausea and vomiting	Obstruction	Discontinue tube feeding.
	Delayed gastric emptying	Check gastric residual; slow administration rate, use continuous drip feedings, or discontinue tube feeding.
	Intolerance to concentration or volume of formula	Use small volume of formula and increase volume and concentration gradually; use continuous drip feedings.
	Psychological reaction to tube feeding	Address patient's concerns.
Skin irritation at enterostomy site	Leakage of GI secretions and friction caused by the tube	Keep site clean; inspect area for redness, tenderness, and drainage; use protective skin cream.

NOTE: Many of the complications presented here can be caused by the patient's primary disorder or drug therapy rather than the tube feeding itself. In such a case, the corrective measure would include treatment of the disorder or a change in drug therapy. Additionally, other corrective measures that require a physician's order are not shown here.

Documentation of Tube Feeding

Chapter 18 emphasized the importance of the medical record as a legal document and communication tool. Before reimbursing the cost of tube feedings, insurance companies and managed care organizations require that the physician appropriately document the patient's need for a tube feeding as well as the justification for using an infusion pump or a special formula, if necessary. The medical record contains the documentation required as well as information that can be used to investigate problems so that corrective measures can be taken promptly. The

TABLE 20-5 Suggested Guidelines for Monitoring Patients on Tube Feedings

Before starting a new feeding:	Complete a nutrition assessment. Check tube placement.
Before each intermittent feeding:	Check patient position. Check gastric residual. Flush feeding tube with water. Check tube placement.
After each intermittent feeding:	Flush feeding tube with water.
Every half hour:	Check gravity drip rate, when applicable.
Every hour:	Check pump drip rate, when applicable.
Every 4 hours:	Check vital signs, including blood pressure, temperature, pulse, and respiration.
Every 6 hours:	Check blood glucose; monitoring blood glucose can be discontinued after 48 hours if test results are consistently negative in a nondiabetic patient.
Every 4 to 6 hours of continuous feeding:	Check patient's position. Check gastric residual. Flush feeding tube with water.
Every 8 hours:	Check intake and output. Check specific gravity of urine. Check tube placement. Chart patient's total intake of, acceptance of, and tolerance to tube feeding.
Every day:	Weigh patient. Change feeding container and attached tubing. Clean feeding equipment.
Every 7 to 10 days:	Reassess nutrition status.
As needed:	Observe patient for any undesirable responses to tube feeding; for example, delayed gastric emptying, nausea, vomiting, or diarrhea. Check nitrogen balance. Check laboratory data. Chart significant details.

health care team should routinely document the following information for patients on tube feedings:

- Nutrition goals for the patient.
- The condition necessitating the tube feeding.
- The feeding route and type of feeding tube used.
- The formula selected to meet nutrition goals and its general nutrient composition.
- The administration schedule (concentration and rate) and method of delivery (bolus, intermittent, or continuous; gravity drip or infusion pump).
- Patient education about nutrition goals and the tube feeding procedure.
- The patient's responses to the tube insertion and feeding procedure.
- The patient's tolerance to the formula and administration schedule, complications (if any), and corrective actions recommended.
- Substances delivered through the feeding tube, including formula, additional water, medications, and any substances used to unclog the feeding tube.
- Changes in the patient's body weight and lab values during the period of tube feeding.
- Reasons why a tube feeding was interrupted or could not be delivered, if applicable.

Transition to Table Foods

Once the medical condition that required a tube feeding resolves, the patient can gradually shift to an oral diet as the volume of formula is tapered off. The patient should be eating about two-thirds of the estimated nutrient needs by mouth before the tube feeding is discontinued. In many cases, a patient can begin to drink the same formula that is being delivered by tube. As patients begin to take more food or formula orally, they can be given less formula by tube. Some people cannot make the transition to oral intake for medical reasons and may need to continue tube feedings at home.

IN SUMMARY To maximize the benefits of tube feedings, formulas must be prepared and administered using food safety techniques that minimize the risk of complications. Tube placement should be verified and monitored to reduce risks of aspiration and inadvertent placement into the respiratory tract. Depending on the feeding route and medical condition, the formula can be delivered in bolus feedings, intermittently, or continuously. Formulas meet a substantial portion of fluid requirements, and supplemental water can be flushed through the feeding tube. Medications should be given separately and accompanied by water flushes to prevent tube clogging. Complications of tube feedings can be gastrointestinal, mechanical, or metabolic in nature.

The accompanying case study can help you consider the many factors involved in tube feedings.

CASE STUDY

Graphics Designer Requiring Enteral Nutrition Support

Nicki is a 24-year-old graphics designer who suffered multiple fractures when she fell from a cliff while hiking. She has been in the hospital for seven days and has no appetite. Nicki has lost 8 pounds over the course of her hospitalization. Due to the nature of her injuries, she is in traction and is immobile, although the head of her bed can be elevated 45 degrees. From the diet history, the dietitian determined that Nicki's nutrition status was adequate prior to hospitalization. The health care team agrees that a nasoduodenal tube feeding should be instituted before nutritional status deteriorates further. The standard formula selected for the feeding is lactose-free, and Nicki's nutrient requirements can be met with 2200 milliliters of the formula per day.

1. What steps can be taken to prepare Nicki for tube feeding? Why might nasoduodenal placement of the feeding tube be preferred to nasogastric placement?
2. The physician's orders specify that the feeding should be given continuously over 18 hours. Develop an appropriate tube feeding schedule.
3. What parameters should be monitored to ensure that Nicki's fluid needs are met? How can additional fluids be given? Describe precautions that should be taken if Nicki is to receive medications through the feeding tube.
4. After three days of feeding, Nicki develops diarrhea. Check Table 20-4 to determine the possible causes. What measures can be taken to correct the diarrhea?
5. What information should be charted in Nicki's medical record? When Nicki is ready to eat table foods again, what steps will the health care team take?

NUTRITION ON THE NET

Access these websites for further study of topics covered in this chapter.

- Find updates and quick links to these and other nutrition-related sites at our website: **www.wadsworth.com/nutrition**
- To find out more about organizations that promote the appropriate use of enteral and parenteral nutrition, visit the:

  American Society for Parenteral and Enteral Nutrition site: **www.clinnutr.org**

  Canadian Parenteral-Enteral Nutrition Association site: **www.cpena.ca/home.html**

  British Association for Parenteral and Enteral Nutrition site: **www.bapen.org.uk/**
- To learn about home enteral nutrition, visit the website of the Oley Foundation, a national, nonprofit organization that provides information, outreach services, and emotional support for consumers of home enteral and parenteral services: **http://c4isr.com/oley/**

STUDY QUESTIONS

These questions will help you review the chapter. You will find the answers in the discussions on the pages provided.

1. Characterize standard formulas, hydrolyzed formulas, modular formulas, and disease-specific formulas, and describe situations in which they are used. (pp. 652–653)
2. Discuss how energy density, nutrient density, osmolality, and fiber content vary in enteral formulas. (p. 653)
3. Identify reasons why oral intake of enteral formulas may be advised. Suggest ways for improving patient acceptance of formulas. (pp. 654–655)
4. List the types of patients who may benefit from tube feedings. Discuss how clinicians can help to relieve anxiety about tube feeding procedures. (pp. 654–655, 661)
5. Describe the different tube feeding routes, and suggest reasons why each might be used. Discuss advantages and disadvantages for each. (pp. 655–657)
6. Identify measures that can help prevent contamination of enteral formulas and equipment. (pp. 659–660)
7. Contrast the different methods of formula delivery, and discuss advantages and disadvantages associated with each. (pp. 660–662)
8. Describe the problems that can occur when medications are delivered through feeding tubes. Suggest guidelines that can prevent these problems. (pp. 663–664)
9. Discuss complications often associated with tube feedings. Summarize possible causes and some measures that can prevent or correct these complications. (pp. 664–665)

These questions will help you prepare for an exam. Answers can be found on p. 669.

1. Which of the following statements is correct?
   a. Standard formulas contain whole proteins or protein isolates.
   b. Standard formulas contain free amino acids or small peptide chains.
   c. Modular formulas contain a mixture of proteins, carbohydrates, and fats.
   d. Hydrolyzed formulas may contain protein isolates or whole proteins.
2. Osmolality refers to an enteral formula's:
   a. energy density.
   b. nutrient density.
   c. fiber content.
   d. concentrations of molecules and ionic particles.
3. For a patient expected to be able to eat table foods in several weeks, but with a high risk of aspiration, an appropriate placement of a feeding tube would be:
   a. nasogastric.
   b. nasoenteric.
   c. gastrostomy.
   d. jejunostomy.
4. In selecting an appropriate enteral formula for a patient, the primary consideration is:
   a. formula osmolality.
   b. the patient's nutrient needs.
   c. availability of infusion pumps.
   d. formula cost.
5. An important measure that can help prevent bacterial contamination of tube feeding formulas is:
   a. nonstop feeding of formula.
   b. using the same feeding bag and tubing each day.
   c. discarding opened containers of formula within 24 hours.
   d. adding formula to the feeding container before it empties completely.
6. Compared to intermittent feedings, continuous feedings:
   a. always require an infusion pump.
   b. allow greater freedom of movement.
   c. are more similar to normal patterns of eating.
   d. are associated with more GI side effects.

7. A patient needs 1800 milliliters of formula a day. If the patient is to receive formula intermittently every 4 hours, he will need _____ milliliters of formula at each feeding.
   a. 225 b. 300 c. 400 d. 425
8. The term that describes the volume of formula remaining in the stomach from a previous feeding is:
   a. residue.
   b. osmolar load.
   c. gastric residual.
   d. intermittent feeding.
9. The nurse using the feeding tube to deliver medications recognizes that:
   a. medications generally do not result in GI complaints.
   b. medications can be added directly to the feeding container.
   c. thick or sticky liquid medications and crushed tablets can clog feeding tubes.
   d. enteral formulas do not interact with medications in the same way that foods do.
10. Tube feedings can gradually be discontinued when:
   a. discharge planning begins.
   b. the patient experiences hunger.
   c. the medical condition resolves.
   d. the patient is able to eat foods or drink formula in sufficient amounts.

REFERENCES

1. American Dietetic Association, *Manual of Clinical Dietetics* (Chicago: American Dietetic Association, 2000).
2. American Dietetic Association, 2000.
3. L. Gramlich and coauthors, Does enteral nutrition compared to parenteral nutrition result in better outcomes in critically ill adult patients? A systematic review of the literature, *Nutrition* 20 (2004): 843–848.
4. J. L. Rombeau and R. H. Rolandelli, eds., *Clinical Nutrition: Enteral and Tube Feeding* (Philadelphia: W.B. Saunders, 1997).
5. L. Matarese, Composite foods and formulas, parenteral and enteral nutrition, in A. M. Coulston, C. L. Rock, and E. R. Monsen, eds., *Nutrition in the Prevention and Treatment of Disease* (San Diego: Academic Press, 2001), pp. 245–260.
6. D. A. Neumann and M. H. DeLegge, Gastric versus small-bowel tube feeding in the intensive care unit: A prospective comparison of efficacy, *Critical Care Medicine* 30 (2002): 1436–1438.
7. L. Klein, Is blue dye safe as a method of detection for pulmonary aspiration? *Journal of the American Dietetic Association* 104 (2004): 1651–1652; J. P. Maloney and T. A. Ryan, Detection of aspiration in enterally fed patients: A requiem for bedside monitors of aspiration, *Journal of Parenteral and Enteral Nutrition* 26 (2002) S34–S42.
8. American Dietetic Association, 2000.
9. American Dietetic Association, 2000.

ANSWERS

Study Questions (multiple choice)

1. a 2. d 3. b 4. b 5. c 6. a 7. b 8. c 9. c 10. d

HIGHLIGHT

Enteral Nutrition and Inborn Errors of Metabolism

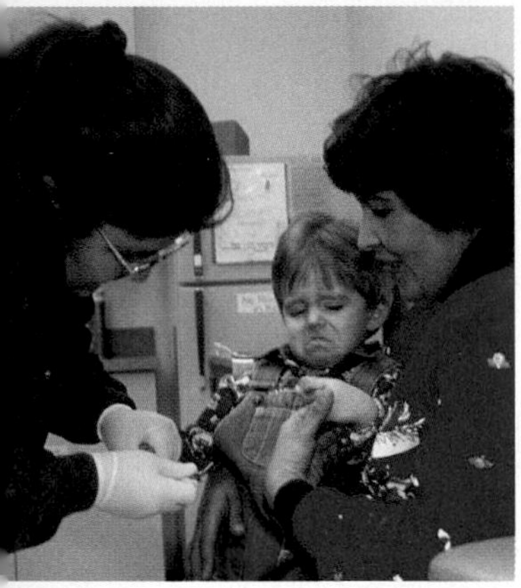
© Miguel Gandert/Corbis

Chapter 20 described the use of enteral formulas for patients who are unable to meet their nutrient needs with conventional foods. Such is the case for individuals with some inborn errors of metabolism; for them, enteral formulas play a vital role in disease management. This highlight describes some inborn errors of metabolism and discusses the role of diet in two of these disorders: phenylketonuria and galactosemia. The accompanying glossary defines terms related to inborn errors of metabolism.

Inborn Errors of Metabolism

An **inborn error of metabolism** is an inherited trait that causes an absence or deficiency of a protein that has a critical metabolic role. The protein may normally function as an enzyme, receptor, transport protein, or structural protein. When the body fails to make a protein, body functions that depend on that protein are impaired. For example, when an enzyme is missing or malfunctioning in a metabolic pathway that typically converts compound A to compound B, then compound A will accumulate and compound B will not be made. The excess of compound A and the lack of compound B may have harmful effects. Furthermore, the imbalances in one pathway may affect other pathways and ultimately cause a number of metabolic and physiologic disturbances.

Inborn errors of metabolism are caused by **mutations** in genes.[1] (Most mutations are responsible for our genetic diversity and do not cause diseases.) The severity of an inborn error of metabolism is related to the degree of impairment caused by the altered or missing protein.

Treatment for Inborn Errors of Metabolism

Successful treatment of an inborn error depends on the ability to screen newborns and diagnose metabolic diseases before irreversible damage can occur. After a genetic defect is identified, family members undergo **genetic counseling** to evaluate the likelihood that they may pass on the disorder to future offspring. During counseling, couples may learn about reproductive options such as artificial insemination, in vitro fertilization, or prenatal monitoring after conception.

Medical nutrition therapy is the primary treatment for many inborn errors. Once the biochemical pathway affected by a genetic mutation is identified, a clinician may be able to manipulate elements of the diet to compensate for deficiencies and excesses. Dietary intervention generally involves re-

GLOSSARY

cystic fibrosis: an inherited disorder that affects the transport of chloride across epithelial cell membranes; primarily affects the gastrointestinal and respiratory systems.

galactosemia (ga-LAK-toe-SEE-me-ah): an inherited disorder that affects galactose metabolism. Accumulated galactose causes damage to the liver, kidney, and brain in untreated patients.

gene therapy: treatment for inherited disorders, in which DNA sequences are introduced into the chromosomes of affected cells, prompting the cells to express the protein needed to correct the disease.

genetic counseling: support for families at risk of genetic disorders; involves diagnosis of disease, identification of inheritance patterns within a family, and review of reproductive options.

hemophilia (HE-moh-FEEL-ee-ah): inherited bleeding disorders characterized by deficiency or absence of plasma proteins needed for clotting blood.

inborn error of metabolism: an inherited trait (present at birth) that causes a deficiency or the absence of a protein that has a critical metabolic role.

metabolites: products of metabolism; the compounds typically produced by a biochemical pathway.

mutations: inheritable alterations in the DNA sequence of a gene.

phenylketonuria (FEN-il-KEY-toe-NU-ree-ah) or **PKU:** an inherited disorder that affects the conversion of the essential amino acid phenylalanine to the amino acid tyrosine.

stricting substances that cannot be properly metabolized and supplying substances that cannot be produced. Thus the goals of medical nutrition therapy are to:

- Prevent the accumulation of toxic metabolites.
- Replace nutrients that are deficient as a result of a defective metabolic pathway.
- Provide a diet that supports normal growth and development and maintains health.

Nondietary therapies are also used to treat many inborn errors of metabolism. In some cases, the missing protein is infused; this is the primary means of treating **hemophilia**, caused by deficiency of one of the plasma proteins needed for clotting blood. Drug therapy is a primary therapy for some inborn errors, as it is with **cystic fibrosis** (discussed in Chapter 24), which is characterized by a protein defect that prevents normal chloride transport across cell membranes.[2] Future approaches to inborn errors may include **gene therapy**, a treatment that will introduce DNA sequences into the chromosomes of affected cells, which will prompt the cells to express the protein needed to correct the disease.

This highlight presents a sampling of inborn errors that benefit primarily from medical nutrition therapy. A classic example is phenylketonuria, a metabolic disorder that affects one's ability to metabolize the essential amino acid phenylalanine.

Phenylketonuria

One of many inborn errors affecting amino acid metabolism, **phenylketonuria (PKU)** affects approximately 1 out of every 10,000 births in the United States each year. The screening of newborns for PKU is one of the most common genetic tests in the United States and many other countries.[3] The early detection and treatment of PKU have prevented many of the damaging consequences of this disorder.

The Error in PKU

In PKU, the liver enzyme that converts the essential amino acid phenylalanine to the amino acid tyrosine is lacking (see Figure H20-1). Without this enzyme, phenylalanine and its **metabolites** (metabolic products) accumulate and damage the developing nervous system. The disruption in the metabolic pathway also prevents liver synthesis of tyrosine and tyrosine-derived compounds (such as the neurotransmitter epinephrine). Under these conditions, tyrosine becomes essential: because the body cannot make tyrosine, the diet must supply it.

Although PKU's most debilitating effect is on brain development, other symptoms may manifest if the condition is untreated. Infants with PKU may have poor appetites and grow slowly. They may be irritable or have tremors or seizures. Their bodies and urine may have a musty odor. Their skin coloring may be unusually pale, and they may develop skin rashes.

FIGURE H20-1 Biochemical Alterations in PKU

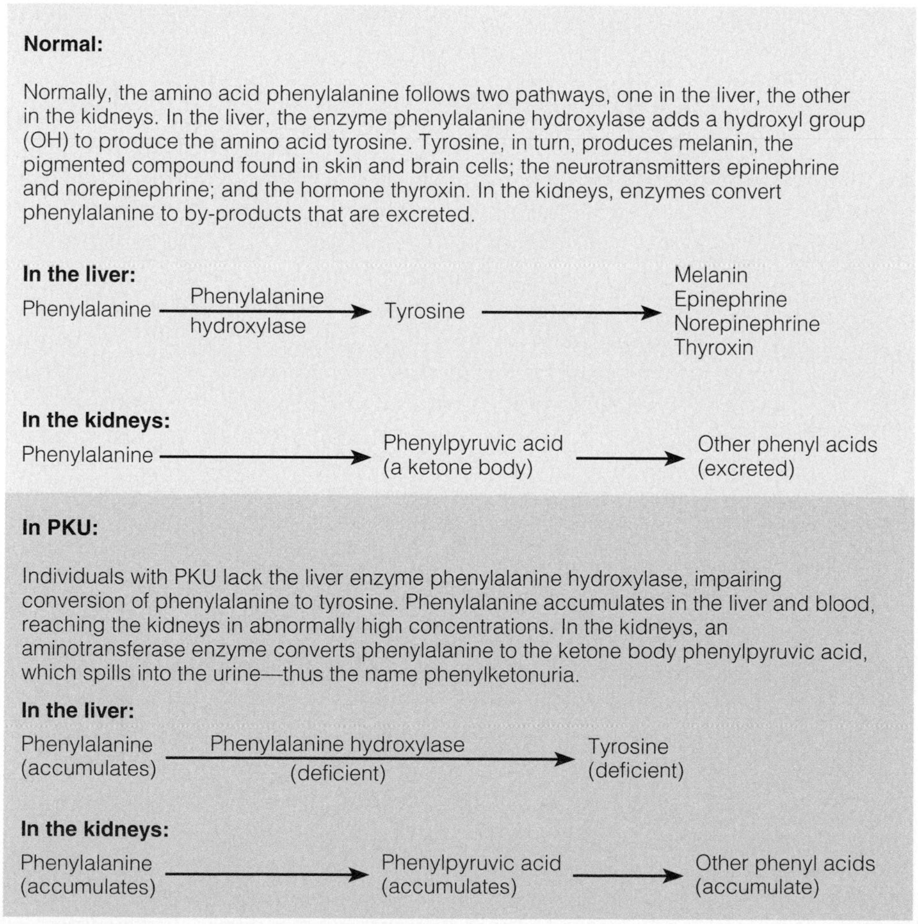
Normal:
Normally, the amino acid phenylalanine follows two pathways, one in the liver, the other in the kidneys. In the liver, the enzyme phenylalanine hydroxylase adds a hydroxyl group (OH) to produce the amino acid tyrosine. Tyrosine, in turn, produces melanin, the pigmented compound found in skin and brain cells; the neurotransmitters epinephrine and norepinephrine; and the hormone thyroxin. In the kidneys, enzymes convert phenylalanine to by-products that are excreted.
In the liver:
Phenylalanine
Phenylalanine hydroxylase
Tyrosine
Melanin
Epinephrine
Norepinephrine
Thyroxin
In the kidneys:
Phenylalanine
Phenylpyruvic acid (a ketone body)
Other phenyl acids (excreted)
In PKU:
Individuals with PKU lack the liver enzyme phenylalanine hydroxylase, impairing conversion of phenylalanine to tyrosine. Phenylalanine accumulates in the liver and blood, reaching the kidneys in abnormally high concentrations. In the kidneys, an aminotransferase enzyme converts phenylalanine to the ketone body phenylpyruvic acid, which spills into the urine—thus the name phenylketonuria.
In the liver:
Phenylalanine (accumulates)
Phenylalanine hydroxylase (deficient)
Tyrosine (deficient)
In the kidneys:
Phenylalanine (accumulates)
Phenylpyruvic acid (accumulates)
Other phenyl acids (accumulate)

Detecting PKU

PKU is not evident at birth, but diagnosis in the first few days of life and early treatment can prevent its devastating effects. For this reason, newborns are routinely screened for PKU in all fifty states.[4] A standard blood test for phenylalanine is typically conducted by heel puncture after the infant has consumed several meals containing protein (usually after 24 hours). Abnormal results require further testing. Before newborn screening, infants with PKU demonstrated developmental delays (for example, inability to crawl) by six to nine

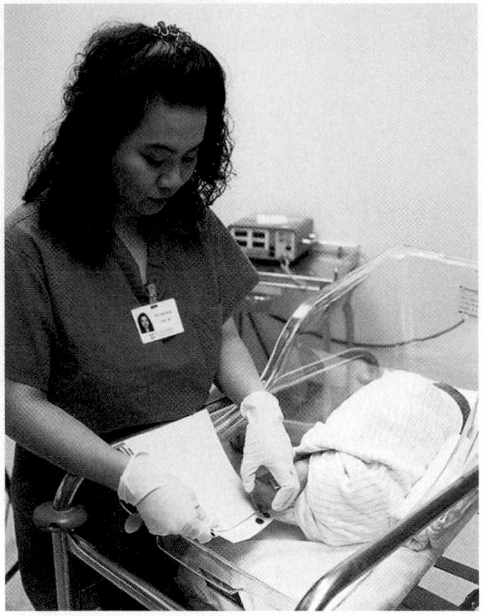
© David Young-Wolff/PhotoEdit
A simple blood test screens newborns for PKU—a common inborn error of metabolism.

months of age. By the time parents recognized the delays, the damage was irreversible.

Medical Nutrition Therapy for PKU

The only current treatment for PKU is a diet that restricts phenylalanine and supplies tyrosine so that blood levels of these amino acids are maintained within safe ranges. If the diet is conscientiously followed, it can prevent the symptoms described earlier.

Because phenylalanine is an essential amino acid, the diet cannot exclude it completely. Children with PKU need phenylalanine to grow, but they cannot handle excesses without detrimental effects. Therefore, their diets must provide enough phenylalanine to support normal growth and health but not enough to cause harm. The diet must also provide tyrosine, which is an essential nutrient for PKU children. To ensure that blood concentrations of phenylalanine and tyrosine are close to normal, blood tests are performed periodically and diets adjusted when necessary.

The PKU Diet

Central to the PKU diet is the use of an enteral formula that supplies a phenylalanine-free source of energy, protein, vitamins, and minerals.[5] Some formulas supply small amounts of phenylalanine and are useful for infants who must meet most of their nutrient needs by consuming formula. Formula requirements need to be recalculated periodically to accommodate the growing infant's shifting needs for protein, phenylalanine, and energy.

Once food consumption begins, a phenylalanine-free formula is used as the main protein source, and foods that contain phenylalanine are carefully monitored. All protein sources contain some phenylalanine; therefore, high-protein foods such as meat, fish, poultry, milk, cheese, legumes, and nuts (including peanut butter) are omitted. Fruits, vegetables, and cereals also contain phenylalanine, so only limited amounts are allowed. Low-protein flours and mixes are available for making low-phenylalanine breads, pasta, cakes, and cookies. Foods that do not contain phenylalanine such as jams, jellies, and most sweeteners can be used freely. Growth rates and nutrition status are monitored to ensure that the diet is adequate.

Parents and children may need to develop creative ways to make the diet enjoyable. The formula can be flavored or combined with fruits or juices to make smoothies or frozen into Popsicles. Sandwiches can be made with low-phenylalanine breads and fillings such as mashed bananas or avocados, shredded carrots and olives, or tomato slices with mayonnaise. Children often enjoy creating special recipes with permitted foods to make their choices more varied and to share with friends.

Continuing Dietary Restrictions

Lifelong adherance to a phenylalanine-restricted diet is currently recommended for all individuals with PKU.[6] Elevated phenylalanine levels can adversely affect cognitive function at any age. Case studies have suggested that PKU patients who discontinue dietary management may have problems with attention span, concentration, and memory. It is especially important that women with PKU maintain safe phenylalanine concentrations during their pregnancies. Elevated phenylalanine levels, especially during the first trimester, have been associated with birth defects, congenital heart disease, and mental retardation in the offspring of PKU mothers who have discontinued dietary treatment.[7]

Galactosemia

Galactosemia is an example of an inborn error of carbohydrate metabolism. Individuals with galactosemia are deficient in one of the enzymes needed to metabolize galactose.[8] An accumulation of galactose can cause damage in multiple tissues. Infants with galactosemia who are given milk react with severe vomiting and liver jaundice within days of the initial feeding (recall that each lactose molecule contains a molecule of galactose). Liver damage can be severe and progress to symptomatic cirrhosis. Other complications may include kidney failure, cataracts, and brain damage. Treatment in the first weeks of life can prevent the most detrimental effects of galactose accumulation, but if treatment is delayed, the damage to the brain is irreversible.

The Galactosemia Diet

The diet for galactosemia is much simpler than the diet for PKU. For one thing, galactose is not an essential nutrient. The galactosemia diet essentially eliminates galactose from the diet and does not require a carefully determined amount of any nutrient, as the PKU diet does. Also, dietary galactose is primarily obtained from lactose (the milk sugar), so the main focus of dietary treatment is the exclusion of milk and milk products. Other foods that contain galactose in substantial amounts, such as organ meats and some legumes, fruits, and vegetables, must also be avoided or restricted. Food lists provided to patients identify the galactose content of many common foods.

Infants diagnosed with galactosemia are given lactose-free formulas to meet their nutrient needs. Once a child begins table foods, special formulas are unnecessary. However, care must be taken to ensure that the diet supplies adequate calcium.

Long-Term Complications

Although the early introduction of a galactose-restricted diet can eliminate the acute toxic effects of galactosemia, complications of the disease may develop despite an individual's compliance with diet therapy. For example, ovarian failure occurs in up to 85 percent of women with galactosemia.[9] Most patients experience delays in speech and language development. Some evidence suggests that IQ declines as a person with galactosemia ages. The reasons for these long-term complications are not fully understood.

Numerous inborn errors of metabolism have been identified. Mainstays of treatment include effective diagnosis, early treatment, and control of environmental factors that may cause toxicity. In some cases, diet is central to treatment and can prevent serious complications. The development and use of enteral formulas to compensate for inborn errors have eased the burden of diet planning and improved the quality of life for many.

REFERENCES

1. L. J. Elsas II, Inborn errors of metabolism, in L. Goldman and D. Ausiello, eds., *Cecil Textbook of Medicine* (Philadelphia: Saunders, 2004), pp. 185–191.
2. L. M. Bellini and M. A. Grippi, Cystic fibrosis, in A. P. Fishman and coeditors, *Fishman's Manual of Pulmonary Disease and Disorders* (New York: McGraw-Hill, 2002), pp. 176–186.
3. C. M. Trahms, Inborn errors of metabolism, in A. M. Coulston, C. L. Rock, and E. R. Monsen, eds., *Nutrition in the Prevention and Treatment of Disease* (San Diego, Academic Press, 2001), pp. 209–225.
4. Trahms, 2001.
5. S. Escott-Stump, *Nutrition and Diagnosis-Related Care* (Baltimore: Lippincott Williams & Wilkins, 2002).
6. S. D. Cederbaum and C. R. Scriver, Disorders of phenylalanine and tyrosine metabolism, in L. Goldman and D. Ausiello, eds., *Cecil Textbook of Medicine* (Philadelphia: Saunders, 2004), pp. 1282–1285.
7. Cederbaum and Scriver, 2004.
8. L. J. Elsas II, Galactosemia, in L. Goldman and D. Ausiello, eds., *Cecil Textbook of Medicine* (Philadelphia: Saunders, 2004), pp. 1268–1270.
9. Elsas, Galactosemia, 2004.

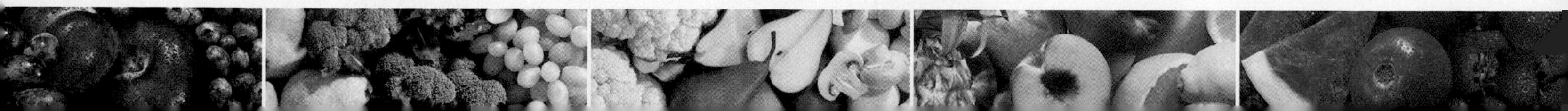

Chapter 21

Parenteral Nutrition Support

Chapter Outline

Indications for Parenteral Support

Parenteral Solutions: *Parenteral Nutrients • Formula Preparation*

Administering Parenteral Nutrition: *Insertion and Care of Intravenous Catheters • Administration of Parenteral Solutions • Managing Metabolic Complications • Discontinuing Intravenous Feedings*

Nutrition Support at Home: *Candidates for Home Nutrition Support • Planning Home Nutrition Care • Quality of Life Issues*

Highlight: *Ethical Issues in Nutrition Care*

Available Online

http://nutrition.wadsworth.com/uncn7

Student Practice Test

Glossary Terms

Nutrition on the Net

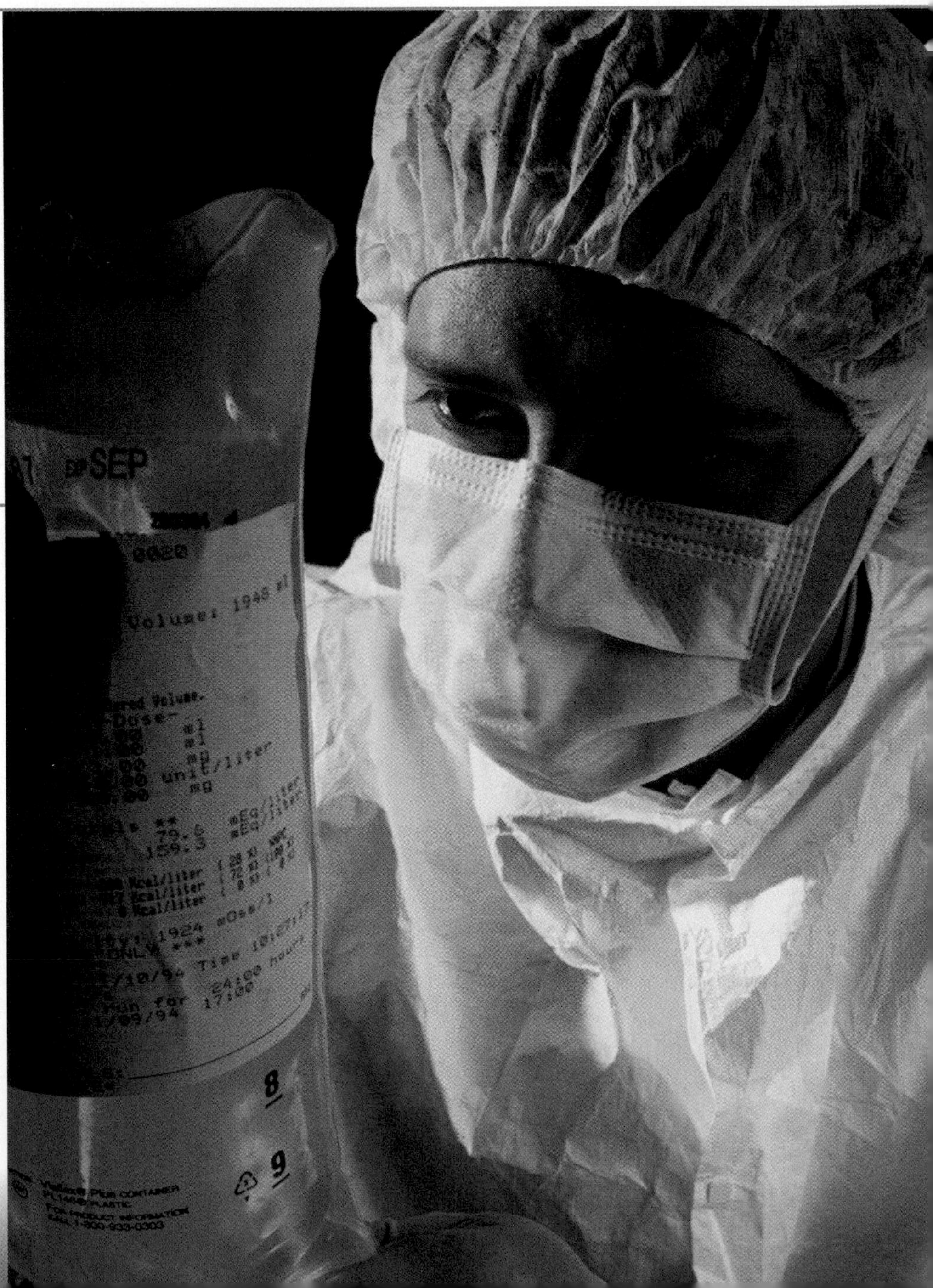

© David Joel/Photographer's Choice/Getty Images

Nutrition in the Professional Setting

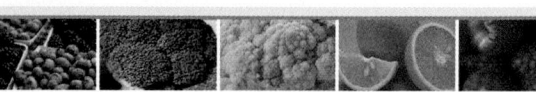

The science of medical nutrition was dramatically changed in 1968 by the demonstration that all nutrient needs could be met by vein. Since then, health practitioners have had a way to feed people who otherwise might have died from malnutrition. Although intravenous feeding techniques have advanced considerably since 1968, parenteral nutrition remains expensive and is sometimes associated with serious complications. For these reasons, clinicians subscribe to the adage, "If the GI tract works, use it."

Chapter 20 described how enteral formulas are used to supplement or replace conventional foods in order to meet nutrition needs. However, enteral formulas cannot be used if intestinal function is inadequate. This chapter discusses parenteral nutrition, the technique of delivering nutrients intravenously.

The ability to meet all nutrient needs by vein is a lifesaving option for critically ill persons. The procedure is costly, however, and associated with many potentially dangerous complications. If the gastrointestinal (GI) tract is functional, enteral nutrition support is preferred, partly to avoid the expense and complications associated with intravenous feedings and partly to preserve healthy GI function. Figure 21-1 on p. 676 summarizes the decision-making process for selecting the most appropriate feeding method.

Indications for Parenteral Support

As is true with other nutrition therapies, the decision to use parenteral nutrition is based on a thorough assessment of the patient's medical condition and nutrient needs. In general, parenteral nutrition is indicated for patients who do not have

FIGURE 21-1 Selecting a Feeding Route

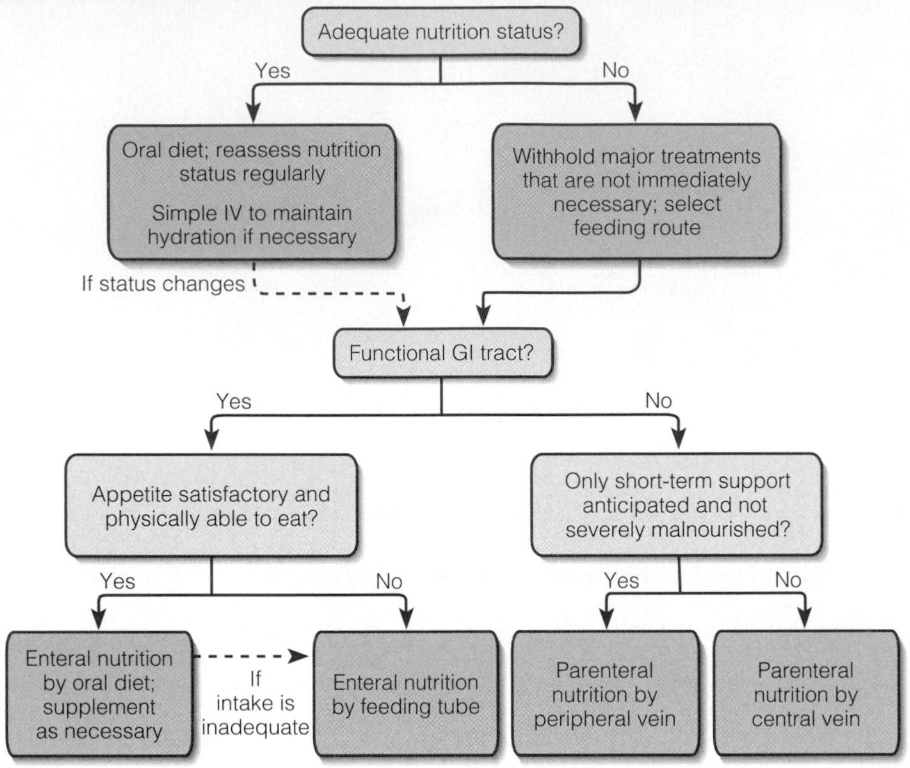
Adequate nutrition status?
Yes
No
Oral diet; reassess nutrition status regularly
Simple IV to maintain hydration if necessary
Withhold major treatments that are not immediately necessary; select feeding route
If status changes
Functional GI tract?
Yes
No
Appetite satisfactory and physically able to eat?
Only short-term support anticipated and not severely malnourished?
Yes
No
Yes
No
Enteral nutrition by oral diet; supplement as necessary
If intake is inadequate
Enteral nutrition by feeding tube
Parenteral nutrition by peripheral vein
Parenteral nutrition by central vein

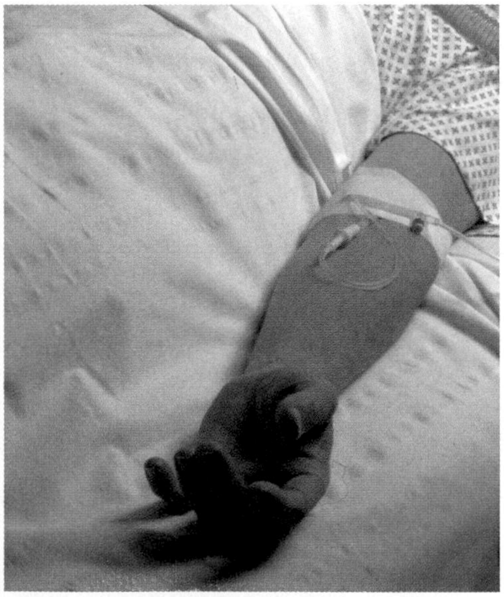

The peripheral veins can provide access to the blood for the delivery of parenteral solutions.

■ Hypertonic solutions cause **phlebitis** (inflammation within the vein) resulting in redness, swelling, and tenderness at the infusion site.

peripheral veins: small-diameter veins that carry blood from the arms and legs.

central veins: large-diameter veins located close to the heart.

peripheral parenteral nutrition (PPN): a type of nutrition support in which intravenous feedings are delivered into peripheral veins.

functioning GI tracts and who are either malnourished or likely to become so. The following conditions may require use of parenteral nutrition:

- Short-bowel syndrome (a portion of the intestine has been removed).
- Severe pancreatitis.
- Malabsorption disorders.
- Intestinal obstructions or fistulas.
- Major trauma or burns.
- Critical illnesses or wasting disorders.
- Bone marrow transplants.
- Being malnourished and having a high risk of aspiration.

Once the decision to use parenteral nutrition has been made, the access site must be selected. The access sites for intravenous feedings fall into two categories: nutrients may be delivered either into the **peripheral veins** located in the arms and legs or into the large-diameter **central veins** located near the heart (see Figure 21-2).

Peripheral Parenteral Nutrition (PPN) In some patients, nutrient needs may be met using peripheral veins only—**peripheral parenteral nutrition (PPN).** Because peripheral veins can be damaged by concentrated solutions,■ PPN can supply only limited amounts of energy and protein. The osmolarity of solutions used in PPN is usually limited to 900 milliosmoles per liter.[1] For this reason, PPN is most often used in patients who need short-term nutrition support (about 7 to 10 days) and who do not have high nutrient needs or fluid restrictions. PPN is not possible if a patient's peripheral veins are not strong enough to tolerate the procedure. In many cases, it is necessary to rotate venous access sites to prevent inflammation.

Total Parenteral Nutrition (TPN) Most patients meet their nutrient needs using the larger, central veins where blood volume is greater and nutrient concen-

FIGURE 21-2 Accessing Central Veins for Total Parenteral Nutrition

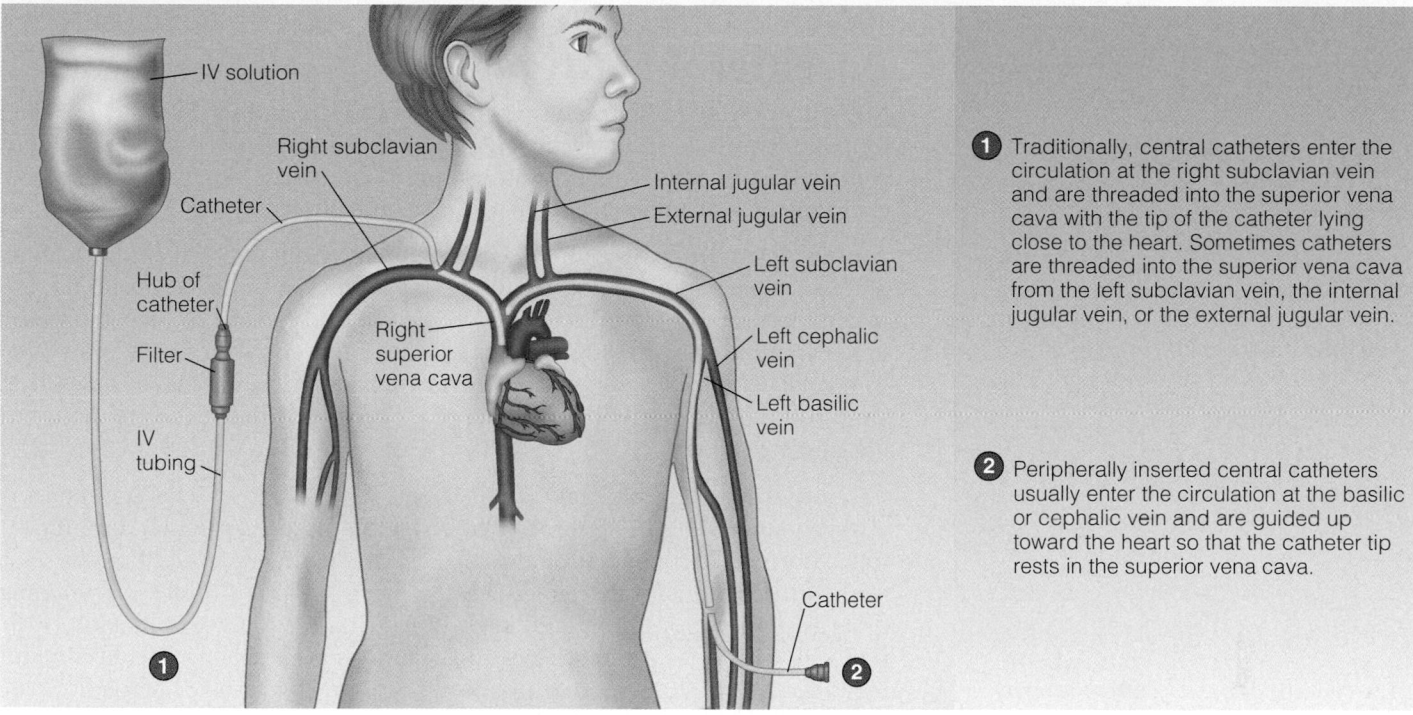

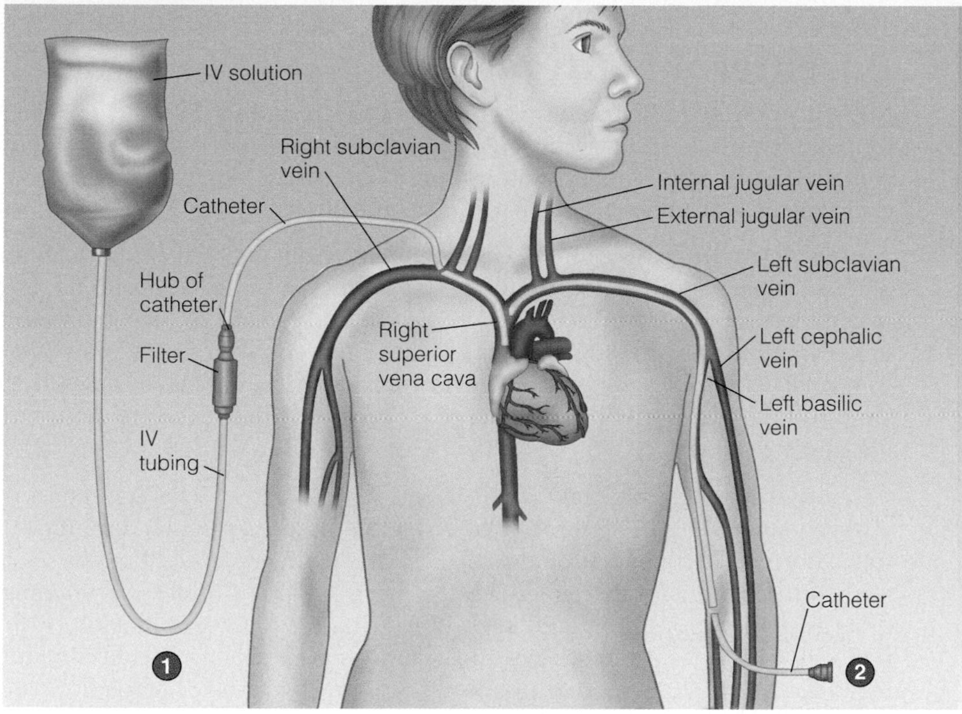
IV solution
Right subclavian vein
Catheter
Internal jugular vein
External jugular vein
Hub of catheter
Left subclavian vein
Filter
Right superior vena cava
Left cephalic vein
Left basilic vein
IV tubing
Catheter
1
2

1 Traditionally, central catheters enter the circulation at the right subclavian vein and are threaded into the superior vena cava with the tip of the catheter lying close to the heart. Sometimes catheters are threaded into the superior vena cava from the left subclavian vein, the internal jugular vein, or the external jugular vein.

2 Peripherally inserted central catheters usually enter the circulation at the basilic or cephalic vein and are guided up toward the heart so that the catheter tip rests in the superior vena cava.

trations do not need to be limited. Because this method can meet a person's complete nutrient requirements, it is called **total parenteral nutrition (TPN).** Central veins lie close to the heart where the large volume of blood rapidly dilutes TPN solutions. Therefore, patients with very high nutrient needs or fluid restrictions are able to receive the nutrient-dense solutions they require. TPN is also preferred for patients who require long-term intravenous feedings.

There are several ways to access central veins. The tip of a central venous **catheter** can be placed directly into a large-diameter central vein or threaded into a central vein through a peripheral vein (review Figure 21-2). Although insertion of peripherally inserted central catheters is less invasive and more easily performed than direct insertion of catheters into larger veins, studies have found higher complication rates associated with peripheral insertion.[2]

IN SUMMARY Parenteral nutrition support delivers nutrients intravenously. It is used in patients whose GI tract is not functioning and who may readily become malnourished. Patients receiving parenteral nutrition frequently have intestinal disorders or are critically ill. If nutrients are infused directly into peripheral veins (peripheral parenteral nutrition), nutrient concentrations must be limited to avoid inflammation of the veins. The infusion of nutrients into central veins (total parenteral nutrition) can supply nutrient-dense solutions and can be used for long-term intravenous feedings.

Parenteral Solutions

The pharmacies located within health care institutions often prepare parenteral solutions. This arrangement is beneficial because the pharmacist can customize formulations to meet patients' nutrient needs and because the solutions have a

total parenteral nutrition (TPN): a type of nutrition support in which intravenous feedings are delivered into a central vein; also called **central parenteral nutrition.**

catheter: a thin tube placed within a narrow lumen (such as a blood vessel) or body cavity; can be used to infuse or withdraw fluids or to keep a passage open.

limited shelf life. This section describes the nutrients and characteristics of parenteral solutions.[3]

Parenteral Nutrients

Nutrients provided intravenously bypass the GI tract and so must be provided in forms that are safe to inject directly into the bloodstream. Parenteral solutions contain the combinations of amino acids, carbohydrate, lipids, vitamins, and minerals that are best suited to meet patients' requirements.

Amino Acids Intravenous solutions contain all of the essential amino acids and different combinations of nonessential amino acids. The amino acid concentrations in commercial preparations range between 3.5 and 15 percent;■ the more concentrated solutions are used only when infusions are delivered into central veins. Just as in regular foods, the amino acids provide 4 kcalories per gram. Disease-specific amino acid solutions have been developed for patients with liver failure, kidney failure, and metabolic stress.

■ A 10% amino acid solution supplies 10 g of amino acids per 100 mL of solution.

Carbohydrate Carbohydrate is usually the main source of energy supplied by intravenous feedings. The form of carbohydrate used in parenteral solutions is called dextrose monohydrate and is made from glucose molecules that are associated with individual water molecules. The energy content of dextrose monohydrate is 3.4 kcalories per gram, slightly less than the glucose in food, which provides 4 kcalories per gram. Dextrose solutions are available in concentrations between 2.5 and 70 percent.■ Concentrations greater than 10 percent are used only when solutions are administered using central veins.

■ The concentration of dextrose is often abbreviated with a "D" followed by its concentration in water (W) or normal saline (NS). For example:

- D5 or D5W means a solution contains 5% dextrose in water.
- D10 or D10W means a solution contains 10% dextrose in water.
- D5/NS means a solution contains 5% dextrose in normal saline.

A 10% dextrose solution provides 10 g of dextrose monohydrate per 100 mL of solution.

Lipids Lipid emulsions supply essential fatty acids and are an important source of energy. They often contain triglycerides from soybean oil and safflower oil, phospholipids to serve as emulsifying agents, and glycerol to make the solutions isotonic. Lipid emulsions are available in 10, 20, and 30 percent solutions, which contain 1.1, 2.0, and 3.0 kcalories per milliliter, respectively. Therefore, a 500-milliliter container of 10 percent lipid emulsion would provide 550 kcalories.■ The same volume of a 20 percent lipid emulsion would provide 1000 kcalories.

Lipid emulsions are often provided daily and may supply 20 to 30 percent of total kcalories. Including lipids as an energy source reduces the need for energy from dextrose and lowers the risk of hyperglycemia in glucose-intolerant patients. Lipid infusions need to be restricted in patients with hypertriglyceridemia, however. There is also concern that lipid emulsions containing an excessive amount of linoleic acid may suppress some aspects of the immune response.

■
- 500 mL of 10% lipid emulsion: 500 mL × 1.1 kcal/mL = 550 kcal.
- 500 mL of 20% lipid emulsion: 500 mL × 2 kcal/mL = 1000 kcal.

Fluids and Electrolytes Daily fluid needs approximate 30 to 40 milliliters per kilogram of body weight in young adults and 30 milliliters per kilogram of body weight in older adults (for a daily average of between 1500 and 2500 milliliters for most people). Adjustments are made according to fluid losses and results of hydration assessment.

The electrolytes added to parenteral solutions include sodium, potassium, chloride, calcium, magnesium, and phosphorus. Requirements for parenteral solutions differ from DRI values because the nutrients are infused directly into the blood and are not influenced by absorption as they are when consumed orally. Generally, blood tests are administered daily to monitor electrolyte status until patients have stabilized. Electrolyte imbalances can be lethal, and therefore electrolyte management by experienced professionals is necessary whenever intravenous therapies are used.

The electrolyte content of parenteral solutions is expressed in *milliequivalents (mEq),* which are units indicating the number of ionic charges provided by electrolytes.■ The body's fluids are neutral solutions that contain equal numbers of positive and negative charges.

■ **Milliequivalents** are determined by dividing an ion's molecular weight by its number of charges. For example:

- 1 mEq of Ca^{++} is equivalent to 20 mg of calcium. For calcium, molecular weight = 40 and its ion has 2 positive charges: 40 ÷ 2 = 20.
- 1 mEq of Na^{+} is equivalent to 23 mg of sodium. For sodium, molecular weight = 23 and its ion has 1 positive charge: 23 ÷ 1 = 23.
- *1 mEq of Ca^{++}* has the same number of charges as *1 mEq of Na^{+}*.

TABLE 21-1 Osmolarity Contribution of Nutrients in Parenteral Solutions

For an estimate of the osmolarity of a 1-liter parenteral solution:

- Multiply the grams of amino acids in the solution by 10.
- Multiply the grams of dextrose in the solution by 5.
- Multiply the millequivalents (mEq) of electrolytes in the solution by 2.
- Multiply the grams of lipids in the solution by 1.5.

Add the values obtained to determine the approximate osmolarity.

Example:
A liter of a TPN solution has the approximate composition shown below. Calculate the osmolarity contribution of each component and estimate the total osmolarity of the solution.

Amino acids: 40 g	Sodium: 40 mEq	Calcium: 4.8 mEq
Dextrose: 250 g	Potassium: 35 mEq	Magnesium: 8 mEq
Lipids: 40 g	Chloride: 77 mEq	Phosphate: 21 mEq

Answer:
Amino acids: 40 g × 10 = 400 mOsm/L.
Dextrose: 250 g × 5 = 1250 mOsm/L.
Electrolytes: (40 + 35 + 77 + 4.8 + 8 + 21) × 2 = 371.6 mOsm/L.
Lipids: 40 g × 1.5 = 60 mOsm/L.
Total osmolarity: 400 + 1250 + 371.6 + 60 = 2081.6 mOsm/L.

SOURCE: Adapted from A. M. Coulston, C. L. Rock, and E. R. Monsen, eds., *Nutrition in the Prevention and Treatment of Disease* (San Diego: Academic Press, 2001), Table 7; p. 254.

Vitamins and Trace Minerals Commercial multivitamin and trace mineral preparations are routinely added to parenteral solutions.[4] All water-soluble vitamins are supplied, as well as vitamins A, D, and E; vitamin K is often omitted and must be added separately. Trace minerals added to parenteral solutions include zinc, copper, chromium, selenium, and manganese. Iron is excluded because it alters the stability of other ingredients in parenteral mixtures; special forms of iron need to be injected separately.

Osmolarity Recall that the **osmolarity**■ of PPN solutions is limited to 900 milliosmoles per liter (because peripheral veins are sensitive to high nutrient concentrations), whereas TPN solutions may be as nutrient-dense as necessary. The components of a solution that contribute most to its osmolarity are amino acids, dextrose, and electrolytes: as concentrations of these nutrients increase, the osmolarity of a solution increases.[5] Because lipids contribute little to osmolarity, lipid emulsions are used to increase the energy provided in PPN solutions. Table 21-1 gives an example of a method of calculating the osmolarity of a parenteral solution.

■ The osmotic property of a solution can be expressed either as *osmolarity* or as *osmolality* (introduced in Chapter 20).
- *Osmolarity* refers to the number of solutes per liter of solution.
- *Osmolality* refers to the number of solutes per kilogram of solvent.

Due to the measurement techniques used in clinical laboratories, the term *osmolality* is often preferred when referring to biological solutions like blood or urine.

Medications To avoid the need for a separate infusion site, medications are occasionally added directly to parenteral solutions or infused through a separate port (attached via a Y-connector). The administration of a second solution using a separate port in a catheter is called a **piggyback.** Insulin, for example, is sometimes added by piggyback to improve glucose tolerance. Heparin (an anticoagulant) may be added to prevent clotting at the catheter tip. In practice, few medications are added to parenteral solutions so that potential drug-nutrient interactions can be avoided.

Formula Preparation

The parenteral solution prescribed depends on a patient's medical condition and nutrition status and whether the solution will be infused into peripheral or central veins. Prescriptions for parenteral solutions are highly individualized and may need to be recalculated daily until the patient's condition is stable. The "How to" on p. 680 describes a method for calculating the macronutrient and energy content when solution ingredients are expressed as percentages.

osmolarity: the concentration of osmotically active particles in a solution, expressed as milliosmoles per liter (mOsm/L). **Osmolality** is an alternative expression of a solution's osmotic properties that is used in clinical practice and uses the units milliosmoles per kilogram (mOsm/kg).

piggyback: the administration of a second solution using a separate port in an intravenous catheter.

HOW TO Calculate the Macronutrient and Energy Content of Parenteral Solutions

Suppose a person is receiving 1800 milliliters of a parenteral solution that contains 16% dextrose, 5% amino acids, and 2.5% lipids. What are the grams of protein, carbohydrate, and fat the person is receiving, and what is the energy content of the solution?

Remember that a percentage is a fraction in which the denominator is always 100. Therefore, a 10% amino acid solution contains 10 grams of amino acids per 100 grams of solution. Note that 1 gram of fluid is equivalent to 1 milliliter.

Step 1: Determine the macronutrient content of the solution.

$$\textbf{16\% dextrose} = \frac{16 \text{ g dextrose}}{100 \text{ mL}}.$$

$$\frac{16 \text{ g dextrose}}{100 \text{ mL}} \times 1800 \text{ mL} = 288 \text{ g of dextrose.}$$

$$\textbf{5\% amino acids} = \frac{5 \text{ g amino acids}}{100 \text{ mL}}$$

$$\frac{5 \text{ g amino acids}}{100 \text{ mL}} \times 1800 \text{ mL} = 90 \text{ g of amino acids.}$$

$$\textbf{2.5\% lipids} = \frac{2.5 \text{ g lipids}}{100 \text{ mL}}.$$

$$\frac{2.5 \text{ g lipids}}{100 \text{ mL}} \times 1800 \text{ mL} = 45 \text{ g of lipids.}$$

Step 2: Determine the energy content of the solution. (Remember that dextrose monohydrate provides 3.4 kcalories per gram.)

$$288 \text{ g dextrose} \times 3.4 \text{ kcal/g} = 979 \text{ kcal.}$$

$$90 \text{ g amino acids} \times 4.0 \text{ kcal/g} = 360 \text{ kcal.}$$

$$45 \text{ g lipid} \times 9.0 \text{ kcal/g}^{a} = 405 \text{ kcal.}$$

Total = 979 kcal + 360 kcal + 405 kcal = 1744 kcal.

[a] Intravenous lipid actually provides more than 9.0 kcalories per gram, but this value is an acceptable estimate.

When a parenteral solution contains dextrose, amino acids, and lipids, it is called a **total nutrient admixture (TNA),** a **3-in-1,** or an **all-in-one** solution. A parenteral solution that excludes lipids is called a **2-in-1 solution,** in which case a lipid emulsion is administered separately, often by piggyback administration. The administration of TNA solutions is simpler because only one infusion pump is required; however, the addition of lipid emulsion to solutions reduces their stability, a major concern when TNA solutions are compounded. Generally, a TNA with a high-lipid concentration is more stable than one with a low-lipid concentration because diluting the lipids reduces the emulsification effect of an emulsion's phospholipids. Lipids are usually administered separately when they are not a major energy source and are used only to provide essential fatty acids.

Intravenous feedings are similar to tube feedings in that careful attention to solution preparation and handling can minimize complications. To prevent bacterial contamination and maintain stability, parenteral solutions are compounded in the pharmacy under aseptic conditions, shielded from light, and refrigerated. Prior to infusion, solutions are removed from the refrigerator and allowed to reach room temperature. During feedings, the solution and catheter need to be checked frequently for signs of contamination.

IN SUMMARY Prescriptions for parenteral solutions are individualized to meet each patient's needs. The solutions, which are compounded in hospital pharmacies using commercial nutrient preparations, include amino acids, dextrose, electrolytes, vitamins, and minerals. Lipid emulsions may be included in the mixture or may be administered separately. A parenteral solution that includes lipids is called a total nutrient admixture, a 3-in-1, or an all-in-one solution. Few medications are added to parenteral solutions due to the potential for drug-nutrient interactions. Parenteral solutions are prepared and handled using aseptic techniques to prevent contamination.

total nutrient admixture (TNA): a parenteral solution that contains dextrose, amino acids, and lipids; also called a **3-in-1** or an **all-in-one** solution.

2-in-1 solution: a parenteral solution that contains dextrose and amino acids, but excludes lipids.

Administering Parenteral Nutrition

Providing parenteral nutrition is complex and requires skills from a variety of disciplines. A nutrition support team,■ made up of physicians, nurses, dietitians, and pharmacists, specializes in the provision of intravenous and tube feedings. Members of the team may serve as advisers to other clinicians or may manage nutrition support directly. They may also have administrative responsibilities, such as receiving patients, purchasing supplies, billing, developing guidelines, and keeping records. Figure 21-3 describes the typical roles of each member of a nutrition support team.

■ Reminder: A *nutrition support team* is a multidisciplinary team of health care professionals who are responsible for the provision of nutrients by tube feedings or intravenous infusion.

Insertion and Care of Intravenous Catheters

Although a skilled nurse can place catheters into peripheral veins, placement of catheters directly into central veins requires insertion by a qualified physician. Patients may be awake for the procedure and given local anesthesia. Unnecessary apprehension can be avoided by explaining the procedure to the patient beforehand.

Catheter-related problems frequently cause complications (see Table 21-2 on p. 682). Catheters are sometimes improperly positioned or may dislodge after placement. Air may leak into catheters, obstructing blood flow. Catheters inserted into

FIGURE 21-3 The Nutrition Support Team

The physician

- Diagnoses medical problems
- Performs medical procedures
- Coordinates and prescribes therapy
- Directs and supervises team
- Approves guidelines and protocols
- Consults with other physicians

The nurse

- Assesses nursing needs
- Performs direct patient care
- Explains medical procedures and treatment plans
- Instructs patients regarding medical care
- Acts as a liaison between team and nursing staff
- Coordinates discharge plans

All team members

- Review current research
- Analyze new products
- Develop guidelines
- Provide in-service training
- Monitor patients
- Correct problems
- Educate patients
- Evaluate the outcome of the care provided and cost savings
- Promote the appropriate use of nutrition support
- Improve communications among team members and between the team and other health care professionals

The dietitian

- Assesses nutrition status
- Determines patients' nutrient needs
- Recommends appropriate diet therapy
- Reevaluates patients regularly
- Instructs patients about their diets
- Acts as a liaison between the team and the dietary department

The pharmacist

- Recommends appropriate drug therapy
- Identifies drug-drug and diet-drug interactions
- Identifies drug-related complications
- Educates patients about their medications
- Acts as a liaison between the team and the pharmacy

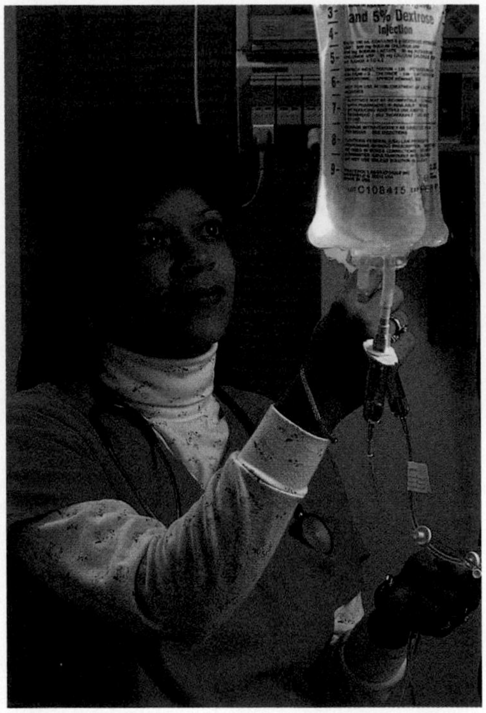
and 5% Dextrose
Injection

Although parenteral solutions may look alike, they are customized to meet patients' needs.

TABLE 21-2 Potential Complications of Parenteral Nutrition

Catheter-Related	Metabolic
Air embolism	Abnormalities in liver function
Blood clotting at catheter tip	Electrolyte imbalances
Clogging of catheter	Gallbladder disease
Dislodgment of catheter	Hyperglycemia, hypoglycemia
Improper placement	Hypertriglyceridemia
Infection, sepsis	Metabolic bone disease
Phlebitis	Nutrient deficiencies
Tissue injury	Refeeding syndrome

peripheral veins may cause phlebitis, requiring reinsertion at an alternate site. A catheter may become clogged from blood clotting or from a buildup of scar tissue around the catheter tip. Catheters are also a leading cause of infection: contamination may be introduced during insertion, at the placement site, or from a contaminated solution.

To reduce complication risk, nurses use aseptic techniques when inserting catheters, changing tubing, or changing a dressing that covers the catheter site. Unusual bleeding or a wet dressing suggests a problem with catheter placement. A change in infusion rate may indicate a clogged catheter. Infection may be indicated by redness or swelling around the catheter site or by an unexplained fever. Thus routine inspections of equipment and frequent monitoring of patients' symptoms help to minimize the problems associated with catheter use.

Administration of Parenteral Solutions

Infusion protocols should be reviewed at individual institutions to identify the preferred methods for initiating parenteral solutions. A common approach is to start solution infusion at a slow rate and gradually increase the infusion rate over a two- to three-day period. For example, 40 milliliters per hour may be infused during the first 24 hours of administration (supplying 960 milliliters) and the rate increased by one liter per day until the goal rate is reached. Another approach is to give the full volume of a nutrient-dilute solution on the first day and advance nutrient concentrations as tolerated. Some clinicians start solutions at full strength unless there is a risk that the patient will become hyperglycemic.

Blood glucose and electrolyte levels are checked regularly to determine tolerance to solutions. Frequent reassessment of nutrient intakes may be necessary until a patient has stabilized. Rapid changes in infusion rate are discouraged in some patients (especially newborn infants) due to a risk of developing hyperglycemia or hypoglycemia (as discussed in the next section). Table 21-3 lists some guidelines for monitoring patients undergoing intravenous feedings.[6]

Parenteral solutions may be infused continuously over 24 hours **(continuous parenteral nutrition)** or during 10- to 16-hour periods only **(cyclic parenteral nutrition).** Continuous feedings are often given to critically ill and malnourished patients who cannot receive adequate nutrition during shorter time periods. Cyclic feedings are often provided at night so that patients can participate in routine activities during the day. This method is especially suited for patients who require long-term parenteral support or for those who will be infusing parenteral solutions at home. Patients may begin with continuous feedings and transition to cyclic feedings as their condition improves.

continuous parenteral nutrition: continuous administration of parenteral solutions over a 24-hour period.

cyclic parenteral nutrition: administration of a parenteral solution over a 10- to 16-hour period.

Managing Metabolic Complications

As discussed in a previous section, the catheters used for parenteral feedings may cause a number of serious complications. This section describes some metabolic complications that may result from intravenous nutrition support (review Table 21-2) and explains how they are managed.[7]

Hyperglycemia Hyperglycemia,■ a common consequence of intravenous feedings, most often occurs in patients who are glucose intolerant or are undergoing severe metabolic stress. It may be prevented by providing insulin along with feedings or by restricting the amount of dextrose in a solution. Dextrose infusions are often limited to less than 5 milligrams per kilogram of body weight per minute in critically ill adult patients so that carbohydrate intakes do not exceed the maximum glucose oxidation rate. Premature infants are especially likely to develop hyperglycemia because their pancreas and liver are not fully functioning.

■ For most patients receiving parenteral nutrition, blood glucose levels should not exceed 200 mg/dL.

Hypoglycemia Although uncommon, hypoglycemia may occur when feedings are interrupted or discontinued. In patients at risk, such as young infants, feedings may be tapered off over several hours before discontinuation.

Hypertriglyceridemia Hypertriglyceridemia may occur in critically ill patients who are unable to tolerate the amount of lipid emulsion that is supplied. It may also result from excessive carbohydrate feedings or from severe infection, which impairs lipid clearance. These conditions may limit the amount of lipid emulsion that can be safely infused. If blood triglyceride levels exceed 350 to 400 milligrams per deciliter, lipid infusions should be reduced or stopped.[8]

Refeeding Syndrome Severely malnourished patients who are fed aggressively (parenterally or otherwise) may exhibit **refeeding syndrome,** characterized by electrolyte and fluid imbalances and hyperglycemia. These effects occur because dextrose infusions raise circulating insulin levels, which promote anabolic processes that quickly remove phosphate, potassium, and magnesium from the blood. The altered electrolyte levels can lead to fluid retention and life-threatening changes in organ systems. To prevent refeeding syndrome, feedings are started slowly and electrolyte levels monitored carefully when malnourished patients begin receiving nutrition support.

Abnormalities in Liver Function Fatty liver often results from parenteral feedings, and therefore serum levels of liver enzymes are routinely monitored. Usually, liver complications are readily reversed when parenteral feedings are discontinued. Long-term parenteral nutrition, however, may result in chronic, irreversible liver disease that may eventually lead to liver failure. The cause of the liver abnormalities is unclear.

Gallbladder Disease Gallbladder problems frequently develop when the GI tract is not used for long periods. When parenteral nutrition is continued for longer than four weeks, sludge (thickened bile) often builds up in the gallbladder and may eventually lead to gallstone formation. Prevention is sometimes possible by initiating enteral feedings before problems develop. Patients who require parenteral nutrition for long periods may be given cholecystokinin injections (to cause gallbladder contraction and bile release) or may have their gallbladders removed surgically.

Metabolic Bone Disease Long-term parenteral nutrition has been associated with decreased bone density and bone mineralization. The occurrence of bone disease may be related to alterations in calcium, phosphorus, and vitamin D metabolism. Another hypothesis is that parenteral feedings alter the function of the parathyroid gland, which then causes disruptions in bone metabolism.[9] Although nutrition status and bone density are carefully monitored during long-term parenteral nutrition, there is no satisfactory remedy for this complication at present.

TABLE 21-3 Patient Monitoring during Parenteral Nutrition

Before Starting

- Complete nutrition assessment.
- Record body height, weight, and body mass index.
- Confirm catheter placement by X-ray.
- Check laboratory tests: blood glucose, sodium, potassium, calcium, phosphorus, magnesium, bicarbonate, serum proteins, liver enzymes, triglycerides, blood urea nitrogen, creatinine, bilirubin, complete blood count.

Every 4 to 8 Hours

- Check vital signs, including body temperature.
- Check blood glucose (once stabilized, check daily).
- Inspect catheter site for signs of inflammation or infection (frequency depends on patient condition).
- Check pump infusion rate and appearance of parenteral solution and tubing.

Daily

- Replace parenteral solution and tubing.
- Check blood glucose and serum electrolytes until stabilized.
- Monitor weight changes.
- Record fluid intake and output.

Several Times Weekly (or as needed)

- Reassess nutrition status.
- Check laboratory tests to monitor blood chemistry (once stabilized, may check less frequently).

Discontinuing Intravenous Feedings

Some patients may require parenteral nutrition for the rest of their lives, but most eventually return to an oral diet. The method used for transitioning patients to oral feedings depends on the patient's overall health and medical condition. Factors to consider include the length of time that the patient was receiving parenteral support and the follow-up treatment planned. Patients must also have

refeeding syndrome: a condition that sometimes develops when a severely malnourished person is aggressively fed; characterized by electrolyte and fluid imbalances and hyperglycemia.

adequate GI function before parenteral feedings can be tapered off and enteral feedings begun.

During the transition from parenteral to oral feedings, a combination of feeding methods is often used. Parenteral feedings are usually tapered off at the same time that tube feedings or oral feedings are begun, such that the two feeding methods supply the needed nutrients. Small enteral feedings may be given at first to determine tolerance. If gastrointestinal symptoms (such as nausea, vomiting, bloating, or diarrhea) develop, the enteral feedings are given more slowly until the intestines adapt. Once two-thirds to three-fourths of nutrient needs can be provided enterally, the intravenous feedings may be discontinued. As discussed in Chapter 18, clear liquid diets (see pp. 611–613) are initially offered following intravenous feedings. Patients can then progress to solid foods as tolerated.

Transitioning directly to an oral diet is often difficult because a person's appetite remains suppressed for several weeks after parenteral nutrition is terminated. Patients receiving continuous parenteral feedings may have better appetites during the day if they are given nocturnal cyclic feedings before beginning oral intakes.

IN SUMMARY A nutrition support team, made up of physicians, nurses, dietitians, and pharmacists, may administer parenteral nutrition support or serve as advisers to other clinicians. Solutions may be initiated gradually or provided full strength in selected patients. Critically ill patients may require continuous feedings, whereas healthier patients and long-term users may prefer cyclic feedings. Catheters are frequently the cause of complications, which include improper placement or dislodgment, infection, clotting, embolism, and phlebitis. Metabolic complications include hyperglycemia and hypoglycemia, hypertriglyceridemia, fluid and electrolyte imbalances, and diseases affecting the liver, gallbladder, and bone. When the need for parenteral nutrition resolves, patients are transitioned to an enteral diet as the volume of parenteral nutrition is gradually reduced. The Case Study can be used to check your understanding of the concepts introduced in this chapter.

Nutrition Support at Home

Occasionally, an individual must continue to receive nutrition support (tube feedings or parenteral nutrition) after a medical condition has stabilized. In such a case, home nutrition support might be an option.

The use of home nutrition support is rapidly expanding. Current technology allows the safe administration of nutrition support in home settings, and insurance coverage often pays a substantial portion of the costs. Home health services and home infusion pharmacies can provide the equipment, enteral formulas or parenteral solutions, and the services necessary for home nutrition care. Most importantly, patients using home nutrition support services can continue to receive specialized nutrition care while leading normal lives.[10]

Candidates for Home Nutrition Support

People who are referred for home nutrition support usually need long-term nutrition care for chronic medical conditions. In the United States, Medicare and Medicaid account for more than half of the payments for parenteral and enteral nutrition services. Medicare reimbursement is possible only if home nutrition support is required for a minimum of 90 days. If patients do not have appropriate clinical diagnoses, reimbursement by government or private insurance companies may be denied.

Home Enteral Nutrition Home enteral nutrition is indicated for people who have functioning GI tracts and illnesses that prevent food from reaching the di-

CASE STUDY

Geologist Requiring Parenteral Nutrition

Adam Taylor, a 27-year-old geologist with an inflammatory intestinal disease, underwent a surgical procedure in which a substantial portion of his small intestine was removed. He had received TPN prior to surgery and continued to receive it afterwards. After ten days, tube feeding was begun, which initially delivered very small feedings.

1. List some reasons why TPN was probably chosen to provide nutrition support in this patient. How would you explain the need for parenteral feedings to Adam?
2. Describe each component of a typical TPN solution. Calculate the energy content of 1 liter of a solution that provides 140 grams of dextrose monohydrate, 45 grams of amino acids, and 20 grams of lipid emulsion. If Adam's energy requirement is 2100 kcalories per day, how many liters of solution will he need each day?
3. Why was it important that Adam begin enteral feedings as soon as possible? Assuming that Adam eventually tolerated a tube feeding, in what ways did the health care team most likely help Adam make the transition from parenteral feedings to tube feeding? Consider some of the physiological problems Adam might face when he begins eating an oral diet.
4. If Adam is unable to meet nutrient needs orally, he may need to continue tube feeding or TPN at home. As you read through the following sections, determine whether Adam would be a good candidate for a home nutrition support program. Consider both the benefits of a proposed program and the problems he could encounter.

gestive tract. Examples include patients with head and neck cancers and patients with neurological impairments that affect swallowing.

Home Parenteral Nutrition Home parenteral nutrition is indicated for people who have illnesses that severely impair nutrient absorption or cause motility problems in the stomach or intestines. Examples include individuals who have had large portions of their small intestine removed and those with intestinal obstructions or malabsorption conditions.

Other Criteria The procedures and risks of home nutrition support need to be acceptable to the patient and caregivers, who are responsible for performing the required techniques. The home should be safe and clean and have adequate storage for formulas or solutions and equipment. The costs of nutrition support should be clearly explained to families who cannot get insurance reimbursement. Users of home nutrition services must be intellectually capable of learning the necessary procedures, monitoring the treatment, and managing complications as necessary.

Planning Home Nutrition Care

As with nutrition support provided in health care facilities, planning for home care involves decisions about access sites, formulas, and nutrient delivery methods. Users of home services should participate in decision making to ensure long-term compliance and satisfaction.

Home Enteral Nutrition Access to the GI tract for home feedings is possible using either nasal tubes or enterostomies (see Chapter 20). Patients sometimes learn to place nasogastric tubes themselves, which may improve acceptance of the therapy. Active children and adults often prefer low-profile gastrostomy tubes, which can allow them to lead a more normal lifestyle. Jejunostomy tubes may be required for some individuals, but are less convenient because the frequent feedings required for jejunostomies can interfere with daytime activities.

The choice of formula for home use is often affected by its cost and availability. Reimbursement for home nutrition support may not include the cost of formula, which is considered to be a "food" product. For this reason, some people may choose to prepare simple formulas at home. The use of blenderized home-cooked foods is possible, but such foods need to be strained to remove particles and

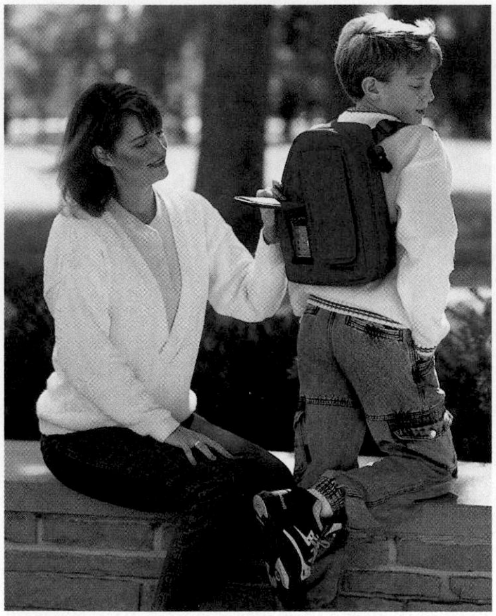
Courtesy of Kendall Healthcare

Portable pumps and convenient carrying cases allow people who require nutrition support at home to move about freely.

clumps that may obstruct the tube. Closed (ready-to-hang) feeding systems may be useful for avoiding contamination risk, but may not be appropriate for intermittent feedings that require smaller amounts of formula.

The advantages and disadvantages associated with different feeding techniques and administration schedules should be fully discussed with patients. Bolus infusions are simplest and can be quickly delivered, but they are not ideal for intestinal feedings. Gravity drip infusions eliminate the need for an infusion pump, but delivery rates are less reliable. Insurance companies may refuse to reimburse the cost of an infusion pump without proof that it is medically necessary.

If intermittent feeding schedules are appropriate, they should be tailored to daily routines. Some people may be able to meet their nutrient needs by eating some foods during the day and infusing formula only at night. Portable pumps can free individuals from the need to infuse formula at home and can also be used when traveling.

Home Parenteral Nutrition Although both peripheral parenteral nutrition and total parenteral nutrition (TPN) may be provided at home, long-term therapy requires access to the larger, central veins that are appropriate for TPN. The catheters used are designed for long-term use and inserted so that the exit site is in an area that is accessible to the patient.

Parenteral solutions need to be sterile and aseptically prepared, and people who plan to mix their own solutions should be carefully trained. Ready-made parenteral solutions require refrigeration and are stable for limited periods; for example, TNA (total nutrient admixture) solutions may be stable for only a week when refrigerated.

Most people prefer cyclic infusions to continuous infusions and often transition to cyclic infusions before discharge from the hospital. Because an infusion pump is required for home TPN, it may need sufficient battery backup in case electrical service is interrupted. Portable pumps are helpful for individuals who lead an active lifestyle or prefer to infuse during the day.

Quality of Life Issues

Although home nutrition programs can help to improve health and extend life, consumers of home services and their families may struggle with the lifestyle adjustments required.[11] In addition to the economic impact of nutrition support, home feedings are often time-consuming and inconvenient. Activities and work schedules must be planned around feedings. Extra planning and precautions must be taken when a person wants to travel or participate in sports activities. Explaining one's medical needs to friends and acquaintances may be embarrassing.

Among physical difficulties, people receiving nocturnal feedings often cite disturbed sleep as a major problem. Disruptions may be due to multiple nighttime bathroom visits, noisy infusion pumps, or difficulty finding a comfortable sleeping position when "hooked up." People using parenteral support sometimes prefer infusing solutions during the day to improve their sleeping patterns.

Among social issues, the inability to consume meals with family and friends is often a great concern. People who need nutrition support may enjoy the social aspects of mealtimes and can be given a place setting at the table. Some individuals may be able to eat small amounts of food and continue to participate in meals despite dietary restrictions. Joining friends at restaurants and attending certain types of social events, however, can be problematic. It is also difficult to explain one's complex medical condition to colleagues or to a new romantic interest.

People who depend on nutrition support face a number of stressful issues that can affect quality of life. Although parenteral and enteral nutrition are life-sustaining therapies, both are associated with serious complications. Many people find that their lifestyles need to be greatly altered to accommodate nutrition therapy and may experience depression, fear, and anxiety. Health practitioners should be ready to recommend support groups or counseling resources to help patients cope with ongoing stresses.■

■ The Oley Foundation is an excellent source of outreach services, emotional support, and current information for people who require home nutrition support (**www.oley.org**).

IN SUMMARY Parenteral and enteral nutrition support can be safely and effectively provided in the home. Candidates for home enteral nutrition services have functional GI tracts but are unable to consume food orally. Parenteral nutrition candidates have illnesses that impair nutrient absorption or cause motility problems. Decisions about access sites, formulas, and nutrient delivery methods should be made with patients and caregivers. Formulas and solutions are often prepared in the home. The use of portable pumps may help individuals lead a normal lifestyle. Nevertheless, lifestyle adjustments to nutrition support may be difficult and stressful.

NUTRITION ON THE NET

Access these websites for further study of topics covered in this chapter.

- Find updates and quick links to these and other nutrition-related sites at our website: **www.wadsworth.com/nutrition**
- To find out more about organizations that promote the appropriate use of enteral and parenteral nutrition, visit the:

  American Society for Parenteral and Enteral Nutrition site: **www.clinnutr.org**

  Canadian Parenteral-Enteral Nutrition Association site: **www.cpena.ca/home.html**

  British Association for Parenteral and Enteral Nutrition site: **www.bapen.org.uk/**
- To learn about home parenteral nutrition, visit the website of the Oley Foundation, a national, nonprofit organization that provides information, outreach services, and emotional support for consumers of home enteral and parenteral services: **http://c4isr.com/oley** or **www.oley.org**

STUDY QUESTIONS

These questions will help you review the chapter. You will find the answers in the discussions on the pages provided.

1. Compare the general characteristics of peripheral parenteral nutrition (PPN) and total parenteral nutrition (TPN). Discuss advantages and disadvantages of each method. (pp. 676–677)
2. Describe how amino acids, carbohydrate, and lipids are provided in parenteral solutions. (pp. 677–678)
3. List vitamins and minerals usually included in parenteral solutions. How are fluid needs estimated? (pp. 678–679)
4. Identify the components of parenteral solutions that contribute to osmolarity. Explain how the osmolarity of a solution can be estimated. (p. 679)
5. Compare components of total nutrient admixtures (TNA) and 2-in-1 solutions. Describe advantages and disadvantages associated with the use of TNA solutions. (p. 680)
6. Discuss potential complications associated with parenteral nutrition. Suggest ways in which complications can be prevented or corrected. (pp. 681–683)
7. Explain how patients make the transition from parenteral to enteral nutrition. (pp. 683–684)
8. Discuss how home nutrition support is administered. Identify ideal candidates for these services and problems that patients may experience. (pp. 684–686)

These questions will help you prepare for an exam. Answers can be found on p. 688.

1. TPN is preferred over PPN for a patient who:
   a. does not have high nutrient requirements.
   b. needs long-term parenteral nutrition support.
   c. has strong peripheral veins and moderate nutrient needs.
   d. needs parenteral feedings as a supplement to tube feedings.
2. Which of the following cannot be delivered intravenously?
   a. dextrose
   b. amino acids
   c. lipid emulsions
   d. hydrolyzed enteral formulas
3. How many kcalories are supplied by 500 milliliters of an 8.5 percent amino acid solution?
   a. 60
   b. 170

   c. 340
   d. 500

4. Compared to solutions delivered by peripheral vein, solutions delivered by central vein provide:
   a. lower osmolarity.
   b. more fat, less dextrose.
   c. more dextrose, less fat.
   d. more vitamins and minerals.

5. For a patient receiving central TPN who also receives intravenous lipid emulsions two or three times a week, the lipid emulsions serve primarily as a source of:
   a. essential fatty acids.
   b. cholesterol.
   c. fat-soluble vitamins.
   d. concentrated energy.

6. Routine monitoring of patients on TPN requires all of the following measures, *except:*
   a. serum electrolytes.
   b. daily weight changes.
   c. indirect calorimetry.
   d. liver function tests.

7. Complications associated with parenteral feedings may include:
   a. hyperglycemia.
   b. hypertriglyceridemia.
   c. infection.
   d. all of the above.

8. Refeeding syndrome causes dangerous fluctuations in:
   a. electrolytes.
   b. liver enzymes.
   c. triglycerides.
   d. ketone bodies.

9. The transition from parenteral feedings to an oral diet is primarily designed to:
   a. improve appetite.
   b. prevent hypoglycemia.
   c. prevent apprehension about eating.
   d. ensure that nutrient needs will continue to be met.

10. Patients using home parenteral nutrition:
   a. are unable to use TNA solutions.
   b. are usually given continuous rather than cyclic infusions.
   c. require infusion pumps for use at home.
   d. are generally unable to work out of the home or travel.

REFERENCES

1. L. Matarese, Composite foods and formulas, parenteral and enteral nutrition, in A. M. Coulston, C. L. Rock, and E. R. Monsen, eds., *Nutrition in the Prevention and Treatment of Disease* (San Diego: Academic Press, 2001), pp. 245–260.
2. L. J. Walshe and coauthors, Complication rates among cancer patients with peripherally inserted central catheters, *Journal of Clinical Oncology* 20 (2002): 3276–3281; C. T. Cowl and coauthors, Complications and cost associated with parenteral nutrition delivered to hospitalized patients through either subclavian or peripherally inserted central catheters, *Clinical Nutrition* 19 (2000): 237–243.
3. Matarese, 2001.
4. Matarese, 2001.
5. B. L. Erstad, Osmolality and osmolarity: Narrowing the terminology gap, *Pharmacotherapy* 23 (2003): 1085–1086.
6. M. M. McMahon, Parenteral nutrition, in L. Goldman and D. Ausiello, eds., *Cecil Textbook of Medicine* (Philadelphia: Saunders, 2004), pp. 1322–1326; A.S.P.E.N. Board of Directors and The Clinical Guidelines Task Force, Guidelines for the use of parenteral and enteral nutrition in adult and pediatric patients, *Journal of Parenteral and Enteral Nutrition* 26 (2002): 1SA–138SA.
7. A.S.P.E.N. Board of Directors and The Clinical Guidelines Task Force, 2002.
8. McMahon, 2004.
9. W. Goodman and coauthors, Altered diurnal regulation of blood ionized calcium and serum parathyroid hormone concentrations during parenteral nutrition, *American Journal of Clinical Nutrition* 71 (2000): 560–568.
10. N. H. Westbrook, Nutrition support in home care, in A. Skipper, ed., *Dietitian's Handbook of Enteral and Parenteral Nutrition* (Gaithersberg, Md.: Aspen Publishers, 1998), pp. 547–576.
11. B. Ehrenpreis and A. Hilf, Home parenteral nutrition: The consumer's perspective, in *Lifeline Letter,* **http://c4isr.com/oley/lifeline/LivingHPN.pdf**, site visited December 11, 2004.

ANSWERS

Study Questions (multiple choice)

1. b 2. d 3. b 4. c 5. a 6. c 7. d 8. a 9. d 10. c

HIGHLIGHT

Ethical Issues in Nutrition Care

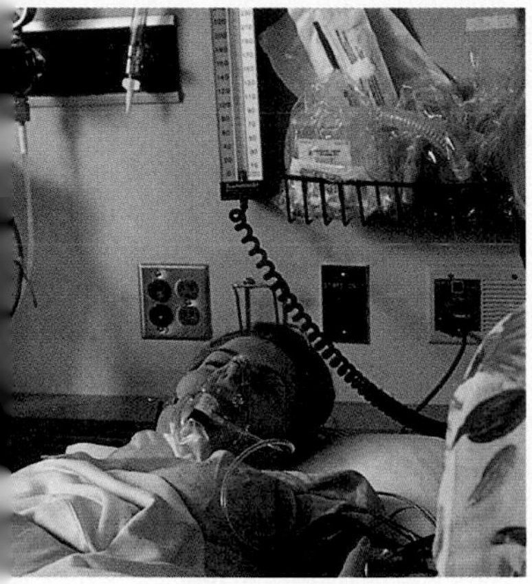

Carolyn A. McKeone/Photo Researchers, Inc.

Like other medical technologies, the availability of specialized nutrition support forces health care professionals and members of our society to face **ethical** issues. When medical treatments prolong life by merely delaying death, the lifetime that remains may be of extremely low quality. This highlight examines the ethical dilemmas that clinicians must face when dealing with patients in critical care. The glossary (p. 690) defines the relevant terms.

Ethical Considerations

If providing nutrition can do little to promote recovery, is it morally and legally appropriate to withhold or to withdraw nutrition support? Do patients and family members have the rights to make these types of decisions themselves? Health care professionals must balance their obligations to provide appropriate care with the following ethical principles:[1]

- The potential benefits **(beneficence)** of any treatment should outweigh its potential harm **(maleficence)**.
- A patient should be fully informed of a treatment's benefits and risks in a fair and honest manner **(disclosure)**. Patient acceptance of a treatment that has been adequately disclosed is considered **informed consent.**
- A patient has the right to make decisions concerning his or her own well-being **(patient autonomy),** even if refusing treatment could result in death. It is generally accepted that a patient's preferences should take precedence over the desires of others.[2]
- A patient must have the mental capacity to make appropriate health care decisions **(decision-making capacity).** If a patient is mentally incapable of doing so, a person designated by the patient should serve as a **surrogate** decision maker.
- Health care providers must determine whether the provision of health care to one patient would unfairly limit the care of other patients **(distributive justice).**

Although the rights of patients and their families may seem simple and obvious, it is often difficult to determine the appropriate action to take during intensive care.[3] When clinicians and families disagree, the courts may be asked to decide.

When a patient's preferences are unknown, a clinician is obligated to provide any and all available care that is likely to sustain the patient's life. Nutrition and hydration are both considered life-sustaining treatments; clearly, withholding or withdrawing either is certain to result in death. Other life-sustaining treatments include **cardiopulmonary resuscitation (CPR),** which supplies oxygen and restores a person's ability to breathe and pump blood; **defibrillation,** in which an electronic device shocks the heart and reestablishes normal contractions; **mechanical ventilation,** which substitutes for lung function; and **dialysis,** which substitutes for kidney function.

Ethical Dilemmas

Although nutrition support is readily provided to patients who have a reasonable chance of recovering from illness, it is sometimes difficult to determine the best course of action for patients who are dying or who are unlikely to regain consciousness. Under such circumstances, a life-sustaining therapy may be considered **futile** because it is unable to improve the outcome of disease or to increase a patient's comfort and well-being. If patients or caregivers demand treatment that health practitioners have determined to be futile, a legal resolution may be required. Conversely, medical personnel may find it objectionable to withdraw life support knowing that the consequence is the death of a patient.

Legal Decisions

One of the most widely publicized cases involving nutrition support was that of Nancy Cruzan.[4] Nancy Cruzan was a young woman who suffered permanent and irreversible brain damage after a car crash in 1983, when she was just 26 years of age. After she had been in a **persistent vegetative state** (awake but unaware) for five years, her parents requested permission to discontinue tube feeding, but hospital staff refused to honor the request and the matter was taken to court. The Missouri Supreme Court determined that Nancy had never

GLOSSARY

advance directive: a written or oral instruction regarding one's preferences for medical treatment to be used in the event of becoming incapacitated.

beneficence (be-NEF-eh-sens): the act of performing beneficial services rather than harmful ones.

cardiopulmonary resuscitation (CPR): life-sustaining treatment that supplies oxygen and restores a person's ability to breathe and pump blood.

conservator: a person who takes responsibility for the person and property of an incompetent individual.

decision-making capacity: the ability to understand pertinent information and make appropriate decisions; known as **decision-making competency** within the legal system.

defibrillation: life-sustaining treatment in which an electronic device is used to shock the heart and reestablish a pattern of normal contractions. Treatment is used when a heart has arrhythmias or has experienced cardiac arrest.

dialysis: life-sustaining treatment in which a patient's blood is filtered using selective diffusion through a semipermeable membrane; substitutes for kidney function.

disclosure: the act of revealing pertinent information. For example, clinicians should accurately describe the proposed tests and procedures, their benefits and risks, and alternative approaches.

distributive justice: the equitable distribution of resources.

do-not-resuscitate (DNR) order: a request by a patient or surrogate to withhold cardiopulmonary resuscitation.

durable power of attorney: a legal document (sometimes called a **health care proxy**) that gives legal authority to another (a *health care agent*) to make medical decisions in the event of incapacitation.

ethical: in accordance with the accepted principles of right and wrong.

futile: medical care that will not improve the medical circumstances of a patient.

health care agent: a person given legal authority to make medical decisions for another in the event of incapacitation.

informed consent: a patient's or caregiver's agreement to undergo a treatment that has been adequately disclosed. Persons must be mentally competent in order to make the decision.

living will: a written statement that specifies the medical procedures desired or not desired in the event that a person is unable to communicate or is incapacitated; also called a **medical directive.**

maleficence (mah-LEF-eh-sens): the performance of evil or harm.

mechanical ventilation: life-sustaining treatment in which a mechanical ventilator is used to substitute for a patient's failing lungs.

patient autonomy: a principle of self-determination, such that patients (or surrogate decision makers) are free to choose the medical interventions that are acceptable to them, even if they choose to refuse interventions that may extend their lives.

persistent vegetative state: a vegetative mental state resulting from brain injury that persists for at least one month. Individuals lose awareness and the ability to think but retain noncognitive brain functions, such as motor reflexes and normal sleep patterns.

surrogate: a substitute; a person who takes the place of another.

definitively stated her "right to die" wishes and that her parents were unable to make such a request for her. The court also stated that preserving life, no matter what its quality, should take precedence over all other considerations. Nancy Cruzan's parents appealed the ruling, but in 1990 the U.S. Supreme Court upheld the Missouri Supreme Court in a five-to-four decision. Three witnesses were eventually found who could testify that Nancy would not desire life-sustaining treatment under the circumstances, and the court finally granted permission to remove the feeding tube. This court decision emphasizes the importance of having an **advance directive** (discussed later in this highlight) that clearly indicates one's preferences for medical treatment in the event of incapacitation.

In another case, family members desired continued care for a patient who was determined to be in a persistent vegetative state by the medical staff. The patient, Helga Wanglie, was an 86-year-old woman who had suffered severe brain damage after a stroke in a nursing home.[5] The medical team was unable to wean her from a respirator, and she was being fed with a feeding tube. Her physicians believed that further medical care was futile and medically inappropriate, but her husband argued that Helen would not have wanted anything done to shorten her life, despite having an irreversible condition. Although the hospital sought the legal appointment of a **conservator** to replace the husband in representing the patient, in 1991 a Minnesota court decided that the husband was the best person to make decisions on Helen's behalf and that his wishes should be followed. Several days after the decision was issued, Helen Wanglie died from multiple organ failure with the respirator and feeding tube in place. This case illustrates the strong consideration given a surrogate decision maker even when medical opinion opposes a demanded treatment.

Religious Viewpoints

The withdrawal of nutrition support and other life-sustaining treatments may not be acceptable to persons of some religious faiths. For example, Orthodox Jews believe that the soul is present in people who are alive (even if permanently unconscious) and disallow actions that would hasten death.[6] If a person's or family's religious beliefs are not in accord with medical recommendations, health practitioners are expected to consider the viewpoint and try to resolve the issue in some way. If practitioners are unable to comply with the wishes of a patient or caregivers, the care of the patient should be transferred elsewhere.

Advance Planning

Health care professionals should discuss the importance of advance directives with competent patients. Individuals are encouraged to discuss their medical preferences with family members and surrogate decision makers so that their wishes will be considered in the event that they become incapacitated. Advance directives are incorporated into the medical record and updated when appropriate. They take effect only if a physician determines that a patient lacks the ability to understand and make decisions about available treatments. If no advance directive is available and a person's preferences are unknown, decisions are based on a patient's best interests as determined by a caregiver or family member.[7]

Advance Directives

A person may declare medical preferences in a **living will**, sometimes called a **medical directive.** Living wills may include detailed instructions about life-sustaining procedures that a person does or does not want. In some states, nutrition and hydration are not considered life-sustaining treatments, and a person's instructions about them may need to be indicated separately. Another important directive is a **durable power of attorney** (sometimes called a **health care proxy**) in which another person (a **health care agent**) is appointed to act as decision maker in the event of incapacitation. The agent should understand one's medical preferences and be absolutely trustworthy. Only one person can be designated, although one or two alternates may also be listed. If an agent is given comprehensive power to supervise care, he or she may make decisions about medical staff, health care facilities, and medical procedures.

Laws regarding advance directives vary from state to state. Some states restrict the use of advance directives to terminal illness or disallow them if a woman is pregnant. State statutes also specify characteristics of people who may serve as health care agents and witnesses. Generally, advance directives created in one state are honored in another.

The Do-Not-Resuscitate Order

A **do-not-resuscitate (DNR) order** is frequently used to withhold cardiopulmonary resuscitation (CPR) in the event of cardiopulmonary arrest, which occurs too suddenly for deliberate decision making.[8] A DNR order is written in the medical record as are other directives, although it is important to advise decision makers that a DNR order does not exclude the use of other life-prolonging measures. A DNR order is most often used in patients with serious illnesses or advanced age. Some institutions allow physicians to write DNR orders for patients who have poor prognoses, but the physician must inform the patient or surrogate if this is done.

Organ and Tissue Donation

End-of-life decisions inevitably raise questions about a dying patient's preferences concerning organ and tissue donation. Even if a donor card has been signed, it is important to let family members know one's wishes, as they may need to sign a consent form in order for donation to occur. Although organ donation is a difficult topic to bring up near the time of death, potential donors can be assured that their gift could greatly enhance or save the lives of others.

Ethical questions sometimes arise when organs are donated. A physician must alert an organ procurement team about a donor's existence and arrange to maintain organ functions until organs are retrieved. Treatments that maintain the viability of organs and tissues cannot be used if they may cause harm to the donor. Sometimes the care of a donor and the needs of a potential recipient may appear to be in conflict, but the care of donors and recipients is always kept separate and performed by different physicians.[9]

Medical decisions that are planned in advance and discussed with close friends and family may help to prevent decision-making dilemmas during emergency situations. Health practitioners should provide the best information possible so that patients are encouraged to consider the medical options that are available and make their preferences known to medical personnel.

REFERENCES

1. M. A. Grippi, Ethics in critical care, in A. P. Fishman and coeditors, *Fishman's Manual of Pulmonary Diseases and Disorders* (New York: McGraw-Hill, 2002), pp. 1111–1114.
2. E. J. Emanuel, Bioethics in the practice of medicine, in L. Goldman and D. Ausiello, eds., *Cecil Textbook of Medicine* (Philadelphia: Saunders, 2004), pp. 5–9.
3. Emanuel, 2004.
4. J. O. Maillet, R. L. Potter, and L. Heller, Position of the American Dietetic Association: Ethical and legal issues in nutrition, hydration, and feeding, *Journal of the American Dietetic Association* 102 (2002): 716–726.
5. Maillet, Potter, and Heller, 2002.
6. Maillet, Potter, and Heller, 2002.
7. American College of Physicians, Ethics manual, *Annals of Internal Medicine* 128 (1998): 576–594.
8. American College of Physicians, 1998.
9. American College of Physicians, 1998.

Chapter 22

Nutrition in Metabolic and Respiratory Stress

Chapter Outline

Available Online

http://nutrition.wadsworth.com/uncn7

Student Practice Test

Glossary Terms

Nutrition on the Net

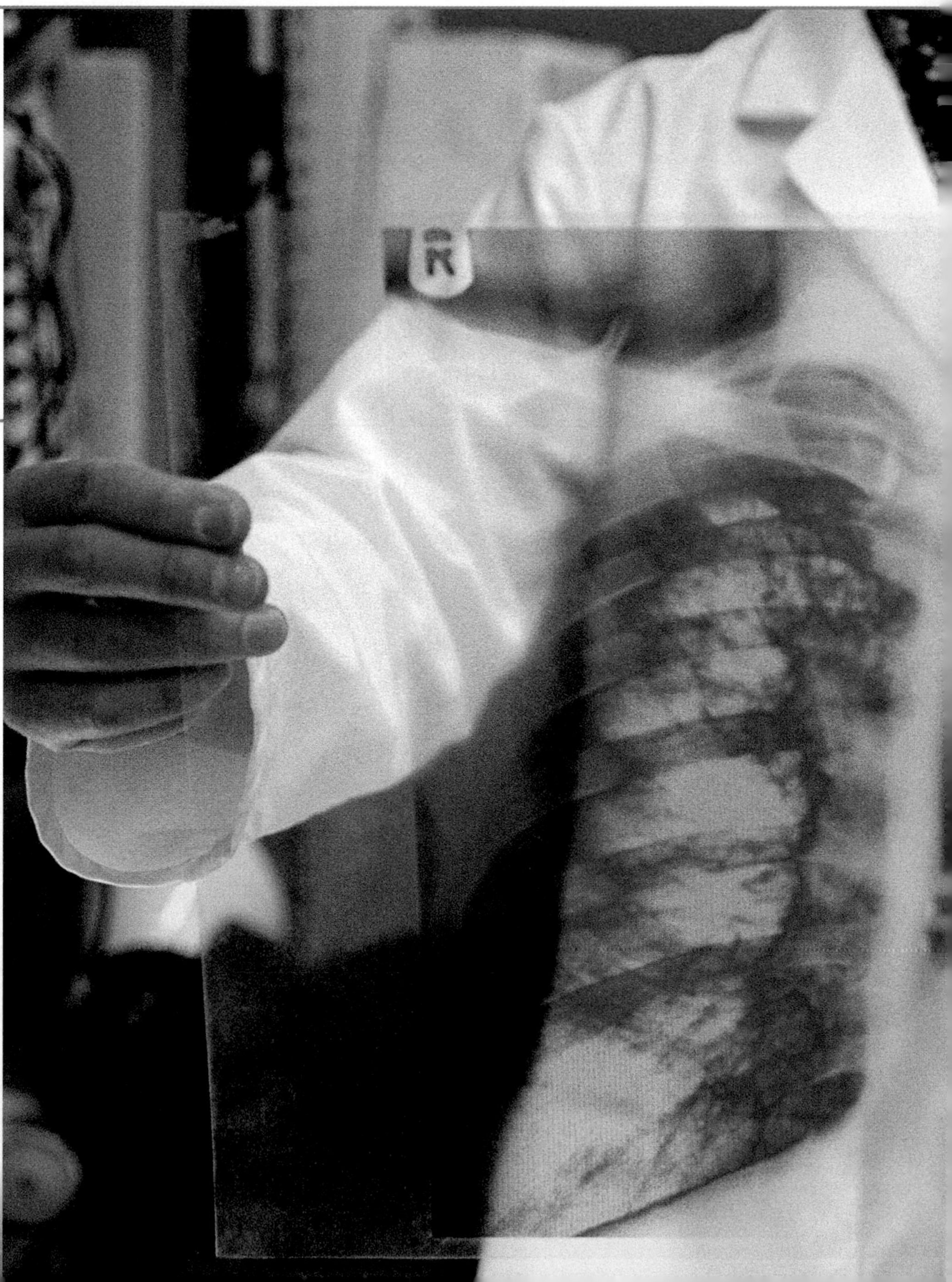

© Mark Douet/The Image Bank/Getty Images

Nutrition in the Professional Setting

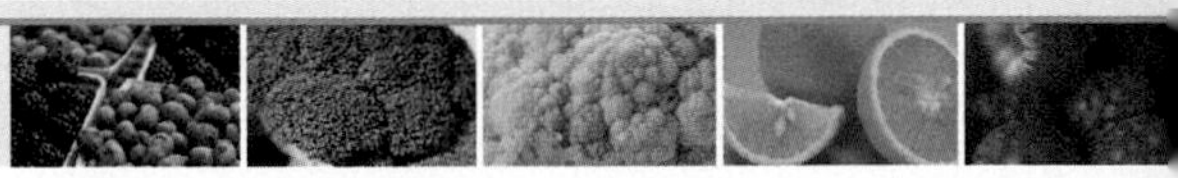

The body's dramatic response to severe stress can alter metabolism enough to threaten survival. Many patients require life support measures and intensive monitoring. Stress also raises nutritional needs considerably—increasing the risk of malnutrition even in previously healthy individuals. Not only is providing nutrition care for these patients challenging, but it is often ineffective for preventing weight loss and lean body losses. Despite these difficulties, the health care professional must determine the best measures to take in order to limit damage and promote recovery.

This chapter focuses on the nutrition care provided to patients who undergo certain types of physiological stress. **Metabolic stress,** a disruption in the body's internal chemical environment, can be caused by uncontrolled infections or extensive tissue damage, such as deep, penetrating wounds or multiple broken bones. As the first sections of the chapter explain, the body's stress response is an attempt to restore balance, but it can have both helpful and harmful effects. The last sections of this chapter deal with **respiratory stress,** characterized by inadequate oxygen and excessive carbon dioxide in the blood and tissues. Both types of stressful conditions may result in **hypermetabolism** (above-normal metabolic rate), **wasting** (breakdown of muscle mass and loss of strength), and, in severe circumstances, life-threatening complications. The highlight following this chapter discusses the causes and consequences of **multiple organ failure,** the simultaneous loss of function of more than one organ system, which is often fatal.

metabolic stress: a disruption in the body's chemical environment due to the effects of disease or injury. Metabolic stress is characterized by changes in metabolic rate, heart rate, blood pressure, hormonal status, and nutrient metabolism.

respiratory stress: inadequate gas exchange between the air and blood, resulting in lower oxygen and higher carbon dioxide levels.

hypermetabolism: a higher-than-normal metabolic rate.

wasting: the breakdown of lean tissue that results from disease or malnutrition.

multiple organ failure: a failure of more than one organ system that occurs during intensive care; often results in death.

The Body's Responses to Stress and Injury

The stress response is the body's *nonspecific* response to a variety of stressors.■ The body's actions focus on immediate survival, while functions of less consequence are delayed. Energy is of primary importance, so energy nutrients are mobilized from storage and made available in the blood. Heart rate and respiration (breathing rate) increase to deliver oxygen and nutrients to cells more quickly, and blood pressure rises. Meanwhile, energy is diverted from processes that are not life sustaining, such as growth, reproduction, and long-term immunity. If stress continues for a long period, interference with these processes begins to cause damage, which can result in growth retardation and illness.

■ Examples of stressors that can lead to metabolic stress include infection, surgery, burns, fractures, extensive bleeding, and deep wounds, such as surgical incisions and gunshot wounds.

Hormonal Responses to Stress

The stress response is mediated by several hormones, which are released into the blood soon after the onset of injury (see Table 22-1).[1] The catecholamines (epinephrine and norepinephrine), often called the "fight-or-flight" hormones, stimulate heart muscle, alter the rate of blood flow, and raise basal metabolic rate. Epinephrine also prompts the secretion of glucagon by the pancreas, causing the release of nutrients from storage. The steroid hormone cortisol enhances protein degradation, which raises amino acid levels in the blood so that they become available for conversion to glucose. All of these hormones result in similar effects on glucose and fat metabolism, causing the breakdown of glycogen (glycogenolysis), the production of glucose from amino acids (gluconeogenesis), and the breakdown of triglycerides in adipose tissue (lipolysis).■ Two other hormones induced by stress, aldosterone and antidiuretic hormone,■ help to maintain blood volume.

Cortisol's effects can be physically detrimental when stress is prolonged. In excess, cortisol causes the depletion of protein in muscle, bone, connective tissue, and skin. It impairs wound healing, and therefore high levels are especially dangerous for a patient with severe injuries. Because cortisol inhibits protein synthesis, eating more protein cannot easily reverse tissue losses. Excess cortisol also disrupts calcium metabolism and causes insulin resistance and abnormal fat deposition. In addition, cortisol suppresses immune responses, increasing susceptibility to infection.■

■ The catecholamines, glucagon, and cortisol have actions opposite those of insulin and are therefore sometimes referred to as **counterregulatory hormones.**

■ Reminder: *Aldosterone* and *antidiuretic hormone* stimulate the kidneys to reabsorb more sodium and water, respectively.

■ Pharmaceutical forms of cortisol are common anti-inflammatory medications (examples include *cortisone* and *prednisone*). Their long-term use may cause undesirable side effects, such as muscle wasting, thinning of the skin, diabetes, and early osteoporosis.

The Inflammatory Response

Cells of the immune system mount a quick, nonspecific response to infection or tissue injury.[2] This **inflammatory response** serves to contain and destroy infectious agents (and their products) and prevent further tissue damage. As in the hormonal response, there is a delicate balance between a response that protects tissues from further injury and an excessive response that can cause additional damage to tissue.

The Inflammatory Process The inflammatory response begins with the dilation of blood vessels that deliver blood to a site of injury (arterioles) and the constriction of small blood vessels that carry blood away from an infected area (venules). Increased permeability of capillaries within the damaged tissue allows inflowing fluid to accumulate, causing localized edema. These changes in blood vessels■ prevent the spread of infection and encourage the entry of immune cells that can destroy foreign agents (see Figure 22-1). The first cells on the scene are the phagocytes (neutrophils and macrophages), which slip through gaps between the endothelial cells that form the vessel walls. The phagocytes engulf microorganisms and destroy them with hydrolytic enzymes and reactive forms of oxygen. When inflammation becomes chronic, these normally useful products of phagocytes can damage healthy tissue.

■ Classic signs of inflammation that accompany altered blood flow:
- **Swelling**—from the accumulation of fluid at the site of injury.
- **Redness**—from the dilation of small blood vessels in the injured area.
- **Heat**—from the influx of warm arterial blood.
- **Pain**—from the pressure of edema within damaged tissue and the actions of certain chemical mediators on pain receptors.

inflammatory response: the metabolic responses of the immune system to infection or injury.

TABLE 22-1 Metabolic Effects of Hormones Released during the Stress Response

Hormone	Metabolic Effects
Catecholamines	• Increase in metabolic rate • Glycogen breakdown in liver and muscle • Glucose production from amino acids • Release of fatty acids from adipose tissue • Glucagon secretion from pancreas
Glucagon	• Glycogen breakdown in liver • Glucose production from amino acids • Release of fatty acids from adipose tissue
Cortisol	• Protein degradation • Enhancement of glucagon's action on liver glycogen • Glucose production from amino acids • Release of fatty acids from adipose tissue
Aldosterone	• Retention of sodium
Antidiuretic hormone	• Retention of water

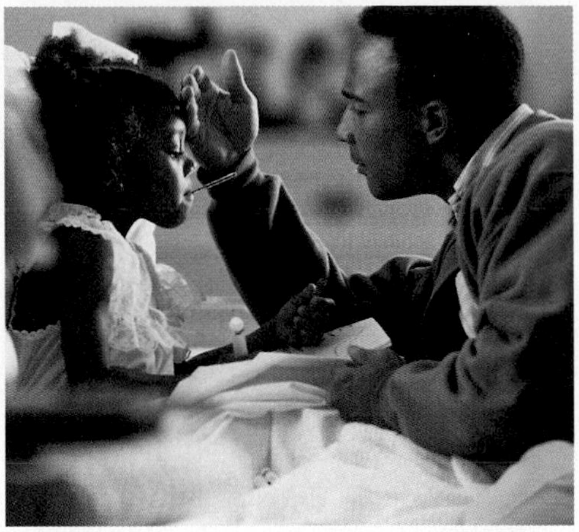

The immune system mounts a quick response to infection and promotes healing of illness and injury.

Mediators of Inflammation Numerous chemical substances control the inflammatory process. These *mediators* are usually released from damaged tissue, blood vessel cells, and activated immune cells. Many of them help to regulate more than one step in the process. Some of the examples that follow were introduced in Highlight 17's discussion of immunity. Histamine, a small molecule similar to an amino acid in structure, is released from granules within **mast cells** and causes vasodilation and capillary permeability.■ Fragments of complement proteins■ trigger histamine release from mast cells and help to recruit and activate phagocytes. The cytokines■ and eicosanoids■ also participate in the inflammatory process. Note that most anti-inflammatory medications, including both steroidal drugs (such as cortisone and prednisone) and nonsteroidal anti-inflammatory drugs (such as aspirin and ibuprofen), act by blocking eicosanoid synthesis.

Changing dietary fat sources can have subtle effects on the inflammatory process.[3] The major precursor for the eicosanoids is arachidonic acid, which is derived from omega-6 fatty acids in vegetable oils. Some omega-3 fatty acids compete

■ *Antihistamines* are medications taken to reduce the effects of histamine.

■ Reminder: *Complement* is a collective term for a group of plasma proteins that assist the activities of antibodies.

■ Reminder: *Cytokines* are proteins produced by white blood cells that regulate immune cell development and activity.

■ Reminder: *Eicosanoids* are derivatives of 20-carbon fatty acids that help to regulate blood pressure, blood clotting, and other body functions.

mast cells: cells within connective tissue that produce and release histamine.

FIGURE 22-1 The Inflammatory Process

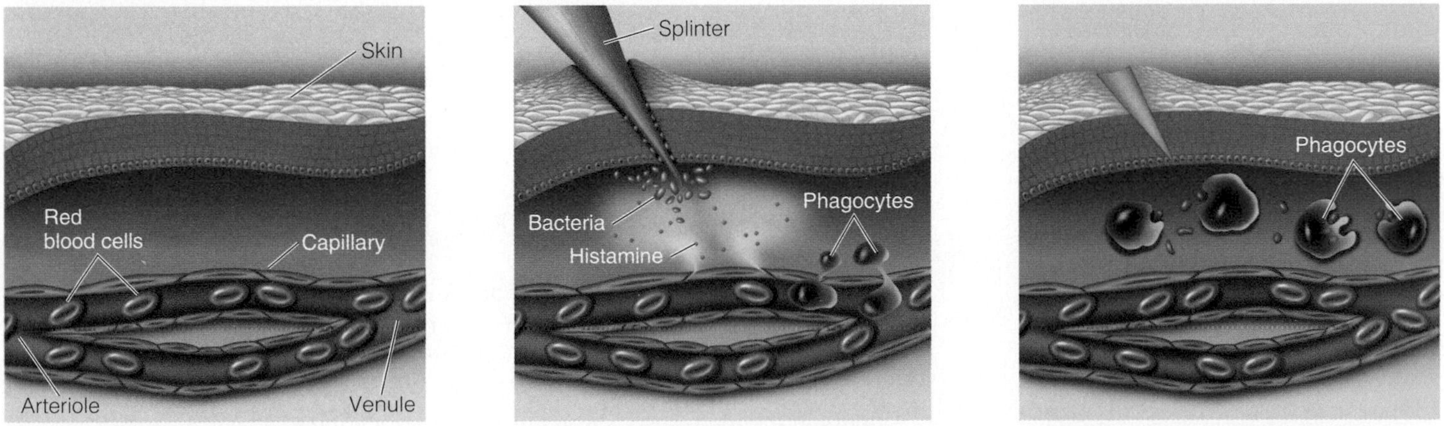
Skin
Red blood cells
Capillary
Arteriole
Venule
Splinter
Bacteria
Histamine
Phagocytes
Phagocytes

Cells lining the blood vessels lie close together, and normally do not allow the contents to cross into tissue.

When tissues are damaged, immune cells release histamine, which dilates some blood vessels, increasing blood flow to the damaged area. Fluid leaks out of capillaries (causing swelling), and phagocytes escape between the small gaps in the blood vessel walls.

Phagocytes engulf bacteria and disable them with hydrolytic enzymes and reactive forms of oxygen.

with arachidonic acid and inhibit the production of the most powerful inflammatory mediators. Partially replacing vegetable oils rich in omega-6 fatty acids with sources high in omega-3 fatty acids (such as fish oil) helps to suppress inflammation, but it is not a reliable treatment.

Systemic Effects of Inflammation Cytokines released during the inflammatory process can also provoke changes in the rest of the body. Within hours (or, in some cases, days) after infection, inflammation, or severe injury, the liver steps up its production of certain proteins in an effort known as the **acute-phase response.**[4] These acute-phase proteins include **C-reactive protein,■** complement, blood-clotting proteins such as fibrinogen and prothrombin, and others. At the same time, plasma concentrations of albumin, iron, and zinc fall (recall from Chapter 17 that albumin levels are often measured to assess health and nutrition status). The acute-phase response is also accompanied by muscle catabolism to make amino acids available for gluconeogenesis, tissue repair, and immune protein synthesis; consequently, negative nitrogen balance (and wasting) frequently results. Other clinical characteristics include an elevated metabolic rate, increased neutrophil numbers, lethargy, anorexia, and often, fever.

■ C-reactive protein, the best clinical indicator of the acute-phase response, also becomes elevated during many chronic diseases.

Severe inflammation that persists for more than a few days can lead to a life-threatening condition: the **systemic inflammatory response syndrome (SIRS).** SIRS is a whole-body response to unresolved inflammation and is diagnosed when a patient's condition becomes severe enough to raise heart rate, respiratory rate, white blood cells, and/or body temperature to critical levels. If identical symptoms result from infection, the condition is called **sepsis.** Complications associated with SIRS or sepsis include excessive fluid retention and tissue edema, low blood pressure, and impaired blood flow. The inability to supply tissues with adequate oxygen and nutrients may eventually cause symptoms of **shock■** and multiple organ failure (see Highlight 22).

■ Shock is a syndrome initiated by an inadequate blood supply that threatens the functioning of multiple organs. It results from injuries, bleeding, sepsis, and other severe conditions and is characterized by reduced blood pressure, rapid heart rate, increased respiration, and muscle weakness.

IN SUMMARY The stress and inflammatory responses are the body's nonspecific responses to stressors that cause infection and injury. The stress response is mediated by the catecholamine hormones, cortisol, and glucagon, which together raise nutrient levels in blood, stimulate heart rate, and constrict blood vessels. Aldosterone and antidiuretic hormone help to maintain adequate blood volume. Chemicals released from damaged tissues, immune cells, and blood vessels mediate the inflammatory response. Signs of inflammation in injured tissues include swelling, redness, heat, and pain. The inflammatory process can also cause systemic effects that alter metabolism, heart rate, blood pressure, body temperature, and immune cell functions. Persistent, severe inflammation may result in shock and lead to multiple organ dysfunction and consequent failure.

acute-phase response: changes in body chemistry resulting from infection, inflammation, or injury; characterized by alterations in plasma proteins.

C-reactive protein: an acute-phase protein released from the liver during acute inflammation or stress.

systemic inflammatory response syndrome (SIRS): a whole-body response to acute inflammation; characterized by raised heart and respiratory rates, abnormal white blood cell counts, and altered body temperature.

sepsis: an acute inflammatory response caused by infection; characterized by symptoms similar to those of SIRS.

shock: a dangerous physiological response to injury, bleeding, or infection that is characterized by an inadequate blood supply; associated with reduced blood pressure, raised heart and respiratory rates, and muscle weakness.

abscesses (ab-SESS-es): accumulated pus that is surrounded by inflamed tissue.

debridement: the surgical removal of dead, damaged, or contaminated tissue resulting from burns or wounds; helps to prevent infection and hasten healing.

Nutrition Support for Acute Stress

As described earlier, the body's responses to metabolic stress may worsen illness and even threaten survival. Therefore, a critical care unit must manage both the acute medical condition that initiated stress and the complications of the stress and inflammatory responses. In addition, many patients have one or more dysfunctional organ systems that require aggressive support.

The immediate concerns during severe stress are usually to restore lost fluids and electrolytes and to remove underlying stressors. Therefore, initial treatments include giving intravenous solutions to correct fluid and electrolyte imbalances, treating infections, repairing wounds, draining **abscesses** (pus), and removing dead tissue **(debridement).** After stabilization, nutrient needs can be estimated and nutrition support provided.

Determining Nutritional Requirements

The most notable metabolic changes in patients undergoing metabolic stress include hypermetabolism, negative nitrogen balance, hyperglycemia, and insulin resistance.[5] Hypermetabolism and negative nitrogen balance can result in wasting, which can worsen organ function and delay recovery. Hyperglycemia increases the risk of infection, a dangerous problem during critical illness. Therefore, the principal nutritional goals are to provide a diet that preserves lean tissue content, maintains immune defenses, and promotes healing.

Feeding an acutely stressed patient is challenging. Overfeeding increases the risks of refeeding syndrome (discussed in Chapter 21)■ and its associated hyperglycemia. Underfeeding worsens nitrogen balance and may increase lean tissue losses. The assessment of nutritional needs is not always straightforward because fluid imbalances prevent accurate measurements of weight and laboratory data reflect the metabolic alterations of illness rather than a person's nutritional status.

■ Reminder: *Refeeding syndrome* leads to electrolyte and fluid imbalances and hyperglycemia.

The amounts of protein and energy to provide during acute illness are controversial and still under investigation. Experimentation is difficult in patients who are critically ill, and therefore research results are mixed. Also, the wide assortment of acute medical conditions that cause metabolic stress makes each patient's situation somewhat unique. The guidelines presented here are subject to change as new findings help to resolve the complex issues related to nutrient intakes and delivery methods. In all cases, clinicians need to closely observe patients' responses to feedings and readjust nutrient intakes as necessary.

Estimation of Energy Needs A common method for determining the energy needs of acutely stressed individuals is to estimate basal energy expenditure (BEE) using the **Harris-Benedict equation** and then multiply the result by a stress factor to account for the increased energy requirements of stress and healing. This method is described in Table 22-2, and the "How to" presents an example. Although a direct measurement of basal metabolism by indirect calorimetry is much preferred, many facilities do not have the proper equipment, personnel, or time to make routine measurements in critically ill patients. Stress factors vary according to the severity of the illness and the patient's nutritional status, and the particular values that are used vary among institutions; those listed in Table 22-2 are given as examples. The energy expenditure of critical care patients may be raised further

TABLE 22-2 Estimating Energy Needs for Acute Metabolic Stress

Step 1. Estimate energy needs to support basal energy expenditure (BEE) using the Harris-Benedict equation.[a]

Women: BEE = 655.1 + [9.563 × weight (kg)] + [1.85 × height (cm)] − [4.676 × age (years)].

Men: BEE = 66.5 + [13.75 × weight (kg)] + [5.003 × height (cm)] − [6.775 × age (years)].

Step 2. Multiply BEE by an appropriate stress factor for acute illness. For example:[b]

- Postoperative (no complications): 1.00 to 1.05
- Peritonitis: 1.05 to 1.25
- Cancer: 1.10 to 1.45
- Long bone fracture: 1.25 to 1.30
- Severe infection: 1.3 to 1.55
- Multiple trauma: 1.3 to 1.55
- Burns (over 40% body surface): 2.0

Adjustment for obesity:

For persons with BMI >30, use an adjusted body weight in the BEE equation. One suggestion is to use an adjusted weight based on ideal body weight (IBW):[c]

Adjusted weight = IBW + [0.5 × (actual body weight − IBW)].

[a]L. J. Hoffer, Protein and energy provision in critical illness. *American Journal of Clinical Nutrition* 78 (2003): 906–911.
[b]W. W. Souba and D. Wilmore, Diet and nutrition in the care of the patient with surgery, trauma, and sepsis, *Modern Nutrition in Health and Disease* (Baltimore: Williams & Wilkins, 1999), p. 1593.
[c]N. Barak and coauthors, Evaluation of stress factors and body weight adjustments currently used to estimate energy expenditure in hospitalized patients, *Journal of Parenteral and Enteral Nutrition* 26 (2002): 231–238.

Harris-Benedict equation: an equation that estimates basal energy expenditure.

HOW TO Estimate Energy and Protein Needs during Acute Stress

Eve is a 39-year-old female who is 5 feet 3 inches tall and weighs 130 pounds. She recently broke a leg and an arm while skiing. Her energy needs may be estimated using the Harris-Benedict equation and a stress factor as follows:

$$\text{Weight in kilograms} = 130 \text{ lb} \div 2.2 \text{ kg/lb} = 59 \text{ kg.}$$

$$\text{Height in centimeters} = 63 \text{ in} \times 2.54 \text{ cm/in} = 160 \text{ cm.}$$

$$\begin{aligned} \text{BEE} &= 655.1 + [9.563 \times \text{weight (kg)}] + [1.85 \times \text{height (cm)}] - [4.676 \times \text{age (years)}] \\ &= 655.1 + (9.563 \times 59) + (1.85 \times 160) - (4.676 \times 39) \\ &= 1333 \text{ kcal.} \end{aligned}$$

Stress factor (see Table 22-2): 1.25.

$$\text{BEE} \times \text{stress factor} = 1333 \times 1.25 = 1666 \text{ kcal.}$$

Eve's energy needs are about 1666 kcalories. Her weight changes can be monitored to determine if her actual needs are higher or lower. In addition, her energy needs are likely to change as stress resolves.

Eve's protein requirements may be estimated using an appropriate protein factor between 1.0 and 2.0 grams per kilogram body weight (g/kg). Assuming that Eve could obtain adequate protein using the factor 1.0 g/kg:

$$\text{Recommended protein intake: } 1.0 \text{ g/kg} \times 59 \text{ kg} = 59 \text{ g protein.}$$

Using the protein factor 1.5 g/kg instead:

$$\text{Protein intake: } 1.5 \text{ g/kg} \times 59 \text{ kg} = 88.5 \text{ g protein.}$$

To calculate the amount of fat and carbohydrate to provide, clinicians usually subtract the protein kcalories from the total energy needs and then supply the remaining kcalories from carbohydrates and fat. Using the second protein prescription in the example, Eve would be given 1312 kcalories from carbohydrate and fat:

$$\text{Carbohydrate and fat kcalories} = 1666 \text{ kcal} - (88.5 \text{ g protein} \times 4 \text{ kcal/g}).$$

$$1666 \text{ kcal (total)} - 354 \text{ kcal (protein)} = 1312 \text{ kcal (carbohydrate and fat).}$$

due to fever, mechanical ventilation, restlessness, and the presence of open wounds.

Another popular method of estimating energy needs is to multiply a patient's body weight by a factor appropriate for the person's medical condition. For example, energy needs for patients with sepsis have been estimated to be 25 to 30 kcalories per kilogram body weight daily;[6] a patient weighing 160 pounds (72.7 kilograms) may therefore require between 1818 and 2181 kcalories per day. The energy intake may be started within this range and then adjusted as the patient's body weight and other determinants of nutrition status change.

■ Reminder: The protein RDA for adults is 0.8 g per kilogram body weight.

Estimation of Protein Needs To protect lean tissue, the protein intakes recommended during acute stress are higher than DRI values.■ Even with adequate protein, however, negative nitrogen balance cannot be prevented because metabolic processes during stress encourage protein catabolism. Protein recommendations vary according to the severity of a condition and are usually estimated to be between 1.0 and 2.0 grams per kilogram body weight for most conditions. The "How to" includes a sample calculation of protein requirements.

The amino acids glutamine and arginine are sometimes added to the diets of acutely stressed and immune-compromised patients. Several studies have suggested that glutamine supplementation is associated with fewer infections, shorter hospital stays, and reduced mortality rates in critically ill patients.[7] Arginine supplementation has been shown to have beneficial effects on the immune responses of postoperative patients.[8] Although glutamine and arginine are often added to enteral formulas promoted for wound healing and enhanced immunity, their use remains controversial.

Carbohydrates and Lipids The bulk of energy needs are supplied from carbohydrate and fat. Carbohydrate is usually the main source of energy and may provide up to 70 percent of kcalories depending on a patient's condition. When parenteral feedings are necessary, dextrose is usually provided to critically ill patients at no more than 5 milligrams per kilogram body weight per minute (see p. 683). Fat provides both energy and essential fatty acids and may supply up to 40 percent of kcalories.

Micronutrients Acutely stressed patients may have increased micronutrient needs, but specific requirements have not been determined. In hypermetabolic patients, the need for B vitamins may be higher to support the increase in energy metabolism. A number of micronutrients, such as zinc, vitamin C, and vitamin A, have critical roles in immunity and wound healing, and their supplementation may speed recovery in certain circumstances. Patients with burns and tissue injury may have increased requirements for trace minerals due to tissue losses; in several studies, supplementation of zinc, copper, and selenium reduced infection rates in burn patients during recovery.[9]

Plasma levels of micronutrients are often altered during critical illness. The acute-phase response causes a redistribution of some micronutrients (such as zinc and iron) that lowers their blood levels; therefore, micronutrient status is sometimes difficult to interpret. Blood concentrations of trace minerals should be monitored in patients receiving parenteral nutrition support to ensure that excessive amounts are not given intravenously.[10]

Nutrient Delivery As Chapter 21 explained, enteral nutrition support is generally preferred over parenteral nutrition in patients with normal intestinal function. Recent studies, however, have not supported earlier beliefs that disuse of the gastrointestinal (GI) tract during parenteral support would lead to intestinal atrophy and increase the risk of **bacterial translocation** from the intestine to the rest of the body.[11] The incidence of bacterial translocation appears to be similar in patients receiving either type of nutrition support. In addition, alterations in intestinal structure and function have been documented in patients receiving enteral nutrition, which raises doubt about the "protection" offered by enteral feedings.[12]

Parenteral nutrition support is indicated in patients who cannot achieve adequate nutrient intakes using enteral feedings. In one study of critically ill patients, only 53 percent were able to obtain adequate nutrient intakes from enteral feedings alone, and energy intakes averaged 77 percent of the amounts prescribed.[13] Therefore, parenteral nutrition is sometimes used to supplement enteral feedings, or it may be used as the main source of nutrients in patients who are likely to become malnourished during critical illness.

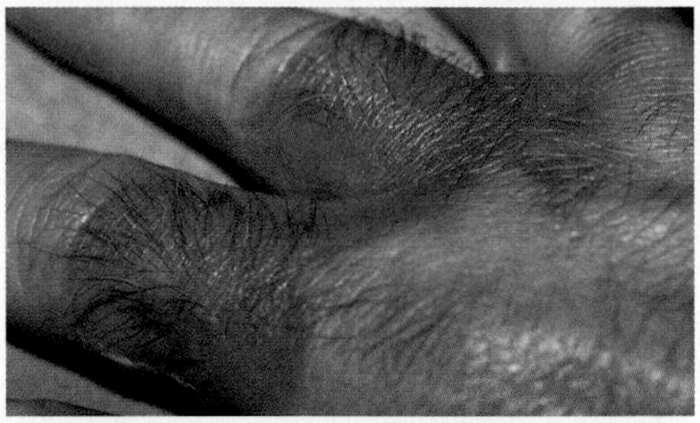

A first-degree burn injures the epidermis and is characterized by pink or reddened skin.

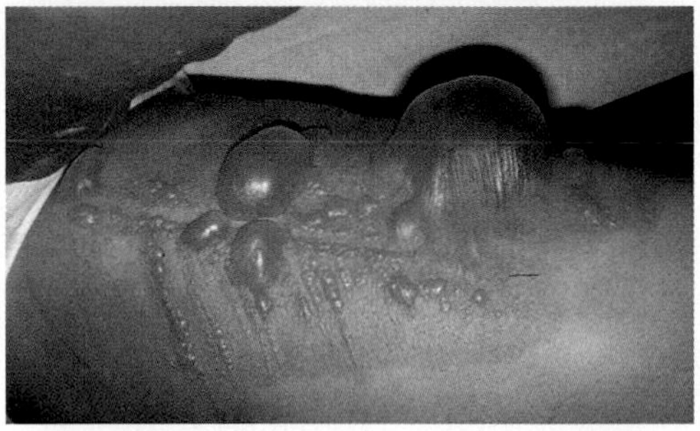

A second-degree burn damages the epidermis and a portion of the dermis and causes redness, swelling, and blistering.

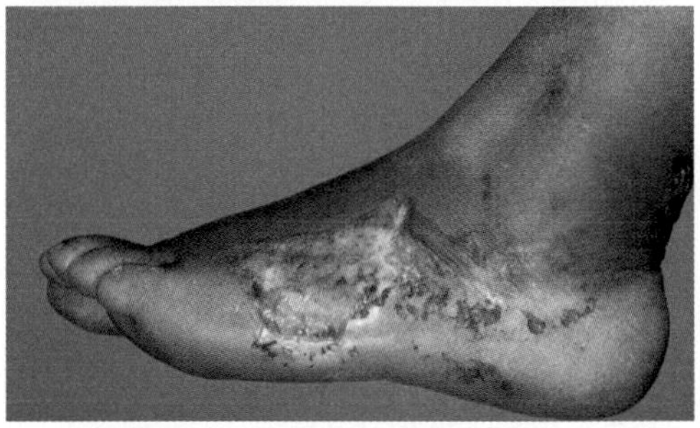

A third-degree burn destroys both the epidermis and dermis and may involve the tissues beneath the skin.

Patients with Burns

Burns are among the most severe injuries that a person may experience. They rank third among the causes of death from accidents in the United States[14] and have destructive effects on growth and health that may persist long after a burn has healed.[15] Causes of burns include flames or scalding water, chemical agents, electricity, and irradiation. When death results, it is usually due to infection.[16]

Burn Classification Burns are classified according to how deeply they penetrate the skin and underlying tissue. First-degree burns affect only the **epidermis** and are pink or red, dry, and painful (for example, a sunburn). Second-degree burns (also called partial-thickness burns) involve both the epidermis and the **dermis** and are red, wet, and blistery; they are extremely painful because nerve endings are exposed. Third-degree burns (also known as full-thickness burns) extend into the tissue below the dermis; they may be white, yellow-brown, or charred and appear dry and leathery. These burns are deep enough to destroy nerves and therefore are not painful.

Burn size in adults is often estimated by dividing the body into 11 parts; each part represents about 9 percent of the total body surface area (TBSA).[17] The head and neck region and each arm are equivalent to about 9 percent TBSA each; the

bacterial translocation: the transfer of bacteria from the intestinal lumen to the bloodstream; increases risks of infection and sepsis.

epidermis (e-pi-DER-miss): the outer layer of the skin.

dermis: the connective tissue layer underneath the epidermis that contains the skin's blood vessels and nerves.

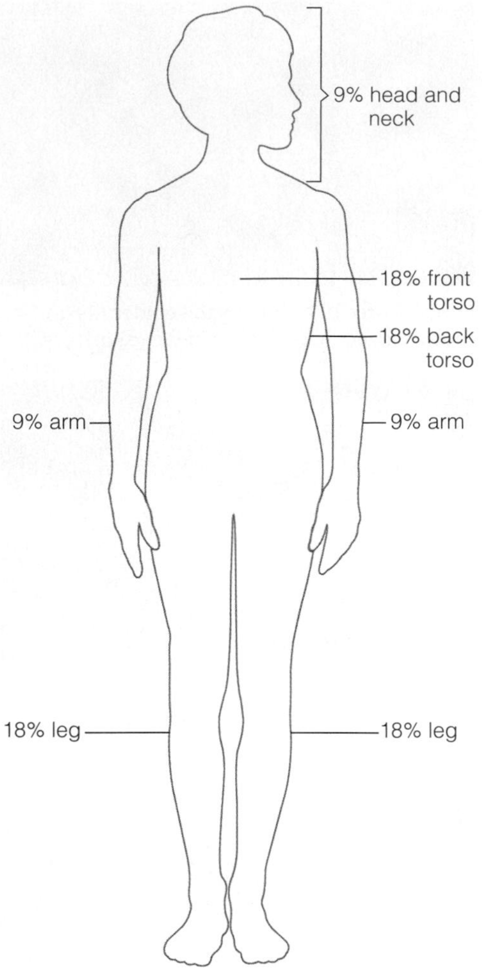
9% head and neck
18% front torso
18% back torso
9% arm
9% arm
18% leg
18% leg

Burn size can be estimated by sectioning the total body surface area (TBSA) as shown.

front torso, the back torso, and each leg represent approximately 18 percent TBSA each (margin drawing). The severity of a burn is based both on its thickness and on the amount of surface area involved.

Treatment Emergency measures after a burn include the removal of clothing, smoldering material, or chemical agents from the skin. The burn is then submerged or flushed with copious amounts of water. Wounds are cleaned and debris removed. The burn area is assessed for possible infection. Blisters and dead tissue are debrided, if necessary. Finally, the surface is covered with topical antibacterial agents and sterile dressings. Immediate care also includes fluid replacement and diagnosis of metabolic disturbances. Some burn victims need immediate oxygen support or mechanical ventilation. Pain relief medication is also required soon after injury.

Metabolic Changes Burns cause severe metabolic stress and the inflammatory response, as discussed earlier in this chapter, and therefore lead to hypermetabolism, tissue breakdown, and alterations in nutrient metabolism. With the protective skin barrier partially destroyed, burns are also accompanied by losses of evaporative water and body heat. Second- and third-degree burns may cause substantial losses of protein and micronutrients. Major burns (25 to 30 percent TBSA) may cause systemic edema. Gastrointestinal function may be disrupted if burns cover 40 to 50 percent TBSA.

Nutrition Support Intravenous fluid and electrolyte replacement is usually maintained during the first 24 to 48 hours after injury.[18] The goals of fluid replacement are to maintain adequate blood volume and blood pressure and to avoid shock; urine and hemoglobin levels are monitored to ensure adequate fluid input. After one or two days, nutrition support is usually needed in patients with burns affecting 20 percent TBSA or more and in those who were malnourished before injury.

The objectives of nutrition care are to achieve nitrogen balance and minimize tissue losses, promote wound healing, and maintain immune defenses.[19] Although energy needs may be calculated as described in Table 22-2 on p. 697, other methods that consider additional factors such as burn severity and ventilator use can be used during peak recovery periods; Table 22-3 shows several popular options. Protein intakes should average 2.0 grams per kilogram body weight or 20 percent of total kcalories, especially if patients have burns greater than 10 percent TBSA. Micronutrient supplements are often provided and may include high amounts of zinc and vitamins A and C, which are thought to support immunity and promote wound healing.

TABLE 22-3 Equations for Calculating Energy Requirements of Burn Patients

Curreri Equation

Energy needs are influenced by the percentage of total body surface area (TBSA) that is burned.

Ages 16–59: [25 kcal × preburn weight (kg)] + (40 kcal × %TBSA*).

Ages 60 and above: [20 kcal × preburn weight (kg)] + (65 kcal × %TBSA*).

*For burns over 50% TBSA, use the value 50% to prevent overestimation of needs.

Modified Harris-Benedict Equation

Use the Harris-Benedict equation to determine BEE and multiply by activity and injury factors as follows:

Energy requirement = BEE × activity factor × injury factor.

- Activity factor: 1.2 if confined to bed; 1.3 if out of bed
- Injury factor: 2.1 (from thermal burn)

SOURCE: Adapted from *Manual of Clinical Dietetics,* 6th edition, © 2000 American Dietetic Association. Reprinted with permission.

CASE STUDY

Journalist with a Severe Burn

Mr. Bray, a 48-year-old journalist, has been admitted to intensive care. He suffered first- and second-degree burns covering over 30 percent of his body when he was trapped inside a burning building. His wife told the nurse that Mr. Bray's height is 6 feet and that he weighed about 175 pounds before he was injured. The physician ordered lab work, including serum protein concentrations, but the results have not yet been received.

1. Describe Mr. Bray's immediate needs after injury. Identify the initial concerns of the health care team and the measures they must take soon after Mr. Bray's arrival at the hospital.
2. Considering Mr. Bray's condition, what problems might the health care team encounter when they attempt to obtain information that can help them assess his nutritional status? What additional concerns might they have if Mr. Bray was malnourished before he experienced the burn?
3. Calculate Mr. Bray's energy and protein needs (use a protein factor of 2 g/kg). Discuss other nutrients that may be of concern during recovery.
4. Due to complications that developed during tube feeding, Mr. Bray was able to obtain only 70 percent of his energy requirements. What other feeding options may be considered?

To help meet energy and protein needs, patients who are able to eat may be given oral supplements and nutrient-dense snacks. Tube feedings are often used to supplement or replace oral feedings if patients cannot obtain the nutrients they need orally. Some burn patients develop gastric ileus and may require nasoenteric feedings (discussed in Chapter 20). Parenteral support may be required if intestinal function is lacking, if complications develop that interfere with enteral feedings, or if nutrient requirements cannot be met by tube feeding alone. The accompanying case study reviews the nutrition care of a burn patient.

IN SUMMARY Severe metabolic stress causes hypermetabolism and negative nitrogen balance and may result in wasting. The main nutrition objectives are to provide a diet that can preserve lean tissue, maintain immune defenses, and promote healing. Energy intake should sustain nitrogen balance but should not result in overfeeding. Protein recommendations are increased to help prevent the loss of lean tissue and allow healing of damaged tissue. Micronutrient requirements may be increased during acute stress and recovery from illness. Enteral and parenteral feedings are sometimes needed to meet the high energy and protein requirements of acutely stressed patients. Burn patients require fluid and electrolyte replacement during the first 24 to 48 hours after injury and also have extremely high energy and protein needs during the recovery period.

Nutrition and Respiratory Stress

The oxidation of nutrients produces carbon dioxide, a waste product that is removed from the body when breath is exhaled. Some medical conditions cause respiratory stress, which upsets the normal gas exchange process between the air and blood. The result is a reduction in the blood's oxygen supply and an increase in carbon dioxide levels. Lung diseases can therefore make exercise difficult and may eventually result in muscle loss. Excess carbon dioxide in blood can disrupt the breathing pattern and may interfere with the food intake of some individuals. Labored breathing entails a higher energy cost than normal breathing does, and this can raise energy needs and increase carbon dioxide production further. Weight loss and malnutrition become dangerous clinical outcomes of some respiratory illnesses, and poor nutritional status, in turn, worsens the progression of lung disease and increases mortality risk.

Chronic Obstructive Pulmonary Disease

Chronic obstructive pulmonary disease (COPD) refers to a group of conditions characterized by persistent obstruction of airflow through the lungs. The two major types of COPD are **chronic bronchitis** and **emphysema,** and many patients display features of both conditions. Figure 22-2 illustrates the main airways **(bronchi** and **bronchioles)** and air sacs **(alveoli)** of the normal respiratory system, and Figure 22-3 shows how they are altered in COPD. Both chronic bronchitis and emphysema reduce the capacity of the lungs to maintain normal oxygen and carbon dioxide levels in blood; shortness of breath **(dyspnea)** results and may eventually cause respiratory or heart failure. COPD ranks as the fourth leading cause of death in the United States.

FIGURE 22-2 The Respiratory System

Inhaled air travels via the trachea to the bronchi and bronchioles, the major airways of the lungs. Oxygen and carbon dioxide are exchanged across the thin-walled alveoli, which are surrounded by capillaries.

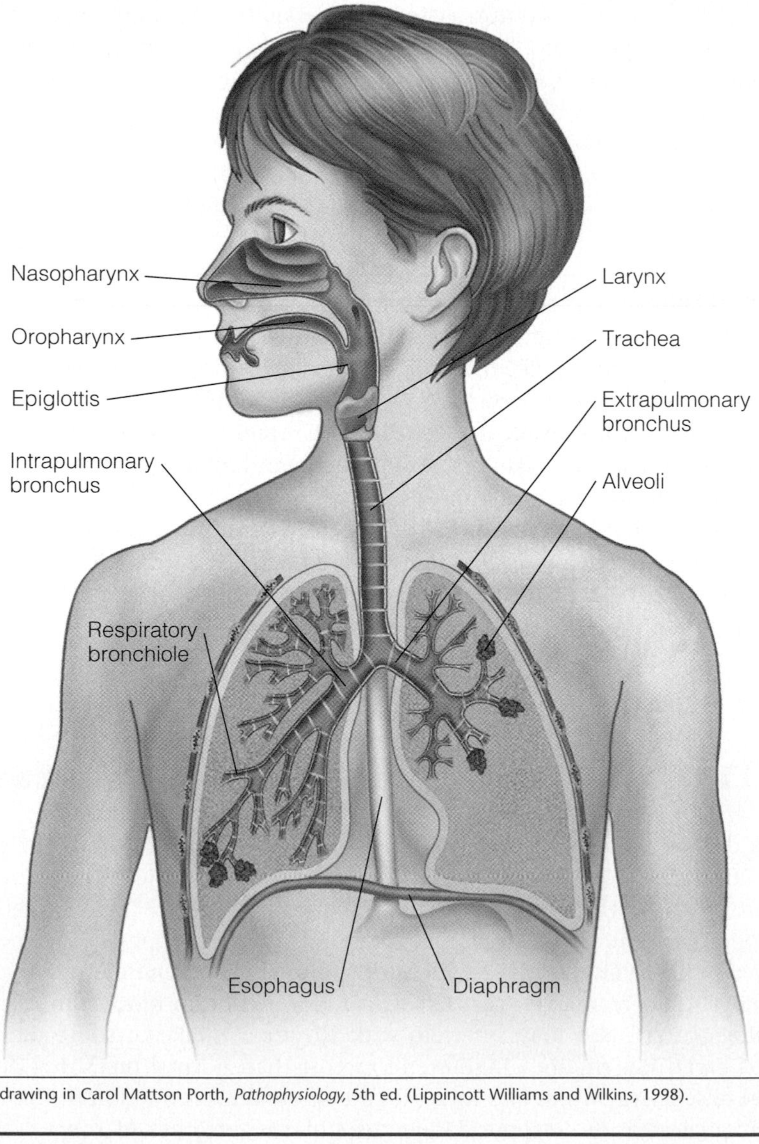
Nasopharynx
Oropharynx
Epiglottis
Intrapulmonary bronchus
Respiratory bronchiole
Larynx
Trachea
Extrapulmonary bronchus
Alveoli
Esophagus
Diaphragm

Based on a drawing in Carol Mattson Porth, *Pathophysiology,* 5th ed. (Lippincott Williams and Wilkins, 1998).

chronic obstructive pulmonary disease (COPD): a group of lung diseases characterized by persistent obstructed airflow through the lungs and airways; include chronic bronchitis and emphysema.

chronic bronchitis (bron-KYE-tis): persistent inflammation of the mucous membranes lining the main airways of the lungs. Chronic inflammation leads to narrower airways and difficulty with breathing.

emphysema (EM-fih-SEE-mah): disease characterized by progressive damage to alveoli (air sacs) in the lungs; causes difficulty with breathing.

bronchi, bronchioles: the main airways of the lungs. The singular form of bronchi is *bronchus.*

alveoli (al-VEE-oh-lie): air sacs in the lungs. One sac is an *alveolus.*

dyspnea (DISP-nee-a): shortness of breath.

FIGURE 22-3 Chronic Obstructive Pulmonary Disease

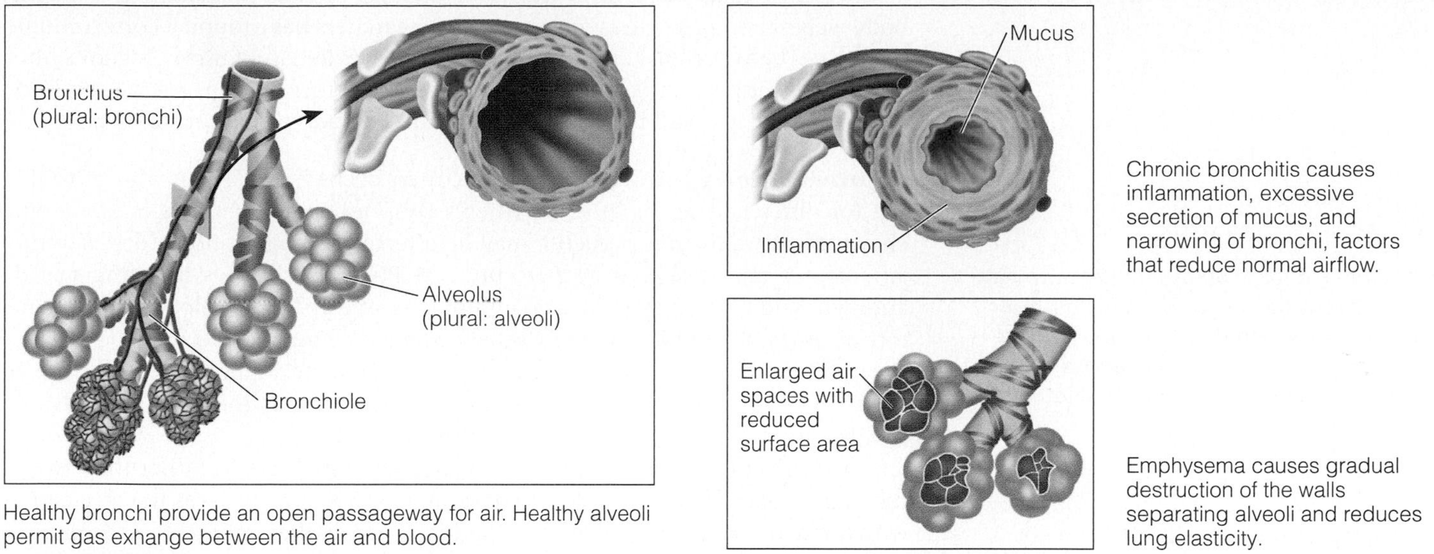
Bronchus
(plural: bronchi)
Alveolus
(plural: alveoli)
Bronchiole
Mucus
Inflammation
Chronic bronchitis causes inflammation, excessive secretion of mucus, and narrowing of bronchi, factors that reduce normal airflow.
Enlarged air spaces with reduced surface area
Emphysema causes gradual destruction of the walls separating alveoli and reduces lung elasticity.

Healthy bronchi provide an open passageway for air. Healthy alveoli permit gas exhange between the air and blood.

Panels 1 and 2 adapted from "Medical Encyclopedia: Bronchitis and Normal Condition in Tertiary Bronchus," MedlinePlus. Copyright 2005, A.D.A.M., Inc. **http://www.nlm.nih.gov/medlineplus/ency/imagepages/19357.htm**. Panel 3 adapted with permission from "Causes and Risk Factors for Emphysema," **Emphysema-Symptoms.com**. Copyright 2005 **Emphysema-Symptoms.com**. All rights reserved. **http://www.emphysema-symptoms.com/html/emphysemacauses.php3**.

Causes of COPD Smoking tobacco is the primary risk factor for COPD and is especially damaging when combined with respiratory infections or an occupational exposure to dusts or chemicals. Only a minority of smokers (15 to 20 percent) develop COPD, however; thus genetic susceptibility also plays a role in its development. Genetic factors are especially likely in patients with early-onset COPD. Alpha-1-antitrypsin deficiency, an inherited disorder, occurs in 1 to 2 percent of patients with COPD. These individuals have inadequate blood levels of alpha-1-antitrypsin, a plasma protein that helps to protect lung tissue.■

The lung damage of COPD is due to a specific type of inflammatory response to irritants in tobacco smoke and other chemicals.■ In chronic bronchitis, excessive mucus is secreted and clogs airways, which ultimately thicken and become too narrow for adequate mucus clearance. A chronic, productive cough is the main symptom. Emphysema is characterized by breakdown of the lungs' elastic structure and destruction of the walls of bronchioles and alveoli, significantly reducing the surface area involved in respiration. Many persons with COPD have elements of both diseases.

The COPD Patient COPD is a debilitating disease. Generally, dyspnea worsens as the condition progresses, resulting in dramatic reductions in physical activity and quality of life. Eventually, routine activities such as bathing or dressing may cause exhaustion or breathlessness. Weight loss is common in long-standing disease and may result from poor food intake, an increased metabolic rate, or the activities of certain inflammatory proteins in the body.[20] Muscle wasting often occurs and is only partially reversible by exercise. As with other chronic illnesses, anxiety and depression are a concern, and psychological distress may reduce a COPD patient's ability to cope with the demands of treatment.

Treatment of COPD Important objectives of COPD treatment are to prevent disease progression and to relieve major symptoms (dyspnea and coughing). People with COPD are encouraged to quit smoking and to get vaccinated against influenza and pneumonia. The most frequently prescribed medications are bronchodilators to improve airflow and corticosteroids (anti-inflammatory medications)■ to prevent symptom recurrence.[21] For people with severe COPD,

■ Alpha-1-antitrypsin inhibits the neutrophil enzyme *elastase,* which can break down connective tissue of lungs.

■ The inflammatory process characteristic of COPD includes the accumulation of neutrophils, a type of white blood cell, in the lungs. When activated, the neutrophils release enzymes and free radicals that can damage lung tissue.

■ The catabolic actions of corticosteroids can exacerbate the loss of muscle mass that accompanies COPD.

supplemental oxygen therapy (12 hours daily) can maintain normal oxygen levels in blood and reduce mortality risk.

The main goals of medical nutrition therapy include maintaining a healthy body weight and preserving muscle mass. Researchers have found a correlation between low body weights and increased mortality.[22] Rehabilitation programs often include exercise training to improve exercise tolerance, thus reducing the likelihood that patients will become sedentary and lose additional muscle mass.

Improving Food Intake Food intake often declines in severe cases of COPD, but for different reasons in each patient. Dyspnea can sometimes interfere with chewing or swallowing. Appetite may be affected by medications, depression or anxiety, or changes in taste perception.■ Physical changes affecting the diaphragm and lungs may reduce abdominal volume and cause bloating or discomfort when eating and lead to early satiety. Some patients may become too disabled to shop for food and prepare it and may lack adequate support at home. A registered dietitian or other medical professional must assess the unique needs of a COPD patient before proposing a nutrition care plan.

■ The altered sense of taste in patients with COPD may be due to chronic mouth breathing, which dries the mouth. Taste is also affected by the use of certain medications, including some bronchodilators.

Some patients may benefit by eating frequent, small meals rather than two or three large ones.[23] Liquids may be consumed between meals so as not to interfere with food intake.■ If bloating is a problem, foods that increase gas formation should be avoided. Eating slowly in a calm environment may help to reduce the amount of air swallowed during a meal. Some individuals may eat better if oxygen is provided at mealtimes. For undernourished patients, a high-energy, high-protein diet may be beneficial, but excessive energy intakes may increase carbon dioxide output and thereby increase respiratory stress. Liquid supplements are sometimes given between meals to improve weight gain or exercise endurance, but high-energy feedings (more than 250 kcalories) may induce satiety and reduce a patient's energy intake at mealtime.[24]

■ Consuming adequate fluids should be encouraged because they help to prevent the secretion of overly thick mucus.

Some patients with COPD may be overweight or obese, which puts an additional strain on the respiratory system. An energy-restricted diet to promote gradual weight loss is encouraged for these individuals.

Incorporating an Exercise Program Loss of muscle can be more readily prevented or reversed if the treatment plan includes a carefully designed exercise program.[25] With exercise, patients are likely to see improvements in their endurance and become less fearful of their physical limitations. For some patients, the combination of an exercise plan and oral supplement may be better for maintaining weight and improving muscle status than either component of treatment alone.[26]

Use of Specialized Formulas Some enteral formulas available for use in pulmonary disease provide more kcalories from fat and fewer from carbohydrate than standard formulas. The ratio of carbon dioxide production to oxygen consumption within cells is lower when fat is consumed, so theoretically these formulas should lower respiratory requirements. However, clinical studies have not confirmed that low-carbohydrate formulas reduce respiratory stress in COPD patients, and they are not currently recommended as a component of treatment.[27]

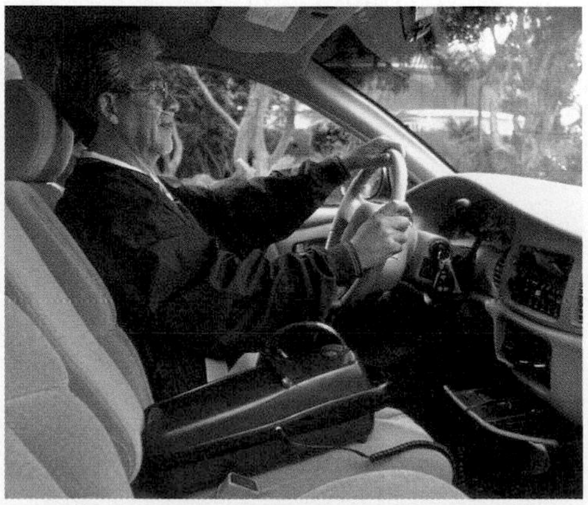

Patients who need supplemental oxygen can use lightweight, portable equipment that allows them to move about freely.

Respiratory Failure

In respiratory failure, the gas exchange between the air and the circulating blood is impaired. This condition can develop from chronic disease (such as COPD) or may arise suddenly (*acute* respiratory failure). Factors affecting any aspect of lung function may be the cause. Respiratory failure may result from obstruction of the upper airways or from weakness or paralysis of the muscles involved in respiration. An embolus lodged within the lungs may prevent blood flow, or toxic substances may damage lung tissue. Surgery sometimes results in respiratory failure due to the depressive effects of anesthesia or because some abdominal procedures can affect breathing.[28] Severe trauma and infection are common triggers of **acute respiratory distress syndrome (ARDS),** which is an acute form of respiratory failure marked by extensive lung damage; it is a life-threatening condition that usually requires the use of **mechanical ventilation** (artificial breathing) to restore normal oxygen and carbon dioxide levels.

Consequences of Respiratory Failure Impaired gas exchange results in **hypoxemia** (low blood levels of oxygen) and **hypercapnia** (excessive carbon dioxide in blood). An inadequate oxygen supply within tissues **(hypoxia)** inhibits cell function and can ultimately cause cell death. Hypercapnia can lead to **acidosis,** which interferes with the functions of the central nervous system and the heart. To compensate for respiratory failure, a person breathes faster, and heart rate quickens. The skin can become sweaty and develop a bluish cast **(cyanosis).** Headache, confusion, and drowsiness may occur. Severe cases of respiratory failure can cause heart arrhythmias and, ultimately, coma.

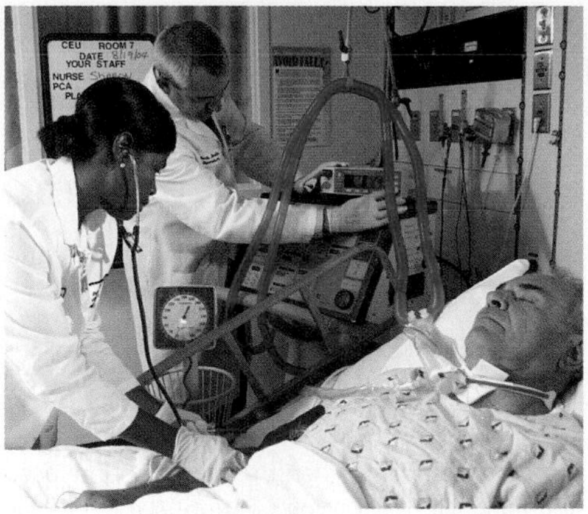

© Yoav Levy/Phototake

Mechanical ventilation controls the rate and amount of oxygen supplied to a patient's airways.

Acute Respiratory Distress Syndrome (ARDS) Acute respiratory distress syndrome (ARDS) typically occurs in individuals who have no history of lung disease and often follows acute lung injury due to sepsis, trauma, severe pneumonia, inhalation of smoke or toxic chemicals, or aspiration of gastric contents.[29] It can develop over 12 to 48 hours or may take several days. The lungs exhibit extensive inflammation and fluid buildup (pulmonary edema) that interferes with lung ventilation and with gas exchange in the alveoli. Blood oxygen levels are typically very low, and patients require mechanical ventilation. The later stages of ARDS are associated with a proliferation of lung cells, which causes fibrosis and disrupts lung structure. Death rates are approximately 50 percent but may be higher in patients over 60 years old or in patients with sepsis. A dangerous complication of ARDS is a progression to multiple organ failure (see the highlight following this chapter).

Treatment of Respiratory Failure Treatment of respiratory failure focuses on supporting lung function and correcting the underlying disorder.[30] Because respiratory failure can be caused by a number of different conditions, the treatment plan can vary greatly. In individuals with chronic lung disease, providing oxygen therapy via face mask or nasal tubing can relieve symptoms, but a patient with ARDS usually requires mechanical ventilation until able to breathe independently. Fluids may need careful monitoring to maintain fluid balance and prevent overload; diuretics are sometimes prescribed to mobilize the fluid that has accumulated in lung tissue. Medications may be needed to treat infections, keep airways open, or relieve inflammation. Complications are common in ARDS and must be forestalled to prevent multiple organ dysfunction.

Nutrition Care during Acute Illness Dietary recommendations are individualized according to the patient's condition. The primary concern is to supply enough energy and protein to support lung function without overtaxing the compromised respiratory system.[31] Fluid restrictions may be necessary to help reverse pulmonary edema. As usual, when nutrition support is necessary, enteral nutrition is preferred over parenteral nutrition.

Energy Usually, energy needs are estimated using the Harris-Benedict equation or other equations. Body weight may need to be corrected for edema, which is often present in patients with acute respiratory failure. A stress factor of 1.2 times BEE may be used initially, although needs may be higher in malnourished patients or if fever or infections are present.■ Energy intakes greater than 1.5 times BEE are not recommended (excessive energy intakes generate extra carbon dioxide) and may increase the risk for complications.

■ Patients on ventilators are usually heavily sedated and are immobile, which lowers their energy requirements.

Fluids Dehydration may arise due to a low fluid intake, an increase in bronchial mucus secretions, and diuretic therapy. Although dehydration may impede the clearance of lung secretions, pulmonary edema is often present, and fluid restriction is required

acute respiratory distress syndrome (ARDS): respiratory failure triggered by acute lung injury; a medical emergency that causes dyspnea and pulmonary edema and usually requires assisted (mechanical) ventilation.

mechanical ventilation: use of a machine to assist or control breathing. In normal respiration, the lungs expand, which draws air into the lungs. With mechanical ventilation, air is forced into the lungs at regular intervals using pressure.

hypoxemia (high-pox-EE-me-ah): a low level of oxygen in the blood.

hypercapnia (high-per-CAP-nee-ah): excess carbon dioxide in the blood.

hypoxia (high-pox-EE-ah): a low amount of oxygen in body tissues.

acidosis: acid accumulation in body tissues; depresses the central nervous system and can lead to disorientation and, eventually, coma.

cyanosis (sigh-ah-NOH-sis): a bluish cast in skin due to the color of deoxygenated hemoglobin. Cyanosis is most evident in persons with lighter, thinner skin; it is mostly seen on lips, cheeks, and ears and under nails.

CASE STUDY

Elderly Person with Emphysema

Mr. Wolf is an 82-year-old man who has emphysema that severely affects both lungs. He is 5 feet 9 inches tall and currently weighs 150 pounds, about 15 pounds less than his weight in earlier years. He lives with a daughter and son-in-law and eats meals with their family. He becomes breathless when eating and when walking around the house, and he feels tired all the time. A medical clinic recently ordered oxygen therapy for home use, but supplies have not yet arrived. Mr. Wolf's daughter is concerned about her father's recent weight loss and breathlessness.

1. Assess Mr. Wolf's risk of malnutrition, using information from Table 17-7 in Chapter 17 (p. 593). What factors may have contributed to his weight loss?
2. Explain possible reasons for Mr. Wolf's difficulty with eating. List some dietary suggestions that may help to improve his appetite and food intake. How might the use of oxygen therapy help?
3. Based on the history given, what factors may account for Mr. Wolf's tiredness? What suggestions would you give Mr. Wolf and his daughter regarding physical activity?

to prevent the additional accumulation of fluids in lung tissue. The edema may also make it difficult to assess whether a critically ill patient is maintaining weight.

Nutrition Support Patients with acute respiratory failure are often unable to eat meals and may need nutrition support. Tube feedings are usually used if the intestine is functioning, and intestinal feedings are preferred over gastric feedings because they reduce the risk of aspiration. Nutrient-dense formulas (2 kcalories per milliliter) are generally used in patients whose fluid is restricted. Pulmonary formulas that provide less carbohydrate and more fat are available (under the assumption that reduced carbohydrate will reduce carbon dioxide production), but these have not been shown to improve outcomes. If risk of aspiration is too high to continue enteral feedings, parenteral nutrition support may be considered. The accompanying case study reviews the nutrition care of a patient with emphysema.

IN SUMMARY Respiratory stress from chronic or acute disease affects body weight, muscle mass, and the normal functioning of all body tissues. Chronic obstructive pulmonary disease (COPD) is a debilitating, progressive illness that causes weakness and fatigue; the hypoxemia and hypercapnia that accompany COPD may lead to tissue death and depress the central nervous system. Although smoking is the primary risk factor for COPD, genetic susceptibility is also an important factor. Depending on patient needs, the goals of nutrition therapy for COPD may be to preserve muscle mass, improve food intake, maintain proper weight, and improve exercise endurance. Acute respiratory failure can develop from COPD or arise in persons with no history of lung disease; it often follows acute lung injury due to severe pneumonia, trauma, or inhalation injury. Nutrition support and fluid restrictions may be required in patients with respiratory failure.

DIET-DRUG INTERACTIONS

Bronchodilators
Bronchodilators can dry the mouth and throat and reduce the ability to taste foods. Some of these agents may increase gastric acid secretion, cause acid reflux, and upset the stomach. Overdoses may cause nausea and vomiting. Caffeine should be avoided if using *theophylline* because it enhances the drug's effects.

Corticosteroids
Prednisone stimulates the appetite, often causing weight gain. Long-term use can lead to negative nitrogen and calcium balances and early osteoporosis: patients using prednisone should consume high-protein, high-calcium, high-potassium diets. Other common effects include glucose intolerance and sodium retention.

NUTRITION ASSESSMENT CHECKLIST for People Experiencing Metabolic or Respiratory Stress

Medical History

Check the medical record to determine:

- ☐ Cause of stress
- ☐ Severity of stress
- ☐ Route of feeding (oral/tube feeding/parenteral)
- ☐ Whether any organ system is compromised

For patients with COPD, check to determine:

- ☐ Degree of breathing difficulty
- ☐ Use of oxygen therapy
- ☐ Exercise tolerance

Review the medical record for complications that may be related to underfeeding or overfeeding, such as:

- ☐ Dehydration or fluid overload
- ☐ Electrolyte imbalances
- ☐ Acid-base imbalances
- ☐ Hyperglycemia
- ☐ Hypertriglyceridemia
- ☐ Fatty liver

Medications

Record all medications and note:

- ☐ Signs that dosages may be inappropriate
- ☐ Signs of nutrient deficiencies
- ☐ Side effects that may alter food intake or nutrition status
- ☐ Use of theophylline, for patients who need to avoid caffeine

Dietary Intake

If the patient is not meeting nutrition goals:

- ☐ Calculate nutrient intake from oral diet, enteral formulas, and parenteral solutions.
- ☐ Investigate appetite difficulties or problems with eating.
- ☐ Consider interventions to improve food intake.
- ☐ Consider need for supplementation.
- ☐ In patients with COPD, consider disabilities that may interfere with the patient's ability to prepare and eat foods.

Anthropometric Data

Measure baseline height and weight and monitor daily weights. Note that body weight may change erratically in acutely ill patients due to the large amounts of fluid required for resuscitation. Once a patient's weight has stabilized:

- ☐ Reestimate protein and energy needs.
- ☐ Ensure that the patient is receiving the diet prescribed.
- ☐ Consider the need to change the energy prescription to meet weight goals.

Laboratory Tests

Laboratory tests that require careful interpretation include:

- ☐ Albumin
- ☐ Transferrin
- ☐ Prealbumin
- ☐ C-reactive protein
- ☐ Serum iron and zinc
- ☐ Total lymphocyte count (white blood counts are often elevated)

Monitor laboratory tests for signs of:

- ☐ Dehydration/fluid overload
- ☐ Electrolyte and acid-base imbalances
- ☐ Acute-phase response
- ☐ Hyperglycemia
- ☐ Hypertriglyceridemia
- ☐ Nutrient deficiencies
- ☐ Negative nitrogen balance
- ☐ Organ dysfunction or organ function that has normalized

Clinical Signs

Regularly assess vital signs including:

- ☐ Blood pressure
- ☐ Pulse
- ☐ Body temperature
- ☐ Respiration

Look for physical signs of:

- ☐ Protein-energy malnutrition
- ☐ Dehydration/fluid overload
- ☐ Nutrient deficiencies and excesses

NUTRITION ON THE NET

Access these websites for further study of topics covered in this chapter.

- Find updates and quick links to these and other nutrition-related sites at our website: **www.wadsworth.com/nutrition**
- To uncover additional information relevant to critical care, visit these sites:

  American Association of Critical Care Nurses: **www.aacn.org**

  American Society for Parenteral and Enteral Nutrition: **www.clinnutr.org**
- These sites provide resources regarding burns for patients and their families:

  American Burn Association: **www.ameriburn.org**

  Burn Survivor Resource Center: **www.burnsurvivor.com**
- This nonprofit group provides comprehensive, up-to-date information for burn care professionals: **www.burnsurgery.org**
- To learn more about lung diseases, visit these sites:

  American Lung Association: **www.lungusa.org**

  Canadian Lung Association: **www.lung.ca**

  National Heart, Lung and Blood Institute: **www.nhlbi.nih.gov**

STUDY QUESTIONS

These questions will help you review the chapter. You will find the answers in the discussions on the pages provided.

1. Describe the effects of the stress response on the body. Specify the main hormones involved and their metabolic effects. (pp. 694–695)
2. Discuss the main effects of the inflammatory response following infection or injury. Identify the chemical mediators involved and explain how they help to regulate the inflammatory process. (pp. 694–695)
3. Characterize the acute-phase response, giving examples of the clinical symptoms and changes in blood chemistry that usually result. (p. 696)
4. How does metabolic stress affect nutrition status? Explain why nutrition status may be difficult to evaluate in an acutely stressed individual. (p. 697)
5. Describe how energy and protein needs are estimated during acute stress. Which micronutrients are sometimes supplemented? (pp. 697–699)
6. Characterize first-degree, second-degree, and third-degree burns. What measures are taken immediately after a burn occurs? (pp. 699–700)
7. Identify the objectives of nutrition care for burn patients. Explain how their energy and protein needs are estimated. What measures are taken to provide adequate nutrient intakes? (pp. 700–701)
8. What is chronic obstructive pulmonary disease (COPD)? Describe its causes and treatment. Discuss the possible effects of COPD on body composition. (pp. 702–704)
9. Describe respiratory failure and its consequences. Identify the key elements of medical treatment and medical nutrition therapy. What are potential causes of acute respiratory distress syndrome (ARDS)? (pp. 704–706)

These questions will help you review for an exam. Answers can be found on p. 709.

1. Which of the following metabolic changes accompany acute stress?
   a. reduced plasma concentrations of glucose and fatty acids
   b. lower blood volume and blood pressure
   c. increased insulin action
   d. catabolism of protein in skeletal muscle and connective tissue
2. Tissue injury is followed by:
   a. fluid accumulation in damaged tissue.
   b. reduced blood flow to injured tissue.
   c. reduced capillary permeability.
   d. decreased body temperature.
3. The acute-phase response results in increased plasma concentrations of:
   a. albumin.
   b. iron.
   c. C-reactive protein.
   d. zinc.
4. Which of the following statements concerning protein and energy recommendations during acute metabolic stress is true?
   a. Protein and energy recommendations are similar to those for healthy people.
   b. Protein and energy recommendations are reduced because a stressed individual cannot metabolize nutrients normally.
   c. Acutely stressed individuals can benefit from as much protein and energy as can be provided.
   d. Protein and energy recommendations are high in order to minimize lean tissue losses.
5. The amount of protein recommended for an acutely stressed individual who weighs 150 pounds ranges from about ________ grams of protein per day.
   a. 55 to 85
   b. 68 to 136
   c. 126 to 158
   d. 150 to 300
6. The most frequent cause of death in burn patients is:
   a. malnutrition.
   b. dehydration.
   c. infection.
   d. hypothermia.
7. During the first 24 to 48 hours after a severe burn, a patient requires:
   a. parenteral feedings.
   b. fluid and electrolyte replacement.
   c. blood transfusions.
   d. micronutrient supplementation.
8. The primary risk factor for COPD is:
   a. alpha-1-antitrypsin deficiency.
   b. occupational exposure to dusts or chemicals.
   c. smoking tobacco.
   d. respiratory infections.
9. The weight loss and wasting that occur during COPD are often caused by:
   a. reduced food intake.
   b. increased metabolic rate.
   c. reduced exercise tolerance.
   d. all of the above.
10. Medical nutrition therapy for a person undergoing respiratory failure includes:
    a. careful attention to providing enough, but not too much, energy.
    b. generous fluid intake to clear the lungs of mucus.
    c. a high-fat intake to prevent weight loss.
    d. a high-carbohydrate intake to limit carbon dioxide production.

REFERENCES

1. S. M. Genuth, The endocrine system, in R. M. Berne and M. N. Levy, eds., *Physiology* (St. Louis, Mo.: Mosby, 1998), pp. 950–960.
2. K. Ley, ed., *Physiology of Inflammation* (New York: Oxford University Press, 2001); J. Phillips, P. Murray, and P. Kirk, eds., *The Biology of Disease* (Oxford: Blackwell Science, 2001).
3. M. J. James, R. A. Gibson, and L. G. Cleland, Dietary polyunsaturated fatty acids and inflammatory mediator production, *American Journal of Clinical Nutrition* 71 (2000): 343S–348S.
4. C. A. Dinarello and R. Porat, The acute phase response, in L. Goldman and D. Ausiello, eds., *Cecil Textbook of Medicine* (Philadelphia: Saunders, 2004), pp. 1733–1735.
5. A.S.P.E.N. Board of Directors and The Clinical Guidelines Task Force, Guidelines for the use of parenteral and enteral nutrition in adult and pediatric patients, *Journal of Parenteral and Enteral Nutrition* 26 (2002): 1–138SA.
6. A.S.P.E.N. Board of Directors and The Clinical Guidelines Task Force, 2002.
7. F. Novak and coauthors, Glutamine supplementation in serious illness: A systematic review of the evidence, *Critical Care Medicine* 30 (2002): 2022–2029.
8. K. C. McCowen and B. R. Bistrian, Immunonutrition: Problematic or problem solving? *American Journal of Clinical Nutrition* 77 (2003): 764–770.
9. A. Shenkin, Micronutrients and outcome, *Nutrition* 13 (1997): 825–828.
10. Shenkin, 1997.
11. A.S.P.E.N. Board of Directors and The Clinical Guidelines Task Force, 2002; K. N. Jeejeebhoy, Total parenteral nutrition: Potion or poison? *American Journal of Clinical Nutrition* 74 (2001): 160–163.
12. A.S.P.E.N. Board of Directors and The Clinical Guidelines Task Force, 2002.
13. A.S.P.E.N. Board of Directors and The Clinical Guidelines Task Force, 2002.
14. S. Escott-Stump, *Nutrition and Diagnosis-Related Care* (Baltimore: Lippincott Williams & Wilkins, 2002), pp. 620–622.
15. A.S.P.E.N. Board of Directors and The Clinical Guidelines Task Force, 2002.
16. M. H. Beers and R. Berkow, eds., *The Merck Manual of Diagnosis and Therapy* (Whitehouse Station, N.J.: Merck Research Laboratories, 1999), pp. 2434–2440.
17. Beers and Berkow, 1999.
18. Beers and Berkow, 1999.
19. American Dietetic Association, *Manual of Clinical Dietetics* (Chicago: American Dietetic Association, 2000).
20. A. G. N. Agusti, Systemic effects of chronic obstructive pulmonary disease, in Novartis Foundation, *Chronic Obstructive Pulmonary Disease: Pathogenesis to Treatment* (New York: John Wiley & Sons, 2001), pp. 245–246.
21. N. Anthonisen, Chronic obstructive pulmonary disease, in L. Goldman and D. Ausiello, eds., *Cecil Textbook of Medicine* (Philadelphia: Saunders, 2004), pp. 509–515; H. R. Gosker and coauthors, Skeletal muscle dysfunction in chronic obstructive pulmonary disease and chronic heart failure: Underlying mechanisms and therapy perspectives, *American Journal of Clinical Nutrition* 71 (2000): 1033–1047.
22. A. M. Schols and E. F. Wouters, Nutritional assessment and support of the stable COPD patient, in T. Similowski, W. A. Whitelaw, and J.-P. Derenne, eds., *Clinical Management of Chronic Obstructive Pulmonary Disease* (New York: Marcel Dekker, 2002), pp. 686–687.
23. Escott-Stump, 2002; American Dietetic Association, 2000.
24. M. A. P. Vermeeren and coauthors, Acute effects of different nutritional supplements on symptoms and functional capacity in patients with chronic obstructive pulmonary disease, *American Journal of Clinical Nutrition* 73 (2001): 295–301.
25. C. F. Donner and A. Patessio, Exercise in stable COPD, in T. Similowski, W. A. Whitelaw, and J.-P. Derenne, eds., *Clinical Management of Chronic Obstructive Pulmonary Disease* (New York: Marcel Dekker, 2002), pp. 731–758; R. M. Senior, Chronic obstructive pulmonary disease: Epidemiology, pathophysiology, pathogenesis, clinical course, management, and rehabilitation, in A. P. Fishman and coeditors, *Fishman's Manual of Pulmonary Diseases and Disorders* (New York: McGraw-Hill, 2002), pp. 118–141.
26. M. C. Steiner and coauthors, Nutritional enhancement of exercise performance in chronic obstructive pulmonary disease: A randomised controlled trial, *Thorax* 58 (2003): 745–751.
27. Schols and Wouters, 2002; Vermeeren and coauthors, 2001.
28. M. A. Grippi, Acute respiratory failure in the surgical patient, in A. P. Fishman and coeditors, *Fishman's Manual of Pulmonary Diseases and Disorders* (New York: McGraw-Hill, 2002), pp. 1034–1043.
29. M. A. Grippi, Acute respiratory distress syndrome, in A. P. Fishman and coeditors, *Fishman's Manual of Pulmonary Diseases and Disorders* (New York: McGraw-Hill, 2002), pp. 1023–1028.
30. Beers and Berkow, 1999.
31. L. M. Bellini, Nutrition in acute respiratory failure, in A. P. Fishman and coeditors, *Fishman's Manual of Pulmonary Diseases and Disorders* (New York: McGraw-Hill, 2002), pp. 1082–1089; American Dietetic Association, 2000.

ANSWERS

Study Questions (multiple choice)

1. d 2. a 3. c 4. d 5. b 6. c 7. b 8. c 9. d 10. a

HIGHLIGHT

Multiple Organ Failure

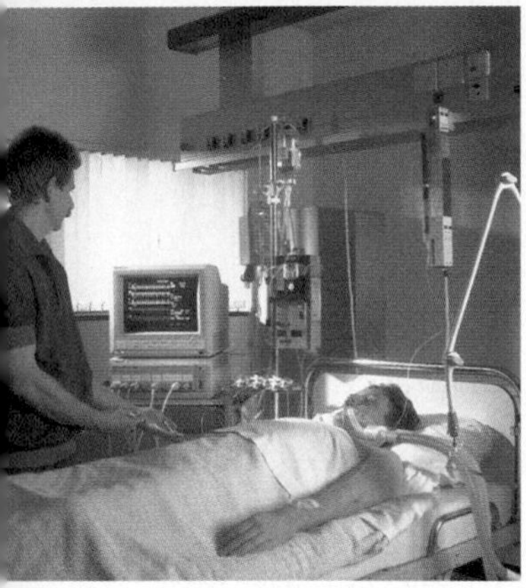

© Hein Hopmans/Phototake

Multiple organ failure is the cause of death in up to one-half of intensive care patients.[1] Described as a failure of two or more of the body's organ systems, multiple organ failure most frequently involves the lungs, liver, kidneys, and gastrointestinal (GI) tract. Involvement of three or more organ systems is associated with a fatality rate of nearly 100 percent. Multiple organ failure is not a disease *per se,* but rather a late stage of severe illness or injury that results from a severe inflammatory response (discussed in the previous chapter). Multiple organ failure is often initiated by a number of very different critical illnesses, including acute respiratory failure, trauma, sepsis, burn injuries, extensive surgery, and pancreatitis. This highlight discusses how multiple organ failure develops, the manner in which it is treated, and the importance of prevention.[2]

As a clinical entity, multiple organ failure was initially recognized only after World War II. Prior to the mid-twentieth century, patients with severe illnesses or multiple injuries frequently died of shock or circulatory failure. After fluid replacement and blood transfusions became standard treatments, the kidneys became the organs at highest risk and kidney failure the most common cause of death. Eventually, physicians learned to better support kidney function by providing appropriate electrolyte solutions and improving urine output. With improved kidney care, the lungs became the most vulnerable organ after severe injury. Improved treatment of respiratory failure eventually led to the current situation: advances in critical care allow patients to survive illnesses and injuries, but the body's responses often overburden organs that were not originally injured.

Development of Multiple Organ Failure

As discussed in Chapter 22, injury and infection cause the release of chemical mediators that have systemic (whole-body) effects. A severe, persistent inflammatory response may cause systemic inflammatory response syndrome (SIRS), which is associated with a constellation of symptoms including fever, raised heart and respiratory rates, and abnormal white blood cell counts. SIRS is a normal adaptive response to a severe insult, but if not reversed quickly enough, it may progress to shock, which is characterized by extremely low blood pressure and an inadequate blood supply to the tissues and organs of the body.

As might be expected from a systemic reduction in blood availability, shock can impair numerous organ systems.[3] The abnormal delivery of oxygen and nutrients to tissues and insufficient removal of wastes results in irreversible injury to cells and tissues. Although each organ system is affected differently, ultimately one or more organs may begin to fail. The failure of one organ may place excessive demands on another, causing the second to fail as well. The progression of SIRS to multiple organ failure reflects the inability of the body's defenses and the medical team to counter the detrimental effects of a sustained and potent inflammatory response.

As mentioned, one failing organ may disrupt the functioning of another. Organ failure seems to occur sequentially and often follows a similar pattern among patients: first the lungs, then the liver, and finally the kidneys, GI tract, or heart.[4] Other organs or systems may also become involved, and each additional failure reduces the likelihood of survival. Table H22-1 lists the organs and systems most often involved in multiple organ failure and the potential consequences of their failure.

TABLE H22-1 Physiological Effects of Organ or System Failure

Organ or System	Effects of Failure
Lungs	Inability to maintain gas exchange
Liver	Altered metabolic processes
Kidneys	Inability to regulate blood volume, maintain electrolytes, remove wastes
Heart	Low cardiac output, low blood pressure, inadequate circulation, shock
GI tract	Impaired digestion and absorption, abnormal bleeding, bacterial translocation
Immune system	Infection, sepsis
Coagulation system	Excessive bleeding or coagulation
Central nervous system	Decreased perceptions, brain injury, coma

Factors That Influence Organ Failure

The pathophysiology of multiple organ failure is complex and poorly understood. Although early reports attempted to link the development of multiple organ failure directly to sepsis, sepsis is not present in all cases.[5] Infection often results from impaired immune function, and therefore is a frequent consequence of multiple organ failure, but it may not necessarily be the underlying trigger of organ dysfunction. Recall from Chapter 22 that sepsis gives rise to the identical symptoms seen in SIRS. Figure H22-1 illustrates the relationships among SIRS, infection, sepsis, and multiple organ failure.

Finding the exact cause of multiple organ failure is difficult because its clinical course differs greatly among patient populations. Epidemiological studies have, however, identified a number of factors that increase risk. For example, patients who develop multiple organ failure are often older, have multiple or severe injuries, and tend to develop severe infections.

FIGURE H22-1 Relationships among SIRS, Sepsis, and Multiple Organ Failure

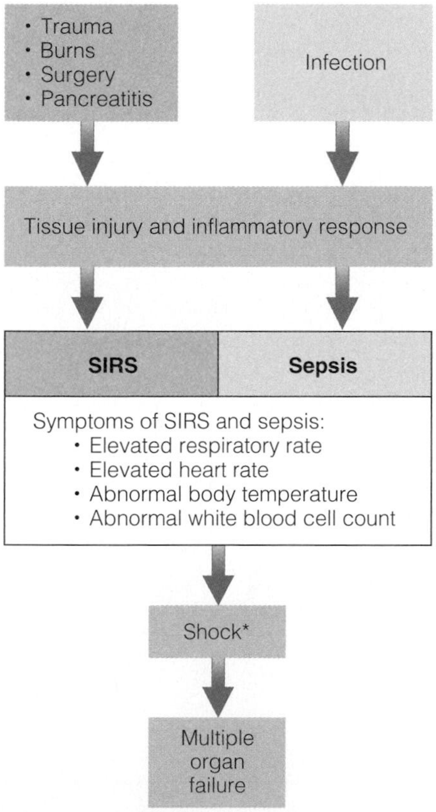

• Trauma
• Burns
• Surgery
• Pancreatitis
Infection
Tissue injury and inflammatory response
SIRS
Sepsis
Symptoms of SIRS and sepsis:
• Elevated respiratory rate
• Elevated heart rate
• Abnormal body temperature
• Abnormal white blood cell count
Shock*
Multiple organ failure

*After critical injury, shock may sometimes precede and be the cause of SIRS.

TABLE H22-2 Factors That Influence Risk of Multiple Organ Failure

- Age over 55 years
- Prior chronic disease
- Persistent SIRS
- Major infection
- Blood transfusions
- Severity of tissue injury
- Length of time between injury and arrival at hospital
- Malnutrition

Table H22-2 lists these and other risk factors frequently associated with multiple organ failure.

Age

Patients over 45 years old are several times more likely to develop multiple organ failure than are younger patients. In elderly patients, this increased risk may be due to the presence of chronic illnesses that directly affect organ function, such as heart disease, lung disease, diabetes, or liver damage. The aging process also decreases the functional reserve of organs, thereby reducing an older patient's ability to deal with the additional stress that arises during critical illness.

Severity of SIRS

The length of time that SIRS persists correlates with the development of multiple organ failure. In one study, patients who had SIRS that persisted for more than three days were more likely to develop multiple organ failure than patients who had SIRS for less than two days.[6]

Infection

Prolonged SIRS may suppress immune function and increase the risk of developing an infection. During hospital stays, critically ill patients frequently contract pneumonia—the principal infection associated with multiple organ failure. The risks of infection and sepsis greatly increase with use of invasive catheters, which are frequently needed during intensive care to provide oxygen support, intravenous fluid resuscitation, nutrition support, and urine clearance.

Blood Transfusions

Blood transfusions are immunosuppressive and may increase a patient's risks of developing infection or sepsis. They frequently have adverse effects that can add further stress. Blood transfusions may cause acute lung injury, allergic reactions, red blood cell hemolysis (breakdown), and other complications.

Treatment of Organ Failure

Once multiple organ failure has developed, extensive medical support is needed until the inflammatory response has abated.[7] Unfortunately, aggressive treatments can have damaging effects of their own and may cause further injury to organs that are already weakened by illness. Clinicians must be aware of the adverse effects of aggressive therapies and alert to a patient's responses to treatments. Examples of therapies that are often used to manage patients with organ failure include:

- *Lung support.* Mechanical ventilation is used to assist injured lungs and sustain gas exchange.
- *Fluid resuscitation.* Fluids and electrolytes are supplied to restore blood volume and maintain electrolyte balance.
- *Heart and blood vessel function.* Medications help to sustain or increase cardiac output and maintain adequate blood pressure.
- *Kidney support.* Hemofiltration or dialysis helps to prevent the buildup of toxic metabolites in blood.
- *Infection.* Antibiotic therapy may reverse or prevent infections.
- *Nutrition support.* Enteral and parenteral nutrition support provide nutrients, help to prevent excessive wasting, and promote recovery.

Because mortality rates for multiple organ failure are so high, prevention is considered at the earliest stages of injury and treatment before an excessive inflammatory response can cause further damage. Clinicians have learned to identify the conditions that may increase organ stress whether they are due to a disease process, an inflammatory response, or an aggressive treatment that is intended to provide organ support. Although improvements in care over the past few decades have reduced some of the complications that arise during intensive care, rates of mortality from multiple organ failure have not changed. Thus, a focus on prevention is critical until the pathophysiology of multiple organ failure is better understood, which may lead to additional therapeutic options.

REFERENCES

1. D. Johnson and I. Mayers, Multiple organ dysfunction syndrome: A narrative review, *Canadian Journal of Anesthesia* 48 (2001): 502–509.
2. J. Parrillo, Approach to the patient with shock, in L. Goldman and D. Ausiello, eds., *Cecil Textbook of Medicine* (Philadelphia: Saunders, 2004), pp. 608–615; Johnson and Mayers, 2001; A. E. Baue, E. Faist, and D. E. Fry, eds., *Multiple Organ Failure: Pathophysiology, Prevention, and Therapy* (New York: Springer-Verlag, 2000); T. W. Evans and M. Smithies, Organ dysfunction, *British Medical Journal* 318 (1999): 1606–1608.
3. Parrillo, 2004.
4. P. J. Offner and E. E. Moore, Risk factors for MOF and pattern of organ failure following severe trauma, in A. E. Baue, E. Faist, and D. E. Fry, eds., *Multiple Organ Failure: Pathophysiology, Prevention, and Therapy* (New York: Springer-Verlag, 2000).
5. Johnson and Mayers, 2001.
6. Offner and Moore, 2000.
7. Johnson and Mayers, 2001.

Chapter 23

Nutrition and Disorders of the Upper Gastrointestinal Tract

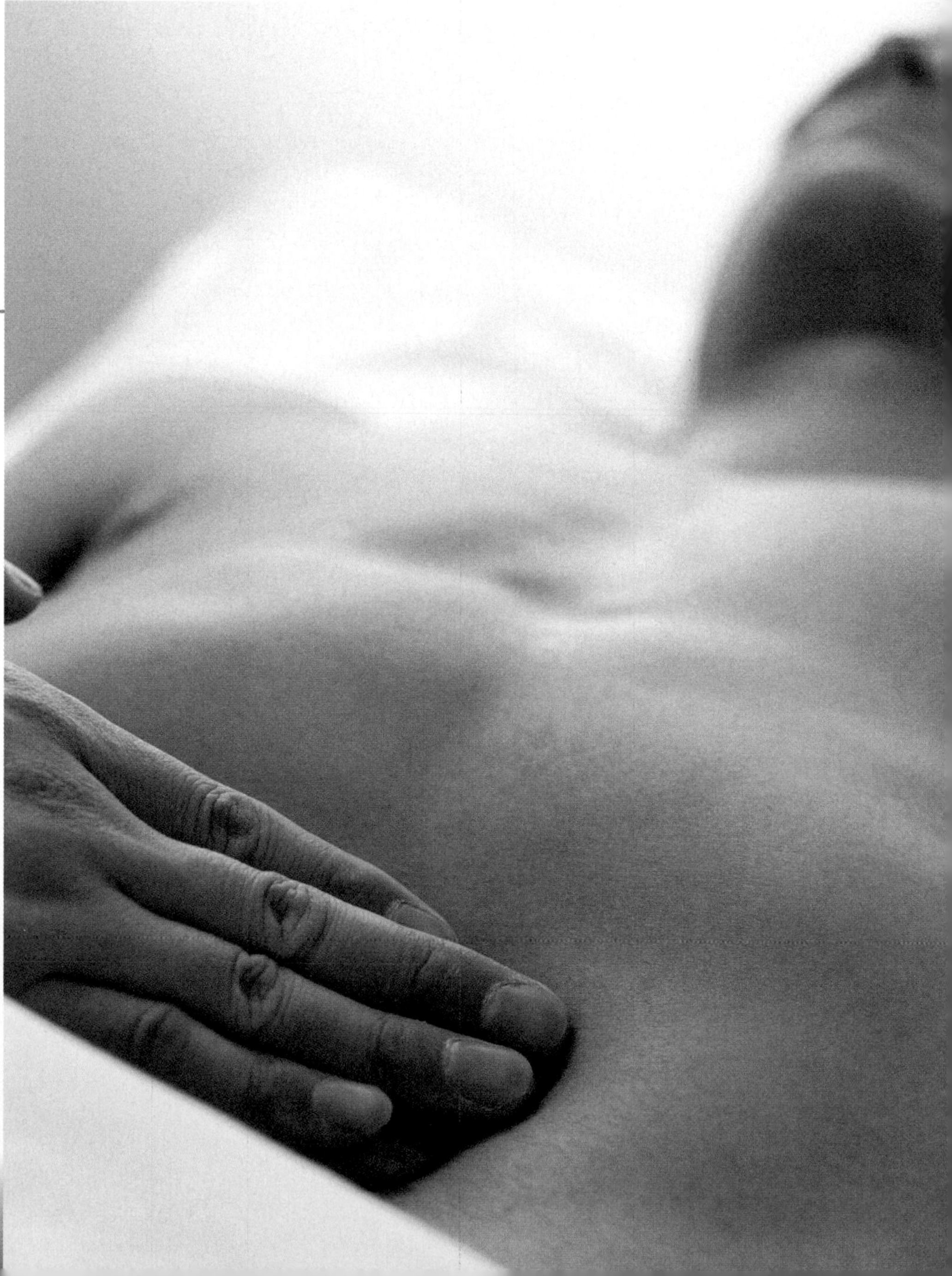

© Photodisc Collection

Chapter Outline

Conditions Affecting The Esophagus:
Dysphagia • Gastroesophageal Reflux Disease

Conditions Affecting The Stomach:
Dyspepsia • Nausea and Vomiting • Gastritis • Peptic Ulcer Disease • Gastric Surgery

Highlight: *Dental Health and Its Relationship with Chronic Illness*

Available Online

http://nutrition.wadsworth.com/uncn7

Student Practice Test

Glossary Terms

Nutrition on the Net

Nutrition in the Professional Setting

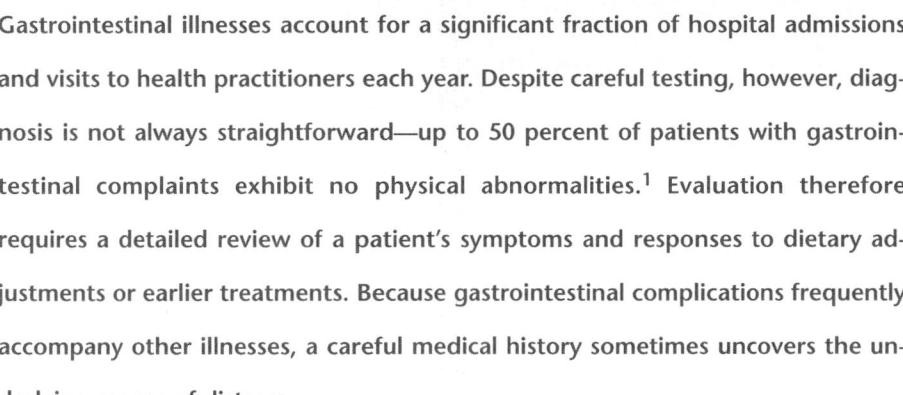

Gastrointestinal illnesses account for a significant fraction of hospital admissions and visits to health practitioners each year. Despite careful testing, however, diagnosis is not always straightforward—up to 50 percent of patients with gastrointestinal complaints exhibit no physical abnormalities.[1] Evaluation therefore requires a detailed review of a patient's symptoms and responses to dietary adjustments or earlier treatments. Because gastrointestinal complications frequently accompany other illnesses, a careful medical history sometimes uncovers the underlying source of distress.

The remarkable gastrointestinal (GI) tract provides a means of delivering nutrients and other food components to the body's interior. When various medical conditions impair some of the GI tract's functions, dietary adjustments can help to ease symptoms and prevent malnutrition. This chapter describes common upper GI tract symptoms and disorders; the next chapter discusses conditions that affect the lower GI tract. Highlight 23 presents several mouth and dental problems and their associations with chronic disease.

Figure 23-1 illustrates the upper GI tract and reviews its functions.■ In the mouth, the teeth and jaw muscles work together to break down food to a consistency that is easily swallowed. Upon swallowing, a bolus of food passes through the pharynx and esophagus to the stomach, assisted by peristalsis. The lower esophageal sphincter relaxes to allow the passage of food to the stomach and closes to prevent reflux (backward flow) of stomach contents.

■ See Chapter 3 for a complete review of the GI tract and its functions; common digestive problems and simple self-help measures were introduced in Highlight 3.

FIGURE 23-1 The Upper GI Tract

Mouth
Chews and mixes food with saliva.

Pharynx
Directs food from mouth to esophagus.

Epiglottis
Protects airway during swallowing.

Upper esophageal sphincter
Allows passage from mouth to esophagus. Prevents backflow from esophagus.

Esophagus
Conducts food to stomach.

Lower esophageal sphincter
Allows passage from esophagus to stomach. Prevents backflow from stomach.

Stomach
Adds acid, enzymes, and fluid. Churns, mixes, and grinds food to a liquid mass.

Pyloric sphincter
Allows passage from stomach to small intestine. Prevents backflow from small intestine.

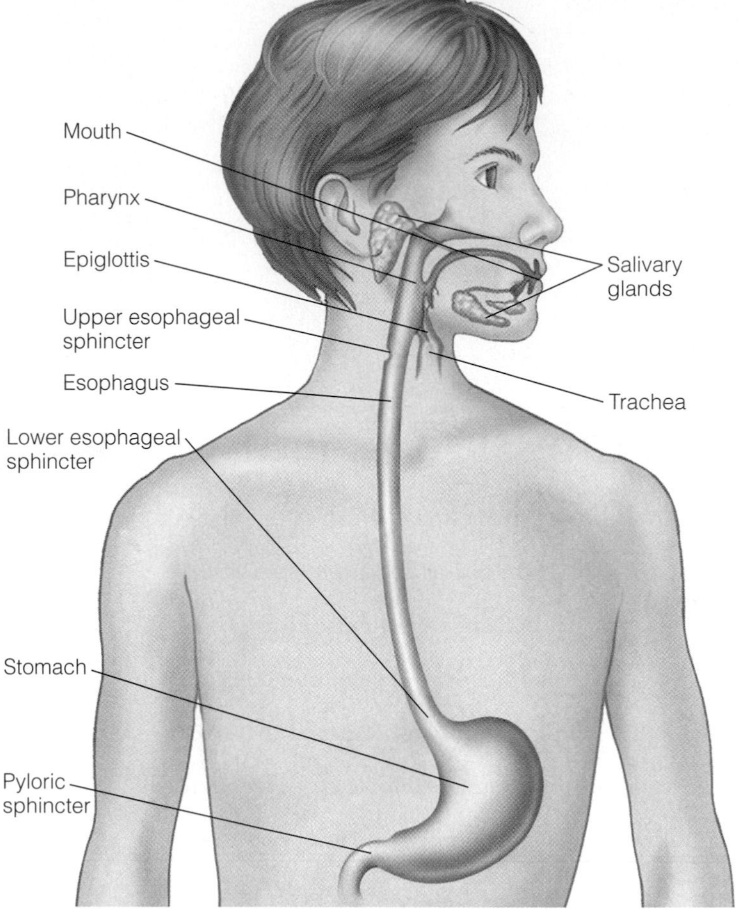
Mouth
Pharynx
Epiglottis
Upper esophageal sphincter
Esophagus
Lower esophageal sphincter
Stomach
Pyloric sphincter
Salivary glands
Trachea

Salivary glands
Secrete saliva (provides moisture and contains starch digesting enzymes).

Trachea
Allows air to pass to and from lungs.

Conditions Affecting the Esophagus

Disorders of the esophagus may be accompanied by difficulty with swallowing, a sensation of something "stuck in the throat," or pain in the chest area. This section examines the causes and treatments of the two most common problems affecting the esophagus.[2] Dysphagia, or difficulty swallowing, was mentioned in earlier chapters, but is discussed in more detail here. Gastroesophageal reflux disease, often referred to as "heartburn," was first introduced and defined in Highlight 3.

Dysphagia

The act of swallowing is complex. In the initial or **oropharyngeal** phase, food is chewed and mixed with saliva and propelled into the pharynx using the tongue. At the same time, the soft palate and larynx close to prevent regurgitation of food material through the nose, and the epiglottis closes over the trachea to prevent aspiration (inhalation) of food substances or saliva into the trachea and lungs. In the second or **esophageal** phase of swallowing, the bolus passes through the esophagus, and the lower esophageal sphincter relaxes to allow passage of the bolus into the stomach.

oropharyngeal (OR-oh-FAIR-in-GEE-al): concerning the mouth and pharynx.

esophageal (ee-SOF-ah-GEE-al): concerning the esophagus.

Types of Dysphagia A person with **oropharyngeal dysphagia** has an impairment that affects the transfer of food from the mouth and pharynx to the esophagus. The problem is often a neuromuscular condition that affects the tongue, other oral tissues, or the swallowing reflex. Symptoms may include an inability to initiate swallowing, coughing during or after swallowing (due to aspiration), and nasal regurgitation. Other signs include bad breath, a gurgling noise after swallowing, a hoarse or "wet" voice, or a speech disorder. Oropharyngeal dysphagia occurs frequently in elderly people and is often caused by stroke.[3] Table 23-1 lists a number of medical conditions that are commonly associated with oropharyngeal dysphagia.

A person with **esophageal dysphagia** has difficulty passing a bolus of food through the esophageal lumen and into the stomach. The main symptom is often the sensation of food "sticking" in the esophagus after it is swallowed. The problem may be caused by either an obstruction in the esophagus or a motility disorder. When dysphagia impairs the passage of solid foods but not liquids, the cause is usually an obstruction in the esophagus resulting from a **stricture** (abnormal narrowing), tumor, or compression of the esophagus by surrounding organs or tissues. If dysphagia occurs with both solids and liquids, the cause is often a motility disorder. **Achalasia,** the most common motility disorder, is a degenerative nerve condition affecting the esophagus; it is characterized by impaired peristalsis and incomplete relaxation of the lower esophageal sphincter when swallowing.[4] Table 23-1 lists additional conditions that may cause esophageal dysphagia.

TABLE 23-1 Causes of Dysphagia

Oropharyngeal Dysphagia

- Brain stem tumors
- Developmental disabilities
- Lou Gehrig's disease (amyotrophic lateral sclerosis)
- Multiple sclerosis
- Myasthenia gravis
- Obstructive structural anomalies
- Obstructive tumors
- Parkinson's disease
- Poliomyelitis
- Severe inflammation
- Stroke
- Thyroid enlargement

Esophageal Dysphagia

- Achalasia
- AIDS
- Esophageal spasm
- Scleroderma
- Strictures (induced by inflammation, medication, radiation)
- Tumors

Complications of Dysphagia Health care providers need to remain alert to various complications that can indicate a dysphagia condition. If food consumption is reduced due to dysphagia, malnutrition and weight loss may occur. People who cannot swallow liquids are at increased risk of dehydration. A serious and potentially life-threatening complication associated with dysphagia is aspiration, which may cause airway obstruction, choking, or respiratory infections, including pneumonia. If a person does not have a normal cough reflex, aspiration is more difficult to diagnose and may go unnoticed.

Evaluating Dysphagia Although the signs and symptoms of dysphagia can help a health care provider recognize the condition, diagnosing the exact cause generally requires further examination.[5] A barium swallow study often reveals the nature of the problem: the patient consumes foods or liquids that contain barium (a metallic element visible on X-rays), and the swallowing process is monitored using a video X-ray technique, known as videofluoroscopy. Another assessment method, endoscopy, uses a thin, flexible tube to examine the esophageal lumen directly. Peristalsis and sphincter pressure can be measured using a manometer, a flexible catheter containing multiple pressure sensors that is passed into the esophagus. A neurological examination may be needed to evaluate mental status, physical reflexes, and the cranial nerves associated with swallowing.

■ Dietary modifications for dysphagia were introduced in Chapter 18 (see p. 611).

Dietary Interventions Because a wide variety of physical, mechanical, and neurological defects can cause dysphagia, finding the best diet is often a challenge.■ Even after careful assessment of a person's swallowing abilities, the foods most easily handled may be determined only by trial and error. Modifying the physical properties of foods and beverages and using alternative feeding methods may help to compensate for swallowing difficulties. A person's swallowing abilities may fluctuate over time, and the dietary plan may need frequent reassessment.

In recent years, there has been an attempt to standardize dysphagia diets so that dietetic practice and terminology would be more similar among institutions in the United States. In 2002, the American Dietetic Association published the National Dysphagia Diet (NDD), which was developed by a panel of dietitians, speech and language therapists, and a food scientist.[6] Table 23-2 presents brief descriptions of the diets and sample meals, and the next section discusses additional dietary considerations. After a diet is selected, it is adjusted to suit the person's swallowing

oropharyngeal dysphagia: an inability to transfer food from the mouth and pharynx to the esophagus; usually due to a neurological or muscular disorder.

esophageal dysphagia: an inability to move a food bolus through the esophagus; usually due to an obstruction or a motility disorder.

stricture: abnormal narrowing of a passageway due to inflammation, scarring, or other structural changes.

achalasia (ack-a-LAY-zhah): an esophageal disorder characterized by weakened peristalsis and impaired relaxation of the lower esophageal sphincter.
- **a** = without
- **chalasia** = relaxation

TABLE 23-2 National Dysphagia Diet

Level 1: Dysphagia Pureed

Foods should be pureed, homogeneous, and cohesive. This diet is for patients with moderate-to-severe dysphagia and poor oral or chewing ability.

Sample meals:

- *Breakfast:* Cream of wheat, pureed pancakes, mashed banana, fruit juice without pulp (thickened as needed), coffee or tea (if thin liquids are acceptable).
- *Lunch or dinner:* Pureed soup, pureed chicken, mashed potatoes with gravy, pureed carrots, broccoli soufflé, applesauce, chocolate pudding.

Level 2: Dysphagia Mechanically Altered

Foods should be moist and soft textured and should easily form a bolus. This diet is for patients with mild-to-moderate dysphagia; some chewing ability is required.

Sample meals:

- *Breakfast:* Scrambled eggs, slightly moistened dry cereals (only those with a simple texture, such as puffed rice cereal or corn flakes), cooked fruit without skin or seeds, fruit juice (thickened as needed), coffee or tea (if thin liquids are allowed).
- *Lunch or dinner:* Soup with easy-to-chew meat and vegetables; well-cooked pasta with moist meatballs and meat sauce; soft, tender vegetables (not fibrous or rubbery); soft fruit pie (with bottom crust only).

Level 3: Dysphagia Advanced

Foods should be moist and be in bite-sized pieces when swallowed. Individuals using this diet need to tolerate mixed textures. This diet is for patients with mild dysphagia.

Sample meals:

- *Breakfast:* Muffin with margarine or butter, cereal and milk (except coarse or dry; milk is restricted if thin liquids are not tolerated), soft peeled fresh fruit or berries, coffee or tea (if thin liquids are tolerated).
- *Lunch or dinner:* Clam chowder; thin-sliced tender meat (can be in sandwich form); rice; cooked, tender vegetables or shredded lettuce with dressing; fresh melon; chocolate chip cookie (without nuts).

Liquid Consistencies (only those that are tolerated are allowed in the diet)

- *Thin:* Watery fluids; may include milk, coffee, tea, juices, carbonated beverages.
- *Nectarlike:* Fluids thicker than water that can be sipped through a straw; may include buttermilk, eggnog, tomato juice.
- *Honeylike:* Fluids that can be eaten with a spoon but do not hold their shape; may include honey, tomato sauce, yogurt.
- *Spoon-thick:* Thick fluids that must be eaten with a spoon and can hold their shape; may include milk pudding, thickened applesauce.

abilities and tolerances. A consultation with a swallowing expert, such as a speech and language therapist, often is necessary.

Food Properties Foods included in dysphagia diets should have easy-to-manage textures and consistencies. Soft, cohesive foods are easier to handle than hard or crumbly foods. Moist foods are preferred over dry foods. Some foods within a category may be acceptable, and others may not; for example, some cookies are soft and tender whereas others are hard and brittle. Sticky or gummy foods, such as peanut butter and cream cheese, may be difficult to clear from the mouth and throat. Foods that have more than one texture, such as vegetable soup or cereal with milk, are harder to handle. Some patients find more viscous beverages like milk shakes easier to manage than thin liquids such as water or juice.

Food Preparation In many cases, the textures of foods need to be altered to make them easier to swallow. Foods are often pureed, mashed, ground, or minced (review Table 18-2 on p. 613 and Table 23-2). A bite of food is more easily tolerated when it has just one consistency, so ingredients are often blended and the addition of items such as nuts and seeds is avoided. Commercial starch thickeners or baby cereals can be used to thicken liquids.

Consuming foods that have a similar consistency can quickly become monotonous. By using commercial thickeners, pureed foods may be formed into attractive

HOW TO Improve Acceptance of Mechanically Altered Foods

Take a moment to think about a meal of pureed or ground foods. A typical dinner of baked chicken, potatoes, carrots, and green beans can look like mounds of differently colored mush. The foods may taste great, but a person may have little appetite before trying a first bite. To improve appetite, be creative when preparing and serving meals:

- Prepare a person's favorite foods and foods that have pleasant smells. The smell and thought of one's favorite foods can help to stimulate the appetite.
- Prepare foods that have strong flavors, for example, curries and chili. Seasonings and spices can enliven food flavors.
- Consider colors and shapes when planning meals and arranging foods on a plate. Substitute brightly colored vegetables for white vegetables; for example, replace mashed potatoes with mashed sweet potatoes. Arranging foods attractively on a plate with colorful garnishes can also add color and eye appeal.
- Try layering ingredients so that the entrée looks like a fancy casserole. For example, recipes can resemble such popular entrées as lasagna, shepherd's pie, and moussaka.

Efforts to improve the visual appearance of foods can go a long way toward helping people to eat nourishing meals and maintain a healthy weight.

shapes. Including a variety of flavors and colors can also make a meal more appealing. The "How to" offers other suggestions that can improve the acceptance of pureed and other mechanically altered diets.

Feeding Strategies Depending on the nature of the disorder, some patients may be able to learn new techniques to help them compensate for their disability. For example, people with oropharyngeal dysphagia may learn exercises that can strengthen the jaws, tongue, or larynx or even new methods of swallowing that can allow them to consume a normal diet. Changing head and neck posture while eating may also minimize some swallowing problems.[7] Speech and language therapists can help patients learn these techniques.

Enteral Nutrition Support Tube feedings are sometimes given to patients with dysphagia who are unable to consume adequate amounts of foods, particularly if they are malnourished or if their swallowing function continues to deteriorate. If an individual is at high risk of aspiration, intestinal feedings are used instead of gastric feedings.

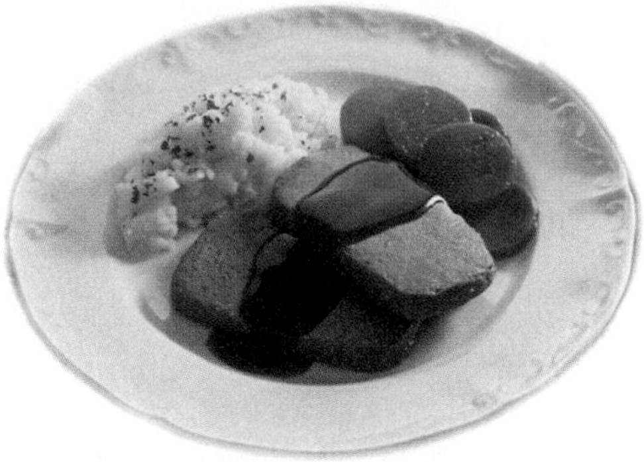

Courtesy Diamond Crystal Specialty Foods

Can you tell that the foods in this photo are pureed foods shaped with commercial thickeners?

Gastroesophageal Reflux Disease

As Highlight 3 mentioned, heartburn is one of the most common gastrointestinal complaints. Sometimes heartburn is accompanied by **regurgitation**, the reflux of small amounts of the stomach's acidic contents into the mouth. These symptoms characterize gastroesophageal reflux disease (GERD), a condition of gastric reflux that causes frequent discomfort and, sometimes, tissue damage. People who suffer from this condition often call it "acid indigestion" as it can be aggravated by the dietary choices a person makes.

Occasional episodes of reflux occur in healthy people and may not necessarily cause symptoms or injury. Reflux is a problem only if it creates complications and requires either lifestyle changes or medical treatment.

Causes of GERD The lower esophageal sphincter is the main barrier to gastric reflux; GERD may result if the sphincter muscle is weak or relaxes inappropriately. In many cases of GERD, the sphincter relaxes more frequently and remains relaxed for longer than usual, thereby opening the path between the esophagus and the stomach. Medical conditions that interfere with the sphincter's mechanism or prevent rapid clearance of acid from the esophagus can predispose a person to GERD.

Conditions associated with high rates of GERD include pregnancy, asthma, and **hiatal hernia,** a condition in which a portion of the stomach protrudes above the

regurgitation: the reflux of small amounts of acidic gastric substances into the mouth.

hiatal hernia: a condition in which the upper portion of the stomach protrudes above the diaphragm. Most cases are asymptomatic.

FIGURE 23-2 The Upper GI Tract, Acid Reflux, and Hiatal Hernia

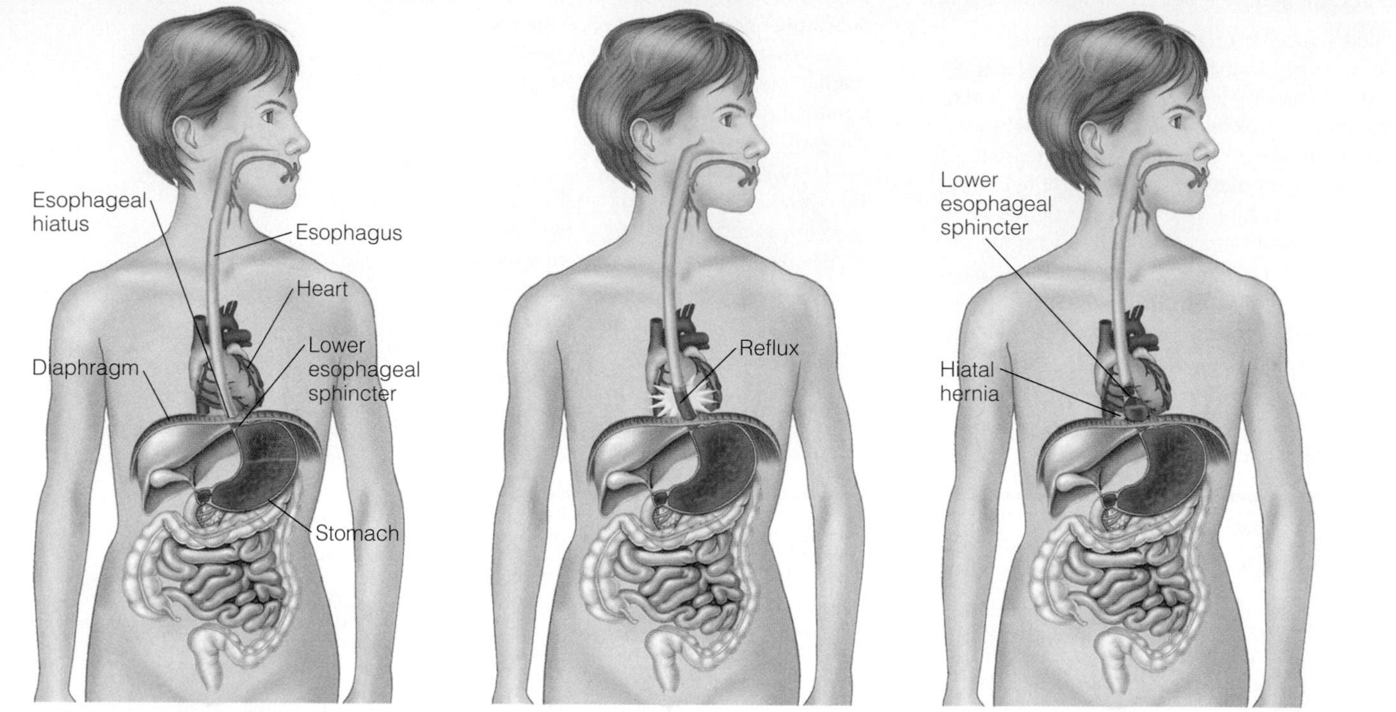
Esophageal hiatus
Esophagus
Heart
Diaphragm
Lower esophageal sphincter
Stomach
Reflux
Lower esophageal sphincter
Hiatal hernia

The stomach normally lies below the diaphragm, and the esophagus passes through the esophageal hiatus. The lower esophageal sphincter prevents reflux of stomach contents.

Whenever the pressure in the stomach exceeds the pressure in the esophagus, as can occur with overeating and overdrinking, the chance of reflux increases. The resulting "heartburn" is so-named because it is felt in the area of the heart.

Risk of acid reflux may increase as a consequence of a hiatal hernia. A "sliding" hiatal hernia occurs when part of the stomach, along with the lower esophageal sphincter, rises above the diaphragm.

diaphragm (see Figure 23-2). Pregnancy is the most common predisposing condition; over 50 percent of pregnant women report heartburn, which often starts in the first trimester (see p. 488). Various other conditions or substances can exacerbate GERD by either weakening the sphincter or raising pressure within the stomach (see Table 23-3 for examples). A number of medications increase the risk of reflux, as does the use of nasogastric tubes in tube feedings.

Consequences of GERD If the acidic contents of the stomach remain in the esophagus long enough to damage its mucosal lining, the resulting inflammation is called **reflux esophagitis.** Severe and chronic inflammation may lead to esophageal ulcers, with consequent bleeding. Healing and scarring of ulcerated tissue may narrow the inner diameter of the esophagus, causing esophageal stricture. The extent of stricture varies: it may affect only a small area or the entire esophagus. A slowly progressive dysphagia for solid foods sometimes results, and swallowing occasionally becomes painful. Chronic reflux is also associated with **Barrett's esophagus,** a condition in which damaged esophageal cells are eventually replaced by cells that resemble those in gastric or intestinal tissue; the cellular changes increase the risk of esophageal cancer. GERD can also lead to reflux damage in the pharynx, larynx, and respiratory tract. Pulmonary disease can develop if gastric contents are aspirated into the lungs.

Treatment of GERD The objectives of treatment are to alleviate symptoms and facilitate the healing of damaged tissue. Severe ulcerative disease may require immediate acid-suppressing medication, whereas a mild case may be managed with dietary and lifestyle modifications.

reflux esophagitis: inflammation in the esophagus related to the reflux of acidic stomach contents.

Barrett's esophagus: a condition in which esophageal cells that have been damaged by chronic exposure to stomach acid are replaced by cells that resemble those in the stomach or small intestine, sometimes becoming cancerous.

Drug Therapy Medications that suppress gastric acid secretion can help the healing process by reducing the damaging effects of acid on esophageal tissue. **Proton-pump inhibitors** are the most effective of the antisecretory agents and are used both for rapid healing of esophagitis and as a maintenance treatment. The other major drugs include **histamine-2-receptor blocking agents** (often referred to as H2-blockers) and antacids, which neutralize gastric acid. Although antacids are frequently used to relieve occasional heartburn, they are not necessarily appropriate for GERD because they have only short-term effects, are associated with gastrointestinal side effects, and may cause some nutrient deficiencies when used long term.

Lifestyle Modifications Management of GERD often requires lifestyle changes to help minimize discomfort and the incidence of acid reflux. Recommendations generally include the following:

- Avoid eating bedtime snacks or lying down after meals. Meals should be consumed at least two to three hours before bedtime.
- Reduce nighttime reflux by elevating the head of the bed on 6-inch blocks, inserting a foam wedge under the mattress, or propping pillows under the head and upper torso.
- Consume only small meals and drink liquids between meals so that the stomach does not become overly distended, which can exert pressure on the lower esophageal sphincter.
- Limit foods that weaken lower esophageal sphincter pressure or increase gastric acid secretion; these include chocolate, fatty foods, spearmint and peppermint, coffee (both caffeinated and decaffeinated), and tea.
- Avoid cigarettes and alcohol; both relax the lower esophageal sphincter.
- Avoid bending over and wearing tight-fitting garments; both can cause pressure in the stomach to increase, heightening the risk of reflux.
- Advise obese patients to lose weight if they are adequately motivated. Obesity can increase abdominal pressure.
- During periods of esophagitis, avoid foods and beverages that may irritate the esophagus, such as citrus fruits and juices, tomato products, pepper, spicy foods, carbonated beverages, and very hot or very cold foods (depending on individual tolerances).
- Avoid using nonsteroidal anti-inflammatory drugs (NSAID) such as aspirin, naproxen, and ibuprofen, which can damage the esophageal mucosa.

Individual food tolerances may vary markedly. Health care providers can help patients pinpoint food intolerances by advising them to keep a record of the foods and beverages consumed and any resulting gastrointestinal symptoms.

Other Interventions Surgery may be required in severe cases of GERD that are unresponsive to medications and lifestyle changes. In one popular procedure (called *fundoplication*), the upper section of the stomach (the fundus) is gathered up around the esophagus and sewn in such a way that the esophagus and sphincter are surrounded by stomach muscle, which increases pressure within the esophagus and fortifies the sphincter muscle. Esophageal strictures are often treated by dilating the esophagus (with an inflatable balloonlike device or with a fixed-size dilator) or by using surgical approaches. The case study on p. 722 includes questions that review the usual treatments for a patient with GERD.

IN SUMMARY Common disorders that affect the esophagus include dysphagia and gastroesophageal reflux, and both are associated with a number of medical conditions. Swallowing disorders may interfere with food intake and increase risk of aspiration. Gastroesophageal reflux disease (GERD) can lead to esophageal ulcers, bleeding, and stricture. Esophageal conditions are

TABLE 23-3 Conditions and Substances Associated with Esophageal Reflux

Conditions That Raise the Likelihood of Reflux

- Ascites (accumulation of fluid in the abdomen)
- Delayed gastric emptying
- Eating large meals
- Lying flat after eating
- Obesity
- Pregnancy
- Wearing clothes that fit tightly across the waist or abdomen

Substances That Weaken Lower Esophageal Sphincter Pressure

- Alcohol
- Anticholinergic agents
- Caffeine
- Calcium channel blockers
- Chocolate
- Cigarette smoking
- Diazepam
- Garlic
- High-fat foods
- Meperidine
- Onions
- Peppermint and spearmint oils
- Progesterone
- Theophylline

proton-pump inhibitors: a class of drugs that inhibit the enzyme that pumps hydrogen ions (protons) into the stomach. Examples include omeprazole (Prilosec) and lansoprazole (Prevacid).

histamine-2-receptor blocking agents: a class of drugs that suppress acid secretion by inhibiting receptors on acid-producing cells (commonly called H2-blockers). Examples include cimetidine (Tagamet), ranitidine (Zantac), and famotidine (Pepcid).

CASE STUDY

Accountant with GERD

Mrs. Rinaldi is a 49-year-old accountant who is 5 feet 4 inches tall and weighs 165 pounds. She recently underwent a complete physical examination. She told her physician that she had been feeling fairly well until she began experiencing heartburn, which has progressively become more frequent and painful. The heartburn often occurs after she eats a large meal and is particularly bad after she goes to bed at night. Direct examination with an endoscope revealed reflux esophagitis and slight narrowing throughout the length of the esophagus.

Mrs. Rinaldi's past health history does not indicate any significant health problems. During her last physical, her physician advised her to stop smoking cigarettes and to lose 20 pounds, but she has not attempted either. The nutrition assessment reveals that Mrs. Rinaldi is feeling very stressed because it is the middle of the tax season. She usually has little time for breakfast, eats a lunch of fast foods while continuing to work, and eats a large dinner at around 8:00 P.M. She generally has wine with dinner and another alcoholic beverage later in the evening.

1. Explain to Mrs. Rinaldi the meaning of her diagnoses of "reflux esophagitis" and "esophageal stricture."
2. From the brief history provided, list the factors and behaviors that increase Mrs. Rinaldi's risks of experiencing reflux. What recommendations can you make to help her change these behaviors?
3. What medications might the physician prescribe and why?

often diagnosed using barium swallow studies and endoscopy. Treatment of dysphagia may include adjusting the diet, doing strengthening exercises, and learning new swallowing techniques. The treatment for GERD usually includes the use of acid-suppressing drugs and lifestyle modifications.

Conditions Affecting the Stomach

Stomach disorders range from occasional bouts of discomfort to conditions that require surgery. This section begins with a discussion of **dyspepsia** (often called "indigestion"), the feeling of pain or discomfort in the upper abdomen that occurs after food consumption. More serious stomach conditions that may benefit from dietary adjustments include **gastritis** and peptic ulcers, which often result from bacterial infection or from the use of medications that damage the stomach lining. Finally, the dietary considerations following gastric surgery are described.[8]

Dyspepsia

Dyspepsia refers to the general symptoms of indigestion in the upper abdominal area, which may include stomach pain, heartburn, fullness, nausea, and bloating. These symptoms sometimes indicate the presence of more serious illnesses, including GERD or peptic ulcer disease. Although a majority of the population experiences occasional dyspepsia, most are unlikely to seek medical attention.

Causes of Dyspepsia Abdominal pain can be difficult to diagnose, and the cause is not always evident from a physical examination. Various medical conditions can cause symptoms: these include peptic ulcers, GERD, motility disorders, malabsorptive disorders (discussed in Chapter 24), gallbladder disease, and tumors in the abdominal region. Some medications, including aspirin and other NSAIDs, antibiotics, glucocorticoids, estrogen, diuretics, digitalis, and theophylline, may cause gastrointestinal distress. Dietary supplements may also be a cause; for example, high-dose iron supplements and some herbal remedies often cause gastrointestinal discomfort. Systemic disorders such as diabetes mellitus, renal disease, thyroid disease, and heart failure may be accompanied by gastric symptoms. Intestinal conditions such as irritable bowel syndrome or lactose intolerance can sometimes mimic dyspepsia. Although pinpointing the cause of gastric symptoms

dyspepsia: a feeling of pain, bloating, or discomfort in the upper abdominal area, often called "indigestion"; a symptom of illness rather than a disease itself.
- **dys** = bad; impaired
- **pepsia** = refers to digestion

gastritis: inflammation of stomach tissue

can be difficult, a complete examination is in order if symptoms include weight loss, persistent vomiting, dysphagia, anemia, or bleeding, which suggest the presence of serious illness.

Bloating and Stomach Gas The feeling of bloating may be caused by excessive gas in the stomach, which accumulates when air is swallowed. Swallowing air often accompanies gum chewing, smoking, rapid eating, drinking carbonated beverages, and using a straw. Omitting these behaviors generally helps to reverse the problem.

Potential Food Intolerances Many people attribute their symptoms to overeating or eating certain foods or spices, although controlled studies have been unable to find associations between specific foods and dyspepsia. Coffee (including decaffeinated) can cause symptoms in many people who complain of dyspepsia and may also increase acid reflux and cause heartburn.[9] Spicy foods may cause some injury to the mucosal lining and exacerbate the pain from a preexisting ulcer. High-fat meals can slow gastric emptying and thereby exacerbate dyspepsia. To minimize symptoms, people with dyspepsia are sometimes advised to consume small meals with well-cooked foods that are not overly seasoned and to consume meals in a relaxed atmosphere.[10]

Nausea and Vomiting

Nausea and vomiting accompany multiple medical conditions.[11] They are also common side effects of medications and can be triggered by motion sickness, food odors, and emotional distress. Nausea and vomiting are common in pregnancy (see p. 488), usually occurring within the first trimester and disappearing by the fourth month. Although occasional vomiting is not dangerous, prolonged vomiting can cause fluid and electrolyte imbalances and may require medical care. Chronic vomiting can also reduce food intake and lead to malnutrition and nutrient deficiencies.

The timing of vomiting gives clues about its cause. Vomiting that occurs within an hour after a meal suggests peptic ulcer or a psychological cause. If it occurs more than one hour after a meal, possible causes include food poisoning, an obstruction that prevents stomach emptying, or a stomach motility disorder.

Treatment of Nausea and Vomiting The main goal of treatment is to find and correct the underlying disorder. Most cases are short-lived and require no treatment. Restoring hydration may be necessary in some cases. If a medication is the cause, taking it with food may help. If the cause is unknown or the underlying disorder cannot be corrected, medications that suppress nausea and vomiting can be prescribed. People with **intractable vomiting**—that is, vomiting that is not easily controlled—may require intravenous nutrition support.

Dietary Interventions Sometimes nausea may be prevented or improved with dietary measures. Eating and drinking slowly may be helpful, as may eating small meals that do not distend the stomach. Drinking clear, cold beverages such as carbonated drinks or fruit juices may ease symptoms. Foods that may reduce nausea include dry, salty foods like crackers or pretzels. Fried or spicy foods and foods with strong odors should be avoided. Foods that are cold or at room temperature may be better tolerated than hot meals. Individuals sometimes have strong food aversions when nauseated, and tolerances vary greatly.

Gastritis

Gastritis is an inflammation of the stomach mucosa and has multiple causes. The term *gastritis*■ is a general one, and therefore more specific diagnoses are preferred.

■ The suffix *-itis* generally indicates the presence of inflammation in an organ or tissue.

intractable vomiting: vomiting that is not easily managed or controlled.

TABLE 23-4 Potential Causes of Gastritis

Infection

- Bacterial: *Helicobacter pylori, Actinomyces israelii*
- Fungal: *Candida albicans*
- Parasitic: Cryptosporidiosis, nematode infection
- Viral: Cytomegalovirus

Chemical Substances

- Alcohol
- Cocaine
- Drugs (especially aspirin and other NSAIDs)
- Ingestion of corrosive materials

Internal (bodily) Causes

- Autoimmune
- Bile reflux
- Stress
- Systemic illness/sepsis

Miscellaneous

- High salt intake
- Food sensitivity (allergy)
- Foreign bodies
- Radiation therapy

Causes and Complications of Gastritis The most common causes of gastritis are ***Helicobacter pylori*** infection and the use of nonsteroidal anti-inflammatory drugs (NSAIDs), which are also primary causes of peptic ulcer. If the gastric mucosa shows signs of **hemorrhage,** tissue erosion, or ulcers, the condition may be called **acute erosive gastritis,** even if inflammation is not present. Acute erosive gastritis can be caused by a variety of factors including alcohol and other chemical substances, radiation treatment, and bile reflux. Chronic gastritis that is characterized by cellular destruction is known as atrophic gastritis. The prevalence of atrophic gastritis increases with aging, perhaps affecting as many as 30 percent of people over the age of 60. Table 23-4 lists some common causes of gastritis.

The extensive tissue damage that sometimes develops in chronic gastritis can disrupt gastric secretory functions. If hydrochloric acid secretions become abnormally low **(hypochlorhydria)** or absent **(achlorhydria),** absorption of nonheme iron and vitamin B_{12} can be impaired and the risk of deficiencies increased.[12] Pernicious anemia, a condition characterized by the destruction of stomach cells that produce intrinsic factor, is a late complication of chronic atrophic gastritis and a primary cause of vitamin B_{12} deficiency (see pp. 341–342).

Dietary Interventions Dietary recommendations vary according to an individual's symptoms. If gastritis is asymptomatic, no dietary adjustments are needed. If pain or discomfort is present, irritating foods and beverages should be avoided; these usually include alcohol, coffee (including decaffeinated), tea, cola beverages, spicy foods, and fatty or greasy foods. If food consumption increases pain or causes nausea and vomiting, food intake should be avoided for 24 to 48 hours to rest the stomach. Nutrition support may be necessary if food is not tolerated for a prolonged period. If gastritis results in hypochlorhydria or achlorhydria, supplementation of iron and vitamin B_{12} may be warranted.

Peptic Ulcer Disease

Ordinarily, the gastrointestinal mucosa has defense mechanisms that protect it from the destructive effects of hydrochloric acid and pepsin. If these defenses are overwhelmed, mucosal tissue can be destroyed, and an ulcer may eventually develop.■ The primary cause of peptic ulcer disease is *Helicobacter pylori* infection, which has been implicated in more than 60 percent of **gastric ulcers** and approximately 80 percent of **duodenal ulcers.**[13]■ The second most-frequent cause of ulcers is the use of nonsteroidal anti-inflammatory drugs (NSAIDs), which have both topical and systemic effects that can damage mucosal tissue. More rarely, ulcers may result from conditions that cause excessive acid secretion: one such condition is **Zollinger-Ellison syndrome,** which is characterized by the presence of gastrin-secreting tumors in the pancreas and duodenum.■ Cigarette smoking and nicotine can contribute to ulcers by increasing gastric secretions, altering mucosal cell populations, and promoting synthesis of hormones and proteins that induce ulcer formation.[14] Ulcer risk is also affected by emotional stress and genetic factors (see the Research Update).

Effects of Emotional Stress Although most ulcers result from either *H. pylori* infection or NSAID use, an estimated 10 to 20 percent of ulcers develop in people who have no exposure to either.[15] Also, the vast majority of people with *H. pylori* infection never develop an ulcer. What, then, is the direct "cause" of an ulcer? Although emotional stress is not believed to cause ulcers *per se,* it has effects on physiological processes and behaviors that may increase a person's vulnerability. Physiological effects of stress vary among individuals, but may include rapid stomach emptying (which increases the acid load in the duodenum), hormonal changes that impair wound healing, and increases in acid and pepsin secretions. Behavioral changes that may result from stress include increased use of alcohol, tobacco, and NSAIDs—all potential risk factors. Although the role of stress in ulcer development is not fully understood, current evidence suggests that it may play a contributory role.

Signs and Symptoms Peptic ulcer symptoms vary. Some people are asymptomatic or experience only mild discomfort. Ulcer "pain" may be experienced as a

■ Reminder: Highlight 3 introduced the topic of peptic ulcers (see p. 99).

■ The specific reasons that ulcers develop have not been determined; fewer than 20% of people with chronic *H. pylori* infection actually develop a peptic ulcer.

■ Reminder: *Gastrin* is a hormone that signals stomach cells to secrete hydrochloric acid (see p. 90).

Helicobacter pylori: a type of bacterium that colonizes gastric mucosa; a major cause of gastritis and peptic ulcer disease.

hemorrhage: extremely severe bleeding; a copious flow of blood from blood vessels.

acute erosive gastritis: a condition in which gastric mucosa is acutely injured, often by the toxic effects of chemical substances or radiation treatment. Damage may include hemorrhages, tissue erosion, and ulcers.

hypochlorhydria (HYE-po-klor-HYE-dree-ah): a reduction in gastric acid secretion.

achlorhydria (AY-klor-HYE-dree-ah): absence of gastric acid secretion.

gastric ulcers: peptic ulcers that develop in stomach tissue.

duodenal ulcers: peptic ulcers that develop in the duodenum.

Zollinger-Ellison syndrome: a syndrome characterized by the development of gastrin-secreting tumors (gastrinomas); most often located in the pancreas and duodenum.

RESEARCH UPDATE Genetic Susceptibility to Peptic Ulcers

As with most complex, multifactorial diseases, the development of peptic ulcer is affected by genetic susceptibility. This relationship has been supported by epidemiological evidence showing that identical twins share a tendency to develop ulcers that is greater than that of fraternal twins. Although research also shows that other first-degree relatives of ulcer patients have high risks of developing ulcers, this could be due in part to the spread of *H. pylori* infection among family members (first-degree relatives are parents, siblings, and children).[a]

Recently, a number of genetic polymorphisms (alterations in genetic structure) have been identified in people who have similar predispositions to developing ulcers. Genetic similarities are especially high among genes for cytokines, which play key roles in regulating immune defenses (against *H. pylori* infection, for example) and in regulating gastric acid secretion.[b] It still is not clear whether an increased genetic vulnerability for peptic ulcer disease is more closely related to a higher susceptibility of the gastric mucosa to ulceration or to a lower resistance to *H. pylori* infection.

a. M. Feldman, L. S. Friedman, and M. H. Sleisenger, eds., *Sleisenger and Fortran's Gastrointestinal and Liver Disease* (Philadelphia: Saunders, 2002).

b. N. Hamajima, Persistent *Helicobacter pylori* infection and genetic polymorphisms of the host, *Nagoya Journal of Medical Science* 66 (2003): 103–117; M. A. Garcia-Gonzalez and coauthors, Association of interleukin 1 gene family polymorphisms with duodenal ulcer disease, *Clinical and Experimental Immunology* 134 (2003): 525–531.

hunger pain, a sensation of gnawing, or a burning pain in the stomach region. The pain or discomfort of ulcers may be relieved by food and recur several hours after a meal, especially if the ulcer is duodenal.■ Gastric ulcers may sometimes be aggravated by food and can cause loss of appetite and eventual weight loss. Ulcer symptoms tend to go into remission regularly and recur every few weeks or months.

■ Approximately 85% of ulcers occur in the duodenum; only about 15% are gastric.

Complications Peptic ulcers are a major cause of gastrointestinal bleeding, which is the first sign of an ulcer in about 10 to 15 percent of cases. Bleeding is suspected if a person feels weak or fatigued or shows other signs of anemia. Severe bleeding or hemorrhage may be evidenced by black, tarry stool samples or, occasionally, vomit that resembles coffee grounds. Hemorrhage requires emergency care, as it is extremely dangerous and can potentially lead to shock and organ dysfunction. Other serious complications of ulcers include perforations of the stomach or duodenum (leading directly into the peritoneal cavity) and gastric outlet obstruction; both types of complications may require surgery.

Drug Therapy The major goals of ulcer treatment are to relieve pain, promote healing, and prevent recurrence. In most cases, treatment requires using antibiotics to eradicate *H. pylori* infection and/or discontinuing the use of aspirin and other NSAIDs, which can irritate the gastric mucosa and delay healing. *H. pylori* infection is difficult to treat: standard treatment requires that two antibiotics be taken simultaneously.■ Antisecretory drugs are also prescribed to relieve pain and allow healing; these may include proton-pump inhibitors, H2-blockers, or antacids (as used in GERD; see the earlier discussion on p. 721). Medications that coat the gastrointestinal lining and prevent further tissue erosion are frequently included in therapy and may include bismuth preparations (Pepto-Bismol) or sucralfate (Carafate). The most frequently prescribed drug regimen is a "triple therapy" that includes two antibiotics and one other type of drug.

■ Antibiotics used in ulcer therapy usually include amoxicillin, tetracycline, metronidazole, and clarithromycin.

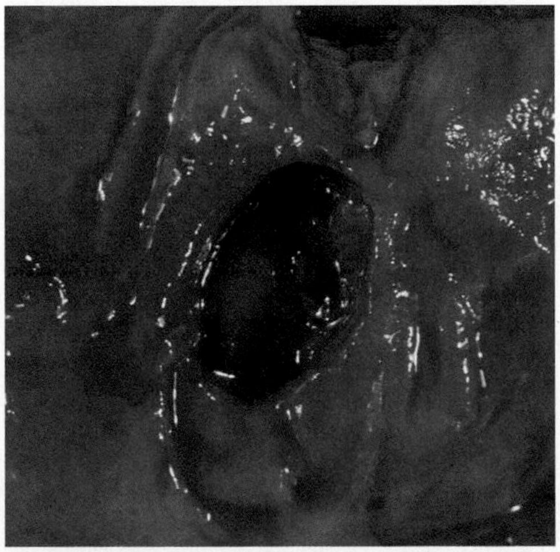

A peptic ulcer, such as the gastric ulcer shown here, damages mucosal tissue and may cause pain and bleeding.

Dietary Considerations Alterations in diet are required only if a person's symptoms are affected by food consumption. As with recommendations for gastritis, dietary adjustments are individualized to personal tolerances. Foods that may irritate the gastrointestinal lining are avoided; these often include alcohol, coffee and caffeine-containing beverages, and spicy foods. Large meals should be avoided so that gastric secretions do not persist for long periods. There is no evidence that dietary adjustments alter the rate of healing.

Gastric Surgery

In recent years, gastric surgery has become extremely popular as an effective treatment for severe obesity. Less frequently, surgery may be used to treat peptic ulcers that are resistant to drug therapy or to correct ulcer complications. Gastric surgery is also necessary for treating stomach cancer. Because gastric surgery interferes with stomach function either temporarily or permanently, dietary adjustments are usually necessary after surgery.

Surgical Procedures Surgical techniques used for severe obesity were initially discussed in Chapter 9. Figure 9-5 (p. 291) illustrates gastroplasty and gastric bypass surgery, two examples of **bariatric surgery.** The gastric pouch that remains after both types of bariatric surgery eventually stretches to hold about a cup of food, thereby restricting meal size. The gastric bypass procedure also restricts absorptive capacity because the digestive route created by the surgery bypasses the duodenum and part of the jejunum.

Although popular in the past, surgical treatment of ulcers is now rarely necessary due to the efficacy of current drug therapies. Peptic ulcer disease is only occasionally treated by **gastrectomy** (see Figure 23-3), a surgical procedure in which diseased portions of the stomach are removed. Gastric **resection** operations are also used to treat ulcer complications, such as gastric outlet obstruction. In a **vagotomy** procedure, the **vagus nerve** is severed in order to suppress gastric acid secretion. Because this procedure may impair gastric motility, it is sometimes followed by a **pyloroplasty,** which widens the pyloric sphincter to ensure drainage from the stomach to the duodenum.

The Postgastrectomy Diet Following surgery, fluids and foods are withheld until some healing has occurred.[16] Initially, fluids are supplied intravenously and fluid balance is carefully monitored. Ice chips or small sips of water (cold or warm) may be allowed 24 to 48 hours after surgery. After several more days, clear liquids (see pp. 611–613) are introduced. Patients can often tolerate solid foods by the fourth or fifth day after surgery, although some patients may need a longer period.

Dietary adjustments after gastrectomy are influenced by the size of the remaining stomach and the more rapid gastric emptying rate that results from this type of surgery. The surgical outcomes not only limit meal size, but also influence food tolerances due to the potential for dumping syndrome, as described in the next section. The diet initially offered is made up of small, frequent meals and snacks and includes mostly soft, low-fat foods. Meals often include foods high in complex carbohydrates (bread, potatoes, and vegetables) and protein (fish, lean meats, and eggs). Sweets and sugars should be avoided because they increase osmolarity in the small intestine. Liquids are restricted during meals (to about ½ cup of fluids) due to the limited stomach capacity and because liquids can speed the emptying rate. Although tolerances vary, some patients may have difficulty with fatty foods, highly spiced foods, carbonated drinks, caffeine-containing beverages, alcohol, extremely hot or cold foods, peppermint, and chocolate. Initially, a dietitian may need to visit a gastrectomy patient after meals to check tolerances for different foods. Table 23-5 lists foods that are permitted and those that are limited in postgastrectomy

FIGURE 23-3 Typical Gastric Surgery Resections

In a gastric resection, part or all of the stomach is surgically removed. The dashed lines show the removed section.

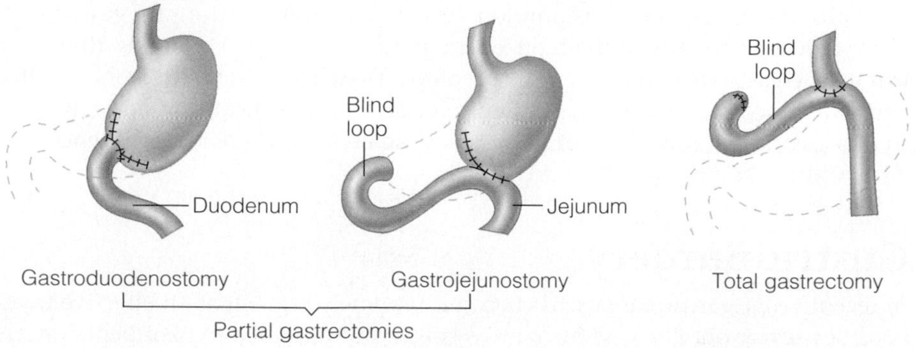
Duodenum
Blind loop
Jejunum
Blind loop
Gastroduodenostomy
Gastrojejunostomy
Total gastrectomy
Partial gastrectomies

bariatric (BAH-ree-AH-trik) **surgery:** surgery that treats obesity.
- **baros** = weight

gastrectomy (gas-TREK-ta-mee): the surgical removal of part of the stomach (partial gastrectomy) or the entire stomach (total gastrectomy).

resection: the surgical removal of part of an organ or body structure.

vagotomy (vay-GOT-oh-mee): surgery that severs the vagus nerve in order to suppress gastric acid secretion. This surgery may impair gastric emptying and require an additional pyloroplasty procedure to allow drainage.

vagus nerve: the cranial nerve that regulates hydrochloric acid secretion and peristalsis. Effects elsewhere in the body include regulation of heart rate and bronchiole constriction.

pyloroplasty (py-LOOR-oh-PLAS-tee): surgery that enlarges the pyloric sphincter.

TABLE 23-5 Postgastrectomy Diet

	Foods Recommended (as tolerated)	Foods to Limit (unless tolerated)
Meat and meat alternates	Lean tender meats, fish, poultry, shellfish, eggs, peanut butter	Fried, highly seasoned, and spicy foods
Milk and milk products	Milk, plain yogurt, mild cheeses	Milk shakes, chocolate milk, heavy cream, fruit yogurt
Breads and cereals	Whole-grain or enriched breads, crackers, bagels, low-fat muffins, dry cereal, oatmeal and other cooked cereals, rice, noodles, pasta	Bread or other baked goods that contain dried fruit, nuts, or seeds; fruitcake; frosted cereals; granola; pastries; doughnuts
Vegetables	Any, as tolerated	Candied yams or sweet potatoes, fried vegetables
Fruit	Fresh fruits, unsweetened canned fruits and fruit juices, fruits canned in light syrup	Dried fruits, sweetened juices, fruits canned in heavy syrup
Desserts	Plain cake, cookies, custard, artificially sweetened pudding and gelatin desserts	Desserts made with chocolate or dried fruit, sweetened gelatin desserts, ice cream and ice milk, candy, marshmallows
Beverages	Milk, diluted or unsweetened fruit drinks, unsweetened carbonated drinks, tea	Coffee, alcoholic beverages, sweetened fruit drinks, sweetened carbonated drinks
Sweeteners and condiments	Sugar substitutes, salt, pepper, mildly flavored sauces and gravies, spices as tolerated	Sugar, syrup, honey, jam, molasses

SOURCE: Adapted from American Dietetic Association, *Manual of Clinical Dietetics* (Chicago: American Dietetic Association, 2000), Chapter 25: Gastric Surgery.

diets. The case study on p. 728 provides the opportunity to design a menu for a postgastrectomy patient.

Dumping Syndrome **Dumping syndrome,** which refers to a group of symptoms resulting from abnormally rapid gastric emptying, is a common complication of both gastrectomy and gastric bypass surgery. Ordinarily, the pyloric sphincter controls the rate of flow from the stomach into the duodenum. After some types of stomach surgery, the hypertonic gastric contents are no longer regulated and can rush into the small intestine after meals, causing a number of unpleasant effects. Early symptoms can occur within 30 minutes and may include nausea, vomiting, abdominal cramping, diarrhea, lightheadedness, rapid heartbeat, and others (see Table 23-6). These symptoms may be due to intestinal distention (which causes the release of an excess amount of vasoactive chemicals), a large fluid shift from blood plasma to the intestine that lowers blood volume, and an increase in peristaltic activity. Several hours later, symptoms of hypoglycemia may occur (see Table 23-6) because the unusually large spike in blood glucose following the meal (due to rapid nutrient influx and absorption) can result in an excessive insulin response.

Dietary adjustments can greatly minimize or prevent dumping syndrome. The dietary goals are to limit the amount of food material that reaches the intestine, slow the rate of gastric emptying, and reduce foods that increase hypertonicity. Therefore, meal size is limited, fluids are restricted during meals, and sugars

TABLE 23-6 Symptoms of Dumping Syndrome

Early Dumping Syndrome	Late Dumping Syndrome
Symptoms may begin within 30 minutes after eating.	Symptoms may begin 1 to 3 hours after eating.
• Abdominal fullness, cramps	• Anxiety
• Diarrhea	• Confusion, difficulty thinking
• Dizziness	• Headache
• Flushing, sweating	• Hunger
• Nausea and vomiting	• Palpitations
• Rapid heartbeat	• Sweating
• Weakness, feeling faint	• Weakness, feeling faint

dumping syndrome: symptoms that result from the rapid emptying of an osmotic load from the stomach into the small intestine. Early symptoms include nausea, abdominal cramps, weakness, and diarrhea; later symptoms are those of hypoglycemia.

CASE STUDY

Commercial Artist Requiring Gastric Surgery

Mr. Toebe, a 58-year-old commercial artist, was admitted to the hospital for gastric surgery after numerous medical treatments failed to manage his severe peptic ulcer disease. A gastrojejunostomy was performed, and after about 24 hours, Mr. Toebe was able to take small sips of warm water. The health care team anticipates multiple nutrition-related problems and is taking measures to prevent them.

1. Review Figure 23-3 to better understand Mr. Toebe's surgical procedure. Consider the possibilities that he might experience the following symptoms: early satiety, nausea and vomiting, weight loss, dumping syndrome, steatorrhea, anemia, and bone disease. Explain why each of these conditions may occur.
2. What type of diet will the physician prescribe for Mr. Toebe after he begins eating solid foods? Create a day's worth of menus, using foods from Table 23-5.
3. What advice can you give Mr. Toebe that will help to prevent dumping syndrome? List several foods from each major food group that may cause dumping symptoms.

(including milk sugar) are restricted. The "How to" lists practical suggestions to reduce the occurrence of dumping syndrome. Sometimes the addition of pectin or guar gum■ can help to control symptoms. In some cases, drugs (for example, octreotide■) or additional surgery may be necessary.

■ Reminder: *Pectin* and *guar gum* are soluble dietary fibers that increase the viscosity of gastric contents and thereby slow the gastric emptying rate.

■ *Octreotide* inhibits gastrointestinal motility, thereby slowing gastric emptying and increasing transit time in the small intestine.

Postsurgical Complications and Nutrition Status Although weight loss is a primary goal for people who elect to have bariatric surgery, substantial weight loss can sometimes be an unintended consequence of gastrectomy.[17] It may take some time for a postgastrectomy patient to learn how much food can be consumed without causing uncomfortable symptoms. The discomfort associated with meals may lead to food avoidance, weight loss, and eventually malnutrition. Another cause of significant weight loss is **steatorrhea.**

Steatorrhea The term *steatorrhea* refers to an excess of fat in the stools due to fat maldigestion and malabsorption.■ Fat maldigestion may occur after surgery due to the accelerated transit of food material, which prevents normal mixing of fat with enzymes and bile. Furthermore, if the duodenum has been removed or bypassed, fewer pancreatic lipases are secreted into the intestine.■ Another potential cause of steatorrhea is **bacterial overgrowth** in the small intestine, which interferes with bile function. Impaired fat digestion, and absorption may result in deficiencies of fat-soluble vitamins and minerals. To improve digestion supplemental pancreatic enzymes are sometimes provided. Medium-chain triglycerides, which are more easily digested and absorbed, can be used to supply additional fat kcalories.

■ Steatorrhea is discussed in more detail in Chapter 24.

■ Reminder: The duodenal hormone secretin stimulates pancreatic enzyme secretion.

Bone Disease The fat malabsorption that results from gastric surgery can cause malabsorption of both calcium■ and vitamin D. Because many gastrectomy patients also avoid milk products to minimize dumping, they are at extremely high risk of calcium and vitamin D deficiencies. The incidence of osteoporosis and osteomalacia is high in gastrectomy patients, and bone density should be monitored during the years following surgery. Supplementation of calcium and vitamin D is often recommended.

■ Fat malabsorption reduces calcium absorption because the negatively charged fatty acids combine with calcium (which is positively charged) and prevent its absorption.

Anemia Gastrectomy patients are at high risk for anemia from iron and vitamin B_{12} deficiencies, although it may take several years to develop. As mentioned earlier, reduced gastric secretions can impair absorption of both iron and vitamin B_{12}. If the duodenum has been removed or is bypassed, iron absorption is greatly reduced because the duodenum is a major site of iron absorption. Supplementation of both iron and vitamin B_{12} is often warranted.

Bariatric Surgery Although bariatric surgeries are extremely effective treatments for morbid obesity, patients need to have realistic expectations about the amount of weight they are likely to lose after surgery, the diet they need to follow, and the complications that may ensue. Bariatric surgery can dramatically affect health and nutrition status, and patients require lifelong management.[18]

steatorrhea (stee-AT-or-REE-ah): excessive fat in the stools resulting from fat malabsorption; characterized by stools that are loose, frothy, and foul smelling due to a high fat content.
- **steat** = fat
- **rheo** = flow

bacterial overgrowth: excessive bacterial colonization of the stomach or small intestine that interferes with normal digestion and absorption; may be caused by low gastric acidity, altered gastrointestinal motility, mucosal damage, or contamination.

HOW TO Alter the Diet to Reduce Symptoms of Dumping Syndrome

Dietary adjustments can minimize or prevent symptoms of dumping syndrome. The following suggestions often help:

- Eat smaller meals to fit the reduced capacity of the stomach. Increase the number of meals consumed daily so that energy intake is adequate.
- Eat in a relaxed setting. Eat slowly and chew food thoroughly.
- Limit the amount of fluid taken with meals. Avoid consuming beverages within 45 minutes before and after meals, but be sure to include adequate fluid intake during the day to avoid dehydration.
- Avoid juices and sweetened beverages and foods that contain high amounts of sugar. Avoid carbonated beverages if they cause bloating.
- Use artificial sweeteners to sweeten beverages and desserts.
- Avoid foods and beverages that are very hot or very cold, unless tolerated.
- Include fiber-rich foods in each meal.
- Avoid milk and most milk products, which are high in lactose. Enzyme-treated milk should also be avoided because the breakdown products of lactose (glucose and galactose) can also cause symptoms. Cheese may be better tolerated because its lactose content is low. An effort should be made to consume nonmilk calcium sources such as green leafy vegetables, tofu, and fish with bones.
- If symptoms of hypoglycemia continue, try including a protein-rich food in each meal.
- Lie down for 20 to 30 minutes (or longer) after eating to help slow the transit of food to the small intestine. While eating a meal, sit upright.

Successful weight loss following bariatric surgery is generally defined as a long-term loss (lasting at least five years) of at least 50 percent of a person's excess weight. The most popular gastric bypass procedure (called a Roux-en-Y gastric bypass) is currently associated with long-term (5- to 14-year) losses averaging between 49 and 62 percent of excess weight.[19] Weight loss is most rapid in the first 6 months after surgery, and weight generally stabilizes after 18 to 24 months.

Dietary Guidelines after Bariatric Surgery Although the gastric pouch created by surgery eventually expands to hold about a cup of food, its initial capacity is only a few tablespoons. As with the postgastrectomy diet, only ice chips and small sips of water are given in the first day or two after bariatric surgery.[20] Afterwards, a full liquid diet is given for one to two weeks; the diet then progresses to pureed foods for a similar time period, then to soft foods, and, finally, to regular foods. Initially, patients receive five to six small meals daily. Some foods may be difficult to manage, especially dry, doughy, or fibrous foods, which may cause pain or vomiting.■ Fluids need to be consumed separately from meals to avoid excessive distention of the gastric pouch.

■ Foods that are potentially problematic after bariatric surgery include chicken, red meat, rice, and white bread.

Patient education and counseling are critical for weight loss and management. Food portion sizes must be carefully controlled to avoid symptoms of dumping syndrome and, later, to maintain weight loss. Patients should learn the elements of a healthy diet as well as the foods that may cause abdominal discomfort, vomiting, or dumping. Dietary supplements need to be taken regularly to avoid nutrient deficiencies. The "How to" on p. 730 includes additional dietary suggestions for patients who have undergone bariatric surgery.

Postsurgical Concerns in Bariatric Surgery The complications that may arise after bariatric surgery are similar to those for gastrectomy patients and may include dumping syndrome, malabsorption, and multiple nutrient deficiencies. Rapid weight loss also increases a person's risk of developing gallbladder disease; patients at especially high risk sometimes have their gallbladders removed during bariatric surgery. After weight loss, plastic surgery may be necessary to remove extra skin, especially on the abdomen, buttocks, hips, and thighs.

HOW TO Alter Dietary Habits to Lose Weight and Maintain Weight Loss after Bariatric Surgery

Patients need to learn new dietary habits after bariatric surgery. The following recommendations may help:

- Chew food thoroughly and consume only small amounts. Use a small spoon, and take small bites. Relax and enjoy the meal, taking at least 20 minutes to eat.
- Understand that at first, the appropriate portion size of each food served at mealtime may be only a few spoonfuls. Learn to recognize the sensations that occur when the gastric pouch is full. Signs of fullness may include pressure in the stomach region, a slight feeling of nausea, or pain in the upper chest or shoulder.
- Learn to recognize foods that cause problems. Foods that are dry, sticky, or fibrous may be difficult to tolerate in the weeks after surgery.
- To control vomiting, try eating smaller volumes of food, eating more slowly, and avoiding foods that are known to cause difficulty. Continued vomiting may be a sign that appropriate food behaviors are not being maintained.
- Eat only at mealtimes. Snacking throughout the day can become a bad habit that causes weight regain.
- Avoid consuming liquids within 45 minutes of mealtime. Consume liquids between meals only. Avoid high-kcalorie drinks like soda, alcoholic beverages, and milk shakes. Carbonated beverages increase stomach gas and may cause bloating.
- Drink adequate fluids between meals to avoid dehydration. Most people meet a substantial portion of their fluid needs by eating foods, but a patient who has had bariatric surgery cannot do this. Therefore, fluid intakes need to be increased after surgery.
- Engage in regular physical activity. Activity is a valuable aid to weight maintenance and can help to maintain lean tissue while weight is being lost.

IN SUMMARY Stomach conditions that sometimes benefit from dietary adjustments include dyspepsia, gastritis, and peptic ulcers. Abdominal pain, nausea, and vomiting can be caused by many different medical conditions, and the primary objective of treatment is to remove the underlying cause. The primary cause of gastritis and peptic ulcer disease is *Helicobacter pylori* infection, which may be eradicated by antibiotic therapy. The second most common cause of these conditions is the use of NSAIDs, which can directly damage the mucosal lining. Extensive damage to the mucosa can reduce gastric secretions and increase risks of iron and vitamin B_{12} deficiencies. Gastric surgeries, used to treat obesity and peptic ulcer disease, are associated with multiple complications and usually require dietary adjustments after surgery. Dumping syndrome is a common complication that results from the rapid influx of nutrients from the stomach into the small intestine.

DIET-DRUG INTERACTIONS

Antacids

Aluminum-containing antacids contribute aluminum to the diet and may cause constipation or lead to phosphorus deficiency. Long-term or inappropriate use can lead to aluminum toxicity.

Calcium-containing antacids contribute calcium to the diet and may cause constipation. Concurrent use with vitamin D supplements or foods containing large amounts of vitamin D can lead to elevated blood calcium levels (hypercalcemia).

Magnesium-containing antacids contribute magnesium to the diet and may cause diarrhea; long-term use may lead to magnesium toxicity.

Sodium bicarbonate, an antacid that contributes sodium to the diet, can alter serum electrolyte levels and raise the pH of the blood. Sodium bicarbonate should not be taken with milk—hypercalcemia can result.

Antibiotics (for *Helicobacter Pylori* Infections)

When *amoxicillin* is given without regard to food, nausea and diarrhea are common side effects. Advise patients to take with food to reduce nausea.

Metronidazole may cause taste alterations (metallic taste), and no alcohol should be used during treatment and for 24 hours afterward. Alcohol can react with metronidazole and result in a disulfram-like reaction with symptoms that include nausea, vomiting, headache, cramps, and flushing of the skin.

Tetracycline and its classic interactions with nutrients were mentioned in Chapter 19. Calcium, magnesium, zinc, aluminum, antacids that contain any of these nutrients, dairy products, and vitamin-mineral supplements should not be used within two hours of a tetracycline dose. Tetracycline can also cause nausea and diarrhea.

Antiemetics, Antinauseants

Antiemetics frequently lead to drowsiness. Two antiemetics, *dronabinol* (a derivative of marijuana) and *prochlorperazine,* stimulate the appetite and can result in weight gain. Prochlorperazine also increases the urinary excretion of riboflavin. Prochlorperazine, *prochloramide,* and *triethylperazine maleate* can lead to mouth dryness. Prochlorperazine, prochloramide, triethylperazine maleate, *granisetron,* and *odansteron* may cause constipation. *Metoclopramide* rarely causes nutrition-related side effects.

Antisecretory Agents

Antisecretory agents may interfere with iron absorption. When iron supplements are necessary, they should be given two hours before or after taking these medications. People taking some antisecretory agents should avoid the use of the herb pennyroyal; antisecretory agents may increase the formation of toxic metabolites from pennyroyal.

NUTRITION ASSESSMENT CHECKLIST for People with Upper GI Tract Disorders

Medical History

Check the patient's health history to uncover medical conditions or treatments that may:

- ☐ Interfere with chewing or swallowing
- ☐ Lead to dyspepsia, nausea, or vomiting

Check for a medical diagnosis of:

- ☐ Hiatal hernia
- ☐ GERD
- ☐ Gastritis or peptic ulcer
- ☐ Pernicious anemia

For a patient who has undergone gastric surgery, check for the following complications:

- ☐ Dumping syndrome
- ☐ Steatorrhea
- ☐ Bone disease
- ☐ Anemia

Medications

Check the medication and dosing schedule for:

- ☐ Medications that may cause dyspepsia, nausea, and vomiting. Note that many medications can cause nausea, especially the first few doses. Suggest that medications be taken with food, when possible, to help alleviate nausea.

Dietary Intake

To devise an acceptable meal plan, obtain:

- ☐ An accurate and thorough record of food intake
- ☐ A record of foods that provoke symptoms of dyspepsia, nausea, GERD, gastritis, peptic ulcers, or dumping syndrome

For patients on long-term dysphagia diets, monitor:

- ☐ Appetite
- ☐ Tolerances to foods
- ☐ Variety of foods offered and regularly consumed

Anthropometric Data

Measure baseline height and weight. Address weight loss early to prevent malnutrition for patients with:

- ☐ Dysphagia or difficulty chewing
- ☐ Dyspepsia or nausea of long duration
- ☐ Malabsorption
- ☐ Dumping syndrome

Laboratory Tests

Check laboratory tests for signs of dehydration for patients with

- ☐ Persistent vomiting
- ☐ Dumping syndrome

Check laboratory tests for nutrition-related anemia in patients with:

- ☐ Gastritis
- ☐ Previous gastric surgeries
- ☐ Conditions that require long-term use of antisecretory medications

Clinical Signs

Look for physical signs of:

- ☐ Dehydration (in patients with persistent vomiting or dumping syndrome)
- ☐ Iron and vitamin B_{12} deficiencies (in patients with hypochlorhydria or achlorhydria)

STUDY QUESTIONS

These questions will help you review the chapter. You will find the answers in the discussions on the pages provided.

1. Provide examples of conditions that can interfere with swallowing. Describe how diets are adjusted to meet the needs of people with dysphagia. (pp. 716–719)
2. Discuss ways to provide appetizing meals for people consuming mechanically altered foods. (p. 719)
3. Identify the symptoms, causes, and complications of gastroesophageal reflux disease (GERD). What lifestyle modifications can benefit patients with GERD? (pp. 719–721)
4. What are possible causes of nausea and vomiting? Discuss interventions that may help. (p. 723)
5. Specify the common causes of gastritis and peptic ulcer disease. Explain the possible consequences of these diseases. Describe the role of diet therapy for both conditions (pp. 723–725)
6. Describe the gastric disorders that may benefit from gastric surgery. What dietary adjustments are usually required after a gastrectomy procedure? (pp. 725–727)
7. What complications may arise after gastric surgery? Discuss the dietary interventions that may help to prevent these consequences. (pp. 727–729)
8. Describe the surgical procedures used to treat morbid obesity. What dietary recommendations may be helpful for patients who have undergone bariatric surgery? (pp. 728–730)

These questions will help you prepare for an exam. Answers can be found on p. 733.

1. If a patient with dysphagia has difficulty swallowing solids but can easily swallow liquids:
   a. the problem is probably a motility disorder.
   b. the patient most likely has achalasia.
   c. the problem is probably an esophageal obstruction.
   d. the patient may also develop oropharyngeal dysphagia.
2. The health care professional working with a patient with dysphagia recognizes that:
   a. only pureed foods should be given to minimize the risk of aspiration.
   b. the patient can have any food that can be comfortably and safely chewed and swallowed.
   c. highly seasoned foods are often restricted.
   d. conventional diets are unable to meet total nutrient needs and supplements are always necessary.
3. Gastroesophageal reflux disease (GERD) is:
   a. characterized by frequent backflow of the stomach's gastric secretions into the esophagus.
   b. a protuberance of a portion of the stomach above the lower esophageal sphincter.
   c. an erosion of the lining of the stomach caused by excess acid in gastric secretions.
   d. an obstruction of the lower esophagus that results in dysphagia.
4. Conditions associated with high rates of GERD include:
   a. hiatal hernia.
   b. Barrett's esophagus.
   c. pregnancy.
   d. all of the above.
5. For the patient with persistent vomiting, the major nutrition-related concern(s) is/are:
   a. dehydration and malnutrition.
   b. reflux esophagitis.
   c. dyspepsia.
   d. peptic ulcers.
6. Chronic gastritis frequently leads to:
   a. dumping syndrome.
   b. bone disease.
   c. iron and vitamin B_{12} deficiencies.
   d. excessive hydrochloric acid secretion.
7. The primary cause of most peptic ulcers is:
   a. consumption of spicy foods.
   b. hypochlorhydria.
   c. smoking cigarettes.
   d. *Helicobacter pylori* infection.
8. Foods discouraged for patients with gastritis or active ulcers include those that:
   a. are high in fiber.
   b. irritate the gastric mucosa.
   c. are easy to swallow.
   d. contain simple sugars.
9. People at risk of dumping syndrome should generally avoid:
   a. high-fiber foods.
   b. sweets and sugars.
   c. beverages.
   d. bread and potatoes.
10. The health care professional assessing a patient who underwent a gastrectomy several years ago should be alert to signs of:
    a. dysphagia.
    b. GERD.
    c. iron-deficiency anemia.
    d. gastritis.

NUTRITION ON THE NET

Access these websites for further study of topics covered in this chapter.

- Find updates and quick links to these and other nutrition-related sites at our website: **www.wadsworth.com/nutrition**
- Visit the websites of these organizations to find information that is helpful both for health practitioners and patients with gastrointestinal problems: American College of Gastroenterology: **www.acg.gi.org**

  American Gastroenterological Association: **www.gastro.org**

  National Institute of Diabetes and Digestive and Kidney Diseases, which is a division of the National Institutes of Health: **www.niddk.nih.gov**
- Visit the website of the North American Society for Pediatric Gastroenterology, Hepatology and Nutrition for information about gastrointestinal disorders affecting children: **www.naspgn.org**
- Find more information about dysphagia at the Dysphagia Resource Center: **www.dysphagia.com**
- Learn more about *Helicobacter pylori* from the Helicobacter Foundation: **www.helico.com**

REFERENCES

1. M. H. Beers and R. Berkow, eds., *The Merck Manual of Diagnosis and Therapy* (Whitehouse Station, N.J.: Merck Research Laboratories, 1999).
2. L. Goldman and D. Ausiello, eds., *Cecil Textbook of Medicine* (Philadelphia: Saunders, 2004); S. L. Friedman, K. R. McQuaid, and J. H. Grendell, eds., *Current Diagnosis and Treatment in Gastroenterology* (New York: Lange Medical Books/McGraw-Hill, 2003); M. Feldman, L. S. Friedman, and M. H. Sleisenger, eds., *Sleisenger and Fordtran's Gastrointestinal and Liver Disease* (Philadelphia: Saunders, 2002); Beers and Berkow, 1999.
3. M. R. Spieker, Evaluating dysphagia, *American Family Physician* 61 (2000): 3639–3648.
4. R. C. Orlando, Diseases of the esophagus, in L. Goldman and D. Ausiello, eds., *Cecil Textbook of Medicine* (Philadelphia: Saunders, 2004), pp. 814–823.
5. D. J. C. Ramsey, D. G. Smithard, and L. Kalra, Early assessments of dysphagia and aspiration risk in acute stroke patients, *Stroke* 34 (2003): 1252–1257; Spieker, 2000.
6. S. L. McCallum, The National Dysphagia Diet: Implementation at a regional rehabilitation center and hospital system, *Journal of the American Dietetic Association* 103 (2003): 381–384; G. McCullough, C. Pelletier, and C. Steele, National Dysphagia Diet: What to swallow? *The ASHA Leader,* November 4, 2003, pp. 16, 27; The National Dysphagia Diet Task Force, *The National Dysphagia Diet: Standardization for Optimal Care* (Chicago: American Dietetic Assocation, 2002).
7. V. Singh and coauthors, Multidisciplinary management of dysphagia: The first 100 cases, *Journal of Laryngology and Otology* 109 (1995): 419–424.
8. Goldman and Ausiello, 2004; Friedman, McQuaid, and Grendell, 2003; Feldman, Friedman, and Sleisenger, 2002; Beers and Berkow, 1999.
9. N. J. Talley, Functional gastrointestinal disorders: Irritable bowel syndrome, nonulcer dyspepsia, and noncardiac chest pain, in L. Goldman and D. Ausiello, eds., *Cecil Textbook of Medicine* (Philadelphia: Saunders, 2004), pp. 806–814.
10. S. Escott-Stump, *Nutrition and Diagnosis-Related Care* (Philadelphia: Lippincott Williams & Wilkins, 2002.)
11. Friedman, McQuaid, and Grendell, 2003; Feldman, Friedman, and Sleisenger, 2002; L. J. Cheskin and D. L. Miller, Nutrition in the prevention and treatment of common gastrointestinal symptoms, in A. M. Coulston, C. L. Rock, and E. R. Monsen, eds., *Nutrition in the Prevention and Treatment of Disease* (San Diego: Academic Press, 2001), pp. 549–562.
12. R. M. Russell, The aging process as a modifier of metabolism, *American Journal of Clinical Nutrition* 72 (2000): 529S–532S; Committee on Dietary Reference Intakes, *Dietary Reference Intakes for Vitamin A, Vitamin K, Arsenic, Boron, Chromium, Copper, Iodine, Iron, Manganese, Molybdenum, Nickel, Silicon, Vanadium, and Zinc* (Washington, D.C.: National Academy Press, 2000).
13. Feldman, Friedman, and Sleisenger, 2002.
14. P. Maity and coauthors, Smoking and the pathogenesis of gastroduodenal ulcer—recent mechanistic update, *Molecular and Cellular Biochemistry* 253 (2003): 329–338.
15. S. Levenstein, The very model of a modern etiology: A biopsychosocial view of peptic ulcer, *Psychosomatic Medicine* 62 (2000): 176–185.
16. American Dietetic Association, *Manual of Clinical Dietetics* (Chicago: American Dietetic Association, 2000).
17. C. R. Parrish, Post-gastrectomy: Managing the nutrition fall-out, *Nutrition Issues in Gastroenterology* 18 (2004): 63–75; American Dietetic Association, 2000.
18. D. R. Ferraro, Management of the bariatric surgery patient: Lifelong postoperative care—Board Review, *Clinician Reviews* 14 (2004): 73–79; W. Marcason, What are the dietary guidelines following bariatric surgery? *Journal of the American Dietetic Association* 104 (2004): 487–488.
19. Ferraro, 2004.
20. Marcason, 2004.

ANSWERS

Study Questions (multiple choice)

1\. c 2. b 3. a 4. d 5. a 6. c 7. d 8. b 9. b 10. c

HIGHLIGHT

Dental Health and Its Relationship with Chronic Illness

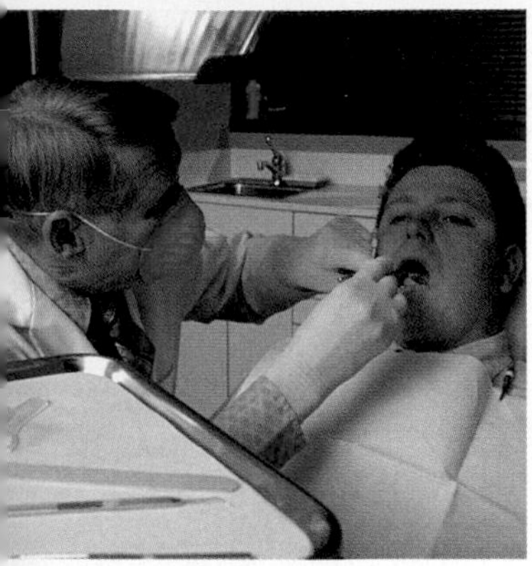

© Ken Sherman/PhotoTake

The relationships between nutrition and dental health were discussed earlier: Chapter 4 described the effects of sugar and other fermentable carbohydrates on tooth decay. Chapter 13 explained how fluoride can help to prevent dental caries. This highlight identifies other dental problems and gives examples of how chronic illnesses may influence the development of dental diseases and, conversely, how dental diseases may increase the risks of developing chronic illnesses. Related terms are defined in the glossary.

Periodontal Disease

Recall from Chapter 4 that dental caries develops when bacteria that reside in dental plaque ferment sugars and produce acid that dissolves tooth enamel (review Figure 4-14 on p. 122). Deposits of plaque can thicken and lead to other dental problems as well.[1] As plaque accumulates on the tooth surface, it fills with calcium and phosphate, eventually forming **dental calculus.** Calculus may develop either at the gum surface or in the crevice between the gum and a tooth; its presence may cause further plaque retention. The buildup of plaque and calculus increases the likelihood of infection and subsequent inflammation.

Periodontal disease refers to inflammatory conditions involving the **periodontium**—the tissues that support the tooth in its bony socket. The periodontium includes the gums (called **gingiva**), other connective tissues surrounding the tooth, and the bone underneath. Inflammation of the gums, called **gingivitis,** is characterized by redness, bleeding, and swelling of gum tissue. **Periodontitis** is an inflammation of the tissues surrounding the tooth. As plaque invades the space below the gum line, the combination of toxic bacterial byproducts and the body's immune response can destroy the tissues holding a tooth in place. Left untreated, the peridontium may be destroyed, leading to permanent tooth loss.

Risk Factors

Dental plaque is the major risk factor associated with periodontal disease, and the severity of the disease is related to the amount of plaque present. Tobacco smoking is another factor, possibly because of its destructive effects on cellular immune responses.[2] Periodontal disease is especially likely if a person has a chronic illness that impairs immune status, such as diabetes mellitus or HIV infection. Other risk factors include genetic susceptibility, stress, and dental conditions that increase plaque accumulation, such as poorly

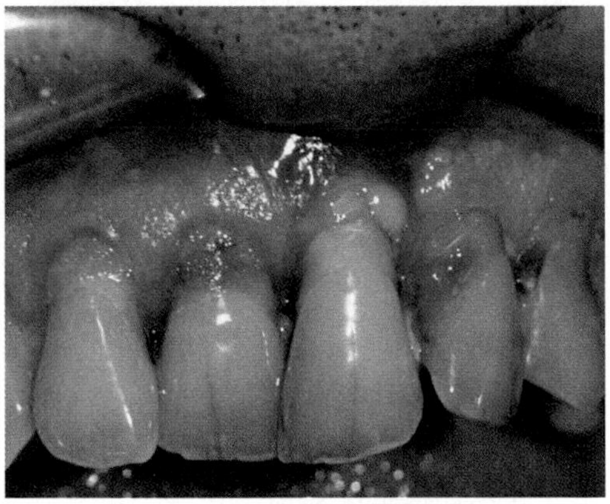

© CNRI/Photo Researchers, Inc.

Periodontal disease destroys the tissues and bones that hold teeth in place.

GLOSSARY

dental calculus: mineralized dental plaque, often associated with inflammation and bleeding.

gingiva (jin-JYE-va, JIN-jeh-va): the gums.

gingivitis (jin-jeh-VYE-tus): inflammation of the gums; characterized by redness, swelling, and bleeding.

periodontal disease: a disease that affects the connective tissue structures that support the teeth.

periodontitis: inflammation or degeneration of the tissues that support the teeth.

periodontium: the tissues that support the teeth, including the gums, cementum (bonelike material covering the dentin layer of the tooth), periodontal ligament, and underlying bone.
- **peri** = around, surrounding
- **odont** = tooth

Sjögren's syndrome: an autoimmune disease characterized by the destruction of secretory glands, especially those that produce saliva and tears resulting in dry mouth and dry eyes.

xerostomia: dry mouth caused by reduced salivary flow.
- **xero** = dry
- **stomia** = mouth

Reminder: *Dental caries* refers to tooth decay. *Dental plaque* is an accumulation of bacteria and their by-products that grow on teeth and can lead to dental caries and gum disease.

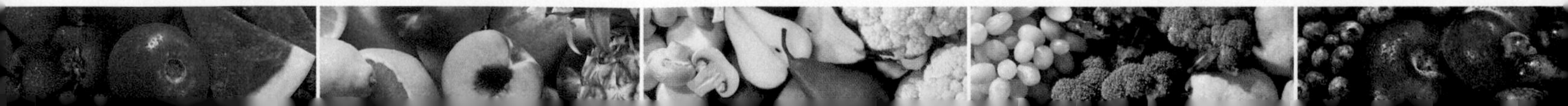

aligned teeth or calculus buildup. Strategies for reducing risk focus on improving oral hygiene (proper brushing and flossing) and encouraging smoking cessation.

Signs and Symptoms

Periodontal disease begins with gingivitis; gums may bleed readily from brushing or flossing and be tender and swollen. The gap between an infected gum and a tooth usually deepens, allowing food particles to get caught easily. A bad taste in the mouth or persistent bad breath is sometimes the first sign of gingivitis. In severe cases, pus may surround the teeth and gums. The teeth may be sensitive and chewing painful. If bone is destroyed, the affected gums usually recede, and teeth may loosen or change position.

Treatment of periodontal disease depends on the extent of damage. In mild cases, deep cleaning and proper oral hygiene may reverse the condition. Antimicrobial mouth rinses and topical antibiotics are often prescribed to control infection. Surgery is sometimes necessary to remove plaque or calculus deposits underneath gum tissue or to replace damaged tissues.

Dry Mouth

Secretions of the salivary glands protect the teeth and the mouth's soft tissues. Saliva lubricates oral tissues and contains antimicrobial proteins to defend against bacteria and fungi. The buffers in saliva raise the mouth's pH protecting tooth enamel from the acid produced by caries-causing bacteria. The calcium and phosphate concentrations of saliva help to prevent dissolution of enamel. Thus saliva helps to control plaque formation, prevent infection, and maintain tooth enamel. If salivary secretions are low or absent, risk of developing dental caries and periodontal disease increases.

Dry mouth **(xerostomia),** caused by reduced salivary flow, is a side effect of many medications and is associated with a number of diseases and disease treatments. Antihistamines, antihypertensive agents, antidepressants, decongestants, and other medications can cause dry mouth. Poorly controlled diabetes is often associated with dry mouth, as are conditions that directly affect salivary gland function, such as **Sjögren's syndrome.** Radiation therapy used to treat head and neck cancers often damages salivary glands, sometimes permanently. Mouth breathing is also a common cause of dry mouth.

A reduction in salivary flow can impair health in other ways as well. Dry mouth may interfere with speech and cause bad breath. Mouth infections are more common. Chewing and swallowing are more difficult, and taste sensation is diminished. Dentures may be uncomfortable to wear, and ulcerations may develop. Dry mouth may cause a person to reduce food intake and thereby increase malnutrition risk. Table H23-1 lists suggestions for managing dry mouth.

TABLE H23-1 Suggestions for Managing Dry Mouth

- Take frequent sips of water, or a sugarless beverage.
- Use sugarless candy or gum to help stimulate salivary flow.
- Suck on ice cubes or frozen fruit juice bars (unless their coldness causes discomfort).
- Avoid citrus juices and spicy or salty foods if they cause mouth irritation.
- Avoid dry foods like toast, chips, and crackers.
- Avoid caffeine, alcohol, and smoking, which may dry the mouth.
- Consume foods that have a high fluid content such as soups, stews, sauces and gravies, yogurt, and pureed fruits.
- Try over-the-counter saliva substitutes (available as gels, sprays, and tablets), especially just before meals and at bedtime.
- Try rinsing the mouth with small amounts of vegetable oil or softened margarine.
- Use a humidifier during the night.
- Pay strict attention to oral hygiene, brushing and flossing at least twice daily. Try to brush immediately after each meal.
- Avoid alcohol- and detergent-containing mouthwashes that may dry and irritate the mouth.
- If dry mouth is caused by a medication, ask your physician about possible alternatives.
- Ask your physician if using a medication to stimulate saliva secretion can be of benefit; examples include nicotinic acid tablets and pilocarpine.

Dental Health and Chronic Illness

Maintaining dental health can be challenging for a person with a chronic illness. As mentioned, many medications can reduce salivary secretions and the immune protection they provide. This section describes how several conditions may increase the risks of developing dental problems.

Diabetes Mellitus

For a number of reasons, periodontal disease is more prevalent among people with diabetes mellitus, especially in those whose diabetes is poorly controlled.[3] People with diabetes often have impaired immune responses and a greater susceptibility for infections. Diabetes also favors the growth of bacteria that tend to infect periodontal tissues.[4] Hyperglycemia weakens the collagen structure of tissues, making them vulnerable. People with diabetes tend to have higher plaque accumulations and dry mouth, predisposing them to periodontal disease.[5]

Because the risk of developing dental caries and oral fungal infections is high for people with diabetes, they must pay strict attention to oral hygiene. Smoking is discouraged because it can increase periodontal disease risk nearly tenfold in people with diabetes.[6] Health care providers should advise patients with diabetes that glucose control and routine dental care are critical to preventing periodontal disease.

Human Immunodeficiency Virus (HIV)/AIDS

HIV infection is characterized by compromised immunity, and the risk of developing periodontal disease is closely linked to the extent of HIV infection. In untreated persons, fungal and viral infections are common and may cause painful ulcerations. The current use of antiretroviral therapies, however, has substantially reduced the incidence of oral infections in HIV-positive persons.[7] Those at greatest risk of developing dental disease include smokers, individuals who decline therapy, and patients in advanced stages of disease.[8] Dry mouth often occurs in HIV-infected individuals as a result of medications or from salivary gland dysfunction.[9]

Oral Cancers

Radiation treatment of oral cancers can cause serious oral and dental complications.[10] Inflammation and tissue damage may be so severe that radiation treatment may need to be halted or the intensity reduced substantially. Radiation can also reduce salivary flow, causing the problem of dry mouth already mentioned. Other complications include fungal and viral infections, changes in taste sensation, and tissue and muscle scarring (which often reduces chewing ability). To minimize complications, dental care is often initiated before radiation therapy begins.

Dental Health and Disease Risk

Dental diseases may have adverse effects on health beyond their effects on teeth.[11] The bacteria that reside on dental tissues can enter the bloodstream and potentially cause infections elsewhere in the body. Evidence supporting a link between dental bacteria and other diseases includes the following:

- *Immune response.* The inflammatory process induced by periodontal disease activates cytokines and other mediators that have systemic effects.
- *Respiratory illnesses.* The teeth of hospital patients often become colonized with bacteria that cause respiratory illnesses. In one study, only patients whose teeth were colonized by respiratory pathogens ended up with pneumonia.[12]
- *Atherosclerosis and heart disease.* Bacteria associated with gingivitis can attack the cells lining the blood vessels, possibly affecting the process of atherosclerosis. In one study, researchers found a significant association between serum antibodies to periodontal bacteria and the incidence of heart disease.[13]
- *Diabetes mellitus.* Periodontal disease can make it more difficult for persons with diabetes to attain glucose control.

Although this evidence is suggestive, researchers studying the effects of periodontal disease have yet to prove cause-and-effect relationships between dental health and other conditions. Additional studies will help clarify the complex interactions between dental disease and chronic illnesses.

REFERENCES

1. American Dietetic Association, Position of the American Dietetic Association: Oral health and nutrition, *Journal of the American Dietetic Association* (2003): 615–625; B. Daly and coauthors, *Essential Dental Public Health* (Oxford: Oxford University Press, 2002); D. P. DePaola, M. P. Faine, and C. A. Palmer, Nutrition in relation to dental medicine, in M. E. Shils and coeditors, *Modern Nutrition in Health and Disease* (Baltimore: Williams & Wilkins, 1999), pp. 1099–1124; D. B. Ferguson, *Oral Bioscience* (London: Churchill Livingstone, 1999).
2. B. Loos and coauthors, Lymphocyte numbers and function in relation to periodontitis and smoking, *Journal of Periodontology* 75 (2004): 557–564.
3. D. C. Matthews, The relationship between diabetes and periodontal disease, *Journal of the Canadian Dental Association* 68 (2002): 161–164; American Association of Periodontology, Position paper: Diabetes and periodontal diseases, *Journal of Periodontology* 71 (2000): 664–678.
4. American Association of Periodontology, 2000.
5. Matthews, 2002.
6. Matthews, 2002.
7. V. Ramirez-Amador and coauthors, The changing clinical spectrum of human immunodeficiency virus (HIV)-related oral lesions in 1,000 consecutive patients: A 12-year study in a referral center in Mexico, *Medicine (Baltimore)* 82 (2003): 39–50; J. D. Eyeson and coauthors, Oral manifestations of an HIV positive cohort in the era of highly active anti-retroviral therapy (HAART) in South London, *Journal of Oral Pathology and Medicine* 31 (2002): 169–174.
8. T. Alpagot and coauthors, Risk factors for periodontitis in HIV patients, *Journal of Periodontal Research* 39 (2004): 149–157.
9. M. Navazesh and coauthors, A 4-year longitudinal evaluation of xerostomia and salivary gland hypofunction in the Women's Interagency HIV Study participants, *Oral Surgery Oral Medicine Oral Pathology Oral Radiology and Endodontics* 95 (2003): 693–698.
10. J. B. Epstein and coauthors, Cancer-related oral health care services and resources: A survey of oral and dental care in Canadian cancer centres, *Journal of the Canadian Dental Association* 70 (2004): 302–304; American Dietetic Association, 2003; P. J. Hancock, J. B. Epstein, and G. R. Sadler, Oral and dental management related to radiation therapy for head and neck cancer, *Journal of the Canadian Dental Association* 69 (2003): 585–590.
11. Y.-T. A. Teng and coauthors, Periodontal health and systemic disorders, *Journal of the Canadian Dental Association* 68 (2002): 188–192.
12. Teng, 2002.
13. Teng, 2002.

Chapter 24

Nutrition and Lower Gastrointestinal Disorders

Chapter Outline

Available Online

http://nutrition.wadsworth.com/uncn7

Student Practice Test

Glossary Terms

Nutrition on the Net

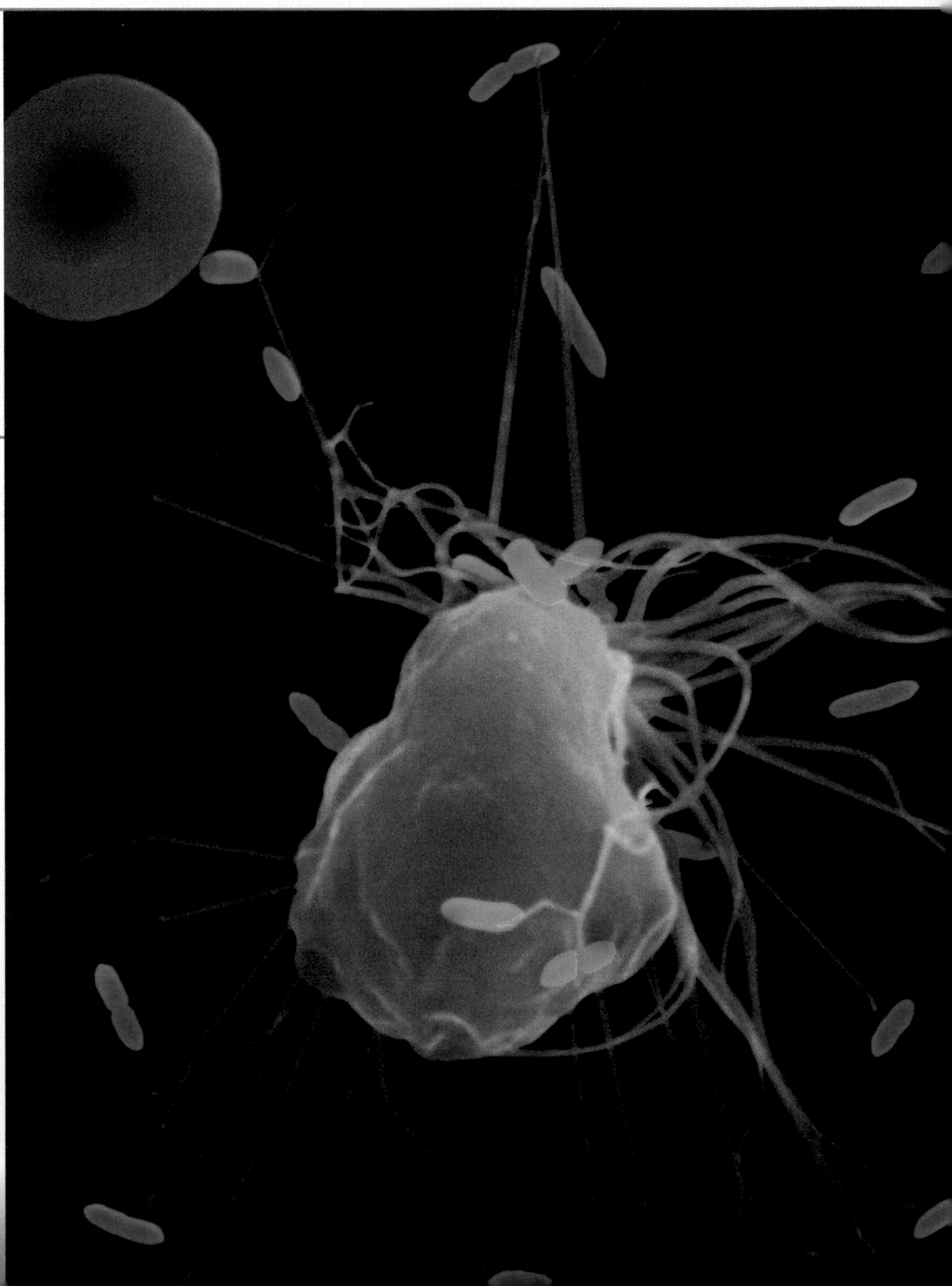

Nutrition in the Professional Setting

Disorders affecting the lower gastrointestinal tract can interfere substantially with a patient's diet and lifestyle. For some diseases, the diets required are complicated and difficult to follow. Furthermore, foods that are tolerated may vary considerably. In follow-up visits with patients, health care professionals can ensure that the diet prescription is understood and can help to pinpoint difficult foods. They can also suggest ways to make restrictive diets more acceptable.

This chapter discusses medical conditions that can upset the digestive and absorptive functions of the lower gastrointestinal (GI) tract. As you may recall from Chapter 3, the lower GI tract consists of the small and large intestines, the rectum, and the anus. The digestion and absorption of nutrients occur primarily in the small intestine. The pancreas and gallbladder support these complex functions, delivering digestive secretions to the duodenum. The large intestine reabsorbs water and facilitates excretion of waste material. Figure 24-1 on p. 740 illustrates the lower GI tract and related organs and reviews the functions of each organ.

Common Intestinal Symptoms and Complications

Intestinal symptoms may result from disorders that affect the lower GI tract or may be due to illnesses and medical treatments that have systemic effects. The discomfort associated with intestinal problems often drives a person to seek medical attention, and symptoms reported to health care providers can help them make more accurate diagnoses of intestinal conditions. The most common intestinal symptoms and their causes and treatments are discussed below.

FIGURE 24-1 The Lower GI Tract and Related Organs

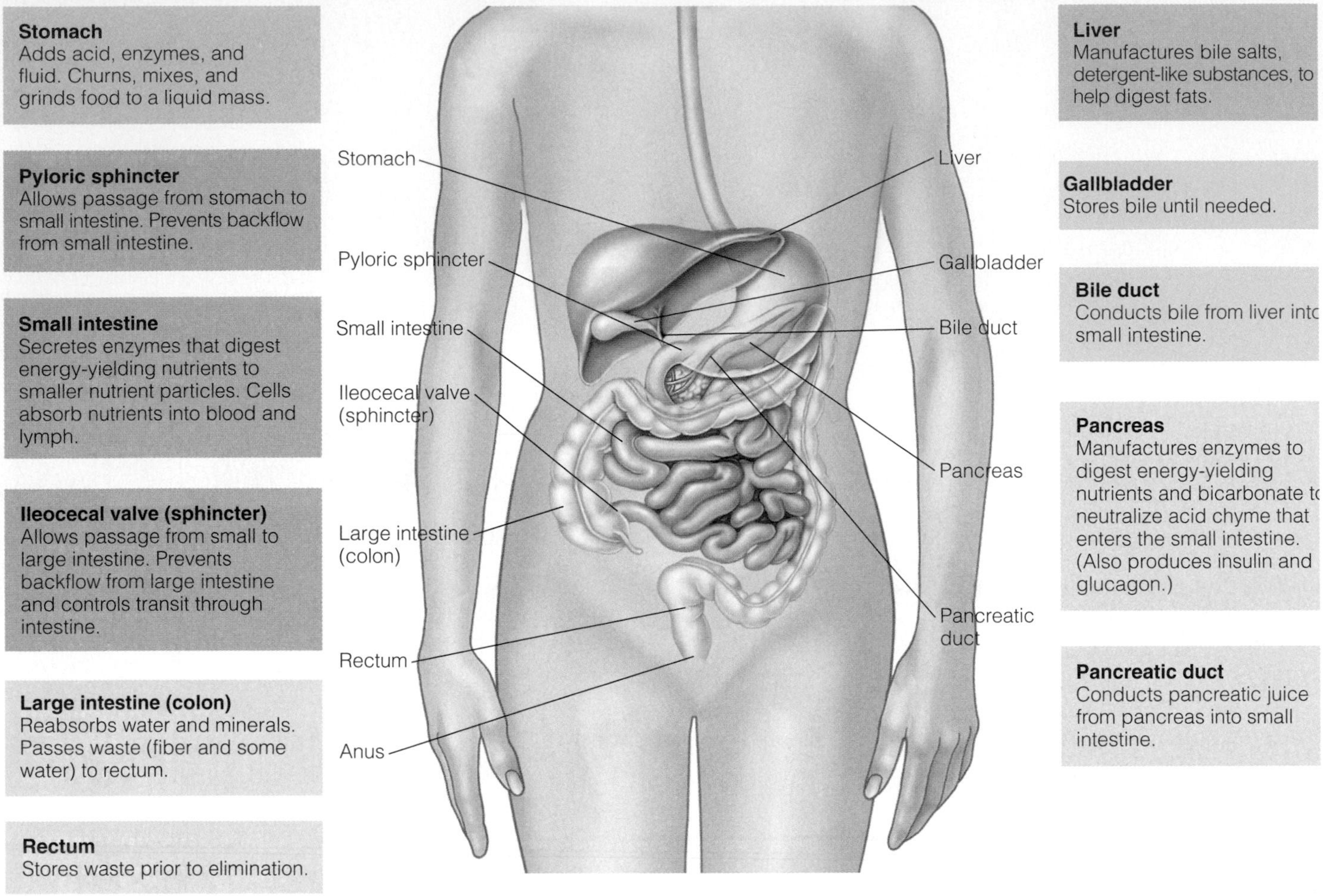
Stomach
Adds acid, enzymes, and fluid. Churns, mixes, and grinds food to a liquid mass.
Pyloric sphincter
Allows passage from stomach to small intestine. Prevents backflow from small intestine.
Small intestine
Secretes enzymes that digest energy-yielding nutrients to smaller nutrient particles. Cells absorb nutrients into blood and lymph.
Ileocecal valve (sphincter)
Allows passage from small to large intestine. Prevents backflow from large intestine and controls transit through intestine.
Large intestine (colon)
Reabsorbs water and minerals. Passes waste (fiber and some water) to rectum.
Rectum
Stores waste prior to elimination.
Stomach
Pyloric sphincter
Small intestine
Ileocecal valve (sphincter)
Large intestine (colon)
Rectum
Anus
Liver
Gallbladder
Bile duct
Pancreas
Pancreatic duct
Liver
Manufactures bile salts, detergent-like substances, to help digest fats.
Gallbladder
Stores bile until needed.
Bile duct
Conducts bile from liver intc small intestine.
Pancreas
Manufactures enzymes to digest energy-yielding nutrients and bicarbonate tc neutralize acid chyme that enters the small intestine. (Also produces insulin and glucagon.)
Pancreatic duct
Conducts pancreatic juice from pancreas into small intestine.

Constipation

An individual who complains of constipation is usually concerned about difficulty passing stools, a sensation of incomplete evacuation, or infrequent bowel movements. Sometimes, however, the perception of constipation is due to a mistaken notion of what constitutes "normal" bowel habits. A medical diagnosis of constipation is based, in part, on a defecation frequency of fewer than three bowel movements per week, which is estimated to affect only about 4 percent of the population.[1] Constipation is much more prevalent among women than men and increases somewhat with aging. Elderly people report greater straining with defecation rather than a reduced frequency of bowel movements. During pregnancy, 40 percent of women report some degree of constipation.

Causes of Constipation In Western societies, constipation generally correlates with low food intake, low-fiber diets, and inactivity. All of these factors can extend transit time, leading to increased water reabsorption within the colon. The result is small, dry, hard stools, which are difficult to pass. As Highlight 3 mentioned, transit time is also prolonged when people ignore the urge to defecate.

Constipation associated with illness may result from the medical condition, accompanying changes in diet or behavior, or the use of medications. Systemic disorders often associated with constipation include hypothyroidism, diabetes mellitus, and chronic renal failure. Neurological conditions such as Parkinson's disease, spinal cord lesions, and multiple sclerosis may cause motor problems that lead to constipation. Psychological problems, like depression and anxiety, may also cause constipation. Constipation is a common side effect of several classes of medications and some dietary supplements, including opiate-containing analgesics, tricyclic antidepressants, antihistamines, calcium channel blockers, aluminum-containing antacids, and iron and calcium supplements.

Treatment of Constipation The initial therapy for constipation is a gradual increase in fiber intake. High-fiber diets increase stool weights and promote a rapid transit of materials through the colon.■ Foods that increase stool weight the most are wheat bran, fruits, and vegetables.[2] Bran intake can be increased by adding bran cereals and whole-wheat bread to the diet or by mixing bran powder with beverages or foods. A transition to a high-fiber diet may be difficult for some people because it may increase intestinal gas; therefore, gradually adding high-fiber foods to the diet may be the best approach. If individuals find it difficult to alter their diets, fiber supplements like methylcellulose (Citrucel), psyllium (Metamucil, Fiberall), and polycarbophil (a synthetic fiber) are also effective; these fiber supplements can be mixed with beverages and taken several times daily (see Table 24-1). Methylcellulose and polycarbophil do not increase gas production in the colon.

Other dietary measures may also help. A person with constipation should make sure that fluid intake is sufficient because dehydration draws water from the colon in order to increase hydration in the rest of the body. Adding prunes or prune juice to the diet is often recommended because prunes contain compounds that have a mild laxative effect. Increasing daily exercise may help to stimulate peristalsis.

Drug Therapies Many types of laxatives can be purchased without prescription. They usually work by increasing stool weight, increasing the water content of the stool, or stimulating peristaltic contractions. Table 24-1 includes examples of the most popular laxatives and describes their modes of action. Enemas and suppositories (chemicals introduced into the rectum) are also used to promote defecation; they work by distending and stimulating the rectum or by lubricating the stool.

Medical Interventions Patients with severe symptoms who do not respond to dietary or laxative treatments may require more aggressive therapies. Some prescription drugs (for example, prucalopride) work by targeting the neural receptors involved with colonic peristalsis. Physical therapy and biofeedback techniques

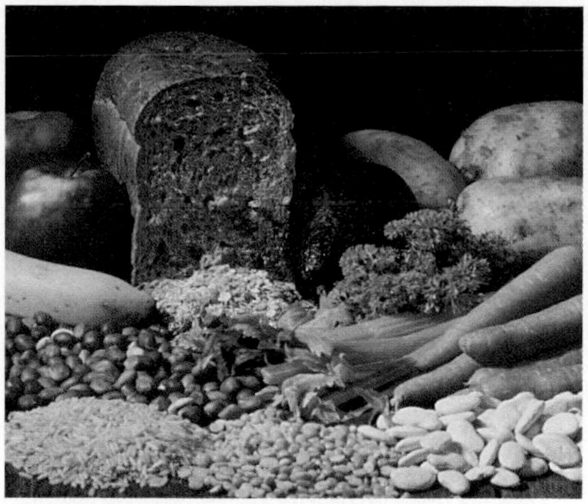

High-fiber foods promote regular bowel movements.

■ Reminder: Fiber-containing foods are listed in Table 4-3 (p. 127), and Appendix H includes the fiber content of most common foods. The fiber DRI for women and men aged 19 to 50 years are 25 and 38 g, respectively.

TABLE 24-1 Laxatives and Bulk-Forming Agents

Laxative Type	Active Ingredients	Product Examples	Method of Action	Cautions
Fiber (bulk formers)	Methylcellulose, polycarbophil, psyllium, malt soup extract	Metamucil, Citrucel, FiberLax	Fiber supplements increase stool weight and aid in formation of soft, bulky stools. Similar effects are achieved by adding bran to the diet. For mild constipation. Safe for long-term use.	Some fiber supplements may increase flatulence. Psyllium may cause an allergic reaction.
Emollient (stool softeners)	Docusate sodium	Colace, Surfak	Detergent action promotes the mixing of water with stools. Prevents formation of dry, hard stools.	Does not increase stool weight. Limited effectiveness.
Nonabsorbable sugars (osmotic laxatives)	Lactulose, sorbitol, mannitol	Chronulac, Cephulac	Unabsorbed sugars attract water to large intestine and promote softer stools. Must be used for several days to take effect. Safe for long-term use.	May cause flatulence and cramps. Can lose effectiveness over time.
Saline laxatives (osmotic laxatives)	Magnesium hydroxide, magnesium citrate, sodium sulfate	Milk of magnesia	Unabsorbed salts attract and retain water in large intestine and stimulate contractions.	May cause bloating and watery stools or diarrhea. Should be used with caution. Avoid using in renal patients and children.
Stimulant or irritant laxatives	Senna, bisacodyl, cascara, castor oil, aloe	Ex-Lax, Correctol, Dulcolax	Act as local irritants to colonic tissue; stimulate peristalsis and mucosal secretions. For moderate-to-severe constipation. Long-term use is discouraged.	Usually given only after milder treatments fail. May alter fluid and electrolyte balance. May lead to laxative dependency.

TABLE 24-2 Dietary Substances That May Increase Intestinal Gas

- Apples
- Beer
- Broccoli
- Brussels sprouts
- Cabbage
- Carbonated beverages
- Cauliflower
- Dried beans and peas
- Fruit juices
- Milk products (if lactose intolerant)
- Onions
- Pears
- Potatoes
- Turnips

have been successful in training patients to relax their pelvic muscles more effectively. Surgical interventions are a last resort for relieving constipation and include colonic resections and colostomy operations (see p. 759).

Intestinal Gas

As mentioned in the previous section, increased intestinal gas **(flatulence)** can be an unpleasant side effect of consuming a high-fiber diet. Because dietary fiber is undigested and unabsorbed, it passes into the colon where it is fermented by bacteria, producing gas as a by-product. Other incompletely digested or absorbed carbohydrates have similar effects; these include fructose, sugar alcohols (sorbitol, mannitol, maltitol), the undigestible carbohydrates in beans (raffinose, stachyose), and some forms of resistant starch, found in grain products and potatoes. Table 24-2 lists some foods commonly associated with excessive gas production.[3] Conditions that cause malabsorption, such as chronic pancreatitis and celiac disease (discussed later in this chapter), also cause flatulence because the undigested nutrients end up in the colon, available for metabolism by bacteria. Another important source of intestinal gas is swallowed air (see Highlight 3). Swallowed air that is not expelled by belching can travel through the intestines and is eventually eliminated via the rectum.

Many people blame their symptoms of abdominal bloating and pain on excessive gas, but these symptoms do not correlate well with increased intestinal gas. In fact, most people who self-diagnose a flatulence problem have no more intestinal gas than others.[4] Individuals who frequently experience symptoms of abdominal bloating and pain are often diagnosed with dyspepsia (see Chapter 23) or irritable bowel syndrome (see pp. 757–758). Removing gas-producing foods from the diet generally does not help alleviate their discomfort.

Diarrhea

Diarrhea is characterized by the passage of frequent, watery stools. In most cases, it lasts for a day or two and subsides without complication. Severe or persistent diarrhea, however, can cause dehydration and electrolyte imbalances. If chronic, it may lead to weight loss and malnutrition. Serious cases of diarrhea are often accompanied by a number of other symptoms, including fever, cramps, dyspepsia, and intestinal bleeding, that help in diagnosing its cause.

Causes of Diarrhea Diarrhea is often classified according to the type of mechanism that causes excessive fluid loss.[5] *Osmotic diarrhea* usually results from nutrient malabsorption, as when poorly absorbed sugars like sorbitol or fructose draw water into the colon and increase fecal water content.■ *Motility disorders* may accelerate the entry of fluids into the colon, where they are inadequately reabsorbed. In many cases of *secretory diarrhea,* the intestines are stimulated to secrete fluid that exceeds the colon's capacity for reabsorption. Secretory diarrhea is often due to bacterial food poisoning but may also be caused by intestinal inflammation, resulting in bloody stools and colonic tissue damage.

■ Osmotic diarrhea is the type of diarrhea associated with lactose intolerance, which was covered in Chapter 4 (see pp. 113–114).

Acute diarrhea often starts abruptly and may last for several weeks. It is frequently caused by viral, bacterial, or protozoal infections or occurs as a side effect of medication use. Diarrhea is a frequent complication of tube feedings or may occur when enteral feedings are resumed after a period of bowel rest.

Chronic diarrhea persists for a month or longer. It is sometimes associated with gastrointestinal disorders that alter GI tract motility or cause intestinal inflammation. Chronic cases may also develop due to malabsorptive and endocrine disorders, infectious diseases, radiation treatment, and many other conditions.

Treatment of Diarrhea Treatment of the underlying medical condition is the first step in treating diarrhea. Infections are treated with appropriate antibiotics. If a medication is responsible, a different medication or form of medication (injectable versus oral, for example) can be used. If a dietary source seems the likely

flatulence: the condition of having excessive intestinal gas, which causes abdominal discomfort.

cause, offending foods are omitted. In cases of chronic diarrhea that do not respond to treatment, antidiarrheal agents may be prescribed to slow GI motility or reduce intestinal secretions. Bulk-forming agents such as psyllium (Metamucil) may help to reduce the liquidity of the stool. Although probiotics■ have been shown to be beneficial for certain types of infectious diarrhea (for example, rotavirus infection), standard protocols for their use have not been developed.

■ Reminder: *Probiotics* are microbial food ingredients that are beneficial to health (see Highlight 13).

Rehydration Therapy A critical element of diarrhea treatment is the replacement of lost fluids and electrolytes. In mild diarrhea, regular beverages and foods may suffice. In more serious cases, oral rehydration solutions can be purchased or easily mixed using water, salts, and glucose or sucrose (see the recipe in the margin).■ The addition of carbohydrate to the rehydration solution facilitates sodium and water absorption. Commercial sports drinks are generally not recommended as oral rehydration solutions because their sodium contents are too low to replace the electrolyte losses that result from severe diarrhea. They can be used if accompanied by salty snack foods.[6] If diarrhea results in severe dehydration, intravenous solutions may be used to quickly replace fluid and electrolyte losses.

■ An oral rehydration solution can be mixed from the following ingredients:
- 2.6 g sodium chloride (table salt).
- 1.5 g potassium chloride.
- 2.9 g sodium bicarbonate (baking soda).
- 13.5 g glucose.
- 1 liter water.

Dietary Adjustments In some cases, avoiding irritating foods may help to improve diarrhea. Table 24-3 lists foods that may aggravate or alleviate diarrhea. Generally, foods and beverages that contain fructose, sugar alcohols, or lactose worsen symptoms, although individual tolerances vary. People with severe, **intractable** diarrhea sometimes require total parenteral nutrition.

Bacterial Overgrowth

Although the colon normally contains a sizable bacterial population, the stomach and small intestine are protected from **bacterial overgrowth** by gastric acid, which destroys bacteria, and peristalsis, which flushes microorganisms through the small intestine before they can multiply. Conditions that disrupt these protective mechanisms can result in bacterial overgrowth in the stomach and small intestine.

The bacteria in the small intestine influence a number of intestinal functions. For example, they partly dismantle bile acids, thereby interfering with fat digestion and absorption. Consequently, malabsorption of fat and fat-soluble vitamins often results from bacterial overgrowth. The bacteria also compete for vitamin B_{12}, impairing its absorption and increasing the risk of vitamin B_{12} deficiency.

TABLE 24-3 Foods That May Affect Diarrhea

Foods That May Worsen Diarrhea	Foods That May Lessen Diarrhea
• Apple juice	• Applesauce
• Caffeine-containing beverages	• Bananas
• Coffee	• Barley
• Dates	• Cheese
• Fried foods	• Oat bran
• Fructose-sweetened drinks	• Oatmeal
• Grapes	• Peanut butter (smooth)
• Honey	• Potatoes
• Milk and milk products	• Rice (boiled)
• Pear juice	• Soda crackers
• Prune juice	• Tapioca
• Sugar-free candies	• Yogurt

NOTE: Individual tolerances vary.
SOURCES: American Dietetic Association, *Manual of Clinical Dietetics* (Chicago: American Dietetic Association, 2000), p. 423; M. H. Beers and R. Berkow, eds., *The Merck Manual of Diagnosis and Therapy* (Whitehouse Station, N.J.: Merck Research Laboratories, 1999), pp. 275–278.

intractable: not easily managed or controlled.

bacterial overgrowth: excessive bacterial colonization of the stomach and small intestine; may be caused by low gastric acidity, altered gastrointestinal motility, mucosal damage, or contamination; interferes with normal digestion and absorption.

Typical symptoms of bacterial overgrowth include chronic diarrhea, abdominal discomfort, bloating, weakness, and weight loss. Fat and carbohydrate malabsorption are common. Vitamin deficiency symptoms often occur and may include night blindness (vitamin A deficiency), bruising (vitamin K deficiency), bone disease (vitamin D deficiency), and megaloblastic anemia (vitamin B_{12} deficiency).

Causes of Bacterial Overgrowth Conditions that impair intestinal motility and allow material to stagnate can predispose a person to bacterial overgrowth. For example, in some types of gastric surgery, a portion of the small intestine is bypassed, causing stasis and allowing bacteria to flourish (see the "blind loop" indicated on Figure 23-3 on p. 726). Intestinal motility can also be slowed by strictures, obstructions, and diverticula (see p. 758), which may develop in the small intestine.

Reduced gastric acid secretions may also lead to bacterial overgrowth. Possible causes include atrophic gastritis (see p. 724), the use of acid-suppressing medications, and acid-reducing surgery (vagotomy) for peptic ulcer disease.

Treatment for Bacterial Overgrowth Treatment usually includes the use of antibiotics to suppress bacterial growth and the surgical correction of anatomical defects that contribute to stasis. Acid-reducing therapies are usually discontinued until the problem is resolved. Dietary supplements are provided to reverse nutrient deficiencies, especially for fat-soluble vitamins, calcium, and vitamin B_{12}. **Medium-chain triglycerides (MCT),** which do not require bile for digestion and absorption, may be used as an alternate source of fat kcalories.

Steatorrhea

Steatorrhea refers to excessive fat in the stools resulting from fat maldigestion or malabsorption. Fat maldigestion is caused by conditions that interfere with the availability of bile or pancreatic lipase. Examples include pancreatitis and cystic fibrosis, which alter pancreatic secretions, and bacterial overgrowth, which disturbs bile function.■ Malabsorption may be caused by conditions that impair mucosal function, such as inflammatory intestinal disorders (including Crohn's disease and celiac disease) or radiation treatment for cancer. Motility disorders that cause rapid gastric emptying or rapid intestinal transit may also result in steatorrhea because they prevent the normal mixing of dietary fat with lipase and bile.

■ Conditions of the liver and gallbladder may affect bile sufficiency and are discussed in Chapter 25.

Consequences of Fat Malabsorption Fat malabsorption is associated with losses of food energy, essential fatty acids, fat-soluble vitamins, and some minerals (see Figure 24-2). Weight loss is possible unless alternate energy sources are provided. Deficiencies of fat-soluble vitamins and essential fatty acids are common in chronic conditions. Absorption of some minerals, including calcium, magnesium, and zinc, may be reduced because they can form **soaps** with unabsorbed fatty acids and bile acids. Calcium deficiency can lead to bone loss, which is further aggravated by the vitamin D deficiency that is common in steatorrhea.

■ Reminder: *Oxalates* are plant compounds that bind with some minerals to form complexes that the body cannot absorb. They are present in green leafy vegetables such as beet greens and spinach.

Oxalate Stones Another complication of steatorrhea is an increased risk of kidney stones, which are most often composed of calcium oxalate (see Figure 24-2). The oxalates■ in foods ordinarily bind to calcium in the small intestine and are excreted in the stool. If calcium instead binds to fatty acids or bile acids, the oxalate is free to be absorbed into the blood and ultimately excreted in urine. The risk of developing oxalate stones increases when urinary oxalate levels are high. Kidney stones are discussed further in Chapter 28.

Dietary Adjustments If steatorrhea does not improve, a fat-restricted diet may be recommended (see Table 24-4, p. 746). The main objectives of fat restriction are to relieve abdominal symptoms that are aggravated by fat intake (usually diarrhea and flatulence) and to reduce vitamin and mineral losses. Fat should not be restricted more than is necessary to relieve symptoms because fat is an important

medium-chain triglycerides (MCT): triglycerides that contain fatty acids that are 8 to 10 carbons in length. MCT do not require digestion and can be absorbed in the absence of lipase or bile.

steatorrhea (stee-AT-or-REE-ah): excessive fat in the stools resulting from fat malabsorption; characterized by stools that are loose, frothy, and foul-smelling due to a high fat content.
- **steat** = fat
- **rheo** = flow

soaps: chemical compounds formed between positively charged minerals and fatty acids.

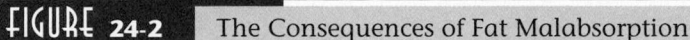

FIGURE 24-2 The Consequences of Fat Malabsorption

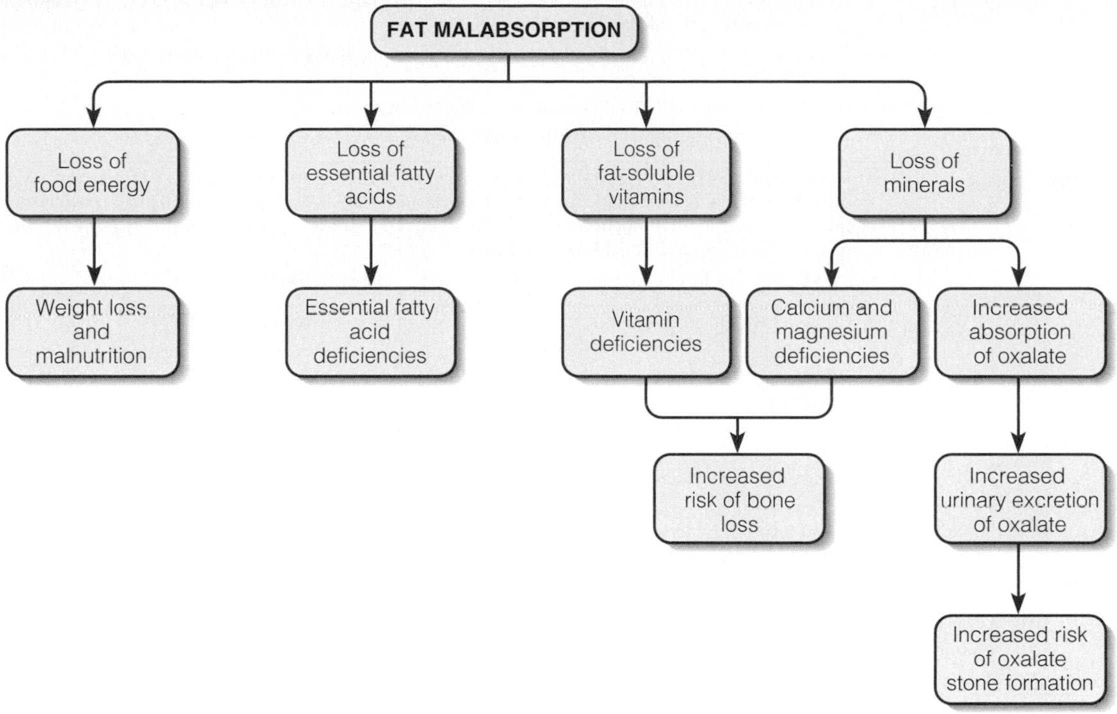
FAT MALABSORPTION
Loss of food energy
Loss of essential fatty acids
Loss of fat-soluble vitamins
Loss of minerals
Weight loss and malnutrition
Essential fatty acid deficiencies
Vitamin deficiencies
Calcium and magnesium deficiencies
Increased absorption of oxalate
Increased risk of bone loss
Increased urinary excretion of oxalate
Increased risk of oxalate stone formation

source of energy. Although MCT oil is sometimes used as a replacement for fat, it does not provide essential fatty acids. The "How to" on p. 747 offers suggestions for following a fat-restricted diet and for using MCT oil.

IN SUMMARY Disorders of the lower GI tract are frequently associated with complications that can cause intestinal discomfort, nutrient deficiencies, and additional illness. Constipation accompanies a wide range of conditions and is often improved with a high-fiber diet or fiber supplements. Diarrhea may result from food poisoning, malabsorption, and motility disorders. Intestinal gas is largely produced by bacteria that colonize the colon and is often associated with nutrient malabsorption. Conditions that reduce gastric acidity or cause intestinal stasis can increase risk of bacterial overgrowth. Steatorrhea may be caused by fat maldigestion or fat malabsorption. Each of these complications may benefit by alterations in dietary intake.

Malabsorption Syndromes

Disorders of the GI tract that cause malabsorption are the most detrimental to nutritional status. Malabsorption syndromes result in multiple nutrient deficiencies and weight loss and are often associated with serious complications. Some conditions disrupt the exocrine■ function of the pancreas, leading to extensive enzyme deficiencies. Others cause severe intestinal inflammation, which interferes with the absorptive functions of intestinal mucosa. Sometimes disease treatments require surgical resection of the small intestine, leaving minimal absorptive capacity in the portion that remains.

■ Reminder: *Exocrine* refers to "outside the body." The exocrine function of the pancreas is to deliver digestive secretions to the small intestine.

TABLE 24-4 Fat-Restricted Diet

General guidelines	• *For fat restriction of 25 grams per day:* Limit meat and meat alternates to 4 ounces daily (cooked weight); limit fat equivalents to 1 per day (see Fats section below). • *For fat restriction of 50 grams per day:* Limit meat and meat alternates to 6 ounces daily (cooked weight); limit fat equivalents to 3 to 5 per day. • *To raise fat content:* Allow additional servings of meat or fat. • *To lower fat content:* Restrict servings of meat or fat.
Meat and meat alternates	• *Recommended:* Choose lean meat, fish, and poultry only. Preparation methods can include broiling, roasting, grilling, or boiling. Trim visible fat and remove poultry skin before consuming. For sandwiches, select turkey breast or other low-fat luncheon meats. Limit eggs to 2 per week or use low-fat egg substitutes. Meat alternates include tofu and dried beans and peas. • *Avoid:* Pork and beans, sausage, bacon, frankfurters, spareribs, duck, goose, tuna packed in oil, fried meats.
Milk and milk products	• Choose milk products that contain less than 1 gram fat per serving. • *Recommended:* Fat-free milk, fat-free yogurt, fat-free sour cream substitutes, fat-free Half-and-Half and cream substitutes, fat-free cheeses. • *Avoid:* Milk products that are not fat-free.
Breads, cereals, rice, and pasta	• Choose breads, cereals, rice, and pasta dishes that contain less than 1 gram fat per serving. • *Recommended:* Whole-grain breads, soda crackers, cooked cereals and most cold cereals, plain tortillas, bagels, English muffins, fat-free muffins, graham crackers, plain rice, plain noodles and pasta. • *Avoid:* Biscuits, pancakes, waffles, doughnuts, granola, snack crackers that contain fat, corn chips, cornbread, fried rice, pasta sauces with added fats.
Vegetables	• Choose vegetables that contain less than 1 gram fat per serving. • *Recommended:* All vegetables prepared without added fats. • *Avoid:* Buttered or fried vegetables, creamed vegetables, au gratin style, french-fried potatoes, olives, sauces with added fats.
Fruit	• Choose fruits that contain less than 1 gram fat per serving. • *Recommended:* All fruits prepared without added fats. • *Avoid:* Avocado, fruit dips made with fat or coconut.
Desserts	• Choose desserts that contain less than 1 gram fat per serving. • *Recommended:* Sherbet, fruit ices, fruit whips, flavored gelatin, angel food cake, meringues, fat-free puddings, fat-free baked products, fat-free ice cream or frozen yogurt, fat-free candies (marshmallows, jelly beans, hard candy). • *Avoid:* Cakes, cookies, pies, and pastries made with fat; puddings made with whole milk or eggs, ice cream, candies made with fat (caramel, chocolates).
Fats	• Choose 1 fat equivalent daily if fat restriction is 25 grams per day, and 3 to 5 fat equivalents daily if fat restriction is 50 grams per day. • *One fat equivalent is equal to:* Vegetable oil: 1 tsp. Butter, margarine: 1 tsp, or 1 tbs diet margarine. Mayonnaise: 1 tsp, or 1 tbs reduced-kcalorie mayonnaise. Salad dressing: 1 tbs, or 2 tbs reduced-kcalorie dressing. Nuts: 6 almonds or cashews, 10 peanuts, 2 tsp peanut butter, 4 halves walnuts or pecans.
Beverages	• Choose beverages that contain less than 1 gram fat per serving. • *Recommended:* Coffee, tea, soft drinks, juices, fat-free milk, coffee substitutes. • *Avoid:* Beverages made with milk (unless fat-free milk) or added cream, chocolate milk, eggnog, milk shakes.

SOURCE: Adapted from American Dietetic Association, *Manual of Clinical Dietetics* (Chicago: American Dietetic Association, 2000), Chapter 58, Fat-restricted diet.

Pancreatitis

Pancreatitis is an inflammatory disorder of the pancreas. Although mild cases may subside in a few days, others may persist for weeks or months. Chronic pancreatitis can cause irreversible damage to pancreatic tissue and permanent loss of function.

Acute Pancreatitis Acute pancreatitis is most often a consequence of gallstones or excessive alcohol use, which account for more than 70 percent of acute cases.[7] Less common causes include hypertriglyceridemia (triglycerides over 1000 mil-

HOW TO Follow a Fat-Restricted Diet

Fat-restricted diets can be difficult to follow. Fats add flavors, aromas, and textures to foods—characteristics that make foods more enjoyable. Unlike some diets that can be introduced gradually, a fat-restricted diet is often implemented immediately, allowing little time for adaptation. These suggestions may help:

- Fat is better tolerated if provided in small portions. Divide the day's allotment into several servings that can be consumed throughout the day.
- Use variety to enhance enjoyment of meals: vary flavors, textures, colors, and seasonings.
- Look for fat-free items when grocery shopping. Incorporate fat-free ingredients when preparing favorite recipes.
- Try fat-free and low-fat condiments to improve the diet's palatability. Experiment with herbs and spices. Instead of butter, use fruit butters on toast. Use butter-flavored granules on vegetables. Replace mayonnaise on sandwiches with spicy mustard. Replace salad dressings with flavored vinegars.
- Avoid products that contain the fat substitute olestra, which may aggravate GI symptoms.

If patients are interested in using MCT oil:

- Explain that MCT products are expensive, but that the cost is sometimes covered by medical insurance.
- Advise patients to add MCT oil to the diet gradually. Diarrhea and abdominal cramps may result if too much is used at once. Tolerance to MCT oil may improve in time.
- Advise patients that MCT oil may have an unpleasant taste when used alone. Suggest using MCT oil in recipes as a substitute for regular oil. MCT oil can replace oil in salad dressings, be incorporated into sauces, and be used in cooking or baking. It can also be added to fat-free milk products to make milk shakes.
- Point out that MCT oil should not be used to fry foods because it decomposes at lower temperatures than most cooking oils.

ligrams per deciliter), exposure to toxins, and the use of some medications. The disease process is thought to begin with the premature activation of digestive enzymes■ within pancreatic tissue, which causes destruction of pancreatic cells. Inflammatory mediators then respond to the injury, starting the inflammatory process (described in Chapter 22). Severe abdominal pain, nausea and vomiting, and abdominal distention are common symptoms. In about 80 percent of patients, the condition is mild and resolves within a week with no complications. Conversely, moderate-to-severe cases may lead to renal failure, sepsis, and other complications that often require prolonged hospitalization.

■ Elevated serum levels of amylase and lipase help to confirm a diagnosis of acute pancreatitis.

Medical Nutrition Therapy for Acute Pancreatitis Oral fluids and food are withheld until pain and tenderness have subsided, and fluids and electrolytes are supplied intravenously. In mild cases, recovery is rapid, and oral intake of a low-fat diet can sometimes begin within 3 to 7 days of disease onset.[8] In more severe cases, an elemental diet delivered by jejunal tube feeding has been shown to effectively provide nourishment and is generally preferred over intravenous nutrition.[9] If the intestine is malfunctioning (due to intestinal **ileus**), intravenous feedings may be preferred.

When oral feedings begin, only small amounts (½ to 1 cup) of fluids may be offered at first. If tolerated, the diet progresses to soft foods and finally to solids, given in small, frequent feedings.[10] As fat has a greater stimulating effect on pancreatic secretions than do carbohydrates or protein, low-fat diets may be better tolerated initially.[11] In severe pancreatitis, protein and energy needs are often high due to the catabolic and hypermetabolic effects of severe inflammation.

Chronic Pancreatitis Chronic pancreatitis results in permanent damage to the structure and function of pancreatic tissue. Alcohol consumption is responsible for 70 percent of chronic cases. Unlike in acute pancreatitis, gallstones are not a cause of chronic pancreatitis.[12] In children, most cases are attributable to cystic fibrosis, discussed in a later section.

In chronic pancreatitis, abdominal pain is often severe and unrelenting and worsens with eating. Analgesics or opiate drugs are often needed for pain control.

ileus: obstruction of the intestine caused by disordered intestinal motility.

■ Reminder: Pancreatic digestive secretions include bicarbonate, which neutralizes the acidic gastric contents, and digestive enzymes, which break down protein, carbohydrate, and fat.

■ Nutrient deficiencies in chronic pancreatitis may be due to malabsorption or may result from the alcohol abuse that caused the disease.

Steatorrhea develops in advanced cases because the pancreas is unable to secrete lipase and bicarbonate; fat maldigestion develops sooner than maldigestion of protein or carbohydrate.■ Food avoidance (due to pain associated with eating) and malabsorption may lead to weight loss and malnutrition. Advanced cases are associated with reductions in both insulin and glucagon secretions, and diabetes eventually develops in up to 30 percent of patients.

Medical Nutrition Therapy for Chronic Pancreatitis The objectives of nutrition therapy are to improve nutritional status, reduce malabsorption, and prevent further damage to the pancreas. Protein and energy needs may be high in patients who have lost weight or are malnourished. Dietary supplements may be needed to correct nutrient deficiencies.■ Patients are cautioned to avoid alcohol completely, as it can worsen pancreatic function.

Steatorrhea is usually treated with pancreatic enzyme replacement. Pancreatic enzymes are often **enteric-coated** to resist the acidity of the stomach and do not dissolve until the pH is above 5.5. If non-enteric-coated preparations are used, acid-suppressing drugs may be required. Fecal fat concentrations are monitored to determine if the enzyme treatment has been effective. A low-fat diet is suggested only if fat malabsorption is resistant to treatment; in that case, MCT oil may also be recommended. The case study describes a patient with chronic pancreatitis.

Cystic Fibrosis

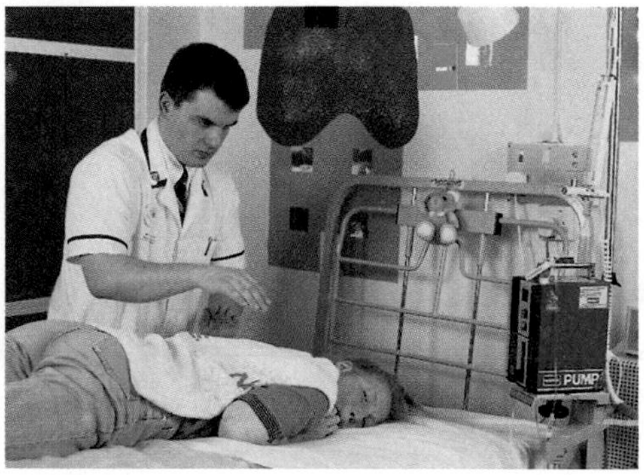
PUMP

Chest physical therapy (postural drainage) promotes maximal lung function for people with cystic fibrosis.

Cystic fibrosis is the most common life-threatening genetic disorder among Caucasians, with an incidence of approximately 1 in 3000 white births. In the United States, about 30,000 people are affected.[13] Cystic fibrosis is caused by a mutation in the gene for a membrane protein that transports chloride ions. The defect causes abnormal secretions by exocrine glands, leading to a broad range of serious complications. Until a few decades ago, few infants born with cystic fibrosis survived to adulthood. Now, with early detection and advances in medical treatment, the average life span is approximately 30 years.[14]

Consequences of Cystic Fibrosis Cystic fibrosis results in abnormal sodium and chloride levels in exocrine secretions. The secretions are unusually viscous and can obstruct the ducts that normally allow their passage. If an exocrine secretion is blocked by obstruction, tissue functions may be disrupted and surrounding tissues damaged. Most people with cystic fibrosis develop complications involving the lungs and pancreas that have serious nutritional implications. Children with cystic fibrosis are chronically undernourished, grow poorly, and have difficulty maintaining normal body weight. Salt losses in sweat are usually excessive, increasing the risk of dehydration.

Lung Disease Patients with cystic fibrosis generally develop persistent respiratory infections, which cause inflammation of the bronchial tissues and progressive airway obstruction. A chronic, productive cough is the initial symptom, but the eventual lung damage leads to breathing difficulties and lower exercise tolerance. Severe obstructive lung disease is generally associated with poor nutritional status due to hypermetabolism, the greater energy cost of labored breathing, and anorexia (loss of appetite).[15]■

■ The nutrition problems associated with chronic obstructive lung diseases were described in Chapter 22 (see pp. 702–704).

Although it has long been assumed that the airways of people with cystic fibrosis secrete greater-than-normal amounts of mucus, a recent report suggests that mucus production is abnormally *low*.[16] The reduced mucus in lung secretions may lower defenses against bacterial infection. The thickened secretions may result from immune processes that may cause white blood cells and their by-products to accumulate.

Pancreatic Disease In approximately 85 percent of patients with cystic fibrosis, the thickened exocrine secretions of the pancreas eventually obstruct the pancreatic ducts, causing digestive enzymes to accumulate in the pancreas and destroy

enteric-coated: refers to medications or enzyme preparations that can withstand gastric acidity and dissolve only at a higher pH.

cystic fibrosis: an inherited disease involving exocrine secretions and characterized by respiratory disease and pancreatic insufficiency.

CASE STUDY

Retired Executive with Chronic Pancreatitis

Mr. Levitt is a 62-year-old man with chronic pancreatitis. He was forced to resign his position as president of an import/export company in his early fifties, when his problems with alcohol and declining health seriously impaired his abilities to run the company. His wife divorced him shortly thereafter, and he currently lives alone. At 5 feet 11 inches tall, Mr. Levitt weighs 145 pounds. He continues to experience frequent, severe abdominal pain and steatorrhea. Mr. Levitt has been advised to follow a high-kcalorie, high-protein diet with no fat restrictions and uses enzyme replacement with meals, but he has difficulty eating enough food. He has not used alcohol for eight months. Mr. Levitt takes pain medications, acid-suppressing drugs, and a multivitamin daily.

1. What are the possible reasons for Mr. Levitt's difficulty with maintaining weight? What suggestions may help? Why was he advised to consume a high-protein diet?
2. What is the reason for malabsorption in chronic pancreatitis? Which nutrients are most likely to be affected?
3. How can Mr. Levitt's physician determine whether enzyme replacement is helping? Explain why Mr. Levitt must continue to use acid suppressants.
4. If Mr. Levitt continues to have problems with steatorrhea, what measures would you suggest? What complications may result if the steatorrhea is not controlled?

---

pancreatic tissue.[17] The inability of pancreatic enzymes to reach the small intestine leads to malabsorption of protein, fat, and fat-soluble vitamins. Complications that may develop over time include pancreatitis, hyperglycemia (from destruction of insulin-producing cells), and diabetes.

Other Complications Cystic fibrosis affects all exocrine secretions, so complications may develop in many tissues or organs. Intestinal obstruction is a common symptom in newborn infants and may also occur in older patients. Gallbladder and liver diseases may result from bile duct obstructions. Abnormalities in genital tissues cause sterility in men and reduced fertility in women.

Medical Nutrition Therapy for Cystic Fibrosis The objectives of nutrition treatment are to improve protein and energy intakes and correct nutrient deficiencies. As described earlier, energy needs are high in patients with cystic fibrosis due to increased requirements, nutrient malabsorption, and reduced food consumption. Malnutrition and impaired growth are often present when cystic fibrosis is diagnosed, and short stature may be an indicator of increased mortality risk.[18] Several studies have indicated that normal growth is possible if the disease is diagnosed early enough and energy intakes are high. Children may need to consume between 120 and 150 percent of recommended energy intakes to achieve normal growth and maintain optimal nutrition status.[19] To obtain sufficient energy, a patient with cystic fibrosis is encouraged to eat high-kcalorie and high-fat foods, eat frequent meals and snacks, and supplement meals with milk shakes or liquid dietary supplements. Supplemental tube feedings are effective for improving nutrition status if energy intakes are inadequate.

Pancreatic enzyme replacement therapy is a central feature of cystic fibrosis treatment. Supplemental enzymes must be included with every meal or snack. When given to infants and small children, the contents of capsules are mixed in small amounts of liquid or a soft food (like applesauce) and fed with a spoon. Enzyme dosages may need to be adjusted if malabsorption continues, as evidenced by poor growth or gastrointestinal symptoms such as steatorrhea, intestinal gas, or abdominal pain.

The risk of micronutrient deficiency in cystic fibrosis patients depends on the degree of malabsorption; nutrients of greatest concern include fat-soluble vitamins, essential fatty acids, and calcium. Multivitamin and fat-soluble vitamin supplements are routinely recommended. The liberal use of table salt and salty foods is encouraged to make up for losses of sodium in sweat. The case study on p. 750 checks your understanding of medical nutrition therapy for a child with cystic fibrosis.

CASE STUDY

Child with Cystic Fibrosis

Julie is a 7-year-old girl diagnosed with cystic fibrosis. Symptoms of steatorrhea and failure to gain weight in infancy prompted the test that led to diagnosis. She is currently 45 inches tall and weighs 42 pounds. Her height-for-age and weight-for-age fall near the 10th percentile (see Appendix E). Julie eats regular foods during the day and receives additional nutrients by tube feedings delivered overnight.

1. What do the height and weight percentiles tell you about her nutritional status? Why is growth failure common in children with cystic fibrosis? Explain to Julie's parents why her weight and height are of concern.
2. Explain why Julie's energy needs are so much higher than normal. Describe the elements of the diet that Julie should follow in order to gain weight. Would her energy requirements change if she developed a respiratory infection?
3. Explain to Julie's parents how to use enzyme replacement therapy effectively.
4. Julie's parents are hoping to discontinue the nightly tube feedings. Do you think the tube feedings are necessary? Why or why not?

Celiac Disease

Celiac disease is characterized by an abnormal immune response to a protein fraction in **wheat gluten**■ and to related proteins found in rye and barley. The reaction to gluten causes severe damage to the intestinal mucosa and subsequent malabsorption. Although celiac disease is considered one of the most prevalent inherited disorders in Europe, its incidence in the United States has been difficult to determine because its symptoms are similar to those of other intestinal disorders and diagnosis requires confirmation with an unpleasant intestinal biopsy. However, blood tests (showing an immunoglobulin response to gliadin) suggest that as many as 1 in every 133 persons in the United States may be at risk.[20]

■ The protein in wheat gluten that has toxic effects in celiac disease is called **gliadin** (GLY-ah-din).

Consequences of Celiac Disease The immune reaction to gluten can cause striking changes in the intestinal mucosa. In affected areas, the absorptive surface appears flattened due to the shortening or absence of villi and overdeveloped crypts.■ The reduction in mucosal surface area and, hence, in mucosa-derived digestive enzymes is often substantial. The damage may be restricted to the duodenum or may involve the full length of the small intestine.[21] The degree of malabsorption depends on the extent and severity of the damage. People with extensive celiac disease may malabsorb all nutrients to some degree, especially the macronutrients, fat-soluble vitamins, electrolytes, calcium, magnesium, zinc, iron, folate, and vitamin B_{12}. As a result of nutrient deficiencies, iron-deficiency anemia is common and bone mineral density is usually low.

■ Reminder: *Crypts* are tubular glands that lie between the intestinal villi and secrete intestinal juices into the small intestine.

Clinical symptoms generally include GI disturbances like diarrhea, steatorrhea, and flatulence. Lactase deficiency can result from intestinal damage, and GI symptoms may be exacerbated if milk products are included in the diet. Children with celiac disease often have stunted growth and are severely underweight. Some gluten-sensitive individuals may have few GI symptoms but react to gluten by developing a severe rash; this condition is called **dermatitis herpetiformis** and requires dietary adjustments similar to those for celiac disease.

celiac (SEE-lee-ack) **disease:** a condition characterized by an abnormal immune reaction to wheat gluten that causes severe intestinal damage and nutrient malabsorption; also called **gluten-sensitive enteropathy** or **celiac sprue.**

wheat gluten (GLU-ten): a family of water-insoluble proteins in wheat; includes gliadin proteins that are toxic to persons with celiac disease.

dermatitis herpetiformis (DERM-ah-TIE-tis HER-peh-tih-FOR-mis): a gluten-sensitive disorder characterized by a severe skin rash. Gastrointestinal symptoms may be mild or absent.

Medical Nutrition Therapy for Celiac Disease The recommended treatment for celiac disease is lifelong adherence to a gluten-free diet. In the majority of cases, improvement in symptoms is evident within several weeks. If lactase deficiency is suspected, lactose-containing foods should be avoided until the intestine has recovered. Dietary supplements can be used to meet micronutrient needs and reverse deficiencies.

The gluten-free diet eliminates all foods that contain wheat, rye, and barley (see Table 24-5). Many common foods contain ingredients derived from these grains, so foods that are problematic are not always obvious. Even small amounts of gluten may cause symptoms in some persons; therefore, ingredient lists on food labels need to be checked carefully. Special gluten-free products can be purchased to replace most common food items, including bread, pasta, and cereals. Although somewhat more expensive, these foods allow celiac patients to expand their food choices and enjoy foods that would otherwise be forbidden.

Not all authorities agree on the foods that are safe to include on gluten-free diets. For example, a survey of celiac organizations and physicians found that only 74 percent believed that buckwheat was acceptable for people with celiac disease.[22] One cause of confusion is that the acceptability of different grains is partly based on the taxonomic relationships among cereal grains, rather than on controlled studies in celiac patients. Another problem is that some foods that are naturally gluten-free may become contaminated with wheat during processing. The use of oats in a gluten-free diet remains controversial in the United States, although a substantial body of evidence supports their safety when used in moderation.[23] A limited intake of oats (40 to 60 grams per day) is currently considered acceptable by celiac organizations in Finland and the United Kingdom (see the Research Update, p. 752).

A gluten-free diet may become monotonous unless care is taken to diversify food choices. The diet can also be a social liability by restricting food choices when eating in restaurants, visiting friends, or traveling. Nonadherence is common when individuals are away from home.[24] Dietetic counseling may help celiac patients learn how to meet their nutrient needs and expand meal options despite dietary constraints.

TABLE 24-5 Gluten-Free Diet

Meat and meat alternates	• *Recommended:* Fresh, frozen, salted, and smoked meats (unless processed meats contain any prohibited grains); products made with hydrolyzed vegetable protein (HVP) or hydrolyzed plant protein (HPP); eggs; dried beans and peas; tofu. • *Questionable:* Luncheon meats, sandwich spreads, meat loaf, frozen burgers, sausage, imitation meat products, meat extenders, egg substitutes, dried egg products, dry roasted nuts, peanut butter. • *Avoid:* Products that are breaded or prepared in cream sauces, gravies.
Milk and milk products	• *Recommended:* Milk, buttermilk, plain yogurt, cheese. • *Questionable:* Milk shakes, cheese spreads, flavored yogurt, frozen yogurt, chocolate milk. • *Avoid:* Malted milk and malted milk powders.
Breads, cereals, rice, and pasta	• *Recommended:* Breads, baked products, and cereals made with corn, rice, soy, potato starch, potato flour, hominy, buckwheat, millet, teff, sorghum, amaranth, quinoa, arrowroot, and tapioca; pasta and noodles made with grains or starches listed above; corn tacos and corn tortillas. • *Questionable:* Oatmeal and oat bran; rice crackers, rice cakes, and corn cakes. • *Avoid:* Breads, baked products, cereals, tortillas, or pastas made with wheat, rye, barley, triticale, spelt, kamut, wheat germ, wheat bran, graham flour, durum flour, wheat starch, bulgur, farina, or semolina from wheat; commercially prepared mixes for biscuits, cornbread, muffins, pancakes, or waffles; malt and malt flavoring; pretzels; matzo.
Fruits and vegetables	• *Recommended:* Any unprocessed fruits or vegetables. • *Questionable:* French fries, especially in fast-food restaurants; commercial salad dressings; fruit pie fillings; dried fruits. • *Avoid:* Scalloped potatoes (with wheat flour), creamed vegetables, vegetables dipped in batters.
Desserts	• *Recommended:* Ice cream, sherbet, egg custards, or gelatin desserts that do not contain gluten; pure baking chocolate; chocolate chips; hard candy. • *Questionable:* Icing, powdered sugar, candies, chocolate bars, marshmallows. • *Avoid:* Puddings thickened with wheat flour; ice cream or sherbets that contain gluten stabilizers; baked products or doughnuts made with wheat, rye, or barley; ice cream cones; licorice.
Beverages	• *Recommended:* Coffee; tea; cocoa; soft drinks; distilled alcoholic beverages such as rum, gin, whisky, and vodka; wine. • *Questionable:* Instant tea or coffee, coffee substitutes, chocolate drinks, hot cocoa mixes. • *Avoid:* Beer, ale, lager, malted beverages, cereal beverages (Postum), beverages that contain nondairy cream substitutes.

SOURCE: Adapted from American Dietetic Association, *Manual of Clinical Dietetics* (Chicago: American Dietetic Association, 2000), Chapter 11, Celiac disease.

RESEARCH UPDATE Use of Oats in Celiac Disease

The suitability of oats for celiac patients has remained controversial despite reports that oats are well tolerated by most persons tested.[a] Although some of the protein fractions in oats are related to the gliadins in wheat, some researchers have found that the amino acid sequences in question are unlikely to stimulate the cellular immune reactions that are typical of celiac disease.[b] Even though sensitivity to oats has been documented in a few patients,[c] results of long-term feeding studies suggest that most people with celiac disease can incorporate moderate amounts of oats into gluten-free diets without harm.[d]

The ingestion of oats has been studied in both adults and children with celiac disease. In the longest-term study to date, adult celiac patients were instructed to include moderate amounts of oats (50 to 70 grams daily) in their diets, while a second group was instructed to avoid oats.[e] After five years, the two groups had similar levels of antibodies against gliadin and similar improvements in their intestinal mucosa. Another study was conducted in children and adolescents (between the ages of 8 months and 17.5 years) who were newly diagnosed with celiac disease. The study was blinded: both the subjects and the controls received unlabeled bread and cereal products. After one year, the group receiving oats exhibited no differences in antibodies or intestinal mucosa when compared with the controls.[f]

The results of these studies have led to a reassessment of the oats restrictions currently recommended by physicians and celiac organizations in the United States.[g] The addition of oats to celiac diets would diversify the dietary choices of celiac patients and potentially improve the acceptability of the gluten-free diet. Nevertheless, concern remains that some individuals would experience additional intestinal symptoms if they included oats in their diets.[h] Another possibility is that oats may become contaminated with gliadins during processing because the equipment used to harvest, transport, and store oats may be used to process several different types of grains.[i] Patients who wish to try oats can be advised to limit their intakes to the amounts found to be safe (about ½ cup of dry rolled oats per day) and to contact product manufacturers to determine whether contamination with gluten-containing products is likely.

[a]T. Thompson, Oats and the gluten-free diet, *Journal of the American Dietetic Association* 103 (2003): 376–379.
[b]L. W. Vader and coauthors, Specificity of tissue transglutaminase explains cereal toxicity in celiac disease, *Journal of Experimental Medicine* 195 (2002): 643–649.
[c]M. Peraaho and coauthors, Effect of an oats-containing gluten-free diet on symptoms and quality of life in coeliac disease. A randomized study, *Scandinavian Journal of Gastroenterology* 39 (2004): 27–33; K. E. Lundin and coauthors, Oats induced villous atrophy in coeliac disease, *Gut* 52 (2003): 1649–1652.
[d]L. Hogberg and coauthors, Oats to children with newly diagnosed coeliac disease: A randomised double blind study, *Gut* 53 (2004): 649–654; E. K. Janatuinen and coauthors, No harm from five year ingestion of oats in coeliac disease, *Gut* 50 (2002): 332–335.
[e]Janatuinen and coauthors, 2002.
[f]Hogberg and coauthors, 2004.
[g]Thompson, 2003.
[h]Peraaho and coauthors, 2004.
[i]Thompson, 2003.

Inflammatory Bowel Diseases

The major forms of **inflammatory bowel disease (IBD)** are **Crohn's disease** and **ulcerative colitis**—distinct disorders that share some common clinical features (see Table 24-6). Both conditions have characteristic patterns of inflammation that result from excessive immune responses in intestinal tissue, although the exact triggers that initiate the diseases are unknown. A complex set of genetic and environmental factors is believed to contribute to the development of IBD. Disease onset occurs most frequently in individuals between 15 and 30 years of age.

Crohn's disease may occur in any region of the GI tract, but most cases involve the ileum and colon. Lesions may be present at several areas within the intestine with normal tissue between the affected regions (called "skip" lesions). The inflammation extends deeply into the tissue, causing ulceration, fissures, and sometimes **fistulas** (abnormal passages between tissues). The main symptoms of disease are diarrhea, abdominal pain, and weight loss.

inflammatory bowel disease (IBD): chronic inflammatory disease of the gastrointestinal tract.

Crohn's disease: inflammatory bowel disease that usually occurs in the lower portion of the small intestine and the colon. Inflammation may pervade the entire intestinal wall.

ulcerative colitis (ko-LY-tis): inflammatory bowel disease that involves the colon. Inflammation affects the mucosa and submucosa.

fistulas (FIST-you-las): abnormal passages between body tissues; may lead from one hollow organ to another or to an organ surface.

TABLE 24-6 Comparison of Crohn's Disease and Ulcerative Colitis

	Crohn's Disease	Ulcerative Colitis
Location of inflammation	Approximately 40% of cases involve ileum and cecum, 30% are in small intestine only, 20% are in colon.	Inflammation is confined to rectum and colon; it begins at rectum and spreads into colon.
Pattern of inflammation	Discrete areas separated by normal tissue ("skip" lesions)	Continuous inflammation that begins at rectum and ends abruptly within colon
Depth of damage	Damage throughout all layers of tissue; causes deep fissures that give intestinal tissue a "cobblestone" appearance	Damage primarily in mucosa and submucosa
Fistulas	Common	Usually do not occur
Cancer risk	Increased	Greatly increased

Ulcerative colitis always involves the rectum and usually extends into the colon. The inflammation is continuous along the length of intestine affected, ending abruptly at the area where healthy tissue begins. Tissue erosion or ulceration develops primarily in the mucosa and submucosa. The major symptoms include diarrhea, rectal bleeding, and abdominal pain during active episodes.

Complications of Inflammatory Bowel Diseases Although the symptoms of Crohn's disease and ulcerative colitis are sometimes similar, the complications associated with each disease can be quite different. Crohn's disease usually involves the small intestine and may cause nutrient malabsorption, whereas ulcerative colitis affects the colon, which is past the absorptive areas. Both diseases may cause nutrient losses due to tissue damage, bleeding, and diarrhea.

Crohn's disease leads to the formation of fibrous scar tissue, which thickens and stiffens the intestine, narrowing the lumen and sometimes causing obstructions. Loops of intestine are often matted together. The strictures that develop may cause severe abdominal pain several hours after meals and also increase the risk of bacterial overgrowth. Malnutrition is common, resulting from reduced food intake, malabsorption, and surgical resections that shorten the bowel. Because extensive disease in the ileum interferes with bile acid reabsorption, bile acid may become depleted, leading to malabsorption of fat, fat-soluble vitamins, calcium, magnesium, and zinc. Vitamin B_{12} deficiency can also develop unless supplements are given.■ If unabsorbed bile acids pass into the colon, they can irritate colonic tissue and cause increased secretions of water and electrolytes. Anemia can result from nutrient malabsorption, blood loss, or the effects of chronic disease (see Highlight 25). Patients with Crohn's disease also have a greater risk of developing intestinal cancers. About 60 to 70 percent of patients require surgical resections during the course of illness, although the disease often recurs in the remaining intestine.[25]

Ulcerative colitis may affect the rectum alone or the entire colon. It usually causes frequent, urgent bowel movements that are small in volume. Stools are often streaked with blood and contain mucus. Although mild disease may cause few complications, weight loss, fever, and weakness are often present when most of the colon is involved. Moderate-to-severe disease is often associated with anemia (due to blood loss), dehydration, and electrolyte imbalances. Protein losses from inflamed tissue may be substantial. Ulcerative colitis patients have a high risk of developing colon cancer. **Colectomy** (removal of the colon) is performed in 20 to 25 percent of patients and prevents future recurrence.[26]

Treatment of Inflammatory Bowel Diseases The objectives of medical treatment for IBD are to control symptoms, reduce inflammation, and minimize complications. Drug treatments include antidiarrheal agents, immunosuppressants, and anti-inflammatory agents (usually corticosteroids and salicylates). The medications help in achieving and maintaining remission, although some may cause gastrointestinal side effects (see the Diet-Drug Interactions box on p. 762). Surgical interventions are frequently necessary.

Medical Nutrition Therapy for Inflammatory Bowel Diseases Crohn's disease often requires active and aggressive dietary management. The effects of the disease may include growth failure in children, protein-energy malnutrition (PEM), and nutrient deficiencies. Nutrition therapy for ulcerative colitis focuses on replacing nutrient losses and correcting deficiencies.

Crohn's Disease The nutrition care of patients with Crohn's disease is highly variable; dietary measures depend on a person's symptoms and the complications that have developed (see Table 24-7). Some people can meet their nutrient needs with unsupplemented conventional diets. Others may require high-kcalorie, high-protein diets to help prevent or treat malnutrition. Liquid supplements added to conventional diets help to increase energy intakes and improve weight gain. Tube feedings may be used to supplement diets and are sometimes the sole

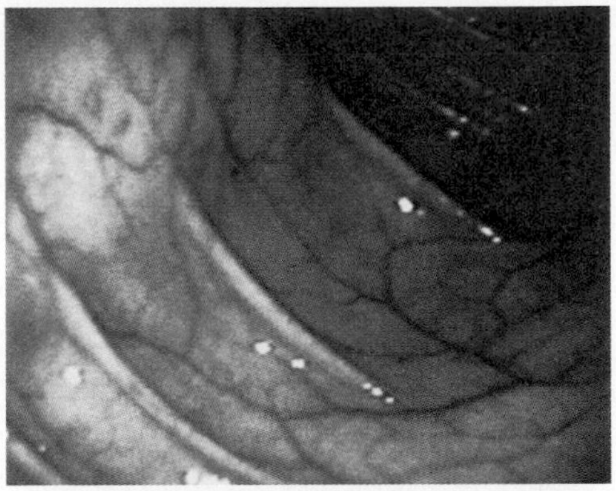

The normal colon has a smooth, shiny surface with a visible pattern of fine blood vessels.

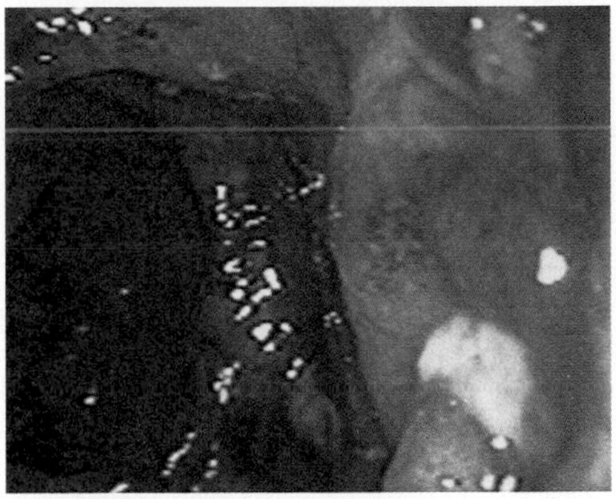

Courtesy of the Crohn's & Colitis Foundation of America Inc. (both)

In ulcerative colitis, the colon appears inflamed and reddened, and ulcers are visible.

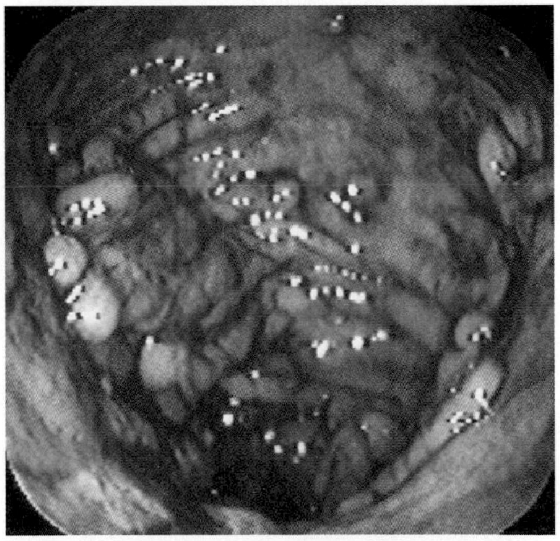

© Albert Paglialunga/PhotoTake

In Crohn's disease, the ulcerated mucosa has a "cobblestone" appearance and is interspersed with narrow sections of healthy tissue.

■ Reminder: Vitamin B_{12} is absorbed only in the ileum. Some patients with Crohn's disease may require regular vitamin B_{12} injections.

colectomy: removal of a portion or all of the colon.

■ Reminder: *Elemental formulas* contain hydrolyzed nutrients that require minimal digestion and are easily absorbed.

means of providing nutrients; elemental formula diets■ are most easily tolerated. If inflammation is severe, oral intakes may exacerbate symptoms. Restriction of high-fiber and lactose-containing foods may benefit some patients. Low-fiber diets are recommended for those with partial intestinal obstructions. Vitamin and mineral supplements are generally recommended, especially if malabsorption is present. Table 24-7 includes examples of other dietary adjustments that are often beneficial.

Ulcerative Colitis In most cases, the diet for ulcerative colitis requires few adjustments. Care should be taken to replace fluid and electrolyte losses and correct deficiencies due to protein and blood losses. A low-fiber diet may reduce irritation by minimizing fecal volume. During exacerbations, food may be withheld to allow bowel rest. As in Crohn's disease, the symptoms and complications that develop can be managed with specific dietary measures (see Table 24-7).

During severe illness, ulcerative colitis often causes substantial losses of fluid, electrolytes, and tissue proteins. Negative nitrogen balance may lead to protein catabolism and weight loss. Fluids and electrolytes may need to be replaced intravenously. Food is often withheld or restricted to clear liquids, and parenteral nutrition may be required. Patients whose conditions deteriorate despite medical management may require a colectomy.

Short-Bowel Syndrome

The treatment of Crohn's disease, cancers of the small intestine, and other intestinal abnormalities may require the surgical removal (resection) of a major portion of the small intestine. **Short-bowel syndrome** is the malabsorption syndrome that results when the absorptive capacity of the remaining intestine is insufficient for meeting nutritional needs. Without adequate nutrition support, short-bowel syndrome can result in fluid and electrolyte imbalances and multiple nutrient deficiencies. Symptoms include diarrhea, steatorrhea, dehydration, weight loss, and growth impairment in children.

TABLE 24-7 Management of Symptoms and Complications in Crohn's Disease

Symptom or Complication	Possible Dietary Measures
Growth failure/weight loss	High-kcalorie diet Enteral supplements Elemental tube feedings
Anorexia/pain with eating	Small, frequent meals Enteral supplements If long-term (> 5 to 7 days): elemental tube feedings
Malabsorption	High-kcalorie diet Nutrient supplementation
Steatorrhea	Fat restriction Medium-chain triglycerides Nutrient supplementation
Diarrhea	Fluid and electrolyte replacement Nutrient supplementation
Lactose intolerance	Avoidance of lactose-containing foods
Nutrient deficiencies	Nutrient-dense diet Nutrient supplementation
Intestinal recovery	High-protein diet Glutamine supplementation
Strictures/fistulas	Low-fiber diet
Severe bowel obstruction/high-output fistulas/severe exacerbations of disease	Total parenteral nutrition

short-bowel syndrome: malabsorption syndrome following small intestinal resection; results from insufficient absorptive capacity in the remaining intestine.

Figure 24-3 reviews nutrient absorption in the GI tract and describes how absorption is affected by surgical resections. Generally, up to 50 percent of the small intestine can be resected without serious nutritional consequences. More extensive resections lead to generalized malabsorption, and patients may need lifelong supplementation of oral intakes with parenteral nutrition.

Intestinal Adaptation After an intestinal resection, the remaining intestine undergoes **intestinal adaptation,** a remarkable adaptive response that dramatically improves its absorptive efficiency. Many patients can eventually return to a normal diet if intestinal adaptation can compensate sufficiently for the removed length of intestine.■ Adaptation begins soon after surgery, but several years may be needed for the full effect. The presence of nutrients in the lumen stimulates adaptation, and therefore oral intakes are begun soon after surgery. A number of dietary and hormonal factors, including the amino acid glutamine, short-chain fatty acids, and a glucagon-like hormone (glucagon-like peptide 2, or GLP-2), are believed to enhance adaptation.

■ The reasons why nutrient absorption improves after intestinal resection are not well understood. In animal studies, resections have resulted in increased villus height and intestinal length, but there is little evidence that similar changes occur in patients with short-bowel syndrome.

The ileum has a greater capacity for adaptation than the jejunum; thus removal of the ileum ultimately has more severe consequences than removal of the jejunum (review Figure 24-3). Resection of the ileum can have permanent consequences on both vitamin B_{12} nutrition and bile acid reabsorption; recall from the discussion of inflammatory bowel disease that bile acid depletion worsens both fat malabsorption and diarrhea. Loss of the ileocecal valve (between the ileum and cecum) increases the likelihood that colonic bacteria will infiltrate the small intestine and cause bacterial overgrowth.

Intestinal adaptation is achieved more easily if both the ileum and the colon remain intact. A functional colon helps to prevent malnutrition because the resident bacteria metabolize unabsorbed nutrients and produce short-chain fatty acids that are readily absorbed. In addition, an intact colon helps to reduce losses of fluids and electrolytes.

intestinal adaptation: after resection, the process of intestinal recovery that leads to improved absorptive capacity.

Treatment of Short-Bowel Syndrome To meet their nutritional needs with enteral (oral) nutrition alone, adults need at least 40 to 80 inches (100 to 200

FIGURE 24-3 Nutrient Absorption and Consequences of Intestinal Surgeries

About 90 to 95 percent of nutrient absorption takes place in the first half of the small intestine. After a resection, nutrient absorption may be reduced.

WHAT IS ABSORBED

Duodenum/ jejunum
- Simple carbohydrates
- Fats
- Amino acids
- Vitamins*
- Minerals*
- Water

Ileum
- Bile salts
- Vitamin B_{12}
- Water

(Assumes absorptive function of duodenum and jejunum with adaptation)

Colon
- Water
- Electrolytes
- Short-chain fatty acids

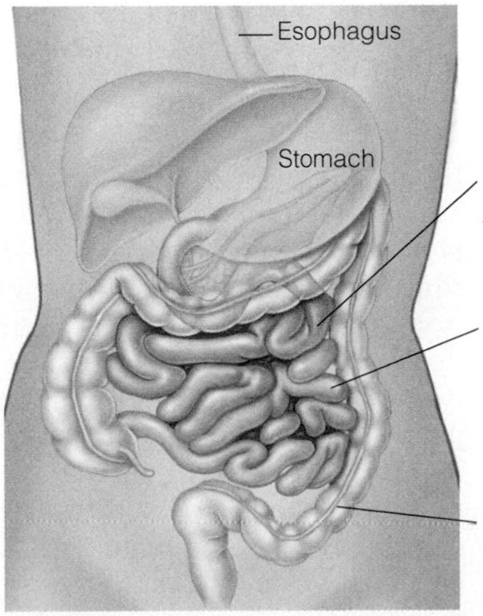
Esophagus
Stomach
Duodenum/ jejunum
Ileum
Colon

POSSIBLE CONSEQUENCES OF RESECTION

Duodenum/ jejunum
- Minimal consequences if the ileum remains intact
- Calcium and iron malabsorption if duodenum resected

Ileum
- Fat malabsorption
- Protein malabsorption
- Malabsorption of fat-soluble vitamins and vitamin B_{12}
- Reduced calcium, magnesium, and zinc absorption
- Fluid losses
- Diarrhea/steatorrhea

Colon
- Fluid and electrolyte losses
- Diarrhea

(Losses are compounded if ileum is also resected)

*The absorption of vitamins and minerals begins in the duodenum and continues throughout the length of the small intestine.

centimeters) of small intestine; the length required depends on the region of intestine that remains.[27] If patients do not have adequate absorptive capacity, the usual treatment is lifelong parenteral nutrition. Intestinal transplantation is an option for patients who cannot continue parenteral nutrition because of life-threatening complications.

Medical Nutrition Therapy Immediately after resection, fluids and electrolytes need to be supplied intravenously. In the first few weeks after surgery, fluid losses from diarrhea can be substantial (sometimes exceeding 2 liters per day), so appropriate rehydration is a central feature of postsurgical management. Antidiarrheal drugs may be needed to limit losses. Clear liquids are usually started orally after diarrhea subsides somewhat and some bowel function is restored. Diarrhea gradually lessens as intestinal adaptation progresses.

Total parenteral nutrition meets nutrient needs after surgery and is gradually reduced as oral feedings increase. Oral feedings are started as soon as possible to promote intestinal adaptation, in as little as five days after surgery in some cases. Initial oral intakes may consist of occasional sips of liquid formulas, progressing to larger amounts, and then to solid foods, as tolerated. Very small, frequent feedings can utilize the remaining intestine most efficiently. Low-fat diets are sometimes suggested to reduce steatorrhea, and a high-carbohydrate diet can help stimulate production of short-chain fatty acids in the colon. Glutamine is often included in feedings to promote adaptation. Intravenous feedings are tapered and gradually discontinued once oral intakes can supply adequate nourishment. Patients with extensive short-bowel resections, however, may require lifelong parenteral support.

Dietary choices are tailored according to individual symptoms and tolerances. Lactose-containing foods are sometimes poorly tolerated. If excessively rapid GI transit leads to dumping symptoms, fluids are restricted during meals, and complex carbohydrates are used in place of simple sugars. In many patients, fat malabsorption is more problematic than protein or carbohydrate malabsorption, and medium-chain triglycerides may be used as an energy source. Patients with short-bowel syndrome have a high risk of developing kidney stones due to calcium malabsorption (see p. 866), and a low-oxalate diet is often suggested.

Vitamin and mineral supplements are generally required. If fat is malabsorbed, increased amounts of the fat-soluble vitamins, calcium, magnesium, and zinc are suggested. If a large portion of the ileum has been removed, vitamin B_{12} must be injected. Iron absorption is usually compromised if upper portions of the small intestine have been removed.

Use the case study on p. 758 to apply the concepts described in this section to a patient with short-bowel syndrome.

IN SUMMARY Widespread malabsorption can be caused by conditions that disrupt normal digestion and absorption. Chronic pancreatitis results in permanent damage to the pancreas. Cystic fibrosis causes pancreatic duct obstructions, leading to destruction of pancreatic tissue. Both pancreatitis and cystic fibrosis lead to enzyme deficiencies, and pancreatic enzyme replacement is central to treatment. Celiac disease and inflammatory bowel conditions cause damage to intestinal mucosa and impair absorption. Although a gluten-free diet can alleviate the symptoms of celiac disease, there is no cure for Crohn's disease, and intestinal resection is often necessary. Ulcerative colitis is an inflammatory bowel condition that affects the colon only, and severe cases can be cured by colectomy. Short-bowel syndrome is a frequent consequence of major resections of the small intestine and may require permanent parenteral nutrition support. In many patients, intestinal adaptation may improve absorptive capacity after surgical resections.

Conditions Affecting the Large Intestine

The large intestine moves undigested materials to the rectum and has a central role in maintaining fluid and electrolyte balances. Its bacterial population ferments the undigested nutrients that reach the colon and produces short-chain fatty acids and some vitamins, which our bodies can absorb and use. This section describes several conditions that may disrupt the normal functioning of the large intestine.

Irritable Bowel Syndrome

People with irritable bowel syndrome■ experience chronic and recurring intestinal symptoms that cannot be explained by specific physical abnormalities. Although irritable bowel syndrome is often described as a motility disorder due to its accompanying symptoms of diarrhea and constipation, motility impairment is not routinely documented in persons diagnosed with the condition. Irritable bowel syndrome is included in this section because it may cause colonic dysfunction; however, the disorder may also involve the small intestine or even areas of the upper GI tract.

■ Reminder: *Irritable bowel syndrome* is an intestinal disorder of unknown cause that affects the functioning of the lower bowel; it is characterized by abdominal pain, flatulence, diarrhea, and constipation.

Irritable bowel syndrome is characterized by alterations in stool frequency and consistency. Both diarrhea and constipation may occur, as well as flatulence, bloating, and distention. Abdominal pain may occur shortly after a meal and be relieved by defecation. In some patients, symptoms may be mild; in others, defecation disturbances can interfere with work and prevent participation in social activities. Irritable bowel syndrome can consume a person's attention and dramatically alter lifestyle and sense of well-being.

The prevalence of irritable bowel syndrome is between 10 and 20 percent worldwide. It occurs more frequently in women and declines with age. Even though symptoms often persist for several months, people with the condition may experience no other health problems.

Causes of Irritable Bowel Syndrome The causes of irritable bowel syndrome remain elusive, but stress and anxiety are among the contributing factors. Symptoms may worsen during periods of psychological stress, and in some cases, stressful life events may trigger the illness. People with irritable bowel syndrome often exhibit hypersensitivity to intestinal distention; for example, they may have an exaggerated response to normal meal transit and rectal distention. Hyperactivity is common outside the GI tract as well, and some studies suggest a generalized abnormality of smooth muscle tissue or of the nervous system. For example, altered reactivity is often seen in bronchial tissue, the gallbladder, and the urinary tract. There is also some evidence that an infection may be the cause of the initial GI disturbances and that tissue sensitization persists after the infection has healed.

Treatment of Irritable Bowel Syndrome Medical treatment of irritable bowel syndrome often includes stress management and behavioral therapies along with dietary adjustments. Medications may be used to treat symptoms but are not always helpful. The drugs generally prescribed include antidiarrheal agents, anticholinergics, antidepressants, and laxatives.

Medical Nutrition Therapy Although dietary changes may be useful, measures that may help one symptom can sometimes make another worse. The usual dietary recommendation is to increase fiber intake, which often helps to reduce constipation and improve stool bulk. To minimize intestinal gas, fiber-containing foods should be added gradually. Other foods that produce gas should be avoided

CASE STUDY

Economist with Short-Bowel Syndrome

Paula Jentamen is a 28-year-old economist with an 8-year history of Crohn's disease. Paula is 5 feet 7 inches tall. Three years ago, she underwent a small bowel resection and remained free of active disease for two years. During that time, her symptoms subsided, she gained weight, and she was able to tolerate most foods without any problem. Ten months ago, Paula experienced a severe flare-up of her Crohn's disease. Since that time, she has lost 15 pounds and currently weighs 118 pounds. She has experienced severe abdominal pain and fatigue that have persisted despite aggressive medical management that included intravenous nutrition. Paula finally underwent another resection five days ago, which left her with 40 percent of healthy small intestine. Her colon is intact. She is experiencing extensive diarrhea.

1. Describe the manifestations of Crohn's disease, and explain why surgery is sometimes necessary as part of the treatment. Describe the complications that may affect nutrient needs in people with Crohn's disease.
2. Calculate Paula's ideal body weight. What nutrition concerns are suggested by her current weight and recent weight loss? What other nutritional problems did Paula probably experience as a consequence of Crohn's disease?
3. Discuss the complications that may follow an extensive intestinal resection. What factors are likely to affect a person's ability to meet nutrient needs with an oral diet?
4. Discuss the dietary progression that is recommended following an intestinal resection. After Paula is able to eat solid foods, what factors may affect the type of diet that is recommended for her?

unless well tolerated (review Table 24-2). If diarrhea persists, a bulking agent (psyllium) may be effective. Avoidance of milk products may benefit those who are lactose intolerant. Caffeine and alcohol may also exacerbate symptoms. The placebo effect has a strong influence on food tolerance, and foods that are perceived to be problematic should be discussed with patients so that the diet is not restricted unnecessarily.

The diet history may reveal dietary behaviors that may worsen symptoms. Generally, small, frequent meals are better tolerated than larger ones. Eating quickly should be discouraged as it may increase the amount of air that is swallowed. Some patients may find a low-fat diet easier to tolerate. Fluid intake should be assessed for adequacy. A careful evaluation of the dietary patterns that exacerbate symptoms may uncover the foods and habits that are most closely associated with intestinal discomfort. The case study on p. 760 can be used to apply this information about irritable bowel syndrome to a clinical situation.

■ Reminder: *Diverticulosis* is characterized by the presence of small outpockets (diverticula) in the intestinal wall; it often develops by middle age.

Diverticular Disease of the Colon

Diverticulosis■ refers to the development of pebble-sized herniations (protrusions) in the intestinal wall, known as diverticula (see Figure 24-4). In Western societies, diverticula occur most often in the sigmoid colon, the portion of the colon just above the rectum. The prevalence of diverticulosis increases with age, occurring in about half of adults over 60 years of age.[28] Most people with diverticulosis are symptom-free and usually remain unaware of the condition until a complication develops.

Epidemiological studies suggest that the development of diverticula is strongly influenced by the amount of dietary fiber a person consumes. By increasing stool weight and bulk, the presence of fiber reduces the amount of work that needs to be performed by the circular muscles that propel fecal matter through the colon. If a low-fiber diet is consumed, more vigorous contractions are needed, and they increase the amount of pressure present in segments immediately adjacent to the circular muscles. The increase in outward pressure during contractions induces small areas of intestinal tissue to balloon outward over time.[29]

FIGURE 24-4 Diverticula in the Colon

Diverticula are small pouches that develop in weakened areas of the intestinal wall. The condition of having diverticula is known as diverticulosis.

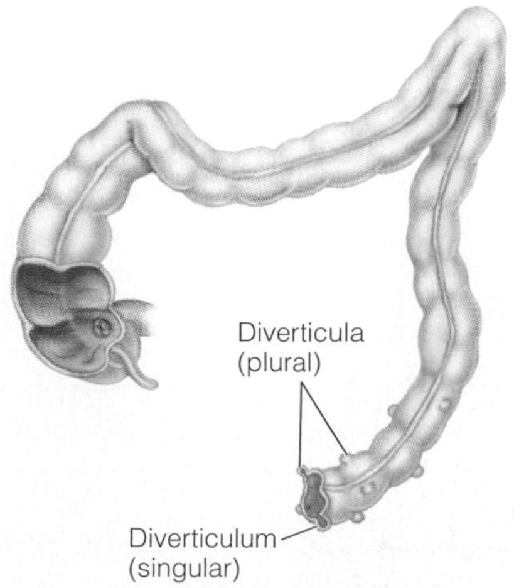
Diverticula
(plural)
Diverticulum
(singular)

Diverticulitis In about 10 to 25 percent of persons with diverticulosis, a localized inflammation or infection develops in the area around a diverticulum. This condition, called diverticulitis,■ is the most common complication of diverticulosis. It is thought to result from hardened or impacted fecal matter that abrades the mucosal lining. The abrasion causes inflammation and may create a microperforation that leads to subsequent infection. The infection may spread to adjacent organs or to the peritoneal cavity. If adjacent organs become involved, fistulas may develop. Peritonitis is uncommon but can be life-threatening, especially if fecal matter spills into the peritoneal cavity. Symptoms of diverticulitis include persistent abdominal pain, fever, and alternating constipation and diarrhea.

■ Reminder: *Diverticulitis* is an inflammation or infection that affects the diverticula.

Treatment for Diverticular Disease Diverticulosis requires treatment only if symptoms develop; in this case, treatment focuses on reducing pain and alleviating constipation. Patients with diverticulosis are usually advised to increase dietary fiber to help prevent disease progression. The addition of wheat bran to meals is often recommended, although bulk-forming agents such as psyllium are equally effective. Dietary advice for diverticulosis sometimes includes a recommendation to avoid nuts, popcorn, and foods that contain seeds, but there is no evidence that these restrictions can reduce complications.[30]

When diverticulitis is present, antibiotics are given to treat infection, and medications may be provided for pain control. In mild cases, a clear liquid diet may be advised initially, with progression to solid foods as tolerated. In more severe cases, bowel rest is necessary (oral fluids and food are withheld), and fluids are given intravenously; dietary intakes are gradually reintroduced as the condition improves. Surgical interventions are sometimes necessary to treat complications of diverticulitis and may include removal of the affected portion of colon (colectomy).

IN SUMMARY Irritable bowel syndrome and diverticular disease are common disorders that affect the colon. Irritable bowel syndrome is often associated with abdominal pain and alternating diarrhea and constipation. Although the causes are unknown, it is influenced by stress and psychological factors. Diverticulosis is often asymptomatic until complications develop; it is affected by factors that influence colon integrity, including aging and fiber intake. Both conditions may benefit from a high-fiber diet.

Ostomies

Treatment for medical conditions that affect the large intestine sometimes requires surgical removal of some or all of the large intestine. In some procedures, the dietary wastes are rerouted so that they exit through a **stoma** (opening) in the abdominal wall. A **colostomy** is a surgical procedure in which a stoma is formed from the final portion of the remaining colon (see Figure 24-5 p. 761). In an **ileostomy,** the entire colon is removed, and the stoma is created from the ileum. To collect wastes, a disposable bag may be worn over the stoma and emptied during the day. Alternatively, a small pouch may be surgically created behind the stoma using intestinal tissue, which eliminates the need for a bag on the outside. The pouch can be emptied when convenient, using a catheter. Colostomies and ileostomies may be either temporary or permanent. Conditions that may require these procedures include inflammatory bowel diseases, diverticulitis, and colorectal cancers.

Removal of part or all of the large intestine reduces the amount of fluid and electrolytes that can be reabsorbed into the body. Stool consistency therefore varies according to the length of colon removed. If a small portion is removed, the effects may be minor and stools may continue to be semisolid. If the entire colon is removed, the output is liquid.

stoma (STOE-ma): a surgical opening made in the abdominal wall.

colostomy (co-LAHS-toe-me): a surgical procedure that creates a stoma from the final segment of colon that remains after a colectomy.

ileostomy (ill-ee-OS-toe-me): a surgical procedure that creates a stoma using the ileum.

CASE STUDY

New College Graduate with Irritable Bowel Syndrome

Meera Gupta is a 22-year-old recent college graduate who began her first professional job in a bank one month ago. As a college student, she occasionally experienced abdominal pain and cramping after eating. She also had frequent bouts of diarrhea and noticed that she felt better after bowel movements. Once Meera began her new job, her symptoms occurred more frequently. At first she attributed her symptoms to job stress, but when the symptoms continued for several months, she decided to see her physician. After taking a careful history and conducting tests to rule out other bowel disorders, the physician diagnosed irritable bowel syndrome. The physician prescribed bulk-forming agents and advised Meera to keep a food intake and symptoms record for one week. Meera was then referred to a dietitian for a review of her dietary records. The dietitian noticed that Meera routinely drank several cups of coffee in the morning and had large meals for lunch and dinner. Meera often ate traditional Indian foods that were highly seasoned and included legumes. Between meals, she snacked on low-carb foods containing sugar alcohols and drank several cans of soda daily. Her dietary fiber intake, however, totaled only about 15 grams daily.

1. Explain the possible causes of irritable bowel syndrome to Meera and indicate the role that stress might play in her illness.
2. How can the dietitian use the food intake and symptoms record to devise an appropriate dietary plan for Meera? Is it likely that any of the foods in Meera's diet may aggravate her symptoms?
3. What type of diet may benefit persons with irritable bowel syndrome? What problems might some of the dietary changes cause?

Medical Nutrition Therapy for Ostomies Following surgery, the diet gradually progresses from clear liquids to a low-fiber diet until healing has occurred. Initially, meals should be small and consist of well-cooked foods.[31] Once a regular diet has resumed, dietary adjustments are made on the basis of individual tolerances. For many, an ostomy diet is less restrictive than the diet they needed to follow during the illness that necessitated the surgery.

People with ileostomies need to chew thoroughly to ensure that foods are adequately digested and to prevent obstructions, which are a common complication. Because the colon is not present to reabsorb water, the diet should provide at least 8 cups of fluid daily to prevent dehydration. Patients are sometimes encouraged to increase intakes of sodium and potassium to offset losses of these minerals in the ileostomy fluid. Foods that are high in insoluble fibers are sometimes avoided because they reduce intestinal transit time and may increase output. If a large portion of the ileum has been removed, fat malabsorption may occur due to bile acid depletion, and vitamin B_{12} injections may be required.

The dietary concerns of persons with colostomies depend on the length of colon removed. If a large portion of the colon is removed, recommendations may be similar to those given to ileostomy patients. A high-fiber diet is generally recommended for colostomy patients to improve stool consistency and promote regularity. Food odors and gas are also frequent concerns.

Obstructions Foods that are incompletely digested can cause obstructions, a primary concern of ileostomy patients. Although almost any food can be consumed if cut into small pieces and carefully chewed, the following foods may cause difficulty: raw vegetables, mushrooms, bean sprouts, lettuce, corn and popcorn, fibrous vegetables like asparagus and celery, dried fruit, fruit skins, pineapple, tough fibrous meats and meats in casings (such as sausage and bratwurst), nuts and seeds, coconut, and very chewy candies.

Diarrhea Diarrhea may be improved by the consumption of foods that tend to thicken stool. Foods that may aggravate or reduce diarrhea were listed in Table 24-3 on p. 743. What works may differ for each individual, however, and is best determined by trial and error.

Reducing Gas and Odors Persons with colostomies may be concerned about foods that increase gas production or cause strong odors. Foods that may cause excessive gas include those listed in Table 24-2 p. 742. Foods that sometimes produce

FIGURE 24-5 Colostomy and Ileostomy

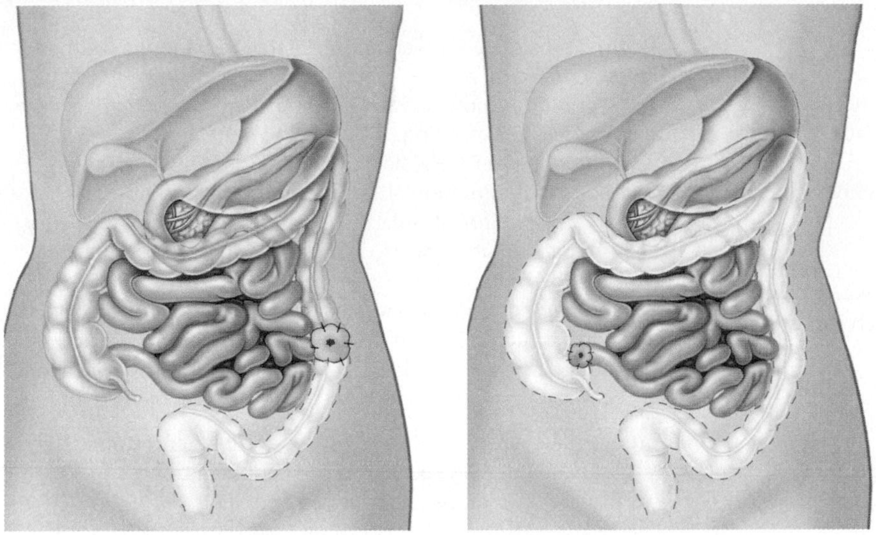
Colostomy
Ileostomy

In a colostomy, the rectum and anus are removed, and the stoma is formed from the remaining colon.

In an ileostomy, the entire colon, rectum, and anus are removed, and the stoma is formed from the ileum.

unpleasant odors include dried beans and peas, fish, garlic and onions, asparagus and turnips, eggs, strong cheeses, and certain spices.[32] Foods that may help to reduce odors include buttermilk, cranberry juice, parsley, and yogurt.

IN SUMMARY Colostomies and ileostomies are surgical procedures in which stomas are created in the abdominal wall using the ileum or colon. Although few foods are restricted after an ostomy, fluid and electrolyte requirements are greater because colon function is reduced or absent. Although foods that are poorly digested may cause obstructions, thorough chewing can reduce risk. Foods are sometimes avoided if they provoke diarrhea or cause excessive gas or strong odors, although individual tolerances differ.

DIET-DRUG INTERACTIONS

Analgesics
Analgesics can cause nausea, vomiting, and stomach cramps. When oral food intake is permitted, giving the medication with food or milk can minimize these effects. Some analgesics may cause gastric bleeding and lead to anemia.
Narcotic analgesics can cause constipation. They can also result in lethargy, which can contribute to reduced food intake.

Antidiarrheals
Antidiarrheals seldom result in significant nutrition-related side effects, with the exception of *opium* and *paregoric,* which can cause nausea and vomiting, constipation, and lethargy.

Anti-Infective Agents
Numerous *anti-infective agents* may be used in the treatment of diarrhea, pulmonary infections (due to cystic fibrosis), bacterial overgrowth, and infections that arise during recovery from surgery; some of these medications may have nutrition-related side effects. Consult a drug guide for information about specific drugs.

Anti-Inflammatory Agents and Immunosuppressants (for Inflammatory Bowel Diseases)
Prednisone can stimulate the appetite and lead to fluid retention, resulting in weight gain. Long-term use also leads to negative nitrogen and calcium balances and osteoporosis. Patients using prednisone are advised to consume high-protein, high-calcium, high-potassium diets. Those who retain fluid may need to limit sodium. The dietary supplement *melatonin* can antagonize the effects of prednisone.

The immunosuppressants *azathioprine* and *6-mercaptopurine* may cause nausea and vomiting.

Sulfasalazine can cause nausea, vomiting, and diarrhea and should be taken with food at regular intervals during the day. Sulfasalazine also inhibits folate absorption; to prevent deficiency, folate supplementation of 1 to 2 milligrams per day is usually recommended.

Mesalamine may cause anorexia and weight loss, but nutrition-related effects are less common than with sulfasalazine. *Infliximab* may cause nausea and abdominal pain and is given by injection.

Laxatives
Common side effects of *laxatives* include nausea and stomach cramps. Patients using laxatives are encouraged to consume high-fiber foods and drink generous amounts of fluids.

Pancreatic Enzyme Replacements
Enzyme replacements sometimes cause nausea and may interfere with iron absorption. Enzyme replacements must be taken with meals and snacks. Enteric-coated forms should not be crushed or chewed. The enteric-coated microspheres (tiny spheres of medication) contained in capsules may be sprinkled on soft foods (such as applesauce), provided they can be swallowed intact and are followed by a glass of water or juice.

NUTRITION ASSESSMENT CHECKLIST for People with Lower GI Tract Disorders

Medical History
Check for a medical diagnosis of diseases that:

- ☐ Interfere with pancreatic enzyme secretion, such as chronic pancreatitis or cystic fibrosis
- ☐ Interfere with nutrient absorption, such as chronic pancreatitis, cystic fibrosis, celiac disease, or Crohn's disease
- ☐ Cause chronic GI symptoms, such as irritable bowel syndrome or ulcerative colitis

Check for surgical procedures involving the lower GI tract, such as:

- ☐ Intestinal resection
- ☐ Ileostomy
- ☐ Colostomy

Check for the following symptoms or complications:

- ☐ Constipation
- ☐ Diarrhea, dehydration
- ☐ Steatorrhea
- ☐ Bacterial overgrowth
- ☐ Lactose intolerance
- ☐ Nutrient deficiencies
- ☐ Bone disease
- ☐ Oxalate kidney stones
- ☐ Anemia
- ☐ Obstructions
- ☐ Fistulas
- ☐ Poor growth, in children

Medications
Check for medications or herbal remedies that may:

- ☐ Cause constipation or diarrhea
- ☐ Interfere with food intake by causing nausea, vomiting, cramps, dry mouth, or drowsiness
- ☐ Alter nutrient needs, including prednisone and sulfasalazine

Dietary Intake
Note the following conditions and contact the dietitian if you suspect a problem with:

- ☐ Poor appetite or limited food intake
- ☐ Food intolerances
- ☐ Inadequate fiber intake, in those with constipation
- ☐ Lactose intolerance, in those with diarrhea
- ☐ Fluid intake

Anthropometric Data
Measure baseline height and weight. Address weight loss early to prevent malnutrition in patients with:

- ☐ Severe or persistent diarrhea
- ☐ Malabsorption

Laboratory Tests
Check laboratory tests for signs of dehydration, nutrient deficiencies, and nutrition-related anemias in patients with:

- ☐ Severe or persistent diarrhea
- ☐ Malabsorption
- ☐ Intestinal resections

Clinical Signs
Look for physical signs of:

- ☐ Dehydration
- ☐ Protein-energy malnutrition
- ☐ Essential fatty acid and fat-soluble vitamin deficiencies
- ☐ Folate and vitamin B_{12} deficiencies
- ☐ Mineral deficiencies

NUTRITION ON THE NET

Access these websites for further study of topics covered in this chapter.

- Find updates and quick links to these and other nutrition-related sites at our website: **www.wadsworth.com/nutrition**
- Visit the websites of these organizations to find information that is helpful for both health practitioners and patients with gastrointestinal problems:

  American College of Gastroenterology: **www.acg.gi.org**

  American Gastroenterological Association: **www.gastro.org**

  National Institute of Diabetes and Digestive and Kidney Diseases, a division of the National Institutes of Health: **www.niddk.nih.gov**
- Find more information about celiac disease by visiting these websites:

  Celiac Disease Foundation: **www.celiac.org**

  Canadian Celiac Association: **www.celiac.ca**

  Celiac Sprue Association: **www.csaceliacs.org**

  Gluten Intolerance Group: **www.gluten.net**
- Learn more about inflammatory bowel diseases at the website of the Crohn's and Colitis Foundation of America: **www.ccfa.org**
- Find additional information about cystic fibrosis at the website of the Cystic Fibrosis Foundation: **www.cff.org/home**

STUDY QUESTIONS

These questions will help you review the chapter. You will find the answers in the discussions on the pages provided.

1. What measures can help to prevent and treat constipation? What are the modes of action of the laxatives used to treat constipation? (pp. 740–742)
2. Describe possible causes of diarrhea and dietary measures that may be included during treatment. (pp. 742–743)
3. Explain why bacterial overgrowth develops and describe its effects on nutrition status. (pp. 743–744)
4. Identify conditions that can cause fat malabsorption, and discuss the primary nutrition problems that can result. (pp. 744–745)
5. Explain how chronic pancreatitis and cystic fibrosis can result in malabsorption. In what ways are their dietary treatments similar? (pp. 747–749)
6. Discuss the cause of celiac disease and describe the diet used in its treatment. Explain why a gluten-free diet may be difficult for patients to follow. (pp. 750–751)
7. Compare the effects of Crohn's disease and ulcerative colitis on nutrition status, and describe the dietary measures that may be required during the course of illness. (pp. 752–754)
8. Identify possible causes of short-bowel syndrome. What nutrition problems often develop? Discuss the adaptive process that occurs in the remaining intestine after a portion of intestine is resected. (pp. 754–756)
9. Describe the irritable bowel syndrome and discuss the ways in which diet can be used in its treatment. (pp. 757–758)
10. Specify the factors that increase the risk of developing diverticular disease. What dietary modification is most useful in its prevention and treatment? (pp. 758–759)
11. Describe the primary nutrition-related concerns of people who have undergone ileostomies and colostomies. (pp. 759–761)

These questions will help you prepare for an exam. Answers can be found on p. 764.

1. The health care professional advising an elderly patient with constipation encourages the patient to:
   a. consume a low-fat diet rich in potassium.
   b. consume a high-protein diet rich in calcium.
   c. gradually add high-fiber foods to the diet.
   d. eliminate gas-forming foods from the diet.
2. Osmotic diarrhea often results from:
   a. excessive motility of fluids within the colon.
   b. excessive fluid secretion by the intestines.
   c. viral, bacterial, or protozoal infections.
   d. nutrient malabsorption.
3. Common nutrition problems associated with bacterial overgrowth in the stomach and small intestine include:
   a. sensitivity to gluten.
   b. fat malabsorption and vitamin B_{12} deficiency.
   c. increased absorption of bile salts and constipation.
   d. permanent loss of digestive enzymes.
4. Nutrition problems that may result from fat malabsorption include all of the following, *except:*
   a. weight loss.
   b. essential amino acid deficiencies.
   c. bone loss.
   d. oxalate kidney stones.
5. The majority of acute pancreatitis cases can be attributed to:
   a. bacterial and viral infections.
   b. cystic fibrosis.
   c. excessive alcohol use and gallstones.
   d. elevated triglyceride levels.
6. The most appropriate diet for a person with cystic fibrosis is a:
   a. high-kcalorie, high-protein diet.
   b. high-fiber diet.

c. gluten-free diet.
d. fat-restricted diet.

7. A person on a gluten-free diet must avoid products containing:
   a. wheat, corn, and rice.
   b. barley, soybeans, and corn.
   c. wheat, barley, and rye.
   d. buckwheat, rice, and millet.

8. A patient with Crohn's disease may develop all of the following nutrition problems, *except:*
   a. fat malabsorption.
   b. dumping syndrome.
   c. vitamin B_{12} deficiency.
   d. anemia.

9. If 80 inches of small intestine remain after a jejunal resection:
   a. lifelong parenteral nutrition is the only option available.
   b. intestinal transplantation is the treatment of choice.
   c. pancreatic enzyme replacement is required.
   d. oral diets are eventually able to meet nutrient needs.

10. After an ileostomy, the most serious concern is:
   a. the diet is too restrictive for meeting nutrient needs.
   b. waste disposal causes frequent daily interruptions.
   c. incompletely digested foods may cause obstructions.
   d. fluid restrictions prevent patients from drinking beverages freely.

REFERENCES

1. S. L. Friedman, K. R. McQuaid, and J. H. Grendell, eds., *Current Diagnosis and Treatment in Gastroenterology* (New York: Lange Medical Books/McGraw-Hill, 2003); M. Feldman, L. S. Friedman, and M. H. Sleisenger, eds., *Sleisenger and Fordtran's Gastrointestinal and Liver Disease: Pathophysiology, Diagnosis, Management* (Philadelphia: Saunders, 2002).
2. Committee on Dietary Reference Intakes, *Dietary Reference Intakes for Energy, Carbohydrate, Fiber, Fat, Fatty Acids, Cholesterol, Protein, and Amino Acids (Macronutrients)* (Washington, D.C.: National Academy Press, 2002).
3. F. L. Suarez and M. D. Levitt, Intestinal gas, in M. Feldman, L. S. Friedman, and M. H. Sleisenger, eds., *Sleisenger and Fordtran's Gastrointestinal and Liver Disease: Pathophysiology, Diagnosis, Management* (Philadelphia: Saunders, 2002); L. J. Cheskin and D. L. Miller, Nutrition in the prevention and treatment of common gastrointestinal symptoms, in A. M. Coulston, C. L. Rock, and E. R. Monsen, eds., *Nutrition in the Prevention and Treatment of Disease* (San Diego: Academic Press, 2001), pp. 549–562; American Dietetic Association, *Manual of Clinical Dietetics* (Chicago: American Dietetic Association, 2000), p. 423.
4. Friedman, McQuaid, and Grendell, 2003; Feldman, Friedman, and Sleisenger, 2002.
5. Friedman, McQuaid, and Grendell, 2003; Feldman, Friedman, and Sleisenger, 2002.
6. Feldman, Friedman, and Sleisenger, 2002.
7. C. Owyang, Pancreatitis, in L. Goldman and D. Ausiello, eds., *Cecil Textbook of Medicine* (Philadelphia: Saunders, 2004), pp. 879–886.
8. C. Dervenis, Enteral nutrition in severe acute pancreatitis: Future development, *Journal of the Pancreas (Online)* 5 (2004): 60–66; E. P. DiMagno and S. Chari, Acute pancreatitis, in M. Feldman, L. S. Friedman, and M. H. Sleisenger, eds., *Sleisenger and Fordtran's Gastrointestinal and Liver Disease: Pathophysiology, Diagnosis, Management* (Philadelphia: Saunders, 2002).
9. Dervenis, 2004; P. E. Marik and G. P. Zaloga, Meta-analysis of parenteral nutrition versus enteral nutrition in patients with acute pancreatitis, *British Medical Journal* 328 (2004): 1407; M. Al-Omran, A. Groof, and D. Wilke, Enteral versus parenteral nutrition for acute pancreatitis (Cochrane Review), *The Cochrane Library,* Issue 2 (2004).
10. DiMagno and Chari, 2002.
11. C. Baum, D. Moxon, and M. Scott, Gastrointestinal disease, in B. A. Bowman and R. M. Russell, eds., *Present Knowledge in Nutrition* (Washington, D.C.: ILSI Press, 2001), pp. 472–482.
12. Owyang, 2004.
13. M. J. Welsh, Cystic fibrosis, in L. Goldman and D. Ausiello, eds., *Cecil Textbook of Medicine* (Philadelphia: Saunders, 2004), pp. 515–519.
14. Welsh, 2004.
15. P. M. Farrell and H.-C. Lai, Nutrition and cystic fibrosis, in A. M. Coulston, C. L. Rock, and E. R. Monsen, eds., *Nutrition in the Prevention and Treatment of Disease* (San Diego: Academic Press, 2001), pp. 549–562.
16. M. O. Henke and coauthors, MUC5AC and MUC5B mucins are decreased in cystic fibrosis airway secretions, *American Journal of Respiratory Cell and Molecular Biology* 31 (2004): 86–91.
17. Welsh, 2004.
18. L. T. Beker, E. Russek-Cohen, and R. J. Fink, Stature as a prognostic factor in cystic fibrosis survival, *Journal of the American Dietetic Association* 101 (2001): 438–442.
19. S. W. Powers and S. R. Patton, A comparison of nutrient intake between infants and toddlers with and without cystic fibrosis, *Journal of the American Dietetic Association* 103 (2003): 1620–1625.
20. A. Fasano and coauthors, Prevalence of celiac disease in at-risk and not-at-risk groups in the United States: A large multicenter study, *Archives of Internal Medicine* 163 (2003): 286–292.
21. Feldman, Friedman, and Sleisenger, 2002.
22. T. Thompson, Questionable foods and the gluten-free diet: Survey of current recommendations, *Journal of the American Dietetic Association* 100 (2000): 463–465.
23. T. Thompson, Oats and the gluten-free diet, *Journal of the American Dietetic Association* 103 (2003): 376–379.
24. A. L. Lee and J. M. Newman, Celiac diet: Its impact on quality of life, *Journal of the American Dietetic Association* 103 (2003): 1533–1535.
25. Friedman, McQuaid, and Grendell, 2003.
26. W. F. Stenson, Inflammatory bowel disease, in L. Goldman and D. Ausiello, eds., *Cecil Textbook of Medicine* (Philadelphia: Saunders, 2004), pp. 861–868.
27. Feldman, Friedman, and Sleisenger, 2002; P. L. Beyer, Nutrient considerations in inflammatory bowel disease and short bowel syndrome, in A. M. Coulston, C. L. Rock, and E. R. Monsen, eds., *Nutrition in the Prevention and Treatment of Disease* (San Diego: Academic Press, 2001), pp. 577–599.
28. C. L. Simmang and G. T. Shires, Diverticular disease of the colon, in M. Feldman, L. S. Friedman, and M. H. Sleisenger, eds., *Sleisenger and Fordtran's Gastrointestinal and Liver Disease: Pathophysiology, Diagnosis, Management* (Philadelphia: Saunders, 2002), pp. 2100–2112.
29. B. E. Stabile and T. D. Arnell, Diverticular disease of the colon, in S. L. Friedman, K. R. McQuaid, and J. H. Grendell, eds., *Current Diagnosis and Treatment in Gastroenterology* (New York: Lange Medical Books/McGraw-Hill, 2003), pp. 436–451; Simmang and Shires, 2002.
30. Stabile and Arnell, 2003.
31. American Dietetic Association, 2000.
32. American Dietetic Association, 2000.

ANSWERS

Study Questions (multiple choice)

1. c 2. d 3. b 4. b 5. c 6. a 7. c 8. b 9. d 10. c

HIGHLIGHT

Food Allergies

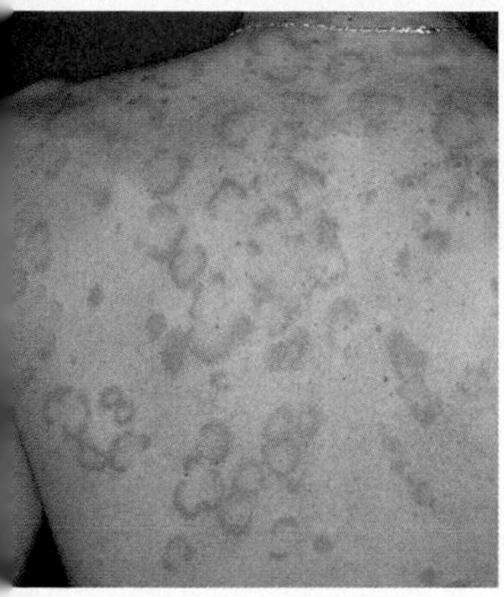
© ISM/Phototake

Some of the intestinal conditions discussed in Chapter 24 involve adverse reactions to specific foods. Chapter 16 explained that such **food hypersensitivities** can be categorized either as *food allergies,* which elicit an immune response, or *food intolerances,* which are caused by other physiological processes.[1] Celiac disease and dermatitis herpetiformis, for example, are characterized by allergic reactions to gluten, whereas lactose intolerance, a result of lactase deficiency, is a type of food intolerance. This highlight focuses on the diagnosis and treatment of food allergies, beginning with a brief review of the body's reactions to an **allergen.** The accompanying glossary defines the relevant terms.

A Review of Food Allergy

A food allergy occurs when a food component, usually an incompletely digested protein strand, is absorbed into the blood and elicits an immune response. The allergen is treated as a foreign particle that needs to be neutralized, and allergen-specific antibodies are produced to mount a defense. These antibodies are attached to specialized cells in mucosal tissue (the mast cells) that release inflammatory mediators when the allergen is encountered. These chemical mediators circulate in the blood and may trigger symptoms in the GI tract, skin, respiratory system, and circulatory system.

Common symptoms of food allergy include skin rashes, itching, abdominal pain, vomiting, and diarrhea. **Hives** occur frequently. These raised, swollen patches of skin or mucous membrane are associated with intense itching. In the condition known as **oral allergy syndrome,** hives, swelling, and itching may be confined to the mouth and throat and usually result after consumption of raw fruits and vegetables. The most dangerous effect of allergy is **anaphylaxis,** a systemic (whole-body) reaction that may cause difficulty breathing and a dangerous fall in blood pressure, potentially leading to shock. People whose food allergies are intense enough to cause anaphylaxis are often prescribed epinephrine, which they can self-inject in an emergency.

Contact dermatitis or hives can also develop on skin after physical contact with food. A rash may appear around the lips and mouth or on the hands. Foods that cause these reactions include raw fruits and vegetables, raw fish and shellfish, meats, and eggs. These symptoms are often seen among food handlers.[2]

Diagnosing Food Allergy

If a food allergy is suspected, an accurate and timely diagnosis can help a person avoid unnecessary dietary restrictions. Parents who believe that food allergy is causing health or behavioral problems may limit their children's food intakes excessively, which can adversely affect growth and nutrition status.[3] A timely diagnosis may also help a person avoid accidental exposure.

GLOSSARY

allergen: a substance that triggers an allergic response.

anaphylaxis: a severe allergic reaction that may include gastrointestinal upset, skin reactions, respiratory symptoms, and low blood pressure, possibly leading to shock.

cross-reactivity: an antibody reaction involving an antigen other than the one that induced the antibody's formation.

food and symptom diaries: records kept by a patient to determine the cause of an adverse reaction; include the specific foods and beverages consumed, symptoms experienced, and the timing of meals and symptom onset.

food hypersensitivities: adverse reactions resulting from ingestion of a specific food.

hives: an allergic reaction characterized by raised, swollen patches of skin or mucous membrane and associated with intense itching; also called **urticaria.**

oral allergy syndrome: an allergic response in which symptoms of hives, swelling, or itching occur only in the mouth and throat; usually a short-lived response that resolves quickly.

Reminder: A *food allergy* is an adverse reaction to food that involves an immune response.

A *food intolerance* is an adverse reaction to food that does not involve an immune response.

A *false positive* indicates that a condition is present (positive) when in fact it is not (therefore false). Conversely, a *false negative* indicates that a condition is not present (negative) when in fact it is (therefore false).

Diagnosis requires a thorough medical history, a physical examination, and selected laboratory studies. **Food and symptom diaries** help to pinpoint the cause of allergic reactions. Although many food allergies cause symptoms soon after food ingestion, in some cases symptoms do not appear until a few hours or days later, when the offending food may be more difficult to identify. Some common diagnostic tools are described in the next paragraphs.

Medical History

A medical history can help to determine which food is responsible for an allergy, the associated symptoms, and the amount of food required for an allergic reaction. It can also help to differentiate whether the symptoms are a response to a food allergy, food intolerance, food poisoning, or food toxicity.

Food and Symptom Diaries

Food and symptom diaries allow patients to record details that are not easily remembered, such as the brands of foods consumed and the exact timing of symptom onset. Food labels can also help to identify food ingredients that may be causing symptoms.

Skin-Prick Testing

To screen for sensitivity to individual foods, commercially prepared food extracts are introduced into the skin (see the photo). Substances that cause redness and swelling greater than 3 millimeters in diameter are considered possible allergens, and larger responses suggest a greater potential for allergy. Although the rate of false positive results for skin tests is about 50 percent (meaning that half of the reactions that appear to be positive are actually negative), the absence of a reaction is fairly good evidence that a substance does not cause allergy.

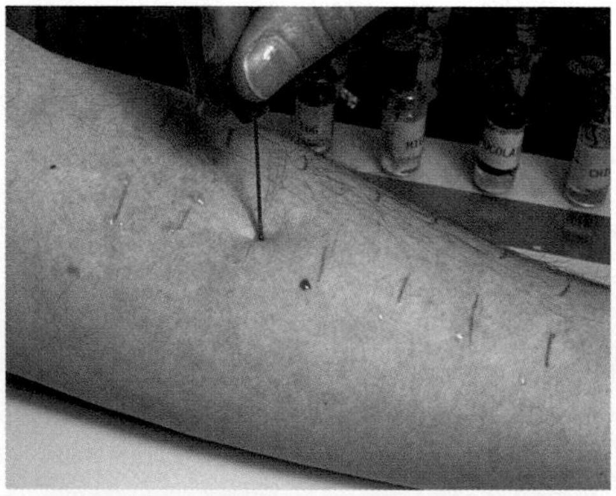

In a skin prick test, extracts containing food allergens are placed on the skin, and the skin is pricked using a lancet or needle, which introduces small amounts of the allergens into the skin.

Antibody Blood Testing

Measures of food-specific serum antibodies are useful for assessing the presence of food allergies; generally, a high antibody level suggests an increased risk of an allergic response to a food. A person with low antibody levels may still have a reaction, however; therefore, antibody test results need to be considered along with other methods of diagnosis.

Oral Food Challenges

When performed properly, food challenges are considered the "gold standard" for diagnosing food allergy. In an oral challenge, a food that is suspected to cause allergy is presented to a patient in a dose suggested by the medical history. If a test substance does not cause symptoms, the challenge is repeated to rule out a false negative result. Ideally, food challenges are double-blinded and placebo controlled: test foods are mixed into other foods or provided in capsules, and placebos are identical in appearance, taste, and texture. A food challenge can be labor-intensive and cannot be performed if a patient has a history of severe anaphylaxis.

Elimination Diets

In an elimination diet, common food allergens are omitted from the diet until symptoms subside, and individual foods are then reintroduced one by one. Although foods that cause symptoms are sometimes easily identified using this method, it may be difficult to identify allergenic substances that are ingredients in packaged foods. Also, allergic reactions sometimes persist after common allergens are removed from the diet; in this case, an elemental formula diet (which contains no intact proteins) may be needed to stabilize the patient before foods are reintroduced.

Dietary Concerns

Food allergies are treated by eliminating all dietary sources of an allergen. Successful treatment depends in part on the patient's ability to identify hidden sources of allergens in foods with multiple ingredients (see Table H24-1). Inadvertent ingestion may occur due to contamination of foods during meal preparation or food processing. Problem foods may also be consumed at restaurants, schools, and other public places. Another dietary concern is that some essential nutrients may be more difficult to obtain due to dietary restrictions. The following sections discuss the foods that account for most allergic reactions in infants and children: cow's milk, eggs, and peanuts.[4]

TABLE H24-1 Food Avoidance in Milk, Egg, and Peanut Allergies

Food Allergy	Excluded Food Ingredients	Hidden Sources
Milk allergy	Milk (including dried, evaporated, and condensed milks), milk solids, buttermilk, yogurt, cheese, butter, artificial butter flavor, Half-and-Half, cream, whipped cream, custard, pudding, ice cream, casein (or caseinates), whey, protein hydrolysates, lactalbumin, lactoferrin, lactaglobulin	Margarine, luncheon meats, frankfurters and sausages, high-protein products (including bars, flours, and beverages), nougat candy, chocolate bars, caramel color or flavorings, coffee whiteners, bakery glazes, salad dressings, sauces. Meats sliced at a delicatessen are subject to cross-contamination from sliced cheeses.
Egg allergy	Eggs (including powdered eggs and egg substitutes), egg white, eggnog, meringue, albumin, globulin, lysozyme, ovalbumin, ovoglobulin, ovomucin, ovomucoid, ovotransferrin, ovovitellin, lecithin (some food labels may indicate that a "binder" or "emulsifier" was added)	Many baked products and baking mixes, noodles and pastas, mayonnaise, béarnaise and hollandaise sauces, breaded meats and vegetables, candies, fondants, marshmallows, frozen desserts, ice cream, custards and puddings, frankfurters and sausages, processed meats, cocoa drinks, salad dressings, bakery glazes
Peanut allergy	Peanuts (also called ground nuts), peanut butter, peanut flour, nut pieces, mixed nuts, beer nuts, artificial nuts, mandalona nuts, peanut sauces (common in Asian cuisine), hydrolyzed vegetable protein (HVP), cold-pressed or gourmet peanut oils (may contain peanut residue)	Chocolate and candy bars, power bars, marzipan, nougat, breakfast cereals, egg rolls, satay sauce, curries, salad dressings. Cross-contamination is possible from food-processing equipment, caution is required when purchasing baked products, ice creams, candies, nut butters, and sunflower seeds

Milk Allergy

Milk and the proteins derived from milk are common ingredients in many prepared and packaged foods (see Table H24-1), so ingredient lists need to be checked carefully. People with milk allergies need to avoid milk from all animals due to the potential for **cross-reactivity.** Foods that are labeled "nondairy" (for example, nondairy creamers) may contain the milk protein casein. Obtaining sufficient calcium and vitamin D from nonmilk sources may be difficult, and supplementation is often warranted. A milk allergy may be difficult to differentiate from lactose intolerance because both conditions may produce gastrointestinal symptoms.

Egg Allergy

Eggs and egg proteins are common ingredients in many recipes and processed foods; Table H24-1 lists terms that may be used on food labels when egg protein is present. Eggs from different species of birds should be avoided to prevent cross-reactivity. Because flu vaccines are prepared using egg embryos, people with egg allergies need to check with their physicians before being vaccinated.

Peanut Allergy

Some people with peanut allergies have severe reactions, including anaphylaxis, to even the smallest quantities of peanuts. Although peanut allergy is not ordinarily associated with other nut allergies, patients may be advised to avoid all nuts due to potential contamination from food-processing equipment (see Table H24-1). Parents often fear that skin contact with peanut butter or inhalation of peanut dust may cause severe allergic reactions, but there is little evidence that this occurs.[5]

In many cases, children and young adults outgrow their food allergies. Those with allergies to peanuts, nuts, and seafood are least likely to develop tolerance.[6] Health care providers advise that allergies be reevaluated periodically so that dietary restrictions are not continued unnecessarily.

REFERENCES

1. H. A. Sampson, Update on food allergy, *Journal of Allergy and Clinical Immunology* 113 (2004): 805–819.
2. Sampson, 2004.
3. L. Christie and coauthors, Food allergies in children affect nutrient intake and growth, *Journal of the American Dietetic Association* 102 (2002): 1648–1651.
4. Sampson, 2004.
5. T. T. Perry and coauthors, Distribution of peanut allergen in the environment, *Journal of Allergy and Clinical Immunology* 113 (2004): 973–976; S. J. Simonte and coauthors, Relevance of casual contact with peanut butter in children with peanut allergy, *Journal of Allergy and Clinical Immunology* 112 (2003): 180–182.
6. Sampson, 2004.

Chapter 25

Nutrition, Liver Disease, and Gallstones

Chapter Outline

Fatty Liver and Hepatitis: *Fatty Liver • Hepatitis*

Cirrhosis: *Consequences of Cirrhosis • Treatment of Cirrhosis*

Liver Transplantation

Gallstone Disease: *Types of Gallstones • Consequences of Gallstones • Risk Factors for Gallstones • Treatment for Gallstones*

Highlight: *Anemia in Illness*

Available Online

http://nutrition.wadsworth.com/uncn7

Student Practice Test

Glossary Terms

Nutrition on the Net

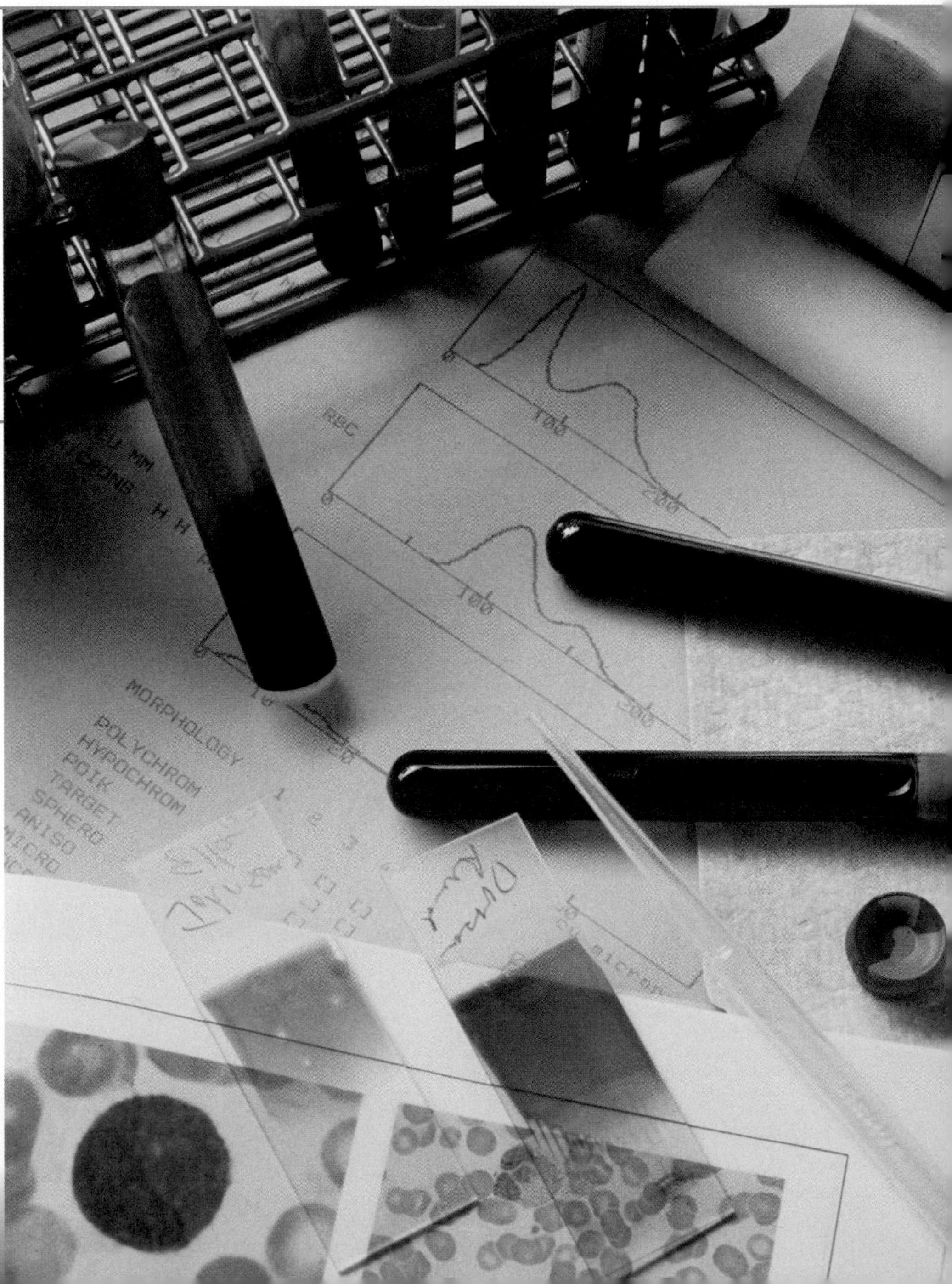
RBC
MORPHOLOGY
POLYCHROM
HYPOCHROM
POIK
TARGET
SPHERO
ANISO

Nutrition in the Professional Setting

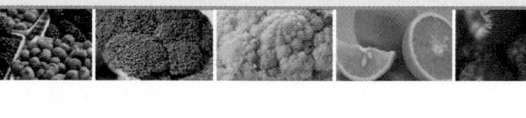

Liver disease progresses slowly. Its primary symptom, fatigue, often goes unnoticed. Other symptoms may be so mild that complications develop before liver disease is diagnosed. At every step of the way, education and support are critical elements of treatment. Health care providers should emphasize the need to preserve remaining liver function, as healthy liver tissue can proliferate, improving prognosis. Preventing additional damage is the principal means of avoiding liver failure or transplantation.

The liver is the most active organ in the body. As you may recall from Chapter 7, the liver plays a central role in processing, storing, and redistributing the nutrients provided by the meals we eat. Table 7-1 on p. 219 summarizes the chemical reactions of liver cells that are related to the metabolism of carbohydrates, lipids, and protein. The liver also produces bile, which is used to emulsify fat during digestion. It synthesizes most of the proteins that circulate in plasma, including albumin, clotting proteins, and transport proteins. The liver detoxifies drugs and alcohol and processes excess nitrogen so that it can be safely excreted as urea. If the liver's numerous roles are upset by liver damage or disease, the effects on health and nutritional status can be profound.

As Figure 25-1, p. 770 shows, the liver is ideally situated for receiving and processing the nutrients absorbed by the small intestine. The portal vein's nutrient-rich blood supplies 70 to 80 percent of the blood that enters liver tissue, whereas the rest arrives via hepatic arteries. Blood is returned to the heart by way of the hepatic vein and then circulates throughout the body. The biliary system of channels and ducts carries bile and other substances from the liver to the gallbladder, where bile is stored and concentrated. The gallbladder releases the bile into the small intestine, where it emulsifies dietary fat.

FIGURE 25-1 The Liver, Biliary System, and Associated Blood Vessels

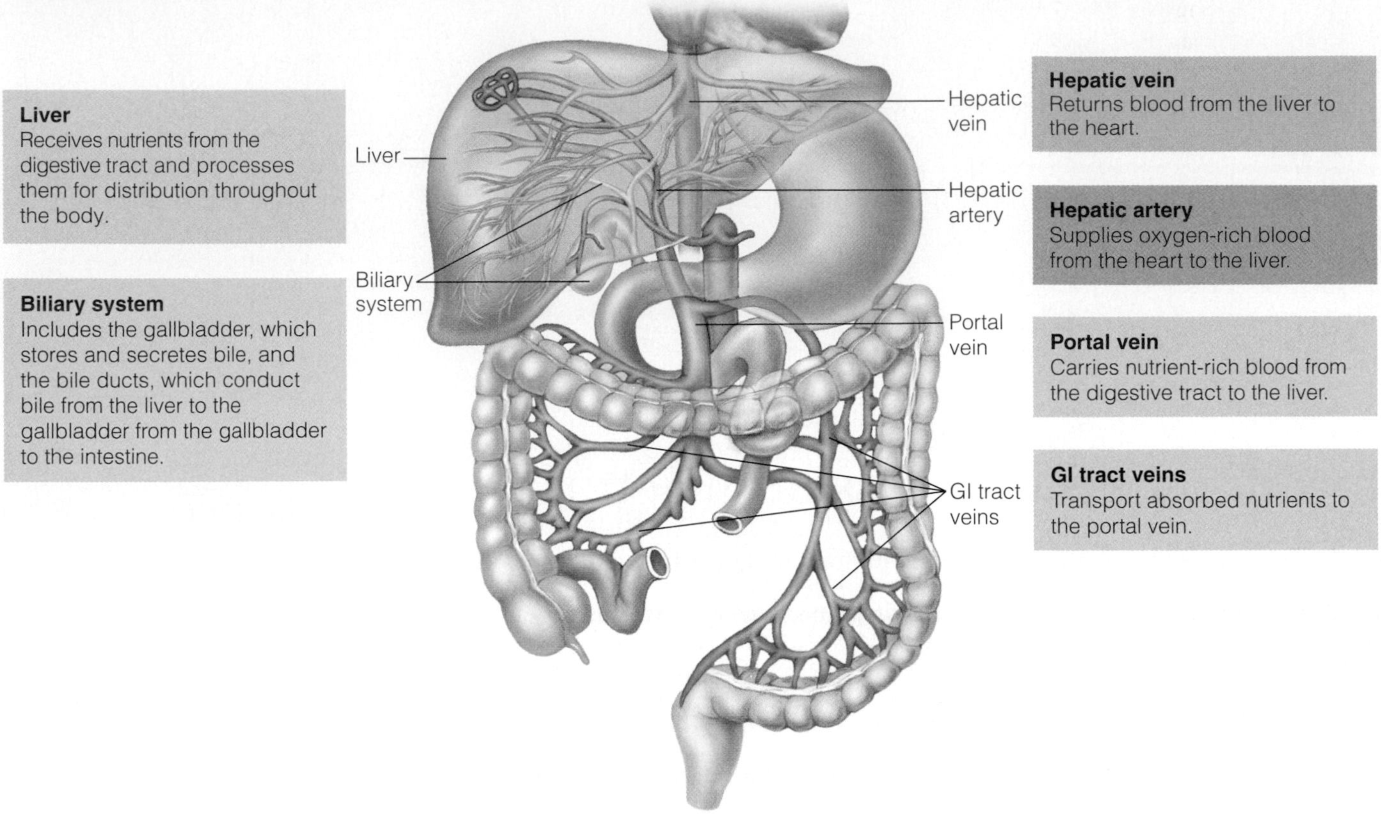
Liver
Receives nutrients from the digestive tract and processes them for distribution throughout the body.
Biliary system
Includes the gallbladder, which stores and secretes bile, and the bile ducts, which conduct bile from the liver to the gallbladder from the gallbladder to the intestine.
Liver
Biliary system
Hepatic vein
Hepatic artery
Portal vein
GI tract veins
Hepatic vein
Returns blood from the liver to the heart.
Hepatic artery
Supplies oxygen-rich blood from the heart to the liver.
Portal vein
Carries nutrient-rich blood from the digestive tract to the liver.
GI tract veins
Transport absorbed nutrients to the portal vein.

Fatty Liver and Hepatitis

Fatty liver and **hepatitis** are the two most common disorders affecting the liver. Although both conditions may be mild and are usually reversible, each may progress to more serious illness and eventually cause liver damage.

Fatty Liver

■ Reminder: *Fatty liver* is an accumulation of triglycerides in the liver; also called **hepatic steatosis** (STEE-ah-TOE-sis).

Fatty liver■ is an accumulation of fat in liver tissue. Normally, the liver's triglycerides are packaged into very-low-density lipoproteins (VLDL) and exported to the bloodstream. Although the exact reasons for fat accumulation are unknown, fatty liver reflects an imbalance between the amount of fat synthesized or picked up from the blood and the amount exported to the blood via VLDL.

Fatty liver is a clinical finding that is common to many conditions. It is present in the majority of patients who have alcoholic liver disease (see p. 243) and can result from exposure to drugs and toxic metals. It is associated with obesity, diabetes mellitus, and diseases of malnutrition, including kwashiorkor and marasmus. Fatty liver may follow gastrointestinal bypass surgery or long-term total parenteral nutrition. Its causes are not always clear, however, as it occurs in as many as 14 percent of adults in the United States.[1]

hepatitis (hep-ah-TIE-tis): inflammation of the liver.
- **hepatic** = pertaining to the liver.

Consequences of Fatty Liver In many individuals, fatty liver is asymptomatic and causes no harm, but it may increase the liver's vulnerability to other metabolic disturbances. Fatty liver is frequently accompanied by other symptoms, such as liver enlargement,■ inflammation,■ and fatigue. If fatty liver is drug induced or associated with certain types of metabolic disorders, it may progress quickly and result in liver damage or even liver failure.[2]

Fatty liver is a major cause of abnormal liver enzyme levels in blood. Laboratory findings may include elevated concentrations of the serum aminotransferase enzymes ALT and AST,■ as well as increased levels of triglycerides, cholesterol, and glucose. Table 17-8 on p. 594 provides normal ranges for these liver enzymes.

Treatment of Fatty Liver The usual therapy for fatty liver is the elimination of the factors that cause it. For example, if fatty liver is due to alcohol abuse or drug therapies, it may improve after the substances are discontinued. In patients with elevated blood lipids, fatty liver may improve upon treatment. An appropriate treatment for obese or diabetic patients might be weight reduction or blood glucose control. Rapid weight loss should be discouraged, however, as it may accelerate the progression of liver disease.[3] It should be noted that lifestyle modifications are not always successful in reversing fatty liver, especially in patients who lack the usual risk factors.

■ Enlargement of the liver is known as **hepatomegaly** (HEP-ah-toe-MEG-ah-lee).

■ Liver inflammation that is associated with fatty liver is called **steatohepatitis** (STEE-ah-toe-HEP-ah-TIE-tis).

■ The aminotransferase enzymes that may be elevated in liver disease are ALT (alanine aminotransferase) and AST (aspartate aminotransferase). Both of these enzymes are involved in amino acid catabolism.

Hepatitis

Although hepatitis can result from any factor that causes damage to liver tissue, it is most often caused by infection with specific viruses, which are designated by the letters A, B, and C. These viruses are primarily spread by blood contact with infected persons or by ingesting contaminated food or water. Hepatitis is also frequently caused by excessive alcohol intake or exposure to certain drugs and toxic chemicals. A number of herbal remedies are reported to cause hepatitis; these include chaparral, germander, ma huang, saw palmetto, and jin bu huan.[4] Less common causes of hepatitis include infection with other viruses and autoimmune disease.

Viral Hepatitis Hepatitis A virus (HAV) is extremely contagious and is the most common cause of acute viral hepatitis (see Table 25-1). It is usually spread by the fecal-oral route, which occurs when foods and beverages become contaminated with fecal material. Outbreaks of hepatitis A are often associated with floods and other natural disasters, when inadequately treated sewage may contaminate water supplies with fecal matter. Less frequently, HAV is spread by the consumption of undercooked shellfish obtained from contaminated waters. Infection with hepatitis A usually resolves within a few months and does not cause chronic illness or permanent liver damage.

About half of viral hepatitis cases are caused by infection with the hepatitis B and C viruses (see Table 25-1). Hepatitis B virus (HBV) is transmitted by infected blood or needles and by sexual contact and is carried by approximately 1.25 million persons in the United States. As a precautionary measure, HBV vaccinations are recommended for health care workers, sexually active adults, and newborn infants

TABLE 25-1 Features of Hepatitis Viruses

Hepatitis Virus	% of Viral Cases	Major Mode of Transmission	Chronic Disease Rate (% of cases)	Vaccination Available
A	48%	Fecal-oral	None	Yes
B	34%	Bloodborne; sexual transmission	<10% of adults >90% of infants	Yes
C	15%	Bloodborne	80–90%	No

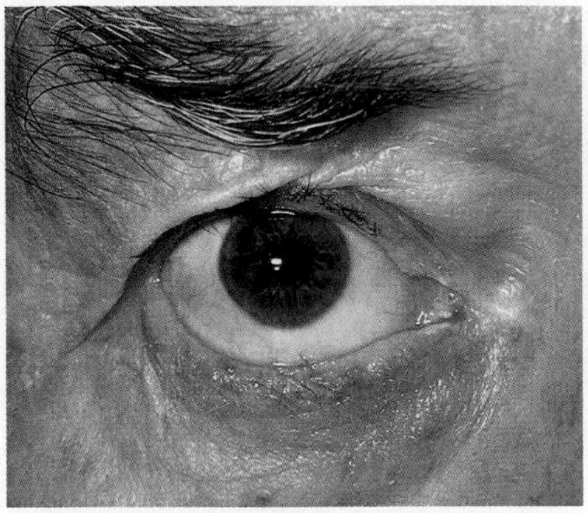

Jaundice is a yellow discoloration of tissues that is most easily seen in the whites of the eyes.

and children. Hepatitis C virus (HCV) is transmitted by blood contact as well, but it is less efficiently spread by sexual contact. It is a major cause of chronic hepatitis and is currently carried by 2.7 million individuals in the United States.■ No vaccine is currently available to protect against HCV infection. Chronic cases of either HBV or HCV infection may lead to cirrhosis (see section below) and liver cancer.

Symptoms of Hepatitis The effects of hepatitis are highly variable and depend on the cause and severity of the disease. Both mild and chronic cases of hepatitis are often asymptomatic. The onset of acute hepatitis may be accompanied by fatigue, nausea, anorexia, and pain in the liver area. The liver is often slightly enlarged. **Jaundice** (yellow pigmentation of tissues) can develop, causing discoloration of the skin, urine, and the whites of the eyes.■ Other symptoms of hepatitis may include fever, diarrhea, muscle pain, and skin rashes. Serum levels of the aminotransferase enzymes (ALT and AST) are typically elevated. Chronic hepatitis can be associated with complications that are typical of liver cirrhosis (described in the next section).

Treatment of Hepatitis The general treatment of hepatitis includes supportive care, such as bed rest and an appropriate diet. The patient should avoid substances that may aggravate the liver, such as alcohol or drugs that cause liver toxicity. Hepatitis A typically resolves without the use of medications. Antiviral agents may be used to treat HBV and HCV infections; these include lamivudine and ribavarin, which block viral replication, and interferon, which both inhibits viral replication and enhances immune responses.[5] Nonviral forms of hepatitis may be treated with anti-inflammatory and immunosuppressant drugs. Hospitalization is rarely needed unless an individual has other medical conditions or complications that may hamper recovery.

Medical Nutrition Therapy for Hepatitis Nutrition therapy is individualized according to a patient's symptoms and nutrition status; for some patients, a conventional diet may suffice. Those who are malnourished or who have lost weight due to illness may require a high-kcalorie, high-protein diet to replenish nutrient stores. A person with mild anorexia or gastrointestinal symptoms may find small, frequent meals easier to tolerate. Fluid and electrolyte replacement may be needed for persistent vomiting. Liquid supplements can help to improve nutrient intakes.

■ Although there are fewer new cases of HCV than of HBV each year (see Table 25-1), more HCV cases become chronic. As a result, there are more HCV carriers than HBV carriers.

■ Jaundice results when liver dysfunction prevents the liver from chemically modifying the bile pigment **bilirubin** to prepare it for elimination from the body via the biliary route. Bilirubin's accumulation in the bloodstream leads to yellow discoloration of tissues.

IN SUMMARY Fatty liver can be a consequence of excessive alcohol intake, drug toxicity, and chronic diseases like diabetes and obesity. Hepatitis is frequently caused by viral infection, but may also result from alcohol abuse and drug use. The treatment for both conditions is variable and depends on the causative factors. Both fatty liver and hepatitis can cause elevations in the liver's aminotransferase enzymes. Although fatty liver is often benign, hepatitis may become chronic and lead to cirrhosis and liver cancer.

Cirrhosis

Cirrhosis■ is an end-stage condition that results from long-term liver disease. Liver disease gradually destroys liver tissue, leading to scarring (fibrosis)■ in some regions and small areas of regenerated, healthy tissue in others. As the disease continues, the scarring becomes more extensive, leaving fewer areas of healthy tissue. A cirrhotic liver is often shrunken in size and has an irregular, nodular appearance (photo, p. 773). Cirrhosis impairs liver function and can eventually lead to liver failure. It is estimated to affect approximately three million people in the United States.[6]

Table 25-2 lists some possible causes of cirrhosis. The most common cause of cirrhosis in the United States is hepatitis C infection, which is responsible for 26

■ Reminder: *Cirrhosis* is an advanced stage of liver disease in which extensive scarring replaces healthy liver tissue, causing impaired liver function and liver failure.

■ Reminder: *Fibrosis* is an intermediate stage of liver disease characterized by scarring of liver tissue.

jaundice (JAWN-dis): yellow discoloration of skin and mucous membranes due to an accumulation of bilirubin—a breakdown product of hemoglobin and other heme-containing proteins that normally exits the body via bile secretions.

percent of cases.[7] Alcoholic liver disease, which develops in approximately 10 to 20 percent of chronic alcoholics, is the second most common cause.[8] Bile duct blockages can lead to cirrhosis by impeding bile flow; the resulting accumulation of toxic bile acids in the liver causes liver injury. All types of chronic hepatitis, if untreated, can eventually lead to cirrhosis. Other causes of cirrhosis include drug-induced liver injury and inherited metabolic disorders that cause toxic substances to accumulate in the liver.

TABLE 25-2 Causes of Cirrhosis

- Alcoholic liver disease
- Autoimmune hepatitis
- Bile duct obstructions (biliary cirrhosis)
  - Diseases that cause bile duct injury
  - Complications of gallbladder surgery
  - Cystic fibrosis
- Drug-induced liver injury
- Inherited disorders
  - Hemochromatosis (causes excessive liver iron)
  - Wilson's disease (causes excessive liver copper)
  - Galactosemia
  - Glycogen storage disease
- Nonalcoholic steatohepatitis (fatty liver disease)
- Viral hepatitis (primarily hepatitis B and C)

Consequences of Cirrhosis

Up to 40 percent of people with cirrhosis are asymptomatic.[9] The effects of cirrhosis may be minimal at first, as liver damage often progresses slowly. Initial symptoms are usually nonspecific and may include fatigue, weakness, anorexia, and weight loss. Later, altered liver function leads to metabolic disturbances; patients may develop anemia, bruise easily, and contract infections readily. If bile obstruction occurs, jaundice and signs of fat malabsorption are likely. Physical changes in liver tissue often disrupt blood flow, leading to abnormal fluid accumulation in body tissues and blood vessels. In advanced cirrhosis, kidney and lung functions may be impaired, and many hormone systems may be disrupted. Figure 25-2, p. 774 illustrates some of the clinical effects of liver cirrhosis, and later sections describe some of these complications in more detail.

Table 25-3 lists laboratory tests that are used to monitor the extent of liver damage. Liver disease destroys liver tissue, causing liver enzymes to spill into the bloodstream. Levels of bilirubin may be elevated if the liver is too damaged to process it or if bile ducts are blocked and prevent its excretion. Reduced synthesis of plasma proteins by the liver lowers albumin levels and extends blood-clotting time. Liver damage also impairs the conversion of ammonia to urea, thereby raising ammonia levels in the blood.

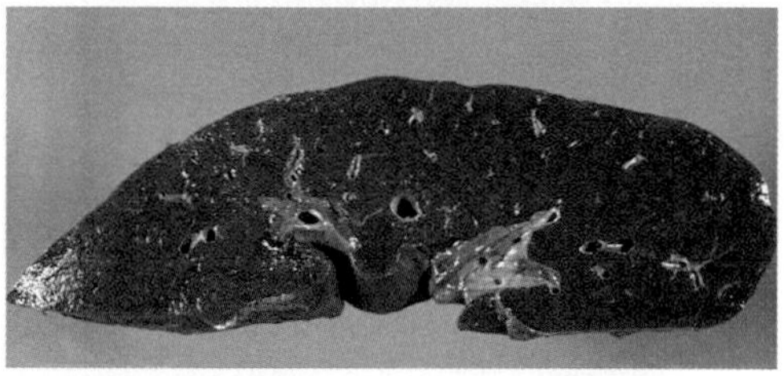

© Martin Rotker/PhotoTake

Normal liver tissue is smooth and has a regular texture.

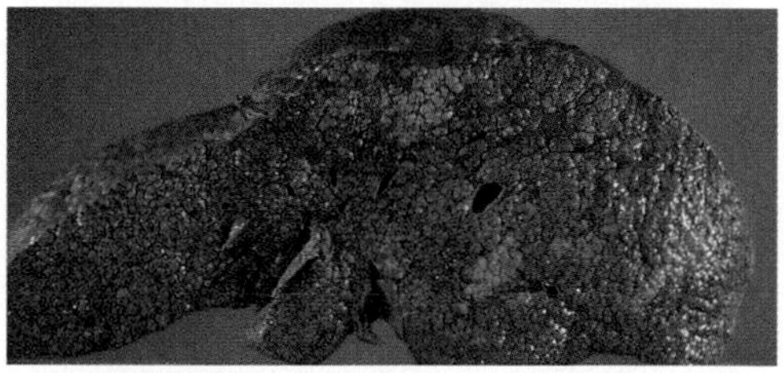

© Dr. Joseph William/PhotoTake

A cirrhotic liver has an irregular, nodular appearance. The nodules that develop in cirrhosis represent clusters of regenerating cells within the damaged liver tissue.

Portal Hypertension A large volume of blood normally flows through the liver. The portal vein and hepatic artery supply approximately 1500 milliliters (about 1.5 quarts) of blood each minute to the extensive network of vessels in the liver. The scarred tissue of a cirrhotic liver impedes this blood flow, which is mostly supplied by the portal vein. The resistance to blood flow within the liver causes a rise in pressure within the portal vein called **portal hypertension.**

Collaterals and Gastroesophageal Varices When blood flow through the portal vein is obstructed, blood is diverted to smaller vessels surrounding the liver. These **collaterals** develop throughout the gastrointestinal (GI) tract and in regions near the abdominal wall. As pressure builds, the collateral vessels become enlarged and engorged, forming **varices.** Esophageal and gastric varices are vulnerable to

TABLE 25-3 Laboratory Tests for Evaluation of Liver Disease

Laboratory Test	Normal Ranges (serum)	Values in Liver Disease
Alanine aminotransferase (ALT)	Male: 10–40 U/L Female: 7–35 U/L	Elevated
Albumin	3.4–4.8 g/dL	Decreased
Alkaline phosphatase	25–100 U/L	Normal or elevated
Ammonia	15–45 μg N/dL	Elevated
Aspartate aminotransferase (AST)	10–30 U/L	Elevated
Bilirubin (total)	0.3–1.2 mg/dL	Elevated
Blood urea nitrogen (BUN)	6–20 mg/dL	Normal or decreased
Prothrombin time[a]	10–13 seconds	Prolonged

[a]The test for prothrombin time evaluates the clotting ability of blood.

portal hypertension: elevated blood pressure in the portal vein; often caused by obstructed blood flow through the liver.

collaterals: blood vessels that enlarge in order to allow an alternate pathway for diverted blood.

varices (VAR-ih-seez): abnormally dilated blood vessels.

FIGURE 25-2 Clinical Effects of Liver Cirrhosis

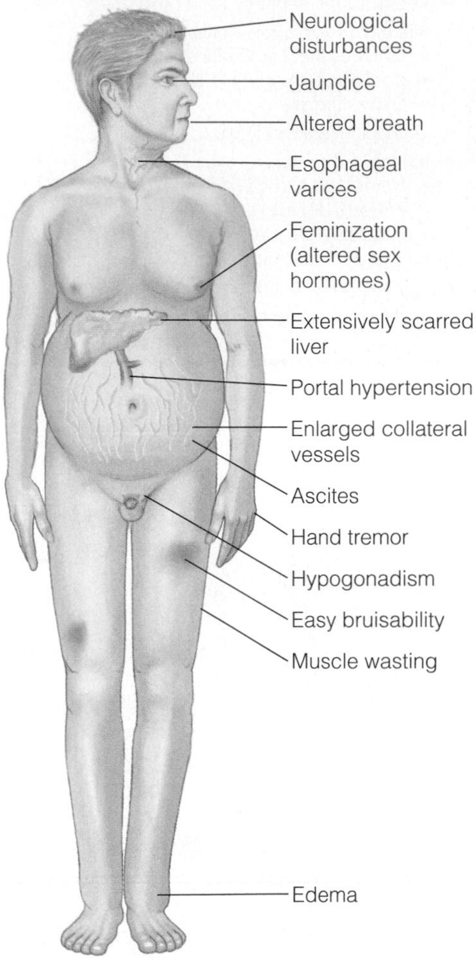
Neurological disturbances
Jaundice
Altered breath
Esophageal varices
Feminization (altered sex hormones)
Extensively scarred liver
Portal hypertension
Enlarged collateral vessels
Ascites
Hand tremor
Hypogonadism
Easy bruisability
Muscle wasting
Edema

rupture, as they have thin walls and often bulge into the lumen. If ruptured, they can cause massive bleeding that is sometimes fatal. The blood loss is exacerbated by the liver's reduced production of blood-clotting factors.

Ascites Within ten years of disease onset, about 50 percent of cirrhosis patients develop ascites.■ The development of ascites indicates that liver dysfunction has reached a critical stage, as half of patients with ascites die within two years.[10]

Ascites is thought to be a consequence of several liver impairments: portal hypertension, water retention due to altered kidney function, and reduced albumin synthesis by the diseased liver. The increased pressure in the portal vein forces fluid from blood plasma into the abdominal cavity, exceeding the capacity of the lymphatic system to return the fluid to the bloodstream. The fluid accumulation is exacerbated by reduced production of albumin, which normally helps to retain fluid in blood vessels. The raised pressure in the portal vein triggers the release of factors (such as nitric oxide) that dilate blood vessels, lowering pressure within vessels elsewhere; this activates sodium and water retention by the kidneys and eventually leads to additional water pooling.[11] The exact mechanisms and the order of events that cause ascites are complex and still under investigation.

Hepatic Encephalopathy Advanced liver disease sometimes leads to **hepatic encephalopathy,** a disorder characterized by abnormal neurological functioning. Symptoms of hepatic encephalopathy include changes in personality, mental abilities, and motor functions (see Table 25-4). At worst, amnesia, seizures, and **hepatic coma** may develop. Although reversible, hepatic encephalopathy is associated with a one-year survival rate of only 40 percent.[12]

The causes of hepatic encephalopathy remain elusive, although elevated blood ammonia levels may be partly responsible due to ammonia's neurotoxicity. Other compounds that are potentially toxic to brain tissue, such as sulfur compounds, short-chain fatty acids, and GABA (a neurotransmitter), may accumulate in brain cells and alter neurotransmitter activity.[13] Another theory is that neurotransmitter functioning is altered by an increased ratio of aromatic amino acids to branched-chain amino acids■ in brain tissue, a result of altered amino acid metabolism in the liver. Most likely, a combination of metabolic abnormalities contribute to disrupted neurological functioning.[14]

Blood Ammonia Levels Much of the body's free ammonia is produced by bacterial action on unabsorbed dietary protein in the colon. Normally, the liver extracts ammonia from portal blood and converts it to urea, most of which is excreted by the kidneys (review Figure 7-17 on p. 229). In advanced liver disease, ammonia-laden portal blood bypasses the liver by way of collateral vessels and reaches the systemic circulation, causing a substantial increase in brain ammonia content. Although there is strong evidence that ammonia contributes to hepatic encephalopathy, blood levels of ammonia do not correlate well with the degree of neurological impairment.

Malnutrition and Wasting Most patients with cirrhosis develop protein-energy malnutrition (PEM) and experience some degree of wasting.[15] Malnutrition is usually caused by a combination of factors (see Table 25-5). Patients often consume less food due to reduced appetite, fatigue, or gastrointestinal symptoms. The

■ Reminder: *Ascites* is the abnormal accumulation of fluid in the abdominal cavity.

■ The aromatic amino acids—phenylalanine, tyrosine, and tryptophan—have carbon rings in their side groups. The branched-chain amino acids include leucine, isoleucine, and valine; their side groups have a branched structure. The chemical structures of these amino acids are shown on p. C-4.

hepatic encephalopathy (en-SEF-ah-LOP-ah-thee): condition characterized by altered neurological functioning, including personality changes, reduced mental abilities, and disturbances in motor function.
- **encephalo** = brain
- **pathy** = disease

hepatic coma: loss of consciousness resulting from severe liver disease.

TABLE 25-4 Symptoms of Hepatic Encephalopathy

Early Stages	Middle Stages	Later Stages
• Lack of attention	• Poor memory	• Disorientation
• Irritability, depression	• Drowsiness	• Amnesia
• Impaired judgment	• Slurred speech	• Muscular rigidity
• Lack of coordination	• Jerking movements	• Abnormal reflexes
• Tremor	• Sleep disorders	• Delirium, stupor

TABLE 25-5 Possible Causes of Malnutrition in Liver Disease

Mechanism	Examples
Reduced nutrient intake	Anorexia, early satiety (due to ascites), nausea and vomiting, restrictive diets, effects of medications (including gastrointestinal disturbances and taste changes), abdominal pain, fatigue, fasting for medical procedures
Malabsorption/nutrient losses	Fat malabsorption (due to reduced bile flow), vomiting, diarrhea, gastrointestinal bleeding, effects of medications (including malabsorption and nutrient losses from diuretic use)
Altered metabolism/increased nutrient needs	Hypermetabolism, catabolism, infections/inflammation, inadequate protein synthesis, reduced nutrient storage and metabolism in the liver

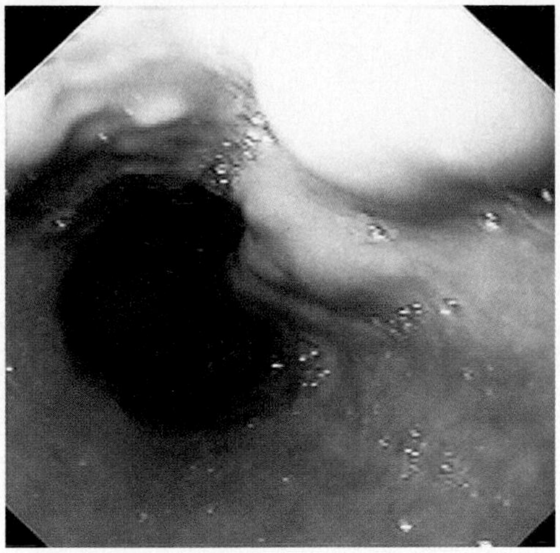

© Camal/PhotoTake

Esophageal varices, such as the one shown here, may protrude into the lumen and be vulnerable to rupture and bleeding.

presence of ascites causes early satiety. If the diet is restricted in sodium to treat ascites, meals may seem monotonous or unpalatable. Fat malabsorption is common, and diarrhea, vomiting, and gastrointestinal bleeding can cause nutrient losses. Patients often are unable to meet their high nutrient needs. If cirrhosis is a consequence of alcohol abuse, multiple nutrient deficiencies may be present.

Treatment of Cirrhosis

Treatment of cirrhosis is highly individualized according to the severity of the illness and the complications that develop. Supportive care, including an appropriate diet and avoidance of liver toxins, can promote recovery and help to prevent further damage. Abstinence from alcohol is critical for preserving liver function and extending survival. Patients who have developed cirrhosis due to viral infection may benefit from the use of antiviral medications.[16] Liver transplantation may be necessary for advanced cirrhosis.

Drug Therapy Drug therapies can be used to treat the symptoms and complications associated with cirrhosis. Drugs to treat portal hypertension and varices either dilate blood vessels (such as nitroglycerin) or constrict them (vasopressin and octreotide). Diuretics may help to control portal hypertension and ascites; common examples include spironolactone and furosemide. To stimulate the appetite and promote weight gain, megestrol acetate or dronabinol is sometimes provided. Drug treatment of hepatic encephalopathy focuses on controlling blood ammonia levels. For example, lactulose, a nonabsorbable disaccharide that is often used as a laxative, helps to reduce ammonia production and absorption in the colon. The antibiotic neomycin is an alternate treatment that works by altering bacterial populations.

Medical Nutrition Therapy for Cirrhosis Medical nutrition therapy for patients with cirrhosis is customized to each person's needs, which vary considerably and depend on accompanying complications. In all cases, avoidance of substances that may cause further liver injury is critical; examples include alcohol, drugs (unless prescribed), herbal supplements, and vitamin or mineral megadoses. Table 25-6, p. 776, lists the general dietary guidelines for liver cirrhosis.

Energy To estimate energy requirements, health providers can use equations such as those presented in Table 22-2 on p. 697. Because energy needs vary substantially among patients with cirrhosis, the use of indirect calorimetry is preferred for estimating basal metabolic rate.[17] Energy recommendations may range from 20 to 75 percent above basal energy expenditure (BEE), depending on complications. Malabsorption, recent weight loss, and infection increase energy needs. In a patient with ascites, energy recommendations should be based on desirable weight or estimated dry weight (weight without ascites) to avoid overestimating requirements.

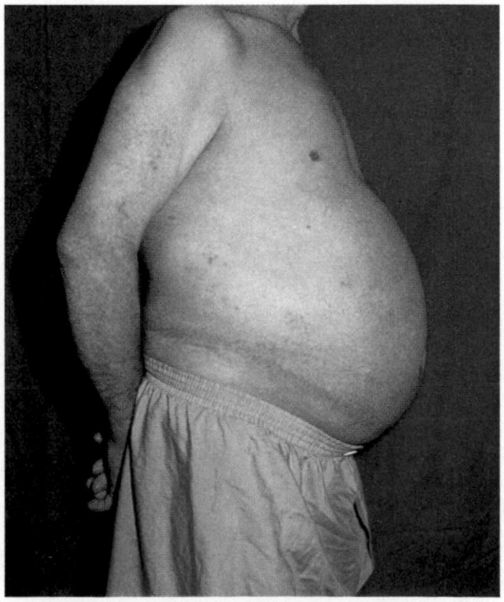

© Garry Watson/Photo Researchers, Inc.

Ascites can be caused by different diseases, but cirrhosis is the underlying cause in most patients with this condition.

TABLE 25-6 Dietary Guidelines for Liver Cirrhosis

Energy	• Without malnutrition, infection, or ascites, energy needs may be 20% above basal energy expenditure (BEE); see Table 22-2 on p. 697. • With malnutrition, infection, or ascites, energy needs may range from 50% to 75% above BEE.
Protein	• Provide 1.2 to 1.5 grams protein per kilogram body weight per day to maintain nitrogen balance and prevent wasting.
Carbohydrate	• No carbohydrate restrictions. • For persons with insulin resistance or diabetes, provide up to 50% to 60% of kcalories from carbohydrates (primarily complex carbohydrates); intake of carbohydrates should be consistent from day to day and at each meal and snack.
Fat	• No fat restrictions unless fat malabsorption is present. • If fat is malabsorbed, restrict fat as necessary to control steatorrhea (see Chapter 24); use medium-chain triglycerides (MCT) to increase kcalories.
Sodium	• Restrict sodium as necessary to control ascites; 2 to 3 grams sodium per day is adequate restriction in most cases.
Vitamins and minerals	• Ensure adequate intake from diet or supplements based on individual needs.

As discussed earlier, some people with cirrhosis have difficulty consuming enough food to achieve good nutritional status. The "How to" offers suggestions for improving the food intake of patients with cirrhosis.

Protein Patients with cirrhosis risk developing PEM and wasting; therefore, protein intakes should be high enough to maintain nitrogen balance. Protein recommendations generally range between 1.2 and 1.5 grams per kilogram body weight per day.■ To prevent protein catabolism, adequate energy is also required.[18]

■ Reminder: The protein RDA for healthy adults is 0.8 g/kg.

Although it was formerly believed that high-protein diets could harm patients with hepatic encephalopathy, protein restrictions are no longer recommended and may worsen malnutrition and wasting.[19] In an attempt to normalize altered amino acid ratios in brain tissue and improve mental status, some clinicians prescribe enteral formulas with added branched-chain amino acids and reduced aromatic amino acids. Clinical studies testing the use of these formulas have yielded mixed results, however, and their routine use is not currently recommended.[20]

Carbohydrate and Fat Carbohydrate provides a substantial proportion of energy needs, and its restriction is not advised.[21] Many patients with cirrhosis have insulin resistance, however, and require medications or insulin to manage their hyperglycemia. Such individuals should follow the dietary guidelines for diabetes: consume mostly complex carbohydrates, and consume them at regular intervals throughout the day. A few small studies have suggested that high-fiber, low glycemic index diets can improve glucose tolerance in patients with cirrhosis, but larger studies are needed to confirm the benefit.[22]

If steatorrhea is present, fat intake is restricted, and medium-chain triglycerides (MCT) may be used to provide additional energy. Essential fatty acids are not present in MCT oils and may need to be supplemented. Severe steatorrhea also warrants supplementation of fat-soluble vitamins, calcium, magnesium, and zinc.

Sodium and Fluid Patients with ascites need to restrict sodium. Ascites is caused by the kidneys' reabsorption of sodium into blood, resulting in sodium and water retention. Therefore, treatment usually combines moderate sodium restriction (2 to 3 grams per day) and diuretic therapy to produce a fluid loss of approximately one pound daily.[23] Potassium intake should be monitored if a potassium-wasting diuretic (such as furosemide) is used.

HOW TO Help the Person with Cirrhosis Eat Enough Food

Individuals with cirrhosis often have difficulty consuming enough food to prevent malnutrition and its consequences. Ascites and gastrointestinal symptoms such as nausea and vomiting may interfere with food intake. Fatigue may cause disinterest in food preparation. Sodium restrictions may make foods unpalatable. To facilitate dietary compliance:

- Individualize the dietary plan based on each person's symptoms and tolerances. The diet should not restrict protein, fat, sodium, or fluids unless such restrictions are warranted.
- Suggest ways to incorporate favorite foods into the diet. Give ideas for recipe modifications that may make foods more palatable.
- Suggest between-meal snacks during the day and a snack at bedtime. An oral supplement like Ensure can substitute for a snack and requires no preparation. Snacks should not be consumed within two hours of meals, or they may reduce appetite at mealtime.
- Recommend energy boosters. Cream sauces and gravies can add kcalories to entrées. Fruit juices and fruit nectars can substitute for drinking water. The following food "additives" can boost the energy content of meals:
  - Sour cream and butter—on vegetables and potatoes.
  - Mayonnaise—in sandwiches and salads.
  - Half-and-Half and light cream—in soups and on cereals.
  - Hard-boiled egg—in casseroles and meat loaf.
  - Cheese—in salads and casseroles and melted on steamed vegetables.
  - Peanut and nut butters, and cream cheese—on crackers or celery, and in milk shakes.
  - Chopped nuts—in salads, cooked cereals, and bakery products.

Low-sodium diets are recommended for treating ascites and other medical conditions, including kidney and heart disorders. The "How to" feature on p. 838 offers suggestions to help patients implement sodium restrictions. To improve the palatability of low-sodium meals:

- Suggest that patients replace the salt they use for cooking and seasoning with strong-flavored herbs and spices like coriander, chili powder, cumin, curry powder, garlic, ginger, mint, lemon, and parsley.
- Advise patients to check food labels to learn the sodium content of the foods they eat. They may be able to find similar products that are lower in sodium. (Persons using potassium-sparing diuretics should be cautioned to avoid salt substitutes that replace sodium with potassium.)

Offer support and encouragement to the patient with cirrhosis. Severe weight loss is less likely to occur if dietary advice is provided before problems progress.

Many patients find low-sodium diets unpalatable, so some clinicians may allow a more liberal sodium intake and depend on diuretics to mobilize excess fluids. If patients do not respond to sodium restriction and diuretic therapy, fluid may be removed directly■ or be diverted to the bloodstream using a catheter.■

■ The surgical puncture used to draw out excess fluid is known as **paracentesis** (PAHR-ah-sen-TEE-sis).

■ The surgical passage created between the peritoneum and jugular vein to divert fluid and relieve ascites is called a **peritoneovenous shunt.**

Vitamins and Minerals Vitamin and mineral deficiencies are common in cirrhosis patients due to the effects of illness, complications of disease, or alcoholism that may have induced the liver disease. Multivitamin supplementation is usually recommended. If steatorrhea is present, fat-soluble nutrients can be provided in water-soluble forms. Patients with esophageal varices may find it easier to ingest supplements in liquid form.

Enteral and Parenteral Nutrition Support If a person with cirrhosis is unable to consume enough food, tube feedings or intravenous feedings may be warranted. Specialized enteral (tube feeding) products are sometimes preferred; these include formulas that are high in kcalories, low in sodium, or high in branched-chain amino acids. If a feeding tube aggravates esophageal varices, the tubing should be as narrow and flexible as possible.

Parenteral nutrition support should be considered for patients who are unable to tolerate enteral feedings due to intestinal obstruction, gastrointestinal bleeding, or uncontrollable vomiting.[24] For those with hyperglycemia,■ the rate of dextrose

■ Reminder: Hyperglycemia is a common complication of both parenteral feedings and liver disease.

infusion should be limited to the amount that can be oxidized within the body, or about 5 milligrams per kilogram body weight per minute. To avoid excessive fluid delivery, concentrated nutrient formulas are recommended for patients with ascites, and central veins are used for feedings. The case study allows you to apply your understanding of cirrhosis to a clinical situation.

IN SUMMARY Liver cirrhosis is characterized by fibrosis and permanent liver dysfunction. In the United States, the primary causes of cirrhosis are hepatitis C infection and alcohol abuse. Symptoms often include fatigue, gastrointestinal disturbances, anorexia, and weight loss. Liver damage may have multiple metabolic consequences, including reduced immunity, anemia, edema, and insulin resistance. Complications associated with cirrhosis include portal hypertension, gastroesophageal varices, ascites, and hepatic encephalopathy. Cirrhosis may also lead to kidney disease, altered hormone function, and wasting. Treatment of cirrhosis is highly individualized and depends on the complications present. Both drug therapies and dietary adjustments are usually necessary. A person with cirrhosis often has a poor food intake and is at high risk of malnutrition.

Liver Transplantation

Acute or chronic liver disease can potentially lead to liver failure, in which case liver transplantation is the only viable treatment option. The most common illnesses that precede liver transplantation are chronic hepatitis C infection and alcoholic liver disease, which account for about 40 percent of liver transplant cases.[25] The five-year survival rate among transplant recipients is 70 to 75 percent, although complications such as ascites and hepatic encephalopathy may worsen the prognosis.[26]

Nutrition Status of Transplant Patients As mentioned earlier, advanced liver disease is usually associated with malnutrition, which can increase the risk of complications following a liver transplant. Evaluating nutrition status in transplant candidates may be difficult because liver dysfunction and malnutrition often have similar metabolic effects. In addition, fluid retention can mask weight loss and alter anthropometric and laboratory values. Correcting malnutrition prior to surgery can help speed recovery after surgery.

Post-Transplantation Concerns The immediate concerns following a transplant are organ rejection and infection. Immunosuppressive drugs■ are given to reduce the immune responses that cause rejection, but they also raise the risk of infection. Infections are the most common cause of death following a liver transplant; therefore, antibiotics and antiviral medications are prescribed to reduce infection risk.[27] To help transplant patients avoid developing foodborne illnesses, dietitians routinely provide information about food safety measures, such as cooking meats adequately and washing fresh produce.[28]

■ Immunosuppressive drugs used after liver transplant include prednisone, cyclosporine, and tacrolimus.

Immunosuppressive drugs can affect nutrition status in numerous ways. Gastrointestinal side effects include nausea, vomiting, diarrhea, abdominal pain, and mouth sores. Some of the drugs may cause hyperglycemia or outright diabetes, which may need to be controlled with insulin. Electrolyte and fluid imbalances are common, and some medications may alter appetite and taste perception. Other possible effects include hypertension, hyperlipidemias, protein catabolism, and increased osteoporosis risk.[29]

Protein and energy requirements are increased after transplantation due to the stress of surgery. High-kcalorie, high-protein snacks and enteral supplements can help the transplant patient meet postsurgical needs. Nutrient supplementation is also an integral part of nutrition care.

CASE STUDY

Carpenter with Cirrhosis

Mark Judd, a 48-year-old carpenter, has just been diagnosed with cirrhosis as a consequence of alcohol abuse over the past 25 years. Although he recognizes that he has an alcohol problem and recently entered an alcohol rehabilitation program, he is still drinking. At 5 feet 7 inches tall, Mark, who formerly weighed 155 pounds, now weighs 125 pounds. Although he is still living at home, he is showing signs of mental deterioration. He is jaundiced and appears thin, although his abdomen is distended with ascites. Laboratory findings indicate elevated serum concentrations of AST, ALT, and ammonia; reduced albumin levels; and hyperglycemia.

1. Do Mark's laboratory values suggest liver disease? Compare the results of his laboratory tests with the values shown in Table 25-3.
2. From the limited information available, evaluate Mark's nutrition status. What medical problem makes it difficult to interpret his present weight? Describe the development of ascites in liver disease and explain how the diet is usually adjusted.
3. Calculate Mark's energy and protein needs. Describe the general diet you might recommend for him. What suggestions do you have for increasing his energy intake?
4. Explain the significance of Mark's elevated blood ammonia levels. What signs might suggest that he is undergoing mental decline?
5. Describe each of the following complications of liver disease: portal hypertension, jaundice, gastroesophageal varices. What complication may result if Mark's esophageal varices are not treated?

IN SUMMARY Liver transplantation has improved the long-term outlook for patients with advanced liver disease. Transplant patients are usually malnourished and have serious complications that may affect transplant success. A major concern is organ rejection, and therefore immunosuppressive drugs are prescribed following surgery. Immunosuppressive drugs can increase the risk of infection and have many side effects that can impair nutrition status and general health.

Gallstone Disease

After bile is produced in the liver, it travels via the bile ducts to the gallbladder where it is concentrated and stored until needed for the digestion of fat. Disorders that obstruct the liver's release of bile can damage the liver. More commonly, disorders of the biliary system result in the formation of **gallstones.** Gallstones affect an estimated 30 million people in the United States, or 10.5 percent of the population.[30]

Types of Gallstones

The formation of gallstones, or **cholelithiasis,** results from excessive concentration and crystallization of the compounds in bile. Bile is a solution of bile salts, cholesterol, proteins, phospholipids (lecithin), and bile pigment (bilirubin). While stored in the gallbladder, bile becomes more concentrated as its water content is extracted. Factors that either increase bile's cholesterol concentration or reduce the gallbladder's motility favor gallstone formation.[31]

Cholesterol Gallstones In about 80 percent of cases, the gallstones are composed primarily of cholesterol, although they also contain calcium salts and bilirubin. The cholesterol in bile precipitates out of solution and forms small crystals, which eventually coalesce to form stones. The stones can be as small as a pea or as large as a ping-pong ball. Some people tend to form many small stones, while others may form only one or two large ones. Cholesterol gallstones often develop because the bile concentrate thickens and forms a **sludge** that cannot be easily expelled by gallbladder contraction. Biliary sludge can develop after rapid weight loss, gastric bypass surgery, and long-term total parenteral nutrition and also occurs during pregnancy.

gallstones: crystalline deposits that form in the gallbladder from cholesterol or bilirubin.

cholelithiasis (KOH-lee-lih-THIGH-ah-sis): formation of gallstones.
- **chole** = bile
- **lithiasis** = formation of stones

sludge: literally, a semisolid mass. Biliary sludge is made up of mucus, cholesterol crystals, and bilirubin granules.

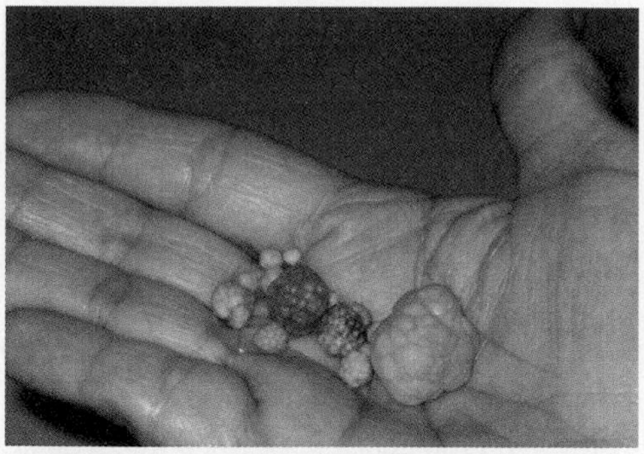
Courtesy of Dr. David King. © Myrna Engler

Most gallstones are made primarily of cholesterol; they can be as small as a pea or as large as a ping-pong ball.

Pigment Gallstones Pigment stones develop in 10 to 25 percent of gallstone cases in the United States, although they are much more common in Asian countries.[32] Pigment stones are primarily made up of the calcium salt of bilirubin (calcium bilirubinate). They often develop as a result of bacterial infection, which alters bilirubin and causes it to precipitate out of bile and form stones. Some cases result from excessive bilirubin accumulation (from red blood cell breakdown). Conditions associated with pigment stone formation include biliary tract infections, pancreatitis, and red blood cell disorders, such as sickle-cell anemia. Pigment stones may form in either the gallbladder or the bile duct. Unlike the crystalline cholesterol stones, pigment stones are soft and easily crushed.

Consequences of Gallstones

About 80 percent of gallstones are asymptomatic■ and are discovered accidentally while testing for other conditions. Many people, however, experience an aggressive course of illness with recurring symptoms.

■ Gallstones that do not cause symptoms are called **silent gallstones.**

Gallstone Symptoms Gallstone pain usually arises when a gallstone temporarily blocks the cystic duct (see Figure 25-3).[33] The pain is steady and severe and may last for several minutes or several hours. Although the pain is usually located in the upper abdomen, it may radiate to the chest or to the back. Nausea, vomiting, and bloating may also be present. Symptoms usually develop after meals, but may occur during the night and awaken a person from sleep.

Complications of Gallstone Disease If a gallstone remains lodged in the cystic duct, it can obstruct bile flow to the duodenum and cause **cholecystitis**—distention and inflammation of the gallbladder. Cholecystitis can lead to infection or to more severe complications, including perforation of the gallbladder, peritonitis, and fistulas.[34] If gallstones obstruct the common bile duct (see Figure 25-3), they can block bile flow from the liver and lead to jaundice or damage to liver tissue. An impacted stone within the common bile duct sometimes results in infection within the duct itself.■ This infection can cause severe pain, sepsis, and fever exceeding 104° Fahrenheit and is often a medical emergency. Gallstones can block the pancreatic duct as well—a primary cause of acute pancreatitis (pp. 746–747). Due to the poten-

■ Bacterial infection of the bile ducts is called **bacterial cholangitis** (KOH-lan-JYE-tis).

FIGURE 25-3 The Gallbladder and Bile Ducts

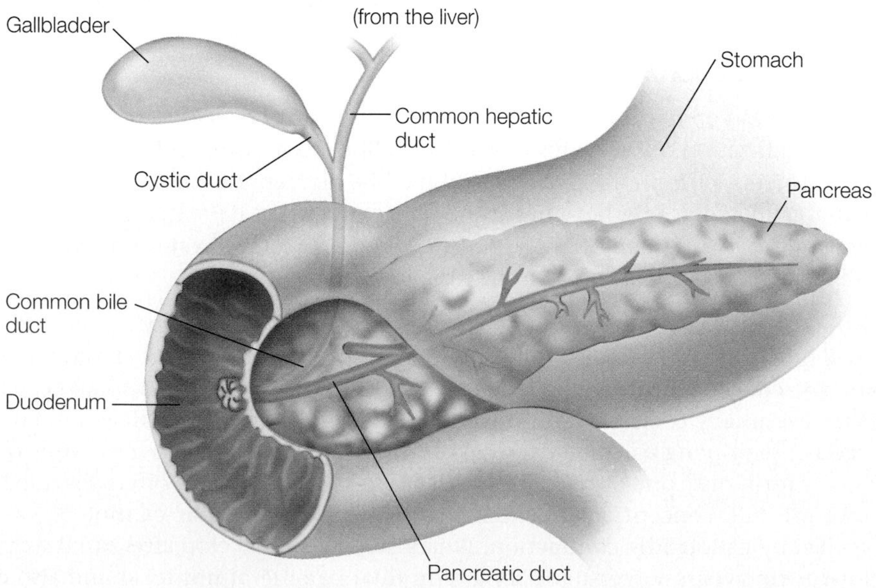
Gallbladder
(from the liver)
Stomach
Common hepatic duct
Cystic duct
Pancreas
Common bile duct
Duodenum
Pancreatic duct

cholecystitis (KOH-lee-sih-STY-tis): inflammation of the gallbladder, usually caused by obstruction of the cystic duct by gallstones.

tial danger of these complications, medical attention should be sought if gallstone pain does not resolve over time or if fever, jaundice, or persistent nausea and vomiting develop.

Risk Factors for Gallstones

The risk of developing gallstones is influenced by a number of genetic and lifestyle factors. Incidence varies among populations, depending on such factors as ethnicity, age, and gender.

Ethnicity Although the genetic factors related to gallstone formation are not yet clear, ethnicity strongly influences gallstone formation. The Pima Indians are an exceptionally high-risk population; gallstones develop in about 70 percent of adult women. Other high-risk populations include Scandinavians, Chileans, and Native Americans in the United States and Canada. In the United States, African Americans have a lower prevalence of gallstones than white populations.[35]

Age and Gender Gallstone prevalence increases with age and is much higher in women than in men. The incidence in women is three times that of men during the reproductive years, but it falls to a similar level after menopause. The reason for the gender difference is that estrogen alters cholesterol metabolism and causes an increased secretion of cholesterol into bile, increasing the likelihood of cholesterol crystallization. The use of estrogen replacement therapy after menopause increases gallstone risk in postmenopausal women.[36]

Pregnancy Some women experience their first gallstone symptoms during pregnancy. Gallstone risk is increased in pregnancy due to hormonal changes: higher serum progesterone levels impair gallbladder motility, and higher estrogen levels increase the secretion of cholesterol into bile.[37]

Obesity and Weight Loss Obesity is associated with increased cholesterol synthesis in the liver, leading to a greater release of cholesterol into bile and an increased risk of gallstone formation. In a cohort study,■ women with a body mass index (BMI) greater than 45 had a risk of gallstone formation seven times that of nonobese women.[38]

■ Reminder: In a *cohort study,* researchers analyze data collected from a selected group of people (a cohort) at intervals over a certain period of time.

Gallstones frequently develop as a result of rapid weight loss, occurring in about 25 percent of obese persons on very-low-kcalorie diets and up to half of those who undergo gastric bypass surgeries.[39] Dieting increases the secretion of cholesterol into bile and may also decrease gallbladder motility. The oral ingestion of bile salts has been shown to reduce the risk of gallstone formation during rapid weight loss.

Other Risk Factors As described earlier, conditions that promote the development of biliary sludge generally increase the risk of gallstone formation. Long-term total parenteral nutrition usually reduces gallbladder motility, an effect that increases sludge and gallstone risk. Some medications (for example, octreotide) may have similar effects. The medication clofibrate, used for heart disease, increases the cholesterol concentration of bile, which promotes cholesterol crystallization and gallstone formation. High triglyceride levels in blood are associated with increased gallstone risk, as are hyperinsulinemia, insulin resistance, and diabetes mellitus.[40]

Treatment for Gallstones

Asymptomatic gallstones generally do not require treatment.[41] Gallstones that cause symptoms or complications are usually treated by gallbladder surgery or by nonsurgical procedures that dissolve or fragment the stones.

Surgery Gallbladder removal, or **cholecystectomy,** is the primary treatment for patients with recurring gallstones. The preferred surgical approach is a **laparoscopic** method, which relies on narrow surgical telescopes to view and perform the

cholecystectomy (KOH-lee-sis-TEK-toe-mee): surgical removal of the gallbladder.

laparoscopic: pertaining to procedures that use a laparoscope for internal examination or surgery. A laparoscope is a narrow surgical telescope that is inserted into the abdominal cavity through a small incision. A video camera is usually attached so that the procedure can be viewed on a television monitor.

necessary procedures via small incisions in the abdomen. The procedure takes less than two hours, and patients are usually discharged within a day or two after surgery.[42] If there are complications such as adhesions (scar tissue) that make organ removal difficult, open cholecystectomy may be performed.

Once the gallbladder has been removed, the common bile duct collects bile between meals, and releases it into the duodenum at mealtimes. Most patients do not experience problems after they recover from surgery, although others may experience abdominal pain, gas, and bloating.[43] A common cause of postsurgical symptoms is the presence of residual stones within the common bile duct that were overlooked during surgery or that formed within the duct itself. Problems may also develop in the cystic duct remnant that remains after surgery.

Nonsurgical Procedures Nonsurgical methods are used primarily in patients who have transient conditions associated with gallstone formation.[44] Gallstones can be treated by oral intake of ursodeoxycholic acid (ursodiol), a bile acid that reduces cholesterol production in the liver and eventually causes the cholesterol crystals in gallstones to dissolve. Ursodeoxycholic acid must be used for 6 to 12 months and is best suited for stones that are 5 millimeters (¼ inch) in diameter or smaller. Recurrence rates after dissolution are as high as 50 percent.[45]

Gallstones can be fragmented by using **shock-wave lithotripsy,** a procedure that is also used to fragment kidney stones. This technique uses high-amplitude shock waves (similar to sound waves) to break gallstones into pieces that are small enough to either pass into the intestine or be dissolved with ursodeoxycholic acid. Shock-wave lithotripsy can be performed only if the gallstones are few in number. Success is highest in patients with solitary stones that are less than 20 millimeters (¾ inch) in diameter.[46] Recurrence of gallstones has been reported in up to 44 percent of patients using this procedure.[47]

IN SUMMARY Gallstones are the most common disorder affecting the gallbladder. They are formed by concentration of the compounds in bile, especially cholesterol and the bile pigment bilirubin. Most people with gallstones have no symptoms. Symptomatic gallstones can cause recurring pain and gastrointestinal problems that usually appear after meals and may persist for several hours. Gallstone complications may cause inflammation or infection in the gallbladder, bile duct, and pancreatic duct. The risk of gallstone formation increases with age and is highest in premenopausal and pregnant women and in persons who are obese or who undergo rapid weight loss. Treatments for gallstones include gallbladder removal and gallstone dissolution or fragmentation.

shock-wave lithotripsy: a nonsurgical procedure that uses high-amplitude sound waves to fragment gallstones.

DIET-DRUG INTERACTIONS

Anti-Infectives

An antibiotic frequently used to control blood ammonia levels in liver disease is *neomycin.* Because neomycin kills bacteria in the intestine, the person may need a vitamin K supplement. The person may be prone to intestinal infections that ordinarily are suppressed by normal bacterial flora. Neomycin can also be toxic to the kidneys.

The antiviral agent *lamivudine* may be used in the treatment of liver diseases: it is described in the box in Chapter 29.

Anti-Inflammatory Agents

For *anti-inflammatory agents,* see p. 762.

Appetite Stimulants

Megestrol acetate and *dronabinol* (a derivative of marijuana) stimulate the appetite and result in weight gain. GI side effects are uncommon, although some people develop nausea, vomiting, and diarrhea. Dronabinol produces euphoria in some people and can reach toxic levels in people with liver dysfunction.

Diuretics

Spironolactone is a potassium-sparing diuretic frequently used to treat ascites. People taking spironolactone should avoid foods high in potassium, potassium supplements, and salt substitutes that contain potassium. Also see p. 841.

Immunosuppressants
Immunosuppressants are used for people who undergo liver transplants. For *cyclosporine* and a general discussion of immunosuppressants, see p. 870.

Another immunosuppressant sometimes used to prevent tissue rejection following a liver transplant is *tacrolimus.* Tacrolimus can be given with food to reduce nausea, vomiting, and GI upsets. Other nutrition-related side effects include anorexia, diarrhea, constipation, anemia, hyperglycemia, potassium imbalances, low blood magnesium levels, and ascites.

Interferon
Interferon can lead to nausea, vomiting, weight loss, fever, fatigue, and depression.

Laxatives
The laxative commonly used in the treatment of liver disease is *lactulose.* Lactulose can cause belching, cramps, and diarrhea. If diarrhea develops, encourage patients to replace fluid and electrolytes.

NUTRITION ASSESSMENT CHECKLIST for People with Liver Disorders

Medical History

Check the medical record to determine:

- ☐ Type of liver disorder
- ☐ Cause of liver disorder
- ☐ If the patient has received a liver transplant
- ☐ If the patient has a history of gallstone disease

Review the medical record for complications that may alter medical nutrition therapy including:

- ☐ Malnutrition
- ☐ Malabsorption
- ☐ Esophageal varices
- ☐ Ascites
- ☐ Hepatic encephalopathy
- ☐ Insulin resistance/diabetes mellitus
- ☐ Infections
- ☐ Anemia
- ☐ Pancreatitis
- ☐ Impaired kidney or lung function

Medications

In patients with liver dysfunction, the risk of diet-drug interactions is very high because most drugs are metabolized in the liver. Risk of interactions is intensified for patients with:

- ☐ Ascites (medications may take a long time to reach the liver)
- ☐ Renal failure (medications are often metabolized further in the kidneys and excreted in the urine)
- ☐ Malnutrition
- ☐ Multiple medication prescriptions
- ☐ Long-term medication use

Dietary Intake

For patients with fatty liver, pay special attention to:

- ☐ Energy intake, if the patient is overweight or malnourished, has diabetes, or is receiving total parenteral nutrition
- ☐ Carbohydrate, if the patient has diabetes or is receiving total parenteral nutrition
- ☐ Alcohol

For patients with hepatitis, cirrhosis, or ascites:

- ☐ Check appetite
- ☐ Ensure that energy and nutrient intakes are adequate
- ☐ Determine alcohol use
- ☐ Determine whether sodium restriction is warranted
- ☐ Base energy needs on desirable or estimated dry weight to avoid overfeeding

Anthropometric Data

Take baseline height and weight measurements and monitor weight regularly. For patients with ascites and edema:

- ☐ Use weight to monitor the degree of fluid retention
- ☐ Remember that the patient may be malnourished, and weight deceptively high

Laboratory Tests

Note that albumin and serum proteins are often reduced in people with liver disease and cannot always be used as indicators of nutrition status. Review the following laboratory test results to assess liver function:

- ☐ Albumin
- ☐ Alkaline phosphatase
- ☐ ALT
- ☐ AST
- ☐ Ammonia
- ☐ Bilirubin
- ☐ Prothrombin time

Check laboratory test results for complications associated with liver failure including:

- ☐ Anemia
- ☐ Fluid retention
- ☐ Hyperglycemia
- ☐ Renal function tests

Clinical Signs

Look for physical signs of:

- ☐ Fluid retention (ascites and edema)
- ☐ PEM (muscle wasting and unintentional weight loss)
- ☐ Nutrient deficiencies

NUTRITION ON THE NET

Access these websites for further study of topics covered in this chapter.

- Find updates and quick links to these and other nutrition-related sites at our website: **www.wadsworth.com/nutrition**
- To obtain additional information about liver diseases, visit the American Liver Foundation and the Canadian Liver Foundation: **www.liverfoundation.org** and **www.liver.ca**

- To find out more about resources and support for children with liver diseases and liver transplants, visit the Children's Liver Alliance: **www.liverkids.org.au**
- To review information about hepatitis, visit the Hepatitis Foundation International: **www.hepfi.org**
- To uncover more information about liver transplants, search the Center Span Transplant News Network: **www.centerspan.org**

STUDY QUESTIONS

These questions will help you review the chapter. You will find the answers in the discussions on the pages provided.

1. Describe fatty liver and identify possible causes. What consequences may develop? What are possible treatments? (pp. 770–771)
2. What is hepatitis, and what are its primary causes? Compare the features of hepatitis virus A, B, and C infections. Identify nutrition concerns for patients with hepatitis. (pp. 771–772)
3. Describe how liver disease can progress to cirrhosis. What are the most common causes of cirrhosis in the United States? (pp. 772–773)
4. Discuss the consequences of cirrhosis, including its clinical effects and complications such as portal hypertension, gastroesophageal varices, ascites, and hepatic encephalopathy. What metabolic changes may result from altered liver function? (pp. 773–774)
5. How does cirrhosis affect nutrition status? Describe the dietary treatment of a patient with cirrhosis. Discuss the special dietary concerns of patients with ascites and esophageal varices. (pp. 774–778)
6. Discuss the problems that arise following liver transplantation that can affect nutrition status. What dietary modifications may be necessary? (pp. 778–779)
7. Explain how gallstones form, and describe the features of the two main types of gallstones. What complications are associated with gallstone disease? (pp. 779–781)
8. Discuss the major risk factors for gallstone disease. Describe the primary methods of treatment. (pp. 781–782)

These questions will help you prepare for an exam. Answers can be found on p. 785.

1. Which of the following dietary strategies would be most appropriate for reversing fatty liver associated with diabetes mellitus?
   a. low-protein diet
   b. fat-restricted diet
   c. fluid- and sodium-restricted diet
   d. modifying energy to achieve a desirable weight and modifying carbohydrates to attain blood glucose control
2. Which of the following statements about hepatitis is true?
   a. Chronic hepatitis can progress to cirrhosis.
   b. Whatever the cause of hepatitis, symptoms are typically severe.
   c. People with hepatitis require high-kcalorie, high-protein diets.
   d. HCV infections can be spread through contaminated foods and water.
3. Esophageal varices are a dangerous complication of liver disease primarily because they:
   a. interfere with food intake.
   b. can lead to massive bleeding.
   c. divert blood flow from the GI tract.
   d. cause portal hypertension and collateral development.
4. A consequence of liver disease that may lead to ascites is:
   a. portal hypertension.
   b. rising blood ammonia levels.
   c. elevated serum albumin levels.
   d. insulin resistance.
5. A patient with cirrhosis may develop personality changes and motor dysfunction, which are signs of:
   a. gallbladder involvement.
   b. encephalopathy.
   c. hyperammonemia.
   d. hepatic coma.
6. With respect to protein intake, patients with cirrhosis should:
   a. consume no more than the protein RDA.
   b. restrict protein intake to 0.6 gram per kilogram body weight.
   c. use formulas with modified amino acids to meet their protein needs.
   d. maintain nitrogen balance by consuming 1.2 to 1.5 grams of protein per kilogram body weight.
7. People with ascites must restrict dietary intake of:
   a. fat.
   b. protein.
   c. sugars.
   d. sodium.
8. For a patient undergoing a liver transplant:
   a. immunosuppressant drugs seldom alter nutrient needs.
   b. enteral nutrition is contraindicated following the transplant.
   c. attention to nutrition before a transplant improves chances of recovery.
   d. provided adequate nutrition care is given after the transplant, nutrition status before surgery has little impact on recovery.

9. Regarding risk factors for gallstone disease:
   a. prevalence is much higher in men than in women.
   b. gallstone risk is increased during pregnancy.
   c. rapid weight loss can temporarily shrink gallstones.
   d. gallstone risk is similar among all ethnicities.
10. Nonsurgical approaches to gallstone treatment include:
    a. cholecystectomy.
    b. weight loss.
    c. dissolution and fragmentation.
    d. immunosuppressant drug therapy.

REFERENCES

1. A. M. Diehl, Alcoholic and nonalcoholic steatohepatitis, in L. Goldman and D. Ausiello, eds., *Cecil Textbook of Medicine* (Philadelphia: Saunders, 2004), pp. 933–936.
2. A. M. Diehl and F. Poordad, Nonalcoholic fatty liver disease, in M. Feldman, L. S. Friedman, and M. H. Sleisenger, eds., *Sleisenger and Fordtran's Gastrointestinal and Liver Disease: Pathophysiology, Diagnosis, Management* (Philadelphia: Saunders, 2002), pp. 1393–1401.
3. Diehl and Poordad, 2002.
4. G. C. Farrell, Liver disease caused by drugs, anesthetics, and toxins, in M. Feldman, L. S. Friedman, and M. H. Sleisenger, eds., *Sleisenger and Fordtran's Gastrointestinal and Liver Disease: Pathophysiology, Diagnosis, Management* (Philadelphia: Saunders, 2002), pp. 1403–1447.
5. R. K. Fox and T. L. Wright, Viral hepatitis, in S. L. Friedman, K. R. McQuaid, and J. H. Grendell, eds., *Current Diagnosis and Treatment in Gastroenterology* (New York: Lange Medical Books/McGraw-Hill, 2003), pp. 546–562.
6. T. D. Schiano and H. C. Bodenheimer, Complications of chronic liver disease, in S. L. Friedman, K. R. McQuaid, and J. H. Grendell, eds., *Current Diagnosis and Treatment in Gastroenterology* (New York: Lange Medical Books/McGraw-Hill, 2003), pp. 639–663.
7. D. C. Wolf, Cirrhosis, available at www.emedicine.com/med/topic3183.htm, visited December 30, 2004.
8. S. H. Rigby and K. B. Schwarz, Nutrition and liver disease, in A. M. Coulston, C. L. Rock, and E. R. Monsen, eds., *Nutrition in the Prevention and Treatment of Disease* (San Diego: Academic Press, 2001), pp. 601–613.
9. S. L. Friedman and T. D. Schiano, Cirrhosis and its sequelae, in L. Goldman and D. Ausiello, eds., *Cecil Textbook of Medicine* (Philadelphia: Saunders, 2004), pp. 936–944.
10. Schiano and Bodenheimer, 2003.
11. B. A. Runyon, Ascites and spontaneous bacterial peritonitis, in M. Feldman, L. S. Friedman, and M. H. Sleisenger, eds., *Sleisenger and Fordtran's Gastrointestinal and Liver Disease: Pathophysiology, Diagnosis, Management* (Philadelphia: Saunders, 2002), pp. 1517–1542.
12. Schiano and Bodenheimer, 2003.
13. J. G. Fitz, Hepatic encephalopathy, hepatopulmonary syndromes, hepatorenal syndrome, coagulopathy, and endocrine complications of liver disease, in M. Feldman, L. S. Friedman, and M. H. Sleisenger, eds., *Sleisenger and Fordtran's Gastrointestinal and Liver Disease: Pathophysiology, Diagnosis, Management* (Philadelphia: Saunders, 2002), pp. 1543–1565.
14. Fitz, 2002.
15. Schiano and Bodenheimer, 2003.
16. Friedman and Schiano, 2004.
17. American Dietetic Association, *Manual of Clinical Dietetics* (Chicago: American Dietetic Association, 2000).
18. American Dietetic Association, 2000.
19. S. Escott-Stump, *Nutrition and Diagnosis-Related Care* (Baltimore: Lippincott Williams & Wilkins, 2002); American Dietetic Association, 2000.
20. B. Als-Nielsen and coauthors, Branched-chain amino acids for hepatic encephalopathy (Cochrane Review), *The Cochrane Library* Issue 3 (2004); American Dietetic Association, 2000.
21. American Dietetic Association, 2000.
22. H. Barkoukis, K. M. Fiedler, and E. Lerner, A combined high-fiber, low-glycemic index diet normalizes glucose tolerance and reduces hyperglycemia and hyperinsulinemia in adults with hepatic cirrhosis, *Journal of the American Dietetic Association* 102 (2002): 1503–1507; D. J. Jenkins and coauthors, Low glycemic index foods and reduced glucose, amino acid, and endocrine responses in cirrhosis, *American Journal of Gastroenterology* 84 (1989): 732–739.
23. Schiano and Bodenheimer, 2003.
24. American Dietetic Association, 2000.
25. E. B. Keeffe, Hepatic failure and liver transplantation, in L. Goldman and D. Ausiello, eds., *Cecil Textbook of Medicine* (Philadelphia: Saunders, 2004), pp. 944–949.
26. J. R. Lake, Liver transplantation, in S. L. Friedman, K. R. McQuaid, and J. H. Grendell, eds., *Current Diagnosis and Treatment in Gastroenterology* (New York: Lange Medical Books/McGraw-Hill, 2003), pp. 813–834.
27. Lake, 2003.
28. D. Shattuck, The dietitian's role on the transplantation team, *Journal of the American Dietetic Association* 102 (2002): 902–903.
29. American Dietetic Association, 2000.
30. N. H. Afdhal, Diseases of the gallbladder and bile ducts, in L. Goldman and D. Ausiello, eds., *Cecil Textbook of Medicine* (Philadelphia: Saunders, 2004), pp. 949–956.
31. J. D. Horton and L. E. Bilhartz, Gallstone disease and its complications, in M. Feldman, L. S. Friedman, and M. H. Sleisenger, eds., *Sleisenger and Fordtran's Gastrointestinal and Liver Disease: Pathophysiology, Diagnosis, Management* (Philadelphia: Saunders, 2002), pp. 1065–1090.
32. Horton and Bilhartz, 2002.
33. I. M. Jacobson, Gallstones, in S. L. Friedman, K. R. McQuaid, and J. H. Grendell, eds., *Current Diagnosis and Treatment in Gastroenterology* (New York: Lange Medical Books/McGraw-Hill, 2003), pp. 772–783.
34. Afdhal, 2004.
35. Horton and Bilhartz, 2002.
36. Horton and Bilhartz, 2002.
37. Jacobson, 2003.
38. Horton and Bilhartz, 2002.
39. Horton and Bilhartz, 2002.
40. Horton and Bilhartz, 2002; G. Misciagna and coauthors, Insulin and gall stones: A population case control study in southern Italy, *Gut* 47 (2000): 144–147.
41. Jacobson, 2003.
42. Jacobson, 2003.
43. R. E. Glasgow and S. J. Mulvihill, Surgical management of gallstone disease and postoperative complications, in M. Feldman, L. S. Friedman, and M. H. Sleisenger, eds., *Sleisenger and Fordtran's Gastrointestinal and Liver Disease: Pathophysiology, Diagnosis, Management* (Philadelphia: Saunders, 2002), pp. 1091–1105.
44. G. Paumgartner, Nonsurgical management of gallstone disease, in M. Feldman, L. S. Friedman, and M. H. Sleisenger, eds., *Sleisenger and Fordtran's Gastrointestinal and Liver Disease: Pathophysiology, Diagnosis, Management* (Philadelphia: Saunders, 2002), pp. 1107–1115.
45. Jacobson, 2003; Paumgartner, 2002.
46. Jacobson, 2003; Paumgartner, 2002.
47. Paumgartner, 2002.

ANSWERS

Study Questions (multiple choice)

1. d 2. a 3. b 4. a 5. b 6. d 7. d 8. c 9. b 10. c

HIGHLIGHT

Anemia in Illness

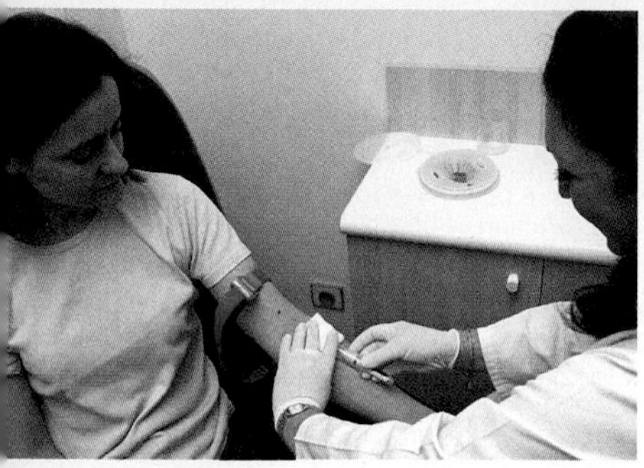

Anemia—the condition of having too few red blood cells—is frequently the first sign of illness and may be the symptom that initially drives an individual to seek medical attention. Though not a disease itself, anemia is a symptom associated with a great number of diseases and treatments: some 20 to 40 percent of hospital patients exhibit some degree of anemia.[1] Earlier chapters in this textbook described some of the relationships between anemia and nutrient deficiencies. This highlight discusses how and why anemia develops during the course of illness. The accompanying glossary defines relevant terms.

Overview of Anemia

Anemia results when red blood cells (also called *erythrocytes*) are not produced in sufficient amounts, when they are too quickly destroyed, or when they are lost due to bleeding. Because red blood cells contain the hemoglobin that supplies oxygen to tissues, their absence can result in fatigue, lack of energy, and reduced stamina. The deficiency of oxygen in tissues is the main stimulus for the production of additional red blood cells.

Red Blood Cell Production

The production of red blood cells **(erythropoiesis)** takes place in bone marrow, which is a soft tissue in the inner cavities of large bones. The process begins when kidney cells sense the low oxygen content of blood and release the hormone **erythropoietin** (see Figure H25-1). Erythropoietin travels to bone marrow where it stimulates precursor cells (stem cells) to divide and differentiate into red blood cells. The cells that are released from bone marrow are immature red blood cells called **reticulocytes.** Reticulocytes develop into mature red blood cells over a 24- to 48-hour period while they circulate in the bloodstream.

Nutritional Anemias

The nutrient deficiencies that most frequently upset red blood cell production are those of iron, folate, and vitamin B_{12}. Iron is required for hemoglobin production, and deficiency results in **microcytic anemia,** characterized by small, hypochromic cells (see pp. 442–443). Vitamin B_{12} and folate participate in DNA synthesis, and deficiency of either nutrient leads to **macrocytic anemia,** characterized by large immature cells (see pp. 339, 342).

Other nutrient deficiencies may also cause anemia, although not as frequently. Vitamin E helps to maintain cell membrane integrity, and its deficiency is associated with hemolytic anemia (red blood cell breakdown). Vitamin B_6 plays a role in hemoglobin production, and a deficiency sometimes

GLOSSARY

anemia of chronic disease: anemia that develops in persons with chronic illness; may resemble iron-deficiency anemia even though iron stores are often adequate.

aplastic anemia: anemia characterized by the inability of bone marrow to produce adequate numbers of blood cells. Causes include genetic defects, viruses, irradiation treatment, and drug toxicity.

erythropoiesis (eh-RIH-throh-poy-EE-sis): production of red blood cells within the bone marrow.

erythropoietin (eh-RIH-throh-POY-eh-tin): a hormone produced by kidney cells that stimulates red blood cell production.

macrocytic anemia: anemia characterized by large red blood cells, as occurs in folate and vitamin B_{12} deficiency; also called **megaloblastic anemia.**

microcytic anemia: anemia characterized by small, hypochromic (pale) red blood cells, as occurs in iron deficiency.

peripheral blood smear: a blood sample spread on a glass slide and stained for analysis under a microscope. *Peripheral* refers to the use of circulating blood rather than tissue blood.

reticulocytes: immature red blood cells released into blood by bone marrow.

Reminder: *Hemolytic anemia* is the condition of having too few red blood cells as a result of erythrocyte hemolysis (breakdown of red blood cells).

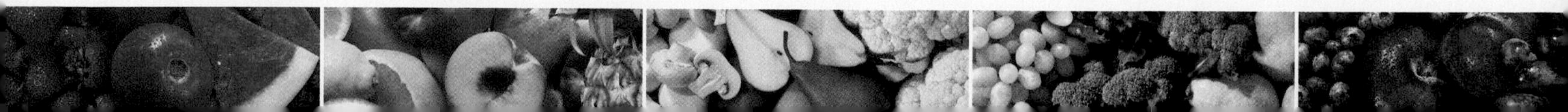

FIGURE H25-1 Erythropoiesis

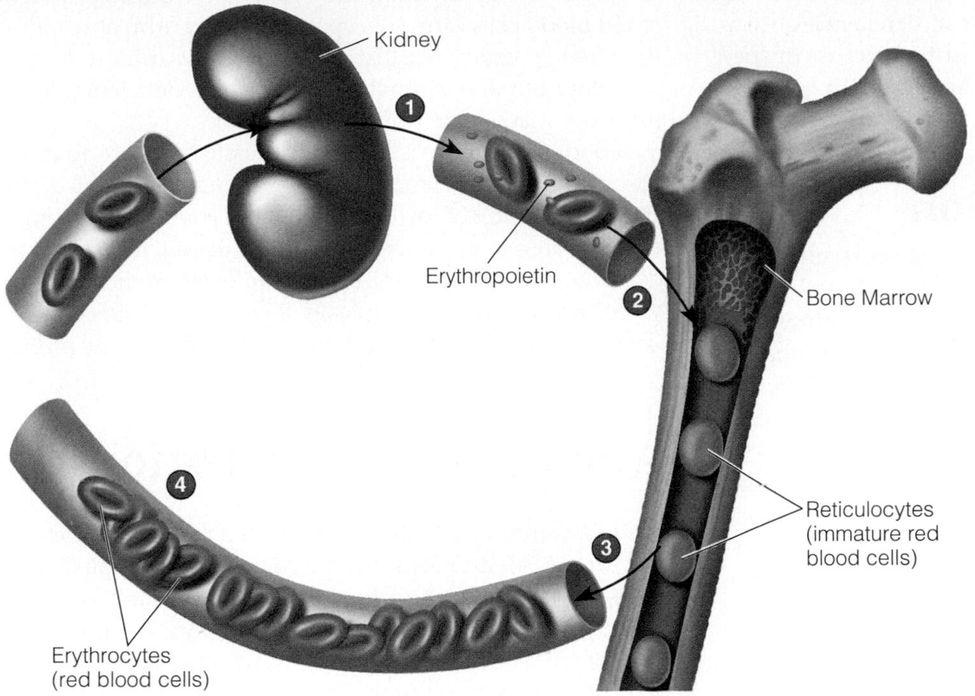
Kidney
1
Erythropoietin
2
Bone Marrow
4
3
Reticulocytes (immature red blood cells)
Erythrocytes (red blood cells)
1 When the kidneys detect reduced oxygen in blood, they secrete the hormone erythropoietin.
2 Erythropoietin stimulates erythropoiesis (red blood cell production) in the bone marrow.
3 Immature red blood cells (called reticulocytes) are released into blood.
4 Reticulocytes mature into red blood cells over a 24- to 48-hour period.

Reprinted with permission from *Human Physiology,* 5th ed., by Sherwood (Brooks/Cole, 2004), Figure 11-4, p. 395.

causes microcytic anemia. Vitamin C supports blood vessel integrity; fragile and bleeding capillaries may result from deficiency. Protein-energy malnutrition leads to anemia because red blood cell development depends on protein synthesis. Although nutrient deficiencies may result from dietary inadequacy, they may also arise during the course of illness due to effects of disease on intestinal absorption, nutrient metabolism, and nutrient losses, as described in the remaining sections.

Identifying Causes of Anemia

Identifying the cause of anemia is sometimes challenging. The results of laboratory tests provide valuable clues, although conditions such as dehydration and inflammation can influence the values. Laboratory results are especially difficult to analyze if several disturbances are present simultaneously. A **peripheral blood smear** (see the photo) is often used to study abnormalities in red blood cell shape and may reveal an underlying cause. Although anemia that develops rapidly usually indicates blood loss, gradual onset can be associated with malnutrition, chronic illness, or slow, chronic bleeding. In some cases, anemia may be a well-known consequence of disease, as when renal failure impairs the synthesis of the hormone erythropoietin.

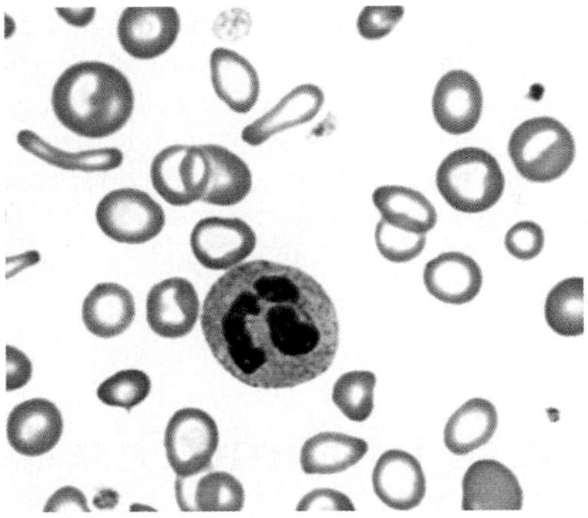

A peripheral blood smear provides information about the number and shape of blood cells.

Nutritional Anemias in Illness

There are numerous ways in which illness can lead to deficiencies of iron, folate, and vitamin B_{12}, the main causes of the nutritional anemias. Illness often leads to a reduction in food intake, as discussed throughout the clinical chapters.

Although liver reserves of iron and vitamin B_{12} may be adequate to prevent deficiencies during transient illness, reserves of folate are limited, and deficiency can develop within a few months if dietary intakes are low. If several deficiencies occur simultaneously, it may be difficult to identify the cause of anemia using standard blood tests (see Appendix E) as both macrocytic and microcytic anemia may be present.

Nutrient Malabsorption

Chapter 24 explained that malabsorption often results from disorders that damage the small intestine. Diseases like Crohn's disease and celiac disease can destroy intestinal mucosa and reduce absorption of all nutrients. Iron is primarily absorbed in the duodenum and upper jejunum, and its absorption is impaired by conditions that reduce hydrochloric acid secretion or result in surgical resection of the upper intestine. Resection of the stomach or ileum can hasten the onset of vitamin B_{12} deficiency because both organs have roles in vitamin B_{12} absorption. Recall from Chapter 10 that the stomach produces a protein called intrinsic factor that is needed for vitamin B_{12} absorption and that the ileum is the site of vitamin B_{12} absorption.

Blood Loss

Blood loss is a primary cause of iron deficiency. Slow, chronic bleeding is sometimes difficult to identify before anemia develops. Excessive bleeding can accompany coagulation disorders, often due to genetic defects, liver disease, or vitamin K deficiency. Conditions that involve the gastrointestinal tract often cause bleeding; examples include peptic ulcers, inflammatory bowel conditions, and gastrointestinal varices that develop in advanced liver disease. Frequent blood draws or surgical procedures can contribute to blood loss and result in iron deficiency.[2]

Anemia of Chronic Disease

The **anemia of chronic disease** is the most common type of anemia affecting hospitalized patients and patients with chronic illnesses.[3] It is sometimes the initial sign that chronic disease is present.[4] The anemia of chronic disease usually occurs in individuals who have chronic infections, inflammatory conditions, autoimmune disorders, or cancer. Although often a mild form of anemia, it can progress and become severe enough to require blood transfusions.[5]

The anemia of chronic disease is characterized by alterations both in the distribution of iron among tissues and in the rates of red blood cell production and destruction. As a result of the inflammatory response, macrophages in the liver, spleen, and bone marrow sequester iron, making it unavailable for erythropoiesis and hence slowing the rate of production of new red blood cells. In addition, red blood cells are destroyed more rapidly than usual, and the reduced production of red blood cells cannot keep pace. Finally, iron absorption is impaired, possibly because intestinal cells inhibit iron's release into blood. Eventually, outright iron deficiency may result from inadequate iron absorption.[6]

Blood tests help to distinguish between the anemia of chronic disease and iron-deficiency anemia (see Table H25-1). The combination of low serum iron and low total iron-binding capacity suggests the anemia of chronic disease rather than iron deficiency. In addition, serum ferritin levels are normal or elevated, whereas they are typically low in iron deficiency. Diagnosis is more complicated if both types of anemia are present.[7]

Anemia and Medication Use

Anemia is among the adverse effects that may result from medication use. Medications can alter nutrient metabolism, influence erythropoiesis and blood coagulation, and sometimes lead to increased red blood cell destruction. Because the life span of red blood cells is about 120 days, long-term use of medications is more likely to result in anemia than short-term use.

Drug-Nutrient Interactions

Table 19-4 on p. 635 listed the general ways in which drugs can alter food intake, nutrient absorption, and nutrient metabolism. As an example, a variety of medications are known to affect the absorption or metabolism of folate and lead to macrocytic anemia. For example, sulfasalazine (for ulcerative colitis) and some anticonvulsant drugs inhibit folate absorption, and methotrexate (an immunosuppressive), triamterene (a diuretic), and pyrimethamine (an antimalarial) interfere with folate metabolism.[8] If a medication is known to result in deficiency, nutrient supplementation is usually recommended as an adjunct therapy.

TABLE H25-1 Laboratory Tests for Evaluating Iron Deficiency and Anemia of Chronic Disease

Laboratory Test	Effect of Iron Deficiency	Effect of Chronic Disease
Red blood cell (RBC) size and number	Microcytic; reduced RBC count	Normocytic or microcytic; reduced RBC count
Serum iron	Low	Low
Serum ferritin	Low	Normal or elevated
Serum transferrin	Elevated	Low
Total iron-binding capacity	High	Low
Bone marrow iron	Low	Normal or elevated

Aplastic Anemia

Many classes of drugs are associated with **aplastic anemia,** a type of anemia that occurs when the bone marrow fails to produce adequate numbers of blood cells. Aplastic anemia can be caused by a genetic defect or may result from viral infections or exposure to toxins. The categories of drugs associated with aplastic anemia include anticonvulsants, antibiotics, antidiabetic drugs, diuretics, antithyroid drugs, and anticancer agents.[9]

Impaired Coagulation

Although anticoagulants are often prescribed specifically to reduce blood clotting, impaired coagulation is sometimes an unwanted effect and can lead to excessive blood loss. Medications can interfere with many of the steps involved in blood clotting, including platelet function, synthesis of clotting proteins, and vitamin K function. Commonly used drugs that impair coagulation include aspirin and other nonsteroidal anti-inflammatory drugs (NSAIDs), acetaminophen, cimetidine (Tagamet), ranitidine (Zantac), and thiazide diuretics.[10] Anticoagulant effects may be augmented if several of these drugs are used simultaneously. Another danger is slow, chronic bleeding that may go unnoticed until excessive blood loss has occurred.

Drug-Induced Hemolytic Anemia

Some patients may develop hemolytic anemia as a result of drug interactions with red blood cells. For example, a drug may alter the red blood cell membrane in such a way that the membrane becomes an antigen, which induces an antibody response that destroys the cell.[11] Several types of antibiotics, including penicillin and cephalosporin, may cause this type of response. Withdrawal of the drug can eventually reverse the anemia, and sometimes medications are given to suppress the immune response.

Anemia is a symptom associated with many diseases and disease treatments. When it occurs during illness, its causes must be investigated before it leads to complications that worsen prognosis. The medical history, blood tests, and peripheral blood smears may all help to determine the reasons why anemia has developed.

REFERENCES

1. K. S. Zuckerman, Approach to the anemias, in L. Goldman and D. Ausiello, eds., *Cecil Textbook of Medicine* (Philadelphia: Saunders, 2004), pp. 963–971.
2. Zuckerman, 2004; J. E. Ansell, Cardinal manifestations of hematologic disease, anemias, and related conditions, in J. Noble and coeditors, *Textbook of Primary Care Medicine* (St. Louis, Mo: Mosby, 2001), pp. 1027–1037.
3. C. N. Roy, D. A. Weinstein, and N. D. Andrews, 2002 E. Mead Johnson Award for Research in Pediatrics lecture: The molecular biology of the anemia of chronic disease: A hypothesis, *Pediatric Research* 53 (2003): 507–512.
4. T. P. Duffy, Microcytic and hypochromic anemias, in L. Goldman and D. Ausiello, eds., *Cecil Textbook of Medicine* (Philadelphia: Saunders, 2004), pp. 1003–1008.
5. Roy, Weinstein, and Andrews, 2003.
6. Duffy, 2004; Roy, Weinstein, and Andrews, 2003; D. A. Weinstein and coauthors, Inappropriate expression of hepcidin is associated with iron refractory anemia: Implications for the anemia of chronic disease, *Blood* 100 (2002): 3776–3781.
7. Roy, Weinstein, and Andrews, 2003.
8. S. P. Stabler and R. H. Allen, Megaloblastic anemias, in L. Goldman and D. Ausiello, eds., *Cecil Textbook of Medicine* (Philadelphia: Saunders, 2004), pp. 1050–1057.
9. H. Castro-Malaspina and R. J. O'Reilly, Aplastic anemia and related disorders, in L. Goldman and D. Ausiello, eds., *Cecil Textbook of Medicine,* (Philadelphia: Saunders, 2004), pp. 1044–1050.
10. M. Shuman, Hemorrhagic disorders: Abnormalities of platelet and vascular function, in L. Goldman and D. Ausiello, eds., *Cecil Textbook of Medicine* (Philadelphia: Saunders, 2004), pp. 1060–1069.
11. A. D. Schreiber, Autoimmune and intravascular hemolytic anemias, in L. Goldman and D. Ausiello, eds., *Cecil Textbook of Medicine* (Philadelphia: Saunders, 2004), pp. 1013–1021.

Chapter 26

Nutrition and Diabetes Mellitus

Chapter Outline

Available Online

http://nutrition.wadsworth.com/uncn7

Student Practice Test

Glossary Terms

Nutrition on the Net

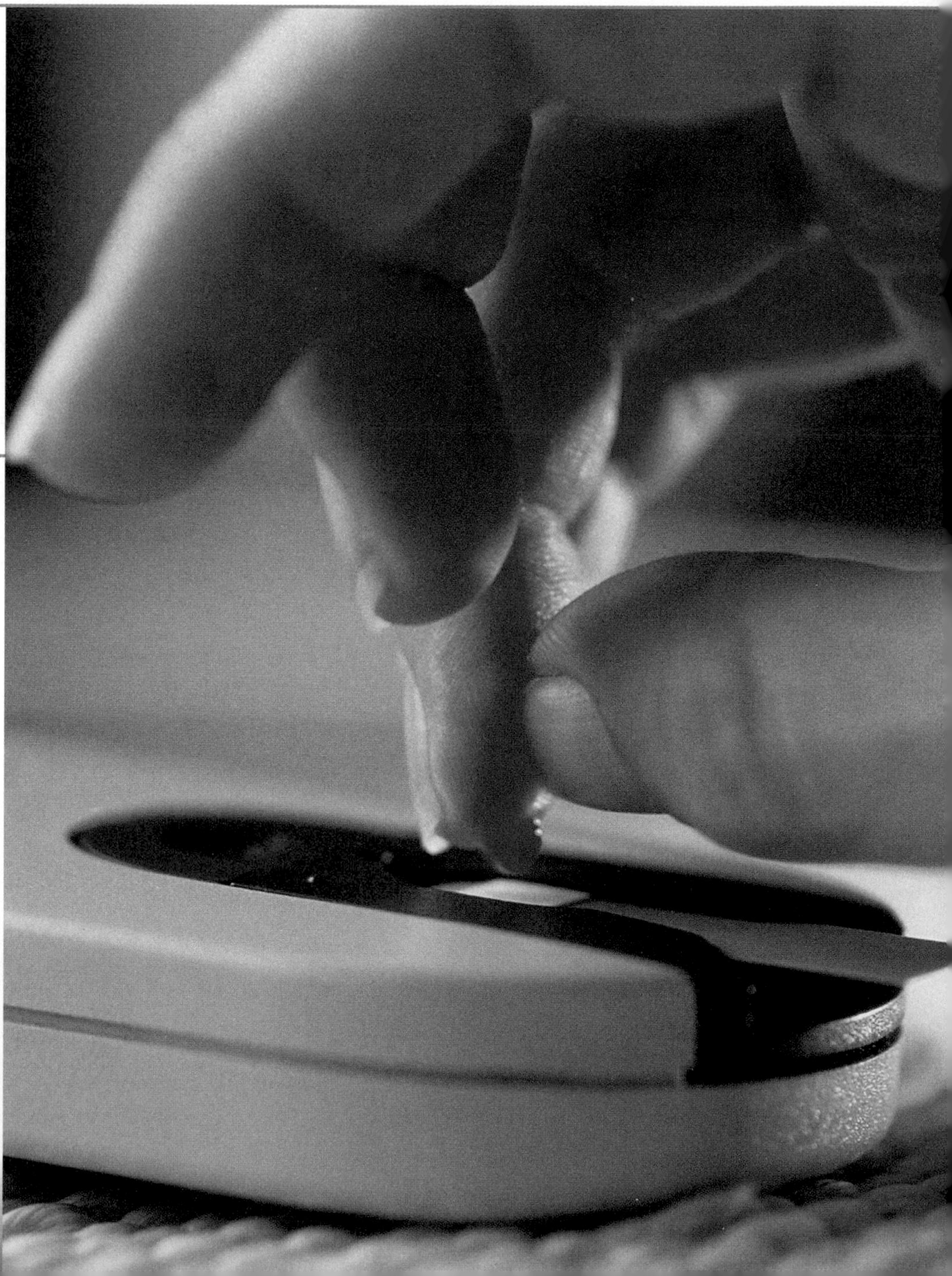

Nutrition in the Professional Setting

Diabetes is often a silent disease. The dangers from high blood glucose can take decades to develop, causing some people to ignore their condition and disregard treatment. If complications develop, there is no way to correct the damage to heart, kidneys, nerves, and eyes that may occur. Because most diabetes care requires self-management, the challenge for health practitioners is to motivate patients to make the dietary and lifestyle changes that are needed. The good news is that careful management allows individuals with diabetes to live long, healthy, and productive lives.

The incidence of **diabetes mellitus**■ is steadily increasing in the United States and in many other countries (see Figure 26-1). It now affects an estimated 6.5 percent of the U.S. population, or more than 17 million people.[1] About one-third of persons with diabetes do not know that they have it; this lack of awareness is especially dangerous because damage to the body often occurs before symptoms develop. Diabetes ranks sixth among the leading causes of death in the United States. It also underlies or contributes to several other major diseases, including heart disease and kidney failure, which are discussed in the two chapters that follow.

■ An unrelated condition with a similar name is *diabetes insipidus,* a pituitary disorder that causes a deficiency of antidiuretic hormone (ADH).

■ *Reminder: Insulin* is a pancreatic hormone that regulates blood glucose concentrations. Its many metabolic actions are countered mainly by the hormone glucagon (see pp. 116–117).

diabetes (DYE-ah-BEE-teez) **mellitus:** a group of metabolic disorders characterized by hyperglycemia and disordered insulin metabolism.
- **diabetes** = siphon (in Greek), referring to the excessive passage of urine that is characteristic of untreated diabetes
- **mellitus** = honey-sweet

Overview of Diabetes Mellitus

The term *diabetes mellitus* refers to a group of disorders characterized by elevated blood glucose concentrations and disordered insulin metabolism. A person with diabetes is unable to secrete sufficient insulin, use insulin effectively, or both.■ Normally, insulin secretions increase after food is ingested and enable muscle and

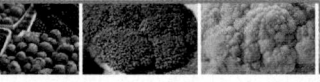

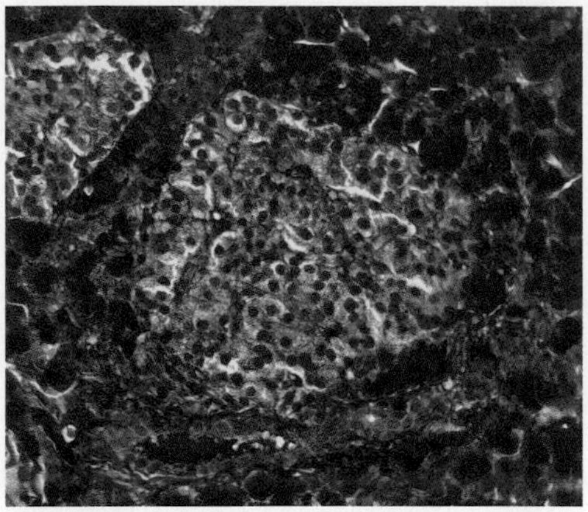

Cross sections of the pancreas reveal distinct areas known as the islets of Langerhans, which contain the alpha cells that produce glucagon and the beta cells that produce insulin.

adipose cells to take up newly absorbed glucose from the blood. Insulin is also secreted between meals in smaller amounts to restrain the glucose-raising actions of glucagon, a hormone that promotes glucose production in the liver (gluconeogenesis) and the breakdown of liver glycogen. In diabetes, insulin secretion may be impaired, and cells that are normally responsive to insulin may become resistant to its effects. This leads to unrestrained glucose production in the liver and abnormal responses to insulin by muscle, adipose, and liver cells. The result is **hyperglycemia,** a marked elevation in blood glucose levels■ that can ultimately cause damage to blood vessels, nerves, and tissues.

■ Normal fasting plasma glucose levels are approximately 74 to 106 mg/dL.

Symptoms of Diabetes

Symptoms of diabetes■ are often related to the degree of hyperglycemia. When the plasma glucose concentration is higher than about 200 milligrams per deciliter (mg/dL), it exceeds the **renal threshold;** that is, the kidneys are unable to reabsorb all of the glucose back into the blood, and some glucose spills into the urine **(glycosuria).** High glucose levels in urine draw additional water out of the blood, increasing the amount of urine produced. Thus the symptoms that arise in diabetes typically include frequent urination **(polyuria),** dehydration, and increased thirst **(polydipsia).** Another potential consequence of hyperglycemia is blurred vision, due to the exposure of eye tissues to hyperosmolar fluids. Increased infections are also common in diabetes and may be due to hyperglycemia or impaired circulation or immune function. Some people experience weight loss and increased appetite **(polyphagia)** as a result of the nutrient depletion that occurs when insulin is deficient. In some cases, constant fatigue is the only symptom and may be related to altered fuel metabolism, dehydration, or other effects of the disease.

■ Symptoms of diabetes mellitus include:
- Frequent urination (polyuria).
- Dehydration, dry mouth.
- Increased thirst (polydipsia).
- Blurred vision.
- Increased infections.
- Weight loss.
- Increased hunger (polyphagia).
- Fatigue.

Diagnosis of Diabetes

The diagnosis of diabetes is based primarily on plasma glucose levels, which can be measured under fasting conditions or at random times during the day. In some cases, an **oral glucose tolerance test** is given in which the patient ingests a 50- or 75-gram glucose load and plasma glucose is measured at one or more time intervals following the glucose ingestion. The presence of symptoms helps to confirm the diagnosis. The following criteria are currently used to diagnose diabetes:

- The plasma glucose concentration of a blood sample obtained at a random time during the day (without regard to food intake) is 200 mg/dL or greater, and classic symptoms of diabetes (such as polyuria, polydipsia, and unexplained weight loss) are present.
- The plasma glucose concentration is 126 mg/dL or greater after a fast of at least eight hours.
- The plasma glucose concentration measured two hours after a 75-gram glucose load is 200 mg/dL or greater.
- Diagnosis is confirmed if a subsequent test yields similar results.

The term **prediabetes** is used to classify blood glucose levels that are between normal and diabetic, that is, between 100 and 125 mg/dL when fasting or between 140 and 200 mg/dL when measured two hours after a 75-gram glucose load. A person with prediabetes is at risk of developing diabetes and cardiovascular diseases.[2]

hyperglycemia: elevated blood glucose concentrations.

renal threshold: blood concentration of a substance that exceeds the kidneys' capacity for reabsorption and leads to appearance of the substance in urine.

glycosuria (GLY-koh-SOOR-ee-ah): an abnormal amount of glucose in urine.

polyuria (pol-lee-YOOR-ee-ah): excessive urine secretion.

polydipsia (pol-lee-DIP-see-ah): excessive thirst.

polyphagia (pol-lee-FAY-jee-ah): excessive appetite or eating.

oral glucose tolerance test: a test that evaluates a person's ability to tolerate a glucose load. A common protocol for diabetes diagnosis is ingestion of a 75 g glucose load followed by measurement of plasma glucose after a two-hour interval.

prediabetes: condition in which blood glucose levels are higher than normal but not high enough to be diagnosed as diabetes; considered a major risk factor for future diabetes and cardiovascular diseases. Also called **impaired glucose tolerance.**

Types of Diabetes

Table 26-1 shows the distinguishing features of the two main types of diabetes, type 1 and type 2 diabetes. Pregnancy can cause abnormal glucose tolerance and the condition known as gestational diabetes, which often resolves after pregnancy but is a risk factor for development of type 2 diabetes (see Chapter 14). Diabetes can also be caused by medical conditions that either damage the pancreas or interfere with insulin function.

Type 1 Diabetes **Type 1 diabetes** accounts for about 5 to 10 percent of diabetes cases. It is usually caused by **autoimmune** destruction of the pancreatic beta cells, which reduces the amount of insulin that can be produced and secreted. By the time type 1 diabetes is diagnosed, the damage to the beta cells has usually reached a point where insulin must be supplied exogenously. Although the trigger for the autoimmune attack is unknown, both inherited and environmental factors are believed to be involved.[3] Individuals who develop type 1 diabetes are at increased risk of developing other autoimmune disorders.

Type 1 diabetes usually occurs during childhood or adolescence, and symptoms may appear abruptly in previously healthy children.[4] Classic symptoms are frequent urination, weight loss, and increased thirst. **Ketoacidosis**—acidosis due to excessive production of ketone bodies—is sometimes the first sign of disease.[5] Disease onset tends to be more gradual in individuals who develop type 1 diabetes in later years. Blood tests that detect antibodies to insulin, pancreatic islet cells, and pancreatic enzymes can confirm the diagnosis and help to predict development of the disease in first-degree relatives.

Type 2 Diabetes **Type 2 diabetes** is the most prevalent form of diabetes, accounting for 90 to 95 percent of cases, and is frequently asymptomatic. The primary defect in type 2 diabetes is **insulin resistance,** a reduced sensitivity to insulin in muscle, adipose, and liver cells. To compensate, the pancreas secretes larger amounts of insulin, and plasma insulin concentrations can rise to abnormally high levels (hyperinsulinemia). Over time, the pancreas becomes less able to compensate for the cells' reduced sensitivity to insulin, and hyperglycemia worsens. The high demand for insulin can eventually exhaust the beta cells of the pancreas and lead to impaired insulin secretion and reduced plasma insulin concentrations. Type 2 diabetes is therefore associated both with insulin resistance and with relative insulin deficiency; that is, the amount of insulin is insufficient to compensate for its diminished effect in cells.

Although the actual causes of type 2 diabetes are unknown, the risk is substantially increased by obesity (especially abdominal obesity), aging, and physical inactivity. An estimated 80 to 90 percent of individuals with type 2 diabetes are obese, and obesity itself can directly cause some degree of insulin resistance.[6] The prevalence of type 2 diabetes increases with age and approaches 20 percent in persons between 65 and 74 years of age; many of these cases, however, remain undiagnosed.[7] Inherited factors strongly influence risk, and type 2 diabetes is more common in certain ethnic populations, including Native Americans, Hispanic Americans, Mexican Americans, African Americans, Asian Americans, and Pacific Islanders.

Although most cases of type 2 diabetes are diagnosed in individuals over 45 years old, children and adolescents who are overweight or have a family history of diabetes are at increased risk. Type 2 diabetes is often asymptomatic, so it is generally detected in children only when high-risk groups are screened for the disease. For example, when 167 obese children of different ethnic groups were screened, prediabetes was detected in 25 percent of children between 4 and 10 years of age and in 21 percent of adolescents between 11 and 18 years of age.[8] Among the Pima Indians in Arizona, a population with one of the highest rates of type 2 diabetes in the world, overt type 2 diabetes was reported in 2.2 percent of 10- to 14-year-old children and in 5 percent of 15- to 19-year-old teens.[9] Routine screening and prevention programs that target food intake and activity patterns can be important safeguards for preventing diabetes in children at risk.

Gestational Diabetes Approximately 7 percent of women who do not have diabetes develop gestational diabetes during pregnancy.[10] Risk is highest in women who have a family history of diabetes, are of certain ethnic groups (listed earlier), are obese, or have given birth to infants weighing over 9 pounds. To ensure that

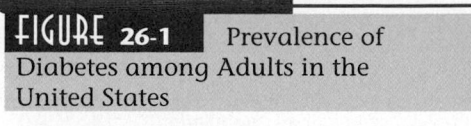

FIGURE 26-1 Prevalence of Diabetes among Adults in the United States

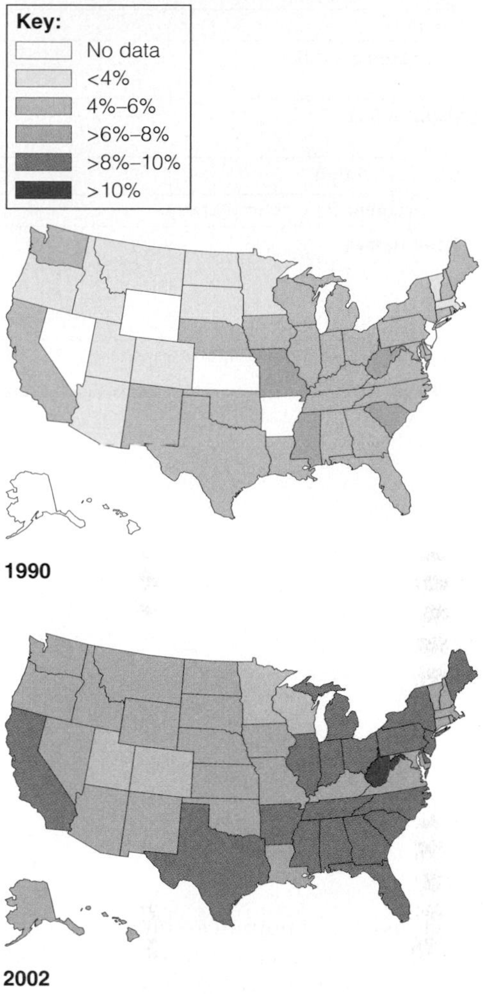
Key:
No data
<4%
4%–6%
>6%–8%
>8%–10%
>10%
1990
2002

SOURCE: Centers for Disease Control and Prevention, www.cdc.gov/nccdphp/aag/aag_ddt.htm.

type 1 diabetes: the type of diabetes that accounts for 5 to 10% of diabetes cases and usually results from autoimmune destruction of pancreatic beta cells. In this type of diabetes, the pancreas produces little or no insulin.

autoimmune: immune response directed against the body's own tissues.
- **auto** = self

ketoacidosis: lowering of pH in blood and tissues due to excessive ketone body production.

type 2 diabetes: the type of diabetes that accounts for 90 to 95% of diabetes cases and usually results from insulin resistance coupled with insufficient insulin secretion. Obesity is present in 80 to 90% of cases.

insulin resistance: reduced sensitivity to insulin in muscle, adipose, and liver cells.

TABLE 26-1 Features of Type 1 and Type 2 Diabetes

	Type 1	Type 2
Prevalence in diabetic population	5 to 10% of cases	90 to 95% of cases
Age of onset	<30 years	>45 years[a]
Associated conditions	Autoimmune diseases, viral infection, inherited factors	Obesity, aging, inherited factors
Major defect	Destruction of pancreatic beta cells; insulin deficiency	Insulin resistance; insulin deficiency (relative to needs)
Insulin secretion	Little or none	Varies; may be normal, increased, or decreased
Requirement for insulin therapy	Always	Sometimes
Other names	Juvenile-onset diabetes	Adult-onset diabetes
	Insulin-dependent diabetes mellitus (IDDM)	Noninsulin-dependent diabetes mellitus (NIDDM)
	Ketosis-prone diabetes	Ketosis-resistant diabetes

[a] Incidence of type 2 diabetes is increasing in children and adolescents; in over 90 percent of these cases, it is associated with overweight or obesity and a family history of type 2 diabetes.

the problems of gestational diabetes are dealt with promptly, physicians routinely test all women between 24 and 28 weeks of gestation. In high-risk women, screening should begin prior to pregnancy or soon after conception. Even mild hyperglycemia can have serious adverse effects on a developing fetus and may lead to complications during pregnancy.[11]

Other Types of Diabetes Diabetes may result from numerous factors that interfere with glucose or insulin sensitivity or pancreatic function. It may be a consequence of genetic defects, diseases that damage the pancreas (including pancreatitis and cystic fibrosis), hormonal imbalances, drug or chemical toxicity, and certain infections.

Acute Complications of Diabetes

Untreated diabetes can result in life-threatening complications. Hyperglycemia has direct effects on blood volume and electrolyte balance, and insulin deficiency can cause severe disturbances in energy metabolism. In treated diabetes, hypoglycemia is a possible complication and develops as a result of inappropriate disease management.

Diabetic Ketoacidosis (Type 1 Diabetes) A severe lack of insulin causes diabetic ketoacidosis. The condition usually develops quickly, within hours or a few days. Without insulin, there is unrestrained breakdown of triglycerides stored in adipose tissue, causing excessive release of fatty acids into the bloodstream. The liver removes these fatty acids from the circulation. The accumulation of fatty acids in the liver together with the lack of insulin results in increased ketone body production (ketosis).■ Ketone bodies, which are acidic, can reach extremely high levels in the bloodstream (ketoacidosis) and spill into the urine **(ketonuria).** Blood pH typically falls below 7.3.■ Blood glucose concentrations are variable and usually exceed 250 mg/dL; in severe cases, they may rise above 1000 mg/dL.[12] The main features of diabetic ketoacidosis thus include ketosis, acidosis, and hyperglycemia.

The clinical manifestations of ketoacidosis include symptoms of acidosis and dehydration. Acidosis is partially corrected by exhalation of carbon dioxide,■ so hyperventilation or deep breathing is characteristic. The loss of fluids (polyuria) that accompanies hyperglycemia lowers blood volume and blood pressure and depletes electrolytes. Ketone accumulation is sometimes evident by a fruity odor on a person's breath **(acetone breath).** Feelings of lethargy or weakness and nausea and vomiting are common symptoms. Mental state may vary from alertness to comatose **(diabetic coma).**[13]■

- Ketosis—the abnormal accumulation of ketone bodies in body tissues—is described in Chapter 7 (see pp. 236–237).
- Normal blood pH is from 7.35 to 7.45.
- Bicarbonate is a major buffer in the bloodstream that can correct acidosis. Acid (H^+) and bicarbonate (HCO_3^-) combine to form carbonic acid (H_2CO_3), which breaks down to water (H_2O) and carbon dioxide (CO_2). The carbon dioxide is subsequently exhaled.
- Diabetic coma was a frequent cause of death before insulin was routinely used to manage diabetes.

ketonuria (kee-toe-NOOR-ee-a): the presence of ketone bodies in urine.

acetone breath: distinctive fruity odor on the breath of a person experiencing ketosis.

diabetic coma: a coma that occurs in uncontrolled diabetes; may be due to diabetic ketoacidosis, the hyperosmolar hyperglycemic state, or excessive doses of insulin or certain antidiabetic drugs.

Diabetic ketoacidosis is the earliest sign leading to diagnosis of type 1 diabetes in about 20 to 25 percent of cases and is sometimes a contributing cause of death.[14] It may result from inappropriate treatment (such as missed insulin injections), concurrent illness or infection, alcohol abuse, and other physiological stressors.[15] Although diabetic ketoacidosis may occur in type 2 diabetes as well, it develops only rarely because even relatively low insulin concentrations can prevent excessive production of ketone bodies. When ketosis occurs in type 2 diabetes, it is usually associated with increased metabolic stress due to infection or serious illness.

Hyperosmolar Hyperglycemic State (Type 2 Diabetes) The **hyperosmolar hyperglycemic state** is a condition of severe hyperglycemia that usually develops in the absence of significant ketosis.■ Unlike diabetic ketoacidosis, it often evolves slowly, over several days or weeks, and is most often associated with type 2 diabetes. Blood glucose levels typically exceed 600 mg/dL and may rise above 2000 mg/dL. The extreme hyperglycemia causes substantial fluid losses, leading to blood volume depletion and electrolyte imbalances. Blood plasma may become so hyperosmolar as to cause neurological abnormalities, such as abnormal reflexes, motor impairments, reduced verbal ability, and seizures; about 10 percent of patients lapse into coma.[16]

■ Ketosis is present in about half of patients with the condition, but it is much milder than in diabetic ketoacidosis.

The hyperosmolar hyperglycemic state is sometimes the first sign of diabetes in older persons. It is usually precipitated by infection, illness, or a drug treatment that impairs insulin action or secretion. The condition often develops because patients are unable to recognize thirst or adequately replace fluid losses due to age, illness, sedation, or incapacity.[17]

Hypoglycemia Hypoglycemia, or low blood glucose, arises from the inappropriate management of diabetes rather than from the disease itself. It can result from using excessive amounts of insulin or antidiabetic drugs, prolonged exercise, skipped or delayed meals, inadequate food intake, or consuming alcohol without food. Hypoglycemia most often occurs in type 1 diabetes and accounts for about 3 to 4 percent of deaths in insulin-treated patients.[18]

Symptoms of hypoglycemia include hunger, sweating, shakiness, heart palpitations, slurred speech, and confusion. Mental confusion may prevent a person from recognizing the problem and taking such corrective action as ingesting glucose tablets, juice, or candy. If hypoglycemia occurs during the night, patients may be completely unaware of its presence. Prolonged hypoglycemia sometimes results in permanent brain damage.

Chronic Complications of Diabetes

Prolonged exposure to high glucose concentrations destroys cells and tissues. Glucose and glucose fragments react with proteins to form **advanced glycation end products (AGEs),** compounds that accumulate and cause damage within cells and blood vessels. Excessive glucose also promotes the production and accumulation of sorbitol, which contributes to cell injury. Complications typically affect the large blood vessels **(macrovascular complications),** arterioles and capillaries **(microvascular complications),** and nervous system **(neuropathy).**

Macrovascular Complications The accumulation of AGEs accelerates the development of atherosclerosis, which affects the coronary arteries and arteries in the limbs. Cardiovascular diseases are the leading cause of death in people with diabetes, accounting for 75 percent of deaths.[19] Type 2 diabetes is often accompanied by multiple risk factors for coronary heart disease, including hypertension, abnormal blood lipids, and obesity.■ People with diabetes also have increased tendencies for thrombosis (blood clot formation) and abnormal ventricle function, both of which can worsen the clinical course of heart disease.[20]

■ People with type 2 diabetes frequently develop the **metabolic syndrome**, a cluster of symptoms associated with insulin resistance (including hyperglycemia, hypertension, and altered blood lipids) that substantially increase cardiovascular disease risk (see Highlight 26).

Impaired blood flow in the arteries of limbs increases the risk of **claudication** (pain while walking) and contributes to the development of foot ulcers. Left

hyperosmolar hyperglycemic state: extreme hyperglycemia that is associated with hyperosmolar blood, dehydration, and altered mental status; formerly called **hyperglycemic hyperosmolar nonketotic coma.**

advanced glycation end products (AGEs): compounds formed when glucose or glucose fragments combine with proteins. AGEs can damage tissues and lead to diabetic complications.

macrovascular complications: disorders that affect the large blood vessels, including cardiovascular diseases and peripheral vascular disease.

microvascular complications: disorders that affect the small blood vessels and capillaries, including retinal damage and kidney disease.

neuropathy: disorders affecting the nervous system.

claudication: pain in the legs while walking; usually due to an inadequate supply of blood to muscles.

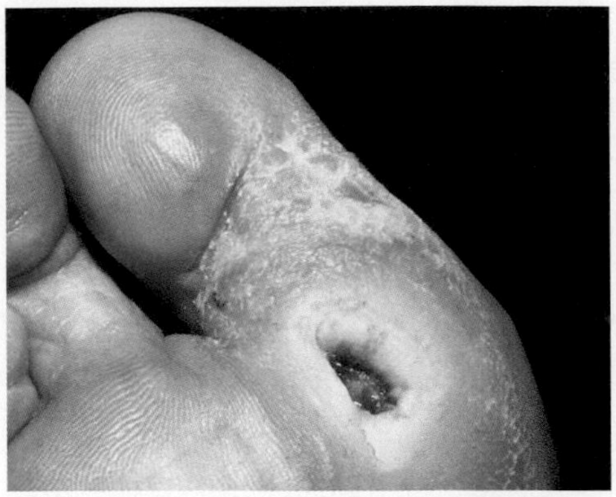

© SPL/Photo Researchers, Inc.

Foot ulcers are a common complication of diabetes because blood circulation is impaired, which slows healing, and nerve damage dampens foot pain, delaying recognition and treatment of cuts and bruises.

untreated, foot ulcers can lead to **gangrene,** and some patients require foot amputation, a major cause of disability in diabetes. About 15 to 20 percent of those with diabetes are hospitalized with foot complications during the course of illness.[21]

Microvascular Complications Damage to small blood vessels in the retina leads to **diabetic retinopathy,** which can impair vision and cause blindness in patients with either type 1 or type 2 diabetes. Retinal damage usually occurs after an individual has had diabetes for many years; for example, 95 percent of persons with type 1 diabetes develop retinopathy by 15 years after diagnosis.[22] Retinopathy progresses most rapidly when diabetes is poorly controlled, and intensive management substantially reduces the risk.[23]

Diabetic nephropathy, a disorder affecting the small blood vessels (glomeruli) of the kidneys, frequently accompanies the later stages of type 1 and type 2 diabetes. Renal failure is a possible consequence and occurs in about 30 to 35 percent of patients with type 1 diabetes. As with retinopathy, intensive diabetes management can help slow the progression of kidney damage.[24]

Diabetic Neuropathy **Diabetic neuropathy,** or nerve degeneration, occurs in about 50 percent of diabetes cases. The extent of nerve damage depends on the severity and duration of hyperglycemia. Clinical effects of neuropathy vary and may be experienced as pain or burning, numbness and tingling in the hands and feet, or loss of sensation. Pain and cramping, especially in the legs, are often severe during the night and may interrupt sleep. Neuropathy can contribute to foot ulcers because cuts and bruises may go unnoticed until wounds are severe. Other manifestations of neuropathy include sweating abnormalities, sexual dysfunction, constipation, and delayed stomach emptying **(gastroparesis).**[25]

IN SUMMARY Diabetes mellitus is a chronic condition characterized by inadequate insulin secretion or impaired insulin action. In type 1 diabetes, the pancreas secretes little or no insulin, and persons with the disease require insulin therapy. Type 2 diabetes is associated with insulin resistance, and disease risk is increased by obesity, aging, and physical inactivity. Acute complications of diabetes result from persistent hyperglycemia coupled with other metabolic abnormalities. In diabetic ketoacidosis, which is more common in type 1 diabetes, hyperglycemia is accompanied by ketosis and acidosis. The hyperosmolar hyperglycemic state, usually a consequence of type 2 diabetes, is associated with severe hyperglycemia and blood volume depletion and may lead to mental impairment and coma. Chronic complications of diabetes include macrovascular disorders like cardiovascular diseases and peripheral vascular disease, microvascular conditions like retinopathy and nephropathy, and diabetic neuropathy.

Treatment of Diabetes Mellitus

Diabetes is a chronic and progressive illness that can cause long-term complications and therefore requires lifelong treatment. Management of blood glucose levels is a delicate balancing act that involves meal planning, proper timing of medications, and physical exercise. Individuals with type 1 diabetes require insulin therapy for survival. Type 2 diabetes is initially treated with diet therapy and exercise, but most patients are eventually treated with oral medications or insulin. Frequent adjustments in treatment are usually necessary to establish good glycemic control. Diabetes management becomes even more difficult once complications develop. Although the health care team must determine an appropriate therapy, an individual with diabetes ultimately assumes much of the responsibility for treatment and therefore requires self-management education.

gangrene: death of tissue due to a deficient blood supply and/or infection.

diabetic retinopathy: retinal damage associated with diabetes.

diabetic nephropathy: kidney damage associated with diabetes.

diabetic neuropathy: nerve degeneration associated with diabetes.

gastroparesis: delayed stomach emptying.

Treatment Goals

The main goal of diabetes treatment is to maintain blood glucose levels within a desirable range to prevent or reduce the risk of complications. In addition, maintaining healthy blood lipid concentrations lowers the risks of developing cardiovascular and peripheral vascular diseases, controlling blood pressure reduces the risk of cardiovascular disease and prevents nephropathy, and managing weight improves insulin resistance. Dietary and lifestyle modifications that support good health are also incorporated into a treatment plan.

Benefits of Intensive Treatment For decades, clinicians assumed that reducing hyperglycemia would help to prevent diabetes complications, and several landmark research studies conducted in the 1980s and 1990s confirmed that keeping blood glucose levels as close to normal as possible offers clear advantages. The Diabetes Control and Complications Trial (DCCT) was a multicenter trial that tested whether *intensive* treatment of diabetes would decrease the frequency and severity of microvascular and neurological complications.[26] In this study, 1441 persons with type 1 diabetes were randomly assigned to receive either conventional or intensive therapy (as summarized in Table 26-2) and were followed for an average of 6.5 years. The study showed that those undergoing intensive therapy had delayed onset and reduced progression of retinopathy, nephropathy, and neuropathy. However, they also experienced increased incidences of severe hypoglycemia and gained more weight. Another trial, the United Kingdom Prospective Diabetes Study, suggested similar advantages to using intensive treatment in type 2 diabetes.[27] The results of these and several follow-up studies have convinced diabetes care providers that attaining near-normal glucose levels should be a fundamental objective of all diabetes treatment plans.

Evaluating Diabetes Treatment The effectiveness of diabetes treatment is largely evaluated by monitoring **glycemic** status. Good glycemic control requires frequent home monitoring of blood glucose using a glucose meter, referred to as **self-monitoring of blood glucose (SMBG).** Glucose testing provides valuable feedback when the patient adjusts food intake, medications, and physical activity and is helpful for preventing hypoglycemia. Ideally, patients with type 1 diabetes should monitor blood glucose three or more times daily—more frequently when therapy is adjusted. Self-monitoring of blood glucose is also useful in type 2 diabetes, although the recommended frequency depends on the specific needs of individual patients.[28]

Health care providers periodically evaluate long-term glycemic control by measuring **glycated hemoglobin** (abbreviated **HbA_{1c}**). The glucose in blood freely enters red blood cells and attaches to hemoglobin molecules in direct proportion to the amount of glucose present. Because the life span of red blood cells averages 120 days, the percentage of HbA_{1c} is a measure of glycemic control during the preceding two to three months. In people without diabetes, HbA_{1c} is less than 6 percent

glycemic: pertaining to blood glucose.

self-monitoring of blood glucose (SMBG): home monitoring of blood glucose levels using a glucose meter.

glycated hemoglobin (HbA_{1c}): hemoglobin molecules to which glucose is attached. The percentage of such molecules is used to evaluate long-term glycemic control. Also called **glycosylated hemoglobin.**

TABLE 26-2 Comparison of Conventional and Intensive Therapies for Diabetes

	Conventional Therapy	Intensive Therapy
Blood glucose monitoring	Monitored daily	Monitored at least 4 times daily
Insulin therapy	1–2 daily injections; no daily adjustments	3 or more daily injections or external insulin pump; dosage adjusted according to results of glucose monitoring and expected carbohydrate intake
Frequency of medical examinations	Every 3 months	Monthly, plus frequent telephone contact
Advantages	Fewer incidences of severe hypoglycemia; less weight gain	Delayed progression of retinopathy, nephropathy, and neuropathy
Disadvantages	More rapid progression of retinopathy, nephropathy, and neuropathy	2- to 3-fold increase in severe hypoglycemia; weight gain; increased risk of becoming overweight

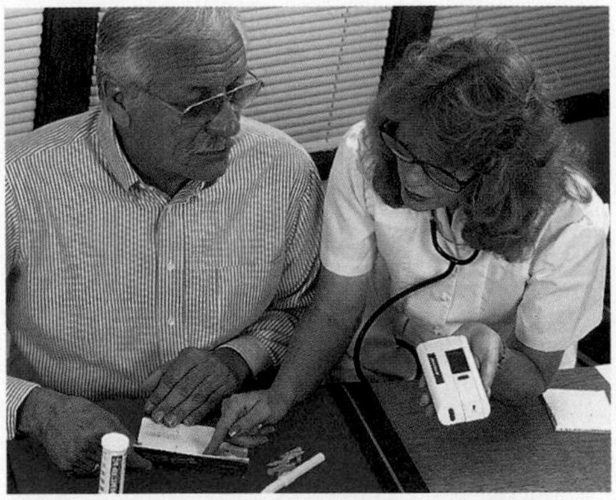

Self-monitoring of blood glucose can help persons with diabetes learn how to maintain blood glucose levels in a desirable range.

■ The small quantities of urinary protein lost during the early stages of diabetic nephropathy are referred to as **microalbuminuria.**

of total hemoglobin. The goal of diabetes treatment is an HbA_{1c} value under 7 percent, but it is often markedly higher in people who are not treated intensively.[29]

Ketone testing is used to check for the development of ketoacidosis if symptoms are present or if risk has increased due to acute illness, stress, or pregnancy. Both blood and urine tests are available for home use, although blood tests are currently more reliable. Ketone testing is most useful for patients who have type 1 diabetes or gestational diabetes.[30]

Individuals with diabetes are routinely monitored for signs of long-term complications. Blood pressure is measured at each checkup. Lipid screening is suggested annually for most adult patients. Routine checks for urinary protein **(albuminuria)** help to determine if nephropathy is present.■ Physical examinations generally screen for signs of retinopathy, neuropathy, and foot problems.[31]

Diabetes Self-Management Education Newly diagnosed patients and their families have much to learn about diabetes and its management. Diabetes education provides an individual with the knowledge and skills necessary to implement treatment. The primary instructor is often a **Certified Diabetes Educator (CDE),** a health care professional who has specialized knowledge about diabetes treatment and the health education process. To manage their diabetes, patients need to learn about appropriate meal planning, medication administration, blood glucose monitoring, weight management, appropriate physical activity, and prevention of complications.

Medical Nutrition Therapy: Nutrient Recommendations

Medical nutrition therapy has a considerable effect on diabetes outcome, as the appropriate dietary choices can improve blood glucose levels and slow the progression of diabetic complications. As always, the nutrition care plan must take personal preferences and lifestyle habits into account. Dietary intakes need to be modified to accommodate growth, lifestyle changes, aging, or the development of complications. Although it is important that all members of the diabetes care team understand the principles of dietary treatment, medical nutrition therapy should be designed and implemented by a skilled registered dietitian.[32]

This section presents the nutrient and energy recommendations for diabetes. A later section describes meal-planning strategies.

Dietary Carbohydrates in Diabetes Treatment Carbohydrate intake is the main influence on blood glucose levels after meals. The total amount of carbohydrate in a meal is more important than the type of carbohydrate consumed; in other words, the more grams of carbohydrate ingested, the greater the glycemic response.[33] The carbohydrate recommendation is based in part on the person's metabolic needs (that is, the type of diabetes or degree of glucose tolerance) and individual preferences. In general, it is recommended that 60 to 70 percent of energy intake should derive from a combination of carbohydrate and monounsaturated fat,[34] suggesting a carbohydrate intake equivalent to about 50 percent of total kcalories.[35]

As discussed in Chapter 4, foods that contain carbohydrate have different effects on blood glucose levels (see pp. 118–119). For example, a portion of white rice may cause blood glucose to rise considerably more than a similar portion of barley (review Figure 4-13 on p. 119). The glycemic response to foods is influenced by a number of factors, including how a food was processed or prepared, its fiber content, the other foods included in a meal, and individual tolerances.[36] Even more confusing, multiple tests of a single type of food sometimes yield a wide range of glycemic values.[37] Studies have not demonstrated consistent improvements in glycemic control when low-glycemic diets were consumed; therefore, the use of the glycemic index is not routinely recommended in diabetes treatment.[38]

albuminuria: the presence of albumin (protein) in the urine, a symptom of kidney disease.

Certified Diabetes Educator (CDE): a health care professional who specializes in diabetes management education. Certification is obtained from the National Certification Board for Diabetes Educators.

However, high-fiber, whole-grain products, which have more moderate effects on blood glucose than do highly processed starchy foods, are among the foods frequently recommended for persons with diabetes.

A common misperception is that persons with diabetes need to avoid sugar and sugar-containing foods. In reality, however, table sugar (sucrose), made up of glucose and fructose, causes a lower glycemic response than starch. This is because the liver metabolizes fructose soon after absorption, thereby reducing its contribution to blood glucose following meals. Clinical studies have confirmed that sugar intakes between 10 and 17 percent of total kcalories (similar to consumption patterns in the United States) do not adversely affect glycemic control in persons with diabetes.[39] Therefore, sugar and sugary foods are not restricted in diabetes diets, although they should be counted as part of the daily carbohydrate allowance.[40] Nevertheless, dietary recommendations for the general population, which suggest choosing foods and beverages with little added sugar or kcaloric sweeteners, also pertain to people with diabetes.

Although fructose has a minimal glycemic effect, its use as an added sweetener is not recommended because excessive dietary fructose may adversely affect blood lipid levels (note that the naturally occurring fructose in fruits and vegetables does not need to be avoided).[41] Sugar alcohols (such as sorbitol and maltitol) have lower glycemic effects than glucose, fructose, or sucrose, but their use has not been found to significantly improve long-term glycemic control. Artificial sweeteners (such as aspartame, saccharin, and sucralose) contain no carbohydrate and can be safely used in place of sugar.

Fiber recommendations for diabetes are similar to those for the general population.■ Although some studies have suggested that very large amounts of fiber (50 grams or more) may improve glycemic control, the benefits have not been consistent across studies, and many persons may have difficulty tolerating such large amounts of fiber.

■ The fiber DRI for adult men and women range from 21 to 38 g. Check the DRI table on the inside front cover for specific DRI values for different age and gender groups.

Dietary Fat and Protein Recommendations As mentioned earlier, people with diabetes are at increased risk of developing cardiovascular diseases; they also tend to be more sensitive to dietary cholesterol than the general population.[42] Guidelines for dietary fat are similar to those for other persons at risk: saturated fat intake should be limited to less than 10 percent of kcalories and cholesterol intake to less than 300 milligrams daily. If an individual's LDL cholesterol levels are elevated, saturated fat should be limited to 7 percent of kcalories and cholesterol intake to 200 milligrams daily. Dietary strategies for cardiovascular disease are discussed further in Chapter 27.

Some evidence suggests that people with diabetes have higher protein requirements than the general population due to the increased protein turnover associated with hyperglycemia.[43] However, protein intakes in the United States generally range from 15 to 20 percent of total kcalories—sufficient to cover any increased needs in diabetes. Although protein intakes within this range have not been found to hasten the development of diabetic nephropathy, higher protein intakes are discouraged because they may be detrimental to kidney function.

Body Weight in Type 1 Diabetes Individuals with newly diagnosed type 1 diabetes are likely to be thin. In growing children, an important dietary concern is to provide adequate energy for normal growth and development.[44] Growth patterns and weight gain are routinely monitored to evaluate whether energy intakes are sufficient.

In some individuals, excessive weight gain is an unwanted side effect of improved glycemic control, especially in patients undergoing intensive insulin therapy. The reasons for weight gain are unclear. Insulin therapy may increase appetite or reduce metabolic rate, which tends to be abnormally high in type 1 diabetes. In addition, energy losses from glycosuria are eliminated by insulin treatment, a change that can contribute to energy excess.[45] Excessive body weight can have adverse effects on blood lipids and blood pressure, counteracting some of the benefits

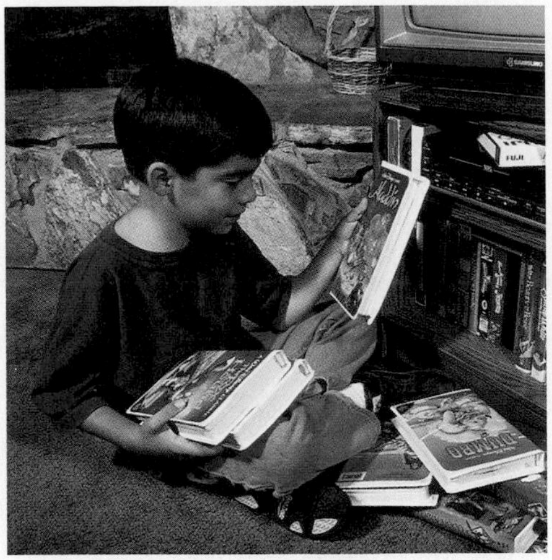

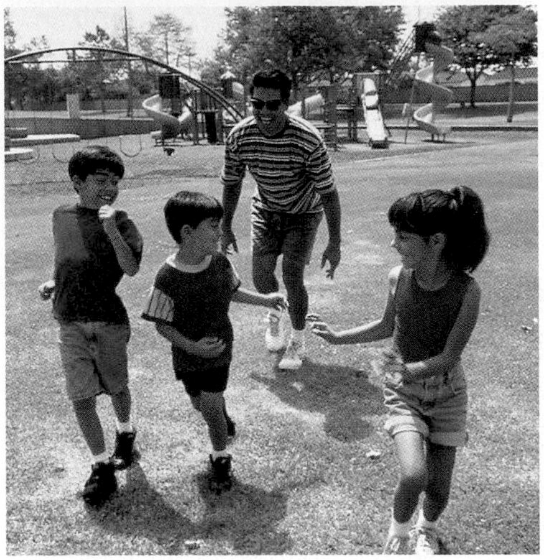

© Tony Freeman/PhotoEdit (both)

A diabetes care plan for a child must be flexible enough to accommodate his or her activity levels and appetite, which can vary considerably from day to day.

■ One drink is equivalent to 12 oz of beer, 5 oz of wine, 10 oz of wine cooler, or 1.5 oz of distilled liquor (80 proof whiskey, scotch, rum, or vodka).

associated with glycemic control.[46] Although efforts should be made to prevent excessive weight gain, concerns about weight should not discourage use of intensive therapy, which is associated with longer life expectancy and fewer complications than occur with conventional therapy. It should also be noted that people with type 1 diabetes are less likely to be overweight than the general population.[47]

Body Weight in Type 2 Diabetes Because excessive body fat can worsen insulin resistance, weight loss is often recommended for people who are overweight or obese. Even moderate weight loss (10 to 20 pounds) can improve glycemic control, blood lipid levels, and blood pressure.[48] Weight loss is most beneficial early in the course of diabetes, before insulin secretion has diminished. The positive effects appear to be related to kcaloric restriction rather than to weight loss itself, and improvements in blood glucose usually appear within days after a weight-loss program is initiated.[49] Clinical studies, however, have indicated that the improved glycemic control often diminishes within a year after weight loss. The reason for this long-term effect may be that subjects are no longer restricting kcalories and have begun to regain the lost weight.[50]

Not all persons with type 2 diabetes are overweight or obese. Older adults and those in long-term care facilities are often underweight and may need to gain weight. Low body weight increases risks of morbidity and mortality in these individuals.[51]

Alcohol Use in Diabetes Adults with diabetes may use alcohol in moderation. Guidelines are similar to those for the general population: daily intake should be limited to one drink for women and two drinks for men.■ People using insulin or medications that stimulate insulin secretion, however, should consume food with alcoholic beverages to avoid hypoglycemia. Alcohol can cause hypoglycemia by interfering with gluconeogenesis in the liver. Conversely, excessive alcohol intakes can worsen hyperglycemia[52] and raise triglyceride levels in susceptible persons.[53] Abstention from alcohol is recommended for pregnant women and people who have pancreatitis, advanced neuropathy, abnormally high triglyercide levels, or a history of alcohol abuse.[54]

Micronutrient Intakes Micronutrient recommendations for persons with diabetes are the same as for the general population. Vitamin and mineral supplementation is not recommended unless nutrient deficiencies are evident. Exceptions include the use of folate supplements during pregnancy to prevent neural tube defects and calcium supplements to reduce osteoporosis risk in older adults.[55]

Although some studies have suggested that chromium supplementation can help to improve glucose tolerance in type 2 diabetes, results have not been consistent.[56] Positive effects of chromium in some studies may have been due to underlying chromium deficiencies in the populations studied.[57] At present, chromium supplementation is not recommended for persons with type 2 diabetes.

Medical Nutrition Therapy: Dietary Strategies

No single approach to meal planning can meet everyone's needs. Dietitians use a number of different strategies to help persons with diabetes maintain glycemic control. To increase the likelihood that a person will adhere to a dietary plan, it should be easy to understand, flexible, and adjusted to personal eating habits. Initial dietary instructions may include a discussion of the *Dietary Guidelines* or other recommendations designed for the general population (see Chapter 2). Providing sample menus that include commonly eaten foods can help to illustrate general principles. Initially, just a few adjustments should be made in a person's current diet, as a complicated dietary plan may be overwhelming to a newly diagnosed individual.

Meal-planning strategies used in diabetes share common themes. Emphasis is often given to controlling carbohydrate intake and portion sizes. A regular eating pattern, with meals spaced throughout the day, is typically recommended. Persons using intensive insulin therapy must coordinate insulin injections with meals and adjust insulin dosages to carbohydrate intake. Although initial attention is given to improving blood glucose levels, dietary interventions that improve blood lipids are frequently included.

Carbohydrate Counting Carbohydrate counting techniques are widely used for planning diabetes diets. Such methods have gained in popularity in recent years, as they are simpler and more flexible than other menu-planning approaches. Carbohydrate counting works as follows: after a dietitian determines a person's dietary needs, the individual is given a daily carbohydrate allowance, often divided into a pattern of meals and snacks according to individual preferences. The carbohydrate allowance can be expressed in grams or as the number of carbohydrate portions allowed per meal (see Table 26-3). The user of such a plan need only be concerned about meeting carbohydrate goals and can select from any of the carbohydrate-containing food groups when planning meals (see Table 26-4 and Figure 26-2). Although encouraged to make healthy food choices (whole-grain breads and cereals, low-fat milk products, fruits and vegetables), an individual has the freedom to choose the foods desired at each meal without risking loss of glycemic control. Some people may need further guidance about noncarbohydrate food portions to help them choose a healthy diet that does not exceed energy needs. The "How to" on pp. 802–803 provides more information about using carbohydrate counting in clinical practice.

Carbohydrate counting is taught at different levels of complexity depending on a person's needs. The basic carbohydrate counting just described can be helpful for most people, although it requires a consistent carbohydrate intake to match the medication or insulin regimen. Advanced carbohydrate counting allows more flexibility but is best suited for patients using intensive insulin therapy. With this method, a person can determine the specific dosage of insulin needed to cover the amount of carbohydrate consumed at a meal. The person is then free to choose the types and portions of food desired without sacrificing glycemic control. Advanced carbohydrate counting requires some training and should be attempted only after more basic methods are mastered.

Exchange Lists for Meal Planning The exchange list system is still popular with some dietitians, although it is more complex and difficult for patients to learn than carbohydrate counting methods. This system of meal planning was introduced in Chapter 2 and is described further in Appendix G (Appendix I for Canadians). The exchange system sorts foods according to their proportions of carbohydrate, fat, and protein so that each item in a food group (or "exchange list") is similar in terms of macronutrient and energy content (see p. G-1). Thus any food on a list can be exchanged, or traded, for any other food on the same list without affecting the macronutrient balance in a day's meals. Table G-3 (p. G-3) shows a sample dietary plan and menu, and the rest of the appendix provides food lists. Although the exchange list system may be helpful for individuals who want a structured dietary plan that provides specific percentages of protein, carbohydrate, and fat, it offers no advantages for maintaining glycemic control and is less flexible than carbohydrate counting.

The exchange lists can be helpful resources for individuals using carbohydrate counting methods because carbohydrate exchanges are interchangeable with the portion sizes used in carbohydrate counting. Foods listed as starch, fruit, or milk exchanges, for example, are equivalent to carbohydrate "portions," as each item contains approximately 15 grams of carbohydrate (see pp. G-4 and G-5; note that the carbohydrate content of milk exchanges can be rounded up to 15 grams). The list labeled "Sweets, Desserts, and Other Carbohydrates" (p. G-6) indicates the number of carbohydrate portions per serving in the far-right column.

HOW TO Use Basic Carbohydrate Counting in Clinical Practice

1. The first step in basic carbohydrate counting is to determine an appropriate carbohydrate intake and suitable distribution pattern (see Table 26-3). A nutrition assessment can help to estimate a person's usual energy and carbohydrate intakes. The carbohydrate level suggested should be acceptable to the person using the plan. Frequent monitoring of blood glucose levels can help determine whether additional carbohydrate restriction would be helpful.

   The example given in Table 26-3 illustrates a meal pattern for a person consuming 2000 kcalories daily with a carbohydrate allowance of 50 percent of kcalories. This is calculated as follows:

   $$50\% \times 2000 \text{ kcal} = 1000 \text{ kcal of carbohydrate.}$$

   $$\frac{1000 \text{ kcal carbohydrate}}{4 \text{ kcal/g carbohydrate}} = 250 \text{ g carbohydrate/day.}$$

   $$\frac{250 \text{ g carbohydrate}}{15 \text{ g/1 carbohydrate portion}} = 16.7 \text{ carbohydrate portions/day.}$$

2. The distribution of carbohydrates among meals and snacks is based on both individual preferences and metabolic needs. In type 1 diabetes, the insulin regimen must coordinate with an individual's dietary and lifestyle choices. People using conventional insulin therapy must have a consistent carbohydrate intake from day to day to match their particular insulin prescription, whereas those using intensive therapy can alter insulin dosages when carbohydrate intakes change. People with type 2 diabetes are encouraged to develop dietary patterns that suit their lifestyle and medication schedules. For all types of diabetes, the carbohydrate recommendation may need to be altered periodically to improve blood glucose control.
3. Carbohydrate counting can be done in one of two ways:
   - Count the grams of carbohydrate provided by foods.
   - Count carbohydrate portions, expressed in terms of servings that contain approximately 15 grams each.

   Success with carbohydrate counting requires knowledge about the food sources of carbohydrates and an understanding of portion control. As shown in Table 26-4, food selections that contain about 15 grams of carbohydrate are interchangeable. However, the size of a portion of food that contains 15 grams may vary substantially, even among foods in a single food group. Accurate carbohydrate counting often requires instruction and practice in portion control using measuring cups, spoons, and a food scale. Food lists that indicate the carbohydrate contents of common foods are available from the American Diabetes Association and the American Dietetic Association; these are helpful resources for learning carbohydrate counting methods.

   Persons using packaged food products can use the "Total Carbohydrate" value on the Nutrition Facts panels of food labels when counting carbohydrate grams. If the fiber content is greater than 5 grams per serving, it should be subtracted from the "Total Carbohydrate" value, as fiber does not contribute to blood glucose. If the sugar alcohol content is greater than 5 grams per

TABLE 26-3 Sample Carbohydrate Distribution for a 2000-kCalorie Diet

Meals	Carbohydrate Allowance In Grams	Carbohydrate Allowance Portions[a]
Breakfast	60	4
Lunch	60	4
Afternoon snack	30	2
Dinner	75	5
Evening snack	30	2
Totals	**255 g**	**17**

NOTE: The carbohydrate allowance in this example is approximately 50 percent of total kcalories.
[a]1 portion = 15 g carbohydrate = 1 portion of starchy food, milk, or fruit.

Insulin Therapy

Insulin therapy is necessary for people who cannot produce enough insulin to meet metabolic needs. They include patients with type 1 diabetes, who require insulin for survival, and patients with type 2 diabetes who are unable to maintain glycemic control with oral medications, diet, and exercise. Normally, pancreatic cells secrete insulin at a low rate between meals and during the night■ and at a much higher rate following a meal. An ideal treatment is one that mimics natural

■ Insulin that is secreted between meals and during the night is called **basal insulin.**

TABLE 26-4 Portion Sizes of Carbohydrate-Containing Foods

Food Groups with Sample Portion Sizes

Bread, cereal, rice, and pasta: 1 portion = 15 g carbohydrate.
- 1 slice of bread or 1 tortilla
- ½ English muffin
- ¾ c unsweetened, ready-to-eat cereal
- ½ c cooked oatmeal
- ⅓ c cooked rice or pasta

Fruit: 1 portion = 15 g carbohydrate.
- 1 medium apple, orange, or peach
- 1 small banana
- ¾ c blueberries or chopped pineapple
- ½ c apple or orange juice

Milk products: 1 portion = 12 g carbohydrate; may be rounded up to 15 g for ease in counting carbohydrate portions.
- 1 c milk (whole, low-fat, or fat-free)
- 1 c buttermilk
- 6 oz plain yogurt

Starchy vegetables: 1 portion = 15 g carbohydrate.
- 1 small (3 oz) potato
- ½ c canned or frozen corn
- ⅓ c baked beans
- 1 c winter squash, cubed

Sweets and desserts: Considerable variation in carbohydrate content; portions listed contain approximately 15 g.
- ½ c ice cream
- 2 sandwich cookies (with cream filling)
- ½ frosted cupcake
- 1 granola bar (1 oz)
- 1 tbs honey

Nonstarchy vegetables: 1 portion = 3 to 6 g carbohydrate; 3 servings are equivalent to 1 carbohydrate portion; can be disregarded if less than 3 servings are consumed.
- 1 c cooked cauliflower
- ½ c cooked cabbage, collards, or kale
- ½ c cooked okra
- ½ c diced or raw tomatoes

NOTE: Unprocessed meats, fish, and poultry contain negligible amounts of carbohydrate.

FIGURE 26-2 Translating Carbohydrate Portions into a Day's Meals

SAMPLE MENU

	Carbohydrate Portions
Breakfast:	
Carbohydrate goal = 4 portions or 60 g.	
¾ c unsweetened, ready-to-eat cereal	1
½ c low-fat milk	½
1 scrambled egg	—
1 slice whole-wheat toast (with margarine or butter)	1
6 oz orange juice	1½
Coffee (without milk or sugar)	—
Lunch:	
Carbohydrate goal = 4 portions or 60 g.	
1 tuna salad sandwich (includes 2 slices whole-grain bread, mayonnaise)	2
6 oz yogurt (plain) with ¾ c blueberries and artificial sweetener	2
Diet cola	—
Afternoon snack:	
Carbohydrate goal = 2 portions or 30 g.	
2 sandwich cookies	1
1 c low-fat milk	1
Dinner:	
Carbohydrate goal = 5 portions or 75 g.	
4 oz grilled steak	—
1 small baked potato (with margarine or butter)	1
Corn on cob, 1 large ear	2
½ c steamed collard greens[a]] 1 c sliced, raw tomatoes[a]]	1
½ c ice cream	1
Evening snack:	
Carbohydrate goal = 2 portions or 30 g.	
1 medium apple	1
1 oz granola bar	1

[a]Three servings of nonstarchy vegetables are equivalent to 1 carbohydrate portion.

serving, half of the grams of sugar alcohol can be subtracted from the "Total Carbohydrate" value.

4. Once they have learned the basic carbohydrate counting method, individuals can select whatever foods they wish, as long as they do not exceed their carbohydrate goals. Figure 26-2 shows a day's menu that follows the dietary plan shown in Table 26-3. Although carbohydrate counting focuses on a single macronutrient, people using this technique should be encouraged to follow a healthy eating plan that meets other dietary objectives as well.

insulin secretion as closely as possible. A variety of insulin preparations have been developed so that several types of insulin can be combined, if necessary, to achieve maximal glycemic control.

Insulin Preparations The forms of insulin available differ by their onset of activity, timing of peak activity, and duration of effects. Table 26-5 and Figure 26-3 show how insulin preparations are classified: they may be rapid-acting (lispro and aspart), short-acting (regular), intermediate-acting (lente and NPH), or long-acting

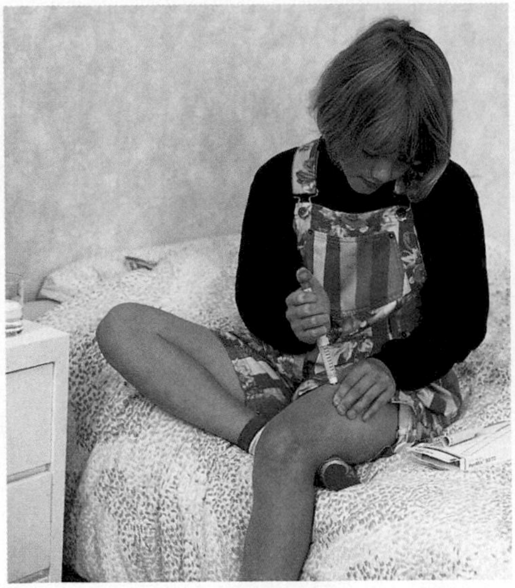

© Mark Clarke/Science Photo Library/Photo Researchers, Inc.

Children often become adept at administering the insulin they require.

TABLE 26-5 Insulin Preparations

Form of Insulin	Common Preparations	Onset of Action	Peak Activity	Duration of Action
Rapid-acting	Lispro Aspart	15 min	30 min to 2 hr	3 to 5 hr
Short-acting	Regular	30 min	2 to 4 hr	5 to 8 hr
Intermediate-acting	Lente NPH	1 to 3 hr	5 to 10 hr	18 to 24 hr
Long-acting	Glargine Ultralente	2 to 4 hr 4 to 6 hr	Steady effects 8 to 12 hr	24 hr Over 30 hr
Insulin mixtures (with sample ratios)	NPH/regular (70:30) NPH/regular (50:50)	Variable; depends on formulation	Variable; depends on formulation	Variable; depends on formulation

(glargine and ultralente), thereby allowing substantial flexibility in finding a suitable insulin regimen. Mixtures of several types of insulin can produce greater glycemic control than any one type alone. Several premixed formulations are commercially available (see Table 26-5).

Most insulin is produced by recombinant DNA techniques that allow the mass production of human insulin by bacteria or yeast. Different forms of insulin are made by chemically modifying insulin's amino acid sequence or by combining insulin with special buffers or peptides. Some formulations of insulin are derived from pork pancreas, although these are less commonly used than human insulin preparations.

Insulin Delivery Because insulin is a protein, it must be delivered by injection—it would be destroyed by digestive processes if taken orally. Injections are usually self-administered or provided by caregivers. Although individual syringes are frequently used, several other options are available. Injection ports can be inserted through the skin and can remain in place for several days, eliminating the need for multiple punctures. Another option is to use an insulin pump, a computerized device that can be programmed to deliver basal levels of insulin continuously and bolus doses at mealtimes. The pump infuses insulin through thin, flexible tubing that remains in the skin. The pump can be worn under clothes, attached to a belt, or kept in a pocket.

Insulin Regimens People with severe insulin deficiency require basal insulin throughout the day and night and larger amounts at mealtimes. Those with milder conditions may use insulin therapy to supplement oral antidiabetic medications. Designing the ideal regimen requires knowledge of a person's usual glucose levels and dietary and exercise habits. Insulin dosages are adjusted according to a person's blood glucose responses.

Insulin Regimen for Type 1 Diabetes Type 1 diabetes is best managed using an insulin pump or multiple daily injections of several different types of insulin. Usually, intermediate- or long-acting insulin is injected to meet basal insulin needs, and rapid- or short-acting insulin is used before meals.■ At least three or four daily injections are required for good glycemic control. Increasing the number of injections allows a more flexible lifestyle but also requires frequent testing of blood glucose levels and a good understanding of carbohydrate counting. Simpler regimens for type 1 diabetes involve twice-daily injections of a mixture of intermediate- and short-acting insulin. These regimens offer less flexibility, however, because meals must be eaten at times of peak insulin activity, and glycemic control may suffer if meals are delayed. With a regimen of twice-daily injections, insulin must be injected at the same time each day to avoid periods of insulin deficiency or excess.[58]

■ Rapid-acting insulin is often preferred at mealtime because its onset of action is only 15 minutes and it can be injected right before a meal. Short-acting insulin requires a half-hour wait before the meal can begin.

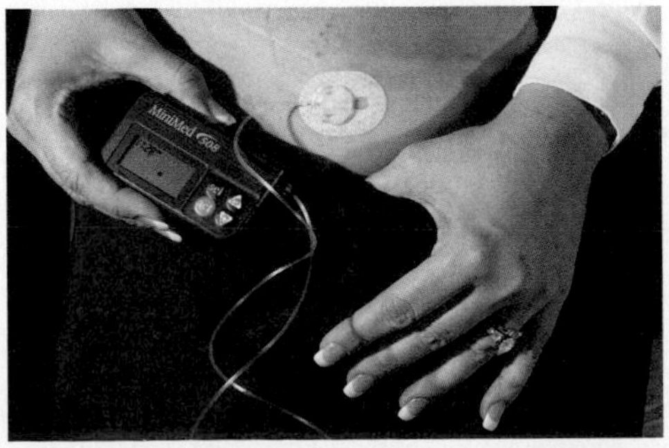
MiniMed 508

© Spencer Grant/Photo Researchers, Inc.

External insulin pumps deliver insulin continuously through thin, flexible tubing inserted into the skin.

Initial treatment of type 1 diabetes is frequently followed by a temporary remission of disease symptoms and a reduced need for insulin treatment, known as

FIGURE 26-3 Effects of Insulin Preparations

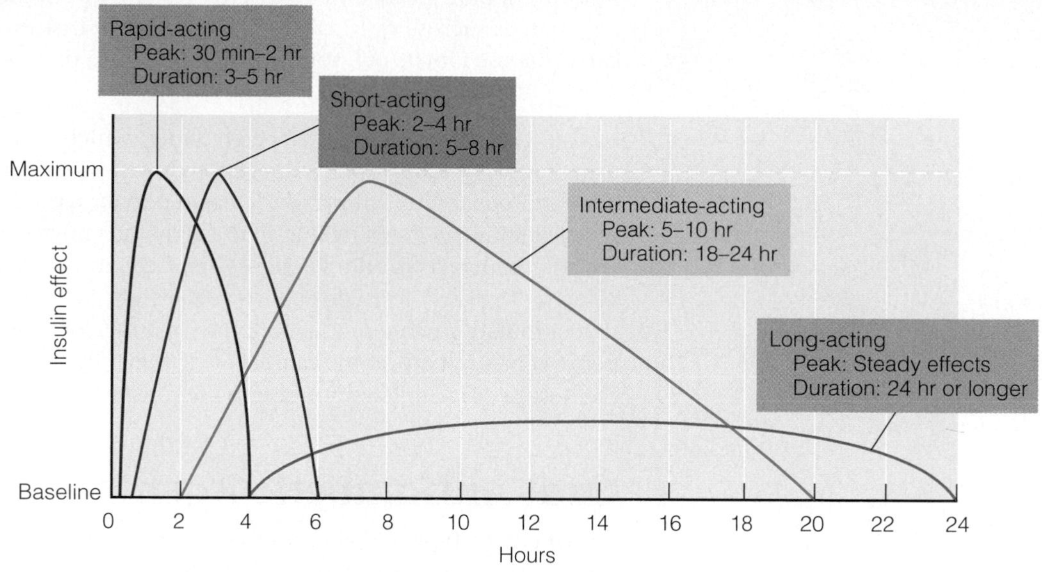
Rapid-acting
Peak: 30 min–2 hr
Duration: 3–5 hr
Short-acting
Peak: 2–4 hr
Duration: 5–8 hr
Intermediate-acting
Peak: 5–10 hr
Duration: 18–24 hr
Long-acting
Peak: Steady effects
Duration: 24 hr or longer
Maximum
Baseline
Insulin effect
0 2 4 6 8 10 12 14 16 18 20 22 24
Hours

the "honeymoon phase." The remission is associated with improved function of the pancreatic beta cells and usually lasts for several weeks or months. It is important to anticipate this period of remission so that insulin excess is avoided. In all cases, diabetes eventually returns and full insulin treatment must be reinstated.

Insulin Regimen for Intensive Therapy A person using intensive therapy must learn to accurately determine the amount of insulin to inject before each meal. The amount required depends on premeal blood glucose levels and the amount of carbohydrate in a meal, and it must also take into account the person's body weight and sensitivity to insulin. To determine insulin sensitivity, a person keeps careful records of food intake, insulin dosages, and blood glucose levels. Eventually, these records are analyzed to determine the appropriate **carbohydrate-to-insulin ratio** for that individual, which can help in calculating insulin dosages at mealtime.[59]

Insulin Regimen for Type 2 Diabetes Approximately 30 percent of persons diagnosed with type 2 diabetes are treated with insulin therapy.[60] Although initial treatment of type 2 diabetes may involve diet therapy, physical activity, and the use of oral antidiabetic agents, long-term results with these treatments are often disappointing. As the disease progresses, persons with type 2 diabetes eventually lose their ability to secrete adequate insulin, and many require insulin therapy to maintain glycemic control.

Many possible regimens may be used to control type 2 diabetes. Some persons may be treated with insulin alone, whereas others may use insulin in combination with oral antidiabetic agents. Often, only one or two daily injections are needed. Some regimens involve a mixture of rapid- and intermediate-acting insulin in the morning and an injection of intermediate- or long-acting insulin at dinner or before bedtime. In some cases, only a single injection of intermediate- or long-acting insulin may be needed at bedtime. Dosages and timing are adjusted according to the results of blood glucose self-monitoring.[61]

Treatment of Hypoglycemia Hypoglycemia is the most common complication of insulin therapy, although it may also result from use of other antidiabetic medications. Hypoglycemia occurs most often in persons using intensive therapy, as the attempt to attain near-normal blood glucose levels increases the risk of overtreatment. Hypoglycemia can be corrected with an immediate intake of glucose or a carbohydrate-containing food. Usually, 15 to 20 grams of carbohydrate■

■ Each of the following sources provides approximately 15 g of carbohydrate:
- Glucose tablets: 2 to 3 tablets.
- Table sugar: 4 tsp.
- Honey: 1 tbs.
- Jellybeans: 15 small.
- Grape juice, unsweetened: ½ c.
- Orange juice, canned: ½ c.

carbohydrate-to-insulin ratio: the amount of carbohydrate that can be handled per unit of insulin. On average, every 15 g of carbohydrate requires about 1 unit of rapid- or short-acting insulin.

can relieve hypoglycemia within 10 to 20 minutes, although blood glucose levels should be reevaluated within an hour in case additional treatment is necessary.[62] A source of pure glucose yields a better response than foods that contain other sugars, such as sucrose or fructose. People who use insulin are typically instructed to carry glucose tablets or a source of carbohydrate that can be readily ingested.

Fasting Hyperglycemia Insulin dosages or preparations sometimes need to be adjusted to prevent fasting hyperglycemia, which has three possible causes. The usual cause is a waning of insulin action during the night due to insufficient insulin. A second possibility, known as the **dawn phenomenon,** is an increase in blood glucose levels in the morning due to the early morning secretion of growth hormone, which counteracts insulin's actions. Less frequently, fasting hyperglycemia may develop in response to nighttime hypoglycemia, which causes hormonal responses that stimulate glucose production; the resulting condition is known as **rebound hyperglycemia.** Whatever the cause, fasting hyperglycemia can be treated by adjusting the dosage or formulation of insulin administered in the evening.

Oral Antidiabetic Agents

Treatment of type 2 diabetes often requires the use of oral medications. These drugs can improve hyperglycemia by four modes of action: they can improve insulin secretion, reduce glucose production by the liver, improve use of glucose by tissues, or delay carbohydrate absorption. Treatment may involve the use of a single medication (monotherapy) or a combination of several (combination therapy). By utilizing several mechanisms at once, combination therapy achieves more rapid and sustained glycemic control than is possible with monotherapy.[63] Table 26-6 lists examples of oral antidiabetic agents and their potential side effects. As medications cannot replace the benefits offered by dietary modifications and physical activity, persons with diabetes should be advised to continue both.

Physical Activity and Diabetes Management

Regular physical activity is a central feature of disease management in type 2 diabetes, as it can substantially improve glycemic control. A regular exercise program improves insulin sensitivity and thereby reduces insulin requirements. It also helps to improve blood lipid levels, lower blood pressure, and promote weight

TABLE 26-6 Oral Antidiabetic Agents

Mode of Action	Drug Category	Common Examples	Possible Side Effects
Stimulates insulin secretion by pancreas	Sulfonylureas	Chlorpropamide Tolbutamide Glyburide Glipizide	Hypoglycemia; weight gain; gastrointestinal side effects like nausea, vomiting, diarrhea, cramps; allergic skin reactions
	Meglitinides	Repaglinide Nateglinide	
Inhibits liver glucose production	Biguanides	Metformin	Anorexia; metallic taste; gastrointestinal side effects like nausea, vomiting, diarrhea, cramps
Increases insulin sensitivity	Thiazolidinediones	Pioglitazone Rosiglitazone	Fluid retention, edema, weight gain, anemia
Delays glucose absorption	Alpha-glucosidase inhibitors	Acarbose Miglitol	Gastrointestinal side effects like nausea, diarrhea, abdominal cramps

dawn phenomenon: morning hyperglycemia that is caused by the early morning release of growth hormone, which counteracts insulin's glucose-lowering effects.

rebound hyperglycemia: hyperglycemia that results from the release of counterregulatory hormones following nighttime hypoglycemia; also called the **Somogyi phenomenon.**

loss. Although exercise is less effective for glycemic control in type 1 diabetes, it helps to maintain other aspects of health, including cardiovascular conditioning. People with type 1 diabetes must carefully adjust food intake and insulin therapy to prevent hypoglycemia during physical activity.

Physical Activity and Insulin Therapy In people without diabetes, blood glucose levels are maintained during exercise because the normal hormonal responses—a fall in insulin levels and increased secretion of glucagon and epinephrine—promote glucose production in the liver. In people who use insulin, the natural hormonal balance is upset: blood glucose levels drop during activity because injected insulin promotes rapid consumption of glucose by exercising muscles and also blocks glucose synthesis by the liver. For this reason, insulin should not be injected immediately before exercise because it can lead to hypoglycemia. Conversely, a complete lack of insulin contributes to hyperglycemia because liver glucose production is unchecked.[64]

The glycemic response to exercise depends on an activity's intensity and duration, the timing of the last insulin injection, and the timing of the previous snack or meal. Insulin dosages that precede exercise often need to be reduced substantially. Persons using insulin pumps, which provide continuous basal infusions, may need to reduce or suspend infusions during exercise. Blood glucose levels should be checked before and after engaging in physical activity. If blood glucose is below 100 milligrams per deciliter, carbohydrate should be consumed before exercise begins. If exercise is prolonged, the person may need to consume carbohydrate during the activity. Hypoglycemia can develop several hours after exercise, so additional food may be needed later in the day. Predicting the precise adjustments in diet and insulin becomes easier as a person gains experience in maintaining glycemic control.[65]

Physical Activity in Type 2 Diabetes Regular physical activity can improve the metabolic outcomes associated with type 2 diabetes, including blood glucose, blood lipids, and blood pressure. A regular exercise program can also prevent or delay the onset of diabetes in persons at risk.[66] People with type 2 diabetes are often overweight and sedentary, however, and many develop complications during the course of disease. Before an exercise program can be planned, a careful medical evaluation should screen for problems that may be worsened by certain activities. Complications involving the heart and blood vessels, eyes, kidneys, feet, and nervous system may limit the types of activity recommended.[67]

An ideal exercise program includes both aerobic exercise and strength training, although only mild or moderate exercise may be prescribed at first. For obese, inactive persons, a short walk at a comfortable pace may be the first activity suggested. Persons with retinopathy should avoid heavy lifting or straining, which may raise blood pressure and damage eye tissue. Persons with nephropathy often have reduced capacity for physical activity, and strenuous exercise is discouraged. Peripheral neuropathy precludes repetitive weight-bearing exercises such as jogging and step exercises, as these activities may lead to foot ulcerations. The use of protective footgear, such as gel or air midsoles and socks that prevent blisters, can help to prevent foot trauma. Proper hydration should be encouraged before and during exercise, as dehydration can adversely affect blood glucose levels and heart function.[68]

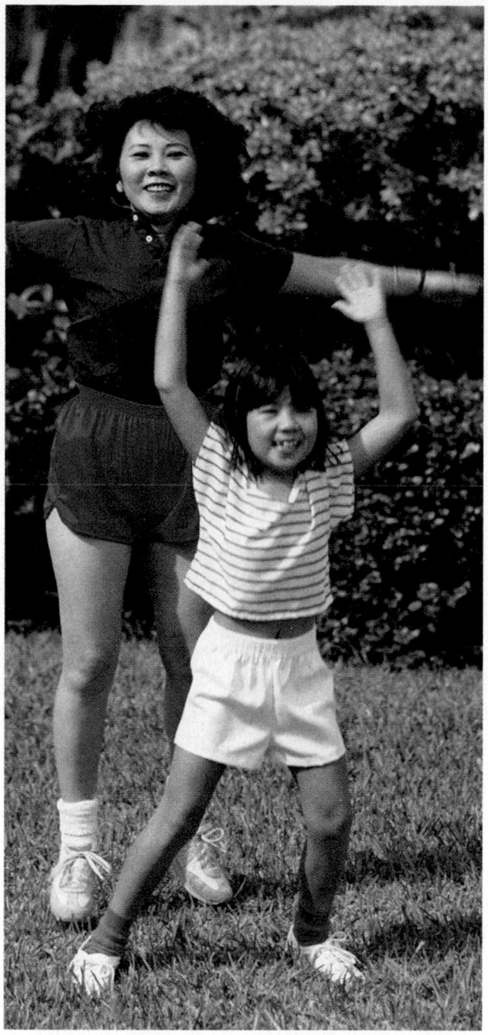

Physical activity plays an important role in the management of diabetes.

Sick-Day Management

The stress of illness, injury, or infection often causes hormonal changes that raise blood glucose levels. Persons with type 1 diabetes must be especially concerned about acute illness, as it increases the risk of diabetic ketoacidosis. Individuals who are too sick to eat often reduce their use of insulin even though they may actually need additional amounts. A patient with type 1 diabetes should be advised to test blood glucose frequently during illness and to test blood or urine for ketones. Insulin doses should be adjusted if blood glucose levels are high. Some carbohydrate should be ingested to avoid ketosis; a daily intake of 150 to 200 grams of carbohydrate (about 45 to 50 grams every three to four hours) is recommended. If appetite is poor, carbohydrate-sweetened beverages or frozen juice bars may be easier to consume than solid foods. Fluid intake should be monitored to prevent dehydration.[69]

IN SUMMARY The goals of diabetes treatment are to maintain glycemic control and reduce the risk of developing microvascular and macrovascular complications. Glycemic control is evaluated by self-monitoring of blood glucose and by measuring glycated hemoglobin. Diabetes treatment often includes diet therapy, insulin or oral medication use, and appropriate physical activity. Blood glucose levels are strongly influenced by carbohydrate intakes. Carbohydrate counting is widely used in menu planning and can be taught at different levels of complexity depending on individual needs. Insulin therapy is required for patients who are unable to produce sufficient insulin and may be used in both type 1 and type 2 diabetes. Oral medications can improve insulin secretion and sensitivity, lower glucose production by the liver, and delay carbohydrate absorption. Physical activity can substantially improve glycemic control in persons with type 2 diabetes. The case study provides an opportunity to review the factors that influence treatment for a 12-year-old with type 1 diabetes.

Diabetes Management in Pregnancy

Women with diabetes face new challenges when they become pregnant. As a result of hormonal changes, pregnancy increases insulin resistance and the need for insulin. Women with type 1 or type 2 diabetes may have greater difficulty maintaining glycemic control during pregnancy. In addition, up to 7 percent of nondiabetic women develop gestational diabetes■ and require treatment during pregnancy. Women with gestational diabetes are at higher risk of developing type 2 diabetes later in life, and their children are at increased risk of developing obesity and type 2 diabetes as they enter into adulthood.

■ Gestational diabetes was introduced in Chapter 14 (see p. 491).

Effect of Diabetes on Pregnancy Pregnancies complicated by diabetes are associated with increased risks for both mother and fetus. Uncontrolled diabetes in early pregnancy is linked with an increased rate of spontaneous abortion (miscarriage). Incidences of birth defects and fetal deaths are much higher than in women without diabetes and are related to poor glycemic control. Newborns are more likely to suffer from respiratory distress syndrome and develop metabolic abnormalities such as hypoglycemia, jaundice, and hypocalcemia. Women with type 2 diabetes and gestational diabetes often deliver babies with macrosomia,■ which makes delivery more difficult or results in birth trauma or cesarean section.[70]

■ Reminder: The term *macrosomia* refers to infant birthweights of 4000 g (9 lb) and above.

Pregnancy in Type 1 or Type 2 Diabetes Women who achieve glycemic control at conception and during the first trimester can substantially reduce the risks of birth defects and spontaneous abortion during pregnancy. For this reason, it is recommended that women contemplating pregnancy receive preconception care to avoid the complications associated with poorly controlled diabetes.[71] Maintaining glycemic control during the second and third trimesters can minimize the risks of macrosomia and morbidity in newborn infants.[72]

Nutrient requirements during pregnancy are generally similar for women with and without diabetes.[73] Dietary adjustments for improving glycemic control are individualized according to a woman's dietary habits and the results of blood glucose monitoring. Regular meals and snacks help to avoid hypoglycemia, which is more likely to occur during pregnancy because glucose is continuously supplied to the fetus. An evening snack is usually necessary to prevent overnight hypoglycemia and ketosis.[74] Insulin and medication changes are often needed during

CASE STUDY

Child with Type 1 Diabetes

Nora is a 12-year-old girl who was diagnosed with type 1 diabetes two years ago. As with most children, Nora's appetite varies from day to day. Nora frequently joins her friends for bicycle rides in the park, although sometimes she prefers to watch TV or surf the Internet. Nora practices intensive therapy and has had the support of her parents and an excellent diabetes management team. With their help, Nora has been able to assume the bulk of the responsibility for her diabetes care and has managed to control her blood glucose remarkably well. In the last few months, however, Nora has been complaining bitterly about the impositions diabetes has placed on her life and her interactions with friends. Sometimes she refuses to monitor her blood glucose levels, and she has skipped insulin injections a few times. Recently, Nora was admitted to the emergency room complaining of fever, nausea, vomiting, and intense thirst. The physician noted that Nora was confused and lethargic. A urine test was positive for ketones, and her blood glucose levels were 400 mg/dL. The diagnosis was diabetic ketoacidosis.

1. Describe the metabolic events that lead to ketoacidosis. Were Nora's symptoms and laboratory tests consistent with the diagnosis?
2. Review Table 26-2 and consider the advantages and disadvantages that intensive therapy might have for Nora.
3. Discuss how Nora's age might influence her ability to cope with and manage her diabetes. Why might she feel that diabetes is disrupting her life? What suggestions may help?
4. Review the list of complications associated with long-term diabetes. How might you explain the importance of glycemic control to a 12-year-old girl?

pregnancy, and these changes may require the woman to adjust her dietary habits further.

Gestational Diabetes Because gestational diabetes usually develops in the later stages of pregnancy, macrosomia and morbidity in the newborn infant are often the greatest concerns. Gestational diabetes can develop earlier in pregnancy, however, and have effects similar to those of type 1 and type 2 diabetes.

Many women who develop gestational diabetes are overweight or obese and may therefore need to adjust their energy intakes during pregnancy. Although adequate energy is needed for fetal development, a modest kcaloric reduction (about 30 percent less than total energy needs) may improve glycemic control without increasing the risk of ketosis.[75] Restricting carbohydrate to 40 to 45 percent of total energy intake can improve blood glucose levels after meals. Because carbohydrate may be poorly tolerated in the morning, reducing carbohydrate at breakfast can be helpful. The remaining carbohydrate intake should be spaced throughout the day into several meals and snacks, including an evening snack to prevent ketosis during the night.[76] Regular aerobic activity is often recommended, as it can help improve glycemic control. Women who fail to achieve glycemic goals by diet and exercise alone may need insulin therapy, which is given to approximately 20 to 25 percent of women with gestational diabetes.[77] Oral antidiabetic drugs generally are not prescribed during pregnancy, pending further research. The case study on p. 810 reviews the connections between gestational diabetes and type 2 diabetes.

IN SUMMARY Careful management of blood glucose levels before and during pregnancy may reduce complications in mother and infant. Most nutrient requirements during pregnancy are similar for women with and without diabetes. Carbohydrate intake should be distributed into several meals and snacks, including an evening snack to prevent overnight ketosis. Carbohydrate restriction may be recommended, especially in women with gestational diabetes. Overweight and obese women may improve glycemic control by moderate energy restriction. Insulin adjustments are frequently necessary and may alter dietary intakes.

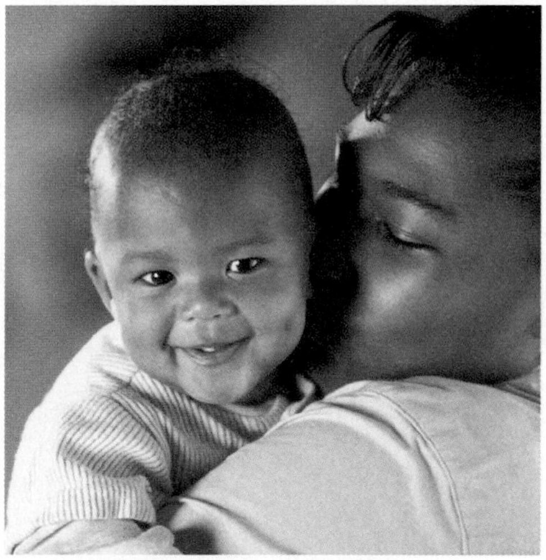

Careful control of blood glucose during pregnancy offers the best chance of a safe delivery and a healthy infant for women with diabetes.

CASE STUDY

School Counselor with Type 2 Diabetes

Mrs. Cordova is a 41-year-old Mexican American woman recently diagnosed with type 2 diabetes. Mrs. Cordova developed gestational diabetes while she was pregnant with her second child. Her blood glucose levels returned to normal following pregnancy, and she was advised to get regular checkups, maintain a desirable weight, and engage in regular physical activity. Although she reports that she does not overeat and that she exercises regularly, she has been unable to maintain a healthy weight. At 5 feet 3 inches tall, Mrs. Cordova currently weighs 155 pounds. She has decided to lose weight and join a gym because she is concerned about the long-term effects of diabetes and the possibility that she may need insulin injections. She is also concerned about her husband and children because they are overweight and not very active. The physician refers Mrs. Cordova to a dietitian to help her plan a diet.

1. What factors in Mrs. Cordova's medical history increase her risk for diabetes? Are her husband and children also at risk?
2. Describe the general characteristics of a diet and exercise program that would be appropriate for Mrs. Cordova. How might weight loss and physical activity benefit her diabetes?
3. If Mrs. Cordova is unable to control her blood glucose with diet and physical activity, what treatment might be suggested? Can you explain to Mrs. Cordova why she would probably not require insulin at this time?
4. What dietary and lifestyle changes may help to prevent diabetes in Mrs. Cordova's husband and children?

DIET-DRUG INTERACTIONS

Alpha-Glucosidase Inhibitors

Alpha-glucosidase inhibitors are taken at the start of each meal. Nutrition-related side effects include abdominal pain, gas, and diarrhea.

Insulin

The timing of *insulin* administration varies, depending on the action of the insulin prescribed. Insulin may cause hypoglycemia.

Insulin Analogs

Lispro and *aspart* can be taken 5 to 10 minutes before meals. Risk of hypoglycemia is lower than with other insulin formulations.

Meglitinides

Repaglinide and *nateglinide* should be taken right before meals; hypoglycemia is a risk if meals are delayed or contain insufficient carbohydrate.

Metformin

Metformin is taken once or twice a day before meals (breakfast or breakfast and dinner). Gastrointestinal side effects include nausea, vomiting, cramps, and diarrhea. Metformin sometimes causes asymptomatic vitamin B_{12} deficiency.

Sulfonylureas

Sulfonylureas are generally taken one or two times a day, before meals. When large amounts of alcohol are taken, a disulfiram-like reaction can occur and cause flushing, throbbing pain in the head and neck, shortness of breath, palpitations, and sweating. Side effects associated with sulfonylureas include hypoglycemia, weight gain, and diarrhea.

Thiazolidinediones

Thiazolidinediones are taken once or twice a day before meals. Weight gain and edema are possible side effects.

NOTE: Ask patients who take insulin or antidiabetic agents about their use of the following dietary supplements, which may affect blood glucose: chromium, fenugreek, garlic, ginger, ginseng, and niacin.

NUTRITION ASSESSMENT CHECKLIST for People with Diabetes

Medical History
Check the medical record to determine:
- ☐ Type of diabetes
- ☐ Duration of diabetes
- ☐ Acute and chronic complications
- ☐ Conditions, including pregnancy, that may alter treatment

Medications
For patients with preexisting diabetes who use antidiabetic agents, insulin, or both, note:
- ☐ Type(s) of antidiabetic agent or insulin
- ☐ Administration schedule
- ☐ Carbohydrate-to-insulin ratio

Check for use of other medications, including:
- ☐ Medications that affect blood glucose levels
- ☐ Cholesterol- and triglyceride-lowering medications
- ☐ Antihypertensive medications

Dietary Intake
To devise an acceptable meal plan and coordinate medications, obtain:
- ☐ An accurate and thorough record of food intake and meal patterns
- ☐ An account of usual physical activities

At medical checkups, reassess the patient's ability to:
- ☐ Maintain appropriate carbohydrate intake
- ☐ Maintain appropriate energy intake
- ☐ Adjust insulin and diet to accommodate sick days
- ☐ Use appropriate foods to treat hypoglycemia

Anthropometric Data
Take accurate baseline height and weight measurements as a basis for:
- ☐ Appropriate energy intake
- ☐ Initial insulin therapy

Periodically reassess height and weight for children and weight for adults and pregnant women to ensure that the meal plan provides an appropriate energy intake.

Laboratory Tests
Monitor the success of diabetes therapy using these tests:
- ☐ Results of self-monitoring of blood glucose
- ☐ Glycated hemoglobin
- ☐ Blood lipid concentrations
- ☐ Blood or urinary ketones
- ☐ Urinary protein (microalbuminuria)

Clinical Signs
Look for signs of:
- ☐ Nerve damage
- ☐ Foot ulcers
- ☐ Dehydration, especially in older adults

NUTRITION ON THE NET

Access these websites for further study of topics covered in this chapter.

- Find updates and quick links to these and other nutrition-related sites at our website: **www.wadsworth.com/nutrition**
- Visit the American Diabetes Association and the Joslin Diabetes Center to find information on a wide range of topics related to diabetes: **www.diabetes.org** and **www.joslin.org**
- Comprehensive and reliable information about diabetes for both health practitioners and consumers is available from the National Institute of Diabetes and Digestive and Kidney Diseases and the Centers for Disease Control: **www.niddk.nih.gov** and **www.cdc.gov/diabetes**
- Find out how to become a diabetes educator by visiting the American Association of Diabetes Educators site: **www.aadenet.org**

STUDY QUESTIONS

These questions will help you review the chapter. You will find the answers in the discussions on the pages provided.

1. Describe the symptoms that develop as a consequence of hyperglycemia. How is diabetes diagnosed? (p. 792)
2. Identify the two major types of diabetes. Which type is more common? Describe the major differences between these two types. What is gestational diabetes? (pp. 792–794)
3. Discuss the acute complications that may arise in uncontrolled diabetes. (pp. 794–795)
4. Describe the macrovascular and microvascular complications that develop from prolonged exposure to high blood glucose concentrations. Discuss the problems associated with diabetic neuropathy. (pp. 795–796)
5. What are the goals of medical and nutrition therapy for people with diabetes? Explain how diabetes treatment is evaluated. (pp. 796–798)
6. Discuss the dietary recommendations for diabetes. Describe the meal-planning strategies that are used for controlling carbohydrate intakes. (pp. 798–801)

7. Describe the insulin regimens for type 1 and type 2 diabetes. Explain how insulin therapy is coordinated with food intake and physical activity. (pp. 802–807)
8. What are oral antidiabetic agents? Describe the ways in which these medications work. (p. 806)
9. What are the risks of poorly controlled diabetes during pregnancy? Describe the dietary adjustments that may be necessary in pregnant women with diabetes. (pp. 808–809)

These questions will help you review for an exam. Answers can be found on p. 813.

1. Which of the following is characteristic of type 1 diabetes?
   a. It frequently goes undiagnosed.
   b. The pancreas makes little or no insulin.
   c. It is the predominant form of diabetes.
   d. It often arises during pregnancy.
2. Which of the following describes type 2 diabetes?
   a. It is usually an autoimmune disease.
   b. The pancreas makes little or no insulin.
   c. Diabetic ketoacidosis is a common complication.
   d. Chronic complications may develop before it is diagnosed.
3. Long-term glycemic control is usually evaluated by:
   a. self-monitoring of blood glucose.
   b. testing urinary ketone levels.
   c. measuring glycated hemoglobin.
   d. testing urinary protein levels (microalbuminuria).
4. The chronic complications associated with all types of diabetes result from:
   a. altered kidney function.
   b. infections that deplete nutrient reserves.
   c. weight gain and hypertension.
   d. damage to blood vessels and nerves.
5. Regarding dietary carbohydrate, a patient with diabetes should be most concerned about:
   a. consuming the correct quantity of carbohydrate at each meal or snack.
   b. consuming the correct proportion of sugars, starches, and fiber in meals.
   c. avoiding added sugars and kcaloric sweeteners.
   d. choosing meals with ideal proportions of protein, carbohydrate, and fat.
6. Which of the following is true regarding the use of alcohol in diabetes?
   a. A serving of alcohol is considered part of the carbohydrate allowance.
   b. Alcohol contributes to hyperglycemia and should be avoided completely.
   c. Alcohol can cause hypoglycemia and should be consumed with food if patients use insulin or medications that stimulate insulin secretion.
   d. Patients can use alcohol in unlimited quantities unless they are pregnant.
7. The meal-planning strategy that is most effective for the person with diabetes is:
   a. carbohydrate counting.
   b. the exchange list system.
   c. dietary guidelines and sample menus.
   d. any approach that best helps the patient control blood glucose levels.
8. A patient using intensive insulin therapy is likely to use a regimen that involves:
   a. twice-daily injections that combine short-, intermediate-, and long-acting insulin in each injection.
   b. a mixture of intermediate- and long-acting insulin injected between meals.
   c. multiple daily injections that supply basal insulin and precise insulin dosages for each meal.
   d. use of both insulin and oral antidiabetic agents.
9. Sudden hyperglycemia in a person who has previously maintained good glycemic control can be precipitated by:
   a. infections or illnesses.
   b. chronic alcohol ingestion.
   c. undertreatment of hypoglycemia.
   d. prolonged exercise.
10. Women with pregnancies complicated by diabetes:
    a. generally benefit from larger meals and a snack at bedtime.
    b. often need less carbohydrate at breakfast.
    c. need more carbohydrate than women with diabetes who are not pregnant.
    d. need more kcalories to support the pregnancy than women without diabetes.

REFERENCES

1. A. Peters Harmel and R. Mathur, eds., *Davidson's Diabetes Mellitus: Diagnosis and Treatment* (Philadelphia: Saunders, 2004).
2. American Diabetes Association, Diagnosis and classification of diabetes mellitus, *Diabetes Care* 27 (2004): S5–S10.
3. K. N. Frayn, *Metabolic Regulation: A Human Perspective* (Oxford, U.K.: Blackwell Science, 2003).
4. R. S. Sherwin, Diabetes mellitus, in L. Goldman and D. Ausiello, eds., *Cecil Textbook of Medicine* (Philadelphia: Saunders, 2004), pp. 1424–1452.
5. Peters Harmel and Mathur, 2004.
6. Peters Harmel and Mathur, 2004; American Diabetes Association, 2004.
7. Peters Harmel and Mathur, 2004.
8. F. R. Kaufman, Diabetes management in children and adolescents, in A. Peters Harmel and R. Mathur, eds., *Davidson's Diabetes Mellitus: Diagnosis and Treatment* (Philadelphia: Saunders, 2004), pp. 299–321.
9. Kaufman, 2004; P. A. Tartaranni and C. Bogardus, Obesity and diabetes mellitus, in D. Porte, Jr., R. S. Sherwin, and A. Baron, eds., *Ellenberg and Rifkin's Diabetes Mellitus* (New York: McGraw-Hill, 2003), pp. 401–413.
10. American Diabetes Association, Gestational diabetes mellitus, *Diabetes Care* 27 (2004): S88–S90.
11. Peters Harmel and Mathur, 2004; Sherwin, 2004.
12. Sherwin, 2004.

13. Peters Harmel and Mathur, 2004.
14. E. D. Ennis and R. A. Kreisberg, Diabetic ketoacidosis, in D. Porte, Jr., R. S. Sherwin, and A. Baron, eds., *Ellenberg and Rifkin's Diabetes Mellitus* (New York: McGraw-Hill, 2003), pp. 573–586.
15. Sherwin, 2004.
16. Peters Harmel and Mathur, 2004; Sherwin, 2004.
17. R. Matz, Hyperglycemic hyperosmolar syndrome, in D. Porte, Jr., R. S. Sherwin, and A. Baron, eds., *Ellenberg and Rifkin's Diabetes Mellitus* (New York: McGraw-Hill, 2003), pp. 587–599.
18. Sherwin, 2004.
19. D. M. Kendall, Reducing cardiovascular risk in type 2 diabetes and the metabolic syndrome: The emerging role of insulin resistance, in A. Peters Harmel and R. Mathur, eds., *Davidson's Diabetes Mellitus: Diagnosis and Treatment* (Philadelphia: Saunders, 2004), pp. 239–257.
20. L. H. Young and D. A. Chyun, Heart disease in patients with diabetes, in D. Porte, Jr., R. S. Sherwin, and A. Baron, eds., *Ellenberg and Rifkin's Diabetes Mellitus* (New York: McGraw-Hill, 2003), pp. 823–844.
21. R. G. Frykberg, Diabetic foot ulcers: Pathogenesis and management, *American Family Physician* 66 (2002): 1655–1662.
22. Sherwin, 2004.
23. Peters Harmel and Mathur, 2004.
24. Peters Harmel and Mathur, 2004.
25. Peters Harmel and Mathur, 2004.
26. Diabetes Control and Complications Trial Research Group, The effect of intensive treatment of diabetes on the development and progression of long-term complications in insulin-dependent diabetes mellitus, *New England Journal of Medicine* 329 (1993): 977–986.
27. American Diabetes Association, Implications of the United Kingdom Prospective Diabetes Study, *Diabetes Care* 21 (1998): 2180–2184.
28. American Diabetes Association, Tests of glycemia in diabetes, *Diabetes Care* 27 (2004): S91–S93.
29. American Diabetes Association, Tests of glycemia in diabetes, 2004.
30. American Diabetes Association, Tests of glycemia in diabetes, 2004.
31. American Diabetes Association, Standards of medical care in diabetes, *Diabetes Care* 27 (2004): S15–S35.
32. American Diabetes Association, Nutrition principles and recommendations in diabetes, *Diabetes Care* 27 (2004): S36–S46.
33. C. A. Beebe, Nutrition and physical activity in diabetes, in A. Peters Harmel and R. Mathur, eds., *Davidson's Diabetes Mellitus: Diagnosis and Treatment* (Philadelphia: Saunders, 2004), pp. 49–69.
34. American Diabetes Association, Nutrition principles and recommendations in diabetes, 2004.
35. Beebe, 2004.
36. American Diabetes Association, Nutrition principles and recommendations in diabetes, 2004.
37. K. Foster-Powell, S. H. A. Holt, and J. C. Brand-Miller, International table of glycemic index and glycemic load values: 2002, *American Journal of Clinical Nutrition* 76 (2002): 5–56.
38. American Diabetes Association, Nutrition principles and recommendations in diabetes, 2004.
39. Beebe, 2004.
40. American Diabetes Association, Nutrition principles and recommendations in diabetes, 2004; Beebe, 2004.
41. American Diabetes Association, Nutrition principles and recommendations in diabetes, 2004; Beebe, 2004.
42. American Diabetes Association, Nutrition principles and recommendations in diabetes, 2004.
43. American Diabetes Association, Nutrition principles and recommendations in diabetes, 2004.
44. American Diabetes Association, Nutrition principles and recommendations in diabetes, 2004.
45. K. V. Williams and coauthors, Improved glycemic control reduces the impact of weight gain on cardiovascular risk factors in type 1 diabetes. The Epidemiology of Diabetes Complications Study, *Diabetes Care* 22 (1999): 1084–1091.
46. A. J. Palmer and coauthors, Deleterious effects of increased body weight associated with intensive insulin therapy for type 1 diabetes: Increased blood pressure and worsened lipid profile partially negate improvements in life expectancy, *Current Medical Research and Opinion* 20 (2004): 67–73.
47. Williams and coauthors, 1999.
48. Beebe, 2004.
49. D. D. Hensrud, Dietary treatment, and long-term weight loss and maintenance in type 2 diabetes, *Obesity Research* 9 (2001): 348S–353S; Beebe, 2004.
50. Hensrud, 2001.
51. American Diabetes Association, Nutrition principles and recommendations in diabetes, 2004.
52. G. Ben and coauthors, Effects of chronic alcohol intake on carbohydrate and lipid metabolism in subjects with type II (non-insulin-dependent) diabetes, *American Journal of Medicine* 90 (1991): 70–76.
53. American Diabetes Association, Nutrition principles and recommendations in diabetes, 2004; Beebe, 2004.
54. American Diabetes Association, Nutrition principles and recommendations in diabetes, 2004.
55. American Diabetes Association, Nutrition principles and recommendations in diabetes, 2004.
56. G. Y. Yeh and coauthors, Systematic review of herbs and dietary supplements for glycemic control in diabetes, *Diabetes Care* 26 (2003): 1277–1294.
57. American Diabetes Association, Nutrition principles and recommendations in diabetes, 2004.
58. Peters Harmel and Mathur, 2004; S. M. Strowig and P. Raskin, Intensive management of type 1 diabetes mellitus, in D. Porte, Jr., R. S. Sherwin, and A. Baron, eds., *Ellenberg and Rifkin's Diabetes Mellitus* (New York: McGraw-Hill, 2003), pp. 501–514.
59. Strowig and Raskin, 2003.
60. D. M. Nathan, Insulin treatment of type 2 diabetes mellitus, in D. Porte, Jr., R. S. Sherwin, and A. Baron, eds., *Ellenberg and Rifkin's Diabetes Mellitus* (New York: McGraw-Hill, 2003), pp. 515–522.
61. Nathan, 2003.
62. M. J. Franz and coauthors, Evidence-based nutrition principles and recommendations for the treatment and prevention of diabetes and related complications, *Diabetes Care* 25 (2002): 148–198.
63. S. Mudaliar and R. R. Henry, The oral antidiabetic agents, in D. Porte, Jr., R. S. Sherwin, and A. Baron, eds., *Ellenberg and Rifkin's Diabetes Mellitus* (New York: McGraw-Hill, 2003), pp. 531–564.
64. Sherwin, 2004; W. Howell, Office management of the diabetic patient, in A. Peters Harmel and R. Mathur, eds., *Davidson's Diabetes Mellitus: Diagnosis and Treatment* (Philadelphia: Saunders, 2004), pp. 259–297.
65. Howell, 2004; D. H. Wasserman, Z.-Q. Shi, and M. Vranic, Metabolic implications of exercise and physical fitness in physiology and diabetes, in D. Porte, Jr., R. S. Sherwin, and A. Baron, eds., *Ellenberg and Rifkin's Diabetes Mellitus* (New York: McGraw-Hill, 2003), pp 453–480.
66. Wasserman,Shi, and Vranic, 2003.
67. American Diabetes Association, Physical activity/exercise and diabetes, *Diabetes Care* 27 (2004): S58–S62.
68. American Diabetes Association, Physical activity/exercise and diabetes, 2004.
69. Franz and coauthors, 2002.
70. Peters Harmel and Mathur, 2004.
71. American Diabetes Association, Preconception care of women with diabetes, *Diabetes Care* 27 (2004): S76–S78.
72. Peters Harmel and Mathur, 2004.
73. Franz and coauthors, 2002.
74. Franz and coauthors, 2002.
75. Franz and coauthors, 2002.
76. American Diabetes Association, Nutrition principles and recommendations in diabetes, 2004.
77. Peters Harmel and Mathur, 2004.

ANSWERS

Study Questions (multiple choice)

1. b 2. d 3. c 4. d 5. a 6. c 7. d 8. c 9. a 10. b

HIGHLIGHT

Metabolic Syndrome

As explained in Chapter 26, insulin resistance—a reduced sensitivity to insulin in muscle, adipose, and liver cells—can contribute to hyperglycemia and hyperinsulinemia and often leads to type 2 diabetes. Insulin resistance is also a central feature of the **metabolic syndrome,** a group of disorders that substantially increase the risk of developing cardiovascular disease (CVD). The metabolic syndrome is a cluster of at least three of the following: insulin resistance, obesity, **hypertriglyceridemia** (elevated blood triglycerides), reduced HDL cholesterol levels, and hypertension (high blood pressure). This highlight describes how the metabolic syndrome is diagnosed, how and why it might develop, its consequences, and current treatment approaches. The accompanying glossary defines the relevant terms.

GLOSSARY

adiponectin (AH-dih-poe-NECK-tin): a hormone produced by adipose cells that improves insulin sensitivity.

fibrinogen (fye-BRIN-oh-jen): a liver protein that promotes blood clot formation.

hypertriglyceridemia (HYE-per-try-GLISS-er-eye-DEEM-ee-ah): elevated blood triglyceride levels.

metabolic syndrome: a cluster of interrelated clinical symptoms, including obesity, insulin resistance, high blood pressure, and abnormal blood lipids, which together increase cardiovascular disease risk two- to threefold; also called **syndrome X** or **insulin resistance syndrome.**

nitric oxide: a compound produced by blood vessel cells that helps to regulate blood vessel activity, including blood vessel dilation and constriction.

plasminogen activator inhibitor-1: a protein that promotes blood clotting by inhibiting blood clot degradation within blood vessels.

resistin (re-ZIST-in): a hormone produced by adipose cells that induces insulin resistance.

Prevalence of the Metabolic Syndrome

Table H26-1 lists the laboratory values used to identify metabolic syndrome, which is currently estimated to affect 24 percent of the adult population in the United States.[1] As Figure H26-1 shows, the prevalence of metabolic syndrome increases with age. Risk also varies among ethnic groups: Hispanic Americans have the highest incidence in the United States, with an overall prevalence of 36 percent.[2] Although the precise cause of metabolic syndrome is not known, the close relationship between abdominal obesity and insulin resistance suggests that the current obesity crisis in the United States may be partly responsible for the high prevalence.

TABLE H26-1 Features of the Metabolic Syndrome

Metabolic syndrome is diagnosed when a person has three or more of the following symptoms.

Symptom	Diagnostic Criteria
Hyperglycemia	Fasting plasma glucose ≥110 mg/dL
Abdominal obesity	Waist circumference >40″ in men, >35″ in women
Hypertriglyceridemia	≥150 mg/dL
Reduced HDL cholesterol	<40 mg/dL in men, <50 mg/dL in women
Hypertension	≥130/85 mm Hg

Obesity and the Metabolic Syndrome

Although the relationship between obesity and the metabolic syndrome is not entirely understood, excessive abdominal fat is known to induce metabolic changes that lead to insulin resistance, which then leads to other abnormalities. The following sections explore these relationships.

Effects of Obesity on Insulin Action

Adipose cells that reside in the abdominal area are more metabolically active than adipose cells elsewhere.[3] Hence, triglycerides break down more rapidly, increasing fatty acid levels in the blood. These higher fatty acid concentrations inhibit the actions of insulin receptors, the proteins that recognize and bind insulin at cell surfaces.[4] Unless the pancreas can secrete enough insulin to compensate, glucose uptake from the blood is reduced, contributing to hyperglycemia.

Secretory Products of Adipose Cells

Obesity alters production of the hormones and proteins made by adipose cells. It causes reduced secretion of **adiponectin,** a hormone that improves insulin sensitivity.[5] Conversely, **resistin,** a hormone that contributes to insulin resistance, is released in greater amounts. Enlarged adipose cells also boost their production of cytokines that induce the synthesis of liver proteins that promote inflammation and blood coagulation.[6] People who are obese often have elevated levels of C-reactive protein,[7] a marker of inflammation linked to an increased risk of CVD.

Obesity and Hypertension

Obesity also increases the risk of developing high blood pressure, a common component of the metabolic syndrome. Both insulin resistance and hyperinsulinemia may be implicated in raising blood pressure.[8] Insulin resistance interferes with the normal relaxation and dilation of blood vessels. Hyperinsulinemia promotes reabsorption of sodium by the kidneys, resulting in fluid retention and increased blood volume. These effects can result in increased blood pressure.

Obesity and Hypertriglyceridemia

Obesity, especially abdominal obesity, is often associated with blood lipid abnormalities.[9] Increases in body weight are linked with higher triglyceride and LDL cholesterol levels and lower HDL cholesterol levels. As a result of obesity, adipose cells are less responsive to insulin and release more fatty acids into the bloodstream. At the same time, they are less able to extract and store triglycerides from chylomicrons and VLDL. To keep up with the greater influx of fatty acids, the liver must accelerate its production of VLDL, and hypertriglyceridemia develops.

FIGURE H26-1 Prevalence of the Metabolic Syndrome in the U.S. Population

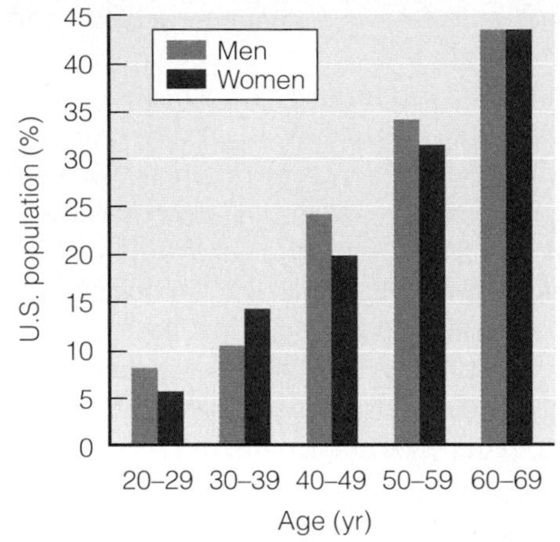
Men
Women
U.S. population (%)
45
40
35
30
25
20
15
10
5
0
20–29
30–39
40–49
50–59
60–69
Age (yr)

Data from E. S. Ford, W. H. Giles, and W. H. Dietz, Prevalence of the metabolic syndrome among U.S. adults: Findings from the third National Health and Nutrition Examination Survey, *Journal of the American Medical Association,* 2002, 287:356–359.

Consequences of the Metabolic Syndrome

A number of factors contribute to CVD risk in individuals with the metabolic syndrome. Obesity, lipid abnormalities, and hypertension are all independent risk factors for CVD. Both insulin resistance and elevated lipoprotein levels can cause damage to blood vessels, accelerating the progression of atherosclerosis.[10] The resulting blood vessel inflammation induces liver secretion of **fibrinogen,** a protein that promotes blood clot formation. C-reactive protein, which is elevated by both inflammation and obesity, inhibits **nitric oxide** production by blood vessel cells, an effect that impairs blood vessel activity and also promotes blood clotting.[11] Another procoagulant factor—**plasminogen activator inhibitor-1**—is overproduced as a consequence of both obesity and hyperinsulinemia. The combined effect of these multiple abnormalities can worsen atherosclerosis and increase the risks of developing heart attack and stroke.[12] Individuals with insulin resistance are also at increased risk of developing diabetes, another major risk factor for CVD.

Treatment Recommendations

The metabolic syndrome is primarily treated with dietary and lifestyle changes, with the goal of correcting abnormalities that increase CVD risk.[13] In most individuals, a combination of weight loss and physical activity can improve insulin resistance, blood pressure, and blood lipid levels. Additional dietary strategies depend on a patient's specific symptoms. If dietary and lifestyle changes are not successful, medications may be prescribed. Because effective treatment requires lifelong commitment, health care providers should work with patients to develop a treatment plan that they are willing to adopt.

Dietary Management

Weight reduction is often recommended for obese patients, and even a small weight loss (10 to 20 pounds) can improve symptoms. Many people find it difficult to achieve and maintain weight loss, however, and should be encouraged to make other dietary changes that can improve their health. Individuals with hypertriglyceridemia are usually advised to reduce their intake of added sugars and refined grain products (soda, juices, white bread, sweetened cereal, desserts) and increase servings of whole grains and foods high in fiber (whole-wheat bread, oatmeal, legumes, fruits, vegetables).[14] Carbohydrate restriction may help to reduce blood triglyceride levels and improve hyperglycemia.[15] Including fish in the diet each week may also improve triglyceride levels.[16] Individuals with hypertension are encouraged to reduce sodium intake and increase consumption of fruits and vegetables and low-fat milk products. A diet low in saturated fat, *trans* fats, and cholesterol can help to reduce LDL cholesterol levels. Chapter 27 includes additional information about dietary modifications that can reduce CVD risk.

Physical Exercise

Regular physical activity helps with weight management and may also improve blood lipid concentrations, hypertension, and insulin resistance—all changes that can reduce CVD risk. A program that includes both aerobic exercise and strength training is best. A minimum of 30 minutes of moderate aerobic activity (brisk walking, jogging, cycling) daily is suggested, although longer periods (one hour daily) are recommended for weight control.[17] A sedentary lifestyle can worsen the progression of metabolic syndrome and should be discouraged.

Drug Therapy

If dietary and lifestyle changes are unsuccessful, medications may be prescribed to correct hypertriglyceridemia and hypertension (Chapter 27 provides details). Insulin resistance is not routinely treated with drug therapy in nondiabetic patients due to insufficient evidence that the medications can benefit individuals with the metabolic syndrome.[18]

As explained in this highlight, the metabolic syndrome consists of a cluster of related disorders that increase the risk for developing CVD. Whereas the common features of the metabolic syndrome are independent risk factors for CVD, in combination they may raise risk two- to threefold. Treatment of the metabolic syndrome emphasizes dietary and lifestyle changes. The following chapter provides additional information about lifestyle changes that can reduce CVD risk.

REFERENCES

1. D. E. Moller and K. D. Kaufman, Metabolic syndrome: A clinical and molecular perspective, *Annual Review of Medicine* 56 (2005): 45–62.
2. Z. T. Bloomgarden, American Association of Clinical Endocrinologists (AACE) consensus conference on the insulin resistance syndrome, *Diabetes Care* 26 (2003): 1297–1303.
3. Moller and Kaufman, 2005.
4. G. A. Bray and C. M. Champagne, Obesity and the metabolic syndrome: Implications for dietetics practitioners, *Journal of the American Dietetic Association* 104 (2004): 86–89.
5. Moller and Kaufman, 2005; P. A. Kern and coauthors, Adiponectin expression from human adipose tissue, *Diabetes* 52 (2003): 1779–1785.
6. Bray and Champagne, 2004; S. M. Grundy, Inflammation, hypertension, and the metabolic syndrome, *Journal of the American Medical Association* 290 (2003): 3000–3002.
7. Grundy, 2003.
8. Grundy, 2003.
9. A. Tiengo and A. Avogaro, Cardiovascular disease, in P. Bjorntorp, ed., *International Textbook of Obesity* (West Sussex, U.K.: John Wiley & Sons, 2001), pp. 365–377.
10. Moller and Kaufman, 2005.
11. S. M. Grundy and coauthors, Clinical management of metabolic syndrome: Report of the American Heart Association/National Heart, Lung, and Blood Institute/American Diabetes Association Conference on Scientific Issues Related to Management, *Circulation* 109 (2004): 551–556.
12. Moller and Kaufman, 2005.
13. Grundy and coauthors, 2004; D. Deen, Metabolic syndrome: Time for action, *American Family Physician* 69 (2004): 2875–2882.
14. Grundy and coauthors, 2004.
15. D. M. Kendall, Reducing cardiovascular risk in type 2 diabetes and the metabolic syndrome: The emerging role of insulin resistance, in A. Peters Harmel and R. Mathur, eds., *Davidson's Diabetes Mellitus: Diagnosis and Treatment* (Philadelphia: Saunders, 2004), pp. 239–257.
16. Deen, 2004.
17. Grundy and coauthors, 2004; Deen, 2004.
18. Grundy and coauthors, 2004.

Chapter 27

Nutrition and Cardiovascular Diseases

Chapter Outline

Available Online

http://nutrition.wadsworth.com/uncn7

Student Practice Test

Glossary Terms

Nutrition on the Net

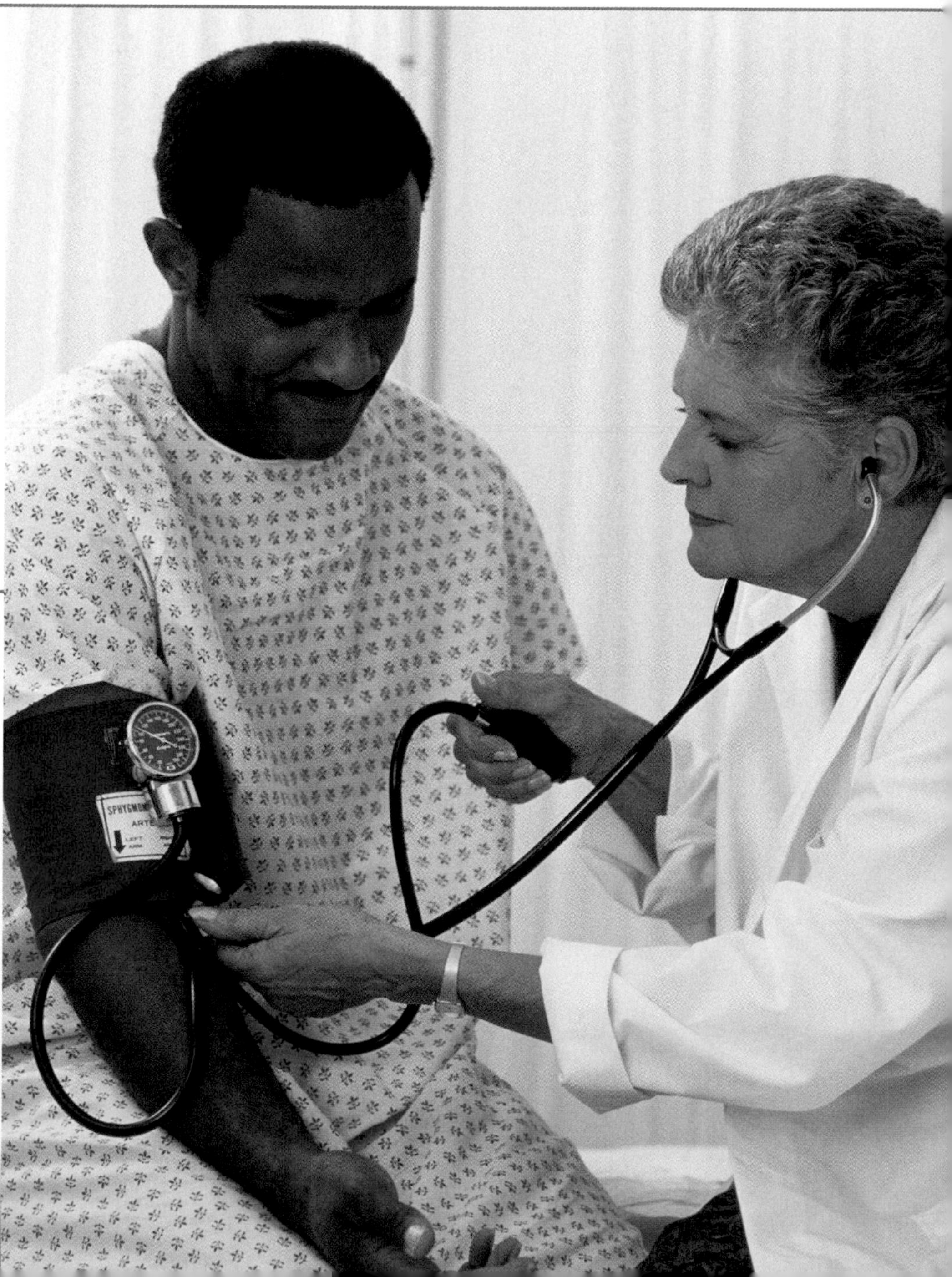
SPHYGMOMANOMETER

Nutrition in the Professional Setting

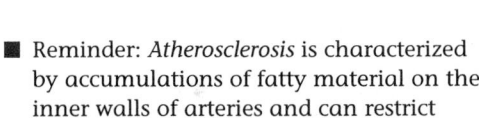

Each heartbeat sends oxygen-rich blood to the body's tissues. A disrupted blood supply hinders the ability of cells to carry out their metabolic functions. This is a frequent consequence of cardiovascular diseases, which disturb the functions of the heart and blood vessels. At first, patients may not realize that their weakness, fatigue, or shortness of breath is due to a cardiovascular condition, but over time the complications can be disabling.

Cardiovascular disease (CVD), a general term describing diseases of the heart and blood vessels, was introduced in Chapter 5 (see p. 159) and discussed further in Highlight 15 (see pp. 547–549). **Coronary heart disease (CHD)** is the most common form of CVD and is caused by atherosclerosis■ in the coronary arteries that supply blood to the heart muscle. If atherosclerosis restricts blood flow in these arteries, the resulting deprivation of oxygen and nutrients can destroy heart tissue and cause a **myocardial infarction (MI)**—a **heart attack.** When the blood supply to brain tissue is blocked, a **stroke** occurs. Both heart attack and stroke may result in disablement or death. This chapter describes these and other cardiovascular disorders. Figure 27-1 shows the percentages of deaths resulting from all types of CVD.

CVD is responsible for nearly 40 percent of deaths in the United States, claiming more lives than the next five leading causes of death combined.[1] Although many people assume that heart problems are men's diseases, CVD deaths in women have exceeded those of men for the past 20 years.[2] CVD is a global health issue; it is the leading cause of death in Europe and contributes to nearly one-third of deaths worldwide.[3]

■ Reminder: *Atherosclerosis* is characterized by accumulations of fatty material on the inner walls of arteries and can restrict blood flow to the surrounding tissues.

cardiovascular disease (CVD): a general term describing diseases of the heart and blood vessels.
- **cardio** = heart
- **vascular** = blood vessels

coronary heart disease (CHD): irregular thickening of the coronary arteries that may eventually disrupt blood flow to heart tissue; also called **coronary artery disease.**

myocardial (my-oh-CAR-dee-al) **infarction** (in-FARK-shun) or **MI:** death of heart muscle caused by a sudden reduction in coronary blood flow; also called a **heart attack** or **cardiac arrest.**
- **myo** = muscle
- **cardial** = heart
- **infarct** = tissue death

stroke: an injury to brain tissue due to disturbed blood flow through arteries that supply blood to the brain; also called a **cerebrovascular accident.**
- **cerebro** = brain

FIGURE 27-1 Percentage Breakdown of Deaths from Cardiovascular Diseases in the United States, 2002

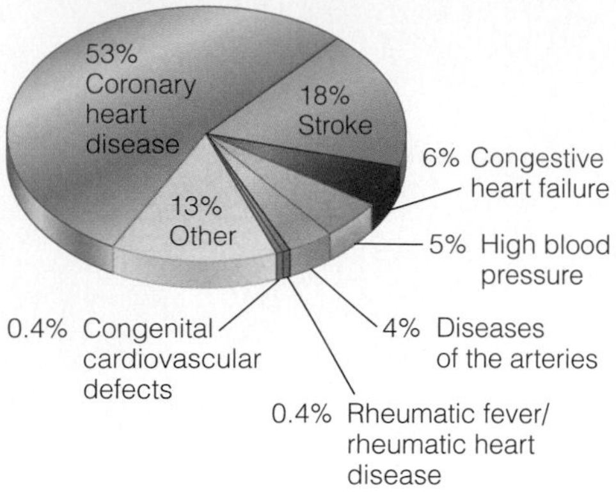
53% Coronary heart disease
18% Stroke
6% Congestive heart failure
5% High blood pressure
4% Diseases of the arteries
0.4% Rheumatic fever/ rheumatic heart disease
0.4% Congenital cardiovascular defects
13% Other

SOURCE: Based on preliminary data for 2002 from the Centers for Disease Control/National Center for Health Statistics and the National Heart, Lung, and Blood Institute.

- Atherosclerosis is the most common form of **arteriosclerosis**, a more general term for arterial diseases characterized by abnormally thickened walls and lost elasticity.

- Reminder: *Monocytes* are phagocytic white blood cells that circulate in blood. Once they enter tissues, they are called macrophages (see Highlight 17).

plaque (PLACK): an abnormal accumulation of fatty deposits, smooth muscle cells, and fibrous connective tissue in blood vessels.

vulnerable plaque: a form of plaque, susceptible to rupture, that is lipid-rich and has only a thin fibrous barrier between the arterial lumen and the plaque's lipid core.

thrombosis (throm-BOH-sis): the formation or presence of a blood clot in blood vessels. A *coronary thrombosis* occurs in a coronary artery, and a *cerebral thrombosis* occurs in an artery that supplies blood to the brain.
• **thrombo** = clot

thrombus: a blood clot formed within a blood vessel that remains attached to its place of origin.

embolus (EM-boh-lus): an abnormal particle, like a blood clot or air bubble, that travels in the blood.
• **embol** = to insert, plug

embolism (EM-boh-lizm): the obstruction of a blood vessel by an embolus, causing sudden tissue death.

ischemia (is-KEY-mee-a): inadequate blood supply to tissues due to obstructed blood flow through arteries.

foam cells: swollen vascular cells that accumulate lipids.

Atherosclerosis

In atherosclerosis, sometimes called "hardening of the arteries," the artery walls become progressively thickened due to an accumulation of fatty deposits, smooth muscle cells, and fibrous connective tissue, collectively known as **plaque.**■ As plaque thickens, it can eventually narrow the lumen of an artery and restrict blood flow.[4] Plaque can exist in a stable form that does not cause complications or an unstable form called **vulnerable plaque.**[5] Vulnerable plaque has only a thin fibrous barrier between its lipid-rich core and the arterial lumen. It is highly susceptible to rupture, which then promotes blood clot formation within the artery **(thrombosis).** A blood clot **(thrombus)** can enlarge in time and ultimately obstruct blood flow. A portion of a clot may also break free **(embolus)** and travel through the circulatory system until it lodges in a narrowed artery and shuts off blood flow to the surrounding tissue **(embolism).** Most complications of atherosclerosis are due to the obstruction of the blood supply to surrounding tissues **(ischemia).**

Stages of Plaque Development

Atherosclerosis begins to develop as early as childhood or adolescence and usually progresses over several decades before symptoms develop.[6] It initially arises in response to minimal but chronic injuries that damage the arterial lining. Damage to the artery causes the immune system to respond, attracting monocytes,■ T cells, and platelets to the region. The monocytes slip under the thin layer of blood vessel cells and engulf LDL cholesterol, becoming **foam cells;** these fat-laden cells are visible as fatty deposits along artery walls, known as *fatty streaks* (see Figure 27-2). Smooth muscle cells are recruited from arterial tissue and stimulated to divide, ingest LDL particles, and produce molecules that form fibrous connective tissue. As the plaque thickens, it also accumulates calcium, and the cholesterol within the lipid core can crystallize and harden.

As atherosclerosis progresses, the artery may expand outward to accommodate the plaque volume (as shown in the third panel of Figure 27-2). Additional lipid accumulation may eventually narrow the diameter of the arterial lumen.[7] Sometimes plaque progression only causes narrowing, rather than expansion, of an artery.

Although arteries that expand are less likely to interfere with blood flow, they usually have an unstable plaque structure (a lipid-rich core covered with a thin fibrous barrier). These vulnerable plaques are more likely to rupture, induce clotting, and increase risk of heart attack or stroke. The arteries that accommodate plaque only by narrowing may impede blood flow, but they generally have a more stable plaque structure (a lower lipid content and a thicker barrier).

The discovery of variations in plaque anatomy has helped to explain why modifying risk factors can dramatically reduce the risk of heart attack and stroke even when plaque volume and the lumen diameter do not change. Researchers now believe that therapeutic interventions can change the structure and composition of plaque and reduce its vulnerability to rupture and thrombosis.[8]

Causes of Atherosclerosis

As discussed in Highlight 15, fatty streaks may appear within the first decade of life. The reasons that atherosclerosis develops and progresses are complex. Generally, the factors that initiate atherosclerosis either cause direct damage to the artery wall or allow lipid materials to penetrate its surface. Other factors promote the progression of atherosclerosis and related complications by inducing plaque rupture[9] or blood coagulation.[10]

Inflammation and Infection Plaque development is an inflammatory response to an injury on the artery wall. As described earlier, the body's immune system is recruited during plaque development.[11] There is also evidence that a

FIGURE 27-2 Stages of Plaque Progression

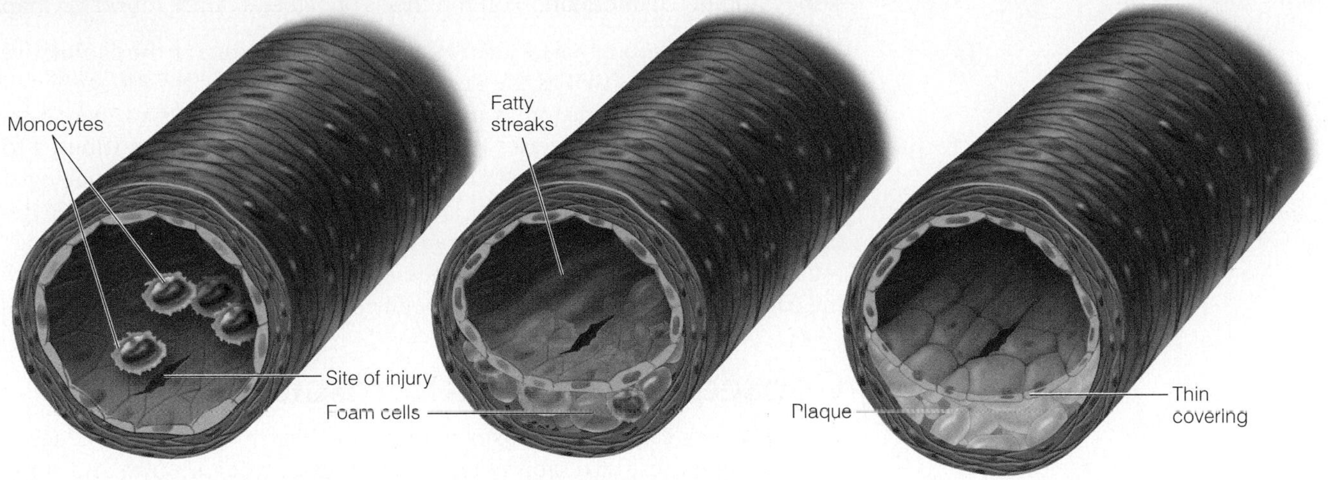
Monocytes
Fatty streaks
Site of injury
Foam cells
Plaque
Thin covering

Monocytes—phagocytic white blood cells—circulate in the bloodstream and respond to injury on the artery wall.

Monocytes slip under blood vessel cells and engulf LDL cholesterol, becoming foam cells. The thin layers of foam cells that develop on artery walls are known as *fatty streaks*.

A fatty streak thickens and forms plaque as it accumulates additional lipids, smooth muscle cells, connective tissue, and cellular debris.

The artery may expand to accommodate plaque. When this occurs, the plaque that develops often contains a large lipid core with a thin fibrous covering and is vulnerable to rupture and thrombosis.

persistent infection within the body may contribute to plaque formation. A number of different bacterial and viral antigens have been identified in plaque.[12]■

Shear Stress The stress of blood flow along the artery walls—called shear stress—can cause mechanical damage within the arteries. Plaque lesions tend to develop at the points where arteries branch or bend because blood flow is disturbed in those regions (see Figure H15-1 on p. 548). High blood pressure intensifies the stress of blood flow on arterial walls.

Smoking Smoking has multiple effects that contribute to plaque development and subsequent disease. Components in smoke impair the normal functions of artery cells and induce vasoconstriction; other toxic substances in smoke increase oxidative stress and promote blood clotting. Passive smoking has similar effects.[13]

Elevated LDL and VLDL High LDL and VLDL■ levels promote atherosclerosis, particularly if the lipoproteins have been oxidized. Oxidation may result from free-radical generation by macrophages and blood vessel cells or from various enzyme reactions.[14] It is not yet known whether dietary intake of oxidized lipids significantly contributes to the levels of oxidized LDL and VLDL in blood.[15]

Oxidized LDL and VLDL are actively taken up and retained in the artery wall.[16] Oxidized LDL have other damaging effects: they activate and recruit the smooth muscle cells involved in plaque formation, induce vasoconstriction, stimulate blood clotting, and inhibit some of the normal protective functions of HDL.[17]■

Elevated concentrations of a variant form of LDL called **lipoprotein(a)** have been found to speed the progression of advanced atherosclerosis[18] and to double the risk of CHD.[19] Abnormally high levels are largely genetically determined and have been associated with premature development of heart disease. Pharmacological doses of niacin and hormone replacement therapy■ in women may lower lipoprotein(a) levels, but the benefits of such treatments are not yet clear.

Diabetes Mellitus Diabetes increases risks of both early and advanced atherosclerosis. Chronic hyperglycemia causes the production of advanced glycation end

■ C-reactive protein, the major blood indicator of an inflammatory response, is associated with increased risk of heart disease (see Chapter 22).

■ Reminder: Cholesterol-carrying lipoproteins that promote atherosclerosis include *low-density lipoproteins (LDL)* and *very-low-density lipoproteins (VLDL)*; see pp. 153–154 for a review of lipoprotein metabolism. Disorders in which blood lipids are abnormally high are called **hyperlipidemias**, or **dyslipidemias.**

■ Reminder: *High-density lipoproteins (HDL)* protect against atherosclerosis by removing cholesterol from circulation and helping to prevent LDL oxidation.

■ Oral estrogen therapy has both positive and negative effects on CHD risk: it can reduce LDL and raise HDL cholesterol, but it can also increase blood-clotting activity.

lipoprotein(a): a variant of LDL associated with a high risk of atherosclerosis and CHD.

■ Reminder: *Advanced glycation end products* are formed when glucose or its fragments combine with protein.

products,■ which damage blood vessels and worsen atherosclerosis.[20] Other effects of diabetes promote blood clot formation, which contributes to plaque progression.[21] Additional information on the effects of diabetes can be found in Chapter 26.

Aging Aging is strongly associated with atherosclerosis due to the cumulative exposure to risk factors as well as the degeneration of arterial cells with age.[22] Aging becomes a significant risk factor for men at age 45 or older, and for women at age 55 or older as they reach menopause. The gender difference has been attributed to estrogen's protective effect on arterial function in women[23] and to the damaging effect of iron overload in men, which can increase oxidative stress.[24] Homocysteine levels (p. 200), which increase with age and are generally higher in men, may damage artery walls and increase oxidative stress, but researchers have not yet determined whether the harmful effects are caused by homocysteine or by something associated with it.[25]

Consequences of Atherosclerosis

Atherosclerosis can affect almost any organ or tissue in the body, and accordingly it is a leading cause of disability and fatal illness. Plaque rupture and subsequent thrombosis can result in pain or discomfort in the chest and surrounding regions **(angina pectoris)** or in death of part of the heart tissue (myocardial infarction or heart attack). Atherosclerosis also causes obstructions in blood flow to the brain, resulting in severe injury to brain tissue (stroke). When peripheral artery disease affects circulation to the legs, it can cause fatigue and pain on walking (intermittent claudication).■ Blockage of the arteries that supply the kidneys can result in kidney disease or even acute kidney failure.

■ Reminder: *Intermittent claudication* is severe pain and weakness in the legs with walking that is associated with an insufficient blood supply.

Atherosclerosis is a risk factor for another type of arterial disease: **aneurysms** (areas of abnormal enlargement within blood vessels).[26] Plaque can weaken the blood vessel wall, allowing it to expand and balloon out. Aneurysms that go undetected can rupture and lead to massive bleeding and death, particularly when a large vessel such as the aorta is affected. In the arteries of the brain, an aneurysm may lead to bleeding within the brain, coma, or stroke.

IN SUMMARY The most common cardiovascular diseases are caused by atherosclerosis, a condition characterized by a buildup of plaque on an artery's wall. Rupture of vulnerable plaque can lead to thrombosis and obstruction of blood flow. Plaque is initiated by factors that damage the artery wall and advanced by plaque rupture and blood coagulation. Leading causes of plaque formation and progression include inflammation, hypertension, smoking, hyperlipidemias, and diabetes. Atherosclerosis can result in complications that include angina pectoris, heart attack, stroke, pain with walking, kidney disease, and development of aneurysms.

Coronary Heart Disease (CHD)

Coronary heart disease (CHD) is the most common type of cardiovascular disease and the leading cause of death in the United States. It is usually caused by atherosclerosis in the large and medium-sized arteries that supply the heart muscle with oxygen and nutrients. The plaque is generally unevenly distributed and vulnerable to rupture, and resulting blood clots can give rise to ischemia and tissue injury. Atherosclerosis can sometimes advance enough to fully block an artery, but most heart attacks occur with less than 50 percent blockage.[27] Occasionally, CHD is due to coronary spasms or inflammatory diseases that affect the coronary arteries.

Although CHD prevalence and mortality are similar in men and women, men suffer more heart attacks than women, whereas more women develop angina pectoris.[28] Women develop heart disease about 10 years later in life than men do, and their in-

angina (an-JYE-nah or AN-ji-nah) **pectoris:** a condition caused by ischemia in the heart muscle that results in discomfort or dull pain in the chest region. The pain often radiates to the left shoulder and arm, to the back, or into the throat, jaws, and teeth.

aneurysms (AN-you-riz-ums): abnormal enlargements or bulging of blood vessels (usually arteries) caused by damage to or weakness in the blood vessel wall.

cidences of serious complications like heart attack and sudden death lag behind men's by about 20 years. In both genders, CHD can lie dormant for years: over half of sudden deaths from CHD occur without prior symptoms in both men and women.[29]

Prevention of CHD

During their lifetimes, most people in the United States develop some degree of coronary atherosclerosis, which largely accounts for the high risk of developing CHD (49 percent for men and 32 percent for women).[30] Because atherosclerosis develops over many years, prevention should begin well before signs and symptoms appear. For most people, prevention of CHD begins by reducing risk. Population studies have suggested that 80 to 90 percent of people with severe heart disease have at least one of the four classic risk factors: smoking, high LDL cholesterol, high blood pressure, and diabetes.[31] These and other major risk factors that can be modified by changes in diet or lifestyle are listed in Table 27-1; only age, gender, and family history cannot be modified.[32]

Blood Cholesterol and CHD Risk Once a person's risks have been identified, treatment focuses on lowering LDL cholesterol. Elevated LDL cholesterol levels are directly related to the development of atherosclerosis, and clinical trials have confirmed that LDL cholesterol–lowering treatments can successfully reduce CHD mortality rates. CHD is seldom seen in populations that maintain desirable LDL levels. Table 27-2 presents standards for LDL cholesterol and other CHD risk factors.

Because HDL protect against atherosclerosis, low HDL cholesterol levels are highly predictive of CHD risk. In addition, low HDL levels often coexist with other risk factors, such as high triglycerides and small, dense LDL (see the Research Update on p. 824). Moreover, some factors that increase CHD risk—obesity, smoking, inactivity, and male gender—also reduce HDL levels. It is not known whether raising HDL will help to reduce CHD risk, but weight loss, physical activity, and smoking cessation can independently help to lower risk.

CHD Risk Assessment The intensity of the LDL cholesterol–lowering treatment depends on a person's level of risk for CHD. The National Cholesterol Education Program (NCEP) periodically issues treatment guidelines that also evaluate an individual's risk status. The most current guidelines, known as Adult Treatment Panel III (ATP III), were released in 2001. ATP III recommends aggressive treatment for patients who already have CHD or a CHD risk equivalent■ and includes guidelines for prevention for people with multiple CHD risk factors. For some people, dietary and lifestyle changes may be the only treatment needed for managing cholesterol levels. (The "How to" box on pp. 826–827 summarizes the use of the ATP III guidelines in clinical practice.)

■ A **CHD risk equivalent** carries the same risk for a major coronary event as established CHD; examples include type 2 diabetes mellitus and diseases caused by atherosclerosis such as stroke or aortic aneurysm.

TABLE 27-1 Risk Factors for CHD

Major Risk Factors for CHD (not modifiable)

- Increasing age.
- Male gender.
- Family history of premature heart disease.

Major Risk Factors for CHD (modifiable)

- High blood LDL cholesterol.
- Low blood HDL cholesterol.
- High blood pressure (hypertension).
- Diabetes.
- Obesity (especially abdominal obesity).
- Physical inactivity.
- Cigarette smoking.
- An "atherogenic" diet (high in saturated fats and low in vegetables, fruits, and whole grains).

NOTE: Risk factors highlighted in color have relationships with diet.
SOURCE: Expert Panel on Detection, Evaluation, and Treatment of High Blood Cholesterol in Adults (Adult Treatment Panel III), *Third Report of the National Cholesterol Education Program (NCEP)*, NIH publication no. 02-5215 (Bethesda, MD.: National Heart, Lung, and Blood Institute, 2002), pp. II-15–II-20.

TABLE 27-2 Standards for CHD Risk Factors

Risk Factors	Desirable	Borderline Risk	High Risk
Total blood cholesterol (mg/dL)	<200	200–239	≥240
LDL cholesterol (mg/dL)	<100[a]	130–159	160–189[b]
HDL cholesterol (mg/dL)	≥60	59–40	<40
Triglycerides, fasting (mg/dL)	<150	150–199	200–499[c]
Body mass index (BMI)[d]	18.5–24.9	25–29.9	≥30
Blood pressure (systolic and/or diastolic pressure)	<120/<80	120–139/80–89[e]	≥140/≥90[f]

[a]100–129 mg/dL LDL indicates a near or above optimal level. <70 mg/dL is a desirable goal for very high-risk persons.
[b]≥190 mg/dL LDL indicates a very high risk.
[c]≥500 mg/dL triglycerides indicates a very high risk.
[d]Body mass index (BMI) was defined in Chapter 8; BMI standards are found on the inside back cover.
[e]These values indicate prehypertension.
[f]These values indicate stage one hypertension; ≥160/≥100 indicates stage two hypertension. Physicians use these classifications to determine medical treatment.

RESEARCH UPDATE LDL Subclasses

LDL "particles" are not all identical, but are made up of distinct subtypes that vary in size and density.[a] LDL diameter is inversely associated with heart disease risk: the smallest, most dense LDL (known as LDL subclass pattern B) are the most atherogenic, and larger, less dense LDL (LDL subclass pattern A) are less atherogenic. People who have "pattern B" frequently have high triglycerides (VLDL) and low HDL levels as well. Epidemiological studies have shown that this lipoprotein profile is associated with a two- to three-fold increased risk of CHD and is also found in families with a genetic predisposition for premature CHD.

LDL particle size is thought to be approximately 35 to 50 percent inherited, and researchers have been working on identifying the genetic mutations that contribute to LDL size.[b] Nongenetic factors that contribute to LDL size include age, gender, adiposity, oral contraceptive use, and diet. The pattern B trait appears in 30 to 35 percent of men over 20 years old but in only 5 to 10 percent of premenopausal women and 20 percent of postmenopausal women. Insulin resistance is strongly associated with LDL subclass pattern B, and the trait is especially prevalent among people with type 2 diabetes mellitus.

Changes in diet can induce expression of the pattern B trait in susceptible individuals. For years, low-fat, high-carbohydrate diets were recommended for lowering cholesterol levels in patients with hyperlipidemias. However, when these diets were tested in experimental subjects who had larger, less dense LDL ("pattern A"), the reduction in LDL cholesterol was often achieved by a depletion of the *cholesterol content* of LDL particles, rather than by a decrease in the *numbers* of circulating LDL. This caused a decrease in LDL diameters and essentially converted the healthier pattern A LDL to the more atherogenic pattern B. In addition, as the fat content in the test diets was lowered, more of the subjects converted to pattern B. Partially as a result of these studies, medical professionals have reconsidered the benefits of using low-fat, high-carbohydrate diets for the control of blood cholesterol.[c] Instead, CHD patients are often advised to modify their diets by replacing foods rich in saturated fats or *trans* fats with foods containing unsaturated fats (see Highlight 5 for more details).[d]

[a] R. M. Krauss, Dietary and genetic effects on low-density lipoprotein heterogeneity, *Annual Reviews of Nutrition* 21 (2001): 283–295.

[b] I. L. Ruel and coauthors, Characterization of LDL particle size among carriers of a defective or a null mutation in the lipoprotein lipase gene, *Arteriosclerosis, Thrombosis, and Vascular Biology* 22 (2002): 1181–1186.

[c] E. J. Parks and M. K. Hellerstein, Carbohydrate-induced hypertriacylglycerolemia: Historical perspective and review of biological mechanisms, *American Journal of Clinical Nutrition* 71(2000): 412–433; S. M. Grundy, The optimal ratio of fat-to-carbohydrate in the diet, *Annual Reviews of Nutrition* 19 (1999): 325–341.

[d] R. M. Krauss and coauthors, Revision 2000: A statement for healthcare professionals from the nutrition committee of the American Heart Association, *Journal of Nutrition* 131 (2001): 132–146.

■ A **lipoprotein profile** provides laboratory values for each type of lipoprotein. It is sometimes called a **blood lipid profile.**

■ Normal blood pressure: <120/<80 mm Hg.

■ Overweight: BMI 25–29.9.
Obesity: BMI ≥30.

■ Abdominal obesity—waist circumference:
Men: >40 in.
Women: >35 in.

Risk assessment requires several key laboratory measures and a medical history. A complete lipoprotein profile,■ which includes measures of total cholesterol, LDL and HDL cholesterol, and triglycerides, should be obtained every 5 years starting at 20 years of age. Sometimes the ratio of total cholesterol to HDL cholesterol is used to predict CHD risk: a high total cholesterol value reflects the magnitude of atherogenic lipoproteins, and a low HDL value is often linked with the multiple risk factors of the metabolic syndrome. A blood pressure measurement is also needed to accurately assess CHD risk.■ For people over 50 years of age, a high systolic blood pressure is more predictive of CHD risk than diastolic blood pressure.[33] Certain diseases, including other disorders caused by atherosclerosis, diabetes mellitus, and the metabolic syndrome, confer high risk for CHD. Overweight and obesity■ also predispose to CHD, particularly when abdominal obesity is present.■ Finally, cigarette smoking strongly contributes to CHD risk. The ATP III guidelines include an algorithm for estimating the ten-year risk of developing CHD that includes some of these risk factors (see the "How to" on p. 828).

Therapeutic Lifestyle Changes for Lowering CHD Risk

People with CHD and those who have multiple risk factors for CHD are usually advised to make dietary and lifestyle changes to reduce their risk before considering drug therapy. The ATP III guidelines recommend an approach to risk reduction called Therapeutic Lifestyle Changes (TLC), which is summarized in Table 27-3.[34] The main features of TLC are a cholesterol-lowering diet, weight reduction, and regular physical activity. If TLC is followed carefully, substantial progress may be seen after six weeks. People with a high risk of CHD should try to lower LDL cholesterol with a three- to six-month trial of TLC before considering drug therapy.[35]

Saturated Fat Of the lipids in our diet, saturated fats have the strongest effect on blood cholesterol levels. Clinical trials have suggested that LDL cholesterol rises

TABLE 27-3 Reducing Risk of CHD with Therapeutic Lifestyle Changes

Dietary Strategies

- Limit saturated fat to less than 7% of total kcalories and cholesterol to less than 200 milligrams a day. Maintaining a fat intake that is 25 to 35% of total kcalories may help with this goal.
- Replace saturated fats with carbohydrates from whole grains, legumes, fruits, and vegetables or with unsaturated fats from fish, vegetable oils, and nuts.
- Avoid food products that contain *trans*-fatty acids. Check package ingredients for "partially hydrogenated vegetable oils." Food labels will be required to list the *trans* fats in food products by January 1, 2006.
- Choose foods high in soluble fibers, including oats, barley, beans, and fruit. Psyllium seed husk can be used as a food supplement to help lower LDL cholesterol levels.
- Regularly consume food products that contain added plant sterols or stanols.
- Regularly consume foods that contain soy protein to replace those that contain animal fat.
- To reduce blood pressure, choose a diet that is high in fruits and vegetables, low-fat milk products, nuts, and whole grains. Limit sodium intake to 2400 milligrams per day.*
- Fish can be consumed regularly as part of a CHD risk-reduction diet.
- If alcohol is consumed, it should be limited to one drink daily for women and two drinks daily for men.

Lifestyle Choices

- Physical activity: At least 30 minutes of moderate-intensity endurance activity should be undertaken on most days of the week. The eventual goal should be an expenditure of at least 2000 kcalories weekly.
- Smoking cessation: Exposure to any form of tobacco smoke should be minimized.

Weight Reduction

- Weight reduction may improve other CHD risk factors. The general goal of a weight-management program should be to prevent weight gain, reduce body weight, and maintain a lower body weight over the long term. The initial goal of a weight-loss program should be to lose no more than 10% of original body weight.

*According to DRI recommendations, sodium intake should be limited to 2300 milligrams daily.

2 percent for every 1 percent increase in kcalories from saturated fat. The major dietary sources of saturated fat in the American diet are whole-milk products, high-fat meats, and baked goods. The TLC's recommendation is to consume less than 7 percent of total kcalories as saturated fat. The American diet provides, on average, about 11 percent of total kcalories from saturated fat.

As Highlight 5 explains, replacing saturated fats with monounsaturated or polyunsaturated fats■ can lower LDL levels. Polyunsaturated fats have a slightly greater effect, but can also promote a slight reduction in HDL cholesterol. TLC recommendations allow up to 20 percent of kcalories from monounsaturated fat, but suggest a maximum of 10 percent of kcalories from polyunsaturated fat due to concerns about the safety of ingesting large quantities over long periods. Cutting down on saturated fats is not as simple as switching from butter to vegetable oil—the main saturated fat sources in most diets are usually high-protein foods served as entrées. Choosing lean meats or fish, using fat-free or low-fat milk products, and avoiding certain types of bakery products may be a more effective means of reducing saturated fat.■

■ Most polyunsaturated fat in the diet consists of omega-6 fatty acids, such as linoleic acid.

■ The TLC recommendation for total fat is 25 to 35% of kcalories. Some persons with the metabolic syndrome may benefit from a slightly higher fat intake of 30 to 35%. Fat intakes higher than this may promote weight gain in some people.

Replacing dietary saturated fats with carbohydrates can also reduce LDL cholesterol, but such a change may lower HDL cholesterol and raise triglycerides. This effect may be offset somewhat by limiting added sugars and including fiber-rich foods; ideally, the diet should include generous amounts of whole grains, legumes, fruits, and vegetables. The TLC diet recommends a carbohydrate intake in the range of 50 to 60 percent of total kcalories.

Dietary Cholesterol High cholesterol intakes have a cholesterol-raising effect, and reducing intakes decreases LDL cholesterol in most people. Some epidemiological studies have suggested that dietary cholesterol may raise CHD risk independently from its effect on blood cholesterol, although this finding has not been seen in all studies. Eggs contribute about one-third of the cholesterol in the American

HOW TO Detect, Evaluate, and Treat High Blood Cholesterol

The most recent NCEP report, Adult Treatment Panel III (ATP III), identifies three categories of risk that affect treatment for LDL cholesterol, based on easily identified risk factors. By using this nine-step risk assessment, a person's risk for an acute coronary event over the next ten years can be identified as being less than 10 percent (low risk), 10 to 20 percent (moderate risk), or over 20 percent (high risk). In addition, treatment goals are set for each risk category. Note that these are guidelines only and should not override the judgment of an attending physician.

Step 1. Obtain a complete lipoprotein profile from blood samples taken after a 9- to 12-hour fast. (Desirable blood lipid levels are shown in Table 27-2.)

Step 2. Identify the presence of diseases that confer high risk for acute CHD events; the following are considered CHD risk equivalents:

- Symptoms of CHD.
- Symptoms of stroke.
- Aortic aneurysm.
- Intermittent claudication.
- Diabetes mellitus.

Step 3. Identify major risk factors other than LDL cholesterol:

- Cigarette smoking.
- Hypertension (blood pressure ≥140/90 mm Hg) or use of an antihypertensive medication.
- Low HDL cholesterol (≤40 mg/dL). If HDL cholesterol is ≥60 mg/dL, substract one risk factor from the total count.
- Family history of premature CHD (CHD in father or brother at younger than 55 years; mother or sister at younger than 65 years).
- Age (if male, 45 years or older; if female, 55 years or older).

Step 4. Assess ten-year CHD risk: high risk (more than 20 percent), moderate risk (10 to 20 percent), and low risk (less than 10 percent).

- If a CHD risk equivalent is present (see Step 2), the person is automatically at high risk (more than 20 percent within next ten years) of an acute coronary event.
- If two or more risk factors (other than LDL) are present (see Step 3), assess ten-year risk according to age, total cholesterol, HDL cholesterol, systolic blood pressure, and smoking habit (see the "How to" on p. 828).
- If one risk factor (or less) is present, a person's ten-year risk is ≤10 percent.

Step 5. Determine LDL goals and treatment options for each risk category:

Risk Category	LDL Goal	LDL Level at Which to Start Therapeutic Lifestyle Changes (TLC)	LDL Level at Which to Consider Drug Therapy
High	<100 mg/dL[a]	≥100 mg/dL	≥130 mg/dL[b]
Moderate	<130 mg/dL[c]	≥130 mg/dL	≥130 mg/dL[b] if 10-year risk 10–20% ≥160 mg/dL if 10-year risk <10%
Low	<160 mg/dL	≥160 mg/dL	≥190 mg/dL

[a]<70 mg/dL is a goal for very high-risk patients.
[b]Drug therapy is sometimes considered for LDL >100 mg/dL.
[c]<100 mg/dL is a goal for some patients.

diet, followed by meats, milk, and cheese. The current daily cholesterol intake in the United States is 256 milligrams, although it is higher in men (331 milligrams) than in women (213 milligrams). The TLC recommendation is to reduce cholesterol to less than 200 milligrams per day.

Trans Fats *Trans*-fatty acids raise LDL cholesterol levels and are also associated with an increased CHD risk. When *trans* fats replace saturated fats in the diet (as when stick margarine replaces butter), they may also cause a decline in HDL cholesterol levels. Most sources of *trans* fats are products made with partially hydrogenated oils: baked goods like crackers, cookies, and doughnuts, and fried foods like french fries and fried chicken. Soft margarines (tub and liquid forms) and other products are now available with little, or no, *trans* fat. Current *trans* fat intakes average about 2.6 percent of kcalories, and the TLC recommendation is to keep it as low as possible.

Soluble Fibers As Chapter 4 explained, soluble, viscous fibers can reduce the absorption of cholesterol and bile by binding them in the intestinal tract and may also influence the liver's production of cholesterol by other means. An extra 5 to 10 grams of soluble fiber daily is associated with an approximately 5 percent reduction in LDL cholesterol. Dietary sources of soluble fibers include oats, barley, legumes, and fruits. The soluble fiber from psyllium seed husks, frequently used as an over-the-counter constipation treatment, is also effective for lowering cholesterol levels when used as a supplement.[36]

Plant Sterols Food manufacturers have designed margarines, cheese, and other products with added plant sterols■ that can lower blood cholesterol levels. Plant sterols work by reducing the intestinal absorption of cholesterol—both dietary cholesterol and the cholesterol in bile. One concern is that plant sterols may also reduce absorption and blood levels of carotenoids, although it is not known

■ Plant sterols are extracted from soybeans and pine-tree oils. They can be hydrogenated to produce *plant stanols,* which are the compounds typically found in commercial products.

Step 6. Initiate Therapeutic Lifestyle Changes (TLC) if the patient's LDL level is above the goal. The main features of TLC include (see the text for details):

- Restricted intake of saturated fat (less than 7 percent of total kcalories) and cholesterol (less than 200 milligrams per day).
- Increased intake of soluble fiber (10–25 grams per day) and plant stanols and sterols (2 grams per day).
- Moderate physical activity (approximately 200 kcalories expended per day).
- Weight reduction, if necessary.

If there is no improvement in LDL after three months, consider drug therapy.

Step 7. Consider adding drug therapy if LDL levels exceed recommendations shown in Step 5. Continue lifestyle changes. Major drugs used for cholesterol lowering include:

- *Statins (include lovastatin, pravastatin):* Reduce cholesterol synthesis in the liver. They reduce LDL and triglycerides and increase HDL.
- *Bile acid sequestrants (include cholestyramine, colestipol):* Bind bile acids in the small intestine, reducing reabsorption. They reduce LDL and raise HDL slightly.
- *Nicotinic acid (a form of niacin):* Reduces triglyceride breakdown in adipose tissue and subsequent VLDL and LDL production. It reduces triglycerides and LDL and raises HDL.
- *Fibric acids (include gemfibrozil, clofibrate):* Affect the production of proteins that help regulate lipoprotein synthesis and breakdown. They reduce triglycerides and raise HDL.

Step 8. Identify metabolic syndrome on the basis of the presence of three or more of the following risk determinants:

- Abdominal obesity (waist measurement of more than 40 inches in men or more than 35 inches in women).
- Elevated triglycerides (≥150 mg/dL).
- Low HDL cholesterol <40 mg/dL in men or <50 mg/dL in women).
- Elevated blood pressure ≥130/≥85 mm Hg).
- Elevated fasting glucose (≥110 mg/dL).

If metabolic syndrome is present, treatment should begin with weight management and moderate physical activity. Aspirin should be recommended for CHD patients. If there is no improvement, elevated blood pressure and dyslipidemias should be actively treated.

Step 9. In general, elevated triglyceride levels (≥150 mg/dL) are treated with weight management and moderate physical activity.

- If they remain above 200 mg/dL, drug therapy should be considered (nicotinic acid and fibric acids).
- If they are above 500 mg/dL, a very-low-fat diet (no more than 15 percent kcalories from fat) may be prescribed to prevent complications.

whether this is harmful and eating more fruits and vegetables could easily compensate for the effect.[37] Clinical trials have shown that a bit more than one tablespoon of margarine daily (containing about 2 grams of plant sterols) can lower LDL cholesterol by 6 to 15 percent without lowering HDL cholesterol.

Soy A number of well-controlled studies have shown that diets low in saturated fat and cholesterol and high in soy protein can reduce LDL cholesterol levels, especially when soy protein replaces foods that contain animal fats. Approximately 25 grams of soy protein daily appears to be needed for significant benefit.[38] Whether the LDL-lowering effect is due to the soy protein alone or to other components of soy, such as isoflavones or saponins, remains unknown.

Sodium/Potassium Ratio Dietary factors may influence the risk of CHD for reasons other than their effect on cholesterol levels. For example, sodium may raise blood pressure in certain people, whereas potassium has blood pressure–lowering effects. The DASH diet introduced in Chapter 12 provides generous amounts of fruits and vegetables, low-fat milk products, nuts, and whole grains. The diet's success in reducing blood pressure is partly due to the generous amounts of potassium and certain other minerals that it supplies. This diet and other factors that affect blood pressure are discussed in detail later in this chapter in the section on hypertension.

Fish and Omega-3 Fatty Acids The omega-3 fatty acids in fish oils, EPA and DHA,■ may benefit people who previously have had a heart attack by suppressing the inflammatory response, reducing blood-clotting time, stabilizing heart rhythm, and lowering triglyceride levels. Large intakes of EPA and DHA, however, may raise LDL cholesterol in some people, and not all studies that have investigated the consumption of fish or fish oil supplements in heart disease patients have reported positive outcomes.[39] The ATP III report states that fish (but not fish oil

■ Reminder: *EPA* and *DHA* are the 20- and 22-carbon omega-3 fatty acids found in fish. See p. 156 for a review of these fatty acids.

HOW TO Assess a Person's Risk of Heart Disease

This assessment estimates a person's ten-year risk for developing a major coronary event associated with CHD, such as a heart attack.* A high score does not mean that the person *will* develop a heart attack, but it warns of the possibility and suggests the need to consult a physician. To use this algorithm, you need to know a person's age, total and HDL cholesterol levels, and blood pressure.

Age (years)

	Men	Women
20–34	−9	−7
35–39	−4	−3
40–44	0	0
45–49	3	3
50–54	6	6
55–59	8	8
60–64	10	10
65–69	11	12
70–74	12	14
75–79	13	16

HDL (mg/dL)

	Men	Women
≥60	−1	−1
50–59	0	0
40–49	1	1
<40	2	2

Systolic Blood Pressure (mm Hg)

	Untreated		Treated	
	Men	Women	Men	Women
<120	0	0	0	0
120–129	0	1	1	3
130–139	1	2	2	4
140–159	1	3	2	5
≥160	2	4	3	6

Total Cholesterol (mg/dL)

	Age 20–39		Age 40–49		Age 50–59		Age 60–69		Age 70–79	
	Men	Women	Men	Women	Men	Women	Men	Women	Men	Women
<160	0	0	0	0	0	0	0	0	0	0
160–199	4	4	3	3	2	2	1	1	0	1
200–239	7	8	5	6	3	4	1	2	0	1
240–279	9	11	6	8	4	5	2	3	1	2
≥280	11	13	8	10	5	7	3	4	1	2

Smoking (any cigarette smoking in the past month)

	Age 20–39 Men	Age 20–39 Women	Age 40–49 Men	Age 40–49 Women	Age 50–59 Men	Age 50–59 Women	Age 60–69 Men	Age 60–69 Women	Age 70–79 Men	Age 70–79 Women
Smoker	8	9	5	7	3	4	1	2	1	1
Nonsmoker	0	0	0	0	0	0	0	0	0	0

Scoring Heart Disease Risk

Add up the total points: ______. Using the table at the right, find the total in the first column and check the second column to learn the percentage risk of developing severe CHD within the next ten years. Recall that the LDL goals and treatment options for people at high risk (more than 20 percent), moderate risk (10 to 20 percent), and low risk (less than 10 percent) are shown in the "How to" on pp. 826–827.

Men		Women	
Total	Risk	Total	Risk
<0	<1%	<9	<1%
0–4	1%	9–12	1%
5–6	2%	13–14	2%
7	3%	15	3%
8	4%	16	4%
9	5%	17	5%
10	6%	18	6%
11	8%	19	8%
12	10%	20	11%
13	12%	21	14%
14	16%	22	17%
15	20%	23	22%
16	25%	24	27%
≥17	≥30%	≥25	≥30%

*An electronic version of this assessment is available on the ATP III page of the National Heart, Lung, and Blood Institute's website (**www.nhlbi.nih.gov/guidelines/cholesterol**). Another risk inventory is available from the American Heart Association (**www.americanheart.org**).

SOURCE: Adapted from Expert Panel on Detection, Evaluation, and Treatment of High Blood Cholesterol in Adults (Adult Treatment Panel III), *Third Report of the National Cholesterol Education Program (NCEP)*, NIH publication no. 02-5216 (Bethesda, MD.: National Heart, Lung, and Blood Institute, 2002), section III.

supplements) should be an optional addition to a CHD risk-reduction diet because fish is low in saturated fat and may provide these potentially protective omega-3 fatty acids.■

■ The American Heart Association recommends consuming two servings of fish per week, with an emphasis on fatty fish (see p. 161).

The 18-carbon omega-3 fatty acids found in flaxseeds and other land plants have lesser or different effects than the omega-3 fatty acids from marine sources. Although limited evidence suggests that moderate increases in these plant sources of omega-3 fatty acids may improve CHD risk, more research is needed to confirm their benefits.[40] Highlight 5 provides additional information about the food sources of omega-3 fatty acids.

Alcohol Moderate consumption of alcohol—from beer, wine, or liquor—has favorable effects on HDL cholesterol levels, atherosclerosis, inflammation, and blood-clotting activity.[41] The use of alcohol is also inversely related to incidence of heart attack. These benefits are most apparent in men and women who are at least 45 and 55 years old, respectively. Of note, only low or moderate amounts of alcohol—no more than one drink daily for women and two for men■—have been found to lower CHD risk, and higher intakes are associated with higher mortality rates. The optimal level of alcohol consumption varies substantially according to a person's age and CHD risk.

■ Reminder: One drink is equivalent to 5 oz of wine, 10 oz of wine cooler, 12 oz of beer, or 1½ oz of hard liquor (80 proof).

For some people, alcohol's negative effects can offset any health advantages. Alcohol consumption is associated with cancers of the gastrointestinal (GI) tract and several other cancers, including liver cancer, breast cancer, and ovarian cancer.[42] It is destructive to the liver and male reproductive system,[43] and high intakes can elevate blood pressure and triglyceride levels. Moreover, up to 10 percent of adults misuse alcohol. For these reasons, nondrinkers are not encouraged to start drinking in an effort to decrease their risk for CHD.

Fish Oil Supplements As mentioned earlier, the omega-3 fatty acids in fish have physiological effects that may benefit heart disease patients, but what about supplements of fish oil? Clinical trials have shown that fish oil supplementation can reduce blood triglyceride levels by approximately 30 percent, with improvements persisting for as long as one year.[44] Additional studies indicate that there is a dose-response effect; that is, low doses of fish oils have less of a triglyceride-lowering effect than high doses.[45] To obtain the amount of fish oil required for maximum benefit (about 3000 to 4000 milligrams of omega-3 fatty acids), a person usually must take 10 to 12 capsules per day—an amount that can cause side effects such as mild gastrointestinal symptoms[46] and a tendency to bleed.[47] Several clinical trials have suggested that fish oil supplements providing a smaller amount of omega-3 fatty acids—about 1000 milligrams per day—may lower the death rate in heart attack patients,[48] but the subjects in the studies continued taking heart medications and did not depend solely on the use of fish oil. Fish oil supplementation also has a blood pressure–lowering effect, but it is not a practical therapy for hypertension because large doses are required to achieve relatively small effects.[49] Fish oil supplements have occasionally been associated with detrimental effects on mortality outcome in CHD patients.[50]

B Vitamin Supplements and Homocysteine Elevated blood homocysteine is a known risk factor for cardiovascular diseases.[51] Whether homocysteine itself is directly damaging or is simply a marker for other abnormalities remains unclear. Possibly, homocysteine has a direct toxic effect on the artery wall or heightens blood-clotting activity that worsens atherosclerosis.[52] Although various combinations of folate, vitamin B_6, and vitamin B_{12} can lower homocysteine levels, it is not yet known whether reducing homocysteine with diet or supplements will reduce the risk of CHD.

Antioxidant Vitamin Supplements As mentioned earlier, oxidized LDL are especially atherogenic, so the value of antioxidant supplements has been a question of enormous interest to researchers. Some epidemiological studies suggest an association between antioxidant-rich diets and reduced incidence of CHD, but antioxidant-rich diets are often linked with a healthy lifestyle, lower body weight, and higher socioeconomic status, making it difficult to determine which factor is responsible for the effect. Carefully controlled trials testing single antioxidant supplements (like vitamins C and E), combinations, or multivitamins have produced results too weak or inconsistent to conclude that they offer any significant benefit for the prevention of CHD,[53] and several studies have suggested possible harm.[54] Major clinical trials of antioxidant use are ongoing, and the results will help to

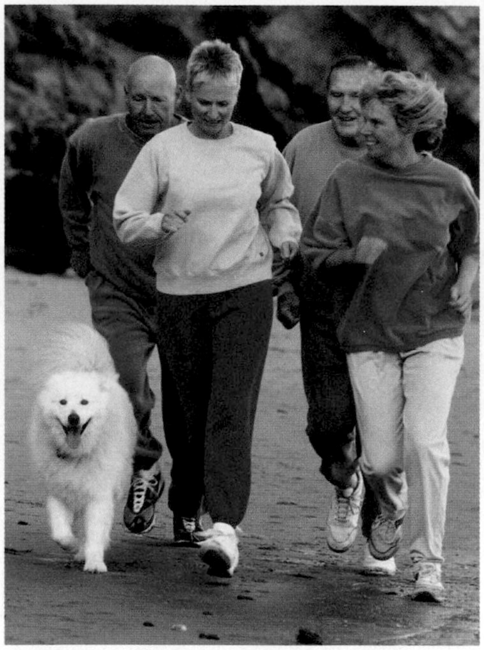
© Ronnie Kaufman/The Stock Market

Regular aerobic exercise can strengthen the cardiovascular system, promote weight loss, reduce blood pressure, and improve blood glucose and lipid levels.

evaluate the potential role of antioxidant supplementation in reducing CHD risk. Until more data are available, there is no recommendation to use antioxidant supplements for heart disease prevention.

Regular Physical Activity Regular physical activity reverses a number of risk factors for CHD. It can lower triglycerides, raise HDL, lower blood pressure, promote weight loss, improve insulin sensitivity, strengthen heart muscle, and increase coronary artery size and tone. Research studies have consistently found that people who engage in regular exercise have a lower incidence of CHD. Generally, the most active persons have a risk of CHD mortality that is about half the risk of those who are least active.[55] Surprisingly, though, exercise remains unpopular in our society: only 25 percent of people in the United States engage in light-to-moderate activity at least five days per week.[56] Exercise is a critical component of cardiac rehabilitation programs for people with established CHD, but only 11 to 38 percent of qualifying patients participate.

The American Heart Association recommends at least 30 minutes of moderate-intensity endurance exercise most days of the week.[57] The activities that help the heart the most are aerobic exercises that use large muscle groups. Such activities include brisk walking, running, swimming, cycling, stair-stepping, and cross-country skiing. Alternatives for busy people may include heavy house cleaning, lawn mowing, raking leaves, and walking to and from work. Some people may find it easier to schedule several short exercise sessions each day, but each should be at least 15 minutes long.[58] The eventual goal should be to expend at least 2000 kcalories in exercise per week. Activity sessions should begin and end with brief "warm-up" and "cool-down" periods that include stretches and low-level aerobic activity, so that there is a gradual transition between rest and vigorous activity. Of note, vigorous activity increases the risk of heart attack and sudden death in individuals with diagnosed heart disease, so sedentary adults should increase their activity levels gradually.

Weight Reduction Obesity, especially abdominal obesity, is a major and independent risk factor for CHD.[59] Metabolic changes that accompany obesity include hypertension, elevated triglycerides, reduced HDL cholesterol, decreased LDL size (see the Research Update on p. 824), and insulin resistance.■ Obesity also alters the concentration and activity of blood-clotting factors to favor coagulation, which can increase risks for both atherosclerosis and heart attack.

■ This pattern of complications associated with obesity characterizes the metabolic syndrome, which is described fully in Highlight 26.

Weight reduction may improve such CHD risk factors as blood pressure, triglyceride levels, and HDL cholesterol levels. The ATP III guidelines recommend that individuals focus on weight reduction *after* they have adopted other dietary measures to lower LDL. This approach ensures that LDL reduction is given priority and that the patient is not provided with a multitude of dietary suggestions at one time. The initial goal of a weight-loss program is no more than 10 percent of a person's original body weight.[60] For some, avoiding additional weight gain may be a desirable starting point.

Smoking Cessation Smoking is a major risk factor for CHD as well as other forms of cardiovascular disease. Compounds in cigarette smoke damage blood vessel cells, decrease the oxygen-carrying capacity of the blood (contributing to ischemia), promote blood coagulation, and raise heart rate and blood pressure.[61] Inadequate oxygen also promotes localized edema and lipid accumulation in blood vessel walls. Passive smoke inhalation can cause these effects as well.

Risk from smoking depends on the amount and duration of exposure: it is related to the age when smoking started, the number of cigarettes smoked daily, and the degree of inhalation. Cigarettes that have low tar and nicotine do not lower the risk. Because overall exposure is the key factor, a long-term habit of smoking only one to four cigarettes daily can still double CHD risk.■

■ Research data concerning cigar and pipe smoking are limited, but these habits can also increase the risk of CHD. The risk may not be quite as great because the smoke is less likely to be inhaled.

Fortunately, quitting smoking can improve CHD risk almost immediately, and quitters can eventually reverse the damage from smoking. One study found that women who had quit for three to four years had a CHD risk identical to that of nonsmokers, regardless of the number of cigarettes or the duration of smoking. It is extremely difficult to stop smoking, however, and the relapse rate is high: only about 8 percent of smokers who want to quit are successful, and only 10 percent of those who quit are likely to maintain their nonsmoking status.[62] Still, the ATP III guidelines specify smoking cessation as a key strategy to reduce CHD risk.

Lifestyle Changes for Hypertriglyceridemia Hypertriglyceridemia is common in people with the metabolic syndrome and diabetes mellitus and may also result from other diseases and the use of various prescription medications. Very high levels of triglycerides can cause serious complications, including fatty deposits in the liver and skin and acute pancreatitis.[63] Diet and lifestyle both contribute to "borderline-high" triglycerides, whereas genetic factors are increasingly important when triglycerides climb to "high" or "very high" levels.■

■ Triglycerides:
Borderline high: 150–199 mg/dL.
High: ≥200 mg/dL.

Changing diet and lifestyle is central to treatment for lowering borderline-high triglycerides. Overweight and obesity, sedentary lifestyle, and cigarette smoking all may raise triglyceride levels. The dietary factors that influence triglycerides the most are high intakes of carbohydrate (60 percent or more of total kcalories) and alcohol. Thus controlling body weight, becoming physically active, quitting smoking, avoiding a high-carbohydrate intake, and restricting alcohol are basic treatments for hypertriglyceridemia. As mentioned earlier, high triglycerides are often associated with low HDL, and the lifestyle changes listed here are likely to improve HDL levels as well.

For patients with high or very high triglyceride levels, medications are prescribed to lower triglycerides alone or to lower both LDL and triglycerides. Weight reduction and physical activity are still emphasized for overweight patients, and a very low-fat diet, providing less than 15 percent of kcalories from fat, may be necessary in extreme cases to prevent dangerous complications. If the dietary fat restriction is severe, medium-chain triglycerides (see pp. 744–745) can be useful for replacing fats and oils in the diet.

Successful Adherence to Lifestyle Changes Incorporating many lifestyle changes at once can be difficult, and instruction and counseling are critical for success. Health professionals need to explain the reasons for each change, set obtainable goals, and provide practical suggestions. An initial diet history can offer clues about a person's behaviors and living situation. Follow-up visits allow an opportunity to determine compliance. Some people may not respond to dietary and lifestyle changes, and high LDL cholesterol levels may persist despite good adherence to a TLC program; drug therapy may be the only effective treatment for such people. Table 27-3 (p. 825) summarizes the Therapeutic Lifestyle Changes discussed in this section, and the "How to" box on p. 832 offers suggestions for implementing a heart-healthy diet.

Drug Therapies Physicians usually prescribe dietary and lifestyle modifications for at least three months before considering drug therapies. If an individual cannot reach LDL goals with lifestyle changes alone, one or more medications may be prescribed. The most common LDL-lowering medications reduce cholesterol synthesis in the liver (statins) or reduce cholesterol and bile absorption in the small intestine (bile acid sequestrants). The nicotinic acid form of the vitamin niacin is highly effective for reducing triglyceride levels and raising HDL cholesterol when taken in pharmacological amounts. Individuals using lipid-lowering medications should continue with the TLC program to ensure that the lowest-possible dosages of the drugs can be used.[64]

In addition to lipid-lowering medications, some people may require drugs that reduce blood pressure (diuretics, beta-blockers, and other antihypertensives) or suppress blood clotting (anticoagulants and aspirin). Nitroglycerin may be given to alleviate angina as needed. People with diabetes may also need glucose-lowering medications or insulin. Some medications may affect nutritional status or food intake (see the Diet-Drug Interactions box on p. 841); the interactions can be even more complicated when multiple medications are used.

HOW TO Implement a Heart-Healthy Diet

Following a heart-healthy diet can require major changes in dietary choices. Patients may find it easier to adopt a new diet if only a few changes are made at a time. Discussing positive choices (what to eat) first, rather than negative ones (what not to eat), may also aid compliance. These suggestions can help patients implement their diet.

Breads, Cereals, and Pasta

- Choose whole-grain breads and cereals. Make sure the first ingredient on bread and cereal labels is "whole wheat" rather than "enriched wheat flour."
- Bakery products often contain *trans*-fatty acids. Choose foods whose labels *do not* list "hydrogenated oil." Crackers, chips, cookies, and doughnuts often include *trans* fats.
- Avoid products that contain tropical oils (coconut, palm, and palm kernel oil), which are high in saturated fat.

Fruits and Vegetables

- Consume fruits and vegetables frequently. Keeping the refrigerator stocked with a variety of colorful fruits and vegetables (baby carrots, grapes, blueberries, melon) makes it easier to choose healthy foods when the urge to nibble arises.
- Incorporate at least one or two servings of fruits and vegetables into each meal. People who rarely eat fruits or vegetables may start by adding at least one of their favorites to each meal.
- Choose canned products carefully. Canned vegetables (especially tomato-based products) may be high in sodium. Fruits that are canned in juice are higher in nutrient density than those canned in syrup.
- Restrict high-sodium foods such as pickles, olives, sauerkraut, and kimchee.
- Avoid french fries from fast-food restaurants, which are often loaded with *trans* fats.

Lunch and Dinner Entrées

- Limit meat, fish, and poultry servings to a maximum intake of 5 ounces per day.
- Select lean cuts of beef, such as sirloin tip, round steak, and arm roast, and lean cuts of pork, such as center-cut ham, loin chops, and tenderloin. Trim visible fat before cooking.
- Select extra-lean ground meat and drain well after cooking. Use lean ground turkey, without skin added, in place of ground beef.
- Limit cholesterol-rich organ meats (liver, brain, sweetbreads) and shrimp.
- Limit egg yolks to no more than two per week because the yolks are high in cholesterol (about 215 milligrams per yolk). Replace whole eggs in recipes with egg whites or commercial egg substitutes or similar reduced-cholesterol products.
- Include more vegetarian entrées or legume dishes to boost soluble fiber and soy protein intakes. Pasta and stir-fry recipes can help to reduce meat intake and increase vegetables in the diet.
- Restrict these high-sodium foods:
  - Cured or smoked meats such as beef jerky, bologna, corned or chipped beef, frankfurters, ham, luncheon meats, salt pork, and sausage.
  - Salty or smoked fish, such as anchovies, caviar, salted or dried cod, herring, sardines, and smoked salmon.
  - Packaged, canned, or frozen soups, sauces, and entrées.

Milk Products

- Milk products can be good sources of protein, calcium, vitamin D, and potassium. To obtain two to three servings daily, include a portion of fat-free or low-fat milk, yogurt, or cottage cheese in each meal.
- Use yogurt or fat-free sour cream to make dips or salad dressings. Substitute evaporated fat-free milk for heavy cream.
- Restrict foods high in saturated fat or sodium, such as cheese, processed cheeses, ice cream, and many other milk-based desserts.

Fats and Oils

- Add nuts (not salted) and avocados to meals to increase monounsaturated fat intakes and make meals more appetizing.
- Include vegetable oils in salad dressings and recipes, such as canola, corn, olive, peanut, safflower, sesame, soybean, and sunflower oils.
- Use margarines with added plant sterols or stanols regularly to lower LDL cholesterol levels.
- Select soft margarines in tubs or liquid form; they are low in *trans* fats. Avoid stick margarines and solid vegetable shortenings.
- Avoid products that contain tropical oils (coconut, palm, and palm kernel oil), which are high in saturated fat.

Spices and Seasonings

- Use salt only at the end of cooking, and you will need to add much less. Use salt substitutes at the table.
- Spices and herbs improve the flavor of foods without adding sodium. Try using more garlic, ginger, basil, curry or chili powder, cumin, pepper, lemon, mint, oregano, rosemary, and thyme.
- Check the sodium content on labels. Flavorings and sauces that are usually high in sodium include bouillon cubes, soy sauce, steak and barbecue sauces, relishes, mustard, and catsup.

Snacks and Desserts

- Select low-sodium and low–saturated fat choices such as unsalted pretzels and nuts, plain popcorn, and unsalted chips and crackers.
- Choose canned or dried fruits and some raw vegetables to boost fruit and vegetable intake.
- Enjoy angel food cake, which is made without egg yolks and added fat.
- Select low-fat frozen desserts such as sherbet, sorbet, fruit bars, and some low-fat ice creams.

The Heart Attack Patient

Over one million people experience a heart attack each year. The death rate is huge: approximately 47 percent of people who experience a first or recurrent heart attack die within a year.[65] Fortunately, the majority of survivors are able to return to work and lead productive lives within months of their illness. Although modern-day emergency procedures are largely responsible for the improved survival rates in the past ten years, much of the rehabilitation effort depends on the patients themselves. The risk-reduction methods discussed earlier are crucial for long-term survival after a life-threatening coronary event has occurred.

Immediate Care after Heart Attack As explained earlier, a heart attack occurs when restricted blood flow in the coronary arteries causes death of heart tissue.■ This typically results from the rupture of coronary plaque and the subsequent formation of a blood clot that blocks the artery. If blood flow within a coronary artery is restored quickly, heart muscle can be saved; if not, muscle tissue dies. Thus medicines that improve immediate survival include clot-busting drugs (called thrombolytics), aspirin, and the anticoagulant heparin.[66] To slow the heart rate and thereby reduce the work of the heart, beta-blockers are usually given. ACE inhibitors■ are often prescribed for high-risk patients to reduce blood pressure and improve blood flow. Although acutely ill patients have little interest in eating, they are typically offered a low-sodium, soft-foods diet during the first few days after a heart attack. The sodium restriction helps to limit fluid retention, but may be lifted after several days if the patient shows no signs of heart failure. A person who has just had a heart attack needs to rest in a quiet, calm room for several days and avoid any activities that increase anxiety and stress.[67]

■ Dead heart tissue releases enzymes and proteins into the blood, so elevated blood levels of these molecules can be used to diagnose a heart attack. These enzymes and proteins include creatine kinase, lactate dehydrogenase, myoglobin, troponin T, and troponin I.

■ *ACE* stands for **angiotensin-converting enzyme.** An ACE inhibitor interferes with the conversion of angiotensin I to angiotensin II, which is a peptide that helps to regulate blood pressure.

Long-Term Management A heart attack patient needs to regain strength and learn strategies that can reduce the risk of a future coronary event. Cardiac rehabilitation programs, found in hospitals and outpatient clinics, may last for several months and typically include exercise therapy, smoking cessation, dietary instruction,■ stress management, and medication counseling. Participation in rehabilitation programs can improve exercise tolerance and compliance with medications and other risk-reduction strategies, thereby lowering the risk of a subsequent heart attack. Unfortunately, these programs are vastly underutilized: only about 15 percent of patients participate due to lack of physician referral, poor motivation, limited financial assistance, or a combination of these factors.[68] Home-based exercise programs are also beneficial, but they are more limited in scope and lack the benefit of group interaction.

■ The dietary strategies that a cardiac patient should adopt are similar to the Therapeutic Lifestyle Changes (TLC) described earlier.

IN SUMMARY Coronary heart disease (CHD) is the leading cause of death in the industrialized world. The reversal of CHD risk factors is a critical aspect of its long-term management and treatment. Modifiable risk factors include blood lipid levels, high blood pressure, cigarette smoking, diabetes, obesity, sedentary lifestyle, and diet. Current treatment guidelines, most notably the ATP III Therapeutic Lifestyle Changes (TLC), emphasize dietary and lifestyle changes that reduce LDL cholesterol levels. The main dietary changes recommended are a reduction of saturated fat, *trans* fats, and cholesterol; an increase in soluble fiber; and incorporation of plant sterols and stanols into the diet. Other essential components of TLC include regular physical activity and weight management. If modifications in diet and lifestyle do not improve blood lipids, drug therapies may be considered. A patient who has had a heart attack needs to adopt the same dietary and lifestyle strategies that are important for risk reduction.

Hypertension

Hypertension affects some 50 million people in the United States and about 1 billion worldwide.[69] Prevalence is especially high among African Americans, who develop hypertension earlier in life and sustain higher average blood pressures throughout their lives.[70] Only 27 percent of people with hypertension take medications to control it, and an estimated 32 percent are completely unaware that they have it. Current classifications for blood pressure are shown in the margin.■

■ Blood pressure is measured when the heart muscle contracts and ejects blood into the aorta (systolic blood pressure) and while the heart muscle is relaxing between beats (diastolic blood pressure):

	Systolic	Diastolic
Normal blood pressure	<120	<80
Prehypertension	120–139	80–89
Hypertension	≥140	≥90

People usually cannot feel the physical effects of high blood pressure, but it is a primary risk factor for atherosclerosis and cardiovascular diseases. For each 20/10 mm Hg increase above normal blood pressure, the risks for CVD double. When blood pressure is high, the heart must work harder to eject blood into the arteries, which can weaken heart muscle and increase risk of heart arrhythmias, congestive heart failure, and even sudden death. Hypertension is also a primary cause of stroke and kidney failure. Therapies that lower blood pressure have been shown to dramatically reduce the incidence of these diseases.

Risk for Developing Hypertension

The underlying causes of most cases of hypertension are not fully understood, but much is known about the physiological factors that affect blood pressure. As shown in Figure 27-3, blood pressure arises from the contractions of heart muscle that pump blood away from the heart **(cardiac output)** and the resistance that blood encounters as it moves through the arterioles **(peripheral resistance).**■

■ The equation describing this relationship is *blood pressure (BP) = CO × PR. Cardiac output (CO)* is influenced by heart rate and the blood volume pumped with each heartbeat. *Peripheral resistance (PR)* is influenced mainly by the diameters of arterioles and blood viscosity.

FIGURE 27-3 Determinants of Blood Pressure

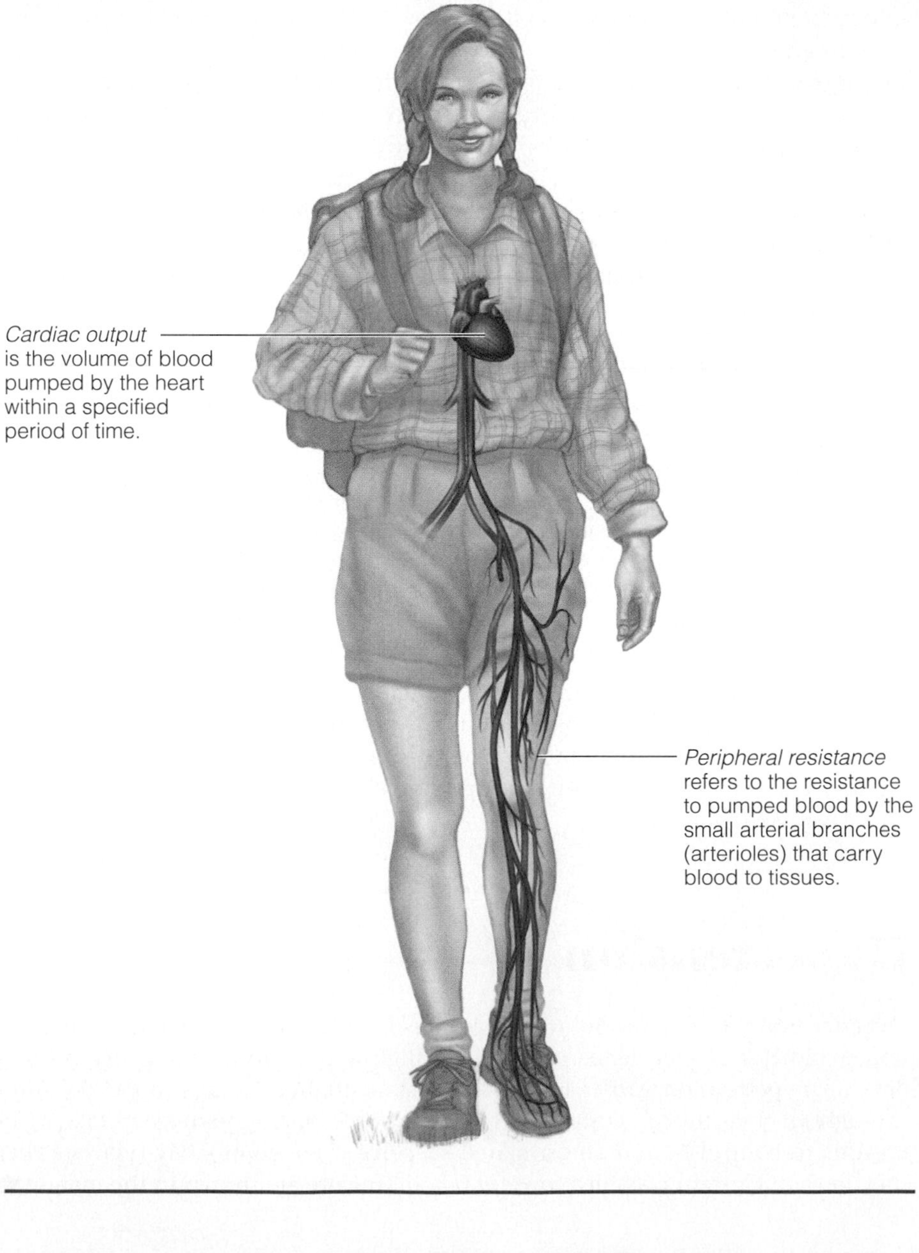
Cardiac output is the volume of blood pumped by the heart within a specified period of time.
Peripheral resistance refers to the resistance to pumped blood by the small arterial branches (arterioles) that carry blood to tissues.

cardiac output: the volume of blood pumped by the heart within a specified period of time.

peripheral resistance: the resistance to pumped blood by the small arterial branches (arterioles) that carry blood to tissues.

When either cardiac output or peripheral resistance increases, blood pressure rises. Cardiac output is raised when heart rate or blood volume increases; peripheral resistance is affected mostly by physical and chemical signals that alter arteriole diameter. Blood pressure responds to signals from the nervous system that influence the heart's pumping activity and the diameters of arterioles and to signals from hormones that promote fluid retention and blood vessel constriction. The kidneys also regulate blood pressure by controlling the secretion of the hormones involved in vasoconstriction and retention of sodium and water.

Hypertension that develops without an identifiable cause, as occurs in 95 percent of cases,[71] is called *primary* or *essential hypertension.* Hypertension that is caused by a specific disorder is called *secondary hypertension;* it usually arises from abnormalities in the organs or hormones involved in blood pressure regulation. For example, chronic kidney disease interferes with the removal of sodium and water from blood, directly increasing blood volume and thus blood pressure. Atherosclerosis in renal arteries may cause increased production of the hormones that stimulate water retention and vasoconstriction. Stiffness and thickening of the aorta or arteries (arteriosclerosis) due to age, diabetes, and other reasons can increase resistance to blood flow, thereby raising blood pressure. A number of hormonal disorders, including some thyroid diseases and adrenal disorders, can also cause hypertension. Most often, however, no direct causes are identified.

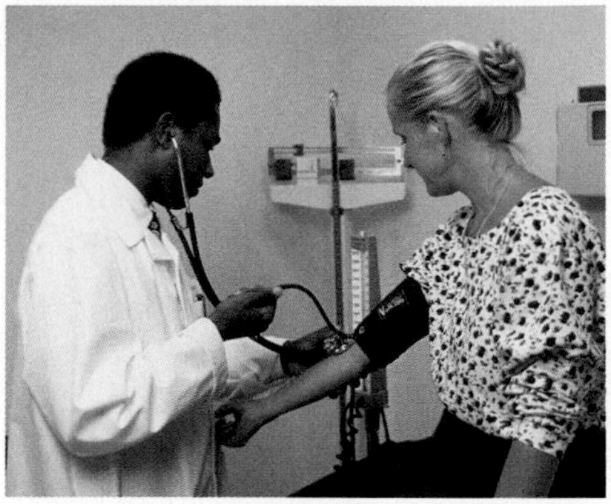

Screening people for hypertension is a first step toward early detection and prevention of complications.

Contributing Factors for Hypertension

Several major risk factors have been implicated in the development of hypertension:

- *Aging.* Hypertension risk increases with age. It has been estimated that individuals who have normal blood pressure at age 55 still have a 90 percent risk of developing high blood pressure during their lifetimes.[72]
- *Genetic.* Hypertension tends to be a family trait. It is also more prevalent and severe within certain ethnic groups; for example, the prevalence in African Americans is about 37 percent, compared with rates of approximately 23 percent in both whites and Mexican Americans.[73]
- *Obesity.* Rates of hypertension in men and women classified as obese (BMI of 30 or higher) are 38.4 percent and 32.2 percent, respectively, compared to 18.2 percent and 16.5 percent in men and women who have healthier weights (BMI below 25).[74]
- *Salt sensitivity.* Among those with hypertension, 55 percent of whites and 73 percent of African Americans have blood pressure that is sensitive to salt and can benefit by reducing salt in their diets.[75]
- *Alcohol.* Heavy alcohol consumption (defined as three or more drinks daily) is strongly associated with hypertension, although alcohol's specific role in blood pressure is unclear. The effect of more moderate alcohol intakes on blood pressure is not known.[76]
- *Diet.* A person's dietary choices may influence hypertension risk. A diet containing generous amounts of fruits, vegetables, nuts, and low-fat milk products can lower blood pressure. These foods provide the major minerals potassium, calcium, and magnesium, which help to reduce blood pressure when included in adequate amounts in the diet.

Treatment of Hypertension

Controlling hypertension■ can reduce the incidence of heart attack by 20 to 25 percent, heart failure by over 50 percent, and stroke by 35 to 40 percent.[77] Usually, both lifestyle modifications and drug therapies are used to treat hypertension. For people with prehypertension,■ changes in diet and lifestyle alone may lower blood pressure to a normal level. In some patients, treatment may focus on systolic

■ The goal of hypertension therapy is to reduce blood pressure to <140/<90 mm Hg (or <130/<80 mm Hg in people with diabetes or kidney disease).

■ Prehypertension: 120–139/80–89 mm Hg.

blood pressure because it is a more important CVD risk factor in people over 50 years of age.

The main lifestyle modifications recommended for lowering blood pressure include weight reduction if overweight or obese, a diet low in sodium and rich in potassium, calcium, and magnesium, regular physical activity, and a moderate alcohol intake (see Table 27-4). Weight reduction and dietary modification have the most dramatic effects. Combining two or more lifestyle modifications can enhance results substantially.

DASH Eating Plan: Dietary Approaches to Stop Hypertension A whole-diet approach to blood pressure management was first recommended after a landmark study showed that subjects achieved substantial reductions in blood pressure by following one of the diets tested.[78] The dietary pattern that proved most successful emphasized fruits, vegetables, and low-fat dairy products and included whole grains, poultry, fish, and nuts. These dietary changes resulted in substantially higher intakes of fiber, potassium, magnesium, and calcium than the standard American dietary pattern that was used as a control diet. The successful DASH pattern, which became known as the "DASH Eating Plan," also limited red meat, sweets, sugar-containing beverages, saturated fat (to 7 percent of kcalories), and cholesterol (to 150 milligrams per day). During the eight-week period when hypertensive subjects consumed the DASH diet, their systolic blood pressures fell by 11.4 mm Hg more than the blood pressures of subjects who remained on the standard American control diet. Table 27-5 shows the DASH Eating Plan, which is currently considered to be an example of a dietary pattern consistent with the recommendations in the 2005 *Dietary Guidelines*.[79]

In a subsequent study, the researchers found that the DASH diet was even more effective when accompanied by lower sodium intakes.[80] After a one-month baseline period during which subjects consumed the DASH diet containing 3300 milligrams of sodium, sodium was reduced to 2400 milligrams for another month, and then reduced further to 1500 milligrams for a final month. Systolic blood pressure decreased only 1.3 mm Hg on average when sodium was reduced from 3300 milligrams to 2400 milligrams, but it dropped another 1.7 mm Hg when sodium was reduced to 1500 milligrams. These results suggest that the optimal sodium intake for treating hypertension may be far lower than is usually recommended.[81]

Sodium restriction by itself may have a modest blood pressure–lowering effect (see Table 27-4), but some people are more responsive than others. A reduced-

TABLE 27-4 Lifestyle Modifications for Blood Pressure Reduction

Modification	Recommendation	Expected Reduction in Systolic Blood Pressure
Weight reduction	Maintain healthy body weight (BMI below 25).	5–20 mm Hg/10 kg lost
DASH eating plan	Adopt a diet rich in fruits, vegetables, and low-fat milk products with reduced saturated fat intake.	8–14 mm Hg
Sodium restriction	Reduce dietary sodium intake to less than 2400 milligrams sodium (less than 6 grams salt) per day.*	2–8 mm Hg
Physical activity	Perform aerobic physical activity for at least 30 minutes per day, most days of the week.	4–9 mm Hg
Moderate alcohol consumption	Men: Limit to 2 drinks per day. Women and lighter-weight men: Limit to 1 drink per day.	2–4 mm Hg

*According to DRI recommendations, sodium intake should be limited to 2300 milligrams daily.
SOURCE: Adapted from *Reference Card from the Seventh Report of the Joint National Committee on Prevention, Detection, Evaluation, and Treatment of High Blood Pressure (JNC 7),* NIH publication no. 03-5231 (Bethesda, Md.: National Institutes of Health, National Heart, Lung, and Blood Institute, and National High Blood Pressure Education Program, May 2003).

TABLE 27-5 The DASH Eating Plan

Food Group	Recommended Servings for Different Energy Intakes (Servings per day except as noted)			
	1600 kcal	2000 kcal	2600 kcal	3100 kcal
Grains and grain products[a] (1 serving = 1 slice bread, 1 oz dry cereal,[b] or ½ cup cooked rice, pasta, or cereal)	6	7–8	10–11	12–13
Vegetables (1 serving = ½ cup cooked vegetables, 1 cup raw leafy vegetables, or 6 oz vegetable juice)	3–4	4–5	5–6	6
Fruits (1 serving = 1 medium fruit; ½ cup fresh, frozen, or canned fruit; ¼ cup dried fruit; or 6 oz fruit juice)	4	4–5	5–6	6
Milk products (low-fat or fat-free) (1 serving = 8 oz milk, 1 cup yogurt, or 1½ oz cheese)	2–3	2–3	3	3–4
Meat, poultry, and fish (1 serving = 3 oz cooked meat, poultry, or fish)	1–2	1–2	2	2–3
Nuts, seeds, and legumes (1 serving = ⅓ cup nuts, 2 tbs seeds, or ½ cup dry beans or peas)	3–4 per week	4–5 per week	1	1
Fats and oils (1 serving = 1 tsp vegetable oil or soft margarine, 1 tbs low-fat mayonnaise, or 2 tbs light salad dressing)	2	2–3	3	4
Sweets (1 serving = 1 tbs sugar, jelly, or jam; ½ oz jelly beans; or 8 oz lemonade)	0	5 per week	2	2

[a]Whole grains are recommended for most servings consumed.
[b]1 oz dry cereal may be equivalent to ½ to 1¼ cups, depending on the cereal. Check the food label for the portion size.
SOURCE: The 2005 *Dietary Guidelines for Americans,* available at **www.healthierus.gov/dietaryguidelines**.

sodium diet is typically recommended for all people with hypertension, but it should be combined with other lifestyle modifications for greater effect. Check the suggestions for reducing sodium intake in the "How to" box on p. 838.

Weight reduction can also reduce blood pressure considerably. In several controlled studies, participants who lost 22 pounds (10 kilograms) lowered systolic blood pressure by an average of 7.0 mm Hg, and greater weight loss was associated with greater reductions in blood pressure.[82] The prevalence of hypertension after a year and a half was 20 to 50 percent lower among subjects who lost weight.

Drug Therapies Most people with hypertension use two or more medications to meet their blood pressure goals. Using a combination of drugs with different modes of action can reduce the dosages of each drug needed and minimize side effects.[83] Most treatments include diuretics, which lower blood pressure by reducing blood volume.■ Other categories of drugs commonly prescribed include ACE inhibitors, beta-blockers, and calcium channel blockers, which are also used to treat various heart conditions. Drug dosages may need to be adjusted in follow-up visits until the blood pressure goal is reached.

■ The diuretics often used to treat hypertension may cause potassium depletion. Blood potassium levels are usually monitored one to two times each year and supplements prescribed as needed.

IN SUMMARY One in every four adults in the United States has hypertension, which frequently contributes to heart disease, heart failure, stroke, and kidney failure. Blood pressure is elevated by factors that increase blood volume, heart rate, and resistance to blood flow. The underlying cause of most cases of hypertension is unknown, but major risk factors include aging, family history, race, obesity, and dietary choices. Treatment usually includes a combination of lifestyle modifications and drug therapies. The case study on p. 839 provides an opportunity to review the risk factors and treatment for CHD and hypertension.

HOW TO Reduce Sodium Intake

- Select fresh, unprocessed foods; packaged products, canned foods, and frozen dinners are often high in sodium.
- Avoid eating at fast-food restaurants; most choices are very high in sodium.
- Do not use salt at the table or while cooking.
- Check food labels. On labels, "low sodium" is a better guide than "reduced sodium" (contains 25 percent less sodium than the regular product) or "light in sodium" (contains 50 percent less sodium). To be labeled "low sodium," a food product must contain less than 140 milligrams of sodium per serving. Keep your goal sodium value of 2000 or 3000 milligrams in mind when you read labels.
- Recognize the high-salt foods in each food category, including:
  - Bakery products made with baking powder or baking soda (sodium bicarbonate); read labels to make sure.
  - Processed meats: ham, corned beef, bologna, salami, sausage, bacon, frankfurters, and pastrami.
  - Fish: salted fish, shellfish, and canned fish.
  - Tomato-based products: tomato sauce, tomato juice, pizza, canned tomatoes, and catsup.
  - Cheese: cottage cheese, American cheese, parmesan, and many other hard cheeses.
  - Condiments and relishes: bouillon cubes, olives, and pickled vegetables.
  - Flavoring sauces: soy sauce, barbecue sauce, and steak sauce.
- Use unsalted snack foods including tortilla chips, popcorn, and nuts. Some snack foods may need to be avoided.
- Check for "sodium" on medication labels. Sodium is often an ingredient in some types of antacids and laxatives.

Congestive Heart Failure (CHF)

Congestive heart failure (CHF) is the failure of the heart to pump adequate blood, causing congestion of fluids in tissues and in the veins leading to the heart. It is often a consequence of other cardiovascular conditions such as hypertension and CHD that create extra work for the heart muscle. To accommodate its extra workload, the overburdened heart can enlarge or pump faster or harder. Although people can live with CHF for years, eventually the heart can weaken and fail completely.

CHF develops mostly in the elderly: approximately 6 to 10 percent of persons older than 65 have CHF. Its incidence is likely to grow as the population ages: at age 80, a person has a 20 percent risk of developing CHF during the remaining years of life.

Consequences of CHF

The symptoms and consequences of CHF depend on which side of the heart fails. The right side of the heart pumps blood from the peripheral tissues to the lungs. If the pump is weak, blood backs up in the peripheral tissues and abdominal organs. Fluid can accumulate in the lower extremities and in the liver and abdomen, causing chest pain, difficulty with digestion and absorption, and swelling in the legs, ankles, and feet. The left side of the heart pumps blood from the lungs to the peripheral tissues. A weakened left heart can increase fluid buildup or congestion in the lungs (pulmonary edema) that can cause extreme shortness of breath and limited exercise tolerance; in severe cases, it can lead to acute respiratory failure. The inadequate blood flow to tissues can impair the functions of other organs such as the liver and kidneys. The effects of CHF also depend on the seriousness of the disease: mild cases may be asymptomatic, but severe cases may restrict activity substantially.

The type of heart failure a person develops has implications that affect food intake and physical activity. Because right-sided heart failure may cause abdominal bloating and an enlarged liver, the pain and discomfort may worsen with meals. Left-sided failure may limit physical activity substantially due to limb weakness and fatigue. End-stage heart failure is often accompanied by **cardiac cachexia,** a condition of malnutrition brought about by changes in body chemistry and worsened by reduced appetite and food intake. Cardiac cachexia causes severe weight loss and tissue wasting. The resultant weakness further lowers the person's activity levels, functional capacity, and strength.[84]

congestive heart failure (CHF): failure of the heart to pump adequate blood, resulting in fluid congestion in tissues and veins leading to the heart.

cardiac cachexia: severe malnutrition associated with heart failure that causes weight loss and tissue wasting.

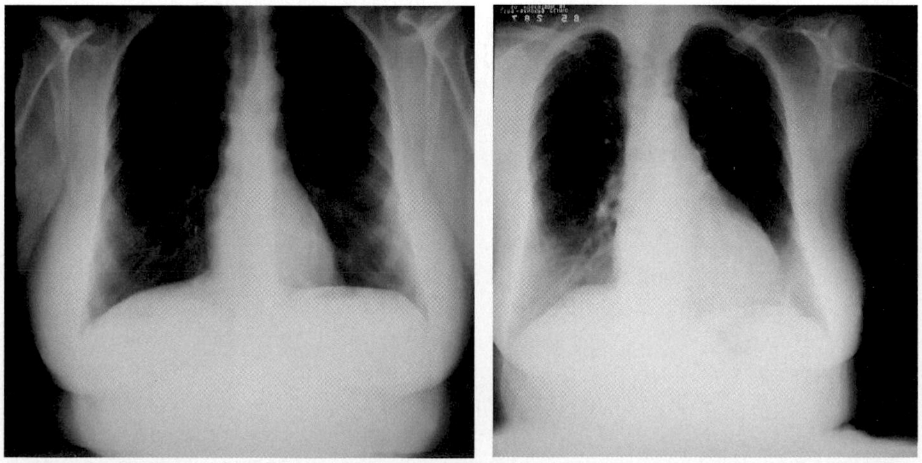

An overburdened heart enlarges in an effort to supply blood to the body's tissues.

CASE STUDY

Computer Programmer with Cardiovascular Disease

Mr. Reid, a 48-year-old African American computer programmer, is 5 feet 9 inches tall and weighs 240 pounds. His work involves sitting for long hours, and he is too tired to exercise when he gets home at night. Meals usually include fatty meats, eggs, and cheese, and he likes dairy desserts like pudding and ice cream. He has a family history of CHD and hypertension. His recent laboratory tests show that his blood pressure is 160/100 mm Hg, his LDL cholesterol is 160 mg/dL, and his HDL is 35 mg/dL. He smokes a pack of cigarettes a day and usually has two glasses of wine at both lunch and dinner.

1. Name Mr. Reid's major risk factors for CHD and hypertension. Which can be modified?
2. What complications might occur if he doesn't seek treatment for his blood lipids and blood pressure?
3. What dietary changes would you recommend that would help to improve Mr. Reid's blood pressure and his LDL and HDL cholesterol? Explain the rationale for each diet change. Prepare a day's menus for Mr. Reid using the DASH diet as an outline for your choices.
4. What other laboratory tests or measurements would you need to better assess his condition? Why?
5. Describe several benefits that Mr. Reid can obtain from a program that includes weight reduction and regular physical activity. Explain why the use of alcohol can be both a protective and a damaging lifestyle habit.
6. Assuming that Mr. Reid does not make any changes in his diet and lifestyle and suffers a heart attack, discuss the elements of a cardiac rehabilitation program that would be critical for his long-term survival.

Medical Management of CHF

There is no cure for CHF. It is a chronic, progressive condition that may require frequent hospitalizations. Many patients face a combination of debilitating symptoms, restrictive treatments, and an uncertain outcome. End-of-life decisions need to be made, as half of all deaths from CHF are sudden. Depression is common and can worsen the course of disease. Important goals of medical therapy are to enhance the patient's quality of life and to stabilize and reduce progression of the disease. Successful treatment also depends on patient participation and compliance with medications and dietary restrictions.[85]

Specific treatment depends on the underlying cause and type of CHF as well as the severity of the disease. In general, drug therapies are used to manage congestion and improve heart function. Dietary sodium and fluid restrictions may help to prevent fluid accumulation. Vaccinations for influenza and pneumonia can reduce the risk of developing respiratory infections.[86] CHF patients are also encouraged to participate in exercise programs to avoid becoming physically disabled and to improve endurance and well-being.[87]

Drug Therapies Four types of drugs are routinely prescribed for CHF: diuretics, ACE inhibitors, beta-blockers, and digitalis. Diuretics are given to reverse or prevent fluid retention. The CHF patient needs to monitor fluid fluctuations by daily weight measurements and can make small adjustments in diuretic therapy as needed. The other drugs listed help to improve heart and blood vessel functioning and blood flow.

Medical Nutrition Therapy The main dietary recommendation for CHF is a moderate sodium intake of 2000 to 3000 milligrams daily, depending on the severity of illness.■ Sodium restriction reduces the likelihood of fluid retention. Patients with more severe cases of CHF may need to reduce sodium intake to 2000 milligrams per day. (Review the "How to" on p. 838.) Salt substitutes often contain potassium, which may not be appropriate for some patients using diuretics.[88] Under some circumstances, fluid restriction may also be needed. For patients who have difficulty eating due to abdominal or chest pain, small, frequent meals may be better tolerated.

■ The 2000 to 3000 mg sodium recommendation is not very restrictive. The current DRI recommendation is to limit sodium intake to 2300 mg daily.

Other Dietary Recommendations Patients with CHF may be prone to constipation due to diuretic use and reduced physical activity. Maintaining an adequate fiber intake can help to minimize constipation problems. Because of alcohol's deleterious effects on blood pressure, heart function, and blood lipids, its use should be avoided.[89]

Cardiac Cachexia There are no known therapies that can reverse cardiac cachexia, and prognosis is poor. Liquid supplements, tube feedings, or parenteral nutrition support can be supportive additions to treatment, however.

IN SUMMARY Congestive heart failure is characterized by a failure of the left or right side of the heart to pump adequate blood to tissues, resulting in backed-up blood (congestion) in veins, lungs, and other organs. It is usually a chronic, progressive heart condition that results from other cardiovascular illnesses. Treatment includes drug therapies that can reduce congestion and strengthen heart function and may also include a moderate sodium restriction.

Stroke

Stroke is the third leading cause of death after heart disease and cancer. It is the second most common cause of neurological disability after Alzheimer's disease. The two main types of strokes are ischemic stroke, which makes up about 88 percent of all strokes, and hemorrhagic stroke, which accounts for 9 percent of strokes.■ Most ischemic strokes are a result of atherosclerotic plaque rupture and thrombosis,■ but an embolus■ may also obstruct the flow of blood. Hemorrhagic strokes often result from rupture of a blood vessel that has been weakened by atherosclerosis and hypertension. Hemorrhagic strokes are more deadly: 38 percent result in death within 30 days.[90]

Strokes that come on suddenly, last for 2 to 30 minutes (or sometimes up to one to two hours), and stop without causing persistent damage, are called **transient ischemic attacks.** These short-lived strokes can be a warning sign that a more severe stroke is to follow, and need to be evaluated quickly. Treatment usually includes the use of aspirin and other drugs that prevent blood clotting.

■ **Ischemic stroke** results from the obstruction of blood flow to brain tissue. **Hemorrhagic stroke** results from bleeding within the brain, which destroys or compresses brain tissue.

■ Reminder: *Thrombosis* is the formation of a blood clot (a *thrombus*).

■ Reminder: *Embolus* is a traveling clot or air bubble that can obstruct a blood vessel and cause sudden tissue death (an *embolism*).

Stroke Prevention

Stroke is largely preventable by recognizing its risk factors and making lifestyle choices that decrease risk. Some risk factors cannot be modified; these include age, family history, and ethnicity. The highest rates of stroke are in the oldest age groups: risk doubles each successive decade after the age of 55.[91] African Americans have a greater risk of stroke than the U.S. white population until age 75, after which stroke risks are similar. A prior history of stroke, transient ischemic attacks, or heart disease also increases risk.

Many of the modifiable risk factors are similar to those for heart disease. Hypertension may be the single greatest risk factor.[92] Other major risk factors include cigarette smoking, diabetes mellitus, and elevated LDL cholesterol. Cocaine use has multiple effects that may promote stroke; it has caused stroke in younger persons, including first-time users and newborn babies whose mothers used cocaine.[93]

Drugs that prevent blood clotting are commonly used to reduce risk of ischemic stroke, especially in people who have suffered a first stroke or a transient ischemic attack. The drugs of choice include aspirin, antiplatelet drugs, and anticoagulants (usually warfarin).■ Anticoagulant therapy requires regular follow-up and occasional adjustments in dosage to prevent excessive bleeding.

■ Warfarin acts by interfering with vitamin K's blood-clotting function (see p. 382).

transient ischemic attacks: temporary reductions in blood flow to the brain, which cause temporary symptoms that vary depending on the part of the brain affected.

Management of Stroke

The effects of a stroke vary according to the area of the brain that has been injured. Body movements, senses, and speech can be impaired. One side of the body may be weakened or paralyzed. Mental disturbances are possible. Early diagnosis and treatment of a stroke are necessary to preserve brain tissue and minimize long-term disability. Ideally, thrombolytic drugs (clot-busting drugs) are used within the first few hours after a stroke to prevent further brain damage.[94]

The main nutritional goals are to maintain nutrition status and overall health despite a patient's disabilities. Dysphagia is a frequent complication of stroke and is associated with poorer prognosis.■ Difficulty with speech prevents patients from describing the problems they may be having with eating and from communicating their food preferences. Coordination problems can make it hard for them to grasp utensils or bring food from table to mouth. In some cases, tube feedings may be necessary until the patient has regained these skills. Highlight 27 gives additional information about feeding people with disabilities such as those that follow stroke.

■ Dysphagia—difficulty swallowing—is discussed in Chapter 23.

IN SUMMARY Strokes are a leading cause of death and disability. The two major types of strokes, ischemic and hemorrhagic stroke, are associated with atherosclerosis, hypertension, or both. Transient ischemic attacks are short-lived "mini"-strokes, and a warning sign that a more severe stroke may occur. Strokes are largely preventable by reversing modifiable risk factors, which include hypertension, cigarette smoking, diabetes mellitus, and elevated LDL cholesterol. Treatment includes anticlotting drugs such as aspirin, antiplatelet drugs, and anticoagulants. A patient who has had a major stroke may have problems eating normally due to lack of coordination and difficulty swallowing.

DIET-DRUG INTERACTIONS

Anticoagulants (including Aspirin)
Aspirin can be taken with food to reduce nausea and GI distress. By damaging mucosal tissue, long-term use of aspirin may reduce iron and calcium absorption and lead to deficiencies. *Ticlopidine* is best absorbed if taken with foods. Ticlopidine may cause nausea, GI distress, and diarrhea. Use of *warfarin* requires a consistent vitamin K intake from day to day to maintain effectiveness. Warfarin may also cause diarrhea. The herbs *danshen, dong quai, feverfew, garlic,* and *ginkgo* and supplements containing coenzyme Q, omega-3 fatty acids, and high doses of vitamin E can affect clotting times and should be avoided by people who are taking anticoagulants.

Antihypertensives
People using *antihypertensives* should avoid natural licorice and limit alcohol. Those using *ACE inhibitors* should avoid salt substitutes containing potassium and use potassium supplements only if prescribed. One ACE inhibitor, *fosinopril,* should not be taken with supplements or antacids that contain calcium or magnesium, as these minerals can reduce the drug's absorption. *Alpha-adrenergic blockers* can cause weight gain and fatigue. *Beta-blockers,* which also act as antianginals, should be taken with foods to reduce nausea and GI distress. People using *calcium channel blockers* should avoid grapefruit juice because it can potentiate the effects of the drugs. *Clonidine* may dry the mouth and lead to constipation and drowsiness.

Antilipemics
Cholestyramine can cause nausea, GI distress, and constipation and reduce absorption of fat-soluble vitamins. *Colestipol* is less likely than cholestyramine to cause nausea and affect fat-soluble vitamins, but can cause constipation. *Gemfibrozil* can cause nausea and GI distress. People using *statins (lovastatin, pravastatin, simvastin)* should avoid grapefruit juice and limit alcohol.

Cardiac Glycosides
Digitoxin, digoxin, and *digitalis* can cause anorexia and nausea. These drugs can be toxic if patients have elevated blood calcium levels or low blood potassium: patients are advised to eat a high-potassium diet and use calcium and vitamin D supplements cautiously. *Cardiac glycosides* should not be taken with supplements or antacids that contain magnesium, which can reduce drug absorption. The herb *hawthorn* can potentiate the effects of cardiac glycosides.

Diuretics
Diuretics can cause potassium imbalances and lead to muscle weakness, numbness and tingling, irregular heartbeats, and cardiac arrest. *Thiazide* and *loop diuretics* increase urinary excretion of potassium, and patients are encouraged to include rich sources of potassium in their diets and are sometimes prescribed potassium supplements. If *aloe vera* is used orally, it can potentiate the loss of potassium. Conversely, potassium-sparing diuretics *(amiloride, spironolactone,* and *triamterene)* can cause potassium retention, and patients should avoid potassium supplements and salt substitutes that contain potassium. Sometimes a combination of both types of diuretics is used to avoid potassium imbalances.

NUTRITION ASSESSMENT CHECKLIST for People with Cardiovascular Diseases

Medical History
Check the medical record for a diagnosis of:

- ☐ Coronary heart disease
- ☐ Hypertension
- ☐ Congestive heart failure
- ☐ Strokes

Review the medical record for complications related to cardiovascular diseases:

- ☐ Heart attacks
- ☐ Transient ischemic attacks
- ☐ Cardiac cachexia

Note risk factors for CHD related to diet, including:

- ☐ Elevated LDL or triglyceride levels
- ☐ Obesity or overweight
- ☐ Diabetes
- ☐ Hypertension

Medications
For patients using drug treatment for cardiovascular diseases, note:

- ☐ Side effects that may alter food intake
- ☐ Medications that may interact with grapefruit juice
- ☐ Use of warfarin, which influences vitamin K intake
- ☐ Use of diuretics associated with potassium imbalances
- ☐ Potential diet-drug or herb-drug interactions

Dietary Intake
For patients with CHD or hypertension, assess the diet for:

- ☐ Total energy intake
- ☐ Saturated fat, *trans* fat, cholesterol, and sodium intakes
- ☐ Soluble fiber and soy protein intakes
- ☐ Consumption of whole grains, fruits, vegetables, legumes, and nuts
- ☐ Alcohol

For patients with complications related to cardiovascular diseases:

- ☐ Check adequacy of food intake in patients with congestive heart failure.
- ☐ Check physical disabilities that may interfere with food preparation or consumption following a stroke.

Anthropometric Data
Measure baseline height and weight and reassess weight at each medical checkup. Note whether patients are meeting weight goals, including:

- ☐ Weight loss or maintenance in patients who are overweight
- ☐ Weight maintenance in patients in later stages of congestive heart failure

Remember that weight may be deceptively high in people who are retaining fluids, especially those with congestive heart failure.

Laboratory Tests
Monitor the following laboratory tests in people with cardiovascular diseases:

- ☐ LDL cholesterol, triglycerides, and HDL cholesterol
- ☐ Blood glucose in those with diabetes
- ☐ Blood potassium in those using diuretics or cardiac glycosides
- ☐ Indicators of fluid retention in those with congestive heart failure
- ☐ Blood-clotting times in those using anticoagulants

Clinical Signs
Blood pressure measurement is routine in physical exams, but is especially important for people who:

- ☐ Have cardiovascular diseases
- ☐ Have experienced a heart attack or stroke
- ☐ Are at risk for CHD or hypertension

Look for signs of:

- ☐ Potassium imbalances (muscle weakness, numbness and tingling, irregular heartbeat) in those using diuretics or cardiac glycosides
- ☐ Fluid overload in patients with congestive heart failure

NUTRITION ON THE NET

Access these websites for further study of topics covered in this chapter.

- Find updates and quick links to these and other nutrition-related sites at our website: **www.wadsworth.com/nutrition**
- To search for additional information about cardiovascular diseases, obtain the American Heart Association dietary guidelines, or find links to other relevant materials, visit the website of the American Heart Association: **www.americanheart.org**
- Information about cardiovascular diseases, the DASH Eating Plan, and implementation of heart-healthy diets is available at the websites of the National Heart, Lung, and Blood Institute and the Heart and Stroke Foundation of Canada: **www.nhlbi.nih.gov** and **ww2.heartandstroke.ca**
- To learn about improving health care and life expectancy of ethnic minority populations at high risk for cardiovascular diseases, visit the website of the International Society on Hypertension in Blacks: **www.ishib.org**

STUDY QUESTIONS

These questions will help you review the chapter. You will find the answers in the discussions on the pages provided.

1. Define atherosclerosis. How can atherosclerosis lead to thrombosis, heart attacks, and strokes? (pp. 820–822)
2. Describe the progression of atherosclerosis. List factors that contribute to the risk of developing atherosclerosis. (pp. 820–822)
3. Discuss the major risk factors for coronary heart disease. Explain how risk is evaluated. (pp. 823–824)
4. Describe each of the Therapeutic Lifestyle Changes that are recommended to reduce risk of coronary heart disease. (pp. 824–831)
5. Describe the medical treatment, medical nutrition therapy, and long-term management required following a heart attack. (pp. 832–833)
6. What complications may result from hypertension? Discuss the major risk factors associated with hypertension and the lifestyle modifications that may lower blood pressure in hypertensive patients. (pp. 834–837)
7. What is congestive heart failure? Discuss its consequences and usual medical treatment. Why is malnutrition a common problem in later stages? What dietary strategies are important in its management? (pp. 838–840)
8. Explain the difference between ischemic stroke and hemorrhagic stroke. What are possible consequences of stroke? How might it affect an individual's nutrition care? (pp. 840–841)

These multiple choice questions will help you prepare for an exam. Answers can be found on p. 845.

1. Monocytes play a role in plaque development by:
   a. causing bleeding and development of blood clots.
   b. engulfing LDL cholesterol and becoming foam cells.
   c. damaging arteries when present in large numbers.
   d. blocking blood flow and causing accumulation of debris.
2. Risk factors for atherosclerosis include all of the following, *except:*
   a. smoking.
   b. shear stress.
   c. diabetes mellitus.
   d. elevated HDL cholesterol and low triglycerides.
3. The dietary lipids that have the strongest influence on blood cholesterol levels are:
   a. monounsaturated fats.
   b. cholesterol.
   c. saturated fats.
   d. plant sterols.
4. The omega-3 fatty acids EPA and DHA, which can improve some risk factors for heart disease, are obtained by consuming:
   a. fish oil.
   b. fruits and vegetables.
   c. egg yolks and organ meats.
   d. soy products and nuts.
5. Moderate alcohol consumption may improve heart disease risk because it:
   a. lowers blood pressure.
   b. improves nutrition status.
   c. offsets the damage from smoking.
   d. increases HDL cholesterol levels.
6. Patients with hypertriglyceridemia may benefit from this dietary change:
   a. reduce sodium intake.
   b. consume one or two alcoholic beverages daily.
   c. avoid a high-carbohydrate intake.
   d. reduce cholesterol intake.
7. In most cases of essential hypertension, the cause is:
   a. excessive alcohol use.
   b. atherosclerosis.
   c. hormonal imbalances.
   d. unknown.
8. Hypertensive patients can benefit from all of the following dietary and lifestyle modifications, *except:*
   a. including nonfat or low-fat milk products in the diet.
   b. reducing total fat intake.
   c. consuming generous amounts of fruits, vegetables, legumes, and nuts.
   d. reducing sodium intake.
9. The medical nutrition therapy for a patient with congestive heart failure is likely to include:
   a. weight loss.
   b. reducing total fat intake.
   c. sodium restriction.
   d. cholesterol restriction.
10. Hemorrhagic stroke:
    a. is the most common type of stroke.
    b. results from obstructed blood flow within brain tissue.
    c. comes on suddenly and usually lasts for up to 30 minutes.
    d. results from bleeding within the brain, which damages brain tissue.

REFERENCES

1. American Heart Association, *Heart Disease and Stroke Statistics—2003 Update* (2003), p. 5, **www.americanheart.org/downloadable/heart/10461207852142003HDSStatsBook.pdf**, site visited July 21, 2003.
2. American Heart Association, 2003.
3. American Heart Association, *International Cardiovascular Disease Statistics* (2003), p. 2, **www.americanheart.org/downloadable/heart/1043250000063IntStats2003.pdf**, site visited July 21, 2003.
4. M. H. Beers and R. Berkow, eds., *The Merck Manual of Diagnosis and Therapy,* 17th ed. (Whitehouse Station, N.J.: Merck Research Laboratories, 1999), pp. 1654–1655.
5. P. Libby, Changing concepts of atherogenesis, *Journal of Internal Medicine* 247 (2000): 349–358; V. Fuster, Z. A. Fayad, and J. J. Badimon, Acute coronary syndromes: Biology, *Lancet* (supplement 2) 353 (1999): 5–9.
6. Libby, 2000.
7. A. M. Varnava, P. G. Mills, and M. J. Davies, Relationship between coronary artery remodeling and plaque vulnerability, *Circulation* 105 (2002): 939–943; J. M. Foody and S. E. Nissen, The unstable plaque, in J. Foody, ed., *Preventive Cardiology* (Totowa, N.J.: Humana Press, 2001), pp. 4–8.
8. Foody and Nissen, 2001; P. K. Shah, Role of inflammation and metalloproteinases in plaque disruption and thrombosis, *Vascular Medicine* 3 (1998): 199–206.
9. A. P. Burke and coauthors, Healed plaque ruptures and sudden coronary death: Evidence that subclinical rupture has a role in plaque progression, *Circulation* 103 (2001): 934–940.
10. J. Willeit and coauthors, Distinct risk profiles of early and advanced atherosclerosis, *Arteriosclerosis, Thrombosis, and Vascular Biology* 20 (2000): 529–537.
11. T. A. Pearson and coauthors, Markers of inflammation and cardiovascular disease, *Circulation* 107 (2003): 499–511.
12. M. A. Lauer, Inflammation and infection in coronary artery disease, in J. Foody, ed., *Preventive Cardiology* (Totowa, N.J.: Humana Press, 2001).
13. R. B. Buchsbaum and J. C. Buchsbaum, Tobacco as a cardiovascular risk factor, J. Foody, ed., *Preventive Cardiology* (Totowa, N.J.: Humana Press, 2001), pp. 178–181.
14. A. Mertens and P. Holvoet, Oxidized LDL and HDL: Antagonists in atherothrombosis, *FASEB Journal* 15 (2001): 2073–2084.
15. I. Staprans and coauthors, Oxidized cholesterol in the diet is a source of oxidized lipoproteins in human serum, *Lipid Research* 44 (2003): 705–715.
16. J. S. Cohn, C. Marcoux, and J. Davignon, Detection, quantification, and characterization of potentially atherogenic triglyceride-rich remnant lipoproteins, *Arteriosclerosis Thrombosis, and Vascular Biology* 19 (1999): 2474–2486; S. C. Whitman and coauthors, Uptake of type III hypertriglyceridemic VLDL by macrophages is enhanced by oxidation, especially after remnant formation, *Arteriosclerosis, Thrombosis, and Vascular Biology* 17 (1997): 1707–1715.
17. Mertens and Holvoet, 2001.
18. Willeit and coauthors, 2000.
19. E. J. Schaefer, Lipoproteins, nutrition, and heart disease, *American Journal of Clinical Nutrition* 75 (2002): 191–212.
20. K. C. B. Tan and coauthors, Advanced glycation end products and endothelial dysfunction in type 2 diabetes, *Diabetes Care* 25 (2002): 1055–1059; A. Chait and J. D. Brunzell, Diabetes mellitus, lipids, and atherosclerosis, in D. LeRoith, S. I. Taylor, and J. M. Olefsky, eds., *Diabetes Mellitus: A Fundamental and Clinical Text,* 2nd ed. (Philadelphia: Lippincott Williams & Wilkins, 2000), pp. 934–939.
21. Willeit and coauthors, 2000.
22. E. H. Lieberman, M. R. Garces, and F. Lopez-Jimenez, Endothelial function and insights for prevention, in J. Foody, ed., *Preventive Cardiology* (Totowa, N.J.: Humana Press, 2001), p. 25.
23. Lieberman, Garces, and Lopez-Jimenez, 2001.
24. Willeit and coauthors, 2000.
25. H. O'Grady and coauthors, Homocysteine and occlusive arterial disease, *British Journal of Surgery* 89 (2002): 838–844.
26. Beers and Berkow, 1999, p. 1777.
27. Libby, 2000.
28. American Heart Association, *Heart Disease and Stroke Statistics—2003 Update,* 2003.
29. American Heart Association, *Heart Disease and Stroke Statistics—2003 Update,* 2003.
30. Expert Panel on Detection, Evaluation, and Treatment of High Blood Cholesterol in Adults (Adult Treatment Panel III), *Third Report of the National Cholesterol Education Program (NCEP),* NIH publication no. 02-5215 (Bethesda, Md.: National Heart, Lung, and Blood Institute, 2002), **www.nhlbi.nih.gov/guidelines/cholesterol/atp3full.pdf**, site visited August 8, 2003.
31. U. N. Khot and coauthors, Prevalence of conventional risk factors in patients with coronary heart disease, *Journal of the American Medical Association* 290 (2003): 898–904.
32. Expert Panel on Detection, Evaluation, and Treatment of High Blood Cholesterol in Adults (Adult Treatment Panel III), 2002.
33. JNC VII Express, Joint National Committee on Prevention, Detection, Evaluation, and Treatment of High Blood Pressure, *Seventh Report,* NIH publication no. 03-5233 (Bethesda, Md.: National Heart, Lung, and Blood Institute, 2003), **www.nhlbi.nih.gov/guidelines/hypertension/express.pdf**, site visited August 10, 2003.
34. Expert Panel on Detection, Evaluation, and Treatment of High Blood Cholesterol in Adults (Adult Treatment Panel III), 2002.
35. L. Van Horn, Therapeutic lifestyle changes, presented at The Challenge of Lipid Management, January 16, 2002, available at American Heart Association Science Online, **www.ahascienceonline.org/atp/summary.asp?sid=1&stid=5**, site visited August 12, 2003.
36. L. Van Horn and coauthors, Other dietary components and cardiovascular risk, in A. M. Coulston, C. L. Rock, and E. R. Monsen, eds., *Nutrition in the Prevention and Treatment of Disease* (San Diego, Academic Press, 2001), pp. 292–293.
37. M. Law, Plant sterol and stanol margarines and health, *British Medical Journal* 320 (2000): 861–864.
38. U.S. Department of Health and Human Services, Food and Drug Administration, Food labeling: Health claims; soy protein and coronary heart disease: Final rule, *Federal Register* 64 (1999): 699–733.
39. P. Marckmann, Fishing for heart protection, *American Journal of Clinical Nutrition* 78 (2003): 1–2; P. M. Kris-Etherton, W. S. Harris, and L. J. Appel, Fish consumption, fish oil, omega-3 fatty acids, and cardiovascular disease, *Circulation* 106 (2002): 2747–2757; D. W. T. Nilsen and coauthors, Effects of a high-dose concentrate of n-3 fatty acids or corn oil introduced early after an acute myocardial infarction on serum triacylglycerol and HDL cholesterol, *American Journal of Clinical Nutrition* 74 (2001): 50–56.
40. S. M. Grundy, N-3 fatty acids: Priority for post-myocardial infarction clinical trials, *Circulation* 107 (2003): 1834–1836.
41. K. J. Mukamai and E. B. Rimm, Alcohol's effects on the risk for coronary heart disease, *Alcohol Research and Health* 25 (2001): 255–261.
42. V. Bagnardi and coauthors, Alcohol consumption and the risk of cancer: A meta-analysis, *Alcohol Research and Health* 25 (2001): 263–270.
43. M. A. Emanuele and N. Emanuele, Alcohol and the male reproductive system, *Alcohol Research and Health* 25 (2001): 282–287.
44. W. S. Harris, n-3 Fatty acids and serum lipoproteins: Human studies, *American Journal of Clinical Nutrition* 65 (1997): 1645S–1654S.
45. E. B. Schmidt and coauthors, n-3 polyunsaturated fatty acid supplementation (Pikasol) in men with moderate and severe hypertriglyceridaemia: A dose-response study, *Annals of Nutrition and Metabolism* 36 (1992): 283–287; M. C. Blonk and coauthors, Dose-response effects of fish-oil supplementation in healthy volunteers, *American Journal of Clinical Nutrition* 52 (1990): 120–127.
46. S. S. Hendler and D. Rorvik, eds., *PDR for Nutritional Supplements* (Montvale, N.J.: Medical Economics Co., 2001), pp. 148–149.
47. J. Eritsland, Safety considerations of polyunsaturated fatty acids, *American Journal of Clinical Nutrition* 71 (2000): 197S–201S.
48. R. Marchioli and coauthors, Early protection against sudden death by n-3 polyunsaturated fatty acids after myocardial infarction: Time-course analysis of the results of the Gruppo Italiano per lo Studio della Sopravvivenza nell'Infarto Miocardico (GISSI)-Prevenzione, *Circulation* 105 (2002): 1897–1903; R. B. Singh and coauthors, Randomized, double-blind, placebo-controlled trial of fish oil and mustard oil in patients with suspected acute myocardial infarction: The Indian experiment of infarct survival—4, *Cardiovascular Drugs and Therapy* 11 (1997): 485–491.
49. M. C. Morris, Dietary fats and blood pressure, *Journal of Cardiovascular Risk* 1 (1994): 21–30.
50. Marckmann, 2003.
51. D. S. Wald, M. Law, and J. K. Morris, Homocysteine and cardiovascular disease: Evidence on causality from a meta-analysis, *British Medical Journal* 325 (2002): 1202.
52. S. Nader and K. Robinson, A recognized risk factor: Homocysteine and coronary artery Disease, in J. Foody, ed., *Preventive Cardiology* (Totowa, N.J.: Humana Press, 2001), pp. 223–226.
53. C. D. Morris and S. Carson, Routine vitamin supplementation to prevent cardiovascular disease: A summary of the evidence for the U.S. preventive services task force, *Annals of Internal Medicine* 139 (2003): 56–57.
54. E. R. Miller and coauthors, Meta-analysis: High-dosage vitamin E supplementation may increase all-cause mortality, *Annals of Internal Medicine* 142 (2005): 37–46; D. H. Lee and coauthors, Does supplemental vitamin C increase cardiovascular disease risk in women with diabetes? *American Journal of Clinical Nutrition* 80 (2004): 1194–1200.
55. P. D. Thompson and coauthors, Exercise and physical activity in the prevention and

treatment of atherosclerotic cardiovascular disease, *Circulation* 107 (2003): 3109–3116.
56. C. A. Schoenborn and coauthors, National Center for Health Statistics, Health behaviors of adults: United States, 1999–2001, *Vital Health Statistics* 10 (2004): 39–40.
57. Thompson and coauthors, 2003.
58. G. G. Blackburn, Exercise in the prevention of coronary artery disease, in J. Foody, ed., *Preventive Cardiology* (Totowa, N.J.: Humana Press, 2001), pp. 144–155.
59. A. Tiengo and A. Avogaro, Cardiovascular disease, in P. Bjorntorp, ed., *International Textbook of Obesity* (West Sussex, U.K.: John Wiley & Sons, 2001), pp. 367–372; K. Napier, Obesity and coronary artery disease: Implications and interventions, in J. Foody, ed., *Preventive Cardiology* (Totowa, N.J.: Humana Press, 2001), pp. 159–169).
60. Obesity Education Initiative, *Clinical Guidelines on the Identification, Evaluation, and Treatment of Overweight and Obesity in Adults: The Evidence Report,* NIH publication no. 98-4083 (Bethesda, Md.: National Heart, Lung, and Blood Institute, 1998).
61. Buchsbaum and Buchsbaum, 2001.
62. Buchsbaum and Buchsbaum, 2001.
63. Expert Panel on Detection, Evaluation, and Treatment of High Blood Cholesterol in Adults (Adult Treatment Panel III), 2002.
64. Expert Panel on Detection, Evaluation, and Treatment of High Blood Cholesterol in Adults (Adult Treatment Panel III), 2002.
65. American Heart Association, *Heart Disease and Stroke Statistics—2003 Update,* 2003.
66. M. A. Militello and T. H. Seo, Pharmacologic agents in preventive cardiology, in J. Foody, ed., *Preventive Cardiology* (Totowa, N.J.: Humana Press, 2001), pp. 243–247.
67. Beers and Berkow, 1999, p. 1676.
68. ACC/AHA Guidelines for the Management of Patients with Acute Myocardial Infarction—Part VII. Long-Term Management (1999), **www.americanheart.org/presenter.jhtml?identifier=1987**, site visited August 20, 2003.
69. JNC VII Express, 2003.
70. American Heart Association, *Heart Disease and Stroke Statistics—2003 Update,* 2003.
71. R. Victor, Arterial hypertension, in L. Goldman and D. Ausiello, eds., *Cecil Textbook of Medicine* (Philadelphia: Saunders, 2004), pp. 346–363.
72. National High Blood Pressure Education Program, *Primary Prevention of Hypertension: Clinical and Public Health Advisory,* NIH publication no. 02-5076 (November 2002).
73. American Heart Association, *Heart Disease and Stroke Statistics—2003 Update,* 2003.
74. Obesity Education Initiative, 1998.
75. W. F. Ganong, Cardiovascular disorders: Vascular disease, in S. J. McPhee and coeditors, *Pathophysiology of Disease,* 2nd ed. (Stamford, Conn.: Appleton and Lange, 1997), p. 271.
76. X. Xin and coauthors, Effects of alcohol reduction on blood pressure: A meta-analysis of randomized controlled trials, *Hypertension* 38 (2001): 1112.
77. JNC VII Express, 2003.
78. L. J. Appel and coauthors, A clinical trial on the effects of dietary patterns on blood pressure, *New England Journal of Medicine* 336 (1997): 1117.
79. U.S. Department of Health and Human Services and U.S. Department of Agriculture, *Dietary Guidelines for Americans, 2005* (Washington, D.C.: Government Printing Office, January 2005).
80. F. M. Sacks and coauthors, Effects on blood pressure of reduced dietary sodium and the Dietary Approaches to Stop Hypertension (DASH) Diet, *New England Journal of Medicine* 344 (2001): 3–10.
81. Sacks and coauthors, 2001.
82. Obesity Education Initiative, 1998.
83. D. G. Vidt, Management of hypertension, in J. Foody, ed., *Preventive Cardiology* (Totowa, N.J.: Humana Press, 2001), p. 105.
84. S. Lutton and N. Anzlovar, Nutrition and congestive heart failure, in A. M. Coulston, C. L. Rock, and E. R. Monsen, *Nutrition in the Prevention and Treatment of Disease* (San Diego: Academic Press, 2001), pp. 325–333.
85. K. L. Grady and coauthors, Team management of patients with heart failure, *Circulation* 102 (2000): 2443–2456.
86. S. A. Hunt and coauthors, ACC/AHA Guidelines for the Evaluation and Management of Chronic Heart Failure in the Adult: Executive Summary, *Journal of the American College of Cardiology* 38 (2001): 2101–2113.
87. G. F. Fletcher and coauthors, Exercise standards for testing and training, *Circulation* 104 (2001):1694–1740.
88. Lutton and Anzlovar, 2001.
89. Lutton and Anzlovar, 2001.
90. American Heart Association, *Heart Disease and Stroke Statistics—2003 Update,* 2003.
91. L. B. Goldstein and coauthors, Primary prevention of ischemic stroke, *Stroke* 32 (2001): 280–299.
92. American Stroke Association, *What Are the Risk Factors of Stroke?* (2002), **www.strokeassociation.org/presenter.jhtml?identifier=1060**, site visited August 24, 2003.
93. C. M. Porth, *Pathophysiology: Concepts of Altered Health States,* 5th ed. (Philadelphia: Lippincott-Raven, 1998), pp. 894–895.
94. Porth, 1998, pp. 897–898.

ANSWERS

Study Questions (multiple choice)

1. b 2. d 3. c 4. a 5. d 6. c 7. d 8. b 9. c 10. d

HIGHLIGHT

Helping People with Feeding Disabilities

Chapter 27 referred to difficulties following a stroke that can interfere with the ability to eat independently. This highlight discusses a broader problem faced by individuals who must cope with disabilities that interfere with the process of eating, such as those that interfere with chewing and swallowing. These obstacles can arise at any time during a person's life and from any number of causes. An infant may be born with a physical impairment such as cleft palate; an adolescent may lose motor control following injuries sustained in an automobile accident; an older adult may struggle with the pain of arthritis or the mental deterioration of dementia. Table H27-1 lists some of the conditions that may lead to feeding problems.

TABLE H27-1 Conditions That May Lead to Feeding Problems

The following conditions may lead to feeding problems by interfering with a person's ability to suck, bite, chew, swallow, or coordinate hand-to-mouth movements.

• Accidents	• Language, visual, or hearing impairment
• Amputations	• Microcephalia
• Arthritis	• Multiple sclerosis
• Birth defects	• Muscle weakness
• Cerebral palsy	• Muscular dystrophy
• Cleft palate	• Neuromotor dysfunction
• Down syndrome	• Parkinson's disease
• Head injuries	• Polio
• Huntington's chorea	• Spinal cord injuries
• Hydrocephalia	• Stroke

Effects of Disabilities on Nutrition Status

Eating and drinking require a surprising number of individual coordinated motions. Consider an infant learning the skills required for feeding: each step—sitting, grasping cups and utensils, bringing food to the mouth, biting, chewing, and swallowing—requires coordinated movements. An injury or disability that interferes with these movements can lead to feeding problems and inadequate food intake. Total food intake is often significantly reduced when individuals with inefficient motor function take a long time to eat.[1] Difficulties that affect procurement of food, such as the inability to drive or walk or carry groceries, can also lower food intake and lead to malnutrition and weight loss.

Energy Requirements

Disabilities may either increase or decrease energy needs. Those that affect muscle tension and mobility can reduce physical activity and, consequently, energy requirements. Other disabilities, such as certain forms of cerebral palsy, cause involuntary muscle activity that raises energy requirements.[2] Loss of a limb due to amputation reduces energy needs in proportion to the weight and metabolism represented by the missing limb, but can result in greater energy needs if an individual increases activity to compensate for the loss, such as by propelling a wheelchair. Because the effects of disabilities are often unpredictable, the health care practitioner may find it difficult to assess energy requirements until weight gain or loss is apparent.

Overweight and obesity often accompany conditions that limit mobility or result in short stature; examples include Down syndrome (see p. 493) and spina bifida (see p. 477). Obesity may also develop because the family or caregiver provides an inappropriate amount of food, sometimes out of sympathy for the disabled individual.[3] In these cases, the health practitioner may need to counsel the family or caregiver about appropriate food choices and portion sizes.

Effects of Disease Symptoms and Medications

Physical symptoms of disease can interfere with eating and nutrition status. Some of these include nausea, frequent coughing or choking, difficulty breathing, and gastroesophageal reflux. Individuals with speech and hearing problems may have a difficult time communicating with caregivers about thirst and hunger. Mobility problems can lead to bone demineralization and pressure sores.

Conditions that require the use of multiple medications can also have a significant impact on nutrition status (see Chapter 19).[4] Medications may alter nutrition status, increase or decrease appetite, or have gastrointestinal effects that cause pain or discomfort with eating.

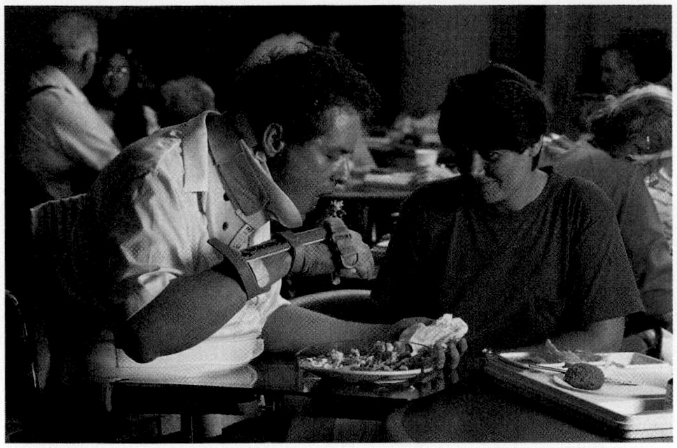
© Charles Gupton/Stock Boston

Adaptive feeding equipment can help patients with feeding disabilities gain independence.

Social Concerns

Because mealtimes are a critical time for social interaction, individuals with feeding problems may encounter emotional and social problems if unable to participate. Children may fail to develop social skills, whereas adults may miss the social stimulation that mealtimes provide. Individuals should be encouraged to sit with family and friends during meals so that they are not deprived of the social and cultural aspects of eating.

Independent Eating for People with Disabilities

The evaluation and treatment of feeding problems may involve the joint efforts of health care professionals from a variety of disciplines including dietitians, occupational and physical therapists, speech-language pathologists, dentists, and nurses. Together, health care professionals evaluate each patient's dietary needs and assess abilities to chew, sip, swallow, grasp utensils, use utensils to pick up foods, and bring foods from the plate to the mouth. A speech-language pathologist most often evaluates chewing and swallowing abilities and trains patients to use lips, tongue, and throat for eating and speaking. An occupational therapist can demonstrate alternate feeding strategies, including changes in body position that improve feeding, handling techniques for utensils and food, and use of special feeding devices.

Feeding Strategies

Direct observation of a patient during mealtimes allows health care providers to evaluate current eating behaviors, demonstrate feeding techniques, monitor the patient's and caregiver's understanding of the techniques, and evaluate how well the care plan is working. To illustrate, consider an example of a child with a feeding problem caused by hypersensitivity to oral stimulation. The health care professional may start by teaching the caregiver to gently and playfully stroke the child's face with a hand, wash cloth, or soft toy. Once the child tolerates touch on less sensitive areas of the face, the health care professional may encourage the caregiver to slowly begin to rub the child's lips, gums, palate, and tongue. With time, the child may be better able to tolerate the presence of food in the mouth. Examples of other strategies that can help feeding problems are listed in Table H27-2.

Adaptive Feeding Equipment

Figure H27-1 shows a few of many special feeding devices that are available and describes their uses. These devices can make a remarkable difference in a person's ability to eat independently.

TABLE H27-2 Interventions for Feeding-Related Problems

Inability to Suck
- Use squeeze bottles, which do not require sucking, to express liquids into the mouth.
- Place a spoon on the center of the tongue and apply downward pressure to stimulate sucking.
- Apply rhythmic, slow strokes on the tongue to alter tongue position and improve sucking response.

Inability to Chew
- Place foods between gums and teeth to promote chewing.
- Improve chewing skills with different textured foods; for example, fruit leathers stimulate jaw movements but dissolve quickly enough to minimize choking.
- Provide soft foods that require minimal chewing or are easily chewed.

Inability to Swallow
- Provide thickened liquids, pureed foods, and moist foods that form boluses easily.
- Provide cold formulas, frozen fruit juice bars, and ice; cold substances promote swallowing movements by the tongue and soft palate.
- Make sure the patient's jaw and lips are closed to facilitate swallowing action.
- Correct posture and head position if they interfere with swallowing ability.

Inability to Grasp or Coordinate Movements
- Provide utensils that have modified handles, or are smaller or larger as necessary.
- Encourage use of hands for feeding if utensils are difficult to maneuver.
- Provide plates with food guards to prevent spilling.
- Supply clothing protection.

Impaired Vision
- Place foods (meats, vegetables) in similar locations at meals.
- Provide plates with food guards to prevent spilling.

SOURCES: J. Case-Smith and R. Humphry, Feeding and oral motor skills, in J. Case-Smith, A. S. Allen, and P. N. Pratt, eds., *Occupational Therapy for Children* (St. Louis: Mosby-Year Book, 1996), pp. 430–460; S. Escott-Stump, *Nutrition and Diagnosis-Related Care* (Baltimore: Lippincott Williams & Wilkins, 2002), pp. 64–65.

FIGURE H27-1 Examples of Adaptive Feeding Devices

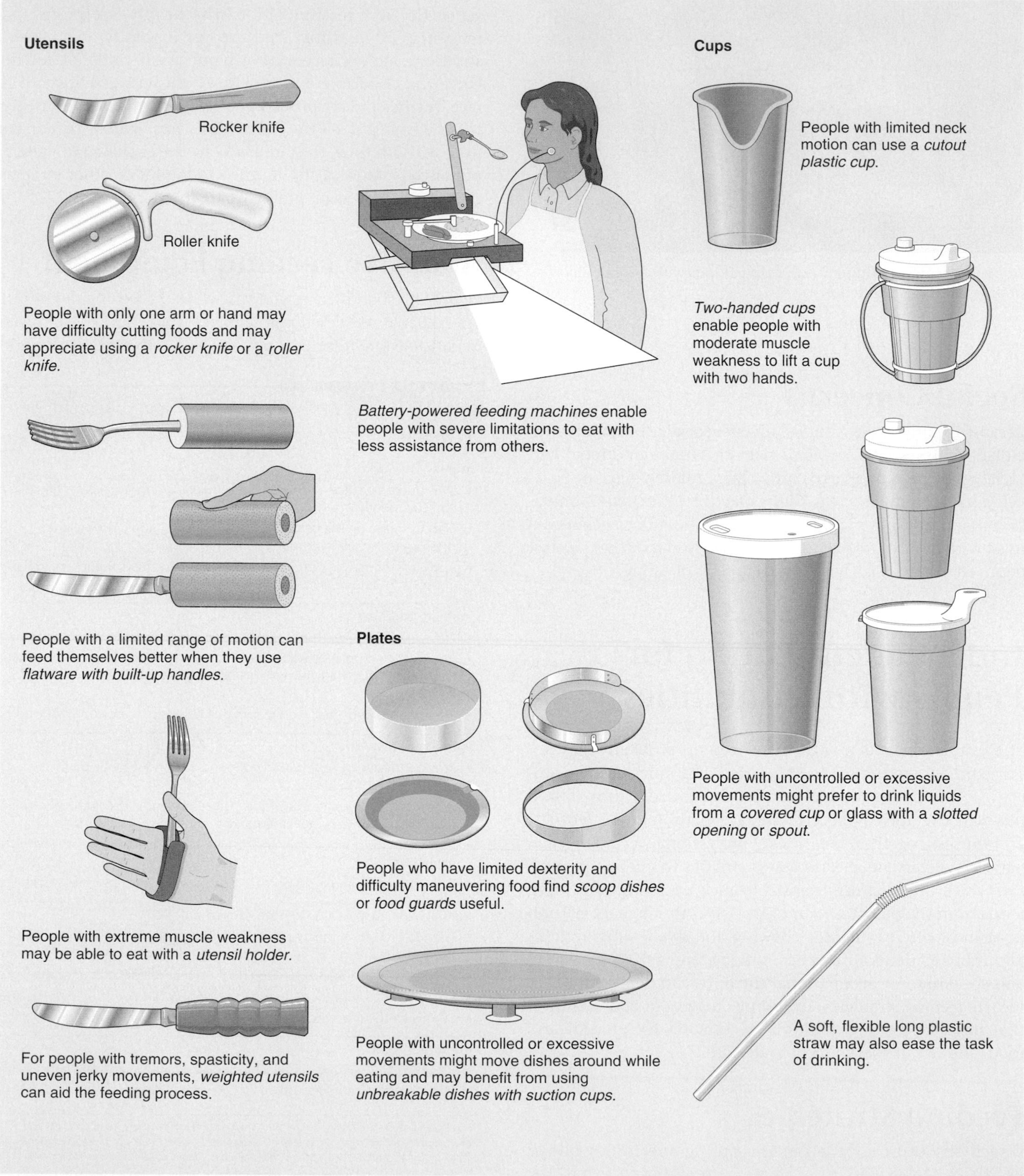
Utensils
Rocker knife
Roller knife
People with only one arm or hand may have difficulty cutting foods and may appreciate using a *rocker knife* or a *roller knife.*
People with a limited range of motion can feed themselves better when they use *flatware with built-up handles.*
People with extreme muscle weakness may be able to eat with a *utensil holder.*
For people with tremors, spasticity, and uneven jerky movements, *weighted utensils* can aid the feeding process.
Battery-powered feeding machines enable people with severe limitations to eat with less assistance from others.
Plates
People who have limited dexterity and difficulty maneuvering food find *scoop dishes* or *food guards* useful.
People with uncontrolled or excessive movements might move dishes around while eating and may benefit from using *unbreakable dishes with suction cups.*
Cups
People with limited neck motion can use a *cutout plastic cup.*
Two-handed cups enable people with moderate muscle weakness to lift a cup with two hands.
People with uncontrolled or excessive movements might prefer to drink liquids from a *covered cup* or glass with a *slotted opening* or *spout.*
A soft, flexible long plastic straw may also ease the task of drinking.

Other examples of adaptive equipment include specialized chairs to improve posture, bolsters inserted under arms to improve elbow stability, and raised trays or eating surfaces to simplify hand-to-mouth movements.[5]

Sometimes, despite the best efforts of all involved, a patient is unable to consume enough food by mouth. In these cases, tube feedings can help to improve nutrition status. Tube feedings are also recommended for patients who have severe dysphagia (difficulty swallowing) or aspiration pneumonia.[6]

A Note for Caregivers

Caring for a disabled person requires time and patience—there are often many new therapies to be learned and administered. The caregiver often spends many hours preparing special foods, monitoring use of adaptive feeding equipment, and helping with feedings. Moreover, a disabled person may need help with many other tasks, and all may require a considerable amount of time. In many cases, a caregiver may receive little or no assistance. Caregivers may feel overwhelmed with responsibility and have little time to care for themselves and other family members. These conditions often lead to strained interactions between caregiver and patient and may cause frustration and depression.[7] Psychologists can offer counseling to patients or caregivers to help them adjust; all members of the health care team can offer emotional support and practical suggestions to ease caregivers' responsibilities and frustrations.

Successful therapy for people with feeding disabilities requires the involvement of many health care professionals and depends on accurate identification of impaired feeding skills and determination of appropriate interventions. Ideally, with training, people with disabilities attain total independence—they are able to prepare, serve, and eat nutritionally adequate food daily without help. In some cases, these goals can be met with the help of caregivers. The combined efforts of the health care team can support both patients and caregivers in enhancing quality of life and in achieving independence to the greatest degree possible.

REFERENCES

1. E. B. Fung and coauthors, Feeding dysfunction is associated with poor growth and health status in children with cerebral palsy, *Journal of the American Dietetic Association* 102 (2002): 361–368.
2. Position of the American Dietetic Association: Providing nutrition services for infants, children, and adults with developmental disabilities and special health care needs, *Journal of the American Dietetic Association* 104 (2004): 97–107.
3. H. H. Cloud, Expanding roles for dietitians working with persons with developmental disabilities, *Journal of the American Dietetic Association* 97 (1997): 129–130.
4. Position of the American Dietetic Association, 2004.
5. J. Case-Smith and R. Humphry, Feeding and oral motor skills, in J. Case-Smith, A. S. Allen, and P. N. Pratt, eds., *Occupational Therapy for Children* (St. Louis: Mosby-Year Book, 1996), pp. 430–460.
6. Position of the American Dietetic Association, 2004.
7. Fung and coauthors, 2002.

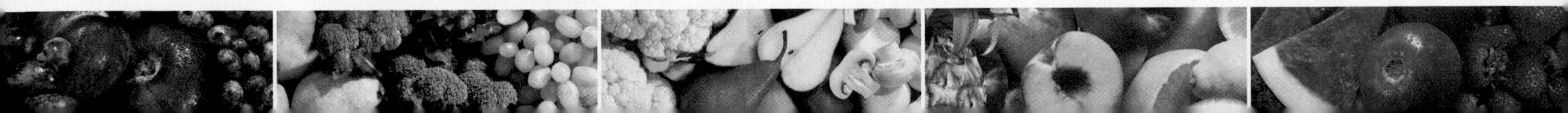

Chapter 28

Nutrition and Renal Diseases

Chapter Outline

Available Online

http://nutrition.wadsworth.com/uncn7

Student Practice Test

Glossary Terms

Nutrition on the Net

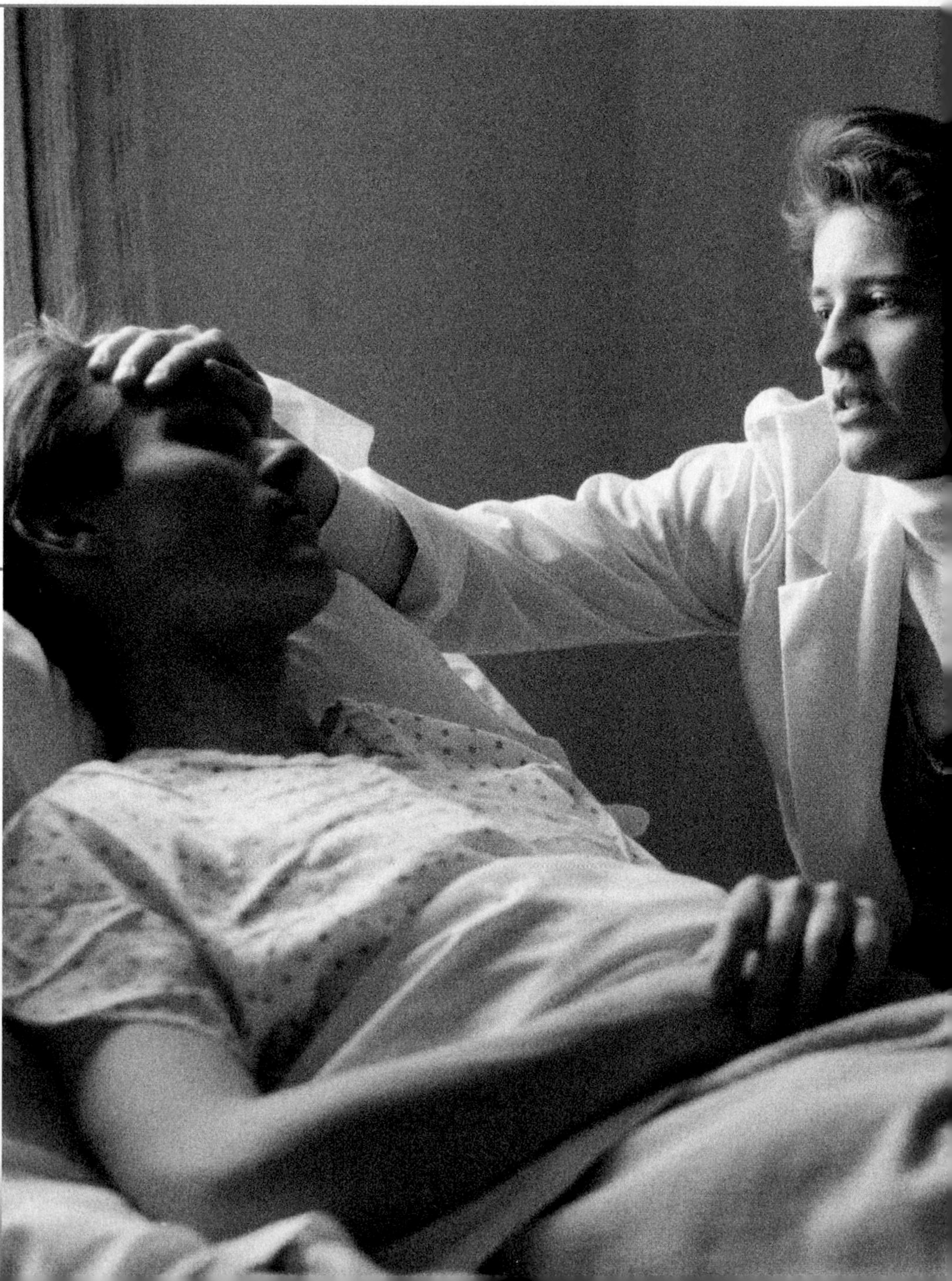

Nutrition in the Professional Setting

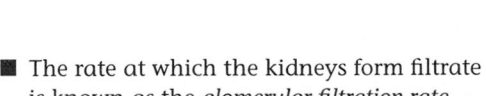

Each bean-shaped kidney is only about the size of a fist, yet the kidneys carry out many critical functions. Among other tasks, the kidneys shoulder much of the responsibility for maintaining the body's chemical balance. If the kidneys fail to function, toxic compounds build up in the blood, causing a wide range of symptoms and life-threatening complications. Health practitioners learn to recognize and treat renal diseases early, before kidney damage progresses and causes serious illness. Unfortunately, acute renal diseases have high mortality rates, and chronic renal disease is underdiagnosed and undertreated.

The two kidneys sit just above the waist on each side of the spinal column. As part of the urinary system (see Figure 28-1), they are responsible for filtering blood and removing excess fluid and wastes for elimination in urine. Many body functions, including the work of the heart, blood vessels, enzymes, and cell membranes, depend on the kidneys to maintain normal fluid volume and composition.[1] Because the kidneys are so proficient at this task, disturbances in body fluids that result from food intake, physical activity, and metabolism are normally corrected within hours. In addition, the kidneys perform a number of other metabolic roles, as discussed in the following section. Thus **renal** disorders not only result in fluid and electrolyte imbalances, but can have widespread effects on health.

What the Kidneys Do

The functional unit of the kidneys is the **nephron,** introduced on p. 400 (see Figure 12-2). Within each nephron, the **glomerulus,** a ball-shaped tuft of capillaries, serves as a gateway through which the components of blood must pass to form **filtrate.**■ The

■ The rate at which the kidneys form filtrate is known as the *glomerular filtration rate,* discussed later in this chapter.

renal (REE-nal): pertaining to the kidneys.

nephron (NEF-ron): the functional unit of the kidneys, consisting of a glomerulus and tubules.
- **nephros** = kidney

glomerulus (gloh-MEHR-yoo-lus): a tuft of capillaries within the nephron that filters water and solutes from blood as urine production begins (plural: *glomeruli*).

filtrate: fluid that passes from blood through the capillaries of the glomeruli, eventually forming urine.

FIGURE 28-1 The Kidneys and Urinary Tract

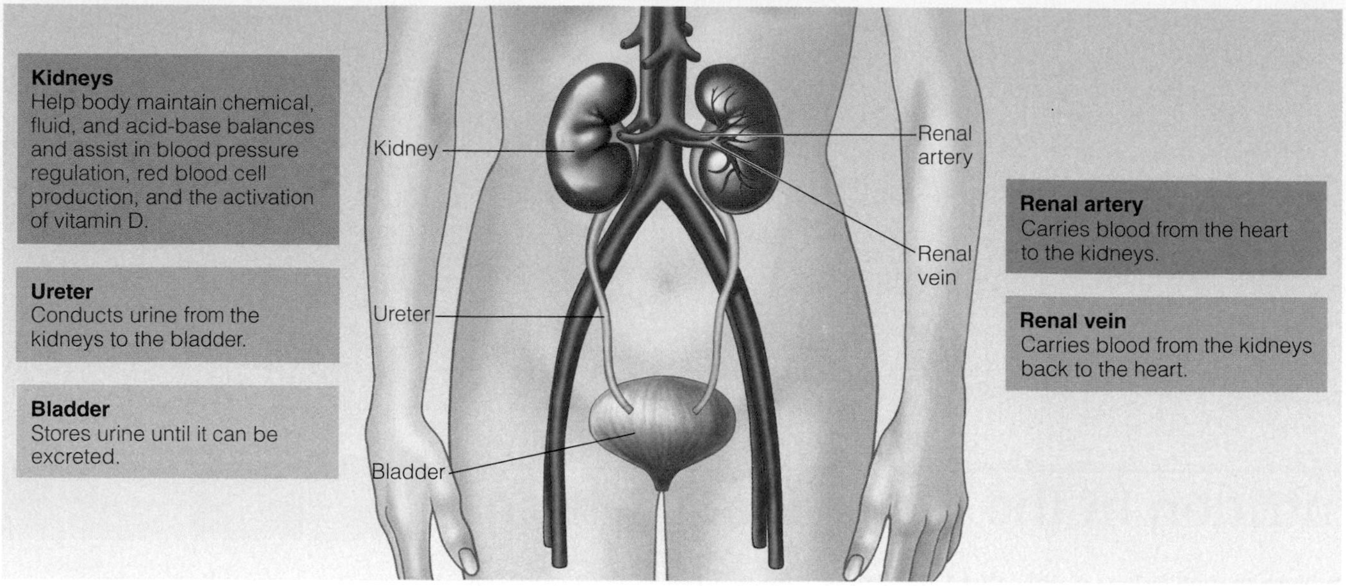
Kidneys
Help body maintain chemical, fluid, and acid-base balances and assist in blood pressure regulation, red blood cell production, and the activation of vitamin D.
Ureter
Conducts urine from the kidneys to the bladder.
Bladder
Stores urine until it can be excreted.
Kidney
Ureter
Bladder
Renal artery
Renal vein
Renal artery
Carries blood from the heart to the kidneys.
Renal vein
Carries blood from the kidneys back to the heart.

glomerulus and surrounding **Bowman's capsule** function like a sieve, retaining blood cells and plasma proteins in blood while allowing fluid and small solutes to enter the nephron's system of **tubules.** As the filtrate passes through the tubules, its composition continuously changes as some of its components are reabsorbed and returned to the body via capillaries surrounding each tubule. Eventually, the remaining filtrate enters a **collecting duct** shared by several nephrons, and additional water is reabsorbed to form the final urine product.■ The urine produced travels through the ureters to the bladder for temporary storage (review Figure 28-1). In this manner, the kidneys regulate extracellular fluid volume and osmolarity, electrolyte concentrations, and acid-base balance. They also excrete metabolic waste products like urea and creatinine, as well as a number of drugs and toxins.

■ About 99% of the substance in filtrate, including water, is reabsorbed, leaving only 1 to 2 L of urine to be excreted daily.

In addition to their remarkable role in maintaining homeostasis, the kidneys have other critical roles:

- The kidneys help to regulate blood pressure by secreting the enzyme renin.■ Renin catalyzes the formation of angiotensin—a potent vasoconstrictor that narrows the diameters of arterioles and thereby raises blood pressure (review pp. 399–400 and Figure 12-3 on p. 401). Angiotensin also stimulates the release of aldosterone, an adrenal hormone that triggers the kidneys to reabsorb more sodium. Sodium reabsorption promotes water retention and increases plasma volume, which raises blood pressure.
- The kidneys produce the hormone **erythropoietin,** which stimulates the production of red blood cells in the bone marrow (see Highlight 25 for details).
- The kidneys convert vitamin D to its active form, 1,25-dihydroxyvitamin D_3 (see Figure 11-9 on p. 376), thereby playing a primary role in calcium regulation and bone formation.

■ Reminder: *Renin* is an enzyme from the kidneys that activates angiotensinogen.

Subsequent sections of this chapter explain how renal diseases interfere with these kidney functions and severely disrupt health.

Bowman's (BO-mins) **capsule:** a cuplike component of the nephron that surrounds the glomerulus and collects the filtrate that is passed to the tubules.

tubules: tubelike structures of the nephron that process filtrate during urine production. The tubules are surrounded by capillaries that reabsorb substances retained by tubule cells.

collecting duct: the last portion of a nephron's tubule, where the final concentration of urine occurs.

erythropoietin (eh-RITH-ro-POY-eh-tin): a hormone made by the kidneys that stimulates red blood cell production.

IN SUMMARY The kidneys are responsible for filtering the blood and removing wastes for excretion in urine. By adjusting the blood's volume and composition, the kidneys help to maintain homeostasis within the body. Other kidney functions include the production of enzymes and hormones that regulate blood pressure, stimulate blood cell production, and activate vitamin D.

The Nephrotic Syndrome

The **nephrotic syndrome** is not a specific disease; rather, the term refers to any kidney disorder that results in urinary protein losses **(proteinuria)** exceeding 3.5 grams per day. It can develop when damage to the glomerular capillaries increases their permeability to plasma proteins, allowing protein to escape into urine. Although various diseases involving the glomeruli are often the cause, the nephrotic syndrome may also be a consequence of diabetes mellitus, immunological and hereditary disorders, infections (involving the kidneys or elsewhere in the body), chemical damage (from medications or illicit drugs), and some cancers. Along with proteinuria, frequent clinical findings include low serum albumin levels, edema, elevated blood lipids, and blood coagulation disorders. Conditions that cause the nephrotic syndrome sometimes progress to renal failure.

Consequences of the Nephrotic Syndrome

Urinary protein losses in the nephrotic syndrome average about 8 grams daily, but additional protein is lost due to protein catabolism within kidney tubules.[2] The liver attempts to compensate for these losses by increasing synthesis of some plasma proteins, but this results in higher concentrations of some proteins and lower levels of others. Thus the complications of the nephrotic syndrome are exacerbated by disturbances in protein metabolism.[3]

Edema Because albumin is the most abundant plasma protein, it is also the major protein lost in urine. Consequently, its blood level is markedly reduced, which contributes to a fluid shift from blood plasma to the interstitial spaces, causing edema.■ In addition, the nephrotic syndrome impairs the kidneys' ability to excrete sodium: the tubules reabsorb sodium in greater amounts than usual, causing sodium and water retention within the body.[4]

■ Reminder: Plasma proteins help to retain fluid within the blood. If their losses are excessive, the fluids in plasma can flow more freely to the interstitial spaces in tissues, causing edema (see p. 190).

Risk of Cardiovascular Disease Patients with the nephrotic syndrome frequently have elevated LDL and VLDL levels and increased risk of developing heart disease and stroke.[5] Levels of the damaging LDL variant known as lipoprotein (a) are also higher (see p. 831). The impaired clearance of VLDL from blood is largely due to reduced lipoprotein lipase■ on blood vessel walls.[6] Furthermore, risk of blood coagulation is greater due to urinary losses of proteins that inhibit blood clotting and higher levels of plasma proteins that favor clotting.[7] Further injury to the kidneys can result if blood clots develop in renal veins.

■ Reminder: *Lipoprotein lipase* is the enzyme that hydrolyzes the triglycerides in lipoproteins (see p. 158).

Other Effects of the Nephrotic Syndrome The proteins lost in urine include immunoglobulins (antibodies) and vitamin D–binding protein. Depletion of immunoglobulins increases susceptibility to bacterial infection. Loss of vitamin D–binding protein results in lower vitamin D and calcium levels and increases the risk of rickets in children. Patients with the nephrotic syndrome frequently develop protein-energy malnutrition (PEM) and muscle wasting from continued proteinuria. Figure 28-2 summarizes the consequences of urinary protein losses in the nephrotic syndrome.

nephrotic (neh-FROT-ik) **syndrome:** a kidney disorder characterized by urinary protein losses exceeding 3.5 g per day. Accompanying symptoms often include low serum albumin, elevated blood lipids, and edema.

proteinuria (PRO-teen-NEW-ree-ah): loss of protein, especially albumin, in the urine; also known as **albuminuria.**

FIGURE 28-2 Consequences of Urinary Protein Losses in the Nephrotic Syndrome

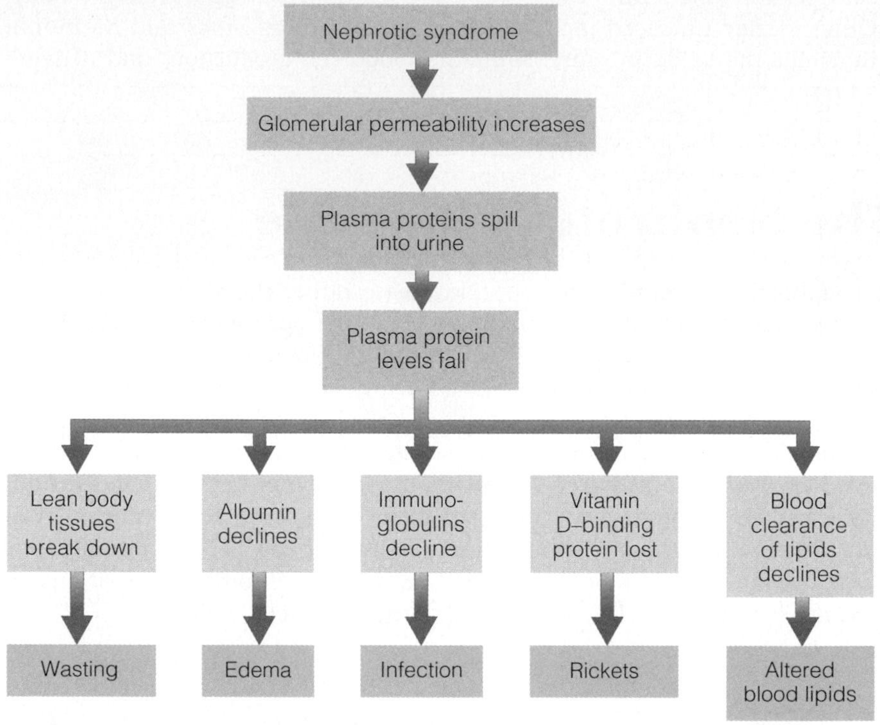
Nephrotic syndrome
Glomerular permeability increases
Plasma proteins spill into urine
Plasma protein levels fall
Lean body tissues break down
Albumin declines
Immuno-globulins decline
Vitamin D–binding protein lost
Blood clearance of lipids declines
Wasting
Edema
Infection
Rickets
Altered blood lipids

Treatment of the Nephrotic Syndrome

Medical treatment of the nephrotic syndrome requires diagnosis and management of the underlying disorder responsible for proteinuria. Complications are managed with medications and medical nutrition therapy. The drugs prescribed may include anti-inflammatory agents, ACE inhibitors (see p. 833), immunosuppressants, antihypertensive agents, diuretics, and lipid-lowering medications. Dietary treatment helps to prevent PEM and alleviate edema.

Protein and Energy Meeting protein and energy needs helps to minimize losses of muscle tissue. High-protein diets are not advised, however, because they can exacerbate urinary protein losses.[8] Instead, protein intake should fall between 0.8 and 1.0 gram per kilogram body weight per day. An adequate energy intake (about 35 kcalories per kilogram body weight daily) sustains weight and spares protein. Weight loss or infections signal the need for additional kcalories.

Fat As Chapter 27 explained, a diet low in saturated fat, cholesterol, and refined sugars helps to control elevated blood lipids. People with the nephrotic syndrome are often unable to control blood lipids adequately by diet alone, however, and physicians may need to prescribe lipid-lowering medications.

Sodium Sodium restriction helps to control edema; an intake of no more than 2 to 3 grams daily is often suggested. Table 28-1 provides guidelines for following a 2-gram sodium-restricted diet. If diuretics prescribed for edema cause potassium wasting, patients are encouraged to select foods rich in potassium.

Vitamins and Minerals Patients with the nephrotic syndrome may require vitamin D and calcium supplementation to prevent bone loss and rickets. Multivitamin supplementation is typically recommended to help prevent additional nutrient deficiencies.[9] ■

■ Nutrient deficiencies may develop if carrier proteins for nutrients are lost in urine.

TABLE 28-1 Two-Gram Sodium-Restricted Diet

General Guidelines

About 75 percent of sodium in the typical diet comes from processed foods, and about 10 percent comes from unprocessed natural foods. About 15 percent of sodium in a typical diet comes from table salt. With this in mind:

- Choose fresh foods and foods frozen or canned without added salt.
- Avoid adding salt to foods while cooking.
- Avoid adding salt to foods at the table.
- When eating out, ask that meals be prepared without salt.

Sodium in Foods

All foods contain sodium, but some contain more than others. Use the information about the average sodium contents of foods to tailor the diet to the individual's preferences.

Food Group	Serving Size	Sodium (mg) per Serving
Fresh meats, poultry, freshwater fish; low-sodium canned meats and fish; low-sodium peanut butter and cheese; unsalted cottage cheese, soybeans, and textured vegetable protein	1 oz	20
Regular fat-free, low-fat, and whole milk and yogurt	8 oz	120
Eggs	1	60
Fresh artichokes, beets, carrots, and celery; beet, collard, dandelion, mustard, and turnip greens	½ c	50
Regular canned vegetables	½ c	300
Regular white and whole-grain bread	1 slice	150
Butter and margarine	1 tsp	50
Salt	½ tsp	1000

Other Foods

These foods can be used freely or with some limits with respect to sodium, although some of these foods may need to be restricted for weight or blood lipid control:

- All fruits and fruit juices.
- Low-sodium canned or frozen vegetables without added salt except those listed above; low-sodium vegetable juices.
- Low-sodium bread and bread products; puffed rice and wheat and shredded wheat cereals; rice; pasta.
- Soups, casseroles, and recipes made with allowed foods and ingredients.
- Unsalted butter, margarine, nuts, and gravy; low-sodium mayonnaise and salad dressing; shortening.
- Low-sodium catsup, mustard, tabasco sauce, and other condiments; low-sodium baking powder.

These foods and dishes prepared with them are high in sodium and should be avoided:

- Cured, canned, salted, or smoked meats, poultry, and fish such as bacon, luncheon meats, corned beef, kosher meats, and canned tuna and salmon; imitation fish products, salted textured vegetable protein, peanut butter, and nuts.
- Buttermilk, regular cheeses.
- Maraschino cherries; crystallized or glazed fruits; dried fruits with sodium sulfite added.
- Pickles, pickled vegetables, sauerkraut, and regular vegetable juices.
- Instant and quick-cooking hot cereals; commercial bread products made from self-rising flour or cornmeal; salted snack foods.
- Salt pork and bacon; commercial salad dressing; olives; regular gravy; catsup, baking powder, soy sauce, bouillon.

A Sample Two-Gram Sodium-Restricted Diet

Using the information above, many diet plans that meet individual needs are possible. Using the guidelines for a heart-healthy diet, a typical plan for a day might look like this:

Food Group	Sodium (mg)
Meat, 6 oz (6 × 20 mg)	120
Milk, 3 c (3 × 120 mg)	360
Fruit, 3 servings	negligible
Vegetables, ½ c vegetables with some sodium (1 × 50)	50
Vegetables, other vegetables and legumes, 2 servings	negligible
Whole-grain bread, 4 slices (4 × 150 mg)	600
Salted margarine, 6 servings (6 × 50 mg)	300
Total	1430

Individuals can use the remainder of the sodium allowance for whatever foods they choose. The sodium content of other foods can be determined by reading food labels or using food composition tables. An individual may choose to use some (¼ teaspoon) table salt or a favorite food that contains sodium.

IN SUMMARY The nephrotic syndrome develops when urinary protein losses exceed 3.5 grams per day. Complications may include edema, lipid abnormalities, blood coagulation disorders, reduced immunity, rickets, and protein-energy malnutrition. Medications treat the underlying condition and help to manage complications. The diet should provide adequate protein and energy to maintain health; however, excess protein intakes should be avoided. Other dietary adjustments may be needed to correct lipid disorders, edema, and nutrient deficiencies.

Acute Renal Failure

In **acute renal failure,** kidney function rapidly deteriorates, over hours or days. The loss of kidney function reduces urine output and causes nitrogenous wastes to build up in blood. The degree of renal dysfunction varies from mild to severe. With prompt treatment, acute renal failure is often reversible, although mortality rates are high, ranging from 35 to 65 percent.[10]

Causes of Acute Renal Failure

Acute renal failure is caused by a wide variety of conditions and often develops as a consequence of severe illness, injury, or surgery. To aid in diagnosis and treatment, its causes are commonly classified as prerenal, intrarenal, or postrenal.[11] *Prerenal* factors are those that cause a sudden reduction in blood flow to the kidneys; they often involve a severe stress such as heart failure, shock, or blood loss. Factors that damage kidney tissue, such as infections, toxins, drugs, or direct trauma, are classified as *intrarenal* causes of failure. *Postrenal* factors are those that prevent excretion of urine due to urinary tract obstructions. Table 28-2 includes specific examples of disorders that cause acute renal failure.

Consequences of Acute Renal Failure

As renal function declines, the composition of blood and urine changes. The kidneys become unable to regulate the levels of electrolytes, acid, and nitrogenous wastes in blood. Urine may be diminished in quantity or absent. Diagnosis is often a complex task, however, because the clinical effects can be subtle and vary according to the underlying cause of disease. This section discusses some common problems that accompany acute renal failure.

TABLE 28-2 Causes of Acute Renal Failure

Prerenal Factors (60 to 70% of cases)	Intrarenal Factors (25 to 40% of cases)	Postrenal Factors (5 to 10% of cases)
• **Low blood volume or pressure:** Hemorrhage, burns, sepsis or shock, anaphylactic reactions, nephrotic syndrome, gastrointestinal losses, diuretics, antihypertensive medications • **Renal artery disorders:** Blood clots or emboli, stenosis, aneurysm, trauma • **Heart disorders:** Congestive heart failure, heart attack, arrhythmias	• **Vascular disorders:** Sickle-cell disease, diabetes mellitus, transfusion reactions • **Obstructions (within kidney):** Inflammation, tumors, stones, scar tissue • **Renal injury:** Infections, environmental contaminants, drugs, medications, *E. coli* food poisoning	• **Obstructions (ureter or bladder):** Strictures, tumors, stones, trauma • **Prostate disorders:** Cancer or hyperplasia • **Renal vein thrombosis** • **Bladder disorders:** Neurological conditions, bladder rupture • **Pregnancy**

acute renal failure: abrupt loss of kidney function over a period of hours or days.

Fluid and Electrolyte Imbalances Edema is frequently an early symptom of acute renal failure, causing puffiness in the face and hands and swelling of the feet and ankles. The edema may be related to a reduction or absence of urine: about half of patients experience **oliguria** during the initial stage of kidney failure, producing less than 400 milliliters of urine per day.[12]■ Because sodium is normally excreted in the urine, sodium retention also contributes to the development of edema. Other electrolytes may be retained as well, resulting in elevated blood levels of potassium, phosphate, and magnesium. In addition to their reduced excretion, excessive amounts of these electrolytes are released into the bloodstream due to the tissue breakdown that accompanies many of the diseases associated with acute renal failure. Elevated potassium **(hyperkalemia)** is of particular concern because potassium imbalances can alter the heart rate and lead to heart failure. Elevated phosphate levels **(hyperphosphatemia)** can cause increased secretion of parathyroid hormone and a reduction in blood calcium levels.

■ Normal urine volume exceeds 800 mL per day, which is equivalent to about 27 fluid ounces or 3.4 cups.

Uremia Reduced kidney function can cause the body's nitrogen-containing waste products—blood urea nitrogen (BUN), creatinine, and uric acid—to accumulate in blood.■ Moreover, a patient who is catabolic has additional nitrogenous wastes. The clinical outcome, called **uremia,** includes symptoms such as fatigue, lethargy, confusion, headache, anorexia, a metallic taste in the mouth, nausea and vomiting, and diarrhea. In more serious cases, rapid pulse, elevated blood pressure, seizures, and delirium or coma may occur. It is sometimes difficult to distinguish the symptoms of uremia from those of an underlying illness.[13]

■ A progressive rise in BUN or creatinine suggests the presence of acute renal failure. Refer to Table 17-8 on p. 594 for normal laboratory values.

Treatment of Acute Renal Failure

The primary goal is to treat the underlying illness in order to prevent further damage to the kidneys. A combination of medical nutrition therapy, drug therapy, and **dialysis** may be undertaken to restore fluid and electrolyte balances and minimize blood concentrations of toxic waste products. Highlight 28 describes common dialysis procedures, including the approach most often used for treating acute renal failure, continuous renal replacement therapy.

In oliguric patients (those unable to produce urine), recovery from renal failure sometimes begins with a period of **diuresis,** in which large amounts of fluid are excreted. Because tubular function is still minimal at this stage, electrolytes cannot be sufficiently reabsorbed; consequently, both fluid depletion and electrolyte imbalances become a concern. Patients with this pattern of recovery need to be monitored closely in case they require replacement of fluids and electrolytes.■

■ The shift from oliguria to diuresis occurs primarily in patients with renal tubular injury, an *intrarenal* cause of acute renal failure.

Drug Therapy Kidney function is normally required for drug excretion. To compensate for limited urine output, patients may require lower dosages of their medications. Conversely, dialysis treatment may increase losses of some drugs, and dosages may need to be increased. Drugs that are **nephrotoxic** (including some antibiotics) or that reduce blood flow to the kidneys (such as nonsteroidal anti-inflammatory drugs) should be avoided.[14]

Patients with edema are prescribed diuretics to mobilize fluids; furosemide (Lasix) is the usual choice. Hyperkalemia is treated with *potassium exchange resins* that bind potassium ions in the gastrointestinal (GI) tract, ensuring excretion in the stool. Rapid correction of hyperkalemia requires the use of insulin, which causes a temporary shift of extracellular potassium into cells. (Note that glucose must be given with insulin to prevent hypoglycemia.) If acidosis is present, bicarbonate may be administered orally or intravenously.[15]

Protein and Energy Although its effects are highly variable, acute renal failure is often a catabolic condition associated with hypermetabolism and muscle wasting. Sufficient protein and energy must be provided to preserve the body's protein content. Because indirect calorimetry is often unavailable for determining specific energy needs, a patient is initially provided with 35 kcalories per kilogram body weight per day, and body weight is monitored to determine if adjustments are needed.

oliguria (OL-leh-GOO-ree-ah): reduced quantity of urine, often less than 400 mL per day.

hyperkalemia (HIGH-per-ka-LEE-me-ah): elevated serum potassium levels.

hyperphosphatemia (HIGH-per-fos-fa-TEE-me-ah): elevated serum phosphate levels.

uremia (you-REE-me-ah): abnormal accumulation of nitrogen-containing substances, especially urea, in the blood; also called **azotemia** (AZE-oh-TEE-me-ah).

dialysis (dye-AL-ih-sis): a process for cleansing the blood using a semipermeable membrane to filter out accumulated wastes. The two main types are *hemodialysis* and *peritoneal dialysis* (see Highlight 28).

diuresis (DYE-uh-REE-sis): excessive urine excretion.

nephrotoxic: toxic to the kidneys.

Protein contributes nitrogen, increasing the kidneys' workload, but it is needed to prevent negative nitrogen balance and additional wasting. Dietary recommendations depend on the degree of catabolism, kidney function, and whether the treatment includes dialysis (dialysis removes nitrogenous wastes). Restricting protein to about 0.6 to 0.8 gram per kilogram body weight per day is suggested for patients with limited kidney function who are not treated with dialysis. Higher intakes (about 1.2 to 1.3 grams per kilogram daily) are recommended if kidney function improves or if dialysis is received. Patients who are catabolic or septic may need additional protein, but require dialysis to accommodate the additional nitrogen load.[16]

Fluids Clinicians assess fluid status by monitoring weight fluctuations, blood pressure, pulse rates, and appearance of the skin and mucous membranes.[17] Another method is to measure serum sodium concentrations: a low sodium level often indicates excessive fluid intake, and a high sodium level suggests inadequate intake.[18]

Fluid balance is carefully restored in patients who are either overhydrated or dehydrated. Thereafter, clinicians determine daily fluid needs by measuring urine output and adding about 500 milliliters to replace the water lost through skin, lungs, and perspiration. An individual with fever, vomiting, or diarrhea requires additional fluid. Fluid intake can be more liberal in patients undergoing dialysis: 1.5 to 2.0 liters per day may be permitted, depending on hydration state.

Electrolytes Sodium restriction may prevent fluid retention and hypertension. Patients with oliguria may need to limit sodium intakes to 2 to 3 grams daily, although lower intakes are sometimes necessary.[19] Generally, potassium and phosphorus are restricted as well; serum electrolyte levels are monitored closely to determine appropriate intakes. Patients undergoing dialysis can generally consume electrolytes more freely. As mentioned previously, oliguric patients who experience diuresis at the beginning of the recovery period may need electrolyte replacement to compensate for urinary losses.

Enteral and Parenteral Nutrition Because acute renal failure causes metabolic stress, some patients need enteral or parenteral nutrition support to obtain adequate energy. A number of enteral products have been specifically designed to meet the nutrient needs of patients with acute renal failure. Compared with standard formulas, renal formulas are more kcalorically dense and have lower concentrations of protein and electrolytes. Enteral support (tube feeding) is generally preferred over parenteral nutrition because it is less likely to cause infection and sepsis. Total parenteral nutrition is provided only if patients are severely malnourished or cannot consume food for more than 14 days.[20]

IN SUMMARY Acute renal failure is characterized by rapid loss in kidney function, causing a buildup of fluid, electrolytes, and nitrogenous wastes in blood. Its causes include prerenal, intrarenal, and postrenal factors. Deterioration in renal function can result in fluid retention, hyperkalemia, and uremia. If hyperkalemia develops, it can have potentially serious consequences on heart function. Acute renal failure is treated with medications, dietary modifications, and dialysis. The accompanying case study checks your understanding of acute renal failure.

Chronic Renal Failure

Unlike acute renal failure, in which kidney function declines suddenly and rapidly, chronic renal failure is characterized by gradual and irreversible deterioration. Because the kidneys have a large functional reserve,■ the disease generally pro-

■ The capacity of the kidneys to function despite loss of some nephrons is referred to as *renal reserve.*

CASE STUDY

Store Manager with Acute Renal Failure

Mrs. Kang is a 63-year-old store manager admitted to the hospital's intensive care unit. She was first seen in the emergency room with severe edema, headache, nausea and vomiting, and a rapid heart rate. She reported an inability to pass more than minimal amounts of urine in the past two days. Her son, who drove her to the emergency room, reported that she had missed work for several days and seemed unusually tired and confused. Laboratory tests revealed elevated serum creatinine, BUN, and potassium levels. After a full accounting of her medical history, the physician learned that she had begun using penicillin earlier in the week and diagnosed acute renal failure, probably caused by a reaction to the medication. Mrs. Kang is 5 feet 3 inches tall and weighs 125 pounds.

1. Describe the probable reason for Mrs. Kang's inability to produce urine. Is her reaction to penicillin considered a prerenal, intrarenal, or postrenal cause of renal failure? What other problems can cause acute renal failure?
2. What medications can the physician prescribe to treat Mrs. Kang's edema and hyperkalemia? What recommendation is likely concerning her continued use of penicillin?
3. What factors should be kept in mind when determining Mrs. Kang's energy, protein, fluid, and electrolyte needs during acute renal failure? How would dialysis treatment alter recommendations?
4. After treatment begins, Mrs. Kang suddenly begins producing copious amounts of urine. How would this development alter dietary treatment?

As you read through the discussion of chronic renal failure, consider how Mrs. Kang's diet would change if her renal failure were to become chronic.

gresses over many years without causing symptoms. Patients are typically diagnosed late in the course of illness, after most kidney function has been lost.[21]

The most common causes of chronic renal failure are diabetes mellitus and hypertension, which are estimated to cause 43 and 26 percent of cases, respectively.[22] Other conditions that result in renal failure include inflammatory, immunological, or hereditary diseases that directly involve the kidneys. In a few cases, chronic renal failure follows acute renal failure.

Consequences of Chronic Renal Failure

In the early stages of chronic renal failure, the nephrons compensate by enlarging so that they can handle the extra workload. Eventually, more nephrons deteriorate, creating additional work for the remaining nephrons. The overburdened nephrons continue to degenerate, until finally the kidneys are unable to function adequately. Symptoms of renal failure may not appear until over 75 percent of kidney function is lost. Once the extent of kidney damage necessitates treatment with dialysis or kidney transplantation, the condition is classified as **end-stage renal disease (ESRD)**.[23]■ Without intervention at this stage, an individual cannot survive. Table 28-3 lists the common clinical effects that occur in both the early and the advanced stages of chronic renal failure.

Renal failure is evaluated using the **glomerular filtration rate (GFR)**, the rate at which the kidneys form filtrate. GFR can be estimated using predictive equations that are based on serum creatinine levels■, age, gender, race, and body size. Table 28-4 shows how kidney disease is classified according to estimated GFR. Other laboratory measures used to assess kidney function include urinary protein levels, BUN, and the ratio of albumin to creatinine in a urine sample.[24]

Altered Electrolytes and Hormones Fluid and electrolyte disturbances usually do not develop until the final stage of renal failure.[25] As GFR falls, the increased activity by the remaining nephrons is sufficient to maintain electrolyte excretion. A number of hormonal adaptations also help to regulate electrolyte levels; these changes may cause complications of their own, however. Increased aldosterone secretion helps to maintain serum potassium levels, but contributes to the development of hypertension (in patients who were not previously hypertensive). Increased

■ The term *end-stage renal disease* is used to classify patients undergoing active treatment and is not synonymous with the term *renal failure.*

■ *Creatinine* is a waste product of creatine, a nitrogen-containing compound in muscle cells.

end-stage renal disease (ESRD): an advanced stage of chronic renal failure in which dialysis or a kidney transplant is necessary to sustain life.

glomerular filtration rate (GFR): the rate at which filtrate is formed within the kidneys, normally approximately 125 mL/min; usually estimated from equations based on serum creatinine levels and several other factors.

TABLE 28-3 Clinical Effects of Chronic Renal Failure

Early Stages

- Anorexia
- Fatigue
- Headache
- Hypertension
- Itching
- Kidney inflammation or nephrotic syndrome
- Nausea and vomiting
- Proteinuria, hematuria (blood in urine)

Advanced Stages

- Anemia, bleeding tendency
- Cardiovascular disease
- Confusion, mental impairments
- Electrolyte abnormalities
- Fluid retention
- Hormonal abnormalities
- Metabolic acidosis
- Peripheral neuropathy
- Protein-energy malnutrition
- Reduced immunity
- Renal osteodystrophy

TABLE 28-4 Evaluation of Chronic Renal Disease

Stage of Disease	Description	GFR[a] (mL/min per 1.73 m^2)
1	Kidney damage with normal or increased GFR	≥90
2	Kidney damage with mildly decreased GFR	60–89
3	Moderately decreased GFR	30–59
4	Severely decreased GFR	15–29
5	Kidney failure	<15 (or undergoing dialysis)

[a] GFR is estimated from the Modification of Diet in Renal Disease study equation and is based on age, gender, race, and calibration for serum creatinine. Normal GFR is approximately 125 milliliters per minute.
SOURCE: A. S. Levey and coauthors, National Kidney Foundation practice guidelines for chronic kidney disease: Evaluation, classification, and stratification, *Annals of Internal Medicine* 139 (2003): 137–147.

■ Elevated parathyroid hormone stimulates bone turnover and the release of calcium from bone into blood, resulting in bone with structural abnormalities and lower mineral content.

secretion of parathyroid hormone keeps serum phosphate levels normal, but contributes to bone loss and development of **renal osteodystrophy,** a bone disorder common in renal patients.■ Electrolyte imbalances may develop when GFR becomes extremely low (less than 5 milliters per minute), when hormonal adaptations are inadequate, or when intakes of water and electrolytes are either very restricted or excessive.

Because the kidneys are responsible for maintaining acid-base balance, acidosis often develops in chronic renal failure. Although usually mild, the acidosis worsens renal bone disease because compounds in bone (protein and phosphates, for example) are released to buffer the acid in blood.

Uremic Syndrome Uremia develops during the final stages of chronic renal failure, when GFR is below 15 milliliters per minute and BUN exceeds 60 milligrams per deciliter.[26] The many symptoms and complications that develop during this stage of illness are collectively known as the **uremic syndrome.** The uremia itself can cause subtle mental dysfunctions and neuromuscular changes such as muscle cramping, twitching, and restless leg syndrome. Other complications result from a wide range of metabolic impairments and include:[27]

- *Impaired hormone synthesis.* Diseased kidneys are unable to produce erythropoietin, causing anemia (see Highlight 25). Reduced production of active vitamin D contributes to bone disease.
- *Impaired hormone degradation.* Numerous clinical disturbances occur as imbalances develop in various hormones including those involved in growth, reproduction, fluid balance, blood glucose regulation, and nutrient metabolism.
- *Bleeding abnormalities.* Defects in platelet function and clotting factors prolong bleeding time and contribute to bruising, gastrointestinal bleeding, and anemia.
- *Increased cardiovascular disease risk.* Risk factors include hypertension, increased insulin resistance, and abnormal blood lipids. Elevated parathyroid hormone levels lead to calcification of blood vessels and heart tissue. Patients are at increased risk of stroke, heart attack, and heart failure.
- *Reduced immunity.* Patients with uremia have poor immune responses and are at high risk of developing infections, a frequent cause of death.

Protein-Energy Malnutrition Patients with chronic renal disease often develop PEM and wasting. Studies suggest that renal patients have energy and protein intakes that are lower than recommended levels, even during early stages of the disease.[28] Anorexia is believed to be a primary cause of poor food intake and may result from hormonal abnormalities, nausea and vomiting, restrictive diets, uremia, and medications. Nutrient losses also contribute to malnutrition and may be a consequence of vomiting, diarrhea, gastrointestinal bleeding, concurrent catabolic disease, and dialysis.

renal osteodystrophy: a bone disorder in patients with chronic renal failure; a consequence of increased parathyroid hormone secretion, reduced serum calcium, acidosis, and impaired vitamin D activation by the kidneys.

uremic syndrome: the cluster of symptoms associated with a GFR below 15 mL/min, including uremia, anemia, bone disease, hormonal imbalances, bleeding impairment, increased cardiovascular disease risk, and reduced immunity.

Treatment of Chronic Renal Failure

The objectives of treatment are to slow disease progression and prevent or alleviate symptoms. A primary goal of nutrition therapy is to prevent PEM and help patients maintain a healthy weight. Once renal failure reaches the final stages, dialysis or a kidney transplant is necessary to sustain life.

Drug Therapy Drug therapies can control some of the complications associated with chronic renal failure. Treatment of hypertension is critical for slowing disease progression and reducing cardiovascular disease risk; patients may require multiple medications, including diuretics, ACE inhibitors,■ angiotensin receptor blockers, calcium channel blockers, and others.[29] Some of the antihypertensive drugs can also reduce proteinuria, helping to slow disease progression. Anemia is usually treated by injection or intravenous administration of erythropoietin (epoetin). Other common drug treatments include phosphate binders (taken with meals) to reduce serum phosphorus levels, sodium bicarbonate to reverse acidosis, and cholesterol-lowering medications. Supplements containing active vitamin D (1,25-dihydroxyvitamin D, or calcitriol) help to raise serum calcium and reduce parathyroid hormone levels.

Dialysis Recall from an earlier section that dialysis can replace kidney function by removing excess fluid and wastes from blood. In **hemodialysis,** the blood is circulated through a **dialyzer** (artificial kidney), where it is bathed by **dialysate,** a solution that selectively removes fluid and wastes. In **peritoneal dialysis,** dialysate is infused into a person's peritoneal cavity, and blood is filtered by the peritoneum (the membrane that surrounds the abdominal cavity); after several hours, the dialysate is drained, removing unneeded fluid and wastes. Additional details about dialysis can be found in Highlight 28.

Medical Nutrition Therapy Medical nutrition therapy profoundly influences the success of medical treatment, as dietary intake can affect disease progression, development of complications, and serum levels of fluids, nitrogenous wastes, and electrolytes. Because the renal diet is complex and dietary needs may change frequently as the disease progresses, a dietitian who specializes in renal disease is best suited to provide medical nutrition therapy. Despite strong evidence that early nutrition care can prevent malnutrition, almost half of the patients beginning dialysis report that they have never seen a dietitian.[30]

Table 28-5 summarizes the general nutrient guidelines for different stages of renal disease. Note that hemodialysis and peritoneal dialysis affect nutrient needs differently. Because patients' needs can vary considerably, actual recommendations should be based on the results of a nutrition assessment. Nutrients not listed in the table should be consumed at levels recommended for the general population.

Energy Energy intake should be high enough to maintain a healthy weight and prevent wasting. Anorexia is a frequent cause of poor food intakes, and dietary restrictions limit food choices. To help prevent malnutrition, foods and beverages of high energy density are recommended.■ Patients are often encouraged to consume high-kcalorie foods and condiments such as hard candy, honey, sugar, jam, salad dressings, and soft margarine. Malnourished patients may require oral supplements or tube feedings to maintain weight.

Patients undergoing peritoneal dialysis can absorb a substantial amount of glucose from the dialysate, which can contribute as many as 800 kcalories daily.■ These kcalories must be included when evaluating intake. Weight gain is sometimes a problem when peritoneal dialysis continues for a long period.

Protein A low-protein diet is often prescribed for predialysis patients to help slow the progression of renal failure: guidelines suggest intakes between 0.6 and 0.75 gram per kilogram body weight per day, just below RDA levels.[31] Low-protein diets produce fewer nitrogenous wastes and therefore reduce the risk of uremia. Furthermore, low-protein diets supply less phosphorus than high-protein diets, reducing risks associated with hyperphosphatemia. Because renal patients often develop

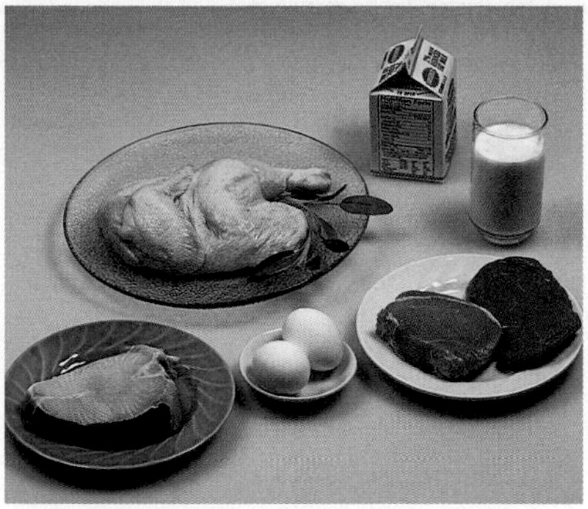

In a renal diet, half of the protein consumed should be from high-quality sources such as eggs, milk, meat, poultry, and fish.

■ Reminder: *ACE* stands for angiotensin-converting enzyme. ACE inhibitors interfere with the activation of angiotensin.

■ Reminder: Foods with high energy density contain a high number of kcalories per unit weight; these foods are generally high in fat and contain little water (see the "How to" on p. 294).

■ A high concentration of glucose in the dialysate draws fluid from the bloodstream to the peritoneal cavity (by osmosis), thereby removing excess fluid from blood.

hemodialysis (HE-moh-dye-AL-ih-sis): removal of fluids and wastes from blood by passing the blood through a dialyzer.

dialyzer (DYE-ah-LIZE-er): a machine used for hemodialysis; also called an *artificial kidney.*

dialysate (dye-AL-ih-sate): solution used during dialysis to draw wastes and fluids from the blood.

peritoneal (PER-ih-toe-NEE-al) **dialysis:** removal of fluids and wastes by using the peritoneal membrane to filter blood.

TABLE 28-5 Dietary Recommendations for Chronic Renal Failure

Nutrient	Predialysis	Hemodialysis	Peritoneal Dialysis
Energy[a] (kcal/kg)	<60 years old: 35 ≥60 years old: 30–35	<60 years old: 35 ≥60 years old: 30–35	<60 years old: 35 ≥60 years old: 30–35 (total kcalories should include those absorbed from dialysate)
Protein (g/kg) (50% from high-quality proteins)	0.6–0.75	1.2	1.2–1.3
Fat	As needed to maintain a healthy lipid profile	As needed to maintain a healthy lipid profile	As needed to maintain a healthy lipid profile
Fluid (mL/day)	Unrestricted if urine output is normal	1000 plus urine output	1500–2000; monitor closely
Sodium (mg/day)	2000	2000	2000
Potassium (mg/day)	Individualized according to laboratory values	2000–3000	3000–4000
Calcium (mg/day)	1200	≤2000 from diet and medications	≤2000 from diet and medications
Phosphorus (mg/day)	Individualized according to laboratory values	800–1000	800–1000

[a] Values listed apply to adults; recommendations for children should not fall below RDA levels.

SOURCE: Reprinted from *Journal of the American Dietetic Association* 104 (2004): 404–409, J. A. Beto and V. K. Bansal, Medical nutrition therapy in chronic kidney failure: Integrating clinical practice guidelines.

■ Reminder: High-quality protein can be obtained from eggs, milk products, meat, poultry, fish, and soybeans.

PEM, however, the diet must be carefully designed to provide enough protein to meet needs and prevent wasting. To ensure that the low-protein diet provides adequate amounts of the essential amino acids, about 50 percent of the protein should be from high-quality sources.■ Low-protein breads, pastas, and other grain-based products are commercially available to help renal patients improve energy intake.

Because low-protein diets are difficult to adhere to and patients are at high risk of wasting, dietitians may suggest consuming higher amounts of protein to preserve health.[32] Once dialysis is begun, protein restrictions can be relaxed, as dialysis removes nitrogenous wastes and some amino acids are lost during the procedure.

Lipids Patients with chronic renal disease are at increased risk of coronary heart disease and are therefore advised to restrict saturated fat and cholesterol to help control elevated blood lipids.[33] Because renal diets include high-fat foods to improve kcaloric intakes, patients should select foods that provide mostly unsaturated fats, such as nuts and seeds, salad dressings and mayonnaise, avocados, and soybean products (see Highlight 5 for more suggestions).

Fluids and Sodium As renal failure progresses, the patient excretes less urine and cannot handle normal amounts of sodium and fluids. Suggested intakes are based on total urine output, changes in body weight and blood pressure, and serum sodium levels. A rise in body weight and blood pressure suggests that the person is retaining sodium and fluid; conversely, declines in these measurements indicate fluid loss. Most persons with renal disease tend to retain sodium and may benefit from mild restriction; less frequently, a patient may have a salt-wasting condition that requires additional dietary sodium.

Fluids are not restricted until urine output decreases. For a person who is neither dehydrated nor overhydrated, daily fluid intake should match the daily urine output. (Obligatory water losses—from skin and lungs—are replaced from water contained in solid foods.) Once a person is on dialysis, sodium and fluid intakes should be controlled so that only about 2 pounds of water weight are gained daily—this excess fluid is removed at the next dialysis treatment.[34] Patients should be advised that foods like flavored gelatin, soups, fruit ices, frozen fruit juice bars, and ice milk contribute to the fluid allowance in fluid-restricted diets.

Potassium Before dialysis treatments begin, renal patients can handle typical intakes of potassium. Although restriction is usually not required, the amount allowed may be adjusted according to serum potassium levels. Some people with diabetic nephropathy are at high risk of hyperkalemia and may need to limit dietary potassium during the early stages of disease. Conversely, supplementation with potassium may be required for persons using potassium-wasting diuretics.

Dialysis patients must control potassium intakes to prevent hyperkalemia or, in some cases, **hypokalemia.**[35] Recommended intakes are based on serum potassium levels, renal function, medications, and the dialysis procedure used. Potassium is generally restricted for patients on hemodialysis and for those producing little or no urine. People undergoing peritoneal dialysis can consume potassium more freely, but must be monitored closely.

All fresh foods supply potassium, but some fruits, vegetables, and juices contain such high amounts that their regular use is discouraged in patients at risk of hyperkalemia; examples include avocados, bananas, brussels sprouts, cantaloupe, dried fruit, prune juice, spinach, swiss chard, and winter squash. Other high-potassium choices include milk, molasses, nuts, and potato chips. People with renal failure should be cautioned that salt substitutes and other low-sodium products often contain potassium chloride, which should be avoided on a potassium-restricted diet. Appendix H provides additional information about the potassium content of common foods.

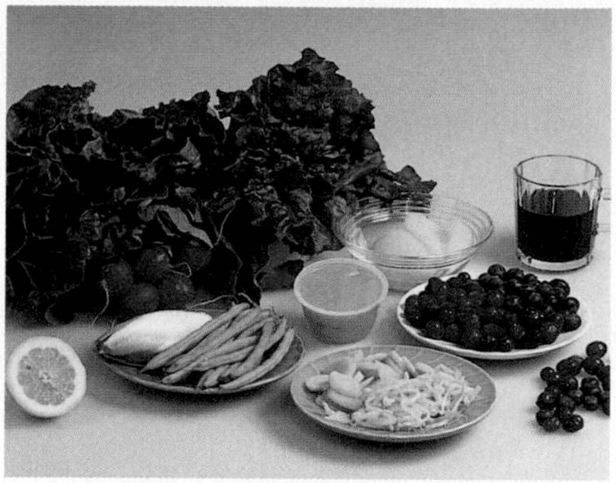
© Craig M. Moore

In limited amounts, the fruits and vegetables pictured here provide a level of potassium acceptable for renal diets.

Calcium, Phosphorus, and Vitamin D Maintaining normal serum calcium and phosphorus levels is critical for preventing bone disease. Furthermore, as mentioned earlier, renal disease reduces the kidneys' ability to produce the active form of vitamin D, so calcium absorption is usually impaired. For these reasons, calcium and phosphorus intakes may need adjustment, even during early stages of renal failure. Serum levels of calcium and phosphorus should be measured regularly once GFR falls below 60 milliliters per minute. Elevations in serum phosphorus indicate a need for dietary phosphorus restriction; in many patients, phosphate binders (taken with meals) are used to control serum levels. Once dialysis begins, phosphorus restrictions and calcium and vitamin D supplementation become standard therapy. Some patients may develop **hypercalcemia** in response to simultaneous vitamin D and calcium supplementation, so serum calcium levels must be monitored.

High-protein foods are typically high in phosphorus, so protein-restricted diets help to curb phosphorus intakes as well. After dialysis treatment begins and protein intakes are liberalized, the use of phosphate binders becomes essential for phosphorus control. Because foods that are rich in calcium (such as milk and milk products) are usually high in phosphorus and therefore restricted, patients must rely upon calcium supplements to meet their calcium needs once phosphorus restrictions are imposed.

Vitamins and Minerals The restrictive diet recommended for renal patients interferes with vitamin and mineral intakes, increasing the risk of deficiencies. Moreover, patients on dialysis lose water-soluble vitamins, and some trace minerals into the dialysate. Dietary supplements designed for renal patients supply generous amounts of folate and vitamin B_6, 1 milligram and 10 milligrams per day, respectively,[36]■ along with recommended levels of the remaining water-soluble vitamins. Supplemental vitamin C should not exceed 100 milligrams per day because excessive amounts can contribute to kidney stone formation in those at risk (see p. 866). Supplements containing vitamins A and E are not recommended because these vitamins sometimes accumulate in patients with renal failure.[37]

■ Supplementation with high doses of folate and vitamin B_6, which are lost during dialysis, help to prevent elevated blood homocysteine levels, a risk factor for heart disease (see p. 829).

Iron deficiency is common in hemodialysis patients and may be due to gastrointestinal bleeding, reduced iron absorption, iron losses into the dialysate, and blood losses associated with dialysis treatment.[38] Intravenous administration of iron, in conjunction with erythropoietin therapy, is more effective than oral iron supplementation for improving iron status.

Enteral and Parenteral Nutrition Enteral and parenteral nutrition support can provide nutrients to renal patients who are unable to eat adequate amounts of food. Suitable formulas for use in renal failure are described on p. 858. **Intradialytic parenteral nutrition** is an option for supplying supplemental nutrients: this technique combines parenteral feedings with hemodialysis treatments. An advantage of this approach is that the volume of fluid infused can be simultaneously removed

hypokalemia (HIGH-po-ka-LEE-me-ah): low serum potassium levels.

hypercalcemia (HIGH-per-kal-SEE-me-ah): elevated serum calcium levels.

intradialytic parenteral nutrition: the infusion of nutrients during hemodialysis, often providing amino acids, dextrose, lipids, and some trace minerals.

(recall that fluid intake is controlled in dialysis patients). Intradialytic parenteral nutrition has been successful for increasing weight gain, muscle mass, and body fat in malnourished hemodialysis patients.[39]

Dietary Compliance Adhering to a renal diet is probably the most difficult aspect of treatment for renal disease patients. Patients often require extensive counseling once multiple dietary restrictions become necessary. Depending on the stage of illness and the patient's laboratory values, the renal diet may limit protein, fluids, sodium, potassium, and phosphorus, thereby affecting food selections from all major food groups. Because these diets have so many restrictions, patient compliance is often a problem. The "How to" provides suggestions to help patients comply with renal diets. The accompanying case study on p. 866 can help you apply your knowledge about chronic renal disease and hemodialysis.

Kidney Transplants

A preferred alternative to dialysis in end-stage renal disease is kidney transplantation.[40] A successful kidney transplant restores kidney function, allows a more liberal diet, and frees the patient from routine dialysis. Given the choice, many patients would prefer transplants, but the demand for suitable kidneys far exceeds the supply. Other barriers to transplantation include age, poor health, financial difficulties, and abnormalities of the urinary tract. Fewer than 20 percent of patients who develop end-stage renal disease receive a kidney transplant.[41]

Immunosuppressive Drug Therapy Following transplant surgery, patients require high doses of immunosuppressive drugs to prevent tissue rejection.■ These drugs have multiple effects that can alter nutrition status. Side effects may include nausea, vomiting, diarrhea, glucose intolerance, altered blood lipids, fluid retention, hypertension, and infection. Because immunosuppressant therapy increases the risk of foodborne infection, food safety guidelines should be discussed with patients and caregivers.

■ Immunosuppressive drugs used after kidney transplant include corticosteroids, cyclosporine, tacrolimus, sirolimus, and mycophenolate mofetil.

Dietary Interventions Protein and energy requirements increase after surgery due to stress and the catabolic effects of drug therapy. Once recovery is under way, side effects from drugs can influence dietary treatment. Typical dietary modifications are shown in Table 28-6. Hyperglycemia can be improved by controlling carbohydrate intake, but oral medications or insulin therapy may also be required. Because blood lipids are frequently elevated, patients should limit saturated fat and cholesterol intakes. Sodium, potassium, and phosphorus intakes are often liberalized following transplant, but serum electrolyte levels must be monitored closely because some drug therapies can cause hyperkalemia or hypophosphatemia. Calcium supplementation is advised due to urinary calcium losses associated with corticosteroids.

TABLE 28-6 Dietary Guidelines following a Kidney Transplant

- **Energy:** Initially 30–35 kcal/kg body weight per day; adjust to maintain reasonable weight.
- **Protein:** Initially 1.3 to 1.5 g/kg body weight per day; reduce to 1.0 g/kg per day after 6–8 weeks.
- **Carbohydrate:** Consistent carbohydrate intake each day; increase fiber.
- **Fat:** Limit saturated fat and cholesterol to help control serum lipids.
- **Sodium:** Restricted (to 2–4 g/day) if fluid retention and hypertension are present.
- **Potassium:** Adjust according to serum potassium levels.
- **Calcium:** 1000 to 1500 mg to minimize bone loss associated with drug therapy.
- **Phosphorus:** 1200 to 1500 mg; supplements needed if serum phosphorus is low.
- **Fluid:** No restrictions.

SOURCE: American Dietetic Association, *Manual of Clinical Dietetics* (Chicago: American Dietetic Association, 2000).

HOW TO Help Patients Comply with a Renal Diet

The challenges faced by dietitians who design renal diets pale in comparison with those encountered by patients and caregivers who must learn and follow a complex set of dietary instructions. The following suggestions can assist patients in complying with dietary recommendations:

1. *To keep track of fluid intake:*
   - Fill a container with an amount of water equal to your total fluid allowance. Each time you use a liquid food or beverage, discard an equivalent amount of water from the container. The amount remaining in the container will show you how much fluid you have left for the day.
   - Be sure to save enough fluid to take medications.
2. *To help control thirst:*
   - Chew gum or suck hard candy.
   - Freeze beverages so that they take longer to consume.
   - Add lemon juice to water to make it more refreshing.
   - Gargle with refrigerated mouthwash.
3. *To add kcalories to meals:*
   - Add extra margarine or butter to rice, noodles, breads, crackers, and cooked vegetables.
   - Add extra salad dressing or oil to salads.
   - Add nondairy whipped toppings to desserts.
   - Include fried foods in your diet.
4. *To prevent the diet from becoming monotonous:*
   - Experiment with new combinations of allowed foods.
   - Substitute nondairy products for milk products. Nondairy products, which are lower in protein, phosphorus, and potassium, can substitute for milk and add energy to the diet.
   - Add zest to foods by seasoning with garlic, onion, chili, curry powder, oregano, pepper, or lemon juice.
   - Consult a dietitian when you want to eat restricted foods. Many restricted foods can be used occasionally and in small amounts if the diet is carefully adjusted.

IN SUMMARY Chronic renal failure causes gradual loss of kidney function, most often resulting from long-standing diabetes mellitus or hypertension. Kidney function is usually evaluated by measuring the glomerular filtration rate (GFR). Depending on the stage of disease, complications may include fluid and electrolyte disturbances, hypertension, renal osteodystrophy, mental impairments, bleeding abnormalities, anemia, reduced immunity, abnormal blood lipids, and insulin resistance. Treatment can help to slow disease progression and correct complications; drug therapies, dietary modifications, and routine dialysis may be required. Medical nutrition therapy usually includes a low-protein diet, controlled fluid and sodium intakes, potassium and phosphorus restrictions, and calcium and vitamin D supplementation. Kidney transplantation can restore renal function and liberalize dietary restrictions.

Kidney Stones

Of the disorders affecting the kidneys and urinary tract, **kidney stones** are the most common: more than 400,000 people in the United States are treated yearly.[42] A kidney stone is a crystalline mass that forms within the urinary tract. Although often asymptomatic, a stone's passage can cause severe pain or block the urinary tract. Stones tend to recur, but can be prevented with dietary and medical treatment.

kidney stones: crystalline masses that form in the urinary tract; also called **renal calculi** and **nephrolithiasis.**

CASE STUDY

Banker with Chronic Renal Failure

Thomas Stone is a 55-year-old banker who developed chronic renal failure as a result of hypertension. His condition was discovered several years ago when routine laboratory tests revealed elevated serum creatinine and BUN levels. Since then, he has been taking antihypertensive medications and restricting dietary sodium, although he reported difficulty following the low-protein diet that was also prescribed. Mr. Stone recently visited his doctor with complaints of low urine output and reduced sensation in his hands and feet. He also reported feeling drowsy at work and mentioned that he was bruising more than usual. The examination revealed a 9-pound weight gain since his last visit and swelling in his ankles and feet. Tests revealed that his GFR had fallen to 10 mg/mL. Mr. Stone is 5 feet 8 inches tall and normally weighs 160 pounds.

1. Explain how chronic renal failure progresses. What happens to GFR, serum creatinine levels, and BUN as renal function declines?
2. What clinical effects would you expect during the final stage of kidney failure? Explain the significance of each of Mr. Stone's physical complaints.
3. Explain why a low-sodium and low-protein diet was prescribed for Mr. Stone at a former visit. What energy and protein intakes were probably recommended?
4. The physician determines that Mr. Stone's kidney failure has reached the final stage and prescribes hemodialysis. How will dialysis alter Mr. Stone's diet? Calculate his new energy and protein needs and compare them to his former diet. What other nutrients will need consideration?

Formation of Kidney Stones

Kidney stones develop when stone constituents become concentrated in urine, allowing crystals to form and grow. About 75 percent of kidney stones are made up primarily of calcium oxalate. Less commonly, stones are composed of uric acid, the amino acid cystine, or magnesium ammonium phosphate (the latter are known as *struvite* stones). Factors that predispose to stone formation include the following:

- *Dehydration* or *low urine volume,* which promotes the crystallization of minerals and other compounds in urine.
- *Obstruction,* which prevents the flow of urine and encourages salt precipitation.
- *Renal disease,* which is associated with calcification of tissues and phosphate accumulation.
- *Urine acidity,* which affects the dissolution of urinary constituents. Some stones form more readily in acidic urine, whereas others form in alkaline urine.
- *Metabolic factors,* which affect the presence of compounds that either promote or inhibit crystal growth.

The most common types of kidney stones are described in this section.

Calcium Oxalate Stones The most common abnormality in people with calcium oxalate stones is **hypercalciuria** (excessive calcium in urine). Hypercalciuria may result from excessive calcium absorption, impaired reabsorption of calcium in kidney tubules, or elevated serum levels of parathyroid hormone or vitamin D. Some people with calcium oxalate stones excrete normal amounts of calcium in urine, however, and the reason they form stones is unknown.

Excessive urinary oxalate, known as **hyperoxaluria,** promotes the formation of calcium oxalate crystals. Oxalate is a normal product of metabolism that readily binds to calcium. Hyperoxaluria may reflect an increase in oxalate synthesis or increased absorption from dietary sources.■ People who form calcium oxalate stones are advised to avoid supplementation with vitamin C, which degrades to oxalate,[43] and to reduce their dietary intake of oxalate (see Table 28-7).[44] Vitamin B_6 deficiency can also increase oxalate production in the body.[45]

■ Reminder: As described in Chapter 24, fat malabsorption promotes oxalate absorption, thereby increasing the risk of oxalate stone formation (see p. 744).

hypercalciuria (HIGH-per-kal-see-YOO-ree-ah): an excessive amount of calcium in urine.

hyperoxaluria (HIGH-per-OX-al-YOO-ree-ah): an excessive amount of oxalate in urine.

TABLE 28-7 Foods High in Oxalate

Vegetables	Fruits	Other
Beans, green and wax	Blackberries	Chocolate and chocolate beverages*
Beets*	Blueberries	Cocoa
Celery	Currants, red	Coffee
Chard, swiss	Gooseberries	Draft beer
Collard greens	Grapes, Concord	Fruit cake
Dandelion greens	Lemon peel	Grits
Eggplant	Lime peel	Nuts, nut butters*
Endive	Orange peel	Peanut butter*
Escarole	Raspberries	Pepper
Leeks	Rhubarb*	Soybean crackers
Legumes	Strawberries*	Tea*
Okra		Tofu
Parsley		Wheat bran*
Potatoes, sweet		Wheat germ
Spinach*		
Squash, summer		

NOTE: The oxalate content of many foods has not been analyzed and even fewer studies have been conducted to determine which foods raise urinary oxalate. The foods marked with an asterisk have been documented to raise urinary oxalate and should be avoided by people who form calcium stones.

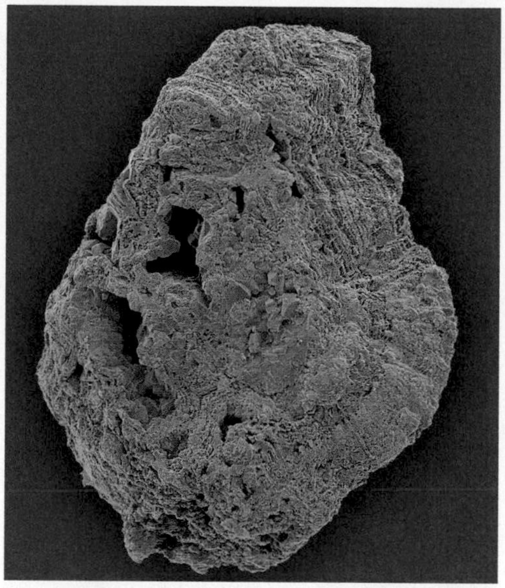

The most common type of kidney stone is composed of calcium oxalate crystals, shown here.

Uric Acid Stones Uric acid stones develop when the urine is abnormally acidic, contains excessive uric acid, or both.[46] These stones are frequently associated with **gout,** a metabolic disorder characterized by elevated uric acid levels in blood and urine. People with gout also tend to have unusually acidic urine, but the cause is unknown. Other diseases that increase the risk of uric acid stones include leukemia, lymphoma, hemolytic anemia, and glycogen storage disease; these conditions are associated with **purine** overproduction, which can increase the uric acid content of urine.[47] A purine-rich diet also contributes to high uric acid levels (see Table 28-8).

Cystine and Struvite Stones Cystine stones form as a consequence of an inherited disorder of amino acid metabolism called **cystinuria.** In this condition, the renal tubules are unable to reabsorb cystine (and several other amino acids) normally. Stones form when the urinary cystine concentration is excessive.

Struvite stones are mainly composed of magnesium ammonium phosphate. These stones form when infectious bacteria degrade urea to ammonia and elevate urinary pH to a level that favors struvite formation. They occur most frequently in patients who have chronic urinary infections or disorders that interfere with urinary flow.

Consequences of Kidney Stones

In most cases, kidney stones do not pose serious medical problems. Small stones may readily pass through the ureters and out of the body with minimal treatment.

Renal Colic A stone passing through the ureter can produce severe, stabbing pain, called **renal colic.** Typically, the pain begins suddenly in the back and intensifies as the stone follows the ureter's course down the abdomen toward the groin (review Figure 28-1 on p. 852). The pain may be severe enough to cause nausea and vomiting and may sometimes require medication. When the stone reaches the bladder, the pain subsides abruptly.

gout: a metabolic disorder that results in excessive uric acid in the blood and urine and the deposition of uric acid in and around the joints, causing acute joint inflammation.

purine (PYOO-reen): an end product of nucleotide metabolism that eventually degrades to form uric acid.

cystinuria (SIS-tin-NOO-ree-ah): an inherited disorder characterized by excessive urinary excretion of several amino acids, including cystine.

struvite (STROO-vite): crystals of magnesium ammonium phosphate.

renal colic: the severe, stabbing pain that occurs when a kidney stone passes through the ureter.

TABLE 28-8 Foods High in Purines

Organ Meats	Meat and Meat Products	Seafood
Brains	Game meat	Anchovies
Kidney	Gravies	Herring
Liver	Meat extracts	Mackerel
Sweetbreads		Sardines
		Scallops

SOURCE: J. A. T. Pennington, *Bowes and Church's Food Values of Portions Commonly Used* (Philadelphia: J. B. Lippincott, 1994), p. 387.

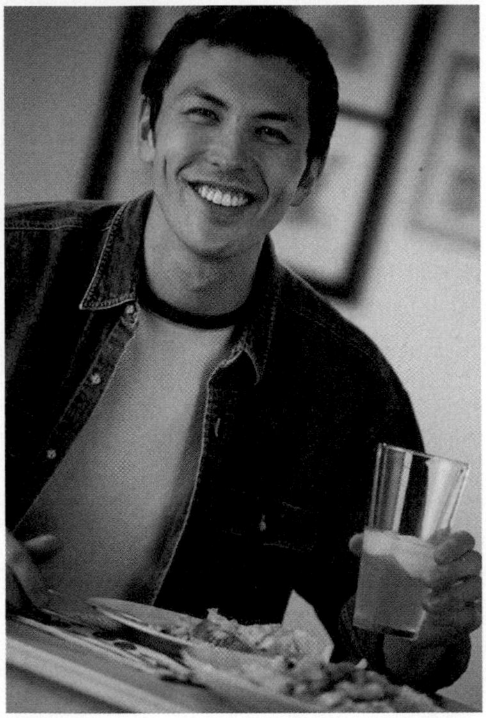

Drinking plenty of water throughout the day is the most important measure for preventing kidney stones.

Urinary Tract Complications Depending on the location of the stone, symptoms may include urination urgency, frequent urination, or inability to urinate. Blood may appear in the urine (called **hematuria**) as a result of damage to the kidney or ureter lining. Stones that are unable to pass through the ureter may cause a urinary tract obstruction and possibly lead to infection.

hematuria (HE-mah-TOO-ree-ah): blood in the urine.

Prevention and Treatment of Kidney Stones

People who form any type of kidney stone should increase fluid intake so that the daily urinary volume remains between 2 and 3 liters.[48] Fluids keep urine dilute so that solutes cannot crystallize and form stones. Patients are generally advised to drink at least 12 to 16 cups of fluid daily; additional amounts may be needed in hot weather or if an individual is extremely active. Acceptable fluid sources include tea, coffee, wine, and beer, but apple and grapefruit juices should be limited because they may increase risk.[49] Dietary measures and drug treatments for the various types of stones are described in the sections that follow.

Calcium Oxalate Stones Dietary and drug treatments aim to reduce urinary calcium and oxalate. Furthermore, the uric acid content of urine must be kept low because uric acid crystals contribute to the formation of these stones.[50] Thiazide diuretics are a mainstay of drug therapy; these help to reduce urinary calcium by enhancing calcium reabsorption by the kidney tubules. Other common medications include cholestyramine, which reduces oxalate absorption, and allopurinol, which reduces uric acid production in the body. Supplementation with potassium citrate inhibits the formation and growth of crystals, but may cause stomach upset and diarrhea.[51]

Medical nutrition therapy includes adjustments in dietary intakes of calcium, oxalate, protein, and sodium. A diet that contains adequate calcium (800 to 1000 milligrams per day) is recommended because dietary calcium combines with oxalate in the intestines, reducing its absorption and helping to control hyperoxaluria.[52] Conversely, low-calcium diets result in increased oxalate absorption and higher urinary oxalate levels. Foods high in oxalate are restricted because dietary oxalate contributes considerably to the amount in urine (see Table 28-7).[53] Because excessive protein and sodium intakes can increase urinary calcium excretion, moderate protein consumption and sodium restriction are advised. See the Research Update feature on p. 869 to learn more about these measures for preventing calcium oxalate stones.

Uric Acid Stones The drug treatments used for uric acid stones include allopurinol to reduce urinary uric acid and potassium citrate to reduce urine acidity. Diets restricted in purines may also help to control urinary uric acid levels (see Table 28-8). Because all meats, poultry, fish, and shellfish contain considerable amounts of purines, strict dietary control over a long period may be difficult to achieve. In addition, the benefits of purine restriction are unknown.

Cystine and Struvite Stones High fluid intakes can prevent the formation of cystine stones in patients who excrete relatively low levels of cystine; others require drug therapy to reduce cystine production in the body.[54] Medications frequently prescribed include penicillamine and tiopronin, which reduce cystine levels, and potassium citrate, which reduces urine acidity.

Preventing urinary tract infections is an important strategy for preventing struvite stones. Patients with these stones may require antibiotic therapy to prevent further stone formation.

IN SUMMARY Kidney stones form when stone constituents become concentrated enough to crystallize in urine. Most stones are made primarily from calcium oxalate; others are made from uric acid, cystine, or struvite. Kidney stones can cause renal colic, difficulty with urination, and obstruction. A principal means of prevention is to maintain urine volumes of 2 to 3 liters daily. Adequate calcium intake can help to control intestinal oxalate absorption. Other dietary measures may include oxalate and purine restrictions, moderate protein intake, and sodium restriction. Medications can help reduce stone formation and maintain ideal urine acidity.

RESEARCH UPDATE Dietary Measures for Calcium Oxalate Stones

Although the ideal treatment for preventing kidney stones continues to be debated, combining several dietary changes may offer the most protection. The most promising of these were tested in a five-year trial that compared two dietary regimens in 120 men, all of whom had hypercalciuria and recurring calcium oxalate stones.[a] In this study, 60 of the men were instructed to follow a low-calcium diet with 400 milligrams of calcium per day. The remaining 60 men consumed a normal-calcium, low-protein, sodium-restricted diet that provided 1200 milligrams of calcium, 52 grams of protein, and 1150 milligrams of sodium per day. (All subjects were instructed to consume 2 to 3 liters of fluids daily and to avoid foods high in oxalate.) After five years, the incidence of recurrent stones in men consuming the latter diet was 49 percent of that experienced by the low-calcium group.

Scientists now realize that a normal calcium intake is much more effective than a low-calcium diet for preventing recurring stones. As explained in the text, calcium binds intestinal oxalate and reduces oxalate absorption. Moreover, a low-calcium intake results in negative calcium balance and increases calcium release from bone, contributing to low bone density and increased osteoporosis risk.[b] Calcium supplements elevate urinary calcium levels and are therefore not as helpful as food sources of calcium.[c]

Excessive protein and sodium in the diet increase calcium losses from bone; therefore, reducing intakes of either can reduce urinary calcium levels. In addition, a low protein intake is beneficial because it increases urinary citrate levels, thereby inhibiting calcium oxalate formation.[d] (Recall that supplementation with potassium citrate is a possible medical treatment.) In addition, protein restriction is associated with both lower urinary oxalate and lower uric acid levels.

Despite the potential effectiveness of dietary modifications, long-term compliance can be a problem. Patients are often unwilling to make lifelong changes to prevent an occasional, transient event like passing a kidney stone.[e] Similarly, the daily use of medications to prevent kidney stones is unacceptable to many patients.

[a] L. Borghi and coauthors, Comparison of two diets for the prevention of recurrent stones in idiopathic hypercalciuria, *New England Journal of Medicine* 346 (2002): 77–84.

[b] A. L. Wasserstein, Nephrolithiasis, in A. Greenberg, ed., *Primer on Kidney Diseases* (San Diego: National Kidney Foundation and Academic Press, 2001), pp. 348–354.

[c] M. S. Parmar, Kidney stones, *British Medical Journal* 328 (2004): 1420–1424.

[d] D. S. Goldfarb, Reconsideration of the 1988 NIH Consensus Statement on prevention and treatment of kidney stones: Are the recommendations out of date? *Reviews in Urology* 4 (2002): 53–60.

[e] Goldfarb, 2002.

DIET-DRUG INTERACTIONS

Antigout
Allopurinol should be taken with meals, although nutrition-related side effects are uncommon. *Colchicine,* used to reduce inflammation, should be taken with meals; it can cause nausea, vomiting, and diarrhea. Colchicine reduces vitamin B_{12} absorption, and the person may need to take vitamin B_{12} supplements.

Antihypertensives
For *antihypertensives,* see p. 841.

Antilipemics
For *antilipemics,* see p. 841.

Diuretics
For *diuretics,* see p. 782 and p. 841.

Exchange Resins
Cellulose sodium phosphate (prescribed for people with hypercalciuria who absorb too much calcium) can alter the sense of taste, cause gastrointestinal distress and diarrhea, and reduce blood magnesium levels. Patients should take the medication with meals and should not take a magnesium supplement for at least one hour before and after taking the resin.

Sodium polystyrene (prescribed to reduce blood potassium levels) can cause anorexia, nausea, vomiting, and constipation and lower blood levels of calcium. The powder can be mixed with sorbitol-containing syrup to prevent constipation. Calcium-containing antacids or calcium supplements should not be taken within several hours of taking sodium polystyrene.

Immunosuppressants
Immunosuppressants have multiple effects on many organ systems, may be toxic to the kidneys and liver, can cause nausea and vomiting, and increase susceptibility to infection. *Cyclosporine* can elevate blood potassium and should not be given with grapefruit or grapefruit juice. The person taking cyclosporine should not use potassium supplements or salt substitutes containing potassium. Other possible side effects of cyclosporine include glucose intolerance and iron-deficiency anemia. *Azathioprine* can cause anemia and lead to pancreatitis. Also see p. 762.

Phosphate Binders
For *calcium acetate, calcium carbonate, calcium citrate, aluminum carbonate,* and *aluminum hydroxide,* see calcium-containing and aluminum-containing antacids on p. 731.

Sevelamer hydrochloride does not contain calcium or aluminum. It is given with meals and can cause nausea, flatulence, gastrointestinal distress, diarrhea, and, less frequently, constipation.

NUTRITION ASSESSMENT CHECKLIST for People with Renal Disorders

Medical History
Check the medical record to determine:

- ☐ Degree of renal function
- ☐ Cause of nephrotic syndrome or renal failure
- ☐ Type of dialysis, if appropriate
- ☐ If patient has received a kidney transplant
- ☐ Type of kidney stone

Review the medical record for complications that may alter nutrient needs:

- ☐ Protein-energy malnutrition
- ☐ Edema or oliguria
- ☐ Metabolic stress or infection
- ☐ Anemia
- ☐ Diabetes mellitus
- ☐ Hyperlipidemia
- ☐ Hypertension

Medications
Assess risks for medication-related malnutrition related to:

- ☐ Long-term use of medications
- ☐ Multiple medication use, especially if medications significantly affect nutrition status
- ☐ Altered renal function, which may alter drug potency

For all patients with renal diseases, note:

- ☐ Whether medications or supplements contain electrolytes that must be controlled
- ☐ Use of drugs or herbs that may be toxic to the kidneys

Dietary Intake
For patients with the nephrotic syndrome, renal failure, or kidney transplants, assess intakes of:

- ☐ Energy
- ☐ Protein
- ☐ Fluid
- ☐ Vitamins, especially vitamin D
- ☐ Minerals, especially calcium, phosphorus, iron, and electrolytes

For patients with kidney stones or a history of kidney stones:

- ☐ Stress the need to drink plenty of fluids throughout the day.
- ☐ Assess intake of calcium, oxalate, sodium, protein, purines, cystine, or vitamin C, as appropriate for the type of stone.

Anthropometric Data
Take accurate baseline height and weight measurements. Keep in mind that:

- ☐ Fluid retention in patients with the nephrotic syndrome or renal failure can mask malnutrition.
- ☐ For patients on dialysis, the weight measured immediately following dialysis treatment, called the "dry weight," most accurately reflects the person's true

weight. Rapid weight gain between dialysis treatments often reflects fluid retention. For patients who regularly have problems with fluid retention, review fluid intake to ensure that the patient understands and is complying with diet recommendations.

- ☐ Weight loss is expected and intentional following a dialysis treatment.

Laboratory Tests

Note that serum protein levels are often low in patients with the nephrotic syndrome or renal failure. Review the following laboratory test results to assess degree of renal function and response to treatments:

- ☐ Glomerular filtration rate (GFR)
- ☐ Creatinine
- ☐ Urinary protein
- ☐ Blood urea nitrogen (BUN)
- ☐ Electrolytes

Check laboratory test results for complications associated with renal disease including:

- ☐ Anemia
- ☐ Hyperglycemia
- ☐ Hyperlipidemia
- ☐ Hyperparathyroidism (bone disease)

Clinical Signs

For patients with the nephrotic syndrome or renal failure, look for physical signs of:

- ☐ Dehydration and fluid retention
- ☐ Iron deficiency
- ☐ Uremia
- ☐ Bone disease
- ☐ Hyperkalemia

NUTRITION ON THE NET

Access these websites for further study of topics covered in this chapter.

- Find updates and quick links to these and other nutrition-related sites at our website: **www.wadsworth.com/nutrition**
- To search for specific topics related to kidney diseases, dialysis, and kidney transplants, visit these sites: National Institute of Diabetes and Digestive and Kidney Diseases: **www.niddk.nih.gov**

  National Kidney Foundation: **www.kidney.org**

  Kidney Foundation of Canada: **www.kidney.ca**

  Renalnet Kidney Information Clearinghouse: **www.renalnet.org**
- To find materials for patients with kidney diseases, visit the American Association of Kidney Patients: **www.aakp.org**
- To find more information about kidney stones, visit the Oxalosis and Hyperoxaluria Foundation: **www.ohf.org**
- To see photographs of kidney stones, visit the website of the Louis C. Herring Laboratory: **www.herringlab.com**

STUDY QUESTIONS

These questions will help you review the chapter. You will find the answers in the discussions on the pages provided.

1. Describe the kidneys' role in maintaining homeostasis. Discuss other functions of the kidneys in the body. (pp. 851–852)
2. Define the nephrotic syndrome and describe the consequences that can develop. Discuss the elements of dietary treatment recommended for the nephrotic syndrome. (pp. 853–855)
3. Describe acute renal failure and list possible causes. Discuss how its consequences—fluid and electrolyte imbalances and waste product accumulation—can disrupt health. Describe the medical treatment of acute renal failure and the elements of medical nutrition therapy. (pp. 856–858)
4. Explain how chronic renal failure differs from acute renal failure. What happens as renal failure progresses? Discuss the symptoms and complications associated with the uremic syndrome. (pp. 858–860)
5. Identify the objectives of treatment for chronic renal failure and discuss the role of dialysis. Describe how dietary recommendations change during the course of illness. Why are protein and phosphorus intakes of particular concern? (pp. 861–863)
6. What are the fluid and electrolyte recommendations for patients with chronic renal failure? What adjustments are needed in vitamin and mineral intakes, and why? (pp. 862–863)
7. Explain why renal patients often have difficulty adhering to a renal diet. Discuss ways to help patients comply with recommendations. (pp. 864–865)
8. Discuss the nutrient needs of a kidney transplant patient. How can immunosuppressive drug therapy affect nutrition status? (p. 864)
9. Identify factors that affect kidney stone formation. Describe the composition of the most common types of kidney stones. Discuss dietary adjustments that may help to prevent kidney stone recurrence. (pp. 866–869)

These questions will help you prepare for an exam. Answers can be found on p. 873.

1. Which of the following is not a function of the kidneys?
   a. activation of vitamin K
   b. maintenance of acid-base balance
   c. elimination of metabolic waste products
   d. maintenance of fluid and electrolyte balance
2. The nephrotic syndrome frequently results in:
   a. the uremic syndrome.
   b. oliguria.
   c. edema.
   d. renal colic.
3. Dietary recommendations for the nephrotic syndrome include:
   a. high-protein intakes.
   b. sodium restrictions.
   c. potassium and phosphorus restrictions.
   d. fluid restrictions.
4. Hyperkalemia is often treated by:
   a. eliminating potassium from the diet.
   b. using diuretics to increase potassium losses.
   c. increasing fluid consumption.
   d. using potassium exchange resins, which bind potassium in the GI tract.
5. Fluid requirements for oliguric patients are estimated by adding about ____ milliliters to the volume of urine output.
   a. 100
   b. 300
   c. 500
   d. 750
6. The most common cause of chronic renal failure is:
   a. diabetes mellitus.
   b. hypertension.
   c. autoimmune disease.
   d. exposure to toxins.
7. Which of the following nutrients may be unintentionally restricted when a patient follows a renal diet?
   a. fluid
   b. calcium
   c. potassium
   d. phosphorus
8. Once dialysis treatment begins, a patient with chronic renal failure is advised to alter dietary intake by:
   a. decreasing protein.
   b. increasing protein.
   c. decreasing potassium and phosphorus.
   d. increasing potassium and phosphorus.
9. Most kidney stones are made primarily from:
   a. struvite.
   b. uric acid.
   c. calcium oxalate.
   d. cystine.
10. Treatment for all kidney stones includes:
    a. dietary oxalate restriction.
    b. dietary protein restriction.
    c. vitamin C supplementation.
    d. a fluid intake that maintains a urine volume of at least 2 liters a day.

REFERENCES

1. J. P. Briggs, W. Kriz, and J. B. Schnermann, Overview of renal function and structure, in A. Greenberg, ed., *Primer on Kidney Diseases* (San Diego: National Kidney Foundation and Academic Press, 2001), pp. 3–19.
2. G. B. Appel, Glomerular disorders, in L. Goldman and D. Ausiello, eds., *Cecil Textbook of Medicine* (Philadelphia: Saunders, 2004), pp. 726–733.
3. G. A. Kaysen, Proteinuria and the nephrotic syndrome, in R. W. Schrier, ed., *Renal and Electrolyte Disorders* (Philadelphia: Lippincott Williams & Wilkins, 2003), pp. 580–622.
4. Kaysen, 2003.
5. Kaysen, 2003.
6. Kaysen, 2003.
7. Kaysen, 2003.
8. Kaysen, 2003; S. Escott-Stump, *Nutrition and Diagnosis-Related Care* (Baltimore: Lippincott Williams & Wilkins, 2002), pp. 665–666.
9. Escott-Stump, 2002.
10. W. E. Mitch, Acute renal failure, in L. Goldman and D. Ausiello, eds., *Cecil Textbook of Medicine* (Philadelphia: Saunders, 2004), pp. 703–708.
11. Mitch, 2004; C. J. Richard, Renal disorders, in L. E. Lancaster, ed., *Core Curriculum for Nephrology Nursing* (Pitman, N.J.: Anthony J. Jannetti, 2001), pp. 85–115.
12. C. L. Edelstein and R. W. Schrier, Acute renal failure: Pathogenesis, diagnosis, and management, in R. W. Schrier, ed., *Renal and Electrolyte Disorders* (Philadelphia: Lippincott Williams & Wilkins, 2003), pp. 401–455.
13. F. N. Hutchison, Management of acute renal failure, in A. Greenberg, ed., *Primer on Kidney Diseases* (San Diego: National Kidney Foundation and Academic Press, 2001), pp. 275–280.
14. Mitch, 2004.
15. Mitch, 2004.
16. J. Stover and G. Morrison, Renal disease, in L. Hark and G. Morrison, eds., *Medical Nutrition and Disease: A Case-Based Approach* (Malden, Mass.: Blackwell Science, 2003), pp. 328–349; Escott-Stump, 2002.
17. Hutchison, 2001.
18. Edelstein and Schrier, 2003.
19. Escott-Stump, 2002.
20. Edelstein and Schrier, 2003.
21. R. G. Luke, Chronic renal failure, in L. Goldman and D. Ausiello, eds., *Cecil Textbook of Medicine* (Philadelphia: Saunders, 2004), pp. 708–716.
22. W. Wang and L. Chan, Chronic renal failure: Manifestations and pathogenesis, in R. W. Schrier, ed., *Renal and Electrolyte Disorders* (Philadelphia: Lippincott Williams & Wilkins, 2003), pp. 456–497.
23. A. S. Levey and coauthors, National Kidney Foundation practice guidelines for chronic kidney disease: Evaluation, classification, and stratification, *Annals of Internal Medicine* 139 (2003): 137–147.
24. Levey and coauthors, 2003.
25. Luke, 2004; Wang and Chan, 2003.
26. Luke, 2004.
27. Luke, 2004; Wang and Chan, 2003.
28. R. Mehrotra and J. D. Kopple, Nutritional management of maintenance dialysis patients: Why aren't we doing better? *Annual Reviews of Nutrition* 21 (2001): 343–379.
29. Luke, 2004.
30. Mehrotra and Kopple, 2001.
31. J. A. Beto and V. K. Bansal, Medical nutrition therapy in chronic kidney failure: Integrating clinical practice guidelines, *Journal of the American Dietetic Association* 104 (2004): 404–409.
32. Beto and Bansal, 2004.
33. Beto and Bansal, 2004.
34. Beto and Bansal, 2004.

35. American Dietetic Association, *Manual of Clinical Dietetics* (Chicago: American Dietetic Association, 2000), p. 458.
36. Stover and Morrison, 2003; American Dietetic Association, 2000.
37. Beto and Bansal, 2004.
38. N. Tolkoff-Rubin and N. Goes, Treatment of irreversible renal failure, in L. Goldman and D. Ausiello, eds., *Cecil Textbook of Medicine* (Philadelphia: Saunders, 2004), pp. 716–726.
39. A. K. Mortelmans and coauthors, Intradialytic parenteral nutrition in malnourished hemodialysis patients: A prospective long-term study, *Journal of Parenteral and Enteral Nutrition* 23 (1999): 90–95; K. Hiroshige and coauthors, Prolonged use of intradialysis parenteral nutrition in elderly malnourished chronic haemodialysis patients, *Nephrology Dialysis Transplantation* 13 (1998): 2081–2087.
40. Tolkoff-Rubin and Goes, 2004.
41 Wang and Chan, 2003.
42. Escott-Stump, 2002.
43. D. G. Assimos, Vitamin C supplementation and urinary oxalate excretion, *Reviews in Urology* 6 (2004): 167.
44. M. S. Parmar, Kidney stones, *British Medical Journal* 328 (2004): 1420–1424.
45. A. G. Wasserstein, Nephrolithiasis, in A. Greenberg, ed., *Primer on Kidney Diseases* (San Diego: National Kidney Foundation and Academic Press, 2001), pp. 348–354.
46. Wasserstein, 2001.
47. F. C. Delvecchio and G. M. Preminger, Management of urinary calculi, in J. Noble, ed., *Textbook of Primary Care Medicine* (St. Louis: Mosby, 2001), pp. 1373–1382.
48. I. Juknevicius and K. A. Hruska, Renal calculi (nephrolithiasis), in L. Goldman and D. Ausiello, eds., *Cecil Textbook of Medicine* (Philadelphia: Saunders, 2004), pp. 761–767.
49. Escott-Stump, 2002.
50. Juknevicius and Hruska, 2004.
51. D. S. Goldfarb, Reconsideration of the 1988 NIH Consensus Statement on prevention and treatment of kidney stones: Are the recommendations out of date? *Reviews in Urology* 4 (2002): 53–60.
52. Escott-Stump, 2002; Goldfarb, 2002.
53. M. S. Krishnamurthy, K. A. Hruska, and P. S. Chandhoke, The urinary response to an oral oxalate load in recurrent calcium stone formers, *Journal of Urology* 169 (2003): 2030–2033.
54. Juknevicius and Hruska, 2004.

ANSWERS

Study Questions (multiple choice)

1. a 2. c 3. b 4. d 5. c 6. a 7. b 8. b 9. c 10. d

HIGHLIGHT

Dialysis

Although there is no perfect substitute for one's own kidneys, dialysis offers a life-sustaining treatment option for people with chronic renal failure. Dialysis can serve as a permanent treatment for kidney failure or as a temporary measure to sustain life until a suitable kidney donor can be found. Dialysis can also restore blood balances in patients with acute renal failure. Clinicians who routinely work with renal patients should understand how dialysis procedures work. This highlight describes the process of dialysis and outlines the different types of procedures used.

The Basics of Dialysis

As described in this section, dialysis removes excess fluids and wastes from the blood by employing the processes of **diffusion, osmosis,** and **ultrafiltration** (see the accompanying glossary and Figure H28-1). In dialysis, the dialysate, a solution similar in composition to normal blood plasma, is delivered to a compartment beside a **semipermeable membrane;** the person's blood flows along the other side of the membrane. The semipermeable membrane acts like a filter: small molecules like urea and glucose can pass through microscopic pores in the membrane, whereas large molecules are unable to cross.

In *hemodialysis,* the tiny tubes that carry blood through the dialyzer are made of materials that serve as semipermeable membranes. In *peritoneal dialysis,* the body's peritoneal membrane, rich with blood vessels, is used to filter blood.

Removal of Solutes

The chemical composition of the dialysate affects the movement of solutes across the membrane. When the concentration of a substance is lower in the dialysate than in the blood, the substance, provided it can cross the membrane, will diffuse out of the blood. To maximally remove waste products like urea from the blood, the dialysate contains no urea. For many other solutes, the dialysate is adjusted so that only excesses will be removed. Potassium can be removed from the blood, for example, by providing a dialysate with a lower concentration of potassium than the person's blood. The dialysate must contain some potassium, however; otherwise the blood potassium would fall too low.

The dialysate can also be used to add needed components back into the blood. For a person with acidosis, for example, bases such as bicarbonate are added to the dialysate and then move by diffusion into the blood to alleviate acidosis.

Removal of Fluid

Because albumin and other plasma proteins are so adept at retaining fluids in blood, osmosis alone is not an efficient process for removing fluid. In hemodialysis, a **pressure gradient** is cre-

GLOSSARY

continuous ambulatory peritoneal dialysis (CAPD): the most common method of peritoneal dialysis; involves frequent exchanges of dialysate, which remains in the peritoneal cavity throughout the day.

continuous renal replacement therapy (CRRT): a slow, continuous method of removing solutes and fluid from blood by gently pumping blood across a filtration membrane over a prolonged time period.

diffusion: movement of solutes from an area of high concentration to one of low concentration.

hemofiltration: removal of fluid and solutes by pumping blood across a membrane; no osmotic gradients are created during the process. Also called **diafiltration.**

oncotic pressure: the pressure exerted by fluid on one side of a membrane as a result of osmosis.

osmosis: movement of water across a membrane toward the side where solutes are more concentrated.

peritonitis: inflammation of the peritoneal membrane.

pressure gradient: change in pressure over a given distance. In dialysis, a pressure gradient is created between the blood and the dialysate.

semipermeable membrane: a membrane that allows some particles to pass through, but not others.

ultrafiltration: removal of fluids and solutes from blood by using pressure to transfer the blood across a semipermeable membrane.

urea kinetic modeling: a method of determining the adequacy of dialysis treatment by calculating urea clearance from blood.

FIGURE H28-1 Diffusion, Osmosis, and Ultrafiltration

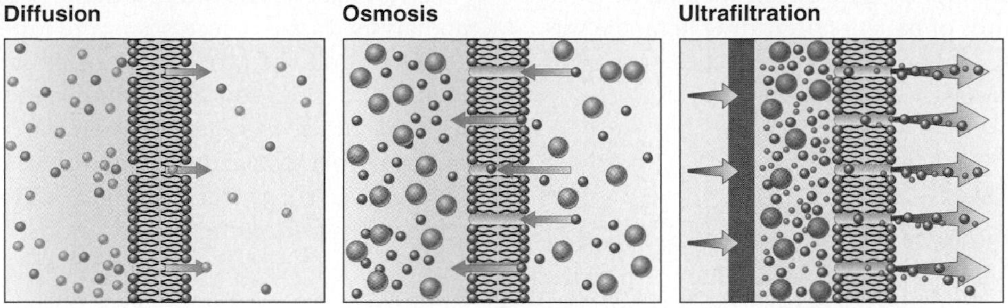
Diffusion
Osmosis
Ultrafiltration

Diffusion: Small molecules (electrolytes and waste products) move from an area of high concentration to an area of low concentration by diffusion.

Osmosis: Water moves from an area of high water concentration to an area of low water concentration. In other words, water moves toward the side where solutes are more concentrated.

Ultrafiltration: Pressure squeezes water and small molecules through the pores of a semipermeable membrane during ultrafiltration.

ated between the blood and the dialysate. Most modern dialyzers produce *positive* pressure in the blood compartment and *negative* pressure in the dialysate compartment,[1] establishing a pressure gradient that "pushes" water (and accompanying solutes) through the pores of the membrane. This process, called ultrafiltration, relies on pumps to establish an appropriate flow rate between the blood and the dialysate.

Evaluation of Dialysis Treatment

A number of methods have been devised for gauging the adequacy of dialysis treatment. The most common method is **urea kinetic modeling,** a technique that evaluates the amount of urea cleared from the blood. The formula used most often is Kt/V, where K is the urea clearance, t is the time on dialysis, and V is the blood volume. The value obtained indicates whether the patient has undergone sufficient dialysis; the goal is a Kt/V result of approximately 1.2. Because technical data need to be incorporated into the calculation (such as dialyzer clearance data, blood flow rate, and dialysate flow rate), the computation is usually done by computer analysis.[2] Current treatment guidelines recommend that hemodialysis adequacy be evaluated at least monthly or more often if problems develop or patients are noncompliant.[3]

Undergoing Dialysis

Three approaches are currently used to remove fluids and wastes from the body. These include hemodialysis, peritoneal dialysis, and continuous renal replacement therapy. The latter procedure is used only to treat acute renal failure.

Hemodialysis

As described previously, hemodialysis utilizes a dialyzer to cleanse the patient's blood. Although dialyzers vary in efficiency, the treatment usually lasts 3 to 4 hours and is required at least three times weekly. Some studies suggest that patients undergoing daily hemodialysis for briefer periods (2 to 2.5 hours) may tolerate dialysis treatment better and have fewer complications, but this approach has not been widely adopted.[4] Most patients visit dialysis centers to obtain treatment: home hemodialysis programs are available, but only about 2 percent of patients use them.

Although lifesaving, hemodialysis is associated with a substantial number of complications.[5] Problems at the vascular access site include infections and blood clotting. Hypotension can

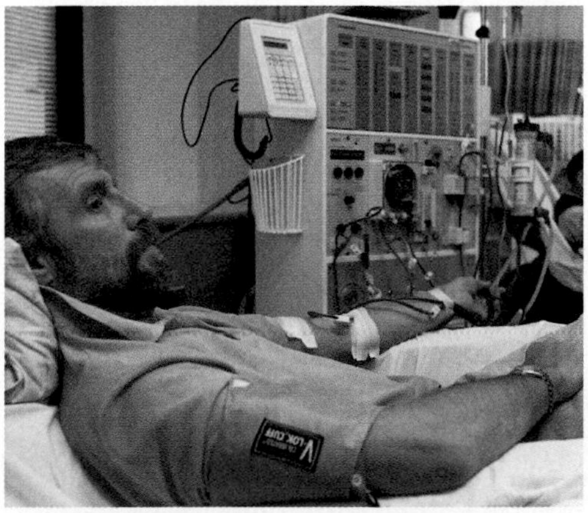

During hemodialysis, blood passes through a dialyzer where wastes are extracted, and the cleansed blood is returned to the body.

develop while blood is circulated through the dialyzer. Muscle cramping often occurs during the procedure, especially in the hands, legs, and feet. Blood losses can worsen anemia, which is already severe in two-thirds of patients beginning hemodialysis treatment.[6] Patients may also experience headaches, weakness, nausea, vomiting, restlessness, and agitation.[7]

Peritoneal Dialysis

In peritoneal dialysis, the peritoneal membrane surrounding the abdominal organs serves as a semipermeable membrane. The dialysate is infused into a catheter that empties into the peritoneal space—the space within the abdomen near the intestines (see Figure H28-2). In the most common procedure, **continuous ambulatory peritoneal dialysis (CAPD),** the dialysate remains in the peritoneal cavity for 4 to 6 hours, after which it is drained and replaced with fresh dialysate (about 2 to 3 liters in adults). Generally, the dialysate solution is exchanged four times daily and requires only about 30 minutes to drain and replace.

Because a pressure gradient cannot be created in the peritoneal cavity as it can in a dialyzer, the glucose concentration in the dialysate must be high enough to create enough **oncotic pressure** to draw fluid from the blood. As indicated in Chapter 28, a substantial amount of glucose can be absorbed into the patient's blood and may contribute to weight gain over time. The high glucose load may also cause hyperglycemia and hypertriglyceridemia in some patients.

Peritoneal dialysis offers a number of advantages over hemodialysis: vascular access is not required, dietary restrictions are fewer, and the procedure can be scheduled when convenient.[8] The most common complication is infection, which can occur at the catheter site or in the peritoneal cavity **(peritonitis).** Other problems that may arise include blood clotting in the catheter, catheter migration, and abdominal hernia due to the dialysate volume.[9]

Continuous Renal Replacement Therapy

In people with acute renal failure, **continuous renal replacement therapy (CRRT)** removes fluids and wastes. CRRT utilizes the process of **hemofiltration,** in which blood is gently pumped across a filtration membrane over a prolonged time period. (This differs from dialysis treatments that rely on the diffusion of wastes across a membrane into dialysate.) Either a pump or the patient's own blood pressure may move the blood across the membrane. The procedure can be used to remove fluids, solutes, or both. Some patients require fluid replacement during the procedure to maintain adequate blood volume, so hydration status must be closely monitored.

FIGURE H28-2 Peritoneal Dialysis

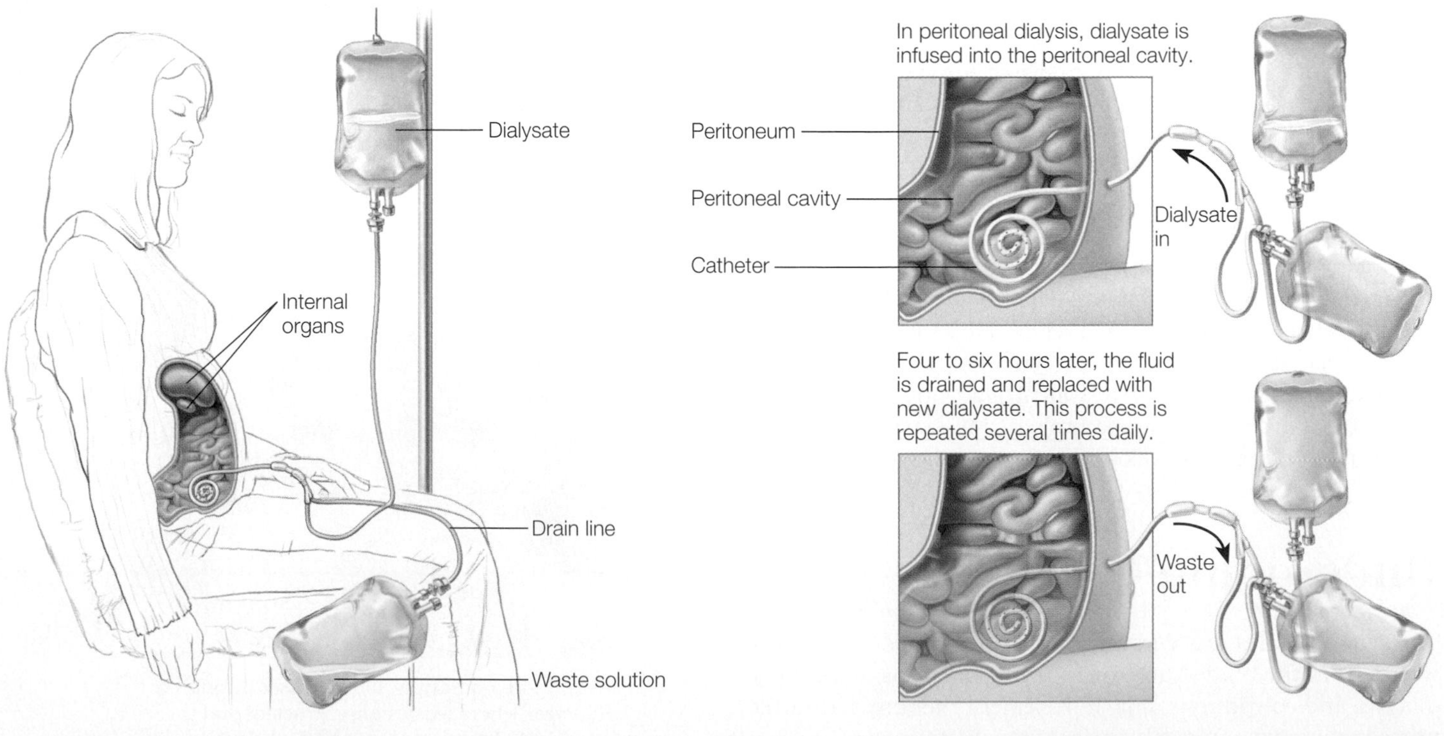
Dialysate
Internal organs
Drain line
Waste solution
In peritoneal dialysis, dialysate is infused into the peritoneal cavity.
Peritoneum
Peritoneal cavity
Catheter
Dialysate in
Four to six hours later, the fluid is drained and replaced with new dialysate. This process is repeated several times daily.
Waste out

The use of CRRT is advantageous in acute care situations because it corrects imbalances without causing sudden shifts in blood volume, which are poorly tolerated in acute care patients.[10] In addition, replacement fluids can include parenteral feedings without upsetting fluid balance. Complications include clotting problems, damage to arteries, and inadequate blood flow rates in hypotensive patients.

Dialysis and CRRT help to remove the wastes and fluids that are normally removed by healthy kidneys. Although these procedures cannot restore the kidneys' hormonal functions, they provide a lifesaving means for alleviating symptoms of uremia, hypertension, and edema.

REFERENCES

1. C. F. Gutch, Principles of hemodialysis, in C. F. Gutch, M. H. Stoner, and A. L. Corea, eds., *Review of Hemodialysis for Nurses and Dialysis Personnel* (St. Louis: Mosby, 1999), pp. 35–45.
2. Gutch, 1999.
3. National Kidney Foundation, K/DOQI Clinical practice guidelines for hemodialysis adequacy: Update 2000, http://kidney.org/professionals/kdoqi/guidelines_updates/doqi_uptoc.html#hd, visited November 17, 2004.
4. A. Pierratos, New approaches to hemodialysis, *Annual Review of Medicine* 55 (2004): 179–189.
5. N. Tolkoff-Rubin and N. Goes, Treatment of irreversible renal failure, in L. Goldman and D. Ausiello, eds., *Cecil Textbook of Medicine* (Philadelphia: Saunders, 2004), pp. 716–726.
6. Tolkoff-Rubin and Goes, 2004.
7. Gutch, 1999.
8. Tolkoff-Rubin and Goes, 2004.
9. Tolkoff-Rubin and Goes, 2004.
10. M. Rolston and coauthors, Dialyzers, dialysate, and delivery systems, in C. F. Gutch, M. H. Stoner, and A. L. Corea, eds., *Review of Hemodialysis for Nurses and Dialysis Personnel* (St. Louis: Mosby, 1999), pp. 46–71.

Chapter 29

Nutrition, Cancer, and HIV Infection

Chapter Outline

Cancer: *How Cancer Develops • Consequences of Cancer • Treatments for Cancer • Medical Nutrition Therapy*

HIV Infection: *How AIDS Develops • Consequences of HIV Infection • Treatments for HIV Infection • Medical Nutrition Therapy*

Highlight: *Illness, Mental Health, and Nutrition*

Available Online

http://nutrition.wadsworth.com/uncn7

Student Practice Test

Glossary Terms

Nutrition on the Net

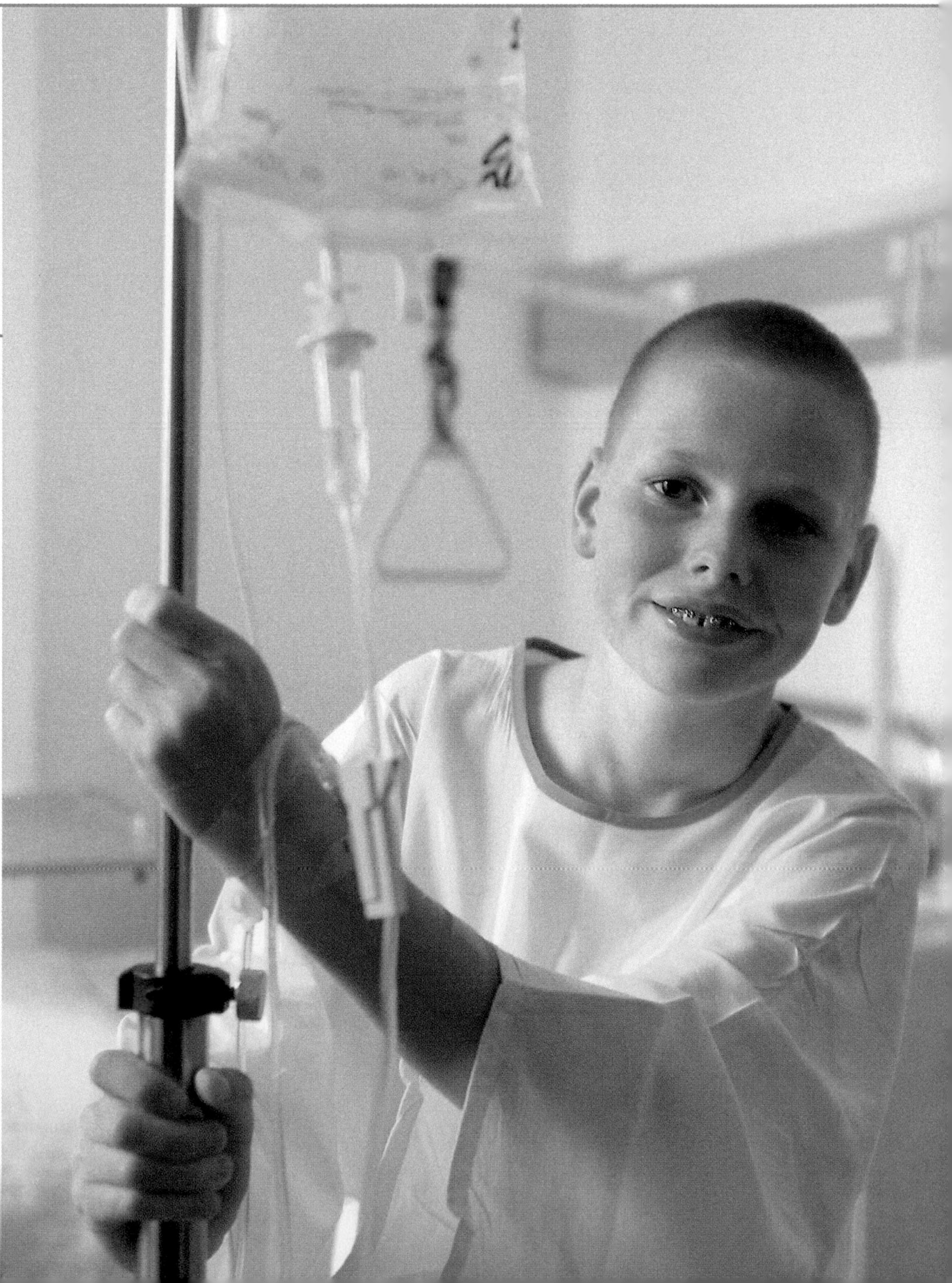

Nutrition in the Professional Setting

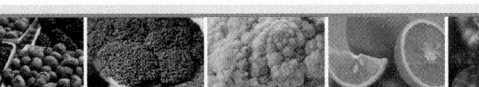

A diagnosis of cancer or HIV infection can be devastating. Patients will likely expect an ever-worsening course of illness and, possibly, death. Medical management soon becomes an ever-present burden, and treatments are often unpleasant. For both illnesses, however, extraordinary therapeutic advances have been made. Treatment options have expanded and patients have benefited by vast improvements in quality of life. The health practitioner's knowledge is the patient's most important resource—and an important source of hope.

Although **cancers** and **HIV (human immunodeficiency virus)** infections are distinct disorders, from a nutritional standpoint, they share many similarities. Both disorders can have effects on many organ systems that influence nutritional needs, and both can lead to severe wasting in advanced cases. Both require medical nutrition therapy that is highly individualized based on the symptoms manifested and the organ systems involved.

Cancer

Cancer ranks just below cardiovascular disease as a cause of death for the entire population, and it is the number one cause of death for those between the ages of 45 and 64. Consequently, many people have personal experiences with cancer. As with cardiovascular disease (and HIV infection, also covered in this chapter), the prognosis for cancer today is far brighter than in the past. Identification of risk factors, new detection techniques, and innovative therapies offer hope and encouragement.

Cancer is not a single disorder. There are many cancers, that is, many different kinds of malignancies.■ They have different characteristics, occur in different

■ Cancers are classified by the tissues or cells from which they develop:
- **Adenomas** (ADD-eh-NO-muz) arise from glandular tissues.
- **Carcinomas** (KAR-sih-NO-muz) arise from epithelial tissues.
- **Gliomas** (gly-OH-muz) arise from glial cells of the central nervous system.
- **Leukemias** (loo-KEE-mee-uz) arise from white blood cell precursors.
- **Lymphomas** (lim-FOE-muz) arise from lymph tissue.
- **Melanomas** (MEL-ah-NO-muz) arise from pigmented skin cells.
- **Sarcomas** (sar-KO-muz) arise from muscle, bone, or connective tissue.

cancers: diseases that result from the unchecked growth of malignant tumors.

HIV (human immunodeficiency virus): the virus that causes AIDS. The infection progresses to become an immune system disorder that leaves its victims defenseless against numerous infections.

locations in the body, take different courses, and require different treatments. Whereas an isolated, nonspreading type of skin cancer may be removed in a physician's office with no effect on nutrition status, advanced cancers, especially those of the gastrointestinal (GI) tract, pancreas, and liver, can seriously impair nutrition status.

How Cancer Develops

The genes in a healthy body work together to regulate cell division and ensure that each new cell is a replica of the parent cell. In this way, the healthy body grows, replacing dead cells and repairing damaged ones. Cancers develop from mutations in the genes that regulate cell division. These mutations silence the genes that ordinarily monitor the errors created by replicating DNA. The affected cells thereby lose their built-in brakes for halting cell division. As the abnormal mass of cells, called a **tumor,** grows, blood vessels form to supply the tumor with the nutrients it needs to support its growth. Eventually, the tumor invades more and more healthy tissue and may **metastasize.** In leukemia (cancer of the blood-forming cells of the bone marrow), the cancer cells do not form a tumor, but rather accumulate in blood and other tissues. Clinicians describe cancers by their location, size, and extent of growth and specify whether the tumor has spread to surrounding lymph nodes or to distant sites in the body. Figure 29-1 illustrates tumor formation and distinguishes between a **benign** and a **malignant** tumor.

tumor: a new growth of tissue forming an abnormal mass with no function; also called a **neoplasm** (NEE-oh-plazm).

metastasize (meh-TAS-tah-size): the spread of cancer cells from one part of the body to another.

benign (bee-NINE): describes tumors that stop growing without intervention or can be removed surgically and most often pose no threat to health.
- **benign** = mild

malignant (ma-LIG-nant): describes tumors that multiply out of control, threaten health, and require treatment.
- **malignus** = of bad kind

Genetic Factors All cancers have a genetic component in that a mutation causes abnormal cell growth, but some cancers have a genetically inherited com-

FIGURE 29-1 Tumor Formation

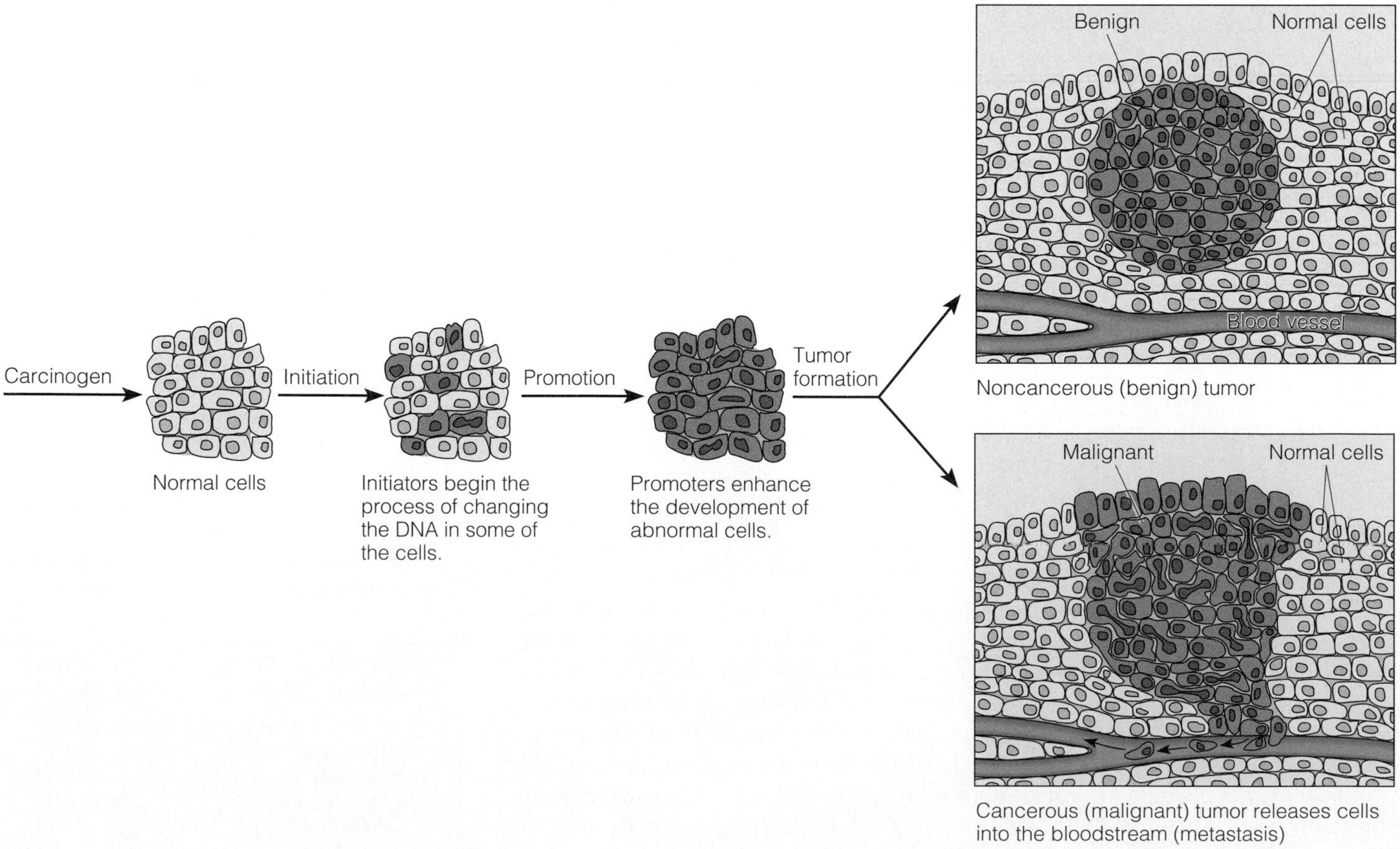

Carcinogen
Initiation
Promotion
Tumor formation
Normal cells
Initiators begin the process of changing the DNA in some of the cells.
Promoters enhance the development of abnormal cells.
Benign
Normal cells
Blood vessel
Noncancerous (benign) tumor
Malignant
Normal cells
Cancerous (malignant) tumor releases cells into the bloodstream (metastasis)

ponent as well. A person with a family history of colon cancer, for example, has a greater risk of developing colon cancer than a person without such a genetic predisposition. This does not mean, however, that the person *will* develop cancer, only that the risk is greater.

Immune Factors A healthy immune system recognizes foreign cells and destroys them. Researchers theorize that an ineffective immune system may not recognize tumor cells as foreign, thus allowing unchecked growth. Aging affects immune function, and the incidence of cancer increases with age. Drugs and diseases that suppress or weaken the immune system can substantially increase the risk of cancer.

Environmental Factors Among environmental factors, exposure to radiation and sunlight, water and air pollution, and smoking are known to cause cancer. Lack of physical activity may also play a role in the development of some types of cancer.[1] Men and women whose lifestyles include regular, vigorous physical activity have the lowest risk of colon cancer.[2] Physical activity may also protect against breast cancer by reducing body weight and by other mechanisms unrelated to body weight.[3]

Obesity is a risk factor for certain types of cancer, including colon, endometrial, kidney, esophageal, and postmenopausal breast cancer.[4] The exact manner in which obesity influences cancer development depends on the cancer site as well as other factors, including hormonal effects. In the case of breast cancer in postmenopausal women, for example, the hormone estrogen is likely involved: obese women have much higher levels of estrogen than do lean women because adipose tissue produces estrogen. The relationships between excessive body weight and some cancers provide yet another reason to adopt a lifestyle that embraces sound nutrition and physical activity.

As Table 29-1 shows, dietary constituents are also associated with an increased risk of certain cancers. Some dietary factors may initiate cancer development **(initiators),** others may promote cancer development once it has started **(promoters),** and still others may protect against the development of cancer **(antipromoters).**

Dietary Factors—Cancer Initiators Although we do not know to what extent the diet contributes to cancer development, some experts estimate that diet may be linked to up to a third of cases. Consequently, people may believe that certain foods, pesticides, and food additives are **carcinogenic.** Although some pesticides may be carcinogenic at extremely high doses, they are safe at the levels permitted on fruits and vegetables. The benefits of eating fruits and vegetables are far greater than any potential risk. As far as food additives are concerned, those approved for use in foods are not carcinogenic.

Cancers of the head and neck correlate strongly with use of alcohol and tobacco (especially when combined) and with low intakes of green and yellow fruits and vegetables. Alcohol intake alone is associated with cancers of the mouth, throat, and breast, and alcoholism often damages the liver and precedes the development of liver cancer. These findings illustrate why the potential benefits of moderate alcohol consumption for cardiovascular disease must be weighed against the potential dangers.

Food preparation methods are responsible for producing certain types of carcinogens in the foods we eat. Cooking meat, poultry, and fish at high temperatures causes carcinogens to form on food surfaces.[5] Carcinogens also accompany the smoke that adheres to foods during grilling and are present in the charred surfaces of meat and fish. The cancer risk from eating such foods is unclear, however, because the biological actions of these carcinogens are modulated by other dietary components, including compounds in vegetables and other plant foods. A number of population studies have linked consumption of well-cooked meats to cancers of the colon, breast, and stomach.[6]

Dietary Factors—Cancer Promoters Unlike carcinogens, which initiate cancers, some dietary components may promote cancers. Once the initiating step has taken place, these components may accelerate tumor development.

initiators: factors that cause mutations that give rise to cancer, such as radiation and carcinogens.

promoters: factors that favor the development of cancers once they have begun.

antipromoters: factors that oppose the development of cancers.

carcinogenic (CAR-sin-oh-JEN-ick): producing cancer. A substance that is capable of causing cancer is called a **carcinogen.**

TABLE 29-1 Factors Associated with Cancer at Specific Sites

Cancer Sites	Associated with:	Probable Protective Effect from:
Bladder cancer	Cigarette smoking and alcohol; weak association with coffee and chlorinated drinking water	Fruits and vegetables (especially fruits); adequate fluid intake
Breast cancer	High intakes of food energy, alcohol intake; low vitamin A intake; obesity, sedentary lifestyle, probably not associated with dietary fat	Monounsaturated fats; physical activity
Cervical cancer	Folate deficiency; viral infection; possibly, cigarette smoking	Adequate folate intake; possibly, fruits and vegetables
Colorectal cancer	High intakes of fat (particularly saturated fat), red meat, alcohol, and supplemental iron; low intakes of fiber, folate, vitamin D, and vegetables; inactivity; cigarette smoking	Vegetables, especially cruciferous (cabbage-type) vegetables; calcium, vitamin D, and dairy intake; possibly, whole wheat, wheat bran; high levels of physical activity
Kidney cancer	Possibly, high intakes of red meat (especially fried, sautéed, charred, burned, or cooked well-done); cigarette smoking; obesity	Fruit and vegetables, especially orange-colored and dark green ones
Mouth, throat, and esophagus cancers	Heavy use of alcohol, tobacco, and especially combined use; heavy use of preserved foods (such as pickles); low intakes of vitamins and minerals; obesity (esophageal)	Fruits and vegetables
Liver cancer	Infection with hepatitis virus; high intakes of alcohol; iron overload; toxins of a mold (aflatoxin) or other toxicity	Vegetables, especially yellow and green ones
Lung cancer	Smoking; low vitamin A; supplements of beta-carotene (in smokers)	Fruits and vegetables
Ovarian cancer	Possibly, high lactose intake from milk products; inversely correlated with oral contraceptive use	Vegetables, especially green leafy ones
Pancreatic and lung cancer	Possibly, high intakes of red meat (pancreatic cancer); correlated with cigarette smoking and air pollution	Fruits and vegetables, especially green and yellow ones
Prostate cancer	High intakes of fats, especially saturated fats from red meats and possibly milk products	Possibly, cooked tomatoes, soybeans, soy products, and flaxseed; adequate selenium intake
Stomach cancer	High intakes of smoke- or salt-preserved foods (such as dried, salted fish); cigarette smoking; possibly, refined flour or starch; infection with ulcer-causing bacteria	Fresh fruits and vegetables, especially tomatoes

SOURCES: National Cancer Policy Board, Institute of Medicine, S. J. Curry, T. Byers, and M. Hewitt, eds., *Fulfilling the Potential of Cancer Prevention and Early Detection* (Washington, D.C.: National Academies Press, 2003), pp. 66–86; S. E. McCann and coauthors, Risk of human ovarian cancer is related to dietary intake of selected nutrients, phytochemicals and food groups, *Journal of Nutrition* 133 (2003): 1937–1942; S. A. Smith-Warner and coauthors, Intake of fruits and vegetables and risk of breast cancer, *Journal of the American Medical Association* 285 (2001): 769–776; R. L. Nelson, Iron and colorectal risk: Human studies, *Nutrition Reviews* 59 (2001): 140–148; M. C. Jansen and coauthors, Dietary fiber and plant foods in relation to colorectal cancer mortality: The Seven Countries Study, *International Journal of Cancer* 81 (1999): 174–179; B. S. Reddy, Role of dietary fiber in colon cancer: An overview, *American Journal of Medicine* 106 (1999): S16–S19.

Studies in animals suggest that high-fat diets may promote cancer. In human studies, however, evidence is mixed.[7] Comparisons of populations around the world reveal that high-fat diets often, but not always, correlate with high cancer rates. Within a single population, however, cancer rates do not reliably reflect fat intakes. Studies of prostate cancer implicate meat fats but not vegetable fats, while consuming fatty fish may be protective.[8]

One attribute of dietary fat is energy density—gram for gram, fat provides more kcalories than either carbohydrate or protein. Diets high in *kcalories* do seem to promote cancer, especially in laboratory settings, so researchers still must untangle the effects of fat alone from those of total energy. The *type* of fat in the diet may also influence cancer promotion or prevention. Some evidence implicates saturated and *trans*-fatty acids in cancer promotion, while suggesting that omega-3 fatty acids from fish may protect against some cancers.[9] Thus the same dietary fat advice applies to cancer protection as to heart disease: reduce saturated and *trans*-fatty acids and increase omega-3 fatty acids.

Protective Dietary Factors Foods also contain anti-initiators and antipromoters. Almost without exception, epidemiological studies find a link between eating plenty of fruits and vegetables and reduced incidence of cancers. Many studies suggest that fiber-rich diets protect against some forms of cancer, including colon cancer.[10] The fiber in fruits and vegetables may protect against colon cancers by speeding up the transit time of materials through the colon so that colon walls are not exposed to cancer-causing substances for long. In addition to fiber, fruits and vegetables contain both nutrients and phytochemicals that are likely to protect against cancer. By acting as scavengers of oxygen-derived free radicals, the antioxidant nutrients vitamin C and vitamin E may help to prevent cell and tissue damage that can give rise to cancer (see Highlight 11). Phytochemicals common to many vegetables, especially cruciferous vegetables, can activate enzymes that destroy carcinogens (see Highlight 13). The recommendations for reducing cancer risk are similar to the recommendations for heart health and are summarized in Table 29-2.[11]

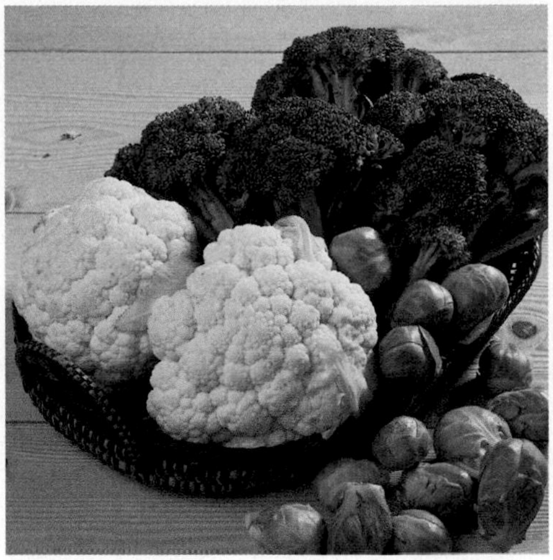

Cruciferous vegetables, such as cauliflower, broccoli, and brussels sprouts, contain nutrients and phytochemicals that inhibit cancer development.

Consequences of Cancer

Once cancer develops, the consequences depend on the location of the tumor, its severity, and the treatment. The complications that arise are often related to the impingement of a tumor on surrounding tissues. Nonspecific effects include anorexia, lethargy, weight loss, night sweats, and fever.[12] The chances of effective treatment are best during cancer's early stages, yet during this time many cancers produce no symptoms and the person may be unaware of any threat to health. Although screening for some cancers, such as prostate, colon, cervical, and breast cancers, has become somewhat routine, other cancers are too rare or screening too expensive to make such measures cost-effective.

TABLE 29-2 Recommendations for Reducing Cancer Risk[a]

Choose a diet rich in a variety of plant-based foods.
• Plant foods, such as vegetables, fruits, whole grains, and beans, should cover two-thirds or more of the plate.
• Fish, poultry, meat, or low-fat milk products should cover one-third or less of the plate.
• Limit consumption of processed foods and refined sugar.
Eat plenty of vegetables and fruits.
• Consume five or more servings of a variety of vegetables and fruits each day.
• Include vegetables that are dark green and leafy, as well as those that are deep orange in color.
• Include citrus fruits and other foods high in vitamin C.
Maintain a healthy weight and be physically active.
• Avoid being underweight or overweight, and limit weight gain during adulthood to less than 11 pounds (5 kilograms).
• If occupational activity is low or moderate, take an hour's brisk walk or participate in a similar exercise daily.
• Exercise vigorously for at least one hour each week.
Drink alcohol in moderation, if at all.
• Avoid alcohol consumption.
• If alcohol is consumed, limit it to less than two drinks a day for men and one for women.
Select foods low in fat and salt.
• Limit consumption of fatty foods, particularly those of animal origin. If red meat is eaten, limit intake to less than 3 ounces daily.
• Choose modest amounts of vegetable oils.
• Limit consumption of salted foods and use of cooking and table salt.
• Use herbs and spices to season foods.
Prepare and store foods safely.
• Use refrigeration and other appropriate methods to preserve perishable foods as purchased and at home.
• Do not eat charred food.
• Consume meat and fish grilled in direct flame and cured and smoked meats only occasionally.
Most importantly, do not smoke or use tobacco in any form.

[a] American Institute for Cancer Research, *The New American Plate,* revised ed. (2004), available at **www.aicr.org/publications/brochures/online/nap.pdf** (site visited February 7, 2005); American Institute for Cancer Research, *Food, Nutrition and the Prevention of Cancer: A Global Perspective (1997).*

Wasting Associated with Cancer Loss of appetite, tissue wasting, weight loss, and fatigue typify **cancer cachexia,** which occurs in as many as 80 percent of people with cancer.[13] Weight loss is often evident at the time cancer is diagnosed, and severe malnutrition, often seen in the later stages of cancer, may be the ultimate cause of death in many cases. Studies have shown that once lean body mass is significantly depleted, regardless of the cause, death will follow. Without adequate energy and nutrients, the body is poorly equipped to maintain immune defenses, support organ function, absorb nutrients, and mend damaged tissues.

Many factors appear to play a role in the wasting associated with cancer. Cytokines, released by both tumor cells and immune cells involved in the inflammatory response (see pp. 694–696), induce a hypermetabolic, catabolic state.[14]■ The combined effects of a poor appetite, accelerated and abnormal metabolism, and diversion of nutrients to support tumor growth result in a lower supply of energy and nutrients at a time when demands are high. Appetite and food intake are further disturbed by the effects of treatments and medications prescribed for cancer patients.

■ Reminder: Chapter 22 describes the immune responses to tissue injury, which include the release of cytokines into the bloodstream. Some of the cytokines that mediate cancer cachexia include tumor necrosis factor, interleukins, and gamma-interferon.

People who develop cachexia swiftly fall into a downward spiral. Once weight loss and wasting have been set into motion, the debilitation and general poor health that follow make it even more difficult for the person to eat. The body is unable to respond to the reduced nutrient supply as it does during fasting and rapidly depletes its nutrient stores.

Metabolic Alterations The metabolic changes that arise in cancer tend to exacerbate the wasting described in the previous section. Cancer patients exhibit increased protein turnover,■ but reduced muscle protein synthesis.[15] Gluconeogenesis increases,■ further straining the supply of body proteins. Triglyceride breakdown increases, but fat synthesis declines; as a consequence, serum lipids may become elevated. Many patients develop insulin resistance. These metabolic abnormalities help to explain why people with cancer fail to regain lean body mass or maintain healthy body weights even when they are receiving adequate energy and nutrients.

■ Reminder: *Protein turnover* refers to the continual degradation and synthesis of the body's proteins (see p. 193).

■ Reminder: *Gluconeogenesis* refers to the production of glucose from amino acids, lactic acid, and glycerol.

Anorexia and Reduced Food Intake Anorexia is a major contributor to the wasting associated with cancer. Some factors that contribute to anorexia or otherwise reduce food intake include:

- *Chronic nausea and early satiety.* People with cancer frequently experience nausea and a premature feeling of fullness after eating small amounts of food.
- *Fatigue.* People with cancer often tire easily and lack the energy to prepare and eat meals. Once cachexia develops, these tasks become even more difficult to handle.
- *Pain.* People in pain may have little interest in eating, particularly if eating makes pain worse.
- *Mental stress.* A cancer diagnosis can cause distress, anxiety, and depression, all of which may reduce appetite. Facing and undergoing cancer treatments causes additional psychological stress.
- *Effects of cancer therapies.* Therapies for cancer (including medications, chemotherapy, radiation therapy, surgery, and bone marrow transplants) can affect food intake by causing nausea, vomiting, altered taste perceptions, food aversions, inflammation of the mouth and esophagus, dry mouth, mouth sores, difficulty swallowing, intestinal cramping, diarrhea, and constipation.
- *Obstructions.* A tumor may partially or completely obstruct a portion of the GI tract, causing complications such as nausea and vomiting, early satiety, delayed gastric emptying, and bacterial overgrowth. Some patients with obstructions are unable to tolerate oral diets.

cancer cachexia (ka-KEK-see-ah): a wasting syndrome associated with cancer and characterized by anorexia, tissue wasting, weight loss, and fatigue.

Treatments for Cancer

The primary medical treatments for cancer—surgery, chemotherapy, radiation therapy, or any combination of the three—aim to remove cancer cells, prevent further tumor growth, and alleviate symptoms. Because treatment decisions are difficult and cancer therapies have considerable side effects, patients rely on the health practitioner to help them make informed decisions.

Surgery Surgery is performed to remove tumors, determine the extent of cancer, and discern whether nearby tissues are involved.[16] Often, surgery must be followed by other cancer treatments to prevent growth of new tumors. The acute metabolic stress caused by surgery raises protein and energy needs and can exacerbate wasting. Surgery may also contribute to pain, fatigue, and anorexia—factors that can reduce food intake at a time when nutritional needs are substantial.[17] Blood loss contributes to nutrient losses and further exacerbates malnutrition. Some surgeries can have long-term effects on nutritional status (see Table 29-3).

Chemotherapy **Chemotherapy** relies on the use of drugs to inhibit tumor growth. Some of these drugs interfere with the **cell cycle** and prevent cell division.[18] Other anticancer drugs sterilize cells that are in a resting phase and not actively dividing. The types of drugs used may include alkaloids, alkylating agents, antibiotics, nitrosoureas, antimetabolites,■ and others.

Ideally, chemotherapy would wipe out cancer cells without destroying healthy ones. Unfortunately, however, most of these drugs have toxic effects on normal cells as well and are especially damaging to rapidly dividing cells, such as those of the GI tract, skin, and bone marrow. Some newer drugs are able to target properties specific to cancer cells and are better tolerated by the body's tissues.[19] Table 29-4 includes a summary of the nutrition-related side effects that may result from chemotherapy.

Radiation Therapy **Radiation** treats cancer by bombarding cancer cells with X-rays, gamma rays, or various atomic particles. These treatments induce the formation of reactive oxygen species,■ such as superoxide and hydroxyl radicals, which can damage cellular DNA and cause cell death.[20] Newer techniques are better able to focus radiation directly at tumors and reduce damage to nearby tissues.

■ One drug in the *antimetabolite* category is methotrexate, which resembles the B vitamin folate. Folate is required for production of DNA and some amino acids (see pp. 335–336). Methotrexate inhibits cancer cell division by competing for the enzyme that converts folate to its active form (see Figure 19-1 on p. 639).

■ Reminder: *Reactive oxygen species,* discussed in Highlight 11, are produced in very small amounts by immune cells, which use them to destroy pathogens.

TABLE 29-3 Possible Effects of Cancer Surgeries on Nutritional Status

Head and Neck Resection	
Difficulty in chewing/swallowing	Inability to chew/swallow
Esophageal Resection	
Diarrhea	Reduced gastric motility
Fistula formation	Steatorrhea (fat malabsorption)
Reduced gastric acid secretion	Stenosis (constriction)
Gastric Resection	
Dumping syndrome	Lack of gastric acid
General malabsorption	Vitamin B_{12} malabsorption
Hypoglycemia	
Intestinal Resection	
Blind loop syndrome	Hyperoxaluria
Diarrhea	Malabsorption
Fluid and electrolyte imbalances	Steatorrhea
Pancreatic Resection	
Diabetes mellitus	Malabsorption

chemotherapy: the use of drugs to arrest or destroy cancer cells; also called **chemotherapeutic** or **antineoplastic agents.**

cell cycle: the phases that a cell goes through from the time it is formed until it divides into two new cells.

radiation therapy: the use of X-rays, gamma rays, or atomic particles to destroy cancer cells.

TABLE 29-4 Nutrition-Related Side Effects of Chemotherapy and Radiation

	Reduced Nutrient Intake	Accelerated Nutrient Losses	Altered Metabolism
Chemotherapy	Abdominal pain Anorexia Mouth ulcers Nausea Taste alterations Vomiting	Diarrhea Intestinal ulcers Malabsorption Vomiting	Fluid and electrolyte imbalances Hyperglycemia Interference with vitamins or other metabolites Negative nitrogen and calcium balances. Secondary effects of malnutrition, infection, or tissue damage (inflammation)
Radiation	Anorexia Damage to teeth and jaws Dysphagia Esophagitis Mouth ulcers Nausea Reduced salivary secretions Taste alterations Thick salivary secretions Vomiting	Blood loss from intestine and bladder Diarrhea Fistulas Intestinal obstructions Malabsorption Radiation enteritis Vomiting	Fluid and electrolyte imbalances as a consequence of vomiting, diarrhea, or malabsorption Secondary effects of malnutrition, infection , or tissue damage (inflammation)

An advantage of radiation therapy over surgery is that it can shrink tumors while preserving organ structure and function. Compared with chemotherapy, it is better able to target specific regions of the body, rather than involving all body cells. Nonetheless, radiation therapy can damage healthy tissues and sometimes has long-term effects on nutritional status. Radiation to the head and neck area may damage salivary glands and taste buds, causing inflammation, dry mouth, and a reduced sense of taste; in severe cases, damage may be permanent. Radiation treatment in the lower abdominal area can cause **radiation enteritis,** an inflammatory condition of the small intestine that causes nausea, vomiting, diarrhea, and malabsorption. Table 29-4 includes additional side effects of radiation treatment that affect nutritional status.

Bone Marrow Transplants **Bone marrow transplants** replace bone marrow that has been destroyed by chemotherapy or radiation treatment and are often the primary treatment for leukemia. If possible, bone marrow cells are collected from the patient before chemotherapy or radiation treatment begins so that it is not necessary to find a separate donor.[21] If another person's cells are used, immunosuppressant drugs are needed to prevent **tissue rejection.**

Bone marrow transplants have a substantial impact on nutritional status. After bone marrow is destroyed, immune function is suppressed, increasing the risk of foodborne illness. Effects of the transplant procedure include anorexia, dry mouth, inflamed mucous membranes, altered taste sensations, and diarrhea.[22] Patients are often unable to consume adequate food and may require nutrition support as described in a later section.

Medications to Combat Anorexia and Wasting To help cancer patients combat anorexia, medications are sometimes prescribed to stimulate the appetite and promote weight gain. One of the most effective medications, megestrol acetate, is a synthetic compound similar in structure to the hormone progesterone.[23] Dronabinol, which resembles the psychoactive ingredient in marijuana, stimulates appetite and helps to reduce nausea and vomiting at doses that have minimal mental effects.[24] Under investigation are medications that may help to restore lean body mass, such as anabolic steroids, growth hormone, and insulin-like growth factor.

Alternative Therapies Many patients turn to *complementary and alternative medicine (CAM)*■ to assist them in their fight against cancer. Although few aban-

■ Reminder: *Complementary and alternative medicine (CAM)* refers to health care systems, practices, and products that have not been proved to be effective. See Highlight 19 for additional information about CAM.

radiation enteritis: inflammation of intestinal tissue caused by exposure to radiation.

bone marrow transplants: procedures that replace bone marrow that has been destroyed by cancer treatments; also used to treat certain types of cancers and blood disorders.

tissue rejection: destruction of donor tissue by the recipient's immune system, which recognizes the donor cells as foreign.

don conventional medicine, 60 to 80 percent of cancer patients combine one or more CAM approaches with standard treatment.[25] People may turn to CAM because they wish to gain more control over treatment or feel more hopeful about their condition, or because they are concerned about the effectiveness of conventional approaches. Few patients discuss their use of CAM with physicians.[26]

Dietary supplements and herbal remedies are among the most frequently used CAM therapies. Although many supplements can be used without risk, others may have adverse effects or interfere with conventional treatments.[27] Use of the herbal remedy St. John's wort, for example, can reduce the effectiveness of some anticancer drugs.[28] As another example, some studies suggest that antioxidant supplementation interferes with chemotherapy and radiation treatment.[29] Clinical trials are currently in progress to learn more about the potential effects and treatment interactions caused by popular supplements.[30]

Medical Nutrition Therapy

The main objectives of medical nutrition therapy are to minimize loss of weight and lean body tissue, correct nutritional deficiencies, and provide a diet that can be tolerated and enjoyed despite the complications of illness. Although diet does not directly influence cancer outcome, attention to nutrition can help people maintain their strength and bolster immune function while they undergo stressful treatments. Moreover, malnourished cancer patients may have a poorer response to treatments and a shorter survival time than healthy patients.[31]

Nutritional needs among cancer patients vary considerably, as there are many forms of cancer and a variety of potential treatments. Furthermore, patients' needs may change at different stages of illness. Patients should be screened for malnutrition when cancer is diagnosed and reassessed during the treatment and recovery periods.[32]

Protein and Energy For patients at risk of weight loss and wasting, protein and energy needs are considerable. Daily protein intake should be 1.0 to 1.5 grams per kilogram body weight for maintenance and 1.5 to 2.0 grams per kilogram for repletion of stores.[33] Energy requirements may reach 145 percent of basal energy expenditure (see Table 22-2 on p. 697).■ Clinicians must regularly monitor patients' weight changes and adjust intake recommendations as necessary. Patients who are unable to eat adequate food may be able to meet needs using nutrient-dense formula supplements.

■ Reminder: The high-kcalorie, high-protein diet was described in Chapter 18. Suggestions for menu planning are provided in Table 18-3 and the "How to" on p. 615.

Breast cancer patients often gain weight. In one survey, 63 percent of women with breast cancer reported weight gains ranging between 5 and 27 pounds.[34] Weight gain occurs most often in premenopausal women and in those undergoing extensive chemotherapy. By discussing weight maintenance soon after diagnosis and encouraging physical activity, health practitioners can help patients avoid unnecessary weight gain.[35]

Managing Symptoms and Complications Medical nutrition therapy depends on the type and severity of cancer, the side effects of treatment, and the patient's nutrition status. In addition, a thorough nutrition assessment may uncover specific symptoms and problems that interfere with eating. Table 29-5 lists dietary considerations for cancers affecting different sites in the body. The "How to" on pp. 888-889 outlines strategies for alleviating symptoms and improving food intake. The suggestions are numerous and detailed, reflecting both the complexity of the problems and the importance of offering specific suggestions for individual problems.

Enteral and Parenteral Nutrition Support In general, tube feedings and parenteral nutrition are not routinely recommended for adequately nourished or mildly malnourished persons with cancer who are unable to eat. Most studies have failed to show that the use of specialized nutrition support reduces complications, shortens hospital stays, or lowers mortality rates. Nonetheless, these approaches

HOW TO Help Patients Handle Food-Related Problems

In people with cancer or HIV infections, many different problems can interfere with eating. Health care providers should try to identify the specific problems that patients are having and offer appropriate solutions. Explain why eating appropriately can help to improve their health. Not all of the suggestions will work for each patient; encourage patients to experiment and find the ones that work best.

I just don't have an appetite.

- Eat small meals and snacks at regular times each day.
- Eat the most food at the time of day when you feel the best.
- Use nutrient-dense foods for meals and snacks. (Suggestions are provided later.)
- Eat nutrient-dense foods first.
- Indulge in favorite foods throughout the day.
- Avoid drinking large amounts of liquids before or with meals.
- Eat in a pleasant and relaxed environment.
- Listen to your favorite music or enjoy a program on TV while you eat.
- Eat with family and friends.
- Serve foods attractively.
- Take a walk before you eat.

I am too tired to fix meals and eat.

- Let friends and family members prepare food for you.
- Use foods that are easy to prepare and eat like sandwiches, frozen dinners, meals from take-out restaurants, instant breakfast drinks, liquid formulas, and supplements in candy bar and pudding form.

Foods just don't taste right.

- Brush your teeth or use a mouthwash before you eat.
- Add sauces and seasonings to meats.
- Eat meats cold or at room temperature.
- Use eggs, fish, poultry, and milk products instead of meats.
- Try new foods and experiment with herbs and spices.
- Use plastic, rather than metal, eating utensils.
- Ask your doctor about zinc supplements. If you have a deficiency, your perception of tastes may change.

I am nauseated a lot of the time, and sometimes I throw up.

- If you experience vomiting, use clear liquids like broths, carbonated beverages, juices, jello, or frozen fruit juice bars to replace fluids and electrolytes.
- If you become nauseated from chemotherapy treatments, avoid eating for at least two hours before treatments.

I can't stand some of the foods I really used to like.

- Save your favorite foods for times when you are not feeling nauseated or sick to your stomach.
- Maintain a food-free "window" of an hour or so before and after you have treatments or take medications that cause nausea or vomiting.

I am having problems chewing and swallowing food.

- Experiment with food consistencies to find the ones you can handle best. Thin liquids, true solids, and sticky foods (like peanut butter) are often difficult to swallow.
- Add sauces and gravies to dry foods.
- Drink fluids with meals to ease chewing and swallowing.
- Try using a straw to drink liquids.
- Tilt your head forward and backward to see if you can swallow easier with the head positioned differently.

I have sores in my mouth and they hurt when I eat.

- Use cold or frozen foods; they are often soothing.
- Try soft, soothing foods like ice cream, milk shakes, bananas, applesauce, mashed potatoes, cottage cheese, and macaroni and cheese.

TABLE 29-5 Dietary Considerations for Specific Cancers

Cancer Sites	Dietary Considerations
Brain/nervous system	Physical feeding disabilities (see Highlight 27); chewing and swallowing problems (see Chapters 18 and 23).
Head/neck	Chewing and swallowing problems.
Mouth/esophagus	Chewing and swallowing problems; vomiting; if obstructed, tube feeding below the obstruction may be necessary.
Stomach	Nausea, vomiting, early satiety; if obstructed, tube feeding below the obstruction or TPN may be necessary; if resection is performed, a postgastrectomy diet (see Chapter 23) may be needed; bacterial overgrowth (Chapter 24) may occur.
Intestine	If obstructed, tube feeding or TPN may be necessary; resections or inflammation may cause multiple nutrition problems (see Chapter 24); fat- and lactose-restricted diet may be useful.
Liver	Protein-, sodium-, and fluid-restricted diet may be necessary (see Chapter 25).
Pancreas	Fat-restricted diet and enzyme replacements may be necessary (see Chapter 24); diabetic diet may be necessary if insulin production is affected (see Chapter 26).
Kidneys	Protein-, electrolyte-, and fluid-controlled diet may be necessary (see Chapter 28).

NOTE: The considerations listed here are specific to the type of cancer; they do not include other nutrition-related effects of treatment.

- Avoid foods that irritate mouth sores like citrus fruits and juices, tomatoes and tomato-based products, spicy foods, foods that are very salty, foods with seeds (like poppy seeds and sesame seeds) that can be trapped in the sore, and coarse foods like raw vegetables and toast.
- Ask your doctor about using a local anesthetic solution like lidocaine before eating to reduce pain.
- Use a straw for drinking liquids to bypass the sores.

My mouth is really dry.

- Rinse your mouth with warm salt water or mouthwash frequently, and drink liquids between meals.
- Ask your doctor or pharmacist about medications that can help with dry mouth.
- Use sour candy or gum to stimulate the flow of saliva.
- Make sure you brush your teeth and floss regularly to prevent cavities and oral infections.

I am having trouble with diarrhea.

- Drink plenty of fluids. Salty broths and soups, diluted fruit juices, and sports drinks are good choices. For severe diarrhea, try commercially prepared oral rehydration formulas.
- Temporarily avoid foods that increase gas, such as legumes, onions, and vegetables of the cabbage family (see Table 24-2 on p. 742).
- Take lactase enzyme replacements when you use milk products because you may also experience lactose intolerance while you are having diarrhea. You may be able to tolerate low-fat yogurt.
- Avoid high-fat foods and foods made with sugar, sugar alcohols, and fructose.
- Avoid caffeine.
- Eat smaller meals more often.
- Check with your doctor about using digestive enzyme replacements if you have had diarrhea for a long time.

I am having trouble with constipation.

- Drink plenty of fluids. Try warm fluids, especially in the morning.
- Eat whole-grain breads and cereals, nuts, fresh fruits, prunes, prune juice, and raw vegetables. Avoid refined carbohydrates like white bread, white rice, and pasta.
- Exercise regularly.

I need to gain weight, but my blood lipids are elevated.

- To gain weight, you will need to eat more fat, but the type of fat you use is important. Use more monounsaturated fats like olive, canola, and peanut oils for baking and frying and in salad dressings and dips. Snack on avocados, nuts, and peanut butter. Make guacamole dip and spread it on vegetables and low-fat crackers. Spread peanut butter on celery, cucumbers, fruit, and low-fat crackers.
- To increase protein in your diet without adding too much of the fat you need to avoid, eat larger-than-usual servings of chicken and fish, especially salmon. Add chicken, fish, or low-fat and fat-free cheeses to sauces, soups, casseroles, and vegetables. Use instant breakfast drinks made with low-fat milk, or use commercially available supplements that contain no more than 30 percent fat. Add low-fat milk or milk powder to meat loaves, casseroles, soups, puddings, and cereals. Use low-fat yogurt.
- Use plenty of dried fruits. Add nuts and dried fruits to desserts, cereals, and salads.

I need help figuring out how to eat more energy and protein.

- Use whole milk and regular yogurt instead of the low-fat or fat-free varieties.
- Use plenty of butter, margarine, mayonnaise, cream cheese, oil, and salad dressings on breads, sandwiches, potatoes, vegetables, salads, pasta, and rice.
- Use yogurt, sour cream, or a sour cream dip with vegetables.
- Add whipping cream to desserts and hot chocolate, or use it to lighten coffee.
- Use cream instead of milk with cereal.

help to maintain nutrition status when anorexia persists or when a patient is severely malnourished and is about to undergo aggressive cancer therapy. Each case is decided individually, and the use of nutrition support is more likely when a person's chances of recovery or of significant response to treatment are good, or when the type of cancer is associated with a high risk of death from malnutrition. Patients requiring head and neck resections, for example, may need long-term tube feedings and may need to continue tube feedings at home. Considering the many adverse effects that cancers can have on GI tract function and immune responses, enteral nutrition is strongly preferred over parenteral nutrition, whenever possible. People with severe radiation enteritis, however, may require home total parenteral nutrition (TPN).

Nutrition Support and Bone Marrow Transplants The person undergoing a bone marrow transplant routinely receives TPN before and after the transplant because the GI tract is severely compromised by the preparatory procedure (which may include high-dose chemotherapy and radiation treatment). When GI function returns, the patient begins to receive foods orally along with TPN, whenever possible. As oral intake improves, TPN is gradually tapered. After a bone marrow transplant, patients may experience severe and debilitating effects on nutrition status, especially if they develop GI complications.■ In some cases, oral intake fails to meet nutrient needs, and TPN is required permanently.

Early oral feedings often start with lactose-free, low-residue, low-fat liquids to maximize absorption and minimize nausea, vomiting, and fat malabsorption. Gradually, solid foods are reintroduced. For about three months after the transplant, the

■ Potential GI complications after a bone marrow transplant include anorexia, bleeding, infections, altered taste sensations, mouth dryness, inflammation of the mucous membranes of the mouth and esophagus, gastroesophageal reflux, early satiety, nausea, vomiting, diarrhea, and malabsorption.

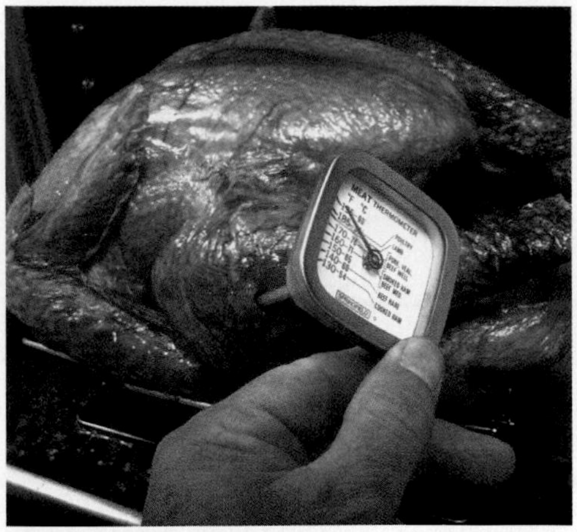
© Tony Freeman/PhotoEdit

Cooking meats, poultry, and fish to the correct internal temperature is an important safeguard against foodborne illness.

diet may exclude most fresh fruits and vegetables, undercooked meats, poultry and eggs, and ground meats to minimize the risk of foodborne infections. Patients are advised to follow safe food-handling practices to minimize the risk of foodborne illness (see the "How to" on pp. 892–893). Fiber, lactose, and fat are gradually added to the diet as individual tolerances allow. Because the transplant recipient often receives immunosuppressants, which may incur negative nitrogen and calcium balances, the final goal is to provide a high-kcalorie, high-protein, high-calcium diet. In addition, physicians often prescribe calcium and vitamin D supplements. Individuals with persistent diarrhea are encouraged to eat high-potassium foods.

Ethical Issues Every malnourished person with cancer (or an HIV infection) who cannot consume an adequate diet orally is a potential candidate for tube feedings or TPN. This chapter describes uses of tube feedings or TPN as they are applied to patients who have a chance of recovery or a reasonable life expectancy. When incurable illness has reached its final stages, however, the patient, caregivers, and the health care team need to make difficult decisions about the continued use of nutrition support.

IN SUMMARY Cancer develops when genes that normally regulate cell division fail to function properly. Dietary factors may initiate cancer, promote cancer once it has begun, or help to prevent cancer. Once cancer develops, effects on nutritional status depend on the type of cancer, its severity, and the treatments used. Cancer cachexia is a frequent complication and may be related to anorexia, altered metabolism, and responses to treatment. Treatments to eradicate cancer include surgery, chemotherapy, and radiation therapy. Bone marrow transplants may be required after some cancer treatments and are also used to cure certain cancers. The case study below helps you apply information about nutrition and cancer.

CASE STUDY

Public Relations Consultant with Cancer

Mrs. Magen is a 54-year-old public relations consultant recently diagnosed with cancer of the colon. Mrs. Magen was feeling well and was unaware of any problem. A fecal occult (hidden) blood test performed as part of a routine medical exam alerted her physician to a potential problem. Mrs. Magen then underwent a colonoscopy, a procedure that allows the physician to examine the colon using a flexible tube attached to an optical device. Mrs. Magen is scheduled to have surgery to remove the cancer and determine if it has spread to the surrounding lymph nodes and other organs. Before surgery, the surgeon explains to Mrs. Magen that most likely a portion of her intestine will be removed and there is a possibility that she will require a temporary colostomy. The severity and extent of the cancer will determine whether radiation therapy or chemotherapy will be required. The dietitian completing the nutrition assessment finds that Mrs. Magen is 5 feet 7 inches tall and weighs 165 pounds. Her typical diet is high in saturated fat and includes meat, poultry, or fish at both lunch and dinner. She eats two to three servings of fruits and vegetables and between three and six servings of grains and starchy vegetables each day. She rarely drinks milk, but often eats cheese.

1. Review Table 29-1 on p. 882 and describe the factors in Mrs. Magen's diet that might have contributed to the development of colon cancer.
2. What nutrition-related problems can occur as a consequence of surgical resection of the colon? Is malabsorption a common problem following surgery of the colon?
3. Describe some of the effects of radiation and chemotherapy on nutrition status.
4. If Mrs. Magen is unresponsive to treatments and her cancer progresses, she may develop cancer cachexia. What is this syndrome, and what are its causes? What are the benefits of preventing or correcting the wasting associated with cancer?
5. Provide suggestions to help Mrs. Magen handle these problems should they develop: poor appetite, fatigue, taste alterations, nausea and vomiting, food aversions, chewing and swallowing difficulties, mouth ulcers, mouth dryness, diarrhea, and weight loss.
6. Under what circumstances might tube feeding or parenteral nutrition be appropriate for Mrs. Magen if she is unable to eat an oral diet?

HIV Infection

Possibly, the most infamous infectious disease today is **AIDS (acquired immune deficiency syndrome).** AIDS develops from infection with HIV (human immunodeficiency virus), which attacks the immune system and disables the body's defenses against other diseases. Then these diseases, which would produce only mild, if any, illness in people with healthy immune systems, destroy health and life.

The HIV/AIDS epidemic continues to sweep across countries, especially in sub-Saharan Africa. Table 29-6 shows its impact worldwide and in the United States. For many years, the devastating effects of HIV infection seemed unstoppable, but in the mid-to-late 1990s, the death rate in the United States from AIDS began to decline, and the progression from HIV to AIDS slowed dramatically. The disease still has no cure, but remarkable progress has been made in understanding and treating HIV infection. Without a cure, the best course is prevention. HIV is transmitted by direct contact with contaminated body fluids, including semen, vaginal secretions, and blood (but not saliva), or by passage of the infection from a mother to her infant during pregnancy, birth, or breastfeeding.

Once a person has been infected with HIV, laboratory tests can detect antibodies within three months, and typically in three to four weeks. Because people remain symptom-free in the early stages of infection, however, they may not even consider being tested for HIV for several years following infection. Thus early detection to prevent the spread of HIV infection and to ensure early treatment for the person infected are important health goals.

TABLE 29-6 HIV and AIDS Epidemic at a Glance, 2004

	World	United States
Living with HIV or AIDS	39,400,000	1,000,000
Newly infected with HIV	4,900,000	44,000
AIDS deaths	3,100,000	16,000

SOURCE: UNAIDS, AIDS epidemic update: 2004, www.unaids.org/wad2004/EPlupdate2004_html_en/epi04_00_en.htm, site visited February 4, 2005.

How AIDS Develops

HIV attacks the immune system and leaves its victims defenseless against **opportunistic infections** and other disorders from which most people are protected. HIV infection progresses in stages, gradually destroying cells that have a specific protein called CD4 on their surfaces. The cells most affected are the *helper T cells,* also called **CD4+ T cells** because the presence of CD4 is a primary characteristic.■ At first, the number of helper T cells declines gradually, and the HIV-infected person remains symptom-free. As the infection continues, depletion of these cells progressively impairs immune function. In later stages, frequent and often fatal complications arise. About half of untreated persons with HIV infection develop AIDS within ten years, although the period varies greatly from person to person depending on such factors as genetic susceptibility, nutrition and health status, and medical interventions. Clinicians evaluate the progression of the disease by measuring the concentrations of helper T cells and circulating virus (called the *viral load*) and by monitoring clinical symptoms.

■ Reminder: *Helper T cells* are a type of lymphocyte that participates in cell-mediated immunity (see Highlight 17).

AIDS (acquired immune deficiency syndrome): the end stage of HIV infection, in which severe complications develop. The cluster of mild symptoms that sometimes occurs early in the course of AIDS is called **AIDS-related complex (ARC).**

opportunistic infections: infections from microorganisms that normally do not cause disease in the general population but can cause great harm in people whose immune systems are compromised (as in HIV infection).

CD4+ T cells: lymphocytes (white blood cells) that have a specific protein receptor (called CD4) on their surfaces; also known as *helper T cells.* Highlight 17 describes T cells and their functions.

AIDS-defining illnesses: complications associated with the later stages of an HIV infection, including wasting; recurrent bacterial pneumonia; infections of the central nervous system, GI tract, and skin; and certain cancers.

HIV-lipodystrophy (LIP-oh-DIS-tro-fee) **syndrome:** a collection of abnormalities in fat and glucose metabolism that result from drug treatments for HIV; includes body fat redistribution, abnormal lipid levels, and insulin resistance. The accumulation of abdominal fat is sometimes called *protease paunch.*

Consequences of HIV Infection

With improved treatments for HIV infection, the progression of the disorder has slowed dramatically. Initial symptoms may include fatigue, skin rashes, fevers, diarrhea, muscle pain, night sweats, weight loss, oral lesions, and infections. In the final stages, the number of helper T cells becomes markedly reduced, and the person develops frequent and eventually fatal complications—called **AIDS-defining illnesses**—such as wasting; recurrent bacterial pneumonia; infections of the central nervous system, GI tract, and skin; and invasive cancers. Improved treatments for HIV infections have significantly reduced the incidences of opportunistic infections.

Lipodystrophy Many of the drug treatments that suppress HIV infection cause abnormalities in glucose and fat metabolism in an estimated 25 to 50 percent of patients. These complications, collectively known as the **HIV-lipodystrophy syndrome,** include body fat redistribution, abnormal lipid levels, and insulin

HOW TO Prevent Foodborne Illness

Most foodborne illness can be prevented by following four simple rules: keep a clean kitchen, avoid cross-contamination, keep hot foods hot, and keep cold foods cold.

Keep a Clean Kitchen

- Wash fruits and vegetables in a clean sink with a scrub brush and warm water; store washed and unwashed produce separately.
- Use hot, soapy water to wash hands, utensils, dishes, nonporous cutting boards, and countertops before handling food and between tasks when working with different foods. Use a bleach solution on cutting boards (one capful per gallon of water).
- Cover cuts with clean bandages before food preparation; dirty bandages carry harmful microorganisms.
- Mix foods with utensils, not hands; keep hands and utensils away from mouth, nose, and hair.
- Anyone may be a carrier of bacteria and should avoid coughing or sneezing over food. A person with a skin infection or infectious disease should not prepare food.
- Wash or replace sponges and towels regularly.
- Clean up food spills and crumb-filled crevices.

Avoid Cross-Contamination

- Wash all surfaces that have been in contact with raw meats, poultry, eggs, fish, and shellfish before reusing.
- Serve cooked foods on a clean plate. Separate raw foods from those that have been cooked.
- Don't use marinade that was in contact with raw meat for basting or sauces.

Keep Hot Foods Hot

- When cooking meats or poultry, use a thermometer to test the internal temperature. Insert the thermometer between the thigh and the body of a turkey or into the thickest part of other meats, making sure the tip of the thermometer is not in contact with bone or the pan. Cook to the temperature indicated for that particular meat; cook hamburgers to at least medium well-done. If you have safety questions, call the USDA Meat and Poultry Hotline: (800) 535-4555.
- Cook stuffing separately, or stuff poultry just prior to cooking.
- Do not cook large cuts of meat or turkey in a microwave oven; it leaves some parts undercooked while overcooking others.
- Cook eggs before eating them (soft-boiled for at least 3½ minutes; scrambled until set, not runny; fried for at least 3 minutes on one side and 1 minute on the other).
- Cook seafood thoroughly. If you have safety questions about seafood call the FDA hotline: (800) FDA-4010.
- When serving foods, maintain temperatures at 140°F or higher.
- Heat leftovers thoroughly to at least 165°F.

Keep Cold Foods Cold

- When running errands, stop at the grocery store last. When you get home, refrigerate the perishable groceries (such as meats and dairy products) immediately. Do not leave perishables in the car any longer than it takes for ice cream to melt.
- Put packages of raw meat, fish, or poultry on a plate before refrigerating to prevent juices from dripping on food stored below.
- Buy only foods that are solidly frozen in store freezers.
- Keep cold foods at 40°F or less; keep frozen foods at 0°F or less (keep a thermometer in the refrigerator).
- Marinate meats in the refrigerator, not on the counter.

resistance.[36] Patients tend to accumulate abdominal fat and lose fat from the face, arms, and legs. Thus they appear to be thin except for a "pot belly." Also observed are breast enlargement (in both men and women), fat accumulation at the base of the neck (called **buffalo hump**), and benign growths composed of fat tissue (called **lipomas**). The changes in body composition are often disfiguring and may cause physical discomfort; moreover, patients often develop hypertriglyceridemia, low HDL cholesterol levels, glucose intolerance, and hyperinsulinemia. The reasons for the development of lipodystrophy are unknown.

Weight Loss and Wasting Even with effective treatment of HIV infection, weight loss and wasting are ongoing problems for HIV-infected patients.[37] Wasting has been linked with accelerated disease progression, reduced strength, and fatigue. In the later stages of AIDS, wasting is severe and increases the risk of death.■ Much as in cancer, the wasting associated with HIV infection has many causes: anorexia and inadequate food intake, altered metabolism, malabsorption, chronic diarrhea, and food-drug interactions.

■ The Centers for Disease Control defines **AIDS-related wasting syndrome** as a 10% weight loss within a six-month period accompanied by diarrhea or fever for more than 30 days without a known cause.

buffalo hump: the accumulation of fatty tissue at the base of the neck.

lipomas (lih-POE-muz): benign tumors composed of fatty tissue.

thrush: a fungal infection of the mouth and esophagus caused by *Candida albicans*. It coats the tongue with a milky film and leads to mouth ulcers, altered taste sensations, and pain on chewing and swallowing. The medical term for this infection is *candidiasis*.

Anorexia and Reduced Food Intake Poor food intake is a key factor in the development of wasting. Anorexia and reduced food intake may result from various factors, including the following:

- *Emotional distress and pain.* The physical and social problems that accompany chronic illness may cause fear, anxiety, and depression, which contribute to anorexia. Pain, which often develops due to disease complications, may cause anorexia and difficulty with eating.
- *Oral infections.* The oral infections associated with HIV infection cause discomfort and interfere with food consumption. One common infection is **thrush,** which alters taste sensitivity, reduces the flow of saliva, and causes

- Refrigerate leftovers promptly; use shallow containers to cool foods faster; use leftovers within three to four days.
- Thaw meats or poultry in the refrigerator, not at room temperature. If you must hasten thawing, use cool water (changed every 30 minutes) or a microwave oven.
- Freeze meat, fish, or poultry immediately if not planning to use within a few days.

In General

- Do not reuse disposable containers; use nondisposable containers or recycle instead.
- Do not taste food that is suspect. "If in doubt, throw it out."
- Throw out foods with danger-signaling odors. Be aware, though, that most food-poisoning bacteria are odorless, colorless, and tasteless.
- Do not buy or use items that have broken seals or mangled packaging; such containers cannot protect against microbes, insects, spoilage, or even vandalism. Check safety seals, buttons, and expiration dates.
- Follow label instructions for storing and preparing packaged and frozen foods; throw out foods that have been thawed or refrozen.
- Discard foods that are discolored, moldy, or decayed or that have been contaminated by insects or rodents.

For Specific Food Items

- *Canned goods.* Carefully discard food from cans that leak or bulge so that other people and animals will not accidentally ingest it; before canning, seek professional advice from the USDA Extension Service (check your phone book under U.S. government listings, or ask directory assistance).
- *Milk and cheeses.* Use only pasteurized milk and milk products. Aged cheeses, such as cheddar and swiss, do well for an hour or two without refrigeration, but should be refrigerated or stored in an ice chest for longer periods.
- *Eggs.* Use clean eggs with intact shells. Do not eat eggs, even pasteurized eggs, raw; raw eggs are commonly found in Caesar salad dressing, eggnog, cookie dough, hollandaise sauce, and key lime pie. Cook eggs until whites are firmly set and yolks begin to thicken.
- *Honey.* Honey may contain dormant bacterial spores, which can awaken in the human body to produce botulism. In adults, this poses little hazard, but infants under one year of age should never be fed honey. Honey can accumulate enough toxin to kill an infant; it has been implicated in several cases of sudden infant death. (Honey can also be contaminated with environmental pollutants picked up by the bees.)
- *Mayonnaise.* Commercial mayonnaise may actually help a food to resist spoilage because of the acid content. Still, keep it cold after opening.
- *Mixed salads.* Mixed salads of chopped ingredients spoil easily because they have extensive surface area for bacteria to invade, and they have been in contact with cutting boards, hands, and kitchen utensils that easily transmit bacteria to food (regardless of their mayonnaise content). Chill them well before, during, and after serving.
- *Picnic foods.* Choose foods that last without refrigeration such as fresh fruits and vegetables, breads and crackers, and canned spreads and cheeses that can be opened and used immediately. Pack foods cold, layer ice between foods, and keep foods out of water.
- *Seafood.* Buy only fresh seafood that has been properly refrigerated or iced. Cooked seafood should be stored separately from raw seafood to avoid cross-contamination.

pain with swallowing. Another, **herpes simplex virus,** causes painful mouth ulcers that interfere with chewing and swallowing. These infections may also contribute to anorexia.

- *Respiratory infections.* Pneumonia and tuberculosis, which frequently occur in patients with HIV infection, cause fever and pain that contribute to anorexia. Some patients find that the supplemental oxygen they need makes eating more difficult.
- *Fatigue, lethargy, and dementia.* Fatigue is a common complication of HIV infection, even during the early stages. Fatigue may be a consequence of weight loss and wasting, infection, or anemia. In the later stages of illness, lethargy and dementia may develop and interfere with food intake.
- *Cancer.* As described earlier in this chapter, cancer leads to anorexia for numerous reasons. In addition, **Kaposi's sarcoma,** a type of cancer frequently associated with HIV infection, can cause lesions and obstructions in the esophagus that make eating painful.
- *Medications.* Medications that treat HIV infection, other infections, and cancer often cause anorexia, taste alterations and food aversions, nausea, vomiting, and diarrhea.

GI Tract Complications Gastrointestinal complications may result from HIV infection (due to immune suppression), opportunistic infections, and medications.[38] In addition to the oral infections described previously, infections commonly develop in the stomach and intestines. Advanced AIDS is often accompanied by characteristic changes in the small intestinal lining, likely caused by GI infection: villi appear shortened and flattened, and the absorptive area is substantially reduced.■ These changes contribute to malabsorption, steatorrhea, and diarrhea.

■ The AIDS-related abnormalities in the intestinal mucosa are sometimes referred to as *HIV enteropathy* (EN-ter-OP-ah-thy).

herpes simplex virus: a common virus that can cause mouth lesions in HIV-infected individuals.

Kaposi's (cap-OH-seez) **sarcoma:** a type of cancer that is rare in the general population but common in people with HIV infections.

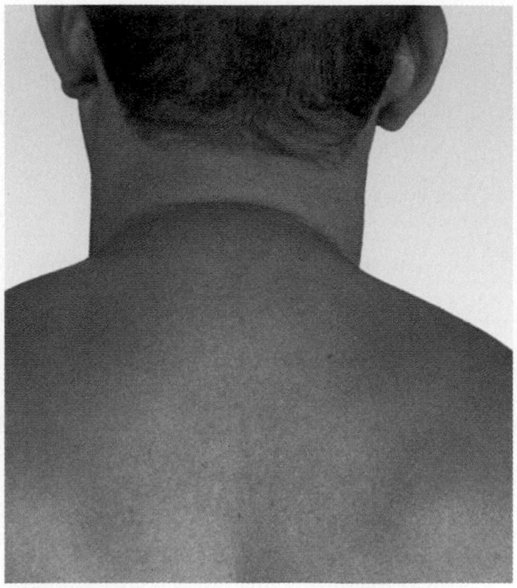

© Mediscan/Visuals Unlimited

HIV-lipodystrophy is sometimes evident by the accumulation of fatty tissue at the base of the neck, referred to as *buffalo hump.*

As described previously, many patients become unable to tolerate the medications used to suppress HIV and develop nausea, vomiting, and diarrhea. Use of medications that treat GI viral, parasitic, and fungal infections contributes to bacterial overgrowth. Thus HIV-infected patients face an extremely high risk of malnutrition due to the combination of intestinal malabsorption, bacterial overgrowth, and nutrient losses from vomiting and diarrhea.

Treatments for HIV Infection

Although there is no cure for HIV infection, treatments can help to slow its progression, reduce complications, and alleviate pain. The standard treatment for suppressing HIV infection is called *highly active antiretroviral therapy (HAART)* and combines two or more antiretroviral drugs. Table 29-7 lists the major drug categories included in antiretroviral therapy and describes the drugs' modes of action.[39] These antiretroviral agents have multiple adverse effects that make their long-term use difficult to tolerate. In addition to the GI effects discussed previously, side effects include rashes, headache, anemia, tingling and numbness, hepatitis, pancreatitis, and kidney stones. Thus, although HAART has improved life span and quality of life for many patients, the drug regimens are difficult to adhere to and cause complications that require continual management.

Control of Anorexia and Wasting Appetite stimulants, physical activity, and anabolic hormones have been successful for reversing weight loss and increasing lean body mass in HIV-infected patients.[40] The medications megestrol acetate and dronabinol (described on p. 886) are sometimes prescribed to stimulate appetite and help with weight gain. Testosterone and human growth hormone have demonstrated positive effects on nitrogen balance and lean tissue mass, especially in combination with resistance training.

Control of Lipodystrophy Treatment strategies for lipodystrophy are under investigation. Both aerobic activity and resistance training may help reduce abdominal fat, although some patients opt for cosmetic surgery.[41] Patients may require alternate antiretroviral drugs to alleviate symptoms. Medications may be needed to treat abnormal blood lipids and insulin resistance.

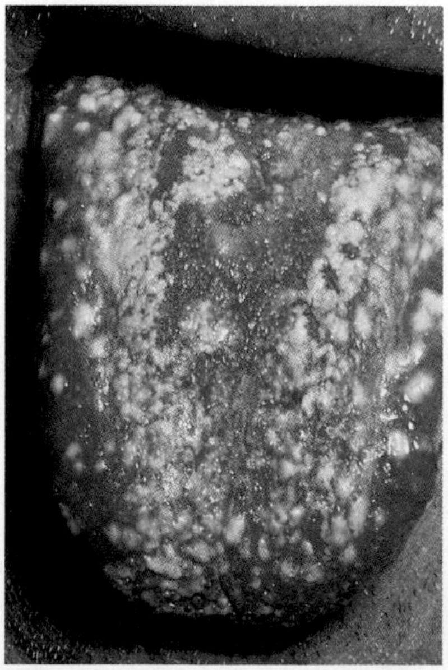

© Biophoto Associates/Photo Researchers, Inc.

The oral infection thrush is easily identified by the characteristic milky white patches on the tongue.

Alternative Therapies Like cancer patients, patients with HIV infection and AIDS are frequently tempted to try unconventional methods of treatment. Although many alternative therapies are harmless, they can be expensive at a time when financial security is of concern. Monitoring patients' use of dietary supplements is essential to reduce the possibility of drug-nutrient and drug-herb interactions.

TABLE 29-7 Antiretroviral Agents for Treatment of HIV Infection

Category	Examples	Mode of Action
Nucleoside reverse transcriptase inhibitors (NRTI)	Zidovudine (AZT) Didanosine Lamivudine	As analogs of the nucleosides needed for DNA synthesis, NRTI impair the ability of HIV's *reverse transcriptase* enzyme to produce usable copies of DNA.
Non-nucleoside reverse transcriptase inhibitors (NNRTI)	Nevirapine Delavirdine Efavirenz	NNRTI bind active sites on HIV's *reverse transcriptase* enzyme, blocking the ability of HIV to produce DNA copies of its genetic material.
Protease inhibitors (PI)	Saquinavir Ritonavir Indinavir	PI inhibit HIV's *protease* enzyme, which cleaves HIV's gene products into usable structural proteins.

Medical Nutrition Therapy

Nutrition assessment and counseling should begin as soon as a patient is diagnosed with HIV infection. The initial evaluation provides baseline data from which to monitor progress throughout the course of the disease. The assessment should include an evaluation of body composition. Follow-up measurements provide the information needed for adjusting diet and drug therapies.

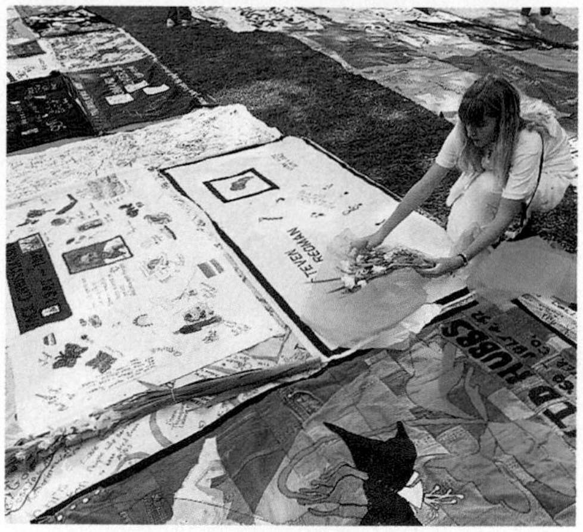

© Lauren Goodsmith/The Image Works

The countless lives touched by AIDS serve as a potent reminder of the need to continue the search for a cure.

Weight Maintenance A primary objective of nutrition therapy is to maintain weight and lean body mass.[42] Daily energy requirements may be 35 to 45 kcalories per kilogram body weight, and protein needs may be as high as 2.0 to 2.5 grams per kilogram. A regular program of resistance exercise can improve lean body mass and strength and correct some of the metabolic abnormalities (altered blood lipids and insulin resistance) that are common in HIV-infected patients.

Because patients are normally seen on an outpatient basis, health practitioners should consider factors that may interfere with food intake, appetite, and exercise and provide suggestions that may prevent future weight problems. If food consumption is difficult, small frequent feedings may be better tolerated than several large meals.[43] Encourage nutrient-dense snacks, protein or energy bars, and oral supplements if needed. Liquid formulas may be especially useful for the person who is too tired to eat or prepare meals. The "How to" on pp. 888–889 offers other suggestions for improving appetite, dealing with complications, and adding kcalories and protein to the diet.

Enteral and Parenteral Nutrition Support People with HIV infections may need aggressive nutrition support if they are unable to consume oral diets that are sufficient to prevent nutritional complications and unintentional weight loss. Tube feedings are preferred whenever the GI tract is functional; they can be given at night to supplement oral diets during the day. Preventing bacterial contamination of the formula is particularly important. Parenteral nutrition is reserved for patients who are unable to tolerate enteral nutrition, such as those with GI obstructions that prevent food intake. For individuals with severe malabsorption, orally administered hydrolyzed formulas containing medium-chain triglycerides may be as effective as parenteral nutrition for reversing weight loss and wasting.

Vitamins and Minerals Vitamin and mineral needs of people with HIV infections are highly variable, and little information is available concerning specific needs. Because nutrient deficiencies are likely to result from reduced food intake, malabsorption, diet-drug interactions, and nutrient losses, multivitamin-mineral supplements are usually recommended.

Metabolic Complications HIV patients using antiretroviral drugs frequently develop elevated triglyceride and LDL cholesterol levels and insulin resistance, and dietary adjustments are usually attempted before medications are prescribed.[44] Patients are advised to achieve or maintain desirable weight, replace saturated fats with monounsaturated and polyunsaturated fats, and limit intakes of *trans*-fatty acids and cholesterol.■ Complex carbohydrates are preferred over foods high in sugars. Regular physical activity is recommended for improving both blood lipid levels and insulin resistance. If problems persist, alternate antiretroviral medications are sometimes attempted.

■ Reminder: Additional suggestions for managing insulin resistance and hyperlipidemias are available in Chapters 26 and 27, respectively. Highlight 5 describes the benefits of replacing saturated and *trans* fats with mono- and polyunsaturated fats.

Food Safety The depressed immunity of people with HIV infections places them at extremely high risk of developing foodborne infections. Patients should be cautioned about their high susceptibility for foodborne illness and given detailed instructions about the safe handling and preparation of foods (review pp. 892–893). Water can also be a source of foodborne illness and is a common cause of **cryptosporidiosis** in HIV-infected individuals. Because water quality varies throughout the United States, local health departments should be consulted to determine if the local tap water is safe for patients to drink. If not, or to take additional safety

cryptosporidiosis (KRIP-toe-spo-rid-ee-OH-sis): a foodborne illness caused by the parasite *Cryptosporidium parvum*.

measures, water used for drinking and making ice cubes should be boiled for one minute. Some types of filtered and bottled waters are also safe, but not all.

IN SUMMARY By primarily attacking helper T cells, HIV causes progressive damage to immune function and may eventually lead to AIDS. Although improved drug therapies have slowed the progression of HIV infection, these drugs can cause the HIV-lipodystrophy syndrome, characterized by body fat redistribution, abnormal lipid levels, and insulin resistance. HIV infection is often associated with weight loss and wasting, anorexia, and various complications that affect food intake. Dietary adjustments, exercise, and medications can improve weight maintenance and prevent wasting, although nutrition support may be needed in some patients. Patients with HIV infections must pay strict attention to food safety guidelines to prevent foodborne infections. The case study below provides an opportunity to review the nutrition concerns of a person with HIV infection.

CASE STUDY

Travel Agent with HIV Infection

Three years ago, Mr. Meckler, a 34-year-old travel agent, sought medical help when he began feeling run-down and developed a painful white coating over his mouth and tongue. The presence of thrush and anemia alerted Mr. Meckler's physician to the possibility of an HIV infection.

When Mr. Meckler tested positive for an HIV infection, he and his family and friends were devastated by the news, but those closest to him have remained supportive. Mr. Meckler has gained weight and developed lipodystrophy and hypertriglyceridemia during the three years since he began antiretroviral drug therapy. Mr. Meckler is 6 feet tall and currently weighs 190 pounds. He occasionally develops diarrhea and sometimes anorexia.

1. What is Mr. Meckler's percent ideal body weight (%IBW)? What is lipodystrophy, and what is its typical pattern in people with HIV infections? Describe an appropriate diet for Mr. Meckler.
2. What suggestions can you give Mr. Meckler for the times he has trouble with diarrhea or anorexia? What factors can lead to diarrhea or contribute to anorexia in people with HIV infections?
3. Describe how HIV infection can lead to wasting as the disease progresses to the later stages.
4. How will Mr. Meckler's diet change if wasting becomes a problem for him?

DIET-DRUG INTERACTIONS

Anabolic Agents
Testosterone, testosterone derivatives (*oxandrolone, nandrolone,* and *oxymetholone*), and *growth hormone* may be used to promote weight gain, specifically a gain of lean body mass. These medications can be taken without regard to food, and nutrition-related side effects are uncommon.

Antidiarrheals
For *antidiarrheals,* see p. 762.

Antinauseants
For *antinauseants,* see p. 731.

Antineoplastics
About 80 antineoplastic agents are in use. Many of these drugs can cause nausea and vomiting, which often begin a few hours after treatment and resolve shortly thereafter. In some cases, the problems may last for several days, and antinauseants may be prescribed. Mouth sores, taste alterations, fatigue, anemia, diarrhea, and constipation are also associated with many antineoplastic drugs.

Megestrol acetate is used as both an antineoplastic agent and an appetite stimulant. Megestrol acetate and some antineoplastic agents that act as hormones (including testosterone) can cause weight gain. Fluid and sodium retention can also occur, although these side effects are not common.

Antiretrovirals
The nucleoside reverse transcriptase inhibitors include *zidovudine (AZT), didanosine,* and *lamivudine.* Zidovudine and lamivudine can be taken without regard to food; zidovudine can cause nausea and vomiting. Patients who use didanosine should avoid aluminum- and

magnesium-containing antacids. Didanosine can lead to nausea and vomiting and should be taken one hour before or two hours after meals.

The non-nucleoside reverse transcriptase inhibitors include *nevirapine* and *delavirdine,* which must be taken one hour apart from antacids. Neither is associated with significant nutrition-related side effects.

The protease inhibitors include *saquinavir, ritonavir,* and *indinavir.* Saquinavir should be taken within two hours of a meal. Ritonavir is better absorbed with food and should be taken with meals. Ritonavir can cause nausea, vomiting, diarrhea, taste alterations, and abdominal pain. Indinavir should be taken one hour before or two hours after meals; however, people who experience nausea and abdominal pain can consume a light meal (less than 300 kcalories) when taking the medication. Indinavir can lead to kidney stones, so patients using this medication are encouraged to consume fluids liberally.

Appetite Stimulants
For *appetite stimulants,* see p. 782.

Immunosuppressants
For *immunosuppressants,* see pp. 762, 783, 870.

NUTRITION ASSESSMENT CHECKLIST for People with Cancer or HIV Infections

Medical History

Check the medical record to determine:

- ☐ Type and extent of cancer
- ☐ Stage of HIV infection

Review the medical record for complications that may alter medical nutrition therapy including:

- ☐ Malnutrition/wasting
- ☐ Anorexia
- ☐ Taste alterations
- ☐ Dry mouth/oral infections
- ☐ GI symptoms/infections
- ☐ Insulin resistance
- ☐ Hyperlipidemias
- ☐ Altered organ function

Medications

For patients with cancer or HIV infections:

- ☐ Check the medications prescribed to identify potential diet-drug interactions.
- ☐ Recommend that antinauseants be used during meals, if needed.
- ☐ Ask about use of dietary supplements, including herbal remedies.

For cancer patients who require chemotherapy:

- ☐ Recommend strategies to prevent food aversions.
- ☐ Offer suggestions for managing drug-related complications.

For HIV-infected patients using antiretroviral drug therapy:

- ☐ Remind patients that some drugs are better absorbed with foods and others must be taken on an empty stomach.
- ☐ Help patients work out a medication schedule that suits their lifestyle and is timed appropriately in regard to food intake.
- ☐ Offer suggestions for managing drug-related complications.

Dietary Intake

For patients with poor food intakes and weight loss:

- ☐ Determine the reasons for reduced food intake.
- ☐ Offer appropriate suggestions to improve food intake.
- ☐ Provide interventions before weight loss progresses too far.

For patients with HIV infections who experience weight gain, elevated triglyceride or LDL cholesterol levels, or hyperglycemia:

- ☐ Assess diet for energy, total fat, types and amounts of specific fats, carbohydrates, fiber, and sugars.
- ☐ For hyperlipidemias, recommend a diet low in saturated fat, *trans*-fatty acids, and sugars.
- ☐ For hyperglycemia, recommend a consistent carbohydrate intake that emphasizes complex carbohydrates.
- ☐ Recommend regular physical activity for weight control and for improving blood lipid levels and insulin resistance.

Anthropometric Data

Take baseline height and weight measurements, monitor weight regularly, and make dietary adjustments promptly, if necessary. Baseline and periodic body composition measurements should be performed in HIV-infected patients using antiretroviral drug therapy.

Laboratory Tests

Note that albumin and serum proteins may be reduced in patients with cancer or HIV infections, especially in those experiencing wasting. Check laboratory tests for indications of:

- ☐ Anemia
- ☐ Dehydration
- ☐ Elevated triglyceride levels
- ☐ Elevated LDL cholesterol levels
- ☐ Hyperglycemia

For patients with HIV infections, disease progression is evaluated by checking:

- ☐ Helper T cell counts
- ☐ Viral load

Clinical Signs

Look for physical signs of:

- ☐ Wasting and protein-energy malnutrition
- ☐ Dehydration (especially for those with fever, vomiting, or diarrhea)
- ☐ Oral infections
- ☐ Karposi's sarcoma

NUTRITION ON THE NET

Access these websites for further study of topics covered in this chapter.

- Find updates and quick links to these and other nutrition-related sites at our website: **www.wadsworth.com/nutrition**
- To learn more about cancer, including risk factors, prevention, screening, detection, treatments (including nutrition), and support networks, visit these sites:

  American Cancer Society: **www.cancer.org**

  National Cancer Institute: **www.nci.nih.gov**

  CancerSource: **www.cancersource.com**

  American Institute for Cancer Research: **www.aicr.org**

  American Association for Cancer Research: **www.aacr.org**
- To find additional information about HIV infection and AIDS, visit these sites:

  The Body: **www.thebody.com**

  AIDS Education Global Information System: **www.aegis.com**

  UCSF Center for HIV Information: **hivinsite.ucsf.edu**
- To review information about safe food handling, visit the FDA's Center for Food Safety and Applied Nutrition: **vm.cfsan.fda.gov**

STUDY QUESTIONS

These questions will help you review the chapter. You will find the answers in the discussions on the pages provided.

1. Describe the process of tumor formation. What factors contribute to cancer development? Discuss the dietary factors that may increase or decrease the risk of cancer. (pp. 880–883)
2. What is cancer cachexia? What factors promote its development? (p. 884)
3. Explain how cancer and its treatments can cause alterations in metabolism, anorexia, and reduced food intake. (pp. 885–886)
4. Discuss the elements of medical nutrition therapy for cancer and strategies that can improve food intake. (pp. 887–890)
5. Explain how HIV affects immune function and how HIV infection progresses to AIDS. (p. 891)
6. Describe the complications associated with HIV infection, such as the HIV-lipodystrophy syndrome, wasting, and complications involving the GI tract. Explain why the complications of HIV infection often result in anorexia and reduced food intake. (pp. 891–894)
7. Discuss the treatment of HIV infection and its complications. What is the medical nutrition therapy for HIV-infected and AIDS patients? (pp. 894–895)
8. Why are people with HIV infections highly susceptible to foodborne illness? Describe the measures that can be taken to prevent foodborne illness. (pp. 895–896)

These questions will help you prepare for an exam. Answers can be found on p. 900.

1. Which dietary substances may help to protect against cancer?
   a. alcohol
   b. well-cooked meats, poultry, and fish
   c. omega-6 fatty acids
   d. phytochemicals from fruits and vegetables
2. The metabolic changes that often result from cancer include:
   a. increased fat synthesis.
   b. increased protein turnover.
   c. reduced gluconeogenesis.
   d. reduced serum lipids.
3. An advantage of radiation therapy over chemotherapy is that:
   a. radiation is not damaging to rapidly dividing cells.
   b. radiation's side effects do not include malnutrition.
   c. radiation can be directed toward the regions affected by cancer.
   d. the radiation used is too weak to damage GI tissues.
4. Although many cancer patients lose weight, which type of cancer is often associated with weight *gain*?
   a. kidney cancer
   b. breast cancer
   c. colon cancer
   d. Karposi's sarcoma
5. Oral diets after bone marrow transplants may restrict:
   a. calcium-rich foods.
   b. carbohydrates.
   c. high-protein foods.
   d. raw fruits and vegetables.
6. The immune cells most seriously damaged by HIV are:
   a. B cells.
   b. helper T cells.
   c. natural killer cells.
   d. neutrophils.

7. Mouth sores in people with HIV infections are most frequently due to:
   a. oral infections.
   b. dehydration.
   c. malabsorption.
   d. foodborne illnesses.
8. HIV-lipodystrophy syndrome is characterized by these changes in body composition:
   a. increased central and peripheral fat.
   b. decreased central and peripheral fat.
   c. increased central and decreased peripheral fat.
   d. decreased central and increased peripheral fat.
9. The medications megestrol acetate and dronabinol:
   a. are used to promote weight gain.
   b. are protease inhibitors that fight HIV infection.
   c. treat common opportunistic infections that develop in AIDS patients.
   d. treat HIV-lipodystrophy syndrome.
10. To prevent cryptosporidiosis, a person with HIV infection may need to:
   a. cook meat, poultry, and fish to an appropriate internal temperature.
   b. avoid consuming undercooked eggs.
   c. avoid consuming foods prepared by people who are sick or who have skin infections.
   d. boil drinking water for one minute.

REFERENCES

1. Y. Mao and coauthors, Physical inactivity, energy intake, obesity and the risk of rectal cancer in Canada, *International Journal of Cancer* 105 (2003): 831–837; A. S. Furberg and I. Thune, Metabolic abnormalities (hypertension, hyperglycemia, and overweight), lifestyle (high energy intake and physical inactivity) and endometrial cancer risk in a Norwegian cohort, *International Journal of Cancer* 104 (2003): 669–676; E. Giovannucci, Diet, body weight, and colorectal cancer: A summary of the epidemiologic evidence, *Journal of Women's Health* 12 (2003): 173–182; H. Vainio, R. Kaaks, and F. Bianchini, Weight control and physical inactivity in cancer prevention: International evaluation of the evidence, *European Journal of Cancer Prevention* 2 (2002): S94–S100.
2. National Cancer Policy Board, Institute of Medicine, S. J. Curry, T. Byers, and M. Hewitt, eds., *Fulfilling the Potential of Cancer Prevention and Early Detection* (Washington, D.C.: National Academies Press, 2003), pp. 58–61; M. L. Slattery and coauthors, Lifestyle and colon cancer: An assessment of factors associated with risk, *American Journal of Epidemiology* 150 (1999): 869–877.
3. National Cancer Policy Board, 2003, pp. 59–60; J. B. Magen, The relationship between obesity and breast cancer risk and mortality, *Nutrition Reviews* 61 (2003): 73–76.
4. E. E. Calle and M. J. Thun, Obesity and cancer, *Oncogene* 23 (2004): 6365–6378; F. Bianchini and coauthors, Overweight, obesity, and cancer risk, *Lancet Oncology* 3 (2002): 565–574.
5. T. Sugimura and coauthors, Heterocyclic amines: Mutagens/carcinogens produced during cooking of meat and fish, *Cancer Science* 95 (2004): 290–299; J. S. Felton and coauthors, Impact of environmental exposures on the mutagenicity/carcinogenicity of heterocyclic amines, *Toxicology* 198 (2004): 135–145; P. Jakszyn and coauthors, Development of a food database of nitrosamines, heterocyclic amines, and polycyclic aromatic hydrocarbons, *Journal of Nutrition* 134 (2004): 2011–2014.
6. G. N. Wogan and coauthors, Environmental and chemical carcinogenesis, *Seminars in Cancer Biology* 14 (2004): 473–486.
7. P. L. Zock, Dietary fats and cancer, *Current Opinions in Lipidology* 12 (2001): 5–10.
8. P. Terry and coauthors, Fatty fish consumption and risk of prostate cancer, *Lancet* 357 (2001): 1764–1766; Zock, 2001.
9. National Cancer Policy Board, 2003, p. 77; P. D. Terry and coauthors, Intakes of fish and marine fatty acids and the risks of cancers of the breast and prostate and of other hormone-related cancers: A review of the epidemiologic evidence, *American Journal of Clinical Nutrition* 77 (2003): 532–543.
10. L. H. Kushi and coauthors, Cereals, legumes, and chronic disease risk reduction: Evidence from epidemiologic studies, *American Journal of Clinical Nutrition* 70 (1999): 451S–458S.
11. American Cancer Society 2001 Nutrition and Physical Activity Guidelines Advisory Committee, *American Cancer Society Guidelines on Nutrition and Physical Activity for Cancer,* available from www.cancer.org or upon request from the American Cancer Society at (800) ACS-2345.
12. H. S. Rugo, Paraneoplastic syndromes and other non-neoplastic effects of cancer, in L. Goldman and D. Ausiello, eds., *Cecil Textbook of Medicine* (Philadelphia: Saunders, 2004), pp. 1124–1131.
13. Rugo, 2004.
14. Rugo, 2004.
15. B. Eldridge and coauthors, Nutrition and the patient with cancer, in A. M. Coulston, C. L. Rock, and E. R. Monsen, eds., *Nutrition in the Prevention and Treatment of Disease* (San Diego: Academic Press, 2001), pp. 397–412.
16. J. R. Bertino and W. Hait, Principles of cancer therapy, in L. Goldman and D. Ausiello, eds., *Cecil Textbook of Medicine* (Philadelphia: Saunders, 2004), pp. 1137–1150.
17. Eldridge and coauthors, 2001.
18. S. E. Salmon and A. C. Sartorelli, Cancer chemotherapy, in B. G. Katzung, ed., *Basic and Clinical Pharmacology* (New York: Lange Medical Books/McGraw-Hill, 2001), pp. 923–958.
19. Bertino and Hait, 2004.
20. Bertino and Hait, 2004.
21. S. Z. Pavletic and J. M. Vose, Hematopoietic stem cell transplantation, in L. Goldman and D. Ausiello, eds., *Cecil Textbook of Medicine* (Philadelphia: Saunders, 2004), pp. 999–1003.
22. Eldridge and coauthors, 2001.
23. M. Tomiska, Palliative treatment of cancer anorexia with oral suspension of megestrol acetate, *Neoplasma* 50 (2003): 227–233.
24. T. R. Kosten and L. E. Hollister, Drugs of abuse, in B. G. Katzung, ed., *Basic and Clinical Pharmacology* (New York: Lange Medical Books/McGraw-Hill, 2001), pp. 532–547.
25. M. A. Richardson and coauthors, Complementary/alternative medicine use in a comprehensive cancer center and the implications for oncology, *Journal of Clinical Oncology* 18 (2000): 2505–2514.
26. Richardson and coauthors, 2000.
27. B. Bruemmer and coauthors, The association between vitamin C and vitamin E supplement use before hematopoietic stem cell transplant and outcomes to two years, *Journal of the American Dietetic Association* 103 (2003): 982–990; H. E. Seifried and coauthors, The antioxidant conundrum in cancer, *Cancer Research* 63 (2003): 4295–4298; M. Markman, Safety issues in using complementary and alternative medicine, *Journal of Clinical Oncology* 20 (2002): 39S–41S.
28. Markman, 2002.
29. Bruemmer and coauthors, 2003; Seifried and coauthors, 2003.
30. M. A. Richardson, Biopharmacologic and herbal therapies for cancer: Research update from NCCAM, *Journal of Nutrition* 131 (2004): 3037S–3040S.
31. Eldridge and coauthors, 2001.
32. Eldridge and coauthors, 2001.
33. S. Escott-Stump, *Nutrition and Diagnosis-Related Care* (Baltimore: Lippincott Williams & Wilkins, 2002), pp. 525–531.
34. J. A. McInnes and M. T. Knobf, Weight gain and quality of life in women treated with adjuvant chemotherapy for early-stage breast cancer, *Oncology Nursing Forum* 28 (2001): 675–684.
35. A. L. Schwartz, Exercise and weight gain in breast cancer patients receiving chemotherapy, *Cancer Practice* 8 (2000): 231–237.
36. P. Koutkia and S. Grinspoon, HIV-associated lipodystrophy: Pathogenesis, prognosis, treatment, and controversies, *Annual Review of Medicine* 55 (2004): 303–317.
37. A. M. Tang and coauthors, Weight loss and survival in HIV-positive patients in the era of highly active antiretroviral therapy, *Journal of Acquired Immune Deficiency Syndromes* 31 (2002): 230–236; C. A. Wanke and coauthors, Weight loss and wasting remain common complications in individuals infected with human immunodeficiency virus in the era of highly active

antiretroviral therapy, *Clinical Infectious Diseases* 31(2000): 803–805.
38. J. G. Bartlett, Gastrointestinal manifestations of AIDS, in L. Goldman and D. Ausiello, eds., *Cecil Textbook of Medicine* (Philadelphia: Saunders, 2004), pp. 2168–2170.
39. Panel on Clinical Practices for Treatment of HIV Infection, *Guidelines for the Use of Antiretroviral Agents in HIV-1-Infected Adults and Adolescents,* October 29, 2004. Available from http://AIDSinfo.nih.gov (site visited November 28, 2004); S. Safrin, Antiviral agents, in B. G. Katzung, ed., *Basic and Clinical Pharmacology* (New York: Lange Medical Books/McGraw-Hill, 2001), pp. 823–844.
40. S. Grinspoon and K. Mulligan, Weight loss and wasting in patients infected with human immunodeficiency virus, *Clinical Infectious Diseases* 36 (2003): S69–S78.
41. Koutkia and Grinspoon, 2004.
42. J. Nerad and coauthors, General nutrition management in patients infected with human immunodeficiency virus, *Clinical Infectious Diseases* 36 (2003): S52–S62; Escott-Stump, 2002, pp. 614–617.
43. Escott-Stump, 2002, pp. 614–617.
44. M. Dube and M. Fenton, Lipid abnormalities, *Clinical Infectious Diseases* 36 (2003): S79–S83; M. C. Gelato, Insulin and carbohydrate dysregulation, *Clinical Infectious Diseases* 36 (2003): S91–S95.

ANSWERS

Study Questions (multiple choice)

1. d 2. b 3. c 4. b 5. d 6. b 7. a 8. c 9. a 10. d

HIGHLIGHT

Illness, Mental Health, and Nutrition

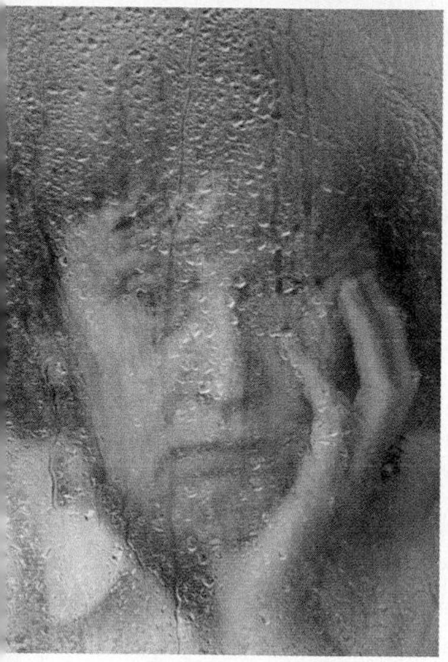

Mentally healthy individuals have the capacity to feed themselves well and maintain healthy lifestyles. People with mental and emotional problems, however, often have poor diets and lifestyle behaviors that contribute to ill health. Many of the conditions discussed in this textbook can lead to emotional distress and loss of hope, causing a person to lose interest in sustaining healthy behaviors. Some illnesses may result in **dementia,** the loss of intellectual function (see the accompanying glossary for *dementia* and other terms). Psychiatric illnesses, described in this highlight, can also have detrimental effects on diet and health. The health care professional who recognizes the relationship between physical illness and mental health is in a better position to offer effective care.

Impact of Emotions on Eating

To understand the connection between mental health and nutrition, consider how depression and anxiety affect your own eating habits. Do you lose your appetite? Overeat? Eat "junk" foods instead of balanced meals? Although transient emotional stress may have little impact on nutrition status, prolonged emotional difficulties can lead to underweight, overweight, or nutrient imbalances.

Mental health problems that are difficult to overcome, such as depression, are likely to lead to nutritional problems. Quite often people who are depressed lose interest in caring for themselves and in participating in usual activities such as eating, socializing, or pursuing hobbies. When these individuals cut themselves off from pleasurable activities and friendships, depression deepens and becomes a self-aggravating condition. Thus people who are depressed may have little interest in preparing and eating food.

GLOSSARY

delusions (dee-LOO-zhuns): false beliefs that are firmly maintained despite lack of proof or evidence to the contrary.

dementia (de-MEN-she-ah): irreversible loss of intellectual function.

mood disorders: mental illness characterized by episodes of severe depression or excessive excitement (mania) or both.

paranoia (PAHR-ah-NOY-ah): mental illness characterized by irrational distrust of others and delusions of persecution.

schizophrenia (SKITZ-oh-FREN-ee-ah): mental illness characterized by an altered concept of reality and, in some cases, delusions and hallucinations.

Reminder: *Alzheimer's disease* is a degenerative disease of the brain involving memory loss and major structural changes in neural networks.

Effect of Illness on Depression

Medical conditions that are strongly linked with depression include asthma, back problems, gastrointestinal disorders, genitourinary conditions, musculoskeletal conditions, and cardiovascular diseases.[1] Depression is most common in hospitalized patients, affecting an estimated 10 to 14 percent.[2] Both treatment outcomes and death rates are worsened by depression.[3]

Factors contributing to depression often include pain, loss of physical independence, and economic hardships imposed by serious illness. Terminal illnesses entail especially difficult emotional adjustments. Furthermore, when people become ill and lose significant amounts of weight, they may develop depression as they lose strength and become unable to perform routine tasks. Depression can be accompanied by anxiety, pessimism, and sleeping difficulties, all of which worsen depression.[4]

Disease treatments are sometimes overlooked as causes of depression. Medications linked to depression include some anticonvulsants, antihistamines, antihypertensives, antibiotics, and immunosuppressant agents.[5] Patients undergoing invasive treatments, recurring pain, and chronic disability are also at risk.

Caring health care professionals should remain alert for signs of depression. If it is recognized early, treatment can be initiated before health status markedly deteriorates. Therapeutic strategies may include support groups, an exercise program, psychotherapy, or, if needed, antidepressant medications.

Depression in the Elderly

Depression is not a normal consequence of aging; in fact, major depression actually becomes less common as people age.[6] When it does occur, disability and the onset of new medical illnesses are likely causes: Approximately 12 to 13 percent of elderly people who are hospitalized or receiving home health care experience depression.[7]

In addition to being associated with illness, depression in the elderly often results from loneliness associated with social isolation and the loss of loved ones, mobility, or a sense of purpose. Many authorities believe that among the elderly, loneliness is particularly relevant to malnutrition. For many individuals, eating is as much a social and psychological event as a biological one. Without companionship, appetite diminishes. Over 9 million elderly people over age 65 live alone.[8] Their most pressing need seems to be for companionship; food takes second place. Social interaction is important to mental health, and elderly people of all classes in our society, both the financially secure and the poverty-stricken, tend to become isolated. Jack Weinberg, professor of psychiatry at the University of Illinois, wrote perceptively of this problem:

> In our efforts to provide the aged with a proper diet, we often fail to perceive it is not what the older person eats but with whom that will be the deciding factor in proper care for him. The oft-repeated complaint of the older patient that he has little incentive to prepare food for only himself is not merely a statement of fact but also a rebuke to the questioner for failing to perceive his isolation and aloneness and to realize that food . . . for one's self lacks the condiment of another's presence which can transform the simplest fare to the ceremonial act with all its shared meaning.[9]

A spiral of sadness can develop when a lonely person neglects to eat well. Malnutrition worsens the apathy that is felt due to loneliness—then the person has even less energy with which to procure and prepare food. Be alert for signs of this problem in elderly people who live alone or who have recently lost a spouse or other loved one.

Nurses, counselors, and social workers can help their elderly patients work through depression and find solutions to their loneliness. Dietitians and diet technicians can help them understand how depression affects food intake and health and how eating a well-balanced diet can prevent additional health and nutrition problems. Meal plans that include easy-to-prepare foods and nutrition supplements can help some people meet their nutrient needs when they lack the motivation to eat. Encouraging patients to eat with family or friends or at congregate meal sites can help combat loneliness.

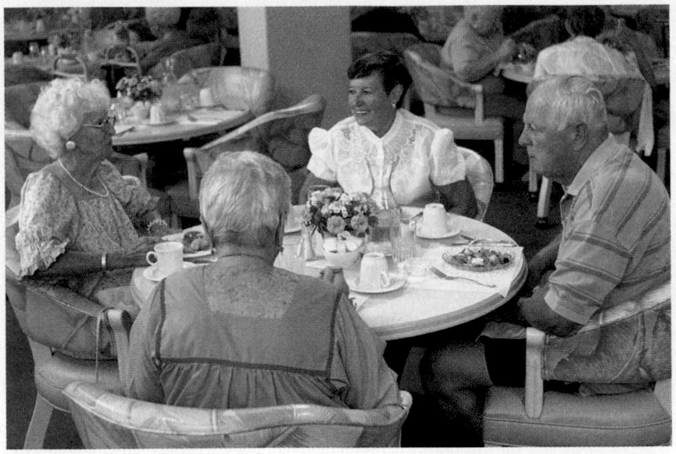

© Thinkstock/SuperStock

Elderly individuals may find companionship to be a more pressing need than food.

Psychiatric Illnesses

Individuals with psychiatric illnesses are likely to develop malnutrition and ill health if their illness affects their ability to take care of themselves. Psychiatric illnesses are often characterized by dementia, illogical thinking, **paranoia, delusions,** depression, or anxiety—any of which may lead to inappropriate eating habits and interfere with nutrition status. Some of these disorders include **schizophrenia,** Alzheimer's disease (see p. 566), **mood disorders,** and substance abuse. People with mental illnesses characterized by illogical thinking or dementia may need assistance in taking care of routine daily activities, including purchasing, preparing, and consuming food. Those who are paranoid may believe that foods are being used to poison them. People suffering from delusions may attribute magical powers to certain foods and insist on eating only those foods. Medications used in the treatment of mental illnesses can also cause weight gain or loss, interact with nutrients, and alter nutrition status.

Nutrition affects the brain and the mind, and the brain and the mind affect the way people eat. All are interrelated, and the wise health care professional will keep these interrelationships in focus.

REFERENCES

1. L. M. Gagnon and S. B. Patten, Major depression and its association with long-term medical conditions, *Canadian Journal of Psychiatry,* March 2002, available at **www.cpa-apc.org/publications/archives/cjp/2002/march/orMajorDepression.asp** (site visited November 29, 2004).
2. W. Katon and M. D. Sullivan, Depression and chronic medical illness, *Journal of Clinical Psychiatry* 51 (1990): 3S–11S.
3. V. Pignay-Demaria and coauthors, Depression and anxiety and outcomes of coronary artery bypass surgery, *Annals of Thoracic Surgery* 75 (2003): 314–321; S. von Ammon and coauthors, Medical illness, past depression, and present depression: A predictive triad for in-hospital mortality, *American Journal of Psychiatry* 158 (2001): 43–48.
4. K. H. Ladwig and coauthors, Gender differences in emotional disability and negative health perception in cardiac patients 6

months after stent implantation, *Journal of Psychosomatic Research* 48 (2000): 501–508.
5. C. Ryan and M. E. Shea, Recognizing depression in older adults: The role of the dietitian, *Journal of the American Dietetic Association* 96 (1996): 1042–1044.
6. Gagnon and Patten, 2002; Ryan and Shea, 1996.
7. M. G. Cole and N. Dendukuri, Risk factors for depression among elderly community subjects: A systematic review and meta-analysis, *American Journal of Psychiatry* 160 (2003): 1147–1156; M. L. Bruce and coauthors, Major depression in elderly home health care patients, *American Journal of Psychiatry* 159 (2002): 1367–1374.
8. National Council on Aging, Facts about older Americans, December 2002, www.ncoa.org/content.cfm?sectionID=106, visited Dececember 1, 2004.
9. J. Weinberg, Psychological implications of the nutritional needs of the elderly, *Journal of the American Dietetic Association* 60 (1972): 293–296.

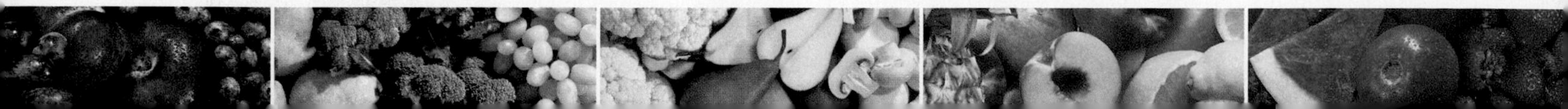

Appendixes

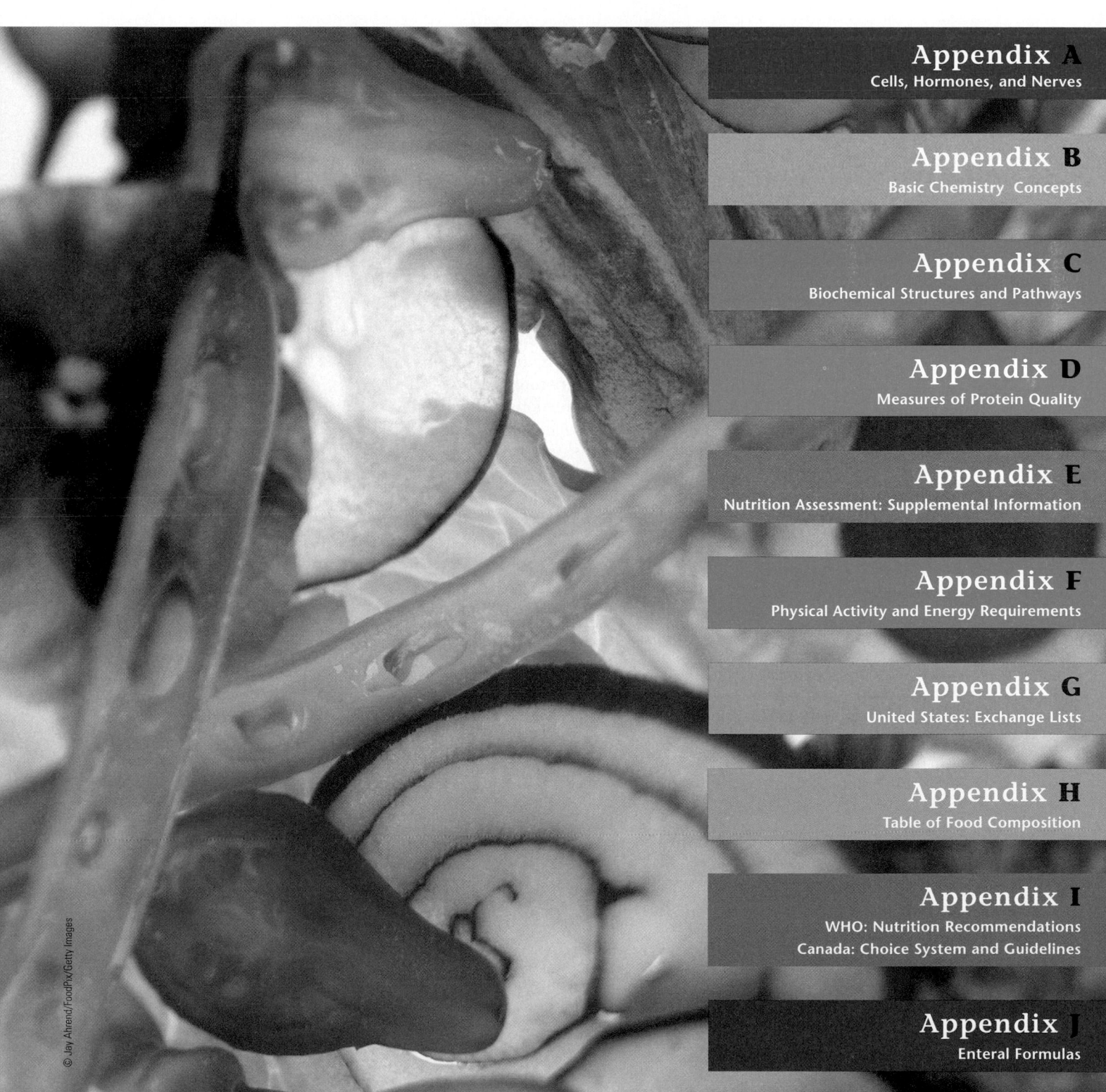

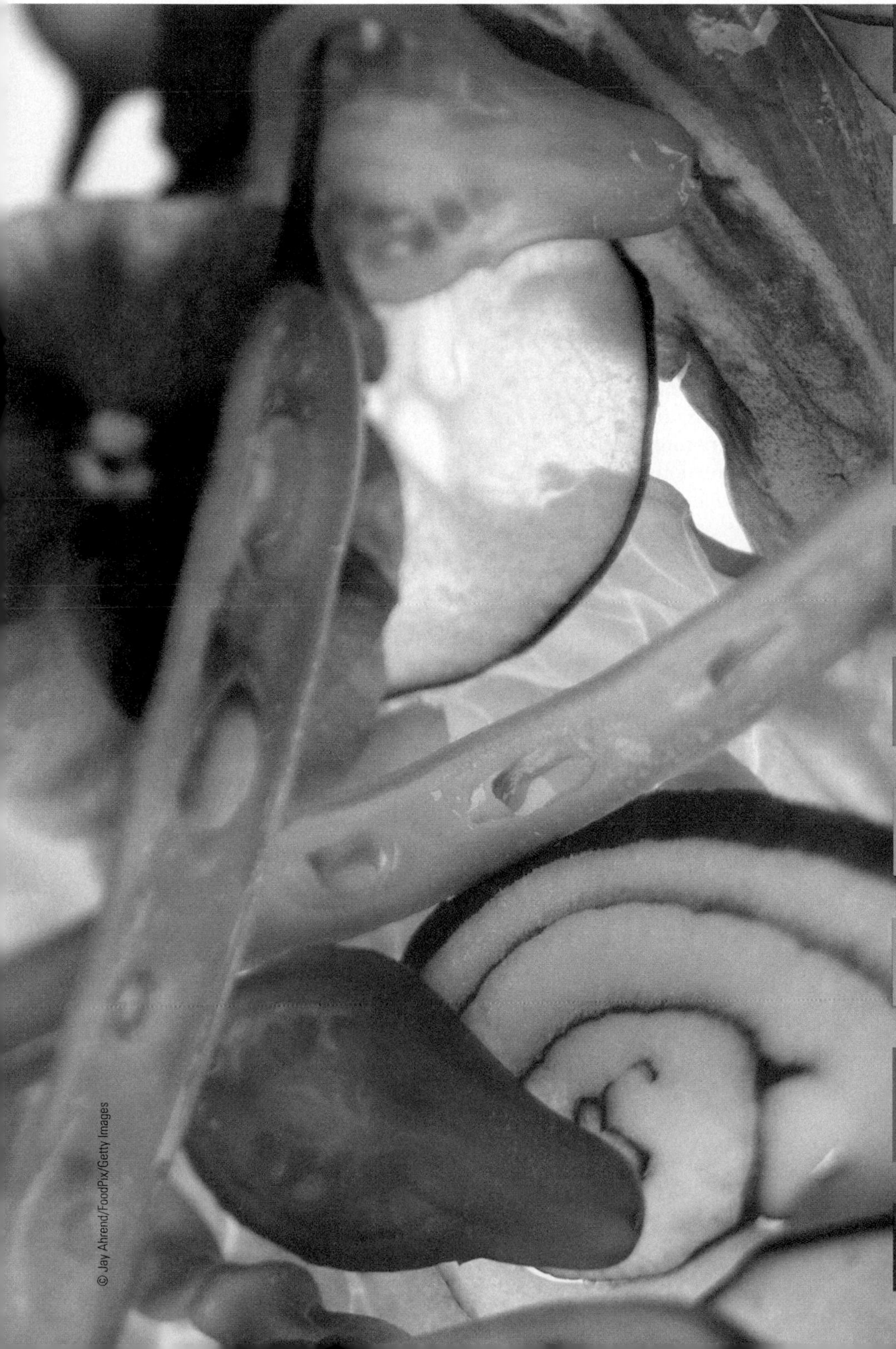
© Jay Ahrend/FoodPix/Getty Images

CONTENTS

Cells, Hormones, and Nerves

This appendix is offered as an optional chapter for readers who want to enhance their understanding of how the body coordinates its activities. The text presents a brief summary of the structure and function of the body's basic working unit (the cell) and of the body's two major regulatory systems (the hormonal system and the nervous system).

The Cell

The body's organs are made up of millions of cells and of materials produced by them. Each **cell** is specialized to perform its organ's functions, but all cells have common structures (see the accompanying glossary and Figure A-1). Every cell is contained within a **cell membrane.** The cell membrane assists in moving materials into and out of the cell, and some of its special proteins act as "pumps" (described in Chapter 6). Some features of cell membranes, such as microvilli (Chapter 3), permit cells to interact with other cells and with their environments in highly specific ways.

Inside the membrane lies the **cytoplasm,** which is filled with **cytosol,** or cell "fluid." The cytoplasm contains much more than just fluid, though. It is a highly organized system of fibers, tubes, membranes, particles, and subcellular **organelles** as complex as a city. These parts intercommunicate, manufacture and exchange materials, package and prepare materials for export, and maintain and repair themselves.

Within each cell is another membrane-enclosed body, the **nucleus.** Inside the nucleus are the **chromosomes,** which contain the genetic material, DNA. The DNA encodes all the instructions for carrying out the cell's activities. The role of DNA in coding for cell proteins is summarized in Figure 6-7 on p. 188. Chapter 6 also describes the variety of proteins produced by cells and the ways they perform the body's work.

Among the organelles within a cell are ribosomes, mitochondria, and lysosomes. Figure 6-7 briefly refers to the **ribosomes;** they assemble amino acids into proteins, following directions conveyed to them by RNA copies from the DNA in the chromosomes.

The **mitochondria** are made of intricately folded membranes that bear thousands of highly organized sets of enzymes on their inner and outer surfaces. Mitochondria are crucial to energy metabolism, described in Chapter 7, and muscles conditioned to work aerobically are packed with them. Their presence is implied whenever the TCA cycle and electron transport chain are mentioned because the mitochondria house the needed enzymes.*

The **lysosomes** are membranes that enclose degradative enzymes. When a cell needs to self-destruct or to digest materials in its surroundings, its lysosomes free their enzymes. Lysosomes are active when tissue repair or remodeling is taking place—for example, in cleaning up infections, healing wounds, shaping embryonic organs, and remodeling bones.

Besides these and other cellular organelles, the cell's cytoplasm contains a highly organized system of membranes, the **endoplasmic reticulum.** The ribosomes may either float free in the cytoplasm or be mounted on these membranes. A membranous surface dotted with ribosomes looks speckled under the microscope and is called "rough" endoplasmic reticulum; such a surface without ribosomes is called "smooth." Some intracellular membranes are organized into tubules that collect cellular materials, merge with the cell membrane, and discharge their contents to the outside of the cell; these

*For the reactions of glycolysis, the TCA cycle, and the electron transport chain, see Chapter 7 and Appendix C. The reactions of glycolysis take place in the cytoplasm; the conversion of pyruvate to acetyl CoA takes place in the mitochondria, as do the TCA cycle and electron transport chain reactions. The mitochondria then release carbon dioxide, water, and ATP as their end products.

GLOSSARY OF CELL STRUCTURES

cell: the basic structural unit of all living things.

cell membrane: the thin layer of tissue that surrounds the cell and encloses its contents; made primarily of lipid and protein.

chromosomes: a set of structures within the nucleus of every cell that contains the cell's genetic material, DNA, associated with other materials (primarily proteins).

cytoplasm (SIGH-toh-plazm): the cell contents, except for the nucleus.
- **cyto** = cell
- **plasm** = a form

cytosol: the fluid of cytoplasm; contains water, ions, nutrients, and enzymes.

endoplasmic reticulum (en-doh-PLAZ-mic reh-TIC-you-lum): a complex network of intracellular membranes. The **rough endoplasmic reticulum** is dotted with ribosomes, where protein synthesis takes place. The **smooth endoplasmic reticulum** bears no ribosomes.
- **endo** = inside
- **plasm** = the cytoplasm

Golgi (GOAL-gee) **apparatus:** a set of membranes within the cell where secretory materials are packaged for export.

lysosomes (LYE-so-zomes): cellular organelles; membrane-enclosed sacs of degradative enzymes.
- **lysis** = dissolution

mitochondria (my-toh-KON-dree-uh); singular **mitochondrion:** the cellular organelles responsible for producing ATP aerobically; made of membranes (lipid and protein) with enzymes mounted on them.
- **mitos** = thread (referring to their slender shape)
- **chondros** = cartilage (referring to their external appearance)

nucleus: a major membrane-enclosed body within every cell, which contains the cell's genetic material, DNA, embedded in chromosomes.
- **nucleus** = a kernel

organelles: subcellular structures such as ribosomes, mitochondria, and lysosomes.
- **organelle** = little organ

FIGURE A-1 The Structure of a Typical Cell

The cell shown might be one in a gland (such as the pancreas) that produces secretory products (enzymes) for export (to the intestine). The rough endoplasmic reticulum with its ribosomes produces the enzymes; the smooth reticulum conducts them to the Golgi region; the Golgi membranes merge with the cell membrane, where the enzymes can be released into the extracellular fluid.

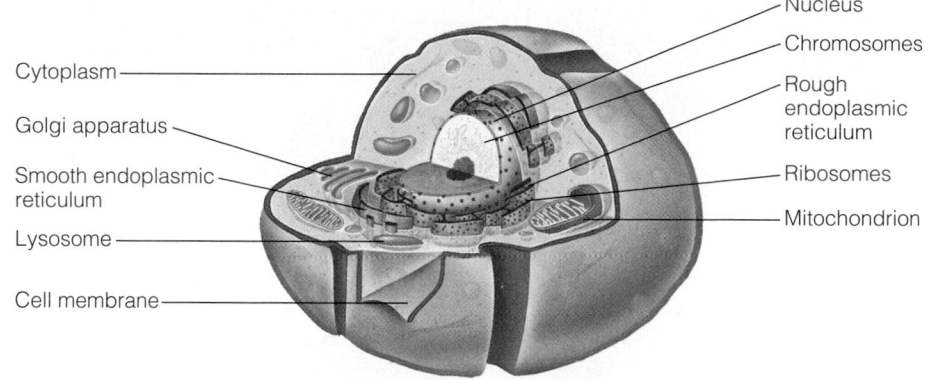

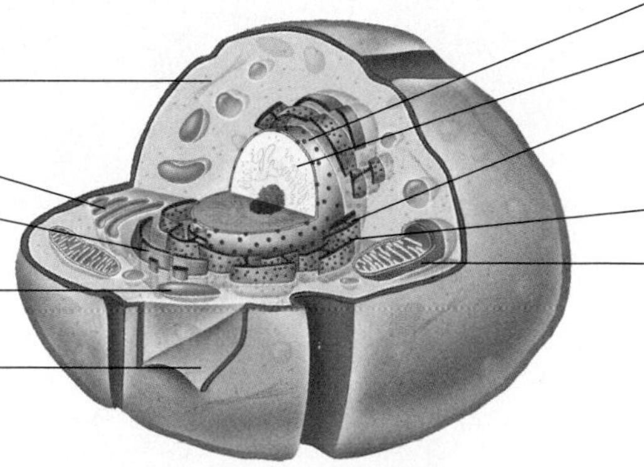
Cytoplasm
Golgi apparatus
Smooth endoplasmic reticulum
Lysosome
Cell membrane
Nucleus
Chromosomes
Rough endoplasmic reticulum
Ribosomes
Mitochondrion

membrane systems are named the **Golgi apparatus,** after the scientist who first described them. The rough and smooth endoplasmic reticula and the Golgi apparatus are continuous with one another, so secretions produced deep in the interior of the cell can be efficiently transported to the outside and released. These and other cell structures enable cells to perform the multitudes of functions for which they are specialized.

The actions of cells are coordinated by both hormones and nerves, as the next sections show. Among the types of cellular organelles are receptors for the hormones delivering instructions that originate elsewhere in the body. Some hormones penetrate the cell and its nucleus and attach to receptors on chromosomes, where they activate certain genes to initiate, stop, speed up, or slow down synthesis of certain proteins as needed. Other hormones attach to receptors on the cell surface and transmit their messages from there. The hormones■ are described in the next section; the nerves, in the one following.

The Hormones

A chemical compound—a **hormone**—originates in a gland and travels in the bloodstream. The hormone flows everywhere in the body, but only its target organs respond to it, because only they possess the receptors to receive it.

The hormones, the glands they originate in, and their target organs and effects are described in this section. Many of the hormones you might be interested in are included, but only a few are discussed in detail. Figure A-2 identifies the glands that produce the hormones, and the accompanying glossary defines the hormones discussed in this section.

Hormones of the Pituitary Gland and Hypothalamus

The anterior pituitary gland■ produces the following hormones, each of which acts on one or more target organs and elicits a characteristic response:

- **Adrenocorticotropin (ACTH)** acts on the adrenal cortex, promoting the production and release of its hormones.
- **Thyroid-stimulating hormone (TSH)** acts on the thyroid gland, promoting the production and release of thyroid hormones.
- **Growth hormone (GH)** acts on all tissues, promoting growth, fat breakdown, and the formation of antibodies.

■ The study of hormones and their effects is **endocrinology.**

■ The **pituitary gland** in the brain has two parts—the **anterior** (front) and the **posterior** (hind) parts.

ribosomes (RYE-boh-zomes): protein-making organelles in cells; composed of RNA and protein.
- **ribo** = containing the sugar ribose (in RNA)
- **some** = body

GLOSSARY OF HORMONES

adrenocorticotropin (ad-REE-noh-KORE-tee-koh-TROP-in) **ACTH:** a hormone, so named because it stimulates *(trope)* the adrenal cortex. The adrenal gland, like the pituitary, has two parts, in this case an outer portion *(cortex)* and an inner core *(medulla)*. The realease of ACTH is mediated by **corticotropin-releasing hormone (CRH).**

aldosterone: a hormone from the adrenal gland involved in blood pressure regulation.
- **aldo** = aldehyde

angiotensin: a hormone involved in blood pressure regulation that is activated by **renin** (REN-in), an enzyme from the kidneys.
- **angio** = blood vessels
- **tensin** = pressure
- **ren** = kidneys

antidiuretic hormone (ADH): the hormone that prevents water loss in urine (also called **vasopressin**).
- **anti** = against
- **di** = through
- **ure** = urine
- **vaso** = blood vessels
- **pressin** = pressure

calcitonin (KAL-see-TOH-nin): a hormone secreted by the thyroid gland that regulates (tones) calcium metabolism.

erythropoietin (eh-REE-throh-POY-eh-tin): a hormone that stimulates red blood cell production.
- **erythro** = red (blood cell)
- **poiesis** = creating (like poetry)

estrogens: hormones responsible for the menstrual cycle and other female characteristics.
- **oestrus** = the egg-making cycle
- **gen** = gives rise to

FIGURE A-2 The Endocrine System

These organs and glands release hormones that regulate body processes. An *endocrine gland* secretes its product directly into *(endo)* the blood; for example, the pancreas cells that produce insulin. An *exocrine gland* secretes its product(s) out *(exo)* to an epithelial surface either directly or through a duct; the sweat glands of the skin and the enzyme-producing glands of the pancreas are both examples. The pancreas is therefore both an endocrine and an exocrine gland.

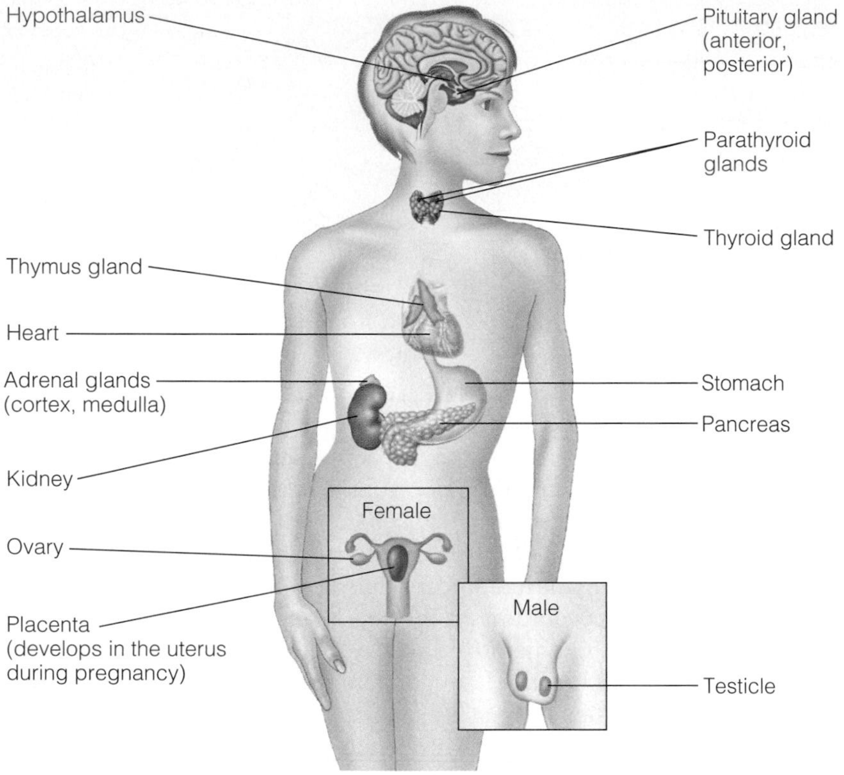

Hypothalamus
Pituitary gland (anterior, posterior)
Parathyroid glands
Thyroid gland
Thymus gland
Heart
Adrenal glands (cortex, medulla)
Stomach
Pancreas
Kidney
Female
Ovary
Male
Placenta (develops in the uterus during pregnancy)
Testicle

Appendix A

■ Hormones that are turned off by their own effects are said to be regulated by **negative feedback.**

follicle-stimulating hormone (FSH): a hormone that stimulates maturation of the ovarian follicles in females and the production of sperm in males. (The ovarian follicles are part of the female reproductive system where the eggs are produced.) The release of FSH is mediated by **follicle-stimulating hormone releasing hormone (FSH–RH).**

glucocorticoids: hormones from the adrenal cortex that affect the body's management of glucose.
- **gluco** = glucose
- **corticoid** = from the cortex

growth hormone (GH): a hormone secreted by the pituitary that regulates the cell division and protein synthesis needed for normal growth. The release of GH is mediated by **GH-releasing hormone (GHRH).**

hormone: a chemical messenger. Hormones are secreted by a variety of endocrine glands in response to altered conditions in the body. Each hormone travels to one or more specific target tissues or organs, where it elicits a specific response to maintain homeostasis.

luteinizing (LOO-tee-in-EYE-zing) **hormone (LH):** a hormone that stimulates ovulation and the development of the corpus luteum (the small tissue that develops from a ruptured ovarian follicle and secretes hormones); so called because the follicle turns yellow as it matures. In men, LH stimulates testosterone secretion. The release of LH is mediated by **luteinizing hormone–releasing hormone (LH–RH).**
- **lutein** = a yellow pigment

- **Follicle-stimulating hormone (FSH)** acts on the ovaries in the female, promoting their maturation, and on the testicles in the male, promoting sperm formation.
- **Luteinizing hormone (LH)** also acts on the ovaries, stimulating their maturation, the production and release of progesterone and estrogens, and ovulation; and on the testicles, promoting the production and release of testosterone.
- **Prolactin,** secreted in the female during pregnancy and lactation, acts on the mammary glands to stimulate their growth and the production of milk.

Each of these hormones has one or more signals that turn it on and another (or others) that turns it off.■ Among the controlling signals are several hormones from the hypothalamus:

- **Corticotropin-releasing hormone (CRH),** which promotes release of ACTH, is turned on by stress and turned off by ACTH when enough has been released.
- **TSH-releasing hormone (TRH),** which promotes release of TSH, is turned on by large meals or low body temperature.
- **GH-releasing hormone (GHRH),** which stimulates the release of growth hormone, is turned on by insulin.
- **GH-inhibiting hormone (GHIH** or **somatostatin),** which inhibits the release of GH and interferes with the release of TSH, is turned on by hypoglycemia

and/or physical activity and is rapidly destroyed by body tissues so that it does not accumulate.

- **FSH/LH–releasing hormone (FSH/LH–RH)** is turned on in the female by nerve messages or low estrogen and in the male by low testosterone.
- **Prolactin-inhibiting hormone (PIH)** is turned on by high prolactin levels and off by estrogen, testosterone, and suckling (by way of nerve messages).

Let's examine some of these controls. PIH, for example, responds to high prolactin levels (remember, prolactin promotes milk production). High prolactin levels ensure that milk is made and—by calling forth PIH—ensure that prolactin levels don't get too high. But when the infant is suckling—and creating a demand for milk—PIH is not allowed to work (suckling turns off PIH). The consequence: prolactin remains high, and milk production continues. Demand from the infant thus directly adjusts the supply of milk. The need is met through the interaction of the nerves and hormones.

As another example, consider CRH. Stress, perceived in the brain and relayed to the hypothalamus, switches on CRH. On arriving at the pituitary, CRH switches on ACTH. Then ACTH acts on its target organ, the adrenal cortex, which responds by producing and releasing stress hormones. The stress hormones trigger a cascade of events involving every body cell and many other hormones.

The numerous steps required to set the stress response in motion make it possible for the body to fine-tune the response; control can be exerted at each step. These two examples illustrate what the body can do in response to two different stimuli—producing milk in response to an infant's need and gearing up for action in an emergency.

The posterior pituitary gland produces two hormones, each of which acts on one or more target cells and elicits a characteristic response:

- **Antidiuretic hormone (ADH),** or **vasopressin,** acts on the arteries, promoting their contraction, and on the kidneys, preventing water excretion. ADH is turned on whenever the blood volume is low, the blood pressure is low, or the salt concentration of the blood is high (see Chapter 12). It is turned off by the return of these conditions to normal.
- **Oxytocin** acts on the uterus, inducing contractions, and on the mammary glands, causing milk ejection. Oxytocin is produced in response to reduced progesterone levels, suckling, or the stretching of the cervix.

Hormones That Regulate Energy Metabolism

Hormones produced by a number of different glands have effects on energy metabolism:

- Insulin from the pancreas beta cells is turned on by many stimuli, including raised blood glucose. It acts on cells to increase glucose and amino acid uptake into them and to promote the secretion of GHRH.
- Glucagon from the pancreas alpha cells responds to low blood glucose and acts on the liver to promote the breakdown of glycogen to glucose, the conversion of amino acids to glucose, and the release of glucose.
- Thyroxin from the thyroid gland responds to TSH and acts on many cells to increase their metabolic rate, growth, and heat production.
- Norepinephrine and epinephrine■ from the adrenal medulla respond to stimulation by sympathetic nerves and produce reactions in many cells that facilitate the body's readiness for fight or flight: increased heart activity, blood vessel constriction, breakdown of glycogen and glucose, raised blood glucose levels, and fat breakdown. Norepinephrine and epinephrine also influence the secretion of the many hormones from the hypothalamus that exert control on the body's other systems.
- Growth hormone (GH) from the anterior pituitary (already mentioned).
- **Glucocorticoids** from the adrenal cortex become active during times of stress and carbohydrate metabolism.

■ Norepinephrine and epinephrine were formerly called **noradrenalin** and **adrenalin,** respectively.

oxytocin (OCK-see-TOH-sin): a hormone that stimulates the mammary glands to eject milk during lactation and the uterus to contract during childbirth.
- **oxy** = quick
- **tocin** = childbirth

progesterone: the hormone of gestation (pregnancy).
- **pro** = promoting
- **gest** = gestation (pregnancy)
- **sterone** = a steroid hormone

prolactin (proh-LAK-tin): a hormone so named because it promotes *(pro)* the production of milk *(lacto).* The release of prolactin is mediated by **prolactin-inhibiting hormone (PIH).**

relaxin: the hormone of late pregnancy.

somatostatin (GHIH): a hormone that inhibits the release of growth hormone; the opposite of **somatotropin (GH).**
- **somato** = body
- **stat** = keep the same
- **tropin** = make more

testosterone: a steroid hormone from the testicles, or testes. The steroids, as explained in Chapter 5, are chemically related to, and some are derived from, the lipid cholesterol.
- **sterone** = a steroid hormone

thyroid-stimulating hormone (TSH): a hormone secreted by the pituitary that stimulates the thyroid gland to secrete its hormones—thyroxine and triiodothyronine. The release of TSH is mediated by **TSH-releasing hormone (TRH).**

Every body part is affected by these hormones. Each different hormone has unique effects; and hormones that oppose each other are produced in carefully regulated amounts, so each can respond to the exact degree that is appropriate to the condition.

Hormones That Adjust Other Body Balances

Hormones are involved in moving calcium into and out of the body's storage deposits in the bones:

- **Calcitonin** from the thyroid gland acts on the bones, which respond by storing calcium from the bloodstream whenever blood calcium rises above the normal range. It also acts on the kidneys to increase excretion of both calcium and phosphorus in the urine. Calcitonin plays a major role in infants and young children, but is less active in adults.
- Parathormone (parathyroid hormone or PTH) from the parathyroid gland responds to the opposite condition—lowered blood calcium—and acts on three targets: the bones, which release stored calcium into the blood; the kidneys, which slow the excretion of calcium; and the intestine, which increases calcium absorption.
- Vitamin D from the skin and activated in the kidneys acts with parathormone and is essential for the absorption of calcium in the intestine.

Figure 12-10 on p. 414 diagrams the ways vitamin D and the hormones calcitonin and parathormone regulate calcium homeostasis.

Another hormone has effects on blood-making activity:

- **Erythropoietin** from the kidneys is responsive to oxygen depletion of the blood and to anemia. It acts on the bone marrow to stimulate the making of red blood cells.

  Another hormone is special for pregnancy:

- **Relaxin** from the ovaries is secreted in response to the raised progesterone and estrogen levels of late pregnancy. This hormone acts on the cervix and pelvic ligaments to allow them to stretch so that they can accommodate the birth process without strain.

  Other agents help regulate blood pressure:

- **Renin** (an enzyme), from the kidneys, in cooperation with **angiotensin** in the blood responds to a reduced blood supply experienced by the kidneys and acts in several ways to increase blood pressure. Renin and angiotensin also stimulate the adrenal cortex to secrete the hormone aldosterone.
- **Aldosterone,** a hormone from the adrenal cortex, targets the kidneys, which respond by reabsorbing sodium. The effect is to retain more water in the bloodstream—thus, again, raising the blood pressure. Figure 12-3 (on p. 401) in Chapter 12 provides more details.

The Gastrointestinal Hormones

Several hormones are produced in the stomach and intestines in response to the presence of food or the components of food:

- Gastrin from the stomach and duodenum stimulates the production and release of gastric acid and other digestive juices and the movement of the GI contents through the system.
- Cholecystokinin from the duodenum signals the gallbladder and pancreas to release their contents into the intestine to aid in digestion.
- Secretin from the duodenum calls forth acid-neutralizing bicarbonate from the pancreas into the intestine and slows the action of the stomach and its secretion of acid and digestive juices.
- Gastric-inhibitory peptide from the duodenum and jejunum inhibits the secretion of gastric acid and slows the process of digestion.

These hormones are defined and presented in more detail in Chapter 3.

The Sex Hormones

There are three major sex hormones:

- **Testosterone** from the testicles is released in response to LH (described earlier) and acts on all the tissues that are involved in male sexuality, promoting their development and maintenance.
- **Estrogens** from the ovary are released in response to both FSH and LH and act similarly in females.
- **Progesterone** from the ovary's corpus luteum and from the placenta acts on the uterus and mammary glands, preparing them for pregnancy and lactation.

This brief description of the hormones and their functions should suffice to provide an awareness of the enormous impact these compounds have on body processes. The other overall regulating agency is the nervous system.

The Nervous System

The nervous system has a central control system—a sort of computer—that can evaluate information about conditions within and outside the body, and a vast system of wiring that receives information and sends instructions. The control unit is the brain and spinal cord, called the **central nervous system;** and the vast complex of wiring between the center and the parts is the **peripheral nervous system.** The smooth functioning that results from the system's adjustments to changing conditions is homeostasis.

The nervous system has two general functions: it controls voluntary muscles in response to sensory stimuli from them, and it controls involuntary, internal muscles and glands in response to nerve-borne and chemical signals about their status. In fact, the nervous system is best understood as two systems that use the same or similar pathways to receive and transmit their messages. The **somatic nervous system** controls the voluntary muscles; the **autonomic nervous system** controls the internal organs.

When scientists were first studying the autonomic nervous system, they noticed that when something hurt one organ of the body, some of the other organs reacted as if in sympathy for the afflicted one. They therefore named the nerve network they were studying the sympathetic nervous system. The term is still used today to refer to that branch of the autonomic nervous system that responds to pain and stress. The other branch is called the parasympathetic nervous system. (Think of the sympathetic branch as the responder when homeostasis needs restoring and the parasympathetic branch as the commander of function during normal times.) Both systems transmit their messages through the brain and spinal cord. Nerves of the two branches travel side by side along the same pathways to transmit their messages, but they oppose each other's actions (see Figure A-3).

An example will show how the sympathetic and parasympathetic nervous systems work to maintain homeostasis. When you go outside in cold weather, your skin's temperature receptors send "cold" messages to the spinal cord and brain. Your conscious mind may intervene at this point to tell you to zip your jacket, but let's say you have no jacket. Your sympathetic nervous system reacts to the external stressor, the cold. It signals your skin-surface capillaries to shut down so that your blood will circulate deeper in your tissues, where it will conserve heat. Your sympathetic nervous system also signals involuntary contractions of the small muscles just under the skin surface. The product of these muscle contractions is heat, and the visible result is goose bumps. If these measures do not raise your body temperature enough, then the sympathetic nerves signal your large muscle groups to shiver; the contractions of these large muscles produce still more heat. All of this activity adds up to a set of adjustments that maintain your homeostasis (with respect

GLOSSARY OF THE NERVOUS SYSTEM

autonomic nervous system: the division of the nervous system that controls the body's automatic responses. Its two branches are the **sympathetic** branch, which helps the body respond to stressors from the outside environment, and the **parasympathetic** branch, which regulates normal body activities between stressful times.
- **autonomos** = self-governing

central nervous system: the central part of the nervous system; the brain and spinal cord.

peripheral (puh-RIFF-er-ul) **nervous system:** the peripheral (outermost) part of the nervous system; the vast complex of wiring that extends from the central nervous system to the body's outermost areas. It contains both somatic and autonomic components.

somatic (so-MAT-ick) **nervous system:** the division of the nervous system that controls the voluntary muscles, as distinguished from the autonomic nervous system, which controls involuntary functions.
- **soma** = body

FIGURE A-3 The Organization of the Nervous System

The brain and spinal cord evaluate information about conditions within and outside the body, and the peripheral nerves receive information and send instructions.

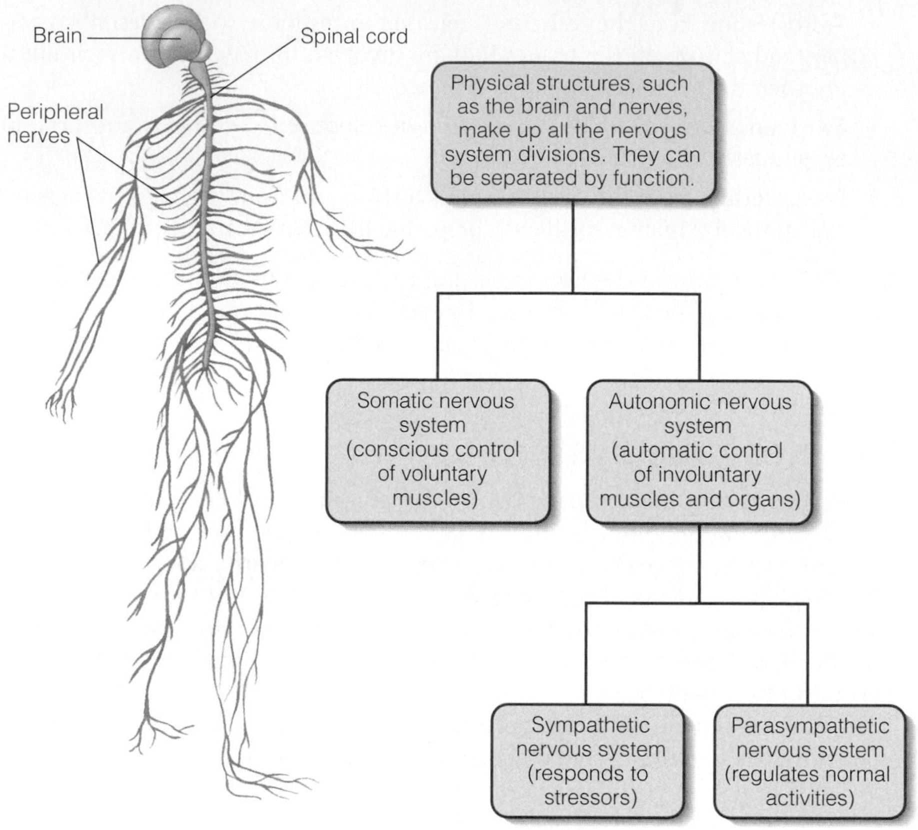
Brain
Spinal cord
Peripheral nerves
Physical structures, such as the brain and nerves, make up all the nervous system divisions. They can be separated by function.
Somatic nervous system (conscious control of voluntary muscles)
Autonomic nervous system (automatic control of involuntary muscles and organs)
Sympathetic nervous system (responds to stressors)
Parasympathetic nervous system (regulates normal activities)

to temperature) under conditions of external extremes (cold) that would throw it off balance. The cold was a stressor; the body's response was resistance.

Now let's say you come in and sit by a fire and drink hot cocoa. You are warm and no longer need all that sympathetic activity. At this point, your parasympathetic nerves take over; they signal your skin-surface capillaries to dilate again, your goose bumps to subside, and your muscles to relax. Your body is back to normal. This is recovery.

Putting It Together

The hormonal and nervous systems coordinate body functions by transmitting and receiving messages. The point-to-point messages of the nervous system travel through a central switchboard (the spinal cord and brain), whereas the messages of the hormonal system are broadcast over the airways (the bloodstream), and any organ with the appropriate receptors can pick them up. Nerve impulses travel faster than hormonal messages do—although both are remarkably swift. Whereas your brain's command to wiggle your toes reaches the toes within a fraction of a second and stops as quickly, a gland's message to alter a body condition may take several seconds or minutes to get started and may fade away equally slowly.

Together, the two systems possess every characteristic a superb communication network needs: varied speeds of transmission, along with private communication lines or public broadcasting systems, depending on the needs of the moment. The hormonal system, together with the nervous system, integrates the whole body's functioning so that all parts act smoothly together.

Basic Chemistry Concepts

This appendix is intended to provide the background in basic chemistry you need to understand the nutrition concepts presented in this book. Chemistry is the branch of natural science that is concerned with the description and classification of **matter,** the changes that matter undergoes, and the **energy** associated with these changes. The accompanying glossary defines matter, energy, and other related terms.

CONTENTS

Matter: The Properties of Atoms

Every substance has physical and chemical properties that distinguish it from all other substances and thus give it a unique identity. The physical properties include such characteristics as color, taste, texture, and odor, as well as the temperatures at which a substance changes its state (from a solid to a liquid or from a liquid to a gas) and the weight of a unit volume (its density). The chemical properties of a substance have to do with how it reacts with other substances or responds to a change in its environment so that new substances with different sets of properties are produced.

A physical change does not change a substance's chemical composition. The three physical states—ice, water, and steam—all consist of two hydrogen atoms and one oxygen atom bound together. In contrast, a chemical change occurs when an electric current passes through water. The water disappears, and two different substances are formed: hydrogen gas, which is flammable, and oxygen gas, which supports life.

Substances: Elements and Compounds

The smallest part of a substance that can exist separately without losing its physical and chemical properties is a **molecule.** If a molecule is composed of **atoms** that are alike, the substance is an **element** (for example, O_2). If a molecule is composed of two or more different kinds of atoms, the substance is a **compound** (for example, H_2O).

Just over 100 elements are known, and these are listed in Table B-1. A familiar example is hydrogen, whose molecules are composed only of hydrogen atoms linked together in pairs (H_2). On the other hand, over a million compounds are known. An example is the sugar glucose. Each of its molecules is composed of 6 carbon, 6 oxygen, and 12 hydrogen atoms linked together in a specific arrangement (as described in Chapter 4).

The Nature of Atoms

Atoms themselves are made of smaller particles. Within the atomic nucleus are protons (positively charged particles), and surrounding the nucleus are electrons (negatively charged particles). The number of protons (+) in the nucleus of an atom determines the number of electrons (−) around it. The positive charge on a proton is equal to the negative charge on an electron, so the charges cancel each other out and leave the atom neutral to its surroundings.

The nucleus may also include neutrons, subatomic particles that have no charge. Protons and neutrons are of equal mass, and together they give an atom its weight. Electrons bond atoms together to make molecules, and they are involved in chemical reactions.

Each type of atom has a characteristic number of protons in its nucleus. The hydrogen atom is the simplest of all. It possesses a single proton, with a single electron associated with it:

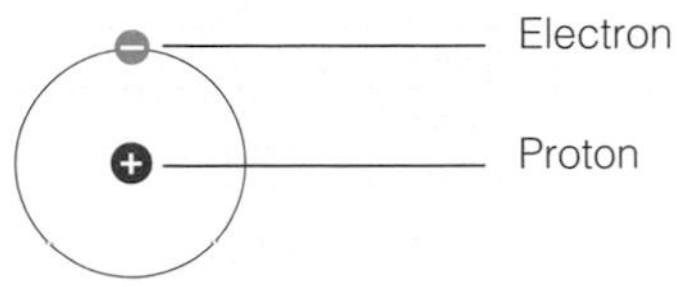
Electron
Proton

Hydrogen atom (H), atomic number 1.

Just as hydrogen always has one proton, helium always has two, lithium three, and so on. The atomic number of each element is the number of protons in the nucleus of that atom, and this never changes in a chemical reaction; it gives the atom its identity. The atomic numbers for the known elements are listed in Table B-1.

GLOSSARY

atoms: the smallest components of an element that have all of the properties of the element.

compound: a substance composed of two or more different atoms—for example, water (H_2O).

element: a substance composed of atoms that are alike—for example, iron (Fe).

energy: the capacity to do work.

matter: anything that takes up space and has mass.

molecule: two or more atoms of the same or different elements joined by chemical bonds. Examples are molecules of the element oxygen, composed of two oxygen atoms (O_2), and molecules of the compound water, composed of two hydrogen atoms and one oxygen atom (H_2O).

Appendix B

TABLE B-1 Chemical Symbols for the Elements

Number of Protons (Atomic Number)	Element	Number of Electrons in Outer Shell	Number of Protons (Atomic Number)	Element	Number of Electrons in Outer Shell
1	Hydrogen (H)	1	52	Tellurium (Te)	6
2	Helium (He)	2	53	Iodine (I)	7
3	Lithium (Li)	1	54	Xenon (Xe)	8
4	Beryllium (Be)	2	55	Cesium (Cs)	1
5	Boron (B)	3	56	Barium (Ba)	2
6	Carbon (C)	4	57	Lanthanum (La)	2
7	Nitrogen (N)	5	58	Cerium (Ce)	2
8	Oxygen (O)	6	59	Praseodymium (Pr)	2
9	Fluorine (F)	7	60	Neodymium (Nd)	2
10	Neon (Ne)	8	61	Promethium (Pm)	2
11	Sodium (Na)	1	62	Samarium (Sm)	2
12	Magnesium (Mg)	2	63	Europium (Eu)	2
13	Aluminum (Al)	3	64	Gadolinium (Gd)	2
14	Silicon (Si)	4	65	Terbium (Tb)	2
15	Phosphorus (P)	5	66	Dysprosium (Dy)	2
16	Sulfur (S)	6	67	Holmium (Ho)	2
17	Chlorine (Cl)	7	68	Erbium (Er)	2
18	Argon (Ar)	8	69	Thulium (Tm)	2
19	Potassium (K)	1	70	Ytterbium (Yb)	2
20	Calcium (Ca)	2	71	Lutetium (Lu)	2
21	Scandium (Sc)	2	72	Hafnium (Hf)	2
22	Titanium (Ti)	2	73	Tantalum (Ta)	2
23	Vanadium (V)	2	74	Tungsten (W)	2
24	Chromium (Cr)	1	75	Rhenium (Re)	2
25	Manganese (Mn)	2	76	Osmium (Os)	2
26	Iron (Fe)	2	77	Iridium (Ir)	2
27	Cobalt (Co)	2	78	Platinum (Pt)	1
28	Nickel (Ni)	2	79	Gold (Au)	1
29	Copper (Cu)	1	80	Mercury (Hg)	2
30	Zinc (Zn)	2	81	Thallium (Tl)	3
31	Gallium (Ga)	3	82	Lead (Pb)	4
32	Germanium (Ge)	4	83	Bismuth (Bi)	5
33	Arsenic (As)	5	84	Polonium (Po)	6
34	Selenium (Se)	6	85	Astatine (At)	7
35	Bromine (Br)	7	86	Radon (Rn)	8
36	Krypton (Kr)	8	87	Francium (Fr)	1
37	Rubidium (Rb)	1	88	Radium (Ra)	2
38	Strontium (Sr)	2	89	Actinium (Ac)	2
39	Yttrium (Y)	2	90	Thorium (Th)	2
40	Zirconium (Zr)	2	91	Protactinium (Pa)	2
41	Niobium (Nb)	1	92	Uranium (U)	2
42	Molybdenum (Mo)	1	93	Neptunium (Np)	2
43	Technetium (Tc)	1	94	Plutonium (Pu)	2
44	Ruthenium (Ru)	1	95	Americium (Am)	2
45	Rhodium (Rh)	1	96	Curium (Cm)	2
46	Palladium (Pd)	—	97	Berkelium (Bk)	2
47	Silver (Ag)	1	98	Californium (Cf)	2
48	Cadmium (Cd)	2	99	Einsteinium (Es)	2
49	Indium (In)	3	100	Fermium (Fm)	2
50	Tin (Sn)	4	101	Mendelevium (Md)	2
51	Antimony (Sb)	5	102	Nobelium (No)	2
			103	Lawrencium (Lr)	2

Key:

- Elements found in energy-yielding nutrients, vitamins, and water.
- Major minerals.
- Trace minerals.

Besides hydrogen, the atoms most common in living things are carbon (C), nitrogen (N), and oxygen (O), whose atomic numbers are 6, 7, and 8, respectively. Their structures are more complicated than that of hydrogen, but each of them possesses the same number of electrons as there are protons in the nucleus. These electrons are found in orbits, or shells (shown below).

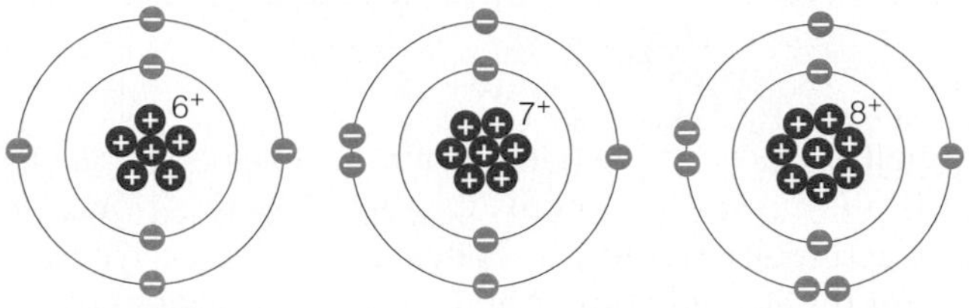
6+
7+
8+

Carbon atom (C), atomic number 6. Nitrogen atom (N), atomic number 7. Oxygen atom (O), atomic number 8.

In these and all diagrams of atoms that follow, only the protons and electrons are shown. The neutrons, which contribute only to atomic weight, not to charge, are omitted.

The most important structural feature of an atom for determining its chemical behavior is the number of electrons in its outermost shell. The first, or innermost, shell is full when it is occupied by two electrons; so an atom with two or more electrons has a filled first shell. When the first shell is full, electrons begin to fill the second shell.

The second shell is completely full when it has eight electrons. A substance that has a full outer shell tends not to enter into chemical reactions. Atomic number 10, neon, is a chemically inert substance because its outer shell is complete. Fluorine, atomic number 9, has a great tendency to draw an electron from other substances to complete its outer shell, and thus it is highly reactive. Carbon has a half-full outer shell, which helps explain its great versatility; it can combine with other elements in a variety of ways to form a large number of compounds.

Atoms seek to reach a state of maximum stability or of lowest energy in the same way that a ball will roll down a hill until it reaches the lowest place. An atom achieves a state of maximum stability:

- By gaining or losing electrons to either fill or empty its outer shell.
- By sharing its electrons through bonding together with other atoms and thereby completing its outer shell.

The number of electrons determines how the atom will chemically react with other atoms. The atomic number, not the weight, is what gives an atom its chemical nature.

Chemical Bonding

Atoms often complete their outer shells by sharing electrons with other atoms. In order to complete its outer shell, a carbon atom requires four electrons. A hydrogen atom requires one. Thus, when a carbon atom shares electrons with four hydrogen atoms, each completes its outer shell (as shown in the next column). Electron sharing binds the atoms together and satisfies the conditions of maximum stability for the molecule. The outer shell of each atom is complete, since hydrogen effectively has the required two electrons in its first (outer) shell, and carbon has eight electrons in its second (outer) shell; and the molecule is electrically neutral, with a total of ten protons and ten electrons.

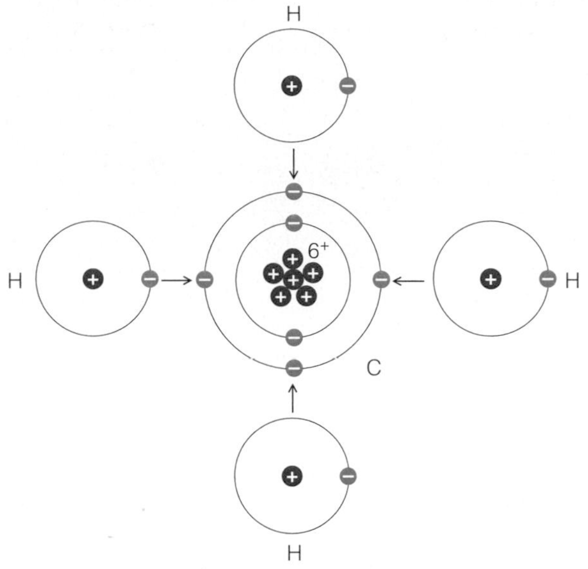
H
H
6+
H
C
H

When a carbon atom shares electrons with four hydrogen atoms, a methane molecule is made.

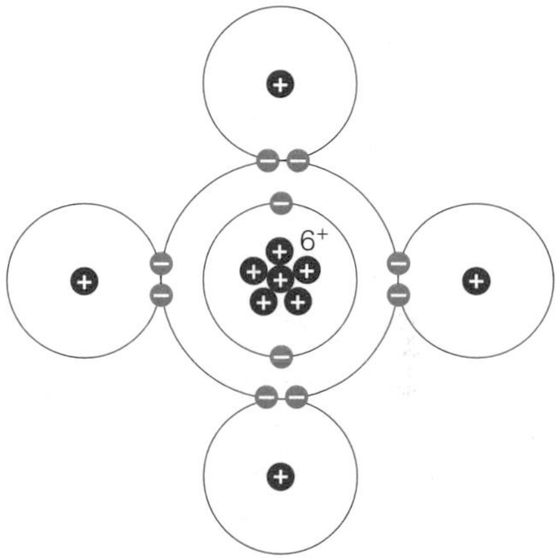
6+

The chemical formula for methane is CH_4. Note that by sharing electrons, every atom achieves a filled outer shell.

Bonds that involve the sharing of electrons, like the bonds between carbon and the four hydrogens, are the most stable kind of association that atoms can form with one another. These bonds are called covalent bonds, and the resulting combination of atoms are called molecules. A single pair of shared electrons forms a single bond. A simplified way to represent a single bond is with a single line. Thus the structure of methane (CH_4) could be represented like this:

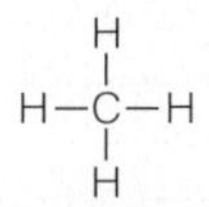

Methane (CH_4).

Similarly, one nitrogen atom and three hydrogen atoms can share electrons to form one molecule of ammonia (NH_3):

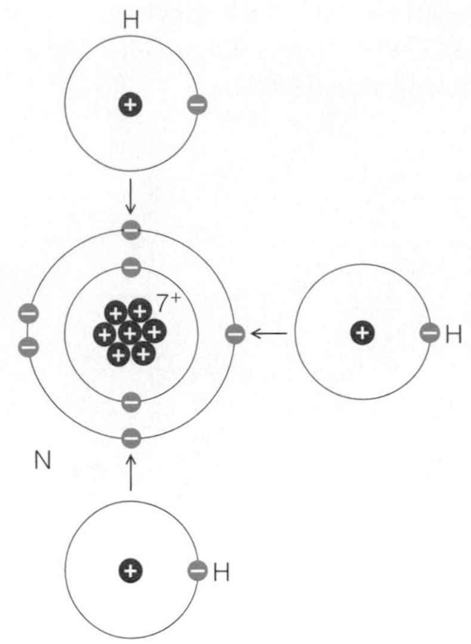
H
7+
H
N
H

When a nitrogen atom shares electrons with three hydrogen atoms, an ammonia molecule is made.

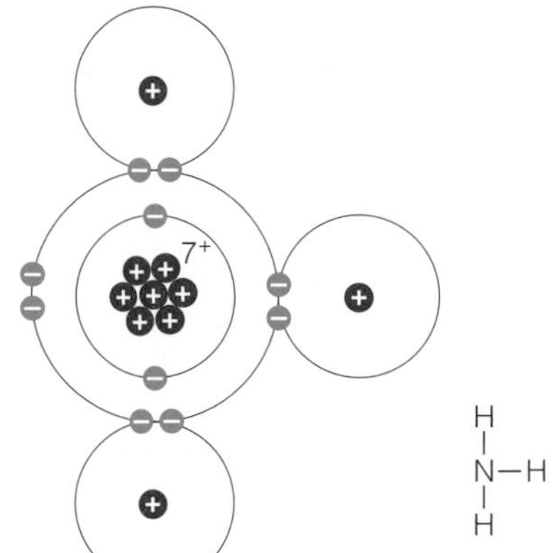
7+
H
N—H
H

Ammonia (NH_3).

The chemical formula for ammonia is NH_3. Count the electrons in each atom's outer shell to confirm that it is filled.

One oxygen atom may be bonded to two hydrogen atoms to form one molecule of water (H_2O):

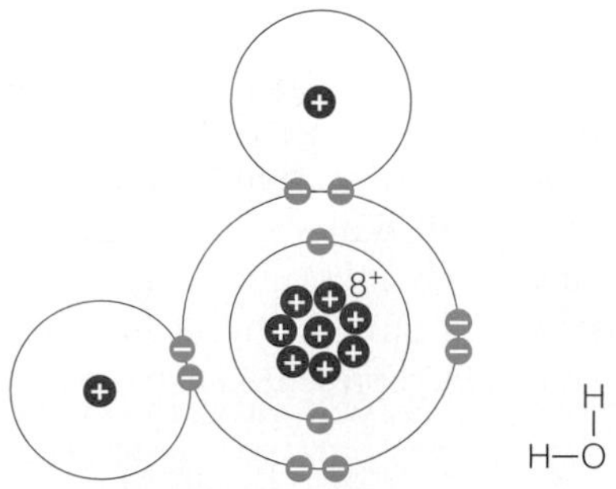
8+
H
H—O

Water molecule (H_2O).

When two oxygen atoms form a molecule of oxygen, they must share two pairs of electrons. This double bond may be represented as two single lines:

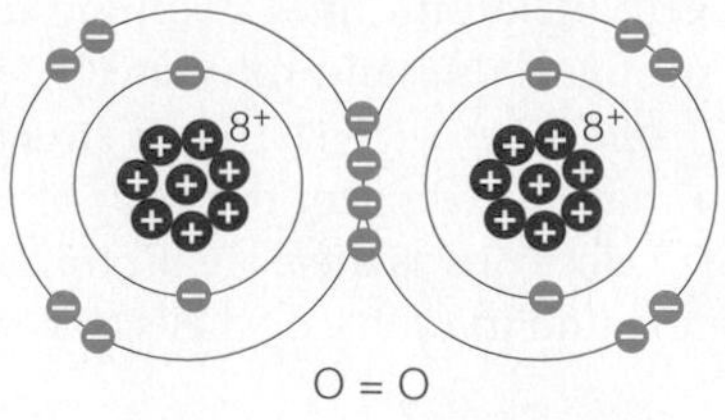
8+
8+
O = O

Oxygen molecule (O_2).

Small atoms form the tightest, most stable bonds. H, O, N, and C are the smallest atoms capable of forming one, two, three, and four electron-pair bonds (respectively). This is the basis for the statement in Chapter 4 that in drawings of compounds containing these atoms, hydrogen must always have one, oxygen two, nitrogen three, and carbon four bonds radiating to other atoms:

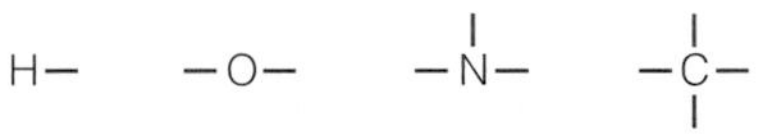
H—
—O—
—N—
—C—

The stability of the associations between these small atoms and the versatility with which they can combine make them very common in living things. Interestingly, all cells, whether they come from animals, plants, or bacteria, contain the same elements in very nearly the same proportions. The elements commonly found in living things are shown in Table B-2.

TABLE B-2 Elemental Composition of the Human Body

Element	Chemical Symbol	By Weight (%)
Oxygen	O	65
Carbon	C	18
Hydrogen	H	10
Nitrogen	N	3
Calcium	Ca	1.5
Phosphorus	P	1.0
Potassium	K	0.4
Sulfur	S	0.3
Sodium	Na	0.2
Chloride	Cl	0.1
Magnesium	Mg	0.1
Total		99.6[a]

[a]The remaining 0.40 percent by weight is contributed by the trace elements: chromium (Cr), copper (Cu), zinc (Zn), selenium (Se), molybdenum (Mo), fluorine (F), iodine (I), manganese (Mn), and iron (Fe). Cells may also contain variable traces of some of the following: boron (B), cobalt (Co), lithium (Li), strontium (Sr), aluminum (Al), silicon (Si), lead (Pb), vanadium (V), arsenic (As), bromine (Br), and others.

Formation of Ions

An atom such as sodium (Na, atomic number 11) cannot easily fill its outer shell by sharing. Sodium possesses a filled first shell of two electrons and a filled second shell of eight; there is only one electron in its outermost shell:

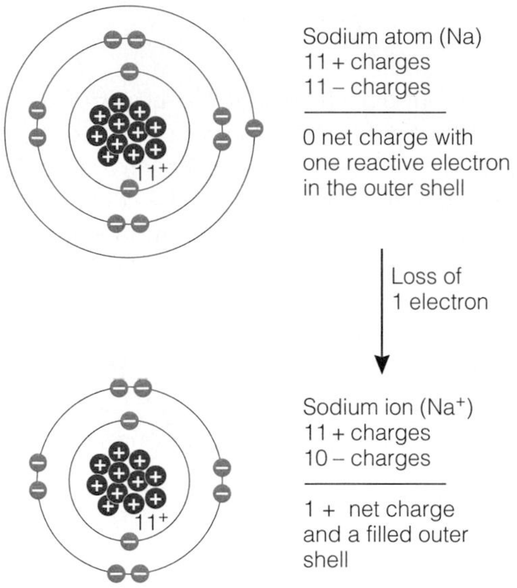

Sodium atom (Na)
11 + charges
11 – charges
0 net charge with one reactive electron in the outer shell
11+
Loss of 1 electron
Sodium ion (Na^+)
11 + charges
10 – charges
1 + net charge and a filled outer shell
11+

If sodium loses this electron, it satisfies one condition for stability: a filled outer shell (now its second shell counts as the outer shell). However, it is not electrically neutral. It has 11 protons (positive) and only 10 electrons (negative). It therefore has a net positive charge. An atom or molecule that has lost or gained one or more electrons and so is electrically charged is called an ion.

An atom such as chlorine (Cl, atomic number 17), with seven electrons in its outermost shell, can share electrons to fill its outer shell, or it can gain one electron to complete its outer shell and thus give it a negative charge:

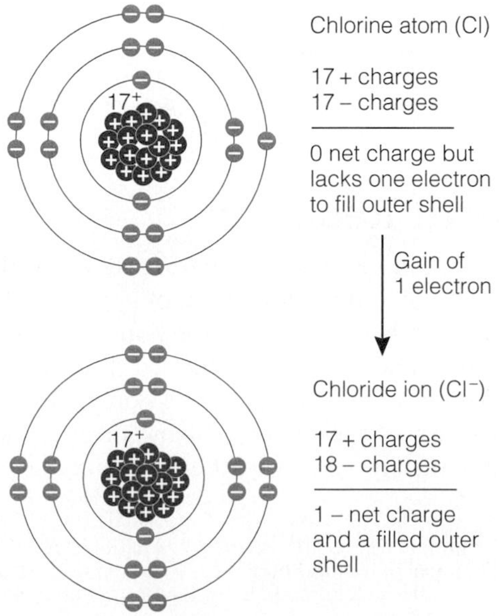

Chlorine atom (Cl)
17 + charges
17 – charges
0 net charge but lacks one electron to fill outer shell
17+
Gain of 1 electron
Chloride ion (Cl^-)
17 + charges
18 – charges
1 – net charge and a filled outer shell
17+

A positively charged ion such as sodium ion (Na^+) is called a cation; a negatively charged ion such as a chloride ion (Cl^-) is called an anion. Cations and anions attract one another to form salts:

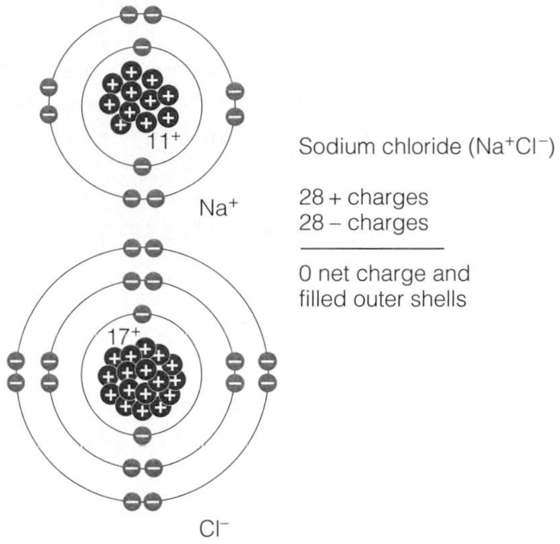

11+
Na^+
Sodium chloride (Na^+Cl^-)
28 + charges
28 – charges
0 net charge and filled outer shells
17+
Cl^-

With all its electrons, sodium is a shiny, highly reactive metal; chlorine is the poisonous greenish yellow gas that was used in World War I. But after sodium and chlorine have transferred electrons, they form the stable white salt familiar to you as table salt, or sodium chloride (Na^+Cl^-). The dramatic difference illustrates how profoundly the electron arrangement can influence the nature of a substance. The wide distribution of salt in nature attests to the stability of the union between the ions. Each meets the other's needs (a good marriage).

When dry, salt exists as crystals; its ions are stacked very regularly into a lattice, with positive and negative ions alternating in a three-dimensional checkerboard structure. In water, however, the salt quickly dissolves, and its ions separate from one another, forming an electrolyte solution in which they move about freely. Covalently bonded molecules rarely dissociate like this in a water solution. The most common exception is when they behave like acids and release H^+ ions, as discussed in the next section.

An ion can also be a group of atoms bound together in such a way that the group has a net charge and enters into reactions as a single unit. Many such groups are active in the fluids of the body. The bicarbonate ion is composed of five atoms—one H, one C, and three Os—and has a net charge of -1 (HCO_3^-). Another important ion of this type is a phosphate ion with one H, one P, and four O, and a net charge of -2 (HPO_4^{-2}).

Whereas many elements have only one configuration in the outer shell and thus only one way to bond with other elements, some elements have the possibility of varied configurations. Iron is such an element. Under some conditions iron loses two electrons, and under other circumstances it loses three. If iron loses two electrons, it then has a net charge of $+2$, and we call it ferrous iron (Fe^{++}). If it donates three electrons to another atom, it becomes the $+3$ ion, or ferric iron (Fe^{+++}).

Ferrous iron (Fe^{++})	Ferric iron (Fe^{+++})
(had 2 outer-shell electrons but has lost them)	(had 3 outer-shell electrons but has lost them)
26 + charges	26 + charges
24 − charges	23 − charges
2 + net charge	3 + net charge

Remember that a positive charge on an ion means that negative charges—electrons—have been lost and not that positive charges have been added to the nucleus.

Water, Acids, and Bases

Water

The water molecule is electrically neutral, having equal numbers of protons and electrons. When a hydrogen atom shares its electron with oxygen, however, that electron will spend most of its time closer to the positively charged oxygen nucleus. This leaves the positive proton (nucleus of the hydrogen atom) exposed on the outer part of the water molecule. We know, too, that the two hydrogens both bond toward the same side of the oxygen. These two facts explain why water molecules are polar: they have regions of more positive and more negative charge.

Polar molecules like water are drawn to one another by the attractive forces between the positive polar areas of one and the negative poles of another. These attractive forces, sometimes known as polar bonds or hydrogen bonds, occur among many molecules and also within the different parts of single large molecules. Although very weak in comparison with covalent bonds, polar bonds may occur in such abundance that they become exceedingly important in determining the structure of such large molecules as proteins and DNA.

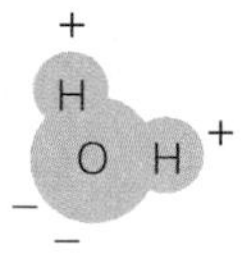
+
H
O
H
+
−
−

This diagram of the polar water molecule shows displacement of electrons toward the O nucleus; thus the negative region is near the O and the positive regions are near the Hs.

Water molecules have a slight tendency to ionize, separating into positive (H^+) and negative (OH^-) ions. In pure water, a small but constant number of these ions is present, and the number of positive ions exactly equals the number of negative ions.

Acid

An acid is a substance that releases H^+ ions (protons) in a water solution. Hydrochloric acid (HCl^-) is such a substance because it dissociates in a water solution into H^+ and Cl^- ions. Acetic acid is also an acid because it dissociates in water to acetate ions and free H^+:

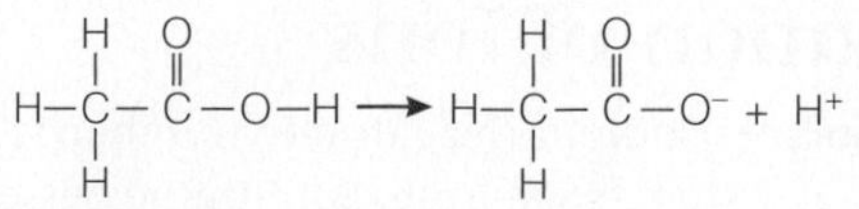

Acetic acid dissociates into an acetate ion and a hydrogen ion.

The more H^+ ions released, the stronger the acid.

pH

Chemists define degrees of acidity by means of the pH scale, which runs from 0 to 14. The pH expresses the concentration of H^+ ions: a pH of 1 is extremely acidic, 7 is neutral, and 13 is very basic. There is a tenfold difference in the concentration of H^+ ions between points on this scale. A solution with pH 3, for example, has *ten times* as many H^+ ions as a solution with pH 4. At pH 7, the concentrations of free H^+ and OH^- are exactly the same—1/10,000,000 moles per liter (10^{-7} moles per liter).* At pH 4, the concentration of free H^+ ions is 1/10,000 (10^{-4}) moles per liter. This is a higher concentration of H^+ ions, and the solution is therefore acidic. Figure 3-7 on p. 81 presents the pH scale.

Bases

A base is a substance that can combine with H^+ ions, thus reducing the acidity of a solution. The compound ammonia is such a substance. The ammonia molecule has two electrons that are not shared with any other atom; a hydrogen ion (H^+) is just a naked proton with no shell of electrons at all. The proton readily combines with the ammonia molecule to form an ammonium ion; thus a free proton is withdrawn from the solution and no longer contributes to its acidity. Many compounds containing nitrogen are important bases in living systems. Acids and bases neutralize each other to produce substances that are neither acid nor base.

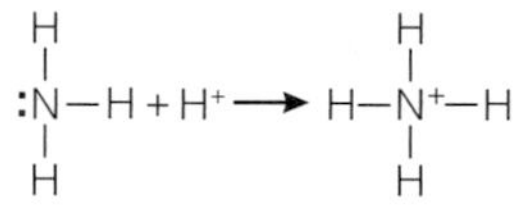

Ammonia captures a hydrogen ion from water. The two dots here represent the two electrons not shared with another atom. These dots are ordinarily not shown in chemical structure drawings. Compare this drawing with the earlier diagram of an ammonia molecule (p. B-4).

Chemical Reactions

A chemical reaction, or chemical change, results in the breakdown of substances and the formation of new ones. Almost all such reactions involve a change in the bonding of atoms. Old bonds are broken, and new ones are formed. The nuclei of atoms are never involved in chemical reactions—only their outer-shell electrons take part. At the end of a chemical reaction, the number of atoms of each type is always the same as at the beginning.

*A mole is a certain number (about 6×10^{23}) of molecules. The pH of a solution is defined as the negative logarithm of the hydrogen ion concentration of the solution. Thus, if the concentration is 10^{-2} (moles per liter), the pH is 2; if 10^{-8}, the pH is 8; and so on.

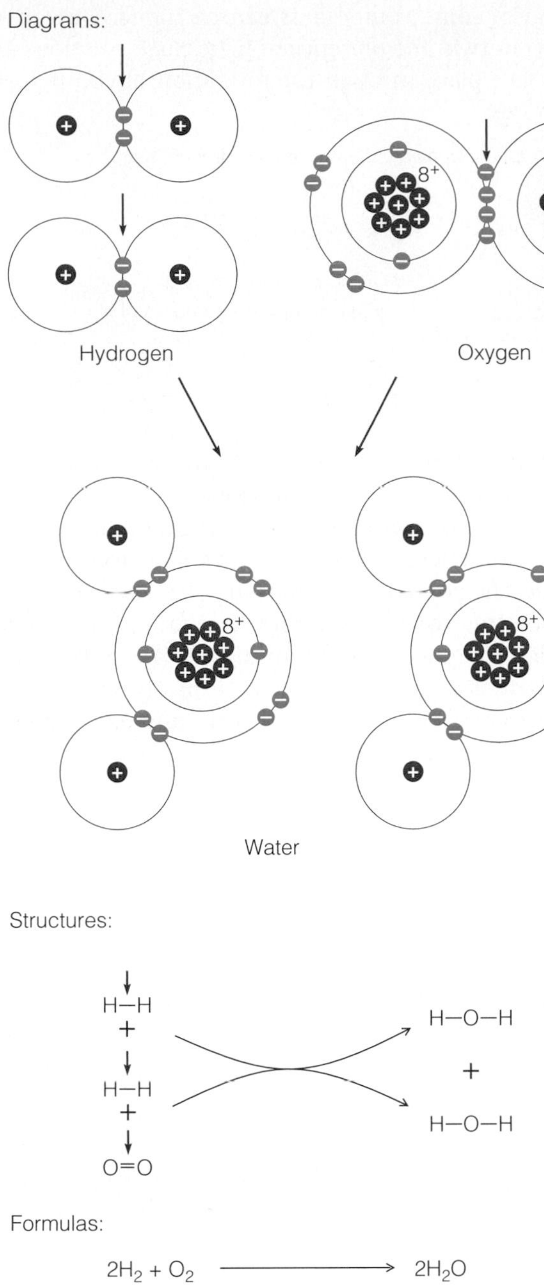
Diagrams:
8+
Hydrogen
Oxygen
Water
Structures:
H—H
+
H—H
+
O=O
H—O—H
+
H—O—H
Formulas:
$2H_2 + O_2 \longrightarrow 2H_2O$

Hydrogen and oxygen react to form water.

For example, two hydrogen molecules ($2H_2$) can react with one oxygen molecule (O_2) to form two water molecules ($2H_2O$). In this reaction two substances (hydrogen and oxygen) disappear, and a new one (water) is formed, but at the end of the reaction there are still four H atoms and two O atoms, just as there were at the beginning. Because the atoms are now linked in a different way, their characteristics or properties have changed.

In many instances chemical reactions involve not the relinking of molecules but the exchanging of electrons or protons among them. In such reactions the molecule that gains one or more electrons (or loses one or more hydrogen ions) is said to be reduced; the molecule that loses electrons (or gains protons) is oxidized. A hydrogen ion is equivalent to a proton. Oxidation and reduction reactions take place simultaneously because an electron or proton that is lost by one molecule is accepted by another. The addition of an atom of oxygen is also oxidation because oxygen (with six electrons in the outer shell) accepts two electrons in becoming bonded. Oxidation, then, is loss of electrons, gain of protons, or addition of oxygen (with six electrons); reduction is the opposite—gain of electrons, loss of protons, or loss of oxygen. The addition of hydrogen atoms to oxygen to form water can thus be described as the reduction of oxygen *or* the oxidation of hydrogen.

If a reaction results in a net increase in the energy of a compound, it is called an endergonic, or "uphill," reaction (energy, *erg,* is added into, *endo,* the compound). An example is the chief result of photosynthesis, the making of sugar in a plant from carbon dioxide and water using the energy of sunlight. Conversely, the oxidation of sugar to carbon dioxide and water is an exergonic, or "downhill," reaction because the end products have less energy than the starting products. Oftentimes, but not always, reduction reactions are endergonic, resulting in an increase in the energy of the products. Oxidation reactions often, but not always, are exergonic.

Chemical reactions tend to occur spontaneously if the end products are in a lower energy state and therefore are more stable than the reacting compounds. These reactions often give off energy in the form of heat as they occur. The generation of heat by wood burning in a fireplace and the maintenance of human body warmth both depend on energy-yielding chemical reactions. These downhill reactions occur easily, although they may require some activation energy to get them started, just as a ball requires a push to start rolling downhill.

Uphill reactions, in which the products contain more energy than the reacting compounds started with, do not occur until an energy source is provided. An example of such an energy source is the sunlight used in photosynthesis, where carbon dioxide and water (low-energy compounds) are combined to form the sugar glucose (a higher-energy compound). Another example is the use of the energy in glucose to combine two low-energy compounds in the body into the high-energy compound ATP (see Chapter 7). The energy in ATP may be used to power many other energy-requiring, uphill reactions. Clearly, any of many different molecules can be used as a temporary storage place for energy.

Energy change as reaction occurs

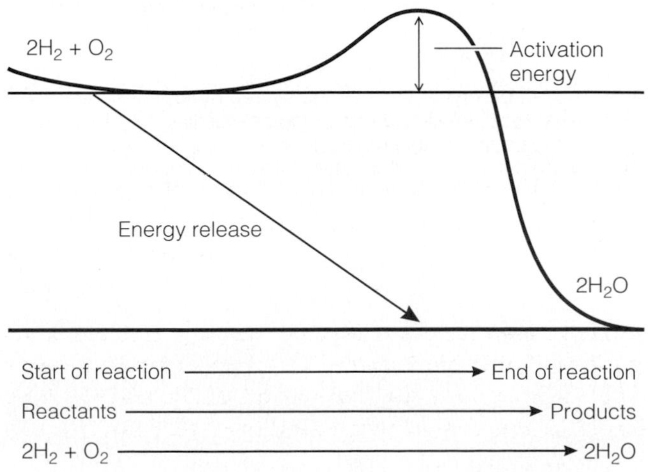
$2H_2 + O_2$
Activation energy
Energy release
$2H_2O$
Start of reaction → End of reaction
Reactants → Products
$2H_2 + O_2 \rightarrow 2H_2O$

Neither downhill nor uphill reactions occur until something sets them off (activation) or until a path is provided for them to follow. The body uses enzymes as a means of providing paths and controlling chemical reactions (see Chapter 6). By controlling the availability and the action of its enzymes, the cells can "decide" which chemical reactions to prevent and which to promote.

Formation of Free Radicals

Normally, when a chemical reaction takes place, bonds break and re-form with some redistribution of atoms and rearrangement of bonds to form new, stable compounds. Normally, bonds don't split in such a way as to leave a molecule with an odd, unpaired electron. When they do, free radicals are formed. Free radicals are highly unstable and quickly react with other compounds, forming more free radicals in a chain reaction. A cascade may ensue in which many highly reactive radicals are generated, resulting finally in the disruption of a living structure such as a cell membrane.

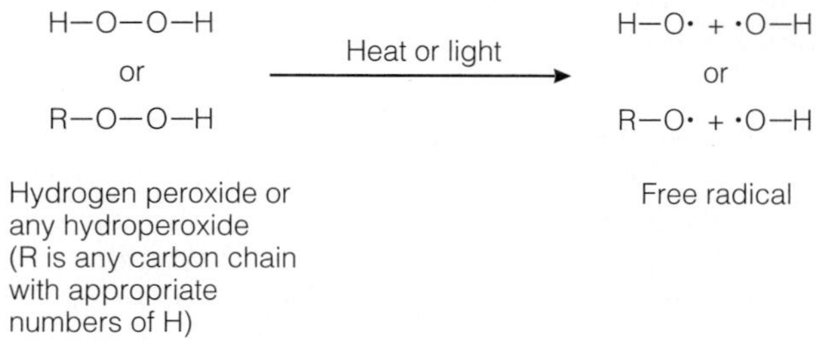
H—O—O—H
or
R—O—O—H
Heat or light
H—O· + ·O—H
or
R—O· + ·O—H
Hydrogen peroxide or any hydroperoxide (R is any carbon chain with appropriate numbers of H)
Free radical

Free radicals are formed. The dots represent single electrons that are available for sharing (the atom needs another electron to fill its outer shell).

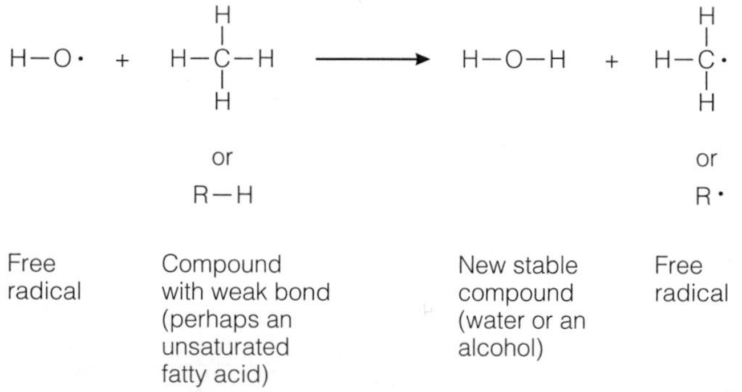
H—O· + H—C—H
or
R—H
H—O—H + H—C·
or
R·
Free radical
Compound with weak bond (perhaps an unsaturated fatty acid)
New stable compound (water or an alcohol)
Free radical

Destruction of biological compounds by free radicals. The free radical attacks a weak bond in a biological compound, disrupting it and forming a new stable molecule and another free radical. This free radical can attack another biological compound, and so on.

Oxidation of some compounds can be induced by air at room temperature in the presence of light. Such reactions are thought to take place through the formation of compounds called peroxides:

Peroxides:

H—O—O—H	Hydrogen peroxide
R—O—O—H	Hydroperoxides (R is any carbon chain with appropriate numbers of H)
R—O—O—R	Peroxide

Some peroxides readily disintegrate into free radicals, initiating chain reactions like those just described.

Free radicals are of special interest in nutrition because the antioxidant properties of vitamins C and E as well as beta-carotene and the mineral selenium are thought to protect against the destructive effects of these free radicals (see Highlight 11). For example, vitamin E on the surface of the lungs reacts with, and is destroyed by, free radicals, thus preventing the radicals from reaching underlying cells and oxidizing the lipids in their membranes.

Biochemical Structures and Pathways

CONTENTS

The diagrams of nutrients presented here are meant to enhance your understanding of the most important organic molecules in the human diet. Following the diagrams of nutrients are sections on the major metabolic pathways mentioned in Chapter 7—glycolysis, fatty acid oxidation, amino acid degradation, the TCA cycle, and the electron transport chain—and a description of how alcohol interferes with these pathways. Discussions of the urea cycle and the formation of ketone bodies complete the appendix.

Carbohydrates

Monosaccharides

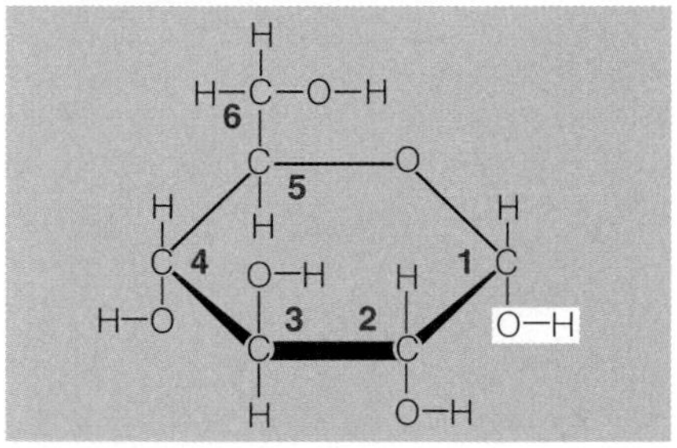

Glucose (alpha form). The ring would be at right angles to the plane of the paper. The bonds directed upward are above the plane; those directed downward are below the plane. This molecule is considered an alpha form because the OH on carbon 1 points downward.

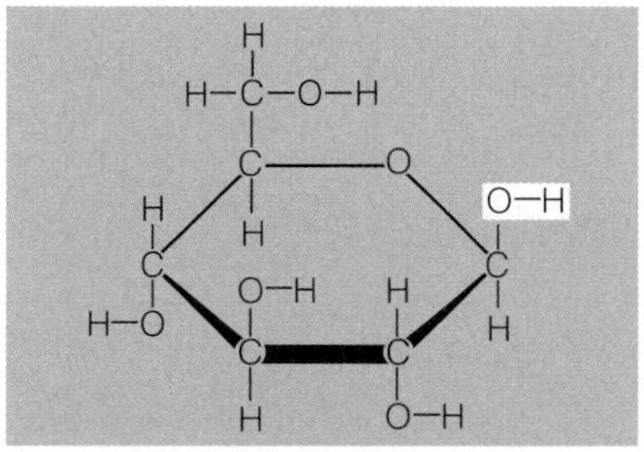

Glucose (beta form). The OH on carbon 1 points upward.
Fructose, galactose: see Chapter 4.

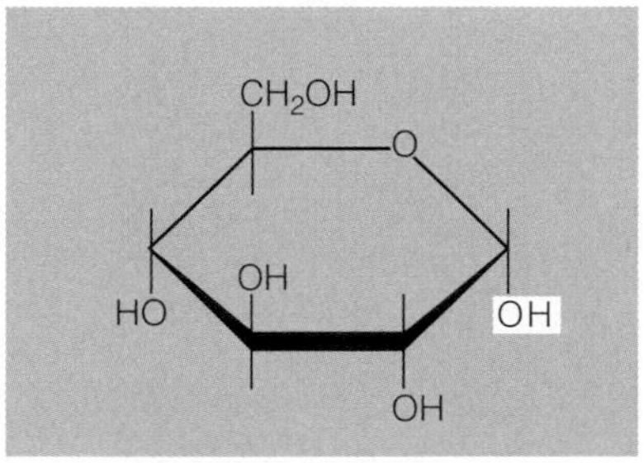

Glucose (alpha form) shorthand notation. This notation, in which the carbons in the ring and single hydrogens have been eliminated, will be used throughout this appendix.

Disaccharides

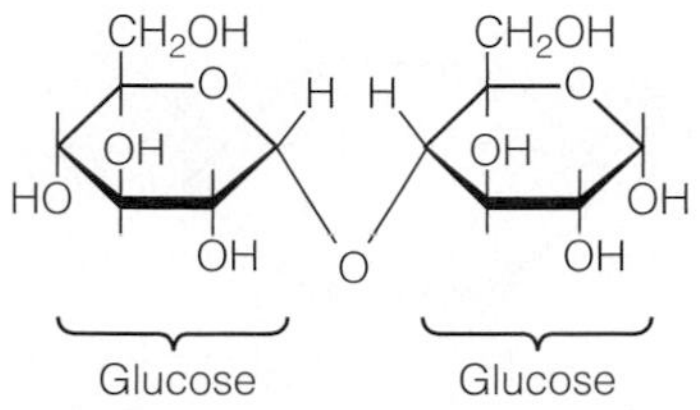
Glucose
Glucose

Maltose.

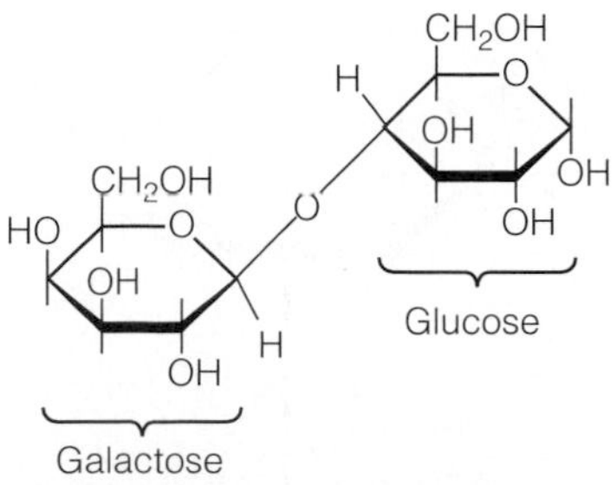
Galactose
Glucose

Lactose (alpha form).

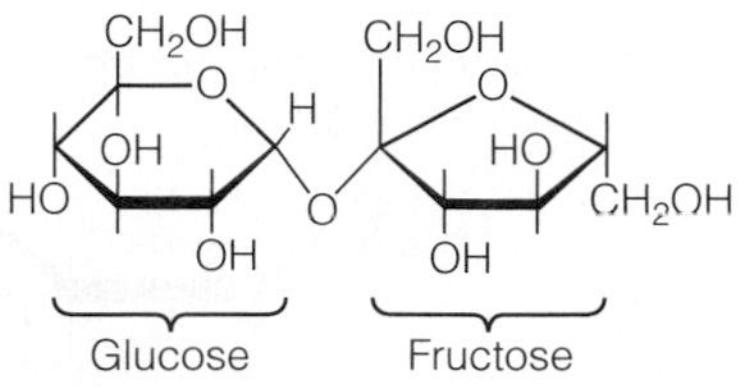
Glucose
Fructose

Sucrose.

Polysaccharides

As described in Chapter 4, starch, glycogen, and cellulose are all long chains of glucose molecules covalently linked together.

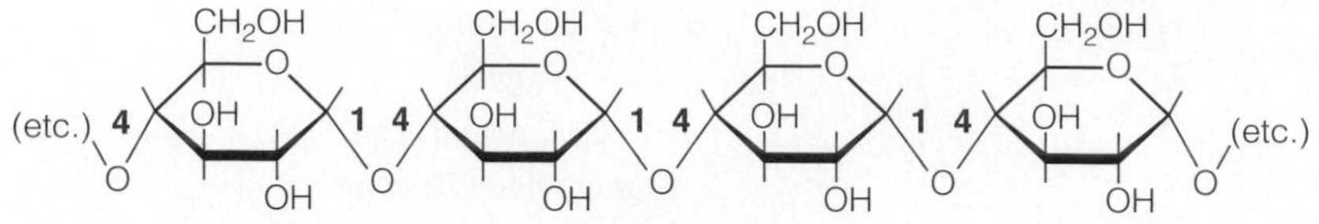

Amylose (unbranched starch)

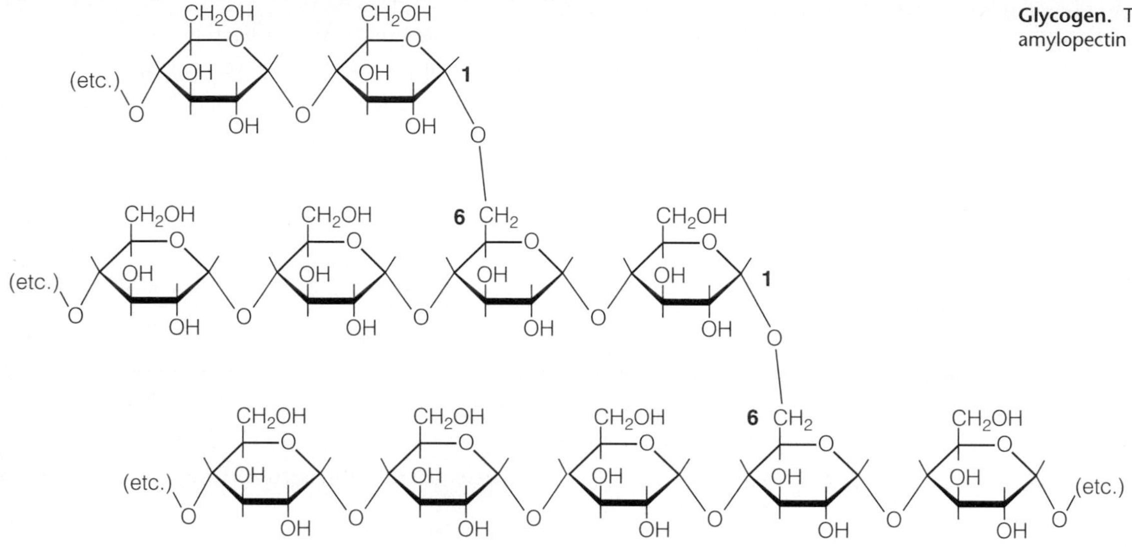

Amylopectin (branched starch)

Starch. Two kinds of covalent linkages occur between glucose molecules in starch, giving rise to two kinds of chains. Amylose is composed of straight chains, with carbon 1 of one glucose linked to carbon 4 of the next (α-1,4 linkage). Amylopectin is made up of straight chains like amylose but has occasional branches arising where the carbon 6 of a glucose is also linked to the carbon 1 of another glucose (α-1,6 linkage).

Glycogen. The structure of glycogen is like amylopectin but with many more branches.

Cellulose. Like starch and glycogen, cellulose is also made of chains of glucose units, but there is an important difference: in cellulose, the OH on carbon 1 is in the beta position (see p. C-1). When carbon 1 of one glucose is linked to carbon 4 of the next, it forms a β-1,4 linkage, which cannot be broken by digestive enzymes in the human GI tract.

Fibers, such as hemicelluloses, consist of long chains of various monosaccharides.

Monosaccharides common in the backbone chain of hemicelluloses:

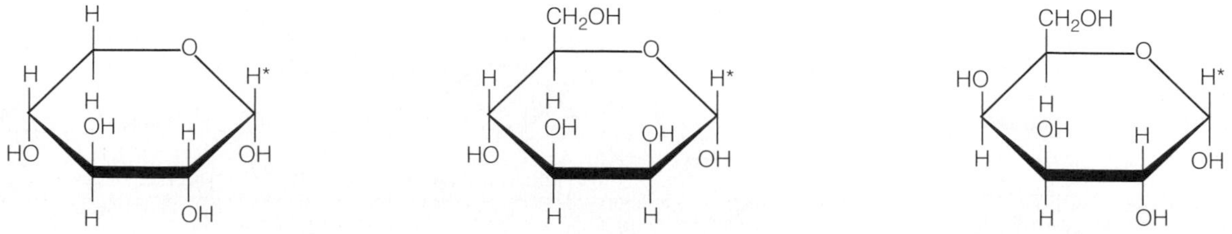

Xylose Mannose Galactose

*These structures are shown in the alpha form with the H on the carbon pointing upward and the OH pointing downward, but they may also appear in the beta form with the H pointing downward and the OH upward.

Monosaccharides common in the side chains of hemicelluloses:

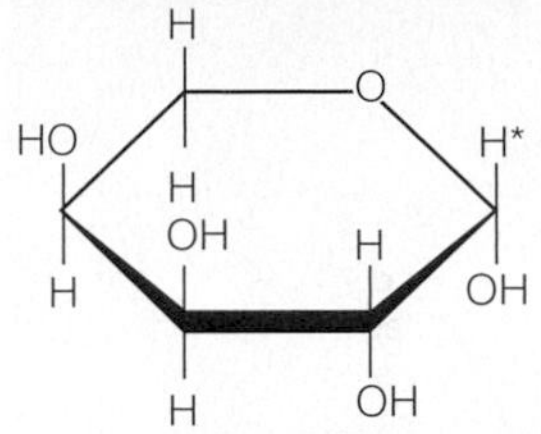
H
HO
H
OH
H
H*
OH
H
OH
O
Arabinose

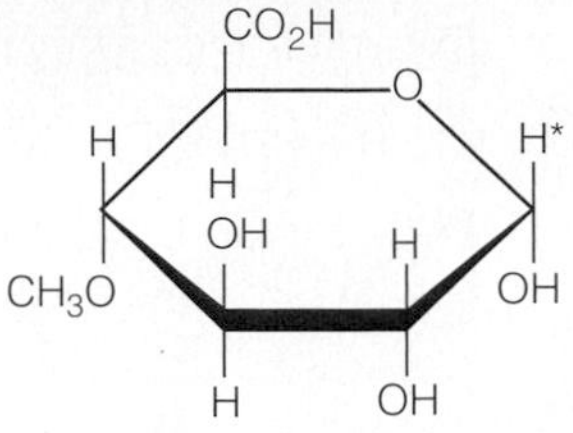
CO_2H
H
H
OH
H
H*
CH_3O
OH
H
OH
O
Glucuronic acid

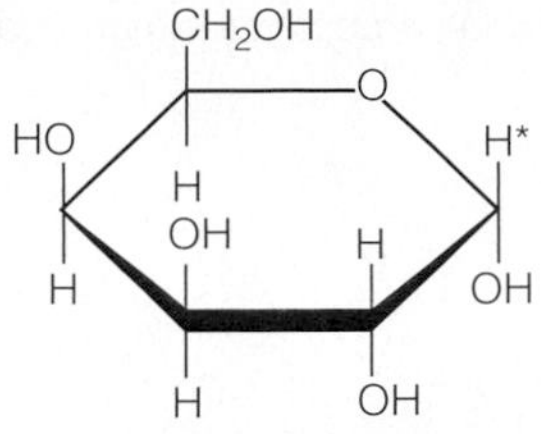
CH_2OH
HO
H
OH
H
H*
H
OH
H
OH
O
Galactose

Hemicelluloses. The most common hemicelluloses are composed of a backbone chain of xylose, mannose, and galactose, with branching side chains of arabinose, glucuronic acid, and galactose.

Lipids

TABLE C-1 Saturated Fatty Acids Found in Natural Fats

Saturated Fatty Acids	Chemical Formulas	Number of Carbons	Major Food Sources
Butyric	C_3H_7COOH	4	Butterfat
Caproic	$C_5H_{11}COOH$	6	Butterfat
Caprylic	$C_7H_{15}COOH$	8	Coconut oil
Capric	$C_9H_{19}COOH$	10	Palm oil
Lauric	$C_{11}H_{23}COOH$	12	Coconut oil, palm oil
Myristic[a]	$C_{13}H_{27}COOH$	14	Coconut oil, palm oil
Palmitic[a]	$C_{15}H_{31}COOH$	16	Palm oil
Stearic[a]	$C_{17}H_{35}COOH$	18	Most animal fats
Arachidic	$C_{19}H_{39}COOH$	20	Peanut oil
Behenic	$C_{21}H_{43}COOH$	22	Seeds
Lignoceric	$C_{23}H_{47}COOH$	24	Peanut oil

[a]Most common saturated fatty acids.

TABLE C-2 Unsaturated Fatty Acids Found in Natural Fats

Unsaturated Fatty Acids	Chemical Formulas	Number of Carbons	Number of Double Bonds	Standard Notation[a]	Omega Notation[b]	Food Sources
Palmitoleic	$C_{15}H_{29}COOH$	16	1	16:1;9	16:1ω7	Seafood, beef
Oleic	$C_{17}H_{33}COOH$	18	1	18:1;9	18:1ω9	Olive oil, canola oil
Linoleic	$C_{17}H_{31}COOH$	18	2	18:2;9,12	18:2ω6	Sunflower oil, safflower oil
Linolenic	$C_{17}H_{29}COOH$	18	3	18:3;9,12,15	18:3ω3	Soybean oil, canola oil
Arachidonic	$C_{19}H_{31}COOH$	20	4	20:4;5,8,11,14	20:4ω6	Eggs, most animal fats
Eicosapentaenoic	$C_{19}H_{29}COOH$	20	5	20:5;5,8,11,14,17	20:5ω3	Seafood
Docosahexaenoic	$C_{21}H_{31}COOH$	22	6	22:6;4,7,10,13,16,19	22:6ω3	Seafood

NOTE: A fatty acid has two ends; designated the methyl (CH_3) end and the carboxyl, or acid (COOH), end.

[a]Standard chemistry notation begins counting carbons at the acid end. The number of carbons the fatty acid contains comes first, followed by a colon and another number that indicates the number of double bonds; next comes a semicolon followed by a number or numbers indicating the positions of the double bonds. Thus the notation for linoleic acid, an 18-carbon fatty acid with two double bonds between carbons 9 and 10 and between carbons 12 and 13, is 18:2;9,12.

[b]Because fatty acid chains are lengthened by adding carbons at the acid end of the chain, chemists use the omega system of notation to ease the task of identifying them. The omega system begins counting carbons at the methyl end. The number of carbons the fatty acid contains comes first, followed by a colon and the number of double bonds; next come the omega symbol (ω) and a number indicating the position of the double bond nearest the methyl end. Thus linoleic acid with its first double bond at the sixth carbon from the methyl end would be noted 18:2ω6 in the omega system.

Protein: Amino Acids

The common amino acids may be classified into the seven groups listed on the next page. Amino acids marked with an asterisk (*) are essential.

1. Amino acids with aliphatic side chains, which consist of hydrogen and carbon atoms (hydrocarbons):

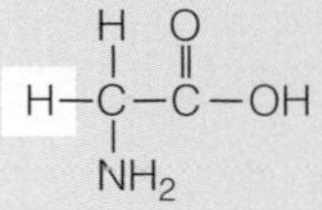

Glycine (Gly)

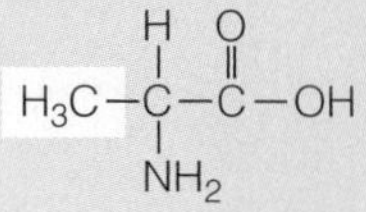

Alanine (Ala)

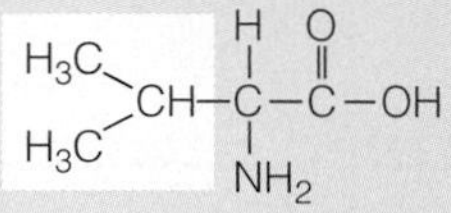

Valine* (Val)

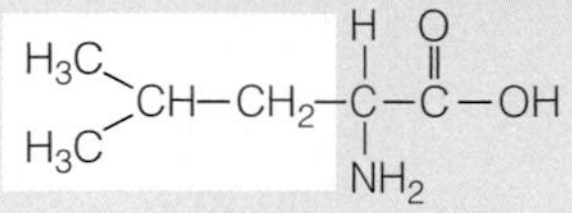

Leucine* (Leu)

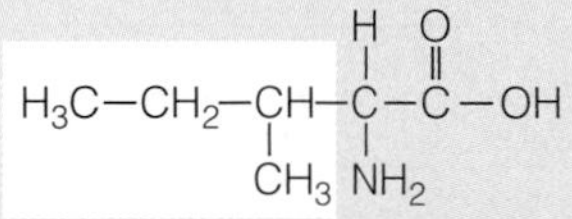

Isoleucine* (Ile)

2. Amino acids with hydroxyl (OH) side chains:

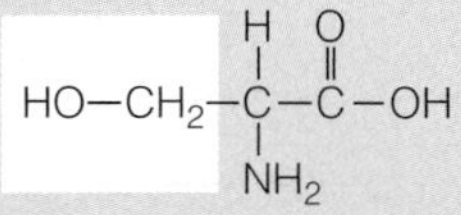

Serine (Ser)

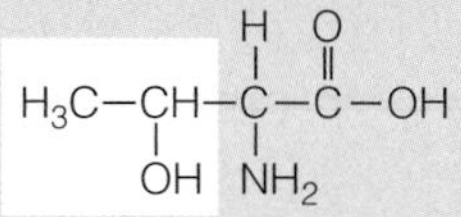

Threonine* (Thr)

3. Amino acids with side chains containing acidic groups or their amides, which contain the group NH_2:

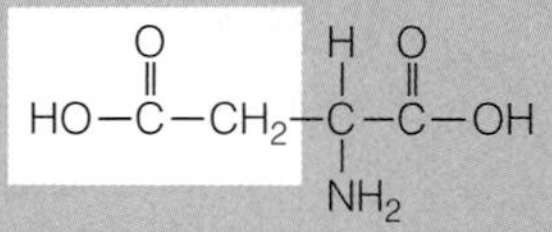

Aspartic acid (Asp)

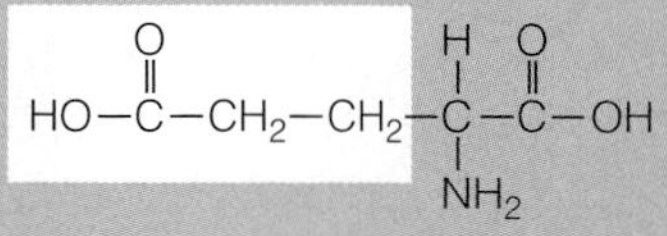

Glutamic acid (Glu)

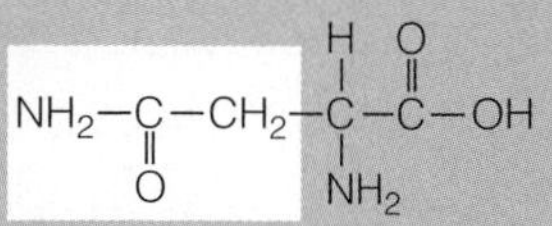

Asparagine (Asn)

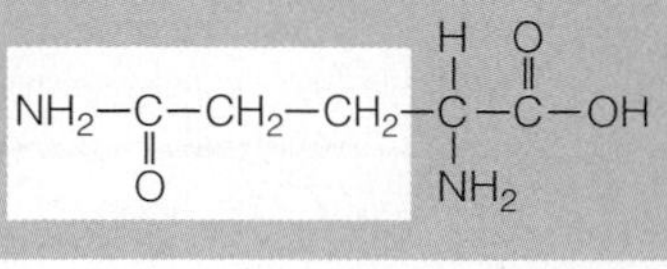

Glutamine (Gln)

4. Amino acids with basic side chains:

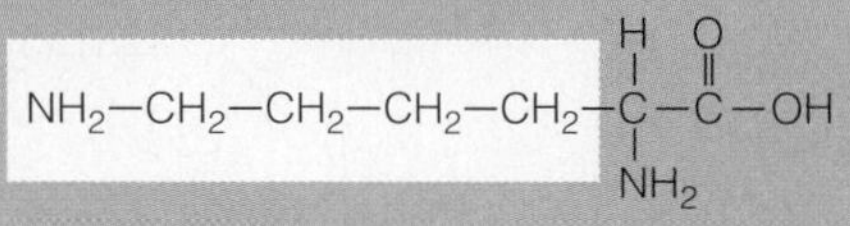

Lysine* (Lys)

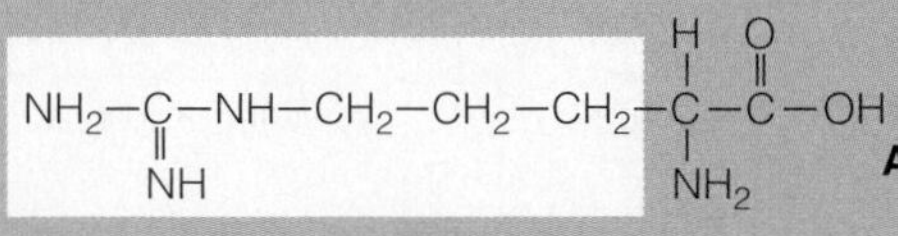

Arginine (Arg)

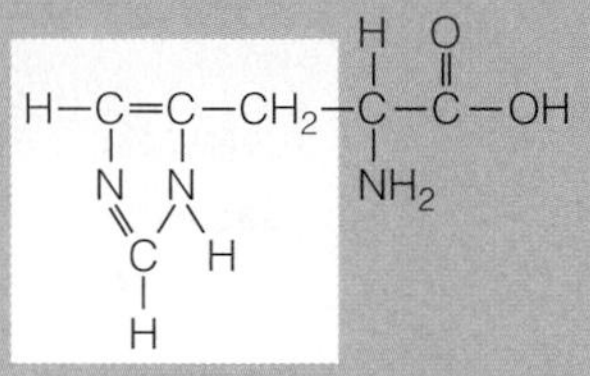

Histidine* (His)

5. Amino acids with aromatic side chains, which are characterized by the presence of at least one ring structure:

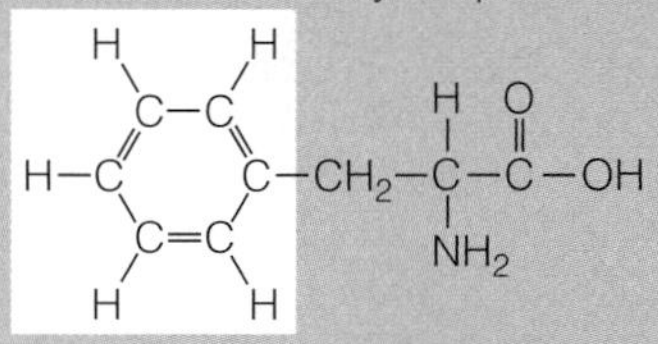

Phenylalanine* (Phe)

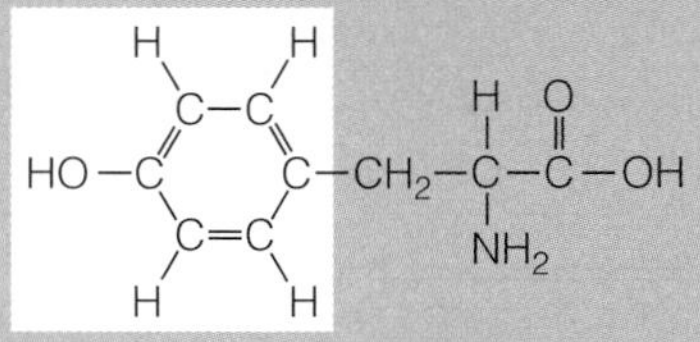

Tyrosine (Tyr)

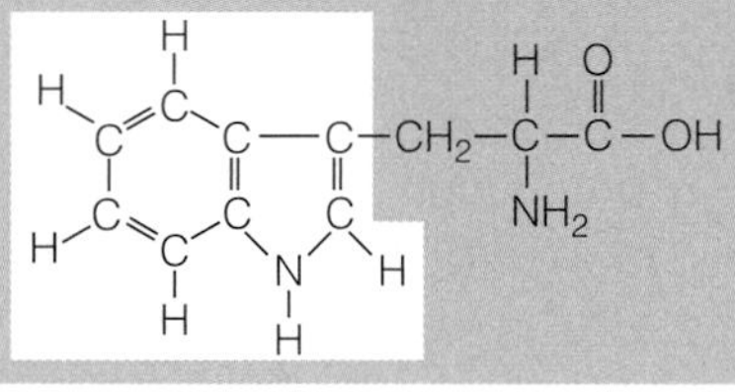

Tryptophan* (Trp)

6. Amino acids with side chains containing sulfur atoms:

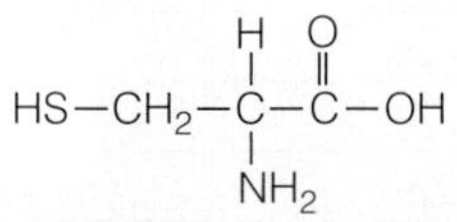

Cysteine (Cys)

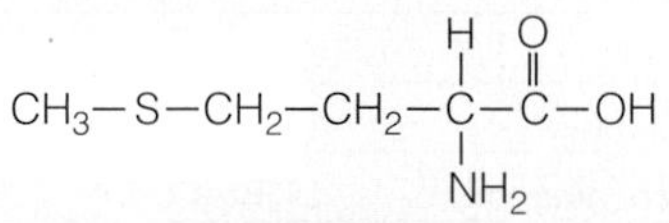

Methionine* (Met)

7. Imino acid:

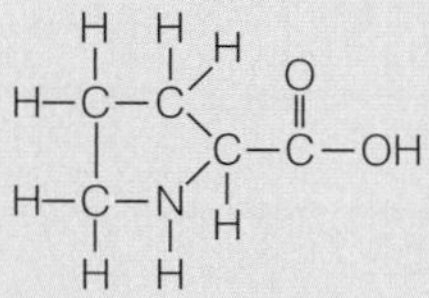

Proline (Pro)

Proline has the same chemical structure as the other amino acids, but its amino group has given up a hydrogen to form a ring.

Appendix C

Vitamins and Coenzymes

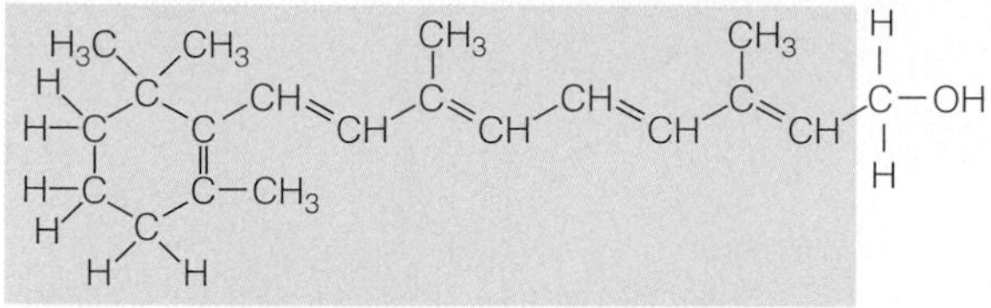

Vitamin A: retinol. This molecule is the alcohol form of vitamin A.

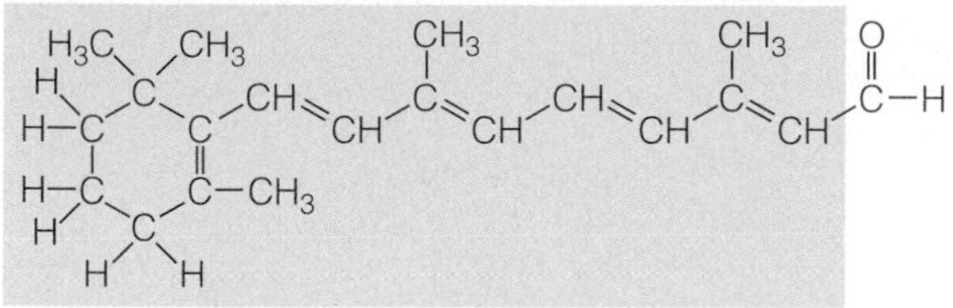

Vitamin A: retinal. This molecule is the aldehyde form of vitamin A.

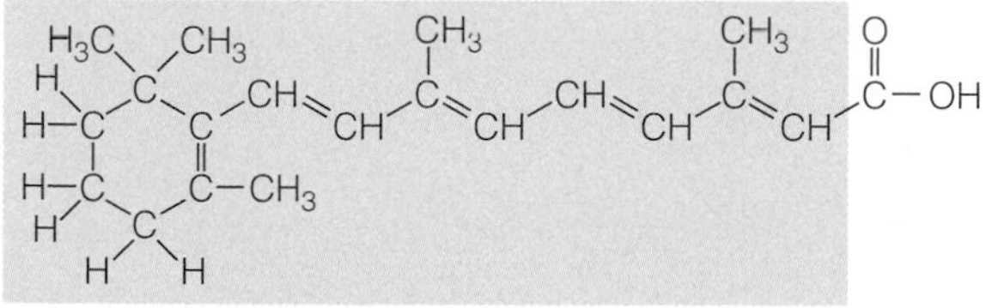

Vitamin A: retinoic acid. This molecule is the acid form of vitamin A.

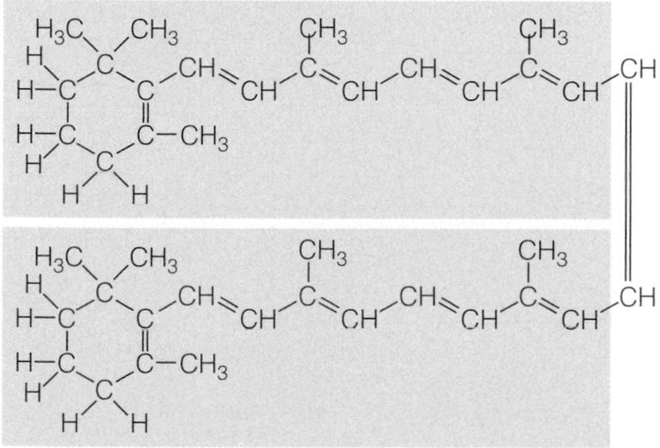

Vitamin A precursor: beta-carotene. This molecule is the carotenoid with the most vitamin A activity.

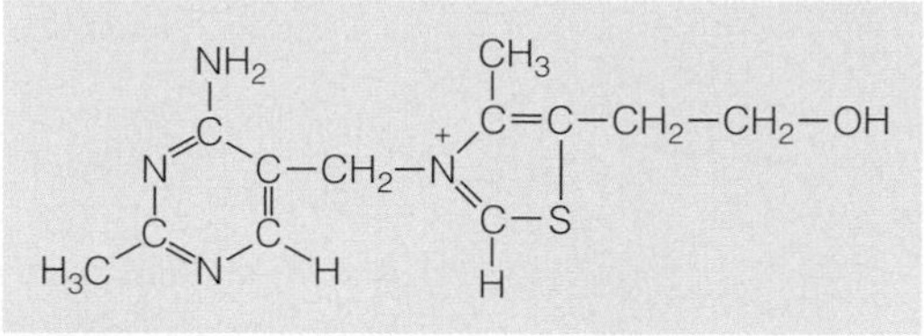

Thiamin. This molecule is part of the coenzyme thiamin pyrophosphate (TPP).

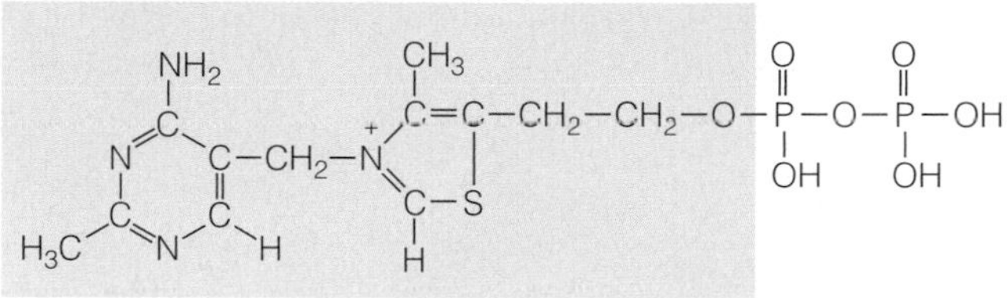

Thiamin pyrophosphate (TPP). TPP is a coenzyme that includes the thiamin molecule as part of its structure.

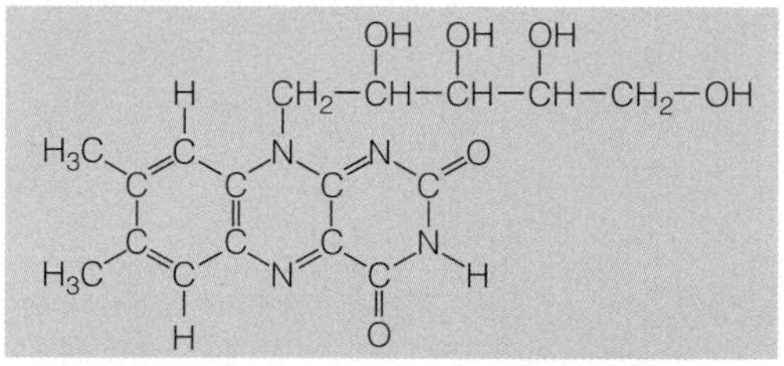

Riboflavin. This molecule is a part of two coenzymes—flavin mononucleotide (FMN) and flavin adenine dinucleotide (FAD).

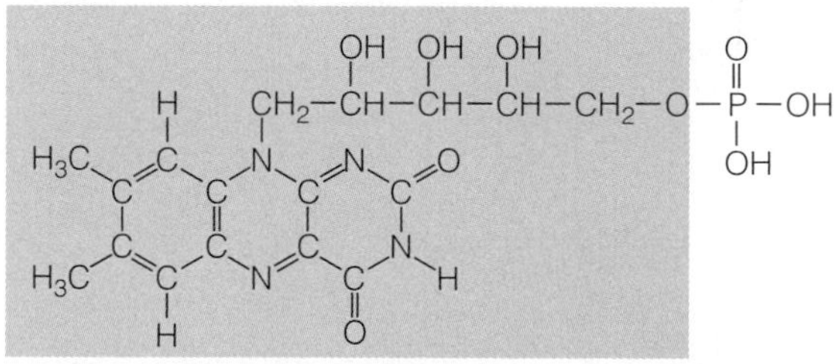

Flavin mononucleotide (FMN). FMN is a coenzyme that includes the riboflavin molecule as part of its structure.

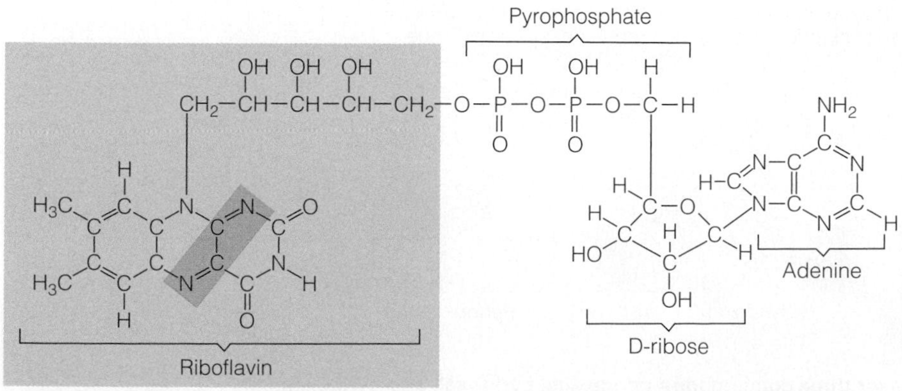
Pyrophosphate
Riboflavin
D-ribose
Adenine

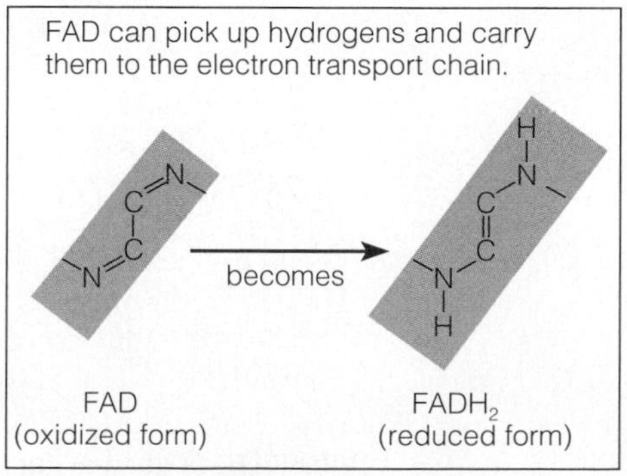
FAD can pick up hydrogens and carry them to the electron transport chain.
becomes
FAD
(oxidized form)
FADH₂
(reduced form)

Flavin adenine dinucleotide (FAD). FAD is a coenzyme that includes the riboflavin molecule as part of its structure.

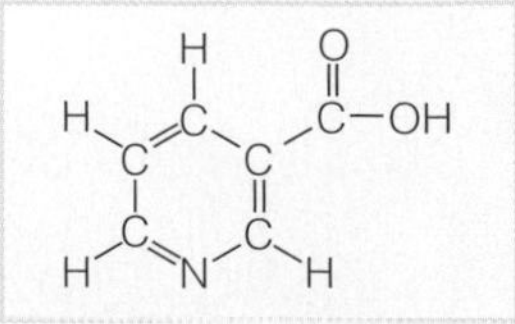

Nicotinic acid

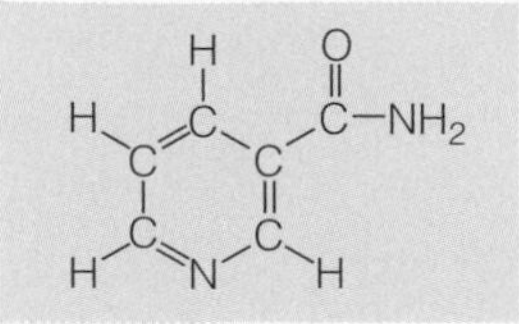

Nicotinamide

Niacin (nicotinic acid and nicotinamide). These molecules are a part of two coenzymes—nicotinamide adenine dinucleotide (NAD^+) and nicotinamide adenine dinucleotide phosphate ($NADP^+$).

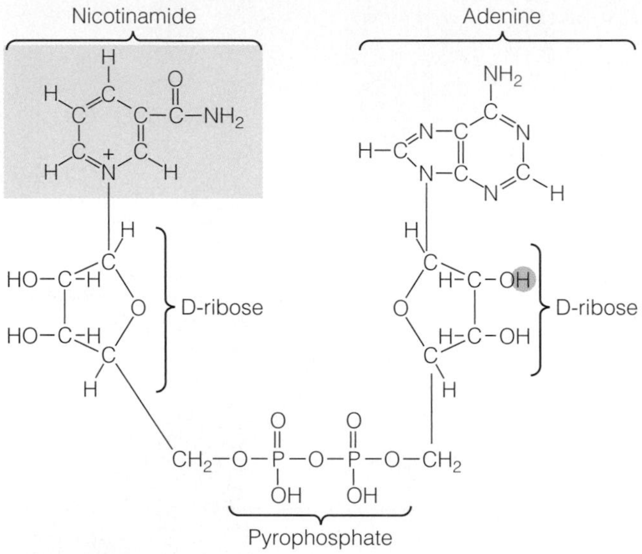
Nicotinamide
Adenine
D-ribose
D-ribose
Pyrophosphate

Nicotinamide adenine dinucleotide (NAD^+) and nicotinamide adenine dinucleotide phosphate ($NADP^+$). NADP has the same structure as NAD but with a phosphate group attached to the O instead of the H.

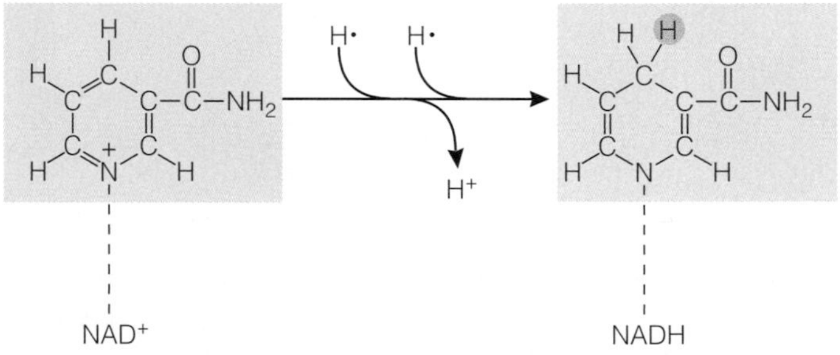
NAD+
NADH

Reduced NAD^+ (NADH). When NAD^+ is reduced by the addition of H^+ and two electrons, it becomes the coenzyme NADH. (The dots on the H entering this reaction represent electrons—see Appendix B.)

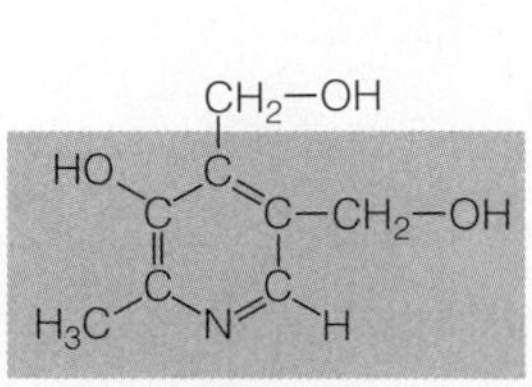

Pyridoxine

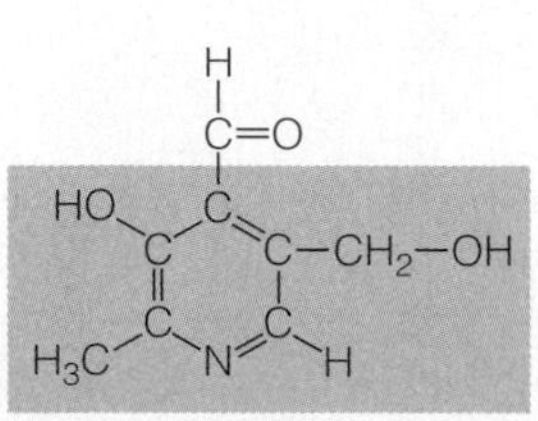

Pyridoxal

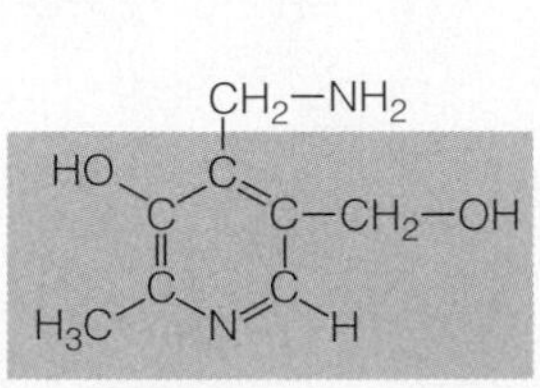

Pyridoxamine

Vitamin B_6 (a general name for three compounds—pyridoxine, pyridoxal, and pyridoxamine). These molecules are a part of two coenzymes—pyridoxal phosphate and pyridoxamine phosphate.

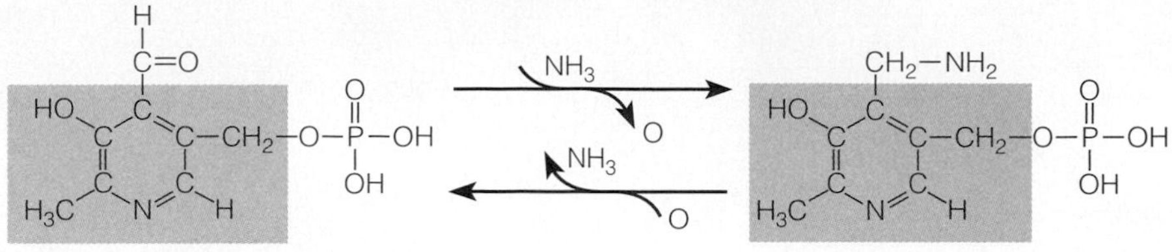
Pyridoxal phosphate
Pyridoxamine phosphate

Pyridoxal phosphate (PLP) and pyridoxamine phosphate. These coenzymes include vitamin B_6 as part of their structures.

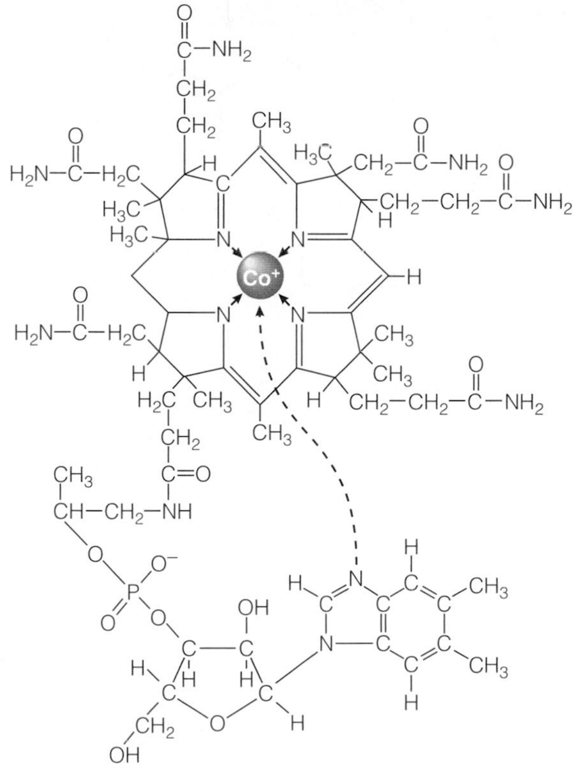

Vitamin B_{12} (cyanocobalamin). The arrows in this diagram indicate that the spare electron pairs on the nitrogens attract them to the cobalt.

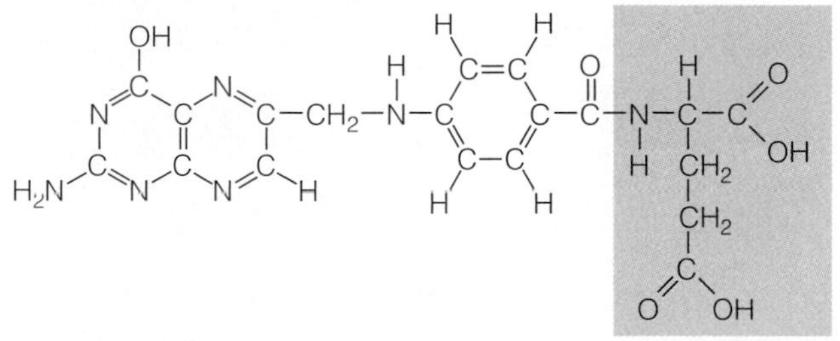

Folate (folacin or folic acid). This molecule consists of a double ring combined with a single ring and at least one glutamate (a nonessential amino acid marked in the box). Folate's biologically active form is tetrahydrofolic acid.

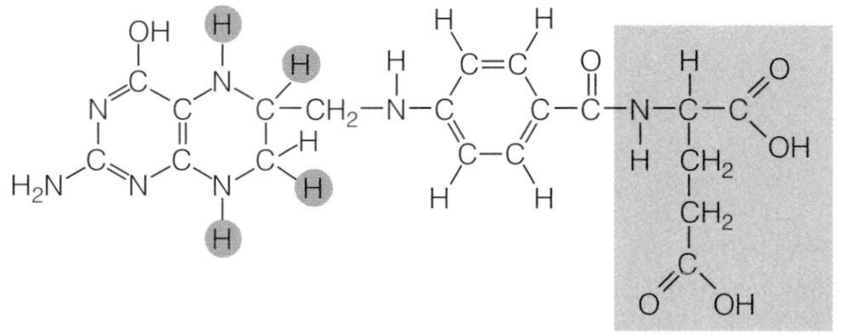

Tetrahydrofolic acid. This active coenzyme form of folate has four added hydrogens. An intermediate form, dihydrofolate, has two added hydrogens.

Appendix C

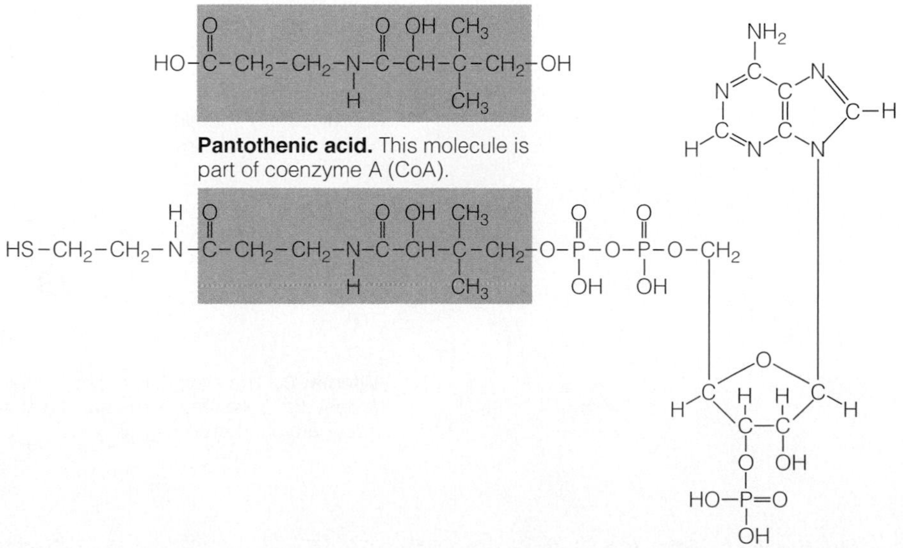

Pantothenic acid. This molecule is part of coenzyme A (CoA).

Coenzyme A (CoA). Coenzyme A is a coenzyme that includes pantothenic acid as part of its structure.

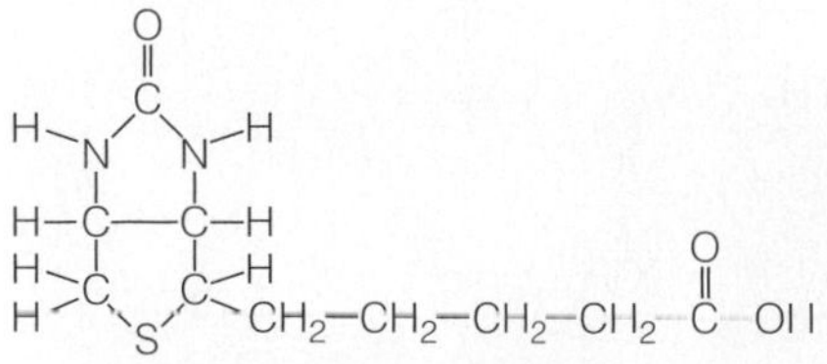

Biotin.

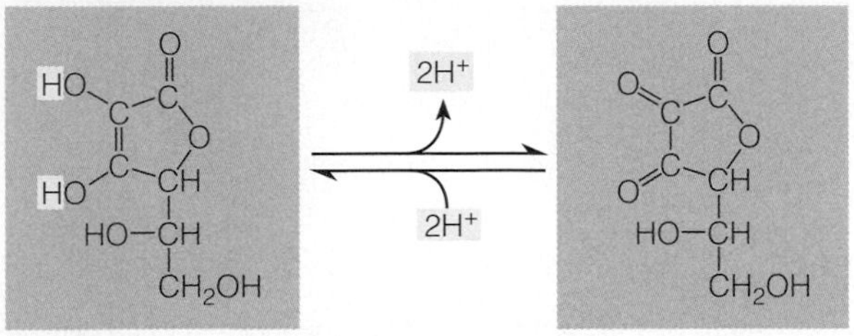
2H+
2H+

Ascorbic acid (reduced form)

Dehydroascorbic acid (oxidized form)

Vitamin C. Two hydrogen atoms with their electrons are lost when ascorbic acid is oxidized and gained when it is reduced again.

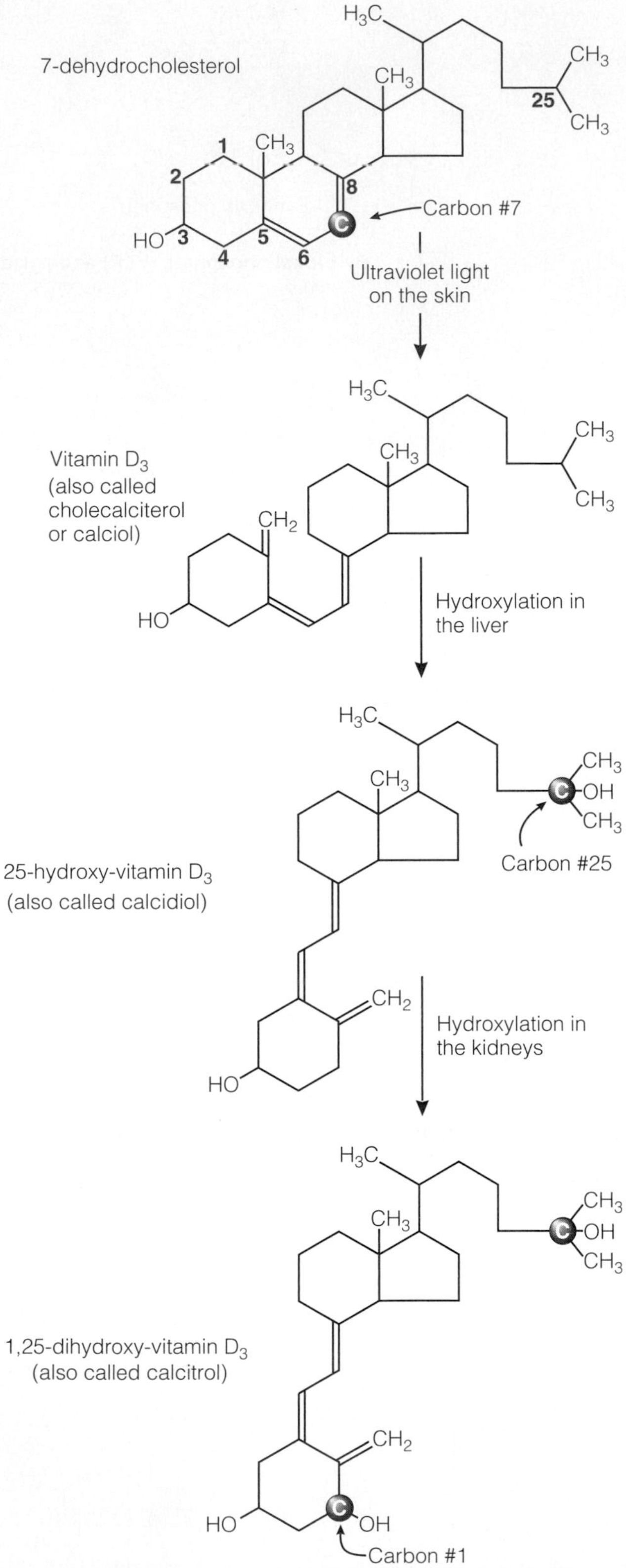
7-dehydrocholesterol
Carbon #7
Ultraviolet light on the skin
Vitamin D3 (also called cholecalciterol or calciol)
Hydroxylation in the liver
25-hydroxy-vitamin D3 (also called calcidiol)
Carbon #25
Hydroxylation in the kidneys
1,25-dihydroxy-vitamin D3 (also called calcitrol)
Carbon #1

Vitamin D. The synthesis of active vitamin D begins with 7-dehydrocholesterol. (The carbon atoms at which changes occur are numbered.)

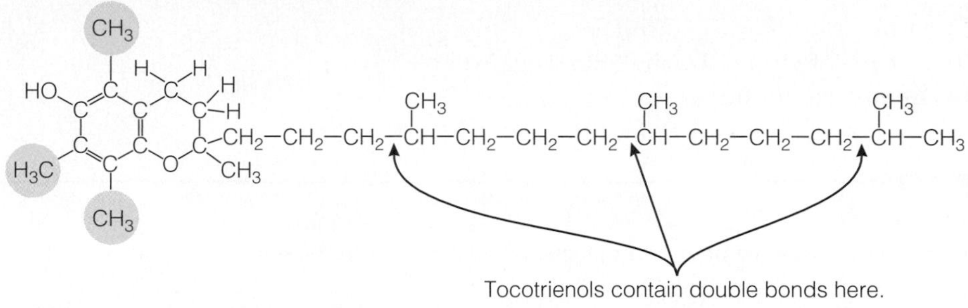
Tocotrienols contain double bonds here.

Vitamin E (alpha-tocopherol). The number and position of the methyl groups (CH_3) bonded to the ring structure differentiate among the tocopherols.

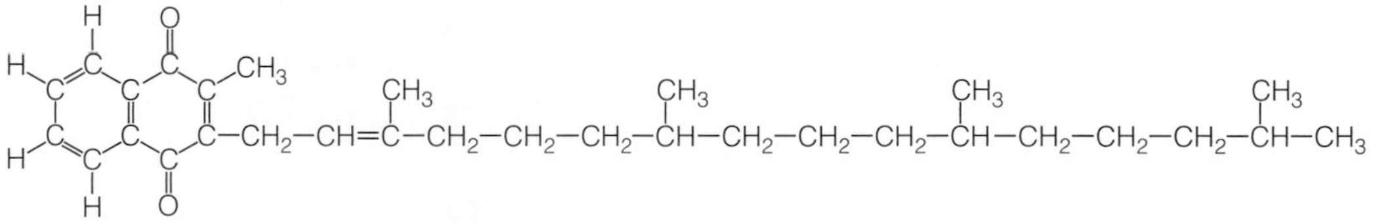

Vitamin K. Naturally occurring compounds with vitamin K activity include phylloquinones (from plants) and menaquinones (from bacteria).

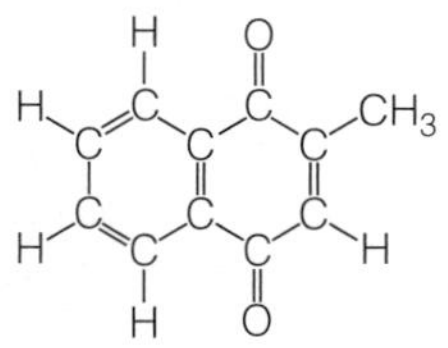

Menadione. This synthetic compound has the same activity as natural vitamin K.

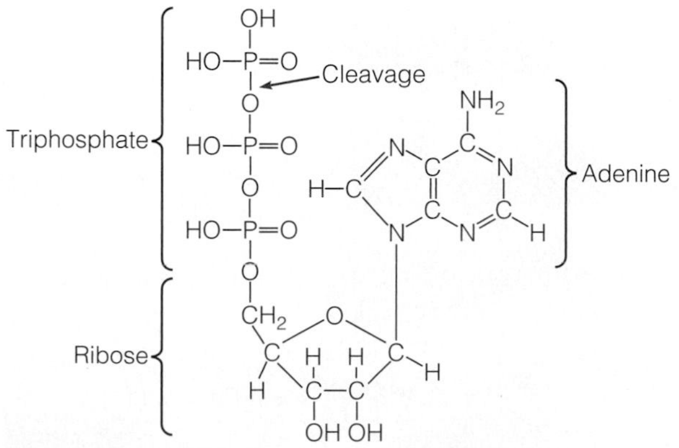
Cleavage
Triphosphate
Adenine
Ribose

Adenosine triphosphate (ATP), the energy carrier. The cleavage point marks the bond that is broken when ATP splits to become ADP + P.

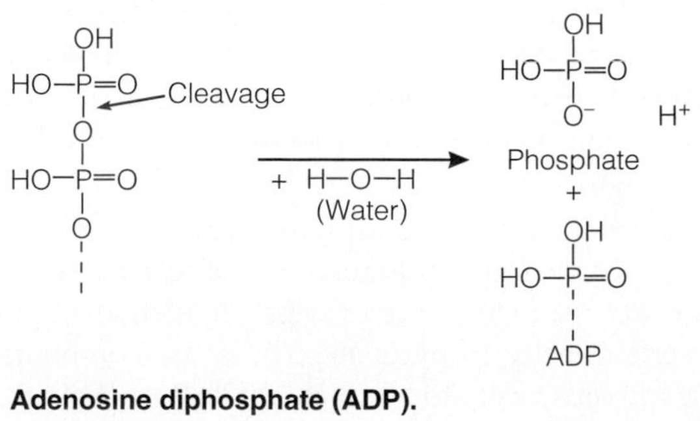
Cleavage
+ H—O—H
(Water)
Phosphate
+
ADP

Adenosine diphosphate (ADP).

Glycolysis

Figure C-1 depicts the events of glycolysis. The following text describes key steps as numbered on the figure.

FIGURE C-1 Glycolysis

Notice that galactose and fructose enter at different places but all continue on the same pathway.

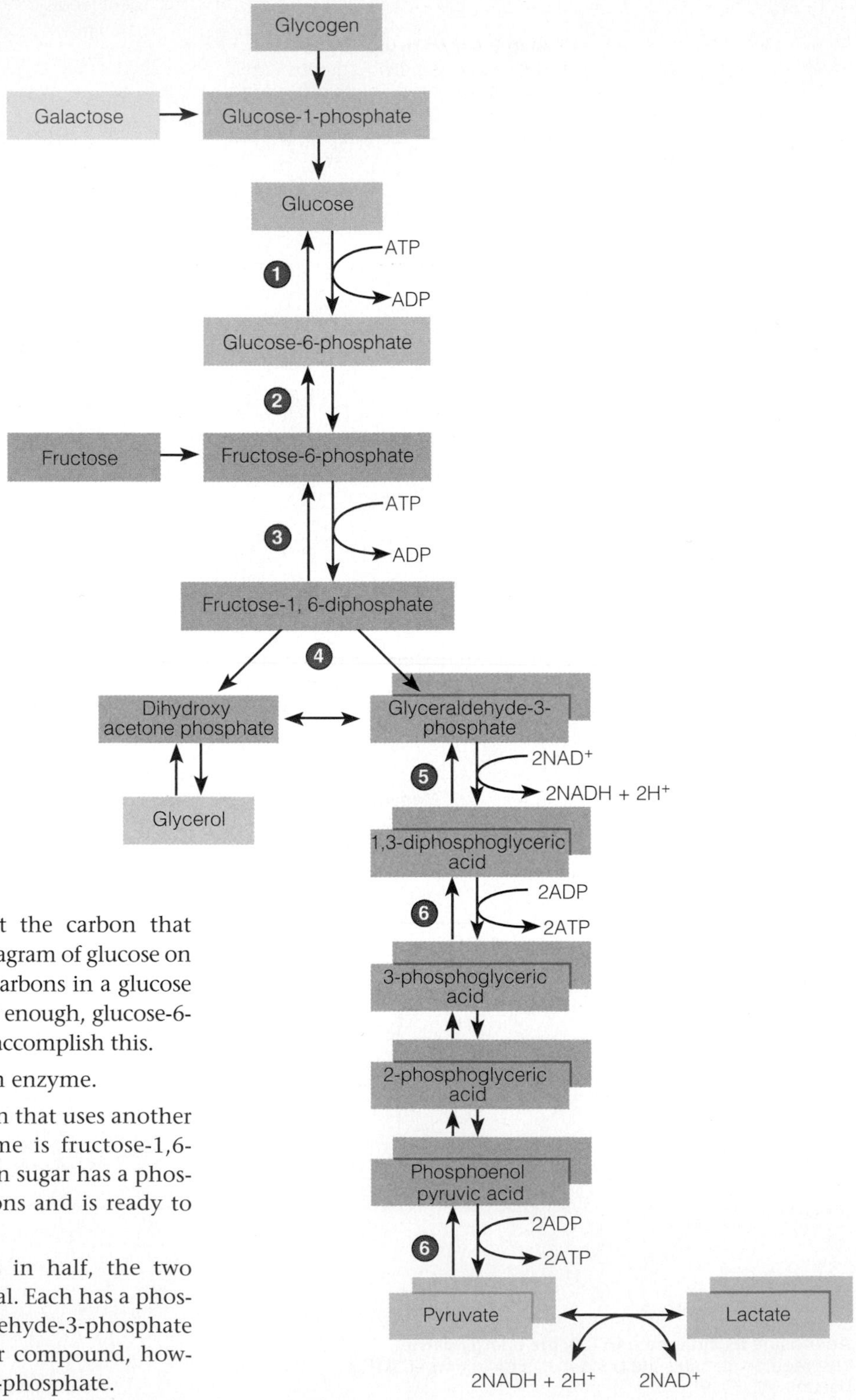

Glycogen
Galactose
Glucose-1-phosphate
Glucose
ATP
1
ADP
Glucose-6-phosphate
2
Fructose
Fructose-6-phosphate
ATP
3
ADP
Fructose-1, 6-diphosphate
4
Dihydroxy acetone phosphate
Glyceraldehyde-3-phosphate
Glycerol
2NAD+
5
2NADH + 2H+
1,3-diphosphoglyceric acid
2ADP
6
2ATP
3-phosphoglyceric acid
2-phosphoglyceric acid
Phosphoenol pyruvic acid
2ADP
6
2ATP
Pyruvate
Lactate
2NADH + 2H+
2NAD+

1. A phosphate is attached to glucose at the carbon that chemists call number 6 (review the first diagram of glucose on p. C-1 to see how chemists number the carbons in a glucose molecule). The product is called, logically enough, glucose-6-phosphate. One ATP molecule is used to accomplish this.
2. Glucose-6-phosphate is rearranged by an enzyme.
3. A phosphate is added in another reaction that uses another molecule of ATP. The product this time is fructose-1,6-diphosphate. At this point the six-carbon sugar has a phosphate group on its first and sixth carbons and is ready to break apart.
4. When fructose-1,6-diphosphate breaks in half, the two three-carbon compounds are not identical. Each has a phosphate group attached, but only glyceraldehyde-3-phosphate converts directly to pyruvate. The other compound, however, converts easily to glyceraldehyde-3-phosphate.

5. In the next step, enough energy is released to convert NAD^+ to $NADH + H^+$.
6. In two of the following steps ATP is regenerated.

Remember that in effect two molecules of glyceraldehyde-3-phosphate are produced from glucose; therefore, four ATP molecules are generated from each glucose molecule. Two ATP were needed to get the sequence started, so the net gain at this point is two ATP and two molecules of $NADH + H^+$. As you will see later, each $NADH + H^+$ moves to the electron transport chain to unload its hydrogens onto oxygen, producing two ATP. Thus the total yield from glucose to pyruvate is eight ATP.

Fatty Acid Oxidation

Figure C-2 presents fatty acid oxidation. The sequence is as follows:

1. The fatty acid is activated by combining with coenzyme A (CoA). In this reaction, ATP loses two phosphorus atoms (PP, or pyrophosphate) and becomes AMP (adenosine monophosphate)—the equivalent of a loss of two ATP.
2. In the next reaction, two H with their electrons are removed and transferred to FAD, forming $FADH_2$.

FIGURE C-2 Fatty Acid Oxidation

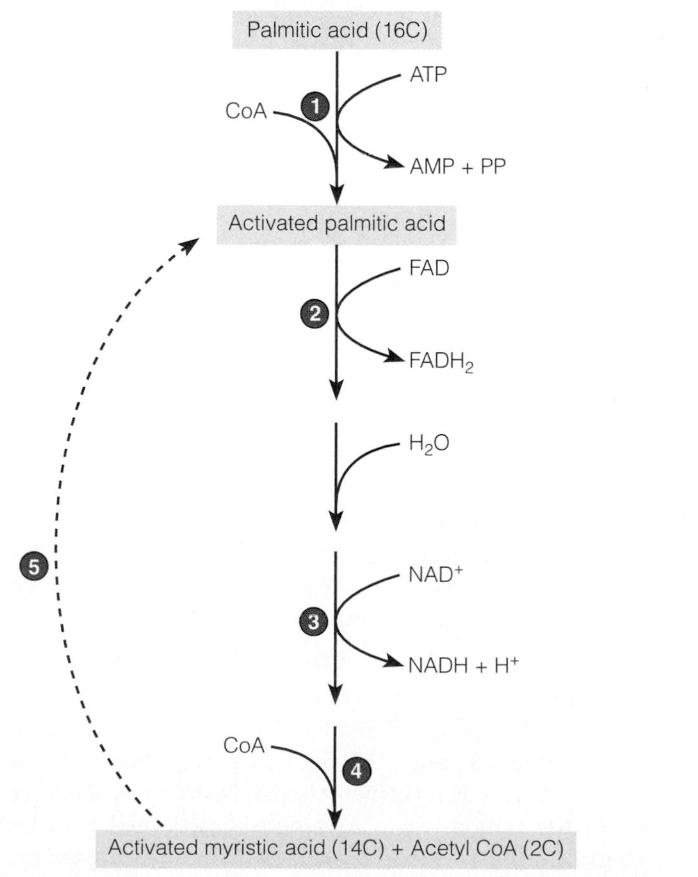
Palmitic acid (16C)
ATP
CoA
1
AMP + PP
Activated palmitic acid
FAD
2
$FADH_2$
H_2O
5
NAD^+
3
$NADH + H^+$
CoA
4
Activated myristic acid (14C) + Acetyl CoA (2C)

3. In a later reaction, two H are removed and go to NAD^+ (forming $NADH + H^+$).
4. The fatty acid is cleaved at the "beta" carbon, the second carbon from the carboxyl (COOH) end. This break results in a fatty acid that is two carbons shorter than the previous one and a two-carbon molecule of acetyl CoA. At the same time, another CoA is attached to the fatty acid, thus activating it for its turn through the series of reactions.
5. The sequence is repeated with each cycle producing an acetyl CoA and a shorter fatty acid until only a 2-carbon fatty acid remains—acetyl CoA.

In the example shown in Figure C-2, palmitic acid (a 16-carbon fatty acid) will go through this series of reactions seven times, using the equivalent of two ATP for the initial activation and generating seven $FADH_2$, seven $NADH + H^+$, and eight acetyl CoA. As you will see later, each of the seven $FADH_2$ will enter the electron transport chain to unload its hydrogens onto oxygen, yielding two ATP (for a total of 14). Similarly, each $NADH + H^+$ will enter the electron transport chain to unload its hydrogens onto oxygen, yielding three ATP (for a total of 21). Thus the oxidation of a 16-carbon fatty acid uses 2 ATP and generates 35 ATP. When the eight acetyl CoA enter the TCA cycle, even more ATP will be generated, as a later section describes.

Amino Acid Degradation

The first step in amino acid degradation is the removal of the nitrogen-containing amino group through either deamination (Figure 7-14 on p. 227) or transamination (Figure 7-15 on p. 228) reactions. Then the remaining carbon skeletons may enter the metabolic pathways at different places, as shown in Figure C-3.

The TCA Cycle

The tricarboxylic acid, or TCA, cycle is the set of reactions that break down acetyl CoA to carbon dioxide and hydrogens. To link glycolysis to the TCA cycle, pyruvate enters the mitochondrion, loses a carbon group, and bonds with a molecule of CoA to become acetyl CoA. The TCA cycle uses any substance that can be converted to acetyl CoA directly or indirectly through pyruvate.

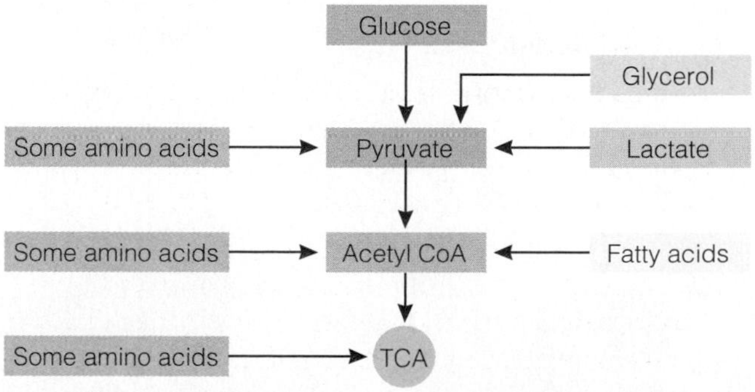
Glucose
Glycerol
Some amino acids
Pyruvate
Lactate
Some amino acids
Acetyl CoA
Fatty acids
Some amino acids
TCA

The step from pyruvate to acetyl CoA is complex. We have included only those substances that will help you understand

C Appendix

FIGURE C-3 Amino Acid Degradation

After losing their amino groups, carbon skeletons can be converted to one of seven molecules that can enter the TCA cycle (presented in Figure C-4).

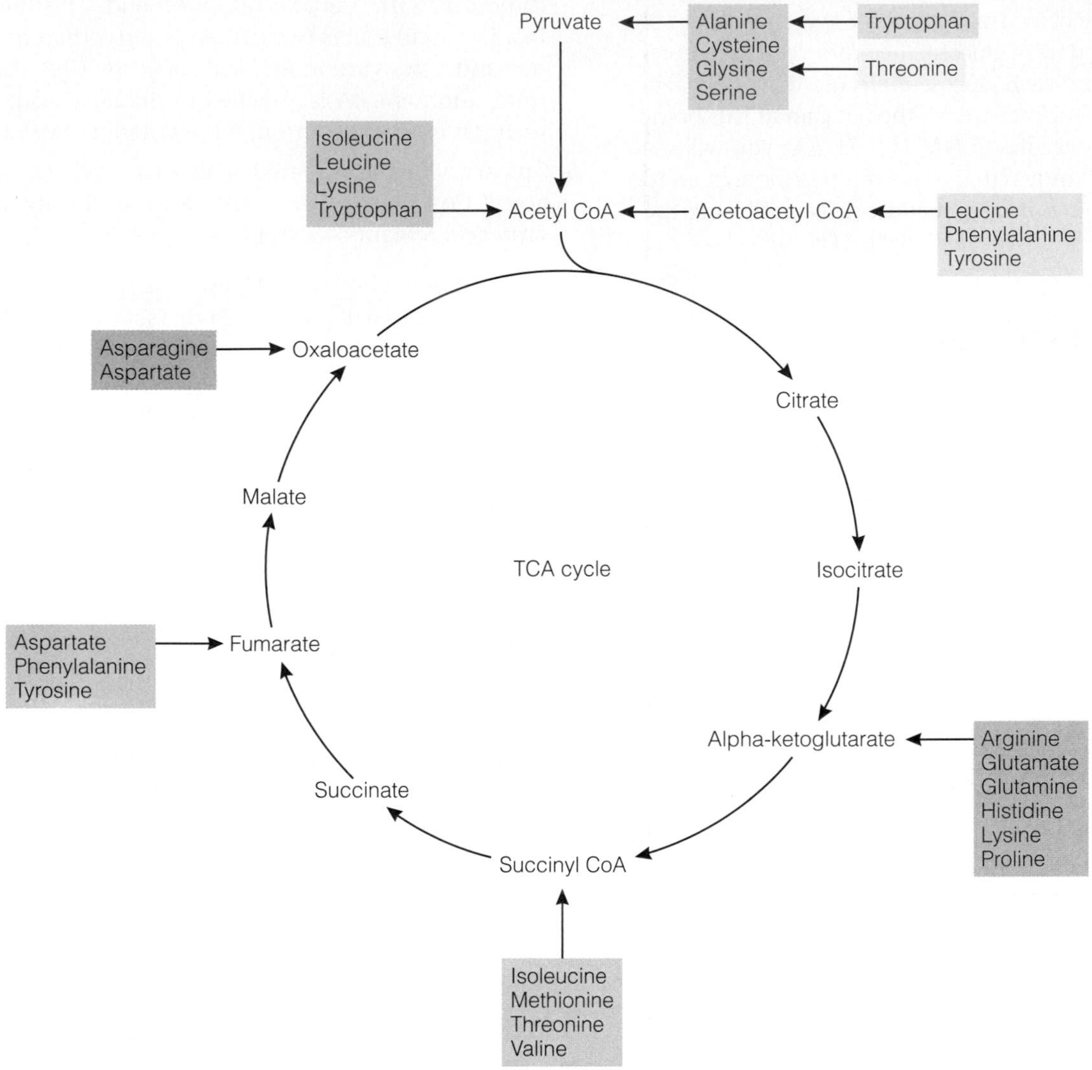

Pyruvate
Alanine
Cysteine
Glysine
Serine
Tryptophan
Threonine
Isoleucine
Leucine
Lysine
Tryptophan
Acetyl CoA
Acetoacetyl CoA
Leucine
Phenylalanine
Tyrosine
Asparagine
Aspartate
Oxaloacetate
Citrate
Malate
TCA cycle
Isocitrate
Aspartate
Phenylalanine
Tyrosine
Fumarate
Alpha-ketoglutarate
Arginine
Glutamate
Glutamine
Histidine
Lysine
Proline
Succinate
Succinyl CoA
Isoleucine
Methionine
Threonine
Valine

Appendix C

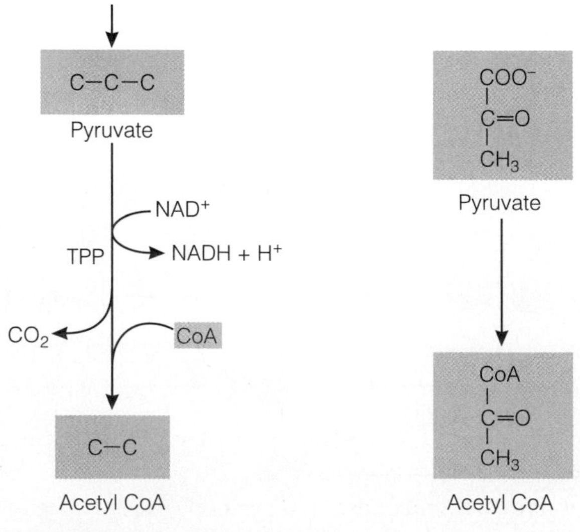

C—C—C
Pyruvate
NAD+
TPP
NADH + H+
CO2
CoA
C—C
Acetyl CoA
COO−
C=O
CH3
Pyruvate
CoA
C=O
CH3
Acetyl CoA

The step from pyruvate to acetyl CoA. (TPP and NAD are coenzymes containing the B vitamins thiamin and niacin, respectively.)

the transfer of energy from the nutrients. Pyruvate loses a carbon to carbon dioxide and is attached to a molecule of CoA. In the process, NAD^+ picks up two hydrogens with their associated electrons, becoming $NADH + H^+$.

Let's follow the steps of the TCA cycle (see the corresponding numbers in Figure C-4).

1. The two-carbon acetyl CoA combines with a four-carbon compound, oxaloacetate. The CoA comes off, and the product is a six-carbon compound, citrate.
2. The atoms of citrate are rearranged to form isocitrate.
3. Now two H (with their two electrons) are removed from the isocitrate. One H becomes attached to the NAD^+ with the two electrons; the other H is released as H^+. Thus NAD^+ becomes $NADH + H^+$. (Remember this $NADH + H^+$, but let's follow the carbons first.) A carbon is combined with two oxygens, forming carbon dioxide (which diffuses away into the blood and is exhaled). What is left is the five-carbon compound alpha-ketoglutarate.

FIGURE C-4 The TCA Cycle

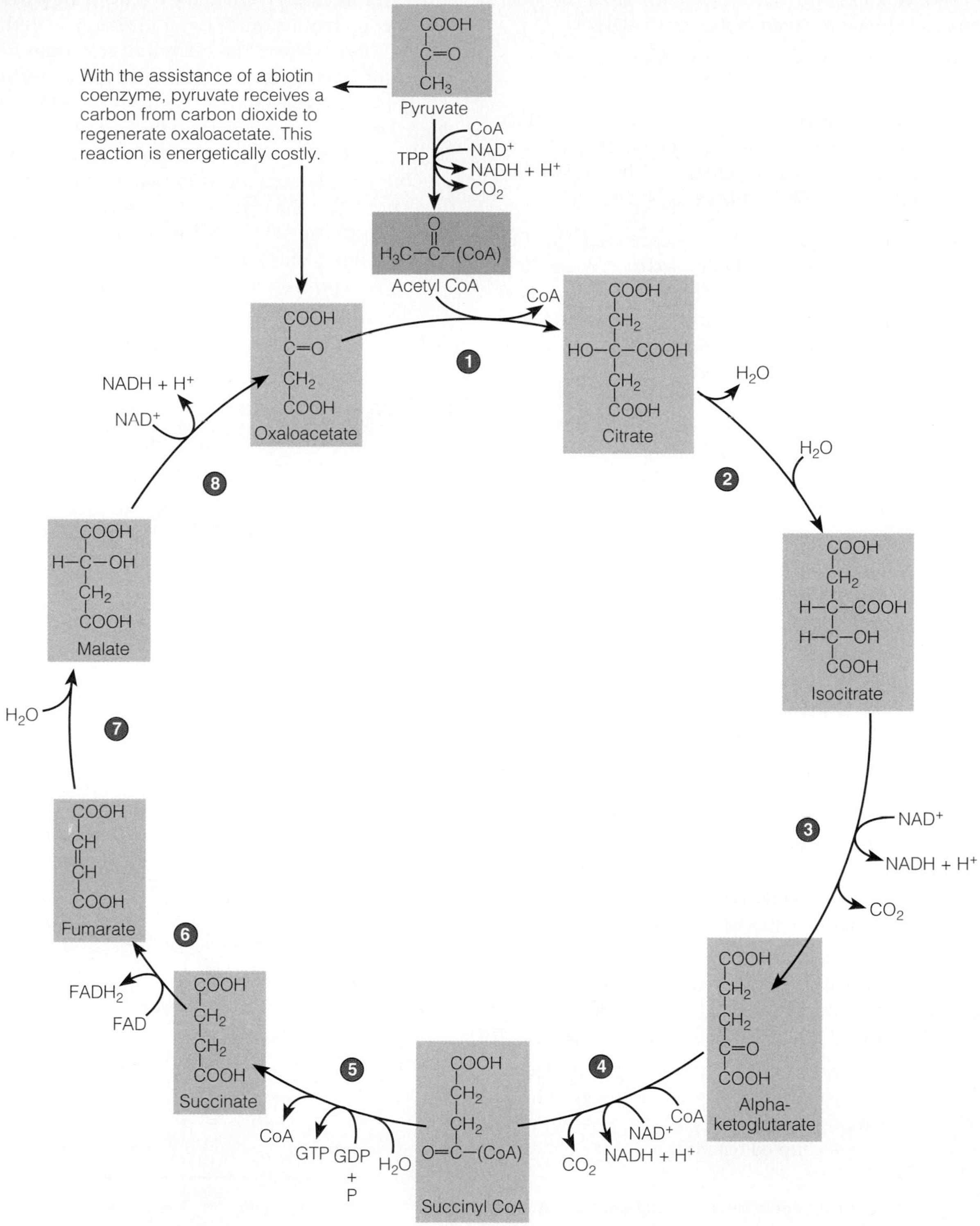

COOH
C=O
CH3
Pyruvate
With the assistance of a biotin coenzyme, pyruvate receives a carbon from carbon dioxide to regenerate oxaloacetate. This reaction is energetically costly.
TPP
CoA
NAD+
NADH + H+
CO2
O
H3C—C—(CoA)
Acetyl CoA
CoA
COOH
CH2
HO—C—COOH
CH2
COOH
Citrate
H2O
H2O
COOH
CH2
H—C—COOH
H—C—OH
COOH
Isocitrate
NAD+
NADH + H+
CO2
COOH
CH2
CH2
C=O
COOH
Alpha-ketoglutarate
CoA
NAD+
NADH + H+
CO2
COOH
CH2
CH2
O=C—(CoA)
Succinyl CoA
H2O
GDP + P
GTP
CoA
COOH
CH2
CH2
COOH
Succinate
FAD
FADH2
COOH
CH
CH
COOH
Fumarate
H2O
COOH
H—C—OH
CH2
COOH
Malate
NAD+
NADH + H+
COOH
C=O
CH2
COOH
Oxaloacetate
1
2
3
4
5
6
7
8

4. Now two compounds interact with alpha-ketoglutarate —a molecule of CoA and a molecule of NAD^+. In this complex reaction, a carbon and two oxygens are removed (forming carbon dioxide); two hydrogens are removed and go to NAD^+ (forming NADH + H^+); and the remaining four-carbon compound is attached to the CoA, forming succinyl CoA. (Remember this NADH + H^+ also. You will see later what happens to it.)

5. Now two molecules react with succinyl CoA—a molecule called GDP and one of phosphate (P). The CoA comes off, the GDP and P combine to form the high-energy compound GTP (similar to ATP), and succinate remains. (Remember this GTP.)

6. In the next reaction, two H with their electrons are removed from succinate and are transferred to a molecule of FAD (a coenzyme like NAD^+) to form $FADH_2$. The product that remains is fumarate. (Remember this $FADH_2$.)
7. Next a molecule of water is added to fumarate, forming malate.
8. A molecule of NAD^+ reacts with the malate; two H with their associated electrons are removed from the malate and form NADH + H^+. The product that remains is the four-carbon compound oxaloacetate. (Remember this NADH + H^+.)

We are back where we started. The oxaloacetate formed in this process can combine with another molecule of acetyl CoA (step 1), and the cycle can begin again, as shown in Figure C-4.

So far, we have seen two carbons brought in with acetyl CoA and two carbons ending up in carbon dioxide. But where are the energy and the ATP we promised?

A review of the eight steps of the TCA cycle shows that the compounds NADH + H^+ (three molecules), $FADH_2$, and GTP capture energy originally found in acetyl CoA. To see how this energy ends up in ATP, we must follow the electrons further—into the electron transport chain.

The Electron Transport Chain

The six reactions described here are those of the electron transport chain, which is shown in Figure C-5. Since oxygen is required for these reactions, and ADP and P are combined to form ATP in several of them (ADP is phosphorylated), these reactions are also called oxidative phosphorylation.

An important concept to remember at this point is that an electron is not a fixed amount of energy. The electrons that bond the H to NAD^+ in NADH have a relatively large amount of energy. In the series of reactions that follow, they release this energy in small amounts, until at the end they are attached (with H) to oxygen (O) to make water (H_2O). In some of the steps, the energy they release is captured into ATP in coupled reactions.

1. In the first step of the electron transport chain, NADH reacts with a molecule called a flavoprotein, losing its electrons (and their H). The products are NAD^+ and reduced flavoprotein. A little energy is released as heat in this reaction.
2. The flavoprotein passes on the electrons to a molecule called coenzyme Q. Again they release some energy as heat, but ADP and P bond together and form ATP, storing much of the energy. This is a coupled reaction: ADP + P $\rightarrow$ ATP.
3. Coenzyme Q passes the electrons to cytochrome *b*. Again the electrons release energy.
4. Cytochrome *b* passes the electrons to cytochrome *c* in a coupled reaction in which ATP is formed: ADP + P $\rightarrow$ ATP.
5. Cytochrome *c* passes the electrons to cytochrome *a*.
6. Cytochrome *a* passes them (with their H) to an atom of oxygen (O), forming water (H_2O). This is a coupled reaction in which ATP is formed: ADP + P $\rightarrow$ ATP.

As Figure C-5 shows, each time NADH is oxidized (loses its electrons) by this means, the energy it releases is captured into three ATP molecules. When the electrons are passed on to water at the end, they are much lower in energy than they were originally. This completes the story of the electrons from NADH.

As for $FADH_2$, its electrons enter the electron transport chain at coenzyme Q. From coenzyme Q to water, ATP is generated in only two steps. Therefore, $FADH_2$ coming out of the TCA cycle yields just two ATP molecules.

One energy-receiving compound of the TCA cycle (GTP) does not enter the electron transport chain but gives its energy directly to ADP in a simple phosphorylation reaction. This reaction yields one ATP.

It is now possible to draw up a balance sheet of glucose metabolism (see Table C-3). Glycolysis has yielded 4 NADH + H^+ and 4 ATP molecules and has spent 2 ATP. The 2 acetyl CoA

FIGURE C-5 The Electron Transport Chain

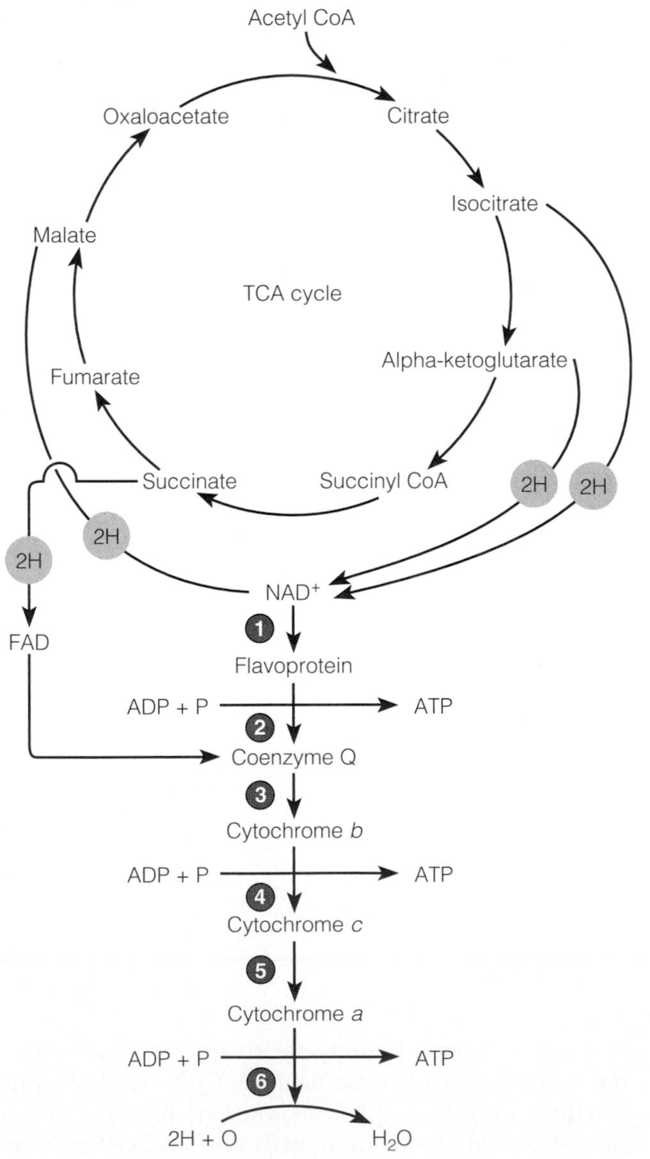
Acetyl CoA
Oxaloacetate
Citrate
Isocitrate
Malate
TCA cycle
Alpha-ketoglutarate
Fumarate
Succinate
Succinyl CoA
2H
2H
2H
2H
2H
NAD+
FAD
1
Flavoprotein
ADP + P
ATP
2
Coenzyme Q
3
Cytochrome b
ADP + P
ATP
4
Cytochrome c
5
Cytochrome a
ADP + P
ATP
6
2H + O
H2O

going through the TCA cycle have yielded 6 NADH + H^+, 2 $FADH_2$, and 2 GTP molecules. After the NADH + H^+ and $FADH_2$ have gone through the electron transport chain, there are 34 ATP. Added to these are the 4 ATP from glycolysis and the 2 ATP from GTP, making the total 40 ATP generated from one molecule of glucose. After the expense of 2 ATP is subtracted, there is a net gain of 38 ATP.*

A similar balance sheet from the complete breakdown of one 16-carbon fatty acid would show a net gain of 129 ATP. As mentioned earlier, 35 ATP were generated from the seven $FADH_2$ and seven NADH + H^+ produced during fatty acid oxidation. The eight acetyl CoA produced will each generate 12 ATP as they go through the TCA cycle and the electron transport chain, for a total of 96 more ATP. After subtracting the 2 ATP needed to activate the fatty acid initially, the net yield from one 16-carbon fatty acid: $35 + 96 - 2 = 129$ ATP.

These calculations help explain why fat yields more energy (measured as kcalories) per gram than carbohydrate or protein. The more hydrogen atoms a fuel contains, the more ATP will be generated during oxidation. The 16-carbon fatty acid molecule, with its 32 hydrogen atoms, generates 129 ATP, whereas glucose, with its 12 hydrogen atoms, yields only 38 ATP.

The TCA cycle and the electron transport chain are the body's major means of capturing the energy from nutrients in ATP molecules. Other means, such as anaerobic glycolysis, contribute energy quickly, but the aerobic processes are the most efficient. Biologists and chemists understand much more about these processes than has been presented here.

TABLE C-3 Balance Sheet for Glucose Metabolism

	Expenditures	Income
Glycolysis:		
1 glucose	2 ATP	4 ATP
1 fructose-1,6-diphosphate		2 NADH + H^+
2 pyruvate		2 NADH + H^+
TCA cycle:		
2 isocitrate		2 NADH + H^+
2 alpha-ketoglutarate		2 NADH + H^+
2 succinyl CoA		2 GTP
2 succinate		2 $FADH_2$
2 malate		2 NADH + H^+
Total ATP collected:		
From glycolysis	2 ATP	4 ATP
From 2 NADH + H^+		4–6 ATP[a]
From 8 NADH + H^+		24 ATP
From 2 GTP		2 ATP
From 2 $FADH_2$		4 ATP
Totals:	2 ATP	38–40 ATP
Balance on hand from 1 molecule of glucose:		36–38 ATP

[a]Each NADH + H^+ from glycolysis can yield 2 or 3 ATP. See the accompanying text.

Alcohol's Interference with Energy Metabolism

Highlight 7 provides an overview of how alcohol interferes with energy metabolism. With an understanding of the TCA cycle, a few more details may be appreciated. During alcohol metabolism, the enzyme alcohol dehydrogenase oxidizes alcohol to acetaldehyde while it simultaneously reduces a molecule of NAD^+ to NADH + H^+. The related enzyme acetaldehyde dehydrogenase reduces another NAD^+ to NADH + H^+ while it oxidizes acetaldehyde to acetyl CoA, the compound that enters the TCA cycle to generate energy. Thus, whenever alcohol is being metabolized in the body, NAD^+ diminishes, and NADH + H^+ accumulates. Chemists say that the body's "redox state" is altered, because NAD^+ can oxidize, and NADH + H^+ can reduce, many other body compounds. During alcohol metabolism, NAD^+ becomes unavailable for the multitude of reactions for which it is required.

As the previous sections just explained, for glucose to be completely metabolized, the TCA cycle must be operating, and NAD^+ must be present. If these conditions are not met (and when alcohol is present, they may not be), the pathway will be blocked, and traffic will back up—or an alternate route will be taken. Think about this as you follow the pathway shown in Figure C-6.

In each step of alcohol metabolism in which NAD^+ is converted to NADH + H^+, hydrogen ions accumulate, resulting in a dangerous shift of the acid-base balance toward acid (Chapter 12 explains acid-base balance). The accumulation of NADH + H^+ depresses TCA cycle activity, so pyruvate and acetyl CoA build up. This condition favors the conversion of pyruvate to lactic acid, which serves as a temporary storage place for hydrogens from NADH + H^+. The conversion of pyruvate to lactic acid restores some NAD^+, but a lactic acid buildup has serious consequences of its own. It adds to the body's acid burden and interferes with the excretion of uric acid, causing goutlike symptoms. Molecules of acetyl CoA become building blocks for fatty acids or ketone bodies. The making of ketone bodies consumes acetyl CoA and generates NAD^+; but some ketone bodies are acids, so they push the acid-base balance further toward acid.

Thus alcohol cascades through the metabolic pathways, wreaking havoc along the way. These consequences have physical effects, which Highlight 7 describes.

The Urea Cycle

Chapter 7 sums up the process by which waste nitrogen is eliminated from the body by stating that ammonia molecules combine with carbon dioxide to produce urea. This is true, but it is not the whole story. Urea is produced in a multistep process within the cells of the liver.

*The total may sometimes be 36 or 37, rather than 38, ATP. The NADH + H^+ generated in the cytoplasm during glycolysis pass their electrons on to shuttle molecules, which move them into the mitochondria. One shuttle, malate, contributes its electrons to the electron transport chain before the first site of ATP synthesis, yielding 3 ATP. Another, glycerol phosphate, adds its electrons into the chain beyond that first site, yielding 2 ATP. Thus sometimes 3, and sometimes only 2, ATP result from the NADH + H^+ that arise from glycolysis. The amount depends on the cell.

FIGURE C-6 Ethanol Enters the Metabolic Path

This is a simplified version of the glucose-to-energy pathway showing the entry of ethanol. The coenzyme NAD (which is the active form of the B vitamin niacin) is the only one shown here; however, many others are involved.

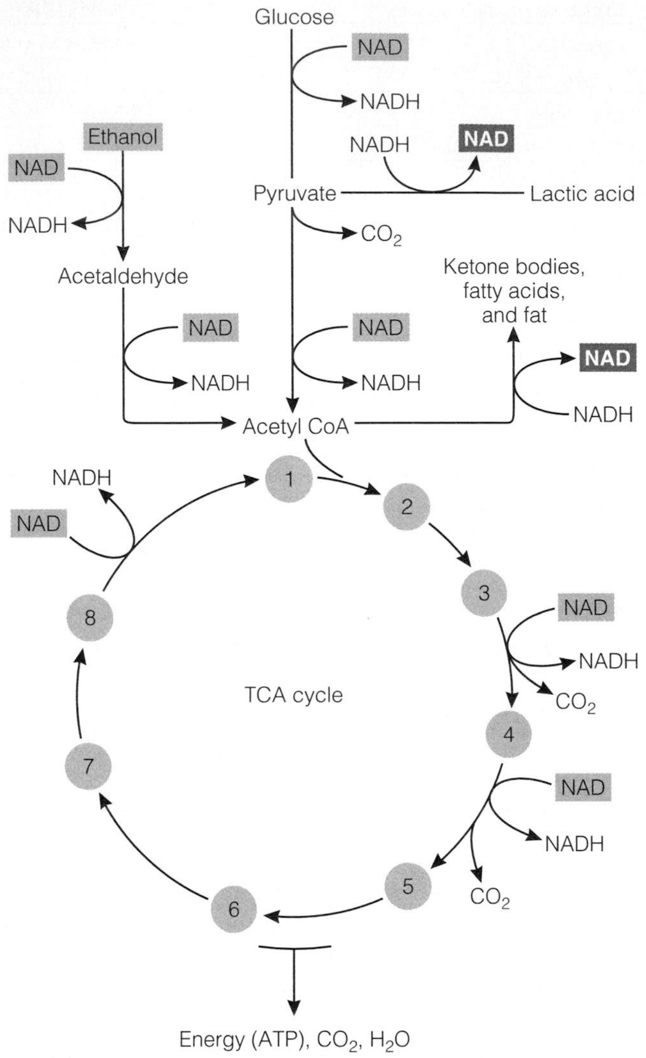

Glucose
NAD
NADH
Ethanol
NAD
NADH
NADH
NAD
Pyruvate
Lactic acid
CO_2
Acetaldehyde
Ketone bodies, fatty acids, and fat
NAD
NADH
NAD
NADH
NAD
NADH
Acetyl CoA
NADH
NAD
1
2
3
8
NAD
NADH
CO_2
TCA cycle
4
7
NAD
NADH
5
CO_2
6
Energy (ATP), CO_2, H_2O

FIGURE C-7 The Urea Cycle

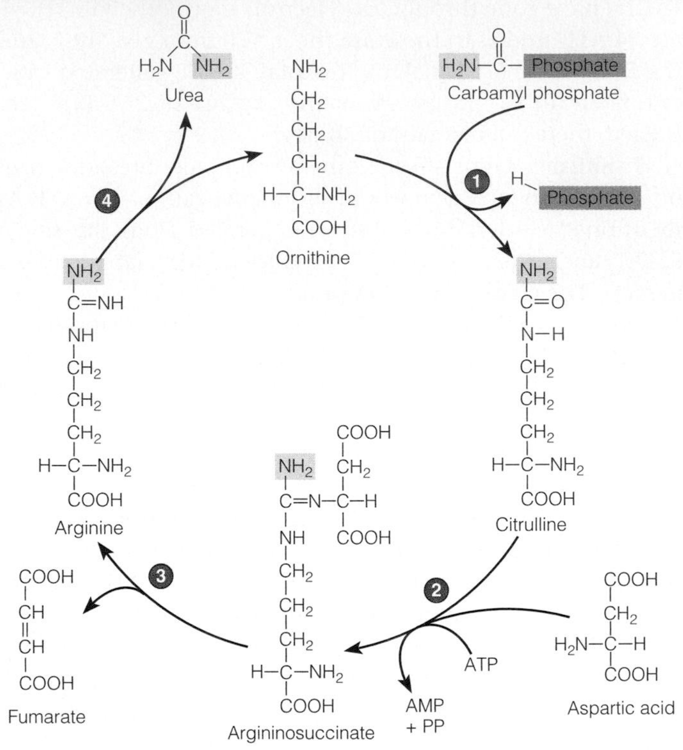

Urea
Carbamyl phosphate
Phosphate
Ornithine
1
4
Phosphate
Arginine
Citrulline
3
2
Fumarate
ATP
AMP + PP
Argininosuccinate
Aspartic acid

Ammonia, freed from an amino acid or other compound during metabolism anywhere in the body, arrives at the liver by way of the bloodstream and is taken into a liver cell. There, it is first combined with carbon dioxide and a phosphate group from ATP to form carbamyl phosphate:

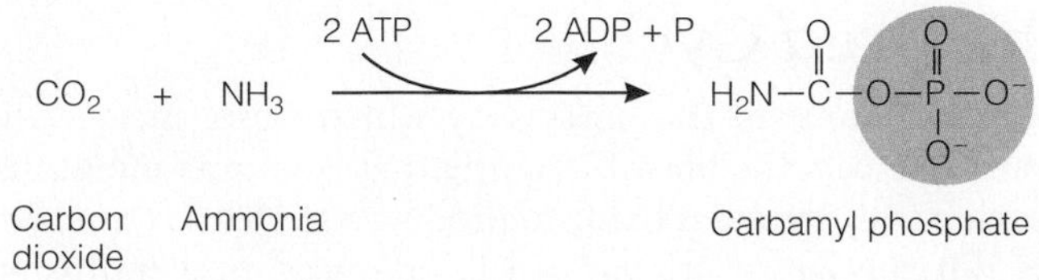

CO_2 + NH_3
2 ATP
2 ADP + P
Carbon dioxide
Ammonia
Carbamyl phosphate

Figure C-7 shows the cycle of four reactions that follow.

1. Carbamyl phosphate combines with the amino acid ornithine, losing its phosphate group. The compound formed is citrulline.
2. Citrulline combines with the amino acid aspartic acid, to form argininosuccinate. The reaction requires energy from ATP. (ATP was shown earlier losing one phosphorus atom in a phosphate group, P, to become ADP. In this reaction, it loses two phosphorus atoms joined together, PP, and becomes adenosine monophosphate, AMP.)
3. Argininosuccinate is split, forming another acid, fumarate, and the amino acid arginine.
4. Arginine loses its terminal carbon with two attached amino groups and picks up an oxygen from water. The end product is urea, which the kidneys excrete in the urine. The compound that remains is ornithine, identical to the ornithine with which this series of reactions began, and ready to react with another molecule of carbamyl phosphate and turn the cycle again.

Formation of Ketone Bodies

Normally, fatty acid oxidation proceeds all the way to carbon dioxide and water. However, in ketosis (discussed in Chapter 7), an intermediate is formed from the condensation of two molecules of acetyl CoA: acetoacetyl CoA. Figure C-8 shows the formation of ketone bodies from that intermediate.

FIGURE C-8 The Formation of Ketone Bodies

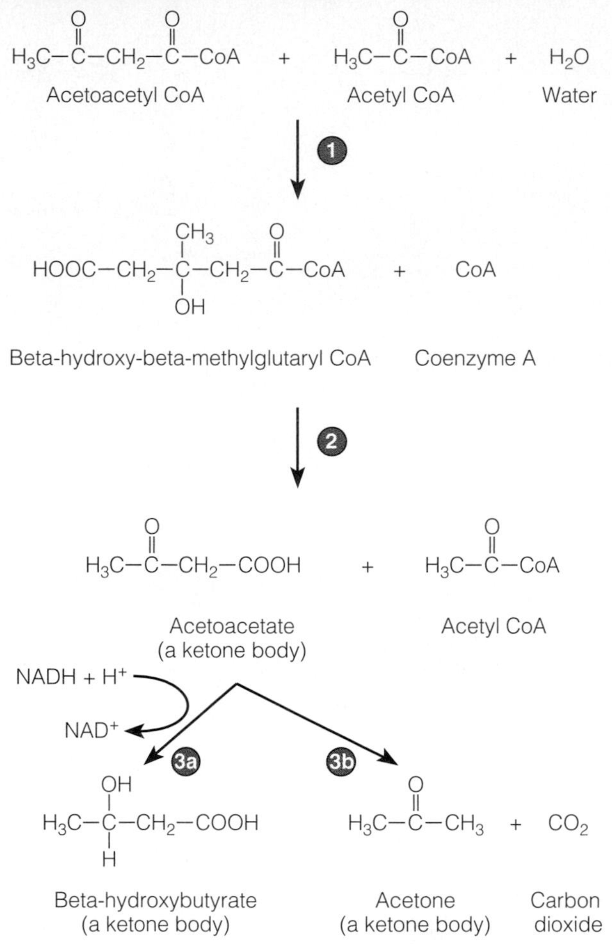

O O
$H_3C-C-CH_2-C-CoA$ + $H_3C-C-CoA$ + H_2O
Acetoacetyl CoA
Acetyl CoA
Water
1
CH_3 O
$HOOC-CH_2-C-CH_2-C-CoA$ + CoA
OH
Beta-hydroxy-beta-methylglutaryl CoA
Coenzyme A
2
$H_3C-C-CH_2-COOH$ + $H_3C-C-CoA$
Acetoacetate
(a ketone body)
Acetyl CoA
NADH + H^+
NAD^+
3a
3b
OH
$H_3C-C-CH_2-COOH$
H
$H_3C-C-CH_3$ + CO_2
Beta-hydroxybutyrate
(a ketone body)
Acetone
(a ketone body)
Carbon
dioxide

1. Acetoacetyl CoA condenses with acetyl CoA to form a six-carbon intermediate, beta-hydroxy-betamethylglutaryl CoA.
2. This intermediate is cleaved to acetyl CoA and acetoacetate.
3. Acetoactate can be metabolized either to beta-hydroxybutyrate acid (step 3a) or to acetone (3b).

Acetoacetate, beta-hydroxybutyrate, and acetone are the so-called ketone bodies of ketosis. Two are real ketones (they have a C=O group between two carbons); the other is an alcohol that has been produced during ketone formation—hence the term *ketone bodies,* rather than ketones, to describe the three of them. There are many other ketones in nature; these three are characteristic of ketosis in the body.

C Appendix

Measures of Protein Quality

CONTENTS

In a world where food is scarce and many people's diets contain marginal or inadequate amounts of protein, it is important to know which foods contain the highest-quality protein. Chapter 6 describes protein quality, and this appendix presents different measures researchers use to assess the quality of a food protein. The accompanying glossary defines related terms.

GLOSSARY

amino acid scoring: a measure of protein quality assessed by comparing a protein's amino acid pattern with that of a reference protein; sometimes called **chemical scoring.**

biological value (BV): a measure of protein quality assessed by measuring the amount of protein nitrogen that is retained from a given amount of protein nitrogen absorbed.

net protein utilization (NPU): a measure of protein quality assessed by measuring the amount of protein nitrogen that is retained from a given amount of protein nitrogen eaten.

PDCAAS (protein digestibility–corrected amino acid score): a measure of protein quality assessed by comparing the amino acid score of a food protein with the amino acid requirements of preschool-age children and then correcting for the true digestibility of the protein; recommended by the FAO/WHO and used to establish protein quality of foods for Daily Value percentages on food labels.

protein efficiency ratio (PER): a measure of protein quality assessed by determining how well a given protein supports weight gain in growing rats; used to establish the protein quality for infant formulas and baby foods.

Amino Acid Scoring

Amino acid scoring evaluates a protein's quality by determining its amino acid composition and comparing it with that of a reference protein. The advantages of amino acid scoring are that it is simple and inexpensive, it easily identifies the limiting amino acid, and it can be used to score mixtures of different proportions of two or more proteins mathematically without having to make up a mixture and test it. Its chief weaknesses are that it fails to estimate the digestibility of a protein, which may strongly affect the protein's quality; it relies on a chemical procedure in which certain amino acids may be destroyed, making the pattern that is analyzed inaccurate; and it is blind to other features of the protein (such as the presence of substances that may inhibit the digestion or utilization of the protein) that would only be revealed by a test in living animals.

Table D-1 shows the reference pattern for the nine essential amino acids. To interpret the table, read, "For every 3210 units of essential amino acids, 145 must be histidine, 340 must be isoleucine, 540 must be leucine," and so on. To compare a test protein with the reference protein, the experimenter first obtains a chemical analysis of the test protein's amino acids. Then, taking 3210 units of the amino acids, the experimenter compares the amount of each amino acid to the amount found in 3210 units of essential amino acids in egg protein. For example, suppose the test protein contained (per 3210 units) 360 units of isoleucine; 500 units of leucine; 350 of lysine; and for each of the other amino acids, more units than egg protein contains. The two amino acids that are low are leucine (500 as compared with 540 in egg) and lysine (350 versus 440 in egg). The ratio, amino acid in the test protein divided by amino acid in egg, is 500/540 (or about 0.93) for leucine and 350/440 (or about 0.80) for lysine. Lysine is the limiting amino acid (the one that falls shortest compared with egg). If the protein's limiting amino acid is 80 percent of the amount found in the reference protein, it receives a score of 80.

TABLE D-1 A Reference Pattern for Amino Acid Scoring of Proteins

Essential Amino Acids	Reference Protein—Whole Egg (mg amino acid/g nitrogen)
Histidine	145
Isoleucine	340
Leucine	540
Lysine	440
Methionine + cystine[a]	355
Phenylalanine + tyrosine[b]	580
Threonine	294
Tryptophan	106
Valine	410
Total	3210

[a]Methionine is essential and is also used to make cystine. Thus the methionine requirement is lower if cystine is supplied.
[b]Phenylalanine is essential and is also used to make tyrosine if not enough of the latter is available. Thus the phenylalanine requirement is lower if tyrosine is also supplied.

PDCAAS

PDCAAS (protein digestibility–corrected amino acid score) takes the amino acid scoring method a step further by correcting for the digestibility of the protein. Chapter 6 presents PDCAAS in detail.

D Appendix

TABLE D-2 Biological Values (BV) of Selected Foods

Egg	100
Milk	93
Beef	75
Fish	75
Corn	72

NOTE: 100 is the maximum BV a food protein can receive.

Biological Value

The **biological value (BV)** of a protein measures its efficiency in supporting the body's needs. In a test of biological value, two nitrogen balance studies are done. In the first, no protein is fed, and nitrogen (N) excretions in the urine and feces are measured. It is assumed that under these conditions, N lost in the urine is the amount the body always necessarily loses by filtration into the urine each day, regardless of what protein is fed (endogenous N). The N lost in the feces (called metabolic N) is the amount the body invariably loses into the intestine each day, whether or not food protein is fed. (To help you remember the terms: endogenous N is "urinary N on a zero-protein diet"; metabolic N is "fecal N on a zero-protein diet.")

In the second study, an amount of protein slightly below the requirement is fed. Intake and losses are measured; then the BV is derived using this formula:

$$BV = \frac{\text{N retained}}{\text{N absorbed}} \times 100.$$

The denominator of this equation expresses the amount of nitrogen *absorbed:* food N minus fecal N (excluding the metabolic N the body would lose in the feces anyway, even without food). The numerator expresses the amount of N *retained* from the N absorbed: absorbed N (as in the denominator) minus the N excreted in the urine (excluding the endogenous N the body would lose in the urine anyway, even without food). The more nitrogen retained, the higher the protein quality. (Recall that when an essential amino acid is missing, protein synthesis stops, and the remaining amino acids are deaminated and the nitrogen excreted.)

Egg protein has a BV of 100, indicating that 100 percent of the nitrogen absorbed is retained. Supplied in adequate quantity, a protein with a BV of 70 or greater can support human growth as long as energy intake is adequate. Table D-2 presents the BV for selected foods.

This method has the advantages of being based on experiments with human beings (it can be done with animals, too, of course) and of measuring actual nitrogen retention. But it is also cumbersome, expensive, and often impractical, and it is based on several assumptions that may not be valid. For example, the physiology, normal environment, or typical food intake of the subjects used for testing may not be similar to those for whom the test protein may ultimately be used. For another example, the retention of protein in the body does not necessarily mean that it is being well utilized. Considerable exchange of protein among tissues (protein turnover) occurs, but is hidden from view when only N intake and output are measured. The test of biological value wouldn't detect if one tissue were shorted.

Net Protein Utilization

Like BV, **net protein utilization (NPU)** measures how efficiently a protein is used by the body and involves two balance studies. The difference is that NPU measures retention of food nitrogen rather than food nitrogen absorbed (as in BV). The formula for NPU is:

$$NPU = \frac{\text{N retained}}{\text{N intake}} \times 100.$$

The numerator is the same as for BV, but the denominator represents food N intake only—not N absorbed.

This method offers advantages similar to those of BV determinations and is used more frequently, with animals as the test subjects. A drawback is that if a low NPU is obtained, the test results offer no help in distinguishing between two possible causes: a poor amino acid composition of the test protein or poor digestibility. There is also a limit to the extent to which animal test results can be assumed to be applicable to human beings.

Protein Efficiency Ratio

The **protein efficiency ratio (PER)** measures the weight gain of a growing animal and compares it to the animal's protein intake. Until recently, the PER was generally accepted in the United States and Canada as the official method for assessing protein quality, and it is still used to evaluate proteins for infants.

Young rats are fed a measured amount of protein and weighed periodically as they grow. The PER is expressed as:

$$PER = \frac{\text{weight gain (g)}}{\text{protein intake (g)}}.$$

This method has the virtues of economy and simplicity, but it also has many drawbacks. The experiments are time-consuming; the amino acid needs of rats are not the same as those of human beings; and the amino acid needs for growth are not the same as for the maintenance of adult animals (growing animals need more lysine, for example). Table D-3 presents PER values for selected foods.

TABLE D-3 Protein Efficiency Ratio (PER) Values of Selected Proteins

Casein (milk)	2.8
Soy	2.4
Glutein (wheat)	0.4

Nutrition Assessment: Supplemental Information

Chapter 17 described data from nutrition assessments that help health professionals evaluate patients' nutrition status and nutrient needs. This appendix provides additional information that may be useful for complete assessments.

CONTENTS

Growth Charts

Health professionals generally evaluate physical development by monitoring the growth rate of a child and comparing this rate with standard charts. Standard charts compare weight to age, height to age, and weight to height; ideally, height and weight are in roughly the same percentile. Although individual growth patterns may vary, a child's growth curve will generally stay at about the same percentile throughout childhood. In children whose growth has been retarded, nutrition rehabilitation will ideally induce height and weight to increase to higher percentiles. In overweight children, the goal is for weight to remain stable as height increases, until weight becomes appropriate for height.

Reminder: The *body mass index (BMI)* is an index of a person's weight in relation to height, determined by dividing the weight in kilograms by the square of the height in meters:

$$BMI = \frac{\text{Weight (kg)}}{\text{Height (m)}^2}.$$

To evaluate growth in infants, an assessor uses charts such as those in Figures E-1 (A and B) through E-6 (A and B).■ The assessor follows these steps to plot a weight measurement on a percentile graph:

■ Chapter 15 presents BMI charts for children and adolescents.

- Select the appropriate chart based on age and gender.
- Locate the child's age along the horizontal axis on the bottom of the chart.
- Locate the child's weight in pounds or kilograms along the vertical axis.
- Mark the chart where the age and weight lines intersect, and read off the percentile.

To assess length, height, or head circumference, the assessor follows the same procedure, using the appropriate chart. (When length is measured, use the chart for birth to 36 months; when height is measured, use the chart for 2 to 20 years.) Head circumference percentile should be similar to the child's height and weight percentiles. With height, weight, and head circumference measures plotted on growth percentile charts, a skilled clinician can begin to interpret the data.

Percentile charts divide the measures of a population into 100 equal divisions. Thus half of the population falls above the 50th percentile, and half falls below. The use of percentile measures allows for comparisons among people of the same age and gender. For example, a six-month-old female infant whose weight is at the 75th percentile weighs more than 75 percent of the female infants her age.

Head circumference is generally measured in children under two years of age. Since the brain grows rapidly before birth and during early infancy, extreme and chronic malnutrition during these times can impair brain development, curtailing the number of brain cells and the size of head circumference. Nonnutritional factors, such as certain disorders and genetic variation, can also influence head circumference.

Appendix E

FIGURE E-1A Weight-for-Age Percentiles: Boys, Birth to 36 Months

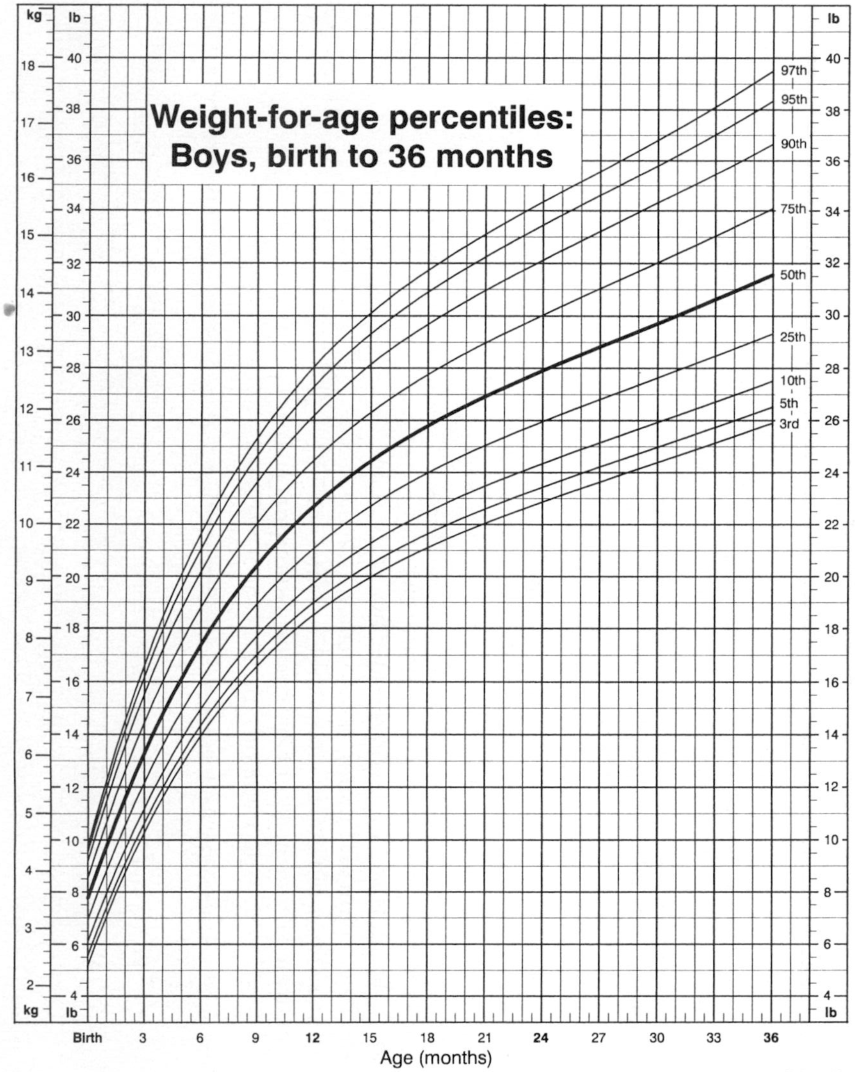
Weight-for-age percentiles:
Boys, birth to 36 months
kg
lb
97th
95th
90th
75th
50th
25th
10th
5th
3rd
Birth
3
6
9
12
15
18
21
24
27
30
33
36
Age (months)
CDC

SOURCE: Developed by the National Center for Health Statistics in collaboration with the National Center for Chronic Disease Prevention and Health Promotion (2000).

Figure 1. Weight-for-age percentiles, boys, birth to 36 months, CDC growth charts: United States

FIGURE E-1B Weight-for-Age Percentiles: Girls, Birth to 36 Months

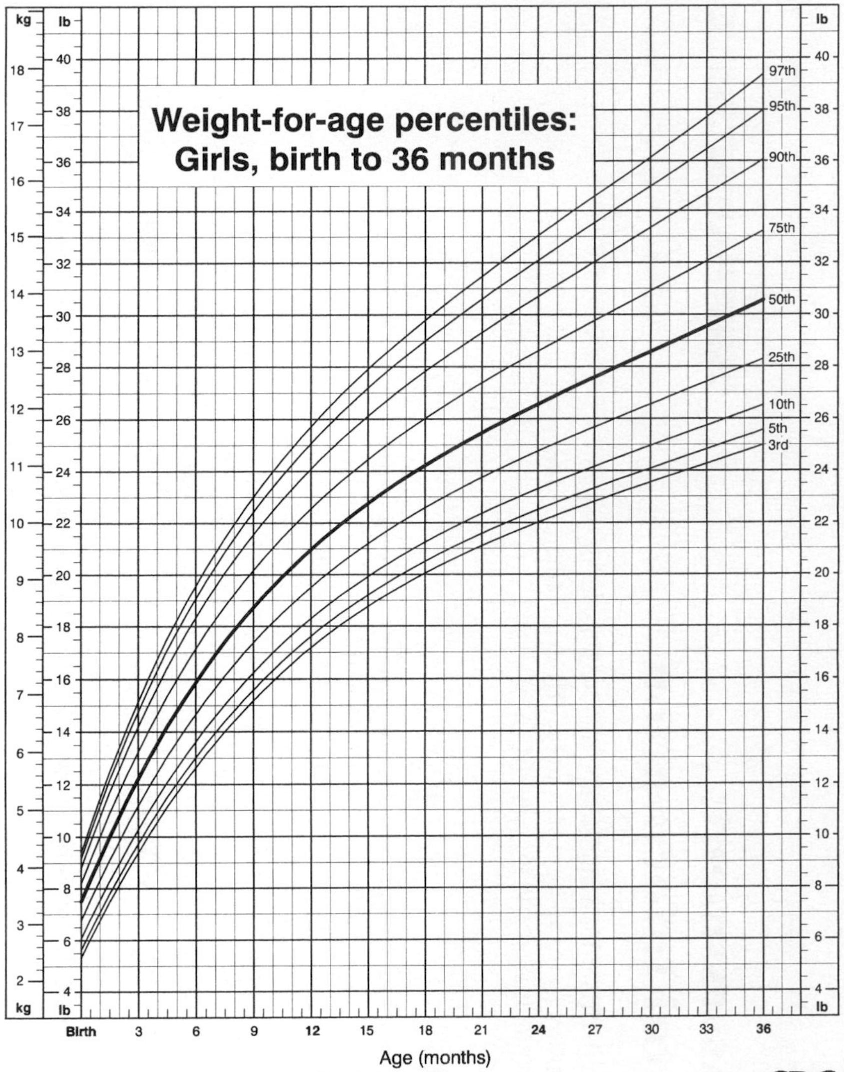
Weight-for-age percentiles:
Girls, birth to 36 months
kg
lb
97th
95th
90th
75th
50th
25th
10th
5th
3rd
Birth
3
6
9
12
15
18
21
24
27
30
33
36
Age (months)
CDC

SOURCE: Developed by the National Center for Health Statistics in collaboration with the National Center for Chronic Disease Prevention and Health Promotion (2000).

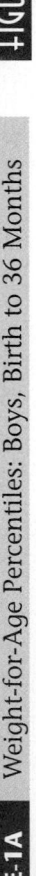

Figure 2. Weight-for-age percentiles, girls, birth to 36 months, CDC growth charts: United States

FIGURE E-2A Length-for-Age Percentiles: Boys, Birth to 36 Months

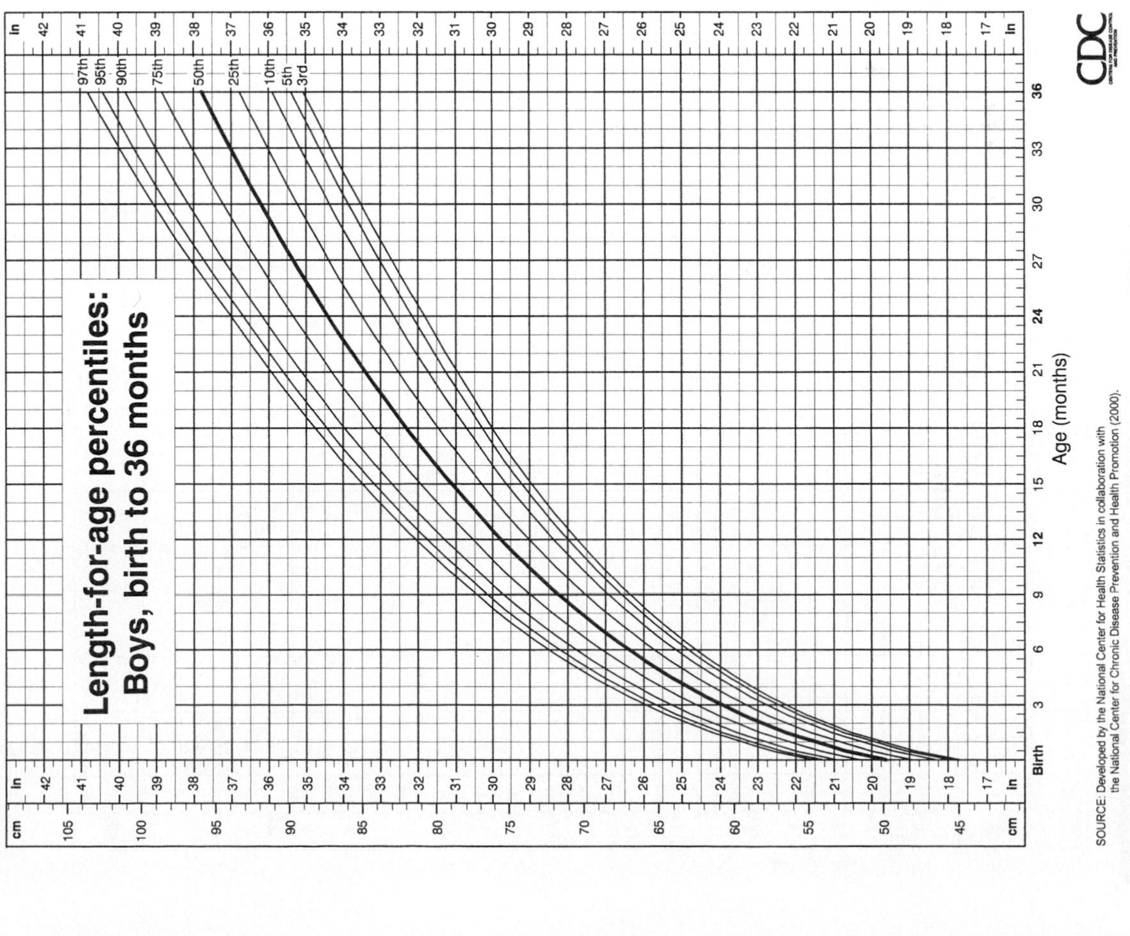
Length-for-age percentiles:
Boys, birth to 36 months
97th
95th
90th
75th
50th
25th
10th
5th
3rd
Age (months)
Birth
3
6
9
12
15
18
21
24
27
30
33
36
cm
in
CDC
SOURCE: Developed by the National Center for Health Statistics in collaboration with the National Center for Chronic Disease Prevention and Health Promotion (2000).
Figure 3. Length-for-age percentiles, boys, birth to 36 months, CDC growth charts: United States

FIGURE E-2B Length-for-Age Percentiles: Girls, Birth to 36 Months

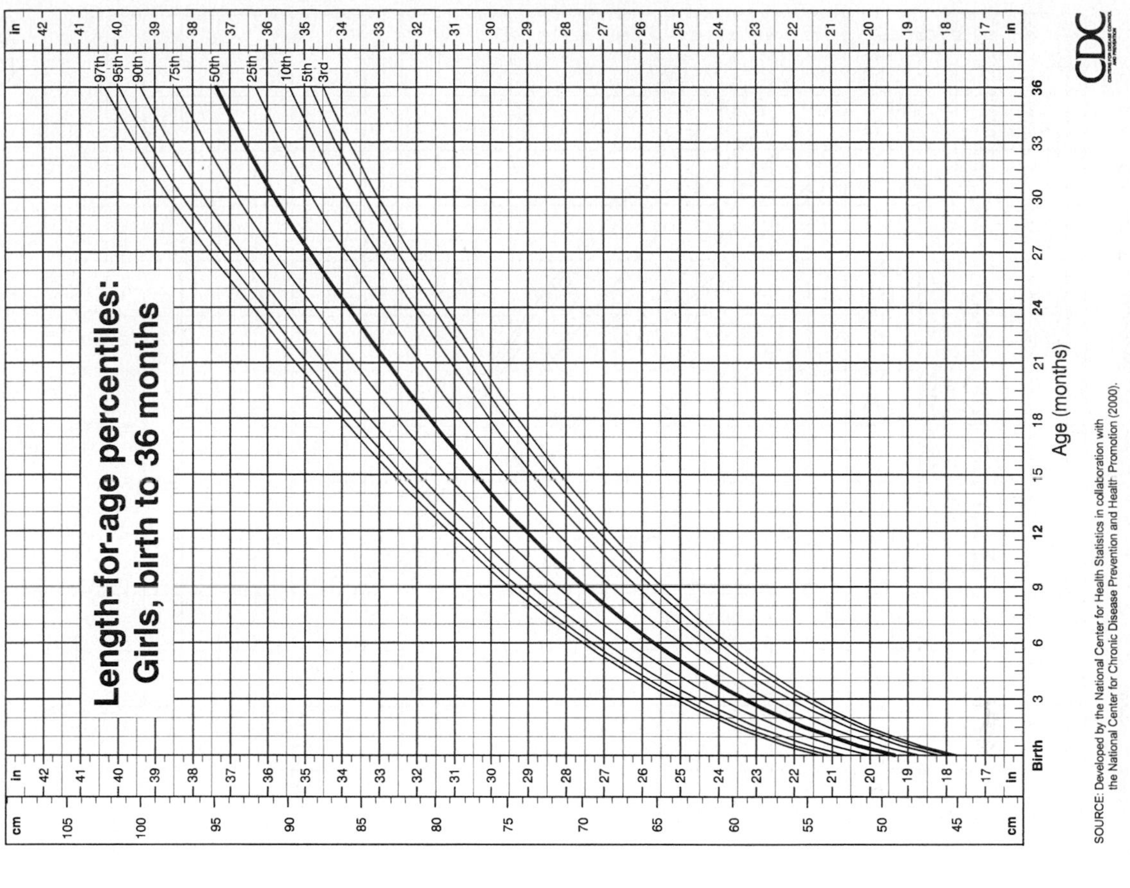
Length-for-age percentiles:
Girls, birth to 36 months
97th
95th
90th
75th
50th
25th
10th
5th
3rd
Age (months)
Birth
3
6
9
12
15
18
21
24
27
30
33
36
cm
in
CDC
SOURCE: Developed by the National Center for Health Statistics in collaboration with the National Center for Chronic Disease Prevention and Health Promotion (2000).
Figure 4. Length-for-age percentiles, girls, birth to 36 months, CDC growth charts: United States

Appendix E

Appendix E

FIGURE E-3A Weight-for-Length Percentiles: Boys, Birth to 36 Months

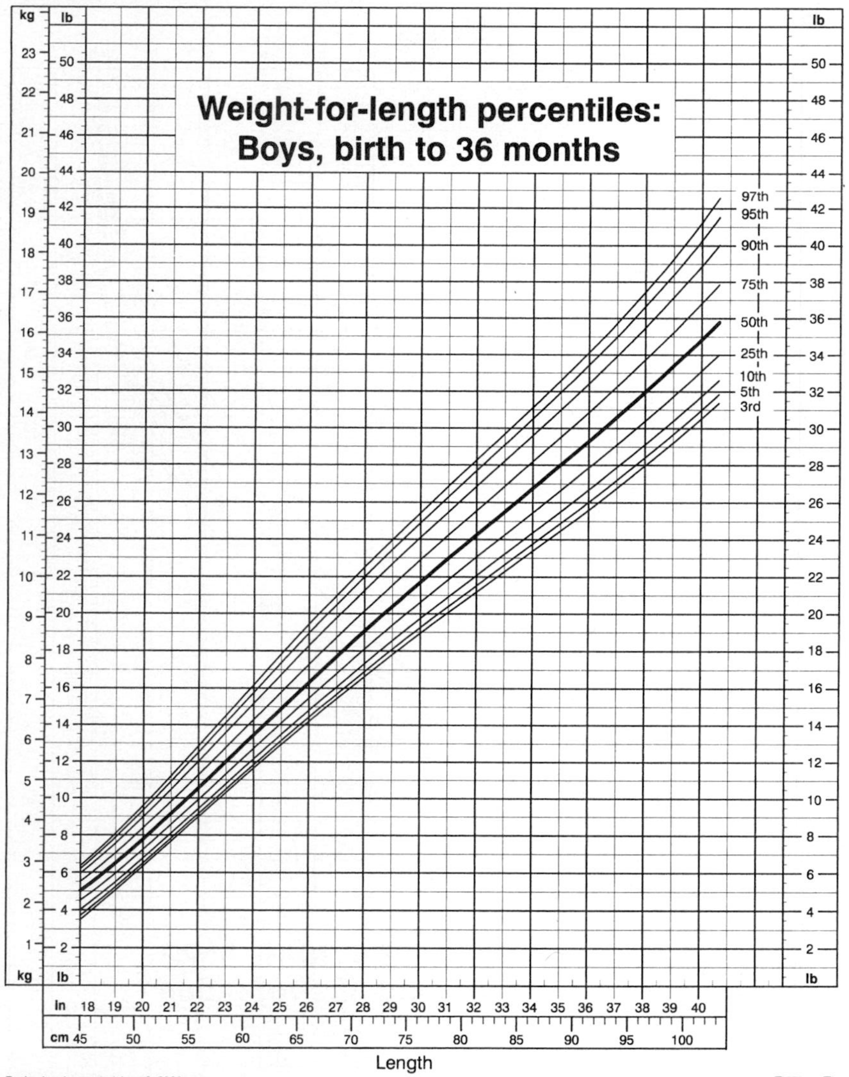
Weight-for-length percentiles:
Boys, birth to 36 months
97th
95th
90th
75th
50th
25th
10th
5th
3rd
kg
lb
in
cm
Length

Revised and corrected June 8, 2000.
SOURCE: Developed by the National Center for Health Statistics in collaboration with the National Center for Chronic Disease Prevention and Health Promotion (2000).

CDC

Figure 5. Weight-for-length percentiles, boys, birth to 36 months, CDC growth charts: United States

FIGURE E-3B Weight-for-Length Percentiles: Girls, Birth to 36 Months

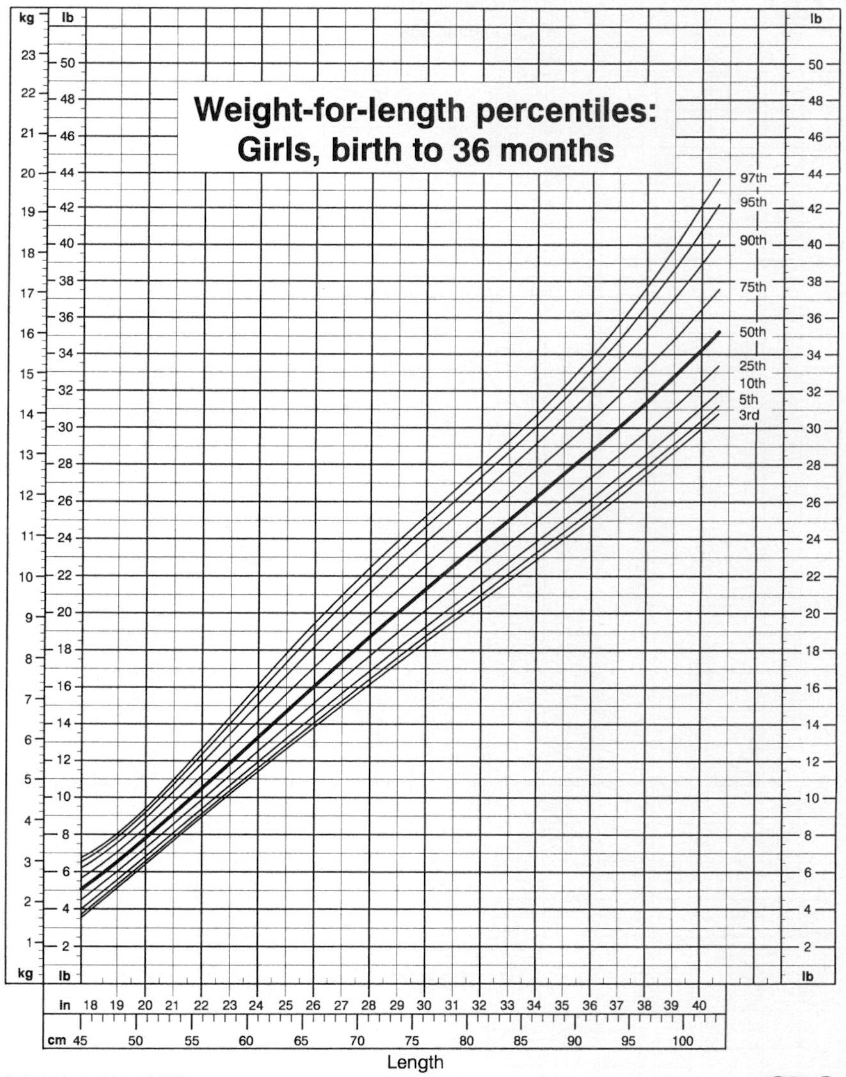
Weight-for-length percentiles:
Girls, birth to 36 months
97th
95th
90th
75th
50th
25th
10th
5th
3rd
kg
lb
in
cm
Length

Revised and corrected June 8, 2000.
SOURCE: Developed by the National Center for Health Statistics in collaboration with the National Center for Chronic Disease Prevention and Health Promotion (2000).

CDC

Figure 6. Weight-for-length percentiles, girls, birth to 36 months, CDC growth charts: United States

FIGURE E-4A Weight-for-Age Percentiles: Boys, 2 to 20 Years

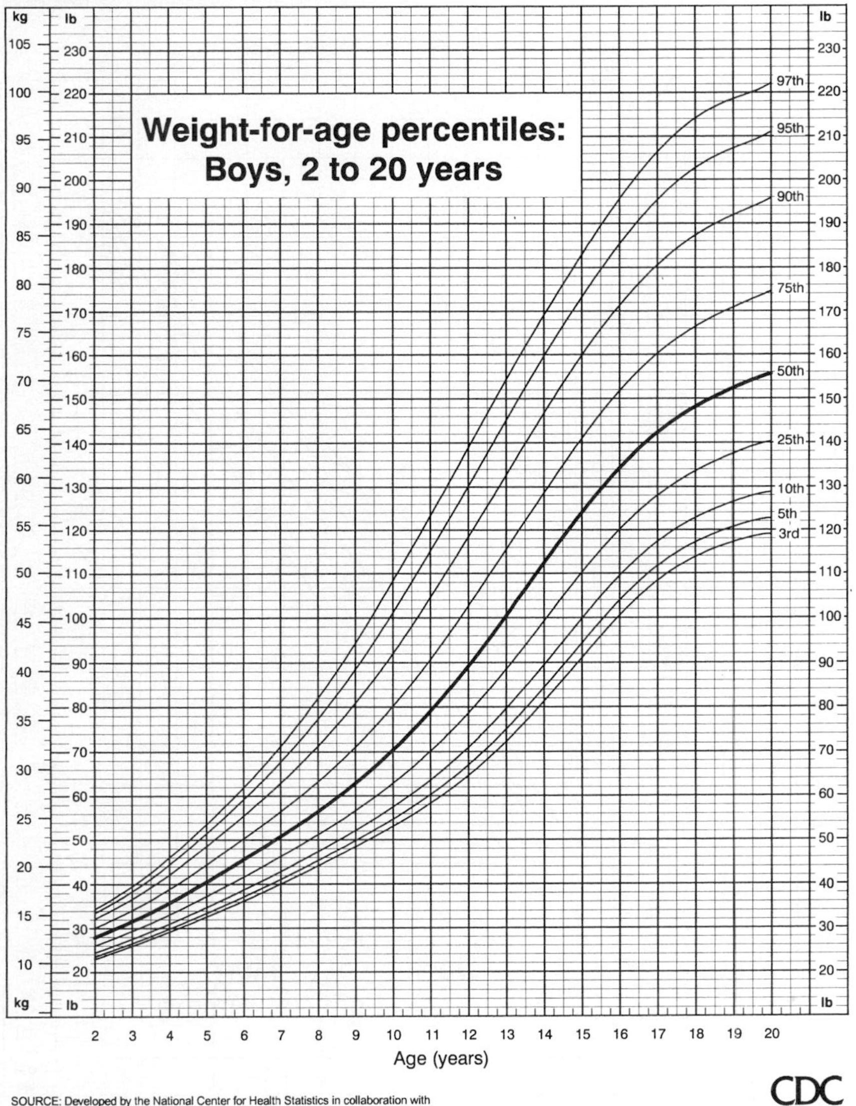
Weight-for-age percentiles:
Boys, 2 to 20 years
kg
lb
97th
95th
90th
75th
50th
25th
10th
5th
3rd
Age (years)
CDC

SOURCE: Developed by the National Center for Health Statistics in collaboration with the National Center for Chronic Disease Prevention and Health Promotion (2000).

Figure 9. Weight-for-age percentiles, boys, 2 to 20 years, CDC growth charts: United States

FIGURE E-4B Weight-for-Age Percentiles: Girls, 2 to 20 Years

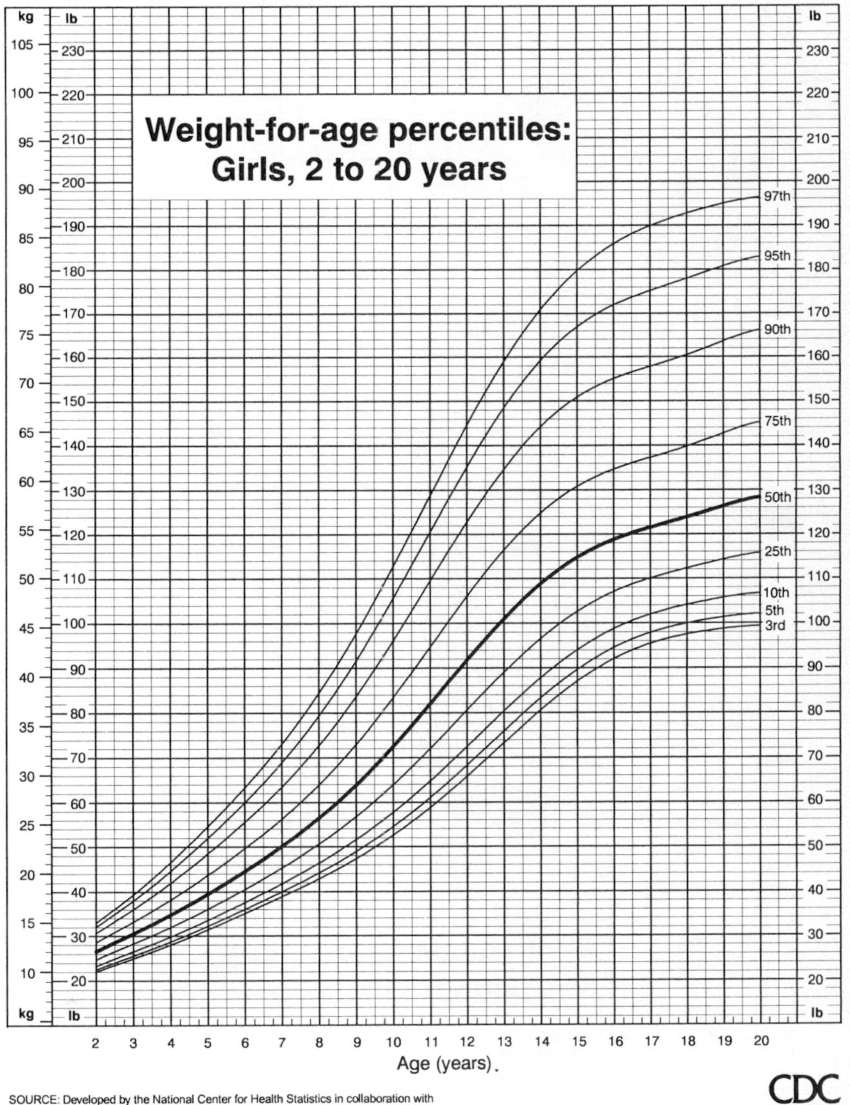
Weight-for-age percentiles:
Girls, 2 to 20 years
kg
lb
97th
95th
90th
75th
50th
25th
10th
5th
3rd
Age (years).
CDC

SOURCE: Developed by the National Center for Health Statistics in collaboration with the National Center for Chronic Disease Prevention and Health Fromotion (2000).

Figure 10. Weight-for-age percentiles, girls, 2 to 20 years, CDC growth charts: United States

FIGURE E-5A Stature-for-Age Percentiles: Boys, 2 to 20 Years

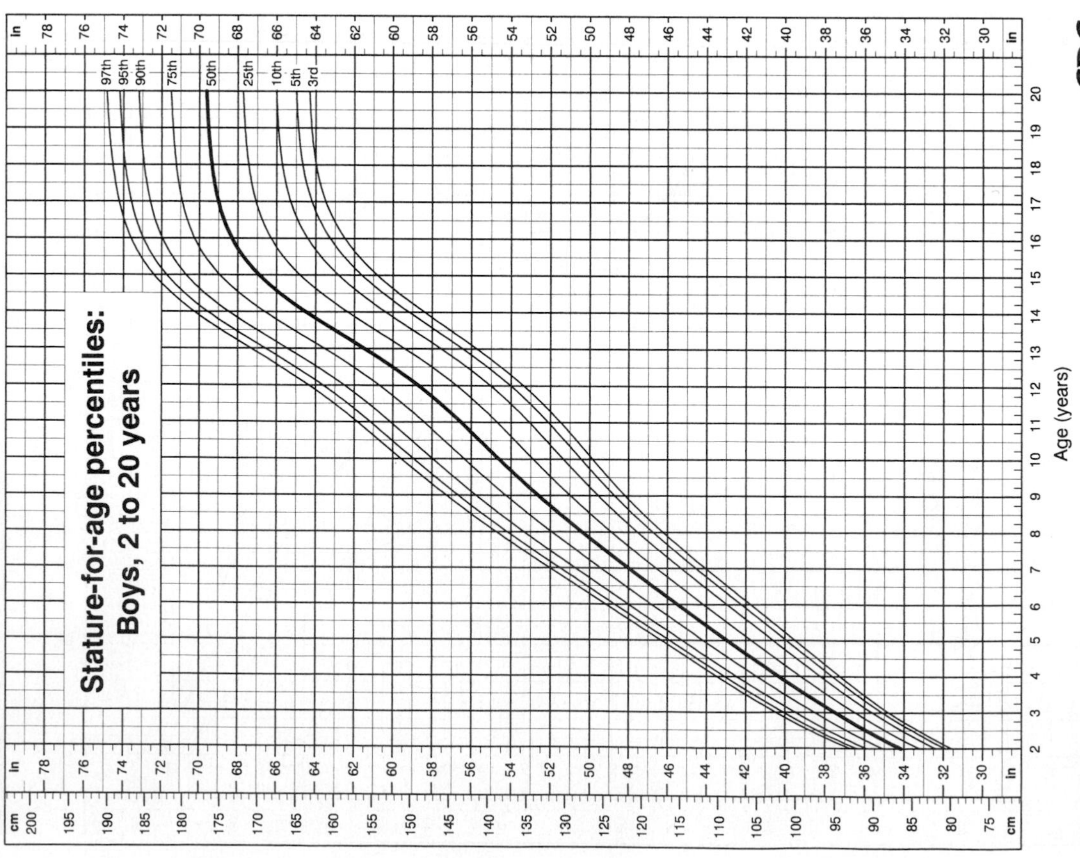
Stature-for-age percentiles:
Boys, 2 to 20 years
97th
95th
90th
75th
50th
25th
10th
5th
3rd
cm
in
Age (years)

SOURCE: Developed by the National Center for Health Statistics in collaboration with the National Center for Chronic Disease Prevention and Health Promotion (2000).

Figure 11. Stature-for-age percentiles, boys, 2 to 20 years, CDC growth charts: United States

FIGURE E-5B Stature-for-Age Percentiles: Girls, 2 to 20 Years

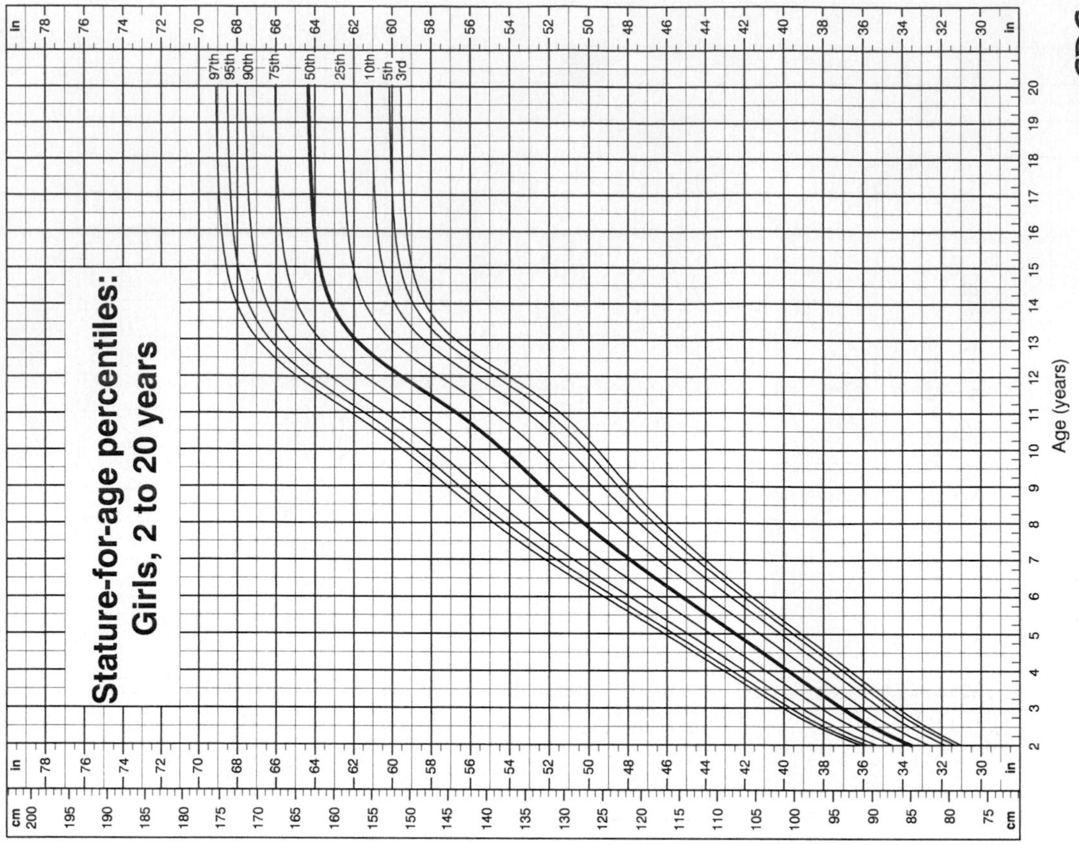
Stature-for-age percentiles:
Girls, 2 to 20 years
97th
95th
90th
75th
50th
25th
10th
5th
3rd
cm
in
Age (years)

SOURCE: Developed by the National Center for Health Statistics in collaboration with the National Center for Chronic Disease Prevention and Health Promotion (2000).

Figure 12. Stature-for-age percentiles, girls, 2 to 20 years, CDC growth charts: United States

FIGURE E-6A Weight-for-Stature Percentiles: Boys, 2 to 20 Years

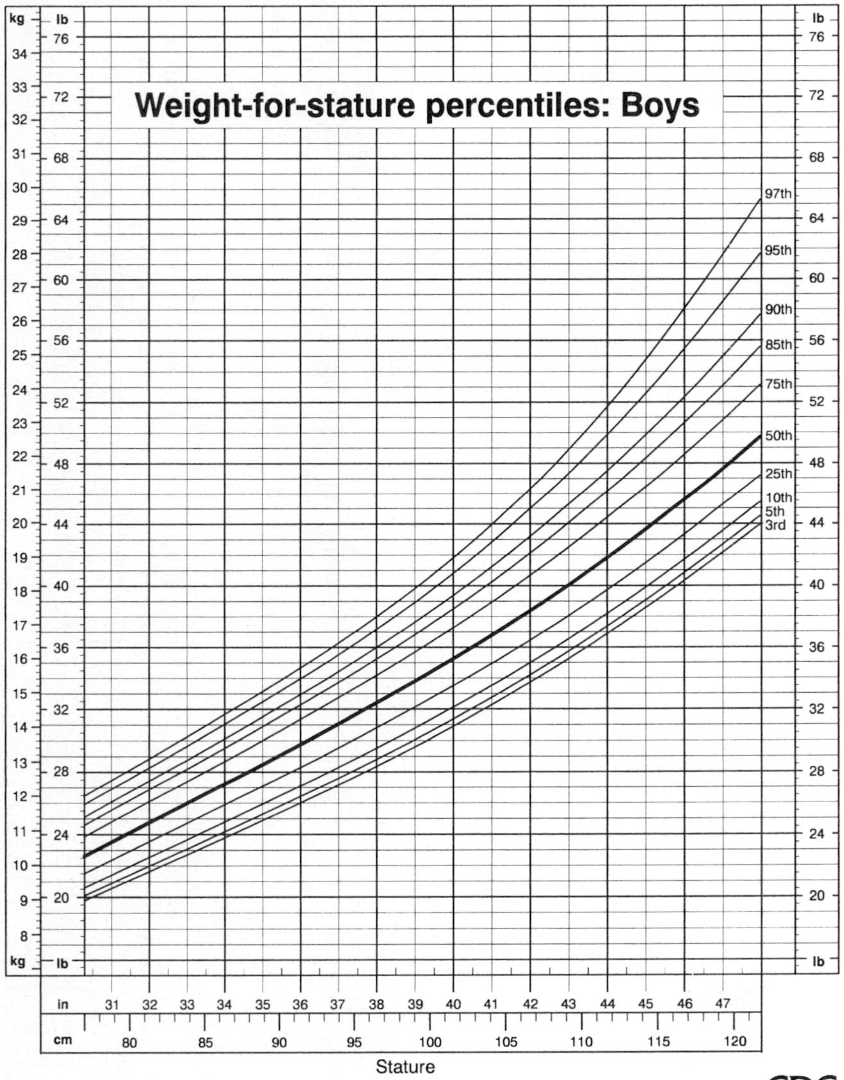
Weight-for-stature percentiles: Boys
kg
lb
97th
95th
90th
85th
75th
50th
25th
10th
5th
3rd
in
cm
Stature
CDC

SOURCE: Developed by the National Center for Health Statistics in collaboration with the National Center for Chronic Disease Prevention and Health Promotion (2000).

Figure 13. Weight-for-stature percentiles, boys, CDC growth charts: United States

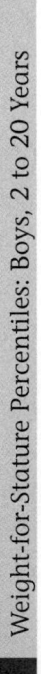

FIGURE E-6B Weight-for-Stature Percentiles: Girls, 2 to 20 Years

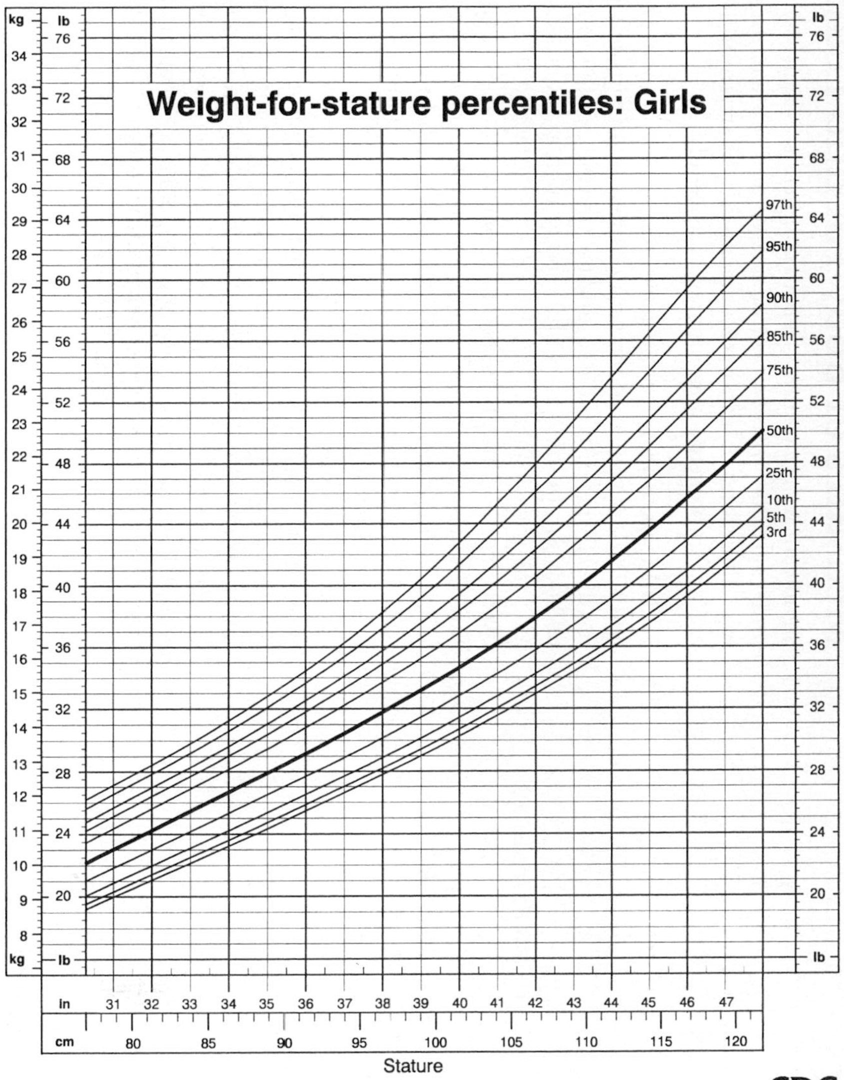
Weight-for-stature percentiles: Girls
kg
lb
97th
95th
90th
85th
75th
50th
25th
10th
5th
3rd
in
cm
Stature
CDC

SOURCE: Developed by the National Center for Health Statistics in collaboration with the National Center for Chronic Disease Prevention and Health Promotion (2000).

Figure 14. Weight-for-stature percentiles, girls, CDC growth charts: United States

Measures of Body Fat and Lean Tissue

Significant weight changes in both children and adults can reflect overnutrition or undernutrition with respect to energy and protein. To estimate the degree to which fat stores or lean tissues are affected by overnutrition or malnutrition, several anthropometric measurements are useful.

Fatfold Measures Fatfold measures provide a good estimate of total body fat and a fair assessment of the fat's location. Approximately half the fat in the body lies directly beneath the skin, and the thickness of this subcutaneous fat reflects total body fat. In some parts of the body, such as the back and the back of the arm over the triceps muscle, this fat is loosely attached;■ a person can pull it up between the thumb and forefinger to obtain a measure of fatfold thickness. To measure the fatfold, a skilled assessor follows a standard procedure using reliable calipers (illustrated in Figure E-7) and then compares the measurement with standards. Triceps fatfold measures greater than 15 millimeters in men or 25 millimeters in women suggest excessive body fat.

■ Common sites for fatfold measures:
- Triceps.
- Biceps.
- Subscapular (below shoulder blade).
- Suprailiac (above hip bone).
- Abdomen.
- Upper thigh.

Fatfold measurements correlate directly with the risk of heart disease. They assess central obesity and its associated risks better than do weight measures alone. If a person gains body fat, the fatfold increases proportionately; if the person loses fat, it decreases. Measurements taken from central-body sites (around the abdomen) better reflect changes in fatness than those taken from upper sites (arm and back). A major limitation of the fatfold test is that fat may be thicker under the skin in one area than in another. A pinch at the side of the waistline may not yield

FIGURE E-7 How to Measure the Triceps Fatfold

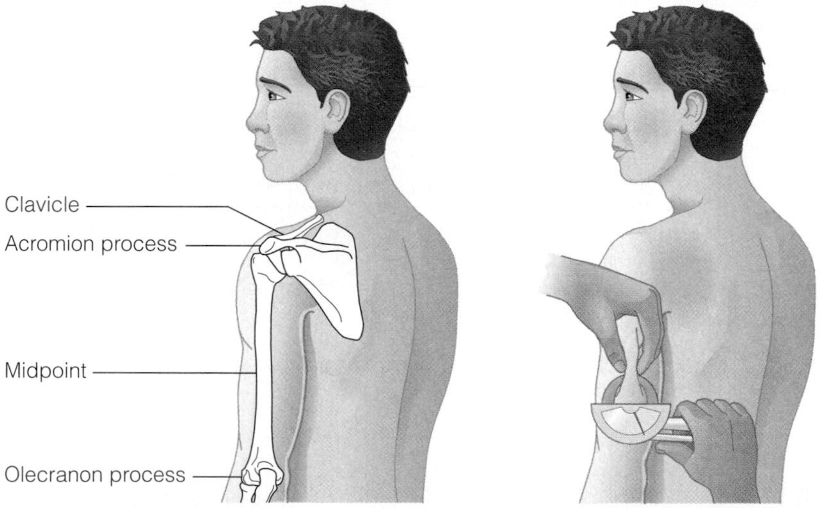
Clavicle
Acromion process
Midpoint
Olecranon process

A. Find the midpoint of the arm:
1. Ask the subject to bend his or her arm at the elbow and lay the hand across the stomach. (If he or she is right-handed, measure the left arm, and vice versa.)
2. Feel the shoulder to locate the acromion process. It helps to slide your fingers along the clavicle to find the acromion process. The olecranon process is the tip of the elbow.
3. Place a measuring tape from the acromion process to the tip of the elbow. Divide this measurement by 2, and mark the midpoint of the arm with a pen.

B. Measure the fatfold:
1. Ask the subject to let his or her arm hang loosely to the side.
2. Grasp a fold of skin and subcutaneous fat between the thumb and forefinger slightly above the midpoint mark. Gently pull the skin away from the underlying muscle. (This step takes a lot of practice. If you want to be sure you don't have muscle as well as fat, ask the subject to contract and relax the muscle. You should be able to feel if you are pinching muscle.)
3. Place the calipers over the fatfold at the midpoint mark, and read the measurement to the nearest 1.0 millimeter in two to three seconds. (If using plastic calipers, align pressure lines, and read the measurement to the nearest 1.0 millimeter in two to three seconds.)
4. Repeat steps 2 and 3 twice more. Add the three readings, and then divide by 3 to find the average.

FIGURE E-8 How to Measure Waist Circumference

Place the measuring tape around the waist just above the bony crest of the hip. The tape runs parallel to the floor and is snug (but does not compress the skin). The measurement is taken at the end of normal expiration.

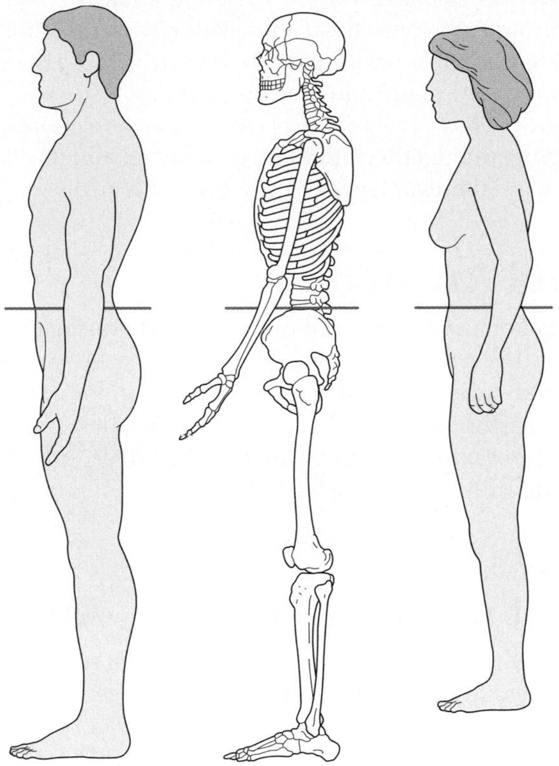

SOURCE: National Institutes of Health Obesity Education Initiative, *Clinical Guidelines on the Identification, Evaluation, and Treatment of Overweight and Obesity in Adults* (Washington, D.C.: U.S. Department of Health and Human Services, 1998), p. 59.

the same measurement as a pinch on the back of the arm. This limitation can be overcome by taking fatfold measurements at several (often three) different places on the body (including upper-, central-, and lower-body sites) and comparing each measurement with standards for that site. Multiple measures are not always practical in clinical settings, however, and most often, the triceps fatfold measurement alone is used because it is easily accessible.

Waist Circumference Chapter 8 described how fat distribution correlates with health risks and mentioned that the waist circumference is a valuable indicator of fat distribution. To measure waist circumference, the assessor places a nonstretchable tape around the person's body, crossing just above the upper hip bones and making sure that the tape remains on a level horizontal plane on all sides (see Figure E-8). The tape is tightened slightly, but without compressing the skin.

Waist-to-Hip Ratio Alternatively, some clinicians measure both the waist and the hips. The waist-to-hip ratio■ also assesses abdominal obesity, but provides no more information than using the waist circumference alone. In general, women with a waist-to-hip ratio of 0.80 or greater and men with a waist-to-hip ratio of 0.90 or greater have a high risk of health problems.

■ To calculate the waist-to-hip ratio, divide the waistline measurement by the hip measurement. For example, a woman with a 28-inch waist and 38-inch hips would have a ratio of 28 ÷ 38 = 0.74.

Hydrodensitometry To estimate body density using hydrodensitometry, the person is weighed twice—first on land and then again when submerged under water. Underwater weighing usually generates a good estimate of body fat and is useful in research, although the technique has drawbacks: it requires bulky, expensive, and nonportable equipment. Furthermore, submerging some people (especially those who are very young, very old, ill, or fearful) under water is not always practical.

Bioelectrical Impedance To measure body fat using the bioelectrical impedance technique, a very-low-intensity electrical current is briefly sent through the body by way of electrodes placed on the wrist and ankle. As is true of other anthropometric techniques, bioelectrical impedance requires standardized procedures and calibrated instruments to provide reliable results. Recent food intake and hydration status, for example, influence results.

Clinicians use many other methods to estimate body fat and its distribution. Each has its advantages and disadvantages as Table E-1 summarizes.

Nutritional Anemias

Anemia, a symptom of a wide variety of nutrition- and nonnutrition-related disorders, is characterized by a reduced number of red blood cells. Iron, folate, and vitamin B_{12} deficiencies caused by inadequate intake, poor absorption, or abnormal metabolism of these nutrients are the most common nutritional anemias. Some nonnutrition-related causes of anemia include massive blood loss, infections, hereditary blood disorders such as sickle-cell anemia, and chronic liver or kidney disease.

Assessment of Iron-Deficiency Anemia

■ Stages of iron deficiency:
1. Iron stores diminish.
2. Transport iron decreases.
3. Hemoglobin production falls.

Iron deficiency, a common mineral deficiency, develops in stages.■ Chapter 13 describes iron deficiency in detail. This section describes tests used to uncover iron deficiency as it progresses. Table E-2 shows which laboratory tests detect various nutrition-related anemias, and Table E-3 provides values used for assessing iron status. Although other tests are more specific in detecting early deficiencies, hemoglobin and hematocrit are the commonly available tests.

TABLE E-1 Methods of Estimating Body Fat and Its Distribution

Method	Cost	Ease of Use	Accuracy	Measures Fat Distribution
Height and weight	Low	Easy	High	No
Fatfolds	Low	Easy	Low	Yes
Circumferences	Low	Easy	Moderate	Yes
Ultrasound	Moderate	Moderate	Moderate	Yes
Hydrodensitometry	Low	Moderate	High	No
Heavy water tritiated	Moderate	Moderate	High	No
Deuterium oxide, or heavy oxygen	High	Moderate	High	No
Potassium isotope (^{40}K)	Very high	Difficult	High	No
Total body electrical conductivity (TOBEC)	High	Moderate	High	No
Bioelectrical impedance (BIA)	Moderate	Easy	High	No
Dual energy X-ray absorptiometry (DEXA)	High	Easy	High	No
Computed tomography (CT)	Very high	Difficult	High	Yes
Magnetic resonance imaging (MRI)	Very high	Difficult	High	Yes

SOURCE: Adapted with permisssion from G. A. Bray, a handout presented at the North American Association for the Study of Obesity and Emory University School of Medicine Conference on Obesity Update: Pathophysiology, Clinical Consequences, and Therapeutic Options, Atlanta, Georgia, August 31–September 2, 1992.

TABLE E-2 Laboratory Tests Useful in Evaluating Nutrition-Related Anemias

Test or Test Result	What It Reflects
For Anemia (general)	
Hemoglobin (Hg)	Total amount of hemoglobin in the red blood cells (RBC)
Hematocrit (Hct)	Percentage of RBC in the total blood volume
Red blood cell (RBC) count	Number of RBC
Mean corpuscular volume (MCV)	RBC size; helps to determine if anemia is microcytic (iron deficiency) or macrocytic (folate or vitamin B_{12} deficiency)
Mean corpuscular hemoglobin concentration (MCHC)	Hemoglobin concentration within the average RBC; helps to determine if anemia is hypochromic (iron deficiency) or normochromic (folate or vitamin B_{12} deficiency)
Bone marrow aspiration	The manufacture of blood cells in different developmental states
For Iron-Deficiency Anemia	
↓ Serum ferritin	Early deficiency state with depleted iron stores
↓ Transferrin saturation	Progressing deficiency state with diminished transport iron
↑ Erythrocyte protoporphyrin	Later deficiency state with limited hemoglobin production
For Folate-Deficiency Anemia	
↓ Serum folate	Progressing deficiency state
↓ RBC folate	Later deficiency state
For Vitamin B_{12}–Deficiency Anemia	
↓ Serum vitamin B_{12}	Progressing deficiency state
Schilling test	Absorption of vitamin B_{12}

Hemoglobin Iron forms an integral part of the hemoglobin molecule that transports oxygen to the cells. In iron deficiency, the body cannot synthesize hemoglobin. Low hemoglobin values signal depleted iron stores. Table E-3 provides hemoglobin values used in nutrition assessment. Hemoglobin's usefulness in evaluating iron status is limited, however, because hemoglobin concentrations drop fairly late in the development of iron deficiency, and other nutrient deficiencies and medical conditions can also alter hemoglobin concentrations.

Hematocrit Hematocrit is commonly used to diagnose iron deficiency, even though it is an inconclusive measure of iron status. To measure the hematocrit, a clinician spins a volume of blood in a centrifuge to separate the red blood cells from the plasma. The hematocrit is the percentage of red blood cells in the total blood volume. Table E-3 includes values used to assess hematocrit status. Low values indicate incomplete hemoglobin formation, which is manifested by microcytic (abnormally small-celled), hypochromic (abnormally lacking in color) red blood cells.

Low hemoglobin and hematocrit values alert the assessor to the possibility of iron deficiency. However, many nutrients and other conditions can affect hemoglobin and hematocrit. The other tests of iron status help pinpoint true iron deficiency.

Serum Ferritin In the first stage of iron deficiency, iron stores diminish. Serum ferritin measures provide a noninvasive estimate of iron stores. Such information is most valuable to iron assessment. Table E-3 shows serum ferritin cutoff values that indicate iron store depletion in children and adults. Serum ferritin is not reliable for diagnosing iron deficiency in infants because normal serum ferritin values are often present in conjunction with iron-responsive anemia.

A decrease in transport iron characterizes the second stage of iron deficiency. This is revealed by an increase in the iron-binding capacity of the protein transferrin and

TABLE E-3 Criteria for Assessing Iron Status

Test	Age (yr)	Gender	Deficiency Value
Hemoglobin (g/dL)	0.5–10	M–F	<11
	11–15	M	<12
		F	<11.5
	>15	M	<13
		F	<12
	Pregnancy		<11
Hematocrit (%)	0.5–4	M–F	<32
	5–10	M–F	<33
	11–15	M	<35
		F	<34
	>15	M	<40
		F	<36
Serum ferritin (μg/L)	0.5–15	M–F	<10
	>15	M–F	<12
Total iron-binding capacity (μg/dL)	>15	M–F	>400
Serum iron (μg/dL)	>15	M–F	<60
Transferrin saturation (%)	0.5–4	M–F	<12
	5–10	M–F	<14
	>10	M–F	<16
Erythrocyte protoporphyrin (μg/dL RBC)	0.5–4	M–F	>80
	>4	M–F	>70

a decrease in serum iron. These changes are reflected by the transferrin saturation, which is calculated from the ratio of the other two values as described in the following paragraphs.

Total Iron-Binding Capacity (TIBC) Iron travels through the blood bound to the protein transferrin. TIBC is a measure of the total amount of iron that transferrin can carry. Lab technicians measure iron-binding capacity directly. Table E-3 includes the value cutoff for TIBC.

Serum Iron Lab technicians can also measure serum iron directly. Elevated values indicate iron overload; reduced values indicate iron deficiency. Table E-3 shows the deficient value for serum iron.

Transferrin Saturation The percentage of transferrin that is saturated with iron is an indirect measure that is derived from the serum iron and total iron-binding capacity measures as follows:

$$\%\text{Transferrin} = \frac{\text{serum iron}}{\text{total iron-binding capacity}} \times 100.$$

Table E-3 shows deficient transferrin saturation values for various age groups.

The third stage of iron deficiency occurs when the supply of transport iron diminishes to the point that it limits hemoglobin production. It is characterized by increases in erythrocyte protoporphyrin, a decrease in mean corpuscular volume, and decreased hemoglobin and hematocrit.

Erythrocyte Protoporphyrin The iron-containing portion of the hemoglobin molecule is heme. Heme is a combination of iron and protoporphyrin. Protoporphyrin accumulates in the blood when iron supplies are inadequate for the formation of heme. Lab technicians can measure erythrocyte protoporphyrin directly in a blood sample. The cutoffs for abnormal values of erythrocyte protoporphyrin are shown in Table E-3.

Mean Corpuscular Volume (MCV) A direct or calculated measure of the mean corpuscular volume (MCV) determines the average size of a red blood cell. Such a measure helps to classify the type of nutrient anemia. In iron deficiency, the red blood cells are smaller than average.

Assessment of Folate and Vitamin B_{12} Anemias

Folate deficiency and vitamin B_{12} deficiency present a similar clinical picture—an anemia characterized by abnormally large red blood cell precursors (megaloblasts) in the bone marrow and abnormally large, mature red blood cells (macrocytic cells) in the blood. Distinguishing between these two deficiencies is particularly important because their treatments differ. Giving folate to a person with vitamin B_{12} deficiency improves many of the lab test results indicative of vitamin B_{12} deficiency, but this is a dangerous error because vitamin B_{12} deficiency causes nerve damage that folate cannot correct. Thus inappropriate folate administration masks vitamin B_{12}–deficiency anemia, and nerve damage worsens. For this reason, it is critical to determine whether the anemia results from a folate deficiency or from a vitamin B_{12} deficiency. The following biochemical assessment techniques help to make this distinction.

Mean Corpuscular Volume (MCV) As previously mentioned, the MCV is a measure of red blood cell size. In folate and vitamin B_{12} deficiencies, the red blood cells are larger than average (macrocytic). Additional tests must be performed to differentiate folate from vitamin B_{12} deficiency.

Folate Levels Serum folate levels fluctuate with changes in folate intake and metabolism. Thus serum folate concentrations reflect current status, but provide little information about folate stores. As folate deficiency progresses and low serum levels persist, folate stores decline, resulting in folate depletion. Folate depletion is characterized by a fall in the folate concentrations of red blood cells (erythrocytes). As erythrocyte folate levels diminish, folate-deficiency anemia develops. Because low erythrocyte folate concentrations also occur with vitamin B_{12} deficiency, serum vitamin B_{12} concentrations must also be measured. Table E-4 shows standards for folate assessment.

Vitamin B_{12} Levels Serum and urinary methylmalonic acid are elevated in vitamin B_{12} deficiency, but not in folate deficiency. Thus this measure is useful in distinguishing between the two. Vitamin B_{12} deficiency usually arises from malabsorption. To determine whether malabsorption is the cause, a small oral dose of vitamin B_{12} is given, and urinary excretion is measured. This procedure measures vitamin B_{12} absorption and is called a Schilling test.

Early stages of vitamin B_{12} deficiency can be detected by a low percentage saturation of its transport protein, a measure similar to iron's transferrin saturation. As the deficiency progresses, serum vitamin B_{12} concentrations fall. Table E-4 shows standards for vitamin B_{12} assessment.

TABLE E-4 Criteria for Assessing Folate and Vitamin B_{12}

	Deficient	Borderline	Acceptable
Serum folate (ng/mL)[a]	<3.0	3.0–5.9	>6.0
Erythrocyte folate (ng/mL)[a]	<140	140–159	>160
Serum vitamin B_{12} (pg/mL)	<150	150–200	≥201
Serum methylmalonic acid (nmol/L)	<376	—	—

NOTE: A nanogram (ng) is one-billionth of a gram; a picogram (pg) is one-trillionth of a gram.
[a]To convert folate values (ng/mL) to international standard units (nmol/L), multiply by 2.266.

Physical Activity and Energy Requirements

CONTENTS

Chapter 8 described how to calculate your estimated energy requirements by using an equation that accounts for your gender, age, weight, height, and physical activity level. This appendix first helps you determine the correct physical activity factor to use in the equation, either by calculating your physical activity level or by guesstimating it. Then the appendix presents tables that provide a shortcut to estimating total energy expenditure.*

Calculating Your Physical Activity Level

To calculate your physical activity level, record all of your activities for a typical 24-hour day, noting the type of activity, the level of intensity, and the duration. Then, using a copy of Table F-1, find your activity in the first column (or an activity that is reasonably similar) and multiply the number of minutes spent on that activity by the factor in the third column. Put your answer in the last column and total the accumulated values for the day. Now add the subtotal of the last column to 1.1 (to account for basal energy and the thermic effect of food) as shown. This score indicates your level of physical activity. Using Table F-2, find the PA (physical activity) factor for your gender that correlates with your physical activity level score and use it in the energy equation presented on p. 260 of Chapter 8.

Guesstimating Your Physical Activity Level

As an alternative to recording your activities for a day, you can use the first two columns of Table F-3 to decide if your daily activity is sedentary, low active, active, or very active. Find the PA factor for your gender that correlates with your typical physical activity level and use it in the energy equation presented on p. 260.

Using a Shortcut to Estimate Total Energy Expenditure

The DRI Committee has developed estimates of total energy expenditure based on the equations presented in Chapter 8. These estimates are presented in Table F-4 for women and Table F-5 for men. You can use these tables to estimate your energy requirement—that is, the number of kcalories needed to maintain your current body weight. On the table appropriate for your gender, find your height in meters (or inches) in the left-hand column. Then follow the row across to find your weight in kilograms (or pounds). (If you can't find your exact height and weight, choose a value between the two closest ones.) Look down the column to find the number of kcalories that corresponds to your activity level.

Importantly, the values given in the tables are for 30-year-old people. Women 19 to 29 should add 7 kcalories per day for each year below age 30; older women should subtract 7 kcalories per day for each year above age 30. Similarly, men 19 to 29 should add 10 kcalories per day for each year below age 30; older men should subtract 10 kcalories per day for each year above age 30.

*This appendix, including the tables, is adapted from Committee on Dietary Reference Intakes, *Dietary Reference Intakes for Energy, Carbohydrate, Fiber, Fat, Fatty Acids, Cholesterol, Protein, and Amino Acids* (Washington, D.C.: National Academies Press, 2002).

TABLE F-1 Physical Activities and Their Scores

If your activity was equivalent to this...	Then list the number of minutes here and ...	Multiply by this factor ...	Add this column to get your physical activity level score:
Activities of Daily Living			
Gardening (no lifting)		0.0032	
Household tasks (moderate effort)		0.0024	
Lifting items continuously		0.0029	
Loading/unloading car		0.0019	
Lying quietly		0.0000	
Mopping		0.0024	
Mowing lawn (power mower)		0.0033	
Raking lawn		0.0029	
Riding in a vehicle		0.0000	
Sitting (idle)		0.0000	
Sitting (doing light activity)		0.0005	
Taking out trash		0.0019	
Vacuuming		0.0024	
Walking the dog		0.0019	
Walking from house to car or bus		0.0014	
Watering plants		0.0014	
Additional Activities			
Billiards		0.0013	
Calisthenics (no weight)		0.0029	
Canoeing (leisurely)		0.0014	
Chopping wood		0.0037	
Climbing hills (carrying 11 lb load)		0.0061	
Climbing hills (no load)		0.0056	
Cycling (leisurely)		0.0024	
Cycling (moderately)		0.0045	
Dancing (aerobic or ballet)		0.0048	
Dancing (ballroom, leisurely)		0.0018	
Dancing (fast ballroom or square)		0.0043	
Golf (with cart)		0.0014	
Golf (without cart)		0.0032	
Horseback riding (walking)		0.0012	
Horseback riding (trotting)		0.0053	
Jogging (6 mph)		0.0088	
Music (playing accordion)		0.0008	
Music (playing cello)		0.0012	
Music (playing flute)		0.0010	
Music (playing piano)		0.0012	
Music (playing violin)		0.0014	
Rope skipping		0.0105	
Skating (ice)		0.0043	
Skating (roller)		0.0052	
Skiing (water or downhill)		0.0055	
Squash		0.0106	
Surfing		0.0048	
Swimming (slow)		0.0033	
Swimming (fast)		0.0057	
Tennis (doubles)		0.0038	
Tennis (singles)		0.0057	
Volleyball (noncompetitive)		0.0018	
Walking (2 mph)		0.0014	
Walking (3 mph)		0.0022	
Walking (4 mph)		0.0033	
Walking (5 mph)		0.0067	
Subtotal			
Factor for basal energy and the thermic effect of food			1.1
Your physical activity level score			

TABLE F-2 Physical Activity Level Scores and Their PA Factors

Physical Activity Level Score	Description	Men: PA Factor	Women: PA Factor
1.0 to 1.39	Sedentary	1.0	1.0
1.4 to 1.59	Low active	1.11	1.12
1.6 to 1.89	Active	1.25	1.27
1.9 and above	Very active	1.48	1.45

TABLE F-3 Physical Activity Equivalents and Their PA Factors

Description	Physical Activity Equivalents	Men: PA Factor	Women: PA Factor
Sedentary	Only those physical activities required for normal independent living	1.0	1.0
	Activities equivalent to walking at a pace of 2–4 mph for the following distances:		
Low active	1.5 to 3.0 miles/day	1.11	1.12
Active	3 to 10 miles/day	1.25	1.27
Very active	10 or more miles/day	1.48	1.45

TABLE F-4 Total Energy Expenditure (TEE in kCalories per Day) for Women 30 Years of Age[a] at Various Levels of Activity and Various Heights and Weights

Heights m (in)	Physical Activity Level	Weight[b] kg (lb)					
1.45 (57)		38.9 (86)	45.2 (100)	52.6 (116)	63.1 (139)	73.6 (162)	84.1 (185)
		kCalories					
	Sedentary	1564	1623	1698	1813	1927	2042
	Low active	1734	1800	1912	2043	2174	2304
	Active	1946	2021	2112	2257	2403	2548
	Very active	2201	2287	2387	2553	2719	2886
1.50 (59)		41.6 (92)	48.4 (107)	56.3 (124)	67.5 (149)	78.8 (174)	90.0 (198)
		kCalories					
	Sedentary	1625	1689	1771	1894	2017	2139
	Low active	1803	1874	1996	2136	2276	2415
	Active	2025	2105	2205	2360	2516	2672
	Very active	2291	2382	2493	2671	2849	3027
1.55 (61)		44.4 (98)	51.7 (114)	60.1 (132)	72.1 (159)	84.1 (185)	96.1 (212)
		kCalories					
	Sedentary	1688	1756	1846	1977	2108	2239
	Low active	1873	1949	2081	2230	2380	2529
	Active	2104	2190	2299	2466	2632	2798
	Very active	2382	2480	2601	2791	2981	3171
1.60 (63)		47.4 (104)	55.0 (121)	64.0 (141)	76.8 (169)	89.6 (197)	102.4 (226)
		kCalories					
	Sedentary	1752	1824	1922	2061	2201	2340
	Low active	1944	2025	2168	2327	2486	2645
	Active	2185	2276	2396	2573	2750	2927
	Very active	2474	2578	2712	2914	3116	3318

continued

[a]For each year below 30, add 7 kcalories/day to TEE. For each year above 30, subtract 7 kcalories/day from TEE.
[b]These columns represent a BMI of 18.5, 22.5, 25, 30, 35, and 40, respectively.

TABLE F-4 Total Energy Expenditure (TEE in kCalories per Day) for Women 30 Years of Age[a] at Various Levels of Activity and Various Heights and Weights—continued

Heights m (in)	Physical Activity Level	Weight[b] kg (lb)					
1.65 (65)		50.4 (111)	58.5 (129)	68.1 (150)	81.7 (180)	95.3 (210)	108.9 (240)
		kCalories					
	Sedentary	1816	1893	1999	2148	2296	2444
	Low active	2016	2102	2556	2425	2594	2763
	Active	2267	2364	2494	2682	2871	3059
	Very active	2567	2678	2824	3039	3254	3469
1.70 (67)		53.5 (118)	62.1 (137)	72.3 (159)	86.7 (191)	101.2 (223)	115.6 (255)
		kCalories					
	Sedentary	1881	1963	2078	2235	2393	2550
	Low active	2090	2180	2345	2525	2705	2884
	Active	2350	2453	2594	2794	2994	3194
	Very active	2662	2780	2938	3166	3395	3623
1.75 (69)		56.7 (125)	65.8 (145)	76.6 (169)	91.9 (202)	107.2 (236)	122.5 (270)
		kCalories					
	Sedentary	1948	2034	2158	2325	2492	2659
	Low active	2164	2260	2437	2627	2817	3007
	Active	2434	2543	2695	2907	3119	3331
	Very active	2758	2883	3054	3296	3538	3780
1.80 (71)		59.9 (132)	69.7 (154)	81.0 (178)	97.2 (214)	113.4 (250)	129.6 (285)
		kCalories					
	Sedentary	2015	2106	2239	2416	2593	2769
	Low active	2239	2341	2529	2731	2932	3133
	Active	2519	2634	2799	3023	3247	3472
	Very active	2855	2987	3172	3428	3684	3940
1.85 (73)		63.3 (139)	73.6 (162)	85.6 (189)	102.7 (226)	119.8 (264)	136.9 (302)
		kCalories					
	Sedentary	2083	2179	2322	2509	2695	2882
	Low active	2315	2422	2624	2836	3049	3262
	Active	2605	2727	2904	3141	3378	3615
	Very active	2954	3093	3292	3562	3833	4103
1.90 (75)		66.8 (147)	77.6 (171)	90.3 (199)	108.3 (239)	126.4 (278)	144.4 (318)
		kCalories					
	Sedentary	2151	2253	2406	2603	2800	2996
	Low active	2392	2505	2720	2944	3168	3393
	Active	2693	2821	3011	3261	3511	3760
	Very active	3053	3200	3414	3699	3984	4270
1.95 (77)		70.3 (155)	81.8 (180)	95.1 (209)	114.1 (251)	133.1 (293)	152.1 (335)
		kCalories					
	Sedentary	2221	2328	2492	2699	2906	3113
	Low active	2470	2589	2817	3053	3290	3526
	Active	2781	2917	3119	3383	3646	3909
	Very active	3154	3309	3538	3838	4139	4439

[a]For each year below 30, add 7 kcalories/day to TEE. For each year above 30, subtract 7 kcalories/day from TEE.
[b]These columns represent a BMI of 18.5, 22.5, 25, 30, 35, and 40, respectively.

TABLE F-5 Total Energy Expenditure (TEE in kCalories per Day) for Men 30 Years of Age[a] at Various Levels of Activity and Various Heights and Weights

Heights m (in)	Physical Activity Level	Weight[b] kg (lb)					
1.45 (57)		38.9 (86)	47.3 (100)	52.6 (116)	63.1 (139)	73.6 (163)	84.1 (185)
		kCalories					
	Sedentary	1777	1911	2048	2198	2347	2496
	Low active	1931	2080	2225	2393	2560	2727
	Active	2127	2295	2447	2636	2826	3015
	Very active	2450	2648	2845	3075	3305	3535
1.50 (59)		41.6 (92)	50.6 (107)	56.3 (124)	67.5 (149)	78.8 (174)	90.0 (198)
		kCalories					
	Sedentary	1848	1991	2126	2286	2445	2605
	Low active	2009	2168	2312	2491	2670	2849
	Active	2215	2394	2545	2748	2951	3154
	Very active	2554	2766	2965	3211	3457	3703
1.55 (61)		44.4 (98)	54.1 (114)	60.1 (132)	72.1 (159)	84.1 (185)	96.1 (212)
		kCalories					
	Sedentary	1919	2072	2205	2376	2546	2717
	Low active	2089	2259	2401	2592	2783	2974
	Active	2305	2496	2646	2862	3079	3296
	Very active	2660	2887	3087	3349	3612	3875
1.60 (63)		47.4 (104)	57.6 (121)	64.0 (141)	76.8 (169)	89.6 (197)	102.4 (226)
		kCalories					
	Sedentary	1993	2156	2286	2468	2650	2831
	Low active	2171	2351	2492	2695	2899	3102
	Active	2397	2601	2749	2980	3210	3441
	Very active	2769	3010	3211	3491	3771	4051
1.65 (65)		50.4 (111)	61.3 (129)	68.1 (150)	81.7 (180)	95.3 (210)	108.9 (240)
		kCalories					
	Sedentary	2068	2241	2369	2562	2756	2949
	Low active	2254	2446	2585	2801	3017	3234
	Active	2490	2707	2854	3099	3345	3590
	Very active	2880	3136	3339	3637	3934	4232
1.70 (67)		53.5 (118)	65.0 (137)	72.3 (159)	86.7 (191)	101.2 (223)	115.6 (255)
		kCalories					
	Sedentary	2144	2328	2454	2659	2864	3069
	Low active	2338	2542	2679	2909	3139	3369
	Active	2586	2816	2961	3222	3483	3743
	Very active	2992	3265	3469	3785	4101	4417
1.75 (69)		56.7 (125)	68.9 (145)	76.6 (169)	91.9 (202)	107.2 (236)	122.5 (270)
		kCalories					
	Sedentary	2222	2416	2540	2757	2975	3192
	Low active	2425	2641	2776	3020	3263	3507
	Active	2683	2927	3071	3347	3623	3900
	Very active	3108	3396	3602	3937	4272	4607
1.80 (71)		59.9 (132)	72.9 (154)	81.0 (178)	97.2 (214)	113.4 (250)	129.6 (285)
		kCalories					
	Sedentary	2301	2507	2628	2858	3088	3318
	Low active	2513	2741	2875	3132	3390	3648
	Active	2782	3040	3183	3475	3767	4060
	Very active	3225	3530	3738	4092	4447	4801

continued

[a]For each year below 30, add 10 kcalories/day to TEE. For each year above 30, subtract 10 kcalories/day from TEE.
[b]These columns represent a BMI of 18.5, 22.5, 25, 30, 35, and 40, respectively.

TABLE F-5 Total Energy Expenditure (TEE in kCalories per Day) for Men 30 Years of Age[a] at Various Levels of Activity and Various Heights and Weights—continued

Heights m (in)	Physical Activity Level	Weight[b] kg (lb)					
1.85 (73)		63.3 (139)	77.0 (162)	85.6 (189)	102.7 (226)	119.8 (264)	136.9 (302)
		kCalories					
	Sedentary	2382	2599	2718	2961	3204	3447
	Low active	2602	2844	2976	3248	3520	3792
	Active	2883	3155	3297	3606	3915	4223
	Very active	3344	3667	3877	4251	4625	4999
1.90 (75)		66.8 (147)	81.2 (171)	90.3 (199)	108.3 (239)	126.4 (278)	144.4 (318)
		kCalories					
	Sedentary	2464	2693	2810	3066	3322	3579
	Low active	2693	2948	3078	3365	3652	3939
	Active	2986	3273	3414	3739	4065	4390
	Very active	3466	3806	4018	4413	4807	5202
1.95 (77)		70.3 (155)	85.6 (180)	95.1 (209)	114.1 (251)	133.1 (293)	152.1 (335)
		kCalories					
	Sedentary	2547	2789	2903	3173	3443	3713
	Low active	2786	3055	3183	3485	3788	4090
	Active	3090	3393	3533	3875	4218	4561
	Very active	3590	3948	4162	4578	4993	5409

[a] For each year below 30, add 10 kcalories/day to TEE. For each year above 30, subtract 10 kcalories/day from TEE.

[b] These columns represent a BMI of 18.5, 22.5, 25, 30, 35, and 40, respectively.

Appendix F

United States: Exchange Lists

CONTENTS

Chapter 2 introduced the exchange system, and this appendix provides details from the 2003 edition. Appendix I presents Canada's choice system for meal planning.

The Exchange Groups and Lists

The exchange system sorts foods into three main groups by their proportions of carbohydrate, fat, and protein. These three groups—the carbohydrate group, the fat group, and the meat and meat substitutes group (protein)—organize foods into several exchange lists (see Table G-1). Then any food on a list can be "exchanged" for any other on that same list. The carbohydrate group covers these exchange lists:

- Starch (cereals, grains, pasta, breads, crackers, snacks, starchy vegetables, and dried beans, peas, and lentils).
- Fruit.
- Milk (fat-free, reduced fat, and whole).
- Other carbohydrates (desserts and snacks with added sugars and fats).
- Vegetables.

The fat group covers this exchange list:

- Fats.

The meat and meat substitutes group (protein) covers these exchange lists:

- Meat and meat substitutes (very lean, lean, medium-fat, and high-fat).

TABLE G-1 The Exchange Groups and Lists

Group/Lists	Typical Item/Portion Size	Carbohydrate (g)	Protein (g)	Fat (g)	Energy[a] (kcal)
Carbohydrate Group					
Starch[b]	1 slice bread	15	3	0–1	80
Fruit	1 small apple	15	—	—	60
Milk					
Fat-free, low-fat	1 c fat-free milk	12	8	0–3	90
Reduced-fat	1 c reduced-fat milk	12	8	5	120
Whole	1 c whole milk	12	8	8	150
Other carbohydrates[c]	2 small cookies	15	varies	varies	varies
Vegetable (nonstarchy)	½ c cooked carrots	5	2	—	25
Meat and Meat Substitute Group[d]					
Meat					
Very lean	1 oz chicken (white meat, no skin)	—	7	0–1	35
Lean	1 oz lean beef	—	7	3	55
Medium-fat	1 oz ground beef	—	7	5	75
High-fat	1 oz pork sausage	—	7	8	100
Fat Group					
Fat	1 tsp butter	—	—	5	45

[a]The energy value for each exchange list represents an approximate average for the group and does not reflect the precise number of grams of carbohydrate, protein, and fat. For example, a slice of bread contains 15 grams of carbohydrate (that's 60 kcalories), 3 grams protein (that's another 12 kcalories), and a little fat—rounded to 80 kcalories for ease in calculating. A half-cup of vegetables (not including starchy vegetables) contains 5 grams carbohydrate (20 kcalories) and 2 grams protein (8 more), which has been rounded down to 25 kcalories.
[b]The starch list includes cereals, grains, breads, crackers, snacks, starchy vegetables (such as corn, peas, and potatoes), and legumes (dried beans, peas, and lentils).
[c]The other carbohydrates list includes foods that contain added sugars and fats such as cakes, cookies, doughnuts, ice cream, potato chips, pudding, syrup, and frozen yogurt.
[d]The meat and meat substitutes list includes legumes, cheeses, and peanut butter.

FIGURE G-1 Seeing Exchanges on a Food Label

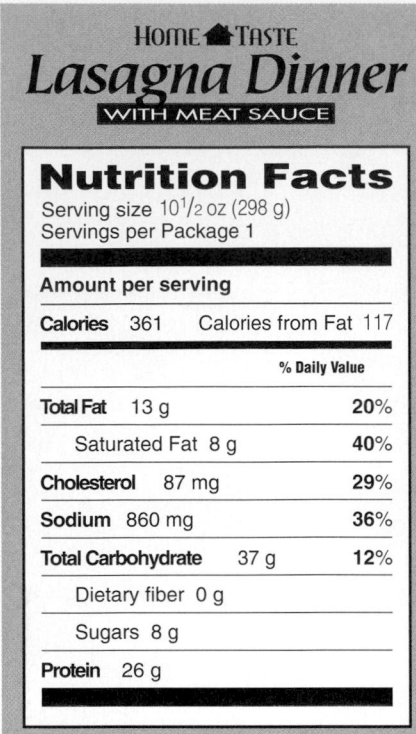

HOME TASTE
Lasagna Dinner
WITH MEAT SAUCE

Nutrition Facts
Serving size 10 1/2 oz (298 g)
Servings per Package 1

Amount per serving	
Calories 361	Calories from Fat 117
	% Daily Value
Total Fat 13 g	**20%**
Saturated Fat 8 g	**40%**
Cholesterol 87 mg	**29%**
Sodium 860 mg	**36%**
Total Carbohydrate 37 g	**12%**
Dietary fiber 0 g	
Sugars 8 g	
Protein 26 g	

Can you "see" these exchanges in the label above?

Exchange	Carbohydrate	Protein	Fat
2 starches	30 g	6 g	—
1 vegetable	5 g	2 g	—
3 medium-fat meats	—	21 g	15 g
Exchange totals	**35**	**29**	**15**
Label totals	**37**	**26**	**13**

Knowing that foods on the starch list provide 15 grams of carbohydrate and those on the vegetable list provide 5, you can count a lasagna dinner that provides 37 grams of carbohydrate as "2 starches and 1 vegetable"; knowing that foods on the meat list provide 7 grams of protein, you might count it as "3 meats"; the grams of fat suggest that the meat (and cheese) is probably medium-fat.

Portion Sizes The exchange system helps people control their energy intakes by paying close attention to portion sizes. The portion sizes have been carefully adjusted and defined so that a portion of any food on a given list provides roughly the same amount of carbohydrate, fat, and protein and, therefore, total kcalories. Any food on a list can then be exchanged, or traded, for any other food on that same list without significantly affecting the diet's balance or total kcalories. For example, a person may select either 17 small grapes or ½ large grapefruit as one fruit portion, and either choice would provide roughly 60 kcalories. A whole grapefruit, however, would count as 2 portions.

A *portion* in the exchange system is not always the same as a *serving* in the Daily Food Guide, especially when it comes to meats. The exchange system lists meats and most cheeses in single ounces; that is, one *portion* (or *exchange*) of meat is 1 ounce, whereas one *serving* in the Daily Food Guide is 2 to 3 ounces. Calculating meat by the ounce encourages a person to keep close track of the exact amounts eaten. This in turn helps control energy and fat intakes. Be aware, too, that most people do not serve foods in carefully measured portions, nor do the amounts reflect the exchange system or Daily Food Guide serving sizes. Many restaurants, for example, offer 8- to 16-ounce steaks that are the equivalent to four or five (2- to 3-ounce) *servings* of meat. Similarly, a bakery may sell muffins or bagels that are two to three times the size of a typical bread serving.

To apply the system successfully, users must become familiar with portion sizes. A convenient way to remember the portion sizes and energy values is to keep in mind a typical item from each list (review Table G-1).

The Foods on the Lists Foods do not always appear on the exchange list where you might first expect to find them. They are grouped according to their energy-nutrient contents rather than by their source (such as milks), their outward appearance, or their vitamin and mineral contents. Notice, for example, that cheeses are grouped with meats (not milk) because, like meats, cheeses contribute energy from protein and fat but provide negligible carbohydrate. Similarly, starchy vegetables such as potatoes are found on the starch list with breads and cereals, not with the vegetables, and bacon is with the fats and oils, not with the meats.

Users of the exchange lists learn to view mixtures of foods, such as casseroles and soups, as combinations of foods from different exchange lists. They also learn to interpret food labels with the exchange system in mind (see Figure G-1).

Controlling Energy and Fat By assigning items like bacon to the fat list, the exchange system alerts consumers to foods that are unexpectedly high in fat. Even the starch list specifies which grain products contain added fat (such as biscuits, muffins, and waffles). In addition, the exchange system encourages users to think of fat-free milk as milk and of whole milk as milk with added fat, and to think of very lean meats as meats and of lean, medium-fat, and high-fat meats as meats with added fat. To that end, foods on the milk and meat lists are separated into categories based on their fat contents. The milk group is classed as fat-free, reduced-fat, and whole; the meat group as very lean, lean, medium-fat, and high-fat.

Control of food energy and fat intake can be highly successful with the exchange system. Exchange plans do not, however, guarantee adequate intakes of vitamins and minerals. Food group plans work better from that standpoint because the food groupings are based on similarities in vitamin-mineral content. In the exchange system, for example, meats are grouped with cheeses, yet the meats are iron-rich and calcium-poor, whereas the cheeses are iron-poor and calcium-rich. To take advantage of the strengths of both food group plans and exchange patterns, and to compensate for their weaknesses, diet planners often combine these two diet-planning tools.

TABLE G-2 Diet Planning with the Exchange System Using the Daily Food Guide Pattern

Patterns from Daily Food Guide Plan	Selections Made Using the Exchange System	Energy Cost (kcal)
Grains (breads and cereals)—6 to 11 servings	Starch list—select 9 exchanges	720
Vegetables—3 to 5 servings	Vegetable list—select 4 exchanges	100
Fruits—2 to 4 servings	Fruit list—select 3 exchanges	180
Meat—2 to 3 servings[a]	Meat list—select 6 lean exchanges	330
Milk—2 servings	Milk list—select 2 fat-free exchanges	180
	Fat list—select 5 exchanges	225
Total		1735

[a]In the food group plan, 1 serving is 2 to 3 ounces; in the exchange system, 1 exchange is 1 ounce. The Daily Food Guide suggests that amounts should total 5 to 7 ounces of meat daily.

Combining Food Group Plans and Exchange Lists

A person may find that using a food group plan together with the exchange lists eases the task of choosing foods that provide all the nutrients. The food group plan ensures the all classes of nutritious foods are included, thus promoting adequacy, balance, and variety. The exchange system classifies the food selections by their energy-yielding nutrients, thus controlling energy and fat intakes.

Table G-2 shows how to use the Daily Food Guide plan together with the exchange lists to plan a diet. The Daily Food Guide ensures that a certain number of servings is chosen from each of the five food groups (see the first column of the table). The second column translates the number of servings (using the midpoint) into exchanges. With the addition of a small amount of fat, this sample diet plan provides abut 1750 kcalories. Most people can meet their needs for all the nutrients within this reasonable energy allowance. The next step in diet planning is to assign the exchanges to meals and snacks. The final plan might look like the one in Table G-3.

Next, a person could begin to fill in the plan with real foods to create a menu (use Tables G-4 through G-12). For example, the breakfast plan calls for 2 starch exchanges, 1 fruit exchange, and 1 fat-free milk exchange. A person might select a bowl of shredded wheat with banana slices and milk:

1 cup shredded wheat = 2 starch exchanges.

1 small banana = 1 fruit exchange.

1 cup fat-free milk = 1 milk exchange.

TABLE G-3 A Sample Diet Plan and Menu

This diet plan is one of many possibilities. It follows the number of servings suggested by the Daily Food Guide and meets dietary recommendations to provide 45 to 65 percent of its kcalories from carbohydrate, 10 to 35 percent from protein, and 20 to 35 percent from fat.

Exchange	Breakfast	Lunch	Snack	Dinner	Snack
9 starch	2	2	1	3	1
4 vegetables				4	
3 fruit	1	1	1		
6 lean meat		2		4	
2 fat-free milk	1				1
5 fat		1		4	

SAMPLE MENU

Breakfast: Cereal with banana and milk
Lunch: Turkey sandwich and a small bunch of grapes
Snack: Popcorn and apple juice
Dinner: Spaghetti with meat sauce; salad with sunflower seeds and dressing; green beans; corn on the cob
Snack: Graham crackers and milk

Or half a bagel and a bowl of cantaloupe pieces topped with yogurt:

½ bagel = 2 starch exchanges.

⅓ cantaloupe melon = 1 fruit exchange.

⅔ cup fat-free plain yogurt = 1 milk exchange.

TABLE G-4 U.S. Exchange System: Starch List

1 starch exchange = 15 g carbohydrate, 3 g protein, 0–1 g fat, and 80 kcal
NOTE: In general, one starch exchange is ½ c cooked cereal, grain, or starchy vegetable; ⅓ c cooked rice or pasta; 1 oz of bread; ¾ to 1 oz snack food.

Serving Size	Food
Bread	
¼ (1 oz)	Bagel, 4 oz
2 slices (1½ oz)	Bread, reduced-kcalorie
1 slice (1 oz)	Bread, white (including French and Italian), whole-wheat, pumpernickel, rye
4 (⅔ oz)	Bread sticks, crisp, 4″ x ½″
½	English muffin
½ (1 oz)	Hot dog or hamburger bun
¼	Naan, 8″ x 2″
1	Pancake, 4″ across, ¼″ thick
½	Pita, 6″ across
1 (1 oz)	Plain roll, small
1 slice (1 oz)	Raisin bread, unfrosted
1	Tortilla, corn, 6″ across
1	Tortilla, flour, 6″ across
⅓	Tortilla, flour, 10″ across
1	Waffle, 4″ square or across, reduced-fat
Cereals and Grains	
½ c	Bran cereals
½ c	Bulgur, cooked
½ c	Cereals, cooked
¾ c	Cereals, unsweetened, ready-to-eat
3 tbs	Cornmeal (dry)
⅓ c	Couscous
3 tbs	Flour (dry)
¼ c	Granola, low-fat
¼ c	Grape nuts
½ c	Grits, cooked
½ c	Kasha
⅓ c	Millet
¼ c	Muesli
½ c	Oats
⅓ c	Pasta, cooked
1½ c	Puffed cereals
⅓ c	Rice, white or brown, cooked
½ c	Shredded wheat
½ c	Sugar-frosted cereal
3 tbs	Wheat germ
Starchy Vegetables	
⅓ c	Baked beans
½ c	Corn
½ cob (5 oz)	Corn on cob, large
1 c	Mixed vegetables with corn, peas, or pasta
½ c	Peas, green
½ c	Plantains
½ medium (3 oz) or ½ c	Potato, boiled
¼ large (3 oz)	Potato, baked with skin
½ c	Potatoes, mashed
1 c	Squash, winter (acorn, butternut, pumpkin)
½ c	Yams, sweet potatoes, plain
Crackers and Snacks	
8	Animal crackers
3	Graham crackers, 2½″ square
¾ oz	Matzoh
4 slices	Melba toast
24	Oyster crackers
3 c	Popcorn (popped, no fat added or low-fat microwave)
¾ oz	Pretzels
2	Rice cakes, 4″ across
6	Saltine-type crackers
15–20 (¾ oz)	Snack chips, fat-free or baked (tortilla, potato)
2–5 (¾ oz)	Whole-wheat crackers, no fat added
Beans, Peas, and Lentils (count as 1 starch + 1 very lean meat)	
½ c	Beans and peas, cooked (garbanzo, lentils, pinto, kidney, white, split, black-eyed)
⅔ c	Lima beans
3 tbs	Miso (400 mg or more of sodium)
Starchy Foods Prepared with Fat (count as 1 starch + 1 fat)	
1	Biscuit, 2½″ across
½ c	Chow mein noodles
1 (2 oz)	Cornbread, 2″ cube
6	Crackers, round butter type
1 c	Croutons
1 c (2 oz)	French-fried potatoes (oven baked)
¼ c	Granola
⅓ c	Hummus
⅕ (1 oz)	Muffin, 5 oz
3 c	Popcorn, microwave
3	Sandwich crackers, cheese or peanut butter filling
9–13 (¾ oz)	Snack chips (potato, tortilla)
⅓ c	Stuffing, bread (prepared)
2	Taco shells, 6″ across
1	Waffle, 4½″ square or across
4–6 (1 oz)	Whole-wheat crackers, fat added

(Salt shaker symbol) = 400 mg or more of sodium per serving.

Then the person could move on to complete the menu for lunch, dinner, and snacks. (Table G-3 includes a sample menu.) As you can see, we all make countless food-related decisions daily—whether we have a plan or not. Following a plan, like the Daily Food Guide, that incorporates health recommendations and diet-planning principles helps a person to make wise decisions.

TABLE G-5 U.S. Exchange System: Fruit List

1 fruit exchange = 15 g carbohydrate and 60 kcal
NOTE: In general, one fruit exchange is 1 small fresh fruit; ½ c canned or fresh fruit or unsweetened fruit juice; ¼ c dried fruit.

Serving Size	Food
1 (4 oz)	Apple, unpeeled, small
½ c	Applesauce, unsweetened
4 rings	Apples, dried
4 whole (5½ oz)	Apricots, fresh
8 halves	Apricots, dried
½ c	Apricots, canned
1 (4 oz)	Banana, small
¾ c	Blackberries
¾ c	Blueberries
⅓ melon (11 oz) or 1 c cubes	Cantaloupe, small
12 (3 oz)	Cherries, sweet, fresh
½ c	Cherries, sweet, canned
3	Dates
1½ large or 2 medium (3½ oz)	Figs, fresh
1½	Figs, dried
½ c	Fruit cocktail
½ (11 oz)	Grapefruit, large
¾ c	Grapefruit sections, canned
17 (3 oz)	Grapes, small
1 slice (10 oz) or 1 c cubes	Honeydew melon
1 (3½ oz)	Kiwi
¾ c	Mandarin oranges, canned
½ (5½ oz) or ½ c	Mango, small
1 (5 oz)	Nectarine, small
1 (6½ oz)	Orange, small
½ (8 oz) or 1 c cubes	Papaya
1 (4 oz)	Peach, medium, fresh
½ c	Peaches, canned
½ (4 oz)	Pear, large, fresh
½ c	Pears, canned
¾ c	Pineapple, fresh
½ c	Pineapple, canned
2 (5 oz)	Plums, small
½ c	Plums, canned
3	Plums, dried (prunes)
2 tbs	Raisins
1 c	Raspberries
1¼ c whole berries	Strawberries
2 (8 oz)	Tangerines, small
1 slice (13½ oz) or 1¼ c cubes	Watermelon
Fruit Juice, unsweetened	
½ c	Apple juice/cider
⅓ c	Cranberry juice cocktail
1 c	Cranberry juice cocktail, reduced-kcalorie
⅓ c	Fruit juice blends, 100% juice
⅓ c	Grape juice
½ c	Grapefruit juice
½ c	Orange juice
½ c	Pineapple juice
⅓ c	Prune juice

TABLE G-6 U.S. Exchange System: Milk List

NOTE: In general, one milk exchange is 1 c milk or yogurt.

Serving Size	Food
Fat-Free and Low-Fat Milk	
1 fat-free/low-fat milk exchange = 12 g carbohydrate, 8 g protein, 0–3 g fat, 90 kcal	
1 c	Fat-free milk
1 c	½% milk
1 c	1% milk
1 c	Fat-free or low-fat buttermilk
½ c	Evaporated fat-free milk
⅓ c dry	Fat-free dry milk
1 c	Soy milk, low-fat or fat-free
⅔ c (6 oz)	Yogurt, fat-free or low-fat, flavored, sweetened with nonnutritive sweetener and fructose
⅔ c (6 oz)	Yogurt, plain fat-free
Reduced-Fat Milk	
1 reduced-fat milk exchange = 12 g carbohydrate, 8 g protein, 5 g fat, 120 kcal	
1 c	2% milk
1 c	Soy milk
1 c	Sweet acidophilus milk
¾ c	Yogurt, plain low-fat
Whole Milk	
1 whole milk exchange = 12 g carbohydrate, 8 g protein, 8 g fat, 150 kcal	
1 c	Whole milk
½ c	Evaporated whole milk
1 c	Goat's milk
1 c	Kefir
¾ c	Yogurt, plain (made from whole milk)

TABLE G-7 U.S. Exchange System: Sweets, Desserts, and Other Carbohydrates List

1 other carbohydrate exchange = 15 g carbohydrate, or 1 starch, or 1 fruit, or 1 milk exchange

Food	Serving Size	Exchanges per Serving
Angel food cake, unfrosted	1/12 cake (2 oz)	2 carbohydrates
Brownies, small, unfrosted	2″ square (1 oz)	1 carbohydrate, 1 fat
Cake, unfrosted	2″ square (1 oz)	1 carbohydrate, 1 fat
Cake, frosted	2″ square (2 oz)	2 carbohydrates, 1 fat
Cookies or sandwich cookies with creme filling	2 small (⅔ oz)	1 carbohydrate, 1 fat
Cookies, sugar-free	3 small or 1 large (¾–1 oz)	1 carbohydrate, 1–2 fats
Cranberry sauce, jellied	¼ c	1½ carbohydrates
Cupcake, frosted	1 small (2 oz)	2 carbohydrates, 1 fat
Doughnut, plain cake	1 medium (1½ oz)	1½ carbohydrates, 2 fats
Doughnut, glazed	3¾″ across (2 oz)	2 carbohydrates, 2 fats
Energy, sport, or breakfast bar	1 bar (1⅓ oz)	1½ carbohydrates, 0–1 fat
Energy, sport, or breakfast bar	1 bar (2 oz)	2 carbohydrates, 1 fat
Fruit cobbler	½ c (3½ oz)	3 carbohydrates, 1 fat
Fruit juice bar, frozen, 100% juice	1 bar (3 oz)	1 carbohydrate
Fruit snacks, chewy (pureed fruit concentrate)	1 roll (¾ oz)	1 carbohydrate
Fruit spreads, 100% fruit	1½ tbs	1 carbohydrate
Gelatin, regular	½ c	1 carbohydrate
Gingersnaps	3	1 carbohydrate
Granola or snack bar, regular or low-fat	1 bar (1 oz)	1½ carbohydrates
Honey	1 tbs	1 carbohydrate
Ice cream	½ c	1 carbohydrate, 2 fats
Ice cream, light	½ c	1 carbohydrate, 1 fat
Ice cream, low-fat	½ c	1½ carbohydrates
Ice cream, fat-free, no sugar added	½ c	1 carbohydrate
Jam or jelly, regular	1 tbs	1 carbohydrate
Milk, chocolate, whole	1 c	2 carbohydrates, 1 fat
Pie, fruit, 2 crusts	⅙ of 8″ commercially prepared pie	3 carbohydrates, 2 fats
Pie, pumpkin or custard	⅛ of 8″ commercially prepared pie	2 carbohydrates, 2 fats
Pudding, regular (made with reduced-fat milk)	½ c	2 carbohydrates
Pudding, sugar-free (made with fat-free milk)	½ c	1 carbohydrate
Reduced-calorie meal replacement (shake)	1 can (10–11 oz)	1½ carbohydrates, 0–1 fats
Rice milk, low-fat or fat-free, plain	1 c	1 carbohydrate
Rice milk, low-fat, flavored	1 c	1½ carbohydrates
Salad dressing, fat-free	¼ c	1 carbohydrate
Sherbet, sorbet	½ c	2 carbohydrates
Spaghetti or pasta sauce, canned	½ c	1 carbohydrate, 1 fat
Sports drinks	8 oz (1 c)	1 carbohydrate
Sugar	1 tbs	1 carbohydrate
Sweet roll or danish	1 (2½ oz)	2½ carbohydrates, 2 fats
Syrup, light	2 tbs	1 carbohydrate
Syrup, regular	1 tbs	1 carbohydrate
Syrup, regular	¼ c	4 carbohydrates
Vanilla wafers	5	1 carbohydrate, 1 fat
Yogurt, frozen	½ c	1 carbohydrate, 0–1 fat
Yogurt, frozen, fat-free	⅓ c	1 carbohydrate
Yogurt, low-fat with fruit	1 c	3 carbohydrates, 0–1 fat

= 400 mg or more sodium per exchange.

TABLE G-8 U.S. Exchange System: Nonstarchy Vegetable List

1 vegetable exchange = 5 g carbohydrate, 2 g protein, 0 g fat, and 25 kcal
NOTE: In general, one vegetable exchange is ½ c cooked vegetables or vegetable juice; 1 c raw vegetables. Starchy vegetables such as corn, peas, and potatoes are on the starch list (Table G-4).

Artichokes	Mushrooms
Artichoke hearts	Okra
Asparagus	Onions
Beans (green, wax, Italian)	Pea pods
Bean sprouts	Peppers (all varieties)
Beets	Radishes
Broccoli	Salad greens (endive, escarole, lettuce, romaine, spinach)
Brussels sprouts	Sauerkraut 🧂
Cabbage	Spinach
Carrots	Summer squash (crookneck)
Cauliflower	Tomatoes
Celery	Tomatoes, canned
Cucumbers	Tomato sauce 🧂
Eggplant	Tomato/vegetable juice 🧂
Green onions or scallions	Turnips
Greens (collard, kale, mustard, turnip)	Water chestnuts
Kohlrabi	Watercress
Leeks	Zucchini
Mixed vegetables (without corn, peas, or pasta)	

🧂 = 400 mg or more sodium per exchange.

G Appendix

TABLE G-9 U.S. Exchange System: Meat and Meat Substitutes List

NOTE: In general, a meat exchange is 1 oz meat, poultry, or cheese; ½ c dried beans (weigh meat and poultry and measure beans after cooking).

Serving Size	Food
Very Lean Meat and Substitutes	
1 very lean meat exchange = 7 g protein, 0–1 g fat, 35 kcal	
1 oz	Poultry: Chicken or turkey (white meat, no skin), Cornish hen (no skin)
1 oz	Fish: Fresh or frozen cod, flounder, haddock, halibut, trout, lox (smoked salmon) ; tuna, fresh or canned in water
1 oz	Shellfish: Clams, crab, lobster, scallops, shrimp, imitation shellfish
1 oz	Game: Duck or pheasant (no skin), venison, buffalo, ostrich
	Cheese with ≤1g fat/oz:
¼ c	Fat-free or low-fat cottage cheese
1 oz	Fat-free cheese
1 oz	Processed sandwich meats with ≤1 g fat/oz (such as deli thin, shaved meats, chipped beef , turkey ham)
2	Egg whites
¼ c	Egg substitutes, plain
1 oz	Hot dogs with ≤1 g fat/oz
1 oz	Kidney (high in cholesterol)
1 oz	Sausage with ≤1 g fat/oz
Count as 1 very lean meat + 1 starch exchange:	
½ c	Beans, peas, lentils (cooked)
Lean Meat and Substitutes	
1 lean meat exchange = 7 g protein, 3 g fat, 55 kcal	
1 oz	Beef: USDA Select or Choice grades of lean beef trimmed of fat (round, sirloin, and flank steak); tenderloin; roast (rib, chuck, rump); steak (T-bone, porterhouse, cubed), ground round
1 oz	Pork: Lean pork (fresh ham); canned, cured, or boiled ham; Canadian bacon ; tenderloin, center loin chop
1 oz	Lamb: Roast, chop, leg
1 oz	Veal: Lean chop, roast
1 oz	Poultry: Chicken, turkey (dark meat, no skin), chicken (white meat, with skin), domestic duck or goose (well drained of fat, no skin)
	Fish:
1 oz	Herring (uncreamed or smoked)
6 medium	Oysters
1 oz	Salmon (fresh or canned), catfish
2 medium	Sardines (canned)
1 oz	Tuna (canned in oil, drained)
1 oz	Game: Goose (no skin), rabbit
	Cheese:
¼ c	4.5%-fat cottage cheese
2 tbs	Grated Parmesan
1 oz	Cheeses with ≤3 g fat/oz
1½ oz	Hot dogs with ≤3 g fat/oz
1 oz	Processed sandwich meat with ≤3 g fat/oz (turkey pastrami or kielbasa)
1 oz	Liver, heart (high in cholesterol)
Medium-Fat Meat and Substitutes	
1 medium-fat meat exchange = 7 g protein, 5 g fat, and 75 kcal	
1 oz	Beef: Most beef products (ground beef, meatloaf, corned beef, short ribs, Prime grades of meat trimmed of fat, such as prime rib)
1 oz	Pork: Top loin, chop, Boston butt, cutlet
1 oz	Lamb: Rib roast, ground
1 oz	Veal: Cutlet (ground or cubed, unbreaded)
1 oz	Poultry: Chicken (dark meat, with skin), ground turkey or ground chicken, fried chicken (with skin)
1 oz	Fish: Any fried fish product
	Cheese with ≤5 g fat/oz:
1 oz	Feta
1 oz	Mozzarella
¼ c (2 oz)	Ricotta
1	Egg (high in cholesterol, limit to 3/week)
1 oz	Sausage with ≤5 g fat/oz
1 c	Soy milk
¼ c	Tempeh
4 oz or ½ c	Tofu
High-Fat Meat and Substitutes	
1 high-fat meat exchange = 7 g protein, 8 g fat, 100 kcal	
1 oz	Pork: Spareribs, ground pork, pork sausage
1 oz	Cheese: All regular cheeses (American , cheddar, Monterey Jack, swiss)
1 oz	Processed sandwich meats with ≤8 g fat/oz (bologna, pimento loaf, salami)
1 oz	Sausage (bratwurst, Italian, knockwurst, Polish, smoked)
1 (10/lb)	Hot dog (turkey or chicken)
3 slices (20 slices/lb)	Bacon
1 tbs	Peanut butter (contains unsaturated fat)
Count as 1 high-fat meat + 1 fat exchange:	
1 (10/lb)	Hot dog (beef, pork, or combination)

= 400 mg or more of sodium per serving.

TABLE G-10 U.S. Exchange System: Fat List

1 fat exchange = 5 g fat and 45 kcal
NOTE: In general, one fat exchange is 1 tsp regular butter, margarine, or vegetable oil; 1 tbs regular salad dressing. Many fat-free and reduced fat foods are on the Free Foods List (Table G-11).

Serving Size	Food
Monounsaturated Fats	
2 tbs (1 oz)	Avocado
1 tsp	Oil (canola, olive, peanut)
8 large	Olives, ripe (black)
10 large	Olives, green, stuffed
6 nuts	Almonds, cashews
6 nuts	Mixed nuts (50% peanuts)
10 nuts	Peanuts
4 halves	Pecans
½ tbs	Peanut butter, smooth or crunchy
1 tbs	Sesame seeds
2 tsp	Tahini or sesame paste
Polyunsaturated Fats	
4 halves	English walnuts
1 tsp	Margarine, stick, tub, or squeeze
1 tbs	Margarine, lower-fat spread (30% to 50% vegetable oil)
1 tsp	Mayonnaise, regular
1 tbs	Mayonnaise, reduced-fat
1 tsp	Oil (corn, safflower, soybean)
1 tbs	Salad dressing, regular
2 tbs	Salad dressing, reduced-fat
2 tsp	Mayonnaise type salad dressing, regular
1 tbs	Mayonnaise type salad dressing, reduced-fat
1 tbs	Seeds (pumpkin, sunflower)
Saturated Fats*	
1 slice (20 slices/lb)	Bacon, cooked
1 tsp	Bacon, grease
1 tsp	Butter, stick
2 tsp	Butter, whipped
1 tbs	Butter, reduced-fat
2 tbs (½ oz)	Chitterlings, boiled
2 tbs	Coconut, sweetened, shredded
1 tbs	Coconut milk
2 tbs	Cream, half and half
1 tbs (½ oz)	Cream cheese, regular
1½ tbs (¾ oz)	Cream cheese, reduced-fat
	Fatback or salt pork†
1 tsp	Shortening or lard
2 tbs	Sour cream, regular
3 tbs	Sour cream, reduced-fat

= 400 mg or more sodium per exchange
*Saturated fats can raise blood cholesterol levels.
†Use a piece 1″ × 1″ × ¼″ if you plan to eat the fatback cooked with vegetables. Use a piece 2″ × 1″ × ½″ when eating only the vegetables with the fatback removed.

G Appendix

TABLE G-11 U.S. Exchange System: Free Foods List

NOTE: A serving of free food contains less than 20 kcalories or no more than 5 grams of carbohydrate; those with serving sizes should be limited to 3 servings a day whereas those without serving sizes can be eaten freely.

Serving Size	Food
Fat-Free or Reduced-Fat Foods	
1 tbs (½ oz)	Cream cheese, fat-free
1 tbs	Creamers, nondairy, liquid
2 tsp	Creamers, nondairy, powdered
4 tbs	Margarine spread, fat-free
1 tsp	Margarine spread, reduced-fat
1 tbs	Mayonnaise, fat-free
1 tsp	Mayonnaise, reduced-fat
1 tbs	Mayonnaise type salad dressing, fat-free
1 tsp	Mayonnaise type salad dressing, reduced-fat
	Nonstick cooking spray
1 tbs	Salad dressing, fat-free or low-fat
2 tbs	Salad dressing, fat-free, Italian
1 tbs	Sour cream, fat-free, reduced-fat
1 tbs	Whipped topping, regular
2 tbs	Whipped topping, light or fat-free
Sugar-Free Foods	
1 piece	Candy, hard, sugar-free
	Gelatin dessert, sugar-free
	Gelatin, unflavored
	Gum, sugar-free
2 tsp	Jam or jelly, light
	Sugar substitutes
2 tbs	Syrup, sugar-free
Drinks	
	Bouillon, broth, consommé
	Bouillon or broth, low-sodium
	Carbonated or mineral water
	Club soda
1 tbs	Cocoa powder, unsweetened
	Coffee
	Diet soft drinks, sugar-free
	Drink mixes, sugar-free
	Tea
	Tonic water, sugar-free
Condiments	
1 tbs	Catsup
	Horseradish
	Lemon juice
	Lime juice
	Mustard
1 tbs	Pickle relish
1½ medium	Pickles, dill
2 slices	Pickles, sweet (bread and butter)
¾ oz	Pickles, sweet (gherkin)
¼ c	Salsa
1 tbs	Soy sauce, regular or light
1 tbs	Taco sauce
	Vinegar
2 tbs	Yogurt
Seasonings	
	Flavoring extracts
	Garlic
	Herbs, fresh or dried
	Hot pepper sauces
	Pimento
	Spices
	Wine, used in cooking
	Worcestershire sauce

= 400 mg or more of sodium per serving.

TABLE G-12 U.S. Exchange System: Combination Foods List

Food	Serving Size	Exchanges per Serving
Entrées		
Tuna noodle casserole, lasagna, spaghetti with meatballs, chili with beans, macaroni and cheese	1 c (8 oz)	2 carbohydrates, 2 medium-fat meats
Chow mein (without noodles or rice)	2 c (16 oz)	1 carbohydrate, 2 lean meats
Tuna or chicken salad	½ c (3½ oz)	½ carbohydrate, 2 lean meats, 1 fat
Frozen Entrées and Meals		
Dinner-type meal	Generally 14–17 oz	3 carbohydrates, 3 medium-fat meats, 3 fats
Entrée or meal with <340 kcal	About 8–11 oz	2–3 carbohydrates, 1–2 lean meats
Meatless burger, soy based	3 oz	½ carbohydrate, 2 lean meats
Meatless burger, vegetable and starch based	3 oz	1 carbohydrate, 1 lean meat
Pizza, cheese, thin crust	¼ of 12″ (6 oz)	2 carbohydrates, 2 medium-fat meats, 1 fat
Pizza, meat topping, thin crust	¼ of 12″ (6 oz)	2 carbohydrates, 2 medium-fat meats, 2 fats
Pot pie	1 (7 oz)	2½ carbohydrates, 1 medium-fat meat, 3 fats
Soups		
Bean	1 c	1 carbohydrate, 1 very lean meat
Cream (made with water)	1 c (8 oz)	1 carbohydrate, 1 fat
Instant	6 oz prepared	1 carbohydrate
Instant with beans/lentils	8 oz prepared	2½ carbohydrates, 1 very lean meat
Split pea (made with water)	½ c (4 oz)	1 carbohydrate
Tomato (made with water)	1 c (8 oz)	1 carbohydrate
Vegetable beef, chicken noodle, or other broth-type	1 c (8 oz)	1 carbohydrate
Fast Foods		
Burrito with beef	1 (5–7 oz)	3 carbohydrates, 1 medium-fat meat, 1 fat
Chicken nuggets	6	1 carbohydrate, 2 medium-fat meats, 1 fat
Chicken breast and wing, breaded and fried	1 each	1 carbohydrate, 4 medium-fat meats, 2 fats
Chicken sandwich, grilled	1	2 carbohydrates, 3 very lean meats
Chicken wings, hot	6 (5 oz)	1 carbohydrate, 3 medium-fat meats, 4 fats
Fish sandwich/tartar sauce	1	3 carbohydrates, 1 medium-fat meat, 3 fats
French fries	1 medium serving (5 oz)	4 carbohydrates, 4 fats
Hamburger, regular	1	2 carbohydrates, 2 medium-fat meats
Hamburger, large	1	2 carbohydrates, 3 medium-fat meats, 1 fat
Hot dog with bun	1	1 carbohydrate, 1 high-fat meat, 1 fat
Individual pan pizza	1	5 carbohydrates, 3 medium-fat meats, 3 fats
Pizza, cheese, thin crust	¼ of 12″ (about 6 oz)	2½ carbohydrates, 2 medium-fat meats
Pizza, meat, thin crust	¼ of 12″ (about 6 oz)	2½ carbohydrates, 2 medium-fat meats, 1 fat
Soft serve cone	1 small (5 oz)	2½ carbohydrates, 1 fat
Submarine sandwich	1 sub (6″)	3 carbohydrates, 1 vegetable, 2 medium-fat meats, 1 fat
Submarine sandwich (<6 g fat)	1 sub (6″)	2½ carbohydrates, 2 lean meats
Taco, hard or soft shell	1 (3–3½ oz)	1 carbohydrate, 1 medium-fat meat, 1 fat

= 400 mg or more sodium per exchange.

G Appendix

CONTENTS

Table of Food Composition

This edition of the table of food composition includes a wide variety of foods from all food groups. It is updated with each edition to reflect nutrient changes for current foods, remove outdated foods, and add foods that are new to the marketplace.*

The nutrient database for this appendix is compiled from a variety of sources, including the USDA Standard Reference database (Release 16), literature sources, and manufacturers' data. The USDA database provides data for a wider variety of foods and nutrients than other sources. Because laboratory analysis for each nutrient can be quite costly, manufacturers tend to provide data only for those nutrients mandated on food labels. Consequently, data for their foods are often incomplete; any missing information is designated in this table as a blank space. Keep in mind that a blank space means only that the information is unknown and should not be interpreted as a zero.

Whenever using nutrient data, remember that many factors influence the nutrient contents of foods, including the mineral content of the soil, the diet of the animal or the fertilizer of the plant, the season of harvest, the method of processing, the length and method of storage, the method of cooking, the method of analysis, and the moisture content of the sample analyzed. With so many factors involved, users must view nutrient data as a close approximation of the actual amount.

For updates, corrections, and a list of 6000 foods and codes found in the diet analysis software that accompanies this text, visit **www.wadsworth.com/nutrition** and click on *Diet Analysis*.

- ***Fats*** Total fats, as well as the breakdown of total fats to saturated, monounsaturated, and polyunsaturated fats, are listed in the table. The fatty acids seldom add up to the total due to rounding and to other fatty acid components that are not included in these basic categories, such as *trans*-fatty acids and glycerol. *Trans*-fatty acids can comprise a large share of the total fat in margarine and shortening (hydrogenated oils) and in any foods that include them as ingredients.
- ***Vitamin A and Vitamin E*** In keeping with the 2001 RDA for vitamin A, which established a new measure of vitamin A activity—retinol activity equivalents (RAE)—this appendix presents data for vitamin A in micrograms (μg) RAE. Similarly, because the 2000 RDA for vitamin E is based only on the alpha-tocopherol form of vitamin E, this appendix reports vitamin E data in milligrams (mg) alpha-tocopherol (listed in the table as mg α).
- ***Bioavailability*** Keep in mind that the availability of nutrients from foods depends not only on the quantity provided by a food, but also on the amount absorbed and used by the body—the bioavailability. The bioavailability of folate from fortified foods, for example, is greater than from naturally occurring sources. Similarly, the body can make niacin from the amino acid tryptophan, but niacin values in this table (and most databases) report preformed niacin only. Chapter 10 provides conversion factors and additional details.
- ***Using the Table*** The items in this table have been organized into several categories, which are listed at the head of each right-hand page. Page numbers have been provided, and each group has been color-coded to make it easier to find individual items.

  In an effort to conserve space, the following abbreviations have been used in the food descriptions and nutrient breakdowns:

  - diam = diameter
  - ea = each

*This food composition table has been prepared for Wadsworth Publishing Company and is copyrighted by ESHA Research in Salem, Oregon—the developer and publisher of the Food Processor and Genesis nutritional software programs. The nutritional data are supported by over 1300 references. Because the list of sources is so extensive, it is not provided here, but is available from the publisher.

- enr = enriched
- f/ = from
- frzn = frozen
- g = grams
- liq = liquid
- pce = piece
- pkg = package
- w/ = with
- w/o = without
- t = trace
- 0 = zero (no nutrient value)
- blank space = information not available

- ***Caffeine Sources*** Caffeine occurs in several plants, including the familiar coffee bean, the tea leaf, and the cocoa bean from which chocolate is made. Most human societies use caffeine regularly, most often in beverages, for its stimulant effect and flavor. Caffeine contents of beverages vary depending on the plants they are made from, the climates and soils where the plants are grown, the grind or cut size, the method and duration of brewing, and the amounts served. The accompanying table shows that in general, a cup of coffee contains the most caffeine; a cup of tea, less than half as much; and cocoa or chocolate, less still. As for cola beverages, they are made from kola nuts, which contain caffeine, but most of their caffeine is added, using the purified compound obtained from decaffeinated coffee beans.

  The FDA lists caffeine as a multipurpose GRAS substance■ that may be added to foods and beverages. Drug manufacturers use caffeine in many kinds of drugs: stimulants, pain relievers, cold remedies, diuretics, and weight-loss aids.

■ Reminder: A GRAS substance is one that is "generally recognized as safe."

TABLE Caffeine Content of Beverages, Foods, and Over-the-Counter Drugs

Beverages and Foods	Average (mg)	Range (mg)
Coffee (5-oz cup)		
Brewed, drip method	130	110–150
Brewed, percolator	94	64–124
Instant	74	40–108
Decaffeinated, brewed or instant	3	1–5
Tea (5-oz cup)		
Brewed, major U.S. brand	40	20–90
Brewed, imported brands	60	25–110
Instant	30	25–50
Iced (12-oz can)	70	67–76
Soft drinks (12-oz can)		
Dr. Pepper	40	
Colas and cherry cola		
Regular		30–46
Diet		2–58
Caffeine-free		0–trace
Jolt	72	
Mountain Dew, Mello Yello	52	
Fresca, Hires Root Beer, 7-Up, Sprite, Squirt, Sunkist Orange	0	
Cocoa beverage (5-oz cup)	4	2–20
Chocolate milk beverage (8 oz)	5	2–7
Milk chocolate candy (1 oz)	6	1–15
Dark chocolate, semisweet (1 oz)	20	5–35
Baker's chocolate (1 oz)	26	
Chocolate flavored syrup (1 oz)	4	

Drugs[a]	Average (mg)
Cold remedies (standard dose)	
Dristan	0
Coryban-D, Triaminicin	30
Diuretics (standard dose)	
Aqua-ban, Permathene H_2Off	200
Pre-Mens Forte	100
Pain relievers (standard dose)	
Excedrin	130
Midol, Anacin	65
Aspirin, plain (any brand)	0
Stimulants	
Caffedrin, NoDoz, Vivarin	200
Weight-control aids (daily dose)	
Prolamine	280
Dexatrim, Dietac	200

NOTE: A pharmacologically active dose of caffeine is defined as 200 milligrams.

[a]Because products change, contact the manufacturer for an update on products you use regularly.

Table H–1

Food Composition (Computer code number is for Wadsworth Diet Analysis program) (For purposes of calculations, use "0" for t, <1, <.1, <.01, etc.)

DA + Code	Food Description	Quantity	Measure	Wt (g)	H_2O (g)	Ener (kcal)	Prot (g)	Carb (g)	Dietary Fiber (g)	Fat (g)	Fat Breakdown (g)		
											Sat	Mono	Poly
	BREADS, BAKED GOODS, CAKES, COOKIES, CRACKERS, CHIPS, PIES												
	Bagels												
8534	Cinnamon & raisin	1	item(s)	71	23	195	7	39	2	1	0.19	0.12	0.48
4910	Enriched, all varieties	1	item(s)	71	23	195	7	38	2	1	0.16	0.09	0.49
4911	Plain, enriched, toasted	1	item(s)	66	18	195	7	38	2	1	0.16	0.09	0.49
8538	Oat bran	1	item(s)	71	23	181	8	38	3	1	0.14	0.18	0.35
12079	Whole grain	1	item(s)	85	—	170	9	35	6	2.5	0	—	—
	Biscuits												
25008	Biscuits	1	item(s)	41	16	121	3	16	1	5	1.40	1.41	1.82
16729	Scone	1	item(s)	42	11	149	4	19	1	6	2.01	2.55	1.26
25166	Wheat biscuits	1	item(s)	55	21	162	4	22	1	7	1.90	1.92	2.51
	Bread												
325	Boston brown, canned	1	slice(s)	45	21	88	2	19	2	1	0.13	0.09	0.25
8716	Bread sticks, plain	4	item(s)	24	1	99	3	16	1	2	0.34	0.86	0.87
25176	Cornbread	1	piece(s)	55	26	141	5	18	1	5	2.09	1.44	1.50
327	Cracked wheat	1	slice(s)	25	9	65	2	12	1	1	0.23	0.48	0.17
9079	Croutons, plain	¼	cup(s)	8	<1	31	1	6	<1	<1	0.11	0.23	0.10
8582	Egg	1	slice(s)	40	14	115	4	19	1	2	0.64	0.92	0.44
8585	Egg, toasted	1	slice(s)	37	10	117	4	19	1	2	0.60	1.11	0.43
329	French	1	slice(s)	25	9	69	2	13	1	1	0.16	0.30	0.17
8591	French, toasted	1	slice(s)	23	7	69	2	13	1	1	0.16	0.30	0.17
8597	Indian fry	1	item(s)	90	24	296	6	48	2	9	2.08	3.59	2.33
332	Italian	1	slice(s)	30	11	81	3	15	1	1	0.26	0.24	0.42
1393	Mixed grain	1	slice(s)	26	10	65	3	12	2	1	0.21	0.40	0.24
8604	Mixed grain, toasted	1	slice(s)	24	8	65	3	12	2	1	0.21	0.40	0.24
8605	Oat bran	1	slice(s)	30	13	71	3	12	1	1	0.21	0.48	0.51
8608	Oat bran, toasted	1	slice(s)	27	10	70	3	12	1	1	0.21	0.47	0.50
8609	Oatmeal	1	slice(s)	27	10	73	2	13	1	1	0.19	0.43	0.46
8613	Oatmeal, toasted	1	slice(s)	25	8	73	2	13	1	1	0.19	0.43	0.46
1409	Pita	1	item(s)	60	19	165	5	33	1	1	0.10	0.06	0.32
7905	Pita, whole wheat	1	item(s)	64	20	170	6	35	5	2	0.26	0.22	0.68
338	Pumpernickel	1	slice(s)	32	12	80	3	15	2	1	0.14	0.30	0.40
334	Raisin, enriched	1	slice(s)	26	9	71	2	14	1	1	0.28	0.60	0.18
8625	Raisin, toasted	1	slice(s)	24	7	71	2	14	1	1	0.28	0.60	0.18
10168	Rice, white	1	slice(s)	42	—	140	1	21	1	6	0.50	—	—
8653	Rye	1	slice(s)	32	12	83	3	15	2	1	0.20	0.42	0.26
8654	Rye, toasted	1	slice(s)	29	9	82	3	15	2	1	0.20	0.42	0.25
336	Rye, light	1	slice(s)	25	9	65	2	12	2	1	0.20	0.30	0.30
8588	Sourdough	1	slice(s)	25	9	69	2	13	1	1	0.16	0.30	0.17
8592	Sourdough, toasted	1	slice(s)	23	7	69	2	13	1	1	0.16	0.30	0.17
491	Submarine or hoagie roll	1	item(s)	135	41	400	11	72	4	8	1.80	3.00	2.20
8596	Vienna, toasted	1	slice(s)	23	7	69	2	13	1	1	0.16	0.30	0.17
8670	Wheat	1	slice(s)	25	9	65	2	12	1	1	0.22	0.43	0.23
8671	Wheat, toasted	1	slice(s)	23	7	65	2	12	1	1	0.22	0.43	0.23
340	White	1	slice(s)	25	9	67	2	13	1	1	0.18	0.17	0.34
1395	Whole wheat	1	slice(s)	46	15	128	4	24	3	2	0.37	0.53	1.35
	Cakes												
386	Angel food, from mix	1	slice(s)	50	16	129	3	29	<1	<1	0.02	0.01	0.06
8772	Butter pound, ready to eat, commercially prepared	1	slice(s)	75	18	291	4	37	<1	15	8.67	4.43	0.80
8737	Carrot, cream cheese frosting, from mix	1	slice(s)	111	23	484	5	52	1	29	5.43	7.24	15.10
4931	Chocolate, chocolate icing, commercially prepared	1	slice(s)	64	15	235	3	35	2	10	3.05	5.61	1.18
8756	Chocolate, from mix	1	slice(s)	95	23	340	5	51	2	14	5.16	5.74	2.62
393	Devil's food cupcake, chocolate frosting	1	item(s)	35	8	120	2	20	1	4	1.80	1.60	0.60
8757	Fruitcake, ready to eat, commercially prepared	1	piece(s)	43	11	139	1	26	2	4	0.45	1.81	1.43
1397	Pineapple upside down, from mix	1	slice(s)	115	37	367	4	58	1	14	3.35	5.97	3.77
411	Sponge, from mix	1	slice(s)	63	19	187	5	36	<1	3	0.82	0.99	0.41
8817	White, coconut frosting, from mix	1	slice(s)	112	23	399	5	71	1	12	4.36	4.14	2.42
8819	Yellow, chocolate frosting, ready to eat, commercially prepared	1	slice(s)	64	14	243	2	35	1	11	2.98	6.14	1.35

PAGE KEY: H–2 = Breads/Baked Goods H–6 = Cereal/Rice/Pasta H–10 = Fruit H–16 = Vegetables/Legumes H–26 = Nuts/Seeds H–28 = Vegetarian H–30 = Dairy H–36 = Eggs H–38 = Seafood H–40 = Meats H–42 = Poultry H–44 = Processed meats H–46 = Beverages H–50 = Fats/Oils H–52 = Sweets H–52 = Sauces/Condiments/Spices H–56 = Mixed Foods/Soups/Sandwiches H–62 = Fast food H–80 = Convenience H–82 = Baby foods

Chol (mg)	Calc (mg)	Iron (mg)	Magn (mg)	Pota (mg)	Sodi (mg)	Zinc (mg)	Vit A (RAE) (µg)	Thia (mg)	Vit E (mg)	Ribo (mg)	Niac (mg)	Vit B_6 (mg)	Fola (µg)	Vit C (mg)	Vit B_{12} (µg)	Sele (µg)
0	13	2.70	20	105	229	0.80	15	0.27	0.11	0.20	2.19	0.04	79	<1	0	22
0	53	2.53	21	72	379	0.62	0	0.38	0.03	0.22	3.24	0.04	75	0	0	23
0	53	2.52	20	72	379	0.62	0	0.31	0.02	0.20	2.91	0.03	64	0	0	23
0	9	2.19	22	82	360	0.64	1	0.24	0.10	0.24	2.10	0.03	70	<1	0	24
0	200	1.08	120	0	200	4.5	0	0.44	0	0.5	8	0.6	—	0	1.79	0
<1	33	1.01	6	37	205	0.27	9	0.13	0.03	0.12	1.08	0.01	26	0	<.1	7
49	80	1.31	7	48	288	0.29	—	0.15	0.72	0.16	1.20	0.03	8	<.1	<1	—
<1	57	1.22	16	81	321	0.42	12	0.16	0.11	0.13	1.49	0.03	29	<.1	<.1	12
<1	32	0.95	28	143	284	0.23	11	0.01	0.25	0.05	0.50	0.04	5	0	<.1	10
0	5	1.03	8	30	158	0.21	0	0.14	0.36	0.13	1.27	0.02	39	0	0	9
21	88	1.01	10	59	209	0.57	38	0.13	0.58	0.16	0.98	0.04	36	2	<1	6
0	11	0.70	13	44	135	0.31	0	0.09	0.15	0.06	0.92	0.08	15	0	<.1	6
0	6	0.31	2	9	52	0.07	0	0.05	—	0.02	0.41	0.00	10	0	0	3
20	37	1.22	8	46	197	0.32	25	0.18	0.24	0.17	1.94	0.03	42	0	<.1	12
21	38	1.24	8	47	200	0.32	26	0.14	0.31	0.16	1.77	0.02	36	0	<.1	12
0	19	0.63	7	28	152	0.22	0	0.13	0.07	0.08	1.19	0.01	37	0	0	8
0	19	0.63	7	28	152	0.22	0	0.10	0.06	0.07	1.07	0.01	22	0	0	8
0	210	3.24	14	67	626	0.45	0	0.39	0.69	0.27	3.27	0.02	67	0	0	21
0	23	0.88	8	33	175	0.26	0	0.14	0.11	0.09	1.31	0.01	57	0	0	8
0	24	0.90	14	53	127	0.33	0	0.11	0.17	0.09	1.13	0.09	31	<.1	<.1	8
0	24	0.90	14	53	127	0.33	0	0.08	0.16	0.08	1.02	0.08	28	<.1	<.1	8
0	20	0.94	11	44	122	0.27	1	0.15	0.19	0.10	1.45	0.02	24	0	0	9
0	19	0.93	9	33	121	0.28	1	0.12	0.12	0.09	1.29	0.01	19	0	0	9
0	18	0.73	10	38	162	0.28	1	0.11	0.16	0.06	0.85	0.02	17	0	<.1	7
0	18	0.74	10	39	163	0.28	1	0.09	0.09	0.06	0.77	0.02	13	<.1	<.1	7
0	52	1.57	16	72	322	0.50	0	0.36	0.02	0.20	2.78	0.02	64	0	0	16
0	10	1.96	44	109	340	0.97	0	0.22	0.58	0.05	1.82	0.17	22	0	0	28
0	22	0.92	17	67	215	0.47	0	0.10	0.14	0.10	0.99	0.04	30	0	0	8
0	17	0.75	7	59	101	0.19	0	0.09	0.13	0.10	0.90	0.02	28	<.1	0	5
0	17	0.76	7	59	102	0.19	0	0.07	0.20	0.09	0.81	0.02	24	<.1	0	5
0	40	1.08	—	45	160	—	0	0.23	—	0.14	1.20	—	40	0	—	—
0	23	0.91	13	53	211	0.36	0	0.14	0.12	0.11	1.22	0.02	35	<1	0	10
0	23	0.90	12	53	210	0.36	0	0.11	0.18	0.10	1.09	0.02	30	<.1	0	10
0	20	0.70	4	51	175	0.18	0	0.10	0.14	0.08	0.80	0.01	5	0	<.1	8
0	19	0.63	7	28	152	0.22	0	0.13	0.07	0.08	1.19	0.01	37	0	0	8
0	19	0.63	7	28	152	0.22	0	0.10	0.06	0.07	1.07	0.01	22	0	0	8
0	100	3.80	—	128	683	—	0	0.54	0.24	0.33	4.50	0.05	—	0	—	42
0	19	0.63	7	28	152	0.22	0	0.10	0.06	0.07	1.07	0.01	22	0	0	8
0	26	0.83	12	50	133	0.26	0	0.10	0.14	0.07	1.03	0.02	23	0	0	8
0	26	0.83	12	50	132	0.26	0	0.08	0.14	0.06	0.93	0.02	19	0	0	8
0	38	0.94	6	25	170	0.19	0	0.11	0.10	0.08	1.10	0.02	28	0	0	4
0	15	1.43	37	144	159	0.69	0	0.14	0.61	0.10	1.83	0.09	30	0	0	18
0	42	0.12	4	68	255	0.07	0	0.05	0.00	0.10	0.09	0.00	10	0	<.1	8
166	26	1.04	8	89	299	0.35	112	0.10	0.17	0.98	0.03	31	0	<1	7	
60	28	1.39	20	124	273	0.54	—	0.15	4.69	0.17	1.13	0.08	13	1	<1	—
27	28	1.41	22	128	214	0.44	—	0.02	1.42	0.09	0.37	0.03	11	<.1	<.1	2
55	57	1.53	30	133	299	0.66	38	0.13	1.51	0.20	1.08	0.04	26	<1	<1	11
19	21	0.70	—	46	92	—	—	0.04	0.63	0.05	0.30	—	2	0	—	2
2	14	0.89	7	66	116	0.12	3	0.02	0.71	0.04	0.34	0.02	9	<1	<.1	1
25	138	1.70	15	129	367	0.36	71	0.18	1.54	0.18	1.37	0.04	30	1	<.1	11
107	26	1.00	6	89	144	0.37	49	0.10	—	0.19	0.76	0.04	25	0	<1	12
1	101	1.30	13	111	318	0.37	13	0.14	0.80	0.21	1.19	0.03	35	<1	<.1	12
35	24	1.33	19	114	216	0.40	21	0.08	1.45	0.10	0.80	0.02	14	0	<1	2

Table H–1

Food Composition (Computer code number is for Wadsworth Diet Analysis program) (For purposes of calculations, use "0" for t, <1, <.1, <.01, etc.)

DA + Code	Food Description	Quantity	Measure	Wt (g)	H_2O (g)	Ener (kcal)	Prot (g)	Carb (g)	Dietary Fiber (g)	Fat (g)	Fat Breakdown (g) Sat	Mono	Poly
	BREADS, BAKED GOODS, CAKES, COOKIES, CRACKERS, CHIPS, PIES—Continued												
8822	Yellow, vanilla frosting, ready to eat, commercially prepared	1	slice(s)	64	14	239	2	38	<1	9	1.52	3.91	3.30
	Snack cakes												
8791	Chocolate snack cake, creme filled, w/frosting	1	item(s)	50	10	188	2	30	<1	7	1.43	2.85	2.62
25010	Cinnamon coffee cake	1	piece(s)	72	23	231	4	36	1	8	2.19	2.65	2.99
16777	Funnel cake	1	item(s)	90	37	278	7	29	1	14	2.77	4.46	6.33
8794	Sponge snack cake, creme filled	1	item(s)	43	9	155	1	27	<1	5	1.09	1.73	1.40
	Snacks, chips, pretzels												
29428	Bagel chips, plain	3	item(s)	29	—	130	3	19	1	5	0.50	—	—
29429	Bagel chips, toasted onion	3	item(s)	29	—	130	4	20	1	5	0.50	—	—
38192	Chex traditional snack mix	1	cup(s)	46	—	198	3	33	2	6	0.76	—	—
654	Potato chips, salted	20	item(s)	28	1	152	2	15	1	10	3.11	2.79	3.46
8816	Potato chips, unsalted	20	item(s)	28	1	152	2	15	1	10	3.11	2.79	3.46
4641	Tortilla chips, plain	6	item(s)	28	1	142	2	18	2	7	1.43	4.39	1.03
5096	Pretzels, plain, hard, twists	5	item(s)	30	1	114	3	24	1	1	0.23	0.41	0.37
4632	Pretzels, whole wheat	1	ounce(s)	28	1	103	3	23	2	1	0.16	0.29	0.24
	Cookies												
8859	Animal crackers	12	piece(s)	30	0	134	2	22	<1	4	1.03	2.29	0.56
8876	Brownie, prepared from mix	1	item(s)	24	3	112	1	12	1	7	1.76	2.60	2.26
25207	Chocolate chip cookies	1	item(s)	30	4	140	2	16	1	8	2.09	3.26	2.09
8915	Chocolate sandwich cookie, extra creme filling	1	item(s)	13	<1	65	<1	9	<1	3	0.50	1.39	1.22
14145	Fig Newtons	1	item(s)	16	—	55	1	10	1	1	0.50	0.50	0.00
8920	Fortune cookie	1	item(s)	8	1	30	<1	7	<1	<1	0.05	0.11	0.04
25208	Oatmeal cookies	1	item(s)	69	12	234	6	45	3	4	0.70	1.28	1.85
25213	Peanut butter cookies	1	item(s)	35	4	163	4	17	1	9	1.65	4.72	2.43
33095	Sugar cookies	1	item(s)	16	4	61	1	7	<1	3	0.63	1.27	0.87
9002	Vanilla sandwich cookie, creme filling	1	item(s)	10	<1	48	<1	7	<1	2	0.30	0.84	0.76
	Crackers												
9008	Cheese crackers (mini)	30	item(s)	30	1	151	3	17	1	8	2.81	3.63	0.74
9010	Cheese crackers (mini), low salt	30	item(s)	30	1	151	3	17	1	8	2.82	2.70	1.44
9012	Cheese cracker sandwich w/peanut butter	4	item(s)	28	1	139	3	16	1	7	1.23	3.64	1.43
8928	Honey graham crackers	4	item(s)	28	1	118	2	22	1	3	0.43	1.14	1.07
9016	Matzo crackers, plain	1	item(s)	28	1	112	3	24	1	<1	0.06	0.04	0.17
9024	Melba toast	3	item(s)	15	1	59	2	11	1	<1	0.07	0.12	0.19
14189	Ritz crackers	5	item(s)	16	<1	80	1	10	1	4	0.50	1.50	0.00
9014	Rye crispbread crackers	1	item(s)	10	1	37	1	8	2	<1	0.01	0.02	0.06
9028	Rye melba toast	3	item(s)	15	1	58	2	12	1	1	0.07	0.14	0.20
9040	Rye wafer	1	item(s)	11	1	37	1	9	3	<.1	0.01	0.02	0.04
432	Saltine crackers	5	item(s)	15	1	65	1	11	<1	2	0.44	0.96	0.25
9046	Saltine crackers, low salt	5	item(s)	15	1	65	1	11	<1	2	0.44	0.96	0.25
9048	Snack crackers, round	10	item(s)	30	1	151	2	18	<1	8	1.13	3.19	2.86
9050	Snack crackers, round, low salt	10	item(s)	30	1	151	2	18	<1	8	1.13	3.19	2.86
9052	Snack cracker sandwich, cheese filling	4	item(s)	28	1	134	3	17	1	6	1.72	3.15	0.72
9054	Snack cracker sandwich, peanut butter filling	4	item(s)	28	1	138	3	16	1	7	1.38	3.86	1.30
9044	Soda crackers	5	item(s)	15	1	65	1	11	<1	2	0.44	0.96	0.25
9055	Wheat crackers	10	item(s)	30	1	142	3	19	1	6	1.55	3.43	0.84
9057	Wheat crackers, low salt	10	item(s)	30	1	142	3	19	1	6	1.55	3.43	0.84
9059	Wheat cracker sandwich, cheese filling	4	item(s)	28	1	139	3	16	1	7	1.16	2.90	2.57
9061	Wheat cracker sandwich, peanut butter filling	4	item(s)	28	1	139	4	15	1	7	1.29	3.29	2.48
9022	Whole wheat crackers	7	item(s)	28	1	124	2	19	3	5	0.95	1.65	1.85
	Pastry												
16754	Apple fritter	1	item(s)	17	6	62	1	6	<1	4	0.87	1.69	1.13
5118	Cinnamon sweet roll w/icing, from refrigerator dough	1	item(s)	30	7	109	2	17	1	4	1.00	2.23	0.52
4945	Croissant, butter	1	item(s)	57	13	231	5	26	1	12	6.59	3.15	0.62
9096	Danish pastry, nut	1	item(s)	65	13	280	5	30	1	16	3.78	8.90	2.78
4947	Doughnut, cake	1	item(s)	47	10	198	2	23	1	11	1.70	4.37	3.70

Chol (mg)	Calc (mg)	Iron (mg)	Magn (mg)	Pota (mg)	Sodi (mg)	Zinc (mg)	Vit A (RAE) (µg)	Thia (mg)	Vit E (mg)	Ribo (mg)	Niac (mg)	Vit B_6 (mg)	Fola (µg)	Vit C (mg)	Vit B_{12} (µg)	Sele (µg)
35	40	0.68	4	34	220	0.16	12	0.06	—	0.04	0.32	0.02	17	0	<.1	4
9	37	1.68	21	61	213	0.26	3	0.11	1.68	0.15	1.21	0.01	20	0	<.1	1
26	50	1.46	10	81	277	0.38	35	0.14	1.06	0.16	1.17	0.02	30	<.1	<1	10
63	128	1.86	18	154	273	0.64	—	0.24	2.54	0.32	1.86	0.05	14	<1	<1	—
7	19	0.55	3	37	155	0.12	2	0.07	0.86	0.06	0.52	0.01	17	<.1	<.1	1
0	0	0.72	—	45	70	—	0	—	—	—	—	—	—	0	0	—
0	0	0.72	—	50	300	—	0	—	—	—	—	—	—	0	0	—
0	0	0.55	0	76	623	0.00	0	0.09	0.00	0.05	1.22	0.00	12	0	—	—
0	7	0.46	19	362	169	0.31	0	0.05	1.39	0.06	1.09	0.19	13	9	0	2
0	7	0.46	19	362	2	0.31	0	0.05	1.39	0.06	1.09	0.19	13	9	0	2
0	44	0.43	25	56	150	0.43	1	0.02	0.39	0.05	0.36	0.08	3	0	0	2
0	11	1.30	11	44	515	0.26	0	0.14	0.06	0.19	1.58	0.03	51	0	0	2
0	8	0.76	9	122	58	0.18	0	0.12	—	0.08	1.86	0.08	15	<1	0	—
0	13	0.82	5	30	1118	0.19	—	0.10	0.44	0.09	1.04	0.00	50	0	<.1	—
18	14	0.44	13	42	82	0.23	42	0.03	—	0.05	0.24	0.02	7	<.1	<.1	3
13	11	0.70	12	62	109	0.24	27	0.07	1.75	0.06	0.82	0.02	16	<.1	<.1	4
0	3	0.37	4	16	64	0.08	0	0.01	0.58	0.02	0.20	0.00	6	0	<.1	<1
0	5	0.36	—	40	60	—	4	0.03	—	0.04	0.22	—	—	<1	—	—
<1	1	0.12	1	3	22	0.01	<.1	0.01	0.03	0.01	0.15	0.00	5	0	<.1	<1
<.1	26	1.94	49	177	311	1.43	48	0.23	0.97	0.12	1.24	0.09	30	<1	<.1	17
13	28	0.67	22	104	157	0.46	51	0.08	3.35	0.09	1.81	0.05	21	<.1	<.1	5
18	5	0.32	2	13	50	0.08	31	0.04	0.45	0.04	0.28	0.01	8	<.1	<.1	3
0	3	0.22	1	9	35	0.04	0	0.03	0.36	0.02	0.27	0.00	5	0	0	<1
4	45	1.43	11	44	299	0.34	9	0.17	0.79	0.13	1.40	0.17	46	0	<1	3
4	45	1.44	11	32	137	0.33	—	0.18	0.30	0.12	1.41	0.18	8	0	<1	—
0	14	0.76	16	61	199	0.29	0	0.15	1.05	0.08	1.63	0.04	26	0	<.1	2
0	7	1.04	8	38	169	0.23	0	0.06	0.57	0.09	1.15	0.02	13	0	0	3
0	4	0.90	7	32	1	0.19	0	0.11	0.02	0.08	1.11	0.03	5	0	0	10
0	14	0.56	9	30	124	0.30	0	0.06	0.01	0.04	0.62	0.01	19	0	0	5
0	20	0.72	3	10	135	0.23	—	0.07	—	0.04	0.45	0.01	10	1	0	—
0	3	0.24	8	32	26	0.24	0	0.02	0.13	0.01	0.10	0.02	5	0	0	4
0	12	0.55	6	29	135	0.20	0	0.07	0.10	0.04	0.71	0.01	13	0	0	6
0	4	0.65	13	54	87	0.31	0	0.05	0.16	0.03	0.17	0.03	5	<.1	0	3
0	18	0.81	4	19	195	0.12	0	0.08	0.23	0.07	0.79	0.01	19	0	0	2
0	18	0.81	4	109	95	0.12	0	0.08	0.23	0.07	0.79	0.01	19	0	0	3
0	36	1.08	8	40	254	0.20	0	0.12	1.36	0.10	1.21	0.02	27	0	0	2
0	36	1.08	8	107	112	0.20	0	0.12	1.36	0.10	1.21	0.02	27	0	0	2
1	72	0.67	10	120	392	0.17	5	0.12	0.72	0.19	1.05	0.01	28	<.1	<.1	6
0	23	0.78	15	60	201	0.32	0	0.14	1.05	0.08	1.71	0.04	24	0	<.1	3
0	18	0.81	4	19	195	0.12	0	0.08	0.23	0.07	0.79	0.01	19	0	0	2
0	15	1.32	19	55	239	0.48	0	0.15	0.97	0.10	1.49	0.04	35	0	0	2
0	15	1.32	19	61	85	0.48	0	0.15	0.97	0.10	1.49	0.04	15	0	0	10
2	57	0.73	15	86	256	0.24	5	0.10	—	0.12	0.89	0.07	18	<1	<.1	7
0	48	0.75	11	83	226	0.23	0	0.11	—	0.08	1.65	0.04	20	0	0	6
0	14	0.86	28	83	185	0.60	0	0.06	0.31	0.03	1.27	0.05	8	0	0	4
14	9	0.25	2	24	7	0.09	—	0.03	0.52	0.04	0.23	0.01	2	<1	<.1	—
0	10	0.80	4	19	250	0.10	—	0.12	0.29	0.07	1.09	0.01	14	<.1	<.1	—
38	21	1.16	9	67	424	0.43	101	0.22	0.25	0.14	1.25	0.03	35	<1	<.1	13
30	61	1.17	21	62	236	0.57	6	0.14	2.37	0.16	1.50	0.07	54	1	<1	9
17	21	0.92	9	60	257	0.26	—	0.10	1.80	0.11	0.87	0.03	22	<.1	<1	0

Table H–1

Food Composition (Computer code number is for Wadsworth Diet Analysis program) (For purposes of calculations, use "0" for t, <1, <.1, <.01, etc.)

DA + Code	Food Description	Quantity	Measure	Wt (g)	H_2O (g)	Ener (kcal)	Prot (g)	Carb (g)	Dietary Fiber (g)	Fat (g)	Fat Breakdown (g) Sat	Mono	Poly
	BREADS, BAKED GOODS, CAKES, COOKIES, CRACKERS, CHIPS, PIES—Continued												
9105	Doughnut, cake, chocolate glazed	1	item(s)	42	7	175	2	24	1	8	2.16	4.74	1.04
9115	Doughnut, creme filling	1	item(s)	85	32	307	5	26	1	21	4.62	10.27	2.62
437	Doughnut, glazed	1	item(s)	60	15	242	4	27	1	14	3.49	7.72	1.74
9117	Doughnut, jelly filling	1	item(s)	85	30	289	5	33	1	16	4.12	8.69	2.02
10617	Toaster pastry, brown sugar cinnamon	1	item(s)	50	5	210	3	35	1	6	1.00	4.00	1.00
30928	Toaster pastry, cream cheese	1	item(s)	54	—	200	3	23	1	11	3.50	—	—
	Muffins												
25015	Blueberry	1	item(s)	63	30	160	3	23	1	6	0.87	1.48	3.25
4997	Bran, from mix	1	item(s)	50	18	138	3	23	2	5	1.18	2.34	0.72
9189	Corn, ready to eat	1	item(s)	57	19	174	3	29	2	5	0.77	1.20	1.83
9121	English muffin, plain, enriched	1	item(s)	57	24	134	4	26	2	1	0.15	0.17	0.51
29582	English, toasted	1	item(s)	50	19	128	4	25	1	1	0.14	0.16	0.48
9145	English, wheat	1	item(s)	57	24	127	5	26	3	1	0.16	0.16	0.48
	Granola bars												
38161	Kudos milk chocolate w/fruit & nuts	1	item(s)	28	—	90	2	15	1	3	1.00	—	—
38196	Nature Valley banana nut crunchy	1	item(s)	21	—	95	2	14	1	4	0.50	—	—
38187	Nature Valley fruit n nut trail mix	1	item(s)	35	—	140	3	25	2	4	0.50	—	—
1383	Plain, hard	1	item(s)	25	1	115	2	16	1	5	0.58	1.07	2.95
4606	Plain, soft	1	item(s)	28	2	126	2	19	1	5	2.06	1.08	1.51
	Pies												
454	Apple pie, from home recipe	1	slice(s)	155	73	411	4	58	2	19	4.73	8.36	5.17
470	Pecan pie, from home recipe	1	slice(s)	122	24	503	6	64	0	27	4.87	13.64	6.97
472	Pumpkin pie, from home recipe	1	slice(s)	155	91	316	7	41	0	14	4.92	5.73	2.81
9007	Pie crust, frozen, ready to bake, enriched, baked	1	slice(s)	16	2	82	1	8	<1	5	1.69	2.51	0.65
5052	Pie crust, prepared w/water, baked	1	slice(s)	20	2	100	1	10	<1	6	1.54	3.46	0.77
	Rolls												
8555	Crescent dinner roll	1	item(s)	28	10	80	2	14	1	1	0.34	0.70	0.25
489	Hamburger roll or bun, plain	1	item(s)	43	15	120	4	21	1	2	0.47	0.48	0.85
490	Hard roll	1	item(s)	57	18	167	6	30	1	2	0.35	0.65	0.98
5127	Kaiser roll	1	item(s)	57	18	167	6	30	1	2	0.35	0.65	0.98
5130	Whole wheat roll or bun	1	item(s)	28	9	76	2	15	2	1	0.24	0.34	0.62
	Sport bars												
37026	Balance original chocolate	1	item(s)	50	—	200	14	22	1	6	3.50	—	—
37024	Balance original peanut butter	1	item(s)	50	—	200	14	22	1	6	2.50	—	—
36580	Clif Bar chocolate brownie energy bar	1	item(s)	68	—	240	10	41	6	4	1.00	—	—
36583	Clif Bar crunchy peanut butter energy bar	1	item(s)	68	—	240	12	39	5	5	0.50	—	—
36584	Clif Luna tropical crisp energy bar	1	item(s)	48	—	180	10	24	2	5	3.50	0.00	0.00
12005	Powerbar apple cinnamon	1	item(s)	65	—	230	10	45	3	3	0.50	1.50	0.50
16078	Powerbar banana	1	item(s)	65	—	230	9	45	3	2	0.50	1.00	0.50
16080	Powerbar chocolate	1	item(s)	65	—	230	10	45	3	2	0.50	0.50	1.00
16079	Powerbar mocha	1	item(s)	65	—	230	10	45	3	3	1.00	1.00	0.50
	Tortillas												
1391	Corn tortillas, soft	1	item(s)	26	11	58	1	12	1	1	0.09	0.17	0.29
1669	Flour tortilla	1	item(s)	32	9	104	3	18	1	2	0.56	1.21	0.34
1390	Taco shells, hard	1	item(s)	13	1	62	1	8	1	3	0.43	1.19	1.13
	Pancakes, waffles												
8926	Pancakes, blueberry, from recipe	3	item(s)	114	61	253	7	33	1	10	2.26	2.64	4.74
5037	Pancakes, from mix w/egg & milk	3	item(s)	114	60	249	9	33	2	9	2.33	2.36	3.33
9219	Waffle, plain, frozen, toasted	2	item(s)	66	28	174	4	27	2	5	0.95	2.12	1.84
500	Waffle, plain, from recipe	1	item(s)	75	<.1	218	6	25	2	11	2.14	2.64	5.08
30311	Waffle, 100% whole grain	1	item(s)	75	32	201	7	25	2	8	2.35	3.38	2.06
	CEREAL, FLOUR, GRAIN, PASTA, NOODLES, POPCORN												
	Grain												
2861	Amaranth, dry	½	cup(s)	98	10	365	14	65	15	6	1.62	1.40	2.82
1953	Barley, pearled, cooked	½	cup(s)	79	54	97	2	22	3	<1	0.07	0.04	0.17
1956	Buckwheat groats, cooked, roasted	½	cup(s)	84	64	77	3	17	2	1	0.11	0.16	0.16
1957	Bulgur, cooked	½	cup(s)	91	71	76	3	17	4	<1	0.04	0.03	0.09
1963	Couscous, cooked	½	cup(s)	79	57	88	3	18	1	<1	0.02	0.02	0.05
1967	Millet, cooked	½	cup(s)	120	86	143	4	28	2	1	0.21	0.22	0.61

PAGE KEY: H–2 = Breads/Baked Goods H–6 = Cereal/Rice/Pasta H–10 = Fruit H–16 = Vegetables/Legumes H–26 = Nuts/Seeds H–28 = Vegetarian H–30 = Dairy H–36 = Eggs H–38 = Seafood H–40 = Meats H–42 = Poultry H–44 = Processed meats H–46 = Beverages H–50 = Fats/Oils H–52 = Sweets H–52 = Sauces/Condiments/Spices H–56 = Mixed Foods/Soups/Sandwiches H–62 = Fast food H–80 = Convenience H–82 = Baby foods

Chol (mg)	Calc (mg)	Iron (mg)	Magn (mg)	Pota (mg)	Sodi (mg)	Zinc (mg)	Vit A (RAE) (μg)	Thia (mg)	Vit E (mg)	Ribo (mg)	Niac (mg)	Vit B_6 (mg)	Fola (μg)	Vit C (mg)	Vit B_{12} (μg)	Sele (μg)
24	89	0.95	14	45	143	0.24	5	0.02	1.13	0.03	0.20	0.01	19	<.1	<.1	2
20	21	1.56	17	68	263	0.68	9	0.29	2.35	0.13	1.91	0.06	60	0	<1	9
4	26	0.36	13	65	205	0.46	2	0.53	1.83	0.04	0.39	0.03	13	<.1	<.1	5
22	21	1.50	17	67	249	0.64	14	0.27	2.09	0.12	1.82	0.09	58	0	<1	11
0	0	1.80	—	70	190	—	—	0.15	0.00	0.17	2.00	0.20	40	0	0	—
15	0	1.08	—	—	230	—	—	—	—	—	—	—	—	0	—	—
20	50	1.15	7	56	288	0.39	20	0.14	1.28	0.15	1.14	0.03	29	<1	<1	9
34	16	1.27	29	74	234	0.57	—	0.10	—	0.12	1.44	0.09	33	0	<.1	—
15	42	1.60	18	39	297	0.31	30	0.16	1.05	0.19	1.16	0.05	46	0	<.1	9
0	30	1.43	12	75	264	0.40	0	0.25	0.10	0.16	2.21	0.02	42	0	<.1	—
0	95	1.36	11	72	252	0.38	0	0.19	0.06	0.14	1.90	0.02	15	<.1	<.1	—
0	101	1.64	21	106	218	0.61	0	0.25	0.28	0.17	1.91	0.05	36	0	0	17
0	200	0.36	—	—	60	—	0	—	—	—	—	—	—	0	0	—
0	10	0.54	—	60	80	—	0	—	—	—	—	—	—	0	—	—
0	0	0.00	—	—	95	—	0	—	—	—	—	—	—	0	—	—
0	15	0.72	24	82	72	0.50	2	0.06	0.00	0.03	0.39	0.02	6	<1	0	4
<1	30	0.73	21	92	79	0.43	0	0.08	—	0.05	0.15	0.03	7	0	<1	5
0	11	1.74	11	122	327	0.29	17	0.23	—	0.17	1.91	0.05	37	3	0	12
106	39	1.81	32	162	320	1.24	100	0.23	—	0.22	1.03	0.07	32	<1	<1	15
65	146	1.97	29	288	349	0.71	660	0.14	—	0.31	1.21	0.07	33	3	<1	11
0	3	0.36	3	18	104	0.05	0	0.04	0.82	0.06	0.39	0.01	9	0	<.1	<1
0	12	0.43	3	12	146	0.08	0	0.06	—	0.04	0.47	0.01	20	0	0	—
0	39	0.89	6	39	157	0.17	0	0.14	—	0.09	1.10	0.01	—	0	<.1	—
0	59	1.43	9	40	206	0.28	0	0.17	0.67	0.14	1.79	0.03	48	0	<.1	8
0	54	1.87	15	62	310	0.54	0	0.27	0.19	0.19	2.42	0.02	54	0	0	22
0	54	1.87	15	62	310	0.54	0	0.27	0.19	0.19	2.42	0.02	54	0	0	22
0	30	0.69	24	78	136	0.57	0	0.07	0.39	0.04	1.05	0.06	9	0	0	14
3	100	4.50	40	160	180	3.75	—	0.38	20.13	0.43	5.00	0.50	100	60	2	18
3	100	4.50	40	130	230	3.75	—	0.38	20.13	0.43	5.00	0.50	100	60	2	18
0	250	5.40	120	260	150	3.75	—	0.38	20.13	0.26	4.00	0.40	80	60	1	18
0	250	5.40	120	300	290	3.75	—	0.38	20.13	0.34	6.00	0.40	100	60	1	14
0	350	6.30	140	120	135	5.25	—	1.50	20.13	1.70	20.00	2.00	400	60	6	25
0	300	6.30	140	110	90	5.25	0	1.50	20.13	1.70	20.00	2.00	400	60	6	—
0	300	6.30	140	200	90	5.25	0	1.50	20.13	1.70	20.00	2.00	400	60	6	—
0	300	6.30	140	150	90	5.25	0	1.50	20.13	1.70	20.00	2.00	400	60	6	—
0	300	6.30	140	150	90	5.25	0	1.50	20.13	1.70	20.00	2.00	400	60	6	—
0	46	0.36	17	40	42	0.24	0	0.03	0.04	0.02	0.39	0.06	26	0	0	1
0	40	1.06	8	42	153	0.23	0	0.17	0.29	0.09	1.14	0.02	33	0	0	7
0	21	0.33	14	24	49	0.19	0	0.03	0.48	0.01	0.18	0.04	17	0	0	2
64	235	1.96	18	157	470	0.62	57	0.22	—	0.31	1.74	0.06	41	3	<1	16
81	245	1.48	25	227	576	0.86	82	0.23	1.29	0.36	1.40	0.12	105	1	<1	—
16	153	2.95	15	84	519	0.38	253	0.25	0.55	0.31	2.93	0.59	36	0	2	11
52	191	1.73	14	119	383	0.50	49	0.19	—	0.26	1.55	0.04	51	<1	<1	35
71	196	1.56	30	173	374	0.85	—	0.15	1.06	0.25	1.47	0.09	14	<1	<1	—
0	149	7.40	259	357	20	3.10	0	0.08	1.00	0.20	1.25	0.22	48	4	0	—
0	9	1.04	17	73	2	0.64	0	0.07	0.04	0.05	1.62	0.09	13	0	0	7
0	6	0.67	43	74	3	0.51	0	0.03	0.20	0.03	0.79	0.06	12	0	0	2
0	9	0.87	29	62	5	0.52	0	0.05	0.03	0.03	0.91	0.08	16	0	0	1
0	6	0.30	6	46	4	0.20	0	0.05	0.01	0.02	0.77	0.04	12	0	0	22
0	4	0.76	53	74	2	1.09	0	0.13	0.07	0.10	1.60	0.13	23	0	0	1

Table H–1

Food Composition (Computer code number is for Wadsworth Diet Analysis program) (For purposes of calculations, use "0" for t, <1, <.1, <.01, etc.)

DA + Code	Food Description	Quantity	Measure	Wt (g)	H_2O (g)	Ener (kcal)	Prot (g)	Carb (g)	Dietary Fiber (g)	Fat (g)	Fat Breakdown (g) Sat	Mono	Poly
	CEREAL, FLOUR, GRAIN, PASTA, NOODLES, POPCORN—Continued												
1969	Oat bran, dry	½	cup(s)	47	3	116	8	31	7	3	0.62	1.12	1.30
1972	Quinoa, dry	½	cup(s)	85	8	318	11	59	5	5	0.50	1.30	1.99
	Rice												
129	Brown, long grain, cooked	½	cup(s)	98	71	108	3	22	2	1	0.18	0.32	0.31
2863	Brown, medium grain, cooked	½	cup(s)	97.5	0.07	109.19	2.26	22.92	1.75	0.8	0.16	0.29	0.28
37488	Jasmine, saffroned, cooked	½	cup(s)	280	—	340	8	78	0	0	0.00	—	—
30280	Pilaf, cooked	½	cup(s)	103	74	129	2	22	1	3	0.67	1.61	0.95
28066	Spanish, cooked	½	cup(s)	120	3	25	2	1	<1	<1	0.33	0.07	18.31
2867	White glutinous, cooked	½	cup(s)	87	67	84	2	18	1	<1	0.03	0.06	0.06
482	White, instant long grain, enriched, boiled	½	cup(s)	83	63	81	2	18	<1	<1	0.04	0.04	0.04
484	White, long grain, boiled	½	cup(s)	79	54	103	2	22	<1	<1	0.06	0.07	0.06
486	White, long grain, enriched, parboiled, cooked	½	cup(s)	88	63	100	2	22	<1	<1	0.06	0.07	0.06
1194	Wild brown, cooked	½	cup(s)	82	0.06	82.81	3.27	17.49	1.47	0.27	0.04	0.04	0.17
	Flour & grain fractions												
505	All purpose flour, self rising, enriched	½	cup(s)	63	7	221	6	46	2	1	0.10	0.05	0.26
503	All purpose flour, white, bleached, enriched	½	cup(s)	63	7	228	6	48	2	1	0.10	0.05	0.26
1643	Barley flour	½	cup(s)	56	6	198	4	45	2	1	0.16	0.10	0.38
383	Buckwheat flour, whole groat	½	cup(s)	60	7	201	8	42	6	2	0.41	0.57	0.57
504	Cake wheat flour, enriched	½	cup(s)	55	7	197	4	43	1	<1	0.07	0.04	0.21
426	Cornmeal, degermed, enriched	½	cup(s)	69	8	253	6	54	5	1	0.16	0.28	0.49
424	Cornmeal, yellow whole grain	½	cup(s)	61	6	221	5	47	4	2	0.31	0.58	1.00
1644	Masa corn flour, enriched	½	cup(s)	57	5	208	5	43	5	2	0.30	0.57	0.98
1976	Rice flour, brown	½	cup(s)	79	9	287	6	60	4	2	0.44	0.80	0.79
1645	Rice flour, white	½	cup(s)	79	9	289	5	63	2	1	0.30	0.35	0.30
1978	Rye flour, dark	½	cup(s)	64	7	207	9	44	14	2	0.20	0.21	0.77
1980	Semolina, enriched	½	cup(s)	84	11	301	11	61	3	1	0.13	0.10	0.36
2827	Soy flour, raw	½	cup(s)	43	2	186	15	15	4	9	1.27	1.94	4.96
1990	Wheat germ, crude	2	tablespoon(s)	14	2	52	3	7	2	1	0.24	0.20	0.86
506	Whole wheat flour	½	cup(s)	60	6	203	8	44	7	1	0.19	0.14	0.47
	Breakfast bars												
39230	Atkins Morning Start apple crisp	1	item(s)	37	—	170	11	12	6	9	4.00	—	—
10574	Health Valley fat free apple	1	item(s)	38	—	110	2	26	3	0	0.00	0.00	0.00
10647	Nutri-Grain blueberry cereal bar	1	item(s)	37	5	140	2	27	1	3	0.50	2.00	0.50
10648	Nutri-Grain raspberry cereal bar	1	item(s)	37	5	140	2	27	1	3	0.50	2.00	0.50
10649	Nutri-Grain strawberry cereal bar	1	item(s)	37	5	140	2	27	1	3	0.50	2.00	0.50
	Breakfast cereals, hot												
363	Corn grits, white, regular & quick, enriched, cooked w/water & salt	½	cup(s)	121	103	71	2	16	<1	<1	0.03	0.06	0.10
8636	Corn grits, yellow, regular & quick, enriched, cooked w/salt	½	cup(s)	121	103	71	2	16	<1	<1	0.03	0.06	0.10
1260	Cream of Wheat, instant, prepared	½	cup(s)	121	106	61	2	13	<1	<.1	0.01	0.01	0.04
365	Farina, enriched, cooked w/water & salt	½	cup(s)	117	102	56	2	12	<1	<.1	0.01	0.01	0.03
8657	Oatmeal, cooked w/water	½	cup(s)	117	100	74	3	13	2	1	0.19	0.37	0.44
5500	Oatmeal, maple & brown sugar, instant, prepared	1	item(s)	198	150	200	5	40	2	2	0.42	0.74	0.85
5510	Oatmeal, ready to serve, packet	1	item(s)	186	158	112	4	20	3	2	0.38	0.66	0.76
	Breakfast cereals, ready to eat												
1197	All-Bran	1	cup(s)	62	2	160	8	46	20	2	0.00	0.00	1.00
1200	All-Bran Buds	1	cup(s)	91	3	212	6	73	42	3	—	—	—
1199	Apple Jacks	1	cup(s)	33	1	130	1	30	1	1	—	—	—
13633	Bran Flakes, Post	1	cup(s)	40	1	133	4	32	7	1	0.00	0.00	0.71
1204	Cap'n Crunch	1	cup(s)	36	1	144	2	30	1	2	0.53	0.39	0.27
1205	Cap'n Crunch Crunchberries w/wildberry colors	1	cup(s)	35	1	139	2	29	1	2	0.49	0.39	0.28
1206	Cheerios	1	cup(s)	30	1	110	3	22	3	2	0.00	0.50	0.50
3415	Cocoa Puffs	1	cup(s)	30	1	120	1	26	0	1	—	—	—
1207	Cocoa Rice Krispies	1	cup(s)	41	1	160	1	36	1	1	0.67	0.00	0.00
5522	Complete wheat bran flakes	1	cup(s)	39	1	120	4	31	7	1	—	—	—
1211	Corn Flakes	1	cup(s)	28	1	100	2	24	1	0	0.00	0.00	0.00

PAGE KEY: H–2 = Breads/Baked Goods H–6 = Cereal/Rice/Pasta H–10 = Fruit H–16 = Vegetables/Legumes H–26 = Nuts/Seeds H–28 = Vegetarian H–30 = Dairy H–36 = Eggs H–38 = Seafood H–40 = Meats H–42 = Poultry H–44 = Processed meats H–46 = Beverages H–50 = Fats/Oils H–52 = Sweets H–52 = Sauces/Condiments/Spices H–56 = Mixed Foods/Soups/Sandwiches H–62 = Fast food H–80 = Convenience H–82 = Baby foods

Chol (mg)	Calc (mg)	Iron (mg)	Magn (mg)	Pota (mg)	Sodi (mg)	Zinc (mg)	Vit A (RAE) (µg)	Thia (mg)	Vit E (mg)	Ribo (mg)	Niac (mg)	Vit B_6 (mg)	Fola (µg)	Vit C (mg)	Vit B_{12} (µg)	Sele (µg)
0	27	2.54	110	266	2	1.46	0	0.55	0.80	0.10	0.44	0.08	24	0	0	21
0	51	7.86	179	629	18	2.81	0	0.17	—	0.34	2.49	0.19	42	0	0	—
0	10	0.41	42	42	5	0.61	0	0.09	0.21	0.02	1.49	0.14	4	0	0	10
0	9.75	0.51	42.9	77.02	0.97	0.6	0	0.09	0.04	0.01	1.29	0.14	3.9	0	0	38
0	—	2.16	—	—	780	—	—	—	—	—	—	—	—	—	—	—
0	13	1.16	9	55	403	0.38	—	0.13	0.53	0.02	1.24	0.06	4	<1	<.1	—
1	47	167.40	48	1	13	0.13	<1	0.03	1.62	0.19	8.71	10.30	<.1	7	<.1	9
0	2	0.12	4	9	4	0.36	0	0.02	0.03	0.01	0.25	0.02	1	0	0	5
0	7	0.52	4	3	2	0.20	0	0.06	0.04	0.04	0.73	0.01	58	0	0	3
0	8	0.95	9	28	1	0.39	0	0.13	0.04	0.01	1.17	0.07	46	0	0	6
0	17	0.99	11	32	3	0.27	0	0.22	0.04	0.02	1.23	0.02	67	0	0	7
0	2.46	0.49	26.23	82.81	2.46	1.09	0	0.04	0.15	0.07	1.05	0.11	21.31	0	0	0.65
0	211	2.92	12	78	794	0.39	0	0.42	0.07	0.26	3.65	0.03	123	0	0	22
0	9	2.90	14	67	1	0.44	0	0.49	0.08	0.31	3.69	0.03	114	0	0	21
0	16	0.71	45	186	4	1.05	0	0.07	0.07	0.03	2.57	0.16	13	0	0	2
0	25	2.44	151	346	7	1.87	0	0.25	0.62	0.11	3.69	0.35	32	0	0	3
0	8	3.99	9	57	1	0.34	0	0.49	0.02	0.23	3.70	0.02	101	0	0	3
0	3	2.85	28	112	2	0.50	8	0.49	0.23	0.28	3.47	0.18	161	0	0	5
0	4	2.10	77	175	21	1.11	7	0.23	0.41	0.12	2.22	0.19	15	0	0	9
0	80	4.11	63	170	3	1.01	0	0.81	0.14	0.43	5.61	0.21	133	0	0	9
0	9	1.56	88	228	6	1.94	0	0.35	0.57	0.06	5.01	0.58	13	0	0	—
0	8	0.28	28	60	0	0.63	0	0.11	0.10	0.02	2.05	0.34	3	0	0	12
0	36	4.13	159	467	1	3.60	1	0.20	1.65	0.16	2.73	0.28	38	0	0	23
0	14	3.64	39	155	1	0.88	0	0.68	0.22	0.48	5.00	0.09	153	0	0	75
0	88	2.71	183	1070	6	1.67	3	0.25	0.83	0.49	1.84	0.20	147	0	0	3
0	6	0.90	34	128	2	1.77	0	0.27	—	0.07	0.98	0.19	40	0	0	11
0	20	2.33	83	243	3	1.76	0	0.27	0.74	0.13	3.82	0.20	26	0	0	42
0	200	—	—	90	70	—	—	0.23	3.02	0.26	3.00	—	—	9	—	—
0	0	0.72	—	160	25	—	—	0.09	—	0.03	0.40	—	—	1	—	—
0	200	1.80	8	75	110	1.50	—	0.38	0.00	0.43	5.00	0.50	40	0	0	—
0	200	1.80	8	70	110	1.50	—	0.38	0.00	0.43	5.00	0.50	40	0	0	—
0	200	1.80	8	55	110	1.50	—	0.38	0.00	0.43	5.00	0.50	40	0	0	—
0	4	0.73	6	25	270	0.08	0	0.10	0.02	0.07	0.87	0.03	40	0	0	4
0	4	0.73	6	25	270	0.08	2	0.10	0.02	0.07	0.87	0.03	40	0	0	3
0	27	8.60	2	17	1	0.10	0	0.07	0.02	0.04	0.60	0.01	357	0	0	—
0	5	0.58	2	15	383	0.09	0	0.07	—	0.05	0.57	0.01	40	0	0	11
0	9	0.80	28	66	1	0.57	0	0.13	0.12	0.02	0.15	0.02	5	0	0	9
0	26	6.84	50	126	404	1.04	0	1.02	0.42	0.05	1.57	0.31	30	0	0	11
0	21	3.96	45	112	241	0.93	0	0.60	0.22	0.05	0.78	0.19	19	0	0	4
0	300	9.00	200	700	160	3.00	300	0.75	—	0.85	10.00	4.00	800	12	12	6
0	0	13.64	182	909	606	4.55	455	1.14	—	1.29	15.15	6.06	1212	18	18	26
0	0	4.50	8	35	150	1.50	150	0.38	—	0.43	5.00	0.50	100	15	2	2
0	0	10.77	80	253	293	2.00	—	0.50	—	0.57	6.65	0.67	133	0	2	—
0	5	6.00	20	72	269	4.99	3	0.51	0.20	0.57	6.66	0.67	133	0	0	7
<.1	7	6.14	19	71	242	5.12	2	0.51	0.23	0.57	6.66	0.67	133	<.1	0	7
0	100	8.10	40	95	280	3.75	150	0.38	0.21	0.43	5.00	0.50	200	6	2	11
0	100	4.50	8	50	170	3.75	0	0.38	0.14	0.43	5.00	0.50	100	6	2	2
0	53	5.99	11	67	253	2.00	200	0.50	—	0.57	6.65	0.67	133	20	2	6
0	0	23.94	53	226	279	19.95	299	2.00	26.78	2.26	26.60	2.66	532	80	8	4
0	0	8.10	3	25	200	0.17	150	0.38	0.04	0.43	5.00	0.50	100	6	2	1

Table H–1

Food Composition (Computer code number is for Wadsworth Diet Analysis program) (For purposes of calculations, use "0" for t, <1, <.1, <.01, etc.)

DA + Code	Food Description	Quantity	Measure	Wt (g)	H_2O (g)	Ener (kcal)	Prot (g)	Carb (g)	Dietary Fiber (g)	Fat (g)	Fat Breakdown (g) Sat	Mono	Poly
	CEREAL, FLOUR, GRAIN, PASTA, NOODLES, POPCORN—Continued												
1247	Corn Pops	1	cup(s)	31	1	120	1	28	0	0	0.00	0.00	0.00
1937	Cracklin' Oat Bran	1	cup(s)	65	0	266	5	47	7	9	2.70	4.70	1.33
1220	Froot Loops	1	cup(s)	32	1	120	1	28	1	1	0.50	0.00	0.00
38214	Frosted Cheerios	1	cup(s)	30	—	120	2	25	1	1	0.00	0.00	0.00
372	Frosted Flakes	1	cup(s)	41	1	160	1	37	1	0	0.00	0.00	0.00
38215	Frosted Mini Chex	1	cup(s)	40	—	146	1	36	0	0	0.00	0.00	0.00
10268	Frosted Mini-Wheats	5	item(s)	51	3	180	5	41	5	1	0.00	0.00	0.50
38216	Frosted Wheaties	1	cup(s)	40	—	146	1	36	<1	0	0.00	0.00	0.00
1223	Granola, prepared	½	cup(s)	61	0	299	9	32	5	15	2.76	4.7	6.53
13334	Granola, Quaker 100% natural, oats & honey	½	cup(s)	48	0	219	5	31	3	9	3.83	4.0	1.19
13335	Granola, Quaker 100% natural, oats, honey & raisins	½	cup(s)	51	0	225	5	34	3	9	3.57	3.80	1.10
2415	Honey Bunches of Oats honey roasted	1	cup(s)	40	1	160	3	33	1	2	0.67	1.20	0.13
1227	Honey Nut Cheerios	1	cup(s)	30	1	120	3	24	2	2	0.00	0.50	0.00
2424	Honeycomb	1	cup(s)	22	<1	83	2	20	<1	<1	0.00	—	—
10286	Kashi puffed	1	cup(s)	25	—	70	3	13	2	1	0.00	—	—
1231	Kix	1	cup(s)	23	<1	90	2	20	1	<1	0.00	0.00	0.00
30569	Life	1	cup(s)	43	2	160	4	33	3	2	0.35	0.64	0.61
1233	Lucky Charms	1	cup(s)	30	1	120	2	25	1	1	0.00	0.00	0.00
1201	Multi-Bran Chex	1	cup(s)	58	1	200	4	49	7	2	0.00	0.00	0.00
38220	Multi Grain Cheerios	1	cup(s)	30	—	110	3	24	3	1	0.00	0.00	0.00
1238	Nutri-Grain golden wheat	1	cup(s)	40	—	133	4	31	5	1	0.00	0.00	0.67
1241	Product 19	1	cup(s)	30	1	100	2	25	1	0	0.00	0.00	0.00
32432	Puffed rice, fortified	1	cup(s)	14	<1	56	1	13	<1	<.1	0.02	—	—
32433	Puffed wheat, fortified	1	cup(s)	12	0	43.68	1.76	9.55	0.52	0.14	0.02	—	—
2420	Raisin Bran	1	cup(s)	59	5	190	4	47	8	1	0.00	0.10	0.36
1244	Rice Chex	1	cup(s)	25	1	96	2	22	<1	0	0.00	0.00	0.00
1245	Rice Krispies	1	cup(s)	26	1	96	2	23	0	0	0.00	0.00	0.00
5593	Shredded Wheat	1	cup(s)	25	1	88	3	20	3	1	0.04	0.01	0.10
1248	Smacks	1	cup(s)	36	1	133	3	32	1	1	0.00	0.00	0.00
1246	Special K	1	cup(s)	31	1	110	7	22	1	0	0.00	0.00	0.00
3428	Total, corn flakes	1	cup(s)	23	1	83	2	18	1	0	0.00	0.00	0.00
1253	Total whole grain	1	cup(s)	40	1	146	3	31	4	1	0.00	0.00	0.00
1254	Trix	1	cup(s)	30	1	120	1	27	1	1	0.00	0.00	0.00
382	Wheat germ, toasted	2	tablespoon(s)	14	0	53.95	4.11	7	2.13	1.51	0.25	0.21	0.93
1257	Wheaties	1	cup(s)	30	1	110	3	24	3	1	0.00	0.00	0.00
	Pasta, noodles												
449	Chinese chow mein noodles, cooked	½	cup(s)	23	<1	119	2	13	1	7	0.99	1.73	3.90
1995	Corn pasta, cooked	½	cup(s)	70	48	88	2	20	3	1	0.07	0.13	0.23
448	Egg noodles, enriched, cooked	½	cup(s)	80	55	106	4	20	1	1	0.25	0.34	0.33
440	Macaroni, enriched, cooked	½	cup(s)	70	46	99	3	20	1	<1	0.07	0.06	0.19
1996	Pasta, plain, fresh-refrigerated, cooked	½	cup(s)	64	44	84	3	16	0	1	0.10	0.08	0.27
1725	Ramen noodles, cooked	½	cup(s)	114	95	104	3	15	1	4	0.19	0.22	0.21
2878	Soba noodles, cooked	½	cup(s)	95	69	94	5	20	0	<.1	0.02	0.02	0.03
2879	Somen noodles, cooked	½	cup(s)	88	60	115	4	24	0	<1	0.02	0.02	0.06
493	Spaghetti, al dente, cooked	½	cup(s)	65	42	95	4	20	1	1	0.05	0.05	0.15
2884	Spaghetti, whole wheat, cooked	½	cup(s)	70	47	87	4	19	3	<1	0.07	0.05	0.15
1563	Spinach egg noodles, enriched, cooked	½	cup(s)	80	55	105	4	19	2	1	0.29	0.39	0.28
2000	Tricolor vegetable macaroni, enriched, cooked	½	cup(s)	67	46	86	3	18	3	<.1	0.01	0.01	0.03
	Popcorn												
476	Air popped	1	cup(s)	8	<1	31	1	6	1	<1	0.05	0.09	0.15
4619	Caramel	1	cup(s)	35	1	152	1	28	2	5	1.27	1.01	1.58
4620	Cheese flavored	1	cup(s)	37	1	196	3	19	4	12	2.38	3.61	5.72
477	Popped in oil	1	cup(s)	33	1	165	3	19	3	9	1.61	2.70	4.43
	FRUIT AND FRUIT JUICES												
	Apples												
223	Raw medium, w/peel	1	item(s)	138	118	72	<1	19	3	<1	0.04	0.01	0.07
224	Slices	½	cup(s)	55	47	29	<1	8	1	<.1	0.02	0.00	0.03

PAGE KEY: H–2 = Breads/Baked Goods H–6 = Cereal/Rice/Pasta H–10 = Fruit H–16 = Vegetables/Legumes H–26 = Nuts/Seeds H–28 = Vegetarian H–30 = Dairy H–36 = Eggs H–38 = Seafood H–40 = Meats H–42 = Poultry H–44 = Processed meats H–46 = Beverages H–50 = Fats/Oils H–52 = Sweets H–52 = Sauces/Condiments/Spices H–56 = Mixed Foods/Soups/Sandwiches H–62 = Fast food H–80 = Convenience H–82 = Baby foods

Chol (mg)	Calc (mg)	Iron (mg)	Magn (mg)	Pota (mg)	Sodi (mg)	Zinc (mg)	Vit A (RAE) (μg)	Thia (mg)	Vit E (mg)	Ribo (mg)	Niac (mg)	Vit B_6 (mg)	Fola (μg)	Vit C (mg)	Vit B_{12} (μg)	Sele (μg)
0	0	1.80	2	25	120	1.50	150	0.38		0.43	5.00	0.50	100	6	2	2
0	27	2.38	80	293	186	2.00	299	0.49	0.33	0.56	6.65	0.67	218	20	2	14
0	0	4.50	8	35	150	1.50	150	0.38	0.12	0.43	5.00	0.50	100	15	2	2
0	100	4.50	16	55	210	3.75	—	0.38	—	0.43	5.00	0.50	100	6	2	—
0	0	5.99	4	27	200	0.21	200	0.50	0.05	0.57	6.65	0.67	133	8	2	2
0	133	11.97	—	33	266	3.99	—	0.50	—	0.57	6.65	0.67	266	8	2	—
0	0	15.30	60	170	5	1.50	0	0.38	0.46	0.43	5.00	0.50	100	0	2	2
0	133	10.77	0	47	266	9.98	—	1.00	—	1.13	13.30	1.33	532	8	4	—
0	48	2.59	107	328	13	2.5	2	0.44	6.28	0.17	1.29	0.18	51	1	0	16.95
1	61	1.21	51	225	20	1.04	1	0.12	0.4	0.11	0.81	0.07	17	<1	0.1	8.3
1	59	1.24	49	250	19	0.99	<1	0.12	0.37	0.11	0.8	0.07	16	<1	0.1	8.82
0	0	3.59	21	67	253	0.40	—	0.50	0.28	0.57	6.65	0.67	133	0	2	—
0	100	4.50	24	95	270	3.75	—	0.38	0.31	0.43	5.00	0.50	200	6	2	7
0	0	2.03	6	26	165	1.13	—	0.28	0.09	0.32	3.74	0.37	75	0	1	—
0	0	0.72	—	35	0	—	0	0.03	—	0.03	0.80	0.00	—	0	—	—
0	113	6.08	6	26	203	2.81	113	0.28	0.06	0.32	3.75	0.38	150	5	1	5
0	124	11.92	41	121	218	5.32	1	0.53	0.23	0.60	7.10	0.70	142	0	0	11
0	100	4.50	16	60	210	3.75	—	0.38	0.13	0.43	5.00	0.50	200	6	2	6
0	100	16.20	60	220	390	3.75	158	0.38	0.67	0.03	5.00	0.50	100	6	2	5
0	100	18.00	24	85	200	15.00	—	1.50	20.13	1.70	20.00	2.00	400	15	6	—
0	0	1.46	32	146	279	4.99	0	0.50	7.14	0.57	6.65	0.67	133	20	2	9
0	0	18.00	16	50	210	15.00	225	1.50	20.13	1.70	20.00	2.00	400	60	6	4
0	1	4.44	4	16	<1	0.14	0	0.36	—	0.25	4.94	0.01	3	0	0	1
0	3.35	3.8	17.39	41.75	0.47	0.28	0	0.31	—	0.21	4.23	0.02	3.83	0	0	14.77
0	20	10.80	80	340	300	2.25	—	0.53	1.37	0.60	7.00	0.70	140	0	2	—
0	80	7.20	7	28	232	3.00	—	0.30	0.03	0.34	4.00	0.40	160	5	1	1
0	0	1.44	13	32	256	0.48	120	0.30	0.03	0.34	4.80	0.40	80	5	1	4
0	10	1.08	31	92	2	0.70	0	0.07	0.13	0.06	1.77	0.10	12	0	0	1
0	0	0.48	11	53	67	0.40	200	0.50	0.18	0.57	6.65	0.67	133	8	2	17
0	0	8.70	16	60	220	0.90	225	0.53	7.05	0.60	7.00	2.00	400	15	6	7
0	750	13.50	0	23	158	11.25	113	1.13	15.00	1.28	15.00	1.50	300	45	5	1
0	1330	23.94	32	120	253	19.95	200	2.00	26.60	2.26	26.60	2.66	532	80	8	2
0	100	4.50	0	15	190	3.75	150	0.38	0.60	0.43	5.00	0.50	100	6	2	6
0	6.35	1.28	45.2	133.76	0.56	2.35	0	0.23	2.04	0.11	0.78	0.13	49.72	0.84	0	9.18
0	0	8.10	32	110	220	7.50	150	0.75	0.37	0.85	10.00	1.00	200	6	3	1
0	5	1.06	12	27	99	0.32	0	0.13	0.04	0.09	1.34	0.02	20	0	0	10
0	1	0.18	25	22	0	0.44	2	0.04	0.23	0.02	0.39	0.04	4	0	0	2
26	10	1.27	15	22	6	0.49	5	0.15	0.04	0.07	1.19	0.03	51	0	<.1	17
0	5	0.98	13	22	1	0.37	0	0.14	0.09	0.07	1.17	0.02	54	0	0	15
21	4	0.73	12	15	4	0.36	4	0.13	—	0.10	0.63	0.02	41	0	<.1	—
18	9	0.89	9	34	415	0.31	—	0.08	0.11	0.05	0.71	0.03	4	<.1	<.1	—
0	4	0.45	9	33	57	0.11	0	0.09	—	0.02	0.48	0.04	7	0	0	—
0	7	0.46	2	25	141	0.19	0	0.02	—	0.03	0.09	0.01	2	0	0	—
0	7	1.00	12	52	1	0.35	0	0.12	0.04	0.07	0.90	0.04	8	0	0	40
0	11	0.74	21	31	2	0.57	0	0.08	0.04	0.03	0.49	0.06	4	0	0	18
26	15	0.87	19	30	10	0.50	4	0.20	0.04	0.10	1.18	0.09	51	0	<1	17
0	7	0.33	13	21	4	0.29	3	0.08	0.03	0.04	0.72	0.02	44	0	0	13
0	1	0.22	11	24	<1	0.28	1	0.02	0.01	0.02	0.16	0.02	2	0	0	1
2	15	0.61	12	38	73	0.20	1	0.02	0.42	0.02	0.77	0.01	2	0	<.1	1
4	42	0.83	34	97	331	0.75	14	0.05	0.04	0.09	0.54	0.09	4	<1	<1	4
0	3	0.92	36	74	292	0.87	3	0.04	0.04	0.04	0.51	0.07	6	<.1	0	2
0	8	0.17	7	148	1	0.06	4	0.02	0.44	0.04	0.13	0.06	4	6	0	0
0	3	0.07	3	59	1	0.02	2	0.01	0.18	0.01	0.05	0.02	2	3	0	0

Table H–1

Food Composition (Computer code number is for Wadsworth Diet Analysis program) (For purposes of calculations, use "0" for t, <1, <.1, <.01, etc.)

DA + Code	Food Description	Quantity	Measure	Wt (g)	H_2O (g)	Ener (kcal)	Prot (g)	Carb (g)	Dietary Fiber (g)	Fat (g)	Fat Breakdown (g) Sat	Mono	Poly
	FRUIT AND FRUIT JUICES—Continued												
946	Slices w/o skin, boiled	½	cup(s)	85	73	45	<1	12	2	<1	0.05	0.01	0.09
948	Dried, sulfured	½	cup(s)	22	7	52	<1	14	2	<.1	0.01	0.00	0.02
952	Juice, from frozen concentrate	½	cup(s)	120	105	56	<1	14	<1	<1	0.02	0.00	0.04
225	Juice, unsweetened, canned	½	cup(s)	124	109	58	<.1	14	<1	<1	0.02	0.01	0.04
226	Applesauce, sweetened, canned	½	cup(s)	128	101	97	<1	25	2	<1	0.04	0.01	0.07
227	Applesauce, unsweetened, canned	½	cup(s)	122	108	52	<1	14	1	<.1	0.01	0.00	0.02
38492	Crabapples	1	item(s)	35	28	27	<1	7	1	<1	0.02	0.00	0.03
	Apricot												
228	Fresh w/o pits	4	item(s)	140	121	67	2	16	3	1	0.04	0.24	0.11
230	Halves, dried, sulfured	¼	cup(s)	33	10	79	1	21	2	<1	0.01	0.02	0.02
229	Halves w/skin, canned in heavy syrup	½	cup(s)	129	100	107	1	28	2	<1	0.01	0.04	0.02
	Avocado												
233	California, whole, w/o skin or pit	1	item(s)	170	<1	284	3	15	12	26	3.59	16.61	3.42
234	Florida, whole, w/o skin or pit	1	item(s)	304	<1	365	7	24	17	31	5.90	16.70	5.00
2998	Pureed	⅛	cup(s)	29	21	46	1	2	2	4	0.61	2.82	0.52
	Banana												
235	Fresh whole, w/o peel	1	item(s)	118	88	105	1	27	3	<1	0.13	0.04	0.09
4580	Dried chips	¼	cup(s)	55	2	287	1	32	4	19	16.00	1.08	0.35
	Blackberries												
237	Raw	½	cup(s)	72	63	31	1	7	4	<1	0.01	0.03	0.20
958	Unsweetened, frozen	½	cup(s)	76	62	48	1	12	4	<1	0.01	0.03	0.18
	Blueberries												
238	Raw	½	cup(s)	72	61	41	1	10	2	<1	0.02	0.03	0.11
959	Canned in heavy syrup	½	cup(s)	128	98	113	1	28	2	<1	0.03	0.06	0.18
960	Unsweetened, frozen	½	cup(s)	78	67	40	1	10	2	1	0.04	0.07	0.22
	Boysenberries												
961	Canned in heavy syrup	½	cup(s)	128	98	113	1	29	3	<1	0.01	0.02	0.09
962	Unsweetened, frozen	½	cup(s)	66	57	33	1	8	3	<1	0.01	0.02	0.10
35576	**Breadfruit**	1	item(s)	384	271	396	4	104	17	1	0.00	0.00	0.00
	Cherries												
3000	Sour red, raw	½	cup(s)	78	67	39	1	9	1	<1	0.05	0.06	0.07
967	Sour red, canned in water	½	cup(s)	122	110	44	1	11	1	<1	0.03	0.03	0.04
240	Sweet, raw	½	cup(s)	73	60	46	1	12	2	<1	0.03	0.03	0.04
3004	Sweet, canned in heavy syrup	½	cup(s)	127	98	105	1	27	2	<1	0.04	0.05	0.06
969	Sweet, canned in water	½	cup(s)	124	108	57	1	15	2	<1	0.03	0.04	0.05
	Cranberries												
3007	Chopped, raw	½	cup(s)	55	48	25	<1	7	3	<.1	0.01	0.01	0.03
1638	Cranberry juice cocktail	½	cup(s)	127	108	72	0	18	<1	<1	0.01	0.02	0.06
241	Cranberry juice cocktail, low calorie, w/saccharin	½	cup(s)	127	120	24	<.1	6	0	<.1	0.00	0.00	0.00
1717	Cranberry apple juice drink	½	cup(s)	123	100	87	<.1	22	<1	<.1	0.00	0.00	0.00
242	Cranberry sauce, sweetened, canned	¼	cup(s)	69	42	105	<1	27	1	<1	0.01	0.01	0.05
	Dates												
244	Domestic, chopped	¼	cup(s)	44.5	0	126	1	33	4	<1	0.01	0.01	0
243	Domestic, whole	¼	cup(s)	44.5	0	126	1	33	4	<1	0.01	0.01	0
	Figs												
973	Raw, medium	2	item(s)	101	80	74	1	19	3	<1	0.06	0.07	0.14
975	Canned in heavy syrup	½	cup(s)	130	99	114	<1	30	3	<1	0.03	0.03	0.06
974	Canned in water	½	cup(s)	124	106	66	<1	17	3	<1	0.02	0.03	0.06
	Fruit cocktail & salad												
245	Fruit cocktail, canned in heavy syrup	½	cup(s)	124	100	91	<1	23	1	<.1	0.01	0.02	0.04
978	Fruit cocktail, canned in juice	½	cup(s)	119	104	55	1	14	1	<.1	0.00	0.00	0.00
977	Fruit cocktail, canned in water	½	cup(s)	119	108	38	<1	10	1	<.1	0.01	0.01	0.02
979	Fruit salad, canned in water	½	cup(s)	123	112	37	<1	10	1	<.1	0.01	0.02	0.03
	Gooseberries												
981	Raw	½	cup(s)	75	66	33	1	8	3	<1	0.03	0.04	0.24
982	Canned in light syrup	½	cup(s)	126	101	92	1	24	3	<1	0.02	0.02	0.14
	Grapefruit												
3022	Raw, pink or red	½	cup(s)	115	<.1	48	1	12	2	<1	0.02	0.02	0.04
247	Raw, white	½	item(s)	118	107	39	1	10	1	<1	0.02	0.02	0.03
251	Juice, pink, sweetened, canned	½	cup(s)	125	109	58	1	14	<1	<1	0.02	0.02	0.03

Appendix H

PAGE KEY: H–2 = Breads/Baked Goods H–6 = Cereal/Rice/Pasta H–10 = Fruit H–16 = Vegetables/Legumes H–26 = Nuts/Seeds H–28 = Vegetarian H–30 = Dairy H–36 = Eggs H–38 = Seafood H–40 = Meats H–42 = Poultry H–44 = Processed meats H–46 = Beverages H–50 = Fats/Oils H–52 = Sweets H–52 = Sauces/Condiments/Spices H–56 = Mixed Foods/Soups/Sandwiches H–62 = Fast food H–80 = Convenience H–82 = Baby foods

Chol (mg)	Calc (mg)	Iron (mg)	Magn (mg)	Pota (mg)	Sodi (mg)	Zinc (mg)	Vit A (RAE) (µg)	Thia (mg)	Vit E (mg)	Ribo (mg)	Niac (mg)	Vit B_6 (mg)	Fola (µg)	Vit C (mg)	Vit B_{12} (µg)	Sele (µg)
0	4	0.16	3	75	1	0.03	2	0.01	0.01	0.01	0.08	0.04	1	<1	0	<1
0	3	0.30	3	97	19	0.04	0	0.00	0.12	0.03	0.20	0.03	0	1	0	<1
0	7	0.31	6	151	8	0.05	0	0.00	0.01	0.02	0.05	0.04	0	1	0	<1
0	9	0.46	4	148	4	0.04	0	0.03	0.01	0.02	0.12	0.04	0	1	0	<1
0	5	0.45	4	78	4	0.05	1	0.02	0.01	0.04	0.24	0.03	1	2	0	<1
0	4	0.15	4	92	2	0.04	1	0.02	0.01	0.03	0.23	0.03	1	1	0	<1
0	6	0.13	2	68	<1	—	0	0.01	0.21	0.01	0.04	—	2	3	0	—
0	18	0.55	14	363	1	0.28	134	0.04	1.25	0.06	0.84	0.08	13	14	0	<1
0	18	0.88	11	383	3	0.13	59	0.00	1.44	0.02	0.85	0.05	3	<1	0	1
0	12	0.39	9	181	5	0.14	80	0.03	1.15	0.03	0.49	0.07	3	4	0	<1
0	22	1.00	49	861	14	1.12	104	0.12	1.77	0.24	3.24	0.47	105	15	0	1
0	30	0.50	73	1067	6	1.20	185	0.00	—	0.10	2.00	0.20	106	53	0	0
0	3	0.16	8	139	2	0.18	2	0.02	0.39	0.04	0.50	0.07	17	3	0	<1
0	6	0.31	32	422	1	0.18	4	0.04	0.32	0.09	0.78	0.43	24	10	0	1
0	10	0.69	42	296	3	0.41	2	0.05	2.98	0.01	0.39	0.14	8	3	0	1
0	21	0.45	14	117	1	0.38	8	0.01	0.51	0.02	0.47	0.02	18	15	0	<1
0	22	0.60	17	106	1	0.19	5	0.02	0.54	0.03	0.91	0.05	26	2	0	<1
0	4	0.20	4	55	1	0.12	2	0.03	0.72	0.03	0.30	0.04	4	7	0	<.1
0	6	0.42	5	51	4	0.09	3	0.04	1.28	0.07	0.14	0.05	3	1	0	<1
0	6	0.14	4	42	1	0.06	2	0.03	0.78	0.03	0.41	0.05	6	2	0	0
0	23	0.55	14	115	4	0.24	3	0.03	0.91	0.04	0.29	0.05	44	8	0	1
0	18	0.56	11	92	1	0.15	2	0.03	0.30	0.02	0.51	0.04	42	2	0	<1
0	65	2.07	96	1882	8	0.46	8	0.42	4.30	0.12	3.46	0.00	54	111	0	2
0	12	0.25	7	134	2	0.08	50	0.02	0.10	0.03	0.31	0.03	6	8	0	0
0	13	1.67	7	120	9	0.09	46	0.02	0.16	0.05	0.22	0.05	10	3	0	0
0	9	0.26	8	161	0	0.05	2	0.02	0.09	0.02	0.11	0.04	3	5	0	0
0	11	0.44	11	183	4	0.13	10	0.03	0.08	0.05	0.50	0.04	5	5	0	0
0	14	0.45	11	162	1	0.10	10	0.03	0.16	0.05	0.51	0.04	5	3	0	0
0	4	0.14	3	47	1	0.06	2	0.01	0.06	0.01	0.06	0.03	1	7	0	<.1
0	4	0.19	3	23	3	0.09	0	0.01	0.00	0.01	0.04	0.02	0	45	0	0
0	11	0.05	3	32	4	0.03	0	0.00	0.00	0.00	0.01	0.00	0	41	0	0
0	6	0.15	2	34	9	0.22	0	0.01	0.00	0.02	0.07	0.03	0	39	0	0
0	3	0.15	2	18	20	0.03	1	0.01	0.07	0.01	0.07	0.01	1	1	0	<1
0	17	0.45	19	292	1	0.12	1	0.02	0.03	0.02	0.56	0.07	9	<1	0	1
0	17	0.45	19	292	1	0.12	1	0.02	0.03	0.02	0.56	0.07	9	<1	0	1
0	35	0.37	17	233	1	0.15	7	0.06	0.89	0.05	0.40	0.11	6	2	0	<1
0	35	0.36	13	128	1	0.14	3	0.03	1.15	0.05	0.55	0.09	3	1	0	<1
0	35	0.36	12	128	1	0.15	2	0.03	1.10	0.05	0.55	0.09	2	1	0	<1
0	7	0.36	6	109	7	0.10	12	0.02	0.36	0.02	0.46	0.06	4	2	0	1
0	9	0.25	8	113	5	0.11	18	0.01	0.24	0.02	0.48	0.06	4	3	0	1
0	6	0.30	8	111	5	0.11	15	0.02	0.34	0.01	0.43	0.06	4	2	0	1
0	9	0.37	6	96	4	0.10	27	0.02	—	0.03	0.46	0.04	4	2	0	1
0	19	0.23	8	149	1	0.09	11	0.03	0.28	0.02	0.23	0.06	5	21	0	<1
0	20	0.42	8	97	3	0.14	9	0.03	0.47	0.07	0.19	0.02	4	13	0	1
0	25	0.09	10	155	0	0.08	30	0.05	—	0.03	0.23	0.06	15	36	0	<1
0	14	0.07	11	175	0	0.08	2	0.04	0.30	0.02	0.32	0.05	12	39	0	2
0	10	0.45	13	203	3	0.08	0	0.05	0.06	0.03	0.40	0.03	13	34	0	<1

Table H–1

Food Composition (Computer code number is for Wadsworth Diet Analysis program) (For purposes of calculations, use "0" for t, <1, <.1, <.01, etc.)

DA + Code	Food Description	Quantity	Measure	Wt (g)	H_2O (g)	Ener (kcal)	Prot (g)	Carb (g)	Dietary Fiber (g)	Fat (g)	Fat Breakdown (g) Sat	Mono	Poly
	FRUIT AND FRUIT JUICES—Continued												
249	Juice, white	½	cup(s)	124	111	48	1	11	<1	<1	0.02	0.02	0.03
248	Sections, canned in light syrup	½	cup(s)	127	106	76	1	20	1	<1	0.02	0.02	0.03
983	Sections, canned in water	½	cup(s)	122	<.1	44	1	11	<1	<1	0.02	0.02	0.03
	Grapes												
255	American, slip skin	½	cup(s)	46	37	31	<1	8	<1	<1	0.05	0.01	0.05
256	European, red or green, adherent skin	½	cup(s)	80	<.1	55	1	14	1	<1	0.04	0.01	0.04
259	Juice, sweetened, added vitamin C, from frozen concentrate	½	cup(s)	125	109	64	<1	16	<1	<1	0.04	0.01	0.03
3159	Juice drink, canned	½	cup(s)	125	109	63	<1	16	0	0	0.00	0.00	0.00
3060	Raisins, seeded, packed	¼	cup(s)	41	7	122	1	32	3	<1	0.07	0.01	0.07
987	**Guava, raw**	1	item(s)	90	77	46	1	11	5	1	0.15	0.05	0.23
35593	**Guava, strawberry**	1	item(s)	6	5	4	<.1	1	<1	<.1	0.01	0.00	0.02
3027	**Jackfruit**	½	cup(s)	83	61	78	1	20	1	<1	0.05	0.04	0.07
8458	**Kiwi fruit**	1	item(s)	77	63	53	1	11	3	1	0.02	0.03	0.19
	Lemon												
992	Raw	1	item(s)	108	94	22	1	12	5	<1	0.04	0.01	0.10
262	Juice	1	tablespoon(s)	15	14	4	<.1	1	<.1	0	0.00	0.00	0.00
993	Peel	1	teaspoon(s)	2	2	1	<.1	<1	<1	<.1	0.00	0.00	0.00
	Lime												
994	Raw	1	item(s)	67	61	15	<1	6	2	<.1	0.01	0.01	0.02
269	Juice	1	tablespoon(s)	15	14	4	<.1	1	<.1	<.1	0.00	0.00	0.00
995	**Loganberries, frozen**	½	cup(s)	74	62	40	1	10	4	<1	0.01	0.02	0.13
	Mandarin orange												
1038	Canned in juice	½	cup(s)	125	111	46	1	12	1	<.1	0.00	0.01	0.01
1039	Canned in light syrup	½	cup(s)	126	105	77	1	20	1	<1	0.02	0.02	0.03
999	**Mango**	½	item(s)	104	85	67	1	18	2	<1	0.07	0.10	0.05
1005	**Nectarine, raw, sliced**	½	cup(s)	69	60	30	1	7	1	<1	0.02	0.06	0.08
	Melons												
271	Cantaloupe	½	cup(s)	80	72	27	1	7	1	<1	0.04	0.00	0.07
1000	Casaba melon	½	cup(s)	85	78	24	1	6	1	<.1	0.02	0.00	0.03
272	Honeydew	½	cup(s)	89	80	32	<1	8	1	<1	0.03	0.00	0.05
318	Watermelon	½	cup(s)	77	71	23	<1	6	<1	<1	0.01	0.03	0.04
	Orange												
273	Raw	1	item(s)	131	114	62	1	15	3	<1	0.02	0.03	0.03
3040	Peel	1	teaspoon(s)	2	1	2	<.1	1	<1	<.1	0.00	0.00	0.00
274	Sections	½	cup(s)	90	78	43	1	11	2	<1	0.01	0.02	0.02
275	Juice	½	cup(s)	124	109	56	1	13	<1	<1	0.03	0.04	0.05
29630	Juice, fresh squeezed	½	cup(s)	124	109	56	1	13	<1	<1	0.03	0.04	0.05
14414	Juice w/calcium & extra vitamin C	½	cup(s)	125	55	1	13	<1	0	0.00	0.00	0.00	0
278	Juice, unsweetened, from frozen concentrate	½	cup(s)	125	110	56	1	13	<1	<.1	0.01	0.01	0.01
	Papaya												
282	Raw	½	cup(s)	70	62	27	<1	7	1	<.1	0.03	0.03	0.02
16830	Dried, strips	2	item(s)	46	12	119	2	30	5	<1	0.13	0.12	0.09
35640	**Passion fruit, purple**	1	item(s)	18	13	17	<1	4	3	<1	0.00	0.00	0.00
	Peach												
283	Raw, medium	1	item(s)	98	87	38	1	9	1	<1	0.02	0.07	0.08
285	Halves, canned in heavy syrup	½	cup(s)	131	104	97	1	26	2	<1	0.01	0.05	0.06
286	Halves, canned in water	½	cup(s)	122	114	29	1	7	2	<.1	0.01	0.03	0.03
290	Slices, sweetened, frozen	½	cup(s)	125	93	118	1	30	2	<1	0.02	0.06	0.08
	Pear												
291	Raw	1	item(s)	166	139	96	1	26	5	<1	0.01	0.04	0.05
8672	Asian	1	item(s)	122	108	51	1	13	4	<1	0.01	0.06	0.07
293	Danjou	1	item(s)	200	168	120	1	30	5	1	0.00	0.20	0.20
294	Halves, canned in heavy syrup	½	cup(s)	133	107	98	<1	25	2	<1	0.01	0.04	0.04
1012	Halves, canned in juice	½	cup(s)	124	107	62	<1	16	2	<.1	0.00	0.02	0.02
1017	**Persimmon**	1	item(s)	25	16	32	<1	8	0	<1	0.01	0.02	0.02
	Pineapple												
295	Raw, diced	½	cup(s)	78	67	37	<1	10	1	<.1	0.01	0.01	0.03
3053	Canned in extra heavy syrup	½	cup(s)	130	101	108	<1	28	1	<1	0.01	0.02	0.05
1019	Canned in juice	½	cup(s)	125	104	75	1	20	1	<.1	0.01	0.01	0.04

Appendix H

PAGE KEY: H–2 = Breads/Baked Goods H–6 = Cereal/Rice/Pasta H–10 = Fruit H–16 = Vegetables/Legumes H–26 = Nuts/Seeds H–28 = Vegetarian H–30 = Dairy H–36 = Eggs H–38 = Seafood H–40 = Meats H–42 = Poultry H–44 = Processed meats H–46 = Beverages H–50 = Fats/Oils H–52 = Sweets H–52 = Sauces/Condiments/Spices H–56 = Mixed Foods/Soups/Sandwiches H–62 = Fast food H–80 = Convenience H–82 = Baby foods

Chol (mg)	Calc (mg)	Iron (mg)	Magn (mg)	Pota (mg)	Sodi (mg)	Zinc (mg)	Vit A (RAE) (µg)	Thia (mg)	Vit E (mg)	Ribo (mg)	Niac (mg)	Vit B_6 (mg)	Fola (µg)	Vit C (mg)	Vit B_{12} (µg)	Sele (µg)
0	11	0.25	15	200	1	0.06	2	0.05	0.06	0.02	0.25	0.05	12	47	0	<1
0	18	0.51	13	164	3	0.10	0	0.05	0.32	0.03	0.31	0.03	11	27	0	1
0	18	0.50	12	161	2	0.11	0	0.05	0.31	0.03	0.30	0.02	11	27	0	1
0	6	0.13	2	88	1	0.02	2	0.04	0.16	0.03	0.14	0.05	2	2	0	<.1
0	8	0.29	6	153	2	0.06	6	0.06	0.45	0.06	0.15	0.07	2	9	0	<.1
0	5	0.13	5	26	3	0.05	0	0.02	0.06	0.03	0.16	0.05	1	30	0	<1
0	4	0.13	4	41	1	0.03	0	0.01	0.00	0.02	0.09	0.02	1	20	0	<1
0	12	1.07	12	340	12	0.07	0	0.05	0.29	0.08	0.46	0.08	1	2	0	<1
0	18	0.28	9	256	3	0.21	28	0.05	1.01	0.05	1.08	0.13	13	165	0	1
0	1	0.01	1	18	2	—	—	0.00	—	0.00	0.04	0.00	—	2	0	—
0	28	0.50	31	251	2	0.35	12	0.02	0.12	0.09	0.33	0.09	12	6	0	<1
0	30	0.38	14	251	2	0.10	4	—	1.17	0.02	0.25	0.05	<.1	74	0	—
0	66	0.76	13	157	3	0.11	2	0.05	—	0.04	0.22	0.12	—	83	0	1
0	1	0.00	1	19	<1	0.01	<1	0.00	0.01	0.00	0.02	0.01	2	7	0	<.1
0	3	0.02	<1	3	<1	0.01	<.1	0.00	0.00	0.00	0.01	0.00	<1	3	0	<.1
0	9	0.06	5	78	1	0.05	1	0.02	0.16	0.01	0.10	0.03	7	20	0	<.1
0	1	0.00	1	17	<1	0.01	<1	0.00	0.01	0.00	0.02	0.01	1	5	0	<.1
0	19	0.47	15	107	1	0.25	1	0.04	1.62	0.02	0.62	0.05	19	11	0	<1
0	14	0.34	14	166	6	0.63	54	0.10	0.62	0.04	0.55	0.05	6	43	0	<1
0	9	0.47	10	98	8	0.30	53	0.07	0.43	0.06	0.56	0.05	6	25	0	1
0	10	0.13	9	161	2	0.04	39	0.06	1.16	0.06	0.60	0.14	14	29	0	1
0	4	0.19	6	139	0	0.12	12	0.02	0.61	0.02	0.78	0.02	3	4	0	0
0	7	0.17	10	215	13	0.14	136	0.03	0.12	0.02	0.59	0.06	17	30	0	<1
0	9	0.29	9	155	8	0.06	0	0.01	0.13	0.03	0.20	0.14	7	19	0	<1
0	5	0.15	9	203	16	0.08	3	0.03	0.13	0.01	0.37	0.08	17	16	0	1
0	5	0.19	8	86	1	0.08	22	0.03	0.12	0.02	0.14	0.03	2	6	0	<1
0	52	0.13	13	237	0	0.09	14	0.11	0.31	0.05	0.37	0.08	39	70	0	1
0	3	0.02	<1	4	<.1	0.01	<1	0.00	0.00	0.00	0.02	0.00	1	3	0	<.1
0	36	0.09	9	164	0	0.06	10	0.08	0.22	0.04	0.26	0.05	27	48	0	<1
0	14	0.25	14	248	1	0.06	12	0.11	0.11	0.04	0.50	0.05	37	62	0	<1
0	14	0.25	14	248	1	0.06	—	0.11	0.11	0.04	0.50	0.05	38	62	0	—
—	175	—	—	225	0	—	5	0.08	—	—	0.40	0.06	30	54	0	—
0	11	0.12	12	237	1	0.06	6	0.10	0.24	0.02	0.25	0.05	55	48	0	<1
0	17	0.07	7	180	2	0.05	39	0.02	0.78	0.02	0.24	0.01	27	43	0	<1
0	73	0.30	30	783	9	0.21	—	0.06	3.41	0.09	0.93	0.05	58	38	0	—
0	2	0.29	5	63	5	—	—	0.00	0.20	0.02	0.27	—	3	5	0	<1
0	6	0.25	9	186	0	0.17	16	0.02	0.69	0.03	0.79	0.02	4	6	0	<.1
0	4	0.35	7	121	8	0.12	22	0.01	1.17	0.03	0.80	0.02	4	4	0	<1
0	2	0.39	6	121	4	0.11	33	0.01	1.09	0.02	0.64	0.02	4	4	0	<1
0	4	0.46	6	163	8	0.06	18	0.02	1.11	0.04	0.82	0.02	4	118	0	1
0	15	0.28	12	198	2	0.17	2	0.02	0.83	0.04	0.26	0.05	12	7	0	<1
0	5	0.00	10	148	0	0.02	0	0.01	0.61	0.01	0.27	0.03	10	5	0	<1
0	22	0.50	12	250	0	0.24	—	0.04	—	0.08	0.20	0.04	15	8	0	1
0	7	0.29	5	86	7	0.11	0	0.01	0.67	0.03	0.32	0.02	1	1	0	0
0	11	0.36	9	119	5	0.11	0	0.01	0.62	0.01	0.25	0.02	1	2	0	0
0	7	0.63	—	78	<1	—	—	—	—	—	—	—	—	17	0	0
0	10	0.22	9	89	1	0.08	2	0.06	0.08	0.02	0.38	0.09	12	28	0	<.1
0	18	0.49	20	133	1	0.14	1	0.12	—	0.03	0.37	0.10	7	9	0	—
0	17	0.35	17	152	1	0.12	2	0.12	0.12	0.02	0.35	0.09	6	12	0	<1

Table H-1

Food Composition (Computer code number is for Wadsworth Diet Analysis program) (For purposes of calculations, use "0" for t, <1, <.1, <.01, etc.)

DA + Code	Food Description	Quantity	Measure	Wt (g)	H_2O (g)	Ener (kcal)	Prot (g)	Carb (g)	Dietary Fiber (g)	Fat (g)	Fat Breakdown (g) Sat	Mono	Poly
	FRUIT AND FRUIT JUICES—Continued												
296	Canned in light syrup	½	cup(s)	126	108	66	<1	17	1	<1	0.01	0.02	0.05
1018	Canned in water	½	cup(s)	123	112	39	1	10	1	<1	0.01	0.01	0.04
299	Juice, unsweetened, canned	½	cup(s)	125	107	70	<1	17	<1	<1	0.01	0.01	0.04
1024	**Plantain, cooked**	½	cup(s)	77	52	89	1	24	2	<1	0.05	0.01	0.03
300	**Plum, raw, large**	1	item(s)	83	72	38	1	9	1	<1	0.01	0.11	0.04
1027	**Pomegranate**	1	item(s)	154	125	105	1	26	1	<1	0.06	0.07	0.10
	Prunes												
5644	Dried	2	item(s)	17	5	40	<1	11	1	<.1	0.01	0.06	0.02
305	Dried, stewed	½	cup(s)	119	<.1	128	1	33	4	<1	0.00	0.15	0.04
306	Juice, canned	1	cup(s)	256	208	182	2	45	3	<.1	0.01	0.05	0.02
	Raisins, *see* grapes												
	Raspberries												
309	Raw	½	cup(s)	62	53	32	1	7	4	<1	0.01	0.04	0.23
310	Red, sweetened, frozen	½	cup(s)	125	91	129	1	33	6	<1	0.01	0.02	0.11
311	**Rhubarb, cooked with sugar**	½	cup(s)	120	82	140	1	38	3	<.1	0.00	0.00	0.05
	Strawberries												
313	Raw	½	cup(s)	72	65	23	<1	6	1	<1	0.01	0.03	0.11
315	Sweetened, frozen, thawed	½	cup(s)	128	100	99	1	27	2	<1	0.01	0.02	0.09
16828	**Tangelo**	1	item(s)	95	82	45	1	11	2	<1	0.01	0.02	0.02
	Tangerine												
316	Raw	1	item(s)	84	74	37	1	9	2	<1	0.02	0.03	0.03
1040	Juice	½	cup(s)	124	110	53	1	12	<1	<1	0.03	0.04	0.05
	VEGETABLES, LEGUMES												
	Amaranth												
1042	Leaves, raw	1	cup(s)	28	26	6	1	1	0	<.1	0.03	0.02	0.04
1043	Leaves, boiled, drained	½	cup(s)	66	60	14	1	3	0	<1	0.03	0.03	0.05
8683	**Arugula leaves, raw**	1	cup(s)	20	18	5	1	1	<1	<1	0.02	0.01	0.06
	Artichoke												
1044	Boiled, drained	1	item(s)	120	101	60	4	13	6	<1	0.04	0.01	0.08
2885	Hearts, boiled, drained	½	cup(s)	84	71	42	3	9	5	<1	0.03	0.00	0.06
	Asparagus												
566	Boiled, drained	½	cup(s)	90	0.08	20	2	4	2	0.19	0.06	0	0.12
568	Canned, drained	½	cup(s)	121	114	23	3	3	2	1	0.18	0.03	0.34
565	Tips, frozen, boiled, drained	½	cup(s)	90	82	25	3	4	1	<1	0.09	0.01	0.17
	Bamboo shoots												
1048	Boiled, drained	½	cup(s)	60	58	7	1	1	1	<1	0.03	0.00	0.06
1049	Canned, drained	½	cup(s)	65	62	12	1	2	1	<1	0.06	0.01	0.12
	Beans												
1801	Adzuki beans, boiled	½	cup(s)	115	76	147	9	28	8	<1	0.04	—	—
511	Baked beans w/franks, canned	½	cup(s)	129	89	182	9	20	9	8	3.02	3.64	1.07
512	Baked beans w/pork in tomato sauce, canned	½	cup(s)	127	92	124	7	25	6	1	0.50	0.56	0.17
513	Baked beans w/pork in sweet sauce, canned	½	cup(s)	127	89	140	7	27	7	2	0.71	0.80	0.24
1805	Black beans, boiled	½	cup(s)	86	57	114	8	20	7	<1	0.12	0.04	0.20
14597	Chickpeas, garbanzo beans, or bengal gram, boiled	½	cup(s)	82	49	134	7	22	6	2	0.22	0.48	0.95
569	Fordhook lima beans, frozen, boiled, drained	½	cup(s)	85	62	88	5	16	5	<1	0.07	0.02	0.14
1806	French beans, boiled	½	cup(s)	89	59	114	6	21	8	1	0.07	0.05	0.40
2773	Great northern beans, boiled	½	cup(s)	89	61	104	7	19	6	<1	0.12	0.02	0.17
2736	Hyacinth beans, boiled, drained	½	cup(s)	44	38	22	1	4	0	<1	0.05	0.06	0.00
515	Lima beans, boiled, drained	½	cup(s)	85	57	105	6	20	5	<1	0.06	0.02	0.13
570	Lima beans, baby, frozen, boiled, drained	½	cup(s)	90	65	95	6	18	5	<1	0.06	0.02	0.13
579	Mung beans, sprouted, boiled, drained	½	cup(s)	62	<.1	13	1	3	<1	<.1	0.02	0.00	0.02
510	Navy beans, boiled	½	cup(s)	91	57	129	8	24	6	1	0.13	0.05	0.22
32816	Pinto beans, boiled, drained, no salt added	½	cup(s)	114	106	25	2	5	0	<1	0.04	0.03	0.21
1052	Pinto beans, frozen, boiled, drained	½	cup(s)	47	27	76	4	15	4	<1	0.03	0.02	0.13
514	Red kidney beans, canned	½	cup(s)	128	99	109	7	20	8	<1	0.06	0.03	0.24

PAGE KEY: H–2 = Breads/Baked Goods H–6 = Cereal/Rice/Pasta **H–10 = Fruit** **H–16 = Vegetables/Legumes** H–26 = Nuts/Seeds H–28 = Vegetarian H–30 = Dairy H–36 = Eggs H–38 = Seafood H–40 = Meats H–42 = Poultry H–44 = Processed meats H–46 = Beverages H–50 = Fats/Oils H–52 = Sweets H–52 = Sauces/Condiments/Spices H–56 = Mixed Foods/Soups/Sandwiches H–62 = Fast food H–80 = Convenience H–82 = Baby foods

Chol (mg)	Calc (mg)	Iron (mg)	Magn (mg)	Pota (mg)	Sodi (mg)	Zinc (mg)	Vit A (RAE) (μg)	Thia (mg)	Vit E (mg)	Ribo (mg)	Niac (mg)	Vit B_6 (mg)	Fola (μg)	Vit C (mg)	Vit B_{12} (μg)	Sele (μg)
0	18	0.49	20	132	1	0.15	3	0.11	0.13	0.03	0.37	0.09	6	9	0	1
0	18	0.49	22	156	1	0.15	2	0.11	0.12	0.03	0.37	0.09	6	9	0	<1
0	21	0.33	16	168	1	0.14	0	0.07	0.03	0.03	0.32	0.12	29	13	0	<1
0	2	0.45	25	358	4	0.10	35	0.04	0.11	0.04	0.58	0.18	20	8	0	1
0	5	0.14	6	130	0	0.08	14	0.02	0.50	0.02	0.34	0.02	4	8	0	0
0	5	0.46	5	399	5	0.18	8	0.05	0.85	0.05	0.46	0.16	9	9	0	1
0	9	0.42	8	125	1	0.09	17	0.01	0.00	0.03	0.33	0.04	1	1	0	<1
0	23	0.46	21	383	1	0.19	37	0.00	0.00	0.12	0.85	0.23	0	3	0	<1
0	31	3.02	36	707	10	0.54	0	0.04	0.03	0.18	2.01	0.56	0	10	0	2
0	15	0.42	14	93	1	0.26	1	0.02	0.28	0.02	0.37	0.03	13	16	0	<1
0	19	0.81	16	143	1	0.23	4	0.02	0.56	0.06	0.29	0.04	33	21	0	<1
0	174	0.25	16	115	1	—	—	0.02	—	0.03	0.25	—	—	4	0	—
0	12	0.30	9	110	1	0.10	1	0.02	0.10	0.02	0.28	0.03	17	42	0	<1
0	14	0.60	8	125	1	0.06	1	0.02	0.34	0.10	0.37	0.04	5	50	0	1
0	38	0.10	10	172	0	0.07	—	0.08	0.23	0.04	0.27	0.06	29	51	0	—
0	12	0.08	10	132	1	0.20	29	0.09	0.20	0.02	0.13	0.06	17	26	0	<1
0	22	0.25	10	220	1	0.04	16	0.07	0.11	0.02	0.12	0.05	6	38	0	<1
0	60	0.65	15	171	6	0.25	0	0.01	0.00	0.04	0.18	0.05	24	12	0	<1
0	138	1.49	36	423	14	0.58	92	0.01	—	0.09	0.37	0.12	38	27	0	1
0	32	0.29	9	74	5	0.09	24	0.01	0.09	0.02	0.06	0.01	19	3	0	<.1
0	54	1.55	72	425	114	0.59	11	0.08	0.23	0.08	1.20	0.13	61	12	0	<1
0	38	1.08	50	297	80	0.41	8	0.05	0.16	0.06	0.84	0.09	43	8	0	<1
0	20.7	0.81	12.6	201.6	12.6	0.54	48.59	0.14	0.27	0.12	0.97	0.07	134.1	6.92	0	5.48
0	19	0.73	12	208	347	0.48	50	0.07	0.52	0.12	1.15	0.13	116	22	0	2
0	21	0.58	12	196	4	0.50	—	0.06	1.13	0.09	0.93	0.02	121	22	0	4
0	7	0.14	2	320	2	0.28	0	0.01	—	0.03	0.18	0.06	1	0	0	<1
0	5	0.21	3	52	5	0.43	1	0.02	0.25	0.02	0.09	0.09	2	1	0	<1
0	32	2.30	60	612	9	2.04	0	0.13	—	0.07	0.82	0.11	139	0	0	1
8	62	2.22	36	302	553	2.40	5	0.07	0.60	0.07	1.16	0.06	39	3	0	8
9	71	4.15	44	380	557	7.41	5	0.07	0.68	0.06	0.63	0.09	29	4	0	6
9	77	2.10	43	336	425	1.90	1	0.06	0.68	0.08	0.44	0.11	47	4	0	6
0	23	1.81	60	305	1	0.96	0	0.21	—	0.05	0.43	0.06	128	0	0	1
0	40	2.37	39	239	6	1.25	1	0.10	0.29	0.05	0.43	0.11	141	1	0	3
0	26	1.55	36	258	59	0.63	9	0.06	0.25	0.05	0.91	0.10	18	11	0	1
0	56	0.96	50	327	5	0.57	0	0.12	—	0.05	0.48	0.09	66	1	0	1
0	60	1.89	44	346	2	0.78	0	0.14	—	0.05	0.60	0.10	90	1	0	4
0	18	0.33	18	114	1	0.17	3	0.02	—	0.04	0.21	0.01	20	2	0	1
0	27	2.08	63	485	14	0.67	16	0.12	0.12	0.08	0.88	0.16	22	9	0	2
0	25	1.76	50	370	26	0.50	7	0.06	0.58	0.05	0.69	0.10	14	5	0	2
0	7	0.40	9	63	6	0.29	1	0.03	0.00	0.06	0.50	0.03	18	7	0	<1
0	64	2.26	54	335	1	0.96	0	0.18	—	0.06	0.48	0.15	127	1	0	5
0	17	0.75	20	111	58	0.19	0	0.08	—	0.07	0.82	0.06	146	7	0	1
0	24	1.27	25	304	39	0.32	0	0.13	—	0.05	0.30	0.09	16	<1	0	1
0	31	1.61	36	329	436	0.70	0	0.13	0.06	0.11	0.58	0.03	65	1	0	2

Table H-1

Food Composition (Computer code number is for Wadsworth Diet Analysis program) (For purposes of calculations, use "0" for t, <1, <.1, <.01, etc.)

DA + Code	Food Description	Quantity	Measure	Wt (g)	H_2O (g)	Ener (kcal)	Prot (g)	Carb (g)	Dietary Fiber (g)	Fat (g)	Fat Breakdown (g) Sat	Mono	Poly
	VEGETABLES, LEGUMES—Continued												
1810	Refried beans, canned	½	cup(s)	127	96	119	7	20	7	2	0.60	0.71	0.19
1053	Shell beans, canned	½	cup(s)	123	111	37	2	8	4	<1	0.03	0.02	0.13
1670	Soybeans, boiled	½	cup(s)	86	54	149	14	9	5	8	1.12	1.70	4.36
1108	Soybeans, green, boiled, drained	½	cup(s)	90	62	127	11	10	4	6	0.67	1.09	2.71
1807	White beans, small, boiled	½	cup(s)	90	57	127	8	23	9	1	0.15	0.05	0.25
575	Yellow snap, string or wax beans, boiled, drained	½	cup(s)	62	<.1	22	1	5	2	<1	0.04	0.00	0.09
576	Yellow snap, string or wax beans, frozen, boiled, drained	½	cup(s)	68	<.1	19	1	4	2	<1	0.02	0.00	0.05
	Beets												
580	Whole, boiled, drained	2	item(s)	100	87	44	2	10	2	<1	0.03	0.04	0.06
581	Sliced, boiled, drained	½	cup(s)	85	74	37	1	8	2	<1	0.02	0.03	0.05
583	Sliced, canned, drained	½	cup(s)	85	77	26	1	6	1	<1	0.02	0.02	0.04
2730	Pickled, canned with liquid	½	cup(s)	114	93	74	1	18	3	<.1	0.01	0.02	0.03
584	Beet greens, boiled, drained	½	cup(s)	72	64	19	2	4	2	<1	0.02	0.03	0.05
585	**Cowpeas or black-eyed peas, boiled, drained**	½	cup(s)	83	0.06	80	2.61	16.76	4.12	0.31	0.07	0.02	0.13
	Broccoli												
587	Raw, chopped	½	cup(s)	44	39	15	1	3	1	<1	0.02	0.00	0.02
588	Chopped, boiled, drained	½	cup(s)	78	70	27	2	6	3	<1	0.06	0.03	0.13
590	Frozen, chopped, boiled, drained	½	cup(s)	92	83	26	3	5	3	<1	0.02	0.01	0.05
16848	**Broccoflower, raw, chopped**	½	cup(s)	32	29	10	1	2	1	<.1	0.01	0.01	0.04
	Brussels sprouts												
591	Boiled, drained	½	cup(s)	78	69	28	2	6	2	<1	0.08	0.03	0.20
592	Frozen, boiled, drained	½	cup(s)	78	67	33	3	6	3	<1	0.06	0.02	0.16
	Cabbage												
594	Raw, shredded	1	cup(s)	70	65	17	1	4	2	<.1	0.01	0.01	0.04
595	Boiled, drained, no salt added	1	cup(s)	150	140	33	2	7	3	1	0.08	0.05	0.29
35611	Chinese (pak choi or bok choy), boiled w/salt, drained	1	cup(s)	170	162	20	3	3	2	<1	0.04	0.02	0.13
16869	Kim chee	1	cup(s)	150	138	31	2	6	2	<1	0.04	0.02	0.15
596	Red, shredded, raw	1	cup(s)	70	63	22	1	5	1	<1	0.02	0.01	0.09
597	Savoy, shredded, raw	1	cup(s)	70	64	19	1	4	2	<.1	0.01	0.00	0.03
11710	**Capers**	1	teaspoon(s)	5	—	0	0	0	0	0	0.00	0.00	0.00
	Carrots												
600	Raw	½	cup(s)	61	54	25	1	6	2	<1	0.02	0.01	0.06
8691	Raw, baby	8	item(s)	80	72	28	1	7	1	<1	0.02	0.01	0.05
601	Grated	½	cup(s)	55	49	23	1	5	2	<1	0.02	0.01	0.06
602	Sliced, boiled, drained	½	cup(s)	78	0.07	27.29	0.59	6.41	2.33	0.14	0.02	0	0.08
1055	Juice, canned	½	cup(s)	123	109	49	1	11	1	<1	0.03	0.01	0.09
32725	**Cassava or manioc**	½	cup(s)	103	61	165	1	39	2	<1	0.08	0.08	0.05
	Cauliflower												
605	Raw, chopped,	½	cup(s)	50	46	13	1	3	1	<1	0.02	0.01	0.05
606	Boiled, drained	½	cup(s)	62	58	14	1	3	2	<1	0.04	0.02	0.13
607	Frozen, boiled, drained	½	cup(s)	90	85	17	1	3	2	<1	0.03	0.01	0.09
	Celery												
609	Diced	½	cup(s)	60	58	8	<1	2	1	<1	0.03	0.02	0.05
608	Stalk	2	item(s)	80	76	11	1	2	1	<1	0.03	0.03	0.06
	Chard												
1056	Swiss chard, raw	1	cup(s)	36	33	7	1	1	1	<.1	0.01	0.01	0.03
1057	Swiss chard, boiled, drained	½	cup(s)	88	81	18	2	4	2	<.1	0.01	0.01	0.02
	Collard greens												
610	Boiled, drained	½	cup(s)	95	87	25	2	5	3	<1	0.04	0.02	0.16
611	Frozen, chopped, boiled, drained	½	cup(s)	85	75	31	3	6	2	<1	0.05	0.02	0.18
	Corn												
29614	Yellow corn, fresh, cooked	1	item(s)	100	0.06	107.37	3.3	24.96	2.78	1.27	0.19	0.37	0.59
612	Yellow sweet corn, boiled, drained	½	cup(s)	82	57	89	3	21	2	1	0.16	0.31	0.49
614	Yellow sweet corn, frozen, boiled, drained	½	cup(s)	82	63	66	2	16	2	1	0.08	0.16	0.26
615	Yellow creamed sweet corn, canned	½	cup(s)	128	101	92	2	23	2	1	0.08	0.16	0.25
618	**Cucumber**	¼	item(s)	75	72	11	<1	3	<1	<.1	0.03	0.00	0.04

PAGE KEY: H–2 = Breads/Baked Goods H–6 = Cereal/Rice/Pasta H–10 = Fruit H–16 = Vegetables/Legumes H–26 = Nuts/Seeds H–28 = Vegetarian H–30 = Dairy H–36 = Eggs H–38 = Seafood H–40 = Meats H–42 = Poultry H–44 = Processed meats H–46 = Beverages H–50 = Fats/Oils H–52 = Sweets H–52 = Sauces/Condiments/Spices H–56 = Mixed Foods/Soups/Sandwiches H–62 = Fast food H–80 = Convenience H–82 = Baby foods

Chol (mg)	Calc (mg)	Iron (mg)	Magn (mg)	Pota (mg)	Sodi (mg)	Zinc (mg)	Vit A (RAE) (µg)	Thia (mg)	Vit E (mg)	Ribo (mg)	Niac (mg)	Vit B_6 (mg)	Fola (µg)	Vit C (mg)	Vit B_{12} (µg)	Sele (µg)
10	44	2.10	42	338	378	1.48	0	0.03	0.00	0.02	0.40	0.18	14	8	0	2
0	36	1.21	18	134	409	0.33	13	0.04	0.04	0.07	0.25	0.06	22	4	0	1
0	88	4.42	74	443	1	0.99	0	0.13	1.68	0.25	0.34	0.20	46	1	0	6
0	131	2.25	54	485	13	0.82	7	0.23	0.01	0.14	1.13	0.05	100	15	0	1
0	65	2.54	61	414	2	0.98	0	0.21	—	0.05	0.24	0.11	123	0	0	1
0	29	0.80	16	187	2	0.22	5	0.05	0.14	0.06	0.38	0.03	21	6	0	<1
0	33	0.59	16	85	6	0.32	7	0.02	0.08	0.06	0.26	0.04	16	3	0	<1
0	16	0.79	23	305	77	0.35	2	0.03	0.30	0.04	0.33	0.07	80	4	0	1
0	14	0.67	20	259	65	0.30	2	0.02	0.26	0.03	0.28	0.06	68	3	0	1
0	13	1.55	14	126	165	0.18	1	0.01	0.26	0.03	0.13	0.05	26	3	0	<1
0	12	0.47	17	168	300	0.30	1	0.01	—	0.05	0.28	0.06	31	3	0	1
0	82	1.37	49	654	174	0.36	276	0.08	0.22	0.21	0.36	0.10	10	18	0	1
0	105.59	0.92	42.9	344.85	3.29	0.84	65.17	0.08	0.14	0.12	1.15	0.05	104.77	1.81	0	2.06
0	21	0.32	9	139	15	0.18	15	0.03	0.73	0.05	0.28	0.08	28	39	0	1
0	31	0.52	16	229	32	0.35	76	0.05	1.32	0.10	0.43	0.16	84	51	0	1
0	30	0.56	12	131	10	0.26	52	0.05	1.52	0.07	0.42	0.12	52	37	0	1
0	11	0.23	6	96	7	0.20	0	0.03	0.01	0.03	0.23	0.07	18	28	0	—
0	28	0.94	16	247	16	0.26	30	0.08	0.66	0.06	0.47	0.14	47	48	0	1
0	20	0.37	14	225	12	0.19	36	0.08	0.45	0.09	0.42	0.22	78	35	0	<1
0	33	0.41	11	172	13	0.13	6	0.04	0.07	0.03	0.21	0.07	30	23	0	1
0	47	0.26	12	146	12	0.14	11	0.09	0.16	0.08	0.42	0.17	30	30	0	1
0	158	1.77	19	631	459	0.29	360	0.05	—	0.11	0.73	0.28	70	44	0	1
0	145	1.28	27	375	995	0.36	—	0.07	0.24	0.10	0.75	0.34	88	80	0	—
0	32	0.56	11	170	19	0.15	39	0.04	0.07	0.05	0.29	0.15	13	40	0	<1
0	25	0.28	20	161	20	0.19	35	0.05	0.07	0.02	0.21	0.13	56	22	0	1
0	—	—	—	—	105	—	—	—	—	—	—	—	—	—	0	—
0	20	0.18	7	195	42	0.15	367	0.04	0.28	0.04	0.60	0.08	12	4	0	<.1
0	26	0.71	8	190	62	0.14	552	0.02	—	0.03	0.44	0.08	26	7	0	1
0	18	0.17	7	177	38	0.13	333	0.04	0.25	0.03	0.54	0.08	11	3	0	<.1
0	23.39	0.26	7.8	183.3	45.24	0.15	1914.9	0.05	0.26	0.03	0.5	0.11	10.92	2.8	0	0.54
0	30	0.57	17	359	36	0.22	1176	0.11	0.01	0.07	0.47	0.27	5	10	0	1
0	16	0.28	22	279	14	0.35	1	0.09	0.20	0.05	0.88	0.09	28	21	0	1
0	11	0.22	8	152	15	0.14	1	0.03	0.02	0.03	0.26	0.11	29	23	0	<1
0	10	0.20	6	88	9	0.11	1	0.03	0.02	0.03	0.25	0.11	27	27	0	<1
0	15	0.37	8	125	16	0.12	0	0.03	0.04	0.05	0.28	0.08	37	28	0	1
0	24	0.12	7	157	48	0.08	13	0.01	0.22	0.03	0.19	0.04	22	2	0	<1
0	32	0.16	9	208	64	0.10	18	0.02	0.29	0.05	0.26	0.06	29	2	0	<1
0	18	0.65	29	136	77	0.13	110	0.01	0.68	0.03	0.14	0.04	5	11	0	<1
0	51	1.98	75	480	157	0.29	268	0.03	1.65	0.08	0.32	0.07	8	16	0	1
0	133	1.10	19	110	15	0.22	386	0.04	0.84	0.10	0.55	0.12	88	17	0	<1
0	179	0.95	26	213	43	0.23	489	0.04	0.43	0.10	0.54	0.10	65	22	0	1
0	2.12	0.6	31.81	247.59	242.45	0.47	21.87	0.21	0.07	0.07	1.6	0.05	—	6.16	0	—
0	2	0.50	26	204	14	0.39	11	0.18	0.07	0.06	1.32	0.05	38	5	0	<1
0	2	0.39	23	191	1	0.52	8	0.02	0.07	0.05	1.08	0.08	29	3	0	1
0	4	0.49	22	172	365	0.68	5	0.03	0.12	0.07	1.23	0.08	58	6	0	1
0	12	0.21	10	111	2	0.15	4	0.02	0.06	0.02	0.07	0.03	5	2	0	<1

Table H–1

Food Composition (Computer code number is for Wadsworth Diet Analysis program) (For purposes of calculations, use "0" for t, <1, <.1, <.01, etc.)

DA + Code	Food Description	Quantity	Measure	Wt (g)	H_2O (g)	Ener (kcal)	Prot (g)	Carb (g)	Dietary Fiber (g)	Fat (g)	Fat Breakdown (g) Sat	Mono	Poly
	VEGETABLES, LEGUMES—Continued												
16870	**Cucumber, kim chee**	½	cup(s)	75	68	16	1	4	1	<.1	0.02	0.00	0.03
	Dandelion greens												
2734	Raw	1	cup(s)	55	47	25	1	5	2	<1	0.09	0.01	0.17
620	Chopped, boiled, drained	½	cup(s)	53	47	17	1	3	2	<1	0.08	0.01	0.14
1066	**Eggplant, boiled, drained**	½	cup(s)	48	43	17	<1	4	1	<1	0.02	0.01	0.04
621	**Endive or escarole, chopped, raw**	1	cup(s)	53	49	9	1	2	2	<1	0.03	0.00	0.05
8784	**Jicama or yambean**	½	cup(s)	65	59	25	<1	6	3	<.1	0.01	0.00	0.03
	Kale												
29313	Raw	1	cup(s)	67	57	34	2	7	1	<1	0.06	0.03	0.23
623	Frozen, chopped, boiled, drained	½	cup(s)	65	59	20	2	3	1	<1	0.04	0.02	0.15
	Kohlrabi												
1071	Raw	1	cup(s)	135	123	36	2	8	5	<1	0.02	0.01	0.06
1072	Boiled, drained	½	cup(s)	83	74	24	1	6	1	<.1	0.01	0.01	0.04
	Leeks												
1073	Raw	1	cup(s)	89	74	54	1	13	2	<1	0.04	0.00	0.15
1074	Boiled, drained	½	cup(s)	52	47	16	<1	4	1	<1	0.01	0.00	0.06
	Lentils												
522	Boiled	½	cup(s)	99	69	115	9	20	8	<1	0.05	0.06	0.17
1075	Sprouted	1	cup(s)	77	52	82	7	17	0	<1	0.04	0.08	0.17
	Lettuce												
624	Butterhead, boston, or bibb	1	cup(s)	55	53	7	1	1	1	<1	0.02	0.00	0.06
625	Butterhead leaves	11	piece(s)	83	79	11	1	2	1	<1	0.02	0.01	0.10
626	Iceberg	1	cup(s)	55	53	6	<1	1	1	<.1	0.01	0.00	0.03
628	Iceberg, chopped	1	cup(s)	55	53	6	<1	1	1	<.1	0.01	0.00	0.03
629	Looseleaf	1	cup(s)	56	54	8	1	2	1	<.1	0.01	0.00	0.05
1665	Romaine, shredded	1	cup(s)	56	53	10	1	2	1	<1	0.02	0.01	0.09
	Mushrooms												
15585	Crimini (about 6)	3	ounce(s)	85	28	4	3	2	0	0.00	0.00	0.00	0
8700	Enoki	30	item(s)	90	80	31	2	6	2	<1	0.04	0.01	0.14
630	Mushrooms, raw	½	cup(s)	35	32	8	1	1	<1	<1	0.02	0.00	0.05
1079	Mushrooms, boiled, drained	½	cup(s)	78	71	22	2	4	2	<1	0.05	0.01	0.14
1080	Mushrooms, canned, drained	½	cup(s)	78	71	20	1	4	2	<1	0.03	0.00	0.09
15587	Portobello, raw	1	item(s)	85	30	3	4	3	0	0.00	0.00	0.00	0
2743	Shiitake, cooked	½	cup(s)	73	61	40	1	10	2	<1	0.04	0.05	0.02
	Mustard greens												
29319	Raw	1	cup(s)	56	51	15	2	3	2	<1	0.01	0.05	0.02
2744	Frozen, boiled, drained	½	cup(s)	75	70	14	2	2	2	<1	0.01	0.08	0.04
	Okra												
632	Sliced, boiled, drained	½	cup(s)	80	74	18	1	4	2	<1	0.04	0.02	0.04
32742	Frozen, boiled, drained, no salt added	½	cup(s)	92	84	26	2	5	3	<1	0.07	0.05	0.07
16866	Batter coated, fried	11	piece(s)	83	55	160	2	13	2	11	1.50	2.80	6.37
	Onions												
633	Raw, chopped	½	cup(s)	80	71	34	1	8	1	<.1	0.02	0.02	0.05
635	Chopped, boiled, drained	½	cup(s)	106	93	47	1	11	1	<1	0.03	0.03	0.08
2748	Frozen, boiled, drained	½	cup(s)	106	98	30	1	7	2	<1	0.02	0.01	0.04
16850	Red onions, sliced, raw	½	cup(s)	58	52	22	1	5	1	<.1	0.02	0.01	0.04
636	Scallions, green or spring onions	2	item(s)	30	27	10	1	2	1	<.1	0.01	0.01	0.02
1081	Onion rings, breaded & pan fried, frozen, heated	11	item(s)	78	22	318	4	30	1	21	6.70	8.49	3.99
16860	**Palm hearts, cooked**	½	cup(s)	73	51	75	2	19	1	<1	0.03	0.00	0.07
637	**Parsley, chopped**	1	tablespoon(s)	4	3	1	<1	<1	<1	<.1	0.01	0.01	0.00
638	**Parsnips, sliced, boiled, drained**	½	cup(s)	78	63	55	1	13	3	<1	0.04	0.09	0.04
	Peas												
639	Green peas, canned, drained	½	cup(s)	85	69	59	4	11	3	<1	0.05	0.03	0.14
641	Green peas, frozen, boiled, drained	½	cup(s)	80	64	62	4	11	4	<1	0.04	0.02	0.10
35694	Pea pods, boiled w/salt, drained	½	cup(s)	80	71	34	3	6	2	<1	0.04	0.02	0.08
1082	Peas & carrots, canned w/liquid	½	cup(s)	128	112	48	3	11	3	<1	0.06	0.03	0.16
1083	Peas & carrots, frozen, boiled, drained	½	cup(s)	80	69	38	2	8	2	<1	0.06	0.03	0.16
640	Snow or sugar peas, raw	½	cup(s)	32	28	13	1	2	1	<.1	0.01	0.01	0.03
2750	Snow or sugar peas, frozen, boiled, drained	½	cup(s)	80	69	42	3	7	2	<1	0.06	0.03	0.13

PAGE KEY: H–2 = Breads/Baked Goods H–6 = Cereal/Rice/Pasta H–10 = Fruit H–16 = Vegetables/Legumes H–26 = Nuts/Seeds H–28 = Vegetarian H–30 = Dairy H–36 = Eggs H–38 = Seafood H–40 = Meats H–42 = Poultry H–44 = Processed meats H–46 = Beverages H–50 = Fats/Oils H–52 = Sweets H–52 = Sauces/Condiments/Spices H–56 = Mixed Foods/Soups/Sandwiches H–62 = Fast food H–80 = Convenience H–82 = Baby foods

Chol (mg)	Calc (mg)	Iron (mg)	Magn (mg)	Pota (mg)	Sodi (mg)	Zinc (mg)	Vit A (RAE) (μg)	Thia (mg)	Vit E (mg)	Ribo (mg)	Niac (mg)	Vit B_6 (mg)	Fola (μg)	Vit C (mg)	Vit B_{12} (μg)	Sele (μg)
0	7	3.62	6	88	766	0.38	—	0.02	0.12	0.02	0.35	0.08	17	3	0	—
0	103	1.71	20	219	42	0.23	137	0.11	1.38	0.14	0.45	0.14	15	19	0	<1
0	74	0.95	13	122	23	0.15	260	0.07	1.31	0.09	0.27	0.08	7	9	0	<1
0	3	0.12	5	59	<1	0.06	1	0.04	0.01	0.01	0.29	0.04	7	1	0	<.1
0	27	0.44	8	165	12	0.41	57	0.04	0.23	0.04	0.21	0.01	75	3	0	<1
0	8	0.39	8	98	3	0.10	1	0.01	0.30	0.02	0.13	0.03	8	13	0	<1
0	90	1.14	23	299	29	0.29	515	0.07	0.54	0.09	0.67	0.18	19	80	0	1
0	90	0.61	12	209	10	0.12	478	0.03	0.12	0.07	0.44	0.06	9	16	0	1
0	32	0.54	26	473	27	0.04	3	0.07	0.65	0.03	0.54	0.20	22	84	0	1
0	21	0.33	16	281	17	0.26	2	0.03	1.38	0.02	0.32	0.13	10	45	0	1
0	53	1.87	25	160	18	0.11	74	0.05	0.82	0.03	0.36	0.21	57	11	0	1
0	16	0.57	7	45	5	0.03	1	0.01	0.00	0.01	0.10	0.06	13	2	0	<1
0	19	3.30	36	365	2	1.26	0	0.17	0.11	0.07	1.05	0.18	179	1	0	3
0	19	2.47	28	248	8	1.16	2	0.18	—	0.10	0.87	0.15	77	13	0	<1
0	19	0.69	7	132	3	0.11	92	0.03	0.24	0.03	0.20	0.05	40	2	0	<1
0	29	1.02	11	196	4	0.17	137	0.05	0.36	0.05	0.29	0.07	60	3	0	<1
0	11	0.19	4	84	5	0.09	9	0.02	0.15	0.01	0.07	0.03	31	2	0	<1
0	11	0.19	4	84	5	0.09	9	0.02	0.15	0.01	0.07	0.03	31	2	0	<1
0	20	0.48	7	109	16	0.10	208	0.04	0.25	0.05	0.21	0.05	21	10	0	<1
0	19	0.55	8	139	5	0.13	163	0.04	0.25	0.04	0.18	0.04	77	14	0	<1
0	0.67	—	—	33	—	0	—	—	—	—	—	—	—	0	0	—
0	1	0.80	14	343	3	0.51	0	0.08	—	0.09	3.28	0.04	27	11	0	14
0	1	0.18	3	110	1	0.18	0	0.03	0.04	0.15	1.35	0.04	6	1	<.1	3
0	5	1.36	9	278	2	0.68	0	0.06	0.09	0.23	3.48	0.07	14	3	0	9
0	9	0.62	12	101	332	0.56	0	0.07	0.09	0.02	1.24	0.05	9	0	0	3
40	0.36	—	—	10	—	0	—	—	—	—	—	—	—	0	0	—
0	2	0.32	10	85	3	0.96	0	0.03	0.09	0.12	1.09	0.12	15	<1	0	18
0	58	0.82	18	199	14	0.11	295	0.05	1.13	0.06	0.45	0.10	105	39	0	1
0	76	0.84	10	104	19	0.15	266	0.03	1.31	0.04	0.19	0.08	53	10	0	<1
0	62	0.22	29	108	5	0.34	11	0.11	0.55	0.04	0.70	0.15	37	13	0	<1
0	88	0.62	47	215	3	0.57	16	0.09	0.63	0.11	0.72	0.04	134	11	0	1
2	54	1.13	32	170	110	0.44	—	0.16	2.72	0.13	1.29	0.11	34	9	<.1	—
0	18	0.15	8	115	2	0.13	0	0.04	0.25	0.02	0.07	0.12	15	5	0	<1
0	23	0.26	12	177	3	0.22	0	0.04	0.14	0.02	0.18	0.14	16	6	0	1
0	17	0.32	6	115	13	0.07	0	0.02	0.20	0.03	0.15	0.07	14	3	0	<1
0	11	0.13	6	90	2	0.11	0	0.02	0.07	0.01	0.09	0.07	11	4	0	—
0	22	0.44	6	83	5	0.12	15	0.02	0.04	0.02	0.16	0.02	19	6	0	<1
0	24	1.32	15	101	293	0.33	9	0.22	—	0.11	2.82	0.06	52	1	0	3
0	13	1.23	7	1318	10	2.72	—	0.03	0.37	0.13	0.62	0.53	15	5	0	—
0	5	0.24	2	21	2	0.04	16	0.00	0.07	0.00	0.05	0.00	6	5	0	<.1
0	29	0.45	23	286	8	0.20	0	0.06	0.78	0.04	0.56	0.07	45	10	0	1
0	17	0.81	14	147	214	0.60	23	0.10	0.32	0.07	0.62	0.05	37	8	0	1
0	19	1.22	18	88	58	0.54	84	0.23	0.14	0.08	1.18	0.09	47	8	0	1
0	34	1.58	21	192	192	0.30	43	0.10	—	0.06	0.43	0.12	23	38	0	1
0	29	0.96	18	128	332	0.74	368	0.09	—	0.07	0.74	0.11	23	8	0	1
0	18	0.75	13	126	54	0.36	374	0.18	0.26	0.05	0.92	0.07	21	6	0	1
0	14	0.66	8	63	1	0.09	17	0.05	0.12	0.03	0.19	0.05	13	19	0	<1
0	47	1.92	22	174	4	0.39	53	0.05	0.17	0.10	0.45	0.14	28	18	0	1

Table H–1

Food Composition (Computer code number is for Wadsworth Diet Analysis program) (For purposes of calculations, use "0" for t, <1, <.1, <.01, etc.)

DA + Code	Food Description	Quantity	Measure	Wt (g)	H_2O (g)	Ener (kcal)	Prot (g)	Carb (g)	Dietary Fiber (g)	Fat (g)	Fat Breakdown (g) Sat	Mono	Poly
	VEGETABLES, LEGUMES—Continued												
29324	Split peas, sprouted	½	cup(s)	60	37	77	5	17	0	<1	0.07	0.04	0.20
	Peppers												
643	Green bell or sweet, raw	½	cup(s)	75	70	15	1	3	1	<1	0.04	0.01	0.05
644	Green bell or sweet, boiled, drained	½	cup(s)	68	62	19	1	5	1	<1	0.02	0.01	0.07
1664	Green hot chili	1	item(s)	45	39	18	1	4	1	<.1	0.01	0.00	0.05
1663	Green hot chili, canned w/liquid	½	cup(s)	68	63	14	1	3	1	<.1	0.01	0.00	0.04
1086	Jalapeno, canned w/liquid	½	cup(s)	68	60	18	1	3	2	1	0.07	0.04	0.35
8703	Yellow bell or sweet	1	item(s)	186	171	50	2	12	2	<1	0.06	0.03	0.21
1087	**Poi**	½	cup(s)	122	87	136	<1	33	<1	<1	0.04	0.01	0.07
	Potatoes												
5791	Baked, flesh & skin	1	item(s)	202	144	220	5	51	4	<1	0.05	0.00	0.09
645	Baked, flesh only	½	cup(s)	61	46	57	1	13	1	<.1	0.02	0.00	0.03
1088	Baked, skin only	1	item(s)	58	27	115	2	27	5	<.1	0.02	0.00	0.02
5794	Boiled, drained, skin & flesh	1	item(s)	150	116	129	3	30	2	<1	0.04	0.00	0.06
647	Boiled, flesh only	½	cup(s)	78	60	67	1	16	1	<.1	0.02	0.00	0.03
5795	Boiled in skin, drained, flesh only	1	item(s)	136	105	118	3	27	2	<1	0.04	0.00	0.06
2759	Microwaved	1	item(s)	202	146	212	5	49	5	<1	0.05	0.00	0.09
5804	Microwaved, skin only	1	item(s)	58	37	77	3	17	4	<.1	0.02	0.00	0.02
2760	Microwaved in skin, flesh only	½	cup(s)	78	57	78	2	18	1	<.1	0.02	0.00	0.03
1089	Au gratin, prepared w/butter	½	cup(s)	123	91	162	6	14	2	9	5.80	2.63	0.34
1090	Au gratin mix, prepared w/water, whole milk, & butter	½	cup(s)	114	90	106	3	15	1	5	2.94	1.34	0.15
648	French fried, deep fried, prepared from raw	14	item(s)	70	32	190	3	24	2	10	1.93	4.21	2.97
649	French fried, frozen, heated	14	item(s)	70	40	140	2	22	2	5	0.88	3.33	0.55
1091	Hashed brown	½	cup(s)	78	37	207	2	27	2	10	1.11	3.13	2.78
653	Mashed, from dehydrated granules w/milk, water, & margarine	½	cup(s)	105	80	122	2	17	1	5	1.27	2.05	1.41
652	Mashed, w/margarine & whole milk	½	cup(s)	105	79	119	2	18	2	4	1.05	1.83	1.27
1097	Potato puffs, frozen, heated	½	cup(s)	64	34	142	2	20	2	7	3.26	2.79	0.51
1093	Scalloped, prepared w/butter	½	cup(s)	123	99	105	4	13	2	5	2.76	1.27	0.20
1094	Scalloped mix, prepared w/water, whole milk, & butter	½	cup(s)	114	90	106	2	15	1	5	2.99	1.38	0.22
	Pumpkin												
1773	Boiled, drained	½	cup(s)	123	115	25	1	6	1	<.1	0.05	0.01	0.00
656	Canned	½	cup(s)	123	110	42	1	10	4	<1	0.18	0.05	0.02
	Radicchio									<.1			
2498	Raw	1	cup(s)	40	37	9	1	2	<1	<1	0.02	0.00	0.04
8731	Raw, leaves	10	item(s)	80	75	18	1	4	1	<1	0.05	0.01	0.09
657	**Radishes**	6	item(s)	27	26	4	<1	1	<1	<.1	0.01	0.00	0.01
1099	**Rutabaga, boiled, drained**	½	cup(s)	85	76	33	1	7	2	<1	0.02	0.02	0.08
658	**Sauerkraut, canned**	½	cup(s)	114	105	22	1	5	3	<1	0.04	0.01	0.07
	Seaweed												
1102	Kelp	½	cup(s)	41	33	17	1	4	1	<1	0.10	0.04	0.02
1104	Spirulina, dried	½	cup(s)	8	<1	22	4	2	<1	1	0.20	0.05	0.16
1106	**Shallots**	3	tablespoon(s)	30	24	22	1	5	0	<.1	0.01	0.00	0.01
	Soybeans												
1670	Boiled	½	cup(s)	86	0.05	148.77	14.31	8.53	5.15	7.71	1.11	1.7	4.35
2825	Dry roasted	½	cup(s)	86	1	388	34	28	7	19	2.69	4.11	10.50
2824	Roasted, salted	½	cup(s)	86	2	405	30	29	15	22	3.16	4.82	12.33
30282	Soup (miso)	1	cup(s)	240	218	85	6	8	2	3	0.59	1.05	1.47
8739	Sprouted, stir fried	3	ounce(s)	85	57	106	11	8	1	6	0.84	1.37	3.41
	Soy products												
1813	Soy milk	1	cup(s)	240	214	118	9	11	3	5	0.51	0.78	2.00
2838	Tofu, dried, frozen (koyadofu)	3	ounce(s)	85	5	408	41	12	6	26	3.73	5.70	14.57
13844	Tofu, extra firm	3	ounce(s)	79	—	80	8	2	1	4	0.50	0.87	2.60
13843	Tofu, firm	3	ounce(s)	79	—	80	8	2	1	4	0.50	0.87	2.17
1816	Tofu, firm, w/calcium sulfate & magnesium chloride (nigari)	3	ounce(s)	85	0.07	65.48	6.83	2.52	0.34	3.79	0.54	0.83	2.14
1817	Tofu, fried	3	ounce(s)	85	43	230	15	9	3	17	2.48	3.79	9.69
13841	Tofu, silken	3	ounce(s)	91	—	30	6	0	1	1	0.50	0.51	1.52
13842	Tofu, soft	3	ounce(s)	91	—	30	6	1	1	1	0.50	1.00	2.00

PAGE KEY: H–2 = Breads/Baked Goods H–6 = Cereal/Rice/Pasta H–10 = Fruit H–16 = Vegetables/Legumes H–26 = Nuts/Seeds H–28 = Vegetarian H–30 = Dairy H–36 = Eggs H–38 = Seafood H–40 = Meats H–42 = Poultry H–44 = Processed meats H–46 = Beverages H–50 = Fats/Oils H–52 = Sweets H–52 = Sauces/Condiments/Spices H–56 = Mixed Foods/Soups/Sandwiches H–62 = Fast food H–80 = Convenience H–82 = Baby foods

Chol (mg)	Calc (mg)	Iron (mg)	Magn (mg)	Pota (mg)	Sodi (mg)	Zinc (mg)	Vit A (RAE) (μg)	Thia (mg)	Vit E (mg)	Ribo (mg)	Niac (mg)	Vit B_6 (mg)	Fola (μg)	Vit C (mg)	Vit B_{12} (μg)	Sele (μg)
0	22	1.36	34	229	12	0.63	5	0.14	—	0.09	1.85	0.16	86	6	0	<1
0	7	0.25	7	130	2	0.10	13	0.04	0.51	0.02	0.36	0.17	8	60	0	0
0	6	0.31	7	113	1	0.08	10	0.04	0.47	0.02	0.32	0.16	11	51	0	<1
0	8	0.54	11	153	3	0.14	27	0.04	0.31	0.04	0.43	0.13	10	109	0	<1
0	5	0.34	10	127	798	0.12	24	0.01	0.47	0.03	0.54	0.10	7	46	0	<1
0	16	1.28	10	131	1136	0.23	58	0.03	0.47	0.03	0.27	0.13	10	7	0	<1
0	20	0.86	22	394	4	0.32	19	0.05	—	0.05	1.66	0.31	48	341	0	1
0	19	1.07	29	223	15	0.27	4	0.16	0.22	0.05	1.34	0.33	26	5	0	1
0	20	2.75	55	844	16	0.65	0	0.22	0.10	0.07	3.32	0.70	22	26	0	2
0	3	0.21	15	239	3	0.18	0	0.06	0.02	0.01	0.85	0.18	5	8	0	<1
0	20	4.08	25	332	12	0.28	1	0.07	0.02	0.06	1.78	0.36	13	8	0	<1
0	13	1.27	34	572	7	0.47	0	0.15	0.08	0.03	2.13	0.44	15	18	0	—
0	6	0.24	16	256	4	0.21	0	0.08	0.04	0.01	1.02	0.21	7	6	0	<1
0	7	0.42	30	515	5	0.41	0	0.14	0.07	0.03	1.96	0.41	14	18	0	<1
0	22	2.50	55	903	16	0.73	0	0.24	—	0.06	3.46	0.69	24	31	0	1
0	27	3.45	21	377	9	0.30	0	0.04	—	0.04	1.29	0.29	10	9	0	<1
0	4	0.32	20	321	5	0.26	0	0.10	—	0.02	1.27	0.25	9	12	0	<1
28	146	0.78	25	485	530	0.85	78	0.08	—	0.14	1.22	0.21	13	12	0	3
17	94	0.36	17	249	499	0.27	59	0.02	—	0.09	1.07	0.05	8	4	0	3
0	9	1.02	28	731	8	0.53	0	0.10	—	0.05	1.90	0.33	13	21	0	—
0	6	0.87	15	293	21	0.28	0	0.08	0.13	0.02	1.46	0.22	8	7	0	<1
0	11	0.43	27	449	267	0.37	0	0.13	0.15	0.03	1.80	0.37	12	10	0	<1
2	34	0.22	21	163	181	0.25	49	0.09	—	0.09	0.91	0.17	8	7	<1	6
1	21	0.27	20	342	350	0.32	43	0.10	0.32	0.05	1.23	0.26	9	11	<.1	1
0	19	1.00	12	243	477	0.19	0	0.13	0.03	0.05	1.38	0.15	11	4	0	<1
15	70	0.70	23	463	410	0.49	39	0.08	—	0.11	1.29	0.22	13	13	0	2
13	41	0.43	16	231	388	0.28	40	0.02	0.17	0.06	1.17	0.05	11	4	0	2
0	18	0.70	11	282	1	0.28	306	0.04	1.30	0.10	0.51	0.05	11	6	0	<1
0	32	1.70	28	252	6	0.21	953	0.03	1.30	0.07	0.45	0.07	15	5	0	<1
0	8	0.23	5	121	9	0.25	<1	0.01	0.90	0.01	0.10	0.02	24	3	0	<1
0	15	0.46	10	242	18	0.50	1	0.01	1.81	0.02	0.20	0.05	48	6	0	1
0	7	0.09	3	63	11	0.08	0	0.00	0.00	0.01	0.07	0.02	7	4	0	<1
0	41	0.45	20	277	17	0.30	0	0.07	0.13	0.03	0.61	0.09	13	16	0	1
0	34	1.67	15	193	751	0.22	1	0.02	0.11	0.02	0.16	0.15	27	17	0	1
0	68	1.16	49	36	94	0.50	2	0.02	0.35	0.06	0.19	0.00	73	1	0	<1
0	9	2.14	15	102	79	0.15	2	0.18	0.38	0.28	0.96	0.03	7	1	0	1
0	11	0.36	6	100	4	0.12	18	0.02	—	0.01	0.06	0.10	10	2	0	<1
0	87.72	4.42	73.95	442.89	0.86	0.98	0.86	0.13	1.34	0.24	0.34	0.2	46.43	1.46	0	6.27
0	120	3.40	196	1173	2	4.10	0	0.37	—	0.65	0.91	0.19	176	4	0	17
0	119	3.35	125	1264	140	2.70	9	0.09	1.68	0.12	1.21	0.18	181	2	0	16
0	64	1.89	37	361	988	0.87	—	0.06	0.69	0.16	2.61	0.17	57	4	<1	—
0	70	0.34	82	482	12	1.79	1	0.36	—	0.16	0.94	0.14	108	10	0	1
0	10	1.39	46	338	29	0.55	5	0.39	0.02	0.17	0.35	0.10	5	0	0	3
0	310	8.28	50	17	5	4.17	22	0.42	—	0.27	1.01	0.24	78	1	0	46
0	60	1.08	78	—	0	—	0	—	0.00	—	—	—	—	0	0	—
0	60	1.08	52	—	0	—	0	—	0.00	—	—	—	—	0	0	—
0	137.78	1.23	39.12	149.68	6.8	0.85	0.85	0.07	—	0.08	0	0.05	28.06	0.17	0	7.99
0	316	4.14	51	124	14	1.69	1	0.14	0.03	0.04	0.09	0.08	23	0	0	24
0	300	0.73	35	—	65	—	0	—	6.04	—	—	—	—	0	2	—
0	300	0.72	33	—	65	—	0	—	6.04	—	—	—	—	0	2	—

Table H–1

Food Composition (Computer code number is for Wadsworth Diet Analysis program) (For purposes of calculations, use "0" for t, <1, <.1, <.01, etc.)

DA + Code	Food Description	Quantity	Measure	Wt (g)	H_2O (g)	Ener (kcal)	Prot (g)	Carb (g)	Dietary Fiber (g)	Fat (g)	Fat Breakdown (g) Sat	Mono	Poly
	VEGETABLES, LEGUMES—Continued												
1671	Tofu, soft, w/calcium sulfate & magnesium chloride (nigari)	3	ounce(s)	85	0.07	51.88	5.57	1.53	0.17	3.13	0.45	0.69	1.76
	Spinach												
659	Raw, chopped	1	cup(s)	30	27	7	1	1	1	<1	0.02	0.00	0.05
663	Canned, drained	½	cup(s)	108	100	25	3	4	3	1	0.09	0.02	0.23
660	Chopped, boiled, drained	½	cup(s)	90	82	21	3	3	2	<1	0.04	0.01	0.10
661	Chopped, frozen, boiled, drained	½	cup(s)	95	84	30	4	5	4	<1	0.09	0.00	0.20
662	Leaf, frozen, boiled, drained	½	cup(s)	95	84	30	4	5	4	<1	0.09	0.00	0.20
8470	Trimmed leaves	1	cup(s)	32	27	3	1	<.1	3	<.1	—	—	—
	Squash												
1662	Acorn, baked	½	cup(s)	103	85	57	1	15	5	<1	0.03	0.01	0.06
29702	Acorn, boiled, mashed	½	cup(s)	123	110	42	1	11	3	<.1	0.02	0.01	0.04
1661	Butternut, baked	½	cup(s)	103	90	41	1	11	3	<.1	0.02	0.01	0.04
29451	Butternut, frozen, boiled	½	cup(s)	132	116	51	2	13	2	<.1	0.02	0.01	0.04
32773	Butternut, frozen, boiled, mashed, no salt added	½	cup(s)	122	<1	47	1	12	0	<.1	0.02	0.00	0.03
29700	Crookneck & straightneck, boiled, drained	½	cup(s)	90	0.08	18	0.81	3.87	1.25	0.27	0.05	0.02	0.11
29703	Hubbard, baked	v	cup(s)	103	87	51	3	11	0	1	0.13	0.05	0.27
1660	Hubbard, boiled, mashed	½	cup(s)	118	107	35	2	8	3	<1	0.09	0.03	0.18
29704	Spaghetti, boiled, drained, or baked	½	cup(s)	78	72	21	1	5	1	<1	0.05	0.02	0.10
664	Summer, all varieties, sliced, boiled, drained	½	cup(s)	90	84	18	1	4	1	<1	0.06	0.02	0.12
665	Winter, all varieties, baked, mashed	½	cup(s)	103	91	38	1	9	3	<1	0.13	0.05	0.27
1112	Zucchini, boiled, drained	½	cup(s)	90	85	14	1	4	1	<.1	0.01	0.00	0.02
1113	Zucchini, frozen, boiled, drained	½	cup(s)	113	107	19	1	4	1	<1	0.03	0.01	0.06
	Sweet potatoes												
666	Baked, peeled	½	cup(s)	100	76	90	2	21	3	<1	0.03	0.00	0.06
667	Boiled, mashed	½	cup(s)	166	133	126	2	29	4	<1	0.05	0.00	0.10
668	Candied, home recipe	½	cup(s)	84	56	115	1	23	2	3	1.13	0.53	0.12
670	Canned, vacuum pack	½	cup(s)	100	76	91	2	21	2	<1	0.04	0.01	0.09
2765	Frozen, baked	½	cup(s)	88	65	88	2	21	2	<1	0.02	0.00	0.05
1136	Yams, baked or boiled, drained	½	cup(s)	68	48	79	1	19	3	<.1	0.02	0.00	0.04
32785	**Taro shoots, cooked, no salt added**	½	cup(s)	70	67	10	1	2	0	<.1	0.01	0.00	0.02
	Tomatillo												
8774	Raw	2	item(s)	68	62	22	1	4	1	1	0.09	0.11	0.28
8777	Raw, chopped	½	cup(s)	66	60	21	1	4	1	1	0.09	0.10	0.28
	Tomato												
671	Fresh, ripe, red	1	item(s)	123	0.11	22.13	1.08	4.82	1.47	0.24	0.05	0.06	0.16
16846	Fresh, cherry	5	item(s)	85	0.07	17.85	0.72	3.94	0.93	0.28	0.03	0.04	0.11
3952	Diced, red	½	cup(s)	90	85	16	1	4	1	<1	0.04	0.05	0.12
1118	Boiled, red	½	cup(s)	120	113	22	1	5	1	<1	0.02	0.02	0.05
675	Juice, canned	½	cup(s)	122	115	21	1	5	<1	<.1	0.01	0.01	0.03
75	Juice, no salt added	½	cup(s)	122	115	21	1	5	<1	<.1	0.01	0.01	0.03
1699	Paste, canned	2	tablespoon(s)	33	24	27	1	6	1	<1	0.04	0.03	0.07
1700	Puree, canned	¼	cup(s)	63	55	24	1	6	1	<1	0.02	0.02	0.05
1125	Sauce, canned	¼	cup(s)	61	55	20	1	5	1	<1	0.02	0.02	0.06
1120	Stewed, canned, red	½	cup(s)	128	117	33	1	8	1	<1	0.03	0.04	0.10
8778	Sun dried	½	cup(s)	27	4	70	4	15	3	1	0.12	0.13	0.30
8783	Sun dried in oil, drained	¼	cup(s)	28	15	59	1	6	2	4	0.52	2.38	0.57
	Turnips												
677	Turnips, cubed, boiled, drained	½	cup(s)	78	73	17	1	4	2	<.1	0.01	0.00	0.03
678	Turnip greens, chopped, boiled, drained	½	cup(s)	72	67	14	1	3	3	<1	0.04	0.01	0.07
679	Turnip greens, frozen, chopped, boiled, drained	½	cup(s)	82	74	24	3	4	3	<1	0.08	0.02	0.14
	Vegetables, mixed												
1132	Canned, drained	½	cup(s)	82	71	40	2	8	2	<1	0.04	0.01	0.10
680	Frozen, boiled, drained	½	cup(s)	91	76	59	3	12	4	<1	0.03	0.01	0.07
7489	Vegetable juice, V8 100%	½	cup(s)	120	113	25	1	5	1	0	0.00	0.00	0.00
7490	Vegetable juice, V8 low sodium	½	cup(s)	120	113	25	0	7	1	0	0.00	0.00	0.00
7491	Vegetable juice, V8 spicy hot	½	cup(s)	120	113	25	1	5	1	0	0.00	0.00	0.00

PAGE KEY: H–2 = Breads/Baked Goods H–6 = Cereal/Rice/Pasta H–10 = Fruit H–16 = Vegetables/Legumes H–26 = Nuts/Seeds H–28 = Vegetarian H–30 = Dairy H–36 = Eggs H–38 = Seafood H–40 = Meats H–42 = Poultry H–44 = Processed meats H–46 = Beverages H–50 = Fats/Oils H–52 = Sweets H–52 = Sauces/Condiments/Spices H–56 = Mixed Foods/Soups/Sandwiches H–62 = Fast food H–80 = Convenience H–82 = Baby foods

Chol (mg)	Calc (mg)	Iron (mg)	Magn (mg)	Pota (mg)	Sodi (mg)	Zinc (mg)	Vit A (RAE) (μg)	Thia (mg)	Vit E (mg)	Ribo (mg)	Niac (mg)	Vit B_6 (mg)	Fola (μg)	Vit C (mg)	Vit B_{12} (μg)	Sele (μg)
0	94.4	0.94	22.96	102.05	6.8	0.54	0.85	0.03	0	0.03	0.45	0.04	37.42	0.17	0	7.56
0	30	0.81	24	167	24	0.16	141	0.02	0.57	0.06	0.22	0.06	58	8	0	<1
0	138	2.49	82	375	29	0.50	531	0.02	1.41	0.15	0.42	0.11	106	16	0	2
0	122	3.21	78	419	63	0.68	472	0.09	0.86	0.21	0.44	0.22	131	9	0	1
0	145	1.86	78	287	92	0.47	573	0.07	0.91	0.17	0.42	0.13	115	2	0	5
0	145	1.86	78	287	92	0.47	573	0.07	0.91	0.17	0.42	0.13	115	2	0	5
0	25	2.13	25	134	38	0.18	—	0.03	—	0.06	0.18	0.07	<.1	8	0	—
0	45	0.95	44	448	4	0.17	22	0.17	—	0.01	0.90	0.20	19	11	0	1
0	32	0.69	32	322	4	0.13	50	0.12	—	0.01	0.65	0.14	13	8	0	<1
0	42	0.62	30	291	4	0.13	572	0.07	—	0.02	0.99	0.13	19	15	0	1
0	25	0.77	12	176	3	0.16	—	0.07	—	0.05	0.61	0.09	22	5	0	1
0	23	0.70	11	162	2	0.14	406	0.05	—	0.05	0.56	0.08	19	4	0	1
0	18.2	0.41	18.2	183.73	1.73	0.25	29.46	0.04	—	0.03	0.39	0.09	19.93	7.28	0	0.17
0	17	0.48	23	367	8	0.15	310	0.08	—	0.05	0.57	0.18	16	10	0	1
0	12	0.33	15	253	6	0.12	236	0.05	0.14	0.03	0.39	0.12	12	8	0	<1
0	16	0.26	9	91	14	0.16	5	0.03	0.09	0.02	0.63	0.08	6	3	0	<1
0	24	0.32	22	173	1	0.35	10	0.04	0.11	0.04	0.46	0.06	18	5	0	<1
0	23	0.45	13	448	1	0.23	268	0.02	0.12	0.07	0.51	0.17	21	10	0	<1
0	12	0.32	20	228	3	0.16	50	0.04	0.11	0.04	0.39	0.07	15	4	0	<1
0	19	0.54	15	219	2	0.23	11	0.05	0.34	0.05	0.44	0.05	9	4	0	<1
0	38	0.69	27	475	36	0.32	961	1.45	0.28	0.11	1.49	0.29	6	20	0	<1
0	45	1.20	30	382	45	0.33	1310	0.09	0.47	0.08	0.89	0.27	10	21	0	<1
7	22	0.95	9	159	59	0.13	176	0.02	0.00	0.04	0.33	0.03	9	6	0	1
0	22	0.89	22	312	53	0.18	399	0.04	0.25	0.06	0.74	0.19	17	26	0	1
0	31	0.48	18	332	7	0.26	722	0.06	0.24	0.05	0.49	0.16	19	8	0	1
0	10	0.36	12	458	5	0.14	4	0.06	0.11	0.02	0.38	0.16	11	8	0	<1
0	10	0.29	6	241	1	0.38	2	0.03	—	0.04	0.57	0.08	2	13	0	1
0	5	0.42	14	182	1	0.15	4	0.03	0.26	0.02	1.26	0.04	5	8	0	<1
0	5	0.41	13	177	1	0.15	4	0.03	0.25	0.02	1.22	0.04	5	8	0	<1
0	12.3	0.33	13.52	291.51	6.15	0.2	76.26	0.04	0.37	0.02	0.73	0.09	18.45	15.62	0	0
0	4.25	0.37	9.35	188.69	7.65	0.07	52.7	0.05	0.25	0.03	0.53	0.07	—	16.23	0	—
0	9	0.24	10	213	5	0.15	38	0.03	0.34	0.02	0.53	0.07	14	11	0	0
0	13	0.82	11	262	13	0.17	29	0.04	0.46	0.03	0.64	0.09	16	27	0	1
0	12	0.52	13	279	328	0.18	28	0.06	1.11	0.04	0.82	0.14	24	22	0	<1
0	12	0.52	13	279	12	0.18	28	0.06	1.11	0.04	0.82	0.14	24	22	0	<1
0	12	0.98	14	333	259	0.21	25	0.02	1.41	0.05	1.01	0.07	4	7	0	2
0	11	1.11	14	274	249	0.23	16	0.02	1.58	0.05	0.92	0.08	7	7	0	3
0	8	0.62	10	203	321	0.12	10	0.01	0.86	0.04	0.60	0.06	6	4	0	<1
0	43	1.70	15	264	282	0.22	11	0.06	0.48	0.04	0.91	0.02	6	10	0	1
0	30	2.45	52	925	566	0.54	12	0.14	0.00	0.13	2.44	0.09	18	11	0	1
0	13	0.74	22	430	73	0.21	18	0.05	—	0.11	1.00	0.09	6	28	0	1
0	26	0.14	7	138	12	0.09	0	0.02	0.02	0.02	0.23	0.05	7	9	0	<1
0	99	0.58	16	146	21	0.10	274	0.03	1.24	0.05	0.30	0.13	85	20	0	1
0	125	1.59	21	184	12	0.34	441	0.04	2.39	0.06	0.38	0.05	32	18	0	1
0	22	0.86	13	237	121	0.33	474	0.04	0.49	0.04	0.47	0.06	20	4	0	<1
0	23	0.75	20	154	32	0.45	195	0.06	0.33	0.11	0.77	0.07	17	3	0	<1
0	20	0.54	13	270	310	0.24	50	0.05	0.38	0.03	0.87	0.17	—	30	0	—
0	20	0.36	—	420	70	—	63	0.02	—	0.02	0.75	—	—	30	0	—
0	20	0.36	13	255	370	0.24	50	0.05	0.38	0.03	0.88	0.17	—	18	0	—

H Appendix

Table H–1

Food Composition (Computer code number is for Wadsworth Diet Analysis program) (For purposes of calculations, use "0" for t, <1, <.1, <.01, etc.)

DA + Code	Food Description	Quantity	Measure	Wt (g)	H_2O (g)	Ener (kcal)	Prot (g)	Carb (g)	Dietary Fiber (g)	Fat (g)	Fat Breakdown (g) Sat	Mono	Poly
	VEGETABLES, LEGUMES—Continued												
	Water chestnuts												
31073	Sliced, drained	½	cup(s)	75	70	20	<1	5	1	0	0.00	0.00	0.00
31087	Whole	½	cup(s)	75	70	20	<1	5	1	0	0.00	0.00	0.00
1135	**Watercress**	1	cup(s)	34	32	4	1	<1	<1	<.1	0.01	0.00	0.01
	NUTS, SEEDS, AND PRODUCTS												
	Almonds												
32886	Blanched	¼	cup(s)	36	2	211	8	7	4	18	1.41	11.70	4.37
32887	Dry roasted, no salt added	¼	cup(s)	35	1	206	8	7	4	18	1.40	11.61	4.36
29724	Dry roasted, salted	¼	cup(s)	35	1	206	8	7	4	18	1.40	11.61	4.36
29725	Oil roasted, salted	¼	cup(s)	39	1	238	8	7	4	22	1.65	13.66	5.31
508	Slivered	¼	cup(s)	34	2	195	7	7	4	17	1.31	10.85	4.12
1137	Almond butter, no salt added	1	tablespoon(s)	16	<1	101	2	3	1	9	0.90	6.14	1.98
32940	Almond butter, salt added	1	tablespoon(s)	16	<1	101	2	3	1	9	0.90	6.14	1.98
1138	**Beechnuts, dried**	¼	cup(s)	57	4	327	4	19	5	28	3.25	12.43	11.41
517	**Brazil nuts, unblanched, dried**	¼	cup(s)	35	1	230	5	4	3	23	5.30	8.59	7.20
1166	**Breadfruit seeds, roasted**	¼	cup(s)	57	28	118	4	23	3	2	0.41	0.20	0.82
1139	**Butternuts, dried**	¼	cup(s)	30	1	184	7	4	1	17	0.39	3.13	12.82
	Cashews												
1140	Dry roasted	¼	cup(s)	34	1	197	5	11	1	16	3.14	9.36	2.68
518	Oil roasted	¼	cup(s)	33	1	189	5	10	1	16	2.76	8.42	2.78
32889	Cashew butter, no salt added	1	tablespoon(s)	16	<1	94	3	4	<1	8	1.56	4.66	1.34
32931	Cashew butter, salt added	1	tablespoon(s)	16	<1	94	3	4	<1	8	1.56	4.66	1.34
	Coconut												
32896	Dried, not sweetened	¼	cup(s)	60	2	393	4	14	10	38	34.06	1.63	0.42
1153	Dried, shredded, sweetened	¼	cup(s)	24	3	122	1	12	1	9	7.68	0.37	0.09
520	Shredded	¼	cup(s)	21	10	75	1	3	2	7	6.27	0.30	0.08
	Chestnuts												
1152	Chinese, roasted	¼	cup(s)	57	23	136	3	30	0	1	0.10	0.35	0.17
32895	European, boiled & steamed	¼	cup(s)	57	39	74	1	16	0	1	0.15	0.27	0.31
32911	European, roasted	¼	cup(s)	57	23	139	2	30	3	1	0.23	0.43	0.49
32922	Japanese, boiled & steamed	¼	cup(s)	57	49	32	<1	7	0	<1	0.02	0.06	0.03
32923	Japanese, roasted	¼	cup(s)	57	28	114	2	26	0	<1	0.07	0.24	0.12
4958	**Flaxseeds or linseeds**	¼	cup(s)	57	5	276	11	19	16	19	1.79	3.85	12.54
32904	**Ginkgo nuts, dried**	¼	cup(s)	57	7	197	6	41	0	1	0.22	0.42	0.42
	Hazelnuts or filberts												
32901	Blanched	¼	cup(s)	57	3	357	8	10	6	35	2.65	27.32	3.15
32902	Dry roasted, no salt added	¼	cup(s)	57	1	366	9	10	5	35	2.56	26.43	4.80
1156	**Hickorynuts, dried**	¼	cup(s)	30	1	197	4	5	2	19	2.11	9.78	6.57
	Macadamias												
1157	Raw	¼	cup(s)	34	<1	241	3	5	3	25	4.04	19.72	0.50
32905	Dry roasted, no salt added	¼	cup(s)	34	1	241	3	4	3	25	4.00	19.86	0.50
32932	Dry roasted, salt added	¼	cup(s)	34	1	240	3	4	3	25	4.00	19.86	0.50
	Mixed nuts												
1159	With peanuts, dry roasted	¼	cup(s)	34	1	203	6	9	3	18	2.36	10.75	3.69
32933	With peanuts, dry roasted, salt added	¼	cup(s)	34	1	203	6	9	3	18	2.36	10.75	3.69
32906	Without peanuts, oil roasted, no salt added	¼	cup(s)	36	1	221	6	8	2	20	3.27	11.93	4.12
	Peanuts												
2807	Dry roasted	¼	cup(s)	37	0	214	9	8	3	18	2.51	8.99	5.72
2806	Dry roasted, salted	¼	cup(s)	37	0	214	9	8	3	18	2.51	8.99	5.72
1763	Oil roasted, salted	¼	cup(s)	36	0	216	10	5	3	19	3.12	9.33	5.49
2804	Raw	¼	cup(s)	37	2	207	9	6	3	18	2.49	8.92	5.68
1884	Peanut butter, chunky	1	tablespoon(s)	16	<1	94	4	3	1	8	1.53	3.77	2.27
30303	Peanut butter, low sodium	1	tablespoon(s)	16	<1	95	4	3	1	8	1.66	3.88	2.21
30305	Peanut butter, reduced fat	1	tablespoon(s)	18	<1	94	5	6	1	6	1.33	2.91	1.85
524	Peanut butter, smooth	1	tablespoon(s)	16	<1	96	4	3	1	8	1.60	3.96	2.38
	Pecans												
32907	Dry roasted, no salt added	¼	cup(s)	57	1	403	5	8	5	42	3.56	24.92	11.66
32936	Dry roasted, salt added	¼	cup(s)	57	1	403	5	8	5	42	3.56	24.92	11.66
1162	Halves, oil roasted	¼	cup(s)	28	<1	197	3	4	3	21	1.99	11.27	6.49

PAGE KEY: H–2 = Breads/Baked Goods H–6 = Cereal/Rice/Pasta H–10 = Fruit H–16 = Vegetables/Legumes H–26 = Nuts/Seeds H–28 = Vegetarian H–30 = Dairy H–36 = Eggs H–38 = Seafood H–40 = Meats H–42 = Poultry H–44 = Processed meats H–46 = Beverages H–50 = Fats/Oils H–52 = Sweets H–52 = Sauces/Condiments/Spices H–56 = Mixed Foods/Soups/Sandwiches H–62 = Fast food H–80 = Convenience H–82 = Baby foods

Chol (mg)	Calc (mg)	Iron (mg)	Magn (mg)	Pota (mg)	Sodi (mg)	Zinc (mg)	Vit A (RAE) (μg)	Thia (mg)	Vit E (mg)	Ribo (mg)	Niac (mg)	Vit B_6 (mg)	Fola (μg)	Vit C (mg)	Vit B_{12} (μg)	Sele (μg)
0	7	0.23	—	—	6	—	0	—	—	—	—	—	—	2	—	—
0	7	0.23	—	—	6	—	0	—	—	—	—	—	—	2	—	—
0	41	0.07	7	112	14	0.04	80	0.03	0.34	0.04	0.07	0.04	3	15	0	<1
0	78	1.35	100	249	10	1.13	0	0.07	9.06	0.20	1.33	0.04	11	0	0	1
0	92	1.56	99	257	<1	1.22	0	0.03	9.07	0.30	1.33	0.04	11	0	0	1
0	92	1.56	99	257	117	1.22	0	0.03	9.07	0.30	1.33	0.04	11	0	0	1
0	114	1.44	108	274	133	1.20	0	0.04	10.31	0.31	1.44	0.05	11	0	0	1
0	84	1.45	93	246	<1	1.13	0	0.08	8.84	0.27	1.32	0.04	10	0	0	1
0	43	0.59	48	121	2	0.49	0	0.02	3.25	0.10	0.46	0.01	10	<1	0	—
0	43	0.59	48	121	72	0.49	0	0.02	3.24	0.10	0.46	0.01	10	<1	0	1
0	1	1.40	0	578	22	0.20	0	0.17	—	0.21	0.50	0.39	64	9	0	4
0	56	0.85	132	231	1	1.42	0	0.22	2.66	0.01	0.10	0.04	8	<1	0	671
0	49	0.51	35	615	16	0.59	9	0.23	—	0.14	4.20	0.24	34	4	0	8
0	16	1.21	71	126	<1	0.94	2	0.11	1.05	0.04	0.31	0.17	20	1	0	5
0	15	2.06	89	194	5	1.92	0	0.07	0.20	0.07	0.48	0.09	24	0	0	4
0	14	1.97	89	205	4	1.74	0	0.12	0.48	0.07	0.56	0.10	8	<.1	0	7
0	7	0.80	41	87	2	0.83	0	0.05	0.25	0.03	0.26	0.04	11	0	0	2
0	7	0.80	41	87	98	0.83	0	0.05	0.25	0.03	0.26	0.04	11	0	0	2
0	15	1.98	54	323	22	1.20	0	0.04	0.80	0.06	0.36	0.18	5	1	0	11
0	4	0.47	12	82	64	0.44	0	0.01	0.33	0.00	0.12	0.07	2	<1	0	4
0	3	0.51	7	75	4	0.23	0	0.01	0.15	0.00	0.11	0.01	5	1	0	2
0	11	0.85	51	271	2	0.53	0	0.09	—	0.05	0.85	0.25	41	22	0	4
0	26	0.98	31	405	15	0.14	1	0.08	0.00	0.06	0.41	0.13	22	15	0	—
0	16	0.52	19	336	1	0.32	1	0.14	0.68	0.10	0.76	0.28	40	15	0	1
0	6	0.30	10	67	3	0.23	1	0.07	—	0.03	0.31	0.06	10	5	0	—
0	20	1.19	36	242	11	0.81	2	0.26	—	—	0.40	0.24	33	16	0	—
0	111	3.48	203	381	19	2.34	0	0.10	2.80	0.09	0.78	0.52	156	1	0	3
0	11	0.91	30	566	7	0.38	31	0.24	—	0.10	6.65	0.36	60	17	0	—
0	84	1.87	91	373	0	1.25	1	0.27	10.15	0.06	0.88	0.33	44	1	0	2
0	70	2.48	98	428	0	1.42	2	0.19	8.75	0.07	1.16	0.35	50	2	0	2
0	18	0.64	52	131	<1	1.29	2	0.26	1.56	0.04	0.27	0.06	12	1	0	2
0	28	1.24	44	123	2	0.44	0	0.40	0.18	0.05	0.83	0.09	4	<1	0	1
0	23	0.89	40	122	1	0.43	0	0.24	0.19	0.03	0.76	0.12	3	<1	0	1
0	23	0.89	40	122	89	0.43	0	0.24	0.19	0.03	0.76	0.12	3	<1	0	4
0	24	1.27	77	204	4	1.30	<1	0.07	2.06	0.07	1.61	0.10	17	<1	0	1
0	24	1.27	77	204	229	1.30	0	0.07	2.06	0.07	1.61	0.10	17	<1	0	3
0	38	0.93	90	196	4	1.68	<1	0.18	2.16	0.17	0.71	0.06	20	<1	0	—
0	20	0.82	64	240	2	1.20	0	0.15	2.27	0.03	4.93	0.09	53	0	0	3
0	20	0.82	64	240	297	1.20	0	0.15	2.16	0.03	4.93	0.09	53	0	0	3
0	22	0.54	63	261	115	1.18	0	0.03	2.13	0.03	4.97	0.16	43	<1	0	1
0	34	1.67	61	257	7	1.19	0	0.23	3.33	0.05	4.40	0.13	88	0	0	3
0	8	0.33	31	101	75	0.52	0	0.02	—	0.02	2.19	0.07	15	0	0	1
0	6	0.29	25	107	3	0.47	0	0.01	1.60	0.02	2.14	0.07	12	0	0	—
0	6	0.34	31	120	97	0.50	0	0.05	1.20	0.01	2.63	0.06	11	0	0	—
0	8	0.30	28	88	80	0.47	0	0.01	1.60	0.02	2.14	0.07	12	0	0	1
0	41	1.59	75	240	1	2.87	4	0.26	2.13	0.06	0.66	0.11	9	<1	0	2
0	41	1.59	75	240	217	2.87	4	0.26	2.13	0.06	0.66	0.11	9	<1	0	2
0	18	0.68	33	108	<1	1.23	1	0.13	1.42	0.03	0.33	0.05	4	<1	0	2

Table H-1

Food Composition (Computer code number is for Wadsworth Diet Analysis program) (For purposes of calculations, use "0" for t, <1, <.1, <.01, etc.)

DA + Code	Food Description	Quantity	Measure	Wt (g)	H_2O (g)	Ener (kcal)	Prot (g)	Carb (g)	Dietary Fiber (g)	Fat (g)	Fat Breakdown (g) Sat	Mono	Poly
	NUTS, SEEDS, AND PRODUCTS—Continued												
526	Raw	¼	cup(s)	27	1	187	2	4	3	19	1.67	11.02	5.84
12973	**Pine nuts or pignolia, dried**	1	tablespoon(s)	9	<1	58	1	1	<1	6	0.42	1.61	2.93
	Pistachios												
1164	Dry roasted	¼	cup(s)	32	1	183	7	9	3	15	1.78	7.75	4.45
32938	Dry roasted, salt added	¼	cup(s)	32	1	182	7	9	3	15	1.78	7.75	4.45
1167	**Pumpkin or squash seeds, roasted**	¼	cup(s)	57	4	296	19	8	2	24	4.52	7.43	10.90
	Sesame												
1169	Sesame seeds, whole, roasted, toasted	3	teaspoon(s)	9	<1	51	2	2	1	4	0.60	1.63	1.89
32912	Sesame butter paste	1	tablespoon(s)	16	<1	95	3	4	1	8	1.14	3.07	3.57
32941	Tahini or sesame butter	1	tablespoon(s)	15	<1	89	3	3	1	8	1.11	3.00	3.48
	Soy nuts												
34173	Deep sea salted	¼	cup(s)	56	—	240	24	18	10	8	2.00	—	—
34174	Unsalted	¼	cup(s)	56	—	240	24	18	10	8	2.00	—	—
	Sunflower seeds												
528	Kernels, dried	¼	cup(s)	36	2	205	8	7	4	18	1.87	3.41	11.78
29721	Kernels, dry roasted, salted	¼	cup(s)	32	<1	186	6	8	3	16	1.67	3.04	10.52
29723	Kernels, toasted, salted	¼	cup(s)	34	<1	207	6	7	4	19	1.99	3.63	12.56
32928	Sunflower seed butter, salt added	1	tablespoon(s)	16	<1	93	3	4	0	8	0.80	1.46	5.04
	Trail mix												
4646	Trail mix	¼	cup(s)	38	3	173	5	17	2	11	2.08	4.70	3.62
4647	Trail mix with chocolate chips	¼	cup(s)	38	2	182	5	17	0	12	2.29	5.08	4.23
4648	Tropical trail mix	¼	cup(s)	35	3	142	2	23	0	6	2.97	0.87	1.81
	Walnuts												
529	Dried black, chopped	¼	cup(s)	31	1	193	8	3	2	18	1.05	4.69	10.96
531	English or persian	¼	cup(s)	30	1	196	5	4	2	20	1.84	2.68	14.15
	VEGETARIAN FOODS												
	Prepared												
34222	Brown rice & tofu stir-fry (vegan)	8	ounce(s)	227	183	228	12	13	3	16	1.25	4.03	9.54
34368	Cheese enchilada casserole (lacto)	8	ounce(s)	227	86	410	18	41	4	19	10.06	6.54	1.24
34247	Five bean casserole (vegan)	8	ounce(s)	228	178	178	6	26	5	6	1.11	2.49	1.96
34261	Lentil stew (vegan)	8	ounce(s)	228	152	125	8	24	7	<1	0.08	0.07	0.21
34397	Macaroni & cheese (lacto)	8	ounce(s)	226	163	181	8	17	<1	9	4.37	2.88	0.89
34238	Steamed rice & vegetables (vegan)	8	ounce(s)	228	100	265	5	40	3	10	1.84	3.91	4.07
34308	Tofu rice burgers (ovo-lacto)	1	piece(s)	218	78	435	22	68	6	8	1.69	2.39	3.52
34276	Vegan spinach enchiladas (vegan)	1	piece(s)	82	59	93	5	15	2	2	0.34	0.55	1.27
34243	Vegetable chow mein (vegan)	8	ounce(s)	227	163	166	6	22	2	6	0.65	2.66	2.47
34454	Vegetable lasagna (lacto)	8	ounce(s)	225	154	177	12	25	2	4	1.92	0.93	0.34
34339	Vegetable marinara (vegan)	8	ounce(s)	229	182	94	3	15	1	3	0.36	1.32	0.92
34356	Vegetable rice casserole (lacto)	8	ounce(s)	227	172	230	9	24	4	12	4.67	3.48	2.96
34311	Vegetable strudel (ovo-lacto)	8	ounce(s)	227	100	756	19	51	4	54	18.24	26.38	6.17
34371	Vegetable taco (lacto)	1	item(s)	227	147	365	13	43	9	17	6.45	5.81	4.02
34282	Vegetarian chili (vegan)	8	ounce(s)	227	196	116	6	21	7	2	0.24	0.29	0.74
34367	Vegetarian vegetable soup (vegan)	8	ounce(s)	226	204	92	3	14	2	4	0.77	1.67	1.30
	Boca burger												
32067	All American flamed grilled patty	1	item(s)	71	—	110	14	6	4	4	1.00	—	—
32070	Bigger chef max's favorite	1	item(s)	99	—	130	18	11	5	4	1.00	1.00	1.50
32069	Bigger vegan	1	item(s)	99	—	120	18	11	6	0	0.00	0.00	0.00
32074	Boca chik'n nuggets	4	item(s)	87	—	190	16	16	2	7	2.00	—	—
32075	Boca meatless ground burger	½	cup(s)	57	—	70	11	7	4	1	0.00	—	—
32073	Boca tenders	1	item(s)	85	—	140	20	9	3	3	0.00	2.00	1.00
32072	Breakfast links	2	item(s)	45	—	100	10	6	5	4	0.00	—	—
32071	Breakfast patties	1	item(s)	38	—	80	8	5	3	4	0.00	—	—
32068	Roasted garlic patty	1	item(s)	71	—	100	14	7	5	2	0.50	—	—
32066	Vegan original patty	1	item(s)	71	—	90	13	4	0	1	0.00	—	—
	Gardenburger												
37810	Bbq chik'n with sauce	1	item(s)	142	—	250	14	30	5	8	1.00	—	—
39661	Black bean burger	1	item(s)	71	—	80	8	11	4	2	0.00	—	—
39666	Buffalo chick'n wing	3	item(s)	95	—	180	9	8	5	12	1.50	—	—
37808	Chik'n grill	1	item(s)	71	—	100	13	5	3	3	0.00	—	—

PAGE KEY: H–2 = Breads/Baked Goods H–6 = Cereal/Rice/Pasta H–10 = Fruit H–16 = Vegetables/Legumes H–26 = Nuts/Seeds H–28 = Vegetarian H–30 = Dairy H–36 = Eggs H–38 = Seafood H–40 = Meats H–42 = Poultry H–44 = Processed meats H–46 = Beverages H–50 = Fats/Oils H–52 = Sweets H–52 = Sauces/Condiments/Spices H–56 = Mixed Foods/Soups/Sandwiches H–62 = Fast food H–80 = Convenience H–82 = Baby foods

Chol (mg)	Calc (mg)	Iron (mg)	Magn (mg)	Pota (mg)	Sodi (mg)	Zinc (mg)	Vit A (RAE) (µg)	Thia (mg)	Vit E (mg)	Ribo (mg)	Niac (mg)	Vit B_6 (mg)	Fola (µg)	Vit C (mg)	Vit B_{12} (µg)	Sele (µg)
0	19	0.68	33	111	0	1.22	1	0.18	1.09	0.04	0.32	0.06	6	<1	0	1
0	1	0.48	22	51	<1	0.55	<.1	0.03	0.30	0.02	0.38	0.01	6	<.1	0	<.1
					<1											
0	35	1.34	38	333	<1	0.74	4	0.27	1.36	0.05	0.46	0.41	16	1	0	3
0	35	1.34	38	333	<1	0.74	4	0.27	1.36	0.05	0.46	0.41	16	1	0	3
0	24	8.48	303	457	10	4.22	11	0.12	0.57	0.18	0.99	0.05	32	1	0	3
0	89	1.33	32	43	1	0.64	0	0.07	—	0.02	0.41	0.07	9	0	0	1
0	154	3.07	58	93	2	1.17	<1	0.04	0.36	0.03	1.07	0.13	16	0	0	1
0	21	0.66	14	69	5	0.69	<1	0.24	0.34	0.02	0.85	0.02	15	1	0	<1
0	120	2.16	—	—	300	—	0	—	—	—	—	—	—	0	—	—
0	120	2.16	—	—	20	—	0	—	—	—	—	—	—	0	—	—
0	42	2.44	127	248	1	1.82	1	0.82	18.10	0.09	1.62	0.28	82	1	0	21
0	22	1.22	41	272	250	1.69	<1	0.03	16.09	0.08	2.25	0.26	76	<1	0	25
0	19	2.28	43	164	205	1.78	0	0.11	—	0.10	1.41	0.27	80	<1	0	21
0	20	0.76	59	12	83	0.85	<1	0.05	—	0.05	0.85	0.13	38	<1	0	—
0	29	1.14	59	257	86	1.21	<1	0.17	—	0.07	1.77	0.11	27	1	0	—
2	41	1.27	60	243	45	1.18	1	0.15	—	0.08	1.65	0.10	24	<1	0	—
0	20	0.92	34	248	4	0.41	1	0.16	—	0.04	0.52	0.11	15	3	0	—
0	19	0.98	63	163	1	1.05	1	0.02	1.47	0.04	0.15	0.18	10	1	0	5
0	29	0.87	47	132	1	0.93	<1	0.10	0.87	0.05	0.34	0.16	29	<1	0	1
0	266	4.73	88	375	112	1.51	121	0.14	1.29	0.12	1.08	0.28	32	18	0	11
42	468	2.58	37	204	1219	1.96	107	0.33	0.96	0.38	2.38	0.11	77	22	<1	22
0	48	1.71	42	367	618	0.60	54	0.09	1.69	0.08	0.93	0.11	33	8	<.1	4
0	23	2.35	31	380	289	0.87	18	0.14	1.08	0.10	1.50	0.16	61	13	0	9
22	187	0.77	20	120	768	1.11	82	0.15	0.46	0.24	1.02	0.04	39	<.1	<1	16
0	41	1.43	68	358	1403	0.91	86	0.16	2.23	0.12	2.76	0.30	28	13	<.1	8
51	468	4.78	90	455	2454	2.07	82	0.27	0.32	0.27	3.43	0.30	99	2	<1	43
0	117	1.13	40	168	134	0.68	26	0.07	0.26	0.07	0.54	0.11	46	1	0	5
0	190	3.65	28	302	371	0.74	8	0.13	1.00	0.12	1.43	0.15	47	7	0	6
10	144	1.91	33	393	637	1.06	31	0.20	1.13	0.27	2.07	0.21	64	15	<1	19
0	15	0.85	17	180	378	0.35	18	0.13	1.31	0.08	1.25	0.11	41	20	0	10
16	176	1.72	28	395	609	1.19	121	0.16	2.18	0.29	1.93	0.18	92	54	<1	6
46	318	3.36	39	299	813	1.98	288	0.45	6.23	0.50	4.52	0.16	123	27	<1	31
21	231	2.58	83	550	893	1.80	81	0.23	2.00	0.18	1.48	0.25	132	12	<1	10
<1	68	2.42	41	532	383	0.78	46	0.13	1.48	0.13	1.26	0.18	58	16	0	5
0	37	1.32	28	443	503	0.44	109	0.11	1.69	0.08	1.54	0.22	38	24	<.1	1
3	150	1.80	—	—	370	—	0	—	—	—	—	—	—	0	—	—
5	150	2.70	—	—	400	—	—	—	—	—	—	—	—	0	—	—
0	60	1.80	—	—	380	—	0	—	—	—	—	—	—	2	—	—
0	80	1.80	—	220	570	—	0	—	—	—	—	—	—	0	—	—
0	80	1.44	—	—	220	—	0	—	—	—	—	—	—	0	—	—
0	80	1.08	—	—	440	—	0	—	—	—	—	—	—	0	—	—
0	60	1.44	—	—	330	—	0	—	—	—	—	—	—	0	—	—
0	60	1.44	—	—	260	—	0	—	—	—	—	—	—	0	—	—
3	100	1.80	—	—	400	—	0	—	—	—	—	—	—	1	—	—
0	80	1.80	—	—	350	—	0	—	—	—	—	—	—	1	—	—
0	150	1.08	—	—	890	—	—	—	—	—	—	—	—	0	—	—
0	40	1.44	—	—	330	—	—	—	—	—	—	—	—	0	—	—
0	40	0.72	—	—	1000	—	—	—	—	—	—	—	—	0	—	—
0	60	3.60	—	—	360	—	—	—	—	—	—	—	—	0	—	—

Table H–1

Food Composition (Computer code number is for Wadsworth Diet Analysis program) (For purposes of calculations, use "0" for t, <1, <.1, <.01, etc.)

DA + Code	Food Description	Quantity	Measure	Wt (g)	H_2O (g)	Ener (kcal)	Prot (g)	Carb (g)	Dietary Fiber (g)	Fat (g)	Fat Breakdown (g) Sat	Mono	Poly
	VEGETARIAN FOODS—Continued												
39665	Country fried chicken w/creamy pepper gravy	1	item(s)	142	—	190	9	16	2	9	1.00	—	—
37805	Crispy nuggets	6	item(s)	82	—	180	4	22	3	9	1.50	—	—
39663	Homestyle classic burger	1	item(s)	71	—	110	12	6	4	5	0.50	—	—
37807	Meatless breakfast sausage	1	item(s)	43	—	50	5	2	2	4	0.00	—	—
37809	Meatless meatballs	6	item(s)	85	—	110	12	8	4	5	1.00	—	—
37806	Meatless riblets w/sauce	1	item(s)	142	—	210	17	11	4	5	0.00	—	—
29913	Original	3	ounce(s)	85	—	132	7	19	4	4	1.80	1.80	0.60
31707	Santa Fe	3	ounce(s)	85	—	156	—	24	5	3	1.20	—	—
29915	Veggie medley	3	ounce(s)	85	—	108	6	22	4	0	0.00	0.00	0.00
	Loma Linda												
9311	Big franks	1	item(s)	51	30	110	10	2	2	7	1.00	2.00	4.00
9315	Chik'n nuggets	5	item(s)	85	40	240	14	13	4	15	2.00	4.50	8.00
9317	Corn dogs	1	item(s)	71	31	150	7	22	3	4	0.50	1.00	2.50
9323	Fried chik'n with gravy	2	piece(s)	80	46	150	12	5	2	10	1.50	2.50	5.00
9326	Linketts, canned	1	item(s)	35	21	70	7	1	1	5	0.50	1.00	2.50
9336	Redi-Burger patties, canned	1	slice(s)	85	50	120	18	7	4	3	0.50	0.50	1.50
9354	Tender Rounds meatball substitute, canned in gravy	6	piece(s)	80	54	120	13	6	1	5	0.50	1.00	2.50
	Morningstar Farms												
33707	America's Original Veggie Dog links	1	item(s)	57	—	80	11	6	1	1	0.00	0.00	0.00
9362	Better n Eggs egg substitute	¼	cup(s)	57	50	20	5	0	0	0	0.00	0.00	0.00
9368	Breakfast links	2	item(s)	45	27	80	9	3	2	3	0.50	0.50	2.00
9371	Breakfast strips	2	item(s)	16	7	60	2	2	1	5	0.50	1.00	3.00
33705	Chik Nuggets	4	piece(s)	86	—	180	13	17	5	6	0.50	1.50	4.00
11587	Chik Patties	1	item(s)	71	36	150	9	16	2	6	1.00	1.50	2.50
2531	Garden veggie patties	1	item(s)	67	40	100	10	9	4	3	0.50	0.50	1.50
9412	Natural Touch low fat vegetarian chili, canned	1	cup(s)	230	173	170	18	21	11	1	—	—	—
33702	Spicy black bean veggie burger	1	item(s)	78	47	150	11	16	5	5	0.50	1.50	2.50
	Worthington												
9422	Chik Stiks	1	item(s)	47	27	110	10	4	2	6	1.00	1.00	3.00
9424	Chili, canned	1	cup(s)	230	167	290	19	21	9	15	2.50	3.50	9.00
9432	Crispychik patties	1	item(s)	71	37	150	9	16	2	6	1.00	1.50	3.50
9440	Dinner roast, frozen	1	slice(s)	85	53	180	12	5	3	12	1.50	5.00	5.00
9442	Fillets, frozen	2	piece(s)	85	48	180	16	8	4	9	1.00	3.50	4.50
9478	Meatless smoked beef, sliced	6	slice(s)	57	—	130	11	7	1	7	1.00	2.00	4.00
9480	Meatless smoked turkey, sliced	3	slice(s)	57	—	140	10	5	0	9	1.00	2.50	5.00
9462	Prosage links	2	item(s)	45	27	80	9	3	2	3	0.50	0.50	2.00
9486	Stripples bacon substitute	2	item(s)	16	7	60	2	2	1	5	0.50	1.00	2.50
9496	Vegetable Skallops	½	cup(s)	85	65	90	15	3	3	2	0.50	0.50	0.00
9434	Vegetarian cutlets	1	slice(s)	61	43	70	11	3	2	1	—	—	—
	DAIRY												
	Butter: *see* Fats & Oils												
	Cheese												
1433	Blue, crumbled	1	ounce(s)	28	12	100	6	1	0	8	5.29	2.21	0.23
884	Brick	1	ounce(s)	28	12	104	7	1	0	8	5.25	2.41	0.22
885	Brie	1	ounce(s)	28	14	94	6	<1	0	8	4.87	2.24	0.23
34821	Camembert	1	ounce(s)	29	15	87	6	<1	0	7	4.43	2.04	0.21
888	Cheddar or colby	1	ounce(s)	28	11	110	7	1	0	9	5.66	2.60	0.27
32096	Cheddar or colby, low fat	1	ounce(s)	28	18	49	7	1	0	2	1.23	0.59	0.06
5	Cheddar, shredded	¼	cup(s)	28	10	114	7	<1	0	9	5.96	2.65	0.27
889	Edam	1	ounce(s)	28	12	100	7	<1	0	8	4.92	2.28	0.19
890	Feta	1	ounce(s)	28	15	74	4	1	0	6	4.18	1.29	0.17
891	Fontina	1	ounce(s)	28	11	109	7	<1	0	9	5.37	2.43	0.46
8527	Goat, soft	1	ounce(s)	28	17	76	5	<1	0	6	4.14	1.37	0.14
893	Gouda	1	ounce(s)	28	12	100	7	1	0	8	4.93	2.17	0.18
894	Gruyere	1	ounce(s)	28	9	116	8	<1	0	9	5.30	2.81	0.49
895	Limburger	1	ounce(s)	28	14	92	6	<1	0	8	4.69	2.41	0.14
896	Monterey jack	1	ounce(s)	28	11	104	7	<1	0	8	5.34	2.45	0.25

PAGE KEY: H–2 = Breads/Baked Goods H–6 = Cereal/Rice/Pasta H–10 = Fruit H–16 = Vegetables/Legumes H–26 = Nuts/Seeds H–28 = Vegetarian H–30 = Dairy H–36 = Eggs H–38 = Seafood H–40 = Meats H–42 = Poultry H–44 = Processed meats H–46 = Beverages H–50 = Fats/Oils H–52 = Sweets H–52 = Sauces/Condiments/Spices H–56 = Mixed Foods/Soups/Sandwiches H–62 = Fast food H–80 = Convenience H–82 = Baby foods

Chol (mg)	Calc (mg)	Iron (mg)	Magn (mg)	Pota (mg)	Sodi (mg)	Zinc (mg)	Vit A (RAE) (µg)	Thia (mg)	Vit E (mg)	Ribo (mg)	Niac (mg)	Vit B_6 (mg)	Fola (µg)	Vit C (mg)	Vit B_{12} (µg)	Sele (µg)
5	40	1.44	—	—	550	—	—	—	—	—	—	—	—	0	—	—
5	60	0.72	—	—	570	—	—	—	—	—	—	—	—	5	—	—
0	80	1.44	—	—	380	—	—	—	—	—	—	—	—	0	—	—
0	20	0.72	—	—	120	—	—	—	—	—	—	—	—	0	—	—
0	60	1.80	—	—	400	—	—	—	—	—	—	—	—	0	—	—
0	60	1.80	—	—	720	—	—	—	—	—	—	—	—	4	—	—
24	72	0.00	37	232	672	1.07	0	0.12	0.24	0.18	1.30	0.10	12	0	<1	8
24	96	0.00	—	—	336	—	0	—	—	—	—	—	—	0		0
0	48	0.00	32	218	336	0.55	—	0.08	0.31	0.10	1.08	0.11	13	0	<.1	5
0	0	0.77	—	50	240	0.89	0	0.23	—	0.43	1.60	0.04	—	0	1	—
0	20	1.44	—	210	410	0.43	0	0.75	—	0.51	6.00	0.90	—	0	3	—
0	0	1.08	—	60	500	0.43	0	0.72	—	0.61	1.47	0.87	—	0	2	—
0	20	1.80	—	70	430	0.34	0	1.05	—	0.34	4.00	0.30	—	0	2	—
0	0	0.36	—	15	160	0.46	0	0.12	—	0.20	0.40	0.20	—	0	1	—
0	0	1.06	—	140	450	1.11	0	0.23	—	0.34	6.00	0.40	—	0	2	—
0	20	1.08	—	80	340	0.66	0	0.75	—	0.17	2.00	0.16	—	0	1	—
0	0	0.72	—	60	580	—	0	—	—	—	—	—	—	0	—	—
0	20	0.63	—	75	90	0.60	75	0.03	0.81	0.34	0.00	0.08	24	0	1	—
0	0	1.44	—	50	320	0.36	0	1.80	—	0.17	2.00	0.30	—	0	3	—
0	0	0.27	—	15	220	0.05	0	0.75	—	0.04	0.40	0.07	—	0	<1	—
0	40	3.60	—	330	590	—	0	1.20	—	0.26	5.00	0.40	—	0	3	—
0	0	1.80	—	210	540	0.31	0	1.80	—	0.17	2.00	0.20	—	0	1	—
0	40	0.72	—	180	350	0.58	—	6.47	—	0.10	0.00	0.00	—	0	0	—
0	40	1.80	—	480	870	1.36	—	0.60	—	0.21	0.00	0.30	—	0	0	—
0	40	1.80	44	320	470	0.93	0	—	—	0.14	0.00	0.21	—	0	<.1	—
0	20	1.80	—	100	300	0.31	0	0.60	—	0.17	6.00	0.40	—	0	2	—
0	40	3.60	—	420	1130	1.24	0	0.06	—	0.07	2.00	0.70	—	0	2	—
0	0	1.80	—	170	440	0.33	0	1.80	—	0.17	2.00	0.20	—	0	1	—
3	40	0.36	—	55	580	0.64	0	1.80	—	0.26	6.00	0.60	—	0	2	—
0	0	1.80	—	130	750	0.92	0	0.68	—	0.14	0.80	0.40	—	0	3	—
0	20	1.80	—	180	510	0.14	0	1.80	—	0.17	6.00	0.40	—	0	2	—
0	100	2.70	—	60	490	0.23	0	1.80	—	0.17	6.00	0.40	—	0	3	—
0	0	1.44	—	50	320	0.36	0	1.80	—	0.17	2.00	0.30	—	0	3	—
0	0	0.36	—	15	220	0.05	0	0.75	—	0.03	0.40	0.08	—	0	<1	—
0	0	0.72	—	10	410	0.67	0	0.03	—	0.03	0.00	0.01	—	0	0	—
0	0	0.00	—	30	340	0.43	0	0.03	—	0.04	0.00	0.04	—	0	0	—
21	150	0.09	7	73	395	0.75	56	0.01	0.18	0.11	0.29	0.05	10	0	<1	4
26	189	0.12	7	38	157	0.73	82	0.00	0.14	0.10	0.03	0.02	6	0	<1	4
28	52	0.14	6	43	176	0.67	49	0.02	0.18	0.15	0.11	0.07	18	0	<1	4
21	112	0.10	6	54	244	0.69	—	0.01	0.19	0.14	0.18	0.07	18	0	<1	4
27	192	0.21	7	36	169	0.86	74	0.00	0.10	0.11	0.03	0.02	5	0	<1	4
6	118	0.12	5	19	174	0.52	17	0.00	0.02	0.06	0.01	0.01	3	0	<1	4
30	204	0.19	8	28	175	0.88	75	0.01	0.10	0.11	0.02	0.02	5	0	<1	4
25	205	0.12	8	53	270	1.05	68	0.01	0.21	0.11	0.02	0.02	4	0	<1	4
25	138	0.18	5	17	312	0.81	35	0.04	0.01	0.24	0.28	0.12	9	0	<1	4
32	154	0.06	4	18	224	0.98	73	0.01	0.10	0.06	0.04	0.02	2	0	<1	4
13	40	0.54	5	7	105	0.26	82	0.02	0.13	0.11	0.12	0.07	3	0	<.1	1
32	196	0.07	8	34	229	1.09	46	0.01	0.10	0.09	0.02	0.02	6	0	<1	4
31	283	0.05	10	23	94	1.09	76	0.02	0.10	0.08	0.03	0.02	3	0	<1	4
25	139	0.04	6	36	224	0.59	95	0.02	0.18	0.14	0.04	0.02	16	0	<1	4
25	209	0.20	8	23	150	0.84	55	0.00	0.10	0.11	0.03	0.02	5	0	<1	4

H Appendix

Table H–1

Food Composition (Computer code number is for Wadsworth Diet Analysis program) (For purposes of calculations, use "0" for t, <1, <.1, <.01, etc.)

DA + Code	Food Description	Quantity	Measure	Wt (g)	H_2O (g)	Ener (kcal)	Prot (g)	Carb (g)	Dietary Fiber (g)	Fat (g)	Fat Breakdown (g) Sat	Mono	Poly
	DAIRY—Continued												
13	Mozzarella, part skim milk	1	ounce(s)	28	15	71	7	1	0	4	2.83	1.26	0.13
12	Mozzarella, whole milk	1	ounce(s)	28	14	84	6	1	0	6	3.68	1.84	0.21
897	Muenster	1	ounce(s)	28	12	103	7	<1	0	8	5.35	2.44	0.19
898	Neufchatel	1	ounce(s)	28	17	73	3	1	0	7	4.14	1.90	0.18
14	Parmesan, grated	1	tablespoon(s)	5	1	22	2	<1	0	1	0.87	0.42	0.06
17	Provolone	1	ounce(s)	28	11	98	7	1	0	7	4.78	2.07	0.22
19	Ricotta, part skim milk	¼	cup(s)	62	46	85	7	3	0	5	3.03	1.42	0.16
18	Ricotta, whole milk	¼	cup(s)	62	44	107	7	2	0	8	5.10	2.23	0.24
20	Romano	1	tablespoon(s)	5	2	19	2	<1	0	1	0.86	0.39	0.03
900	Roquefort	1	ounce(s)	28	11	103	6	1	0	9	5.39	2.37	0.37
21	Swiss	1	ounce(s)	28	10	106	8	2	0	8	4.98	2.04	0.27
	Imitation cheese												
7998	Shredded imitation cheddar	¼	cup(s)	28	—	90	5	2	0	7	1.50	—	—
8028	Shredded imitation mozzarella	¼	cup(s)	28	—	80	6	1	0	6	1.00	—	—
	Cottage Cheese												
9	Low fat, 1% fat	½	cup(s)	113	93	81	14	3	0	1	0.73	0.33	0.04
8	Low fat, 2% fat	½	cup(s)	113	90	102	16	4	0	2	1.38	0.62	0.07
	Cream cheese												
11	Cream cheese	2	tablespoon(s)	29	16	101	2	1	0	10	6.37	2.85	0.37
17366	Fat free cream cheese	2	tablespoon(s)	30	23	29	4	2	0	<1	0.27	0.10	0.02
10438	Tofutti Better Than Cream Cheese	2	tablespoon(s)	30	—	80	1	1	0	8	2.00	—	6.00
	Processed cheese												
22	American cheese, processed	1	ounce(s)	28	11	106	6	<1	0	9	5.58	2.54	0.28
24	American cheese food, processed	1	ounce(s)	28	12	94	5	2	0	7	4.23	2.05	0.31
25	American cheese spread, processed	1	ounce(s)	28	14	82	5	2	0	6	3.78	1.77	0.18
9110	Kraft deluxe singles pasteurized process American cheese	1	ounce(s)	28	—	110	5	1	0	9	6.00	—	—
23	Swiss cheese, processed	1	ounce(s)	28	12	95	7	1	0	7	4.55	2.00	0.18
	Soy cheese												
10430	Nu Tofu cheddar flavored cheese alternative	1	ounce(s)	28	—	70	6	1	0	4	0.50	2.50	1.00
10435	Nu Tofu mozzarella flavored cheese alternative	1	ounce(s)	28	—	70	6	2	0	4	0.50	2.50	1.00
	Cream												
26	Half & half	1	tablespoon(s)	15	12	20	<1	1	0	2	1.07	0.50	0.06
28	Light coffee or table, liquid	1	tablespoon(s)	15	11	29	<1	1	0	3	1.80	0.84	0.11
30	Light whipping cream, liquid	1	tablespoon(s)	15	10	44	<1	<1	0	5	2.90	1.36	0.13
32	Heavy whipping cream, liquid	1	tablespoon(s)	15	9	52	<1	<1	0	6	3.45	1.60	0.21
34	Whipped cream topping, pressurized	1	tablespoon(s)	4	2	10	<1	<1	0	1	0.52	0.24	0.03
	Sour cream												
36	Sour cream	2	tablespoon(s)	24	17	51	1	1	0	5	3.13	1.45	0.19
30556	Fat free sour cream	2	tablespoon(s)	32	26	24	1	5	0	0	0.00	0.00	0.00
	Imitation cream												
3659	Coffeemate nondairy creamer, liquid	1	tablespoon(s)	16	—	20	0	2	0	1	0.00	0.50	0.00
40	Cream substitute, powder	1	teaspoon(s)	2	<.1	11	<.1	1	0	1	0.65	0.02	0.00
35972	Nondairy coffee whitener, liquid, frozen	1	tablespoon(s)	16	12	22	<1	2	0	2	0.31	1.20	0.00
35975	Nondairy dessert topping, pressurized	1	tablespoon(s)	5	3	12	<.1	1	0	1	0.88	0.09	0.01
35976	Nondairy dessert topping, frozen	1	tablespoon(s)	5	3	16	<.1	1	0	1	1.09	0.08	0.03
904	Imitation sour cream	2	tablespoon(s)	24	17	50	1	2	0	5	4.27	0.14	0.01
	Fluid milk												
57	Fat free, nonfat, or skim	1	cup(s)	245	223	83	8	12	0	<1	0.29	0.12	0.02
58	Fat free, nonfat, or skim, w/nonfat milk solids	1	cup(s)	245	221	91	9	12	0	1	0.40	0.16	0.02
54	Low fat, 1%	1	cup(s)	244	219	102	8	12	0	2	1.54	0.68	0.09
55	Low fat, 1%, w/nonfat milk solids	1	cup(s)	245	220	105	9	12	0	2	1.48	0.69	0.09
60	Low fat buttermilk	1	cup(s)	245	221	98	8	12	0	2	1.34	0.62	0.08
51	Reduced fat, 2%	1	cup(s)	244	218	122	8	11	0	5	2.35	2.04	0.17
52	Reduced fat, 2%, w/nonfat milk solids	1	cup(s)	245	218	125	9	12	0	5	2.93	1.36	0.17
50	Whole, 3.3%	1	cup(s)	244	216	146	8	11	0	8	4.55	1.98	0.48
	Canned												
61	Whole evaporated	2	tablespoon(s)	32	23	42	2	3	0	2	1.45	0.74	0.08

PAGE KEY: H–2 = Breads/Baked Goods H–6 = Cereal/Rice/Pasta H–10 = Fruit H–16 = Vegetables/Legumes H–26 = Nuts/Seeds H–28 = Vegetarian H–30 = Dairy H–36 = Eggs H–38 = Seafood H–40 = Meats H–42 = Poultry H–44 = Processed meats H–46 = Beverages H–50 = Fats/Oils H–52 = Sweets H–52 = Sauces/Condiments/Spices H–56 = Mixed Foods/Soups/Sandwiches H–62 = Fast food H–80 = Convenience H–82 = Baby foods

Chol (mg)	Calc (mg)	Iron (mg)	Magn (mg)	Pota (mg)	Sodi (mg)	Zinc (mg)	Vit A (RAE) (µg)	Thia (mg)	Vit E (mg)	Ribo (mg)	Niac (mg)	Vit B_6 (mg)	Fola (µg)	Vit C (mg)	Vit B_{12} (µg)	Sele (µg)
18	219	0.06	6	24	173	0.77	36	0.01	0.12	0.08	0.03	0.02	3	0	<1	4
22	141	0.12	6	21	176	0.82	50	0.01	0.10	0.08	0.03	0.01	2	0	1	5
27	201	0.11	8	38	176	0.79	83	0.00	0.13	0.09	0.03	0.02	3	0	<1	4
21	21	0.08	2	32	112	0.15	83	0.00	—	0.05	0.04	0.01	3	0	<.1	1
4	55	0.05	2	6	76	0.19	6	0.00	0.04	0.02	0.01	0.00	1	0	<1	1
19	212	0.15	8	39	245	0.90	66	0.01	0.10	0.09	0.04	0.02	3	0	<1	4
19	167	0.27	9	77	77	0.82	66	0.01	0.13	0.11	0.05	0.01	8	0	<1	10
31	127	0.23	7	65	52	0.71	74	0.01	0.22	0.12	0.06	0.03	7	0	<1	9
5	53	0.04	2	4	60	0.13	5	0.00	0.04	0.02	0.00	0.00	<1	0	<.1	1
25	185	0.16	8	25	507	0.58	82	0.01	0.18	0.16	0.21	0.03	14	0	<1	4
26	221	0.06	11	22	54	1.22	62	0.02	0.14	0.08	0.03	0.02	2	0	1	5
0	150	0.00	—	—	420	—	—	—	—	—	—	—	—	0	—	—
0	150	0.00	8	—	320	1.20	—	0.00	—	0.26	0.00	0.00	40	0	<1	—
5	69	0.16	6	97	459	0.43	12	0.02	0.12	0.19	0.14	0.08	14	0	1	10
9	78	0.18	7	108	459	0.47	24	0.03	0.06	0.21	0.16	0.09	15	0	1	12
32	23	0.35	2	35	86	0.16	106	0.00	0.27	0.06	0.03	0.01	4	0	<1	1
2	56	0.05	4	49	164	0.26	84	0.02	0.01	0.05	0.05	0.02	11	0	<1	1
0	0	0.00	—	—	135	—	0	—	—	—	—	—	—	0	—	—
27	156	0.05	8	48	422	0.81	72	0.01	0.13	0.10	0.02	0.02	2	0	<1	4
23	162	0.16	9	83	359	0.91	57	0.02	0.20	0.15	0.05	0.02	2	0	<1	5
16	160	0.09	8	69	382	0.74	49	0.01	0.20	0.12	0.04	0.03	2	0	<1	3
25	150	0.00	0	25	450	0.90	84	—	—	0.10	—	—	—	0	<1	—
24	219	0.17	8	61	388	1.02	56	0.00	0.19	0.08	0.01	0.01	2	0	<1	5
0	200	0.36	—	—	190	—	—	—	—	—	—	—	—	0	—	—
0	150	0.36	—	—	190	—	—	—	—	—	—	—	—	0	—	—
6	16	0.01	2	20	6	0.08	15	0.01	0.02	0.02	0.01	0.01	<1	<1	<.1	<1
10	14	0.01	1	18	6	0.04	27	0.00	0.02	0.02	0.01	0.00	<1	<1	<.1	<.1
17	10	0.00	1	15	5	0.04	42	0.00	0.09	0.02	0.01	0.00	1	<.1	<.1	<.1
21	10	0.00	1	11	6	0.03	62	0.00	0.09	0.02	0.01	0.00	1	<.1	<.1	<.1
3	4	0.00	<1	6	5	0.01	7	0.00	0.02	0.00	0.00	0.00	<1	0	<.1	<.1
11	28	0.01	3	35	13	0.06	42	0.01	0.14	0.04	0.02	0.00	3	<1	<.1	1
3	40	0.00	3	41	45	0.16	—	0.01	0.00	0.05	0.02	0.01	4	0	<.1	—
0	0	0.00	—	30	0	—	0	0.02	—	0.02	0.20	—	—	0	—	—
0	<1	0.02	<.1	16	4	0.01	<.1	0.00	0.01	0.00	0.00	0.00	0	0	0	<.1
0	1	0.00	<.1	30	13	0.00	—	0.00	0.26	0.00	0.00	0.00	0	0	0	<1
0	<1	0.00	<.1	1	3	0.00	—	0.00	0.01	0.00	0.00	0.00	0	0	0	<.1
0	<1	0.01	<.1	1	1	0.00	—	0.00	0.01	0.00	0.00	0.00	0	0	0	<1
0	1	0.09	1	39	24	0.28	0	0.00	0.04	0.00	0.00	0.00	0	0	0	1
5	223	1.23	22	238	108	2.08	149	0.11	0.10	0.45	0.23	0.09	12	0	1	8
5	316	0.12	37	419	130	1.00	149	0.10	0.10	0.43	0.22	0.11	12	2	1	5
12	264	0.85	27	290	122	2.12	142	0.05	0.10	0.45	0.23	0.09	12	0	1	8
10	314	0.12	34	397	127	0.98	145	0.10	0.10	0.42	0.22	0.11	12	2	1	6
10	284	0.12	27	370	257	1.03	17	0.08	0.15	0.38	0.14	0.08	12	2	1	5
20	271	0.24	27	342	115	1.17	134	0.10	0.17	0.45	0.22	0.09	12	<1	1	6
20	314	0.12	34	397	127	0.98	137	0.10	0.17	0.42	0.22	0.11	12	2	1	6
24	246	0.07	24	325	105	0.93	68	0.11	0.24	0.45	0.26	0.09	12	0	1	9
9	82	0.06	8	95	33	0.24	20	0.01	0.06	0.10	0.06	0.02	3	1	<.1	1

Table H–1

Food Composition (Computer code number is for Wadsworth Diet Analysis program) (For purposes of calculations, use "0" for t, <1, <.1, <.01, etc.)

DA + Code	Food Description	Quantity	Measure	Wt (g)	H_2O (g)	Ener (kcal)	Prot (g)	Carb (g)	Dietary Fiber (g)	Fat (g)	Fat Breakdown (g) Sat	Mono	Poly
	DAIRY—Continued												
62	Fat free, nonfat, or skim evaporated	2	tablespoon(s)	32	25	25	2	4	0	<.1	0.04	0.02	0.00
63	Sweetened condensed	2	tablespoon(s)	38	10	123	3	21	0	3	2.10	0.93	0.13
	Dried Milk												
64	Dried buttermilk	¼	cup(s)	30	1	118	10	15	0	2	1.09	0.51	0.07
65	Instant nonfat dry milk w/added vitamin A	¼	cup(s)	17	1	63	6	9	0	<1	0.08	0.03	0.00
5234	Skim milk powder	¼	cup(s)	18	1	64	6	9	0	<1	0.08	0.03	0.01
907	Whole dry milk	¼	cup(s)	32	1	161	9	12	0	9	5.43	2.57	0.22
909	**Goat milk**	1	cup(s)	244	212	168	9	11	0	10	6.51	2.71	0.36
	Chocolate milk												
69	Low fat	1	cup(s)	250	211	158	8	26	1	3	1.54	0.75	0.09
68	Reduced fat	1	cup(s)	250	209	180	8	26	1	5	3.10	1.47	0.18
67	Whole milk	1	cup(s)	250	206	208	8	26	2	8	5.26	2.48	0.31
33156	Chocolate syrup, fortified, prepared w/milk	1	cup(s)	263	220	197	8	24	<1	8	5.22	2.44	0.31
908	Cocoa, hot, prepared w/milk	1	cup(s)	250	206	193	9	27	3	6	3.58	1.69	0.09
33184	Cocoa mix with aspartame, added sodium & vitamin A, no added calcium or phosphorus, prepared with water	1	cup(s)	192	177	56	2	10	1	<1	0.00	0.15	0.01
70	**Eggnog**	1	cup(s)	254	189	343	10	34	0	19	11.29	5.67	0.86
	Breakfast drinks												
10093	Carnation Instant Breakfast classic chocolate malt, prepared w/skim milk, no sugar added	1	cup(s)	243	—	142	11	21	<1	1	0.89	—	—
10091	Carnation Instant Breakfast strawberry creme, prepared w/skim milk	1	cup(s)	273	—	220	13	39	0	<1	0.40	—	—
10094	Carnation Instant Breakfast strawberry creme, prepared w/skim milk, no sugar added	1	cup(s)	243	—	134	12	21	0	<1	0.45	—	—
10092	Carnation Instant Breakfast vanilla creme, prepared w/skim milk, no sugar added	1	cup(s)	273	—	220	13	39	0	<1	0.40	—	—
1417	Ovaltine rich chocolate flavor, prepared w/skim milk	1	cup(s)	243	—	134	12	21	0	<1	0.45	—	—
8539	**Malted milk, chocolate mix, fortified, prepared w/milk**	1	cup(s)	265	216	223	9	29	1	9	4.95	2.17	0.54
	Milkshakes												
73	Chocolate	1	cup(s)	227	164	270	7	48	1	6	3.81	1.77	0.23
74	Vanilla	1	cup(s)	227	169	254	9	40	0	7	4.28	1.98	0.26
	Ice cream												
4776	Chocolate	½	cup(s)	66	37	143	3	19	1	7	4.49	2.12	0.27
16514	Chocolate, soft serve	½	cup(s)	87	50	177	3	24	1	8	5.17	2.43	0.31
12137	Chocolate fudge, fat free no sugar added	½	cup(s)	71	—	100	4	22	0	0	0.00	0.00	0.00
82	Light vanilla	½	cup(s)	66	42	109	4	18	<1	3	1.71	0.57	0.10
78	Light vanilla, soft serve	½	cup(s)	86	60	108	4	19	0	2	1.40	0.65	0.09
16523	Sherbet, all flavors	½	cup(s)	97	64	133	1	29	<1	2	1.12	0.51	0.08
4778	Strawberry	½	cup(s)	66	40	127	2	18	1	6	3.43	—	—
76	Vanilla	½	cup(s)	66	40	133	2	16	<1	7	4.48	1.96	0.30
12146	Vanilla chocolate swirl, fat free, no sugar added	½	cup(s)	71	—	100	4	20	0	0	0.00	0.00	0.00
	Soy desserts												
10694	Tofutti low fat vanilla fudge nondairy frozen dessert	½	cup(s)	70	—	120	2	24	0	2	1.00	—	—
15721	Tofutti premium chocolate supreme nondairy frozen dessert	½	cup(s)	60	—	180	3	18	0	11	2.00	—	—
15720	Tofutti premium vanilla nondairy frozen dessert	½	cup(s)	60	—	190	2	20	0	11	2.00	—	—
	Ice milk												
16516	Flavored, not chocolate	½	cup(s)	66	45	91	2	15	0	3	1.72	0.81	0.11
16517	Chocolate	½	cup(s)	66	43	95	3	17	<1	2	1.29	0.61	0.08
	Pudding												
25032	Chocolate	½	cup(s)	144	110	154	5	23	1	5	2.78	1.94	0.23
1923	Chocolate, sugar free, prepared w/2% milk	½	cup(s)	133	—	100	5	14	<1	3	1.50	—	—

PAGE KEY: H–2 = Breads/Baked Goods H–6 = Cereal/Rice/Pasta H–10 = Fruit H–16 = Vegetables/Legumes H–26 = Nuts/Seeds H–28 = Vegetarian H–30 = Dairy H–36 = Eggs H–38 = Seafood H–40 = Meats H–42 = Poultry H–44 = Processed meats H–46 = Beverages H–50 = Fats/Oils H–52 = Sweets H–52 = Sauces/Condiments/Spices H–56 = Mixed Foods/Soups/Sandwiches H–62 = Fast food H–80 = Convenience H–82 = Baby foods

Chol (mg)	Calc (mg)	Iron (mg)	Magn (mg)	Pota (mg)	Sodi (mg)	Zinc (mg)	Vit A (RAE) (µg)	Thia (mg)	Vit E (mg)	Ribo (mg)	Niac (mg)	Vit B_6 (mg)	Fola (µg)	Vit C (mg)	Vit B_{12} (µg)	Sele (µg)
1	93	0.09	9	106	37	0.29	38	0.01	0.00	0.10	0.06	0.02	3	<1	<.1	1
13	109	0.07	10	142	49	0.36	28	0.03	0.08	0.16	0.08	0.02	4	1	<1	6
21	360	0.09	33	484	157	1.22	15	0.12	0.12	0.48	0.27	0.10	14	2	1	6
3	215	0.05	20	298	96	0.77	124	0.07	0.00	0.30	0.16	0.06	9	1	1	5
3	222	0.06	21	307	99	0.79	0	0.07	0.00	0.31	0.16	0.06	9	1	1	5
31	296	0.15	28	431	120	1.08	83	0.09	0.35	0.39	0.21	0.10	12	3	1	5
27	327	0.12	34	498	122	0.73	139	0.12	0.22	0.34	0.68	0.11	2	3	<1	3
8	288	0.60	33	425	153	1.03	145	0.10	0.07	0.42	0.32	0.10	13	2	1	5
18	285	0.60	33	423	150	1.03	138	0.09	0.13	0.41	0.32	0.10	13	2	1	5
30	280	0.60	33	418	150	1.03	65	0.09	0.23	0.41	0.31	0.10	13	2	1	5
34	292	2.68	32	460	147	0.92	—	0.09	—	0.55	6.53	0.11	13	2	1	5
20	263	1.20	58	493	110	1.58	128	0.10	0.26	0.46	0.33	0.10	13	1	1	7
<1	90	0.75	33	405	171	0.52	27	0.04	0.06	0.21	0.16	0.05	2	<1	<1	2
150	330	0.51	48	419	137	1.17	114	0.09	0.58	0.48	0.27	0.13	3	4	1	11
9	445	4.01	89	632	196	3.38	—	0.35	4.48	0.45	4.45	0.45	4	27	1	8
9	500	4.47	100	638	360	3.75	—	0.38	5.03	0.51	5.08	0.48	100	30	1	9
9	445	4.01	89	570	187	3.38	—	0.33	4.48	0.45	4.45	0.45	89	27	1	8
9	500	4.50	100	630	240	3.75	—	0.38	5.03	0.51	5.00	0.50	100	30	2	9
9	445	4.01	89	570	187	3.38	—	0.33	4.48	0.45	4.45	0.45	89	27	1	8
27	339	3.76	45	578	231	1.17	904	0.76	0.33	1.32	11.08	1.01	19	32	1	12
25	299	0.70	36	508	252	1.09	41	0.11	0.23	0.50	0.28	0.06	11	0	1	4
27	331	0.23	27	415	215	0.88	57	0.07	0.23	0.44	0.33	0.10	16	0	1	5
22	72	0.61	19	164	50	0.38	78	0.03	0.22	0.13	0.15	0.04	11	<1	<1	2
22	103	0.33	19	192	44	0.48	—	0.04	0.23	0.13	0.11	0.03	5	1	<1	—
0	80	0.36	—	—	60	—	—	—	—	—	—	—	—	0	—	—
17	77	0.05	9	137	49	0.48	91	0.02	0.00	0.11	0.06	0.02	3	<1	<1	1
10	135	0.05	12	190	60	0.46	25	0.04	0.00	0.17	0.10	0.04	5	1	<1	3
5	52	0.14	8	93	44	0.46	—	0.02	0.06	0.07	0.09	0.03	4	4	<1	—
19	79	0.14	9	124	40	0.22	63	0.03		0.17	0.11	0.03	8	5	<1	1
29	84	0.06	9	131	53	0.46	78	0.03	0.14	0.16	0.08	0.03	3	<1	<1	1
0	80	0.00	50	0												
0	0	0.00	—	8	90	—	0	—	—	—	—	—	—	0	—	—
0	0	0.00	—	7	180	—	0	—	—	—	—	—	—	0	—	—
0	0	0.00	—	2	210	—	0	—	—	—	—	—	—	0	—	—
9	91	0.07	10	138	56	0.29	—	0.04	0.00	0.17	0.06	0.04	4	1	<1	—
6	94	0.17	13	155	41	0.38	—	0.03	0.06	0.12	0.09	0.03	4	<1	<1	—
35	138	1.04	29	211	135	1.07	73	0.04	0.20	0.25	0.18	0.03	7	<1	<1	5
10	150	0.72	—	330	310	—	—	0.06	—	0.26	—	—	—	0	—	—

H Appendix

Table H–1

Food Composition (Computer code number is for Wadsworth Diet Analysis program) (For purposes of calculations, use "0" for t, <1, <.1, <.01, etc.)

DA + Code	Food Description	Quantity	Measure	Wt (g)	H_2O (g)	Ener (kcal)	Prot (g)	Carb (g)	Dietary Fiber (g)	Fat (g)	Fat Breakdown (g) Sat	Mono	Poly
	DAIRY—Continued												
1722	Rice	½	cup(s)	113	73	175	6	26	1	6	1.99	2.14	0.88
4747	Tapioca, ready to eat	1	item(s)	142	105	169	3	28	<1	5	0.85	2.24	1.93
25031	Vanilla	½	cup(s)	136	110	116	5	17	<.1	3	1.31	1.21	0.16
1924	Vanilla, sugar free, prepared w/2% milk	½	cup(s)	133	90	4	12	<1	2	1.50	10	150	0.00
	Frozen yogurt												
4785	Chocolate, soft serve	½	cup(s)	72	46	115	3	18	2	4	2.61	1.26	0.16
1747	Fruit varieties	½	cup(s)	113	80	144	3	24	0	4	2.63	1.11	0.11
4786	Vanilla, soft serve	½	cup(s)	72	47	117	3	17	0	4	2.46	1.14	0.15
	Milk substitutes												
	Lactose free												
16081	Fat free calcium fortified milk	1	cup(s)	240	—	90	9	13	0	0	0.00	—	—
36486	Low fat milk	1	cup(s)	240	—	110	8	13	0	3	1.50	—	—
36487	Reduced fat milk	1	cup(s)	240	—	130	8	13	0	5	3.00	—	—
36488	Whole milk	1	cup(s)	240	—	160	8	12	0	9	5.00	—	—
	Rice												
10083	Rice Dream carob rice beverage	1	cup(s)	240	—	150	1	32	0	3	0.00	—	—
10087	Rice Dream vanilla enriched rice beverage	1	cup(s)	240	—	130	1	28	0	2	0.00	—	—
17089	Rice Dream original rice beverage, enriched	1	cup(s)	240	—	120	1	25	0	2	0.00	—	—
	Soy												
34750	Soy Dream chocolate enriched soy beverage	1	cup(s)	240	—	210	7	37	1	4	0.50	—	—
34749	Soy Dream vanilla enriched soy beverage	1	cup(s)	240	—	150	7	22	0	4	0.50	—	—
13840	Vitasoy light chocolate soymilk	1	cup(s)	237	—	100	4	17	0	2	0.50	0.50	1.00
13839	Vitasoy light vanilla soymilk	1	cup(s)	237	—	70	4	10	0	2	0.50	0.50	1.00
13836	Vitasoy rich chocolate soymilk	1	cup(s)	237	—	160	7	24	1	4	0.50	1.00	2.50
13835	Vitasoy vanilla delite soymilk	1	cup(s)	237	—	120	8	13	1	4	0.50	1.00	2.50
	Yogurt												
3615	Custard style, fruit flavors	6	ounce(s)	170	127	190	7	32	0	4	2.00	—	—
3617	Custard style, vanilla	6	ounce(s)	170	134	190	7	32	0	4	2.00	0.94	0.10
32101	Fruit, low fat	1	cup(s)	245	184	243	10	46	0	3	1.82	0.77	0.08
29638	Fruit, nonfat, sweetened w/low calorie sweetener	1	cup(s)	241	208	122	11	19	1	<1	0.21	0.10	0.04
93	Plain, low fat	1	cup(s)	245	208	154	13	17	0	4	2.45	1.04	0.11
94	Plain, nonfat	1	cup(s)	245	209	137	14	19	0	<1	0.28	0.12	0.01
32100	Vanilla, low fat	1	cup(s)	245	194	208	12	34	0	3	1.97	0.84	0.09
5242	Yogurt beverage	1	cup(s)	245	200	172	6	33	0	2	1.39	0.59	0.06
38202	Yogurt smoothie, nonfat, all flavors	1	item(s)	325	—	290	10	60	6	0	0.00	0.00	0.00
	Soy yogurt												
10453	White Wave plain silk cultured	8	ounce(s)	227	—	120	5	22	1	3	0.00	—	—
34616	Stonyfield Farm Osoy chocolate-vanilla pack organic cultured	1	serving(s)	113	—	90	4	15	3	2	0.00	—	—
34617	Stonyfield Farm Osoy strawberry-peach pack organic cultured	1	serving(s)	113	—	90	4	15	3	2	0.00	—	—
	EGGS												
96	Raw, whole	1	item(s)	50	38	74	6	<1	0	5	1.55	1.91	0.68
97	Raw, white	1	item(s)	33	29	17	4	<1	0	<.1	0.00	0.00	0.00
98	Raw, yolk	1	item(s)	17	9	53	3	1	0	4	1.59	1.95	0.70
99	Fried	1	item(s)	46	32	92	6	<1	0	7	1.98	2.92	1.22
100	Hard boiled	1	item(s)	50	37	78	6	1	0	5	1.63	2.04	0.71
101	Poached	1	item(s)	50	38	74	6	<1	0	5	1.54	1.90	0.68
102	Scrambled, prepared w/milk & butter	2	item(s)	122	89	203	14	3	0	15	4.49	5.82	2.62
	Egg Substitute												
920	Frozen	¼	cup(s)	60	44	96	7	2	0	7	1.16	1.46	3.74
918	Liquid	¼	cup(s)	63	52	53	8	<1	0	2	0.41	0.56	1.01
4028	Egg Beaters	¼	cup(s)	61	—	30	6	1	0	0	0.00	0.00	0.00

PAGE KEY: H–2 = Breads/Baked Goods H–6 = Cereal/Rice/Pasta H–10 = Fruit H–16 = Vegetables/Legumes H–26 = Nuts/Seeds H–28 = Vegetarian H–30 = Dairy H–36 = Eggs H–38 = Seafood H–40 = Meats H–42 = Poultry H–44 = Processed meats H–46 = Beverages H–50 = Fats/Oils H–52 = Sweets H–52 = Sauces/Condiments/Spices H–56 = Mixed Foods/Soups/Sandwiches H–62 = Fast food H–80 = Convenience H–82 = Baby foods

Chol (mg)	Calc (mg)	Iron (mg)	Magn (mg)	Pota (mg)	Sodi (mg)	Zinc (mg)	Vit A (RAE) (μg)	Thia (mg)	Vit E (mg)	Ribo (mg)	Niac (mg)	Vit B_6 (mg)	Fola (μg)	Vit C (mg)	Vit B_{12} (μg)	Sele (μg)
71	130	1.21	21	250	253	0.61	—	0.10	0.60	0.26	0.73	0.08	14	1	<1	—
1	119	0.33	11	136	226	0.38	0	0.03	0.13	0.14	0.44	0.03	4	1	<1	2
35	133	0.25	14	173	134	0.63	73	0.03	0.14	0.24	0.11	0.03	6	<1	<1	5
—	190	380	—	—	0.03	—	—	0.17	—	—	—	0	—	—		
4	106	0.90	19	188	71	0.35	32	0.03	0.10	0.15	0.22	0.05	8	<1	<1	2
15	113	0.52	11	176	71	0.32	—	0.05	0.09	0.20	0.08	0.05	5	1	<.1	—
1	103	0.22	10	152	63	0.30	42	0.03	0.04	0.16	0.21	0.06	4	1	<1	2
3	500	0.00	—	—	130	—	100	—	0.10	—	—	—	—	0	—	—
15	300	0.00	—	—	125	—	100	—	—	—	—	—	—	0	—	—
20	300	0.00	—	—	125	—	98	—	—	—	—	—	—	0	—	—
35	300	0.00	—	—	125	—	58	—	—	—	—	—	—	0	—	—
0	20	0.72	—	—	100	—	—	—	0.81	—	—	—	—	1	—	—
0	300	0.00	—	—	90	—	—	—	0.81	—	—	—	—	0	2	—
0	300	0.00	13	60	90	0.24	—	0.07	0.81	0.00	0.84	0.08	—	0	2	—
0	300	1.80	60	350	160	0.60	33	0.15	5.03	0.07	0.80	0.12	60	0	3	—
0	300	1.80	40	260	140	0.60	33	0.15	5.03	0.07	0.80	0.12	60	0	3	—
0	300	0.72	24	200	140	0.90	0	0.09	—	0.34	—	—	24	0	1	—
0	300	0.72	24	200	110	0.90	0	0.09	—	0.34	—	—	24	0	1	—
0	300	1.08	40	320	150	0.90	0	0.15	—	0.34	—	—	60	0	1	—
0	40	0.72	—	320	115	—	0	—	—	—	—	—	—	0	—	—
15	200	0.00	16	310	90	—	0	—	0.05	0.26	—	—	—	0	—	—
15	200	0.00	16	300	90	—	0	—	0.08	0.26	—	—	—	0	—	—
12	338	0.15	32	434	130	1.64	27	0.08	0.08	0.40	0.21	0.09	22	1	1	7
3	370	0.62	41	550	139	1.83	0.10	0.17	0.45	0.50	0.11	32	26	1		
15	448	0.20	42	573	172	2.18	34	0.11	0.10	0.52	0.28	0.12	27	2	1	8
5	488	0.22	47	625	189	2.38	5	0.12	0.01	0.57	0.30	0.13	29	2	1	9
12	419	0.17	39	537	162	2.03	29	0.10	0.08	0.49	0.26	0.11	27	2	1	12
13	260	0.22	39	399	98	1.10	—	0.11	0.01	0.51	0.30	0.15	29	2	2	—
5	300	2.70	100	580	290	2.25	—	0.38	5.03	0.43	5.00	0.50	100	15	2	—
0	700	0.90	—	—	30	—	—	—	—	—	—	—	—	0	0	—
0	100	0.72	—	—	20	—	0	—	—	—	—	—	—	0	—	—
0	100	0.72	—	—	20	—	0	—	—	—	—	—	—	0	—	—
212	27	0.92	6	67	70	0.56	70	0.03	0.53	0.24	0.04	0.07	24	0	1	16
0	2	0.03	4	54	55	0.01	0	0.00	0.00	0.15	0.04	0.00	1	0	<.1	7
205	21	0.45	1	18	8	0.38	63	0.03	0.52	0.09	0.00	0.06	24	0	<1	9
210	27	0.91	6	68	94	0.55	91	0.03	0.75	0.24	0.04	0.07	23	0	1	16
212	25	0.60	5	63	62	0.53	85	0.03	0.53	0.26	0.03	0.06	22	0	1	15
211	27	0.92	6	67	147	0.55	70	0.03	0.53	0.24	0.04	0.07	24	0	1	16
429	87	1.46	15	168	342	1.22	174	0.06	1.60	0.53	0.10	0.14	37	<1	1	27
1	44	1.19	9	128	119	0.59	7	0.07	1.27	0.23	0.08	0.08	10	<1	<1	25
1	33	1.32	6	207	111	0.82	11	0.07	0.30	0.19	0.07	0.00	9	0	<1	16
0	20	1.08	4	85	115	0.60	113	0.15	0.81	0.85	0.20	0.08	60	0	1	—

Table H–1

Food Composition (Computer code number is for Wadsworth Diet Analysis program) (For purposes of calculations, use "0" for t, <1, <.1, <.01, etc.)

DA + Code	Food Description	Quantity	Measure	Wt (g)	H_2O (g)	Ener (kcal)	Prot (g)	Carb (g)	Dietary Fiber (g)	Fat (g)	Fat Breakdown (g) Sat	Mono	Poly
	SEAFOOD												
	Fish												
	Cod												
6040	Atlantic cod or scrod, baked or broiled	3	ounce(s)	44	34	46	10	0	0	<1	0.07	0.05	0.13
1573	Atlantic cod, cooked, dry heat	3	ounce(s)	85	65	89	19	0	0	1	0.14	0.11	0.25
2905	**Eel, raw**	3	ounce(s)	85	58	156	16	0	0	10	2.01	6.12	0.81
	Fish fillets												
25079	Baked	3	ounce(s)	84	80	99	22	0	0	1	0.08	0.07	0.26
8615	Batter coated or breaded, fried	3	ounce(s)	85	0.04	197.19	12.46	14.42	0.42	10.44	2.39	2.19	5.32
25082	Broiled fish steaks	3	ounce(s)	86	69	129	24	0	0	3	0.37	0.87	0.84
25083	Poached fish steaks	3	ounce(s)	86	68	112	21	0	0	2	0.33	0.76	0.74
25084	Steamed fish fillets	3	ounce(s)	86	73	80	17	0	0	1	0.12	0.08	0.22
25089	**Flounder, baked**	3	ounce(s)	85	65	114	15	<1	<.1	6	1.15	2.17	1.44
1825	**Grouper, cooked, dry heat**	3	ounce(s)	85	62	100	21	0	0	1	0.25	0.23	0.34
	Haddock												
6049	Baked or broiled	3	ounce(s)	44	33	50	11	0	0	<1	0.07	0.07	0.14
1578	Cooked, dry heat	3	ounce(s)	85	63	95	21	0	0	1	0.14	0.13	0.26
1886	**Halibut, Atlantic & Pacific, cooked, dry heat**	3	ounce(s)	85	61	119	23	0	0	2	0.35	0.82	0.80
1582	**Herring, Atlantic, pickled**	4	piece(s)	60	33	157	9	6	0	11	1.43	7.17	1.01
1587	**Jack mackerel, solids, canned, drained**	2	ounce(s)	57	39	88	13	0	0	4	1.05	1.26	0.94
8580	**Octopus, common, cooked, moist heat**	3	ounce(s)	85	51	139	25	4	0	2	0.39	0.28	0.41
1831	**Perch, mixed species, cooked, dry heat**	3	ounce(s)	85	62	99	21	0	0	1	0.20	0.17	0.40
1592	**Pacific rockfish, cooked, dry heat**	3	ounce(s)	85	62	103	20	0	0	2	0.40	0.38	0.50
	Salmon												
29727	Smoked chinook (lox)	2	ounce(s)	57	<.1	66	10	0	0	2	0.52	1.14	0.56
1594	Broiled or baked w/butter	3	ounce(s)	85	54	155	23	0	0	6	1.16	2.29	2.33
2938	Coho, farmed, raw	3	ounce(s)	85	60	136	18	0	0	7	1.54	2.83	1.58
154	**Sardines, Atlantic, with bones, canned in oil**	2	item(s)	24	<.1	50	6	0	0	3	0.36	0.92	1.23
	Scallops												
155	Mixed species, breaded, fried	3	item(s)	47	<.1	100	8	5	0	5	1.24	2.09	1.32
1599	Steamed	3	ounce(s)	85	65	90	14	2	0	3	—	—	—
1839	**Snapper, mixed species, cooked, dry heat**	3	ounce(s)	85	60	109	22	0	0	1	0.31	0.27	0.50
	Squid												
1868	Mixed species, fried	3	ounce(s)	85	55	149	15	7	0	6	1.60	2.34	1.82
16617	Steamed or boiled	3	ounce(s)	85	63	90	15	3	0	1	0.35	0.11	0.51
1570	**Striped bass, cooked, dry heat**	3	ounce(s)	85	62	105	19	0	0	3	0.55	0.72	0.85
1601	**Sturgeon, steamed**	3	ounce(s)	85	59	111	17	0	0	4	0.97	2.04	0.73
1840	**Surimi, formed**	3	ounce(s)	85	65	84	13	6	0	1	0.16	0.13	0.38
1842	**Swordfish, cooked, dry heat**	3	ounce(s)	85	58	132	22	0	0	4	1.20	1.68	1.00
1846	**Tuna, yellowfin or ahi, raw**	3	ounce(s)	85	60	92	20	0	0	1	0.20	0.13	0.24
	Tuna, canned												
159	Light, canned in oil, drained	2	ounce(s)	57	34	113	17	0	0	5	0.87	1.68	1.64
355	Light, canned in water, drained	2	ounce(s)	57	42	66	14	0	0	<1	0.13	0.09	0.19
33211	Light, no salt, canned in oil, drained	2	ounce(s)	57	34	112	17	0	0	5	0.87	1.67	1.64
33212	Light, no salt, canned in water, drained	2	ounce(s)	57	43	66	14	0	0	<1	0.13	0.09	0.19
2961	White, canned in oil, drained	2	ounce(s)	57	36	105	15	0	0	5	0.73	1.85	1.69
351	White, canned in water, drained	2	ounce(s)	57	41	73	13	0	0	2	0.45	0.44	0.63
33213	White, no salt, canned in oil, drained	2	ounce(s)	57	36	105	15	0	0	5	0.94	1.41	1.92
33214	White, no salt, canned in water, drained	2	ounce(s)	57	42	73	13	0	0	2	0.45	0.44	0.63
	Yellowtail												
2970	Mixed species, raw	2	ounce(s)	57	42	83	13	0	0	3	0.73	1.13	0.81
8548	Mixed species, cooked, dry heat	3	ounce(s)	85	0.05	158.94	25.21	0	0	5.71	1.44	2.21	1.52
	Shellfish, meat only												
1857	Abalone, mixed species, fried	3	ounce(s)	85	51	161	17	9	0	6	1.40	2.33	1.42
16618	Abalone, steamed or poached	3	ounce(s)	85	41	177	29	10	0	1	0.25	0.18	0.18
	Crab												
1851	Blue crab, canned	2	ounce(s)	57	43	56	12	0	0	1	0.14	0.12	0.25
1852	Blue crab, cooked, moist heat	3	ounce(s)	85	66	87	17	0	0	2	0.19	0.24	0.58
8562	Dungeness crab, cooked, moist heat	3	ounce(s)	85	62	94	19	1	0	1	0.14	0.18	0.35

PAGE KEY: H–2 = Breads/Baked Goods H–6 = Cereal/Rice/Pasta H–10 = Fruit H–16 = Vegetables/Legumes H–26 = Nuts/Seeds H–28 = Vegetarian H–30 = Dairy H–36 = Eggs H–38 = Seafood H–40 = Meats H–42 = Poultry H–44 = Processed meats H–46 = Beverages H–50 = Fats/Oils H–52 = Sweets H–52 = Sauces/Condiments/Spices H–56 = Mixed Foods/Soups/Sandwiches H–62 = Fast food H–80 = Convenience H–82 = Baby foods

Chol (mg)	Calc (mg)	Iron (mg)	Magn (mg)	Pota (mg)	Sodi (mg)	Zinc (mg)	Vit A (RAE) (μg)	Thia (mg)	Vit E (mg)	Ribo (mg)	Niac (mg)	Vit B_6 (mg)	Fola (μg)	Vit C (mg)	Vit B_{12} (μg)	Sele (μg)
24	6	0.22	19	108	35	0.26	—	0.04	0.13	0.03	1.11	0.13	5	<1	<1	17
47	12	0.42	36	207	66	0.49	12	0.07	0.26	0.07	2.14	0.24	7	1	1	32
107	17	0.43	17	231	43	1.38	887	0.13	3.40	0.03	2.98	0.06	13	2	3	6
44	8	0.32	29	489	86	0.49	10	0.03	0.28	0.05	2.48	0.46	8	3	1	44
28.89	15.3	1.79	20.39	272	452.2	0.37	10.19	0.09	—	0.09	1.78	0.08	17	0	0.94	7.73
37	55	0.99	98	529	64	0.49	55	0.06	1.00	0.08	6.88	0.36	13	0	1	43
33	48	0.86	85	460	55	0.43	48	0.06	0.87	0.08	5.97	0.33	12	0	1	37
42	13	0.30	25	323	42	0.35	12	0.07	0.22	0.06	1.92	0.22	6	1	1	32
44	19	0.35	47	225	281	0.21	39	0.06	1.84	0.08	2.03	0.19	7	3	2	34
40	18	0.97	31	404	45	0.43	43	0.07	—	0.01	0.32	0.30	9	0	1	40
33	19	0.60	22	177	39	0.21	—	0.02	0.41	0.02	2.05	0.15	4	0	1	18
63	36	1.15	43	339	74	0.41	16	0.03	—	0.04	3.94	0.29	11	0	1	34
35	51	0.91	91	490	59	0.45	46	0.06	0.93	0.08	6.05	0.34	12	0	1	40
8	46	0.73	5	41	522	0.32	155	0.02	0.60	0.08	1.98	0.10	1	0	3	35
45	137	1.16	21	110	215	0.58	74	0.02	0.79	0.12	3.50	0.12	3	1	4	21
82	90	8.11	51	536	391	2.86	77	0.05	1.02	0.06	3.21	0.55	20	7	31	76
98	87	0.99	32	292	67	1.22	9	0.07	—	0.10	1.62	0.12	5	1	2	14
37	10	0.45	29	442	65	0.45	60	0.04	1.06	0.07	3.33	0.23	9	0	1	40
13	6	0.48	10	99	1134	0.17	15	0.01	—	0.05	2.67	0.15	1	0	2	22
40	15	1.02	27	377	99	0.56	—	0.14	1.54	0.05	8.33	0.19	4	2	2	41
43	10	0.29	26	383	40	0.37	48	0.08	—	0.09	5.79	0.56	11	1	2	11
34	108	0.70	9	95	121	0.31	16	0.01	0.05	0.05	1.25	0.04	3	0	2	13
28	20	0.38	27	155	216	0.49	10	0.01	—	0.05	0.69	0.06	23	1	1	13
27	21	0.22	—	238	366	—	—	—	—	—	—	—	—	2	—	—
40	34	0.20	31	444	48	0.37	30	0.05	—	0.00	0.29	0.39	5	1	3	42
221	33	0.86	32	237	260	1.48	9	0.05	—	0.39	2.21	0.05	12	4	1	44
227	31	0.63	29	192	356	1.49	—	0.02	1.17	0.32	1.70	0.04	4	3	1	—
88	16	0.92	43	279	75	0.43	26	0.10	—	0.03	2.17	0.29	9	0	4	40
63	11	0.59	30	239	389	0.36	—	0.07	—	0.07	8.31	0.19	14	0	2	—
26	8	0.22	37	95	122	0.28	17	0.02	—	0.02	0.19	0.03	2	0	1	24
43	5	0.88	29	314	98	1.25	35	0.04	—	0.10	10.02	0.32	2	1	2	52
38	14	0.62	43	378	31	0.44	15	0.37	0.43	0.04	8.33	0.77	2	1	<1	31
10	7	0.79	18	118	202	0.51	13	0.02	0.68	0.07	7.06	0.06	3	0	1	43
17	6	0.87	15	134	192	0.44	10	0.02	0.30	0.04	7.53	0.20	2	0	2	46
10	7	0.79	18	117	28	0.51	13	0.02	—	0.07	7.03	0.06	3	0	1	43
17	6	0.87	15	134	28	0.44	10	0.02	0.30	0.04	7.53	0.20	2	0	2	46
18	2	0.37	19	189	225	0.27	3	0.01	—	0.04	6.63	0.24	3	0	1	34
24	8	0.55	19	134	214	0.27	3	0.00	0.90	0.02	3.29	0.12	1	0	1	37
18	2	0.37	19	189	28	0.27	14	0.01	—	0.04	6.63	0.24	3	0	1	34
24	8	0.55	19	134	28	0.27	3	0.00	0.90	0.02	3.29	0.12	1	0	1	37
31	13	0.28	17	238	22	0.29	16	0.08	—	0.02	3.86	0.09	2	2	1	21
60.34	24.64	0.53	32.29	457.29	42.5	0.56	26.35	0.14	—	0.04	7.41	0.15	3.4	2.46	1.06	39.77
80	31	3.23	48	241	502	0.81	2	0.19	—	0.11	1.62	0.13	12	2	1	44
143	50	4.85	69	295	980	1.38	—	0.29	6.74	0.13	1.90	0.22	6	3	1	—
50	57	0.48	22	212	189	2.28	1	0.05	0.57	0.05	0.78	0.09	24	2	<1	18
85	88	0.77	28	275	237	3.59	2	0.09	0.85	0.04	2.81	0.15	43	3	6	34
65	50	0.37	49	347	321	4.65	26	0.05	—	0.17	3.08	0.15	36	3	9	40

Table H–1

Food Composition (Computer code number is for Wadsworth Diet Analysis program) (For purposes of calculations, use "0" for t, <1, <.1, <.01, etc.)

DA + Code	Food Description	Quantity	Measure	Wt (g)	H_2O (g)	Ener (kcal)	Prot (g)	Carb (g)	Dietary Fiber (g)	Fat (g)	Fat Breakdown (g) Sat	Mono	Poly
	SEAFOOD—Continued												
1860	**Clams, cooked, moist heat**	3	ounce(s)	85	54	126	22	4	0	2	0.16	0.15	0.47
1853	**Crayfish, farmed, cooked, moist heat**	3	ounce(s)	85	69	74	15	0	0	1	0.18	0.21	0.35
	Oysters												
8720	Baked or broiled	3	ounce(s)	85	69	90	6	3	0	6	1.38	2.18	1.88
152	Eastern, farmed, raw	3	ounce(s)	85	73	50	4	5	0	1	0.38	0.13	0.50
8715	Eastern, wild, cooked, moist heat	3	ounce(s)	85	60	116	12	7	0	4	1.31	0.53	1.65
8584	Pacific, cooked, moist heat	3	ounce(s)	85	55	139	16	8	0	4	0.87	0.66	1.52
1865	Pacific, raw	3	ounce(s)	85	70	69	8	4	0	2	0.43	0.30	0.76
1854	**Lobster, northern, cooked, moist heat**	3	ounce(s)	85	65	83	17	1	0	1	0.09	0.14	0.08
1862	**Mussels, blue, cooked, moist heat**	3	ounce(s)	85	52	146	20	6	0	4	0.72	0.86	1.03
	Shrimp												
1855	Mixed species, cooked, moist heat	3	ounce(s)	85	66	84	18	0	0	1	0.25	0.17	0.37
158	Mixed species, breaded, fried	3	ounce(s)	85	0.04	205.69	18.18	9.74	0.34	10.43	1.77	3.24	4.32
	BEEF, LAMB, PORK												
	Beef												
4450	Breakfast strips, cooked	2	slice(s)	23	0	101.47	7.07	0.31	0	7.77	3.24	3.8	0.35
174	Corned, canned	3	ounce(s)	85	49	213	23	0	0	13	5.25	5.07	0.54
33147	Cured, thin sliced	2	ounce(s)	57	31	87	18	2	0	1	0.54	0.48	0.04
4581	Jerky	1	ounce(s)	28	0	116.44	9.42	3.12	0.51	7.27	3.08	3.21	0.28
	Ground												
4411	Extra lean, broiled, well	3	ounce(s)	85	46	225	24	0	0	13	5.28	5.88	0.50
4417	Lean, broiled, medium	3	ounce(s)	85	47	231	21	0	0	16	6.16	6.87	0.59
4418	Lean, broiled, well	3	ounce(s)	85	45	238	24	0	0	15	5.89	6.56	0.56
4423	Regular, broiled, medium	3	ounce(s)	85	46	246	20	0	0	18	6.91	7.70	0.65
	Rib												
4183	Rib, whole, lean & fat, ¼" fat, roasted	3	ounce(s)	85	39	320	19	0	0	27	10.71	11.42	0.94
	Roast												
4264	Bottom round, lean & fat, ¼" fat, braised	3	ounce(s)	85	44	241	24	0	0	15	5.71	6.63	0.58
169	Bottom round, separable lean, ¼" fat, roasted	3	ounce(s)	85	0.05	160.64	24.45	0	0	6.26	2.13	2.83	0.24
4147	Chuck, arm pot roast, lean & fat, ¼" fat, braised	3	ounce(s)	85	41	282	23	0	0	20	7.97	8.68	0.77
4161	Chuck, blade roast, lean & fat, ¼" fat, braised	3	ounce(s)	85	40	293	23	0	0	22	8.70	9.44	0.78
5853	Chuck, blade roast, separable lean, ¼" trim, pot roasted	3	ounce(s)	85	0.04	209.1	27.45	0	0	10.15	3.94	4.37	0.33
4295	Eye of round, lean, ¼" fat, roasted	3	ounce(s)	85	55	149	25	0	0	5	1.76	2.06	0.15
4285	Eye of round, lean & fat, ¼" fat, roasted	3	ounce(s)	85	51	195	23	0	0	11	4.23	4.66	0.39
	Steak												
1757	Rib, small end, lean, ¼" fat, broiled	3	ounce(s)	85	49	188	24	0	0	10	3.84	4.01	0.27
4349	Short loin, T-bone steak, lean, ¼" fat, broiled	3	ounce(s)	85	52	174	23	0	0	9	3.05	4.23	0.26
4348	Short loin, T-bone steak, lean & fat, ¼" fat, broiled	3	ounce(s)	85	43	274	19	0	0	21	8.29	9.58	0.75
4360	Top loin, prime, lean & fat, ¼" fat, broiled	3	ounce(s)	85	43	275	22	0	0	20	8.16	8.61	0.73
	Variety												
188	Liver, pan fried	3	ounce(s)	85	53	149	23	4	0	4	1.27	0.56	0.49
4447	Tongue, simmered	3	ounce(s)	85	49	236	16	0	0	19	6.91	8.59	0.56
	Lamb												
	Chop												
3275	Loin, domestic, lean & fat, ¼" fat, broiled	3	ounce(s)	85	44	269	21	0	0	20	8.36	8.25	1.43
3287	Shoulder, arm, domestic, lean & fat, ¼" fat, braised	3	ounce(s)	85	38	294	26	0	0	20	8.39	8.65	1.45
3290	Shoulder, arm, domestic, lean, ¼" fat, braised	3	ounce(s)	85	42	237	30	0	0	12	4.28	5.24	0.78
	Leg												
3264	Domestic, lean & fat, ¼" fat, cooked	3	ounce(s)	85	46	250	21	0	0	18	7.51	7.50	1.28

PAGE KEY: H–2 = Breads/Baked Goods H–6 = Cereal/Rice/Pasta H–10 = Fruit H–16 = Vegetables/Legumes H–26 = Nuts/Seeds H–28 = Vegetarian H–30 = Dairy H–36 = Eggs H–38 = Seafood H–40 = Meats H–42 = Poultry H–44 = Processed meats H–46 = Beverages H–50 = Fats/Oils H–52 = Sweets H–52 = Sauces/Condiments/Spices H–56 = Mixed Foods/Soups/Sandwiches H–62 = Fast food H–80 = Convenience H–82 = Baby foods

Chol (mg)	Calc (mg)	Iron (mg)	Magn (mg)	Pota (mg)	Sodi (mg)	Zinc (mg)	Vit A (RAE) (μg)	Thia (mg)	Vit E (mg)	Ribo (mg)	Niac (mg)	Vit B_6 (mg)	Fola (μg)	Vit C (mg)	Vit B_{12} (μg)	Sele (μg)
57	78	23.77	15	534	95	2.32	145	0.13	—	0.36	2.85	0.09	25	19	84	54
116	43	0.94	28	202	82	1.26	13	0.04	—	0.07	1.42	0.11	9	<1	3	29
42	37	5.30	38	126	418	72.22	60	0.07	1.27	0.06	1.04	0.05	8	3	15	—
21	37	4.91	28	105	151	32.23	7	0.09	—	0.06	1.08	0.05	15	4	14	54
89	77	10.19	81	239	359	154.37	46	0.16	—	0.15	2.11	0.10	12	5	30	61
85	14	7.82	37	257	180	28.25	124	0.11	—	0.38	3.08	0.08	13	11	24	131
43	7	4.35	19	143	90	14.14	69	0.06	0.72	0.20	1.71	0.04	9	7	14	65
61	52	0.33	30	299	323	2.48	22	0.01	0.85	0.06	0.91	0.07	9	0	3	36
48	28	5.71	31	228	314	2.27	77	0.26	—	0.36	2.55	0.09	65	12	20	76
166	33	2.63	29	155	190	1.33	58	0.03	0.43	0.03	2.20	0.11	3	2	1	34
150.44	56.95	1.07	34	191.25	292.39	1.17	47.59	0.1	—	0.11	2.6	0.08	20.39	1.27	1.58	35.44
26.89	2.03	0.7	6.1	93.11	509.17	1.43	0	0.02	0.03	0.05	1.46	0.07	1.8	0	0.77	6.05
73	10	1.77	12	116	855	3.03	0	0.02	0.13	0.12	2.07	0.11	8	0	1	36
45	3	1.58	11	140	1582	2.49	0	0.03	0.08	0.12	1.85	0.16	5	0	1	13
13.63	5.67	1.53	14.48	169.54	628.49	2.3	0	0.04	0.11	0.04	0.49	0.05	38.05	0	0.28	3.03
84	8	2.35	21	314	70	5.47	0	0.06	0.15	0.27	4.97	0.27	9	0	2	19
74	9	1.79	18	256	65	4.56	0	0.04	0.17	0.18	4.39	0.22	8	0	2	25
86	10	2.08	20	297	76	5.27	0	0.05	0.17	0.20	5.07	0.26	9	0	2	22
77	9	2.07	17	248	71	4.40	0	0.03	0.20	0.16	4.90	0.23	8	0	2	16
72	9	1.96	16	252	54	4.45	0	0.06	0.20	0.14	2.86	0.20	6	0	2	19
82	5	2.65	19	240	43	4.17	0	0.06	0.15	0.20	3.17	0.28	9	0	2	27
66.3	4.25	2.66	23.79	332.35	56.09	3.92	0	0.06	—	0.2	3.45	0.31	10.19	0	2.29	23.29
84	9	2.64	16	209	51	5.81	0	0.06	0.19	0.20	2.70	0.24	8	0	3	21
88	11	2.64	16	196	54	7.07	0	0.06	0.17	0.20	2.06	0.22	4	0	2	21
73.94	11.05	3.12	19.54	223.55	60.34	8.72	0	0.06	0.09	0.23	0	0.24	—	0	2.09	22.69
59	4	1.66	23	336	53	4.03	0	0.08	—	0.14	3.19	0.32	6	0	2	23
61	5	1.56	20	308	50	3.69	0	0.07	0.15	0.14	2.97	0.30	6	0	2	22
68	11	2.18	23	335	59	5.94	0	0.09	0.12	0.19	4.08	0.34	7	0	3	19
50	5	3.11	22	278	65	4.34	0	0.09	0.12	0.21	3.94	0.33	7	0	2	9
58	7	2.56	18	234	58	3.56	0	0.08	0.19	0.18	3.29	0.28	6	0	2	10
67	8	1.89	20	294	54	3.85	0	0.07	—	0.15	3.96	0.31	6	0	2	19
324	5	5.24	19	298	65	4.45	6582	0.15	0.54	2.91	14.85	0.87	221	1	71	28
112	4	2.22	13	156	55	34.77	0	0.02	0.30	0.25	2.97	0.13	6	1	3	11
85	17	1.54	20	278	65	2.96	0	0.09	0.11	0.21	6.04	0.11	15	0	2	23
102	21	2.03	22	260	61	5.17	0	0.06	0.13	0.21	5.66	0.09	15	0	2	32
103	22	2.30	25	287	65	6.21	0	0.06	0.15	0.23	5.38	0.11	19	0	2	32
82	14	1.60	20	264	61	3.79	0	0.09	0.12	0.21	5.66	0.11	15	0	2	22

Table H–1

Food Composition (Computer code number is for Wadsworth Diet Analysis program) (For purposes of calculations, use "0" for t, <1, <.1, <.01, etc.)

DA + Code	Food Description	Quantity	Measure	Wt (g)	H_2O (g)	Ener (kcal)	Prot (g)	Carb (g)	Dietary Fiber (g)	Fat (g)	Fat Breakdown (g) Sat	Mono	Poly
	BEEF, LAMB, PORK—Continued												
	Rib												
183	Domestic, lean, ¼" fat, broiled	3	ounce(s)	85	50	200	24	0	0	11	3.95	4.43	1.00
182	Domestic, lean & fat, ¼" fat, broiled	3	ounce(s)	85	40	307	19	0	0	25	10.80	10.30	2.01
	Shoulder												
187	Arm & blade, domestic, choice, lean, ¼" fat, roasted	3	ounce(s)	85	54	173	21	0	0	9	3.47	3.71	0.81
186	Arm & blade, domestic, choice, lean & fat, ¼" fat, roasted	3	ounce(s)	85	48	235	19	0	0	17	7.17	6.94	1.38
	Variety												
3375	Brain, pan fried	3	ounce(s)	85	52	232	14	0	0	19	4.82	3.42	1.94
3406	Tongue, braised	3	ounce(s)	85	49	234	18	0	0	17	6.66	8.50	1.06
	Pork												
	Cured												
161	Bacon, cured, broiled, pan fried or roasted	2	slice(s)	13	2	68	5	<1	0	5	1.73	2.33	0.57
29229	Bacon, Canadian style, cured	2	ounce(s)	57	38	89	12	1	0	4	1.26	1.79	0.36
35422	Breakfast strips, cured, cooked	3	slice(s)	34	9	156	10	<1	0	12	4.34	5.58	1.92
16561	Ham, smoked or cured, lean, cooked	1	slice(s)	42	28	66	11	0	0	2	0.77	1.06	0.27
189	Ham, cured, boneless, 11% fat, roasted	3	ounce(s)	85	55	151	19	0	0	8	2.65	3.77	1.20
1316	Ham, cured, extra lean, 5% fat, roasted	3	ounce(s)	85	58	123	18	1	0	5	1.54	2.23	0.46
29215	Ham, cured, extra lean, 4% fat, canned	2	ounce(s)	57	42	68	10	0	0	3	0.86	1.25	0.22
	Chop												
32671	Loin, blade, lean & fat, pan fried	3	ounce(s)	85	42	291	18	0	0	24	8.65	9.97	2.64
32672	Loin, center cut, lean & fat, pan fried	3	ounce(s)	85	45	236	25	0	0	14	5.11	6.00	1.62
32682	Loin, center rib, boneless, lean & fat, braised	3	ounce(s)	85	49	217	22	0	0	13	5.21	6.13	1.12
32603	Loin, center rib, lean, broiled	3	ounce(s)	85	48	186	26	0	0	8	2.94	3.78	0.53
32481	Loin, whole, lean, braised	3	ounce(s)	85	52	174	24	0	0	8	2.87	3.54	0.60
32478	Loin, whole, lean & fat, braised	3	ounce(s)	85	50	203	23	0	0	12	4.35	5.15	1.00
	Leg or ham												
32471	Rump portion, lean & fat, roasted	3	ounce(s)	85	48	214	25	0	0	12	4.47	5.42	1.17
32468	Whole, lean & fat, roasted	3	ounce(s)	85	47	232	23	0	0	15	5.50	6.70	1.43
	Ribs												
32696	Loin, country style, lean, roasted	3	ounce(s)	85	49	210	23	0	0	13	4.52	5.49	0.94
32693	Loin, country style, lean & fat, roasted	3	ounce(s)	85	43	279	20	0	0	22	7.83	9.36	1.71
	Shoulder												
32629	Arm picnic, lean, roasted	3	ounce(s)	85	51	194	23	0	0	11	3.66	5.09	1.02
32626	Arm picnic, lean & fat, roasted	3	ounce(s)	85	44	270	20	0	0	20	7.47	9.12	2.00
	Rabbit												
3366	Domesticated, roasted	3	ounce(s)	85	52	167	25	0	0	7	2.04	1.84	1.33
3367	Domesticated, stewed	3	ounce(s)	85	50	175	26	0	0	7	2.13	1.93	1.39
	Veal												
3391	Liver, braised	3	ounce(s)	85	51	163	24	3	0	5	1.69	0.97	0.88
3319	Rib, lean only, roasted	3	ounce(s)	85	55	150	22	0	0	6	1.77	2.26	0.57
1732	**Deer or venison, roasted**	3	ounce(s)	85	55	134	26	0	0	3	1.06	0.75	0.53
	POULTRY												
	Chicken												
29562	Flaked, canned	2	ounce(s)	57	0.03	97.47	10.37	0.05	0	5.87	1.62	2.32	1.29
	Fried												
29632	Breast, meat only, breaded, baked or fried	3	ounce(s)	85	44	193	25	7	<1	7	1.62	2.66	1.73
35327	Broiler breast, meat only, fried	3	ounce(s)	85	51	159	28	<1	0	4	1.10	1.46	0.91
36413	Broiler breast, meat & skin, flour coated, fried	3	ounce(s)	85	48	189	27	1	<.1	8	2.08	2.98	1.67
35389	Broiler drumstick, meat only, fried	3	ounce(s)	85	53	166	24	0	0	7	1.81	2.50	1.68
36414	Broiler drumstick, meat & skin, flour coated, fried	3	ounce(s)	85	48	208	23	1	<.1	12	3.11	4.61	2.75
35406	Broiler leg, meat only, fried	3	ounce(s)	85	52	177	24	1	0	8	2.12	2.92	1.89
35484	Broiler wing, meat only, fried	3	ounce(s)	85	51	179	26	0	0	8	2.13	2.62	1.76
29580	Patty, fillet, or tenders, breaded, cooked	3	ounce(s)	85	42	241	14	13	<1	15	4.62	7.25	1.87

PAGE KEY: H–2 = Breads/Baked Goods H–6 = Cereal/Rice/Pasta H–10 = Fruit H–16 = Vegetables/Legumes H–26 = Nuts/Seeds H–28 = Vegetarian H–30 = Dairy H–36 = Eggs H–38 = Seafood H–40 = Meats H–42 = Poultry H–44 = Processed meats H–46 = Beverages H–50 = Fats/Oils H–52 = Sweets H–52 = Sauces/Condiments/Spices H–56 = Mixed Foods/Soups/Sandwiches H–62 = Fast food H–80 = Convenience H–82 = Baby foods

Chol (mg)	Calc (mg)	Iron (mg)	Magn (mg)	Pota (mg)	Sodi (mg)	Zinc (mg)	Vit A (RAE) (μg)	Thia (mg)	Vit E (mg)	Ribo (mg)	Niac (mg)	Vit B_6 (mg)	Fola (μg)	Vit C (mg)	Vit B_{12} (μg)	Sele (μg)
77	14	1.88	25	266	72	4.48	0	0.09	0.15	0.21	5.57	0.13	18	0	2	26
84	16	1.60	20	230	65	3.40	0	0.08	0.10	0.19	5.95	0.09	12	0	2	20
74	16	1.81	21	225	58	5.13	0	0.08	0.15	0.22	4.90	0.13	21	0	2	24
78	17	1.67	20	213	56	4.45	0	0.08	0.12	0.20	5.23	0.11	18	0	2	22
2128	18	1.73	19	304	133	1.70	0	0.14	—	0.31	3.87	0.20	6	20	20	10
161	9	2.24	14	134	57	2.54	0	0.07	—	0.36	3.14	0.14	3	6	5	24
14	1	0.18	4	71	291	0.44	1	0.05	0.07	0.03	1.40	0.04	<1	0	<1	8
28	5	0.39	10	195	799	0.79	0	0.43	0.15	0.10	3.53	0.22	2	0	<1	14
36	5	0.67	9	158	714	1.25	0	0.25	0.10	0.13	2.58	0.12	1	0	1	8
23	3	0.40	9	133	557	1.08	0	0.29	0.11	0.11	2.11	0.20	2	0	<1	—
50	7	1.14	19	348	1275	2.10	0	0.62	0.22	0.28	5.23	0.26	3	0	1	17
45	7	1.26	12	244	1023	2.45	0	0.64	0.22	0.17	3.42	0.34	3	0	1	17
22	3	0.53	10	206	712	1.09	0	0.47	0.15	0.13	3.01	0.26	3	0	<1	8
72	26	0.75	18	282	57	2.71	3	0.53	0.22	0.25	3.36	0.29	3	1	1	30
78	23	0.77	25	361	68	1.96	2	0.97	0.22	0.26	4.76	0.40	5	1	1	33
62	4	0.78	14	329	34	1.76	2	0.45	—	0.21	3.67	0.26	3	<1	<1	28
69	26	0.70	24	357	55	2.02	2	0.95	0.22	0.28	5.25	0.40	3	<1	1	40
67	15	0.96	17	329	43	2.11	2	0.56	0.22	0.23	3.90	0.33	3	1	<1	41
68	18	0.91	16	318	41	2.02	2	0.54	0.22	0.22	3.76	0.31	3	1	<1	39
82	10	0.89	23	318	53	2.40	3	0.64	0.22	0.28	3.96	0.27	3	<1	1	40
80	12	0.86	19	299	51	2.52	3	0.54	0.22	0.27	3.89	0.34	9	<1	1	39
79	25	1.10	20	297	25	3.24	2	0.49	—	0.29	3.97	0.37	4	<1	1	36
78	21	0.90	20	293	44	2.01	3	0.76	—	0.29	3.67	0.38	4	<1	1	32
81	8	1.21	17	299	68	3.46	2	0.49	—	0.30	3.67	0.35	4	<1	1	33
80	16	1.00	14	276	60	2.93	2	0.44	—	0.26	3.33	0.30	3	<1	1	29
70	16	1.93	18	326	40	1.93	0	0.08	—	0.18	7.17	0.40	9	0	7	33
73	17	2.01	17	255	31	2.01	0	0.05	0.67	0.14	6.09	0.29	8	0	6	33
434	5	4.34	17	280	66	9.55	17973	0.15	0.29	2.43	11.18	0.78	281	1	72	16
98	10	0.82	20	264	82	3.82	0	0.05	0.31	0.25	6.38	0.23	12	0	1	9
95	6	3.80	20	285	46	2.34	0	0.15	—	0.51	5.70	—	—	0	—	11
35.34	7.98	0.9	6.84	148.19	410.39	0.8	19.37	0	—	0.07	3.6	0.19	—	0	0.16	—
67	19	1.05	25	223	450	0.84	—	0.08	0.72	0.10	10.98	0.47	4	0	<1	—
77	14	0.97	26	235	67	0.92	—	0.07	0.36	0.11	12.57	0.54	3	0	<1	22
76	14	1.01	26	220	65	0.94	—	0.07	0.39	0.11	11.69	0.49	5	0	<1	20
80	10	1.12	20	212	82	2.74	—	0.07	0.42	0.20	5.23	0.33	8	0	<1	17
77	10	1.14	20	195	76	2.46	—	0.07	0.66	0.19	5.13	0.30	9	0	<1	16
84	11	1.19	21	216	82	2.53	—	0.07	0.38	0.21	5.69	0.33	8	0	<1	16
71	13	0.97	18	177	77	1.80	—	0.04	0.41	0.11	6.16	0.50	3	0	<1	22
51	14	1.06	17	209	452	0.88	—	0.08	1.66	0.12	5.71	0.26	9	<1	<1	—

Table H–1

Food Composition (Computer code number is for Wadsworth Diet Analysis program) (For purposes of calculations, use "0" for t, <1, <.1, <.01, etc.)

DA + Code	Food Description	Quantity	Measure	Wt (g)	H_2O (g)	Ener (kcal)	Prot (g)	Carb (g)	Dietary Fiber (g)	Fat (g)	Fat Breakdown (g) Sat	Mono	Poly
	POULTRY—Continued												
	Roasted, meat only												
35409	Broiler chicken leg	3	ounce(s)	85	55	162	23	0	0	7	1.95	2.59	1.68
35486	Broiler chicken wing	3	ounce(s)	85	53	173	26	0	0	7	1.92	2.22	1.51
35138	Roasting chicken, dark meat	3	ounce(s)	85	57	151	20	0	0	7	2.07	2.82	1.70
35136	Roasting chicken, light meat	3	ounce(s)	85	58	130	23	0	0	3	0.92	1.29	0.79
35132	Roasting chicken	3	ounce(s)	85	57	142	21	0	0	6	1.54	2.13	1.28
	Stewed												
3174	Meat only, stewed	3	ounce(s)	85	0.05	150.44	23.19	0	0	5.7	1.56	2.03	1.3
1268	Gizzard, simmered	3	ounce(s)	85	58	124	26	0	0	2	0.57	0.45	0.30
1270	Liver, simmered	3	ounce(s)	85	57	142	21	1	0	6	1.75	1.20	1.08
	Duck												
1286	Domesticated, meat & skin, roasted	3	ounce(s)	85	44	286	16	0	0	24	8.22	10.97	3.10
1287	Domesticated, meat only, roasted	3	ounce(s)	85	55	171	20	0	0	10	3.54	3.15	1.22
	Goose												
35507	Domesticated, meat & skin, roasted	3	ounce(s)	85	44	259	21	0	0	19	5.84	8.72	2.14
35524	Domesticated, meat only, roasted	3	ounce(s)	85	49	202	25	0	0	11	3.88	3.69	1.31
1297	Liver pâté, smoked, canned	4	tablespoon(s)	52	19	240	6	2	0	23	7.51	13.32	0.44
	Turkey												
3256	Ground turkey, cooked	3	ounce(s)	85	51	200	23	0	0	11	2.88	4.16	2.75
222	Roasted, fryer roaster breast, meat only	3	ounce(s)	85	58	115	26	0	0	1	0.20	0.11	0.17
219	Roasted, dark meat, meat only	3	ounce(s)	85	54	159	24	0	0	6	2.06	1.39	1.84
220	Roasted, light meat, meat only	3	ounce(s)	85	56	133	25	0	0	3	0.88	0.48	0.73
3263	Patty, batter coated, breaded, fried	1	item(s)	94	47	266	13	15	<1	17	4.41	7.02	4.43
1302	Turkey roll, light meat	2	slice(s)	57	41	83	11	<1	0	4	1.15	1.42	0.99
1303	Turkey roll, light & dark meat	2	slice(s)	57	40	84	10	1	0	4	1.16	1.30	1.01
	PROCESSED MEATS												
	Beef												
1331	Corned beef loaf, jellied, sliced	2	slice(s)	57	39	87	13	0	0	3	1.47	1.52	0.18
	Bologna												
13458	Made w/chicken, pork, & beef	1	slice(s)	28	15	90	3	1	0	8	3.00	4.05	1.10
13461	Light, made w/pork, chicken, & beef	1	slice(s)	28	18	60	3	2	0	4	1.50	2.04	0.43
13459	Beef	1	slice(s)	28	15	90	3	1	0	8	3.50	4.26	0.31
13565	Turkey	1	slice(s)	28	19	50	3	1	0	4	1.00	1.09	0.98
	Chicken												
13562	Oven roasted white chicken	1	slice(s)	28	20	40	4	1	0	3	0.50	—	—
	Ham												
13581	Honey glazed, traditional carved	2	slice(s)	45	—	50	8	1	0	2	0.50	0.68	0.18
13777	Deli sliced cooked	1	slice(s)	28	—	30	5	1	0	1	0.50	0.39	0.11
13778	Deli sliced honey	1	slice(s)	28	—	35	5	1	0	1	0.50	0.39	0.11
8614	**Pork & beef mortadella, sliced**	2	slice(s)	46	24	143	8	1	0	12	4.37	5.23	1.44
1323	**Pork olive loaf**	2	slice(s)	57	33	133	7	5	0	9	3.32	4.47	1.10
1324	**Pork pickle & pimento loaf**	2	slice(s)	57	32	149	7	3	0	12	4.45	5.45	1.47
	Sausages & frankfurters												
37296	Beerwurst beef beer salami (bierwurst)	1	slice(s)	29	17	74	4	1	0	6	2.50	2.69	0.21
37257	Beerwurst pork beer salami	1	slice(s)	21	13	50	3	<1	0	4	1.32	1.89	0.50
35338	Berliner, pork & beef	1	ounce(s)	28	17	65	4	1	0	5	1.72	2.27	0.45
37299	Braunschweiger pork liver sausage	1	slice(s)	15	0	51.34	1.97	0.34	0	4.48	1.52	2.08	0.52
37298	Bratwurst pork, cooked	1	piece(s)	74	42	181	10	2	0	14	5.15	6.73	1.51
1329	Cheesefurter or cheese smokie, beef & pork	1	item(s)	43	23	141	6	1	0	12	4.52	5.89	1.30
1330	Chorizo, beef & pork	2	ounce(s)	57	18	258	14	1	0	22	8.15	10.43	1.96
8600	Frankfurter, beef	1	item(s)	45	23	149	5	2	0	13	5.26	6.44	0.53
202	Frankfurter, beef & pork	1	item(s)	57	32	174	7	1	1	16	6.14	7.79	1.56
1293	Frankfurter, chicken	1	item(s)	45	26	116	6	3	0	9	2.49	3.82	1.82
3261	Frankfurter, turkey	1	item(s)	45	28	102	6	1	0	8	2.65	2.51	2.25
37275	Italian sausage, pork, cooked	1	item(s)	68	34	220	14	1	0	17	6.14	8.13	2.23
37307	Kielbasa, kolbassa, pork & beef	2⅛	ounce(s)	61	37	135	10	2	0	9	3.40	4.44	1.06
1333	Knockwurst or knackwurst, beef & pork	2	ounce(s)	57	31	174	6	2	0	16	5.79	7.26	1.66
37285	Pepperoni, beef & pork	1	slice(s)	11	3	55	2	<1	0	5	1.77	2.32	0.48

PAGE KEY: H–2 = Breads/Baked Goods H–6 = Cereal/Rice/Pasta H–10 = Fruit H–16 = Vegetables/Legumes H–26 = Nuts/Seeds H–28 = Vegetarian H–30 = Dairy H–36 = Eggs H–38 = Seafood H–40 = Meats H–42 = Poultry H–44 = Processed meats H–46 = Beverages H–50 = Fats/Oils H–52 = Sweets H–52 = Sauces/Condiments/Spices H–56 = Mixed Foods/Soups/Sandwiches H–62 = Fast food H–80 = Convenience H–82 = Baby foods

Chol (mg)	Calc (mg)	Iron (mg)	Magn (mg)	Pota (mg)	Sodi (mg)	Zinc (mg)	Vit A (RAE) (µg)	Thia (mg)	Vit E (mg)	Ribo (mg)	Niac (mg)	Vit B_6 (mg)	Fola (µg)	Vit C (mg)	Vit B_{12} (µg)	Sele (µg)
80	10	1.11	20	206	77	2.43	—	0.06	0.23	0.20	5.37	0.32	7	0	<1	19
72	14	0.99	18	179	78	1.82	—	0.04	0.23	0.11	6.22	0.50	3	0	<1	21
64	9	1.13	17	191	81	1.81	14	0.05	—	0.16	4.88	0.26	6	0	<1	17
64	11	0.92	20	201	43	0.66	7	0.05	0.23	0.08	8.90	0.46	3	0	<1	22
64	10	1.03	18	195	64	1.29	10	0.05	—	0.13	6.70	0.35	4	0	<1	21
70.55	11.89	0.99	17.85	153	59.5	1.69	12.75	0.04	0.18	0.13	5.19	0.22	5.09	0	0.18	17.76
315	14	2.71	3	152	48	3.76	0	0.02	1.01	0.18	2.65	0.06	4	0	1	35
479	9	9.89	21	224	65	3.38	3384	0.25	1.22	1.69	9.39	0.64	491	24	14	70
71	9	2.30	14	173	50	1.58	54	0.15	0.60	0.23	4.10	0.15	5	0	<1	17
76	10	2.30	17	214	55	2.21	20	0.22	0.60	0.40	4.34	0.21	9	0	<1	19
77	11	2.41	19	280	60	2.23	18	0.07	1.48	0.28	3.55	0.32	2	0	<1	19
82	12	2.44	21	330	65	2.70	10	0.08	—	0.33	3.47	0.40	10	0	<1	22
78	36	2.86	7	72	362	0.48	521	0.05	—	0.16	1.31	0.03	31	0	5	23
87	21	1.64	20	230	91	2.43	0	0.05	0.29	0.14	4.10	0.33	6	0	<1	32
71	10	1.30	25	248	44	1.48	0	0.04	0.08	0.11	6.37	0.48	5	0	<1	27
72	27	1.98	20	247	67	3.79	0	0.05	0.54	0.21	3.10	0.31	8	0	<1	35
59	16	1.15	24	259	54	1.73	0	0.05	0.08	0.11	5.81	0.46	5	0	<1	27
58	13	2.07	14	259	752	1.35	10	0.09	2.25	0.18	2.16	0.19	26	0	<1	19
24	23	0.73	9	142	277	0.88	0	0.05	0.08	0.13	3.97	0.18	2	0	<1	13
31	18	0.77	10	153	332	1.13	0	0.05	0.19	0.16	2.72	0.15	3	0	<1	17
27	6	1.16	6	57	540	2.32	0	0.00	0.11	0.06	1.00	0.07	5	0	1	10
30	0	0.36	6	43	290	0.40	0	—	—	—	—	—	—	0	—	—
15	0	0.36	6	46	310	0.45	0	—	—	—	—	—	—	0	—	—
20	0	0.36	4	47	310	0.57	0	0.01	—	0.03	0.68	0.05	4	0	<1	—
20	40	0.36	6	43	270	0.52	0	—	—	—	—	—	—	0	—	—
15	0	0.36	7	85	350	0.32	0	—	—	—	—	—	—	0	—	—
25	0	0.72	—	—	560	—	0	—	—	—	—	—	—	0	—	—
15	0	0.00	—	—	240	—	0	—	—	—	—	—	—	0	—	—
15	0	0.00	—	—	240	—	0	—	—	—	—	—	—	0	—	—
26	8	0.64	5	75	573	0.97	0	0.05	0.10	0.07	1.23	0.06	1	0	1	10
22	62	0.31	11	169	843	0.78	34	0.17	0.14	0.15	1.04	0.13	1	0	1	9
21	54	0.58	10	193	789	0.80	12	0.17	0.14	0.14	1.17	0.11	3	0	1	8
18	3	0.44	4	67	265	0.71	0	0.02	0.06	0.04	0.99	0.05	1	0	1	5
12	2	0.16	3	53	261	0.36	0	0.12	—	0.04	0.69	0.07	1	0	<1	—
13	3	0.33	4	80	368	0.70	0	0.11	0.06	0.06	0.88	0.06	1	0	1	4
23.69	1.36	1.42	1.67	27.49	131.54	0.42	641.01	0.03	0.04	0.23	1.27	0.05	—	0	3.05	8.81
44	33	0.96	11	157	412	1.70	0	0.37	0.19	0.14	2.37	0.16	1	1	1	16
29	25	0.46	6	89	465	0.97	20	0.11	0.14	0.07	1.25	0.06	1	0	1	7
50	5	0.90	10	226	700	1.93	0	0.36	0.12	0.17	2.91	0.30	1	0	1	12
24	6	0.68	6	70	513	1.11	0	0.02	0.09	0.07	1.07	0.04	2	0	1	4
29	6	0.66	6	95	638	1.05	10	0.11	0.14	0.07	1.50	0.07	2	0	1	8
45	43	0.90	5	38	617	0.47	18	0.03	0.10	0.05	1.39	0.14	2	0	<1	8
48	48	0.83	6	81	642	1.40	0	0.02	0.28	0.08	1.86	0.10	4	0	<1	7
53	16	1.02	12	207	627	1.62	0	0.42	0.17	0.16	2.83	0.22	3	1	1	15
41	27	0.88	10	169	566	1.23	0	0.14	0.13	0.13	1.75	0.11	3	0	1	11
34	6	0.37	6	113	527	0.94	0	0.19	0.32	0.08	1.55	0.10	1	0	1	8
9	1	0.15	2	38	224	0.28	0	0.04	0.02	0.03	0.55	0.03	<1	0	<1	—

Table H–1

Food Composition (Computer code number is for Wadsworth Diet Analysis program) (For purposes of calculations, use "0" for t, <1, <.1, <.01, etc.)

DA + Code	Food Description	Quantity	Measure	Wt (g)	H_2O (g)	Ener (kcal)	Prot (g)	Carb (g)	Dietary Fiber (g)	Fat (g)	Fat Breakdown (g) Sat	Mono	Poly
	PROCESSED MEATS—Continued												
37313	Polish sausage, pork	2	slice(s)	57	31	163	8	2	—	14	4.91	6.42	1.46
206	Salami, beef, cooked, sliced	2	slice(s)	46	28	119	6	1	0	10	4.54	4.90	0.48
37272	Salami, pork, dry or hard	1	slice(s)	13	5	52	3	<1	0	4	1.52	2.05	0.48
3262	Salami, turkey	2	slice(s)	57	31	125	8	11	<.1	5	1.98	1.80	1.43
7162	Sausage, breakfast, turkey	2½	ounce(s)	100	67	190	17	<1	0	13	3.90	6.23	3.33
8620	Smoked sausage, beef & pork	2	ounce(s)	57	31	181	7	1	0	16	5.54	6.94	2.23
8619	Smoked, sausage, pork	2	ounce(s)	57	22	221	13	1	0	18	6.42	8.30	2.13
37273	Smoked, sausage, pork link	1	piece(s)	76	30	295	17	2	—	24	8.58	11.09	2.85
1336	Summer sausage, thuringer, or cervelat, beef & pork	2	ounce(s)	57	29	190	9	<1	0	17	6.82	7.35	0.68
37294	Vienna sausage, cocktail, beef & pork, canned	1	piece(s)	16	10	45	2	<1	0	4	1.49	2.01	0.27
	Spreads												
32419	Pork & beef sandwich spread	4	tablespoon(s)	60	36	141	5	7	<1	10	3.59	4.57	1.54
1318	Ham salad spread	¼	cup(s)	60	38	130	5	6	0	9	3.04	4.32	1.62
	Turkey												
16049	Breast, hickory smoked, slices	1	slice(s)	56	—	50	11	1	0	0	0.00	0.00	0.00
13606	Breast, hickory smoked fat free	1	slice(s)	28	—	25	4	1	0	0	0.00	0.00	0.00
16047	Breast, honey roasted, slices	1	slice(s)	56	—	60	11	2	0	0	0.00	0.00	0.00
16048	Breast, oven roasted, slices	1	slice(s)	56	—	50	11	1	0	0	0.00	0.00	0.00
13583	Breast, traditional carved	2	slice(s)	45	—	40	9	0	0	1	0.00	0.07	0.14
13604	Breast, oven roasted, fat free	1	slice(s)	28	—	25	4	1	0	0	0.00	0.00	0.00
13567	Turkey ham, 10% water added	1	slice(s)	28	20	35	5	0	0	1	0.00	0.22	0.31
13596	Turkey pastrami	2	ounce(s)	56	—	70	11	1	0	2	1.00	—	—
13597	Turkey salami	2	ounce(s)	56	—	120	8	1	0	9	2.50	2.92	2.30
	BEVERAGES												
	Alcoholic												
	Beer												
866	Ale, mild	12	fluid ounce(s)	360	332	148	1	13	1	0	0.00	0.00	0.00
686	Beer	12	fluid ounce(s)	356	336	118	1	6	<1	<1	0.00	0.00	0.00
869	Beer, light	12	fluid ounce(s)	354	337	99	1	5	0	0	0.00	0.00	0.00
16886	Beer, nonalcoholic	12	fluid ounce(s)	360	353	32	1	5	0	0	0.00	0.00	0.00
31608	Budweiser beer	12	fluid ounce(s)	355	328	143	1	11	0	0	0.00	0.00	0.00
31609	Bud Light beer	12	fluid ounce(s)	355	335	110	1	7	0	0	0.00	0.00	0.00
31613	Michelob Beer	12	fluid ounce(s)	355	323	155	1	13	0	0	0.00	0.00	0.00
31614	Michelob Light beer	12	fluid ounce(s)	355	330	134	1	12	0	0	0.00	0.00	0.00
	Gin, rum, vodka, whiskey												
687	Distilled alcohol, 80 proof	1	fluid ounce(s)	28	19	64	0	0	0	0	0.00	0.00	0.00
688	Distilled alcohol, 86 proof	1	fluid ounce(s)	28	18	70	0	<.1	0	0	0.00	0.00	0.00
689	Distilled alcohol, 90 proof	1	fluid ounce(s)	28	17	73	0	0	0	0	0.00	0.00	0.00
856	Distilled alcohol, 94 proof	1	fluid ounce(s)	28	17	76	0	0	0	0	0.00	0.00	0.00
857	Distilled alcohol, 100 proof	1	fluid ounce(s)	28	16	82	0	0	0	0	0.00	0.00	0.00
	Liqueurs												
3142	Coffee liqueur, 63 proof	1	fluid ounce(s)	35	14	107	<.1	11	0	<1	0.04	0.01	0.04
33187	Coffee liqueur, 53 proof	1	fluid ounce(s)	35	11	117	<.1	16	0	<1	0.04	0.01	0.04
736	Cordials, 54 proof	1	fluid ounce(s)	30	9	106	<.1	13	0	<.1	0.02	0.01	0.04
	Wine												
858	Champagne, domestic	5	fluid ounce(s)	150	—	105	<1	4	0	0	0.00	0.00	0.00
861	Red wine, California	5	fluid ounce(s)	150	133	125	<1	4	0	0	0.00	0.00	0.00
690	Sweet dessert wine	5	fluid ounce(s)	150	106	240	<1	21	0	0	0.00	0.00	0.00
1481	White wine	5	fluid ounce(s)	148	132	100	<1	1	0	0	0.00	0.00	0.00
1811	Wine cooler	10	fluid ounce(s)	300	270	150	<1	18	<.1	<.1	0.01	0.00	0.02
	Carbonated												
692	Club soda	12	fluid ounce(s)	355	355	0	0	0	0	0	0.00	0.00	0.00
12010	Coca-Cola Classic cola soda	12	fluid ounce(s)	360	—	146	0	41	0	0	0.00	0.00	0.00
12031	Coke diet cola soda	12	fluid ounce(s)	360	—	2	0	<1	0	0	0.00	0.00	0.00
693	Cola	12	fluid ounce(s)	426	380	179	<1	46	0	0	0.00	0.00	0.00
9522	Cola soda, decaffeinated	12	fluid ounce(s)	372	331	156	<1	40	0	0	0.00	0.00	0.00
1415	Cola, low calorie w/aspartame	12	fluid ounce(s)	355	354	4	<1	<1	0	0	0.00	0.00	0.00

PAGE KEY: H–2 = Breads/Baked Goods H–6 = Cereal/Rice/Pasta H–10 = Fruit H–16 = Vegetables/Legumes H–26 = Nuts/Seeds H–28 = Vegetarian H–30 = Dairy H–36 = Eggs H–38 = Seafood H–40 = Meats H–42 = Poultry H–44 = Processed meats H–46 = Beverages H–50 = Fats/Oils H–52 = Sweets H–52 = Sauces/Condiments/Spices H–56 = Mixed Foods/Soups/Sandwiches H–62 = Fast food H–80 = Convenience H–82 = Baby foods

Chol (mg)	Calc (mg)	Iron (mg)	Magn (mg)	Pota (mg)	Sodi (mg)	Zinc (mg)	Vit A (RAE) (µg)	Thia (mg)	Vit E (mg)	Ribo (mg)	Niac (mg)	Vit B_6 (mg)	Fola (µg)	Vit C (mg)	Vit B_{12} (µg)	Sele (µg)
40	7	0.82	8	102	546	1.10	0	0.29	—	0.08	1.96	0.11	1	1	1	10
33	3	1.01	6	86	524	0.81	0	0.05	0.09	0.09	1.49	0.08	1	0	1	7
10	2	0.17	3	48	289	0.54	0	0.12	0.04	0.04	0.72	0.07	<1	0	<1	3
45	42	0.87	15	225	616	1.76	1	0.24	0.32	0.17	2.26	0.24	6	12	1	11
92	57	2.20	18	188	665	2.07	0	0.04	0.24	0.12	3.55	0.29	5	1	<1	—
33	7	0.43	7	101	517	0.71	7	0.11	0.12	0.06	1.67	0.09	1	0	<1	0
39	17	0.66	11	191	851	1.60	0	0.40	0.14	0.15	2.57	0.20	3	1	1	12
52	23	0.88	14	255	1137	2.14	0	0.53	0.19	0.20	3.43	0.27	4	0	1	16
43	7	1.44	8	154	704	1.45	0	0.09	0.12	0.19	2.44	0.15	1	0	3	12
8	2	0.14	1	16	152	0.26	0	0.01	0.04	0.02	0.26	0.02	1	0	<1	3
23	7	0.47	5	66	608	0.61	16	0.10	1.04	0.08	1.04	0.07	1	0	1	6
22	5	0.35	6	90	547	0.66	0	0.26	1.04	0.07	1.26	0.09	1	0	<1	11
25	0	0.72	—	—	730	—	0	—	—	—	—	—	—	0	—	—
10	0	0.00	—	—	300	—	0	—	—	—	—	—	—	0	—	—
20	0	0.72	—	—	640	—	0	—	—	—	—	—	—	0	—	—
20	0	0.72	—	—	620	—	0	—	—	—	—	—	—	0	—	—
20	0	0.72	—	—	540	—	0	—	—	—	—	—	—	0	—	—
10	0	0.00	—	—	330	—	0	—	—	—	—	—	—	0	—	—
20	0	0.36	6	81	310	0.73	0	—	—	—	—	—	—	0	—	—
40	0	0.72	—	—	590	—	0	—	—	—	—	—	—	0	—	—
50	40	0.72	—	—	500	—	0	—	—	—	—	—	—	0	—	—
0	18	0.11	—	—	18	—	0	0.02	—	0.10	1.63	—	—	0	<.1	—
0	18	0.07	21	89	14	0.04	0	0.02	0.00	0.09	1.61	0.18	21	0	<.1	2
0	18	0.14	18	64	11	0.11	0	0.03	0.00	0.11	1.39	0.12	14	0	<.1	2
0	25	0.04	32	90	18	0.04	—	0.02	0.00	0.10	1.63	0.18	22	0	<.1	—
0	18	0.11	21	89	9	0.07	0	0.02	0.00	0.09	1.61	0.18	21	0	<.1	4
0	18	0.14	18	64	9	0.11	0	0.03	0.00	0.11	1.39	0.12	15	0	<.1	4
0	18	0.11	21	89	9	0.07	0	0.02	0.00	0.09	1.61	0.18	21	0	<.1	4
0	18	0.14	18	64	9	0.11	0	0.03	0.00	0.11	1.39	0.12	15	0	<.1	4
0	0	0.01	0	1	<1	0.01	0	0.00	0.00	0.00	0.00	0.00	0	0	0	0
0	0	0.01	0	1	<1	0.01	0	0.00	0.00	0.00	0.00	0.00	0	0	0	0
0	0	0.01	0	1	<1	0.01	0	0.00	0.00	0.00	0.00	0.00	0	0	0	0
0	0	0.01	0	1	<1	0.01	0	0.00	—	0.00	0.00	0.00	0	0	0	0
0	0	0.01	0	1	<1	0.01	0	0.00	—	0.00	0.00	0.00	0	0	0	0
0	<1	0.02	1	10	3	0.01	0	0.00	—	0.00	0.05	0.00	0	0	0	<1
0	<1	0.02	1	10	3	0.01	0	0.00	0.00	0.00	0.05	0.00	0	0	0	<1
0	<1	0.02	<1	5	2	0.01	0	0.00	—	0.00	0.02	0.00	0	0	0	—
0	—	—	—	—	—	—	—	—	—	—	0.00	—	—	—	0	—
0	12	1.43	16	171	15	0.15	0	0.02	0.00	0.04	0.12	0.05	1	0	<.1	—
0	12	0.36	14	138	14	0.11	0	0.03	0.00	0.03	0.32	0.00	0	0	0	1
0	13	0.47	15	118	7	0.10	0	0.01		0.01	0.10	0.02	0	0	0	<1
0	17	0.81	16	135	25	0.17		0.01	0.02	0.02	0.13	0.04	4	5	<.1	—
0	18	0.04	4	7	75	0.36	0	0.00	0.00	0.00	0.00	0.00	0	0	0	0
0	—	—	—	0	50	—	0	—	0.00	—	—	—	—	0	—	—
0	—	—	—	18	42	—	0	—	0.00	—	—	—	—	0	—	—
0	13	0.09	4	4	17	0.04	0	0.00	0.00	0.00	0.00	0.00	0	0	0	<1
0	11	0.07	4	4	15	0.04	0	0.00	0.00	0.00	0.00	0.00	0	0	0	<1
0	11	0.11	4	21	18	0.00	0	0.02	0.00	0.08	0.00	0.00	0	0	0	0

Table H–1

Food Composition (Computer code number is for Wadsworth Diet Analysis program) (For purposes of calculations, use "0" for t, <1, <.1, <.01, etc.)

DA + Code	Food Description	Quantity	Measure	Wt (g)	H_2O (g)	Ener (kcal)	Prot (g)	Carb (g)	Dietary Fiber (g)	Fat (g)	Fat Breakdown (g) Sat	Mono	Poly
	BEVERAGES—Continued												
9524	Cola, decaffeinated, low calorie w/aspartame	12	fluid ounce(s)	355	354	4	<1	<1	0	0	0.00	0.00	0.00
1412	Cream soda	12	fluid ounce(s)	371	321	189	0	49	0	0	0.00	0.00	0.00
31899	Diet 7 Up	12	fluid ounce(s)	360	—	0	0	0	0	0	0.00	0.00	0.00
695	Ginger ale	12	fluid ounce(s)	366	334	124	0	32	0	0	0.00	0.00	0.00
694	Grape soda	12	fluid ounce(s)	372	330	160	0	42	0	0	0.00	0.00	0.00
1876	Lemon lime soda	12	fluid ounce(s)	368	330	147	0	38	0	0	0.00	0.00	0.00
29392	Mountain Dew diet soda	12	fluid ounce(s)	360	—	0	0	0	0	0	0.00	0.00	0.00
29391	Mountain Dew soda	12	fluid ounce(s)	360	—	170	0	46	0	0	0.00	0.00	0.00
3145	Orange soda	12	fluid ounce(s)	372	326	179	0	46	0	0	0.00	0.00	0.00
1414	Pepper-type soda	12	fluid ounce(s)	368	329	151	0	38	0	<1	0.26	0.00	0.00
2391	Pepper-type or cola soda, low calorie w/saccharin	12	fluid ounce(s)	355	354	0	0	<1	0	0	0.00	0.00	0.00
29389	Pepsi diet cola soda	12	fluid ounce(s)	360	—	0	0	0	0	0	0.00	0.00	0.00
29388	Pepsi regular cola soda	12	fluid ounce(s)	360	—	150	0	41	0	0	0.00	0.00	0.00
696	Root beer	12	fluid ounce(s)	370	330	152	0	39	0	0	0.00	0.00	0.00
31898	7 Up	12	fluid ounce(s)	360	—	240	0	59	0	0	0.00	0.00	0.00
12034	Sprite diet soda	12	fluid ounce(s)	360	—	4	0	0	0	0	0.00	0.00	0.00
12044	Sprite soda	12	fluid ounce(s)	360	—	144	0	39	0	0	0.00	0.00	0.00
	Coffee												
731	Brewed	8	fluid ounce(s)	237	236	9	<1	0	0	2	0.00	0.00	0.00
9520	Brewed, decaffeinated	8	fluid ounce(s)	237	235	5	<1	1	0	0	0.00	0.00	0.00
16882	Cappuccino	8	fluid ounce(s)	240	224	78	4	6	<1	4	2.53	1.18	0.15
16883	Cappuccino, decaffeinated	8	fluid ounce(s)	240	224	78	4	6	<1	4	2.53	1.18	0.15
16880	Espresso	8	fluid ounce(s)	237	235	5	<1	1	0	0	0.00	0.00	0.00
16881	Espresso, decaffeinated	8	fluid ounce(s)	237	235	5	<1	1	0	0	0.00	0.00	0.00
732	Instant, prepared	8	fluid ounce(s)	239	237	5	<1	1	0	0	0.00	0.00	0.00
	Fruit drinks												
29357	Crystal Light low calorie lemonade drink	8	fluid ounce(s)	240	—	5	0	0	0	0	0.00	0.00	0.00
6012	Fruit punch drink w/added vitamin C, canned	8	fluid ounce(s)	276	242	129	0	33	<1	<.1	0.01	0.01	0.01
260	Grape drink, canned	8	fluid ounce(s)	250	221	113	<.1	29	0	0	0.00	0.00	0.00
266	Lemonade, from frozen concentrate	8	fluid ounce(s)	248	213	131	<1	34	<1	<1	0.02	0.00	0.04
268	Limeade, from frozen concentrate	8	fluid ounce(s)	247	220	104	<.1	26	0	<.1	0.00	0.00	0.00
31143	Gatorade Thirst Quencher, all flavors	8	fluid ounce(s)	240	—	50	0	14	0	0	0.00	0.00	0.00
17372	Kool-Aid (lemonade/punch/fruit drink)	8	fluid ounce(s)	248	220	108	<1	28	<1	<.1	0.01	0.01	0.02
17225	Kool-Aid sugar free, low calorie tropical punch mix, prepared	8	fluid ounce(s)	240	—	5	0	0	0	0	0.00	0.00	0.00
14266	Odwalla strawberry 'c' monster fruit drink	8	fluid ounce(s)	240	—	150	2	34	1	1	0.00	—	—
10080	Odwalla strawberry lemonade quencher	8	fluid ounce(s)	240	—	120	1	28	1	0	0.00	0.00	0.00
10099	Snapple fruit punch	8	fluid ounce(s)	240	—	110	0	29	0	0	0.00	0.00	0.00
10096	Snapple kiwi strawberry	8	fluid ounce(s)	240	211	110	0	28	0	0	0.00	0.00	0.00
	Slim Fast ready to drink shake												
16056	Dark chocolate fudge	11	fluid ounce(s)	325	—	220	10	42	5	3	1.00	1.50	0.50
16054	French vanilla	11	fluid ounce(s)	325	—	220	10	40	5	3	0.50	1.50	0.50
16055	Strawberries n cream	11	fluid ounce(s)	325	—	220	10	40	5	3	0.50	1.50	0.50
	Tea												
733	Tea, prepared	8	fluid ounce(s)	237	236	2	0	1	0	0	0.00	0.00	0.01
33179	Decaffeinated, prepared	8	fluid ounce(s)	237	236	2	0	1	0	0	0.00	0.00	0.01
1877	Herbal, prepared	8	fluid ounce(s)	237	236	2	0	<1	0	0	0.00	0.00	0.01
734	Instant tea mix, unsweetened, prepared	8	fluid ounce(s)	237	236	2	<.1	<1	0	0	0.00	0.00	0.00
735	Instant lemon flavored tea mix w/sugar, prepared	8	fluid ounce(s)	259	236	88	<1	22	0	<.1	0.01	0.00	0.02
	Water												
1413	Mineral water, carbonated	8	fluid ounce(s)	237	237	0	0	0	0	0	0.00	0.00	0.00
33183	Poland spring water, bottled	8	fluid ounce(s)	237	237	0	0	0	0	0	0.00	0.00	0.00
1	Tap water	8	fluid ounce(s)	237	237	0	0	0	0	0	0.00	0.00	0.00
1879	Tonic water	8	fluid ounce(s)	244	222	83	0	21	0	0	0.00	0.00	0.00

PAGE KEY: H–2 = Breads/Baked Goods H–6 = Cereal/Rice/Pasta H–10 = Fruit H–16 = Vegetables/Legumes H–26 = Nuts/Seeds H–28 = Vegetarian H–30 = Dairy H–36 = Eggs H–38 = Seafood H–40 = Meats H–42 = Poultry H–44 = Processed meats H–46 = Beverages H–50 = Fats/Oils H–52 = Sweets H–52 = Sauces/Condiments/Spices H–56 = Mixed Foods/Soups/Sandwiches H–62 = Fast food H–80 = Convenience H–82 = Baby foods

Chol (mg)	Calc (mg)	Iron (mg)	Magn (mg)	Pota (mg)	Sodi (mg)	Zinc (mg)	Vit A (RAE) (µg)	Thia (mg)	Vit E (mg)	Ribo (mg)	Niac (mg)	Vit B_6 (mg)	Fola (µg)	Vit C (mg)	Vit B_{12} (µg)	Sele (µg)
0	14	0.11	4	0	21	0.28	0	0.02	0.00	0.08	0.00	0.00	0	0	0	<1
0	19	0.19	4	4	44	0.26	0	0.00	0.00	0.00	0.00	0.00	0	0	0	0
0	—	—	—	116	53	—	—	—	—	—	—	—	—	—	—	—
0	11	0.66	4	4	26	0.18	0	0.00	0.00	0.00	0.00	0.00	0	0	0	<1
0	11	0.30	4	4	56	0.26	0	0.00	0.00	0.00	0.00	0.00	0	0	0	0
0	7	0.26	4	4	41	0.18	0	0.00	0.00	0.00	0.06	0.00	0	0	0	0
0	—	—	—	70	35	—	—	—	—	—	—	—	—	—	—	—
0	—	—	—	0	70	—	—	—	—	—	—	—	—	—	—	—
0	19	0.22	4	7	45	0.37	0	0.00	0.00	0.00	0.00	0.00	0	0	0	0
0	11	0.15	0	4	37	0.15	0	0.00	0.00	0.00	0.00	0	0	0	<1	
0	14	0.07	4	14	57	0.11	0	0.00	0.00	0.00	0.00	0.00	0	0	0	<1
0	—	—	—	30	35	—	—	—	—	—	—	—	—	—	—	—
0	—	—	—	0	35	—	—	—	—	—	—	—	—	—	—	—
0	18	0.18	4	4	48	0.26	0	0.00	0.00	0.00	0.00	0.00	0	0	0	<1
0	—	—	—	0	113	—	—	—	—	—	—	—	—	—	—	—
0	—	—	—	110	36	—	0	—	0.00	—	—	—	—	0	—	—
0	—	—	—	0	71	—	0	—	0.00	—	—	—	—	0	—	—
0	2	0.02	5	114	2	0.02	0	0.00	0.00	0.12	0.00	0.00	5	0	0	0
0	5	0.12	12	128	5	0.05	0	0.00	0.00	0.00	0.53	0.00	<1	0	0	0
17	152	0.26	22	250	62	0.50	—	0.04	0.12	0.20	0.37	0.05	5	1	<1	—
17	152	0.26	22	250	62	0.50	—	0.04	0.12	0.20	0.37	0.05	5	1	<1	—
0	5	0.12	12	128	5	0.05	0	0.00	0.00	0.00	0.53	0.00	<1	0	0	—
0	5	0.12	12	128	5	0.05	0	0.00	0.00	0.00	0.53	0.00	<1	0	0	—
0	10	0.10	7	72	5	0.02	0	0.00	0.00	0.00	0.56	0.00	0	0	0	<1
0	0	0.00	—	160	20	—	0	—	—	—	—	—	—	0	—	—
0	22	0.58	6	69	61	0.33	—	0.06	0.00	0.06	0.06	0.00	4	99	0	0
0	5	0.45	3	30	15	0.30	0	0.00	0.00	0.01	0.03	0.01	0	85	0	<1
0	10	0.52	5	50	7	0.07	0	0.02	—	0.07	0.05	0.02	2	13	0	<1
0	7	0.02	2	22	5	0.02	0	0.00	—	0.01	0.02	0.01	2	6	0	<1
0	10	0.18	—	30	110	—	—	—	—	—	—	—	—	1	—	—
0	14	0.46	5	50	31	0.20	—	0.04	—	0.05	0.05	0.01	4	42	0	1
0	0	0.00	—	10	10	—	0	—	—	—	—	—	—	6	—	—
0	20	1.44	—	330	40	—	—	—	—	—	—	—	—	600	0	—
0	20	0.00	—	70	30	—	0	—	—	—	—	—	—	60	0	—
0	0	0.00	—	20	10	—	0	—	—	—	—	—	—	0	0	—
0	0	0.00	—	40	10	—	0	—	—	—	—	—	—	0	0	—
5	400	2.70	140	600	220	2.25	—	0.53	20.13	0.60	7.00	0.70	120	60	2	18
5	400	2.70	140	600	220	2.25	—	0.53	20.13	0.60	7.00	0.70	120	60	2	18
5	400	2.70	140	600	220	2.25	—	0.53	20.13	0.60	7.00	0.70	120	60	2	18
0	0	0.05	7	88	7	0.05	0	0.00	0.00	0.03	0.00	0.00	12	0	0	0
0	0	0.05	7	88	7	0.05	0	0.00	0.00	0.03	0.00	0.00	12	0	0	0
0	5	0.19	2	21	2	0.09	0	0.02	0.00	0.01	0.00	0.00	2	0	0	0
0	7	0.05	5	47	7	0.02	0	0.00	0.00	0.00	0.09	0.00	0	0	0	0
0	5	0.05	5	49	8	0.03	0	0.00	—	0.04	0.09	0.01	0	<1	0	<1
0	33	0.00	0	0	2	0.00	0	0.00	—	0.00	0.00	0.00	0	0	0	0
0	2	0.02	2	0	2	0.00	0	0.00	—	0.00	0.00	0.00	0	0	0	0
0	4.74	0.00	2.37	0	4.74	0	0	0	0	0	0	0	0	0	0	0
0	2	0.02	0	0	10	0.24	0	0.00	0.00	0.00	0.00	0.00	0	0	0	0

Table H–1

Food Composition (Computer code number is for Wadsworth Diet Analysis program) (For purposes of calculations, use "0" for t, <1, <.1, <.01, etc.)

DA + Code	Food Description	Quantity	Measure	Wt (g)	H_2O (g)	Ener (kcal)	Prot (g)	Carb (g)	Dietary Fiber (g)	Fat (g)	Fat Breakdown (g)		
											Sat	Mono	Poly
	FATS AND OILS												
	Butter												
104	Butter	1	tablespoon(s)	15	2	108	<1	<.1	0	12	6.13	5.00	0.43
921	Unsalted	1	tablespoon(s)	15	3	108	<1	<.1	0	12	7.71	3.15	0.46
107	Whipped	1	tablespoon(s)	11	2	82	<.1	<.1	0	9	5.76	2.67	0.34
944	Whipped, unsalted	1	tablespoon(s)	11	2	82	<.1	<.1	0	9	5.76	2.67	0.34
2522	Butter Buds, dry butter substitute	1	teaspoon(s)	2	—	8	0	2	0	0	0.00	0.00	0.00
	Fats, cooking												
2671	Beef tallow, semisolid	1	tablespoon(s)	13	0	115	0	0	0	13	6.37	5.35	0.51
922	Chicken fat	1	tablespoon(s)	13	<.1	115	0	0	0	13	3.81	5.72	2.68
5454	Household shortening w/vegetable oil	1	tablespoon(s)	13	0	115	0	0	0	13	3.39	5.56	2.75
111	Lard	1	tablespoon(s)	13	0	114	0	0	0	13	4.94	5.68	1.41
	Margarine												
114	Margarine	1	tablespoon(s)	14	2	101	<1	<1	0	11	2.23	5.05	3.58
116	Soft	1	tablespoon(s)	14	2	101	<1	<.1	0	11	1.95	4.02	4.88
117	Soft, unsalted	1	tablespoon(s)	14	3	101	<1	<1	0	11	1.95	5.26	3.62
928	Unsalted	1	tablespoon(s)	14	3	101	<.1	<.1	0	11	2.12	5.17	3.53
119	Whipped	1	tablespoon(s)	9	1	64	<.1	<.1	0	7	1.17	3.25	2.51
	Spreads												
16164	I Can't Believe It's Not Butter! whipped spread	1	tablespoon(s)	14	4	60	0	0	0	7	1.50	1.50	2.50
16157	Promise vegetable oil spread, stick	1	tablespoon(s)	14	4	90	0	0	0	10	2.50	2.00	4.00
	Oils												
2681	Canola	1	tablespoon(s)	14	0	120	0	0	0	14	0.97	8.01	4.03
120	Corn	1	tablespoon(s)	14	0	120	0	0	0	14	1.73	3.29	7.98
122	Olive	1	tablespoon(s)	14	0	119	0	0	0	14	1.82	9.98	1.35
124	Peanut	1	tablespoon(s)	14	0	119	0	0	0	14	2.28	6.24	4.32
2693	Safflower	1	tablespoon(s)	14	0	120	0	0	0	14	0.84	10.15	1.95
923	Sesame	1	tablespoon(s)	14	0	120	0	0	0	14	1.93	5.40	5.67
130	Soybean w/cottonseed oil	1	tablespoon(s)	14	0	120	0	0	0	14	2.45	4.01	6.54
128	Soybean, hydrogenated	1	tablespoon(s)	14	0	120	0	0	0	14	2.03	5.85	5.11
2700	Sunflower	1	tablespoon(s)	14	0	120	0	0	0	14	1.77	6.28	4.95
357	**Pam original no stick cooking spray**	1	serving(s)	0	—	0	0	0	0	0	0.00	0.00	0.00
	Salad dressing												
132	Blue cheese	2	tablespoon(s)	31	10	154	1	2	0	16	3.03	3.76	8.51
133	Blue cheese, low calorie	2	tablespoon(s)	32	25	32	2	1	0	2	0.82	0.57	0.78
1764	Caesar	2	tablespoon(s)	30	10	158	<1	1	<.1	17	2.64	4.05	9.86
29654	Creamy, reduced calorie, fat free, cholesterol free, sour cream and/or buttermilk & oil	2	tablespoon(s)	32	24	34	<1	6	0	1	0.16	0.21	0.46
29617	Creamy, reduced calorie, sour cream and/or buttermilk & oil	2	tablespoon(s)	30	22	48	<1	2	0	4	0.63	0.98	2.40
134	French	2	tablespoon(s)	31	11	143	<1	5	0	14	1.76	2.63	6.56
135	French, low fat	2	tablespoon(s)	33	18	76	<1	10	<1	4	0.36	1.92	1.64
136	Italian	2	tablespoon(s)	29	17	86	<1	3	0	8	1.32	1.86	3.80
137	Italian, diet	2	tablespoon(s)	30	25	23	<1	1	0	2	0.14	0.66	0.51
139	Mayonnaise type	2	tablespoon(s)	29	12	115	<1	7	0	10	1.44	2.65	5.29
942	Oil & vinegar	2	tablespoon(s)	31	15	140	0	1	0	16	2.84	4.62	7.52
1765	Ranch	2	tablespoon(s)	30	12	146	<1	2	<.1	16	2.32	3.85	8.92
3666	Ranch, reduced calorie	2	tablespoon(s)	30	21	62	<1	2	<.1	6	1.13	1.79	2.89
940	Russian	2	tablespoon(s)	31	11	151	<1	3	0	16	2.23	3.61	9.00
939	Russian, low calorie	2	tablespoon(s)	33	21	46	<1	9	<.1	1	0.20	0.29	0.75
941	Sesame seed	2	tablespoon(s)	31	12	136	1	3	<1	14	1.90	3.64	7.68
142	Thousand island	2	tablespoon(s)	31	15	115	<1	5	<1	11	1.59	2.46	5.68
143	Thousand island, low calorie	2	tablespoon(s)	31	19	62	<1	7	<1	4	0.23	1.98	0.82
	Sandwich spreads												
138	Mayonnaise w/soybean oil	1	tablespoon(s)	14	2	99	<1	1	0	11	1.64	2.70	5.89
2708	Mayonnaise w/soybean & safflower oils	1	tablespoon(s)	14	0	98.94	0.15	0.37	0	10.95	1.18	1.79	7.59
140	Mayonnaise, low calorie	1	tablespoon(s)	16	10	37	<.1	3	0	3	0.53	0.72	1.70
141	Tartar sauce	2	tablespoon(s)	28	9	144	<1	4	<.1	14	2.14	4.13	7.57

PAGE KEY: H–2 = Breads/Baked Goods H–6 = Cereal/Rice/Pasta H–10 = Fruit H–16 = Vegetables/Legumes H–26 = Nuts/Seeds H–28 = Vegetarian H–30 = Dairy H–36 = Eggs H–38 = Seafood H–40 = Meats H–42 = Poultry H–44 = Processed meats H–46 = Beverages H–50 = Fats/Oils H–52 = Sweets H–52 = Sauces/Condiments/Spices H–56 = Mixed Foods/Soups/Sandwiches H–62 = Fast food H–80 = Convenience H–82 = Baby foods

Chol (mg)	Calc (mg)	Iron (mg)	Magn (mg)	Pota (mg)	Sodi (mg)	Zinc (mg)	Vit A (RAE) (μg)	Thia (mg)	Vit E (mg)	Ribo (mg)	Niac (mg)	Vit B_6 (mg)	Fola (μg)	Vit C (mg)	Vit B_{12} (μg)	Sele (μg)
32	4	0.00	<1	4	86	0.01	103	0.00	0.24	0.01	0.01	0.00	<1	0	<.1	<1
32	4	0.00	<1	4	2	0.01	103	0.00	0.24	0.01	0.01	0.00	<1	0	<.1	<1
25	3	0.02	<1	3	94	0.01	78	0.00	0.18	0.00	0.00	0.00	<1	0	<.1	<1
25	3	0.02	<1	3	1	0.01	—	0.00	0.18	0.00	0.01	0.00	<1	0	<.1	—
0	0	0.00	0	2	70	0.00	0	0.00	0.00	0.00	0.00	0.00	<1	0	0	—
14	0	0.00	0	0	0	0.00	0	0.00	0.35	0.00	0.00	0.00	0	0	0	<.1
11	0	0.00	0	0	0	0.00	0	0.00	0.35	0.00	0.00	0.00	0	0	0	<.1
0	0	0.00	0	0	0	0.00	0	0.00	2.10	0.00	0.00	0.00	0	0	0	—
12	0	0.00	0	0	0	0.01	0	0.00	0.15	0.00	0.00	0.00	0	0	0	<.1
0	4	0.01	<1	6	133	0.00	115	0.00	1.80	0.01	0.00	0.00	<1	<.1	<.1	0
0	4	0.00	<1	5	152	0.00	103	0.00	1.69	0.00	0.00	0.00	<1	<.1	<.1	0
0	4	0.00	<1	5	4	0.00	103	0.00	1.23	0.00	0.00	0.00	<1	<.1	<.1	0
0	2	0.00	<1	4	<1	0.00	115	0.00	1.80	0.00	0.00	0.00	<1	<.1	<.1	0
0	2	0.00	<1	3	97	0.00	—	0.00	1.08	0.00	0.00	0.00	<.1	<.1	<.1	—
0	10	0.18	—	4	70	—	—	1.65	0.00	0.00	0.00	—	—	1	—	—
0	10	0.18	—	9	90	—	—	0.00	3.02	0.00	0.00	—	—	1	—	—
0	0	0.00	0	0	0	0.00	0	0.00	2.85	0.00	0.00	0.00	0	0	0	0
0	0	0.00	0	0	0	0.00	0	0.00	2.87	0.00	0.00	0.00	0	0	0	0
0	<1	0.09	0	<1	<1	0.00	0	0.00	1.67	0.00	0.00	0.00	0	0	0	0
0	0	0.00	0	0	0	0.00	0	0.00	1.74	0.00	0.00	0.00	0	0	0	0
0	0	0.00	0	0	0	0.00	0	0.00	4.68	0.00	0.00	0.00	0	0	0	0
0	0	0.00	0	0	0	0.00	0	0.00	0.56	0.00	0.00	0.00	0	0	0	0
0	0	0.00	0	0	0	0.00	0	0.00	3.84	0.00	0.00	0.00	0	0	0	0
0	0	0.00	0	0	0	0.00	0	0.00	2.47	0.00	0.00	0.00	0	0	0	0
0	0	0.00	0	0	0	0.00	0	0.00	6.94	0.00	0.00	0.00	0	0	0	0
0	0	0.00	—	0	0	—	0	—	—	—	—	—	—	0	0	—
5	25	0.06	0	11	335	0.08	21	0.00	2.85	0.03	0.03	0.01	9	1	<.1	<1
<1	28	0.16	2	2	384	0.08	—	0.01	0.29	0.03	0.02	0.01	1	<.1	<.1	—
1	7	0.05	1	9	323	0.03	—	0.00	1.56	0.00	0.01	0.00	1	0	<.1	—
0	12	0.08	2	43	320	0.06	0	0.00	0.21	0.02	0.01	0.01	1	0	0	—
0	2	0.04	1	11	307	0.01	—	0.00	0.57	0.00	0.01	0.01	4	<1	<.1	—
0	7	0.25	2	21	261	0.09	7	0.01	2.63	0.02	0.06	0.00	0	0	<.1	0
0	4	0.28	3	35	262	0.07	9	0.01	0.39	0.02	0.15	0.02	1	0	0	1
0	2	0.19	1	14	486	0.04	1	0.00	3.05	0.01	0.00	0.02	0	0	0	1
2	3	0.20	1	26	410	0.06	<1	0.00	0.45	0.00	0.00	0.02	0	0	0	2
8	4	0.06	1	3	209	0.05	19	0.00	1.18	0.01	0.00	0.00	2	0	<.1	<1
0	0	0.00	0	2	<1	0.00	0	0.00	2.75	0.00	0.00	0.00	0	0	0	0
1	4	0.03	1	8	354	0.01	—	0.00	3.22	0.00	0.00	0.00	<1	<.1	<.1	—
<1	5	0.01	1	8	414	0.02	—	0.00	0.28	0.01	0.01	0.00	<1	<1	<.1	—
6	6	0.18	1	48	266	0.13	5	0.02	3.12	0.02	0.18	0.01	3	2	<.1	<1
2	6	0.20	1	51	283	0.03	1	0.00	0.25	0.00	0.00	0.00	1	2	<.1	1
0	6	0.18	0	48	306	0.03	1	0.00	1.53	0.00	0.00	0.00	0	0	0	<1
8	5	0.37	2	33	269	0.08	3	0.45	0.36	0.02	0.13	0.00	0	0	0	<1
<1	5	0.28	2	62	254	0.06	5	0.01	0.36	0.01	0.13	0.00	0	0	0	0
5	2	0.07	<1	5	78	0.02	12	0.00	0.32	0.00	0.00	0.08	1	0	<.1	<1
8.14	2.48	0.06	0.13	4.69	78.38	0.01	11.59	0	2.42	0	0	0.07	1.1	0	0.03	0.22
4	<.1	0.00	<.1	2	80	0.02	0	0.00	1.03	0.00	0.00	0.00	0	0	0	—
11	6	0.21	1	10	200	0.05	—	0.00	2.04	0.00	0.01	0.08	2	<1	<.1	—

Table H–1

Food Composition (Computer code number is for Wadsworth Diet Analysis program) (For purposes of calculations, use "0" for t, <1, <.1, <.01, etc.)

DA + Code	Food Description	Quantity	Measure	Wt (g)	H_2O (g)	Ener (kcal)	Prot (g)	Carb (g)	Dietary Fiber (g)	Fat (g)	Fat Breakdown (g) Sat	Mono	Poly
	SWEETS												
4799	**Butterscotch or caramel topping**	2	tablespoon(s)	41	13	103	1	27	<1	<.1	0.05	0.01	0.00
	Candy												
1786	Almond Joy candy bar	1	item(s)	49	5	240	2	29	2	13	9.00	3.63	0.74
1785	Bit-o-Honey candy	6	item(s)	40	2	170	1	34	0	3	2.00	0	20
33375	Butterscotch candy	2	piece(s)	12	1	47	<.1	11	0	<1	0.25	0.10	0.01
1701	Chewing gum, stick	1	item(s)	3	<.1	7	0	2	<.1	<.1	0.00	0.00	0.00
33378	Chocolate fudge w/nuts, prepared	2	piece(s)	38	3	175	2	26	1	7	2.29	1.41	2.81
1787	Jelly beans	15	item(s)	43	3	159	0	40	<.1	<.1	0.00	0.00	0.00
1784	Kit Kat wafer bar	1	item(s)	42	1	220	3	27	1	11	7.00	3.53	0.34
4674	Krackel candy bar	1	item(s)	41	1	220	3	26	1	11	6.00	3.94	0.37
4934	Licorice	4	piece(s)	44	7	147	1	34	1	1	0.18	0.07	0.00
1780	Life Savers candy	1	item(s)	2	—	8	0	2	0	<.1	0.00	—	—
1790	Lollipop	1	item(s)	28	—	108	0	28	0	0	0.00	0.00	0.00
4679	M & Ms peanut chocolate candy, small bag	1	item(s)	49	1	250	5	30	2	13	5.00	5.42	2.07
1781	M & Ms plain chocolate candy, small bag	1	item(s)	48	1	240	2	34	1	10	6.00	3.30	0.30
4673	Milk chocolate bar	1	item(s)	91	1	483	8	53	2	28	16.69	7.20	0.63
1783	Milky Way bar	1	item(s)	58	4	270	2	41	1	10	5.00	3.50	0.35
1788	Peanut brittle	1½	ounce(s)	43	<1	206	3	30	1	8	1.76	3.43	1.94
1789	Reese's peanut butter cups	2	piece(s)	45	1	250	5	25	1	14	5.00	6.17	2.34
4689	Reese's pieces candy, small bag	1	item(s)	46	1	230	6	26	1	11	7.00	0.97	0.46
33399	Semisweet chocolate candy, made w/butter	½	ounce(s)	14	<.1	68	1	9	1	4	2.49	1.41	0.13
1782	Snickers bar	1	item(s)	59	3	280	4	35	1	14	5.00	6.13	2.89
4694	Special Dark chocolate bar	1	item(s)	41	<1	220	2	24	3	13	8.00	4.59	0.41
4695	Starburst fruit chews, original fruits	1	package	59	4	240	0	48	0	5	1.00	2.10	1.83
4698	Taffy	3	piece(s)	45	2	169	<.1	41	0	1	0.92	0.43	0.05
4699	Three Musketeers bar	1	item(s)	60	4	260	2	46	1	8	4.50	2.59	0.27
4702	Twix caramel cookie bars	2	item(s)	58	2	280	3	37	1	14	5.00	7.75	0.49
4705	York peppermint pattie	1	item(s)	42	4	170	1	34	1	3	2.00	1.32	0.12
	Frosting, icing												
4760	Chocolate frosting, ready to eat	2	tablespoon(s)	28	5	112	<1	18	<1	5	1.55	2.54	0.60
4771	Creamy vanilla frosting, ready to eat	2	tablespoon(s)	28	4	118	0	19	<.1	5	0.84	1.37	2.24
17291	Dec-a-Cake variety pack candy decoration	1	teaspoon(s)	4	—	15	0	3	0	1	0.00	—	—
536	White icing	2	tablespoon(s)	40	3	163	<1	32	0	4	0.86	2.07	1.19
	Gelatin												
13697	Gelatin snack, all flavors	1	item(s)	99	97	70	1	17	0	0	0.00	0.00	0.00
2616	Mixed fruit gelatin mix, sugar free, low calorie, prepared	½	cup(s)	121	—	10	1	0	0	0	0.00	0.00	0.00
548	**Honey**	1	tablespoon(s)	21	4	64	<.1	17	<.1	0	0.00	0.00	0.00
545	**Marshmallows**	4	item(s)	29	5	92	1	23	<.1	<.1	0.02	0.02	0.01
4800	**Marshmallow cream topping**	2	tablespoon(s)	28	6	91	<1	22	<.1	<.1	0.02	0.02	0.01
555	**Molasses**	1	tablespoon(s)	20	4	58	0	15	0	<.1	0.00	0.01	0.01
4780	**Popsicle or ice pop**	1	item(s)	59	47	42	0	11	0	0	0.00	0.00	0.00
	Sugar												
559	Brown, packed	1	teaspoon(s)	5	<.1	17	0	4	0	0	0.00	0.00	0.00
563	Powdered, sifted	⅓	cup(s)	33	<.1	130	0	33	0	<.1	0.01	0.01	0.02
561	White granulated	1	teaspoon(s)	4	<.1	15	0	4	0	0	0.00	0.00	0.00
	Sugar Substitute												
1760	Equal sweetener, packet	1	item(s)	1	<.1	4	<.1	1	0	0	0.00	0.00	0.00
13029	Splenda granular no calorie sweetener	1	teaspoon(s)	1	—	2	0	1	0	0	0.00	0.00	0.00
1759	Sweet n Low sugar substitute, packet	1	item(s)	1	<.1	4	0	1	0	0	0.00	0.00	0.00
	Syrup												
3148	Chocolate	2	tablespoon(s)	38	12	105	1	24	1	<1	0.19	0.11	0.01
29676	Maple	¼	cup(s)	80	26	209	0	54	0	<1	0.03	0.05	0.08
4795	Pancake	¼	cup(s)	80	30	187	0	49	1	0	0.00	0.00	0.00
	SAUCES, SPICES, CONDIMENTS												
	Spices												
807	Allspice, ground	1	teaspoon(s)	2	<1	5	<1	1	<1	<1	0.05	0.01	0.04

PAGE KEY: H–2 = Breads/Baked Goods H–6 = Cereal/Rice/Pasta H–10 = Fruit H–16 = Vegetables/Legumes H–26 = Nuts/Seeds H–28 = Vegetarian H–30 = Dairy H–36 = Eggs H–38 = Seafood H–40 = Meats H–42 = Poultry H–44 = Processed meats H–46 = Beverages H–50 = Fats/Oils H–52 = Sweets H–52 = Sauces/Condiments/Spices H–56 = Mixed Foods/Soups/Sandwiches H–62 = Fast food H–80 = Convenience H–82 = Baby foods

Chol (mg)	Calc (mg)	Iron (mg)	Magn (mg)	Pota (mg)	Sodi (mg)	Zinc (mg)	Vit A (RAE) (µg)	Thia (mg)	Vit E (mg)	Ribo (mg)	Niac (mg)	Vit B_6 (mg)	Fola (µg)	Vit C (mg)	Vit B_{12} (µg)	Sele (µg)
<1	22	0.08	3	34	143	0.08	11	0.00	—	0.04	0.02	0.01	1	<1	<.1	0
3	20	0.36	33	138	70	0.40	0	0.02	—	0.08	0.24	—	—	0	—	—
0.00	—	—	85	—	0	—	—	—	—	—	—	0	—	—		
1	<1	0.00	<1	<1	47	0.00	3	0.00	0.01	0.00	0.00	0.00	0	0	0	<.1
0	0	0.00	0	<.1	<.1	0.00	0	0.00	0.00	0.00	0.00	0.00	0	0	0	<.1
5	21	0.75	21	68	16	0.54	14	0.03	0.25	0.04	0.12	0.03	6	<.1	<.1	1
0	1	0.06	1	16	21	0.02	0	0.00	0.00	0.00	0.00	0.00	0	0	0	<1
3	40	0.36	16	126	25	0.52	8	0.07	—	0.23	1.07	0.05	60	0	<.1	2
3	60	0.37	—	169	80	—	0	—	—	—	—	—	—	0	—	—
0	3	0.13	3	28	109	0.07	0	0.01	0.08	0.02	0.04	0.00	0	0	0	—
0	<1	0.04	—	0	1	—	0	0.00	—	0.00	0.00	—	—	0	—	0
0	0	0.00	—	—	11	—	0	0.00	—	0.00	0.00	—	—	0	—	1
5	40	0.36	36	171	25	1.13	15	0.03	1.06	0.07	1.60	0.04	17	1	<.1	2
5	40	0.36	20	127	30	0.46	15	0.03	0.41	0.07	0.11	0.01	3	1	<1	1
22	228	0.83	61	399	92	1.00	20	0.06	0.19	0.26	0.15	0.10	11	2	<1	—
5	60	0.18	20	140	95	0.41	15	0.02	0.40	0.07	0.20	0.03	6	1	<1	3
5	11	0.52	18	71	189	0.37	17	0.06	1.17	0.02	1.13	0.03	20	0	<.1	1
3	20	0.36	40	233	140	0.82	7	0.11	—	0.08	2.08	0.07	25	0	<.1	2
0	40	0.00	20	182	90	0.35	25	0.04	—	0.07	1.31	0.03	13	0	<.1	1
3	5	0.44	16	52	2	0.23	<1	0.01	—	0.01	0.06	0.01	<1	0	0	<1
5	40	0.36	42	—	140	1.38	15	0.03	1.53	0.07	1.60	0.05	23	1	<.1	3
3	0	0.72	46	136	0	0.60	0	0.01	—	0.03	0.16	0.01	1	0	0	1
0	10	0.18	1	1	0	0.00	—	0.00	0.89	0.00	0.00	0.00	0	30	0	<1
4	1	0.03	<1	2	40	0.02	—	0.00	—	0.01	0.01	0.00	0	0	<.1	—
5	20	0.36	18	80	110	0.33	14	0.02	0.28	0.03	0.20	0.01	0	1	<1	2
5	40	0.36	18	117	115	0.45	15	0.09	0.40	0.13	0.69	0.02	14	1	<1	1
0	0	0.36	25	71	10	0.31	0	0.01	—	0.04	0.34	0.01	2	0	<.1	—
0	2	0.40	6	55	51	0.08	0	0.00	0.67	0.00	0.03	0.00	<1	0	0	<1
0	1	0.04	<1	10	52	0.02	0	0.00	1.33	0.08	0.06	0.00	2	0	0	<.1
0	0	0.00	—	—	15	—	0	—	—	—	—	—	—	0	—	—
<1	5	0.02	—	7	92	—	—	0.00	—	0.01	0.00	—	—	<.1	—	—
0	0	0.00	—	0	40	—	0	—	—	—	—	—	—	0	—	—
0	0	0.00	0	0	50	0.00	0	0.00	0.00	0.00	0.00	0.00	0	0	0	—
0	1	0.09	<1	11	1	0.05	0	0.00	0.00	0.01	0.03	0.01	<1	<1	0	<1
0	1	0.07	1	1	23	0.01	0	0.00	0.00	0.00	0.02	0.00	<1	0	0	<1
0	1	0.06	1	1	23	0.01	0	0.00	0.00	0.00	0.02	0.00	<1	0	0	1
0	41	0.94	48	293	7	0.06	0	0.01	0.00	0.00	0.19	0.13	0	0	0	4
0	0	0.00	1	2	7	0.01	0	0.00	0.00	0.00	0.00	0.00	0	0	0	0
0	4	0.09	1	16	2	0.01	0	0.00	0.00	0.00	0.00	0.00	<.1	0	0	<.1
0	<1	0.01	0	1	<1	0.00	0	0.00	0.00	0.01	0.00	0.00	0	0	0	<1
0	<.1	0.00	0	<.1	0	0.00	0	0.00	0.00	0.00	0.00	0.00	0	0	0	<.1
0	0	0.00	0	0	0	0.00	0	0.00	0.00	0.00	0.00	0.00	0	0	0	0
0	10	0.18	—	—	<1	—	—	0.02	—	0.02	0.20	—	—	1	0	—
0	0	0.00	0	—	0	0.00	0	0.00	0.00	0.00	0.00	0.00	0	0	0	0
0	5	0.79	24	84	27	0.27	0	0.00	0.01	0.02	0.12	0.00	1	<.1	0	1
0	54	0.96	11	163	7	3.33	0	0.00	0.00	0.01	0.02	0.00	0	0	0	<1
0	2	0.02	2	12	66	0.06	0	0.00	0.00	0.01	0.01	0.00	0	0	0	0
0	13	0.13	3	20	1	0.02	1	0.00	0.02	0.00	0.05	0.00	1	1	0	<.1

Table H–1

Food Composition (Computer code number is for Wadsworth Diet Analysis program) (For purposes of calculations, use "0" for t, <1, <.1, <.01, etc.)

DA + Code	Food Description	Quantity	Measure	Wt (g)	H_2O (g)	Ener (kcal)	Prot (g)	Carb (g)	Dietary Fiber (g)	Fat (g)	Fat Breakdown (g) Sat	Mono	Poly
	SAUCES, SPICES, CONDIMENTS—Continued												
1171	Anise seeds	1	teaspoon(s)	2	<1	7	<1	1	<1	<1	0.01	0.21	0.07
729	Baker's yeast active	1	teaspoon(s)	4	<1	12	2	2	1	<1	0.02	0.10	0.00
683	Baking powder, double acting, w/phosphate	1	teaspoon(s)	5	<1	2	<.1	1	<.1	0	0.00	0.00	0.00
1611	Baking soda	1	teaspoon(s)	5	<.1	0	0	0	0	0	0.00	0.00	0.00
8552	Basil	1	teaspoon(s)	1	1	<1	<.1	<.1	<.1	<.1	0.00	0.00	0.00
34959	Basil, fresh	1	piece(s)	1	<1	<1	<.1	<.1	<.1	<.1	0.00	0.00	0.00
808	Basil, ground	1	teaspoon(s)	1	<.1	4	<1	1	1	<.1	0.00	0.01	0.03
809	Bay leaf	1	teaspoon(s)	1	<.1	2	<.1	<1	<1	<.1	0.01	0.01	0.01
11720	Betel leaves	1	ounce(s)	28	—	17	2	2	0	<.1	—	—	—
818	Black pepper	1	teaspoon(s)	2	<1	5	<1	1	1	<.1	0.02	0.02	0.02
730	Brewer's yeast	1	teaspoon(s)	3	<1	8	1	1	1	0	0.00	0.00	0.00
35417	Capers	1	teaspoon(s)	4	—	2	0	0	0	0	0.00	0.00	0.00
1172	Caraway seeds	1	teaspoon(s)	2	<1	7	<1	1	1	<1	0.01	0.15	0.07
819	Cayenne pepper	1	teaspoon(s)	2	<1	6	<1	1	<1	<1	0.06	0.05	0.15
1173	Celery seeds	1	teaspoon(s)	2	<1	8	<1	1	<1	1	0.04	0.32	0.07
1174	Chervil, dried	1	teaspoon(s)	1	<.1	1	<1	<1	<.1	<.1	0.00	0.01	0.01
810	Chili powder	1	teaspoon(s)	3	<1	8	<1	1	1	<1	0.08	0.09	0.19
8553	Chives, chopped	1	teaspoon(s)	1	1	<1	<.1	<.1	<.1	<.1	0.00	0.00	0.00
8556	Cilantro	1	teaspoon(s)	2	1	<1	<.1	<.1	<.1	<.1	0.00	0.00	0.00
811	Cinnamon, ground	1	teaspoon(s)	2	<1	6	<.1	2	1	<.1	0.01	0.01	0.01
812	Cloves, ground	1	teaspoon(s)	2	<1	7	<1	1	1	<1	0.11	0.03	0.15
1175	Coriander leaf, dried	1	teaspoon(s)	1	<.1	2	<1	<1	<.1	<.1	0.00	0.01	0.00
1176	Coriander seeds	1	teaspoon(s)	2	<1	5	<1	1	1	<1	0.02	0.24	0.03
1706	Cornstarch	1	tablespoon(s)	8	1	30	<.1	7	<.1	<.1	0.00	0.00	0.00
11729	Cumin, ground	1	teaspoon(s)	5	—	11	<1	1	1	<1	—	—	—
1177	Cumin seeds	1	teaspoon(s)	2	<1	8	<1	1	<1	<1	0.03	0.29	0.07
1178	Curry powder	1	teaspoon(s)	2	<1	7	<1	1	1	<1	0.04	0.11	0.05
1179	Dill seeds	1	teaspoon(s)	2	<1	6	<1	1	<1	<1	0.02	0.20	0.02
1180	Dill weed, dried	1	teaspoon(s)	1	<.1	3	<1	1	<1	<.1	0.00	0.01	0.00
34949	Dill weed, fresh	5	piece(s)	1	1	<1	<.1	<.1	<.1	<.1	0.00	0.01	0.00
4949	Fennel leaves, fresh	1	teaspoon(s)	1	1	<1	<.1	<.1	0	<.1	0.00	0.00	0.00
1181	Fennel seeds	1	teaspoon(s)	2	<1	7	<1	1	1	<1	0.01	0.20	0.03
1182	Fenugreek seeds	1	teaspoon(s)	4	<1	12	1	2	1	<1	0.05	—	—
11733	Garam masala, powder	1	ounce(s)	28	—	107	4	13	0	4	—	—	—
1067	Garlic clove	1	item(s)	3	2	4	<1	1	<.1	<.1	0.00	0.00	0.01
813	Garlic powder	1	teaspoon(s)	3	<1	9	<1	2	<1	<.1	0.00	0.00	0.01
1183	Ginger, ground	1	teaspoon(s)	2	<1	6	<1	1	<1	<1	0.03	0.02	0.02
1068	Ginger root	2	teaspoon(s)	4	3	3	<.1	1	<.1	<.1	0.01	0.01	0.01
35497	Leeks, bulb & lower leaf, freeze-dried	¼	cup(s)	1	<.1	3	<1	1	<.1	<.1	0.00	0.00	0.01
1184	Mace, ground	1	teaspoon(s)	2	<1	8	<1	1	<1	1	0.16	0.19	0.07
1185	Marjoram, dried	1	teaspoon(s)	1	<.1	2	<.1	<1	<1	<.1	0.00	0.01	0.03
1186	Mustard seeds, yellow	1	teaspoon(s)	3	<1	15	1	1	<1	1	0.05	0.65	0.18
814	Nutmeg, ground	1	teaspoon(s)	2	<1	12	<1	1	<1	1	0.57	0.07	0.01
2747	Onion flakes, dehydrated	1	teaspoon(s)	2	<.1	6	<1	1	<1	<.1	0.00	0.00	0.00
1187	Onion powder	1	teaspoon(s)	2	<1	7	<1	2	<1	<.1	0.00	0.00	0.01
815	Oregano, ground	1	teaspoon(s)	2	<1	5	<1	1	1	<1	0.04	0.01	0.08
816	Paprika	1	teaspoon(s)	2	<1	6	<1	1	1	<1	0.04	0.03	0.17
817	Parsley, dried	1	teaspoon(s)	0	<.1	1	<.1	<1	<.1	<.1	0.00	0.01	0.00
1189	Poppy seeds	1	teaspoon(s)	3	<1	15	1	1	<1	1	0.14	0.18	0.86
1190	Poultry seasoning	1	teaspoon(s)	2	<1	5	<1	1	<1	<1	0.05	0.02	0.03
1191	Pumpkin pie spice, powder	1	teaspoon(s)	2	<1	6	<.1	1	<1	<1	0.11	0.02	0.01
1192	Rosemary, dried	1	teaspoon(s)	1	<1	4	<.1	1	1	<1	0.09	0.04	0.03
11723	Rosemary, fresh	1	teaspoon(s)	1	<1	1	<.1	<1	<.1	<.1	0.02	0.01	0.01
2722	Saffron powder	1	teaspoon(s)	1	<.1	2	<.1	<1	<.1	<.1	0.01	0.00	0.01
11724	Sage	1	ounce(s)	28	—	34	1	4	0	1	—	—	—
1193	Sage, ground	1	teaspoon(s)	1	<.1	2	<.1	<1	<1	<.1	0.05	0.01	0.01
822	Salt, table	¼	teaspoon(s)	2	<.1	0	0	0	0	0	0.00	0.00	0.00
30189	Salt substitute	¼	teaspoon(s)	1	—	<.1	0	<.1	0	0	0.00	0.00	0.00
30190	Salt substitute, seasoned	¼	teaspoon(s)	1	—	1	<.1	<1	0	<.1	0.00	—	—
1194	Savory, ground	1	teaspoon(s)	1	<1	4	<.1	1	1	<.1	0.05	—	—

PAGE KEY: H–2 = Breads/Baked Goods H–6 = Cereal/Rice/Pasta H–10 = Fruit H–16 = Vegetables/Legumes H–26 = Nuts/Seeds H–28 = Vegetarian H–30 = Dairy H–36 = Eggs H–38 = Seafood H–40 = Meats H–42 = Poultry H–44 = Processed meats H–46 = Beverages H–50 = Fats/Oils H–52 = Sweets H–52 = Sauces/Condiments/Spices H–56 = Mixed Foods/Soups/Sandwiches H–62 = Fast food H–80 = Convenience H–82 = Baby foods

Chol (mg)	Calc (mg)	Iron (mg)	Magn (mg)	Pota (mg)	Sodi (mg)	Zinc (mg)	Vit A (RAE) (µg)	Thia (mg)	Vit E (mg)	Ribo (mg)	Niac (mg)	Vit B_6 (mg)	Fola (µg)	Vit C (mg)	Vit B_{12} (µg)	Sele (µg)
0	14	0.78	4	30	<1	0.11	<1	0.01	0.02	0.01	0.06	0.01	<1	<1	0	<1
0	3	0.66	4	80	2	0.26	0	0.09	0.00	0.22	1.59	0.06	94	<.1	<.1	1
0	339	0.52	2	<1	363	0.00	0	0.00	0.00	0.00	0.00	0.00	0	0	0	<.1
0	0	0.00	0	0	1259	0.00	0	0.00	0.00	0.00	0.00	0.00	0	0	0	<.1
0	1	0.03	1	4	<.1	0.01	2	0.00	0.00	0.00	0.01	0.00	1	<1	0	<.1
0	1	—	<1	2	<.1	0.00	—	0.00	0.00	0.00	0.01	0.00	<1	—	0	<.1
0	30	0.59	6	48	<1	0.08	7	0.00	0.02	0.00	0.10	0.03	4	1	0	<.1
0	5	0.26	1	3	<1	0.02	2	0.00	0.01	0.00	0.01	0.01	1	<1	0	<.1
0	110	2.29	—	156	2	—	—	0.04	—	0.07	0.20	—	—	1	0	—
0	9	0.61	4	26	1	0.03	<1	0.00	0.02	0.01	0.02	0.01	<1	<1	0	<.1
0	6	0.47	6	51	3	0.21	0	0.42	0.00	0.11	1.00	0.07	104	0	0	0
0	0	0.00	—	—	140	—	0	—	—	—	—	—	—	0	—	—
0	14	0.34	5	28	<1	0.12	<1	0.01	0.05	0.01	0.08	0.01	<1	<1	0	<1
0	3	0.14	3	36	1	0.04	37	0.01	0.09	0.02	0.16	0.04	2	1	0	<1
0	35	0.90	9	28	3	0.14	<.1	0.01	0.02	0.01	0.06	0.02	<1	<1	0	<1
0	8	0.19	1	28	<1	0.05	2	0.00	0.01	0.00	0.03	0.01	2	<1	0	<1
0	7	0.37	4	50	26	0.07	39	0.01	0.03	0.02	0.21	0.10	3	2	0	<1
0	1	0.02	<1	3	<.1	0.01	2	0.00	0.00	0.00	0.01	0.00	1	1	0	<.1
0	1	0.03	<1	8	1	0.00	—	0.00	0.03	0.00	0.02	0.00	1	1	0	<.1
0	28	0.88	1	12	1	0.05	<1	0.00	0.00	0.00	0.03	0.01	1	1	0	<.1
0	14	0.18	6	23	5	0.02	1	0.00	0.04	0.01	0.03	0.01	2	2	0	<1
0	7	0.25	4	27	1	0.03	2	0.01	0.01	0.01	0.06	0.00	2	3	0	<1
0	13	0.29	6	23	1	0.08	0	0.00	—	0.01	0.04	—	0	<1	0	<1
0	<1	0.04	<1	<1	1	0.00	0	0.00	0.00	0.00	0.00	0.00	0	0	0	<1
0	20	—	—	44	5	—	—	—	—	—	—	—	—	—	—	—
0	20	1.39	8	38	4	0.10	1	0.01	0.02	0.01	0.10	0.01	<1	<1	0	<1
0	10	0.59	5	31	1	0.08	1	0.01	0.01	0.01	0.07	0.02	3	<1	0	<1
0	32	0.34	5	25	<1	0.11	<.1	0.01	0.02	0.01	0.06	0.01	<1	<1	0	<1
0	18	0.49	5	33	2	0.03	3	0.00	—	0.00	0.03	0.02	2	1	0	0
0	2	—	1	7	1	0.01	—	0.00	—	0.00	0.02	0.00	2	—	0	—
0	1	0.03	—	4	<.1	—	—	0.00	—	0.00	0.01	0.00	—	<1	0	—
0	24	0.37	8	34	2	0.07	<1	0.01	—	0.01	0.12	0.01	—	<1	0	0
0	7	1.24	7	28	2	0.09	<1	0.01	—	0.01	0.06	0.02	2	<1	0	<1
0	215	9.25	94	411	28	1.07	—	0.10	—	0.09	0.71	—	0	0	0	—
0	5	0.05	1	12	1	0.03	0	0.01	0.00	0.00	0.02	0.04	<.1	1	0	<1
0	2	0.08	2	31	1	0.07	0	0.01	0.00	0.00	0.02	0.08	<.1	1	0	1
0	2	0.21	3	24	1	0.08	<1	0.00	0.01	0.00	0.09	0.02	1	<1	0	1
0	1	0.02	2	17	1	0.01	0	0.00	0.01	0.00	0.03	0.01	<1	<1	0	<.1
0	3	0.06	1	19	<1	0.01	<1	0.01	—	0.00	0.03	0.01	3	1	0	<.1
0	4	0.24	3	8	1	0.04	1	0.01	0.04	0.01	0.02	0.00	1	<1	0	<.1
0	12	0.50	2	9	<1	0.02	2	0.00	0.01	0.00	0.02	0.01	2	<1	0	<.1
0	17	0.33	10	23	<1	0.19	<.1	0.02	0.08	0.01	0.26	0.01	3	<.1	0	4
0	4	0.07	4	8	<1	0.05	<1	0.01	0.06	0.00	0.03	0.00	2	<.1	0	<.1
0	4	0.03	2	27	<1	0.03	<.1	0.01	0.02	0.00	0.02	0.03	3	1	0	<.1
0	8	0.05	3	20	1	0.05	0	0.01	0.00	0.00	0.01	0.03	3	<1	0	<.1
0	24	0.66	4	25	<1	0.07	5	0.01	0.03	0.00	0.09	0.02	4	1	0	<.1
0	4	0.50	4	49	1	0.09	55	0.01	0.01	0.04	0.32	0.08	2	1	0	<.1
0	4	0.29	1	11	1	0.01	2	0.00	0.01	0.00	0.02	0.00	1	<1	0	<.1
0	41	0.26	9	20	1	0.29	0	0.02	0.08	0.00	0.03	0.01	2	<.1	0	<.1
0	15	0.53	3	10	<1	0.05	2	0.00	0.02	0.00	0.04	0.02	2	<1	0	<1
0	12	0.34	2	11	1	0.04	<1	0.00	0.01	0.00	0.04	0.01	1	<1	0	<1
0	15	0.35	3	11	1	0.04	2	0.01	0.02	0.01	0.01	0.02	4	1	0	<.1
0	2	0.05	1	5	<1	0.01	1	0.00	0.01	0.00	0.01	0.00	1	<1	0	—
0	1	0.08	2	12	1	0.01	<1	0.00	0.01	0.00	0.01	0.01	1	1	0	<.1
0	170	—	45	110	1	0.48	—	0.03	—	—	—	—	—	—	0	—
0	12	0.20	3	7	<.1	0.03	2	0.01	0.01	0.00	0.04	0.02	2	<1	0	<.1
0	<1	0.00	<.1	<1	581	0.00	0	0.00	0.00	0.00	0.00	0.00	0	0	0	<.1
0	7	0.00	<.1	604	<.1	—	0	—	—	—	—	—	—	0	—	—
0	0	0	476	<1	—	0	—	—	—	—	—	—	0	—	—	
0	30	0.53	5	15	<1	0.06	4	0.01	—	—	0.06	0.03	—	1	0	<.1

H Appendix

Table H–1

Food Composition (Computer code number is for Wadsworth Diet Analysis program) (For purposes of calculations, use "0" for t, <1, <.1, <.01, etc.)

DA + Code	Food Description	Quantity	Measure	Wt (g)	H_2O (g)	Ener (kcal)	Prot (g)	Carb (g)	Dietary Fiber (g)	Fat (g)	Fat Breakdown (g) Sat	Mono	Poly
	SAUCES, SPICES, CONDIMENTS—Continued												
820	Sesame seed kernels, toasted	1	teaspoon(s)	3	<1	15	<1	1	<1	1	0.18	0.49	0.57
11725	Sorrel	1	tablespoon(s)	9	—	2	<1	<1	<.1	<.1	0.00	—	—
11721	Spearmint	1	teaspoon(s)	2	2	1	<.1	<1	<1	<.1	0.00	0.00	0.01
35498	Sweet green peppers, freeze-dried	¼	cup(s)	2	<.1	5	<1	1	<1	<.1	0.01	0.00	0.03
11726	Tamarind leaves	1	ounce(s)	28	—	33	2	5	0	1	—	—	—
11727	Tarragon	1	ounce(s)	28	—	14	1	2	0	<1	—	—	—
1195	Tarragon, ground	1	teaspoon(s)	2	<1	5	<1	1	<1	<1	0.03	0.01	0.06
11728	Thyme, fresh	1	teaspoon(s)	1	1	1	<.1	<1	<1	<.1	0.00	0.00	0.00
821	Thyme, ground	1	teaspoon(s)	1	<1	4	<1	1	1	<1	0.04	0.01	0.02
1196	Turmeric, ground	1	teaspoon(s)	2	<1	8	<1	1	<1	<1	0.07	0.04	0.05
11995	Wasabi	1	tablespoon(s)	14	11	11	1	2	<1	<.1	—	—	—
1188	White pepper	1	teaspoon(s)	2	<1	7	<1	2	1	<.1	0.02	0.02	0.01
	Condiments												
674	Catsup or ketchup	1	tablespoon(s)	15	11	14	<1	4	<1	<.1	0.01	0.01	0.04
703	Dill pickle	1	ounce(s)	28	26	5	<1	1	<1	<.1	0.01	0.00	0.02
1641	Horseradish sauce, prepared	1	teaspoon(s)	5	3	10	<1	<1	<.1	1	0.59	0.28	0.04
140	Mayonnaise, low calorie	1	tablespoon(s)	16	10	37	<.1	3	0	3	0.53	0.72	1.70
138	Mayonnaise w/soybean oil	1	tablespoon(s)	14	2	99	<1	1	0	11	1.64	2.70	5.89
1682	Mustard, brown	1	teaspoon(s)	5	4	5	<1	<1	<.1	<1	—	—	—
700	Mustard, yellow	1	teaspoon(s)	5	4	3	<1	<1	<1	<1	0.01	0.11	0.03
706	Sweet pickle relish	1	tablespoon(s)	15	9	20	<.1	5	<1	<.1	0.01	0.03	0.02
141	Tartar sauce	2	tablespoon(s)	28	9	144	<1	4	<.1	14	2.14	4.13	7.57
	Sauces												
685	Barbecue sauce	2	tablespoon(s)	31	25	23	1	4	<1	1	0.08	0.24	0.21
834	Cheese sauce	¼	cup(s)	70	49	121	5	5	<1	9	4.19	2.67	1.81
32123	Chili enchilada sauce, green	2	tablespoon(s)	57	53	15	1	3	1	<1	0.04	0.04	0.13
32122	Chili enchilada sauce, red	2	tablespoon(s)	32	24	27	1	5	2	1	0.08	0.05	0.43
29688	Hoisin sauce	1	tablespoon(s)	16	7	35	1	7	<1	1	0.09	0.15	0.27
16670	Mole poblano sauce	½	cup(s)	133	103	155	5	11	2	11	2.67	5.15	2.91
29689	Oyster sauce	1	tablespoon(s)	16	13	8	<1	2	<.1	<.1	0.01	0.01	0.01
1655	Pepper sauce or tabasco	1	teaspoon(s)	5	5	1	<.1	<.1	<.1	<.1	0.01	0.00	0.02
347	Salsa	2	tablespoon(s)	16	14	4	<1	1	<1	<.1	0.00	0.00	0.02
841	Soy sauce	1	tablespoon(s)	18	13	10	1	2	0	<.1	0.00	0.00	0.01
839	Sweet & sour sauce	2	tablespoon(s)	39	30	37	<.1	9	<.1	<.1	0.00	0.00	0.00
1613	Teriyaki sauce	1	tablespoon(s)	18	12	15	1	3	<.1	0	0.00	0.00	0.00
25294	Tomato sauce	½	cup(s)	112	100	46	2	8	2	1	0.18	0.29	0.72
728	White sauce, medium	¼	cup(s)	63	47	92	2	6	<1	7	1.78	2.78	1.79
1654	Worcestershire sauce	1	teaspoon(s)	6	4	4	0	1	0	0	0.00	0.00	0.00
	Vinegar												
30853	Balsamic	1	tablespoon(s)	15	—	10	0	2	0	0	0.00	0.00	0.00
727	Cider	1	tablespoon(s)	15	14	2	0	1	0	0	0.00	0.00	0.00
1673	Distilled	1	tablespoon(s)	15	14	2	0	1	0	0	0.00	0.00	0.00
15439	Tarragon	1	tablespoon(s)	16	—	0	0	0	0	0	0.00	0.00	0.00
	MIXED FOODS, SOUPS, SANDWICHES												
	Mixed Dishes												
16652	Almond chicken	1	cup(s)	242	186	280	22	16	3	15	1.91	6.07	5.62
25224	Barbecued chicken	2	piece(s)	177	100	325	27	15	<1	17	4.63	6.78	3.71
25227	Bean burrito	1	item(s)	149	82	327	17	33	6	15	8.30	4.73	0.85
9516	Beef & vegetable fajita	1	item(s)	223	144	397	23	35	3	18	5.50	7.53	3.45
16796	Beef or pork egg roll	2	item(s)	128	85	227	10	19	1	12	2.88	5.96	2.64
177	Beef stew w/vegetables, prepared	1	cup(s)	245	201	220	16	15	3	11	4.40	4.50	0.50
30233	Beef stroganoff w/noodles	1	cup(s)	256	190	343	20	23	2	19	7.37	5.62	4.47
16651	Cashew chicken	1	cup(s)	242	131	644	43	17	3	46	7.75	20.83	14.47
475	Cheese pizza	2	slice(s)	126	60	281	15	41	0	6	3.08	1.98	0.98
30330	Cheese quesadilla	1	item(s)	54	19	183	6	18	1	10	3.49	3.42	2.16
215	Chicken & noodles, prepared	1	cup(s)	240	170	365	22	26	1	18	5.10	7.10	3.90
30239	Chicken & vegetables w/broccoli, onion, bamboo shoots in soy based sauce	1	cup(s)	162	112	287	22	6	1	19	5.13	7.65	4.68
25093	Chicken cacciatore	1	cup(s)	230	166	266	28	5	1	14	3.98	5.78	3.11

Appendix H

PAGE KEY: H–2 = Breads/Baked Goods H–6 = Cereal/Rice/Pasta H–10 = Fruit H–16 = Vegetables/Legumes H–26 = Nuts/Seeds H–28 = Vegetarian H–30 = Dairy H–36 = Eggs H–38 = Seafood H–40 = Meats H–42 = Poultry H–44 = Processed meats H–46 = Beverages H–50 = Fats/Oils H–52 = Sweets H–52 = Sauces/Condiments/Spices H–56 = Mixed Foods/Soups/Sandwiches H–62 = Fast food H–80 = Convenience H–82 = Baby foods

Chol (mg)	Calc (mg)	Iron (mg)	Magn (mg)	Pota (mg)	Sodi (mg)	Zinc (mg)	Vit A (RAE) (µg)	Thia (mg)	Vit E (mg)	Ribo (mg)	Niac (mg)	Vit B_6 (mg)	Fola (µg)	Vit C (mg)	Vit B_{12} (µg)	Sele (µg)
0	4	0.21	9	11	1	0.28	<.1	0.03	0.06	0.01	0.15	0.00	3	0	0	<.1
0	—	—	—	—	<1	—	—	—	—	—	—	—	—	—	—	—
0	4	0.23	1	9	1	0.02	4	0.00	0.01	0.00	0.02	0.00	2	<1	0	—
0	2	0.17	3	51	3	0.04	3	0.02	0.06	0.02	0.12	0.04	4	30	0	<.1
0	85	1.48	20	—	—	—	—	0.07	—	0.03	1.16	—	—	1	0	—
0	48	—	14	128	3	0.17	—	0.04	—	—	—	—	—	1	0	—
0	18	0.52	6	48	1	0.06	3	0.00	0.03	0.02	0.14	0.04	4	1	0	<.1
0	3	0.14	1	5	<.1	0.01	2	0.00	—	0.00	0.01	0.00	<1	1	0	—
0	26	1.73	3	11	1	0.09	3	0.01	0.02	0.01	0.07	0.01	4	1	0	<.1
0	4	0.91	4	56	1	0.10	0	0.00	0.00	0.01	0.11	0.04	1	1	0	<.1
0	13	0.11	—	—	—	—	—	0.02	—	0.01	0.07	—	—	11	0	—
0	6	0.34	2	2	<1	0.03	0	0.00	0.06	0.00	0.01	0.00	<1	1	0	<.1
0	3	0.08	3	57	167	0.04	7	0.00	0.22	0.07	0.23	0.02	2	2	0	<.1
0	3	0.15	3	33	363	0.04	3	0.00	0.05	0.01	0.02	0.00	<1	1	0	0
2	5	0.00	1	7	15	0.01	—	0.00	0.03	0.01	0.00	0.00	1	<.1	<.1	—
4	<.1	0.00	<.1	2	80	0.02	0	0.00	1.03	0.00	0.00	0.00	0	0	0	—
5	2	0.07	<1	5	78	0.02	12	0.00	0.32	0.00	0.00	0.08	1	0	<.1	<1
0	6	0.09	1	7	68	0.02	0	0.00	0.22	0.00	0.01	0.00	<1	<.1	0	—
0	4	0.09	2	8	56	0.03	<1	0.00	0.09	0.00	0.02	0.00	<1	<1	0	2
0	<1	0.13	1	4	122	0.02	1	0.00	0.01	0.00	0.03	0.00	<1	<1	0	0
11	6	0.21	1	10	200	0.05	—	0.00	2.04	0.00	0.01	0.08	2	<1	<.1	—
0	6	0.28	6	54	255	0.06	<1	0.01	0.35	0.01	0.28	0.02	1	2	0	<1
20	128	0.15	6	21	578	0.68	56	0.00	0.22	0.08	0.02	0.01	3	<1	<.1	2
0	5	0.36	9	126	62	0.11	—	0.03	0.21	0.02	0.63	0.06	6	44	0	0
0	7	1.05	11	231	114	0.15	—	0.02	0.42	0.22	0.61	0.34	7	<1	0	<1
<1	5	0.16	4	19	258	0.05	0	0.00	0.00	0.03	0.19	0.01	4	<.1	0	<1
1	37	1.51	57	283	305	0.95	—	0.07	1.77	0.09	1.82	0.09	14	5	<.1	—
0	5	0.03	1	9	437	0.01	0	0.00	0.01	0.02	0.24	0.00	2	<.1	<.1	1
0	1	0.06	1	6	32	0.01	4	0.00	0.69	0.00	0.01	0.01	<.1	<1	0	—
0	5	0.16	2	34	69	0.04	5	0.01	0.10	0.01	0.13	0.02	3	2	0	<.1
0	3	0.36	6	32	1029	0.07	0	0.01	0.00	0.02	0.61	0.03	3	0	0	—
0	5	0.20	1	8	98	0.01	0	0.00		0.01	0.12	0.04	<1	0	0	—
0	5	0.31	11	41	690	0.02	0	0.01	0.00	0.01	0.23	0.02	4	0	0	<1
0	21	1.08	19	431	199	0.30	48	0.05	1.55	0.05	1.18	0.13	15	15	0	1
4	74	0.21	9	98	221	0.26	—	0.04	0.85	0.12	0.25	0.03	3	1	<1	—
0	6	0.30	1	45	56	0.01	—	0.00	0.00	0.01	0.04	0.00	0	1	0	—
0	0	0.00	—	—	0	—	0	—	—	—	—	—	—	0	—	—
0	1	0.09	3	15	<1	0.00	0	0.00	0.00	0.00	0.00	0.00	0	0	0	<.1
0	1	0.09	0	2	<1	0.00	0	0.00	0.00	0.00	0.00	0.00	0	0	0	5
0	0	0.00	—	0	0	—	0	—	—	—	—	—	—	0	0	—
40	69	1.97	60	549	526	1.62	—	0.09	3.80	0.20	9.48	0.44	26	7	<1	—
120	26	1.64	31	387	477	2.69	69	0.07	1.12	0.37	6.92	0.39	15	5	<1	19
38	331	2.95	45	384	514	1.92	119	0.24	1.52	0.29	1.82	0.15	115	4	<1	18
45	84	3.74	37	476	757	3.51	—	0.39	1.73	0.30	5.37	0.38	23	27	2	—
74	30	1.66	20	248	547	0.91	—	0.32	1.66	0.25	2.55	0.19	20	4	<1	—
71	29	2.90	—	613	292	—	—	0.15	1.35	0.17	4.70	—	—	17	<.1	15
74	70	3.26	37	393	818	3.66	—	0.21	1.64	0.31	3.80	0.21	17	1	2	—
96	74	2.92	94	640	1355	2.24	—	0.23	5.83	0.22	19.76	0.88	64	11	<1	—
19	233	1.16	32	219	672	1.63	147	0.37	—	0.33	4.96	0.09	69	3	1	27
13	132	1.21	13	77	230	0.64	—	0.13	1.05	0.14	1.09	0.04	6	15	<.1	—
103	26	2.20	—	149	600	—	—	0.05	0.43	0.17	4.30	—	—	0	—	29
84	22	1.38	29	344	962	1.70	—	0.08	0.94	0.17	7.90	0.32	13	8	<1	—
103	45	2.21	37	444	451	2.01	53	0.10	1.18	0.21	9.20	0.54	15	8	<1	22

H Appendix

Table H-1

Food Composition (Computer code number is for Wadsworth Diet Analysis program) (For purposes of calculations, use "0" for t, <1, <.1, <.01, etc.)

DA + Code	Food Description	Quantity	Measure	Wt (g)	H_2O (g)	Ener (kcal)	Prot (g)	Carb (g)	Dietary Fiber (g)	Fat (g)	Fat Breakdown (g) Sat	Mono	Poly
	MIXED FOODS, SOUPS, SANDWICHES—Continued												
28020	Chicken fried turkey steak	3	ounce(s)	85	48	122	13	12	1	2	0.59	0.37	0.78
218	Chicken pot pie	1	cup(s)	252	154	542	23	42	3	31	9.79	12.52	7.03
30240	Chicken teriyaki	1	cup(s)	244	163	339	51	13	1	7	1.78	2.03	1.71
25119	Chicken waldorf salad	½	cup(s)	100	68	178	14	6	1	11	1.76	3.18	5.05
25099	Chili con carne	¾	cup(s)	215	175	197	14	21	7	7	2.55	2.83	0.54
1062	Coleslaw	¾	cup(s)	90	73	62	1	11	1	2	0.35	0.64	1.22
1896	Combination pizza, w/meat & vegetables	2	slice(s)	158	75	368	26	43	5	11	3.07	5.09	1.83
1574	Crab cakes, from blue crab	1	item(s)	60	43	93	12	<1	0	5	0.89	1.69	1.36
32144	Enchiladas w/green chili sauce (enchiladas verdes)	1	item(s)	144	104	207	9	18	3	12	6.35	3.65	0.96
2793	Falafel patty	3	item(s)	51	18	170	7	16	0	9	1.22	5.19	2.12
28546	Fettuccine alfredo	1	cup(s)	222	81	247	11	42	1	3	1.61	0.79	0.43
32146	Flautas	3	item(s)	162	78	438	25	36	4	22	8.22	8.80	2.29
29629	Fried rice w/meat or poultry	1	cup(s)	198	129	329	12	41	1	12	2.27	3.53	5.69
16649	General tso chicken	1	cup(s)	146	91	293	19	16	1	17	3.98	6.27	5.27
1826	Green salad	¾	cup(s)	104	99	17	1	3	2	<.1	0.01	0.00	0.04
1814	Hummus	½	cup(s)	123	80	218	6	25	5	11	1.38	6.04	2.56
16650	Kung pao chicken	1	cup(s)	162	88	431	29	11	2	31	5.19	13.95	9.69
16622	Lamb curry	1	cup(s)	236	188	256	28	3	1	14	3.93	4.92	3.35
25253	Lasagna w/ground beef	1	cup(s)	237	157	288	18	22	2	15	7.47	4.84	0.84
442	Macaroni & cheese	1	cup(s)	200	122	393	15	40	1	19	8.18	6.72	2.66
25105	Meat loaf	1	slice(s)	115	85	244	17	7	<1	16	6.15	6.89	0.83
16646	Moo shi pork	1	cup(s)	151	77	512	19	5	1	46	6.84	14.80	22.07
16788	Nachos w/beef, beans, cheese, tomatoes, & onions	7	item(s)	551	284	1496	40	119	19	99	22.34	40.19	30.69
1668	Pepperoni pizza	2	slice(s)	142	66	362	20	40	1	14	4.47	6.28	2.33
655	Potato salad	½	cup(s)	125	95	179	3	14	2	10	1.79	3.10	4.67
29637	Ravioli, meat filled, w/tomato or meat sauce, canned	1	cup(s)	251	196	220	9	38	2	4	1.58	1.49	0.41
25109	Salisbury steaks w/mushroom sauce	1	serving(s)	135	102	251	17	9	1	15	5.98	6.67	0.76
16637	Shrimp creole w/rice	1	cup(s)	243	176	311	27	28	1	9	1.83	3.79	2.88
497	Spaghetti & meat balls w/tomato sauce, prepared	1	cup(s)	248	174	330	19	39	3	12	3.90	4.40	2.20
28585	Spicy thai noodles (pad thai)	8	ounce(s)	231	74	222	9	36	3	6	0.83	3.33	1.83
33073	Stir fried pork & vegetables w/rice	1	cup(s)	235	173	349	15	34	2	16	5.55	6.87	2.62
28588	Stuffed shells	2½	item(s)	299	189	292	18	33	3	10	3.81	3.57	1.62
16821	Sushi w/egg in seaweed	6	piece(s)	156	117	190	9	20	<1	8	2.09	3.02	1.55
16819	Sushi w/vegetables & fish	6	piece(s)	156	102	217	8	44	2	1	0.16	0.14	0.20
16820	Sushi w/vegetables in seaweed	6	piece(s)	156	110	182	3	41	1	<1	0.10	0.11	0.11
25266	Sweet & sour pork	¾	cup(s)	249	206	264	29	17	1	8	2.59	3.51	1.48
16824	Tabouli, tabbouleh, or tabuli	1	cup(s)	160	124	199	3	16	4	15	2.04	10.83	1.37
25276	Three bean salad	½	cup(s)	99	82	95	2	10	3	6	0.76	1.41	3.48
160	Tuna salad	½	cup(s)	103	65	192	16	10	0	9	1.58	2.96	4.23
25241	Turkey & noodles	1	cup(s)	319	228	271	24	21	1	9	2.39	3.48	2.27
16794	Vegetable egg roll	2	item(s)	128	90	202	5	20	2	12	2.46	5.71	2.65
16818	Vegetable sushi, no fish	6	piece(s)	156	99	225	5	50	2	<1	0.11	0.10	0.14
	Sandwiches												
1744	Bacon, lettuce & tomato w/mayonnaise	1	item(s)	164	97	349	11	34	2	19	4.54	7.22	6.07
30287	Bologna & cheese w/margarine	1	item(s)	111	46	350	13	28	1	20	8.55	8.40	2.28
30286	Bologna w/margarine	1	item(s)	83	34	256	7	26	1	13	4.08	6.31	2.07
16546	Cheese	1	item(s)	83	31	262	10	27	1	13	5.59	4.77	1.67
8789	Cheeseburger, large, plain	1	item(s)	185	72	609	30	47	0	33	14.84	12.74	2.44
8624	Cheeseburger, large, w/bacon, vegetables, & condiments	1	item(s)	195	85	608	32	37	2	37	16.24	14.49	2.71
1745	Club w/bacon, chicken, tomato, lettuce, & mayonnaise	1	item(s)	246	137	555	31	48	3	26	5.94	—	—
1908	Cold cut submarine w/cheese & vegetables	1	item(s)	228	132	456	22	51	2	19	6.81	8.23	2.28
30247	Corned beef	1	item(s)	130	75	268	19	25	2	10	3.75	3.96	0.80
25283	Egg salad	1	item(s)	126	72	278	10	29	1	13	2.96	3.97	4.79
16686	Fried egg	1	item(s)	96	50	226	10	26	1	9	2.29	3.51	1.64

PAGE KEY: H–2 = Breads/Baked Goods H–6 = Cereal/Rice/Pasta H–10 = Fruit H–16 = Vegetables/Legumes H–26 = Nuts/Seeds H–28 = Vegetarian H–30 = Dairy H–36 = Eggs H–38 = Seafood H–40 = Meats H–42 = Poultry H–44 = Processed meats H–46 = Beverages H–50 = Fats/Oils H–52 = Sweets H–52 = Sauces/Condiments/Spices H–56 = Mixed Foods/Soups/Sandwiches H–62 = Fast food H–80 = Convenience H–82 = Baby foods

Chol (mg)	Calc (mg)	Iron (mg)	Magn (mg)	Pota (mg)	Sodi (mg)	Zinc (mg)	Vit A (RAE) (µg)	Thia (mg)	Vit E (mg)	Ribo (mg)	Niac (mg)	Vit B_6 (mg)	Fola (µg)	Vit C (mg)	Vit B_{12} (µg)	Sele (µg)
27	69	1.34	19	197	139	1.08	5	0.15	0.08	0.18	3.46	0.22	21	<1	<1	16
69	64	3.38	38	393	651	1.93	607	0.40	2.73	0.40	7.24	0.24	31	11	<1	—
157	52	3.27	67	589	3209	3.75	—	0.15	0.67	0.37	16.69	0.89	23	6	1	—
42	20	0.78	24	197	246	1.13	21	0.04	1.04	0.10	4.05	0.25	15	2	<1	11
27	43	3.16	50	646	865	2.44	25	0.13	1.65	0.23	3.01	0.18	56	10	1	10
7	41	0.53	9	163	21	0.18	48	0.06	—	0.06	0.24	0.11	24	29	0	1
41	202	3.07	36	357	765	2.23	117	0.43	—	0.35	3.92	0.19	65	3	1	22
90	63	0.65	20	194	198	2.45	34	0.05	—	0.05	1.74	0.10	32	2	4	24
27	266	1.08	38	251	276	1.27	—	0.07	0.46	0.16	1.28	0.18	45	59	<1	6
0	28	1.74	42	298	150	0.77	1	0.07	—	0.08	0.53	0.06	47	1	0	1
9	153	1.88	32	123	386	1.48	51	0.35	0.17	0.34	2.60	0.06	103	1	<1	35
73	146	2.66	61	223	886	3.44	0	0.10	0.33	0.17	3.00	0.27	96	0	1	37
102	36	2.66	31	182	821	1.42	—	0.30	2.19	0.19	3.51	0.24	24	3	<1	—
65	27	1.49	24	250	906	1.40	—	0.10	1.78	0.19	6.28	0.28	17	12	<1	—
0	13	0.65	11	178	27	0.22	59	0.03	—	0.05	0.57	0.08	38	24	0	<1
0	60	1.93	36	213	298	1.34	0	0.11	1.23	0.06	0.49	0.49	73	10	0	3
64	49	1.96	63	428	907	1.50	—	0.15	3.90	0.15	13.23	0.59	43	8	<1	—
89	36	2.97	40	495	495	6.62	—	0.09	1.20	0.28	8.05	0.20	27	1	3	—
68	222	2.33	40	437	493	2.81	108	0.19	1.15	0.29	3.02	0.20	50	10	1	22
30	323	2.26	42	263	800	1.95	327	0.25	1.45	0.40	2.18	0.10	12	<1	<1	—
85	54	2.09	21	278	423	3.55	27	0.08	0.28	0.29	3.77	0.13	20	<1	2	17
172	30	1.45	26	330	1078	1.83	—	0.50	8.51	0.38	2.90	0.31	22	8	1	—
82	699	6.71	205	1067	1611	7.55	—	0.31	14.23	0.50	5.62	0.85	59	14	1	—
28	129	1.87	17	305	534	1.04	105	0.27	—	0.47	6.09	0.11	74	3	<1	26
85	24	0.81	19	318	661	0.39	40	0.10	—	0.08	1.11	0.18	9	13	0	5
17	28	2.04	23	337	1354	1.19	—	0.22	0.41	0.20	2.88	0.14	17	22	<1	—
60	64	2.21	23	282	370	3.66	27	0.11	0.22	0.30	4.00	0.13	22	<1	2	17
181	101	4.44	64	439	381	1.73	—	0.29	3.99	0.10	4.77	0.22	12	18	1	—
89	124	3.70	—	665	1009	—	82	0.25	1.94	0.30	4.00	—	—	22	—	22
37	32	1.58	50	187	598	1.08	38	0.18	1.31	0.13	1.88	0.17	44	22	<.1	3
46	39	2.65	32	394	574	2.07	80	0.51	1.19	0.20	5.07	0.30	102	18	<1	23
35	241	3.18	63	462	543	1.68	280	0.32	1.30	0.36	4.64	0.30	109	15	<1	36
217	42	1.63	18	128	527	0.98	—	0.12	0.89	0.29	1.33	0.13	29	2	<1	—
11	24	2.18	25	204	340	0.79	—	0.26	0.58	0.07	2.77	0.15	14	4	<1	—
0	20	1.54	20	99	153	0.70	—	0.20	0.13	0.04	1.86	0.14	10	2	0	—
74	41	1.78	35	622	624	2.53	64	0.80	0.98	0.37	6.69	0.65	14	10	1	50
0	29	1.25	36	246	799	0.48	—	0.08	2.10	0.05	1.14	0.11	31	29	0	—
0	26	0.96	15	144	224	0.31	12	0.04	1.41	0.06	0.26	0.06	31	9	0	3
13	17	1.03	19	182	412	0.57	25	0.03	—	0.07	6.87	0.08	8	2	1	42
77	60	2.69	33	379	576	2.64	108	0.23	1.30	0.32	6.40	0.30	60	1	1	34
60	29	1.61	18	193	548	0.51	—	0.16	1.77	0.21	1.59	0.10	27	6	<1	—
0	23	2.40	23	158	369	0.84	—	0.28	0.19	0.06	2.44	0.13	15	4	0	—
20	76	2.54	27	328	837	0.98	—	0.39	1.87	0.27	3.81	0.20	31	15	<1	—
35	221	2.18	24	185	940	1.68	—	0.30	0.95	0.33	2.77	0.12	21	<.1	1	—
16	60	1.96	15	112	598	0.85	—	0.29	0.76	0.21	2.73	0.08	19	<.1	<1	—
19	216	1.75	20	135	655	1.14	—	0.25	0.92	0.29	2.04	0.07	19	<.1	<1	—
96	91	5.46	39	644	1589	5.55	185	0.48	—	0.57	11.17	0.28	74	0	3	39
111	162	4.74	45	332	1043	6.83	82	0.31	—	0.41	6.63	0.31	86	2	2	33
72	116	4.05	47	463	855	1.65	—	0.61	2.59	0.44	11.92	0.59	48	9	1	—
36	189	2.51	68	394	1651	2.58	71	1.00	—	0.80	5.49	0.14	87	12	1	31
46	67	2.67	20	187	1177	2.24	—	0.24	0.26	0.25	3.23	0.10	22	2	1	—
217	107	2.60	18	147	494	0.94	94	0.26	0.95	0.43	2.27	0.16	82	1	1	24
207	80	2.25	17	120	433	0.85	—	0.27	0.89	0.41	2.06	0.10	34	0	<1	—

Table H–1

Food Composition (Computer code number is for Wadsworth Diet Analysis program) (For purposes of calculations, use "0" for t, <1, <.1, <.01, etc.)

DA + Code	Food Description	Quantity	Measure	Wt (g)	H_2O (g)	Ener (kcal)	Prot (g)	Carb (g)	Dietary Fiber (g)	Fat (g)	Fat Breakdown (g) Sat	Mono	Poly
	MIXED FOODS, SOUPS, SANDWICHES—Continued												
16547	Grilled cheese	1	item(s)	83	27	292	10	27	1	16	6.22	6.29	2.54
16659	Gyro w/onion & tomato	1	item(s)	105	67	170	12	21	1	4	1.53	1.41	0.43
1906	Ham & cheese	1	item(s)	146	74	352	21	33	2	15	6.44	6.74	1.38
31890	Ham w/mayonnaise	1	item(s)	112	55	282	14	27	1	13	3.06	5.04	3.79
756	Hamburger, double patty, large, w/condiments & vegetables	1	item(s)	226	121	540	34	40	0	27	10.52	10.33	2.80
8793	Hamburger, large, plain	1	item(s)	137	58	426	23	32	2	23	8.38	9.88	2.14
8795	Hamburger, large, w/vegetables & condiments	1	item(s)	218	121	512	26	40	3	27	10.42	11.42	2.20
25134	Hot chicken salad	1	item(s)	98	49	239	16	23	1	9	2.83	2.61	2.76
1411	Hot dog w/bun, plain	1	item(s)	98	53	242	10	18	2	15	5.11	6.85	1.71
25133	Hot turkey salad	1	item(s)	98	50	221	16	23	1	7	2.23	1.76	2.28
30249	Pastrami	1	item(s)	134	71	331	14	27	2	18	6.18	8.74	1.02
16701	Peanut butter	1	item(s)	93	24	344	13	37	3	17	3.55	8.16	4.58
30306	Peanut butter & jelly	1	item(s)	93	24	330	11	42	3	15	3.00	6.87	3.82
1910	Roast beef, plain	1	item(s)	139	68	346	22	33	1	14	3.61	6.80	1.71
1909	Roast beef submarine w/mayonnaise & vegetables	1	item(s)	216	127	410	29	44	—	13	7.09	1.84	2.61
1907	Steak w/mayonnaise & vegetables	1	item(s)	204	104	459	30	52	2	14	3.81	5.34	3.35
25288	Tuna salad	1	item(s)	179	102	414	24	29	2	22	3.61	5.46	11.43
31891	Turkey w/mayonnaise	1	item(s)	143	75	330	29	26	1	11	2.61	3.25	4.40
30283	Turkey submarine w/cheese, lettuce, tomato, & mayonnaise	1	item(s)	277	156	583	37	51	3	25	7.15	8.03	7.81
	Soups												
25296	Bean	1	cup(s)	301	253	191	14	29	6	2	0.67	0.83	0.53
711	Bean with pork, condensed, prepared w/water	1	cup(s)	265	223	180	8	24	9	6	1.59	2.28	1.91
713	Beef noodle, condensed, prepared w/water	1	cup(s)	244	224	83	5	9	1	3	1.15	1.24	0.49
825	Cheese, condensed, prepared w/milk	1	cup(s)	251	207	231	9	16	1	15	9.11	4.09	0.45
826	Chicken broth, condensed, prepared w/water	1	cup(s)	244	234	39	5	1	0	1	0.39	0.59	0.27
25297	Chicken noodle	1	cup(s)	286	258	117	11	11	1	3	0.78	1.10	0.66
827	Chicken noodle, condensed, prepared w/water	1	cup(s)	241	222	75	4	9	1	2	0.65	1.11	0.55
724	Chicken noodle, dehydrated, prepared w/water	1	cup(s)	252	237	58	2	9	<1	1	0.31	0.52	0.39
823	Cream of asparagus, condensed, prepared w/milk	1	cup(s)	248	213	161	6	16	1	8	3.32	2.08	2.23
824	Cream of celery, condensed, prepared w/milk	1	cup(s)	248	214	164	6	15	1	10	3.94	2.46	2.65
708	Cream of chicken, condensed, prepared w/milk	1	cup(s)	248	210	191	7	15	<1	11	4.64	4.46	1.64
715	Cream of chicken, condensed, prepared w/water	1	cup(s)	244	221	117	3	9	<1	7	2.07	3.27	1.49
709	Cream of mushroom, condensed, prepared w/milk	1	cup(s)	248	210	203	6	15	<1	14	5.13	2.98	4.61
716	Cream of mushroom, condensed, prepared w/water	1	cup(s)	244	220	129	2	9	<1	9	2.44	1.71	4.22
25298	Cream of vegetable	1	cup(s)	285	251	165	7	15	2	9	1.56	4.62	1.92
16689	Egg drop	1	cup(s)	244	229	73	8	1	0	4	1.15	1.52	0.59
25138	Golden squash	1	cup(s)	258	224	144	8	21	2	4	0.84	2.18	0.88
16663	Hot & sour	1	cup(s)	244	210	161	15	5	1	8	2.72	3.40	1.20
28054	Lentil chowder	1	cup(s)	229	188	150	11	27	12	<1	0.09	0.08	0.22
28560	Macaroni & bean	1	cup(s)	229	129	136	6	21	5	3	0.48	2.06	0.59
714	Manhattan clam chowder, condensed, prepared w/water	1	cup(s)	244	224	78	2	12	1	2	0.38	0.38	1.29
28561	Minestrone	1	cup(s)	230	177	99	4	16	5	2	0.32	1.30	0.43
717	Minestrone, condensed, prepared w/water	1	cup(s)	241	220	82	4	11	1	3	0.55	0.70	1.11
28038	Mushroom & wild rice	1	cup(s)	230	188	81	4	12	2	<1	0.05	0.02	0.15
828	New England clam chowder, condensed, prepared w/milk	1	cup(s)	248	211	164	9	17	1	7	2.95	2.26	1.09
28036	New England style clam chowder	1	cup(s)	229	207	83	3	15	2	<1	0.08	0.03	0.05

PAGE KEY: H–2 = Breads/Baked Goods H–6 = Cereal/Rice/Pasta H–10 = Fruit H–16 = Vegetables/Legumes H–26 = Nuts/Seeds H–28 = Vegetarian H–30 = Dairy H–36 = Eggs H–38 = Seafood H–40 = Meats H–42 = Poultry H–44 = Processed meats H–46 = Beverages H–50 = Fats/Oils H–52 = Sweets H–52 = Sauces/Condiments/Spices H–56 = Mixed Foods/Soups/Sandwiches H–62 = Fast food H–80 = Convenience H–82 = Baby foods

Chol (mg)	Calc (mg)	Iron (mg)	Magn (mg)	Pota (mg)	Sodi (mg)	Zinc (mg)	Vit A (RAE) (µg)	Thia (mg)	Vit E (mg)	Ribo (mg)	Niac (mg)	Vit B_6 (mg)	Fola (µg)	Vit C (mg)	Vit B_{12} (µg)	Sele (µg)
19	219	1.76	21	137	696	1.15	—	0.19	1.38	0.28	1.86	0.06	13	<.1	<1	—
34	46	1.85	21	209	272	2.30	—	0.24	0.29	0.21	3.14	0.13	18	4	1	—
58	130	3.24	16	291	771	1.37	96	0.31	0.29	0.48	2.69	0.20	76	3	1	23
36	59	2.10	23	245	1033	1.50	—	0.71	1.09	0.31	4.89	0.26	19	0	<1	—
122	102	5.85	50	570	791	5.67	5	0.36	—	0.38	7.57	0.54	77	1	4	26
71	74	3.58	27	267	474	4.11	0	0.29	—	0.29	6.25	0.23	60	0	2	27
87	96	4.93	44	480	824	4.88	24	0.41	—	0.37	7.28	0.33	83	3	2	34
39	114	1.93	20	150	470	1.22	28	0.20	1.09	0.23	4.93	0.20	54	<1	<1	17
44	24	2.31	13	143	670	1.98	0	0.24	—	0.27	3.65	0.05	48	<.1	1	26
37	113	2.04	22	167	459	1.09	23	0.19	1.04	0.21	4.36	0.23	54	<1	<1	20
51	68	2.64	23	243	1335	2.69	—	0.29	0.33	0.27	4.77	0.13	21	2	1	—
1	80	2.47	62	272	479	1.25	0	0.33	3.12	0.25	6.46	0.17	43	0	<.1	—
1	68	2.11	53	239	409	1.06	—	0.27	2.63	0.21	5.45	0.15	37	<1	<.1	—
51	54	4.23	31	316	792	3.39	11	0.38	—	0.31	5.87	0.26	57	2	1	29
73	41	2.81	67	330	845	4.38	30	0.41	—	0.41	5.96	0.32	71	6	2	26
73	92	5.16	49	524	798	4.53	20	0.41	—	0.37	7.30	0.37	90	6	2	42
53	100	3.29	35	302	795	1.08	46	0.26	1.27	0.26	12.29	0.48	70	1	2	71
69	78	3.10	34	315	490	2.94	—	0.30	1.23	0.33	6.64	0.46	24	0	<1	—
70	324	3.88	51	552	2408	2.66	—	0.53	2.67	0.49	12.50	0.54	46	5	2	—
5	80	3.08	61	590	690	1.41	26	0.27	0.28	0.15	3.61	0.23	139	3	<1	8
3	85	2.15	48	421	996	1.09	48	0.09	0.08	0.03	0.59	0.04	34	2	<.1	8
5	15	1.10	5	100	952	1.54	7	0.07	0.00	0.06	1.07	0.04	20	<1	<1	7
48	289	0.80	20	341	1019	0.68	359	0.06	0.25	0.33	0.50	0.08	10	1	<1	7
0	10	0.51	2	210	776	0.24	0	0.01	0.04	0.07	3.35	0.02	5	0	<1	0
24	26	1.34	16	335	776	0.77	49	0.15	0.20	0.16	5.57	0.13	40	1	<1	10
7	17	0.77	5	55	1106	0.39	36	0.05	0.07	0.06	1.39	0.03	22	<1	<1	6
10	5	0.50	8	33	577	0.20	3	0.20	0.10	0.08	1.09	0.03	18	0	<.1	10
22	174	0.87	20	360	1042	0.92	62	0.10	0.84	0.28	0.88	0.06	30	4	<1	8
32	186	0.69	22	310	1009	0.20	114	0.07	0.97	0.25	0.44	0.06	7	1	<1	5
27	181	0.67	17	273	1047	0.67	179	0.07	0.24	0.26	0.92	0.07	7	1	1	8
10	34	0.61	2	88	986	0.63	163	0.03	0.20	0.06	0.82	0.02	2	<1	<.1	7
20	179	0.60	20	270	918	0.64	35	0.08	1.34	0.28	0.91	0.06	10	2	<1	4
2	46	0.51	5	100	881	0.59	15	0.05	1.24	0.09	0.72	0.01	5	1	<.1	1
1	68	1.38	17	312	784	0.74	100	0.12	5.13	0.20	3.27	0.12	37	10	<1	5
103	21	0.75	5	220	729	0.48	—	0.02	0.29	0.19	3.03	0.05	15	0	<1	—
4	203	1.63	39	412	500	1.72	454	0.17	2.46	0.38	1.15	0.15	32	10	1	8
34	29	1.89	29	382	1561	1.51	—	0.27	0.15	0.25	4.97	0.20	13	1	<1	—
<1	47	4.07	55	590	26	1.44	163	0.21	0.54	0.12	1.69	0.30	164	13	0	3
<1	64	1.86	32	254	489	0.46	174	0.15	0.73	0.13	1.36	0.09	59	7	0	9
2	27	1.63	12	188	578	0.98	56	0.03	0.73	0.04	0.82	0.10	10	4	4	9
0	68	1.76	31	273	423	0.38	138	0.10	0.57	0.10	0.69	0.07	47	12	0	4
2	34	0.92	7	313	911	0.75	118	0.05	0.07	0.04	0.94	0.10	36	1	0	8
0	27	1.08	26	332	267	0.87	4	0.06	0.22	0.21	2.97	0.14	18	4	<.1	4
22	186	1.49	22	300	992	0.79	57	0.07	0.15	0.24	1.03	0.13	10	3	10	13
2	69	1.29	26	430	236	0.66	34	0.07	0.61	0.12	1.02	0.20	17	12	3	4

Table H–1

Food Composition (Computer code number is for Wadsworth Diet Analysis program) (For purposes of calculations, use "0" for t, <1, <.1, <.01, etc.)

DA + Code	Food Description	Quantity	Measure	Wt (g)	H_2O (g)	Ener (kcal)	Prot (g)	Carb (g)	Dietary Fiber (g)	Fat (g)	Fat Breakdown (g) Sat	Mono	Poly
	MIXED FOODS, SOUPS, SANDWICHES—Continued												
28566	Old country pasta	1	cup(s)	228	164	135	6	20	3	3	1.17	1.60	0.63
725	Onion, dehydrated, prepared w/water	1	cup(s)	246	237	27	1	5	1	1	0.12	0.32	0.07
16667	Shrimp gumbo	1	cup(s)	244	206	171	10	19	3	7	1.34	3.02	2.05
28037	Southwestern corn chowder	1	cup(s)	229	202	102	5	18	2	<1	0.12	0.12	0.20
25140	Split pea	1	cup(s)	165	117	85	4	19	2	<1	0.07	0.03	0.18
718	Split pea with ham, condensed, prepared w/water	1	cup(s)	253	207	190	10	28	2	4	1.77	1.80	0.63
710	Tomato, condensed, prepared w/milk	1	cup(s)	248	210	161	6	22	3	6	2.90	1.61	1.12
719	Tomato, condensed, prepared w/water	1	cup(s)	244	220	85	2	17	<1	2	0.37	0.44	0.95
726	Tomato vegetable, dehydrated, prepared w/water	1	cup(s)	253	237	56	2	10	1	1	0.38	0.30	0.08
28595	Turkey noodle	1	cup(s)	228	203	106	8	14	2	2	0.27	1.06	0.67
28051	Turkey vegetable	1	cup(s)	227	203	98	11	8	2	1	0.32	0.17	0.30
720	Vegetable beef, condensed, prepared w/water	1	cup(s)	244	224	78	6	10	<1	2	0.85	0.81	0.12
28598	Vegetable gumbo	1	cup(s)	229	168	153	4	26	3	4	0.61	2.93	0.56
25141	Vegetable	1	cup(s)	252	225	96	5	20	4	—	0.06	0.04	0.16
721	Vegetarian vegetable, condensed, prepared w/water	1	cup(s)	241	223	72	2	12	—	2	0.29	0.82	0.72
	FAST FOOD												
	Arby's												
36094	Au jus sauce	1	serving(s)	85	—	5	<1	1	<.1	<.1	0.02	—	—
751	Beef 'n cheddar sandwich	1	item(s)	198	—	480	23	43	2	24	8.00	—	—
9279	Cheddar curly fries	1	serving(s)	170	—	460	6	54	4	24	6.00	—	—
36131	Chocolate shake	1	serving(s)	397	—	480	10	84	0	16	8.00	—	—
36045	Curly fries, large	1	serving(s)	198	—	620	8	78	7	30	7.00	—	—
36044	Curly fries, medium	1	serving(s)	128	—	400	5	50	4	20	5.00	—	—
9265	Fish fillet sandwich	1	item(s)	220	—	529	23	50	2	27	7.00	9.20	10.60
752	Ham 'n cheese sandwich	1	item(s)	170	—	340	23	35	1	13	4.50	—	—
36048	Homestyle fries, large	1	serving(s)	213	—	560	6	79	6	24	6.00	—	—
36047	Homestyle fries, medium	1	serving(s)	142	—	370	4	53	4	16	4.00	—	—
33465	Homestyle fries, small	1	serving(s)	113	—	300	3	42	3	13	3.50	—	—
9267	Italian sub sandwich	1	item(s)	312	—	780	29	49	3	53	15.00	—	—
36041	Market Fresh grilled chicken caesar salad w/o dressing	1	serving(s)	338	—	230	33	8	3	8	3.50	—	—
9291	Roast beef deluxe sandwich, light	1	item(s)	182	—	296	18	33	6	10	3.00	5.00	2.00
9251	Roast beef sandwich, giant	1	item(s)	228	—	480	32	41	3	23	10.00	—	—
9249	Roast beef sandwich, junior	1	item(s)	129	—	310	16	34	2	13	4.50	—	—
750	Roast beef sandwich, regular	1	item(s)	157	—	350	21	34	2	16	6.00	—	—
2009	Roast beef sandwich, super	1	item(s)	245	—	470	22	47	3	23	7.00	—	—
9269	Roast beef sub sandwich	1	item(s)	334	—	760	35	47	3	48	16.00	—	—
9295	Roast chicken deluxe sandwich, light	1	item(s)	194	—	260	23	33	3	5	1.00	—	—
9293	Roast turkey deluxe sandwich, light	1	item(s)	194	—	260	23	33	3	5	0.50	—	—
36132	Strawberry shake	1	serving(s)	397	—	500	11	87	0	13	8.00	—	—
9273	Turkey sub sandwich	1	item(s)	306	—	630	26	51	2	37	9.00	—	—
36130	Vanilla shake	1	serving(s)	397	—	470	10	83	0	15	7.00	—	—
	Auntie Anne's												
35371	Cheese dipping sauce	1	serving(s)	35	—	100	3	4	0	8	4.00	—	—
35353	Cinnamon sugar soft pretzel	1	item(s)	120	—	350	9	74	2	2	0.00	—	—
35354	Cinnamon sugar soft pretzel w/butter	1	item(s)	120	—	450	8	83	3	9	5.00	—	—
35372	Marinara dipping sauce	1	serving(s)	35	—	10	0	4	0	0	0.00	0.00	0.00
35357	Original soft pretzel	1	item(s)	120	—	340	10	72	3	1	0.00	—	—
35358	Original soft pretzel w/butter	1	item(s)	120	—	370	10	72	3	4	2.00	—	—
35359	Parmesan herb soft pretzel	1	item(s)	120	—	390	11	74	4	5	2.50	—	—
35360	Parmesan herb soft pretzel w/butter	1	item(s)	120	—	440	10	72	9	13	7.00	—	—
35361	Sesame soft pretzel	1	item(s)	120	—	350	11	63	3	6	1.00	—	—
35362	Sesame soft pretzel w/butter	1	item(s)	120	—	410	12	64	7	12	4.00	—	—
35364	Sour cream & onion soft pretzel	1	item(s)	120	—	310	9	66	2	1	0.00	—	—
35366	Sour cream & onion soft pretzel w/butter	1	item(s)	120	—	340	9	66	2	5	3.00	—	—
35373	Sweet mustard dipping sauce	1	serving(s)	35	—	60	1	8	0	2	1.00	—	—

PAGE KEY: H–2 = Breads/Baked Goods H–6 = Cereal/Rice/Pasta H–10 = Fruit H–16 = Vegetables/Legumes H–26 = Nuts/Seeds H–28 = Vegetarian H–30 = Dairy H–36 = Eggs H–38 = Seafood H–40 = Meats H–42 = Poultry H–44 = Processed meats H–46 = Beverages H–50 = Fats/Oils H–52 = Sweets H–52 = Sauces/Condiments/Spices H–56 = Mixed Foods/Soups/Sandwiches H–62 = Fast food H–80 = Convenience H–82 = Baby foods

Chol (mg)	Calc (mg)	Iron (mg)	Magn (mg)	Pota (mg)	Sodi (mg)	Zinc (mg)	Vit A (RAE) (µg)	Thia (mg)	Vit E (mg)	Ribo (mg)	Niac (mg)	Vit B_6 (mg)	Fola (µg)	Vit C (mg)	Vit B_{12} (µg)	Sele (µg)
6	51	2.32	47	434	319	0.69	114	0.20	0.85	0.15	2.42	0.23	65	17	<.1	9
0	12	0.15	5	64	849	0.05	0	0.03	0.10	0.06	0.48	0.00	2	<1	0	2
51	99	2.34	51	515	515	0.93	—	0.19	2.38	0.10	2.54	0.19	59	26	<1	—
1	65	1.10	24	374	200	0.73	46	0.08	0.20	0.14	1.65	0.22	27	37	<1	2
0	30	1.25	33	352	608	0.57	112	0.12	0.13	0.09	1.67	0.21	61	9	0	<1
8	23	2.28	48	400	1007	1.32	23	0.15	—	0.08	1.47	0.07	3	2	<1	8
17	159	1.81	22	449	744	0.30	64	0.13	2.60	0.25	1.52	0.16	17	68	<1	2
0	12	1.76	7	264	695	0.24	29	0.09	2.49	0.05	1.42	0.11	15	66	0	<1
0	8	0.63	20	104	1146	0.18	10	0.06	0.81	0.05	0.79	0.05	10	6	0	5
24	27	1.40	22	200	372	0.67	81	0.20	0.54	0.11	2.68	0.15	45	5	<1	13
20	36	1.30	22	383	328	0.90	110	0.08	0.19	0.09	3.33	0.27	21	10	<1	9
5	17	1.12	5	173	791	1.54	95	0.04	0.32	0.05	1.03	0.08	10	2	<1	4
0	52	1.90	35	313	471	0.56	15	0.17	1.13	0.07	1.59	0.16	51	18	0	4
0	41	2.45	38	688	674	0.78	118	0.12	2.32	0.13	2.37	0.27	33	23	0	5
0	22	1.08	7	210	822	0.46	116	0.05	0.80	0.05	0.92	0.06	10	1	0	4
0	0	0.00	—	—	386	—	0	—	—	—	—	—	—	0	—	—
90	100	3.60	—	—	1240	—	0	—	0.41	—	—	—	—	1	—	—
5	60	1.80	—	—	1290	—	0	—	—	—	—	—	—	15	—	—
45	500	0.72	—	—	370	—	38	—	—	—	—	—	—	2	—	—
0	0	2.70	—	—	1540	—	0	—	—	—	—	—	—	21	—	—
0	0	1.80	—	—	990	—	0	—	—	—	—	—	—	15	—	—
43	90	3.78	—	450	864	—	10	0.35	—	0.31	5.60	—	—	1	—	—
90	150	2.70	—	—	1450	—	20	—	—	—	—	—	—	1	—	—
0	0	1.80	—	—	1070	—	0	—	—	—	—	—	—	30	—	—
0	0	1.08	—	—	710	—	0	—	—	—	—	—	—	21	—	—
0	0	0.72	—	—	570	—	0	—	—	—	—	—	—	15	—	—
120	250	2.70	—	—	2440	—	—	—	—	—	—	—	—	2	—	—
80	200	1.80	—	—	920	—	—	—	—	—	—	—	—	42	—	—
42	130	4.50	—	392	826	—	40	0.27	—	0.49	8.40	—	—	8	—	—
110	60	5.40	—	—	1440	—	0	—	—	—	—	—	—	0	—	—
70	60	2.70	—	—	740	—	0	—	—	—	—	—	—	0	—	—
85	60	3.60	—	—	950	—	0	—	—	—	—	—	—	0	—	—
85	80	3.60	—	—	1130	—	40	—	—	—	—	—	—	1	—	—
130	300	4.50	—	—	2230	—	40	—	—	—	—	—	—	4	—	—
40	100	2.70	—	—	1010	—	—	—	—	—	—	—	—	2	—	—
40	80	1.80	—	—	980	—	—	—	—	—	—	—	—	1	—	—
15	350	0.36	—	—	340	—	36	—	—	—	—	—	—	1	—	—
100	200	0.36	—	—	2170	—	—	—	—	—	—	—	—	2	—	—
45	500	1.08	—	—	360	—	39	—	—	—	—	—	—	2	—	—
10	100	0.00	—	—	510	—	—	—	—	—	—	—	—	0	—	—
0	20	1.98	—	—	410	—	0	—	—	—	—	—	—	0	—	—
25	30	2.34	—	—	430	—	—	—	—	—	—	—	—	0	—	—
0	0	0.00	—	—	180	—	0	—	—	—	—	—	—	0	—	—
0	30	2.34	—	—	900	—	0	—	—	—	—	—	—	0	—	—
10	30	2.16	—	—	930	—	—	—	—	—	—	—	—	0	—	—
10	80	1.80	—	—	780	—	—	—	—	—	—	—	—	1	—	—
30	60	1.80	—	—	660	—	—	—	—	—	—	—	—	1	—	—
0	20	2.88	—	—	840	—	0	—	—	—	—	—	—	0	—	—
15	20	2.70	—	—	860	—	—	—	—	—	—	—	—	0	—	—
0	30	1.98	—	—	920	—	—	—	—	—	—	—	—	0	—	—
10	40	2.16	—	—	930	—	—	—	—	—	—	—	—	0	—	—
40	0	0.00	—	—	120	—	0	—	—	—	—	—	—	0	—	—

Table H–1

Food Composition (Computer code number is for Wadsworth Diet Analysis program) (For purposes of calculations, use "0" for t, <1, <.1, <.01, etc.)

DA + Code	Food Description	Quantity	Measure	Wt (g)	H_2O (g)	Ener (kcal)	Prot (g)	Carb (g)	Dietary Fiber (g)	Fat (g)	Fat Breakdown (g) Sat	Mono	Poly
	FAST FOOD—Continued												
35367	Whole wheat soft pretzel	1	item(s)	120	—	350	11	72	7	2	0.00	—	—
35368	Whole wheat soft pretzel w/butter	1	item(s)	120	—	370	11	72	7	5	1.50	—	—
	Boston Market												
34975	Bbq baked beans	¾	cup(s)	201	—	270	8	48	12	5	2.00	—	—
34976	Black beans & rice	1	cup(s)	227	—	300	8	45	5	10	1.50	—	—
34978	Butternut squash	¾	cup(s)	193	—	150	2	25	6	6	4.00	—	—
35006	Caesar side salad	1	serving(s)	119	—	300	5	13	1	26	4.50	—	—
34979	Chicken gravy	1	ounce(s)	28	—	15	0	2	0	1	0.00	—	—
34973	Chicken pot pie	1	item(s)	425	—	750	26	57	2	46	14.00	—	—
35007	Cole slaw	¾	cup(s)	184	—	300	2	30	3	19	3.00	—	—
35057	Cornbread	1	item(s)	68	—	200	3	33	1	6	1.50	—	—
35008	Cranberry walnut relish	¾	cup(s)	210	—	350	3	75	3	5	0.00	—	—
34980	Creamed spinach	¾	cup(s)	181	—	260	9	11	2	20	13.00	—	—
34981	Glazed carrots	¾	cup(s)	153	—	280	1	35	4	15	3.00	—	—
34983	Green bean casserole	¾	cup(s)	170	—	80	1	9	2	5	1.50	—	—
34982	Green beans	¾	cup(s)	85	—	70	1	6	2	4	0.50	—	—
34967	Half chicken, w/skin	1	item(s)	277	—	590	70	4	0	33	10.00	—	—
34984	Homestyle mashed potatoes	¾	cup(s)	173	—	210	4	30	2	9	5.00	—	—
34985	Homestyle mashed potatoes & gravy	1	cup(s)	201	—	230	4	32	3	9	5.00	—	—
34969	Honey glazed ham	5	ounce(s)	142	—	210	24	10	0	8	3.00	—	—
34988	Hot cinnamon apples	¾	cup(s)	181	—	250	0	56	3	5	0.50	—	—
34989	Macaroni & cheese	¾	cup(s)	192	—	280	13	33	1	11	6.00	—	—
34970	Meatloaf	5	ounce(s)	142	—	282	20	15	1	17	7.28	—	—
35012	Old-fashioned potato salad	¾	cup(s)	150	—	200	3	22	2	12	2.00	—	—
34965	Quarter chicken, dark meat, no skin	1	item(s)	95	—	190	22	1	0	10	3.00	—	—
34966	Quarter chicken, dark meat, w/skin	1	item(s)	125	—	320	30	2	0	21	6.00	—	—
34963	Quarter chicken, white meat, no skin or wing	1	item(s)	140	—	170	33	2	0	4	1.00	—	—
34964	Quarter chicken, white meat, w/skin & wing	1	item(s)	152	—	280	40	2	0	12	3.50	—	—
34993	Rice pilaf	1	cup(s)	137	—	140	2	24	1	4	0.50	—	—
34968	Rotisserie turkey breast, skinless	5	ounce(s)	142	—	170	36	3	0	1	0.00	—	—
34998	Savory stuffing	1	cup(s)	132	—	190	4	27	2	8	1.50	—	—
34999	Squash casserole	¾	cup(s)	187	—	330	7	20	3	24	13.00	—	—
35003	Steamed vegetables	1	cup(s)	102	—	30	2	6	2	0	0.00	—	—
35004	Sweet potato casserole	¾	cup(s)	181	—	280	3	39	2	13	4.50	—	—
35005	Whole kernel corn	¾	cup(s)	146	—	180	5	30	2	4	0.50	—	—
	Burger King												
29731	Biscuit with sausage, egg, & cheese	1	item(s)	189	—	650	20	38	1	46	14.00	—	—
3739	BK Broiler chicken sandwich	1	item(s)	258	—	550	30	52	3	25	5.00	—	—
14249	Cheeseburger	1	item(s)	133	—	360	19	31	2	17	8.00	—	—
14251	Chicken sandwich	1	item(s)	224	—	660	25	53	3	39	8.00	—	—
3808	Chicken Tenders, 8 pieces	1	serving(s)	123	—	340	22	20	1	19	5.00	—	—
14259	Chocolate shake, small	1	item(s)	333	—	620	12	72	2	32	21.00	—	—
29732	Croissanwich w/sausage & cheese	1	item(s)	107	—	420	14	23	1	31	11.00	—	—
14261	Croissanwich w/sausage, egg, & cheese	1	item(s)	157	—	520	19	24	1	39	14.00	—	—
3809	Double cheeseburger	1	item(s)	189	—	540	32	32	2	31	15.00	—	—
14244	Double Whopper	1	item(s)	374	—	980	52	52	4	62	22.00	—	—
14245	Double Whopper w/cheese	1	item(s)	399	—	1070	57	53	4	70	27.00	—	—
14250	Fish Fillet sandwich	1	item(s)	185	—	520	18	44	2	30	8.00	—	—
14255	French fries, medium, salted	1	item(s)	117	—	360	4	46	4	18	5.00	—	—
14262	French toast sticks	1	serving(s)	112	—	390	6	46	2	20	4.50	—	—
14248	Hamburger	1	item(s)	121	—	310	17	31	2	13	5.00	—	—
14263	Hash brown rounds, small	1	serving(s)	75	—	230	2	23	2	15	4.00	—	—
14256	Onion rings, medium	1	serving(s)	91	—	320	4	40	3	16	4.00	—	—
39000	Tendercrisp chicken sandwich	1	item(s)	310	—	810	28	72	6	47	8.00	—	—
14258	Vanilla shake, small	1	item(s)	305	—	560	11	56	1	32	21.00	—	—
1736	Whopper	1	item(s)	291	—	710	31	52	4	43	13.00	—	—
14243	Whopper w/cheese	1	item(s)	316	—	800	36	53	4	50	18.00	—	—
	Carl's Jr												
10801	Carl's Catch fish sandwich	1	item(s)	201	—	530	18	55	2	28	7.00	—	1.89

PAGE KEY: H–2 = Breads/Baked Goods H–6 = Cereal/Rice/Pasta H–10 = Fruit H–16 = Vegetables/Legumes H–26 = Nuts/Seeds H–28 = Vegetarian H–30 = Dairy H–36 = Eggs H–38 = Seafood H–40 = Meats H–42 = Poultry H–44 = Processed meats H–46 = Beverages H–50 = Fats/Oils H–52 = Sweets H–52 = Sauces/Condiments/Spices H–56 = Mixed Foods/Soups/Sandwiches H–62 = Fast food H–80 = Convenience H–82 = Baby foods

Chol (mg)	Calc (mg)	Iron (mg)	Magn (mg)	Pota (mg)	Sodi (mg)	Zinc (mg)	Vit A (RAE) (µg)	Thia (mg)	Vit E (mg)	Ribo (mg)	Niac (mg)	Vit B_6 (mg)	Fola (µg)	Vit C (mg)	Vit B_{12} (µg)	Sele (µg)
0	30	1.98	—	—	1100	—	0	—	—	—	—	—	—	0	—	—
10	30	2.34	—	—	1120	—	—	—	—	—	—	—	—	0	—	—
0	100	3.60	—	—	540	—	42	—	—	—	—	—	—	6	—	—
0	40	1.80	—	—	1050	—	0	—	—	—	—	—	—	4	—	—
20	80	1.08	—	—	560	—	1150	—	—	—	—	—	—	30	—	—
15	100	0.72	—	—	690	—	—	—	—	—	—	—	—	9	—	—
0	0	0.00	—	—	180	—	0	—	—	—	—	—	—	0	—	—
110	40	4.50	—	—	1530	—	—	—	—	—	—	—	—	1	—	—
20	60	0.72	—	—	540	—	108	—	—	—	—	—	—	36	—	—
25	0	1.08	—	—	390	—	0	—	—	—	—	—	—	0	—	—
0	0	5.40	—	—	0	—	0	—	—	—	—	—	—	0	—	—
55	250	2.70	—	—	740	—	—	—	—	—	—	—	—	9	—	—
0	40	1.08	—	—	80	—	1000	—	—	—	—	—	—	1	—	—
5	20	0.72	—	—	670	—	—	—	—	—	—	—	—	2	—	—
0	40	0.36	—	—	250	—	30	—	—	—	—	—	—	5	—	—
290	0	2.70	—	—	1010	—	0	—	—	—	—	—	—	0	—	—
25	40	0.36	—	—	590	—	53	—	—	—	—	—	—	15	—	—
25	60	0.36	—	—	780	—	—	—	—	—	—	—	—	15	—	—
75	0	1.08	—	—	1460	—	0	—	—	—	—	—	—	0	—	—
0	20	0.36	—	—	45	—	—	—	—	—	—	—	—	0	—	—
30	300	1.44	—	—	890	—	—	—	—	—	—	—	—	0	—	—
68	91	2.46	—	—	592	—	—	—	—	—	—	—	—	1	—	—
15	60	1.08	—	—	450	—	0	—	—	—	—	—	—	6	—	—
115	0	1.08	—	—	440	—	0	—	—	—	—	—	—	0	—	—
155	0	1.80	—	—	500	—	0	—	—	—	—	—	—	0	—	—
85	0	0.72	—	—	480	—	0	—	—	—	—	—	—	0	—	—
135	0	1.08	—	—	510	—	0	—	—	—	—	—	—	0	—	—
0	20	1.08	—	—	520	—	—	—	—	—	—	—	—	4	—	—
100	20	1.80	—	—	850	—	0	—	—	—	—	—	—	0	—	—
5	40	1.44	—	—	620	—	—	—	—	—	—	—	—	2	—	—
70	200	0.72	—	—	1110	—	—	—	—	—	—	—	—	5	—	—
0	40	0.35	—	—	135	—	389	—	—	—	—	—	—	18	—	—
10	40	1.08	—	—	190	—	—	—	—	—	—	—	—	9	—	—
0	0	0.36	—	—	170	—	20	—	—	—	—	—	—	5	—	—
190	150	2.70	—	—	1600	—	90	—	—	—	—	—	—	0	—	—
105	60	3.60	—	—	1110	—	—	0.46	3.81	0.23	10.50	—	—	6	—	—
50	150	3.60	—	—	790	—	63	0.25	—	0.32	4.18	—	—	1	—	—
70	80	2.70	—	—	1330	—	—	0.47	—	0.30	9.59	—	—	0	—	—
50	20	0.72	—	—	840	—	—	0.14	0.41	0.12	10.93	—	—	0	—	—
95	350	1.08	—	—	310	—	42	0.11	—	0.56	0.24	—	—	0	—	—
45	100	3.60	—	—	840	—	—	—	—	—	—	—	—	0	—	—
210	300	4.50	—	—	1090	—	140	0.36	—	0.42	4.35	—	—	0	—	—
100	250	4.50	—	—	1050	—	100	0.26	1.89	0.45	6.37	—	—	1	—	—
160	150	9.00	—	—	1070	—	—	0.40	—	0.60	11.08	—	—	9	—	—
185	300	9.00	—	—	1500	—	—	0.40	—	0.67	11.07	—	—	9	—	—
55	150	2.70	—	—	840	—	14	—	—	—	—	—	—	1	—	—
0	20	0.72	—	—	640	—	0	0.16	—	0.48	2.32	—	—	9	—	—
0	60	1.80	—	—	440	—	0	0.19	—	0.22	2.86	—	—	0	—	—
40	76	3.60	—	—	580	—	9	0.25	—	0.29	4.26	—	—	1	—	—
0	0	0.36	—	—	450	—	0	0.11	—	0.07	2.11	—	—	1	—	—
0	97	0.00	—	—	460	—	0	0.14	—	0.09	2.33	—	—	0	—	—
60	80	4.50	—	—	1800	—	—	—	—	—	—	—	—	9	—	—
95	300	0.36	—	—	220	—	39	0.11	—	0.64	0.22	—	—	0	—	—
85	150	6.30	—	—	980	—	52	0.39	4.25	0.44	7.33	—	—	9	—	—
110	250	6.30	—	—	1420	—	157	0.39	—	0.51	7.31	—	—	9	—	—
80	150	1.80	—	—	1030	—	60	—	—	—	—	—	—	2	—	—

H Appendix

Table H–1

Food Composition (Computer code number is for Wadsworth Diet Analysis program) (For purposes of calculations, use "0" for t, <1, <.1, <.01, etc.)

DA + Code	Food Description	Quantity	Measure	Wt (g)	H_2O (g)	Ener (kcal)	Prot (g)	Carb (g)	Dietary Fiber (g)	Fat (g)	Fat Breakdown (g) Sat	Mono	Poly
	FAST FOOD—Continued												
10862	Carl's Famous Star hamburger	1	item(s)	254	—	590	24	50	3	32	9.00	—	—
10866	Charboiled chicken salad-to-go	1	item(s)	350	—	200	25	12	4	7	3.00	—	1.02
10855	Charboiled Sante Fe chicken sandwich	1	item(s)	220	—	540	28	37	2	31	8.00	—	—
10790	Chicken stars (6 pieces)	6	item(s)	90	—	260	13	14	1	16	4.50	—	1.71
34864	Chocolate shake, small	1	item(s)	595	—	530	14	96	0	10	7.00	—	—
10797	Crisscut fries	1	serving(s)	139	—	410	5	43	4	24	5.00	—	—
10799	Double western bacon cheeseburger	1	item(s)	308	—	920	51	65	3	50	21.00	—	6.55
34855	Famous bacon cheeseburger	1	item(s)	279	—	700	31	51	3	41	13.00	—	—
14238	French fries, small	1	serving(s)	92	—	290	5	37	3	14	3.00	—	—
10798	French toast dips w/o syrup	1	serving(s)	105	—	370	6	42	1	20	2.50	—	1.35
34856	Hamburger	1	item(s)	119	—	280	14	36	1	9	3.50	—	—
10802	Onion rings	1	serving(s)	127	—	430	7	53	3	22	5.00	—	0.84
38925	Six Dollar burger	1	item(s)	539	—	1000	39	72	6	82	25.00	—	—
34858	Spicy chicken sandwich	1	item(s)	198	—	480	14	47	2	26	5.00	—	—
34867	Strawberry shake, small	1	item(s)	595	—	510	14	91	0	10	7.00	—	—
10865	Super Star hamburger	1	item(s)	345	—	790	41	51	3	47	15.00	—	—
10818	Vanilla shake, small	1	item(s)	595	—	470	15	78	0	11	7.00	—	—
10770	Western bacon cheeseburger	1	item(s)	225	—	660	31	64	3	30	12.00	—	4.85
	Chick Fil-A												
38746	Biscuit w/bacon, egg, & cheese	1	item(s)	155	—	430	16	38	1	24	9.00	—	—
38747	Biscuit w/egg	1	item(s)	135	—	340	11	38	1	16	4.50	—	—
38748	Biscuit w/egg & cheese	1	item(s)	148	—	390	13	38	1	21	7.00	—	—
38753	Biscuit w/gravy	1	item(s)	191	—	310	5	44	1	13	3.50	—	—
38752	Biscuit w/sausage, egg, & cheese	1	item(s)	189	—	540	18	43	1	33	13.00	—	—
38741	Biscuit, plain	1	item(s)	78	—	260	4	38	1	11	2.50	—	—
38771	Carrot & raisin salad	1	item(s)	91	—	130	1	22	2	5	1.00	—	—
38761	Chargrilled chicken cool wrap	1	item(s)	245	—	380	29	54	3	6	3.00	—	—
38766	Chargrilled chicken garden salad	1	item(s)	275	—	180	22	9	3	6	3.00	—	—
38758	Chargrilled chicken sandwich	1	item(s)	157	—	280	26	30	1	7	1.50	—	—
38759	Chargrilled deluxe chicken sandwich	1	item(s)	195	—	290	27	31	2	7	1.50	—	—
38742	Chicken biscuit	1	item(s)	137	—	400	16	43	2	18	4.50	—	—
38743	Chicken biscuit w/cheese	1	item(s)	151	—	450	19	43	2	23	7.00	—	—
38762	Chicken caesar wrap	1	item(s)	227	—	460	36	52	2	10	6.00	—	—
38757	Chicken deluxe sandwich	1	item(s)	208	—	420	28	39	2	16	3.50	—	—
38764	Chicken salad sandwich	1	item(s)	153	—	350	20	32	5	15	3.00	—	—
38756	Chicken sandwich	1	item(s)	170	—	410	28	38	1	15	3.50	—	—
38768	Chick-n-Strip salad	1	item(s)	331	—	390	34	22	4	18	5.00	—	—
38763	Chick-n-Strips	4	item(s)	127	—	290	29	14	1	13	2.50	—	—
38770	Coleslaw	1	item(s)	105	—	210	1	14	2	17	2.50	—	—
38755	Hash browns	1	serving(s)	84	—	170	2	20	2	9	4.50	—	—
38765	Hearty breast of soup	1	cup(s)	241	—	140	8	18	1	4	1.00	—	—
38778	Icedream, small cone	1	item(s)	135	—	160	4	28	0	4	2.00	—	—
38774	Icedream, small cup	1	serving(s)	213	—	230	5	38	0	6	3.50	—	—
38775	Lemonade	1	cup(s)	255	—	170	0	41	0	1	0.00	—	—
38776	Lemonade, diet	1	cup(s)	255	—	25	0	5	0	0	0.00	0.00	0.00
38777	Nuggets	8	item(s)	113	—	260	26	12	1	12	2.50	—	—
38769	Side salad	1	item(s)	108	—	60	3	4	2	3	1.50	—	—
38767	Southwest chargrilled salad	1	item(s)	303	—	240	22	17	5	8	3.50	—	—
38772	Waffle potato fries, small, salted	1	serving(s)	85	—	280	3	37	5	14	5.00	—	—
	Cinnabon												
39569	Caramel Pecanbon	1	item(s)	272	—	1100	16	141	8	56	10.00	—	—
39572	Caramellata Chill w/whipped cream	16	fluid ounce(s)	480	—	406	10	61	0	14	8.00	—	—
39571	Cinnapoppers	1	serving(s)	74	—	368	4	41	2	21	11.00	—	—
39567	Classic roll	1	item(s)	221	—	813	15	117	4	32	8.00	—	—
39568	Minibon	1	item(s)	92	—	339	6	49	2	13	3.00	—	—
39573	Mochalatta chill w/whipped cream	16	fluid ounce(s)	480	—	362	9	55	0	13	8.00	—	—
39570	Stix	5	item(s)	85	—	379	6	41	1	21	6.00	—	—
	Dairy Queen												
1466	Banana split	1	item(s)	369	—	510	8	96	3	12	8.00	3.00	0.50
38552	Brownie Earthquake	1	serving(s)	304	—	740	10	112	0	27	16.00	—	—

PAGE KEY: H–2 = Breads/Baked Goods H–6 = Cereal/Rice/Pasta H–10 = Fruit H–16 = Vegetables/Legumes H–26 = Nuts/Seeds H–28 = Vegetarian H–30 = Dairy H–36 = Eggs H–38 = Seafood H–40 = Meats H–42 = Poultry H–44 = Processed meats H–46 = Beverages H–50 = Fats/Oils H–52 = Sweets H–52 = Sauces/Condiments/Spices H–56 = Mixed Foods/Soups/Sandwiches H–62 = Fast food H–80 = Convenience H–82 = Baby foods

Chol (mg)	Calc (mg)	Iron (mg)	Magn (mg)	Pota (mg)	Sodi (mg)	Zinc (mg)	Vit A (RAE) (µg)	Thia (mg)	Vit E (mg)	Ribo (mg)	Niac (mg)	Vit B_6 (mg)	Fola (µg)	Vit C (mg)	Vit B_{12} (µg)	Sele (µg)
70	100	4.50	—	—	910	—	—	—	—	—	—	—	—	6	—	—
75	150	1.80	—	—	440	—	—	—	—	—	—	—	—	5	—	—
95	200	2.70	—	—	1210	—	—	—	—	—	—	—	—	6	—	—
40	20	1.08	—	—	480	—	0	—	—	—	—	—	—	0	—	—
45	600	1.08	—	—	350	—	0	—	—	—	—	—	—	0	—	—
0	20	1.80	—	—	950	—	0	—	—	—	—	—	—	12	—	—
155	300	7.20	—	—	1770	—	—	—	—	—	—	—	—	1	—	—
95	200	5.40	—	—	1310	—	102	—	—	—	—	—	—	6	—	—
0	0	1.08	—	—	180	—	0	—	—	—	—	—	—	21	—	—
0	40	1.08	—	—	430	—	0	0.26	—	0.24	2.00	—	—	0	—	—
35	80	2.70	—	—	480	—	0	—	—	—	—	—	—	1	—	—
0	20	0.72	—	—	700	—	0	—	—	—	—	—	—	4	—	—
135	350	5.40	—	—	1690	—	—	—	—	—	—	—	—	21	—	—
40	100	2.70	—	—	1220	—	—	—	—	—	—	—	—	6	—	—
45	600	0.00	—	—	330	—	0	—	—	—	—	—	—	0	—	—
130	100	7.20	—	—	980	—	—	—	—	—	—	—	—	9	—	—
50	600	0.00	—	—	350	—	0	—	—	—	—	—	—	0	—	—
85	200	5.40	—	—	1410	—	40	—	—	—	—	—	—	1	—	—
265	150	3.60	—	—	1070	—	—	—	—	—	—	—	—	0	—	—
245	80	2.70	—	—	740	—	—	—	—	—	—	—	—	0	—	—
260	150	2.70	—	—	960	—	—	—	—	—	—	—	—	0	—	—
5	60	1.80	—	—	930	—	0	—	—	—	—	—	—	0	—	—
280	150	3.60	—	—	1030	—	—	—	—	—	—	—	—	0	—	—
0	60	1.80	—	—	670	—	0	—	—	—	—	—	—	0	—	—
0	20	0.36	—	—	90	—	—	—	—	—	—	—	—	4	—	—
70	200	2.70	—	—	1060	—	—	—	—	—	—	—	—	6	—	—
70	150	0.72	—	—	660	—	—	—	—	—	—	—	—	30	—	—
70	80	1.80	—	—	980	—	0	—	—	—	—	—	—	2	—	—
70	80	1.80	—	—	990	—	—	—	—	—	—	—	—	5	—	—
30	60	2.70	—	—	1200	—	0	—	—	—	—	—	—	0	—	—
45	150	2.70	—	—	1430	—	—	—	—	—	—	—	—	0	—	—
80	500	2.70	—	—	1390	—	—	—	—	—	—	—	—	1	—	—
60	100	2.70	—	—	1300	—	—	—	—	—	—	—	—	2	—	—
65	150	1.80	—	—	880	—	—	—	—	—	—	—	—	0	—	—
60	100	2.70	—	—	1300	—	—	—	—	—	—	—	—	0	—	—
80	200	0.36	—	—	860	—	—	—	—	—	—	—	—	30	—	—
65	20	0.36	—	—	730	—	—	—	—	—	—	—	—	1	—	—
20	40	0.36	—	—	180	—	—	—	—	—	—	—	—	27	—	—
10	0	0.72	—	—	350	—	—	—	—	—	—	—	—	0	—	—
25	40	1.08	—	—	900	—	—	—	—	—	—	—	—	0	—	—
15	100	0.36	—	—	80	—	—	—	—	—	—	—	—	0	—	—
25	150	0.00	—	—	100	—	—	—	—	—	—	—	—	0	—	—
0	0	0.36	—	—	10	—	0	—	—	—	—	—	—	15	—	—
0	0	0.36	—	—	5	—	0	—	—	—	—	—	—	15	—	—
70	40	1.08	—	—	1090	—	0	—	—	—	—	—	—	0	—	—
10	100	0.00	—	—	75	—	—	—	—	—	—	—	—	15	—	—
60	200	1.08	—	—	770	—	—	—	—	—	—	—	—	24	—	—
15	20	0.00	—	—	105	—	0	—	—	—	—	—	—	21	—	—
63	—	—	—	—	600	—	—	—	—	—	—	—	—	—	—	—
46	—	—	—	—	187	—	—	—	—	—	—	—	—	—	—	—
62	—	—	—	—	104	—	—	—	—	—	—	—	—	—	—	—
67	—	—	—	—	801	—	—	—	—	—	—	—	—	—	—	—
27	—	—	—	—	337	—	—	—	—	—	—	—	—	—	—	—
46	100	0.00	—	—	252	—	—	—	—	—	—	—	—	0	—	—
16	—	—	—	—	413	—	—	—	—	—	—	—	—	—	—	—
30	250	1.80	—	860	180	—	—	0.15	—	0.60	0.20	—	—	15	—	—
50	250	1.80	—	—	350	—	—	—	—	—	—	—	—	0	—	—

H Appendix

Table H–1

Food Composition (Computer code number is for Wadsworth Diet Analysis program) (For purposes of calculations, use "0" for t, <1, <.1, <.01, etc.)

DA + Code	Food Description	Quantity	Measure	Wt (g)	H_2O (g)	Ener (kcal)	Prot (g)	Carb (g)	Dietary Fiber (g)	Fat (g)	Fat Breakdown (g) Sat	Mono	Poly
	FAST FOOD—Continued												
38561	Chocolate chip cookie dough blizzard, small	1	item(s)	319	—	720	12	105	0	28	14.00	—	—
1464	Chocolate malt, small	1	item(s)	418	—	650	15	111	0	16	10.00	—	—
38541	Chocolate shake, small	1	item(s)	397	—	560	13	93	1	15	10.00	—	—
17257	Chocolate soft serve	½	cup(s)	94	—	150	4	22	0	5	3.50	—	—
1463	Chocolate sundae, small	1	item(s)	163	—	280	5	49	0	7	4.50	1.00	1.00
1462	Dipped cone, small	1	item(s)	156	—	340	6	42	1	17	9.00	4.00	3.00
38555	Oreo cookies blizzard, small	1	item(s)	283	—	570	11	83	1	21	10.00	—	—
38547	Royal Treats Peanut Buster parfait	1	item(s)	305	—	730	16	99	2	31	17.00	—	—
17256	Vanilla soft serve	½	cup(s)	94	—	140	3	22	0	5	3.00	—	—
	Domino's												
31606	Barbeque wings	1	item(s)	25	—	50	6	2	<1	2	0.65	—	—
31604	Breadsticks	1	item(s)	37	—	116	3	18	1	4	0.79	—	—
37551	Buffalo chicken kickers	1	item(s)	24	14	47	4	3	<1	2	0.39	—	—
37548	Cinnastix	1	item(s)	32	8	122	2	15	1	6	1.15	—	—
	Classic hand tossed pizza												
31573	America's favorite feast, 12"	2	slice(s)	205	99	508	22	57	4	22	9.20	—	—
31574	America's favorite feast, 14"	2	slice(s)	283	138	697	30	79	5	30	12.70	—	—
37543	Bacon cheeseburger feast, 12"	2	slice(s)	198	60	549	25	55	3	26	11.62	—	—
37545	Bacon cheeseburger feast, 14"	2	slice(s)	275	121	762	35	75	4	36	16.10	—	—
37546	Barbeque feast, 12"	2	slice(s)	192	85	506	22	62	3	20	9.08	—	—
37547	Barbeque feast, 14"	2	slice(s)	262	115	691	30	85	4	27	12.24	—	—
31569	Cheese, 12"	2	slice(s)	159	—	375	15	55	3	11	4.81	—	—
31570	Cheese, 14"	2	slice(s)	219	—	516	21	75	4	15	6.72	—	—
37538	Deluxe feast, 12"	2	slice(s)	201	102	465	20	57	3	18	7.66	—	—
37540	Deluxe feast, 14"	2	slice(s)	273	138	627	26	78	5	24	10.20	—	—
31685	Deluxe, 12"	2	slice(s)	213	—	465	20	57	3	18	7.65	—	—
31694	Deluxe, 14"	2	slice(s)	273	—	627	26	78	5	24	10.20	—	—
31686	Extravaganzza, 12"	2	slice(s)	245	127	576	27	59	4	27	11.56	—	—
31695	Extravaganzza, 14"	2	slice(s)	329	171	773	36	88	5	36	15.42	—	—
31575	Hawaiian feast, 12"	2	slice(s)	204	105	450	21	58	3	16	7.20	—	—
31576	Hawaiian feast, 14"	2	slice(s)	283	147	623	29	80	5	22	10.09	—	—
31687	Meatzza, 12"	2	slice(s)	213	—	560	26	57	3	26	11.40	—	—
31696	Meatzza, 14"	2	slice(s)	293	139	753	35	78	5	34	15.24	—	—
31571	Pepperoni feast, extra pepperoni & cheese, 12"	2	slice(s)	196	87	534	24	56	3	25	10.92	—	—
31572	Pepperoni feast, extra pepperoni & cheese, 14"	2	slice(s)	270	121	732	33	77	4	34	15.00	—	—
31577	Vegi feast, 12"	2	slice(s)	203	107	439	19	57	4	16	7.09	—	—
31578	Vegi feast, 14"	2	slice(s)	278	147	304	27	78	5	22	9.89	—	—
37549	Dot cinnamon	1	item(s)	28	8	99	2	15	1	4	0.68	—	—
31605	Double cheesy bread	1	item(s)	35	11	123	4	13	1	6	2.06	—	—
31607	Hot wings	1	item(s)	25	—	45	5	1	<1	2	0.65	—	—
	Thin crust pizza												
31583	America's favorite, 12"	¼	item(s)	159	—	408	19	34	2	23	9.77	—	—
31584	America's favorite, 14"	¼	item(s)	202	—	557	26	47	3	31	13.19	—	—
31579	Cheese, 12"	¼	item(s)	106	—	273	12	31	2	12	9.37	—	—
31580	Cheese, 14"	¼	item(s)	148	—	382	17	43	2	17	6.72	—	—
31688	Deluxe, 12"	¼	item(s)	159	—	363	16	34	2	19	7.64	—	—
31697	Deluxe, 14"	¼	item(s)	202	—	494	22	47	3	25	10.20	—	—
31689	Extravaganzza, 12"	¼	item(s)	159	—	425	20	34	3	24	9.41	—	—
31698	Extravaganzza, 14"	¼	item(s)	202	—	571	27	48	4	31	12.44	—	—
31585	Hawaiian, 12"	¼	item(s)	159	—	349	18	35	2	16	7.20	—	—
31586	Hawaiian, 14"	¼	item(s)	202	—	489	25	48	3	23	10.09	—	—
31690	Meatzza, 12"	¼	item(s)	159	—	458	23	33	2	27	11.39	—	—
31699	Meatzza, 14"	¼	item(s)	202	—	619	31	46	3	36	15.24	—	—
31581	Pepperoni, extra pepperoni & cheese 12"	¼	item(s)	159	—	420	20	32	2	24	10.46	—	—
31582	Pepperoni, extra pepperoni & cheese 14"	¼	item(s)	202	—	586	28	45	3	34	14.55	—	—
31587	Vegi, 12"	¼	item(s)	159	—	338	16	34	3	17	7.08	—	—
31588	Vegi, 14"	¼	item(s)	202	—	471	22	47	3	23	9.89	—	—

Appendix H

PAGE KEY: H–2 = Breads/Baked Goods H–6 = Cereal/Rice/Pasta H–10 = Fruit H–16 = Vegetables/Legumes H–26 = Nuts/Seeds H–28 = Vegetarian H–30 = Dairy H–36 = Eggs H–38 = Seafood H–40 = Meats H–42 = Poultry H–44 = Processed meats H–46 = Beverages H–50 = Fats/Oils H–52 = Sweets H–52 = Sauces/Condiments/Spices H–56 = Mixed Foods/Soups/Sandwiches H–62 = Fast food H–80 = Convenience H–82 = Baby foods

Chol (mg)	Calc (mg)	Iron (mg)	Magn (mg)	Pota (mg)	Sodi (mg)	Zinc (mg)	Vit A (RAE) (μg)	Thia (mg)	Vit E (mg)	Ribo (mg)	Niac (mg)	Vit B_6 (mg)	Fola (μg)	Vit C (mg)	Vit B_{12} (μg)	Sele (μg)
50	350	2.70	—	—	370	—	—	—	—	—	—	—	—	1	—	—
55	450	1.80	—	—	370	—	—	—	—	—	—	—	—	2	—	—
50	450	1.44	—	—	280	—	—	0.12	—	—	—	—	—	2	—	—
15	100	0.72	—	—	75	—	—	—	—	—	—	—	—	0	—	—
20	200	1.08	—	278	140	—	—	0.06	—	0.24	0.20	—	—	0	—	—
20	200	1.08	—	290	130	—	—	0.06	—	0.26	0.20	—	—	1	—	—
40	350	2.70	—	—	430	—	—	—	—	—	—	—	—	1	—	—
35	300	1.80	—	—	400	—	—	—	—	—	—	—	—	1	—	—
15	150	0.72	—	—	70	—	150	—	—	—	—	—	—	0	—	—
26	6	0.32	—	—	175	—	—	—	—	—	—	—	—	<.1	—	—
0	<.1	0.87	—	—	152	—	—	—	—	—	—	—	—	6	—	—
9	3	0.00	—	—	163	—	—	—	—	—	—	—	—	0	—	—
0	6	0.70	—	—	110	—	—	—	—	—	—	—	—	<.1	—	—
49	202	3.70	—	—	1221	—	—	—	—	—	—	—	—	1	—	—
68	281	5.10	—	—	1685	—	—	—	—	—	—	—	—	1	—	—
60	293	3.56	—	—	1274	—	—	—	—	—	—	—	—	0	—	—
84	395	4.96	—	—	1809	—	—	—	—	—	—	—	—	0	—	—
46	—	—	—	—	1206	—	—	—	—	—	—	—	—	—	—	—
63	393	4.42	—	—	1672	—	—	—	—	—	—	—	—	2	—	—
23	187	2.99	—	—	776	—	131	—	—	—	—	—	—	0	—	—
32	261	4.13	—	—	1080	—	184	—	—	—	—	—	—	0	—	—
40	199	3.56	—	—	1063	—	—	—	—	—	—	—	—	1	—	—
53	276	4.84	—	—	1432	—	—	—	—	—	—	—	—	2	—	—
40	199	3.56	—	—	1063	—	—	—	—	—	—	—	—	1	—	—
53	276	4.85	—	—	1432	—	—	—	—	—	—	—	—	2	—	—
60	290	4.08	—	—	1348	—	—	—	—	—	—	—	—	1	—	—
89	403	5.48	—	—	1780	—	—	—	—	—	—	—	—	2	—	—
41	274	3.30	—	—	1102	—	—	—	—	—	—	—	—	2	—	—
57	384	4.57	—	—	1544	—	—	—	—	—	—	—	—	3	—	—
344	282	3.71	—	—	1463	—	—	—	—	—	—	—	—	<1	—	—
85	393	5.04	—	—	1947	—	—	—	—	—	—	—	—	<1	—	—
57	279	3.36	—	—	1349	—	155	—	—	—	—	—	—	<1	—	—
78	390	4.66	—	—	1855	—	233	—	—	—	—	—	—	<1	—	—
34	279	3.44	—	—	987	—	—	—	—	—	—	—	—	1	—	—
47	389	4.71	—	—	1369	—	—	—	—	—	—	—	—	2	—	—
0	6	0.59	—	—	86	—	—	—	—	—	—	—	—	<.1	—	—
6	47	0.66	—	—	164	—	—	—	—	—	—	—	—	<1	—	—
26	5	0.30	—	—	354	—	—	—	—	—	—	—	—	1	—	—
51	318	1.52	—	—	1285	—	—	—	—	—	—	—	—	<1	—	—
69	444	2.07	—	—	1751	—	—	—	—	—	—	—	—	1	—	—
23	225	0.97	—	—	835	—	125	—	—	—	—	—	—	0	—	—
32	315	1.36	—	—	1172	—	175	—	—	—	—	—	—	0	—	—
40	237	1.54	—	—	1123	—	—	—	—	—	—	—	—	1	—	—
53	330	2.08	—	—	1523	—	—	—	—	—	—	—	—	2	—	—
53	245	1.95	—	—	1408	—	—	—	—	—	—	—	—	1	—	—
69	340	2.59	—	—	1871	—	—	—	—	—	—	—	—	2	—	—
41	312	1.28	—	—	1162	—	—	—	—	—	—	—	—	2	—	—
57	437	1.80	—	—	1635	—	—	—	—	—	—	—	—	3	—	—
64	320	1.69	—	—	1523	—	—	—	—	—	—	—	—	<1	—	—
454	446	2.27	—	—	2039	—	—	—	—	—	—	—	—	<1	—	—
54	316	1.34	—	—	1362	—	162	—	—	—	—	—	—	<1	—	—
76	442	1.87	—	—	1900	—	227	—	—	—	—	—	—	<1	—	—
34	317	1.42	—	—	1047	—	—	—	—	—	—	—	—	1	—	—
47	442	1.94	—	—	1460	—	—	—	—	—	—	—	—	2	—	—

Table H–1

Food Composition (Computer code number is for Wadsworth Diet Analysis program) (For purposes of calculations, use "0" for t, <1, <.1, <.01, etc.)

DA + Code	Food Description	Quantity	Measure	Wt (g)	H_2O (g)	Ener (kcal)	Prot (g)	Carb (g)	Dietary Fiber (g)	Fat (g)	Fat Breakdown (g) Sat	Mono	Poly
	FAST FOOD—Continued												
	Ultimate deep dish pizza												
31596	America's favorite, 12"	2	slice(s)	235	—	617	26	59	4	33	12.88	—	—
31702	America's favorite, 14"	2	slice(s)	311	—	851	36	84	5	44	17.35	—	—
31590	Cheese, 12"	2	slice(s)	181	—	482	19	56	3	22	7.91	—	—
31591	Cheese, 14"	2	slice(s)	257	—	677	26	80	5	30	10.88	—	—
31589	Cheese, 6"	1	item(s)	215	—	598	23	68	4	28	9.94	—	—
31691	Deluxe, 12"	2	slice(s)	235	—	527	23	59	4	29	10.75	—	—
31700	Deluxe, 14"	2	slice(s)	311	—	788	31	84	5	38	14.36	—	—
31692	Extravaganzza, 12"	2	slice(s)	235	—	635	27	59	4	34	12.52	—	—
31701	Extravaganzza, 14"	2	slice(s)	311	—	866	36	85	6	45	16.60	—	—
31599	Hawaiian, 12"	2	slice(s)	235	—	558	24	60	4	26	10.31	—	—
31600	Hawaiian, 14"	2	slice(s)	311	—	784	35	85	5	36	14.25	—	—
31693	Meatzza, 12"	2	slice(s)	235	—	667	30	58	4	37	14.50	—	—
31703	Meatzza, 14"	2	slice(s)	311	—	914	40	83	5	49	19.40	—	—
31593	Pepperoni, extra pepperoni & cheese 12"	2	slice(s)	235	—	629	26	57	4	34	13.57	—	—
31594	Pepperoni, extra pepperoni & cheese 14"	2	slice(s)	311	—	880	37	82	5	47	18.71	—	—
31602	Vegi, 12"	2	slice(s)	235	—	547	22	59	4	26	10.19	—	—
31603	Vegi, 14"	2	slice(s)	311	—	765	32	84	6	36	14.05	—	—
31598	With ham & pineapple tidbits, 6"	1	item(s)	430	—	619	25	70	4	28	10.19	—	—
31595	With Italian sausage, 6"	1	item(s)	430	—	642	25	70	4	31	11.33	—	—
31592	With pepperoni, 6"	1	item(s)	430	—	647	25	69	4	32	11.70	—	—
31601	With vegetables, 6"	1	item(s)	430	—	619	23	71	5	29	10.11	—	—
	In-n-Out Burger												
34374	Cheeseburger	1	item(s)	268	—	480	22	39	3	27	10.00	—	—
34391	Cheesburger w/mustard & ketchup	1	item(s)	268	—	400	22	41	3	18	9.00	—	—
34390	Cheeseburger, lettuce leaves instead of buns	1	item(s)	300	—	330	18	11	2	25	9.00	—	—
34377	Chocolate shake	1	item(s)	425	—	690	9	83	0	36	24.00	—	—
34375	Double-Double cheeseburger	1	item(s)	328	—	670	37	40	3	41	18.00	—	—
34393	Double-Double cheeseburger w/mustard & ketchup	1	item(s)	328	—	590	37	42	3	32	17.00	—	—
34392	Double-Double cheeseburger, lettuce leaves instead of buns	1	item(s)	361	—	520	33	11	2	39	17.00	—	—
34376	French fries	1	item(s)	125	—	400	7	54	2	18	5.00	—	—
34373	Hamburger	1	item(s)	243	—	390	16	39	3	19	5.00	—	—
34389	Hamburger w/mustard & ketchup	1	item(s)	243	—	310	16	41	3	10	4.00	—	—
34388	Hamburger, lettuce leaves instead of buns	1	item(s)	275	—	240	12	10	2	17	4.50	—	—
34379	Strawberry shake	1	item(s)	425	—	690	8	91	2	33	22.00	—	—
34378	Vanilla shake	1	item(s)	425	—	680	9	78	2	37	25.00	—	—
	Jack in the Box												
30392	Bacon ultimate cheeseburger	1	item(s)	353	—	1120	52	59	2	55	28.00	—	—
1740	Breakfast Jack	1	item(s)	133	—	310	14	34	1	14	5.00	—	—
14074	Cheeseburger	1	item(s)	116	—	300	14	31	2	13	6.00	—	—
14106	Chicken breast pieces	5	piece(s)	150	—	360	27	24	1	17	3.00	—	—
37241	Chicken club salad	1	item(s)	535	—	310	28	15	5	16	6.00	—	—
14111	Chocolate ice cream shake	1	item(s)	315	—	660	11	89	1	29	18.00	—	—
14075	Double cheeseburger	1	item(s)	155	—	410	20	32	1	22	11.00	—	—
14098	French fries, jumbo	1	serving(s)	142	—	410	4	55	4	20	4.50	—	—
14099	French fries, super scoop	1	serving(s)	198	—	580	6	77	6	28	6.00	—	—
14073	Hamburger	1	item(s)	104	—	250	12	30	2	9	3.50	—	—
14090	Hash browns	1	serving(s)	57	—	150	1	13	2	10	2.50	—	—
14072	Jack's Spicy Chicken sandwich	1	item(s)	253	—	580	24	53	3	31	6.00	—	—
1468	Jumbo Jack hamburger	1	item(s)	269	—	600	22	58	3	31	11.00	—	—
1469	Jumbo Jack hamburger w/cheese	1	item(s)	294	—	690	26	60	3	38	16.00	—	—
1470	Onion rings	1	serving(s)	119	—	500	6	51	3	30	5.00	—	—
33141	Sausage, egg, & cheese biscuit	1	item(s)	223	—	760	25	33	2	60	20.00	—	—
14095	Seasoned curly fries	1	serving(s)	125	—	400	6	45	5	23	5.00	—	—
14077	Sourdough Jack	1	item(s)	244	—	700	30	36	3	49	16.00	—	—
37249	Southwest chicken salad	1	serving(s)	598	—	340	28	31	9	13	6.00	—	—

PAGE KEY: H–2 = Breads/Baked Goods H–6 = Cereal/Rice/Pasta H–10 = Fruit H–16 = Vegetables/Legumes H–26 = Nuts/Seeds H–28 = Vegetarian H–30 = Dairy H–36 = Eggs H–38 = Seafood H–40 = Meats H–42 = Poultry H–44 = Processed meats H–46 = Beverages H–50 = Fats/Oils H–52 = Sweets H–52 = Sauces/Condiments/Spices H–56 = Mixed Foods/Soups/Sandwiches H–62 = Fast food H–80 = Convenience H–82 = Baby foods

Chol (mg)	Calc (mg)	Iron (mg)	Magn (mg)	Pota (mg)	Sodi (mg)	Zinc (mg)	Vit A (RAE) (µg)	Thia (mg)	Vit E (mg)	Ribo (mg)	Niac (mg)	Vit B_6 (mg)	Fola (µg)	Vit C (mg)	Vit B_{12} (µg)	Sele (µg)
58	334	4.43	—	—	1573	—	—	—	—	—	—	—	—	1	—	—
78	464	6.24	—	—	2155	—	—	—	—	—	—	—	—	1	—	—
30	241	3.88	—	—	1123	—	151	—	—	—	—	—	—	<1	—	—
41	335	5.53	—	—	1575	—	210	—	—	—	—	—	—	1	—	—
36	295	4.67	—	—	1341	—	174	—	—	—	—	—	—	1	—	—
47	253	4.45	—	—	1410	—	—	—	—	—	—	—	—	2	—	—
62	349	6.25	—	—	1927	—	—	—	—	—	—	—	—	2	—	—
60	261	4.86	—	—	1696	—	—	—	—	—	—	—	—	2	—	—
78	359	6.76	—	—	2275	—	—	—	—	—	—	—	—	2	—	—
48	328	4.19	—	—	1449	—	—	—	—	—	—	—	—	2	—	—
67	457	5.97	—	—	2039	—	—	—	—	—	—	—	—	3	—	—
379	336	4.60	—	—	1810	—	—	—	—	—	—	—	—	1	—	—
501	466	6.44	—	—	2443	—	—	—	—	—	—	—	—	1	—	—
61	332	4.25	—	—	1650	—	187	—	—	—	—	—	—	1	—	—
85	462	6.04	—	—	2304	—	260	—	—	—	—	—	—	1	—	—
41	333	4.33	—	—	1334	—	—	—	—	—	—	—	—	2	—	—
57	462	6.11	—	—	1864	—	—	—	—	—	—	—	—	2	—	—
43	298	4.84	—	—	1498	—	—	—	—	—	—	—	—	1	—	—
45	302	4.89	—	—	1478	—	—	—	—	—	—	—	—	1	—	—
47	299	4.81	—	—	1524	—	168	—	—	—	—	—	—	1	—	—
36	307	5.10	—	—	1472	—	—	—	—	—	—	—	—	5	—	—
60	200	3.60	—	—	1000	—	188	—	—	—	—	—	—	15	—	—
55	200	3.60	—	—	1080	—	182	—	—	—	—	—	—	15	—	—
60	200	1.08	—	—	720	—	—	—	—	—	—	—	—	18	—	—
95	300	0.72	—	—	350	—	143	—	—	—	—	—	—	0	—	—
120	350	5.40	—	—	1430	—	184	—	—	—	—	—	—	15	—	—
115	350	5.40	—	—	1510	—	229	—	—	—	—	—	—	15	—	—
120	350	1.08	—	—	1160	—	275	—	—	—	—	—	—	18	—	—
0	20	1.80	—	—	245	—	0	—	—	—	—	—	—	0	—	—
40	40	3.60	—	—	640	—	50	—	—	—	—	—	—	15	—	—
35	40	3.60	—	—	720	—	75	—	—	—	—	—	—	15	—	—
40	40	1.08	—	—	370	—	—	—	—	—	—	—	—	18	—	—
85	250	0.00	—	—	280	—	134	—	—	—	—	—	—	0	—	—
90	300	0.00	—	—	390	—	145	—	—	—	—	—	—	0	—	—
160	300	7.20	—	600	2260	—	—	—	—	—	—	—	—	1	—	—
210	150	3.60	—	210	770	—	—	—	—	—	—	—	—	4	—	—
40	150	3.60	—	180	840	—	40	—	—	—	—	—	—	0	—	—
80	20	1.80	—	430	970	—	—	—	—	—	—	—	—	1	—	—
65	300	3.60	—	1010	890	—	—	—	—	—	—	—	—	54	—	—
110	350	0.36	—	720	270	—	215	—	—	—	—	—	—	0	—	—
70	250	4.50	—	280	920	—	—	—	—	—	—	—	—	1	—	—
0	20	1.08	—	550	690	—	0	—	—	—	—	—	—	6	—	—
0	20	1.44	—	770	960	—	0	—	—	—	—	—	—	9	—	—
30	100	3.60	—	155	610	—	0	—	—	—	—	—	—	0	—	—
0	10	0.18	—	190	230	—	0	—	—	—	—	—	—	0	—	—
60	150	1.80	—	470	950	—	—	—	—	—	—	—	—	9	—	—
45	164	4.92	—	390	980	—	—	—	—	—	—	—	—	10	—	—
75	250	4.50	—	420	1360	—	—	—	—	—	—	—	—	9	—	—
0	40	2.70	—	140	420	—	40	—	—	—	—	—	—	18	—	—
280	100	2.70	—	240	1390	—	—	—	—	—	—	—	—	0	—	—
0	40	1.80	—	580	890	—	—	—	—	—	—	—	—	0	—	—
80	200	4.50	—	450	1220	—	—	—	—	—	—	—	—	9	—	—
60	300	4.50	—	1020	920	—	—	—	—	—	—	—	—	48	—	—

H Appendix

Table H–1

Food Composition (Computer code number is for Wadsworth Diet Analysis program) (For purposes of calculations, use "0" for t, <1, <.1, <.01, etc.)

DA + Code	Food Description	Quantity	Measure	Wt (g)	H_2O (g)	Ener (kcal)	Prot (g)	Carb (g)	Dietary Fiber (g)	Fat (g)	Fat Breakdown (g) Sat	Mono	Poly
	FAST FOOD—Continued												
14112	Strawberry ice cream shake	1	item(s)	313	—	640	10	84	0	28	18.00	—	—
14078	Ultimate cheeseburger	1	item(s)	328	—	990	41	59	2	66	28.00	—	—
14110	Vanilla ice cream shake	1	item(s)	285	—	570	12	65	0	29	18.00	—	—
	Jamba Juice												
31646	Banana berry smoothie	24	fluid ounce(s)	719	—	470	5	112	5	2	0.50	—	—
31647	Caribbean passion smoothie	24	fluid ounce(s)	730	—	440	4	102	4	2	1.00	—	—
38422	Carrot juice	16	fluid ounce(s)	472	—	100	3	23	0	1	0.00	—	—
31648	Chocolate mood smoothie	24	fluid ounce(s)	612	—	690	16	142	2	8	4.50	—	—
31649	Citrus squeeze smoothie	24	fluid ounce(s)	729	—	450	4	105	5	2	1.00	—	—
31650	Coffee mood smoothie	24	fluid ounce(s)	560	—	596	13	121	1	6	4.00	—	—
31651	Coldbuster smoothie	24	fluid ounce(s)	724	—	430	5	100	5	3	1.00	—	—
31652	Cranberry craze smoothie	24	fluid ounce(s)	731	—	420	6	97	4	2	1.00	—	—
31654	Jamba powerboost smoothie	24	fluid ounce(s)	730	—	440	6	103	7	2	0.00	—	—
38423	Lemonade	16	fluid ounce(s)	483	—	300	1	75	0	0	0.00	0.00	0.00
31656	Lime sublime smoothie	24	fluid ounce(s)	721	—	450	3	104	6	2	1.00	—	—
31657	Mango-a-go-go smoothie	24	fluid ounce(s)	739	—	500	4	117	4	2	1.00	—	—
38424	Orange juice, freshly squeezed	16	fluid ounce(s)	496	—	220	3	52	1	1	0.00	—	—
38426	Orange/carrot juice	16	fluid ounce(s)	484	—	160	3	37	0	1	0.00	—	—
31660	Orange-a-peel smoothie	24	fluid ounce(s)	726	—	440	9	102	5	1	0.00	—	—
31665	Protein berry pizzaz smoothie	24	fluid ounce(s)	710	—	440	20	92	6	2	0.00	—	—
31667	Raspberry refresher smoothie	24	fluid ounce(s)	636	—	442	3	101	8	3	0.90	—	—
31668	Razzmatazz smoothie	24	fluid ounce(s)	730	—	480	3	112	4	2	1.00	—	—
31669	Strawberries wild smoothie	24	fluid ounce(s)	725	—	450	6	105	4	0	0.00	—	—
38421	Strawberry tsunami smoothie	24	fluid ounce(s)	740	—	530	4	128	4	2	1.00	—	—
38427	Vibrant C juice	16	fluid ounce(s)	448	—	210	2	50	1	0	0.00	0.00	0.00
38428	Wheatgrass juice, freshly squeezed	1	ounce(s)	32	—	5	1	1	0	0	0.00	0.00	0.00
	Kentucky Fried Chicken (KFC)												
31850	BBQ baked beans	1	serving(s)	156	—	190	6	33	6	3	1.00	—	—
31853	Biscuit	1	item(s)	56	—	180	4	20	1	10	2.50	—	—
31851	Coleslaw	1	serving(s)	142	—	232	2	26	3	14	2.00	—	—
31842	Colonel's Crispy Strips	3	item(s)	150	—	340	28	20	0	16	4.50	—	—
31849	Corn on the cob	1	item(s)	162	—	150	5	35	2	2	0.00	—	—
3761	Extra Crispy chicken, breast	1	item(s)	162	—	470	34	19	0	28	8.00	—	—
3762	Extra Crispy chicken, drumstick	1	item(s)	60	—	160	12	5	0	10	2.50	—	—
3763	Extra Crispy chicken, thigh	1	item(s)	114	—	370	21	12	0	26	7.00	—	—
3764	Extra Crispy chicken, whole wing	1	item(s)	52	—	190	10	10	0	12	3.50	—	—
31833	Honey BBQ wing pieces	6	item(s)	189	—	607	33	33	1	38	10.00	—	—
10810	Hot & spicy chicken, breast	1	item(s)	179	—	450	33	20	0	27	8.00	—	—
10813	Hot & spicy chicken, drumstick	1	item(s)	60	—	140	13	4	0	9	2.50	—	—
10811	Hot & spicy chicken, thigh	1	item(s)	128	—	390	22	14	0	28	8.00	—	—
10812	Hot & spicy chicken, whole wing	1	item(s)	55	—	180	11	9	0	11	3.00	—	—
10859	Hot wings pieces	6	piece(s)	135	—	471	27	18	2	33	8.00	—	—
31848	Macaroni & cheese	1	serving(s)	153	—	180	7	21	2	8	3.00	—	—
31847	Mashed potatoes with gravy	1	serving(s)	136	—	120	1	17	2	6	1.00	—	—
10825	Original Recipe chicken, breast	1	item(s)	161	—	370	40	11	0	19	6.00	—	—
10826	Original Recipe chicken, drumstick	1	item(s)	59	—	140	14	4	0	8	2.00	—	—
10827	Original Recipe chicken, thigh	1	item(s)	126	—	360	22	12	0	25	7.00	—	—
10828	Original Recipe chicken, whole wing	1	item(s)	47	—	145	11	5	0	9	2.50	—	—
3760	Original Recipe chicken sandwich w/sauce	1	item(s)	200	—	450	29	33	2	22	5.00	—	—
31834	Original Recipe chicken sandwich w/o sauce	1	item(s)	187	—	360	29	21	1	13	3.50	—	—
31852	Potato salad	1	serving(s)	160	—	230	4	23	3	14	2.00	—	—
10845	Potato wedges	1	serving(s)	156	—	376	6	53	5	15	4.20	—	—
10853	Rotisserie Gold chicken, breast & wing w/skin	4	ounce(s)	114	—	218	26	1	0	12	3.51	—	—
10851	Rotisserie Gold chicken, thigh & leg w/skin	4	ounce(s)	114	—	260	23	1	0	18	5.15	—	—
10852	Rotisserie Gold chicken, thigh & leg w/o skin	4	ounce(s)	117	—	217	27	0	0	12	3.50	—	—
31843	Spicy Crispy Strips	3	item(s)	115	—	335	25	23	1	15	4.00	—	—
10854	Tender Roast chicken, breast w/o skin	1	item(s)	118	—	169	31	1	0	4	1.20	—	—

PAGE KEY: H–2 = Breads/Baked Goods H–6 = Cereal/Rice/Pasta H–10 = Fruit H–16 = Vegetables/Legumes H–26 = Nuts/Seeds H–28 = Vegetarian H–30 = Dairy H–36 = Eggs H–38 = Seafood H–40 = Meats H–42 = Poultry H–44 = Processed meats H–46 = Beverages H–50 = Fats/Oils H–52 = Sweets H–52 = Sauces/Condiments/Spices H–56 = Mixed Foods/Soups/Sandwiches H–62 = Fast food H–80 = Convenience H–82 = Baby foods

Chol (mg)	Calc (mg)	Iron (mg)	Magn (mg)	Pota (mg)	Sodi (mg)	Zinc (mg)	Vit A (RAE) (µg)	Thia (mg)	Vit E (mg)	Ribo (mg)	Niac (mg)	Vit B_6 (mg)	Fola (µg)	Vit C (mg)	Vit B_{12} (µg)	Sele (µg)
110	350	0.00	—	610	220	—	202	—	—	—	—	—	—	0	—	—
130	300	7.20	—	480	1670	—	—	—	—	—	—	—	—	1	—	—
115	400	0.00	—	630	220	—	218	—	—	—	—	—	—	0	—	—
5	200	1.08	32	1000	85	0.30	—	0.06	0.40	0.26	1.20	0.40	33	15	0	0
5	100	1.80	24	810	60	0.30	—	0.09	0.81	0.26	5.00	0.50	100	78	0	1
0	150	2.70	80	1030	250	0.90	0	0.53	1.61	0.26	5.00	0.70	80	18	0	6
25	500	1.08	32	760	280	0.60	0	0.09	0.00	0.85	0.40	0.08	9	6	1	4
5	150	1.80	60	1150	50	0.30	—	0.30	0.50	0.26	1.90	0.40	100	168	0	1
28	455	0.30	49	634	429	1.50	—	0.10	0.20	0.60	0.30	0.10	18	7	1	3
5	100	1.08	60	1240	35	15.00	—	0.38	22.15	0.34	3.00	0.40	122	1302	0	1
5	250	1.44	16	500	90	0.30	—	0.03	0.80	0.26	5.00	0.50	100	54	0	1
0	1100	1.44	480	1110	40	15.00	—	5.25	22.15	5.78	66.00	6.80	640	294	10	70
0	20	0.00	8	200	10	0.00	0	0.03	0.00	0.17	14.00	1.80	320	36	0	0
5	150	1.80	32	660	75	0.60	—	0.12	0.40	0.26	7.00	0.80	160	66	<1	1
5	100	1.08	24	800	60	0.30	—	0.15	2.01	0.26	5.00	0.70	120	72	0	1
0	60	1.08	60	990	0	0.30	0	0.45	0.40	0.14	2.00	0.20	160	246	0	0
0	100	1.80	60	1010	125	0.60	0	0.45	0.81	0.26	3.00	0.50	120	132	0	3
0	250	1.80	60	1350	100	0.30	—	0.38	0.81	0.43	3.00	0.40	140	240	0	1
0	1100	2.62	39	650	240	0.58	0	0.09	0.39	0.10	1.55	0.40	58	60	0	4
3	104	2.20	56	806	47	0.80	—	0.10	0.50	0.30	1.60	0.40	43	35	<1	1
5	150	1.80	32	790	70	0.60	—	0.09	0.40	0.26	6.00	0.90	160	60	0	1
0	250	1.80	32	1020	115	0.30	—	0.03	0.40	0.34	1.20	0.20	32	60	0	1
5	100	1.08	24	480	10	0.30	0	0.06	0.81	0.34	14.00	1.80	320	90	0	1
0	20	1.08	40	720	0	0.30	0	0.30	0.40	0.10	1.60	0.40	80	678	0	0
0	0	1.80	8	80	0	0.00	0	0.03	0.00	0.03	0.40	0.04	16	4	0	3
5	80	1.80	—	—	760	—	—	—	—	—	—	—	—	1	—	—
0	20	1.08	—	—	560	—	—	—	—	—	—	—	—	1	—	—
8	30	0.18	—	—	284	—	65	—	—	—	—	—	—	34	—	—
70	10	0.72	—	—	1140	—	—	—	—	—	—	—	—	1	—	—
0	10	0.18	—	—	20	—	10	—	—	—	—	—	—	4	—	—
135	19	1.44	—	—	1230	—	—	—	0.91	—	—	—	—	1	—	—
70	9	0.65	—	—	415	—	—	—	0.46	—	—	—	—	1	—	—
120	19	1.04	—	—	710	—	—	—	0.53	—	—	—	—	1	—	—
55	9	0.34	—	—	390	—	—	—	0.48	—	—	—	—	1	—	—
193	40	1.44	—	—	1145	—	—	—	—	—	—	—	—	5	—	—
130	10	1.07	—	—	1450	—	—	—	—	—	—	—	—	1	—	—
65	20	0.68	—	—	380	—	—	—	—	—	—	—	—	1	—	—
125	10	1.44	—	—	1240	—	—	—	—	—	—	—	—	1	—	—
60	10	0.72	—	—	420	—	—	—	—	—	—	—	—	1	—	—
150	40	1.44	—	—	1230	—		—	—	—	—	—	—	1	—	—
10	150	0.18	—	—	860	—	350	—	—	—	—	—	—	1	—	—
1	10	0.36	—	—	440	—	—	—	—	—	—	—	—	1	—	—
145	20	1.14	—	—	1145	—	—	—	—	—	—	—	—	1	—	—
75	10	0.70	—	—	440	—	—	—	—	—	—	—	—	1	—	—
165	10	1.00	—	—	1060	—	—	—	—	—	—	—	—	1	—	—
60	10	0.36	—	—	370	—	—	—	—	—	—	—	—	1	—	—
70	40	1.80	—	—	940	—	—	—	2.81	—	—	—	—	1	—	—
60	40	1.80	—	—	890	—	—	—	—	—	—	—	—	1	—	—
15	20	2.70	—	—	540	—	100	—	—	—	—	—	—	1	—	—
4	36	1.55	—	—	1323	—	—	—	—	—	—	—	—	8	—	—
102	7	0.12	—	—	718	—	—	—	—	—	—	—	—	1	—	—
127	8	0.14	—	—	764	—	—	—	—	—	—	—	—	1	—	—
128	10	0.18	—	—	772	—	—	—	—	—	—	—	—	1	—	—
70	20	0.90	—	—	1140	—	—	—	—	—	—	—	—	1	—	—
112	10	0.18	—	—	797	—	—	—	—	—	—	—	—	1	—	—

Table H–1

Food Composition (Computer code number is for Wadsworth Diet Analysis program) (For purposes of calculations, use "0" for t, <1, <.1, <.01, etc.)

DA + Code	Food Description	Quantity	Measure	Wt (g)	H_2O (g)	Ener (kcal)	Prot (g)	Carb (g)	Dietary Fiber (g)	Fat (g)	Fat Breakdown (g) Sat	Mono	Poly
	FAST FOOD—Continued												
	Long John Silver												
39392	Baked cod	1	serving(s)	101	—	120	22	1	0	5	1.00	—	—
3777	Batter dipped fish sandwich	1	item(s)	177	—	440	17	48	3	20	5.00	—	—
37568	Battered fish	1	item(s)	92	—	230	11	16	0	13	4.00	—	—
37569	Breaded clams	1	serving(s)	85	—	240	8	22	1	13	2.00	—	—
39404	Clam chowder	1	item(s)	227	—	220	9	23	0	10	4.00	—	—
39398	Cocktail sauce	1	ounce(s)	28	—	25	0	6	0	0	0.00	0.00	0.00
3770	Coleslaw	1	serving(s)	113	—	200	1	15	4	15	2.50	1.76	4.10
39394	Crunchy shrimp basket	21	item(s)	114	—	340	12	32	2	19	5.00	—	—
39400	French fries, large	1	item(s)	142	—	390	4	56	5	17	4.00	—	—
3774	Fries regular	1	serving(s)	85	—	230	3	34	3	10	2.50	7.40	5.10
3779	Hushpuppy	1	piece(s)	23	—	60	1	9	1	3	0.50	—	—
3781	Shrimp batter-dipped	1	piece(s)	14	—	45	2	3	0	3	1.00	—	—
39399	Tartar sauce	1	ounce(s)	28	—	100	0	4	0	9	1.50	—	—
39395	Ultimate fish sandwich	1	item(s)	199	—	500	20	48	3	25	8.00	—	—
	McDonald's												
2247	Barbecue sauce	1	serving(s)	28	—	45	0	10	0	0	0.00	0.00	0.00
737	Big Mac hamburger	1	item(s)	216	—	590	24	47	3	34	11.00	—	—
738	Cheeseburger	1	item(s)	121	—	330	15	36	2	14	6.00	—	—
29775	Chicken McGrill sandwich	1	item(s)	213	—	400	25	37	2	17	3.00	—	—
3792	Chicken McNuggets	4	item(s)	72	—	210	10	12	1	13	2.50	—	—
1873	Chicken McNuggest	6	item(s)	108	—	310	15	18	2	20	4.00	—	—
73	Chocolate milkshake	8	fluid ounce(s)	227	164	270	7	48	1	6	3.81	1.77	0.23
29774	Crispy chicken sandwich	1	item(s)	219	—	500	22	46	2	26	4.50	—	—
743	Egg McMuffin	1	item(s)	138	—	300	18	29	2	12	4.50	—	—
742	Filet-o-fish sandwich	1	item(s)	156	—	470	15	45	1	26	5.00	—	—
2257	French fries, large	1	serving(s)	176	—	540	8	68	6	26	4.50	—	—
1872	French fries, small	1	serving(s)	68	—	210	3	26	2	10	1.50	—	—
2244	French fries, super size	1	serving(s)	198	—	610	9	77	7	29	5.00	—	—
33822	Fruit n' yogurt parfait	1	item(s)	338	—	380	10	76	2	5	2.00	—	—
2251	Garden salad	1	item(s)	177	—	35	2	7	3	0	0.00	0.00	0.00
739	Hamburger	1	item(s)	107	—	280	12	35	2	10	4.00	—	—
2003	Hash browns	1	item(s)	53	—	130	1	14	1	8	1.50	—	—
2249	Honey sauce	1	item(s)	14	—	45	0	12	0	0	0.00	0.00	0.00
33816	McSalad Shaker chef salad	1	item(s)	206	—	150	17	5	2	8	3.50	—	—
33817	McSalad Shaker garden salad	1	item(s)	149	—	100	7	4	2	6	3.00	—	—
33818	McSalad Shaker grilled chicken caesar salad	1	item(s)	163	—	100	17	3	2	3	1.50	—	—
38396	Newman's Own cobb salad dressing	1	item(s)	59	—	120	1	9	0	9	1.50	—	—
38397	Newman's Own creamy caesar salad dressing	1	item(s)	59	—	190	2	4	0	18	3.50	—	—
38398	Newman's Own low fat balsamic vinaigrette salad dressing	1	item(s)	44	—	40	0	4	0	3	0.00	—	—
38399	Newman's Own ranch salad dressing	1	item(s)	59	—	290	1	4	0	30	4.50	—	—
1874	Plain hotcakes w/syrup & margarine	3	item(s)	228	—	600	9	104	0	17	3.00	—	—
740	Quarter Pounder hamburger	1	item(s)	172	—	430	23	37	2	21	8.00	—	—
741	Quarter Pounder hamburger w/cheese	1	item(s)	200	—	530	28	38	2	30	13.00	—	—
2005	Sausage McMuffin w/egg	1	item(s)	164	—	450	20	29	2	28	10.00	—	—
3163	Strawberry milkshake	8	fluid ounce(s)	226	168	256	8	43	1	6	3.93	—	—
74	Vanilla milkshake	8	fluid ounce(s)	227	169	254	9	40	0	7	4.28	1.98	0.26
	Pizza Hut												
39009	Hot chicken wings	2	item(s)	57	—	110	11	1	0	6	2.00	—	—
14025	Meat Lovers hand tossed pizza	1	slice(s)	125	—	320	16	30	2	15	7.00	—	—
14026	Meat Lovers pan pizza	1	slice(s)	130	—	360	16	29	2	20	7.00	—	—
31009	Meat Lovers stuffed crust pizza	1	slice(s)	188	—	500	25	44	3	25	11.00	—	—
14024	Meat Lovers thin 'n crispy pizza	1	slice(s)	112	—	310	15	22	2	18	8.00	—	—
14031	Pepperoni Lovers hand tossed pizza	1	slice(s)	114	—	300	15	30	2	14	7.00	—	—
14032	Pepperoni Lovers pan pizza	1	slice(s)	119	—	350	15	29	2	19	8.00	—	—
31011	Pepperoni Lovers stuffed crust pizza	1	slice(s)	171	—	480	23	44	3	24	11.00	—	—
14030	Pepperoni Lovers thin 'n crispy pizza	1	slice(s)	94	—	270	13	22	2	14	7.00	—	—
10834	Personal Pan pepperoni pizza	1	slice(s)	59	—	150	7	18	—	6	2.50	—	—

PAGE KEY: H–2 = Breads/Baked Goods H–6 = Cereal/Rice/Pasta H–10 = Fruit H–16 = Vegetables/Legumes H–26 = Nuts/Seeds H–28 = Vegetarian H–30 = Dairy H–36 = Eggs H–38 = Seafood H–40 = Meats H–42 = Poultry H–44 = Processed meats H–46 = Beverages H–50 = Fats/Oils H–52 = Sweets H–52 = Sauces/Condiments/Spices H–56 = Mixed Foods/Soups/Sandwiches H–62 = Fast food H–80 = Convenience H–82 = Baby foods

Chol (mg)	Calc (mg)	Iron (mg)	Magn (mg)	Pota (mg)	Sodi (mg)	Zinc (mg)	Vit A (RAE) (µg)	Thia (mg)	Vit E (mg)	Ribo (mg)	Niac (mg)	Vit B_6 (mg)	Fola (µg)	Vit C (mg)	Vit B_{12} (µg)	Sele (µg)
90	20	0.72	—	—	240	—	—	—	—	—	—	—	—	0	—	—
35	60	3.60	—	—	1120	—	—	—	—	—	—	—	—	9	—	—
30	20	1.80	—	—	700	—	—	—	—	—	—	—	—	5	—	—
10	20	1.08	—	—	1110	—	—	—	—	—	—	—	—	0	—	—
25	150	0.72	—	—	810	—	—	—	—	—	—	—	—	0	—	—
0	0	0.00	—	—	250	—	—	—	—	—	—	—	—	0	—	—
20	40	0.36	—	223	340	0.70	34	0.07	—	0.08	2.35	—	—	18	—	—
105	500	1.80	—	—	720	—	—	—	—	—	—	—	—	1	—	—
0	0	0.00	—	—	580	—	—	—	—	—	—	—	—	24	—	—
0	0	0.00	—	370	350	0.30	—	0.09	—	0.02	1.60	—	—	15	—	—
0	20	0.36	—	—	200	—	—	—	—	—	—	—	—	0	—	—
15	0	0.00	—	—	125	—	—	—	—	—	—	—	—	1	—	—
15	0	0.00	—	—	250	—	—	—	—	—	—	—	—	0	—	—
50	150	3.60	—	—	1310	—	—	—	—	—	—	—	—	9	—	—
0	10	0.18	—	45	250	—	3	—	1.53	—	—	—	—	4	—	—
85	300	4.50	—	430	1090	—	60	—	—	—	—	—	—	4	—	—
45	250	2.70	—	250	830	—	60	—	0.57	—	—	—	—	2	—	—
60	200	2.70	—	440	890	—	—	—	—	—	—	—	—	6	—	—
35	20	0.72	—	180	460	—	—	—	—	—	—	—	—	1	—	—
50	20	0.72	—	260	680	—	—	—	—	—	—	—	—	1	—	—
25	299	0.70	36	508	252	1.09	41	0.11	0.23	0.50	0.28	0.06	11	0	1	4
50	200	2.70	—	400	1100	—	—	—	—	—	—	—	—	6	—	—
235	300	2.70	—	210	830	—	—	—	0.56	—	—	—	—	1	—	—
50	200	1.80	—	280	890	—	40	—	—	—	—	—	—	1	—	—
0	20	1.44	—	1210	350	—	—	—	0.30	—	—	—	—	21	—	—
0	10	0.36	—	470	135	—	—	—	—	—	—	—	—	9	—	—
0	20	1.44	—	1370	390	—	—	—	—	—	—	—	—	24	—	—
15	300	1.80	—	550	240	—	—	—	—	—	—	—	—	24	—	—
0	40	1.09	—	410	20	—	—	—	0.61	—	—	—	—	24	—	—
30	200	2.70	—	230	590	—	5	—	0.43	—	—	—	—	2	—	—
0	10	0.36	—	210	330	—	—	—	0.10	—	—	—	—	2	—	—
0	10	0.18	—	7	0	—	—	—	—	—	—	—	—	1	—	—
95	150	1.44	—	360	740	—	323	—	—	—	—	—	—	15	—	—
75	150	1.08	—	290	120	—	273	—	—	—	—	—	—	15	—	—
40	100	1.08	—	420	240	—	—	—	—	—	—	—	—	12	—	—
10	40	0.18	—	13	440	—	—	—	—	—	—	—	—	1	—	—
20	60	0.18	—	16	500	—	—	—	—	—	—	—	—	1	—	—
0	10	0.18	—	9	730	—	—	—	—	—	—	—	—	2	—	—
20	40	0.18	—	64	530	—	—	—	—	—	—	—	—	1	—	—
20	100	4.50	—	280	770	—	—	—	—	—	—	—	—	1	—	—
70	200	4.50	—	370	840	—	10	—	—	—	—	—	—	2	—	—
95	350	4.50	—	420	1310	—	100	—	—	—	—	—	—	2	—	—
255	300	2.70	—	260	930	—	115	—	2.30	—	—	—	—	1	—	—
25	256	0.25	29	412	188	0.82	59	0.10	—	0.44	0.40	0.10	7	2	1	5
27	331	0.23	27	415	215	0.88	57	0.07	0.23	0.44	0.33	0.10	16	0	1	5
70	0	0.36	—	—	450	—	—	—	—	—	—	—	—	0	—	—
40	150	1.80	—	—	830	—	—	—	—	—	—	—	—	6	—	—
40	150	2.70	—	—	810	—	—	—	—	—	—	—	—	6	—	—
65	250	2.70	—	—	1450	—	—	—	—	—	—	—	—	9	—	—
45	150	1.80	—	—	880	—	—	—	—	—	—	—	—	9	—	—
40	200	1.80	—	—	730	—	58	—	—	—	—	—	—	2	—	—
40	200	2.70	—	—	710	—	58	—	—	—	—	—	—	2	—	—
65	300	2.70	—	—	1300	—	—	—	—	—	—	—	—	4	—	—
40	200	1.44	—	—	700	—	58	—	—	—	—	—	—	2	—	—
15	80	1.44	—	—	340	—	38	—	—	—	—	—	—	1	—	—

Table H–1

Food Composition (Computer code number is for Wadsworth Diet Analysis program) (For purposes of calculations, use "0" for t, <1, <.1, <.01, etc.)

DA + Code	Food Description	Quantity	Measure	Wt (g)	H_2O (g)	Ener (kcal)	Prot (g)	Carb (g)	Dietary Fiber (g)	Fat (g)	Fat Breakdown (g) Sat	Mono	Poly
	FAST FOOD—Continued												
10842	Personal Pan supreme pizza	1	slice(s)	73	—	170	8	19	1	7	3.00	—	—
39013	Personal Pan Veggie Lovers pizza	1	slice(s)	69	—	150	6	19	1	6	2.00	—	—
14028	Veggie Lovers hand tossed pizza	1	slice(s)	120	—	220	10	31	2	6	3.00	—	—
14029	Veggie Lovers pan pizza	1	slice(s)	125	—	260	10	31	2	12	4.00	—	—
31010	Veggie Lovers stuffed crust pizza	1	slice(s)	181	—	370	17	45	3	14	7.00	—	—
14027	Veggie Lovers thin 'n crispy pizza	1	slice(s)	110	—	190	8	23	2	7	3.00	—	—
39012	Wing blue cheese dipping sauce	1	item(s)	43	—	230	2	2	0	24	5.00	—	—
39011	Wing ranch dipping sauce	1	item(s)	43	—	210	1	4	0	22	3.50	—	—
	Starbucks												
38042	Apple cider, tall steamed	12	fluid ounce(s)	360	—	180	0	45	0	0	0.00	0.00	0.00
38052	Cappuccino, tall	12	fluid ounce(s)	360	—	120	7	10	0	6	4.00	—	—
38053	Cappuccino, tall nonfat	12	fluid ounce(s)	360	—	80	7	11	0	0	0.00	0.00	0.00
38054	Cappuccino, tall soy milk	12	fluid ounce(s)	360	—	100	5	13	1	3	0.00	—	—
38059	Cinnamon spice mocha, tall nonfat w/o whipped cream	12	fluid ounce(s)	360	—	170	11	32	0	0	0.50	0.00	0.00
38057	Cinnamon spice mocha, tall w/whipped cream	12	fluid ounce(s)	360	—	320	10	31	0	17	11.00	—	—
38051	Espresso, single shot	1	fluid ounce(s)	30	—	5	0	1	0	0	0.00	0.00	0.00
38088	Flavored syrup, 1 pump	1	serving(s)	10	—	20	0	5	0	0	0.00	0.00	0.00
32562	Frappuccino coffee drink, lite mocha	9½	fluid ounce(s)	281	—	100	7	12	3	3	2.00	—	—
38079	Frappuccino, grande chocolate malt	16	fluid ounce(s)	480	—	470	15	87	2	10	3.50	—	—
38075	Frappuccino, grande mocha malt	12	fluid ounce(s)	360	—	430	14	91	1	7	4.00	—	—
32561	Frappuccino low fat coffee drink, all flavors	9½	fluid ounce(s)	281	—	190	6	39	0	3	2.00	—	—
38067	Frappuccino, tall caramel	12	fluid ounce(s)	360	—	210	4	43	0	3	1.50	—	—
38078	Frappuccino, tall chocolate	12	fluid ounce(s)	360	—	290	13	52	1	5	1.00	—	—
38069	Frappuccino, tall chocolate brownie	12	fluid ounce(s)	360	—	270	5	51	1	7	4.50	—	—
38070	Frappuccino, tall coffee	12	fluid ounce(s)	360	—	190	4	38	0	3	1.50	—	—
38071	Frappuccino, tall espresso	12	fluid ounce(s)	360	—	160	4	33	0	2	1.50	—	—
38073	Frappuccino, mocha	12	fluid ounce(s)	360	—	220	5	44	0	3	1.50	—	—
38072	Frappuccino, tall mocha coconut	12	fluid ounce(s)	360	—	300	5	58	2	7	5.00	—	—
38080	Frappuccino, tall vanilla	12	fluid ounce(s)	360	—	260	11	47	0	4	1.00	—	—
38074	Frappuccino, tall white chocolate	12	fluid ounce(s)	360	—	240	5	48	0	4	2.50	—	—
33111	Latte, tall w/nonfat milk	12	fluid ounce(s)	360	335	123	12	17	0	1	0.40	0.16	0.02
33112	Latte, tall w/whole milk	12	fluid ounce(s)	360	325	212	11	17	0	11	6.90	3.24	0.42
33109	Macchiato, tall caramel w/nonfat milk	12	fluid ounce(s)	360	—	140	7	27	0	1	0.40	—	—
33110	Macchiato, tall caramel w/whole milk	12	fluid ounce(s)	360	—	190	6	27	0	7	4.00	—	—
33107	Mocha coffee drink, tall nonfat, w/o whipped cream	12	fluid ounce(s)	360	—	180	12	33	1	2	1.50	0.68	0.08
38089	Mocha syrup	1	serving(s)	17	—	25	1	6	0	1	0.00	—	—
33108	Mocha, tall w/whole milk	12	fluid ounce(s)	360	—	340	12	33	1	20	12.00	3.48	0.44
38084	Tazo chai black tea, tall	12	fluid ounce(s)	360	—	210	6	36	0	5	3.50	—	—
38083	Tazo chai black tea, tall nonfat	12	fluid ounce(s)	360	—	170	6	37	0	0	0.00	0.00	0.00
38087	Tazo chai black tea, tall soy milk	12	fluid ounce(s)	360	—	190	4	39	1	2	0.00	—	—
38063	Tazo chai creme frappuccino, tall	12	fluid ounce(s)	360	—	280	11	51	0	4	1.00	—	—
38076	Tazo iced tea, tall	12	fluid ounce(s)	360	—	60	0	16	0	0	0.00	0.00	0.00
38077	Tazo tea, grande lemonade	16	fluid ounce(s)	480	—	120	0	31	0	0	0.00	0.00	0.00
38065	Tazoberry creme frappuccino, tall	12	fluid ounce(s)	360	—	240	4	54	1	1	0.00	—	—
38066	Tazoberry frappuccino, tall	12	fluid ounce(s)	360	—	140	1	36	1	0	0.00	0.00	0.00
38045	Vanilla creme steamed nonfat milk, tall w/whipped cream	12	fluid ounce(s)	360	—	180	12	32	0	0	0.00	0.00	0.00
38046	Vanilla creme steamed soy milk, tall w/whipped cream	12	fluid ounce(s)	360	—	300	8	37	1	12	6.00	—	—
38044	Vanilla creme steamed whole milk, tall w/whipped cream	12	fluid ounce(s)	360	—	340	10	31	0	18	12.00	—	—
38090	Whipped cream	1	serving(s)	27	—	100	0	2	0	9	6.00	—	—
38062	White chocolate mocha, tall nonfat w/o whipped cream	12	fluid ounce(s)	360	—	260	12	45	0	4	3.00	—	—
38061	White chocolate mocha, tall w/whipped cream	12	fluid ounce(s)	360	—	410	11	44	0	20	13.00	—	—
38048	White hot chocolate, tall w/o whipped cream	12	fluid ounce(s)	360	—	300	15	51	0	5	3.50	—	—

PAGE KEY: H–2 = Breads/Baked Goods H–6 = Cereal/Rice/Pasta H–10 = Fruit H–16 = Vegetables/Legumes H–26 = Nuts/Seeds H–28 = Vegetarian H–30 = Dairy H–36 = Eggs H–38 = Seafood H–40 = Meats H–42 = Poultry H–44 = Processed meats H–46 = Beverages H–50 = Fats/Oils H–52 = Sweets H–52 = Sauces/Condiments/Spices H–56 = Mixed Foods/Soups/Sandwiches H–62 = Fast food H–80 = Convenience H–82 = Baby foods

Chol (mg)	Calc (mg)	Iron (mg)	Magn (mg)	Pota (mg)	Sodi (mg)	Zinc (mg)	Vit A (RAE) (μg)	Thia (mg)	Vit E (mg)	Ribo (mg)	Niac (mg)	Vit B_6 (mg)	Fola (μg)	Vit C (mg)	Vit B_{12} (μg)	Sele (μg)
15	80	1.86	—	—	400	—	—	—	—	—	—	—	—	4	—	—
10	80	1.80	—	—	280	—	—	—	—	—	—	—	—	4	—	—
15	150	1.80	—	—	490	—	—	—	—	—	—	—	—	9	—	—
15	150	2.70	—	—	470	—	—	—	—	—	—	—	—	9	—	—
35	250	2.70	—	—	980	—	—	—	—	—	—	—	—	12	—	—
15	150	1.44	—	—	480	—	—	—	—	—	—	—	—	12	—	—
25	20	0.00	—	—	550	—	0	—	—	—	—	—	—	0	—	—
10	0	0.00	—	—	340	—	0	—	—	—	—	—	—	0	—	—
0	0	1.08	—	—	15	—	0	—	—	—	—	—	—	0	0	—
25	250	0.00	—	—	95	—	0	—	—	—	—	—	—	1	0	—
3	200	0.00	—	—	100	—	0	—	—	—	—	—	—	0	0	—
0	250	0.72	—	—	75	—	0	—	—	—	—	—	—	0	0	—
5	300	0.72	—	—	150	—	0	—	—	—	—	—	—	0	0	—
70	350	1.08	—	—	140	—	0	—	—	—	—	—	—	2	0	—
0	0	0.00	—	—	0	—	0	—	—	—	—	—	—	0	0	—
0	0	0.00	—	—	0	—	0	—	—	—	—	—	—	0	0	—
13	200	1.08	—	—	80	—	—	—	—	—	—	—	—	0	—	—
15	250	2.70	—	—	420	—	0	—	—	—	—	—	—	12	0	—
20	250	1.08	—	—	390	—	0	—	—	—	—	—	—	0	0	—
12	220	0.00	—	—	110	—	—	—	—	—	—	—	—	0	—	—
10	150	0.00	—	—	180	—	0	—	—	—	—	—	—	0	0	—
3	400	1.80	—	—	300	—	0	—	—	—	—	—	—	5	0	—
10	150	1.44	—	—	220	—	0	—	—	—	—	—	—	0	0	—
10	150	0.00	—	—	180	—	0	—	—	—	—	—	—	0	0	—
10	100	0.00	—	—	160	—	0	—	—	—	—	—	—	0	0	—
10	150	0.72	—	—	180	—	0	—	—	—	—	—	—	0	0	—
10	150	1.08	—	—	220	—	0	—	—	—	—	—	—	0	0	—
3	400	0.00	—	—	280	—	0	—	—	—	—	—	—	4	0	—
10	150	0.00	—	—	210	—	0	—	—	—	—	—	—	0	0	—
6	420	0.18	40	—	174	1.35	—	0.12	0.20	0.47	0.36	0.14	18	4	1	—
46	400	0.18	47	254	165	1.28	—	0.13	0.40	0.54	0.35	0.14	17	3	1	—
25	250	0.36	—	—	110	—	—	—	—	—	—	—	—	2	—	—
25	200	0.36	—	—	105	—	—	—	—	—	—	—	—	1	—	—
5	350	2.70	—	—	150	—	—	—	—	—	—	—	—	2	—	—
0	0	0.72	—	—	0	—	0	—	—	—	—	—	—	0	0	—
47	300	0.18	—	—	169	—	—	—	—	—	—	—	—	2	—	—
20	200	0.36	—	—	85	—	0	—	—	—	—	—	—	1	0	—
5	200	0.36	—	—	95	—	0	—	—	—	—	—	—	0	0	—
0	200	0.72	—	—	70	—	0	—	—	—	—	—	—	0	0	—
3	400	0.00	—	—	280	—	0	—	—	—	—	—	—	4	0	—
0	0	0.00	—	—	0	—	0	—	—	—	—	—	—	0	0	—
0	0	0.00	—	—	15	—	0	—	—	—	—	—	—	5	0	—
0	150	0.00	—	—	125	—	0	—	—	—	—	—	—	1	0	—
0	0	0.00	—	—	30	—	0	—	—	—	—	—	—	0	0	—
5	350	0.00	—	—	170	—	0	—	—	—	—	—	—	0	0	—
30	400	1.44	—	—	130	—	0	—	—	—	—	—	—	0	0	—
75	40	0.00	—	—	160	—	0	—	—	—	—	—	—	2	0	—
40	0	0.00	—	—	10	—	0	—	—	—	—	—	—	0	0	—
5	400	0.00	—	—	210	—	0	—	—	—	—	—	—	0	0	—
70	400	0.00	—	—	210	—	0	—	—	—	—	—	—	2	0	—
10	450	0.00	—	—	250	—	0	—	—	—	—	—	—	0	0	—

Table H–1

Food Composition (Computer code number is for Wadsworth Diet Analysis program) (For purposes of calculations, use "0" for t, <1, <.1, <.01, etc.)

DA + Code	Food Description	Quantity	Measure	Wt (g)	H_2O (g)	Ener (kcal)	Prot (g)	Carb (g)	Dietary Fiber (g)	Fat (g)	Fat Breakdown (g) Sat	Mono	Poly
	FAST FOOD—Continued												
38047	White hot chocolate, tall w/whipped cream	12	fluid ounce(s)	360	—	460	13	50	0	22	15.00	—	—
38050	White hot chocolate soy milk, tall w/whipped cream	12	fluid ounce(s)	360	—	420	11	56	1	16	9.00	—	—
	Subway												
34023	Asiago caesar chicken wrap	1	item(s)	244	—	413	22	47	2	15	3.00	—	—
38622	Atkins-friendly chicken bacon ranch wrap	1	item(s)	213	—	480	40	19	11	27	9.00	—	—
38623	Atkins-friendly turkey bacon melt wrap	1	item(s)	199	—	430	32	22	12	25	9.00	—	—
34029	Bacon & egg breakfast sandwich	1	item(s)	127	—	302	14	29	1	15	4.00	—	—
32045	Chocolate chip cookie	1	item(s)	48	—	209	3	29	1	10	3.50	—	—
32048	Chocolate chip M&M cookie	1	item(s)	48	—	210	2	29	1	10	3.00	—	—
32049	Chocolate chunk cookie	1	item(s)	48	—	210	2	30	1	10	3.00	—	—
4024	Classic Italian B.M.T. sandwich, 6", white bread	1	item(s)	250	—	453	21	40	3	24	8.00	—	—
16397	Club salad	1	item(s)	323	—	145	17	12	3	4	1.00	—	—
3422	Club sandwich, 6", white bread	1	item(s)	253	—	294	22	40	3	5	1.50	—	—
4030	Cold cut trio sandwich, 6", white bread	1	item(s)	254	—	415	19	40	3	20	7.00	—	—
34030	Ham & egg breakfast sandwich	1	item(s)	147	—	291	15	30	1	12	3.00	—	—
3885	Ham sandwich, 6", white bread	1	item(s)	219	—	261	17	39	3	5	1.50	—	—
34026	Honey mustard melt sandwich, 6", Italian bread	1	item(s)	258	—	373	23	47	3	11	5.00	—	—
34027	Horseradish roast beef sandwich, 6", Italian bread	1	item(s)	230	—	401	18	42	3	17	3.00	—	—
4651	Meatball sandwich, 6", white bread	1	item(s)	284	—	501	23	46	4	25	10.00	—	—
15839	Melt sandwich, 6", white bread	1	item(s)	256	—	380	23	41	3	15	5.00	—	—
32046	Oatmeal raisin cookie	1	item(s)	48	—	197	3	29	1	8	2.00	—	—
32047	Peanut butter cookie	1	item(s)	48	—	220	3	26	1	12	3.00	—	—
3957	Roast beef sandwich, 6", white bread	1	item(s)	220	—	264	18	39	3	5	1.00	—	—
16403	Roasted chicken breast salad	1	item(s)	304	—	137	16	12	3	3	0.50	—	—
16378	Roasted chicken breast sandwich, 6", white bread	1	item(s)	234	—	311	25	40	3	6	1.50	—	—
34028	Southwest steak & cheese sandwich, 6", Italian bread	1	item(s)	255	—	412	23	42	4	18	6.00	—	—
4032	Spicy italian sandwich, 6", white bread	1	item(s)	213	—	458	19	42	2	24	9.00	—	—
4031	Steak & cheese sandwich, 6", white bread	1	item(s)	253	—	362	23	41	4	13	4.50	—	—
34024	Steak & cheese wrap	1	item(s)	245	—	353	22	46	3	9	4.00	—	—
32050	Sugar cookie	1	item(s)	48	—	222	2	28	1	12	3.00	—	—
16402	Tuna salad	1	item(s)	314	—	238	13	11	3	16	4.00	—	—
15844	Tuna sandwich, 6", white bread	1	item(s)	252	—	419	18	39	3	21	5.00	—	—
15834	Turkey breast & ham sandwich, 6", white bread	1	item(s)	229	—	267	18	40	3	5	1.00	—	—
34025	Turkey breast & bacon wrap	1	item(s)	228	—	318	19	45	2	7	2.50	—	—
16376	Turkey breast sandwich, 6", white bread	1	item(s)	220	—	254	16	39	3	4	1.00	—	—
16375	Veggie delite, 6", white bread	1	item(s)	163	—	200	7	37	3	3	0.50	—	—
32051	White macadamia nut cookie	1	item(s)	48	—	221	2	27	1	12	3.00	—	—
	Taco Bell												
29906	7-layer burrito	1	item(s)	283	—	530	18	67	10	22	8.00	—	—
744	Bean burrito	1	item(s)	198	—	370	14	55	8	10	3.50	—	—
749	Beef burrito supreme	1	item(s)	248	—	440	18	51	7	18	8.00	—	—
33417	Beef chalupa supreme	1	item(s)	153	—	390	14	31	3	24	10.00	—	—
29910	Beef gordita supreme	1	item(s)	153	—	310	14	30	3	16	7.00	—	—
2014	Beef soft taco	1	item(s)	99	—	210	10	21	2	10	4.50	—	—
10860	Beef soft taco supreme	1	item(s)	134	—	260	11	22	3	14	7.00	—	—
2018	Big beef burrito supreme	1	item(s)	291	—	510	23	52	11	23	9.00	6.55	1.61
14467	Big chicken burrito supreme	1	item(s)	255	—	460	27	50	3	17	6.00	—	—
34472	Chicken burrito supreme	1	item(s)	248	—	410	21	50	5	14	6.00	—	—
33418	Chicken chalupa supreme	1	item(s)	153	—	370	17	30	1	20	8.00	—	—
29900	Chicken fajita wrap supreme	1	item(s)	255	—	510	20	53	3	24	7.76	—	—
29895	Choco taco ice cream dessert	1	item(s)	113	—	310	3	37	1	17	10.00	—	—
10794	Cinnamon twists	1	serving(s)	35	—	160	0	28	0	5	1.00	—	—

Appendix H

PAGE KEY: H–2 = Breads/Baked Goods H–6 = Cereal/Rice/Pasta H–10 = Fruit H–16 = Vegetables/Legumes H–26 = Nuts/Seeds H–28 = Vegetarian H–30 = Dairy H–36 = Eggs H–38 = Seafood H–40 = Meats H–42 = Poultry H–44 = Processed meats H–46 = Beverages H–50 = Fats/Oils H–52 = Sweets H–52 = Sauces/Condiments/Spices H–56 = Mixed Foods/Soups/Sandwiches H–62 = Fast food H–80 = Convenience H–82 = Baby foods

Chol (mg)	Calc (mg)	Iron (mg)	Magn (mg)	Pota (mg)	Sodi (mg)	Zinc (mg)	Vit A (RAE) (µg)	Thia (mg)	Vit E (mg)	Ribo (mg)	Niac (mg)	Vit B_6 (mg)	Fola (µg)	Vit C (mg)	Vit B_{12} (µg)	Sele (µg)
75	500	0.00	—	—	250	—	0	—	—	—	—	—	—	4	0	—
35	500	1.44	—	—	210	—	0	—	—	—	—	—	—	0	0	—
46	40	2.70	—	—	1320	—	—	—	—	—	—	—	—	15	—	—
90	350	2.70	—	—	1340	—	—	—	—	—	—	—	—	7	—	—
65	300	2.70	—	—	1650	—	—	—	—	—	—	—	—	5	—	—
185	60	1.80	—	—	480	—	—	—	—	—	—	—	—	15	—	—
12	0	1.00	—	—	135	—	0	—	—	—	—	—	—	0	—	—
13	0	1.00	—	—	135	—	0	—	—	—	—	—	—	0	—	—
12	0	1.00	—	—	150	—	0	—	—	—	—	—	—	0	—	—
56	100	2.70	—	—	1740	—	—	—	—	—	—	—	—	24	—	—
30	40	1.80	—	—	1070	—	—	—	—	—	—	—	—	30	—	—
30	40	3.60	—	—	1250	—	60	—	—	—	—	—	—	24	—	—
57	150	3.60	—	—	1670	—	100	—	—	—	—	—	—	24	—	—
189	60	2.70	—	—	700	—	67	—	—	—	—	—	—	15	—	—
25	40	2.70	—	—	1260	—	—	—	—	—	—	—	—	24	—	—
41	100	2.70	—	—	1570	—	—	—	—	—	—	—	—	24	—	—
27	40	3.60	—	—	880	—	—	—	—	—	—	—	—	24	—	—
56	100	3.60	—	—	1350	—	—	—	—	—	—	—	—	24	—	—
41	100	2.70	—	—	1690	—	—	—	—	—	—	—	—	24	—	—
14	0	1.00	—	—	180	—	0	—	—	—	—	—	—	0	—	—
0	0	1.00	—	—	200	—	0	—	—	—	—	—	—	0	—	—
20	40	3.60	—	—	840	—	60	—	—	—	—	—	—	24	—	—
36	40	1.08	—	—	730	—	—	—	—	—	—	—	—	30	—	—
48	60	3.60	—	—	880	—	—	—	—	—	—	—	—	24	—	—
44	100	6.30	—	—	1120	—	—	—	—	—	—	—	—	24	—	—
57	30	3.00	—	—	1498	—	—	—	—	—	—	—	—	13	—	—
37	100	6.30	—	—	1200	—	—	—	—	—	—	—	—	24	—	—
37	150	7.20	—	—	1400	—	—	—	—	—	—	—	—	15	—	—
18	0	1.00	—	—	170	—	0	—	—	—	—	—	—	0	—	—
42	100	1.08	—	—	880	—	177	—	—	—	—	—	—	30	—	—
42	100	2.70	—	—	1180	—	100	—	—	—	—	—	—	24	—	—
23	40	2.70	—	—	1210	—	—	—	—	—	—	—	—	24	—	—
24	60	2.70	—	—	1490	—	—	—	—	—	—	—	—	15	—	—
15	40	2.70	—	—	1000	—	—	—	—	—	—	—	—	24	—	—
0	40	1.80	—	—	500	—	—	—	—	—	—	—	—	24	—	—
13	0	1.00	—	—	140	—	0	—	—	—	—	—	—	0	—	—
25	300	3.59	—	—	1360	—	—	—	—	—	—	—	—	5	—	—
10	200	2.69	—	—	1200	—	53	—	—	—	—	—	—	5	—	—
40	200	2.70	—	—	1330	—	351	—	—	—	—	—	—	9	—	—
40	150	1.80	—	—	600	—	—	—	—	—	—	—	—	5	—	—
35	150	2.70	—	—	590	—	—	—	—	—	—	—	—	5	—	—
25	100	1.80	—	—	620	—	44	—	—	—	—	—	—	2	—	—
40	150	1.80	—	—	630	—	73	—	—	—	—	—	—	5	—	—
60	150	2.70	—	493	1500	—	877	—	0.79	0.07	—	—	—	5	—	—
70	101	1.46	—	—	1200	—	—	—	—	—	—	—	—	2	—	—
45	200	2.70	—	—	1270	—	—	—	—	—	—	—	—	9	—	—
45	100	1.08	—	—	530	—	—	—	—	—	—	—	—	5	—	—
57	165	1.52	—	—	1182	—	—	—	—	—	—	—	—	7	—	—
20	60	0.72	—	—	100	—	—	—	—	—	—	—	—	0	—	—
0	0	0.37	—	—	150	—	0	—	—	—	—	—	—	0	—	—

H Appendix

Table H–1

Food Composition (Computer code number is for Wadsworth Diet Analysis program) (For purposes of calculations, use "0" for t, <1, <.1, <.01, etc.)

DA + Code	Food Description	Quantity	Measure	Wt (g)	H_2O (g)	Ener (kcal)	Prot (g)	Carb (g)	Dietary Fiber (g)	Fat (g)	Fat Breakdown (g) Sat	Mono	Poly
	FAST FOOD—Continued												
14465	Grilled chicken burrito	1	item(s)	198	—	390	19	49	3	13	4.00	—	—
29911	Grilled chicken gordita supreme	1	item(s)	153	—	290	17	28	2	12	5.00	—	—
14463	Grilled chicken soft taco	1	item(s)	99	—	190	14	19	0	6	2.50	—	—
29912	Grilled steak gordita supreme	1	item(s)	153	—	290	16	28	2	13	6.00	—	—
29904	Grilled steak soft taco	1	item(s)	127	—	280	12	21	1	17	4.50	—	—
29905	Grilled steak soft taco supreme	1	item(s)	135	—	240	15	20	2	11	5.00	—	—
2021	Mexican pizza	1	serving(s)	216	—	550	21	46	7	31	11.00	—	—
2011	Nachos	1	serving(s)	99	—	320	5	33	2	19	4.50	—	—
2012	Nachos bellgrande	1	serving(s)	308	—	780	20	80	12	43	13.00	—	—
34473	Steak burrito supreme	1	item(s)	248	—	420	19	50	6	16	7.00	—	—
33419	Steak chalupa supreme	1	item(s)	153	—	370	15	29	2	22	8.00	—	—
29899	Steak fajita wrap supreme	1	item(s)	255	—	510	21	52	3	25	8.00	—	—
747	Taco	1	item(s)	78	—	170	8	13	3	10	4.00	—	—
2015	Taco salad w/salsa, with shell	1	serving(s)	533	—	790	31	73	13	42	15.00	—	—
14459	Taco supreme	1	item(s)	113	—	220	9	14	3	14	7.00	—	—
748	Tostada	1	item(s)	170	—	250	11	29	7	10	4.00	—	—
29901	Veggie fajita wrap supreme	1	item(s)	255	—	470	11	55	3	22	7.00	—	—
	CONVENIENCE MEALS												
	Banquet												
29961	Barbeque chicken meal	1	item(s)	281	—	330	16	37	2	13	3.00	—	—
14788	Boneless white fried chicken meal	1	item(s)	234	—	490	14	49	2	27	7.00	—	—
29960	Fish sticks meal	1	item(s)	187	—	270	13	31	3	10	3.00	—	—
29957	Lasagna with meat sauce meal	1	item(s)	312	—	320	15	46	7	9	4.00	—	—
14777	Macaroni & cheese meal	1	item(s)	340	—	420	15	57	5	14	8.00	—	—
1741	Meatloaf meal	1	item(s)	269	—	240	14	20	4	11	4.00	—	—
39418	Pepperoni pizza meal	1	item(s)	191	—	480	11	56	5	23	8.00	—	—
33759	Roasted white turkey meal	1	item(s)	255	—	230	14	30	5	6	2.00	—	—
1743	Salisbury steak meal	1	item(s)	269	197	380	12	28	3	24	12.00	—	—
	Budget Gourmet												
1914	Cheese manicotti w/meat sauce	1	item(s)	284	194	420	18	38	4	22	11.00	6.00	1.34
1915	Chicken w/fettucini	1	item(s)	284	—	380	20	33	3	19	10.00	—	—
3986	Light beef stroganoff	1	item(s)	248	177	290	20	32	3	7	4.00	—	—
3996	Light sirloin of beef in herb sauce	1	item(s)	269	214	260	19	30	5	7	4.00	2.30	0.31
3987	Light vegetable lasagna	1	item(s)	298	227	290	15	36	5	9	1.79	0.89	0.60
	Healthy Choice												
36979	Bowls chicken teriyaki with rice	1	item(s)	298	—	330	19	50	5	6	2.00	2.00	2.00
9425	Cheese French bread pizza	1	item(s)	170	—	360	20	57	5	5	1.50	—	—
9306	Chicken enchilada suprema meal	1	item(s)	320	252	360	13	59	8	7	3.00	2.00	2.00
9316	Lemon pepper fish meal	1	item(s)	303	—	280	11	49	5	5	2.00	1.00	2.00
9322	Traditional salisbury steak meal	1	item(s)	354	250	360	23	45	5	9	3.50	4.00	1.00
9359	Traditional turkey breasts meal	1	item(s)	298	—	330	21	50	4	5	2.00	1.50	1.50
9451	Zucchini lasagna	1	item(s)	383	—	280	13	47	5	4	2.50	—	—
	Stouffers												
2363	Cheese enchiladas with mexican rice	1	serving(s)	276	—	370	12	48	5	14	5.00	—	—
2313	Cheese French bread pizza	1	serving(s)	294	—	370	14	43	3	16	6.00	—	—
11138	Cheese manicotti w/tomato sauce	1	item(s)	255	—	330	17	35	3	13	8.00	—	—
2366	Chicken pot pie	1	item(s)	284	—	740	23	56	4	47	18.00	12.41	10.48
11116	Homestyle baked chicken breast w/mashed potatoes & gravy	1	item(s)	252	—	260	19	21	1	11	3.00	—	—
11146	Homestyle beef pot roast & potatoes	1	item(s)	252	—	270	16	25	3	12	4.50	—	—
11152	Homestyle roast turkey breast w/stuffing & mashed potatoes	1	item(s)	273	—	300	16	34	2	11	3.00	—	—
11043	Lean Cuisine Cafe Classics baked chicken & whipped potatoes w/stuffing	1	item(s)	227	—	240	17	33	3	5	1.50	1.50	1.00
11046	Lean Cuisine Cafe Classics honey mustard chicken	1	item(s)	213	—	260	18	37	1	4	1.50	1.00	1.00
360	Lean Cuisine Everyday Favorites chicken chow mein w/rice	1	item(s)	255	—	210	12	33	2	3	1.00	1.00	0.50
9467	Lean Cuisine Everyday Favorites fettucini alfredo	1	item(s)	262	—	280	13	40	2	7	3.50	2.00	1.00

PAGE KEY: H–2 = Breads/Baked Goods H–6 = Cereal/Rice/Pasta H–10 = Fruit H–16 = Vegetables/Legumes H–26 = Nuts/Seeds H–28 = Vegetarian H–30 = Dairy H–36 = Eggs H–38 = Seafood H–40 = Meats H–42 = Poultry H–44 = Processed meats H–46 = Beverages H–50 = Fats/Oils H–52 = Sweets H–52 = Sauces/Condiments/Spices H–56 = Mixed Foods/Soups/Sandwiches H–62 = Fast food H–80 = Convenience H–82 = Baby foods

Chol (mg)	Calc (mg)	Iron (mg)	Magn (mg)	Pota (mg)	Sodi (mg)	Zinc (mg)	Vit A (RAE) (µg)	Thia (mg)	Vit E (mg)	Ribo (mg)	Niac (mg)	Vit B_6 (mg)	Fola (µg)	Vit C (mg)	Vit B_{12} (µg)	Sele (µg)
40	151	1.44	—	—	1240	—	—	—	—	—	—	—	—	2	—	—
45	100	1.80	—	—	530	—	—	—	—	—	—	—	—	5	—	—
30	100	1.08	—	—	550	—	15	—	—	—	—	—	—	1	—	—
35	100	2.70	—	—	520	—	—	—	—	—	—	—	—	4	—	—
30	100	1.44	—	—	650	—	29	—	—	—	—	—	—	4	—	—
35	100	1.08	—	—	510	—	29	—	—	—	—	—	—	4	—	—
45	350	3.60	—	—	1030	—	—	—	—	—	—	—	—	6	—	—
4	80	0.72	—	—	530	—	0	—	—	—	—	—	—	0	—	—
35	200	2.70	—	—	1300	—	162	—	—	—	—	—	—	6	—	—
35	200	2.70	—	—	1260	—	789	—	—	—	—	—	—	9	—	—
35	100	1.44	—	—	520	—	—	—	—	—	—	—	—	4	—	—
50	150	1.80	—	—	1200	—	—	—	—	—	—	—	—	6	—	—
25	60	1.08	—	—	350	—	44	—	—	—	—	—	—	2	—	—
65	400	6.23	—	—	1670	—	—	—	—	—	—	—	—	21	—	—
40	80	1.44	—	—	360	—	73	—	—	—	—	—	—	5	—	—
15	150	1.44	—	—	710	—	281	—	—	—	—	—	—	5	—	—
30	150	1.44	—	—	990	—	—	—	—	—	—	—	—	6	—	—
50	40	1.08	—	—	1210	—	0	—	—	—	—	—	—	5	—	—
65	60	1.08	—	—	1150	—	—	—	—	—	—	—	—	0	—	—
30	60	1.44	—	—	690	—	—	—	—	—	—	—	—	2	—	—
20	100	2.70	—	—	1170	—	—	—	—	—	—	—	—	0	—	—
20	150	1.44	—	—	1330	—	0	—	—	—	—	—	—	0	—	—
30	0	1.80	—	—	1040	—	0	—	—	—	—	—	—	0	—	—
35	150	1.80	—	—	870	—	0	—	—	—	—	—	—	0	—	—
25	60	1.80	—	—	1070	—	—	—	—	—	—	—	—	4	—	—
60	40	1.44	—	—	1140	—	0	—	—	—	—	—	—	0	—	—
85	300	2.70	45	484	810	2.29	—	0.45	1.95	0.51	4.00	0.23	31	0	1	—
85	100	2.70	—	—	810	—	—	0.15	—	0.43	6.00	—	—	0	—	—
35	40	1.80	39	280	580	4.71	—	0.17	2.16	0.37	4.28	0.27	19	2	3	—
30	40	1.80	58	540	850	4.81	—	0.16	0.62	0.29	5.53	0.37	38	6	2	—
15	283	3.03	79	420	780	1.39	—	0.22	2.42	0.45	3.13	0.32	75	59	<1	—
40	20	0.72	—	—	600	—	—	—	—	—	—	—	—	15	—	—
10	350	3.60	—	—	600	—	—	—	—	—	—	—	—	12	—	—
30	40	1.44	—	—	580	—	—	—	—	—	—	—	—	4	—	—
30	40	0.36	—	—	580	—	—	—	—	—	—	—	—	30	—	—
45	80	2.70	—	—	580	—	—	—	—	—	—	—	—	21	—	—
35	40	1.44	—	—	600	—	—	—	—	—	—	—	—	0	—	—
10	200	1.80	—	—	310	—	—	—	—	—	—	—	—	0	—	—
25	200	1.44	—	360	890	—	—	—	—	—	—	—	—	12	—	—
15	200	1.80	—	240	880	—	—	—	—	—	—	—	—	0	—	—
40	350	1.08	—	430	810	—	—	—	—	—	—	—	—	1	—	—
65	150	2.70	—	—	1170	—	—	—	—	—	—	—	—	2	—	—
50	20	0.72	—	500	760	—	0	—	—	—	—	—	—	0	—	—
35	20	1.80	—	790	820	—	—	—	—	—	—	—	—	6	—	—
35	40	0.72	—	450	1190	—	0	—	—	—	—	—	—	0	—	—
30	80	0.72	—	480	690	—	—	—	—	—	—	—	—	0	—	—
35	60	0.36	—	370	640	—	—	—	—	—	—	—	—	0	—	—
30	20	0.36	—	310	620	—	—	—	—	—	—	—	—	0	—	—
20	200	0.36	—	260	670	—	0	—	—	—	—	—	—	0	—	—

H Appendix

Table H–1

Food Composition (Computer code number is for Wadsworth Diet Analysis program) (For purposes of calculations, use "0" for t, <1, <.1, <.01, etc.)

DA + Code	Food Description	Quantity	Measure	Wt (g)	H_2O (g)	Ener (kcal)	Prot (g)	Carb (g)	Dietary Fiber (g)	Fat (g)	Fat Breakdown (g) Sat	Mono	Poly
	CONVENIENCE MEALS—Continued												
11055	Lean Cuisine Everyday Favorites lasagna w/meat sauce	1	item(s)	291	—	300	19	41	3	8	4.00	2.00	0.50
9479	Lean Cuisine French bread deluxe pizza	1	item(s)	174	—	330	18	44	3	9	3.50	1.50	1.00
	Weight Watchers												
11164	Smart Ones chicken enchiladas suiza entree	1	serving(s)	255	—	270	15	33	2	9	3.50	—	—
11155	Smart Ones garden lasagna entree	1	item(s)	312	—	270	14	36	5	7	3.50	—	—
11187	Smart Ones pepperoni pizza	1	item(s)	158	—	390	23	46	4	12	4.00	—	—
31514	Smart Ones spicy penne pasta & ricotta	1	item(s)	289	—	280	11	45	4	6	2.00	—	—
31512	Smart Ones spicy szechuan style vegetables & chicken	1	item(s)	255	—	220	11	39	3	2	0.50	—	—
	BABY FOODS												
787	Apple juice	4	fluid ounce(s)	127	112	60	0	15	<1	<1	0.02	0.00	0.04
778	Applesauce, strained	4	tablespoon(s)	64	55	31	<1	8	1	<1	0.02	0.01	0.04
779	Bananas w/tapioca, strained	4	tablespoon(s)	60	50	34	<1	9	1	<.1	0.02	0.01	0.01
604	Carrots, strained	4	tablespoon(s)	56	52	15	<1	3	1	<.1	0.01	0.00	0.03
770	Chicken noodle dinner, strained	4	tablespoon(s)	64	55	42	2	6	1	1	0.38	0.55	0.30
801	Green beans, strained	4	tablespoon(s)	60	0.05	15	0.77	3.53	1.13	0.05	0.01	0	0.03
910	Human milk, mature	2	fluid ounce(s)	62	54	43	1	4	0	3	1.24	1.02	0.31
760	Mixed cereal, prepared w/whole milk	4	ounce(s)	114	85	128	5	18	1	4	2.19	1.25	0.43
772	Mixed vegetable dinner, strained	2	ounce(s)	57	50	23	1	5	1	<.1	0.00	0.00	0.06
762	Rice cereal, prepared w/whole milk	4	ounce(s)	114	85	131	4	19	<1	4	2.64	1.02	0.16
758	Teething biscuits	1	item(s)	11	1	43	1	8	<1	<1	0.17	0.16	0.09

PAGE KEY: H–2 = Breads/Baked Goods H–6 = Cereal/Rice/Pasta H–10 = Fruit H–16 = Vegetables/Legumes H–26 = Nuts/Seeds H–28 = Vegetarian H–30 = Dairy H–36 = Eggs H–38 = Seafood H–40 = Meats H–42 = Poultry H–44 = Processed meats H–46 = Beverages H–50 = Fats/Oils H–52 = Sweets H–52 = Sauces/Condiments/Spices H–56 = Mixed Foods/Soups/Sandwiches H–62 = Fast food H–80 = Convenience H–82 = Baby foods

Chol (mg)	Calc (mg)	Iron (mg)	Magn (mg)	Pota (mg)	Sodi (mg)	Zinc (mg)	Vit A (RAE) (μg)	Thia (mg)	Vit E (mg)	Ribo (mg)	Niac (mg)	Vit B_6 (mg)	Fola (μg)	Vit C (mg)	Vit B_{12} (μg)	Sele (μg)
30	200	1.08	—	590	650	—	—	—	—	—	—	—	—	5	—	—
20	100	1.80	—	390	630	—	—	—	—	—	—	—	—	9	—	—
50	250	1.08	—	—	660	—	—	—	—	—	—	—	—	4	—	—
30	350	1.80	—	—	610	—	—	—	—	—	—	—	—	6	—	—
45	450	1.80	—	320	650	—	55	—	—	—	—	—	—	5	—	—
5	150	2.70	—	250	400	—	—	—	—	—	—	—	—	6	—	—
10	150	1.80	—	—	730	—	—	—	—	—	—	—	—	2	—	—
0	5	0.72	4	115	4	0.04	1	0.01	0.76	0.02	0.11	0.04	0	73	0	<1
0	3	0.14	2	45	1	0.01	1	0.01	0.38	0.02	0.04	0.02	1	25	0	<1
0	3	0.12	6	53	5	0.04	1	0.01	0.36	0.02	0.11	0.07	4	10	0	<1
0	12	0.21	5	110	21	0.08	321	0.01	0.29	0.02	0.26	0.04	8	3	0	<1
10	17	0.41	9	89	15	0.35	70	0.03	0.14	0.04	0.46	0.04	7	<.1	<.1	2
0	23.39	0.44	14.39	94.8	1.2	0.12	27	0.01	0.24	0.05	0.2	0.02	21	3.11	0	0.18
9	20	0.02	2	31	10	0.10	38	0.01	0.55	0.02	0.11	0.01	3	3	<.1	1
12	250	11.85	31	226	53	0.81	28	0.49	—	0.66	6.56	0.07	12	1	<.1	—
0	12	0.19	6	69	5	0.09	77	0.01	—	0.02	0.29	0.04	5	2	0	<1
12	272	13.85	51	216	52	0.73	25	0.53	—	0.57	5.91	0.13	9	1	<1	4
0	29	0.39	4	36	40	0.10	3	0.03	0.05	0.06	0.48	0.01	5	1	<.1	3

H Appendix

WHO: Nutrition Recommendations Canada: Guidelines and Meal Planning

CONTENTS

This appendix first presents nutrition recommendations from the World Health Organization (WHO) and then provides details for Canadians on Canada's *Guide to Healthy Eating* and meal planning system.

Nutrition Recommendations from WHO

The World Health Organization (WHO) has assessed the relationships between diet and the development of chronic diseases. Its recommendations include:

- Total energy: sufficient to support normal growth, physical activity, and healthy body weight (body mass index = 20 to 22).
- Total fat: 15 to 30 percent of total energy.
- Saturated fat: less than 10 percent of total energy.
- Total carbohydrate: 55 to 75 percent of total energy.
- Added sugars: less than 10 percent of total energy.
- Protein: 10 to 15 percent of total energy.
- Salt: less than 5 grams/day, preferably iodized.
- Fruit and vegetables: at least 400 grams (almost 1 pound) daily.
- Physical activity: one hour per day of moderate intensity on most days of the week.

Canada's *Food Guide to Healthy Eating*

Figure I-1 presents the 1992 Canada's *Food Guide to Healthy Eating,* which interprets Canada's *Guidelines for Healthy Eating* (see Table 2-2 on p. 43) for consumers and recommends a range of servings to consume daily from each of the four food groups. The following publications, which are available from Health Canada, through its website, explain how to use the *Guide: Using the Food Guide; Food Guide Facts: Background for Educators and Communicators; Canada's Food Guide to Healthy Eating—Focus on Preschoolers: Background for Educators and Communicators;* and *Canada's Food Guide to Healthy Eating—Focus on Children Six to Twelve Years: Background for Educators and Communicators*. Figure I-2 presents Canada's Physical Activity Guide.

Canada's *Guidelines for Healthy Eating* and Canada's *Food Guide to Healthy Eating* are being reviewed for consistency with the new Dietary Reference Intakes. Check the website for the Health Canada Office of Nutrition Policy and Promotion, **www.hc-sc.gc.ca/hpfb-dgpsa/onpp-bppn/**, for the status of the review.

FIGURE I-1 Canada's *Food Guide to Healthy Eating*

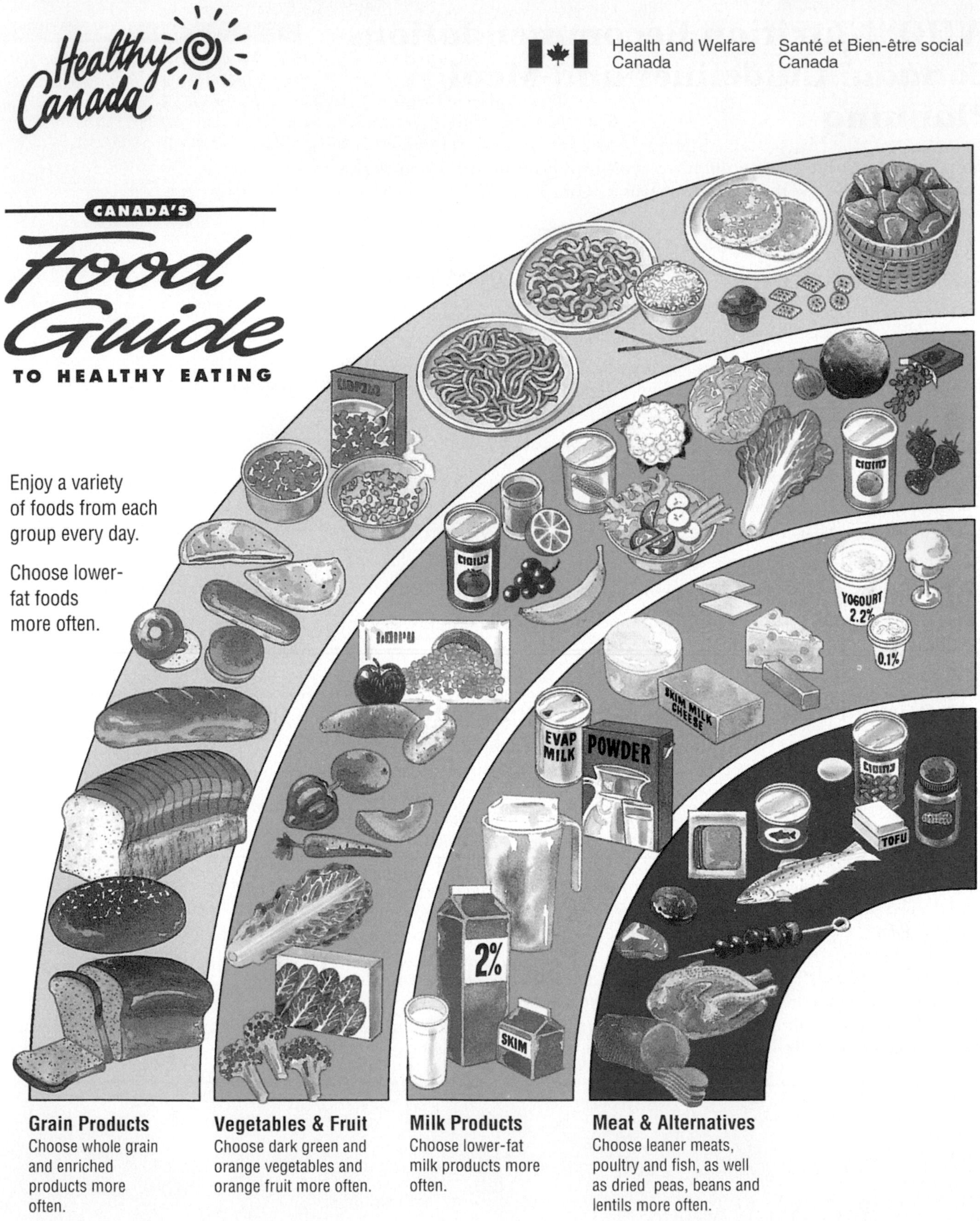

Healthy Canada
Health and Welfare Canada
Santé et Bien-être social Canada
CANADA'S
Food Guide
TO HEALTHY EATING
Enjoy a variety of foods from each group every day.
Choose lower-fat foods more often.
YOGOURT 2.2%
0.1%
SKIM MILK CHEESE
EVAP MILK
POWDER
TOFU
2%
SKIM
Grain Products
Choose whole grain and enriched products more often.
Vegetables & Fruit
Choose dark green and orange vegetables and orange fruit more often.
Milk Products
Choose lower-fat milk products more often.
Meat & Alternatives
Choose leaner meats, poultry and fish, as well as dried peas, beans and lentils more often.

FIGURE I-1 Canada's *Food Guide to Healthy Eating*—continued

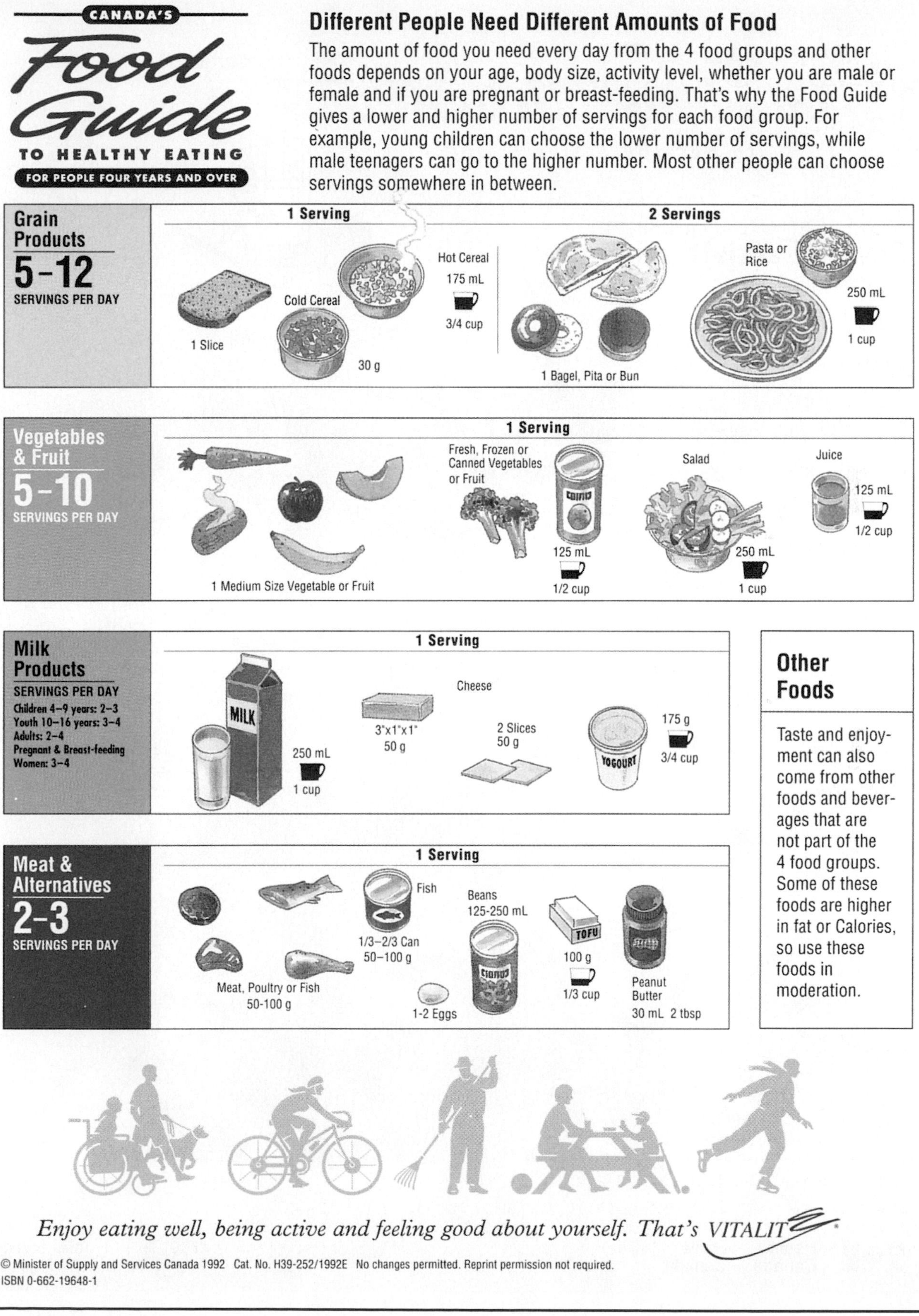

CANADA'S
Food Guide
TO HEALTHY EATING
FOR PEOPLE FOUR YEARS AND OVER
Different People Need Different Amounts of Food
The amount of food you need every day from the 4 food groups and other foods depends on your age, body size, activity level, whether you are male or female and if you are pregnant or breast-feeding. That's why the Food Guide gives a lower and higher number of servings for each food group. For example, young children can choose the lower number of servings, while male teenagers can go to the higher number. Most other people can choose servings somewhere in between.
Grain Products
5–12
SERVINGS PER DAY
1 Serving
1 Slice
Cold Cereal
30 g
Hot Cereal
175 mL
3/4 cup
2 Servings
1 Bagel, Pita or Bun
Pasta or Rice
250 mL
1 cup
Vegetables & Fruit
5–10
SERVINGS PER DAY
1 Serving
1 Medium Size Vegetable or Fruit
Fresh, Frozen or Canned Vegetables or Fruit
125 mL
1/2 cup
Salad
250 mL
1 cup
Juice
125 mL
1/2 cup
Milk Products
SERVINGS PER DAY
Children 4–9 years: 2–3
Youth 10–16 years: 3–4
Adults: 2–4
Pregnant & Breast-feeding Women: 3–4
1 Serving
MILK
250 mL
1 cup
Cheese
3"x1"x1"
50 g
2 Slices
50 g
YOGOURT
175 g
3/4 cup
Meat & Alternatives
2–3
SERVINGS PER DAY
1 Serving
Meat, Poultry or Fish
50-100 g
Fish
1/3–2/3 Can
50–100 g
1-2 Eggs
Beans
125-250 mL
TOFU
100 g
1/3 cup
Peanut Butter
30 mL 2 tbsp
Other Foods
Taste and enjoyment can also come from other foods and beverages that are not part of the 4 food groups. Some of these foods are higher in fat or Calories, so use these foods in moderation.
Enjoy eating well, being active and feeling good about yourself. That's VITALITÉ
© Minister of Supply and Services Canada 1992 Cat. No. H39-252/1992E No changes permitted. Reprint permission not required.
ISBN 0-662-19648-1

FIGURE I-2 Canada's Physical Activity Guide

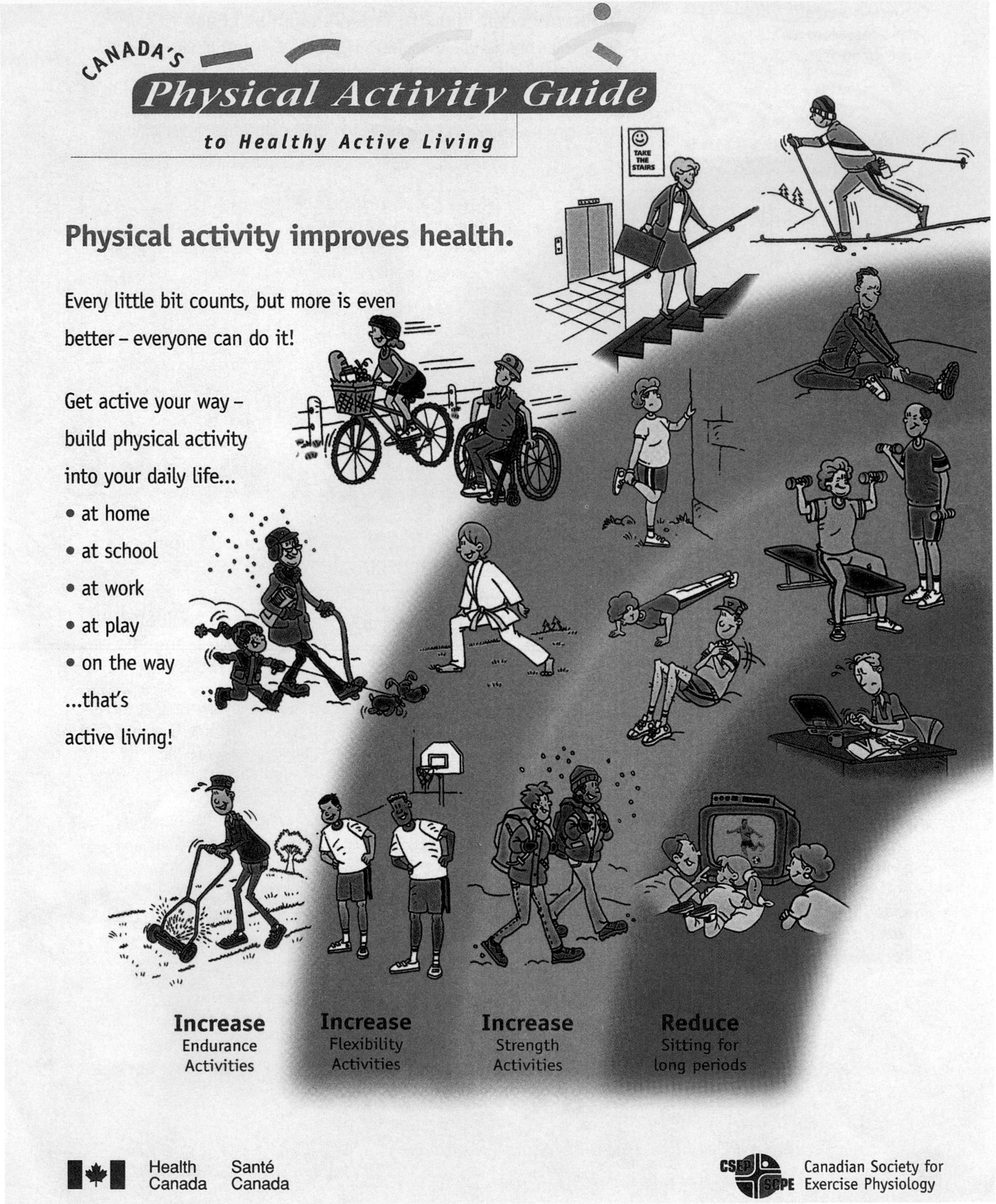
CANADA'S
Physical Activity Guide
to Healthy Active Living
TAKE THE STAIRS
Physical activity improves health.
Every little bit counts, but more is even better – everyone can do it!
Get active your way – build physical activity into your daily life...
• at home
• at school
• at work
• at play
• on the way
...that's active living!
Increase
Endurance Activities
Increase
Flexibility Activities
Increase
Strength Activities
Reduce
Sitting for long periods
Health Canada
Santé Canada
CSEP SCPE
Canadian Society for Exercise Physiology

FIGURE I-2 Canada's Physical Activity Guide—continued

Choose a variety of activities from these three groups:

Endurance

4-7 days a week
Continuous activities for your heart, lungs and circulatory system.

Flexibility

4-7 days a week
Gentle reaching, bending and stretching activities to keep your muscles relaxed and joints mobile.

Strength

2-4 days a week
Activities against resistance to strengthen muscles and bones and improve posture.

Starting slowly is very safe for most people. Not sure? Consult your health professional.

For a copy of the *Guide Handbook* and more information: **1-888-334-9769**, or **www.paguide.com**

Eating well is also important. Follow *Canada's Food Guide to Healthy Eating* to make wise food choices.

Get Active Your Way, Every Day—For Life!

Scientists say accumulate 60 minutes of physical activity every day to stay healthy or improve your health. As you progress to moderate activities you can cut down to 30 minutes, 4 days a week. Add-up your activities in periods of at least 10 minutes each. Start slowly... and build up.

Time needed depends on effort

Very Light Effort	Light Effort *60 minutes*	Moderate Effort *30-60 minutes*	Vigorous Effort *20-30 minutes*	Maximum Effort
• Strolling • Dusting	• Light walking • Volleyball • Easy gardening • Stretching	• Brisk walking • Biking • Raking leaves • Swimming • Dancing • Water aerobics	• Aerobics • Jogging • Hockey • Basketball • Fast swimming • Fast dancing	• Sprinting • Racing

Range needed to stay healthy

You Can Do It – Getting started is easier than you think

Physical activity doesn't have to be very hard. Build physical activities into your daily routine.

- Walk whenever you can – get off the bus early, use the stairs instead of the elevator.
- Reduce inactivity for long periods, like watching TV.
- Get up from the couch and stretch and bend for a few minutes every hour.
- Play actively with your kids.
- Choose to walk, wheel or cycle for short trips.
- Start with a 10 minute walk – gradually increase the time.
- Find out about walking and cycling paths nearby and use them.
- Observe a physical activity class to see if you want to try it.
- Try one class to start, you don't have to make a long-term commitment.
- Do the activities you are doing now, more often.

Benefits of regular activity:

- better health
- improved fitness
- better posture and balance
- better self-esteem
- weight control
- stronger muscles and bones
- feeling more energetic
- relaxation and reduced stress
- continued independent living in later life

Health risks of inactivity:

- premature death
- heart disease
- obesity
- high blood pressure
- adult-onset diabetes
- osteoporosis
- stroke
- depression
- colon cancer

ACTIVE LIVING

Cat. No. H39-429/1998-1E ISBN 0-662-86627-7

Canada's Physical Activity Guide to Healthy Active Living

Canada's Meal Planning for Healthy Eating

Beyond the Basics: Meal Planning for Healthy Eating, Diabetes Prevention and Management is Canada's system of meal planning.[1] Similar to the U.S. exchange system, *Beyond the Basics* sorts foods into groups and defines portion sizes to help people manage their blood glucose and maintain a healthy weight. Because foods that contain carbohydrate raise blood glucose, the food groups are organized into two sections—those that contain carbohydrate (presented in Table I-1) and those that contain little or no carbohydrate (shown in Table I-2). One portion from any of the food groups listed in Table I-1 provides about 15 grams of available carbohydrate (total carbohydrate minus fiber) and counts as one carbohydrate choice. Within each group, foods are identified as those to "choose more often" (generally higher in vitamins, minerals, and fiber) and those to "choose less often" (generally higher in sugar, saturated fat, or *trans* fat).

[1]The tables for the Canadian meal planning system are adapted from *Beyond the Basics: Meal Planning for Healthy Eating, Diabetes Prevention and Management,* copyright 2005, with permission of the Canadian Diabetes Association. Additional information is available from **www.diabetes.ca**.

● = choose more often
▲ = choose less often

TABLE I-1 Food Groups that Contain Carbohydrate

1 serving = 15 g carbohydrate or 1 carbohydrate choice

Food	Measure
Grains and starches: 15 g carbohydrate, 2 g protein, 0 g fat, 286 kJ (68 kcal)	
▲ Bagel, large	¼
▲ Bagel, small	½
▲ Bannock, fried	1.5″ × 2.5″
● Bannock, whole grain baked	1.5″ × 2.5″
● Barley, cooked	125 mL (½ c)
▲ Bread, white	30 g (1 oz)
● Bread, whole grain	30 g (1 oz)
● Bulgur, cooked	125 mL (½ c)
▲ Bun, hamburger or hotdog	½
▲ Cereal, flaked unsweetened	125 mL (½ c)
● Cereal, hot	¾ c
● Chapati, whole wheat (6″)	1
● Corn	125 mL (½ c)
● Couscous, cooked	125 mL (½ c)
▲ Crackers, soda type	7
▲ Croutons	⅔ c
● English muffin, whole grain	½
▲ French fries	10
● Millet, cooked	⅓ c
▲ Naan bread (6″)	¼
▲ Pancake (4″)	1
● Pasta, cooked	125 mL (½ c)
▲ Pita bread, white (6″)	1
● Pita bread, whole wheat (6″)	1
▲ Pizza crust (12″)	1/12
● Plantain, mashed	⅓ c
● Potatoes, boiled or baked	½ medium

(continued on the next page)

TABLE I-1 Food Groups that Contain Carbohydrate—continued

1 serving = 15 g carbohydrate or 1 carbohydrate choice

Food	Measure
Grains and starches: 15 g carbohydrate, 2 g protein, 0 g fat, 286 kJ (68 kcal)	
● Rice, cooked	⅓ c
● Roti, whole wheat (6″)	1
● Soup, thick type	250 mL (1 c)
● Sweet potato, mashed	⅓ c
▲ Taco shells (5″)	2
● Tortilla, whole wheat (6″)	1
▲ Waffle (4″)	1
Fruits:15 g carbohydrate, 1 g protein, 0 g fat, 269 kJ (64 kcal)	
● Apple	1 medium
● Apple sauce, unsweetened	125 mL (½ c)
● Banana	1 small
● Blackberries	500 mL (2 c)
● Cherries	15
● Fruit, canned in juice	125 mL (½ c)
▲ Fruit, dried	50 mL (¼ c)
● Grapefruit	1 small
● Grapes	15
● Kiwi	2 medium
▲ Juice	125 mL (½ c)
● Mango	½ medium
● Melon	250 mL (1 c)
● Orange	1 medium
● Other berries	250 mL (1 c)
● Pear	1 medium
● Pineapple	¾ c
● Plum	2 medium
● Raspberries	500 mL (2 c)
● Strawberries	500 mL (2 c)
Milk and alternatives: 15 g carbohydrate, 8 g protein, variable fat, 386-651 kJ (92-155 kcal)	
● Chocolate milk, 1%	125 mL (½ c)
● Evaporated milk, canned	125 mL (½ c)
● Milk, fluid	250 mL (1 c)
● Milk powder, skim	30 mL (2 tbs)
● Soy beverage, flavored	125 mL (½ c)
● Soy beverage, plain	250 mL (1 c)
● Soy yogurt, flavored	⅓ c
● Yogurt, nonfat, plain	¾ c
● Yogurt, skim, artificially sweetened	250 mL (1 c)
Other choices (sweet foods and snacks): 15 g carbohydrate, variable protein and fat	
▲ Brownies, unfrosted	2″ × 2″
▲ Cake, unfrosted	2″ × 2″
▲ Cookies, arrowroot or gingersnap	3–4
▲ Jam, jelly, marmalade	15 mL (1 tbs)
● Milk pudding, skim, no sugar added	125 mL (½ c)
▲ Muffin	1 small (2″)
▲ Oatmeal granola bar	1 (28 g)
● Popcorn, low fat	750 mL (3 c)
▲ Pretzels, low fat, large	7
▲ Pretzels, low fat, sticks	30
▲ Sugar, white	15 mL (3 tsp or packets)

TABLE I-2 Food Groups that Contain Little or No Carbohydrate

Food	Measure
Vegetables: To encourage consumption, most vegetables are considered "free"	
● Asparagus	
● Beans, yellow or green	
● Bean sprouts	
● Beets	
● Broccoli	
● Cabbage	
● Carrots	
● Cauliflower	
● Celery	
● Cucumber	
● Eggplant	
● Greens	
● Leeks	
● Mushrooms	
● Okra	
▲ Parsnips[a]	
▲ Peas[a]	
● Peppers	
▲ Rutabagas (turnips)[a]	
● Salad vegetables	
● Snow peas	
▲ Squash, winter[a]	
● Tomatoes	
Meat and alternatives: 0 g carbohydrate, 7 g protein, 3–5 g fat, 307 kJ (73 kcal)	
● Cheese, skim (<7% milk fat)	30 g (1 oz)
● Cheese, light (<17% milk fat)	30 g (1 oz)
▲ Cheese, regular (17–33% milk fat)	30 g (1 oz)
● Cottage cheese (1–2% milk fat)	50 mL (¼ c)
● Egg	1 large
▲ Fish, canned in oil	50 mL (¼ c)
● Fish, canned in water	50 mL (¼ c)
● Fish, fresh, cooked	30 g (1 oz)
● Hummus[b]	⅓ c
● Legumes, cooked[b]	125 mL (½ c)
● Meat, game, cooked	30 g (1 oz)

[a] These vegetables provide significant carbohydrate when more than 125 mL (½ c) is eaten.
[b] Legumes contain 15 g carbohydrate in a 125 mL (½ c) serving.

(continued on the next page)

TABLE I-2 Food Groups that Contain Little or No Carbohydrate—continued

Food	Measure
Meat and alternatives: 0 g carbohydrate, 7 g protein, 3–5 g fat, 307 kJ (73 kcal)	
● Meat, ground, lean, cooked	30 g (1 oz)
▲ Meat, ground, medium-regular, cooked	30 g (1 oz)
● Meat, lean, cooked	30 g (1 oz)
● Meat, organ or tripe, cooked	30 g (1 oz)
● Meat, prepared, low fat	30 g (1 oz)
▲ Meat, prepared, regular fat	30 g (1 oz)
▲ Meat, regular, cooked	30 g (1 oz)
● Peameal/back bacon, cooked	30 g (1 oz)
● Poultry, ground, lean, cooked	30 g (1 oz)
● Poultry, skinless, cooked	30 g (1 oz)
▲ Poultry/wings, skin on, cooked	30 g (1 oz)
● Shellfish, cooked	30 g (1 oz)
● Tofu (soybean)	½ block (100 g)
● Vegetarian meat alternatives	30 g (1 oz)
Fats: 0 g carbohydrate, 0 g protein, 5 g fat, 189 kJ (45 kcal)	
● Avocado	⅙
▲ Bacon	30 g (1 oz)
● Butter	5 mL (1 tsp)
▲ Cheese, spreadable	15 mL (1 tbs)
● Margarine, non-hydrogenated	5 mL (1 tsp)
▲ Mayonnaise, light	30 mL (2 tbs)
● Nuts	15 mL (1 tbs)
● Oil, canola or olive	5 mL (1 tsp)
● Salad dressing, regular	15 mL (1 tbs)
● Seeds	15 mL (1 tbs)
● Tahini	7.5 mL (½ tbs)
Extras: <5 g carbohydrate, 84 kJ (20 kcal)	
Broth	
Coffee	
Herbs and spices	
Ketchup	
Mustard	
Sugar-free soft drinks	
Sugar-free gelatin	
Tea	

Enteral Formulas

The large number of enteral formulas available allows health care professionals to meet a variety of their patients' medical needs, but also complicates the process of selecting an appropriate formula. The first step in narrowing the choice of formulas is to determine the patient's ability to digest and absorb nutrients. Table J-1 on pp. J-2 through J-3 lists examples of standard formulas for patients who can adequately digest and absorb nutrients, and Table J-2 on p. J-4 provides examples of hydrolyzed formulas for patients with limited ability to digest or absorb nutrients. Products promoted to the general public and intended primarily as oral supplements, such as Carnation Instant Breakfast® (Nestlé), Boost® (Mead Johnson), and Ensure (Ross), are not included as examples. Each formula is listed only once, although a formula may have more than one use. A high-protein formula, for example, may also be a fiber-containing formula. Tables J-3 through J-5 on p. J-5 list modular formulas.

The information listed in this appendix reflects the literature provided by manufacturers and does not suggest endorsement by the authors. Manufacturers frequently add new formulas, discontinue old ones, and change formula composition. Consult the manufacturers' literature and websites for updates and additional examples of enteral formulas. The following products are listed in this appendix:

- Mead Johnson Nutritionals:[a]
  - Kindercal® TF
- Nestlé Nutrition:[b]
  - Crucial®
  - Glytrol®
  - Nutren® 1.0
  - Nutren® 1.5
  - Nutren® 2.0
  - Nutren® Fiber
  - Nutren® Junior
  - NutriHep®
  - NutriRenal®
  - NutriVent®
  - Peptamen®
  - Peptamen Junior®
  - Probalance®
  - Replete®
- Novartis Medical Nutrition:[c]
  - Casec®
  - Choice DM® TF
  - Compleat® Pediatric
  - Comply®
  - Criticare HN®
  - Deliver® 2.0
  - Impact®
  - Impact® 1.5
  - Impact® Glutamine
  - Isocal®
  - Isocal® HN
  - Isocal® HN Plus
  - Isosource® Standard
  - Magnacal®
  - Renal®
  - MCT Oil®
  - Microlipid®
  - Novasource® Pulmonary
  - Novasource® Renal
  - Protain XL®
  - Resource® Diabetic
  - Ultracal® HN Plus
  - Vivonex® Pediatric
  - Vivonex® Plus
  - Vivonex® T.E.N.
- Ross Medical Nutritionals:[d]
  - Advera®
  - Alitraq®
  - Glucerna®
  - Jevity®
  - Nepro®
  - Optimental®
  - Osmolite®
  - Oxepa®
  - PediaSure®
  - Perative®
  - Polycose Liquid®
  - Polycose Powder®
  - ProMod®
  - Promote®
  - Promote® with Fiber
  - Pulmocare®

[a]Mead Johnson Nutritionals, www.meadjohnson.com, visited March 9, 2005.
[b]Nestlé Nutrition, www.nestleclinicalnutrition.com, visited March 9, 2005.
[c]Novartis Medical Nutrition, www.novartis.com, visited March 9, 2005.
[d]Ross Medical Nutritionals, www.ross.com, visited March 9, 2005.

TABLE J-1 Standard Formulas

Product[a]	Volume to Meet 100% RDI[b] (mL)	Energy (kcal/mL)	Protein or Amino Acids (g/L)	Carbohydrate (g/L)	Fat (g/L)	Osmolality[c] (mOsm/kg)	Notes
Lactose-Free, Standard Formulas							
Isocal®	1890	1.06	34	135	44	270	20% fat from MCT
Isosource® Standard	1165	1.20	43	170	39	490	50% fat from MCT
Nutren® 1.0	1500	1.00	40	127	38	315	25% fat from MCT
Osmolite®	2000	1.06	37	151	35	300	20% fat from MCT
Lactose-Free, Fiber-Containing Formulas							
Jevity®	1321	1.06	44	155	35	300	14 g fiber/L
Nutren® Fiber	1500	1.00	40	127	38	330	14 g fiber/L
ProBalance®	1000	1.20	54	156	41	350	10 g fiber/L
Promote® with Fiber	1000	1.00	63	138	28	380	14 g fiber/L
Lactose-Free, High-kCalorie Formulas							
Comply®	830	1.50	60	180	61	460	20% fat from MCT
Deliver® 2.0	1000	2.00	75	200	101	640	30% fat from MCT
Nutren® 1.5	1000	1.50	60	169	68	430	50% fat from MCT
Nutren® 2.0	750	2.00	80	196	104	745	75% fat from MCT
Lactose-Free, High-Protein Formulas							
Isocal® HN	1180	1.06	44	124	45	270	Low residue
Isocal® HN Plus	1000	1.20	54	156	40	400	Low residue
Promote®	1000	1.00	63	130	26	340	20% fat from MCT, low residue
Ultracal® HN Plus	1000	1.20	54	156	40	370	30% fat from MCT, 10 g fiber/L
Special-Use Formulas: Pediatric (1 to 10 years)							
Compleat® Pediatric	Varies[d]	1.00	38	130	39	380	Blenderized formula, 6.8 g fiber/L
Kindercal® TF	Varies[d]	1.06	30	135	44	345	12% fat from MCT
Nutren Junior®	Varies[d]	1.00	30	110	50	350	21% fat from MCT
PediaSure®	Varies[d]	1.00	30	110	50	430	
Special-Use Formulas: Glucose Intolerance							
Choice DM® TF	1120	1.06	45	119	51	300	14 g fiber/L
Glucerna®	1420	1.00	42	96	54	355	14 g fiber/L
Glytrol®	1400	1.00	45	100	48	380	15 g fiber/L; 20% fat from MCT
Resource® Diabetic	1180	1.06	63	100	47	300	13 g fiber/L
Special-Use Formulas: Immune System Support							
Impact®	1500	1.00	56	130	28	375	Enriched with arginine, nucleic acids, and omega-3 fatty acids
Impact® 1.5	1250	1.50	84	140	69	550	Same as above
Impact® Glutamine	1000	1.30	78	150	43	630	Same as above and enriched with glutamine; 10 g fiber/L

NOTE: MCT = Medium-chain triglycerides.
[a]Formulas come in ready-to-use (liquid) form unless specified under "Notes."
[b]RDI = Reference Daily Intakes, which are labeling standards for vitamins, minerals, and protein. Consuming 100 percent of the RDI will meet the nutrient needs of most people using the product.
[c]Osmolality may vary, depending on the flavorings added to a product.
[d]Depends on age of child.

TABLE J-1 Standard Formulas—continued

Product[a]	Volume to Meet 100% RDI[b] (mL)	Energy (kcal/ mL)	Protein or Amino Acids (g/L)	Carbohydrate (g/L)	Fat (g/L)	Osmolality[c] (mOsm/ kg)	Notes
Special-Use Formulas: Renal Failure							
Magnacal® Renal	1000	2.00	75	200	101	570	20% fat from MCT; intended for use once hemodialysis has been instituted
Nepro®	947	2.00	70	222	96	665	High-calcium, low-phosphorus; intended for use once dialysis has been instituted
Novasource® Renal	1000	2.00	74	200	100	700	Low in electrolytes; intended for use once dialysis has been instituted
NutriRenal®	750	2.00	70	205	104	650	50% fat from MCT; enriched with vitamins C and B_6, folate, zinc, and selenium; intended for use once dialysis has been instituted
Special-Use Formulas: Respiratory Insufficiency							
Novasource® Pulmonary	933	1.50	75	150	68	650	8 g fiber/L
NutriVent®	1000	1.50	68	100	94	330	55% kcal from fat, 40% fat from MCT
Oxepa	1420	1.50	63	106	94	493	55% kcal from fat, enriched with antioxidant nutrients
Pulmocare®	1420	1.50	63	106	93	475	55% kcal from fat, 20% fat from MCT, enriched with antioxidant nutrients
Special-Use Formulas: Wound Healing							
Protain XL®	1250	1.00	57	145	30	340	9 g fiber/L, 20% fat from MCT, enriched with vitamins A and C and zinc
Replete®	1000	1.00	62	113	34	300	Enriched with vitamins A and C and zinc; 25% fat from MCT

TABLE J-2 Hydrolyzed Protein Formulas

Product	Volume to Meet 100% RDI[a] (mL)	Energy (kcal/mL)	Protein or Amino Acids (g/L)	Carbohydrate (g/L)	Fat (g/L)	Osmolality[b] (mOsm/kg)	Notes
Special-Use Hydrolyzed Formulas: Hepatic Insufficiency							
NutriHep®	1000	1.50	40	290	21	790	Free amino acids, high in branched-chain amino acids, low in aromatic amino acids
Special-Use Hydrolyzed Formulas: HIV Infection or AIDS							
Advera®	1184	1.28	60	216	23	680	78% hydrolyzed and 22% intact protein, low fat, fiber added, enriched with vitamins E, C, B_6, B_{12}, and folate
Special-Use Hydrolyzed Formulas: Immune System Support							
Alitraq®	1500	1.00	53	165	16	575	Powder form; 47% free amino acids, 42% small peptides, enriched with glutamine and arginine
Crucial®	1000	1.50	94	135	68	490	Enriched with arginine, glutamine, antioxidant nutrients, and zinc
Perative®	1500	1.30	67	180	37	460	Enriched with arginine and beta-carotene
Vivonex® Plus	1800	1.00	45	190	7	650	Powder form; 100% free amino acids, enriched with glutamine, arginine, and branched-chain amino acids
Special-Use Hydrolyzed Formulas: Malabsorption							
Criticare HN®	1890	1.06	38	220	5	650	Mix of free amino acids and small peptides
Optimental®	1422	1.00	51	139	28	540	Contains MCT and arginine; enriched with vitamins C and E and beta-carotene
Peptamen®	1500	1.00	40	127	39	270	70% fat from MCT
Vivonex® T.E.N.	2000	1.00	38	210	3	630	Powder form; 100% free amino acids, enriched with glutamine
Special-Use Hydrolyzed Formulas: Pediatric (1 to 10 years)							
Peptamen Junior®	Varies[c]	1.0	30	138	39	260	60% fat from MCT; contains glutamine
Vivonex® Pediatric	Varies[c]	0.8	24	130	24	360	Powder form; 100% free amino acids

[a]RDI = Reference Daily Intakes, which are labeling standards for vitamins, minerals, and protein. Consuming 100 percent of the RDI will meeet the nutrient needs of most people using the product.
[b]Osmolality may vary depending on the flavorings added to a product.
cDepends on age of child.

TABLE J-3 Protein Modules

Product	Form	Major Protein Source	Energy (kcal/g)	Protein (g/100 g)
Casec®	Powder	Calcium caseinate	3.8	90
ProMod®	Powder	Whey protein	4.2	75

TABLE J-4 Carbohydrate Modules

Product	Form	Major Carbohydrate Source	Energy (kcal/mL or g)
Polycose Liquid®	Liquid	Hydrolyzed cornstarch	2.0 kcal/ml
Polycose Powder®	Powder	Hydrolyzed cornstarch	3.8 kcal/g

TABLE J-5 Fat Modules

Product	Form	Major Fat Source	Energy (kcal/mL)	Protein (g/100 mL)
MCT Oil®	Liquid	Medium-chain triglycerides	7.7	86
Microlipid®	Liquid	Safflower oil	4.5	51

Glossary

GENERAL

a- or *an-* = not or without
ana- = up
ant- or *anti-* = against
ante- or *pre-* or *pro-* = before
cata- = down
co- = with or together
bi- or *di-* = two, twice
dys- or *mal-* = bad, difficult, painful
endo- = inner or within
epi- = upon
extra- = outside of, beyond, or in addition
exo- = outside of or without
gen- or *-gen* = gives rise to, producing
homeo- = like, similar, constant unchanging state
hyper- = over, above, excessive
hypo- = below, under, beneath
in- = not
inter- = between, in the midst
intra- = within
-itis = infection or inflammation
-lysis = break
macro- = large or long
micro- = small
mono- = one, single
neo- = new, recent
oligo- = few or small
-osis or *-asis* = condition
para- = near
peri- = around, about
poly- = many or much
semi- = half
-stat or *-stasis-* = stationary
tri- = three

BODY

angi- or *vaso-* = vessel
arterio- = artery
cardiac or *cardio-* = heart
-cyte = cell
enteron = intestine
gastro- = stomach
hema- or *-emia* = blood
hepatic = liver
myo- or *sarco-* = muscle
nephr- or *renal* = kidney
neuro- = nerve
osteo- = bone
pulmo- = lung
ure- or *-uria* = urine
vena = vein

CHEMISTRY

-al = aldehyde
-ase = enzyme
-ate = salt
glyc- or *gluc-* = sweet (glucose)
hydro- or *hydrate* = water
lipo- = lipid
-ol = alcohol
-ose = carbohydrate
saccha- = sugar

Many medical terms have their origins in Latin or Greek. By learning a few common derivations, you can glean the meaning of words you have never heard of before. For example, once you know that "hyper" means above normal, "glyc" means glucose, and "emia" means blood, you can easily determine that "hyperglycemia" means high blood glucose. The derivations at left will help you to learn many terms presented in this glossary.

A

abscesses (ab-SESS-es): accumulated pus that is surrounded by inflamed tissue.

absorption: the uptake of nutrients by the cells of the small intestine for transport into either the blood or the lymph.

Acceptable Daily Intake (ADI): the estimated amount of a sweetener that individuals can safely consume each day over the course of a lifetime without adverse effect.

Acceptable Macronutrient Distribution Ranges (AMDR): ranges of intakes for the energy nutrients that provide adequate energy and nutrients and reduce the risk of chronic diseases.

accredited: approved; in the case of medical centers or universities, certified by an agency recognized by the U.S. Department of Education.

acesulfame (AY-sul-fame) **potassium:** an artificial sweetener composed of an organic salt that has been approved for use in both the United States and Canada; also known as **acesulfame-K** because K is the chemical symbol for potassium.

acetaldehyde (ass-et-AL-duh-hide): an intermediate in alcohol metabolism.

acetone breath: distinctive fruity odor on the breath of a person experiencing ketosis.

acetyl CoA (ASS-eh-teel, or ah-SEET-il, coh-AY): a 2-carbon compound (**acetate,** or **acetic acid,** shown in Figure 5-1 on p. 142) to which a molecule of CoA is attached.

achalasia (ack-a-LAY-zhah): an esophageal disorder characterized by weakened peristalsis and impaired relaxation of the lower esophageal sphincter.

achlorhydria (AY-klor-HYE-dree-ah): absence of gastric acid secretion.

acid controllers: medications used to prevent or relieve indigestion by suppressing production of acid in the stomach; also called **H2 blockers.** Common brands include Pepcid AC, Tagamet HB, Zantac 75, and Axid AR.

acid-base balance: the equilibrium in the body between acid and base concentrations (see Chapter 12).

acidophilus (ASS-ih-DOF-ih-lus) **milk:** a cultured milk created by adding *Lactobacillus acidophilus,* a bacterium that breaks down lactose to glucose and galactose, producing a sweet, lactose-free product.

acidosis (assi-DOE-sis): above-normal acidity in the blood and body fluids, which can depress the central nervous system and lead to disorientation and, eventually, coma.

acids: compounds that release hydrogen ions in a solution.

acne: a chronic inflammation of the skin's follicles and oil-producing glands, which leads to an accumulation of oils inside the ducts that surround hairs; usually associated with the maturation of young adults.

acupuncture (AK-you-PUNK-cher): a therapy that involves inserting thin needles into the skin at specific anatomical points, allegedly to correct disruptions in the flow of energy within the body.

acute erosive gastritis: a condition in which gastric mucosa is acutely injured, often by the toxic effects of chemical substances or radiation treatment. Damage may include hemorrhages, tissue erosion, and ulcers.

acute PEM: protein-energy malnutrition caused by recent severe food restriction; characterized in children by thinness for height (wasting).

acute renal failure: abrupt loss of kidney function over a period of hours or days.

acute respiratory distress syndrome (ARDS): respiratory failure triggered by acute lung injury; a medical emergency that causes dyspnea and pulmonary edema and usually requires assisted (mechanical) ventilation.

acute-phase proteins: plasma proteins released from the liver at the onset of acute infection. An example is **C-reactive protein,** which is considered one of the main indicators of severe infection and has antimicrobial effects.

acute-phase response: changes in body chemistry resulting from infection, inflammation, or injury; characterized by alterations in plasma proteins.

adaptive immunity: immunity that is specific for particular antigens; adapts to antigens in an individual's environment and is characterized by "memory" for particular antigens. Also called **acquired immunity.**

adaptive thermogenesis: adjustments in energy expenditure related to changes in environment such as extreme cold and to physiological events such as overfeeding, trauma, and changes in hormone status.

added sugars: sugars and syrups used as an ingredient in the processing and preparation of foods such as breads, cakes, beverages, jellies, and ice cream as well as sugars eaten separately or added to foods at the table.

adequacy (dietary): providing all the essential nutrients, fiber, and energy in amounts sufficient to maintain health.

Adequate Intake (AI): the average daily amount of a nutrient that appears sufficient to maintain a specified criterion; a value used as a guide for nutrient intake when an RDA cannot be determined.

adiponectin (AH-dih-poe-NECK-tin): a hormone produced by adipose cells that improves insulin sensitivity.

adipose (ADD-ih-poce) **tissue:** the body's fat tissue; consists of masses of triglyceride-storing cells.

adolescence: the period from the beginning of puberty until maturity.

adrenal glands: glands adjacent to, and just above, each kidney.

adrenocorticotropin (ad-REE-noh-KORE-tee-koh-TROP-in) **ACTH:** a hormone, so named because it stimulates *(trope)* the adrenal cortex. The adrenal gland, like the pituitary, has two parts, in this case an outer portion *(cortex)* and an inner core *(medulla)*. The realease of ACTH is mediated by **corticotropin-releasing hormone (CRH).**

advance directive: a written or oral instruction regarding one's preferences for medical treatment to be used in the event of becoming incapacitated.

advanced glycation end products (AGEs): compounds formed when glucose or glucose fragments combine with proteins. AGEs can damage tissues and lead to diabetic complications.

adverse reactions: unusual responses to food (including intolerances and allergies).

aerobic (air-ROE-bic): requiring oxygen.

AIDS (acquired immune deficiency syndrome): the end stage of HIV infection, in which severe complications develop. The cluster of mild symptoms that sometimes occurs early in the course of AIDS is called **AIDS-related complex (ARC).**

AIDS-defining illnesses: complications associated with the later stages of an HIV infection, including wasting; recurrent bacterial pneumonia; infections of the central nervous system, GI tract, and skin; and certain cancers.

albuminuria: the presence of albumin (protein) in the urine, a symptom of kidney disease.

alcohol: a class of organic compounds containing hydroxyl (OH) groups.

alcohol abuse: a pattern of drinking that includes failure to fulfill work, school, or home responsibilities; drinking in situations that are physically dangerous (as in driving while intoxicated); recurring alcohol-related legal problems (as in aggravated assault charges); or continued drinking despite ongoing social problems that are caused by or worsened by alcohol.

alcohol dehydrogenase (dee-high-DROJ-eh-nayz): an enzyme active in the stomach and the liver that converts ethanol to acetaldehyde.

alcoholism: a pattern of drinking that includes a strong craving for alcohol, a loss of control and an inability to stop drinking once begun, withdrawal symptoms (nausea, sweating, shakiness, and anxiety) after heavy drinking, and the need for increasing amounts of alcohol in order to feel "high."

alcohol-related birth defects (ARBD): malformations in the skeletal and organ systems (heart, kidneys, eyes, ears) associated with prenatal alcohol exposure.

alcohol-related neurodevelopmental disorder (ARND): abnormalities in the central nervous system and cognitive development associated with prenatal alcohol exposure.

aldosterone (al-DOS-ter-own): a hormone secreted by the adrenal glands that stimulates the reabsorption of sodium by the kidneys; involved in blood pressure regulation.

alitame (AL-ih-tame): an artificial sweetener composed of two amino acids (alanine and aspartic acid); FDA approval pending.

alkalosis (alka-LOE-sis): above-normal alkalinity (base) in the blood and body fluids.

allergen: any substance that triggers an inappropriate immune response.

allergy: an excessive and inappropriate immune reaction to a harmless substance.

alpha-lactalbumin (lact-AL-byoo-min): a major protein in human breast milk, as opposed to **casein** (CAY-seen), a major protein in cow's milk.

alpha-tocopherol: the active vitamin E compound.

alternative medicine: an approach that uses unconventional therapies *in place of* conventional medicine.

alveoli (al-VEE-oh-lie): air sacs in the lungs. One sac is an *alveolus.*

Alzheimer's disease: a degenerative disease of the brain involving memory loss and major structural changes in neuron networks; also known as *senile dementia of the Alzheimer's type (SDAT), primary degenerative dementia of senile onset,* or *chronic brain syndrome.*

amenorrhea (ay-MEN-oh-REE-ah): the absence of or cessation of menstruation. **Primary amenorrhea** is menarche delayed beyond 16 years of age. **Secondary amenorrhea** is the absence of three to six consecutive menstrual cycles.

American Dietetic Association (ADA): the professional organization of dietitians in the United States. The Canadian equivalent is Dietitians of Canada, which operates similarly.

amino acid pool: the supply of amino acids derived from either food proteins or body proteins that collect in the cells and circulating blood and stand ready to be incorporated in proteins and other compounds or used for energy.

amino acid scoring: a measure of protein quality assessed by comparing a protein's amino acid pattern with that of a reference protein; sometimes called **chemical scoring.**

amino (a-MEEN-oh) **acids:** building blocks of proteins. Each contains an amino group, an acid group, a hydrogen atom, and a distinctive side group, all attached to a central carbon atom.

ammonia: a compound with the chemical formula NH_3; produced during the deamination of amino acids.

amniotic (am-nee-OTT-ic) **sac:** the "bag of waters" in the uterus, in which the fetus floats.

amylase (AM-ih-lace): an enzyme that hydrolyzes amylose (a form of starch). Amylase is a *carbohydrase,* an enzyme that breaks down carbohydrates.

anabolism (an-ABB-o-lism): reactions in which small molecules are put together to build larger ones. Anabolic reactions require energy.

anaerobic (AN-air-ROE-bic): not requiring oxygen.

anaphylactic (an-AFF-ill-LAC-tic) **shock:** a life-threatening whole-body allergic reaction.

anaphylaxis: a severe allergic reaction that may include gastrointestinal upset, skin reactions, respiratory symptoms, and low blood pressure, possibly leading to shock.

anemia (ah-NEE-me-ah): literally, "too little blood." Anemia is any condition in which too few red blood cells are present, or the red blood cells are immature (and therefore large) or too small or contain too little hemoglobin to carry the normal amount of oxygen to the tissues. It is not a disease itself but can be a symptom of many different disease conditions, including many nutrient deficiencies, bleeding, excessive red blood cell destruction, and defective red blood cell formation.

anemia of chronic disease: anemia that develops in persons with chronic illness; may resemble iron-deficiency anemia even though iron stores are often adequate.

anencephaly (AN-en-SEF-a-lee): an uncommon and always fatal type of neural tube defect; characterized by the absence of a brain.

aneurysms (AN-you-riz-ums): abnormal enlargements or bulging of blood vessels (usually arteries) caused by damage to or weakness in the blood vessel wall.

angina (an-JYE-nah or AN-ji-nah) **pectoris:** a condition caused by ischemia in the heart muscle that results in discomfort or dull pain in the chest region. The pain often radiates to the left shoulder and arm, to the back, or into the throat, jaws, and teeth.

angiotensin (AN-gee-oh-TEN-sin): a hormone involved in blood pressure regulation. Its precursor protein is called **angiotensinogen;** is activated by **renin** (REN-in), an enzyme from the kidneys.

anions (AN-eye-uns): negatively charged ions.

anorexia (an-oh-RECK-see-ah) **nervosa:** an eating disorder characterized by a refusal to maintain a minimally normal body weight and a distortion in perception of body shape and weight.

antacids: medications used to relieve indigestion by neutralizing acid in the stomach. Common brands include Alka-Seltzer, Maalox, Rolaids, and Tums.

antagonist: a competing factor that counteracts the action of another factor. When a drug displaces a vitamin from its site of action, the drug renders the vitamin ineffective and thus acts as a vitamin antagonist.

anthropometric (AN-throw-poe-MET-rick): relating to measurement of the physical characteristics of the body, such as height and weight.

antibodies: large proteins produced by the immune system in response to the invasion of the body by foreign molecules (usually proteins called *antigens*). Antibodies combine with and inactivate the foreign invaders, thus protecting the body.

antidiuretic hormone (ADH): a hormone produced by the pituitary gland in response to dehydration (or a high sodium concentration in the blood). It stimulates the kidneys to reabsorb more water and therefore prevents water loss in urine (also called **vasopressin**). (This ADH should not be confused with the enzyme alcohol dehydrogenase, which is also sometimes abbreviated ADH.)

antigens: substances that elicit the formation of antibodies or an inflammation reaction from the immune system. A bacterium, a virus, a toxin, and a protein in food that causes allergy are all examples of antigens.

antioxidants: in the body, compounds that protect others from oxidation by being oxidized themselves, thereby decreasing the adverse effects of free radicals on normal physiological functions.

antipromoters: factors that oppose the development of cancers.

antiscorbutic (AN-tee-skor-BUE-tik) **factor:** the original name for vitamin C.

anus (AY-nus): the terminal outlet of the GI tract.

aplastic anemia: anemia characterized by the inability of bone marrow to produce adequate numbers of blood cells. Causes include genetic defects, viruses, irradiation treatment, and drug toxicity.

appendix: a narrow blind sac extending from the beginning of the colon that stores lymph cells.

appetite: the integrated response to the sight, smell, thought, or taste of food that initiates or delays eating.

arachidonic (a-RACK-ih-DON-ic) **acid:** an omega-6 polyunsaturated fatty acid with 20 carbons and four double bonds; present in small amounts in meat and other animal products and synthesized in the body from linoleic acid.

aromatherapy: inhalation of oil extracts from plants to cure illness or enhance health.

arteries: vessels that carry blood from the heart to the tissues.

artesian water: water drawn from a well that taps a confined aquifer in which the water is under pressure.

arthritis: inflammation of a joint, usually accompanied by pain, swelling, and structural changes.

artificial fats: zero-energy fat replacers that are chemically synthesized to mimic the sensory and cooking qualities of naturally occurring fats, but are totally or partially resistant to digestion.

artificial sweeteners: sugar substitutes that provide negligible, if any, energy; sometimes called **nonnutritive sweeteners.**

ascites: an accumulation of fluid in the abdominal cavity.

ascorbic acid: one of the two active forms of vitamin C (see Figure 10-15). Many people refer to vitamin C by this name.

-ase (ACE): a word ending denoting an enzyme. The word beginning often identifies the compounds the enzyme works on.

aspartame (ah-SPAR-tame or ASS-par-tame): an artificial sweetener composed of two amino acids (phenylalanine and aspartic acid); approved for use in both the United States and Canada.

aspiration: drawing in by suction or breathing; a common complication of enteral feedings in which foreign material enters the lungs, often from reflux of stomach contents.

aspiration pneumonia: a lung condition resulting from the abnormal entry of foreign material; caused by either bacterial infection or irritation of the lower airways.

atherosclerosis (ATH-er-oh-scler-OH-sis): a type of artery disease characterized by accumulations of lipid-containing material on the inner walls of the arteries (see Chapter 27).

atoms: the smallest components of an element that have all of the properties of the element.

ATP or **adenosine** (ah-DEN-oh-seen) **triphosphate** (try-FOS-fate): a common high-energy compound composed of a purine (adenine), a sugar (ribose), and three phosphate groups.

atrophic (a-TRO-fik) **gastritis** (gas-TRY-tis): chronic inflammation of the stomach accompanied by a diminished size and functioning of the mucous membrane and glands.

autoimmune: immune response directed against the body's own tissues.

autoimmune diseases: diseases characterized by an attack of immune defenses on the body's own cells.

autonomic nervous system: the division of the nervous system that controls the body's automatic responses. Its two branches are the **sympathetic** branch, which helps the body respond to stressors from the outside environment, and the **parasympathetic** branch, which regulates normal body activities between stressful times.

ayurveda: a traditional medical system from India that promotes the use of diet, herbs, meditation, massage, and yoga for preventing and treating illness.

B

B cells: lymphocytes that produce antibodies.

bacterial overgrowth: excessive bacterial colonization of the stomach or small intestine that interferes with normal digestion and absorption; may be caused by low gastric acidity, altered gastrointestinal motility, mucosal damage, or contamination.

bacterial translocation: the transfer of bacteria from the intestinal lumen to the bloodstream; increases risks of infection and sepsis.

balance (dietary): providing foods in proportion to each other and in proportion to the body's needs.

bariatric (BAH-ree-AH-trik) **surgery:** surgery that treats obesity

Barrett's esophagus: a condition in which esophageal cells that have been damaged by chronic exposure to stomach acid are replaced by cells that resemble those in the stomach or small intestine, sometimes becoming cancerous.

basal metabolic rate (BMR): the rate of energy use for metabolism under specified conditions: after a 12-hour fast and restful sleep, without any physical activity or emotional excitement, and in a comfortable setting. It is usually expressed as kcalories per kilogram body weight per hour.

basal metabolism: the energy needed to maintain life when a body is at complete digestive, physical, and emotional rest.

bases: compounds that accept hydrogen ions in a solution.

beer: an alcoholic beverage brewed by fermenting malt and hops.

behavior modification: the changing of behavior by the manipulation of antecedents (cues or environmental factors that trigger behavior), the behavior itself, and consequences (the penalties or rewards attached to behavior).

belching: the expulsion of gas from the stomach through the mouth.

beneficence (be-NEF-eh-sens): the act of performing beneficial services rather than harmful ones.

benign (bee-NINE): describes tumors that stop growing without intervention or can be removed surgically and most often pose no threat to health.

beriberi: the thiamin-deficiency disease.

beta-carotene (BAY-tah KARE-oh-teen): one of the carotenoids; an orange pigment and vitamin A precursor found in plants.

bicarbonate: an alkaline compound with the formula HCO_3 that results from the dissociation of carbonic acid; of particular importance in maintaining the body's acid-base balance. (Bicarbonate is also an alkaline secretion of the pancreas, part of the pancreatic juice.)

bifidus (BIFF-id-us, by-FEED-us) **factors:** factors in colostrum and breast milk that favor the growth of the "friendly" bacterium *Lactobacillus* (lack-toh-ba-SILL-us) *bifidus* in the infant's intestinal tract, so that other, less desirable intestinal inhabitants will not flourish.

bile: an emulsifier that prepares fats and oils for digestion; an exocrine secretion made by the liver, stored in the gallbladder, and released into the small intestine when needed.

binders: chemical compounds in foods that combine with nutrients (especially minerals) to form complexes the body cannot absorb. Examples include **phytates** (FYE-tates) and **oxalates** (OCK-sa-lates).

binge-eating disorder: an eating disorder whose criteria are similar to those of bulimia nervosa, excluding purging or other compensatory behaviors.

bioavailability: the rate at and the extent to which a nutrient is abosrbed and used.

bioelectrical or **bioelectromagnetic therapies:** therapies that involve the unconventional use of electric or magnetic fields to cure illness.

biofeedback: a technique in which individuals are trained to gain voluntary control of certain physiological processes, such as skin temperature or brain wave activity, to help reduce stress and anxiety.

biofield therapies: healing methods based on the belief that illnesses can be healed by manipulating energy fields that purportedly surround and penetrate the body. Examples include *acupuncture, qi gong,* and *therapeutic touch.*

biological value (BV): a measure of protein quality assessed by measuring the amount of protein nitrogen that is retained from a given amount of protein nitrogen absorbed.

biotin (BY-oh-tin): a B vitamin that functions as a coenzyme in metabolism.

blenderized formulas: dietary formulas that are made by blenderizing whole foods.

blind experiment: an experiment in which the subjects do not know whether they are members of the experimental group or the control group.

blood lipid profile: results of blood tests that reveal a person's total cholesterol, triglycerides, and various lipoproteins.

body composition: the proportions of muscle, bone, fat, and other tissue that make up a person's total body weight.

body mass index (BMI): an index of a person's weight in relation to height; determined by dividing the weight (in kilograms) by the square of the height (in meters).

bolus (BOH-lus): a portion; with respect to food, the amount swallowed at one time.

bolus (BOH-lus) **feeding:** delivery of about 250 to 500 mL of formula in less than 15 minutes.

bomb calorimeter (KAL-oh-RIM-eh-ter): an instrument that measures the heat energy released when foods are burned, thus providing an estimate of the potential energy of the foods.

bone density: a measure of bone strength. When minerals fill the bone matrix (making it dense), they give it strength.

bone marrow transplants: procedures that replace bone marrow that has been destroyed by cancer treatments; also used to treat certain types of cancers and blood disorders.

bone meal or **powdered bone:** crushed or ground bone preparations intended to supply calcium to the diet. Calcium from bone is not well absorbed and is often contaminated with toxic minerals such as arsenic, mercury, lead, and cadmium.

bottled water: drinking water sold in bottles.

botulism (BOT-chew-lism): an often fatal foodborne illness caused by the ingestion of foods containing a toxin produced by bacteria that grow without oxygen.

Bowman's (BO-mins) **capsule:** a cuplike component of the nephron that surrounds the glomerulus and collects the filtrate that is passed to the tubules.

bronchi, bronchioles: the main airways of the lungs. The singular form of bronchi is *bronchus.*

brown adipose tissue: masses of specialized fat cells packed with pigmented mitochondria that produce heat instead of ATP.

brown sugar: refined white sugar crystals to which manufacturers have added molasses syrup with natural flavor and color; 91 to 96% pure sucrose.

buffalo hump: the accumulation of fatty tissue at the base of the neck.

bulimia (byoo-LEEM-ee-ah) **nervosa:** an eating disorder characterized by repeated episodes of binge eating usually followed by self-induced vomiting, misuse of laxatives or diuretics, fasting, or excessive exercise.

C

calcitonin (KAL-see-TOH-nin): a hormone secreted by the thyroid gland that regulates (tones) calcium metabolism by lowering it when levels rise too high.

calcium: the most abundant mineral in the body; found primarily in the body's bones and teeth.

calcium rigor: hardness or stiffness of the muscles caused by high blood calcium concentrations.

calcium tetany (TET-ah-nee): intermittent spasm of the extremities due to nervous and muscular excitability caused by low blood calcium concentrations.

calcium-binding protein: a protein in the intestinal cells, made with the help of vitamin D, that facilitates calcium absorption.

calmodulin (cal-MOD-you-lin): an inactive protein that becomes active when bound to calcium. Once activated, it becomes a messenger that tells other proteins what to do. The system serves as an interpreter for hormone- and nerve-mediated messages arriving at cells.

calories: units by which energy is measured. Food energy is measured in **kilocalories** (1000 calories equal 1 kilocalorie), abbreviated **kcalories** or **kcal.** One kcalorie is the amount of heat necessary to raise the temperature of 1 kilogram (kg) of water 1°C. The scientific use of the term *kcalorie* is the same as the popular use of the term *calorie.*

cancer cachexia (ka-KEK-see-ah): a wasting syndrome associated with cancer and characterized by anorexia, tissue wasting, weight loss, and fatigue.

cancers: diseases that result from the unchecked growth of malignant tumors.

capillaries (CAP-ill-aries): small vessels that branch from an artery. Capillaries connect arteries to veins. Exchange of oxygen, nutrients, and waste materials takes place across capillary walls.

carbohydrates: compounds composed of carbon, oxygen, and hydrogen arranged as monosaccharides or multiples of monosaccharides. Most, but not all, carbohydrates have a ratio of one carbon molecule to one water molecule: $(CH_2O)_n$.

carbohydrate-to-insulin ratio: the amount of carbohydrate that can be handled per unit of insulin. On average, every 15 g of carbohydrate requires about 1 unit of rapid- or short-acting insulin.

carbonated water: water that contains carbon dioxide gas, either naturally occurring or added, that causes bubbles to form in it; also called *bubbling* or *sparkling water.* Seltzer, soda, and tonic waters are legally soft drinks and are not regulated as water.

carbonic acid: a compound with the formula H_2CO_3 that results from the combination of carbon dioxide (CO_2) and water (H_2O); of particular importance in maintaining the body's acid-base balance.

carcinogenic (CAR-sin-oh-JEN-ick): producing cancer. A substance that is capable of causing cancer is called a **carcinogen.**

cardiac cachexia: severe malnutrition associated with heart failure that causes weight loss and tissue wasting.

cardiac output: the volume of blood pumped by the heart within a specified period of time.

cardiopulmonary resuscitation (CPR): life-sustaining treatment that supplies oxygen and restores a person's ability to breathe and pump blood.

cardiovascular disease (CVD): a general term describing diseases of the heart and blood vessels.

carnitine (CAR-neh-teen): a nonessential nutrient made in the body from the amino acid lysine that helps transport long-chain fatty acids from the cytosol to the mitochondria for oxidation.

carotenoids (kah-ROT-eh-noyds): pigments commonly found in plants and animals, some of which have vitamin A activity. The carotenoid with the greatest vitamin A activity is beta-carotene.

carpal tunnel syndrome: a pinched nerve at the wrist, causing pain or numbness in the hand. It is often caused by repetitive motion of the wrist.

catabolism (ca-TAB-o-lism): reactions in which large molecules are broken down to smaller ones. Catabolic reactions release energy.

catalyst (CAT-uh-list): a compound that facilitates chemical reactions without itself being changed in the process.

cataracts (KAT-ah-rakts): thickenings of the eye lenses that impair vision and can lead to blindness.

cathartic (ka-THAR-tik): a strong laxative.

catheter: a thin tube placed within a narrow lumen (such as a blood vessel) or body cavity; can be used to infuse or withdraw fluids or to keep a passage open.

cations (CAT-eye-uns): positively charged ions.

CD4+ T cells: lymphocytes (white blood cells) that have a specific protein receptor (called CD4) on their surfaces; also known as *helper T cells.*

celiac (SEE-lee-ack) **disease:** a condition characterized by an abnormal immune reaction to wheat gluten that causes severe intestinal damage and nutrient malabsorption; also called **gluten-sensitive enteropathy** or **celiac sprue.**

cell: the basic structural unit of all living things.

cell cycle: the phases that a cell goes through from the time it is formed until it divides into two new cells.

cell differentiation (DIF-er-EN-she-AY-shun): the process by which immature cells develop specific functions different from those of the original that are characteristic of their mature cell type.

cell membrane: the thin layer of tissue that surrounds the cell and encloses its contents; made primarily of lipid and protein.

cell-mediated immunity: immunity conferred by T cells and macrophages.

cellulite (SELL-you-light or SELL-you-leet): supposedly, a lumpy form of fat; actually, a fraud. Fatty areas of the body may appear lumpy when the strands of connective tissue that attach the skin to underlying muscles pull tight where the fat is thick. The fat itself is the same as fat anywhere else in the body. If the fat in these areas is lost, the lumpy appearance disappears.

central nervous system: the central part of the nervous system; the brain and spinal cord.

central obesity: excess fat around the trunk of the body; also called **abdominal fat** or **upper-body fat.**

central veins: large-diameter veins located close to the heart.

Certified Diabetes Educator (CDE): a health care professional who specializes in diabetes management education. Certification is obtained from the National Certification Board for Diabetes Educators.

cesarean section: a surgically assisted birth involving removal of the fetus by an incision into the uterus, usually by way of the abdominal wall.

chelate (KEY-late): a substance that can grasp the positive ions of a metal.

chemotherapy: the use of drugs to arrest or destroy cancer cells; also called **chemotherapeutic** or **antineoplastic agents.**

chiropractic (KYE-roh-PRAK-tic): an alternative medical system based on the unproven theory that spinal manipulation can restore health.

chloride (KLO-ride): the major anion in the extracellular fluids of the body. Chloride is the ionic form of chlorine, Cl^-; see Appendix B for a description of the chlorine-to-chloride conversion.

chlorophyll (KLO-row-fil): the green pigment of plants, which absorbs light and transfers the energy to other molecules, thereby initiating photosynthesis.

cholecystectomy (KOH-lee-sis-TEK-toe-mee): surgical removal of the gallbladder.

cholecystitis (KOH-lee-sih-STY-tis): inflammation of the gallbladder, usually caused by obstruction of the cystic duct by gallstones.

cholecystokinin (coal-ee-sis-toe-KINE-in), or **CCK:** a hormone produced by cells of the intestinal wall. Target organ: the gallbladder. Response: release of bile and slowing of GI motility.

cholelithiasis (KOH-lee-lih-THIGH-ah-sis): formation of gallstones.

cholesterol (koh-LESS-ter-ol): one of the sterols containing a four-carbon ring structure with a carbon side chain.

cholesterol-free: less than 2 mg cholesterol per serving and 2 g or less saturated fat and *trans* fat combined per serving.

choline (KOH-leen): a nitrogen-containing compound found in foods and made in the body from the amino acid methionine. Choline is used to make the phospholipid lecithin and the neurotransmitter acetylcholine.

chromosomes: a set of structures within the nucleus of every cell that contains the cell's genetic material, DNA, associated with other materials (primarily proteins).

chronic bronchitis (bron-KYE-tis): persistent inflammation of the mucous membranes lining the main airways of the lungs. Chronic inflammation leads to narrower airways and difficulty with breathing.

chronic diseases: diseases characterized by a slow progression and long duration. Examples include heart disease, cancer, and diabetes.

chronic obstructive pulmonary disease (COPD): a group of lung diseases characterized by persistent obstructed airflow through the lungs and airways; include chronic bronchitis and emphysema.

chronic PEM: protein-energy malnutrition caused by long-term food deprivation; characterized in children by short height for age (stunting).

chronological age: a person's age in years from his or her date of birth.

chylomicrons (kye-lo-MY-cronz): the class of lipoproteins that transport lipids from the intestinal cells to the rest of the body.

chyme (KIME): the semiliquid mass of partly digested food expelled by the stomach into the duodenum.

cirrhosis (seer-OH-sis): advanced liver disease in which liver cells turn orange, die, and harden, permanently losing their function; often associated with alcoholism.

claudication: pain in the legs while walking; usually due to an inadequate supply of blood to muscles.

clear liquid diet: a diet that consists of foods that are liquid at room temperature and leaves almost no residue (undigested material) in the intestines after digestion and absorption.

clinically severe obesity: a BMI of 40 or greater or a BMI of 35 or greater with additional risk factors. A less preferred term used to describe the same condition is *morbid obesity.*

closed feeding systems: delivery systems in which formula comes prepackaged in containers that are ready to be attached to feeding tubes for administration.

CoA (coh-AY): coenzyme A; the coenzyme derived from the B vitamin pantothenic acid and central to energy metabolism.

coenzymes: complex organic molecules that work with enzymes to facilitate the enzymes' activity. Many coenzymes have B vitamins as part of their structures (Figure 10-1 in Chapter 10 illustrates coenzyme action).

colectomy: removal of a portion or all of the colon.

colitis (ko-LYE-tis): inflammation of the colon.

collagen (KOL-ah-jen): the protein from which connective tissues such as scars, tendons, ligaments, and the foundations of bones and teeth are made.

collaterals: blood vessels that enlarge in order to allow an alternate pathway for diverted blood.

collecting duct: the last portion of a nephron's tubule, where the final concentration of urine occurs.

colonic irrigation: the popular, but potentially harmful practice of "washing" the large intestine with a powerful enema machine.

colostomy (co-LAHS-toe-me): a surgical procedure that creates a stoma from the final segment of colon that remains after a colectomy.

colostrum (ko-LAHS-trum): a milklike secretion from the breast, present during the first day or so after delivery before milk appears; rich in protective factors.

complement: a group of plasma proteins that assist the activities of antibodies.

complementary and alternative medicine (CAM): diverse medical and health care systems, practices, and products that currently are not considered part of conventional medicine; also called *unconventional* or *unorthodox therapies.*

complementary medicine: an approach that uses unconventional therapies *in addition to,* and not simply as a replacement for, conventional medicine.

complementary proteins: two or more dietary proteins whose amino acid assortments complement each other in such a way that the essential amino acids missing from one are supplied by the other.

complex carbohydrates (starches and **fibers):** polysaccharides composed of straight or branched chains of monosaccharides.

compound: a substance composed of two or more different atoms—for example, water (H_2O).

conception: the union of the male sperm and the female ovum; fertilization.

condensation: a chemical reaction in which two reactants combine to yield a larger product.

conditionally essential amino acid: an amino acid that is normally nonessential, but must be supplied by the diet in special circumstances when the need for it exceeds the body's ability to produce it.

confectioners' sugar: finely powdered sucrose, 99.9% pure.

congestive heart failure (CHF): failure of the heart to pump adequate blood, resulting in fluid congestion in tissues and veins leading to the heart.

congregate meals: nutrition programs that provide food for the elderly in conveniently located settings such as community centers.

conservator: a person who takes responsibility for the person and property of an incompetent individual.

constipation: the condition of having infrequent or difficult bowel movements.

contamination iron: iron found in foods as the result of contamination by inorganic iron salts from iron cookware, iron-containing soils, and the like.

continuous ambulatory peritoneal dialysis (CAPD): the most common method of peritoneal dialysis; involves frequent exchanges of dialysate, which remains in the peritoneal cavity throughout the day.

continuous feedings: slow delivery of formula at a constant rate over an 8- to 24-hour period.

continuous parenteral nutrition: continuous administration of parenteral solutions over a 24-hour period.

continuous renal replacement therapy (CRRT): a slow, continuous method of removing solutes and fluid from blood by gently pumping blood across a filtration membrane over a prolonged time period.

control group: a group of individuals similar in all possible respects to the experimental group except for the treatment. Ideally, the control group receives a placebo while the experimental group receives a real treatment.

conventional medicine: diagnosis and treatment of diseases as practiced by medical doctors (M.D.) and doctors of osteopathy (D.O.) and assisted by allied health professionals such as registered nurses, pharmacists, and physical therapists; also called *Western, mainstream,* or *orthodox medicine.*

Cori cycle: the path from muscle lactic acid (which travels to the liver) to glucose (which can travel back to the muscle); named after the scientist who elucidated this pathway.

corn sweeteners: corn syrup and sugars derived from corn.

corn syrup: a syrup made from cornstarch that has been treated with acid, high temperatures, and enzymes that produce glucose, maltose, and dextrins. See also *high-fructose corn syrup (HFCS).*

cornea (KOR-nee-uh): the transparent membrane covering the outside of the eye.

coronary heart disease (CHD): irregular thickening of the coronary arteries that may eventually disrupt blood flow to heart tissue; also called **coronary artery disease.**

correlation (CORE-ee-LAY-shun): the simultaneous increase, decrease, or change in two variables. If A increases as B increases, or if A decreases as B decreases, the correlation is **positive.** (This does not mean that A causes B or vice versa.) If A increases as B decreases, or if A decreases as B increases, the correlation is **negative.** (This does not mean that A prevents B or vice versa.) Some third factor may account for both A and B.

correspondence schools: schools that offer courses and degrees by mail. Some correspondence schools are accredited; others are not.

cortical bone: the very dense bone tissue that forms the outer shell surrounding trabecular bone and comprises the shaft of a long bone.

coupled reactions: pairs of chemical reactions in which some of the energy released from the breakdown of one compound is used to create a bond in the formation of another compound.

covert (KOH-vert): hidden, as if under covers.

C-reactive protein: an acute-phase protein released from the liver during acute inflammation or stress.

cretinism (CREE-tin-ism): a congenital disease characterized by mental and physical retardation and commonly caused by maternal iodine deficiency during pregnancy.

critical pathways (or **clinical pathways**): interdisciplinary care plans for specific diagnoses, treatments, or procedures that merge the medical and nursing plans with those of other disciplines, such as physical therapy, nutrition, and mental health.

critical periods: finite periods during development in which certain events occur that will have irreversible effects on later developmental stages; usually a period of rapid cell division.

Crohn's disease: inflammatory bowel disease that usually occurs in the lower portion of the small intestine and the colon. Inflammation may pervade the entire intestinal wall.

cross-reactivity: an antibody reaction involving an antigen other than the one that induced the antibody's formation.

cryptosporidiosis (KRIP-toe-spo-rid-ee-OH-sis): a foodborne illness caused by the parasite *Cryptosporidium parvum.*

crypts (KRIPTS): tubular glands that lie between the intestinal villi and secrete intestinal juices into the small intestine.

cyanosis (sigh-ah-NOH-sis): a bluish cast in skin due to the color of deoxygenated hemoglobin. Cyanosis is most evident in persons with lighter, thinner skin; it is mostly seen on lips, cheeks, and ears and under nails.

cyberspace: a term coined by William Gibson referring to the nonphysical place where all Internet activity occurs.

cyclamate (SIGH-kla-mate): an artificial sweetener that is being considered for approval in the United States and is available in Canada as a tabletop sweetener, but not as an additive.

cyclic parenteral nutrition: administration of a parenteral solution over a 10- to 16-hour period.

cystic fibrosis: an inherited disorder that affects the transport of chloride across epithelial cell membranes; characterized by respiratory disease and pancreatic insufficiency.

cystinuria (SIS-tin-NOO-ree-ah): an inherited disorder characterized by excessive urinary excretion of several amino acids, including cystine.

cytokines (SIGH-toe-kines): proteins produced by white blood cells that regulate immune cell development and immune responses.

cytoplasm (SIGH-toh-plazm): the cell contents, except for the nucleus.

cytosol: the fluid of cytoplasm; contains water, ions, nutrients, and enzymes.

D

Daily Values (DV): reference values developed by the FDA specifically for use on food labels.

dawn phenomenon: morning hyperglycemia that is caused by the early morning release of growth hormone, which counteracts insulin's glucose-lowering effects.

deamination (dee-AM-eh-NAY-shun): removal of the amino (NH_2) group from a compound such as an amino acid.

debridement: the surgical removal of dead, damaged, or contaminated tissue resulting from burns or wounds; helps to prevent infection and hasten healing.

decision-making capacity: the ability to understand pertinent information and make appropriate decisions; known as **decision-making competency** within the legal system.

defecate (DEF-uh-cate): to move the bowels and eliminate waste.

defibrillation: life-sustaining treatment in which an electronic device is used to shock the heart and reestablish a pattern of normal contractions. Treatment is used when a heart has arrhythmias or has experienced cardiac arrest.

deficient: the amount of a nutrient below which almost all healthy people can be expected, over time, to experience deficiency symptoms.

dehydration: the condition in which body water output exceeds water input. Symptoms include thirst, dry skin and mucous membranes, rapid heartbeat, low blood pressure, and weakness.

delusions (dee-LOO-zhuns): false beliefs that are firmly maintained despite lack of proof or evidence to the contrary.

dementia (de-MEN-she-ah): irreversible loss of intellectual function.

denaturation (dee-NAY-chur-AY-shun): the change in a protein's shape and consequent loss of its function brought about by heat, agitation, acid, base, alcohol, heavy metals, or other agents.

dental calculus: mineralized dental plaque, often associated with inflammation and bleeding.

dental caries: decay of teeth.

dental plaque: a gummy mass of bacteria that grows on teeth and can lead to dental caries and gum disease.

dermatitis herpetiformis (DERM-ah-TIE-tis HER-peh-tih-FOR-mis): a gluten-sensitive disorder characterized by a severe skin rash. Gastrointestinal symptoms may be mild or absent.

dermis: the connective tissue layer underneath the epidermis that contains the skin's blood vessels and nerves.

dextrose: an older name for glucose.

DHA, or **docosahexaenoic** (DOE-cossa-HEXA-ee-NO-ick) **acid:** an omega-3 polyunsaturated fatty acid with 22 carbons and six double bonds; present in fish and synthesized in limited amounts in the body from linolenic acid.

diabetes (DYE-ah-BEE-teez) **mellitus:** a disorder of carbohydrate metabolism characterized by hyperglycemia and disordered insulin metabolism, usually resulting from inadequate or ineffective insulin.

diabetic coma: a coma that occurs in uncontrolled diabetes; may be due to diabetic ketoacidosis, the hyperosmolar hyperglycemic state, or excessive doses of insulin or certain antidiabetic drugs.

diabetic nephropathy: kidney damage associated with diabetes.

diabetic neuropathy: nerve degeneration associated with diabetes.

diabetic retinopathy: retinal damage associated with diabetes.

dialysate (dye-AL-ih-sate): solution used during dialysis to draw wastes and fluids from the blood.

dialysis: life-sustaining treatment in which a patient's blood is filtered using selective diffusion through a semipermeable membrane; substitutes for kidney function.

dialyzer (DYE-ah-LIZE-er): a machine used for hemodialysis; also called an *artificial kidney.*

diarrhea: the frequent passage of watery bowel movements.

diet: the foods and beverages a person eats and drinks.

diet history: a comprehensive record of a person's food intake and dietary practices.

diet manual: a book that specifies the foods allowed and restricted on modified diets and provides sample menus.

diet orders: specific instructions for dietary management; also called **diet prescriptions.**

diet progression: a change in diet as a patient's tolerances permit.

dietary folate equivalents (DFE): the amount of folate available to the body from naturally occurring sources, fortified foods, and supplements, accounting for differences in the bioavailability from each source.

Dietary Reference Intakes (DRI): a set of nutrient intake values for healthy people in the United States and Canada. These values are used for planning and assessing diets and include:

- Estimated Average Requirements (EAR).
- Recommended Dietary Allowances (RDA).
- Adequate Intakes (AI).
- Tolerable Upper Intake Levels (UL).

dietetic technician: a person who has completed a minimum of an associate's degree from an accredited university or college and an approved dietetic technician program that includes a supervised practice experience. See also *dietetic technician, registered (DTR).*

dietetic technician, registered (DTR): a dietetic technician who has passed a national examination and maintains registration through continuing professional education.

dietitian: a person trained in nutrition, food science, and diet planning. See also *registered dietitian.*

diffusion: movement of solutes from an area of high concentration to one of low concentration.

digestion: the process by which food is broken down into absorbable units.

digestive enzymes: proteins found in digestive juices that act on food substances, causing them to break down into simpler compounds.

digestive system: all the organs and glands associated with the ingestion and digestion of food.

dipeptide (dye-PEP-tide): two amino acids bonded together.

disaccharides (dye-SACK-uh-rides): pairs of monosaccharides linked together. See Appendix C for the chemical structures of the disaccharides.

disclosure: the act of revealing pertinent information. For example, clinicians should accurately describe the proposed tests and procedures, their benefits and risks, and alternative approaches.

discretionary kcalorie allowance: the kcalories remaining in a person's energy allowance after consuming enough nutrient-dense foods to meet all nutrient needs for a day.

disease-specific formulas: dietary formulas designed to meet the nutrient needs of patients with specific illnesses.

disordered eating: eating behaviors that are neither normal nor healthy, including restrained eating, fasting, binge eating, and purging.

dissociates (dis-SO-see-ates): physically separates.

distilled liquor or **hard liquor:** an alcoholic beverage made by fermenting and distilling grains; sometimes called *distilled spirits.*

distilled water: water that has been vaporized and recondensed, leaving it free of dissolved minerals.

distributive justice: the equitable distribution of resources.

diuresis (DYE-uh-REE-sis): excessive urine excretion.

diverticula (dye-ver-TIC-you-la): sacs or pouches that develop in the weakened areas of the intestinal wall (like bulges in an inner tube where the tire wall is weak).

diverticulitis (DYE-ver-tic-you-LYE-tis): infected or inflamed diverticula.

diverticulosis (DYE-ver-tic-you-LOH-sis): the condition of having diverticula. About one in every six people in Western countries develops diverticulosis in middle or later life.

dolomite: a compound of minerals (calcium magnesium carbonate) found in limestone and marble. Dolomite is powdered and is sold as a calcium-magnesium supplement, but may be contaminated with toxic minerals, is not well absorbed, and interacts adversely with absorption of other esssential minerals.

do-not-resuscitate (DNR) order: a request by a patient or surrogate to withhold cardiopulmonary resuscitation.

double-blind experiment: an experiment in which neither the subjects nor the researchers know which subjects are members of the experimental group and which are serving as control subjects, until after the experiment is over.

Down syndrome: a genetic abnormality that causes mental retardation, short stature, and flattened facial features.

drink: a dose of any alcoholic beverage that delivers ½ oz of pure ethanol.

drug: a substance that can modify one or more of the body's functions.

DTR: see *dietetic technician, registered.*

dumping syndrome: symptoms that result from the rapid emptying of an osmotic load from the stomach into the small intestine. Early symptoms include nausea, abdominal cramps, weakness, and diarrhea; later symptoms are those of hypoglycemia.

duodenal ulcers: peptic ulcers that develop in the duodenum.

duodenum (doo-oh-DEEN-um, doo-ODD-num): the top portion of the small intestine (about "12 fingers' breadth" long in ancient terminology).

durable power of attorney: a legal document (sometimes called a **health care proxy**) that gives legal authority to another (a *health care agent*) to make medical decisions in the event of incapacitation.

dysentery (DISS-en-terry): an infection of the digestive tract that causes diarrhea.

dyspepsia: a feeling of pain, bloating, or discomfort in the upper abdominal area, often called "indigestion"; a symptom of illness rather than a disease itself.

dysphagia (dis-FAY-gee-ah): difficulty in swallowing.

dyspnea (DISP-nee-a): shortness of breath.

E

eating disorders: disturbances in eating behavior that jeopardize a person's physical or psychological health.

eclampsia (eh-KLAMP-see-ah): a severe stage of preeclampsia characterized by convulsions.

edema (eh-DEEM-uh): the swelling of body tissue caused by excessive amounts of fluid in the interstitial spaces; seen in protein deficiency (among other conditions).

eicosanoids (eye-COSS-uh-noyds): derivatives of 20-carbon fatty acids; biologically active compounds that help to regulate blood pressure, blood clotting, and other body functions. They include *prostaglandins* (PROS-tah-GLAND-ins), *thromboxanes* (throm-BOX-ains), and *leukotrienes* (LOO-ko-TRY-eens).

electrolyte solutions: solutions that can conduct electricity.

electrolytes: salts that dissolve in water and dissociate into charged particles called ions.

electron transport chain: the final pathway in energy metabolism that transports electrons from hydrogen to oxygen and captures the energy released in the bonds of ATP.

element: a substance composed of atoms that are alike—for example, iron (Fe).

embolism (EM-boh-lizm): the obstruction of a blood vessel by an embolus, causing sudden tissue death.

embolus (EM-boh-lus): an abnormal particle, like a blood clot or air bubble, that travels in the blood.

embryo (EM-bree-oh): the developing infant from two to eight weeks after conception.

emergency kitchens: programs that provide prepared meals to be eaten on site; often called *soup kitchens.*

emetic (em-ETT-ic): an agent that causes vomiting.

emphysema (EM-fih-SEE-mah): disease characterized by progressive damage to alveoli (air sacs) in the lungs; causes difficulty with breathing.

empty-kcalorie foods: a popular term used to denote foods that contribute energy but lack protein, vitamins, and minerals.

emulsifier (ee-MUL-sih-fire): a substance with both water-soluble and fat-soluble portions that promotes the mixing of oils and fats in a watery solution.

endoplasmic reticulum (en-doh-PLAZ-mic reh-TIC-you-lum): a complex network of intracellular membranes. The **rough endoplasmic reticulum** is dotted with ribosomes, where protein synthesis takes place. The **smooth endoplasmic reticulum** bears no ribosomes.

end-stage renal disease (ESRD): an advanced stage of chronic renal failure in which dialysis or a kidney transplant is necessary to sustain life.

enemas: solutions inserted into the rectum and colon to stimulate a bowel movement and empty the lower large intestine.

energy: the capacity to do work. The energy in food is chemical energy. The body can convert this chemical energy to mechanical, electrical, or heat energy.

energy density: a measure of the energy a food provides relative to the amount of food (kcalories per gram).

energy-yielding nutrients: the nutrients that break down to yield energy the body can use.

enriched: the addition to a food of nutrients that were lost during processing so that the food will meet a specified standard.

enteral (EN-ter-al) **nutrition:** provision of nutrients using the GI tract, including the use of tube feedings and oral diets.

enteric-coated: refers to medications or enzyme preparations that can withstand gastric acidity and dissolve only at a higher pH.

enteropancreatic (EN-ter-oh-PAN-kree-AT-ik) **circulation:** the circulatory route from the pancreas to the intestine and back to the pancreas.

enterostomy (EN-ter-OSS-toe-mee): an opening into the GI tract through which a feeding tube can be passed.

enzymes: proteins that facilitate chemical reactions without being changed in the process; protein catalysts.

EPA, or **eicosapentaenoic** (EYE-cossa-PENTA-ee-NO-ick) **acid:** an omega-3 polyunsaturated fatty acid with 20 carbons and five double bonds; present in fish and synthesized in limited amounts in the body from linolenic acid.

epidemic (EP-ee-DEM-ick): the appearance of a disease (usually infectious) or condition that attacks many people at the same time in the same region.

epidermis (e-pi-DER-miss): the outer layer of the skin.

epiglottis (epp-ee-GLOTT-iss): cartilage in the throat that guards the entrance to the trachea and prevents fluid or food from entering it when a person swallows.

epinephrine (EP-ih-NEFF-rin): a hormone of the adrenal gland that modulates the stress response; formerly called **adrenaline.** When administered by injection, it counteracts anaphylactic shock by opening the airways and maintaining heartbeat and blood pressure.

epithelial (ep-i-THEE-lee-ul) **cells:** cells on the surface of the skin and mucous membranes.

epithelial tissue: the layer of the body that serves as a selective barrier between the body's interior and the environment (examples are the cornea, the skin, the respiratory lining, and the lining of the digestive tract).

erythrocyte (eh-RITH-ro-cite) **hemolysis** (he-MOLL-uh-sis): the breaking open of red blood cells (erythrocytes); a symptom of vitamin E–deficiency disease in human beings.

erythrocyte protoporphyrin (PRO-toe-PORE-fe-rin): a precursor to hemoglobin.

erythropoiesis (eh-RIH-throh-poy-EE-sis): production of red blood cells within the bone marrow.

erythropoietin (eh-RITH-ro-POY-eh-tin): a hormone made by the kidneys that stimulates red blood cell production.

esophageal (ee-SOF-ah-GEE-al): concerning the esophagus.

esophageal (ee-SOF-ah-GEE-al) **sphincter:** a sphincter muscle at the upper or lower end of the esophagus. The *lower esophageal sphincter* is also called the *cardiac sphincter.*

esophageal dysphagia: an inability to move a food bolus through the esophagus; usually due to an obstruction or a motility disorder.

esophagus (ee-SOFF-ah-gus): the food pipe; the conduit from the mouth to the stomach.

essential amino acids: amino acids that the body cannot synthesize in amounts sufficient to meet physiological needs (see Table 6-1).

essential fatty acids: fatty acids needed by the body, but not made by it in amounts sufficient to meet physiological needs.

essential nutrients: nutrients a person must obtain from food because the body cannot make them for itself in sufficient quantity to meet physiological needs; also called **indispensable nutrients.** About 40 nutrients are currently known to be essential for human beings.

Estimated Average Requirement (EAR): the average daily amount of a nutrient that will maintain a specific biochemical or physiological function in half the healthy people of a given age and gender group.

Estimated Energy Requirement (EER): the average dietary energy intake that maintains energy balance and good health in a person of a given age, gender, weight, height, and level of physical activity.

estrogens: hormones responsible for the menstrual cycle and other female characteristics.

ethanol: a particular type of alcohol found in beer, wine, and distilled liquor; also called *ethyl alcohol* (see Figure H7-1). Ethanol is the most widely used—and abused—drug in our society. It is also the only legal, nonprescription drug that produces euphoria.

ethical: in accordance with the accepted principles of right and wrong.

exchange lists: diet-planning tools that organize foods by their proportions of carbohydrate, fat, and protein. Foods on any single list can be used interchangeably.

experimental group: a group of individuals similar in all possible respects to the control group except for the treatment. The experimental group receives the real treatment.

extra lean: less than 5 g of fat, 2 g of saturated fat and *trans* fat combined, and 95 mg of cholesterol per serving and per 100 g of meat, poultry, and seafood.

extracellular fluid: fluid outside the cells. Extracellular fluid includes two main components—the interstitial fluid and plasma. Extracellular fluid accounts for approximately one-third of the body's water.

F

fad diets: popular eating plans that promise quick weight loss. Most fad diets severely limit certain foods or overemphasize others (for example, never eat potatoes or pasta or eat cabbage soup daily).

faith healing: the use of prayer or belief in divine intervention to promote healing.

false negative: a test result indicating that a condition is not present (negative) when in fact it is present (therefore false).

false positive: a test result indicating that a condition is present (positive) when in fact it is not (therefore false).

fat replacers: ingredients that replace some or all of the functions of fat and may or may not provide energy.

fat-free: less than 0.5 g of fat per serving (and no added fat or oil); synonyms include "zero-fat," "no-fat," and "nonfat."

fats: lipids that are solid at room temperature (70°F or 25°C).

fatty acid: an organic compound composed of a carbon chain with hydrogens attached and an acid group (COOH) at one end and a methyl group (CH_3) at the other end.

fatty acid oxidation: the metabolic breakdown of fatty acids to acetyl CoA; also called **beta oxidation.**

fatty liver: an early stage of liver deterioration seen in several diseases, including kwashiorkor and alcoholic liver disease. Fatty liver is characterized by an accumulation of fat in the liver cells.

fatty streaks: accumulations of cholesterol and other lipids along the walls of the arteries.

FDA (Food and Drug Administration): a federal agency that is responsible for, among other things, supplement safety, manufacturing, and information, including product labeling, package inserts, and accompanying literature. Another federal agency, the **FTC (Federal Trade Commission),** is responsible for, among other things, supplement advertising.

female athlete triad: a potentially fatal combination of three medical problems: disordered eating, amenorrhea, and osteoporosis.

fermentable: the extent to which bacteria in the GI tract can break down fibers to fragments that the body can use.

ferritin (FAIR-ih-tin): the iron storage protein.

fertility: the capacity of a woman to produce a normal ovum periodically and of a man to produce normal sperm; the ability to reproduce.

fetal alcohol effects (FAE): an older, less preferred, term used to describe both ARBD and ARND.

fetal alcohol syndrome (FAS): a cluster of physical, behavioral, and cognitive abnormalities associated with prenatal alcohol exposure, including facial malformations, growth retardation, and central nervous disorders.

fetal programming: the influence of substances during fetal growth on the development of diseases in later life.

fetus (FEET-us): the developing infant from eight weeks after conception until term.

fibers: in plant foods, the *nonstarch polysaccharides* that are not digested by human digestive enzymes, although some are digested by GI tract bacteria. Fibers include cellulose, hemicelluloses, pectins, gums, and mucilages and the nonpolysaccharides lignins, cutins, and tannins.

fibrinogen (fye-BRIN-oh-jen): a liver protein that promotes blood clot formation.

fibrocystic (FYE-bro-SIS-tik) **breast disease:** a harmless condition in which the breasts develop lumps, sometimes associated with caffeine consumption. In some, it responds to abstinence from caffeine; in others, it can be treated with vitamin E.

fibrosis (fye-BROH-sis): an intermediate stage of liver deterioration seen in several diseases, including viral hepatitis and alcoholic liver disease. In fibrosis, the liver cells lose their function and assume the characteristics of connective tissue cells (fibers).

filtered water: water treated by filtration, usually through *activated carbon filters* that reduce the lead in tap water, or by *reverse osmosis* units that force pressurized water across a membrane removing lead, arsenic, and some microorganisms from tap water.

filtrate: fluid that passes from blood through the capillaries of the glomeruli, eventually forming urine.

fistulas (FIST-you-las): abnormal passages between body tissues; may lead from one hollow organ to another or to an organ surface.

flatulence: the condition of having excessive intestinal gas, which causes abdominal discomfort.

flavonoids (FLAY-von-oyds): yellow pigments in foods; phytochemicals that may exert physiological effects on the body.

flaxseed: the small brown seed of the flax plant; used in baking, cereals, or other foods and valued by industry as a source of linseed oil and fiber.

fluid balance: maintenance of the proper types and amounts of fluid in each compartment of the body fluids (see also Chapter 12).

fluorapatite (floor-APP-uh-tite): the stabilized form of bone and tooth crystal, in which fluoride has replaced the hydroxyl groups of hydroxyapatite.

fluorosis (floor-OH-sis): discoloration and pitting of tooth enamel caused by excess fluoride during tooth development.

foam cells: swollen vascular cells that accumulate lipids.

folate (FOLE-ate): a B vitamin; also known as folic acid, folacin, or pteroylglutamic (tare-o-EEL-glue-TAM-ick) acid (PGA). The coenzyme forms are **DHF (dihydrofolate)** and **THF (tetrahydrofolate).**

follicle-stimulating hormone (FSH): a hormone that stimulates maturation of the ovarian follicles in females and the production of sperm in males. (The ovarian follicles are part of the female reproductive system where the eggs are produced.) The release of FSH is mediated by **follicle-stimulating hormone releasing hormone (FSH–RH).**

food allergy: an adverse reaction to food that involves an immune response; also called **food-hypersensitivity reaction.**

food and symptom diaries: records kept by a patient to determine the cause of an adverse reaction; include the specific foods and beverages consumed, symptoms experienced, and the timing of meals and symptom onset.

food aversions: strong desires to avoid particular foods.

food bank: a facility that collects and distributes food donations to authorized organizations feeding the hungry.

food cravings: strong desires to eat particular foods.

food frequency questionnaire: a survey of foods routinely consumed. Some questionnaires ask about the types of food eaten and yield only qualitative information, whereas others include questions about portions consumed and yield semi-quantitative data as well.

food group plans: diet-planning tools that sort foods into groups based on nutrient content and specify the amounts of foods that people should eat from each group.

food hypersensitivities: adverse reactions resulting from ingestion of a specific food.

food insecurity: limited or uncertain access to foods of sufficient quality or quantity to sustain a healthy and active life.

food insufficiency: an inadequate amount of food due to a lack of resources.

food intolerances: adverse reactions to foods that do not involve the immune system.

food pantries: programs that provide groceries to be prepared and eaten at home.

food poverty: hunger resulting from inadequate access to available food for various reasons, including inadequate resources, political obstacles, social disruptions, poor weather conditions, and lack of transportation.

food record: a detailed log of food eaten during a specified time period, usually several days. A food record may also include information regarding disease symptoms, physical activity, emotions, or medication use; also called a **food diary.**

food recovery: collecting wholesome food for distribution to low-income people who are hungry.

food security: certain access to enough food for all people at all times to sustain a healthy and active life.

food substitutes: foods that are designed to replace other foods.

foods: products derived from plants or animals that can be taken into the body to yield energy and nutrients for the maintenance of life and the growth and repair of tissues.

fortified: the addition to a food of nutrients that were either not originally present or present in insignificant amounts. Fortification can be used to correct or prevent a widespread nutrient deficiency or to balance the total nutrient profile of a food.

fraud or **quackery:** the promotion, for financial gain, of devices, treatments, services, plans, or products (including diets and supplements) that alter or claim to alter a human condition without proof of safety or effectiveness. (The word *quackery* comes from the term *quacksalver,* meaning a person who quacks loudly about a miracle product—a lotion or a salve.)

free radicals: unstable and highly reactive atoms or molecules that have one or more unpaired electrons in the outer orbital (see Appendix B for a review of basic chemistry concepts).

free: "nutritionally trivial" and unlikely to have a physiological consequence; synonyms include "without," "no," and "zero." A food that does not contain a nutrient naturally may make such a claim, but only as it applies to all similar foods (for example, "applesauce, a fat-free food").

French sizes: units of measure used for a feeding tube's outer diameter. One French unit is one-third of a millimeter.

fructose (FRUK-tose or FROOK-tose): a monosaccharide. Sometimes known as fruit sugar or **levulose,** fructose is found abundantly in fruits, honey, and saps.

fuel: compounds that cells can use for energy. The major fuels include glucose, fatty acids, and amino acids; other fuels include ketone bodies, lactic acid, glycerol, and alcohol.

functional foods: foods that contain physiologically active compounds that provide health benefits beyond basic nutrition; sometimes called *designer foods* or *nutraceuticals.*

futile: medical care that will not improve the medical circumstances of a patient.

G

galactose (ga-LAK-tose): a monosaccharide; part of the disaccharide lactose.

galactosemia (ga-LAK-toe-SEE-me-ah): an inherited disorder that affects galactose metabolism. Accumulated galactose causes damage to the liver, kidney, and brain in untreated patients.

gallbladder: the organ that stores and concentrates bile. When it receives the signal that fat is present in the duodenum, the gallbladder contracts and squirts bile through the bile duct into the duodenum.

gallstones: crystalline deposits that form in the gallbladder from cholesterol or bilirubin.

gangrene: death of tissue due to a deficient blood supply and/or infection.

gastrectomy (gas-TREK-ta-mee): the surgical removal of part of the stomach (partial gastrectomy) or the entire stomach (total gastrectomy).

gastric decompression: the use of suction to remove the stomach contents (including swallowed saliva, stomach secretions, and gas) of patients who have motility disorders or obstructions that prevent stomach emptying.

gastric glands: exocrine glands in the stomach wall that secrete gastric juice into the stomach.

gastric juice: the digestive secretion of the gastric glands of the stomach.

gastric residual: the volume of formula that remains in the stomach from a previous feeding.

gastric ulcers: peptic ulcers that develop in stomach tissue.

gastric-inhibitory peptide: a hormone produced by the intestine. Target organ: the stomach. Response: slowing of the secretion of gastric juices and of GI motility.

gastrin: a hormone secreted by cells in the stomach wall. Target organ: the glands of the stomach. Response: secretion of gastric acid.

gastritis: inflammation of stomach tissue

gastroesophageal reflux: the backflow of stomach acid into the esophagus, causing damage to the cells of the esophagus and the sensation of heartburn. **Gastroesophageal reflux disease (GERD)** is characterized by symptoms of reflux occurring two or more times a week.

gastrointestinal (GI) tract: the digestive tract. The principal organs are the stomach and intestines

gastroparesis: delayed stomach emptying.

gastrostomy (gas-TROSS-toe-mee): an opening into the stomach through which a feeding tube can be passed. A nonsurgical technique for creating a gastrostomy under local anesthesia is called **percutaneous endoscopic gastrostomy (PEG).**

gatekeepers: with respect to nutrition, key people who control other people's access to foods and thereby exert profound impacts on their nutrition. Examples are the spouse who buys and cooks the food, the parent who feeds the children, and the caregiver in a day-care center.

gene expression: the process by which a cell converts the genetic code into RNA and protein.

gene pool: all the genetic information of a population at a given time.

gene therapy: treatment for inherited disorders, in which DNA sequences are introduced into the chromosomes of affected cells, prompting the cells to express the protein needed to correct the disease.

genes: segments of DNA that contain the information needed to make proteins.

genetic counseling: support for families at risk of genetic disorders; involves diagnosis of disease, identification of inheritance patterns within a family, and review of reproductive options.

genome (GEE-nome): the full complement of genetic material (DNA) in the chromosomes of a cell. In human beings, the genome consists of 23 pairs of chromosomes.

genomics: the study of genomes.

gestation (jes-TAY-shun): the period from conception to birth. For human beings, the average length of a healthy gestation is 40 weeks. Pregnancy is often divided into thirds, called **trimesters.**

gestational diabetes: abnormal glucose tolerance during pregnancy.

ghrelin (GRELL-in): a protein produced by the stomach cells that enhances appetite and decreases energy expenditure.

gingiva (jin-JYE-va, JIN-jeh-va): the gums.

gingivitis (jin-jeh-VYE-tus): inflammation of the gums; characterized by redness, swelling, and bleeding.

gland: a cell or group of cells that secretes materials for special uses in the body. Glands may be **exocrine** (EKS-oh-crin) **glands,** secreting their materials "out" (into the digestive tract or onto the surface of the skin), or **endocrine** (EN-doe-crin) **glands,** secreting their materials "in" (into the blood).

glomerular filtration rate (GFR): the rate at which filtrate is formed within the kidneys, normally approximately 125 mL/min; usually estimated from equations based on serum creatinine levels and several other factors.

glomerulus (gloh-MEHR-yoo-lus): a tuft of capillaries within the nephron that filters water and solutes from blood as urine production begins (plural: *glomeruli*).

glucagon (GLOO-ka-gon): a hormone that is secreted by special cells in the pancreas in response to low blood glucose concentration and elicits release of glucose from liver glycogen stores.

glucocorticoids: hormones from the adrenal cortex that affect the body's management of glucose.

gluconeogenesis (gloo-co-nee-oh-GEN-ih-sis): the making of glucose from a noncarbohydrate source (described in more detail in Chapter 7).

glucose (GLOO-kose): a monosaccharide; sometimes known as blood sugar or **dextrose.**

glycated hemoglobin (HbA_{1c}): hemoglobin molecules to which glucose is attached. The percentage of such molecules is used to evaluate long-term glycemic control. Also called **glycosylated hemoglobin.**

glycemic: pertaining to blood glucose.

glycemic (gligh-SEEM-ic) **response:** the extent to which a food raises the blood glucose concentration and elicits an insulin response.

glycemic index: a method of classifying foods according to their potential for raising blood glucose.

glycerol (GLISS-er-ol): an alcohol composed of a three-carbon chain, which can serve as the backbone for a triglyceride.

glycogen (GLY-co-gen): an animal polysaccharide composed of glucose; manufactured and stored in the liver and muscles as a storage form of glucose. Glycogen is not a significant food source of carbohydrate and is not counted as one of the complex carbohydrates in foods.

glycolysis (gligh-COLL-ih-sis): the metabolic breakdown of glucose to pyruvate. Glycolysis does not require oxygen (anaerobic).

glycosuria (GLY-koh-SOOR-ee-ah): an abnormal amount of glucose in urine.

goblet cells: cells of the GI tract (and lungs) that secrete mucus.

goiter (GOY-ter): an enlargement of the thyroid gland due to an iodine deficiency, malfunction of the gland, or overconsumption of a goitrogen. Goiter caused by iodine deficiency is **simple goiter.**

goitrogen (GOY-troh-jen): a substance that enlarges the thyroid gland and causes **toxic goiter**. Goitrogens occur naturally in such foods as cabbage, kale, brussels sprouts, cauliflower, broccoli, and kohlrabi.

Golgi (GOAL-gee) **apparatus:** a set of membranes within the cell where secretory materials are packaged for export.

good source of: the product provides between 10 and 19% of the Daily Value for a given nutrient per serving.

gout: a metabolic disorder that results in excessive uric acid in the blood and urine and the deposition of uric acid in and around the joints, causing acute joint inflammation.

granulated sugar: crystalline sucrose; 99.9% pure.

growth hormone (GH): a hormone secreted by the pituitary that regulates the cell division and protein synthesis needed for normal growth. The release of GH is mediated by **GH-releasing hormone (GHRH).**

H

HACCP (Hazard Analysis and Critical Control Point): systems of food or formula preparation that identify food safety hazards and critical control points during foodservice procedures; pronounced *hassip.*

hard water: water with a high calcium and magnesium content.

Harris-Benedict equation: an equation that estimates basal energy expenditure.

HDL (high-density lipoprotein): the type of lipoprotein that transports cholesterol back to the liver from the cells; composed primarily of protein.

health care agent: a person given legal authority to make medical decisions for another in the event of incapacitation.

health claims: statements that characterize the relationship between a nutrient or other substance in a food and a disease or health-related condition.

healthy: a food that is low in fat, saturated fat, cholesterol, and sodium and that contains at least 10% of the Daily Values for vitamin A, vitamin C, iron, calcium, protein, or fiber.

Healthy Eating Index: a measure developed by the USDA for assessing how well a diet conforms to the recommendations of the USDA Food Guide and the *Dietary Guidelines for Americans.*

Healthy People: a national public health initiative under the jurisdiction of the U.S. Department of Health and Human Services (DHHS) that identifies the most significant preventable threats to health and focuses efforts toward eliminating them.

heartburn: a burning sensation in the chest area caused by backflow of stomach acid into the esophagus.

heavy metals: any of a number of mineral ions such as mercury and lead, so called because they are of relatively high atomic weight. Many heavy metals are poisonous.

Heimlich (HIME-lick) **maneuver (abdominal thrust maneuver):** a technique for dislodging an object from the trachea of a choking person (see Figure H3-2); named for the physician who developed it.

Helicobacter pylori: a type of bacterium that colonizes gastric mucosa; a major cause of gastritis and peptic ulcer disease.

hematocrit (hee-MAT-oh-krit): measurement of the volume of the red blood cells packed by centrifuge in a given volume of blood.

hematuria (HE-mah-TOO-ree-ah): blood in the urine.

heme (HEEM): the iron-holding part of the hemoglobin and myoglobin proteins. About 40% of the iron in meat, fish, and poultry is bound into heme; the other 60% is **nonheme** iron.

hemochromatosis (HE-moh-KRO-ma-toe-sis): a hereditary defect in iron absorption characterized by deposits of iron-containing pigment in many tissues, with tissue damage.

hemodialysis (HE-moh-dye-AL-ih-sis): removal of fluids and wastes from blood by passing the blood through a dialyzer.

hemofiltration: removal of fluid and solutes by pumping blood across a membrane; no osmotic gradients are created during the process. Also called **diafiltration.**

hemoglobin (HE-moh-GLOW-bin): the globular protein of the red blood cells that carries oxygen from the lungs to the cells throughout the body.

hemolytic (HE-moh-LIT-ick) **anemia:** the condition of having too few red blood cells as a result of erythrocyte hemolysis.

hemophilia (HE-moh-FEEL-ee-ah): inherited bleeding disorders characterized by deficiency or absence of plasma proteins needed for clotting blood.

hemorrhage: extremely severe bleeding; a copious flow of blood from blood vessels.

hemorrhagic (hem-oh-RAJ-ik) **disease:** a disease characterized by excessive bleeding.

hemorrhoids (HEM-oh-royds): painful swelling of the veins surrounding the rectum.

hemosiderin (heem-oh-SID-er-in): an iron storage protein primarily made in times of iron overload.

hemosiderosis (HE-moh-sid-er-OH-sis): a condition characterized by the deposition of hemosiderin in the liver and other tissues.

hepatic coma: loss of consciousness resulting from severe liver disease.

hepatic encephalopathy (en-SEF-ah-LOP-ah-thee): condition characterized by altered neurological functioning, including personality changes, reduced mental abilities, and disturbances in motor function.

hepatic vein: the vein that collects blood from the liver capillaries and returns it to the heart.

hepatitis (hep-ah-TIE-tis): inflammation of the liver.

herpes simplex virus: a common virus that can cause mouth lesions in HIV-infected individuals.

hiatal hernia: a condition in which the upper portion of the stomach protrudes above the diaphragm. Most cases are asymptomatic.

hiccups (HICK-ups): repeated cough-like sounds and jerks that are produced when an involuntary spasm of the diaphragm muscle sucks air down the windpipe; also spelled *hiccoughs.*

high: 20% or more of the Daily Value for a given nutrient per serving; synonyms include "rich in" or "excellent source."

high fiber: 5 g or more fiber per serving. A high-fiber claim made on a food that contains more than 3 g fat per serving and per 100 g of food must also declare total fat.

high potency: 100% or more of the Daily Value for the nutrient in a single supplement and for at least two-thirds of the nutrients in a multinutrient supplement.

high-fructose corn syrup (HFCS): a syrup made from cornstarch that has been treated with an enzyme that converts some of the glucose to the sweeter fructose; made especially for use in processed foods and beverages, where it is the predominant sweetener. With a chemical structure similar to sucrose, HFCS has a fructose content of 42, 55, or 90%, with glucose making up the remainder.

high-quality proteins: dietary proteins containing all the essential amino acids in relatively the same amounts that human beings require. They may also contain nonessential amino acids.

high-risk pregnancy: a pregnancy characterized by indicators that make it likely the birth will be surrounded by problems such as premature delivery, difficult birth, retarded growth, birth defects, and early infant death.

histamine (HISS-tah-mean or HISS-tah-men): a substance produced by cells of the immune system as part of a local immune reaction to an antigen; participates in causing inflammation.

histamine-2-receptor blocking agents: a class of drugs that suppress acid secretion by inhibiting receptors on acid-producing cells (commonly called H2-blockers). Examples include cimetidine (Tagamet), ranitidine (Zantac), and famotidine (Pepcid).

HIV (human immunodeficiency virus): the virus that causes AIDS. The infection progresses to become an immune system disorder that leaves its victims defenseless against numerous infections.

hives: an allergic reaction characterized by raised, swollen patches of skin or mucous membrane and associated with intense itching; also called **urticaria.**

HIV-lipodystrophy (LIP-oh-DIS-tro-fee) **syndrome:** a collection of abnormalities in fat and glucose metabolism that result from drug treatments for HIV; includes body fat redistribution, abnormal lipid levels, and insulin resistance. The accumulation of abdominal fat is sometimes called *protease paunch.*

homeopathic (HO-mee-oh-PATH-ic) **medicine:** a practice based on the theory that "like cures like"; that is, substances believed to cause certain symptoms are prescribed for curing the same symptoms, but are given in extremely diluted amounts.

homeostasis (HOME-ee-oh-STAY-sis): the maintenance of constant internal conditions (such as blood chemistry, temperature, and blood pressure) by the body's control systems. A homeostatic system is constantly reacting to external forces so as to maintain limits set by the body's needs.

honey: sugar (mostly sucrose) formed from nectar gathered by bees. An enzyme splits the sucrose into glucose and fructose. Composition and flavor vary, but honey always contains a mixture of sucrose, fructose, and glucose.

hormones: chemical messengers. Hormones are secreted by a variety of glands in response to altered conditions in the body. Each hormone travels to one or more specific target tissues or organs, where it elicits a specific response to maintain homeostasis.

hormone-sensitive lipase: an enzyme inside adipose cells that responds to the body's need for fuel by hydrolyzing triglycerides so that their parts (glycerol and fatty acids) escape into the general circulation and thus become available to other cells for fuel. The signals to which this enzyme responds include epinephrine and glucagon, which oppose insulin (see Chapter 4).

humoral immunity: immunity conferred by B cells, which produce and release antibodies into body fluids.

hunger: the painful sensation caused by a lack of food that initiates food-seeking behavior.

hydrochloric acid: an acid composed of hydrogen and chloride atoms (HCl). The gastric glands normally produce this acid.

hydrogenation (HIGH-dro-gen-AY-shun or high-DROJ-eh-NAY-shun): a chemical process by which hydrogens are added to monounsaturated or polyunsaturated fatty acids to reduce the number of double bonds, making the fats more saturated (solid) and more resistant to oxidation (protecting against rancidity). Hydrogenation produces *trans*-fatty acids.

hydrolysis (high-DROL-ih-sis): a chemical reaction in which a major reactant is split into two products, with the addition of a hydrogen atom (H) to one and a hydroxyl group (OH) to the other (from water, H_2O). (The noun is **hydrolysis;** the verb is **hydrolyze.**)

hydrolyzed formulas: dietary formulas that contain macronutrients that have been partially or fully hydrolyzed; also called **monomeric, defined,** or **elemental formulas.**

hydrophilic (high-dro-FIL-ick): a term referring to water-loving, or water-soluble, substances.

hydrophobic (high-dro-FOE-bick): a term referring to water-fearing, or non-water-soluble, substances; also known as **lipophilic** (fat loving).

hydroxyapatite (high-drox-ee-APP-ah-tite): crystals made of calcium and phosphorus.

hyperactivity: inattentive and impulsive behavior that is more frequent and severe than is typical of others a similar age; professionally called **attention-deficit/ hyperactivity disorder (ADHD).**

hypercalcemia (HIGH-per-kal-SEE-me-ah): elevated serum calcium levels.

hypercalciuria (HIGH-per-kal-see-YOO-ree-ah): an excessive amount of calcium in urine.

hypercapnia (high-per-CAP-nee-ah): excess carbon dioxide in the blood.

hyperglycemia: elevated blood glucose concentrations.

hyperkalemia (HIGH-per-ka-LEE-me-ah): elevated serum potassium levels.

hypermetabolism: a higher-than-normal metabolic rate.

hyperosmolar hyperglycemic state: extreme hyperglycemia that is associated with hyperosmolar blood, dehydration, and altered mental status; formerly called **hyperglycemic hyperosmolar nonketotic coma.**

hyperoxaluria (HIGH-per-OX-al-YOO-ree-ah): an excessive amount of oxalate in urine.

hyperphosphatemia (HIGH-per-fos-fa-TEE-me-ah): elevated serum phosphate levels.

hypersensitivity: immune responses that are excessive or inappropriate. One type of hypersensitivity is *allergy.*

hypertonic formula: a formula with an osmolality greater than that of blood serum.

hypertriglyceridemia (HYE-per-try-GLISS-er-eye-DEEM-ee-ah): elevated blood triglyceride levels.

hypnotherapy: a technique that uses hypnosis and the power of suggestion to improve health behaviors, relieve pain, and promote healing.

hypoallergenic formulas: clinically tested infant formulas that do not provoke reactions in 90% of infants or children with confirmed cow's milk allergy. Like all infant formulas, hypoallergenic formulas must demonstrate nutritional suitability to support infant growth and development. Extensively hydrolyzed and free amino acid–based formulas are examples.

hypochlorhydria (HYE-po-klor-HYE-dree-ah): a reduction in gastric acid secretion.

hypoglycemia (HIGH-po-gligh-SEE-me-ah): an abnormally low blood glucose concentration.

hypokalemia (HIGH-po-ka-LEE-me-ah): low serum potassium levels.

hypothalamus (high-po-THAL-ah-mus): a brain center that controls activities such as maintenance of water balance, regulation of body temperature, and control of appetite.

hypothesis (hi-POTH-eh-sis): an unproven statement that tentatively explains the relationships between two or more variables.

hypoxemia (high-pox-EE-me-ah): a low level of oxygen in the blood.

hypoxia (high-pox-EE-ah): a low amount of oxygen in body tissues.

I

ileocecal (ill-ee-oh-SEEK-ul) **valve:** the sphincter separating the small and large intestines.

ileostomy (ill-ee-OS-toe-me): a surgical procedure that creates a stoma using the ileum.

ileum (ILL-ee-um): the last segment of the small intestine.

ileus: obstruction of the intestine caused by disordered intestinal motility.

imagery: the use of mental images of things or events to aid relaxation or promote self-healing.

imitation foods: foods that substitute for and resemble another food, but are nutritionally inferior to it with respect to vitamin, mineral, or protein content. If the substitute is not inferior to the food it resembles and if its name provides an accurate description of the product, it need not be labeled "imitation."

immune system: the body's defense system against foreign substances.

immunity: the body's ability to defend itself against diseases; see Highlight 17.

immunoglobulins (IM-you-no-GLOB-you-linz): proteins produced by B cells that function as antibodies.

implantation: the stage of development in which the zygote embeds itself in the wall of the uterus and begins to develop; occurs during the first two weeks after conception.

inborn error of metabolism: an inherited trait (present at birth) that causes a deficiency or the absence of a protein that has a critical metabolic role.

indigestion: incomplete or uncomfortable digestion, usually accompanied by pain, nausea, vomiting, heartburn, intestinal gas, or belching.

inflammation: a nonspecific response to injury or infection; a type of innate immune response.

inflammatory bowel disease (IBD): chronic inflammatory disease of the gastrointestinal tract.

inflammatory response: the metabolic responses of the immune system to infection or injury.

informed consent: a patient's or caregiver's agreement to undergo a treatment that has been adequately disclosed. Persons must be mentally competent in order to make the decision.

inherited disorders: medical conditions resulting from genetic defects.

initiators: factors that cause mutations that give rise to cancer, such as radiation and carcinogens.

innate immunity: immunity that is present at birth, unchanging throughout life, and nonspecific for particular antigens; also called **natural immunity.**

inorganic: not containing carbon or pertaining to living things.

inositol (in-OSS-ih-tall): a nonessential nutrient that can be made in the body from glucose. Inositol is a part of cell membrane structures.

insoluble fibers: indigestible food components that do not dissolve in water. Examples include the tough, fibrous structures found in the strings of celery and the skins of corn kernels.

insulin (IN-suh-lin): a hormone secreted by special cells in the pancreas in response to (among other things) increased blood glucose concentration. The primary role of insulin is to control the transport of glucose from the bloodstream into the muscle and fat cells.

insulin resistance: reduced sensitivity to insulin in muscle, adipose, and liver cells.

integrative medicine: an approach to medical care that combines mainstream medical therapies and CAM therapies for which there is some high-quality scientific evidence of safety and effectiveness.

intermittent claudication (klaw-dih-KAY-shun): severe calf pain caused by inadequate blood supply. It occurs when walking and subsides during rest.

intermittent feedings: delivery of about 250 to 400 mL of formula over 20 to 40 minutes.

Internet (the Net): a worldwide network of millions of computers linked together to share information.

interstitial (IN-ter-STISH-al) **fluid:** fluid between the cells (intercellular), usually high in sodium and chloride. Interstitial fluid is a large component of extracellular fluid.

intestinal adaptation: after resection, the process of intestinal recovery that leads to improved absorptive capacity.

intra-abdominal fat: fat stored within the abdominal cavity in association with the internal abdominal organs, as opposed to the fat stored directly under the skin (subcutaneous fat).

intracellular fluid: fluid within the cells, usually high in potassium and phosphate. Intracellular fluid accounts for approximately two-thirds of the body's water.

intractable: not easily managed or controlled.

intractable vomiting: vomiting that is not easily managed or controlled.

intradialytic parenteral nutrition: the infusion of nutrients during hemodialysis, often providing amino acids, dextrose, lipids, and some trace minerals.

intravenous feedings: the provision of nutrients through a vein, bypassing the intestine.

intrinsic factor: a glycoprotein (a protein with short polysaccharide chains attached) manufactured in the stomach that aids in the absorption of vitamin B_{12}.

invert sugar: a mixture of glucose and fructose formed by the hydrolysis of sucrose in a chemical process; sold only in liquid form and sweeter than sucrose. Invert sugar is used as a food additive to help preserve freshness and prevent shrinkage.

ions (EYE-uns): atoms or molecules that have gained or lost electrons and therefore have electrical charges. Examples include the positively charged sodium ion (Na^+) and the negatively charged chloride ion (Cl^-). For a closer look at ions, see Appendix B.

iron deficiency: the state of having depleted iron stores.

iron overload: toxicity from excess iron.

iron-deficiency anemia: severe depletion of iron stores that results in low hemoglobin and small, pale red blood cells. Anemias that impair hemoglobin synthesis are **microcytic.**

irritable bowel syndrome: an intestinal disorder of unknown cause. Symptoms include abdominal discomfort and cramping, diarrhea, constipation, or alternating diarrhea and constipation.

ischemia (is-KEY-mee-a): inadequate blood supply to tissues due to obstructed blood flow through arteries.

isotonic formula: a formula with an osmolality similar to that of blood serum (300 mOsm/kg).

J

jaundice (JAWN-dis): yellow discoloration of skin and mucous membranes due to an accumulation of bilirubin—a breakdown product of hemoglobin and other heme-containing proteins that normally exits the body via bile secretions.

jejunostomy (JE-ju-NOSS-toe-mee): an opening in the jejunum through which a feeding tube can be passed. A nonsurgical technique for creating a jejunostomy is called **percutaneous endoscopic jejunostomy (PEJ).** The tube can either be guided into the jejunum via a gastrostomy or passed directly into the jejunum **(direct PEJ).**

jejunum (je-JOON-um): the first two-fifths of the small intestine beyond the duodenum.

Joint Commission on Accreditation of Healthcare Organizations (JCAHO): a nonprofit organization that sets standards for health care performance and safety and awards accreditation to health care organizations that meet these standards.

K

Kaposi's (cap-OH-seez) **sarcoma:** a type of cancer that is rare in the general population but common in people with HIV infections.

kcalorie (energy) control: management of food energy intake.

kcalorie-free: fewer than 5 kcal per serving.

keratin (KARE-uh-tin): a water-insoluble protein; the normal protein of hair and nails. Keratin-producing cells may replace mucus-producing cells in vitamin A deficiency.

keratinization: accumulation of keratin in a tissue; a sign of vitamin A deficiency.

keratomalacia (KARE-ah-toe-ma-LAY-shuh): softening of the cornea that leads to irreversible blindness; seen in severe vitamin A deficiency.

keto (KEY-toe) **acid:** an organic acid that contains a carbonyl group (C=O).

ketoacidosis: lowering of pH in blood and tissues due to excessive ketone body production.

ketone (KEE-tone) **bodies:** the product of the incomplete breakdown of fat when glucose is not available in the cells.

ketonuria (kee-toe-NOOR-ee-a): the presence of ketone bodies in urine.

ketosis (kee-TOE-sis): an undesirably high concentration of ketone bodies in the blood and urine.

kidney stones: crystalline masses that form in the urinary tract; also called **renal calculi** and **nephrolithiasis.**

kwashiorkor (kwash-ee-OR-core, kwash-ee-or-CORE): a form of PEM that results either from inadequate protein intake or, more commonly, from infections.

L

lactadherin (lack-tad-HAIR-in): a protein in breast milk that attacks diarrhea-causing viruses.

lactase: an enzyme that hydrolyzes lactose.

lactase deficiency: a lack of the enzyme required to digest the disaccharide lactose into its component monosaccharides (glucose and galactose).

lactation: production and secretion of breast milk for the purpose of nourishing an infant.

lactic acid: a 3-carbon compound produced from pyruvate during anaerobic metabolism.

lactoferrin (lack-toh-FERR-in): a protein in breast milk that binds iron and keeps it from supporting the growth of the infant's intestinal bacteria.

lacto-ovo-vegetarians: people who include milk, milk products, and eggs, but exclude meat, poultry, fish, and seafood from their diets.

lactose (LAK-tose): a disaccharide composed of glucose and galactose; commonly known as milk sugar.

lactose intolerance: a condition that results from inability to digest the milk sugar lactose; characterized by bloating, gas, abdominal discomfort, and diarrhea. Lactose intolerance differs from milk allergy, which is caused by an immune reaction to the protein in milk.

lactovegetarians: people who include milk and milk products, but exclude meat, poultry, fish, seafood, and eggs from their diets.

laparoscopic: pertaining to procedures that use a laparoscope for internal examination or surgery. A laparoscope is a narrow surgical telescope that is inserted into the abdominal cavity through a small incision. A video camera is usually attached so that the procedure can be viewed on a television monitor.

large intestine or **colon** (COAL-un): the lower portion of intestine that completes the digestive process. Its segments are the ascending colon, the transverse colon, the descending colon, and the sigmoid colon.

larynx: the voice box (see Figure H3-1).

laxatives: substances that loosen the bowels and thereby prevent or treat constipation.

LDL (low-density lipoprotein): the type of lipoprotein derived from very-low-density lipoproteins (VLDL) as VLDL triglycerides are removed and broken down; composed primarily of cholesterol.

lean: less than 10 g of fat, 4.5 g of saturated fat and *trans* fat combined, and 95 mg of cholesterol per serving and per 100 g of meat, poultry, and seafood.

lean body mass: the weight of the body minus the fat content.

lecithin (LESS-uh-thin): one of the phospholipids. Both nature and the food industry use lecithin as an emulsifier to combine water-soluble and fat-soluble ingredients that do not ordinarily mix, such as water and oil.

legumes (lay-GYOOMS, LEG-yooms): plants of the bean and pea family, with seeds that are rich in protein compared with other plant-derived foods.

leptin: a protein produced by fat cells under direction of the *ob* gene that decreases appetite and increases energy expenditure; sometimes called the ***ob* protein.**

less: at least 25% less of a given nutrient or kcalories than the comparison food (see individual nutrients); synonyms include "fewer" and "reduced."

less cholesterol: 25% or less cholesterol than the comparison food (reflecting a reduction of at least 20 mg per serving), and 2 g or less saturated fat and *trans* fat combined per serving.

less fat: 25% or less fat than the comparison food.

less saturated fat: 25% or less saturated fat and *trans* fat combined than the comparison food.

let-down reflex: the reflex that forces milk to the front of the breast when the infant begins to nurse.

leukocytes: blood cells that function in immunity; also called **white blood cells.**

levulose: an older name for fructose.

license to practice: permission under state or federal law, granted on meeting specified criteria, to use a certain title (such as dietitian) and offer certain services. **Licensed dietitians** may use the initials **LD** after their names.

life expectancy: the average number of years lived by people in a given society.

life span: the maximum number of years of life attainable by a member of a species.

light in sodium: no more than 50% of the sodium of the comparison food.

light: one-third fewer kcalories than the comparison food; 50% or less of the fat or sodium than in the comparison food any use of the term other than as defined must specify what it is referring to (for example, "light in color" or "light in texture").

lignans: phytochemicals present in flaxseed, but not in flax oil, that are converted to phytosterols by intestinal bacteria and are under study as possible anticancer agents.

limiting amino acid: the essential amino acid found in the shortest supply relative to the amounts needed for protein synthesis in the body.

linoleic (lin-oh-LAY-ick) **acid:** an essential fatty acid with 18 carbons and two double bonds.

linolenic (lin-oh-LEN-ick) **acid:** an essential fatty acid with 18 carbons and three double bonds.

lipids: a family of compounds that includes triglycerides, phospholipids, and sterols. Lipids are characterized by their insolubility in water. (Lipids also include the fat-soluble vitamins, described in Chapter 11.)

lipomas (lih-POE-muz): benign tumors composed of fatty tissue.

lipoprotein lipase (LPL): an enzyme that hydrolyzes triglycerides passing by in the bloodstream and directs their parts into the cells, where they can be metabolized for energy or reassembled for storage.

lipoprotein(a): a variant of LDL associated with a high risk of atherosclerosis and CHD.

lipoproteins (LIP-oh-PRO-teenz): clusters of lipids associated with proteins that serve as transport vehicles for lipids in the lymph and blood.

listeriosis: an infection caused by eating food contaminated with the bacterium *Listeria monocytogenes,* which can be killed by pasteurization and cooking, but can survive at refrigerated temperatures; certain ready-to-eat foods, such as hot dogs and deli meats, may become contaminated after cooking or processing, but before packaging.

liver: the organ that manufactures bile. (The liver's many other functions are described in Chapter 7.)

living will: a written statement that specifies the medical procedures desired or not desired in the event that a person is unable to communicate or is incapacitated; also called a **medical directive.**

longevity: long duration of life.

low birthweight (LBW): a birthweight of 5½ lb (2500 g) or less; indicates probable poor health in the newborn and poor nutrition status in the mother during pregnancy, before pregnancy, or both. Normal birthweight for a full-term baby is 6½ to 8¾ lb (about 3000 to 4000 g).

low cholesterol: 20 mg or less cholesterol per serving and 2 g or less saturated fat and *trans* fat combined per serving.

low: an amount that would allow frequent consumption of a food without exceeding the Daily Value for the nutrient. A food that is naturally low in a nutrient may make such a claim, but only as it applies to all similar foods (for example, "fresh cauliflower, a low-sodium food"); synonyms include "little," "few," and "low source of."

low fat: 3 g or less fat per serving.

low kcalorie: 40 kcal or less per serving.

low saturated fat: 1 g or less saturated fat and less than 0.5 g of *trans* fat per serving.

low sodium: 140 mg or less per serving.

low-risk pregnancy: a pregnancy characterized by indicators that make a normal outcome likely.

lumen (LOO-men): the space within a vessel, such as the intestine.

lutein (LOO-teen): a plant pigment of yellow hue; a phytochemical believed to play roles in eye functioning and health.

luteinizing (LOO-tee-in-EYE-zing) **hormone (LH):** a hormone that stimulates ovulation and the development of the corpus luteum (the small tissue that develops from a ruptured ovarian follicle and secretes hormones); so called because the follicle turns yellow as it matures. In men, LH stimulates testosterone secretion. The release of LH is mediated by **luteinizing hormone–releasing hormone (LH–RH).**

lycopene (LYE-koh-peen): a pigment responsible for the red color of tomatoes and other red-hued vegetables; a phytochemical that may act as an antioxidant in the body.

lymph (LIMF): a clear yellowish fluid that is almost identical to blood except that it contains no red blood cells or platelets. Lymph from the GI tract transports fat and fat-soluble vitamins to the bloodstream via lymphatic vessels.

lymphatic (lim-FAT-ic) **system:** a loosely organized system of vessels and ducts that convey fluids toward the heart. The GI part of the lymphatic system carries the products of fat digestion into the bloodstream.

lymphatic vessels: vessels through which lymph travels.

lymphocytes (LIM-foe-sites): white blood cells that recognize specific antigens and therefore function in adaptive immunity; include *T cells* and *B cells.*

lymphoid tissues: tissues that contain lymphocytes.

lysosomes (LYE-so-zomes): cellular organelles; membrane-enclosed sacs of degradative enzymes.

lysozyme (LYE-so-zyme): enzyme with antibacterial properties found in immune cells and body secretions such as tears, saliva, and sweat.

M

macrobiotic diets: extremely restrictive diets limited to a few grains and vegetables; based on metaphysical beliefs and not on nutrition.

macrocytic anemia: anemia characterized by large red blood cells, as occurs in folate and vitamin B_{12} deficiency; also called **megaloblastic anemia.**

macrophages (MAK-roe-fay-jez): monocytes that have left circulation and settled in a tissue, where they serve as scavengers and activate the immune response.

macrovascular complications: disorders that affect the large blood vessels, including cardiovascular diseases and peripheral vascular disease.

macular (MACK-you-lar) **degeneration:** deterioration of the macular area of the eye that can lead to loss of central vision and eventual blindness. The **macula** is a small, oval, yellowish region in the center of the retina that provides the sharp, straight-ahead vision so critical to reading and driving.

magnesium: a cation within the body's cells, active in many enzyme systems.

major minerals: essential mineral nutrients found in the human body in amounts larger than 5 g; sometimes called **macrominerals.**

maleficence (mah-LEF-eh-sens): the performance of evil or harm.

malignant (ma-LIG-nant): describes tumors that multiply out of control, threaten health, and require treatment.

malnutrition: any condition caused by excess or deficient food energy or nutrient intake or by an imbalance of nutrients.

maltase: an enzyme that hydrolyzes maltose.

maltose (MAWL-tose): a disaccharide composed of two glucose units; sometimes known as malt sugar.

mammary glands: glands of the female breast that secrete milk.

maple sugar: a sugar (mostly sucrose) purified from the concentrated sap of the sugar maple tree.

marasmus (ma-RAZ-mus): a form of PEM that results from a severe deprivation, or impaired absorption, of energy, protein, vitamins, and minerals.

massage therapy: manual manipulation of muscles to reduce tension, increase blood circulation, improve joint mobility, and promote healing of injuries.

mast cells: cells within connective tissue that produce and release histamine.

matrix (MAY-tricks): the basic substance that gives form to a developing structure; in the body, the formative cells from which teeth and bones grow.

matter: anything that takes up space and has mass.

Meals on Wheels: a nutrition program that delivers food for the elderly to their homes.

meat replacements: products formulated to look and taste like meat, fish, or poultry; usually made of textured vegetable protein.

mechanical ventilation: use of a machine to assist or control breathing. In normal respiration, the lungs expand, which draws air into the lungs. With mechanical ventilation, air is forced into the lungs at regular intervals using pressure.

medical nutrition therapy: nutrition care provided by a registered dietitian; includes diagnosing nutrition problems, prescribing diet plans, and providing dietary counseling.

meditation: a self-directed technique of calming the mind and relaxing the body.

medium-chain triglycerides (MCT): triglycerides that contain fatty acids that are 8 to 10 carbons in length. MCT do not require digestion and can be absorbed in the absence of lipase or bile.

MEOS or **microsomal** (my-krow-SO-mal) **ethanol-oxidizing system:** a system of enzymes in the liver that oxidize not only alcohol, but also several classes of drugs.

metabolic stress: a disruption in the body's chemical environment due to the effects of disease or injury. Metabolic stress is characterized by changes in metabolic rate, heart rate, blood pressure, hormonal status, and nutrient metabolism.

metabolic syndrome: a cluster of interrelated clinical symptoms, including obesity, insulin resistance, high blood pressure, and abnormal blood lipids, which together increase cardiovascular disease risk two- to threefold; also called **syndrome X** or **insulin resistance syndrome.**

metabolism: the sum total of all the chemical reactions that go on in living cells. Energy metabolism includes all the reactions by which the body obtains and spends the energy from food.

metabolites: products of metabolism; the compounds typically produced by a biochemical pathway.

metalloenzymes (meh-TAL-oh-EN-zimes): enzymes that contain one or more minerals as part of their structures.

metallothionein (meh-TAL-oh-THIGH-oh-neen): a sulfur-rich protein that avidly binds with and transports metals such as zinc.

metastasize (meh-TAS-tah-size): the spread of cancer cells from one part of the body to another.

MFP factor: a factor associated with the digestion of **m**eat, **f**ish, and **p**oultry that enhances nonheme iron absorption.

micelles (MY-cells): tiny spherical complexes of emulsified fat that arise during digestion; most contain bile salts and the products of lipid digestion, including fatty acids, monoglycerides, and cholesterol.

microarray technology: research technology that monitors the expression of thousands of genes simultaneously.

microcytic anemia: anemia characterized by small, hypochromic (pale) red blood cells, as occurs in iron deficiency.

microvascular complications: disorders that affect the small blood vessels and capillaries, including retinal damage and kidney disease.

microvilli (MY-cro-VILL-ee, MY-cro-VILL-eye): tiny, hairlike projections on each cell of every villus that can trap nutrient particles and transport them into the cells; singular **microvillus.**

milk anemia: iron-deficiency anemia that develops when an excessive milk intake displaces iron-rich foods from the diet.

milliequivalents (mEq): the concentration of electrolytes in a volume of solution. Milliequivalents are a useful measure when considering ions because the number of charges reveals characteristics about the solution that are not evident when the concentration is expressed in terms of weight.

mineral oil: a purified liquid derived from petroleum and used to treat constipation.

mineral water: water from a spring or well that typically contains 250 to 500 parts per million (ppm) of minerals. Minerals give water a distinctive flavor. Many mineral waters are high in sodium.

mineralization: the process in which calcium, phosphorus, and other minerals crystallize on the collagen matrix of a growing bone, hardening the bone.

minerals: inorganic elements. Some minerals are essential nutrients required in small amounts by the body for health.

misinformation: false or misleading information.

mitochondria (my-toh-KON-dree-uh); singular **mitochondrion:** the cellular organelles responsible for producing ATP aerobically; made of membranes (lipid and protein) with enzymes mounted on them.

moderation: in relation to alcohol consumption, not more than two drinks a day for the average-sized man and not more than one drink a day for the average-sized woman.

moderation (dietary): providing enough but not too much of a substance.

modified diet: a diet that is adjusted to meet medical needs. Such diets may be adjusted in consistency, in level of energy or nutrient content, or by the inclusion or elimination of certain foods.

modular formulas: dietary formulas that contain only one or two macronutrients; used to enhance other formulas, meet specific nutrient needs, or create individualized formulas for people with unique needs.

molasses: the thick brown syrup produced during sugar refining. Molasses retains residual sugar and other by-products and a few minerals; blackstrap molasses contains significant amounts of calcium and iron—the iron comes from the *machinery* used to process the sugar.

molecule: two or more atoms of the same or different elements joined by chemical bonds. Examples are molecules of the element oxygen, composed of two oxygen atoms (O_2), and molecules of the compound water, composed of two hydrogen atoms and one oxygen atom (H_2O).

molybdenum (mo-LIB-duh-num): a trace element.

monocytes (MON-oh-sites): cells released from the bone marrow that move into tissues and mature into macrophages.

monoglycerides: molecules of glycerol with one fatty acid attached. A molecule of glycerol with two fatty acids attached is a **diglyceride.**

monosaccharides (mon-oh-SACK-uh-rides): carbohydrates of the general formula $C_nH_{2n}O_n$ that consist of a single ring. See Appendix C for the chemical structures of the monosaccharides.

monounsaturated fatty acid: a fatty acid that lacks two hydrogen atoms and has one double bond between carbons—for example, oleic acid. A **monounsaturated fat** is composed of triglycerides in which most of the fatty acids are monounsaturated.

mood disorders: mental illness characterized by episodes of severe depression or excessive excitement (mania) or both.

more: at least 10% more of the Daily Value for a given nutrient than the comparison food; synonyms include "added" and "extra."

mouth: the oral cavity containing the tongue and teeth.

mucous (MYOO-kus) **membranes:** the membranes, composed of mucus-secreting cells, that line the surfaces of body tissues.

mucus (MYOO-kus): a slippery substance secreted by cells of the GI lining (and other body linings) that protects the cells from exposure to digestive juices (and other destructive agents). The lining of the GI tract with its coat of mucus is a **mucous membrane**. (The noun is **mucus;** the adjective is **mucous.**)

multigene or **polygenic:** involving a number of genes, rather than a single gene.

multiple organ failure: a failure of more than one organ system that occurs during intensive care; often results in death.

muscle dysmorphia (dis-MORE-fee-ah): a newly coined psychiatric disorder characterized by a preoccupation with building body mass.

muscular dystrophy (DIS-tro-fee): a hereditary disease in which the muscles gradually weaken. Its most debilitating effects arise in the lungs.

mutations: inheritable alterations in the DNA sequence of a gene.

myocardial (my-oh-CAR-dee-al) **infarction** (in-FARK-shun) or **MI:** death of heart muscle caused by a sudden reduction in coronary blood flow; also called a **heart attack** or **cardiac arrest.**

myoglobin: the oxygen-holding protein of the muscle cells.

N

NAD (nicotinamide adenine dinucleotide): the main coenzyme form of the vitamin niacin. Its reduced form is NADH.

narcotic (nar-KOT-ic): a drug that dulls the senses, induces sleep, and becomes addictive with prolonged use.

nasoduodenal (ND): tube is placed into the duodenum via the nose.

nasoenteric: tube is placed into the GI tract via the nose. *(Nasoenteric feedings* usually refer to *nasoduodenal* and *nasojejunal* feedings.)

nasogastric (NG): tube is placed into the stomach via the nose.

nasojejunal (NJ): tube is placed into the jejunum via the nose.

National Center for Complementary and Alternative Medicine (NCCAM): a federal agency that researches and provides information about complementary and alternative therapies.

natural killer cells: lymphocytes that confer nonspecific immunity by destroying a wide array of viruses and tumor cells.

natural water: water obtained from a spring or well that is certified to be safe and sanitary. The mineral content may not be changed, but the water may be treated in other ways such as with ozone or by filtration.

naturopathic (NAY-chur-oh-PATH-ic) **medicine:** an approach to medical care using practices alleged to enhance the body's natural healing abilities. Treatments may include a variety of alternative therapies including dietary supplements, herbal remedies, exercise, and homeopathy.

neotame (NEE-oh-tame): an artificial sweetener composed of two amino acids (phenylalanine and aspartic acid); approved for use in the United States.

nephron (NEF-ron): the functional unit of the kidneys, consisting of a glomerulus and tubules.

nephrotic (neh-FROT-ik) **syndrome:** a kidney disorder characterized by urinary protein losses exceeding 3.5 g per day. Accompanying symptoms often include low serum albumin, elevated blood lipids, and edema.

nephrotoxic: toxic to the kidneys.

net protein utilization (NPU): a measure of protein quality assessed by measuring the amount of protein nitrogen that is retained from a given amount of protein nitrogen eaten.

neural tube defects: malformations of the brain, spinal cord, or both during embryonic development that often result in lifelong disability or death. The two main types of neural tube defects are **spina bifida** (literally, "split spine") and **anencephaly** ("no brain").

neurons: nerve cells; the structural and functional units of the nervous system. Neurons initiate and conduct nerve transmissions.

neuropathy: disorders affecting the nervous system.

neuropeptide Y: a chemical produced in the brain that stimulates appetite, diminishes energy expenditure, and increases fat storage.

neurotransmitters: chemicals that are released at the end of a nerve cell when a nerve impulse arrives there. They diffuse across the gap to the next cell and alter the membrane of that second cell to either inhibit or excite it.

neutrophils (NEW-tro-fills): the most common type of white blood cell. Neutrophils destroy antigens by phagocytosis.

niacin (NIGH-a-sin): a B vitamin. The coenzyme forms are **NAD (nicotinamide adenine dinucleotide)** and **NADP (the phosphate form of NAD).** Niacin can be eaten preformed or made in the body from its precursor, tryptophan, one of the amino acids.

niacin equivalents (NE): the amount of niacin present in food, including the niacin that can theoretically be made from its precursor, tryptophan, present in the food.

niacin flush: a temporary burning, tingling, and itching sensation that occurs when a person takes a large dose of nicotinic acid; often accompanied by a headache and reddened face, arms, and chest.

night blindness: slow recovery of vision after flashes of bright light at night or an inability to see in dim light; an early symptom of vitamin A deficiency.

nitric oxide: a compound produced by blood vessel cells that helps to regulate blood vessel activity, including blood vessel dilation and constriction.

nitrogen balance: the amount of nitrogen consumed (N in) as compared with the amount of nitrogen excreted (N out) in a given period of time.

noncoding sequences: regions of DNA that do not code for proteins. Some noncoding sequences may have regulatory or structural properties, but most have no known function.

nonessential amino acids: amino acids that the body can synthesize (see Table 6-1).

nonnutrients: compounds in foods that do not fit within the six classes of nutrients.

nonselective menus: menus that do not allow choices and list only preselected food items.

nucleotides: the subunits of DNA and RNA molecules. These compounds—cytosine (C), thymine (T), uracil (U), guanine (G), and adenine (A)—are each composed of a phosphate group, a 5-carbon sugar (ribose), and a nitrogen-containing base. A DNA molecule is made up of two long chains of nucleotides held together by hydrogen bonding between nucleotide bases on opposing strands; each hydrogen-bonded nucleotide couple is called a **base pair.**

nucleus: a major membrane-enclosed body within every cell, which contains the cell's genetic material, DNA, embedded in chromosomes.

nursing bottle tooth decay: extensive tooth decay due to prolonged tooth contact with formula, milk, fruit juice, or other carbohydrate-rich liquid offered to an infant in a bottle.

nutrient claims: statements that characterize the quantity of a nutrient in a food.

nutrient density: a measure of the nutrients a food provides relative to the energy it provides. The more nutrients and the fewer kcalories, the higher the nutrient density.

nutrients: chemical substances obtained from food and used in the body to provide energy, structural materials, and regulating agents to support growth, maintenance, and repair of the body's tissues. Nutrients may also reduce the risks of some diseases.

nutrition: the science of foods and the nutrients and other substances they contain, and of their actions within the body (including ingestion, digestion, absorption, transport, metabolism, and excretion). A broader definition includes the social, economic, cultural, and psychological implications of food and eating.

nutrition assessment: a comprehensive analysis of a person's nutrition status that uses health, socioeconomic, drug, and diet histories; anthropometric measurements; physical examinations; and laboratory tests.

nutrition care plans: strategies for meeting an individual's nutritional needs.

nutrition care process: an organized approach to nutrition care that consists of assessing, diagnosing, intervening, monitoring, and evaluating the patient's problems and progress.

nutrition screening: an examination process that identifies patients who require intervention for existing or potential nutritional problems.

Nutrition Screening Initiative: a collaboration by health, social service, and medical organizations that promotes nutrition screening in the elderly.

nutrition support: the delivery of formulated nutrients by feeding tube or intravenous infusion.

nutrition support teams: health care professionals responsible for the provision of nutrients by tube feedings or intravenous infusion.

nutritional genomics: the science of how nutrients affect the activities of genes and how genes affect the activities of nutrients; also known as **nutrigenomics.**

nutritionist: a person who specializes in the study of nutrition. Note that this definition does not specify qualifications and may apply not only to registered dietitians but also to self-described experts whose training is questionable. Most states have licensing laws that define the scope of practice for those calling themselves nutritionists.

nutritive sweeteners: sweeteners that yield energy, including both sugars and sugar replacers.

O

oils: lipids that are liquid at room temperature (70°F or 25°C).

olestra: a synthetic fat made from sucrose and fatty acids that provides 0 kcalories per gram; also known as **sucrose polyester.**

oliguria (OL-leh-GOO-ree-ah): reduced quantity of urine, often less than 400 mL per day.

omega: the last letter of the Greek alphabet (ω), used by chemists to refer to the position of the first double bond from the methyl end of a fatty acid.

omega-3 fatty acid: a polyunsaturated fatty acid in which the first double bond is three carbons away from the methyl (CH_3) end of the carbon chain.

omega-6 fatty acid: a polyunsaturated fatty acid in which the first double bond is six carbons from the methyl (CH_3) end of the carbon chain.

omnivores: people who have no formal restriction on the eating of any foods.

oncotic pressure: the pressure exerted by fluid on one side of a membrane as a result of osmosis.

open feeding systems: delivery systems that require formula to be transferred from the original packaging to feeding containers before being administered through feeding tubes.

opportunistic infections: infections from microorganisms that normally do not cause disease in the general population but can cause great harm in people whose immune systems are compromised (as in HIV infection).

opsin (OP-sin): the protein portion of the visual pigment molecule.

oral allergy syndrome: an allergic response in which symptoms of hives, swelling, or itching occur only in the mouth and throat; usually a short-lived response that resolves quickly.

oral glucose tolerance test: a test that evaluates a person's ability to tolerate a glucose load. A common protocol for diabetes diagnosis is ingestion of a 75 g glucose load followed by measurement of plasma glucose after a two-hour interval.

organelles: subcellular structures such as ribosomes, mitochondria, and lysosomes.

organic: in chemistry, a substance or molecule containing carbon-carbon bonds or carbon-hydrogen bonds. In agriculture, growing crops and raising livestock according to U.S. Department of Agriculture (USDA) standards. On food labels, that at least 95% of the product's ingredients have been grown and processsed according to USDA regulations defining the use of fertilizers, herbicides, insecticides, fungicides, preservatives, and other chemical ingredients.

orlistat (OR-leh-stat): a drug used in the treatment of obesity that inhibits the absorption of fat in the GI tract, thus limiting kcaloric intake.

orogastric: tube is placed into the GI tract via the mouth. This method is often used to feed infants because a nasogastric tube can hinder the infant's breathing.

oropharyngeal (OR-oh-FAIR-in-GEE-al): concerning the mouth and pharynx.

oropharyngeal dysphagia: an inability to transfer food from the mouth and pharynx to the esophagus; usually due to a neurological or muscular disorder.

osmolality (OZ-moh-LAL-eh-tee): the osmotic property of a solution, based on its concentrations of molecules and ionic particles. Osmolality is expressed as milliosmoles (mOsm) per kilogram.

osmolarity: the concentration of osmotically active particles in a solution, expressed as milliosmoles per liter (mOsm/L). **Osmolality** is an alternative expression of a solution's osmotic properties that is used in clinical practice and uses the units milliosmoles per kilogram (mOsm/kg).

osmosis: the movement of water across a membrane *toward* the side where the solutes are more concentrated.

osmotic pressure: the amount of pressure needed to prevent the movement of water across a membrane.

osteoarthritis: a painful, degenerative disease of the joints that occurs when the cushioning cartilage in a joint deteriorates; joint structure is damaged, with loss of function; also called **degenerative arthritis.**

osteomalacia (OS-tee-oh-ma-LAY-shuh): a bone disease characterized by softening of the bones. Symptoms include bending of the spine and bowing of the legs. The disease occurs most often in adult women.

osteopathic (AHS-tee-oh-PATH-ic) **manipulation:** a manipulative technique performed by osteopaths that includes deep tissue massage and manipulation of joints, spine, and soft tissues. Doctors of Osteopathic Medicine (D.O.s) are fully trained and licensed medical physicians.

osteoporosis (OS-tee-oh-pore-OH-sis): a disease in which the bones become porous and fragile due to a loss of minerals; also called **adult bone loss.**

overnutrition: excess energy or nutrients.

overt (oh-VERT): out in the open and easy to observe.

overweight: body weight above some standard of acceptable weight that is usually defined in relation to height (such as BMI).

ovum (OH-vum): the female reproductive cell, capable of developing into a new organism upon fertilization; commonly referred to as an egg.

oxaloacetate (OKS-ah-low-AS-eh-tate): a carbohydrate intermediate of the TCA cycle.

oxidants (OK-see-dants): compounds (such as oxygen itself) that oxidize other compounds. Compounds that prevent oxidation are called *anti*oxidants, whereas those that promote it are called *pro*oxidants.

oxidation (OKS-ee-day-shun): the process of a substance combining with oxygen; oxidation reactions involve the loss of electrons.

oxidative stress: an imbalance between the production of free radicals and the body's ability to handle them and prevent damage.

oxytocin (OCK-see-TOH-sin): a hormone that stimulates the mammary glands to eject milk during lactation and the uterus to contract during childbirth.

oyster shell: a product made from the powdered shells of oysters that is sold as a calcium supplement, but is not well absorbed by the digestive system.

P

pancreas: a gland that secretes digestive enzymes and juices into the duodenum.

pancreatic (pank-ree-AT-ic) **juice:** the exocrine secretion of the pancreas, containing enzymes for the digestion of carbohydrate, fat, and protein as well as bicarbonate, a neutralizing agent. The juice flows from the pancreas into the small intestine through the pancreatic duct. (The pancreas also has an endocrine function, the secretion of insulin and other hormones.)

pantothenic (PAN-toe-THEN-ick) **acid:** a B vitamin. The principal active form is part of coenzyme A, called "CoA" throughout Chapter 7.

paranoia (PAHR-ah-NOY-ah): mental illness characterized by irrational distrust of others and delusions of persecution.

parathormone (PAIR-ah-THOR-moan): a hormone from the parathyroid glands that regulates blood calcium by raising it when levels fall too low; also known as **parathyroid hormone.**

parenteral (par-EN-ter-al) **nutrition:** intravenous provision of nutrients that bypasses the GI tract.

patient autonomy: a principle of self-determination, such that patients (or surrogate decision makers) are free to choose the medical interventions that are acceptable to them, even if they choose to refuse interventions that may extend their lives.

PDCAAS (protein digestibility–corrected amino acid score): a measure of protein quality assessed by comparing the amino acid score of a food protein with the amino acid requirements of preschool-age children and then correcting for the true digestibility of the protein; recommended by the FAO/WHO and used to establish protein quality of foods for Daily Value percentages on food labels.

peak bone mass: the highest attainable bone size and density for an individual, developed during the first three decades of life.

peer review: a process in which a panel of scientists rigorously evaluates a research study to assure that the scientific method was followed.

pellagra (pell-AY-gra): the niacin-deficiency disease.

pepsin: a gastric enzyme that hydrolyzes protein. Pepsin is secreted in an inactive form, **pepsinogen,** which is activated by hydrochloric acid in the stomach.

peptic ulcer: a lesion in the mucous membrane of either the stomach (a gastric ulcer) or the duodenum (a duodenal ulcer).

peptidase: a digestive enzyme that hydrolyzes peptide bonds. *Tripeptidases* cleave tripeptides; *dipeptidases* cleave dipeptides. *Endopeptidases* cleave peptide bonds within the chain to create smaller fragments, whereas *exopeptidases* cleave bonds at the ends to release free amino acids.

peptide bond: a bond that connects the acid end of one amino acid with the amino end of another, forming a link in a protein chain.

percent fat-free: may be used only if the product meets the definition of *low fat* or *fat-free* and must reflect the amount of fat in 100 g (for example, a food that contains 2.5 g of fat per 50 g can claim to be "95 percent fat free").

periodontal disease: a disease that affects the connective tissue structures that support the teeth.

periodontitis: inflammation or degeneration of the tissues that support the teeth.

periodontium: the tissues that support the teeth, including the gums, cementum (bonelike material covering the dentin layer of the tooth), periodontal ligament, and underlying bone.

peripheral blood smear: a blood sample spread on a glass slide and stained for analysis under a microscope. *Peripheral* refers to the use of circulating blood rather than tissue blood.

peripheral (puh-RIFF-er-ul) **nervous system:** the peripheral (outermost) part of the nervous system; the vast complex of wiring that extends from the central nervous system to the body's outermost areas. It contains both somatic and autonomic components.

peripheral parenteral nutrition (PPN): a type of nutrition support in which intravenous feedings are delivered into peripheral veins.

peripheral resistance: the resistance to pumped blood by the small arterial branches (arterioles) that carry blood to tissues.

peripheral veins: small-diameter veins that carry blood from the arms and legs.

peristalsis (per-ih-STALL-sis): wavelike muscular contractions of the GI tract that push its contents along.

peritoneal (PER-ih-toe-NEE-al) **dialysis:** removal of fluids and wastes by using the peritoneal membrane to filter blood.

peritonitis: inflammation of the peritoneal membrane.

pernicious (per-NISH-us) **anemia:** a blood disorder that reflects a vitamin B_{12} deficiency caused by lack of intrinsic factor and characterized by abnormally large and immature red blood cells. Other symptoms include muscle weakness and irreversible neurological damage.

persistent vegetative state: a vegetative mental state resulting from brain injury that persists for at least one month. Individuals lose awareness and the ability to think but retain noncognitive brain functions, such as motor reflexes and normal sleep patterns.

pH: the unit of measure expressing a substance's acidity or alkalinity. The lower the pH, the higher the H^+ ion concentration and the stronger the acid. A pH above 7 is alkaline, or base (a solution in which OH^- ions predominate).

phagocytes (FAG-oh-sites): white blood cells (neutrophils and macrophages) that have the ability to engulf and destroy antigens.

phagocytosis (FAG-oh-sigh-TOE-sis): the process by which phagocytes engulf and destroy antigens.

pharynx (FAIR-inks): the passageway leading from the nose and mouth to the larynx and esophagus, respectively.

phenylketonuria (FEN-il-KEY-toe-NU-ree-ah) or **PKU:** an inherited disorder that affects the conversion of the essential amino acid phenylalanine to the amino acid tyrosine.

phospholipid (FOS-foe-LIP-id): a compound similar to a triglyceride but having a phosphate group (a phosphorus-containing salt) and choline (or another nitrogen-containing compound) in place of one of the fatty acids.

phosphorus: a major mineral found mostly in the body's bones and teeth.

photosynthesis: the process by which green plants use the sun's energy to make carbohydrates from carbon dioxide and water.

physiological age: a person's age as estimated from her or his body's health and probable life expectancy.

phytic (FYE-tick) **acid:** a nonnutrient component of plant seeds; also called **phytate** (FYE-tate). Phytic acid occurs in the husks of grains, legumes, and seeds and is capable of binding minerals such as zinc, iron, calcium, magnesium, and copper in insoluble complexes in the intestine, which the body excretes unused.

phytochemicals (FIE-toe-KEM-ih-cals): nonnutrient compounds found in plant-derived foods that have biological activity in the body.

phytoestrogens: plant-derived compounds that have structural and functional similarities to human estrogen. Phytoestrogens include genistein, daidzein, and glycitein.

phytosterols: plant-derived compounds that have structural similarities to cholesterol and lower blood cholesterol by competing with cholesterol for absorption. Phytosterols include sterol esters and stanol esters.

pica (PIE-ka): a craving for nonfood substances. Also known as **geophagia** (gee-oh-FAY-gee-uh) when referring to clay eating and **pagophagia** (pag-oh-FAY-gee-uh) when referring to ice craving.

piggyback: the administration of a second solution using a separate port in an intravenous catheter.

pigment: a molecule capable of absorbing certain wavelengths of light so that it reflects only those that we perceive as a certain color.

placebo (pla-SEE-bo): an inert, harmless medication given to provide comfort and hope; a sham treatment used in controlled research studies.

placebo effect: the result of expectations in the effectiveness of a medicine, even medicine without pharmaceutical effects.

placenta (plah-SEN-tuh): the organ that develops inside the uterus early in pregnancy, through which the fetus receives nutrients and oxygen and returns carbon dioxide and other waste products to be excreted.

plaque (PLACK): an accumulation of fatty deposits, smooth muscle cells, and fibrous connective tissue that develops in the artery walls in atherosclerosis.

plasminogen activator inhibitor-1: a protein that promotes blood clotting by inhibiting blood clot degradation within blood vessels.

point of unsaturation: the double bond of a fatty acid, where hydrogen atoms can easily be added to the structure.

polydipsia (pol-lee-DIP-see-ah): excessive thirst.

polymorphisms: differences in the DNA sequences among individuals. A **single-nucleotide polymorphism** involves a single nucleotide at a particular area in the DNA strand.

polypeptide: many (ten or more) amino acids bonded together.

polyphagia (pol-lee-FAY-jee-ah): excessive appetite or eating.

polysaccharides: compounds composed of many monosaccharides linked together. An intermediate string of three to ten monosaccharides is an **oligosaccharide.**

polyunsaturated fatty acid (PUFA): a fatty acid that lacks four or more hydrogen atoms and has two or more double bonds between carbons—for example, linoleic acid (two double bonds) and linolenic acid (three double bonds). A **polyunsaturated fat** is composed of triglycerides in which most of the fatty acids are polyunsaturated.

polyuria (pol-lee-YOOR-ee-ah): excessive urine secretion.

portal hypertension: elevated blood pressure in the portal vein; often caused by obstructed blood flow through the liver.

portal vein: the vein that collects blood from the GI tract and conducts it to capillaries in the liver.

post term (infant): an infant born after the 42nd week of pregnancy.

postpartum amenorrhea: the normal temporary absence of menstrual periods immediately following childbirth.

potassium: the principal cation within the body's cells; critical to the maintenance of fluid balance, nerve impulse transmissions, and muscle contractions.

precursors: substances that precede others; with regard to vitamins, compounds that can be converted into active vitamins; also known as **provitamins.**

prediabetes: condition in which blood glucose levels are higher than normal but not high enough to be diagnosed as diabetes; considered a major risk factor for future diabetes and cardiovascular diseases. Also called **impaired glucose tolerance.**

preeclampsia (PRE-ee-KLAMP-see-ah): a condition characterized by hypertension, fluid retention, and protein in the urine; formerly known as *pregnancy-induced hypertension.** (*The Working Group on High Blood Pressure in Pregnancy, convened by the National High Blood Pressure Education Program of the National Heart, Lung, and Blood Institute, suggested abandoning the term *pregnancy-induced hypertension* because it failed to differentiate between the mild, transient hypertension of pregnancy and the life-threatening hypertension of preeclampsia.)

preformed vitamin A: dietary vitamin A in its active form.

prenatal alcohol exposure: subjecting a fetus to a pattern of excessive alcohol intake characterized by substantial regular use or heavy episodic drinking.

pressure gradient: change in pressure over a given distance. In dialysis, a pressure gradient is created between the blood and the dialysate.

pressure ulcers: damage to the skin and underlying tissues as a result of compression and poor circulation; commonly seen in people who are bedridden or chairbound.

preterm (infant): an infant born prior to the 38th week of pregnancy; also called a **premature infant.** A **term** infant is born between the 38th and 42nd week of pregnancy.

primary deficiency: a nutrient deficiency caused by inadequate dietary intake of a nutrient.

probiotics: microbial food ingredients that are beneficial to health. Nondigestible food ingredients that encourage the growth of favorable bacteria are called **prebiotics.**

processed foods: foods that have been treated to change their physical, chemical, microbiological, or sensory properties.

progesterone: the hormone of gestation (pregnancy).

prolactin (pro-LAK-tin): a hormone secreted from the anterior pituitary gland that acts on the mammary glands to initiate and sustain milk production.

promoter: a region of DNA involved with gene activation.

promoters: factors that favor the development of cancers once they have begun.

proof: a way of stating the percentage of alcohol in distilled liquor. Liquor that is 100 proof is 50% alcohol; 90 proof is 45%, and so forth.

prooxidants: substances that significantly induce oxidative stress.

proteases (PRO-tee-aces): enzymes that hydrolyze protein.

protein digestibility: a measure of the amount of amino acids absorbed from a given protein intake.

protein digestibility–corrected amino acid score (PDCAAS): a measure of protein quality assessed by comparing the amino acid score of a food protein with the amino acid requirements of preschool-age children and then correcting for the true digestibility of the protein.

protein efficiency ratio (PER): a measure of protein quality assessed by determining how well a given protein supports weight gain in growing rats; used to establish the protein quality for infant formulas and baby foods.

protein isolates: proteins that have been separated from foods. Examples include casein from milk and soy protein from soybeans.

protein turnover: the degradation and synthesis of protein.

protein-energy malnutrition (PEM), also called **protein-kcalorie malnutrition (PCM):** a deficiency of protein, energy, or both, including kwashiorkor, marasmus, and instances in which they overlap (see p. 198).

proteins: compounds composed of carbon, hydrogen, oxygen, and nitrogen atoms, arranged into amino acids linked in a chain. Some amino acids also contain sulfur atoms.

protein-sparing action: the action of carbohydrate (and fat) in providing energy that allows protein to be used for other purposes.

proteinuria (PRO-teen-NEW-ree-ah): loss of protein, especially albumin, in the urine; also known as **albuminuria.**

proton-pump inhibitors: a class of drugs that inhibit the enzyme that pumps hydrogen ions (protons) into the stomach. Examples include omeprazole (Prilosec) and lansoprazole (Prevacid).

puberty: the period in life in which a person becomes physically capable of reproduction.

public health dietitians: dietitians who specialize in providing nutrition services through organized community efforts.

public water: water from a municipal or county water system that has been treated and disinfected.

purified water: water that has been treated by distillation or other physical or chemical processes that remove dissolved solids. Because purified water contains no minerals or contaminants, it is useful for medical and research purposes.

purine (PYOO-reen): an end product of nucleotide metabolism that eventually degrades to form uric acid.

pyloric (pie-LORE-ic) **sphincter:** the circular muscle that separates the stomach from the small intestine and regulates the flow of partially digested food into the small intestine; also called *pylorus* or *pyloric valve.*

pyloroplasty (py-LOOR-oh-PLAS-tee): surgery that enlarges the pyloric sphincter.

pyruvate (PIE-roo-vate): a 3-carbon compound that plays a key role in energy metabolism.

Q

qi gong (chee GUNG): a Chinese system that combines movement, meditation, and breathing techniques and allegedly cures illness by enhancing the flow of "qi" energy within the body.

quality of life: a person's perceived physical and mental well-being.

R

radiation enteritis: inflammation of intestinal tissue caused by exposure to radiation.

radiation therapy: the use of X-rays, gamma rays, or atomic particles to destroy cancer cells.

randomization (RAN-dom-ih-ZAY-shun): a process of choosing the members of the experimental and control groups without bias.

raw sugar: the first crop of crystals harvested during sugar processing. Raw sugar cannot be sold in the United States because it contains too much filth (dirt, insect fragments, and the like). Sugar sold as "raw sugar" domestically has actually gone through over half of the refining steps.

RD: see *registered dietitian.*

rebound hyperglycemia: hyperglycemia that results from the release of counterregulatory hormones following nighttime hypoglycemia; also called the **Somogyi phenomenon.**

Recommended Dietary Allowance (RDA): the average daily amount of a nutrient considered adequate to meet the known nutrient needs of practically all healthy people; a goal for dietary intake by individuals.

rectum: the muscular terminal part of the intestine, extending from the sigmoid colon to the anus.

reduced kcalorie: at least 25% fewer kcalories per serving than the comparison food.

refeeding syndrome: a condition that sometimes develops when a severely malnourished person is aggressively fed; characterized by electrolyte and fluid imbalances and hyperglycemia.

reference protein: a standard against which to measure the quality of other proteins.

refined: the process by which the coarse parts of a food are removed. When wheat is refined into flour, the bran, germ, and husk are removed, leaving only the endosperm.

reflexology: a technique that applies pressure or massage on areas of the hands or feet to allegedly cure disease or relieve pain in other areas of the body; sometimes called **zone therapy.**

reflux esophagitis: inflammation in the esophagus related to the reflux of acidic stomach contents.

reflux: a backward flow.

registered dietitian (RD): a person who has completed a minimum of a bachelor's degree from an accredited university or college, has completed approved course work and a supervised practice program, has passed a national examination, and maintains registration through continuing professional education.

registration: listing; with respect to health professionals, listing with a professional organization that requires specific course work, experience, and passing of an examination.

regurgitation: the reflux of small amounts of acidic gastric substances into the mouth.

relaxin: the hormone of late pregnancy.

remodeling: the dismantling and re-formation of a structure, in this case, bone.

renal (REE-nal): pertaining to the kidneys.

renal colic: the severe, stabbing pain that occurs when a kidney stone passes through the ureter.

renal osteodystrophy: a bone disorder in patients with chronic renal failure; a consequence of increased parathyroid hormone secretion, reduced serum calcium, acidosis, and impaired vitamin D activation by the kidneys.

renal threshold: blood concentration of a substance that exceeds the kidneys' capacity for reabsorption and leads to appearance of the substance in urine.

renin (REN-in): an enzyme from the kidneys that activates angiotensin.

replication (REP-lee-KAY-shun): repeating an experiment and getting the same results. The skeptical scientist, on hearing of a new, exciting finding, will ask, "Has it been replicated yet?" If it hasn't, the scientist will withhold judgment regarding the finding's validity.

requirement: the lowest continuing intake of a nutrient that will maintain a specified criterion of adequacy.

resection: the surgical removal of part of an organ or body structure.

residue: material left in the intestine after digestion; includes mostly dietary fiber and undigested starches and proteins.

resistant starches: starches that escape digestion and absorption in the small intestine of healthy people.

resistin (re-ZIST-in): a hormone produced by adipose cells that induces insulin resistance.

respiratory stress: inadequate gas exchange between the air and blood, resulting in lower oxygen and higher carbon dioxide levels.

resting metabolic rate (RMR): similar to the BMR, a measure of the energy use of a person at rest in a comfortable setting, but with less stringent criteria for recent food intake and physical activity. Consequently, the RMR is slightly higher than the BMR.

reticulocytes: immature red blood cells released into blood by bone marrow.

retina (RET-in-uh): the layer of light-sensitive nerve cells lining the back of the inside of the eye; consists of rods and cones.

retinoids (RET-ih-noyds): chemically related compounds with biological activity similar to that of retinol; metabolites of retinol.

retinol activity equivalents (RAE): a measure of vitamin A activity; the amount of retinol that the body will derive from a food containing preformed retinol or its precursor beta-carotene.

retinol-binding protein (RBP): the specific protein responsible for transporting retinol.

rheumatoid (ROO-ma-toyd) **arthritis:** a disease of the immune system involving painful inflammation of the joints and related structures.

rhodopsin (ro-DOP-sin): a light-sensitive pigment of the retina; contains the retinal form of vitamin A and the protein opsin.

riboflavin (RYE-boh-flay-vin): a B vitamin. The coenzyme forms are **FMN (flavin mononucleotide)** and **FAD (flavin adenine dinucleotide).**

ribosomes (RYE-boh-zomes): protein-making organelles in cells; composed of RNA and protein.

rickets: the vitamin D–deficiency disease in children characterized by inadequate mineralization of bone (manifested in bowed legs or knock-knees, outward-bowed chest, and knobs on ribs). A rare type of rickets, not caused by vitamin D deficiency, is known as *vitamin D–refractory rickets.*

risk factor: a condition or behavior associated with an elevated frequency of a disease but not proved to be causal. Leading risk factors for chronic diseases include obesity, cigarette smoking, high blood pressure, high blood cholesterol, physical inactivity, and a diet high in saturated fats and low in vegetables, fruits, and whole grains.

S

saccharin (SAK-ah-ren): an artificial sweetener that has been approved for use in the United States. In Canada, approval for use in foods and beverages is pending; currently available only in pharmacies and only as a tabletop sweetener, not as an additive.

saliva: the secretion of the salivary glands. Its principal enzyme begins carbohydrate digestion.

salivary glands: exocrine glands that secrete saliva into the mouth.

salt: a compound composed of a positive ion other than H^+ and a negative ion other than OH^-. An example is sodium chloride ($Na^+ Cl^-$).

salt sensitivity: a characteristic of individuals who respond to a high salt intake with an increase in blood pressure or to a low salt intake with a decrease in bloood pressure.

sarcopenia (SAR-koh-PEE-nee-ah): loss of skeletal muscle mass, strength, and quality.

satiating: having the power to suppress hunger and inhibit eating.

satiation (say-she-AY-shun): the feeling of satisfaction and fullness that occurs during a meal and halts eating. Satiation determines how much food is consumed during a meal.

satiety (sah-TIE-eh-tee): the feeling of satisfaction that occurs after a meal and inhibits eating until the next meal. Satiety determines how much time passes between meals.

saturated fat-free: less than 0.5 g of saturated fat and 0.5 g of *trans* fat per serving.

saturated fatty acid: a fatty acid carrying the maximum possible number of hydrogen atoms—for example, stearic acid. A **saturated fat** is composed of triglycerides in which most of the fatty acids are saturated.

schizophrenia (SKITZ-oh-FREN-ee-ah): mental illness characterized by an altered concept of reality and, in some cases, delusions and hallucinations.

scurvy: the vitamin C–deficiency disease.

secondary deficiency: a nutrient deficiency caused by something other than an inadequate intake such as a disease condition or drug interaction that reduces absorption, accelerates use, hastens excretion, or destroys the nutrient.

secretin (see-CREET-in): a hormone produced by cells in the duodenum wall. Target organ: the pancreas. Response: secretion of bicarbonate-rich pancreatic juice.

segmentation (SEG-men-TAY-shun): a periodic squeezing or partitioning of the intestine at intervals along its length by its circular muscles.

selective menus: menus with two or more choices in some or all menu categories.

selenium (se-LEEN-ee-um): a trace element.

self-monitoring of blood glucose (SMBG): home monitoring of blood glucose levels using a glucose meter.

semipermeable membrane: a membrane that allows some particles to pass through, but not others.

semiselective menus: menus that combine aspects of both selective and nonselective menus.

senile dementia: the loss of brain function beyond the normal loss of physical adeptness and memory that occurs with aging.

sepsis: an acute inflammatory response caused by infection; characterized by symptoms similar to those of SIRS.

serotonin (SER-oh-tone-in): a neurotransmitter important in sleep regulation, appetite control, and sensory perception among other roles.

set point: the point at which controls are set (for example, on a thermostat). The set-point theory that relates to body weight proposes that the body tends to maintain a certain weight by means of its own internal controls.

shock: a dangerous physiological response to injury, bleeding, or infection that is characterized by an inadequate blood supply; associated with reduced blood pressure, raised heart and respiratory rates, and muscle weakness.

shock-wave lithotripsy: a nonsurgical procedure that uses high-amplitude sound waves to fragment gallstones.

short-bowel syndrome: malabsorption syndrome following small intestinal resection; results from insufficient absorptive capacity in the remaining intestine.

sibutramine (sigh-BYOO-tra-mean): a drug used in the treatment of obesity that slows the reabsorption of serotonin in the brain, thus suppressing appetite and creating a feeling of fullness.

sickle-cell anemia: a hereditary form of anemia characterized by abnormal sickle- or crescent-shaped red blood cells. Sickled cells interfere with oxygen transport and blood flow. Symptoms are precipitated by dehydration and insufficient oxygen (as may occur at high altitudes) and include hemolytic anemia (red blood cells burst), fever, and severe pain in the joints and abdomen.

simple carbohydrates (sugars): monosaccharides and disaccharides.

Sjögren's syndrome: an auto-immune disease characterized by the destruction of secretory glands, especially those that produce saliva and tears resulting in dry mouth and dry eyes.

sludge: literally, a semisolid mass. Biliary sludge is made up of mucus, cholesterol crystals, and bilirubin granules.

small intestine: a 10-foot length of small-diameter intestine that is the major site of digestion of food and absorption of nutrients. Its segments are the duodenum, jejunum, and ileum.

soaps: chemical compounds formed between positively charged minerals and fatty acids.

sodium: the principal cation in the extracellular fluids of the body; critical to the maintenance of fluid balance, nerve impulse transmissions, and muscle contractions.

sodium-free and **salt-free:** less than 5 mg of sodium per serving.

soft water: water with a high sodium or potassium content.

soluble fibers: indigestible food components that dissolve in water to form a gel. An example is pectin from fruit, which is used to thicken jellies.

solutes (SOLL-yutes): the substances that are dissolved in a solution. The number of molecules in a given volume of fluid is the **solute concentration.**

somatic (so-MAT-ick) **nervous system:** the division of the nervous system that controls the voluntary muscles, as distinguished from the autonomic nervous system, which controls involuntary functions.

somatostatin (GHIH): a hormone that inhibits the release of growth hormone; the opposite of **somatotropin (GH).**

sperm: the male reproductive cell, capable of fertilizing an ovum.

sphincter (SFINK-ter): a circular muscle surrounding, and able to close, a body opening. Sphincters are found at specific points along the GI tract and regulate the flow of food particles.

spina (SPY-nah) **bifida** (BIFF-ih-dah): one of the most common types of neural tube defects; characterized by the incomplete closure of the spinal cord and its bony encasement.

spring water: water originating from an underground spring or well. It may be bubbly (carbonated), or "flat" or "still," meaning not carbonated. Brand names such as "Spring Pure" do not necessarily mean that the water comes from a spring.

standard formulas: general-purpose dietary formulas that contain intact proteins and polysaccharides; also called **polymeric** or **intact formulas.**

standard or **regular diet:** a diet that includes all foods and meets the nutrient needs of healthy people.

starches: plant polysaccharides composed of glucose.

steatorrhea (stee-AT-or-REE-ah): excessive fat in the stools resulting from fat malabsorption; characterized by stools that are loose, frothy, and foul-smelling due to a high fat content.

sterile: free of microorganisms, such as bacteria.

sterols (STARE-ols or STEER-ols): compounds containing a four-carbon ring structure with any of a variety of side chains attached.

stevia (STEE-vee-ah): a South American shrub whose leaves are used as a sweetener; sold in the United States as a dietary supplement that provides sweetness without kcalories.

stoma (STOE-ma): a surgical opening made in the abdominal wall.

stomach: a muscular, elastic, saclike portion of the digestive tract that grinds and churns swallowed food, mixing it with acid and enzymes to form chyme.

stools: waste matter discharged from the colon; also called **feces** (FEE-seez).

stress: any threat to a person's well-being; a demand placed on the body to adapt.

stress fractures: bone damage or breaks caused by stress on bone surfaces during exercise.

stress response: the body's response to stress, mediated by both nerves and hormones.

stressors: environmental elements, physical or psychological, that cause stress.

stricture: abnormal narrowing of a passageway due to inflammation, scarring, or other structural changes.

stroke: an injury to brain tissue due to disturbed blood flow through arteries that supply blood to the brain; also called a **cerebrovascular accident.**

structure-function claims: statements that characterize the relationship between a nutrient or other substance in a food and its role in the body.

struvite (STROO-vite): crystals of magnesium ammonium phosphate.

subclinical deficiency: a deficiency in the early stages, before the outward signs have appeared.

Subjective Global Assessment (SGA): a technique for assessing malnutrition that uses historical and physical information.

subjects: the people or animals participating in a research project.

successful weight-loss maintenance: achieving a weight loss of at least 10 percent of initial body weight and maintaining the loss for at least one year.

sucralose (SUE-kra-lose): an artificial sweetener approved for use in the United States and Canada.

sucrase: an enzyme that hydrolyzes sucrose.

sucrose (SUE-krose): a disaccharide composed of glucose and fructose; commonly known as table sugar, beet sugar, or cane sugar. Sucrose also occurs in many fruits and some vegetables and grains.

sudden infant death syndrome (SIDS): the unexpected and unexplained death of an apparently well infant; the most common cause of death of infants between the second week and the end of the first year of life; also called *crib death.*

sugar replacers: sugarlike compounds that can be derived from fruits or commercially produced from dextrose; also called **sugar alcohols** or **polyols.** Sugar alcohols are absorbed more slowly than other sugars and metabolized differently in the human body; they are not readily utilized by ordinary mouth bacteria. Examples are **maltitol, mannitol, sorbitol, xylitol, isomalt,** and **lactitol.**

sugar-free: less than 0.5 g of sugar per serving.

sulfate: the oxidized form of sulfur.

sulfur: a mineral present in the body as part of some proteins.

supplements: pills, capsules, tablets, liquids, or powders that contain vitamins, minerals, herbs, or amino acids; intended to increase dietary intake of these substances.

surrogate: a substitute; a person who takes the place of another.

systemic inflammatory response syndrome (SIRS): a whole-body response to acute inflammation; characterized by raised heart and respiratory rates, abnormal white blood cell counts, and altered body temperature.

T

T cells: lymphocytes that attack antigens.

tagatose (TAG-ah-tose): a monosaccharide structurally similar to fructose that is incompletely absorbed and thus provides only 1.5 kcalories per gram; approved for use as a "generally recognized as safe" ingredient.

TCA cycle or **tricarboxylic** (try-car-box-ILL-ick) **acid cycle:** a series of metabolic reactions that break down molecules of acetyl CoA to carbon dioxide and hydrogen atoms; also called the **Kreb's cycle** after the biochemist who elucidated its reactions.

tempeh (TEM-pay): a fermented soybean food, rich in protein and fiber.

teratogenic (ter-AT-oh-jen-ik): causing abnormal fetal development and birth defects.

testosterone: a steroid hormone from the testicles, or testes. The steroids, as explained in Chapter 5, are chemically related to, and some are derived from, the lipid cholesterol.

textured vegetable protein: processed soybean protein used in vegetarian products such as soy burgers; see also *meat replacements.*

theory: a tentative explanation that integrates many and diverse findings to further the understanding of a defined topic.

therapeutic touch: a technique of passing hands over a patient to purportedly identify energy imbalances and transfer healing power from therapist to patient; also called **laying on of hands.**

thermic effect of food (TEF): an estimation of the energy required to process food (digest, absorb, transport, metabolize, and store ingested nutrients); also called the **specific dynamic effect (SDE)** of food or the **specific dynamic activity (SDA)** of food. The sum of the TEF and any increase in the metabolic rate due to overeating is known as **diet-induced thermogenesis (DIT).**

thermogenesis: the generation of heat; used in physiology and nutrition studies as an index of how much energy the body is expending.

thiamin (THIGH-ah-min): a B vitamin. The coenzyme form is **TPP (thiamin pyrophosphate).**

thirst: a conscious desire to drink.

thrombosis (throm-BOH-sis): the formation or presence of a blood clot in blood vessels. A *coronary thrombosis* occurs in a coronary artery, and a *cerebral thrombosis* occurs in an artery that supplies blood to the brain.

thrombus: a blood clot formed within a blood vessel that remains attached to its place of origin.

thrush: a fungal infection of the mouth and esophagus caused by *Candida albicans.* It coats the tongue with a milky film and leads to mouth ulcers, altered taste sensations, and pain on chewing and swallowing. The medical term for this infection is *candidiasis.*

thyroid-stimulating hormone (TSH): a hormone secreted by the pituitary that stimulates the thyroid gland to secrete its hormones—thyroxine and triiodothyronine. The release of TSH is mediated by **TSH-releasing hormone (TRH).**

tissue rejection: destruction of donor tissue by the recipient's immune system, which recognizes the donor cells as foreign.

tocopherol (tuh-KOFF-er-ol): a general term for several chemically related compounds, one of which has vitamin E activity (see Appendix C for chemical structures).

tofu (TOE-foo): a curd made from soybeans, rich in protein and often fortified with calcium; used in many Asian and vegetarian dishes in place of meat.

Tolerable Upper Intake Level (UL): the maximum daily amount of a nutrient that appears safe for most healthy people and beyond which there is an increased risk of adverse health effects.

tolerance level: the maximum amount of a residue permitted in a food when a pesticide is used according to the label directions.

total nutrient admixture (TNA): a parenteral solution that contains dextrose, amino acids, and lipids; also called a **3-in-1** or an **all-in-one** solution.

total parenteral nutrition (TPN): a type of nutrition support in which intravenous feedings are delivered into a central vein; also called **central parenteral nutrition.**

trabecular (tra-BECK-you-lar) **bone:** the lacy inner structure of calcium crystals that supports the bone's structure and provides a calcium storage bank.

trace minerals: essential mineral nutrients found in the human body in amounts smaller than 5 g; sometimes called **microminerals.**

trachea (TRAKE-ee-uh): the windpipe; the passageway from the mouth and nose to the lungs.

traditional Chinese medicine (TCM): an approach to medical care based on the concept that illness can be cured by enhancing the flow of "qi" energy within a person's body. Treatments may include herbal therapies, physical exercises, meditation, acupuncture, and remedial massage.

***trans* fat-free:** less than 0.5 g of *trans* fat and less than 0.5 g of saturated fat per serving.

transamination (TRANS-am-ih-NAY-shun): the transfer of an amino group from one amino acid to a keto acid, producing a new nonessential amino acid and a new keto acid.

transcription factors: proteins that bind DNA at specific sequences to regulate gene expression.

***trans*-fatty acids:** fatty acids with hydrogens on opposite sides of the double bond.

transferrin (trans-FAIR-in): the iron transport protein.

transient hypertension of pregnancy: high blood pressure that develops in the second half of pregnancy and resolves after childbirth, usually without affecting the outcome of the pregnancy.

transient ischemic attacks: temporary reductions in blood flow to the brain, which cause temporary symptoms that vary depending on the part of the brain affected.

transnasal: through the nose. A **transnasal feeding tube** is one that is inserted through the nose.

triglycerides (try-GLISS-er-rides): the chief form of fat in the diet and the major storage form of fat in the body; composed of a molecule of glycerol with three fatty acids attached; also called **triacylglycerols** (try-ay-seel-GLISS-er-ols).

tripeptide: three amino acids bonded together.

tube feedings: liquid formulas delivered through a tube placed in the stomach or intestine.

tubules: tubelike structures of the nephron that process filtrate during urine production. The tubules are surrounded by capillaries that reabsorb substances retained by tubule cells.

tumor: a new growth of tissue forming an abnormal mass with no function; also called a **neoplasm** (NEE-oh-plazm).

turbinado (ter-bih-NOD-oh) **sugar:** sugar produced using the same refining process as white sugar, but without the bleaching and anti-caking treatment. Traces of molasses give turbinado its sandy color.

24-hour recall: a record of foods consumed in the previous 24 hours; sometimes modified to include foods consumed in a typical day.

2-in-1 solution: a parenteral solution that contains dextrose and amino acids, but excludes lipids.

type 1 diabetes: the type of diabetes that accounts for 5 to 10% of diabetes cases and usually results from autoimmune destruction of pancreatic beta cells. In this type of diabetes, the pancreas produces little or no insulin.

type 2 diabetes: the type of diabetes that accounts for 90 to 95% of diabetes cases and usually results from insulin resistance coupled with insufficient insulin secretion. Obesity is present in 80 to 90% of cases.

type I osteoporosis: osteoporosis characterized by rapid bone losses, primarily of trabecular bone.

type II osteoporosis: osteoporosis characterized by gradual losses of both trabecular and cortical bone.

U

ulcer: a lesion of the skin or mucous membranes characterized by inflammation and damaged tissues. See also *peptic ulcer.*

ulcerative colitis (ko-LY-tis): inflammatory bowel disease that involves the colon. Inflammation affects the mucosa and submucosa.

ultrafiltration: removal of fluids and solutes from blood by using pressure to transfer the blood across a semipermeable membrane.

umbilical (um-BILL-ih-cul) **cord:** the ropelike structure through which the fetus's veins and arteries reach the placenta; the route of nourishment and oxygen to the fetus and the route of waste disposal from the fetus. The scar in the middle of the abdomen that marks the former attachment of the umbilical cord is the **umbilicus** (um-BILL-ih-cus), commonly known as the "belly button."

undernutrition: deficient energy or nutrients.

underweight: body weight below some standard of acceptable weight that is usually defined in relation to height (such as BMI).

unsaturated fatty acid: a fatty acid that lacks hydrogen atoms and has at least one double bond between carbons (includes monounsaturated and polyunsaturated fatty acids). An **unsaturated fat** is composed of triglycerides in which most of the fatty acids are unsaturated.

unspecified eating disorders: eating disorders that do not meet the defined criteria for specific eating disorders.

urea (you-REE-uh): the principal nitrogen-excretion product of protein metabolism. Two ammonia fragments are combined with carbon dioxide to form urea.

urea kinetic modeling: a method of determining the adequacy of dialysis treatment by calculating urea clearance from blood.

uremia (you-REE-me-ah): abnormal accumulation of nitrogen-containing substances, especially urea, in the blood; also called **azotemia** (AZE-oh-TEE-me-ah).

uremic syndrome: the cluster of symptoms associated with a GFR below 15 mL/min, including uremia, anemia, bone disease, hormonal imbalances, bleeding impairment, increased cardiovascular disease risk, and reduced immunity.

uterus (YOU-ter-us): the muscular organ within which the infant develops before birth.

V

vagotomy (vay-GOT-oh-mee): surgery that severs the vagus nerve in order to suppress gastric acid secretion. This surgery may impair gastric emptying and require an additional pyloroplasty procedure to allow drainage.

vagus nerve: the cranial nerve that regulates hydrochloric acid secretion and peristalsis. Effects elsewhere in the body include regulation of heart rate and bronchiole constriction.

validity (va-LID-ih-tee): having the quality of being founded on fact or evidence.

variables: factors that change. A variable may depend on another variable (for example, a child's height depends on his age), or it may be independent (for example, a child's height does not depend on the color of her eyes). Sometimes both variables correlate with a third variable (a child's height and eye color both depend on genetics).

varices (VAR-ih-seez): abnormally dilated blood vessels.

variety (dietary): eating a wide selection of foods within and among the major food groups.

vasoconstrictor (VAS-oh-kon-STRIK-tor): a substance that constricts or narrows the blood vessels.

vegans (VEE-guns, VAY-guns, or VEJ-ans): people who exclude all animal-derived foods (including meat, poultry, fish, eggs, and dairy products) from their diets; also called **pure vegetarians, strict vegetarians,** or **total vegetarians.**

vegetarians: a general term used to describe people who exclude meat, poultry, fish, or other animal-derived foods from their diets.

veins (VANES): vessels that carry blood to the heart.

very low sodium: 35 mg or less per serving.

villi (VILL-ee, VILL-eye): fingerlike projections from the folds of the small intestine; singular **villus.**

viscous: a gel-like consistency.

vitamin A: all naturally occurring compounds with the biological activity of retinol (RET-ih-nol), the alcohol form of vitamin A.

vitamin A activity: a term referring to both the active forms of vitamin A and the precursor forms in foods without distinguishing between them.

vitamin B_6: a family of compounds—pyridoxal, pyridoxine, and pyridoxamine. The primary active coenzyme form is **PLP (pyridoxal phosphate).**

vitamin B_{12}: a B vitamin characterized by the presence of cobalt (see Figure 13-12 in Chapter 13). The active forms of coenzyme B_{12} are **methylcobalamin** and **deoxyadenosylcobalamin.**

vitamins: organic, essential nutrients required in small amounts by the body for health.

VLDL (very-low-density lipoprotein): the type of lipoprotein made primarily by liver cells to transport lipids to various tissues in the body; composed primarily of triglycerides.

vomiting: expulsion of the contents of the stomach up through the esophagus to the mouth.

vulnerable plaque: a form of plaque, susceptible to rupture, that is lipid-rich and has only a thin fibrous barrier between the arterial lumen and the plaque's lipid core.

W

waist circumference: an anthropometric measurement used to assess a person's abdominal fat.

wasting: the gradual atrophy (loss) of body tissues; associated with protein-energy malnutrition or chronic disease.

water balance: the balance between water intake and output (losses).

water intoxication: the rare condition in which body water contents are too high in all body fluid compartments.

wean: gradually replacing breast milk with infant formula or other foods appropriate to an infant's diet.

websites: Internet resources composed of text and graphic files, each with a unique URL (Uniform Resource Locator) that names the site (for example, www.usda.gov).

well water: water drawn from ground water by tapping into an aquifer.

Wernicke-Korsakoff (VER-nee-key KORE-sah-kof) **syndrome:** a neurological disorder typically associated with chronic alcoholism and caused by a deficiency of the B vitamin thiamin; also called *alcohol-related dementia.*

wheat gluten (GLU-ten): a family of water-insoluble proteins in wheat; includes gliadin proteins that are toxic to persons with celiac disease.

white sugar: pure sucrose or "table sugar," produced by dissolving, concentrating, and recrystallizing raw sugar.

whole grain: a grain milled in its entirety (all but the husk), not refined.

wine: an alcoholic beverage made by fermenting grape juice.

World Wide Web (the Web, commonly abbreviated **www**): a graphical subset of the Internet.

X

xanthophylls (ZAN-tho-fills): pigments found in plants; responsible for the color changes seen in autumn leaves.

xerophthalmia (zer-off-THAL-mee-uh): progressive blindness caused by severe vitamin A deficiency.

xerosis (zee-ROW-sis): abnormal drying of the skin and mucous membranes; a sign of vitamin A deficiency.

xerostomia: dry mouth caused by reduced salivary flow.

Y

yogurt: milk fermented by specific bacterial cultures.

Z

Zollinger-Ellison syndrome: a syndrome characterized by the development of gastrin-secreting tumors (gastrinomas); most often located in the pancreas and duodenum.

zygote (ZY-goat): the product of the union of ovum and sperm; so-called for the first two weeks after fertilization.

Index

Page references in **bold** *indicate definitions of terms. (See also* Glossary, GL to GL-21)
Page references followed by the letter "f" indicate figures.
Page references followed by the letter "t" indicate tables.
Page references followed by the letter "n" indicate footnotes.
Page references consisting of a single letter (A, B, C or X, Y, Z) refer to the inside front and back covers respectively.
Page references with combined letter and number (A-1) refer to the appendixes.

C

E

M

Aids to Calculation

Many mathematical problems have been worked out in the "How to" and "Nutrition Calculations" sections of the text. These pages provide additional help and examples.

Conversion Factors

A conversion factor is a fraction in which the numerator (top) and the denominator (bottom) express the same quantity in different units. For example, 2.2 pounds (lb) and 1 kilogram (kg) are equivalent; they express the same weight. The conversion factors used to change pounds to kilograms and vice versa are:

$$\frac{1 \text{ kg}}{2.2 \text{ lb}} \text{ and } \frac{2.2 \text{ lb}}{1 \text{ kg}}.$$

Because a conversion factor equals 1, measurements can be multiplied by the factor to change the *unit* of measure without changing the *value* of the measurement. To change one unit of measurement to another, use the factor with the unit you are seeking in the numerator (top) of the fraction.

Example 1 Convert the weight of 130 pounds to kilograms.

- Choose the conversion factor in which the kilograms are on top and multiply by 130 pounds:

$$\frac{1 \text{ kg}}{2.2 \text{ lb}} \times 130 \text{ lb} = \frac{130 \text{ kg}}{2.2} = 59 \text{ kg}.$$

Example 2 Consider a 4-ounce (oz) hamburger that contains 7 grams (g) of saturated fat. How many grams of saturated fat are contained in a 3-ounce hamburger?

- Because you are seeking grams of saturated fat, the conversion factor is:

$$\frac{7 \text{ g saturated fat}}{4 \text{ oz hamburger}}.$$

- Multiply 3 ounces of hamburger by the conversion factor:

$$3 \text{ oz hamburger} \times \frac{7 \text{ g saturated fat}}{4 \text{ oz hamburger}} = \frac{3 \times 7}{4} = \frac{21}{4} =$$

5 g saturated fat (rounded off).

Percentages

A percentage is a comparison between a number of items (perhaps the number of kcalories in your daily energy intake) and a standard number (perhaps the number of kcalories used for Daily Values on food labels). To find a percentage, first divide by the standard number and then multiply by 100 to state the answer as a percentage (*percent* means "per 100").

Example 3 Suppose your energy intake for the day is 1500 kcalories (kcal): What percentage of the Daily Value (DV) for energy does your intake represent? (Use the Daily Value of 2000 kcalories as the standard.)

- Divide your kcalorie intake by the Daily Value:

  1500 kcal (your intake) ÷ 2000 kcal (DV) = 0.75.

- Multiply your answer by 100 to state it as a percentage:

  0.75 × 100 = 75% of the Daily Value.

Example 4 Sometimes the percentage is more than 100. Suppose your daily intake of vitamin C is 120 milligrams (mg) and your RDA (male) is 90 milligrams. What percentage of the RDA for vitamin C is your intake?

120 mg (your intake) ÷ 90 mg (RDA) = 1.33.

1.33 × 100 = 133% of the RDA.

Example 5 Sometimes the comparison is between a part of a whole (for example, your kcalories from protein) and the total amount (your total kcalories). In this case, the total is the number you divide by. If you consume 60 grams (g) protein, 80 grams fat, and 310 grams carbohydrate, what percentages of your total kcalories for the day come from protein, fat, and carbohydrate?

- Multiply the number of grams by the number of kcalories from 1 gram of each energy nutrient (conversion factors):

$$60 \text{ g protein} \times \frac{4 \text{ kcal}}{1 \text{ g protein}} = 240 \text{ kcal}.$$

$$80 \text{ g fat} \times \frac{9 \text{ kcal}}{1 \text{ g fat}} = 720 \text{ kcal}.$$

$$310 \text{ g carbohydrate} \times \frac{4 \text{ kcal}}{1 \text{ g carbohydrate}} = 1240 \text{ kcal.}$$

- Find the total kcalories:

  240 + 720 + 1240 = 2200 kcal.

- Find the percentage of total kcalories from each energy nutrient (see Example 3):

  Protein: 240 ÷ 2200 = 0.109 × 100 = 10.9 = 11% of kcal.

  Fat: 720 ÷ 2200 = 0.327 × 100 = 32.7 = 33% of kcal.

  Carbohydrate: 1240 ÷ 2200 = 0.563 × 100 = 56.3 = 56% of kcal.

  Total: 11% + 33% + 56% = 100% of kcal.

In this case, the percentages total 100 percent, but sometimes they total 99 or 101 because of rounding—a reasonable estimate.

Ratios

A ratio is a comparison of two (or three) values in which one of the values is reduced to 1. A ratio compares identical units and so is expressed without units.

Example 6 Suppose your daily intakes of potassium and sodium are 3000 milligrams (mg) and 2500 milligrams, respectively. What is the potassium-to-sodium ratio?

- Divide the potassium milligrams by the sodium milligrams:

  3000 mg potassium ÷ 2500 mg sodium = 1.2.

The potassium-to-sodium ratio is 1.2:1 (read as "one point two to one" or simply "one point two"), which means there are 1.2 milligrams of potassium for every 1 milligram of sodium. A ratio greater than 1 means that the first value (in this case, potassium) is greater than the second (sodium). When the ratio is less than 1, the second value is larger.

Weights and Measures

LENGTH

1 meter (m) = 39 in.
1 centimeter (cm) = 0.4 in.
1 inch (in) = 2.5 cm.
1 foot (ft) = 30 cm.

TEMPERATURE

	Celsius*	Fahrenheit	
Steam	100°C	212°F	Steam
Body temperature	37°C	98.6°F	Body temperature
Ice	0°C	32°F	Ice

- To find degrees Fahrenheit (°F) when you know degrees Celsius (°C), multiply by 9/5 and then add 32.
- To find degrees Celsius (°C) when you know degrees Fahrenheit (°F), subtract 32 and then multiply by 5/9.

VOLUME

1 liter (L) = 1000 mL, 0.26 gal, 1.06 qt, or 2.1 pt.
1 milliliter (mL) = 1/1000 L or 0.03 fluid oz.
1 gallon (gal) = 128 oz, 8 c, or 3.8 L.
1 quart (qt) = 32 oz, 4 c, or 0.95 L.
1 pint (pt) = 16 oz, 2 c, or 0.47 L.
1 cup (c) = 8 oz, 16 tbs, about 250 mL, or 0.25 L.
1 ounce (oz) = 30 mL.
1 tablespoon (tbs) = 3 tsp or 15 mL.
1 teaspoon (tsp) = 5 mL.

WEIGHT

1 kilogram (kg) = 1000 g or 2.2 lb.
1 gram (g) = 1/1000 kg, 1000 mg, or 0.035 oz.
1 milligram (mg) = 1/1000 g or 1000 µg.
1 microgram (µg) = 1/1000 mg.
1 pound (lb) = 16 oz, 454 g, or 0.45 kg.
1 ounce (oz) = about 28 g.

ENERGY

1 kilojoule (kJ) = 0.24 kcal.
1 millijoule (mJ) = 240 kcal.
1 kcalorie (kcal) = 4.2 kJ.
1 g carbohydrate = 4 kcal = 17 kJ.
1 g fat = 9 kcal = 37 kJ.
1 g protein = 4 kcal = 17 kJ.
1 g alcohol = 7 kcal = 29 kJ.

*Also known as *centigrade*.

Daily Values for Food Labels

The Daily Values are standard values developed by the Food and Drug Administration (FDA) for use on food labels. The values are based on 2000 kcalories a day for adults and children over 4 years old. Chapter 2 provides more details.

Nutrient	Amount
Protein[a]	50 g
Thiamin	1.5 mg
Riboflavin	1.7 mg
Niacin	20 mg NE
Biotin	300 µg
Pantothenic acid	10 mg
Vitamin B_6	2 mg
Folate	400 µg
Vitamin B_{12}	6 µg
Vitamin C	60 mg
Vitamin A	5000 IU[b]
Vitamin D	400 IU[b]
Vitamin E	30 IU[b]
Vitamin K	80 µg
Calcium	1000 mg
Iron	18 mg
Zinc	15 mg
Iodine	150 µg
Copper	2 mg
Chromium	120 µg
Selenium	70 µg
Molybdenum	75µg
Manganese	2 mg
Chloride	3400 mg
Magnesium	400 mg
Phosphorus	1000 mg

[a]The Daily Values for protein vary for different groups of people: pregnant women, 60 g; nursing mothers, 65 g; infants under 1 year, 14 g; children 1 to 4 years, 16 g.
[b]Equivalent values for nutrients expressed as IU are: vitamin A, 1500 RAE (assumes a mixture of 40% retinol and 60% beta-carotene); vitamin D, 10 µg; vitamin E, 20 mg.

Food Component	Amount	Calculation Factors
Fat	65 g	30% of kcalories
Saturated fat	20 g	10% of kcalories
Cholesterol	300 mg	Same regardless of kcalories
Carbohydrate (total)	300 g	60% of kcalories
Fiber	25 g	11.5 g per 1000 kcalories
Protein	50 g	10% of kcalories
Sodium	2400 mg	Same regardless of kcalories
Potassium	3500 mg	Same regardless of kcalories

GLOSSARY OF NUTRIENT MEASURES

kcal: kcalories; a unit by which energy is measured (Chapter 1 provides more details).

g: grams; a unit of weight equivalent to about 0.03 ounces.

mg: milligrams; one-thousandth of a gram.

µg: micrograms; one-millionth of a gram.

IU: international units; an old measure of vitamin activity determined by biological methods (as opposed to new measures that are determined by direct chemical analyses). Many fortified foods and supplements use IU on their labels.
- For vitamin A, 1 IU = 0.3 µg retinol, 3.6 µg β-carotene, or 7.2 µg other vitamin A carotenoids.
- For vitamin D, 1 IU = 0.025 µg cholecalciferol.
- For vitamin E, 1 IU = 0.67 natural α-tocopherol (other conversion factors are used for different forms of vitamin E).

mg NE: milligrams niacin equivalents; a measure of niacin activity (Chapter 10 provides more details).
- 1 NE = 1 mg niacin.
  = 60 mg tryptophan (an amino acid).

µg DFE: micrograms dietary folate equivalents; a measure of folate activity (Chapter 10 provides more details).
- 1 µg DFE = 1 µg food folate.
  = 0.6 µg fortified food or supplement folate.
  = 0.5 µg supplement folate taken on an empty stomach.

µg RAE: micrograms retinol activity equivalents; a measure of vitamin A activity (Chapter 11 provides more details).
- 1 µg RAE = 1 µg retinol.
  = 12 µg β-carotene.
  = 24 µg other vitamin A carotenoids.

mmol: millimoles; one-thousanth of a mole, the molecular weight of a substance. To convert mmol to mg, multiply by the atomic weight of the substance.
- For sodium, mmol × 23 = mg Na.
- For chloride, mmol × 35.5 = mg Cl.
- For sodium chloride, mmol × 58.5 = mg NaCl.